2016

T0121123

Procedural Coding

EXPERT

Ensuring CPT® coding and billing compliance

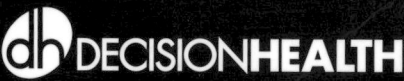

www.codingbooks.com

Type of Service (TOS) Indicators

Type of Service (TOS) is an indicator that the contractor places on the Form CMS-1500 paper form or electronic format. The indicator is mainly used for data purposes. However, in some instances it affects payment. All HCPCS codes have a corresponding TOS indicator.

Medicare administrative contractors must assign the proper TOS using the annual HCPCS update from the CMS mainframe. Changes to this list are issued annually via a Recurring Update Notification. Some procedures may have more than one applicable TOS. For claims received on or after April 3, 1995, CWF produced alerts on codes with incorrect TOS designations. Effective July 3, 1995, CWF began rejecting codes with incorrect TOS designations.

The only exceptions to this annual update are:

- Surgical services billed for dates of service through December 31, 2007, containing the ASC facility service modifier SG must be reported as TOS F. Effective for services on or after January 1, 2008, the SG modifier is no longer applicable for Medicare services. ASC providers should discontinue applying the SG modifier on ASC facility claims. The indicator 'F' does not appear in the TOS table because its use depends upon claims submitted with POS 24 (ASC Facility) from an ASC (specialty 49). This became effective for dates of service January 1, 2008 and after.

- Surgical services billed with an assistant-at-surgery modifier (80-82, AS,) must be reported with TOS 8. The 8 indicator does not appear on the TOS table because its use is dependent upon the use of the appropriate modifier. (See Pub. 100-04, Medicare Claims Processing Manual, Chapter 12, "Physician/Nonphysician Practitioner," for instructions on when assistant-at-surgery is allowable.)

- TOS H appears in the list of descriptors. However, it does not appear in the table. In CWF, "H" is used only as an indicator for hospice. The contractor should not submit TOS H to CWF at this time.

- For outpatient services, when a transfusion medicine code appears on a claim that also contains a blood product, the service is paid under reasonable charge at 80%, coinsurance and deductible apply. When transfusion medicine codes are paid under the clinical laboratory fee schedule pay at 100%, coinsurance and deductible do not apply.

***NOTE**: For injection codes with more than one possible TOS designation, use the following guidelines when assigning the TOS:*

When the choice is L or 1:

- Use TOS L when the drug is used related to ESRD; or
- Use TOS 1 when the drug is not related to ESRD and is administered in the office.

When the choice is G or 1:

- Use TOS G when the drug is an immunosuppressive drug; or
- Use TOS 1 when the drug is used for other than immunosuppression.

When the choice is P or 1:

- Use TOS P if the drug is administered through durable medical equipment (DME); or
- Use TOS 1 if the drug is administered in the office.

The place of service or diagnosis may be considered when determining the appropriate TOS. The descriptors for each of the TOS codes listed in the annual HCPCS update are:

Type of Service Indicators

0	Whole Blood
1	Medical Care
2	Surgery
3	Consultation
4	Diagnostic Radiology
5	Diagnostic Laboratory
6	Therapeutic Radiology
7	Anesthesia
8	Assistant at Surgery
9	Other Medical Items or Services
A	Used DME
B	High Risk Screening Mammography
C	Low Risk Screening Mammography
D	Ambulance
E	Enteral/Parenteral Nutrients/Supplies
F	Ambulatory Surgical Center (Facility Usage for Surgical Services)
G	Immunosuppressive Drugs
H	Hospice
J	Diabetic Shoes
K	Hearing Items and Services
L	ESRD Supplies
M	Monthly Capitation Payment for Dialysis
N	Kidney Donor
P	Lump Sum Purchase of DME, Prosthetics, Orthotics
Q	Vision Items or Services
R	Rental of DME
S	Surgical Dressings or Other Medical Supplies
T	Outpatient Mental Health Treatment Limitation
U	Occupational Therapy
V	Pneumococcal/Flu Vaccine
W	Physical Therapy

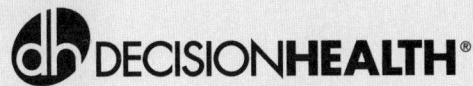

HCPCS Level II Expert

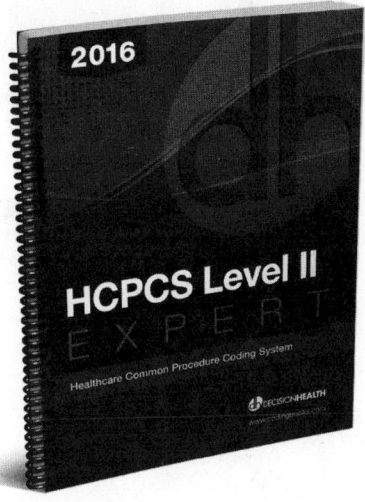

Do you bill for durable medical equipment (DME), injections, Medicare services, drugs and other medical supplies? Keep this book close and use it to help reduce claims denials, comply with HIPAA and get paid quicker. Don't settle for less reimbursement than you deserve.

$109.95 | Item: MPB-HCPCS-16
Available: December 28, 2015

■ **UPDATED! New, Revised and Deleted HCPCS Level II Codes** — quickly spot code changes thanks to code change icons.

■ **UPDATED! Expanded Alphabetical Index** — DecisionHealth's proprietary index gives you multiple ways to find a drug, device or supply quickly.

■ **UPDATED! DMEPOS icons identify reimbursement opportunities** — spot Medicare allowed billing opportunities for certain durable medical equipment, prosthetics, orthotics and supplies.

■ **UPDATED! Deleted codes crosswalk** — quickly identify new valid codes that have replaced temporary codes and other deleted codes.

■ **G Codes for PQRS** — clarifies requirements for your PQRS reporting program.

■ **NEW! National Coverage Determination (NCD) policy citations at the code level** — ensure compliance with Medicare coverage policy for certain HCPCS procedures and professional services.

■ **UPDATED! Medicare Pub. 100 information** — included with associated code and full descriptions in Appendix in the back of the book.

■ **UPDATED! Table of Drugs Appendix** — find J codes more quickly with cross- referenced Brand names.

■ **UPDATED! APC and ASC Payment Icons** — quickly identify reimbursement opportunity. Icons identify 23 specific OutPatient Prospective Payment System (OPPS) payment statuses, as well as 18 ASC groupings to improve reimbursement.

■ **UPDATED! AHA Coding Clinic for HCPCS** — identify where to find critical guidance on challenging HCPCS Level II codes or sections.

■ **HCPCS Level II modifiers** — ensure that required modifiers are appended to codes reducing delays and denials.

For more information, call toll-free **1-855-CALL-DH1**
or visit **www.codingbooks.com**

Procedural Coding Expert

The Ultimate Guide to CPT® Coding

2016

2016 Procedural Coding Expert

Published by DecisionHealth, LLC

9737 Washingtonian Blvd.
Suite 200
Gaithersburg, MD 20878
1-855-CALL-DH1

Copyright © 2016 DecisionHealth
All rights reserved

Printed in the United States of America

ISBN: 978-1-58383-845-7

Item ID: MPB-PCE-16

DISCLAIMER

No part of this publication may be reproduced, stored in a retrieval system, or transmitted, in any form or by any means, electronic, mechanical, photocopy, recording, or otherwise, without the prior written permission of the publisher. Any five digit numeric Physicians' Current Procedural Terminology, Fourth Edition (CPT) codes, service descriptions, instructions and/or guidelines are Copyright 2015 American Medical Association (or such other date of publication of CPT as defined in the Federal copyright laws). All rights reserved. No fee schedules, basic unit values, relative value guides, conversion factors, or scales or components thereof are included in the CPT. Additional proprietary guidance contained herein are derived by DecisionHealth coding and reimbursement experts, in consultation CMS, MACs, and other official, published guidance. The AMA assumes no responsibility for the consequences attributable to, related to any use or interpretation of any information or views contained in, or not contained in this publication. This publication is sold with the understanding that the publisher is not engaged in rendering legal, medical, accounting, or other professional service in specific situations. Although prepared for professionals, this publication should not be utilized as a substitute for professional service in specific situations. If legal or medical advice is required, the services of a professional should be sought. No part of this publication may be reproduced, stored in a retrieval system, or transmitted, in any form, by any means. Copyright violations will be prosecuted. To report violations, contact Steve McVearry at 1-301-287-2266 or smcvearry@ucg.com.

Contents

Surgical Procedures 169

Radiological Procedures 614

Laboratory/Pathology Services............... 674

Medicine Procedures/Services................ 780

Preface

The *Procedural Coding Expert* was created to be the best resource in its class to make CPT® coding as accurate as possible. As a result of the input and guidance from experienced coding and billing professionals, as well as staff subject matter experts with years of coding experience, the user will find the *Procedural Coding Expert* to be easy-to-use and loaded with the help on Medicare coverage, global billing, modifier usage and other fundamental information needed to code on a daily basis. Some of the features in the *Procedural Coding Expert* include:

- **Color anatomical illustrations** – more than 650 illustrations to provide greater insight to specific procedures and help interpret clinical notes more effectively

- **Full codes and descriptions** – all 2016 CPT codes with entire code description listed so you can avoid any confusion

- **Introduction** loaded with essential information such as coding fundamentals, description of modifiers, common medical abbreviations, prefixes, suffixes and roots, coding terms glossary, detailed explanation of all icons and data elements and multiple summary tables including code additions, deletions and revisions

- **Coding Tips and Guidance** accompanies selective codes providing additional information on coding more accurately and efficiently

- **Documentation Tips** accompany selective codes highlighting synonyms and/or supporting chart references essential to medical necessity for the respective procedure.

- **Hundreds of references for guidance from the AMA's *CPT®Assistant* and Medicare's Pub 100 manuals** integrated with the relevant codes to help you validate code choices

- **Relative Value Units (RVUs)**, Medicare global follow-up days and modifier rules for each code

- **Extra help on new, revised and deleted codes** – icons identify new procedure codes, revised code descriptions and text. Deleted codes are highlighted with a strikethrough and cross-referenced to valid codes when a valid replacement code exists

- **Coverage Determination Alerts identify National Coverage Policies** in existence at the time of publication to alert you to Medicare restrictions.

- **Age and sex edit icons** help prevent claim denials and delays.

- **Additional symbols** noting ASC, APC, as well as moderate/conscious sedation and denial risk

- **Color-coded page ends** to provide easy distinction of procedural sections in the Tabular list

Sources and Contributors

This book contains CPT codes effective for January 1, 2016 through December 31, 2016, as maintained and released by the American Medical Association. The following individuals have contributed to the development and layout of this book:

Tonya Nevin, *Vice President, Medical Practice Group*
Carol Brault, MA, *Product Manager*
Lori Becks, RHIA *Clinical Technical Editor*
Michelle L. Suitor, CPC, *Clinical Technical Editor*
Ruby Woodward, CPC, *Clinical Technical Editor*
Juli Folk, *Books Manager*
Lori Cipro, *Production Manager*
Bethany Angleberger, *Desktop Publisher*
Jennifer Fairman, *Certified Medical Illustrator*
Bradley Clark, *Illustrator*
Jonas A. Croft, *Illustrator*
Justin Clark, *Illustrator*

Introduction

Procedural coding is the translation of medical services, procedures, events, and circumstances into numeric and alphanumeric codes to facilitate insurance billing. Core coding reference books, specifically the CPT book and derivative works, are the key to understanding these codes. The ***Procedural Coding Expert*** was developed to enhance the coding information of the AMA's CPT code set with critical billing guidance.

The family of codes used to report medical or surgical services and procedures, products and supplies is collectively referred to as HCPCS (Healthcare Common Procedural Coding System). HCPCS Level I codes consist of five-digit numeric codes from the physician's *Current Procedural Terminology* (CPT®) as published and maintained by the American Medical Association (AMA). HCPCS Level II is a standardized coding system that is used primarily to identify products, supplies, and services not included in the CPT codes, such as ambulance services and durable medical equipment, prosthetics, orthotics, and supplies (DMEPOS). Because Medicare and other insurers cover a variety of services, supplies, and equipment that are not identified by CPT codes, the Level II HCPCS codes were established for submitting claims for these items. CPT codes are the focus of ***Procedural Coding Expert*** because these codes are the most frequently used codes for reporting physician services and procedures.

CPT (HCPCS Level I) Codes

CPT codes consist of the five-digit numeric codes listed in the Physicians' Current Procedural Terminology published by the American Medical Association. The codes are updated annually, and the new codes for the upcoming year are available at the end of the preceding year for use on January 1, 2016.

Organization of CPT Book

The CPT book is organized into three code categories. Category I codes make up the main body of the book. These codes must meet two criteria:

- The service or procedure must be performed by many health care professionals in clinical practice in multiple locations
- FDA approval, if required, must already have been received

Category II codes are a set of supplementary tracking codes that are used for performance measurement and quality reporting. These codes are not required for correct reporting of services and procedures and may not be used in place of Category I codes.

Category III codes are temporary codes that are used to report emerging technologies, services, and procedures. These codes allow data to be collected about new and emerging medical technologies, services and procedures that do not meet the criteria described above for Category I codes. That is, these technologies, services and procedures are not yet in widespread use and/or are not FDA approved.

Category I Codes

The main body of the book is organized into 6 sections by type of service which includes:

- Evaluation and Management Services
- Anesthesia
- Surgery
- Radiology
- Laboratory
- Medicine

Within each section, codes are sequenced in the following order:

- Top to bottom of body (head to toe)
- Central to peripheral in some subsections (i.e., cardiovascular and nervous system codes)
- Outside to inside of body (incision/excision)

CPT Coding Conventions

CPT coding conventions differ slightly from those used in the ***Procedural Coding Expert*** text. CPT coding conventions are reviewed here to illustrate how they differ from ***Procedural Coding Expert*** coding conventions.

Indented Format

The AMA's CPT book uses an indented format. Codes with a common element are listed sequentially. The first code provides the full description with the common element in the procedure listed in the first part of the descriptor followed by a semicolon and the unique elements of the service described after the semicolon. In ***Procedural Coding Expert***, the full code description is listed for all codes.

CPT Symbols

In addition to understanding the layout of CPT and knowing how to reference the book, the user must also understand symbols and their meanings.

● Indicates a new code has been added to the edition the coder is referencing. For example:

> ● 39401   Mediastinoscopy; includes biopsy(ies) of mediastinal mass (eg, lymphoma), when performed

▲ Indicates the code number is the same, but the definition or description has changed since the last edition

> ▲ 65855   Trabeculoplasty by laser surgery

Deleted Codes

The AMA's CPT book omits deleted codes from the tabular, listing them instead only in Appendix B. In Procedural Coding Expert, the deleted codes for the 2016 code year remain within the tabular with a strikethrough over the code description for easier identification. A list of this year's new and revised codes, as well as a Deleted Code Crosswalk, is also available in the front section of our manual.

⊘ Identifies codes that are exempt from the use of modifier 51, but have not been designated as add-on procedures/ services.

> ⊘ 99143   Moderate sedation services (other than those services described by codes 00100-01999) provided by the same physician performing the diagnostic or therapeutic service that the sedation supports, requiring the presence of an independent trained observer to assist in the monitoring of the patient's level of consciousness and physiological status; under 5 years of age, first 30 minutes intra-service time

Note: For more information on modifier 51, see the Modifier chapter.

⊙ Identifies codes that include conscious sedation.

> ⊙ 92960   Cardioversion, elective, electrical conversion of arrhythmia; external

Add-on Codes

Add-on procedures or services are ones that are performed in addition to the primary procedure/service. In the CPT book, a ✚ indicates a CPT add-on code.

CPT © 2015 American Medical Association. All rights reserved.
© 2016 DecisionHealth

99291   Critical care, evaluation and management of the critically ill or critically injured patient; first 30-74 minutes

+ 99292   each additional 30 minutes (List separately in addition to code for primary service)

The add-on procedure is performed on the same day by the same provider that performed the primary procedure/service. These codes should never be reported alone and should not be reported with modifier 51.

Resequenced Codes

The AMA's CPT book resequences codes to place like procedures together. Codes that are out of numeric sequence are identifed by the # symbol. The code along with a note is placed where the code would be located if it were in numerical sequence.

Codes that are out of numeric sequence are identified by the # symbol. The code along with a note is also placed where the code would be located if it were in numerical sequence.

In *Procedural Coding Expert,* all codes are organized by numeric sequence.

Modifiers

Modifiers consist of two numeric or alphanumeric digits appended to a code to indicate when a service or procedure that still fits the code description was altered by a specific circumstance or when additional information about the procedure performed needs to be provided. See the Modifier chapter for an in-depth breakdown of modifiers and their usage.

Unlisted Procedure or Service

The procedure performed may not always be found with a designated code assignment in CPT. Unlisted procedure codes are provided in every section to be used in these cases. An accompanying operative report or other visit documentation is required when reporting unlisted codes in order for the payer to identify what the procedure entailed and determine its eligibility for reimbursement. An unlisted procedure code should not be used when a Category III code better describes the procedure performed.

Surgical Package

The concept of a global fee for surgical procedures is a long-established concept under which a single fee is billed that pays for all necessary services normally furnished by the surgeon before, during, and after the procedure. Since the fee schedule is based on uniform national relative values, it is necessary to have a uniform national definition of global surgery to assure that equivalent payment is made for the same amount of work and resources.

The following items are included in the global package reimbursement:

- Local anesthesia, digital block, or topical anesthesia
- After the decision for surgery is made, one E/M service one day before or the day of surgery
- Postoperative care that occurs directly after the procedure
- Examining the patient in the recovery area
- Any postoperative care occurring during the designated postoperative period

To assist in this uniform implementation, the CPT Editorial Panel created five modifiers (24, 25, 59, 78, and 79) to identify a service or procedure furnished during a global period that is not a part of the global surgery fee, such as a service unrelated to the condition requiring surgery or for treating the underlying condition and not for normal recovery from the surgery. These types of services may be reported in addition to the global fee.

Category II Codes

The Category II section of CPT contains a set of supplemental tracking codes that can be used for performance measurement. This section of codes was implemented in 2004 to facilitate data collection about the quality of care rendered for specific conditions by coding certain services and test results that support nationally established performance measures with evidence of contributing to increased quality patient care. It is not required for providers to report these codes; the use of these codes is optional.

Category II codes consist of five numeric-alpha codes that end in an F and the following categories are included in this code set:

- Composite Codes
- Patient Management
- Patient History
- Physical Examination
- Diagnostic/Screening Processes or Results
- Therapeutic, Preventive or Other Interventions
- Follow-up or Other Outcomes
- Patient Safety
- Structural Measures

Category III Codes

Category III codes are temporary codes that identify emerging technologies, services, and procedures, and allow for data collection to determine clinical efficacy, utilization, and outcomes. They consist of four numbers, followed by the letter.

A Category III code should be reported instead of an unlisted code if it better describes the procedure that was performed. These temporary codes may or may not be assigned a Category I CPT code in the future.

Using the *Procedural Coding Expert*

The *Procedural Coding Expert* uses some of the same conventions as the AMA's CPT code book, but there are some differences. The next section on *Procedural Coding Expert* Conventions should be reviewed prior to using the reference book. In addition, some instructions are found below on locating codes in the *Procedural Coding Expert.*

Locating a CPT Code

To code appropriately, it is necessary to have a working knowledge of medical terminology and anatomy. Translating verbal descriptions of procedures and services into the most appropriate numerical code(s) is a complex activity that was originally undertaken to provide access to data in medical records according to diagnoses and operations for medical research, education, and administrative purposes. Medical codes today are utilized to facilitate payment of health services, to evaluate utilization patterns, and to study the appropriateness of healthcare costs. Coding provides the basis for epidemiological studies and research into the quality of healthcare.

There are two ways to locate a code in the *Procedural Coding Expert* book:

- By anatomical site (numerically)
- The Index (alphabetically)

A code can be located simply by knowing the site or body system. For example, if a patient had an EKG performed in the emergency department, the user may try to locate a code using the Index. Alternatively, the coder may know that the patient's heart was being monitored, which means a code from the Medicine (90000) section in the Cardiovascular subsection should be used to report this procedure. In this case, the coder may prefer to go directly to the Medicine section and look in the Cardiovascular subsection for the code.

Organization of the Index

The Index is organized by main terms, shown in bold typeface. There are four primary classes of main entries:

- Procedure or service – Laparoscopy, Angioplasty
- Organ or other anatomic site – Arm, Chest, Abdomen
- Condition – Angina, Lesion
- Synonyms, eponyms and abbreviations – EKG, ABG, HDL

Each main term may stand alone or it may be followed by additional levels called sub-terms that add further specificity or clarification. When more specific levels of terms appear, these subterms need to be reviewed before selecting the code to be assigned.

Whenever more than one code applies to a given index entry, a code range is listed. If two or more nonsequential codes apply, they will be separated by a comma. For example:

Brachytherapy
supply placement, 19298, 57160, 58346, 92974

If more than one sequential code applies, they will be separated by a hyphen. For example:

Office and/or Other Outpatient Services
Established patient 99211-99215

The alphabetic index is not a substitute for the main text of CPT. The user must always refer to the main text to ensure that the code selection is accurate and not assign any codes from the Index entry alone.

Procedural Coding Expert Conventions

The Tabular List of Procedures in the *Procedural Coding Expert* makes use of certain punctuation and symbol conventions that need to be understood for efficient and effective coding.

Punctuation

; In the AMA's CPT manuals, a semicolon is used as a space-saving convention. Some code descriptions are not reprinted in their entirety to avoid repetition. However, in the *Procedural Coding Expert*, full descriptions are included for all CPT codes to minimize confusion and the need to flip backwards in the manual to comprehend the full intent of a code description. For example, in AMA's CPT products, codes 20100 and 20101 would appear as:

20100	Exploration of penetrating wound (separate procedure); neck
20101	chest

In the *Procedural Coding Expert*, codes 20100 and 20101 contain full descriptions for every code and appear as follows:

20100	Exploration of penetrating wound (separate procedure); neck
20101	Exploration of penetrating wound (separate procedure); chest

Text Formatting

References to Medicare's Pub 100 manuals and gap-filled RVU data are in italics.

Symbols

●   A circle denotes a new code.

▲   The triangle denotes a revised code description. The code number itself has not changed.

✖   The 'x' indicates that a code was deleted and should not be used for the current year. The full description of the code will be included, but with a strikethrough throughout the description.

~~word~~   A strikethrough highlights a word(s) that has been deleted from a particular code description. If a cross-reference to a valid code is available, it will be noted underneath the deleted description.

⊙   The bullseye indicates procedures that include the administration of moderate (conscious) sedation as part of the procedure. Codes for conscious sedation (99143-99150) are not reported separately.

✚   This plus sign indicates an add-on code that should not be reported as a stand-alone code under any circumstance. It is always reported with another code as the primary procedure, with the add-on code as a secondary procedure. Add-on codes also contain a parenthetical statement as part of the code description that reads "List separately in addition to the primary procedure."

⊘   Codes that are exempt from modifier 51. This symbol identifies codes that are typically not subject to multiple procedure payment reductions. These codes have not been designated as add-on codes. They are usually performed with another procedure; however, they may also be performed alone.

⊖   Codes that are exempt from modifier 63. This symbol identifies codes that are typically not used in conjuction with other procedure codes.

Ⓐ (red)   Age edit. Age edits apply for codes that have specific age designations within the code description.

Ⓜ (green)   Maternity

⊗   High Risk Denial Alert. Identifies when a diproportionate percentage of the total services billed are denied.

♀ (red)   Female. Procedures and services that are only performed on females are designated with this symbol.

♂ (red)   Male. Procedures and services that are only performed on males are designated with this symbol.

AMA (purple)   *CPT® Assistant* References

⊠ (black)   Unlisted code. Unlisted codes are available for reporting procedures and services that do not have a more specific code listed in the CPT book. These codes should only be used when there is not a current Category I or Category III code that would better describe the procedure or service.

A2–**Z3** (blue)   ASC Payment Indicators. Certain HCPCS Level II codes are reimbursable when provided in an Ambulatory Surgical Center (ASC) under the Outpatient Prospective Payment System (OPPS). Under the ASC reimbursement system, a payment indicator is assigned to each HCPCS code. The payment indicator directs how payment is made or not made under OPPS for each individual code submitted.

Indicator	Payment Indicator Definition
A2	Surgical procedure on ASC list in CY 2007; payment based on OPPS relative payment weight.
D5	Deleted/discontinued code; no payment made.
F4	Corneal tissue acquisition, hepatitis B vaccine; paid at reasonable cost.
G2	Non office-based surgical procedure added in CY 2008 or later; payment based on OPPS relative payment weight.
H2	Brachytherapy source paid separately when provided integral to a surgical procedure on ASC list; payment based on OPPS rate.
J7	OPPS pass-through device paid separately when provided integral to a surgical procedure on ASC list; payment contractor-priced.
J8	Device-intensive procedure; paid at adjusted rate.
K2	Drugs and biologicals paid separately when provided integral to a surgical procedure on ASC list; payment based on OPPS rate.
K7	Unclassified drugs and biologicals; payment contractor-priced.
L1	Influenza vaccine; pneumococcal vaccine. Packaged item/service; no separate payment made.
L6	New Technology Intraocular Lens (NTIOL); special payment.
N1	Packaged service/item; no separate payment made.
P2	Office-based surgical procedure added to ASC list in CY 2008 or later with MPFS nonfacility PE RVUs; payment based on OPPS relative payment weight.
P3	Office-based surgical procedure added to ASC list in CY 2008 or later with MPFS nonfacility PE RVUs; payment based on MPFS nonfacility PE RVUs.
R2	Office-based surgical procedure added to ASC list in CY 2008 or later without MPFS nonfacility PE RVUs; payment based on OPPS relative payment weight.
Z2	Radiology service paid separately when provided integral to a surgical procedure on ASC list; payment based on OPPS relative payment weight.
Z3	Radiology service paid separately when provided integral to a surgical procedure on ASC list; payment based on MPFS nonfacility PE RVUs.

A – Y (red) OPPS Status Indicators. The Ambulatory Payment Classification (APC) system is a Medicare-based fee schedule for outpatient hospital reimbursement under the Outpatient Prospective Payment System (OPPS). Procedures and services are grouped, or assigned to APC codes for fee calculation. Under the APC system, a status indicator is assigned each line item. The status indicator directs how payment is made or not made under OPPS for each individual code submitted and describes the type of service, procedure, device, or supply being reported. The same indicator applies to all codes within an APC.

Indicator	Item/Code/Service	OPPS Payment Status
A	Services furnished to a hospital outpatient that are paid under a fee schedule or payment system other than OPPS, for example:	Not paid under OPPS. Paid by MACs under a fee schedule or payment system other than OPPS.
		Services are subject to deductible or coinsurance unless indicated otherwise.
	• Ambulance Services	
	• Separately Payable Clinical Diagnostic Laboratory Services	Not subject to deductible or coinsurance.
	• Separately Payable Non-Implantable Prosthetics and Orthotics	
	• Physical, Occupational, and Speech Therapy	
	• Diagnostic Mammography	
	• Screening Mammography	Not subject to deductible or coinsurance.
B	Codes that are not recognized by OPPS when submitted on an outpatient hospital Part B bill type (12x and 13x).	Not paid under OPPS.
		• May be paid by MACs when submitted on a different bill type, for example, 75x (CORF), but not paid under OPPS.
		• An alternate code that is recognized by OPPS when submitted on an outpatient hospital Part B bill type (12x and 13x) may be available.
C	Inpatient Procedures	Not paid under OPPS. Admit patient. Bill as inpatient.
D	Discontinued Codes	Not paid under OPPS or any other Medicare payment system.
E	Items, Codes, and Services:	Not paid by Medicare when submitted on outpatient claims (any outpatient bill type).
	• For which pricing information is not available	
	• Not covered by any Medicare outpatient benefit category	
	• Statutorily excluded by Medicare	
	• Not reasonable and necessary	
F	Corneal Tissue Acquisition; Certain CRNA Services and Hepatitis B Vaccines	Not paid under OPPS. Paid at reasonable cost.
G	Pass-Through Drugs and Biologicals	Paid under OPPS; separate APC payment.
H	Pass-Through Device Categories	Separate cost-based pass-through payment; not subject to copayment.
J1	Hospital Part B services paid through a comprehensive APC	Paid under OPPS; all covered Part B services on the claim are packaged with the primary "J1" service for the claim, except services with OPPS SI=F,G, H, L and U; ambulance services; diagnostic and screening mammography; all preventive services; and certain Part B inpatient services.

Indicator	Item/Code/Service	OPPS Payment Status
J2	Hospital Part B Services That May Be Paid Through a Comprehensive APC	Paid under OPPS; Addendum B displays APC assignments when services are separately payable.
		(1) Comprehensive APC payment based on OPPS comprehensive-specific payment criteria. Payment for all covered Part B services on the claim is packaged into a single payment for specific combinations of services, except services with OPPS SI=F,G, H, L and U; ambulance services; diagnostic and screening mammography; all preventive services; and certain Part B inpatient services.
		(2) Packaged APC payment if billed on the same claim as a HCPCS code assigned status indicator "J1."
		(3) In other circumstances, payment is made through a separate APC payment or packaged into payment for other services.
K	Nonpass-Through Drugs and Nonimplantable Biologicals, Including Therapeutic Radiopharmaceuticals	Paid under OPPS; separate APC payment.
L	Influenza Vaccine; Pneumococcal Pneumonia Vaccine	Not paid under OPPS. Paid at reasonable cost; not subject to deductible or coinsurance.
M	Items and Services Not Billable to the MAC	Not paid under OPPS.
N	Items and Services Packaged into APC Rates	Paid under OPPS; payment is packaged into payment for other services. Therefore, there is no separate APC payment.
P	Partial Hospitalization	Paid under OPPS; per diem APC payment.
Q1	STV-Packaged Codes	Paid under OPPS; Addendum B displays APC assignments when services are separately payable.
		(1) Packaged APC payment if billed on the same date of service as a HCPCS code assigned status indicator "S," "T," or "V."
		(2) In other circumstances, payment is made through a separate APC payment.
Q2	T-Packaged Codes	Paid under OPPS; Addendum B displays APC assignments when services are separately payable.
		(1) Packaged APC payment if billed on the same date of service as a HCPCS code assigned status indicator "T."
		(2) In other circumstances, payment is made through a separate APC payment.
Q3	Codes That May Be Paid Through a Composite APC	Paid under OPPS; Addendum B displays APC assignments when services are separately payable.
		Addendum M displays composite APC assignments when codes are paid through a composite APC.
		(1) Composite APC payment based on OPPS composite-specific payment criteria. Payment is packaged into a single payment for specific combinations of services.
		(2) In other circumstances, payment is made through a separate APC payment or packaged into payment for other services.
Q4	Conditionally packaged laboratory tests	Paid under OPPS or CLFS.
		(1) Packaged APC payment if billed on the same claim as a HCPCS code assigned published status indicator "J1," "J2," "S," "T," "V," "Q1," "Q2," or "Q3."
		(2) In other circumstances, laboratory tests should have an SI=A and payment is made under the CLFS.
R	Blood and Blood Products	Paid under OPPS; separate APC payment.
S	Procedure or Service, Not Discounted When Multiple	Paid under OPPS; separate APC payment.
T	Procedure or Service, Multiple Procedure Reduction Applies	Paid under OPPS; separate APC payment.
U	Brachytherapy Sources	Paid under OPPS; separate APC payment.
V	Clinic or Emergency Department Visit	Paid under OPPS; separate APC payment.
Y	Non-Implantable Durable Medical Equipment	Not paid under OPPS. All institutional providers other than home health agencies bill to DMERC.

CPT © 2015 American Medical Association. All rights reserved.

Documentation Finder

Tips for code documentation are defined in narrative form, explaining possible gaps and noting important components for coding.

National Coverage Determinations (NCD)

NCDs are provided to aid in avoiding medical necessity denials for specific contractors. Use policy title citation to reference the complete policy document on respective payers' website.

Code Level Enhancements

To facilitate the coding process, and to add emphasis and enhance its utility, critical value-added data at the code-level has been incorporated into the body of the *Procedural Coding Expert*. This additional data is found only in the Tabular List of Procedures. The next few pages explain, in detail, the code-specific data elements found throughout this guide.

Medicare Physician Fee Schedule and RVUs

Beneath each code, Medicare's total Relative Value Unit (RVU) amounts from the MPFS are provided for the facility and non-facility settings. Facility RVUs should be used for services and procedures performed in inpatient hospitals, outpatient hospitals, emergency rooms, skilled nursing facilities, ambulatory surgical centers, and any other setting where the facility receives a separate payment for the service. Nonfacility RVUs are used for physician office settings and other outpatient settings not listed above. Not all codes on the MPFS have RVUs assigned. Codes without RVUs generally fall into two categories, Medicare noncovered services and contractor priced services. Some codes on the MPFS have three RVU values, one for the technical component (TC), one for the professional component (PC) (modifier 26), and one for the global value (sum of the TC and PC). For codes with both a technical and professional component, the *Procedural Coding Expert* provides three values, the value for the global service identified without a modifier, the professional component identified as 26 and the technical component identified as TC. For RVU values, with breakdowns by work, practice expense, and gap-filled data, please refer to the 2016 *RBRVS Sourcebook*.

Global Periods

Medicare's global periods are provided at the code level. The global period represents the number of post-procedure days during which services related to the procedure are not separately reimbursed. Both CMS and the AMA provide definitions of the global package, and it should be noted that these definitions differ. The global package refers to the services included in the reimbursement for the surgical or other procedure. Services listed as included in the global package are not reimbursed separately unless an exception exists. Any exceptions are listed in CMS manuals or in the AMA guidelines. Many private payers use the global periods and guidelines provided by CMS. The global periods and definitions listed below are those found in the MPFS. There are seven global periods defined by CMS which are as follows:

000 Payment for codes with a global period of "0" do not include payment for any follow-up services or other related procedures/services. However, reimbursement for these codes does include payment for E/M and other usual services related to the original procedure when performed on the same date of service. The 0-day global period tends to be reserved for minor or endoscopic procedures.

010 10-day global periods apply to minor procedures that require a minimal amount of post-surgical follow-up. Again, related E/M services and procedures performed on the day of the surgery and the subsequent 10-day period would not be considered separately billable.

090 The 90-day global period is reserved for the major surgeries. Not only does payment for codes with this designation include all related services performed the day of the surgery, but also 1 day prior and 90 days afterwards.

MMM Maternity care and delivery codes in the CPT range 59400-59622 (with the exception of add-on code 59525) follow different global package rules than typical procedures. Because these codes are governed by special global billing rules set for antepartum, delivery and postpartum care, they do not adhere to the typical 0, 10, 90 day surgical periods. View the coding guidance prior to these code ranges for more specifics on correct maternity care package billing.

XXX An "X" in the global period area signifies that the global concept does not apply to this particular code and that even related services performed on the same date of service can potentially be billed and reimbursed separately. As indicated by the definition of the global package, codes with "X" designation are typically, but not always, non-surgical in nature (e.g., anesthesia administration, diagnostic radiology and lab tests, and medical services).

YYY Codes with the "Y" global indicator have their global periods set by individual insurance carriers, rather than on a national level. Most of the CPT codes with a "Y" indicator are unlisted procedures or services for which there is no specific assigned CPT code, hence carriers review the billing and determine pricing for these codes on a case-by-case basis.

ZZZ The "Z" global indicator applies to add-on CPT codes. Because these codes can only be used as supplemental codes to another CPT code, the global periods for the primary procedure code always take precedence. To eliminate any confusion by potentially having differing global periods than the primary codes, add-on codes are assigned the status "Z."

Modifier Rules

Another enhancement provided at the code level is modifier information. Medicare's rules regarding the applicability of the modifiers for multiple procedures (51), bilateral procedures (50), assistant surgeon (80) and co-surgeons (62) are listed. On the MPFS, the applicable modifier rules for each modifier are designated by a number. These number designations are defined in supplementary information provided with the MPFS RVU table. In the *Procedural Coding Expert*, each of the four modifiers is listed at the code level with the number that identifies the MPFS reimbursement rules for the listed code. The meaning of the number for each modifier is explained below:

Mult Proc = Multiple Procedure (Modifier 51)

Indicates applicable payment adjustment rule for multiple procedures:

0 No payment adjustment rules for multiple procedures apply. If procedure is reported on the same day as another procedure, base the payment on the lower of (a) the actual charge, or (b) the fee schedule amount for the procedure.

1 Standard payment adjustment rules in effect before January 1, 1995 for multiple procedures apply. In the 1995 file, this indicator only applies to codes with a status code of "D". If procedure is reported on the same day as another procedure that has an indicator of 1, 2, or 3, rank the procedures by fee schedule amount and apply the appropriate reduction to this code (100%, 50%, 25%, 25%, 25%, and by report). Base the payment on the lower of (a) the actual charge, or (b) the fee schedule amount reduced by the appropriate percentage.

2 Standard payment adjustment rules for multiple procedures apply. If procedure is reported on the same day as another procedure with an indicator of 1, 2, or 3, rank the procedures by fee schedule amount and apply the appropriate reduction to this code (100%, 50%, 50%, 50%, 50% and by report). Base the payment on the lower of (a) the actual charge, or (b) the fee schedule amount reduced by the appropriate percentage.

3 Special rules for multiple endoscopic procedures apply if procedure is billed with another endoscopy in the same family (i.e., another endoscopy that has the same base procedure). Apply the multiple endoscopy rules to a family before ranking the family with the other procedures performed on the same day (for example, if multiple endoscopies in the same family are reported on the same day as endoscopies in another family or on the same day as a non-endoscopic procedure). If an endoscopic procedure

is reported with only its base procedure, do not pay separately for the base procedure. Payment for the base procedure is included in the payment for the other endoscopy.

5   Subject to 25% of the practice expense component for certain therapy services (effective for services January 1, 2011, and after).

9   Concept does not apply.

Bilat Surg = Bilateral Surgery (Modifier 50)

Indicates services subject to payment adjustment.

0   150% payment adjustment for bilateral procedures **does not** apply. If procedure is reported with modifier 50 or with modifiers RT and LT, base the payment for the two sides on the lower of: (a) the total actual charge for both sides or (b) 100% of the fee schedule amount for a single code. Example: The fee schedule amount for code XXXXX is $125. The physician reports code XXXXX-LT with an actual charge of $100 and XXXXX-RT with an actual charge of $100. Payment should be based on the fee schedule amount ($125) since it is lower than the total actual charges for the left and right sides ($200). The bilateral adjustment is inappropriate for codes in this category (a) because of physiology or anatomy, or (b) because the code description specifically states that it is a unilateral procedure and there is an existing code for the bilateral procedure.

1   150% payment adjustment for bilateral procedures applies. If the code is billed with the bilateral modifier or is reported twice on the same day by any other means (e.g., with RT and LT modifiers, or with a 2 in the units field), base the payment for these codes when reported as bilateral procedures on the lower of: (a) the total actual charge for both sides or (b) 150% of the fee schedule amount for a single code. If the code is reported as a bilateral procedure and is reported with other procedure codes on the same day, apply the bilateral adjustment before applying any multiple procedure rules.

2   150% payment adjustment **does not** apply. RVUs are already based on the procedure being performed as a bilateral procedure. If the procedure is reported with modifier 50 or is reported twice on the same day by any other means (e.g., with RT and LT modifiers or with a 2 in the units field), base the payment for both sides on the lower of (a) the total actual charge by the physician for both sides, or (b) 100% of the fee schedule for a single code. Example: The fee schedule amount for code YYYYY is $125. The physician reports code YYYYY-LT with an actual charge of $100 and YYYYY-RT with an actual charge of $100. Payment should be based on the fee schedule amount ($125) since

it is lower than the total actual charges for the left and right sides ($200). The RVUs are based on a bilateral procedure because (a) the code descriptor specifically states that the procedure is bilateral, (b) the code descriptor states that the procedure may be performed either unilaterally or bilaterally, or (c) the procedure is usually performed as a bilateral procedure.

3   The usual payment adjustment for bilateral procedures **does not** apply. If the procedure is reported with modifier 50 or is reported for both sides on the same day by any other means (e.g., with RT and LT modifiers or with a 2 in the units field), base the payment for each side or organ or site of a paired organ on the lower of (a) the actual charge for each side or (b) 100% of the fee schedule amount for each side. If the procedure is reported as a bilateral procedure and with other procedure codes on the same day, determine the fee schedule amount for a bilateral procedure before applying any multiple procedure rules. Services in this category are generally radiology procedures or other diagnostic tests which are not subject to the special payment rules for other bilateral surgeries.

9   Concept does not apply.

Asst Surg = Assistant at Surgery (Modifier 80)

Indicates services where an assistant at surgery is never paid for per ***Medicare Claims Manual***.

0   Payment restriction for assistants at surgery applies to this procedure unless supporting documentation is submitted to establish medical necessity.

1   Statutory payment restriction for assistants at surgery applies to this procedure. Assistant at surgery may not be paid.

2   Payment restriction for assistants at surgery does not apply to this procedure. Assistant at surgery may be paid.

9   Concept does not apply.

Co Surg = Co-surgeons (Modifier 62)

Indicates services for which two surgeons, each in a different specialty, may be paid.

0   Co-surgeons not permitted for this procedure.

1   Co-surgeons could be paid, though supporting documentation is required to establish the medical necessity of two surgeons for the procedure.

2   Co-surgeons permitted and no documentation required if the two-specialty requirement is met.

9   Concept does not apply.

CPT © 2015 American Medical Association. All rights reserved.

CPT Modifiers

This section contains a list of CPT modifiers and accompanying coding tips that provide further clarification on using modifiers for claims submission.

Modifiers and Coding Tips

22   **Increased Procedural Services** – When the work required to provide a service is substantially greater than typically required, it may be identified by adding modifier 22 to the usual procedure code. Documentation must support the substantial additional work and the reason for the additional work (ie, increased intensity, time, technical difficulty of procedure, severity of patient's condition, physical and mental effort required). Note: This modifier should not be appended to an E/M service.

     Coding Guidance: Claims submitted to Medicare, Medicaid, and other payers containing modifier 22 for unusual procedural services that do not have attached supporting documentation that illustrates the unusual distinction of the services will be processed as if the procedure codes were not appended with this modifier. Some payers might suspend the claims and request additional information from the provider, but this is the exception rather than the rule. For most payers, this modifier includes additional reimbursement to the provider for the additional work.

23   **Unusual Anesthesia** – Occasionally, a procedure which usually requires either no anesthesia or local anesthesia, because of unusual circumstances must be done under general anesthesia. This circumstance may be reported by adding the modifier 23 to the procedure code of the basic service.

     Coding Guidance: This modifier is most commonly appended to procedures performed on children or handicapped individuals.

24   **Unrelated Evaluation and Management Service by the Same Physician or Other Qualified Health Care Professional During a Postoperative Period** – The physician or other qualified health care professional may need to indicate that an evaluation and management service was performed during a postoperative period for a reason(s) unrelated to the original procedure. This circumstance may be reported by adding modifier 24 to the appropriate level of E/M service.

     Coding Guidance: A postoperative period is one that has been determined to be included in the payment for the procedure that was performed. During this time, the provider renders follow-up care related to the procedure in follow-up visits, which is not reimbursed separately. Appending modifier 24 indicates that the evaluation and management service provided during the follow-up period for a surgical procedure is not related to the surgery and therefore should be reimbursed separately. Medicare has postoperative periods for procedures of 0, 10, or 90 days (number of days applicable for each procedure can be found in the Federal Register or Physician Fee Schedule (RBRVS) released by CMS. Commercial payers may have variable numbers of postoperative days for procedures; check with each to determine the appropriate number of global days for a given procedure.

25   **Significant, Separately Identifiable Evaluation and Management Service by the Same Physician or Other Qualified Health Care Professional on the Same Day of the Procedure or Other Service** – It may be necessary to indicate that on the day a procedure or service identified by a CPT code was performed, the patient's condition required a significant, separately identifiable E/M service above and beyond the other service provided or beyond the usual preoperative and postoperative care associated with the procedure that was performed. A significant, separately identifiable E/M service is defined or substantiated by documentation that satisfies the relevant criteria for the respective E/M service to be reported (see Evaluation and Management Services Guidelines of CPT for instructions on determining level of E/M service). The E/M service may be prompted by the symptom or condition for which the procedure and/or service was provided. As such, different diagnoses are not required for reporting of the E/M services on the same date. This circumstance may be reported by adding modifier 25 to the appropriate level of E/M service. Note: This modifier is not used to report an E/M service that resulted in a decision to perform surgery. See modifier 57. For significant, separately identifiable non-E/M services, see modifier 59.

     Coding Guidance:

1. *Modifier 25 should be used only when a visit is separately payable when billed in addition to a minor surgical procedure (any surgery with a 0- or 10-day postoperative period per Medicare). Payment for pre- and postoperative work in minor procedures is included in the payment for the procedure. Where the decision to perform the minor procedure is typically made immediately before the service (e.g., sutures are needed to close a wound), it is considered to be a routine preoperative service and visit should not be billed in addition to the minor procedure. In circumstances in which the physician provides an E/M service that is beyond the usual pre- and post-operative work for the service, the visit may be billed with a modifier 25. A modifier is not needed if the visit was performed the day before a minor surgery because the global period for minor procedures does not include the day prior to the surgery.*

2. *The global surgery policy does not apply to services of other physicians who may be rendering services during the pre- or postoperative period unless the physician is a member of the same group as the operating physician.*

3. *The provider must determine if the E/M service for which they are billing is clearly distinct from the surgical service. When the decision to perform the minor procedure is typically done immediately before the procedure is rendered, the visit should not be billed separately.*

26   **Professional Component** – Certain procedures are a combination of a physician or other qualified health care professional component and a technical component. When the physician or other qualified health care professional component is reported separately, the service may be identified by adding the modifier 26 to the usual procedure number.

     Coding Guidance: Use of modifier 26 indicates the provider performed the professional component of a service that has both a professional and technical component, and provided a written report including an interpretation of findings to document the service in the medical record. The technical component is reported with modifier TC appended to the code. Reimbursement will be split between the professional and technical components if this is applied to the code.

     To determine which codes have both a professional and technical component for Medicare, review the Federal Register and/or the Physician Fee Schedule for a breakdown. Usually commercial payers follow CMS determinations of professional and technical components. Some CPT codes are already broken down into professional and technical components by definition and do not require the 26 modifier. For example:

93005   Electrocardiogram, routine ECG with at least 12 leads; tracing only, without interpretation and report (technical component)

93010   Electrocardiogram, routine ECG with at least 12 leads; interpretation and report only

32   Mandated Services – Services related to mandated consultation and/or related services (eg, third party payer, governmental, legislative or regulatory requirement) may be identified by adding modifier 32 to the basic procedure.

Coding Guidance Modifier 32 is considered informational and will have no effect on reimbursement.

33   Preventive Services – When the primary purpose of the service is the delivery of an evidence based service in accordance with the US Preventive Services Task Force A or B rating in effect and other preventive services identified in preventive services mandates (legislative or regulatory), the service may be identified by adding modifier 33 to the procedure. For separately reported services specifically identified as preventive, the modifier should not be used.

47   Anesthesia by Surgeon – Regional or general anesthesia provided by the surgeon may be reported by adding modifier 47 to the basic service. (This does not include local anesthesia.) Note: Modifier 47 would not be used as a modifier for the anesthesia procedures.

Coding Guidance This service is not covered by Medicare and many state Medicaid programs. Commercial payers and managed care organizations may cover this additional service.

50   Bilateral Procedure – Unless otherwise identified in the listings, bilateral procedures that are performed at the same session should be identified by adding modifier 50 to the appropriate five digit code.

Coding Guidance Reported as a one-line item for Medicare claims with modifier 50 appended to the end of the code, although, some payers request that bilateral procedures be reported with the LT and RT HCPCS Level II modifiers reported as two-line items.

51   Multiple Procedures – When multiple procedures, other than E/M services, Physical Medicine and Rehabilitation services or provision of supplies (eg, vaccines), are performed at the same session by the same individual, the primary procedure or service may be reported as listed. The additional procedure(s) or service(s) may be identified by appending modifier 51 to the additional procedure or service code(s). Note: This modifier should not be appended to designated "add-on" codes.

Coding Guidance Applicable Modifier 51 Exempt codes are noted at the code level by the icon ⊘. This signifies that the procedure should not be appended a modifier 51 at the end of the code.

52   Reduced Services – Under certain circumstances a service or procedure is partially reduced or eliminated at the discretion of the physician or other qualified health care professional. Under these circumstances the service provided can be identified by its usual procedure number and the addition of modifier 52, signifying that the service is reduced. This provides a means of reporting reduced services without disturbing the identification of the basic service. Note: For hospital outpatient reporting of a previously scheduled procedure/service that is partially reduced or cancelled as a result of extenuating circumstances or those that threaten the well-being of the patient prior to or after administration of anesthesia, see modifiers 73 and 74.

Coding Guidance: Procedures reported with this modifier should include the following documentation:

- *A concise statement about how the service or procedure differs from the usual or normal*
- *The operative (or other) report*

Claims reported with modifier 52 that do not include

documentation that serves to clarify the use of this modifier will be processed as if there were no modifiers reported. Most payers will reduce reimbursement if this code is used.

53   Discontinued Procedure – Under certain circumstances, the physician or other qualified health care professional may elect to terminate a surgical or diagnostic procedure. Due to extenuating circumstances or those that threaten the well being of the patient, it may be necessary to indicate that a surgical or diagnostic procedure was started but discontinued. This circumstance may be reported by adding modifier 53 to the code reported by the individual for the discontinued procedure.

Note: This modifier is not used to report the elective cancellation of a procedure prior to the patient's anesthesia induction and/or surgical preparation in the operating suite. For outpatient hospital/ambulatory surgery center (ASC) reporting of a previously scheduled procedure/service that is partially reduced or cancelled as a result of extenuating circumstances or those that threaten the well being of the patient prior to or after administration of anesthesia, see modifiers 73 and 74.

54   Surgical Care Only – When one physician or other qualified health care professional performs a surgical procedure and another provides preoperative and/or postoperative management, surgical services may be identified by adding modifier 54 to the usual procedure number.

Coding Guidance:
- *Both claims submitted by the surgeon and the other provider must report the date patient care was assumed and relinquished in block 19 of the CMS-1500 or electronic equivalent.*
- *Both the surgeon and the other provider must keep a copy of the written transfer agreement in the patient's medical record.*
- *Both providers will use the same CPT code, but they will use different modifiers that identify which portion of care they provided.*

When more than one physician provides care for a procedure, the care is split between the providers. The providers will use the same CPT code, but attach a modifier to the end of the code. The modifiers that indicate split care has taken place are:

54   Surgical care only
55   Postoperative management only
56   Preoperative management only

The global payment of the surgery is distributed between the providers according to the procedure percentages as determined by CMS and most payers follow the same rules. Workers Compensation payers use different percentage amounts for split care reimbursement. Medicare payment for postoperative care by more than one physician will be apportioned according to the number of the 90 days each doctor renders care. In most cases, the surgeon will perform the in-hospital care, but may turn over the out-of-hospital or postoperative care to another physician.

55   Postoperative Management Only – When one physician or other qualified health care professional performed the postoperative management and another physician performed the surgical procedure, the postoperative component may be identified by adding modifier 55 to the usual procedure number.

Coding Guidance: Both providers will use the same CPT code, but they will use different modifiers that identify which portion of care they provided.

56   Preoperative Management Only – When one physician or other qualified health care professional performed the preoperative care and evaluation and another performed the surgical procedure, the preoperative component may be identified by adding modifier 56 to the usual procedure number.

CPT © 2015 American Medical Association. All rights reserved.
© 2016 DecisionHealth

Coding Guidance: Both providers will use the same CPT code, but will they will use different modifiers that identify which portion of care they provided. Some payers do not allow modifier 56 as they consider all preoperative management to be included in the global payment.

57   Decision for Surgery – An evaluation and management service that resulted in the initial decision to perform the surgery may be identified by adding modifier 57 to the appropriate level of E/M service. .

Coding Guidance: When billing Medicare, this modifier should only be used when the surgery being discussed qualifies as a major surgery. E/M visits by the same physician on the day before or the same day as a major surgery are included in the payment for the procedure, unless the visit establishes the decision to operate. Major Surgery with a global period of 90 days (as defined by Medicare) includes the day before and the day of surgery. For example, a visit the day before or the same day could be properly billed in addition to a cholecystotomy if the need for the surgery was found during the encounter; modifier 57 should be added to the E/M code. Billing for a visit would not be appropriate if the physician was only discussing the upcoming surgical procedure.

58   Staged or Related Procedure or Service by the Same Physician or Other Qualified Health Care Professional During the Postoperative Period – It may be necessary to indicate that the performance of a procedure or service during the postoperative period was: a) planned or anticipated (staged); b) more extensive than the original procedure; or c) for therapy following a surgical procedure. This circumstance may be reported by adding modifier 58 to the staged or related procedure. Note: For treatment of a problem that requires a return to the operating/procedure room (e.g., unanticipated clinical condition), see modifier 78.

Coding Guidance: Modifier 58 must be used for purposes of identifying procedures performed by the original physician during the postoperative period of the original procedure, within the constraints of the modifier's definition. These procedures cannot be repeat operations (unless the procedures are more extensive than the original procedure) and cannot be for the treatment of complications requiring a return trip to the operating room.

The existence of modifier 58 does not negate the global fee concept. Services that are included in CPT as multiple sessions or are defined as including multiple services or events may not be billed with this modifier. This modifier is designed to allow a method of reporting additional, related surgeries that are due to a progression of the disease and are not to be used to avoid global surgery edits applicable to staged procedures.

Modifier 58 should be used on surgical codes only and has no effect on the payment amount. It should not be used with codes defined as "one or more sessions or stages."

59   Distinct Procedural Service – Under certain circumstances, it may be necessary to indicate that a procedure or service was distinct or independent from other non-E/M services performed on the same day. Modifier 59 is used to identify procedures/services, other than E/M services, that are not normally reported together, but are appropriate under the circumstances. Documentation must support a different session, different procedure or surgery, different site or organ system, separate incision/excision, separate lesion, or separate injury (or area of injury in extensive injuries) not ordinarily encountered or performed on the same day by the same individual. However, when another already established modifier is appropriate it should be used rather than modifier 59. Only if no more descriptive modifier is available, and the use of modifier 59 best explains the circumstances, should modifier 59 be used. Note: Modifier 59 should not be appended to an E/M service. To report a separate and distinct E/M service with a non-E/M service performed on the same date, see modifier 25.

Coding Guidance: Modifier 59 was established to demonstrate that multiple, yet distinct, services were provided to a patient on the same date of service by the same provider. Because distinct procedures or services rendered on the same day by the same physician cannot be easily identified and properly adjudicated by simply listing the CPT procedure codes, modifier 59 assists the payer or Medicare carrier in applying the appropriate reimbursement protocol. If the modifier is not used in these circumstances, services may be denied, with the explanation of benefits stating that the payer does not reimburse for this service because it is part of another service that was performed at the same time.

62   Two Surgeons – When two surgeons work together as primary surgeons performing distinct part(s) of a procedure, each surgeon should report his/her distinct operative work by adding modifier 62 to the procedure code and any associated add-on code(s) for that procedure as long as both surgeons continue to work together as primary surgeons. Each surgeon should report the co-surgery once using the same procedure code. If additional procedure(s) (including add-on procedure(s) are performed during the same surgical session, separate code(s) may also be reported with modifier 62 added. Note: If a co-surgeon acts as an assistant in the performance of additional procedure(s) during the same surgical session, those services may be reported using separate procedure code(s) with modifier 80 or modifier 82 added, as appropriate.

Coding Guidance: Under Medicare, payment for the two physicians is based on the two physicians splitting 125 percent of the allowed charge(s). Check with other payers to determine payment based on this modifier. This modifier should not be confused with modifier 80 (assistant surgeon).

63   Procedure Performed on Infants Less than 4 kg – Procedures performed on neonates and infants up to a present body weight of 4 kg may involve significantly increased complexity and physician work commonly associated with these patients. This circumstance may be reported by adding modifier 63 to the procedure number. **Note**: Unless otherwise designated, this modifier may only be appended to procedures/services listed in the 20005-69990 code series. Modifier 63 should not be appended to any CPT codes listed in the Evaluation and Management Services, Anesthesia, Radiology, Pathology/Laboratory, or Medicine sections.

Coding Guidance: Applicable Modifier 63 exempt codes are noted at the code level by the icon ⊖. These signify that modifier 63 should not be appended at the end of the procedure code.

66   Surgical Team – Under some circumstances, highly complex procedures (requiring the concomitant services of several physicians or other qualified health care professionals, often of different specialties, plus other highly skilled, specially trained personnel, various types of complex equipment) are carried out under the "surgical team" concept. Such circumstances may be identified by each participating physician with the addition of modifier 66 to the basic procedure number used for reporting services.

Coding Guidance: Each surgeon that participates in the procedure would report the same CPT code with the 66 modifier. Only surgical CPT codes (10021-69990) should be used with modifier 66 unless otherwise stated by the payer.

76   Repeat Procedure or Service by Same Physician or Other Qualified Health Care Professional – It may be necessary to indicate that a procedure or service was repeated by the same physician or other qualified health care professional, subsequent to the original procedure or service. This circumstance may be reported by adding modifier 76 to the repeated procedure/service. Note: This modifier should not be appended to an E/M service.

Coding Guidance: This is usually due to the patient's medical condition, requiring the need for additional diagnostic testing or further therapeutic intervention. If repeat laboratory tests are performed, report modifier 91 instead of modifier 76.

77   Repeat Procedure by Another Physician or Other Qualified Health Care Professional – It may be necessary to indicate that a basic procedure or service was repeated by another physician or other qualified health care professional subsequent to the original procedure or service. This circumstance may be reported by adding modifier 77 to the repeated procedure/service. Note: This modifier should not be appended to an E/M service.

Coding Guidance: Appending this modifier does not guarantee payment of the repeat procedure, but will assist in determining duplicate billings for the procedure.

78   Unplanned Return to the Operating/Procedure Room by the Same Physician or Other Qualified Health Care Professional Following Initial Procedure for a Related Procedure During the Postoperative Period – It may be necessary to indicate that another procedure was performed during the postoperative period of the initial procedure (unplanned procedure following initial procedure). When this procedure is related to the first, and requires the use of an operating/ procedure room, it may be reported by adding modifier 78 to the related procedure. (For repeat procedures, see modifier 76.)

Coding Guidance: Medicare includes specific medical and/or surgical care for postoperative complications as included within the global surgical package, for which there is no additional payment. Included in the global surgical package is defined as, "additional medical and surgical services required of the surgeon during the postoperative period of the surgery because of complications which do not require additional trips to the operating room."

79   Unrelated Procedure or Service by the Same Physician or Other Qualified Health Care Professional During the Postoperative Period – The individual may need to indicate that the performance of a procedure or service during the postoperative period was unrelated to the original procedure. This circumstance may be reported by using modifier 79. (For repeat procedures on the same day, see modifier 76.)

Coding Guidance: When billing for an unrelated procedure by the same physician during the postoperative period of an original procedure, a new postoperative period will begin with the subsequent procedure. A different ICD-9-CM diagnosis should be indicated on the claim.

80   Assistant Surgeon – Surgical assistant services may be identified by adding modifier 80 to the usual procedure number(s).

Coding Guidance: Some surgical procedures are not eligible for this modifier; check the Medicare physician

fee schedule or with other payers to determine payment eligibility.

81   Minimum Assistant Surgeon – Minimum surgical assistant services are identified by adding modifier 81 to the usual procedure number.

82   Assistant Surgeon (when qualified resident surgeon not available) – The unavailability of a qualified resident surgeon is a prerequisite for use of modifier 82 appended to the usual procedure code number(s).

Coding Guidance: In some hospitals with residency programs, Medicare pays through the medical program or graduate medical education (GME) program. Because of this, they will not reimburse for a resident when they are used as an assistant surgeon. Although under special circumstances, payment may be made if there is a emergent situation that is life-threatening.

90   Reference (Outside) Laboratory – When laboratory procedures are performed by a party other than the treating or reporting physician or other qualified health care professional, the procedure may be identified by adding modifier 90 to the usual procedure number.

Coding Guidance: Check with payers to determine if the provider may bill for the laboratory procedure if performed incident to his/her services by an ancillary staff member.

91   Repeat Clinical Diagnostic Laboratory Test – In the course of treatment of the patient, it may be necessary to repeat the same laboratory test on the same day to obtain subsequent (multiple) test results. Under these circumstances, the laboratory test performed can be identified by its usual procedure number and the addition of modifier 91. Note: This modifier may not be used when tests are rerun to confirm initial results; due to testing problems with specimens or equipment; or for any other reason when a normal, one-time, reportable result is all that is required. This modifier may not be used when other code(s) describe a series of test results (eg, glucose tolerance tests, evocative/suppression testing). This modifier may only be used for laboratory test(s) performed more than once on the same day on the same patient.

92   Alternative Laboratory Platform Testing – When laboratory testing is being performed using a kit or transportable instrument that wholly or in part consists of a single use, disposable analytical chamber, the service may be identified by adding modifier 92 to the usual laboratory procedure code (HIV testing 86701-86703 and 87389). The test does not require permanent dedicated space, hence by its design may be hand carried or transported to the vicinity of the patient for immediate testing at that site, although location of the testing is not in itself determinative of the use of this modifier.

Coding Guidance: This modifier should only be appended to HIV testing codes 86701-86703 and 87389.

99   Multiple Modifiers – Under certain circumstances two or more modifiers may be necessary to completely delineate a service. In such situations modifier 99 should be added to the basic procedure, and other applicable modifiers may be listed as part of the description of the service.

CPT © 2015 American Medical Association. All rights reserved.   © 2016 DecisionHealth

Coding Reference Information

Root Words

Root Words	Combining Forms
abdomin/o	abdomen
acous/o	hearing
acr/o	extremities, top, extreme point
aden/o	gland
adip/o	fat
andr/o	male
ankyl/o	stiff, bent, crooked
anter/o	front
arthr/o	joint
ather/o	yellowish, fatty plaque
audi/o	hearing
aur/o	ear
aut/o	self
axill/o	armpit
balan/o	glans penis
bi/o	life
blast/o	developing cell
blephr/o	eyelid
brach/o	arm
bronch/o	bronchial tubes
carcin/o	cancer
card/o	heart
cheil/o	lip
chol/o	gall, bile
cholangi/o	bile duct
chondr/o	cartilage
cis/o	to cut
colp/o	vagina
coron/o	heart
cost/o	ribs
crani/o	skull
cry/o	cold
cutane/o	skin
cyan/o	blue
cyt/o	cell
cyst/o	urinary bladder
dacry/o	tear duct, tear
derm/o	skin
dermat/o	skin
dipl/o	double, two
dips/o	thirst
dist/o	distant, far
ech/o	sound
encephal/o	brain
enter/o	intestine
erythr/o	red

erythem/o	red
eti/o	cause of disease
galact/o	milk
gastr/o	stomach
gloss/o	tongue
gluc/o	sugar
glyc/o	sugar
gon/o	seed
gravid/o	pregnancy
gynec/o	female, woman
hemat/o	blood
hepat/o	liver
hidr/o	sweat
hist/o	tissue
home/o	sameness
inguin/o	groin
isch/o	to hold back
kal/o	potassium
kerat/o	horny tissue, hard
labi/o	lip
lapar/o	abdomen, abdominal
laryng/o	larynx
lei/o	smooth
leuk/o	white
lingu/o	tongue
lith/o	stone
lord/o	swayback, curvature in lumbar region
mamm/o	breast
mast/o	breast
melan/o	black
ment/o	mind
metr/o	uterus
morph/o	shape, form
my/o	muscle
myc/o	fungus
myel/o	spinal cord
myring/o	eardrum
natr/o	sodium
necr/o	death (of cells or all of the body)
nephr/o	kidney
neur/o	nerve
noct/o	night
odont/o	tooth
olig/o	few, scanty
omphal/o	naval, umbilicus
onc/o	tumor
onych/o	nail
oophor/o	ovary

opt/o	eye
ophthalm/o	eye
or/o	mouth
orch/o	testis
orchi/o	testis
orchid/o	testis
orth/o	straight
oste/o	bone
ot/o	ear
ov/o	egg
ovul/o	egg
pachy/o	thick
path/o	disease
phag/o	to eat, swallow
phleb/o	vein
phon/o	voice
phot/o	light
phren/o	diaphragm
plas/o	formation, development
pneumon/o	lungs
poli/o	gray matter
proct/o	rectum and anus
pulmon/o	lungs
psych/o	mind
py/o	pus
quadr/o	four
ren/o	kidney
rhin/o	nose
rhytid/o	wrinkle
rhiz/o	nerve root
salping/o	fallopian tubes
sial/o	salivary gland
sarc/o	flesh
sect/o	to cut
spir/o	breathing
spondyl/o	vertebra
squam/o	scale-like
staphyl/o	clusters
steat/o	fat
strept/o	twisted chains
terat/o	monster
thec/o	sheath
thorac/o	chest
thromb/o	clot
trich/o	hair
tympan/o	eardrum
ung/o	nail
vas/o	vessel
ven/o	vein

viscer/o	internal organs
xanth/o	yellow
xer/o	dry

Prefixes

a(d)-	towards
a(n)-	without
ab-	from
ab(s)-	away from
ad-	towards
allo-	other, another
ambi-	both
amphi-	on both sides, around
ana-	up to, back, again, movement from
aniso-	different, unequal
ante-	before, forwards
anti-	against, opposite
ap-, apo-	from, back, again
bi(s)-	twice, double
bio-	life
brachy-	short
cata-	down
circum-	around
con-	together
contra-	against
cyte-	cell
de-	from, away from, down from
deca-	ten
di(s)-	two
dia-	through, complete
di(a)s	separation
diplo-	double
dolicho-	long
dur-	hard, firm
dys-	bad, abnormal
e-, ec-	out, from out of
ecto-	outside, external
ek-	out
em-	in
en-	into
endo-	into
ent-	within
epi-	on, up, against, high
eso-	will carry
eu-	well, abundant, prosperous
eury-	broad, wide
ex-, exo-	out, from out of
extra-	outside, beyond, in addition
haplo-	single
hapto-	bind to

hemi-	half
hept-	seven
hetero-	ifferent
hex-	six
homo-	same
hyper-	above, excessive
hypo-	below, deficient
im-, in-	not
in-	into, to
infra-	below, underneath
inter-	among, between
intra-	within, inside, during
intro-	inward, during
iso-	equal, same
juxta-	adjacent to
kata-	down, down from
macro-	large
magno-	large
medi-	middle
mega-	large
megalo-	very large
meso-	middle
meta-	beyond, between
micro-	small
neo-	new
non-	not
ob-	before, against
octa-	eight
octo-	eight
oligo-	few
pachy-	thick
pan-	all
para-	beside, to the side of, wrong
pent-	five
per-	by, through, throughout
peri-	around, round-about
pleo-	more than usual
poly	many
post-	behind, after
pre-	before, in front, very
pros-	besides
prox-	besides
pseudo-	false, fake
quar(r)-	four
re, red-	back, again
retro-	backwards, behind
semi-	half
sex-	six
sept-	seven
sub-	under, beneath
super-	above, in addition, over
supra-	above, on the upper side

syn-	together, with
sys-	together, with
tetra-	four
thio-	sulfur
trans-	across, beyond
tri-	three
uni-	one
ultra-	beyond, besides, over

Suffixes

-ase	fermenter
-ate	do
-cide	killer
-c(o)ele	cavity, hollow
-ectomy	removal of, cut out
-form	shaped like
-ia	got
-iasis	full of
-ile	little version
-illa	little version
-illus	little version
-in	stuff
-ism	theory, characteristic of
-itis	inflammation
-ity	makes a noun of quality
-ium	thing
-ize	do
-logy	study of, reasoning about
-megaly	large
-noid	mind, spirit
-oid	resembling, image of
-ogen	precursor
-ol(e)	alcohol
-ole	little version
-oma	tumor (usually)
-osis	full of
-ostomy	"mouth-cut"
-pathy	disease of, suffering
-penia	lack
-pexy	fix in place
-plasty	re-shaping
-philia	affection for
-rhage	burst out
-rhea	discharge, flowing out
-rhexis	shredding
-pagus	Siamese twins
-sis	idea (makes a noun, typically abstract)
-thrix	hair
-tomy	cut
-ule	little version
-um	thing (makes a noun, typically abstract)

CPT © 2015 American Medical Association. All rights reserved.   © 2016 DecisionHealth

Abbreviations

The following definitions are medical terms commonly seen while coding/billing for primary care:

a	before meals
A	without, lack of, apathy
A & P	anterior and posterior; auscultation and percussion abd abdomen
AA	aortic aneurysm; ascending aorta
AAA	abdominal aortic aneurysm
AAR	aortic arch syndrome
AAT	atrial demand triggered pacemaker
Ab	antibody
Ab	away from
ABE	acute bacterial endocarditis
ABG	arterial blood gases
ABP	arterial blood pressure
ac	before meals
ACBG	aortocoronary bypass graft
ACD	absolute cardiac dullness
ACE	angiotensin converting enzyme
ACG	angiocardiography
ACI	acute coronary insufficiency
ACL	anterior cruciate ligament
ACT	anticoagulant therapy; active motion
ACTH	adrenocorticotropic hormone
ad	to, toward, near to
Ad lib	as desired
ADG	atrial diastolic gallop
ADH	antidiuretic hormone
ADL	activities of daily living
AED	automatic external defibrillator
AEI	atrial escape interval
AEP	average evoked potential
AER	average evoked response
AF	aortic flow; atrial fibrillation
AFB	acid-fast bacilli
AFIB	atrial fibrillation
AFP	alpha-fetoprotein
AGA	appropriate for gestational age
AI	aortic insufficiency
AICD	automated implantable cardio-defibrillator
AIDS	acquired immune deficiency syndrome
AKA	above knee amputation
ALMI	anterior lateral myocardial infarction
ALP	alkaline phosphatase
ALT	alanine transaminase, alanine aminotransferase
AMA	against medical advice
AMB	ambulatory
Ambi	both, ambidextrous
AMI	acute myocardial infarction
amphi	about, on both sides, both
ampho	both, amphogenic
ana	up, back, again, excessive, anatomy
ant	before, forward
anti	against, opposed to, reversed
AO	angle of; aorta
AOD	arteriosclerotic occlusive disease
AP	apical pulse
apo	from, away from
APSGN	acute poststreptococcal glomerulonephritis
ARF	acute renal failure
AS	aortic stenosis
ASCVD	arteriosclerotic cardiovascular disease
ASD	atrial septal defect
ASHD	arteriosclerotic heart disease
AST	aspartate aminotransferase
ATN	acute tubular necrosis
AU	both ears
AV	aortic valve
AVB	atrio-ventricular block
AVR	aortic valve replacement
B/K	below knee
BBS	bilateral breath sounds
BE	barium enema
BG	blood glucose
BI	brain injury
Bi	twice, double
BID	twice a day
bilat	bilateral
BM	bowel movement; breast milk
BMR	basal metabolic rate
BP	blood pressure
BPH	benign prostatic hypertrophy
BRM	biologic response modifiers
BRP	bathroom privileges
BS	bowel sounds
BSA	body surface area
BSE	breast self examination

BT	bowel tones
BUN	blood urea nitrogen
bx	biopsy
C	Celsius(centigrade)
c (C)	with
C&S	culture and sensitivity
c/o	complaint of
Ca	calcium, cancer, carcinoma
CA	cardiac arrest
CABG	coronary artery bypass graft
CAD	coronary artery disease
CAPD	continuous ambulatory peritoneal dialysis
CAT	computerized tomography scan
cata	down
CATH LAB	cardiac catheterization lab
CBC	complete blood count
CBD	common bile duct
CBE	clinical breast examination
CBG	corticosteroid-binding globulin
CBI	continuous bladder irrigation
CBR	complete bed rest
CC	chief complaint
CCK	cholecystokinin
CCPD	continuous cyclic peritoneal dialysis
CCU	cardiac care unit
CD	cardiovascular disease
CEA	cultured epithelial autograft
CFT	complement-fixation test
CHD	coronary heart disease
CHF	congestive heart failure
CI	cardiac insufficiency
CICU	cardiac intensive care unit
CIHD	chronic ischemic heart disease
CIN	cervical intraepithelial neoplasm
circum	around, about circumflex
CMS	circulation, motion, sensation
CO	cardiac output
CO2	carbon dioxide
Com	with, together
Con	with, together
Contra	against, opposite
COPD	chronic obstructive pulmonary disease
CP	chest pain; cleft palate
CPAP	continuous positive airway pressure
CPD	cephalo-pelvic disproportion
CPP	cerebral perfusion pressure
CPPD	chest percussion and post drainage
CPR	cardiopulmonary resuscitation
CRF	chronic renal failure
CRRT	continuous renal replacement therapy
CRT	capillary refill time
CSF	cerebrospinal fluid; colony stimulating factors
CT	chest tube; computed tomography
CVA	cerebral vascular accident; costovertebral angle
CVEA	complex ventricular ectopy
CVP	central venous pressure
CX	circumflex
Cx'd	cancelled
CXR	chest x-ray
D5LR	Dextrose 5% with lactated ringers
D5W	Dextose 5% in water
DAT	diet as tolerated
DBP	diastolic blood pressure
DC (dc)	discontinue
DCCT	diabetes control and complication trials
De	away from
DEX (DXT)	dextrose
Di	twice, double
Dia	through, apart, across
DIC	disseminated intravascular coagulation
Dis	reversal, apart from, separation
DKA	diabetic ketoacidosis
DM	diabetes mellitus
DNA	deoxyribonucleic acid
DNR	do not resuscitate
DTR	deep tendon reflex
DVT	deep vein thrombosis
Dx	diagnosis
Dys	bad, difficult, disordered
E, ex	out, away from
EBV	Epstein-Barr Virus
Ec	out from, ectopic; eccentric; ectasia
ECF	extracellular fluid; extended care facility
ECG (EKG)	electrocardiogram/electrocardiograph
Ecto	on outer side, situated on
EENT	eye, ear, nose and throat
EM	erythema multiform
EMC	ensephalomyocarditis

CPT © 2015 American Medical Association. All rights reserved.
© 2016 DecisionHealth

EMG	electromyogram
en (em)	in
Endo	within
Epi	upon, on
ERCP	endoscopic retrograde cholangiopancreatography
ESRD	end stage renal disease
ET	endotracheal tube
Exo	outside, on outer side, outer layer
extra	outside
F & R	force and rhythm
FA	fatty acid
FBS	fasting blood sugar
FD	fatal dose, focal distance
FDA	Food and Drug Administration
FUO	fever of unknown origin
FVD	fluid volume deficit
fx	fracture
GB	gallbladder
GFR	glomerular filtration rate
GGT	gamma-glutamyl transferase
GI	gastrointestinal
GOT	glutamic oxalic transaminase
GU	genitourinary
GVHD	graft-versus-host-disease
h/o	history of
HA	headache
Hb	hemoglobin
HCG	human chorionic gonadotropin
HCO3	bicarbonate
HCT	hematocrit
HCVD	hypertensive cardiovascular disease
HD	heart disease, hemodiaysis
HDL	high density lipoprotein
HEENT	head, eye, ear, nose and throat
hemi	half
Hgb	hemoglobin
HIV	human immunodeficiency virus
HM	heart murmur
HPI	history of present illness
HRT	hormone replacement therapy
HS	hour of sleep
HTN (BP)	hypertension
Hx	history
hyper	over, above, excessive

hypo	under, below, deficient
I&O	intake and output
IBC	iron binding capacity
IBD	inflammatory bowel disease
IBS	irritable bowel syndrome
IBW	ideal body weight
ICCE	intracapsular cataract extraction
ICF	intermediate care facility
ICP	intracranial pressure
ICS	intercostal space
ICT	inflammation of connective tissue
ICU	intensive care unit
IDDM	insulin dependent diabetes mellitus
IDM	infant of diabetic mother
IE	inspiratory exerciser
IH	infectious hepatitis
IHD	ischemic heart disease
IHR	intrinsic heart rate
IIP	implantable insulin pump
IM	intramuscular
Im, in	in, into; not
Imp	impression
IMV	intermittent mandatory ventilation
infra	below
INR	international normalization ratio
inter	between
intra	within
intro	into, within
IPD	intermittent peritoneal dialysis
IPPB	intermittent positive pressure breathing
ITP	immune thrombocytopenic purpura
IV	intravenous
IVF	in vitro fertilization
IVP	intravenous pyelography
JAMA	Journal of the American Medical Association
JVP	jugular venous pressure
K	potassium
KCl	potassium chloride
KI	potassium iodide
KUB	kidney, ureter, bladder
KVO	keep vein open
L & A	light and accommodation
LB	large bowel
LDL	low density lipoprotein

LE	lupus erythematosus		ORIF	open reduction internal fixation
LFTs	liver function tests		OS	left eye
LLQ	left lower quadrant		OT	occupational therapy
LMP	last menstrual period		OU	both eyes
LP	lumbar puncture		p	after
LUQ	left upper quadrant		P	pulse
Lytes	electrolytes		P.T.	physical therapy
MAP	mean arterial pressure		PABA	para-aminobenzoic acid
MAR	medication administration record		para	beside, beyond, near to
MDI	multiple daily vitamin		PCA	patient controlled analgesia; posterior communicating artery
meta	beyond, after, change		PCN	penicillin; primary care nurse
MI	myocardial infarction		PCV	packed cell volume
MLC	midline catheter		PD	peritoneal dialysis
MM	mucous membrane		PDA	patent ductus arteriosus
MoAbs	monoclonal antibodies		PDD	pervasive development disorder
MOM	Milk of Magnesia		PDR	physician's desk reference
MRDD	mental retarded/developmentally disabled		PE	physical examination
MRI	magnetic resonance imaging		PEG	percutaneous endoscopic gastrostomy
MRM	modified radical mastectomy		PEJ	percutaneous endoscopic jejunostomy
MS	multiple sclerosis; morphine sulfate		peri	around
MV	mitral valve		PERL	pupils equal, react to light
MVP	mitral valve prolapse		PERRLA	pupils equal, round, react to light, accommodation
Na	sodium		PET	positron emission tomography
NaCl	sodium chloride		PFT	pulmonary function test
NAD	no apparent distress		PG	prostaglandin
NED	no evidence of disease		PH	past history
Neg	negative		PI	present illness
NICU	neonatal intensive care unit		PICC	peripherally inserted central venous catheter
NIDDM	noninsulin dependent diabetes mellitus		PID	pelvic inflammatory disease
NKA	no known allergies		PMH	past medical history
NKDA	non-ketotic diabetic acidosis		PMI	point of maximal impulse
NKMA	no known medication allergies		PNH	paroxysmal nocturnal hemoglobinuria
noc	night		PO	by mouth
NPD	nightly peritoneal dialysis		Post	after, behind
NPO	nothing by mouth		post op	post-operative
NS (NIS)	normal saline		PRBC	packed red blood cells
NSAID	nonsteroidal anti-inflammatory drug		Pre	before, in front of
NSR	normal sinus rhythm		pre op	pre-operative
NTD	neural tube defect		prep	preparation
NV	nausea and vomiting		PRN	as needed
NYD	not yet diagnosed		Pro	before, in front of
O2	oxygen		PS	pyloric stenosis
OOB	out of bed		PSA	prostate specific antigen
opistho	behind, backward			

CPT © 2015 American Medical Association. All rights reserved.

© 2016 DecisionHealth

PT	prothrombin time		SOP	standard operating procedure
PTT	partial thromboplastin time		SR	sinus rhythm
PUD	peptic ulcer disease		SS	social services
PVD	peripheral vascular disease		STAT	immediately
Px	pneumothorax		STD	sexually transmitted disease
Q	every		STH	somatotropic hormone
Q2H	every two hours		STM	short term memory
QD	everyday		sub	under
QH	every hour		SUI	stress urinary incontinence
QID	four times a day		super	above, upper, excessive
qns	quantity not sufficient		supra	above, upper, excessive
QOD	every other day		SVR	systemic vascular resistance
Qs	quantity sufficient, quantity required		Sx	symptoms
R	respirations		sym	together, with
RAD	reactive airway disease		T	temperature
RAI	radioactive iodine		T3	triiodothyronine
RAIU	radioactive iodine uptake		T4	thyroxine
RBC	red blood cells		TBSA	total body surface area
RDW	red cell distribution width		TCDB	turn, cough, deep breathe
Re	back, again, contrary		TDM	treadmill
REEDA	redness, edema, ecchymosis, drainage, approximation		TED (hose)	thrombo-embolism deterrent
Retro	backward, located behind		TEP	transesophageal puncture
RHD	rheumatic heart disease, relative hepatic dullness		THR	total hip replacement
			THTM	thallium treadmill
RLQ	right lower quadrant		TIA	transient ischemic attack
RM	respiratory movement		TIBC	total iron binding capacity
RO	rule out		TID	three times a day
ROM	range of motion		TIL	tumor infiltrating lymphocytes
ROS	review of systems		TKR	total knee replacement
RT or R	right		TNF	tumor necrosis factor
RUQ	right upper quadrant		TNM	tumor, node, metastases
Rx	prescription, pharmacy		TNTC	too numerous to count
S (s)	without		TP	tuberculin precipitation
S/S	signs and symptoms		TPN	total parenteral nutrition
SAB	spontaneous abortion		TPR	temperature, pulse, respiration
SAST	serum aspartate aminotransferase		trans	across, through, beyond
SB	spina bifida		TTN	transient tachypnea of the newborn
SBO	small bowel obstruction		TTP	thrombotic thrombocytopenia purpura
semi	half		TUPR	trans-urethral prostatic resection
SGPT	serum glutamic-pyruvic transaminase		TUR (TURP)	trans-urethral resection of the prostate
SLE	systemic lupus erythematosus			
SNF	skilled nursing facility		TWB	touch weight bear
SOB	shortness of breath		TWE	tap water enema
			Tx	treatment, traction
SOBOE	shortness of breath on exertion		UA	urinalysis

UAO	upper airway obstruction
UBW	usual body weight
UGA	under general anesthesia
UGI	upper gastrointestinal
ultra	beyond, in excess
up ad lib	up as desired
UPJ	ureteropelvic junction
URI	upper respiratory infection
US	ultrasonic, ultrasound
USA	unstable angina
UTI	urinary tract infection
UVJ	ureterovesical junction
VA	visual acuity
VBAC	vaginal birth after caesarean
VBP	venous blood pressure
VC	ventricular contraction
VENT	ventral
VF/Vfib	ventricular fibrillation
VLDL	very low density lipoprotein
VMA	vanillylmandelic acid
VP	venous pressure; venipuncture
VPB	ventricular premature beats
VPC	ventricular premature contractions
VS	vital signs
VSD	ventricular septal defect
VT/Vtach	ventricular tachycardia
VW	vessel wall
W/C	wheelchair
WBC	white blood cell
WD	well developed
WHO	World Health Organization
WN	well nourished
WNL	within normal limits
WPW	Wolff-Parkinson - White Syndrome
X	times

Coding Terms Glossary

The following definitions are medical terms commonly seen while coding and billing the healthcare field:

Abdominal Aorta – The portion of the aorta (main blood vessel of the body) in the abdomen.

Ablation – Destruction of selected portions of tissue.

Abscess – A localized collection of pus in any part of the body, usually surrounded by inflamed tissue.

ACE (Angiotensin-Converting Enzyme) Inhibitor – A drug that lowers blood pressure by interfering with the breakdown of a substance involved in blood pressure regulation.

Acute Sinusitis – Inflammation of the paranasal sinuses that begins suddenly.

Adenoma – Benign tumor of glandular origin (e.g., parathyroid adenoma).

Adhesion – Fibrous scars caused when body tissues that are normally separate are joined. Abdominal adhesions may be painful when stretched because fibrous tissue is not elastic.

Adrenal Glands – Two glands (located above each kidney), of which the cortex (outer portion) produces cortisone-like hormones and the medulla (inner portion) produces adrenalin and noradrenalin. Adrenal glands help the body's metabolism and help regulate sodium, potassium, and blood pressure.

Adrenaline – The hormone secreted by the central part (medulla) of the adrenal gland.

Aldosterone – Produced by the adrenal glands. Helps to regulate salt and water balance by holding on to salt and water and removing potassium.

Allergen – A substance (e.g., food, fur, pollen, or dust) that is normally harmless but causes an allergic reaction in susceptible people.

Allergic Conjunctivitis – Red, itchy, watery eyes resulting from an exposure to an allergen or an irritant.

Allergy – Reaction of the immune system to substances that, in the majority of people, do not cause symptoms.

Alveoli – Air sacs in the lungs where oxygen and carbon dioxide are exchanged to and from the bloodstream.

Amenorrhea – Complete absence of menstruation.

Amniocentesis – The suction of fluid from the amniotic sac through the use of a needle inserted through the abdomen.

Analgesia – Loss of sensibility to pain, and/or loss of response to a painful stimulus.

Analgesic – A medication that reduces or eliminates pain.

Anaphylaxis – A severe and life-threatening allergic reaction to a substance.

Anaplastic Thyroid Cancer – A rare type of thyroid cancer that spreads rapidly. This is the least common but most deadly of all thyroid cancers.

Androgens – Hormones responsible for facial hair and other secondary masculine characteristics

Anemia – A condition of too few red blood cells in the blood.

Anesthesia – Loss of sensation of a body part when induced by the administration of a drug.

Anesthetic – An agent that causes loss of sensation with or without the loss of consciousness.

Aneurysm – A sac-like protrusion from a blood vessel or the heart, resulting from a weakening of the vessel wall or heart muscle.

Angina (or Angina Pectoris) – Pain, discomfort, pressure or squeezing, usually centered in the chest that results from diseased blood vessels restricting blood and oxygen flow to the heart. Tightness or heaviness in the arms, neck or jaw, shortness of breath, nausea, sweating, weakness or palpitations may also be present. This is usually due to a clogged artery to the heart.

Angiography – An x-ray technique that makes use of contrast injected into the arteries to study blood circulation through the vessels. This test allows physicians to measure the degrees of obstruction to blood flow.

Angioplasty – A non-surgical technique for treating diseased arteries by temporarily inflating a tiny balloon inside an artery to push aside plaque build-up.

Anterior – Front of the body or situated nearer the front of the body.

Anterolateral – Situated or occurring in front of and to the side.

Antibiotic – A substance that combats bacterial infection.

Antibody – A protein manufactured by white blood cells to neutralize an antigen or foreign protein.

Anticoagulant – A drug that keeps blood from clotting.

Anticonvulsant – A medication that prevents or relieves seizures.

Antidepressant – A medication that prevents or treats depression.

Antidiuretic Hormone (Vasopressin) – Causes the kidneys to hold on to water and helps to control blood pressure, produced by the pituitary gland.

Antiemetic – A medication that prevents or alleviates nausea or vomiting.

Antifungal – A medication that combats fungal infections.

Antiglucocorticoid – A drug that suppresses glucocorticoid activity in the body. These drugs are also referred to as glucocorticoid antagonists. Glucocorticoids are steroid hormones produced in the adrenal cortex that affect metabolism of carbohydrates, proteins, and fats.

Antihistamine – A category of drugs that block the effects of histamine, a chemical released in body fluids during an allergic reaction. Antihistamines reduce itching, sneezing and runny nose.

Antihypertensives – Any drugs or other therapy that lowers blood pressure.

Anti-Inflammatory Drug – A drug that reduces signs and symptoms of inflammation.

Antiseptic – Any substance that kills infectious agents. Antiseptics are too strong to be swallowed or injected into the body.

Antithyroid Drug – A medication that slows down the thyroid gland's ability to produce thyroid hormone, which interferes with the thyroid's ability to synthesize hormone.

Aorta – The largest artery in the body and the initial blood-supply vessel from the heart to the rest of the body.

Aortic Valve – The valve that prevents blood flowing backwards from the aorta into the heart.

Aphakia – The loss or absence of the lens of an eye

Aphasia – The inability to speak, write or understand spoken or written language because of brain injury or disease.

Apnea – Cessation of respiration; inability to get one's breath.

Arrhythmia – An abnormal rhythm of the heart. Symptoms are a skipped beat, prolonged fluttering or pounding in the chest. Serious arrhythmias cause lightheadedness, syncope, or a myocardial infarction. Also called dysrhythmia.

Arterial Blood Gas (ABG) – A blood test drawn from an artery to measure the amount of oxygen, carbon dioxide and acid in the blood. Changes in respiratory care can be made on the basis of this test.

Arteries – Vessels that carry oxygen-rich blood to the body.

Arterioles – Small, muscular branches of arteries. Arterioles are the terminal branches of arteries that divide to form the capillary network.

Arteriosclerosis – A disease process, commonly called hardening of the arteries, which causes artery walls to thicken and lose elasticity. Also called narrowing of the arteries.

Arteritis – An inflammation of the arteries.

Arthralgia – Joint pain.

Arthritis – Inflammation of a joint or a state characterized by inflammation of joints.

Ascending Aorta – The first portion of the aorta, emerging from the heart's left ventricle.

Aspiration – Withdrawal of a fluid from the body by suction, usually through a needle or syringe.

Asthma – A chronic inflammatory lung disease characterized by recurrent breathing problems.

Atelectasis – An incomplete expansion or collapse of a segment of the lung.

Atherosclerosis – A disease process that leads to the accumulation of a waxy substance (plaque) inside blood vessels.

Atopic Dermatitis – Red, itchy, dry skin most common in infants, which is a result of an exposure to an allergen or an irritant.

Atria – The two (right and left) upper collecting chambers of the heart.

Atrial Fibrillation – A condition in which the heart contracts and relaxes at an irregular and sometimes rapid rate.

Atrium – One of the heart's two upper chambers.

Atrophy – A wasting of tissues, organs, or the entire body.

Attention Deficit Hyperactivity Disorder (ADHD) – A syndrome that is characterized by serious and persistent difficulties resulting in inattentiveness, impulsivity, and hyperactivity.

Audiologist – A professional trained in assessing hearing. In an assessment, an audiologist would look for signs of whether or not there are any hearing impairments or loss, usually by placing earphones through which sounds are transmitted at various frequencies. Audiologists often work closely with speech and language specialists to address problems in communication.

Autoimmune – A condition in which the body makes antibodies against its own tissues and damages itself.

Axillary Lymph Nodes – Numerous nodes around the axillary veins (below the shoulder joint) which receive the lymphatic drainage from the upper limb, scapular region and pectoral region (including mammary gland). They drain into the subclavian trunk.

Bacterium – A single celled organism that has a cell wall and typically multiples by cell division. Some types of bacteria have the potiential to cause disease.

Bagging – Pumping air or oxygen into the lungs by squeezing a rubber bag attached to a soft mask placed over the nose and mouth. This is also known as bag and mask ventilation.

Basal – The lowest body temperature, used to determine ovulation.

Benign – Describing an abnormal growth that will neither spread nor recur after removal.

Beta Blocker – An antihypertensive drug that limits the activity of epinephrine, a hormone that increases blood pressure.

Bililights – Lights used to assist in the breakdown of bilirubin and decrease jaundice in newborns.

Binocular Vision – The blending of the separate images seen by each eye into a single image, allowing images to be seen with depth.

Biopsy – The process by which a small sample of tissue is taken for examination.

Blood Clot – A jelly-like mass of blood tissue formed by clotting factors in the blood, which help stop the flow of blood from an injury. They can also form inside an artery whose walls are damaged by plaque build-up and can cause a myocardial infarction or stroke.

Blood Pressure – The force or pressure exerted by the heart and arteries in pumping blood.

Bradycardia – An abnormally slow heartbeat (usually less than 50 beats per minute).

Bradykinesia – Slowness in movement.

Bronchitis – An inflammation of the mucous membranes of the bronchi (lung airways).

Bronchodilator – A group of drugs that widen the airways in the lungs.

Bundle Branch Block – A condition in which portions of the heart's conduction system are defective and unable to conduct electrical signals normally.

Bursa – A closed fluid-filled sac that functions as a gliding surface to reduce friction between tissues.

Bursectomy – Surgical removal of the bursa or bursal sac.

Calcitonin – A peptide hormone produced by the parathyroid, thyroid, and thymus that acts to increase deposition of calcium and phosphate in bone and decrease levels of calcium in the blood.

Calcium Channel Blockers – Drugs that lower blood pressure by regulating calcium-related electrical activity in the heart.

Candida – A group of yeast-like fungi that may produce infection.

Capillaries – Microscopic blood vessels between arteries and veins that distribute oxygenated blood to body tissues.

Carbon Dioxide (CO2) – Gas that is produced by the cells of the body. It is carried by the blood to the lungs, where it is exhaled.

Carcinogen – Any substance that can cause cancer.

Carcinoma – A malignant growth composed of epithelial cells.

Cardiac – Pertaining to the heart.

Cardiac Arrest – The stopping of the heart, caused by interference with the electrical signal that regulates the heartbeat.

Cardiac Catheterization – A procedure that involves inserting a fine, flexible, catheter into an artery, usually in the groin area and passing it into the heart. Cardiac catheterization has become a key procedure for visualizing the heart and blood vessels to diagnose and treat heart disease.

Cardiac Enzymes – Complex substances found in cardiac muscles that are capable of speeding up certain biochemical processes. Abnormal blood levels of these enzymes may signal a myocardial infarction.

Cardiac Output – The amount of blood the heart pumps through the circulatory system in one minute.

Cardiomyopathy – A disease of the heart muscle that leads to deteriorization of the muscle and its pumping ability.

Cardiopulmonary Resuscitation (CPR) – An emergency method consisting of artificial respirations and chest compressions, used to restart the heart and lungs.

Cardiovascular (CV) – Pertaining to the heart and blood vessels.

Cardioversion – A technique of applying an electrical shock to the chest in order to convert an abnormal heartbeat to a normal rhythm.

Carotid Artery – A major artery (right and left) in the neck that supplies blood to the brain.

Cartilage – The hard, thin layer of white glossy tissue that covers the end of bone at a joint. This tissue allows motion to take place with a minimal amount of friction.

Cataract – An opacity or haziness of the lens of the eye. It may or may not reduce the vision depending on size, density and location.

Catheter – A tube used to remove or infuse fluid in a body cavity or blood vessel.

Cauterization – Destruction of tissue by burning it away with a caustic chemical, a red-hot instrument, or electricity. Cauterization can be used to remove growths on the skin (e.g., warts) or mucous membrane.

Central Nervous System – Part of the nervous system which consists of the brain and spinal cord, to which sensory impulses are transmitted. It supervises and coordinates the activity of the entire nervous system.

Cerebral Embolism – A blood clot or plaque formed in one part of the body and carried by the bloodstream to the brain, where it blocks an artery.

Cerebral Hemorrhage – Bleeding within the brain resulting from a ruptured blood vessel, aneurysm, or head injury.

Cerebral Thrombosis – The formation of a blood clot in an artery that supplies part of the brain.

Cerebrospinal Fluid (CSF) – Water-like fluid produced in the brain that circulates around and protects the brain and spinal cord.

CPT © 2015 American Medical Association. All rights reserved.

© 2016 DecisionHealth

Shrinking or expanding of the cranial contents is usually quickly balanced by the increase or decrease of this fluid.

Cerebrovascular – Pertaining to the blood vessels of the brain.

Cerebrovascular Accident – An impeded blood supply to some part of the brain, resulting in injury to brain tissue. Also known as a stroke.

Cervical – Relating to the neck.

Cholesterol – A steroid that occurs naturally in the human body and that is also present in food, particularly animal fats and dairy products. It circulates in the blood and excessive amounts play a role in atheroma (plaque) formation in the arteries. Limited quantities are required for the normal development of cell membranes.

Chronic Sinusitis – Inflammation of the paranasal sinuses, with symptoms that typically persist for greater than 12 weeks despite medical treatment.

Circulatory System – Pertains to the heart, blood vessels, and circulation of blood.

Claudication – A tiredness or pain in the arms and legs caused by an inadequate supply of oxygen to the muscles, due to narrowed arteries.

Coagulation – The process of clotting.

Cold Nodule – A lump in the thyroid gland or surrounding tissue that does not take up iodine on a scan.

Collagen – A fibrous protein which is a major constituent of connective tissue, skin, tendons, ligaments, cartilage, and bones.

Colon – Large intestine.

Coma – State of profound unconsciousness.

Compensatory Goiter – Thyroid enlargement due to inefficient thyroid tissue that compensates by enlarging.

Complete Blood Count (CBC) – Tests to measure the number and types of cells in the blood.

Computed Tomography (CT) – X-ray technique that uses a computer to create cross-sectional images of the body.

Concusssion – A disruption of neurological function, typically temporary, resulting from a blow to the head or violent shaking.

Congenital – Referring to conditions that are present at birth.

Congestive Heart Failure (CHF) – When the heart cannot pump all the blood returning to it efficiently, leading to a back-up of blood in vessels, and accumulation of fluid in body tissues, lungs and abdominal organs.

Conjunctivitis – Inflammation of the membrane covering the surface of the eyeball. It can be a result of infection, irritation, or related to systemic diseases, such as Reiter's syndrome.

Conscious Sedation – Intravenous medication used to help relax a patient during a procedure, without putting them to sleep.

Contact Dermatitis – Inflammation of the skin or a rash caused by external substances coming in contact with the skin.

Contagious – A term applied to diseases that can spread from person to person.

Contrast Medium – Any material (usually opaque to x-rays) employed to delineate or define a structure during a radiologic procedure.

Contusion – A bruise; an area in which blood that has leaked out of blood vessels is mixed with surrounding tissue.

Cornea – The clear front window of the eye that transmits and focuses light into the eye.

Coronary Artery Bypass Grafting (CABG) – A surgical rerouting (bypassing) of blood around a diseased vessel that supplies the heart by grafting either a piece of vein from the leg or the artery from under the breastbone or another location.

Coronary Artery Disease (CAD), or Coronary Atherosclerosis – Occurs when there is a buildup of cholesterol rich plaque along the lining of the coronary arteries, greatly increasing a person's risk of having a heart attack.

Coronary Heart Disease – Caused by the atherosclerotic narrowing of the coronary arteries, likely to produce angina pectoris or myocardial infarction.

Coronary Occlusion – An obstruction of one of the coronary arteries that hinders blood flow to some parts of the heart muscle.

Coronary Thrombosis – The formation of a clot in one of the arteries that carry blood to the heart muscle. Also known as coronary occlusion.

Cortex – The outer portion of an organ such as surface of the brain.

Corticosteroid – A group of anti-inflammatory drugs similar to the natural corticosteroid hormones produced by the cortex of the adrenal glands.

Cortisol – A steroid hormone produced by the adrenal glands. The blood levels of this hormone typically follow a pattern throughout the day, with the lowest levels occurring around four in the afternoon. More cortisol is released during times of stress (biological and psychological). Cortisol strongly influences the metabolism of glucose and other vital bodily functions.

Creatinine Clearance – Kidney function test determined by 12 or 24 hour urine collection.

CT Scan (Computed Tomography Scan) – A diagnostic imaging technique in which a computer reads x-rays to create a three-dimensional map of soft tissue or bone.

Cyanosis – Blueness of skin caused by insufficient oxygen in the blood.

Cyst – A sac or vesicle in the body

Cystitis – Inflammation of the bladder, usually caused by a bacterial infection.

Deciduous Teeth – Also known as baby or primary teeth.

Deep Vein Thrombosis – A blood clot in a deep vein in the calf, thigh, arm or pelvis.

Defibrillation – Delivery of a large electrical current to the heart when it is beating erratically. The purpose is to restore a regular heartbeat.

Defibrillator (Implantable Defibrillator/ICD) – A surgically implantable electronic device designed to provide an electric shock at the appropriate time to regularize abnormal heart rhythms in a malfunctioning heart.

Dehydration – Excessive loss of water from the body, often due to severe vomiting or diarrhea.

Detached Retina – A condition in which the retina separates from another layer of cells in the back of the eye, resulting in a decrease in nutrition and visual function. It may be due to a hemorrhage, trauma, tumor, vascular malformation or from traction of the vitreous to which it is attached.

DeQuervain's Thyroiditis – Inflammation of the thyroid gland causing enlargement and pain. It often causes fever and symptoms of hyperthyroidism.

Development – The process of how a child acquires skills in the areas of social, emotional, intellectual, speech, language, and physical development including fine and gross motor skills. Developmental stages refer to the expected, sequential order of acquiring skills that children typically go through. For example, most children crawl before they walk, or use their fingers to feed themselves before they use utensils.

Developmental Assessment – An ongoing process of observing and thinking about a child's current competencies (including knowledge, skills, and personality), and the best ways to help the child develop further.

Developmental Domains – Term used by professionals to describe areas of a child's development, for example: gross motor development – large muscle movement and control; fine motor development – hand and finger skills, and hand-eye coordination; speech and language/communication; the child's relationship to toys and other objects, to people and to the larger world around them; and the child's emotions and feeling states, coping behavior and self-help skills.

Developmental History – Term used by many professionals for the story of a child's development, beginning before birth.

Developmental Milestone – Term frequently used to describe a memorable accomplishment on the part of a baby or young child -- for example, rolling over, sitting up without support, crawling, pointing to get an adult's attention, walking.

Diabetes (Diabetes Mellitus) – A disease in which the body doesn't produce or properly use insulin. Insulin is needed to convert sugar and starch into the energy needed in daily life.

Diarrhea – A condition characterized by watery stool or increased frequency (or both) when compared to a normal amount.

Diastolic Blood Pressure – The lowest blood pressure measured in the arteries, occurring when the heart muscle is relaxed, between beats.

Diffuse Goiter – Generalized enlargement of the entire thyroid gland with a smooth surface.

Dilation – Enlargement of an opening or hollow structure in the body, such as dilation of a blood vessel.

Diplopia – Commonly known as double vision. In children, diplopia is often associated with a muscle imbalance such as esotropia. A refractive error may also cause enough blurring that a person sees two objects.

Distal – Situated away from the center of the body.

Diuretics – Drugs that lower blood pressure by stimulating fluid loss, promoting urine production.

Doppler Ultrasound – A technology that uses sound waves to assess internal structures and their function, such as blood flow within the heart and blood vessels.

Drip – The common name for an intravenous infusion (IV). A catheter is inserted into a vein, through which the liquid runs from an elevated sterile container.

Dye (Contrast) – In radiology, a radiopaque substance used during an x-ray exam to provide contrast in the different tissues and organs. Dye refers to the contrast media given intravenously.

Dysarthria – The imperfect articulation of speech resulting from muscular problems caused by damage to the brain or nervous system.

Dyslexia – A learning problem in which a person has difficulty with letter or word recognition. Evidence suggests that dyslexia is a decoding problem based on phonemes (basic language components). This is a higher cortical processing problem, not a vision or eye problem.

Dysmenorrhea – Painful periods.

Dyspnea – Shortness of breath.

Echocardiogram (Echo) – A method of studying the heart's structure and function by analyzing sound waves (similar to those used to visualize a baby in the womb) bounced off the heart and recorded by an electronic sensor placed on the chest. A computer processes the information to produce a one-, two- or three-dimensional moving picture that shows how the heart and valves are functioning.

E. Coli (Escherichia Coli) – Species of bacteria found in the intestines of humans, which is often the cause of urinary tract infections, diarrhea in infants, and wound infections.

Edema – Swelling caused by fluid accumulation in body tissues.

Electrocardiogram (ECG/EKG) – A test that measures the electrical output of the heart. It is a simple procedure that will allow a physician to make decisions regarding the health of the heart's muscle, arteries, and electrical system.

Electroencephalogram (EEG) – A graphic record of the electrical impulses produced by the brain.

Electromyography (EMG) – A method of recording the electrical currents generated in a muscle during its contraction.

Electrophysiology Studies (EPS) – An electrical current stimulates the heart in an effort to provoke an arrhythmia. EPS is used primarily to identify the origin of arrhythmias and to test the effectiveness of treatment.

Embolization – The insertion of a substance through a catheter into a blood vessel to stop hemorrhaging or excessive bleeding.

Embolus (Embolism) – A blood clot or plaque that forms in the blood vessel in one part of the body and travels to another part.

Endocarditis – A bacterial infection of the heart's inner lining (endothelium) or heart valves.

Endocrine Modulator – Any chemical that affects the normal operation of the endocrine system.

Endocrinology – The science that deals with the study of the endocrine glands and secretion, and the hormones.

Endoscope – A medical device for viewing internal portions of the body. It is comprised of fiber optic tubes and video display instruments.

Endoscopy – Inspection of internal body structures or cavities using an endoscope.

Endothelium – The smooth inner lining of many body structures, including the heart (endocardium) and blood vessels.

CPT © 2015 American Medical Association. All rights reserved.

Endotracheal Tube (ET Tube) – A plastic tube inserted into the trachea (windpipe) to deliver air and/or oxygen to the lungs.

Enlarged Heart – A state in which the heart is larger than normal due to heredity, long-term heavy exercise, or diseases and disorders such as obesity, high blood pressure, and coronary artery disease.

Enzymes – Complex chemicals capable of speeding up specific biochemical processes in the body.

Eosinophil – A type of white blood cell that usually comprises < 5% of all white blood cells in the blood. Eosinophils are found in increased numbers in chronic sinusitis, nasal polyps, and asthma. They contribute to inflammation by production of inflammatory mediators, such as leukotriene C4.

Epinephrine – A naturally occurring hormone that dilates the airways to improve breathing. It also narrows blood vessels in the skin and intestines so that an increased flow of blood reaches the muscles and allows them to cope with the demands of exercise. Also known as adrenaline.

Erythropoietin – Produced by the kidneys, it stimulates red blood cell production.

Estrogen – A female hormone, produced by the ovaries, that protects women against heart disease. Estrogen is not produced after menopause.

Etiology – The cause or origin of a disabling condition.

Excision – Removal by cutting away material.

Exercise Stress Test (Exercise Test/Stress Test/Treadmill Test) – A common test for diagnosing coronary artery disease, especially in patients who have symptoms of heart disease. This test helps physicians assess blood flow through coronary arteries in response to exercise, usually walking at varied speeds and for various lengths of time on a treadmill. A stress test may include use of electrocardiography, echocardiography, and injection of radioactive substances.

Exogenous – Originating outside of the body.

Extubation – Removal of the endotracheal tube.

Familial Hypercholesterolemia – A genetic predisposition to dangerously high cholesterol levels.

Farsightedness – The ability to see distant objects more clearly than close objects. Also known as hyperopia.

Fatty Acids (Fats) – Substances that occur in several forms in foods. Different fatty acids have different effects on lipid profiles.

Fenestration – Surgical creation of a window-like opening.

Fever (also Pyrexia) – An abnormal temperature of the body. A fever generally indicates that there is an abnormal process occurring in the body.

Fibrillation – Rapid, uncoordinated contractions of individual heart muscle fibers. The heart chamber involved does not contract all at once and pumps blood ineffectively.

Fibrinolysis – The process in which enzymes in the blood dissolve blood clots.

Fibroid Tumors – Benign tumors of the muscle of the uterus.

Fluoride – A natural chemical that strengthens enamel (hard outer coating on teeth), helps prevent tooth decay, and repairs early damage to teeth.

Flutter – The rapid, ineffective contraction of any heart chamber. A flutter is considered to be more coordinated than fibrillation.

Fracture – A disruption of the normal continuity of bone.

Follicle-Stimulating Hormone – Sex hormone that stimulates the production of follicles in the female and stimulates the seminiferous tubules to produce sperm in the male.

Follicular Thyroid Cancer – The second most common form of thyroid cancer.

Foramen – A natural opening or passage in bone.

Gallbladder Series – A series of x-rays of the gallbladder, taken after the gallbladder has been outlined with a special x-ray dye. The dye is taken by mouth the night prior to the study.

Gastroesophageal Reflex Disease (GERD) – The backward flow of stomach acid into the esophagus.

Gastrostomy Tubes – A gastrostomy tube (feeding tube) is inserted into the stomach if the patient is unable to take food by mouth.

Gavage Feeding – A method of feeding milk or formula through a small tube which is passed through the nose or mouth into the stomach. Also known as tube feeding.

Gland – A cell, group of cells, or organ producing a secretion.

Glaucoma – An eye condition in which the fluid pressure inside the eyes rises because of slowed fluid drainage from the eye. Untreated, it may damage the optic nerve and other parts of the eye, leading to vision loss or even blindness.

Glucagon – A hormone produced by the pancreas, which raises the blood sugar level.

Glucose – A sugar that supplies the body with energy.

Goiter – Enlargement of the thyroid gland. It may be generalized enlargement (diffuse) or asymmetric (nodular).

Gonadotropins – Consisting of the two hormones from the pituitary gland that stimulate the gonads or sex glands.

Gonads – Sex glands. (e.g., testes, ovaries).

Graves' Disease – Hyperthyroidism caused by an overactive diffuse goiter often associated with exophthalmos.

Growth Hormone – A hormone produced by the pituitary gland, which controls growth and development and promotes protein production.

Hashimoto's Thyroiditis – Inflammation of the thyroid gland, which causes diffuse enlargement (goiter), destruction of the functional cells of the thyroid, and eventually hypothyroidism.

Heart Attack (myocardial infarction) – Occurs when one of the arteries which supplies blood to the heart muscle becomes suddenly blocked. Symptoms are usually severe and sudden in onset. They may include fullness, discomfort or squeezing in the chest area radiating to the arms, throat, neck, or jaw, with nausea and sweating.

Heart Block – A condition in which the electrical impulses that activate the heart muscle cells are delayed or interrupted somewhere along their path.

Heart-Lung Machine – An apparatus that oxygenates and pumps blood to the body during open heart surgery.

Heelstick – Method of obtaining samples of blood by pricking the heel of the foot.

Hemangioma – A benign tumor consisting of a mass of blood vessels.

Hematocrit – Test that measures the percentage of red blood cells in the blood.

Hematoma – A blood clot.

Hemiplegia – Paralysis of one side of the body.

Hemorrhage – Bleeding due to the escape of blood from a blood vessel.

Heredity – The genetic transmission of a particular quality or trait from parent to offspring.

Hernia – Inguinal: A lump under the skin in the groin caused by a portion of the intestine protruding through a weak place in the abdominal muscle wall. Umbilical: a lump under the skin at the navel caused by a portion of the intestine protruding through a weak place in the abdominal wall.

High Blood Pressure – A chronic increase in blood pressure above its normal range.

High Density Lipoprotein (HDL) – A component of cholesterol that helps protect against heart disease by promoting cholesterol breakdown and removal from the blood; hence, also called "good cholesterol."

Histamine – A chemical present in cells throughout the body that is released during an allergic reaction.

Histologic – Pertaining to the study of microscopic structures of tissue.

Holter Monitor – A portable device for recording heartbeats over a period of 24 hours or more.

Homeostatic – The body's ability to maintain a regulated temperature, heart rate, or another body function.

Hormone – A chemical produced by an endocrine gland and released into the blood. It travels to other organs where it produces its effect.

Hot Nodule – A lump in the thyroid gland that concentrates iodine on a scan more than the normal surrounding thyroid tissue.

Hydrocephalus – An increased amount of fluid within the spaces of the brain.

Hyperopia – The ability to see things in the distance better than close up. Also known as farsightedness.

Hyperparathyroidism – Overproduction of parathyroid hormone (PTH) by a diseased parathyroid gland. The excess PTH causes the calcium to be too high, leading to kidney stones, osteoporosis, and several nervous system complications.

Hypertension – High blood pressure.

Hyperthyroidism – Symptoms of increased metabolism due to excess thyroid hormone in the blood. It may be due to an abnormal thyroid gland or from taking thyroid medication.

Hypoglycemia – Low levels of glucose in the blood.

Hypotension – Abnormally low blood pressure.

Hypothalamus – Part of the brain that directs the nervous system, endocrine system, and other parts of the body.

Hypothyroidism – Symptoms of decreased metabolism due to a deficiency of thyroid hormone in the blood.

Hypoxia – Less than the normal content of oxygen in the organs and tissues of the body.

Hysterectomy – Removal of the uterus.

Iliac – Part of the pelvic bone that is above the hip joint and from which autogenous bone grafts are frequently obtained.

Iliac Crest – The large, prominent portion of the pelvic bone at the belt line of the body.

Immobilization – Limitation of motion or fixation of a body part usually to promote healing.

Immunosuppressive Medications – Any drug that suppresses the body's immune system. These medications are used to minimize the chances that the body will reject a newly transplanted organ, such as a heart.

Immunotherapy – Gradual, increased doses of an allergen, which causes the immune system to become less sensitive to the substance. It reduces the symptoms of the allergy when the substance is encountered in the future.

Incubation Period – The time lag between infection and appearance of symptoms. During this time, infectious agents are multiplying but are insufficient in number to cause symptoms. Incubation periods range from a few days (influenza) to months (hepatitis).

Inderal – A beta-blocking drug.

Inferior – Situated below or directed downward.

Inferior Vena Cava – The large vein returning blood from the legs and abdomen to the heart.

Infuse – To introduce a solution into the body through a vein.

Inotropic Medications – Drugs that increase the strength of the heart's contraction.

Insulin – Produced by the pancreas, it lowers the blood sugar level, affects the metabolism of blood sugar, protein, and fat throughout the body.

Insulin-Like Growth Factor (IGF-1) – A blood test of the level of growth hormone production. Growth hormone stimulates growth and regulates metabolism.

Interstitial – Small space between two parts.

Intraocular Pressure (IOP) – The pressure that the fluid (vitreous) contained within the eye exerts on the globe (lining of the eyeball). Increased intraocular pressure is a symptom of glaucoma.

Intravascular Echocardiography – A combination of echocardiography and cardiac catheterization, in which a miniature echo device on the tip of a catheter is used to generate images inside the heart and blood vessels.

Intravenous Pyelogram – Test that examines the urinary system using a contrast medium that can be seen on x-rays to show possible obstructions, tumors, cysts, stones, and other abnormalities.

Intraventricular Hemorrhage – Bleeding in or around the brain.

Intrinsic – Situated entirely within or pertaining exclusively to a part.

Intubation – The placement of an endotracheal tube into the trachea to allow air to reach the lungs.

 CPT © 2015 American Medical Association. All rights reserved.

Iodine – A non-metallic element found in food. It is necessary for normal thyroid function.

Iodine-Induced Goiter – A goiter caused by excess iodine or by a sensitivity to iodine.

Iris – The colored part of the eye that helps regulate the amount of light that enters the eye.

Ischemia – Decreased blood flow to an organ, usually due to constriction or obstruction of an artery.

Isthmus – A small piece of thyroid tissue that connects the right and left lobes of the thyroid gland.

Jaundice – The temporary yellow coloring of the skin or the whites of the eyes caused by elevated blood levels of bilirubin.

Joint – The junction or articulation of two or more bones that permits varying degrees of motion.

Jugular Veins – Veins that carry blood back from the head to the heart.

Kidney – Pair of small oval glandular organs in the back part of the abdominal cavity that maintain water balance, regulate acid/base concentrations, and excrete urine.

Kidney Function Tests – Blood tests that show how well the kidneys are working to remove waste. Kidney function blood tests include BUN (blood urea nitrogen) and Cr (creatinine).

Kyphosis – An abnormal increase in the normal kyphotic curvature of the thoracic spine.

Lacrimal Gland – The tear gland located under the upper eyelid at the outer corner of the eye. The fluid it secretes cleans and provides moisture for the cornea. It is responsible for tearing following corneal irritation by a foreign body or chemical during emotional stimulation.

Lamina – The flattened or arched part of the vertebral arch, forming the roof of the spinal canal.

Larynx – The top of the trachea containing the vocal cords. Also known as the voice box.

Laser – Light amplification by stimulated emission of radiation. The device that produces a focused beam of light at a defined wavelength that can vaporize tissue. In surgery, lasers can be used to operate on small areas without damaging delicate surrounding tissue.

Lateral – Situated away from the midline of the body.

Learning Disability (LD) – A disorder that affects the ability to either interpret what is seen and heard or to link information from different parts of the brain. These limitations are characterized by difficulty in reading, writing, and arithmetic.

Lens – The lens is the transparent structure inside the eye that focuses light rays onto the retina.

Lesion – An injury, wound, or other abnormality on the skin.

Ligament – A band of flexible, fibrous connective tissue that is attached at the end of a bone near a joint. The main functions of a ligament are to attach bones to one another, to provide stability of a joint, and to prevent or limit some joint motion.

Lipids – Fatty substances insoluble in blood.

Lipoproteins – Lipids surrounded by a protein, making the lipid soluble in blood.

Lithium – A metal, the salt of which is used in treating depression. It sometimes interferes with thyroid function and can cause goiter.

Liver Function Tests – Blood tests that measure how well the liver is producing and processing many of the things needed by the body (e.g., vitamins, fats, iron, protein, and sugar).

Lordosis – Curvature of the spine with the convexity forward.

Low Birthweight Infant – Baby who weighs less than 5 1/2 pounds at birth (2500g), which may be premature or full-term at birth.

Low Density Lipoprotein (LDL) – A type of cholesterol in blood. Also known as bad cholesterol.

Lugole's Solution – A liquid medication containing iodine.

Lumbar – The lower part of the spine between the thoracic region and the sacrum. The lumbar spine consists of five vertebrae.

Lumbar Puncture (Spinal Tap) – A procedure in which a short, narrow needle is placed between two lumbar vertebrae into the area where there is spinal fluid. The fluid is removed for testing.

Lumen – The hollow area within a tube, such as a blood vessel.

Luteinizing Hormone (LH) and Follicle Stimulating Hormone – Produced by the pituitary gland, these hormones work together to control reproductive functions including the production of sperm and semen, the maturing of the female's eggs, and the menstrual cycle. They control male and female characteristics such as body hair, muscle formation, skin texture, and thickness, and voice.

Magnetic Resonance Angiography (MRA) – A non-invasive study which is conducted in a magnetic resonance imager (MRI). Contrast is injected and magnetic images are assembled by a computer to provide an image of the arteries.

Magnetic Resonance Imaging (MRI) – A technique that produces images of the heart and other body structures by measuring the response of certain elements (such as hydrogen) in the body to a magnetic field. When stimulated by radio waves, the elements emit distinctive signals in a magnetic field.

Malignant Neoplasm – Designating an abnormal growth that tends to spread (metastasize), and which may eventually cause death. Malignant tumors sometimes recur after apparent removal

Mammography/Mammogram – An x-ray of the breast used to detect breast cancer and other abnormalities of the breast.

Meconium – The dark green or blackish bowel movements that infants have in the first days of life.

Medial – Toward the inside or center of the body.

Medulla – The central part of a gland, such as the adrenal medulla.

Medullary Thyroid Carcinoma – A rare form of thyroid cancer that causes overproduction of the hormone calcitonin. This form of thyroid cancer is often hereditary.

Menorrhalgia – Pelvic pain, PMS, and dysmenorrhea with menstruation.

Metabolism – The use of calories and oxygen to produce energy.

Methimazole – An antithyroid medication used to treat hyperthyroidism.

Microalbumin – Urine test for protein, which may indicate an early stage of kidney disease

Mitral Valve – The structure that controls blood flow between the heart's left atrium (upper chamber) and left ventricle (lower chamber).

Mitral Valve Prolapse – A condition that occurs when the leaflets of the mitral valve between the left atrium (upper chamber) and left ventricle (lower chamber) are longer than needed, thereby allowing bulging into the ventricle, which may allow some backflow of blood into the atrium (mitral regurgitation).

Monounsaturated Fats – Types of fat found in many foods, but predominantly in avocados, and canola, olive, and peanut oils. Monounsaturated fats tend to lower LDL cholesterol levels, and some studies suggest that it may do so without also lowering HDL cholesterol levels.

Multi-Nodular Goiter – Enlarged thyroid gland with two or more nodules.

Murmur – The noises superimposed on normal heart sounds. They are caused by congenital defects or damaged heart valves that do not close properly and allow blood to leak back into the chamber from which it has come.

Myocardial Infarction (MI) – The damage or death of an area of the heart muscle (myocardium) resulting from a blocked blood supply to the area. The affected tissue dies, injuring the heart. Symptoms include prolonged, intensive chest pain and a decrease in blood pressure that often causes shock.

Mydriatic – A drug that dilates the pupil (cycloplegia).

Myocardium – The muscular wall of the heart. It contracts to pump blood out of the heart and then relaxes as the heart refills with returning blood.

Myopia – A refractive error in which the light rays focus in front of the retina producing blurry distance vision. If the myopia is greater than six diopters, a condition known as high myopia, the possibility of retinal detachment is increased. Also known as nearsightedness.

Myringotomy – A surgical opening of the eardrum to release pressure on the middle ear.

Myxedema – Severe hypothyroidism.

Nasogastric Tube (NG) – A small tube inserted through the nose down the esophagus, and into the stomach. Used to gavage-feed and/or to stop air from collecting in the stomach.

Necrosis – Refers to the death of tissue within a certain area.

Necrotizing Enterocolitis (NEC) – An inflammatory disease affecting the intestinal tract, causing death of intestinal tissue. The condition is most often a complication seen in premature infants.

Needle Biopsy – A small needle is inserted into the abnormal area in almost any part of the body, guided by imaging techniques, to obtain a tissue biopsy. This type of biopsy can provide a diagnosis without surgical intervention.

Neoplasm – Any new or abnormal growth, specifically a new growth of tissue in which the growth is uncontrolled.

Neuralgia – A paroxysmal pain extending along the course of one or more nerves.

Nitroglycerin (NTG) – A drug that helps relax and dilate arteries, often used to treat cardiac chest pain (angina).

Nodular Goiter – Enlarged thyroid gland with one or more nodules.

Nodule – A lump or growth of tissue within the thyroid gland.

Non-Invasive Procedures – Any diagnostic or treatment procedures in which an instrument does not enter the body.

Nystagmus – Rapid, rhythmic, repetitious, and involuntary eye movements. Nystagmus can be horizontal, vertical, or rotary.

Obesity – The condition of being significantly overweight. It is usually applied to a condition of 30% or more over ideal body weight. Obesity puts a strain on the heart and can increase the chance of developing high blood pressure, diabetes, and heart disease.

Occluded Artery – An artery in which the blood flow has been impaired by a blockage.

Ophthalmoscope – A lighted instrument used to examine the inside of the eye, including the retina and the optic nerve.

Orthopaedics – The medical specialty involved in the preservation and restoration of function of the musculoskeletal system that includes treatment of spinal disorders and peripheral nerve lesions.

Osteoma – A benign tumor of bone.

Osteoporosis – A disorder in which bone is abnormally brittle, less dense, and is the result of a number of different diseases and abnormalities.

Otitis Media – An infection or inflammation located in the middle ear.

Otoacoustic Emissions (OAE) – A method of hearing screening in newborn infants.

Otoscope – A lighted instrument that allows the physician to see inside the ear.

Ovaries – Female sex glands.

Pacemakers – Small, surgically implantable devices, which can control the heart's rhythm when it has a tendency to beat too slowly. Most pacemakers will last 5–10 years before generator replacement is necessary.

Palpate – To touch or feel.

Palpitations – Uncomfortable sensations within the chest caused by an irregular heartbeat.

Pancreas – The abdominal organ that secretes insulin and glucagon, which control the utilization of sugar, the body's chief source of energy.

Papillary Thyroid Carcinoma – The most common form of thyroid cancer, usually curable by surgery.

Paraplegia – Paralysis of the lower part of the body including the legs.

Parathyroid Glands – Four small glands located in the neck, near the thyroid gland. They produce parathyroid hormone which controls calcium metabolism. Production of too much parathyroid hormone causes primary hyperparathyroidism and osteoporosis.

Parathyroid Hormone – Hormone secreted by the parathyroid glands that regulates the level of calcium circulating in the blood.

Patent Ductus Arteriosus – A congenital defect in which the opening between the aorta and the pulmonary artery does not close after birth.

Percuss – To tap firmly on the body with the fingers, used to map out the area of an organ and detect possible changes in the consistency of its tissues.

Percutaneous Transluminal Coronary Angioplasty (PTCA) – A procedure performed to open heart muscle arteries blocked by atherosclerosis inflating a tiny balloon in the vessel, pushing the plaque aside.

Pericardiocentesis – A diagnostic procedure using a needle to withdraw fluid from the sac or membrane surrounding the heart (pericardium).

Pericarditis – Inflammation of the outer membrane surrounding the heart. Rheumatic fever, heart surgery, viral and bacterial infections are some of its possible causes.

Pericardium – The outer fibrous sac that surrounds the heart.

Peripheral Vision – The ability to see objects and movement outside of the direct line of vision. Also known as side vision.

Pheochromocytoma – A tumor of the adrenal medulla which secretes adrenaline.

Photophobia – Severe discomfort to bright lights. Usually a symptom of eye disease in an infant or retinal disease in a child or adult. Sometimes treated with dark sunglasses.

Physical Therapy – The treatment consisting of exercising specific parts of the body such as the legs, arms, hands or neck, in an effort to strengthen, regain range of motion, relearn movement and/or rehabilitate the musculoskeletal system to improve function.

Physiology – The science of the functioning of living organisms, and of their component systems or parts.

Pineal Gland – Cone-shaped gland at the base of the brain that secretes the hormone melatonin, which may help to synchronize biorhythms and mark the passage of time.

Pituitary Gland – A small gland the size of a peanut that is located behind the eyes at the base of the brain. It secretes hormones that control other glands (thyroid, adrenal, testicles and ovaries) as well as growth. It secretes throid stimulating hormone (TSH) which helps control thyroid function.

Plaque – A deposit of fatty (and other) substances in the inner lining of the artery wall, which is a characteristic of atherosclerosis.

Platelets – A type of cell found in the blood that aids in clotting of the blood.

Pneumatic Otoscope – An instrument that blows a puff of air into the ear to test eardrum movement.

Pneumonia – An infection in the lungs.

Pneumothorax – An abnormal collection of air between the chest wall and the lungs that causes one or both lungs to collapse.

Polyunsaturated Fat – The major fat constituent in most vegetable oils including corn, safflower, sunflower and soybean. Polyunsaturated fat actually tends to lower LDL cholesterol levels but may also reduce HDL cholesterol levels as well.

Positron Emission Tomography (PET SCAN) – An imaging test that uses positron emitting substances to assess information about the metabolism of elements that can be used to indicate how well tissues and organs are functioning.

Posterior – The back of the body or situated nearer the back of the body.

Post-Ictal – State following a seizure, often characterized by altered function of the limbs and/or mentation.

Presbyopia – The normal decrease in focusing power (accommodation) of the eye which occurs with aging. It begins about age twelve but becomes most noticeable to the average farsighted person after age forty. Bifocals or reading glasses are required for clear near vision.

Progesterone – A hormone produced by the ovaries that prepares the lining of the uterus (womb) for the fertilized egg and breasts for milk production.

Prolactin – A hormone produced by the pituitary gland, which starts and maintains milk production in the female.

Propylthiouracil – An antithyroid medication which prevents thyroid cells from producing thyroid hormone. Used to control hyperthyroidism.

Prosthetic Valve – An artificial heart valve.

Proximal – Nearest the center of the body.

Pulmonary – Refers to the lungs and respiratory system.

Pulmonary Valve – The heart valve between the right ventricle and the pulmonary artery that controls blood flow from the right ventricle into the pulmonary artery.

Pulmonary Vein – The blood vessel that carries newly oxygenated blood from the lungs back to the left atrium of the heart.

Pupil – The pupil is the dark aperture in the iris that determines how much light is let into the eye.

Pyelogram, IV Urogram, IVP – An x-ray of the renal pelvis, showing the kidney and associated structures, after injection of a radiopaque dye.

Pyelonephritis – An infection of the kidney.

Quadriplegia – Paralysis of all four limbs.

Radioactive Iodine – An isotope of iodine used in the diagnosis and treatment of the thyroid lesions and thyroid cancers.

Refraction – In ophthamology, the bending of light that takes place within the human eye. Refractive errors include nearsightedness (myopia), farsightedness (hyperopia), and astigmatism. Lenses can be used to control the amount of refraction, correcting those errors.

Renal – Pertaining to the kidneys.

Respiratory Distress Syndrome (RDS) – A breathing disorder that primarily affects premature infants where the tiny air sacs of the lungs tend to collapse at the end of each breath, due to a lack of a substance called surfactant. This condition is also referred to as hyaline membrane disease (HMD).

Retina – The retina is the nerve layer that lines the back of the eye that senses light and creates impulses that travel through the optic nerve to the brain.

Retinopathy of Prematurity (ROP) – An eye disease in which abnormal blood vessels and scar tissue grow within and over the retina, the light detecting layer of cells inside the eye. ROP mainly effects premature babies.

Retraction – The sucking in of the chest wall during breathing; a common symptom of respiratory distress.

Reye's Syndrome – A potentially serious or deadly disorder in children; characterized by a rash, vomiting, and confusion soon after the onset.

CPT © 2015 American Medical Association. All rights reserved.

Rheumatic Fever – A disease, usually occurring in childhood, that may follow a streptococcal infection. Symptoms may include fever, sore or swollen joints, skin rash, involuntary muscle twitching, and development of nodules under the skin. If the infection involves the heart, scars may form on heart valves and the heart's outer lining may be damaged.

Rhinitis – An inflammation of the mucous membrane that lines the nose; often due to allergy to pollen, dust, or other airborne substances; causes sneezing, itching, a runny nose, and nasal congestion.

Risk Factor – An element or condition involving a certain hazard or danger.

Rods – The visual cells of the retina that are important for night vision and peripheral vision. The rods are the first cells affected in rod-cone degenerations.

Sagittal – Longitudinal.

Saturated Fat – A type of fat found in foods of animal origin and a few of vegetable origin that is usually solid at room temperature. Abundant in meat and dairy products, saturated fats tend to increase LDL cholesterol levels and they may raise the risk of certain types of cancer.

Sciatica – Pain along the course of a sciatic nerve, especially noted in the back of the thigh and below the knee.

Sclera – The tough white outer coat of the eyeball.

Sepsis – A complication of an infection characterized by a severe whole body inflammatory response that has the potential to cause organ failure and death.

Septal Defect – A hole in the wall of the heart separating the atria and/or ventricles.

Septum – The muscular wall dividing the chamber on the left side of the heart from the chamber on the right.

Shock – A life-threatening condition caused by circulatory failure. The condition may be caused by blood loss, a disturbance in the function of the circulatory system, infection, or a severe hypersensitivity reaction.

Shunt – A connector that allows blood to flow between two locations.

Sick Sinus Syndrome – The failure of the sinus node to regulate the heart's rhythm.

Silent Ischemia – An episode of cardiac ischemia not accompanied by chest pain.

Sinusitis – An inflammation of the membrane lining the paranasal sinuses, often caused by bacterial or viral infections.

Sinus (SA) Node – The "natural" pacemaker of the heart. The node is a group of specialized cells in the top of the right atrium which produces the electrical impulses that travel down to eventually reach the ventricular muscle, causing the heart to contract.

Skeleton – The rigid framework of bones that gives form to the body, protects and supports the soft organs and tissues, and provides attachments for muscles.

Snellen Chart – The familiar eye chart with larger letters at the top and smaller ones at the bottom. It is used for measuring central vision.

Sodium – A mineral essential to life found in nearly all plant and animal tissue. Table salt (sodium chloride) is nearly half sodium.

Sperm – A mature male reproductive cell. Synonymous with spermatozoum.

Sphygmomanometer – An instrument used to measure blood pressure.

Spinal Canal – The bony channel that is formed by the intravertebral foramen of the vertebrae and which surrounds and protects the spinal cord.

Spinal Cord – The longitudinal cord of nerve tissue that is enclosed in the spinal canal. It serves not only as a pathway for nervous impulses to and from the brain, but as a center for carrying out and coordinating many reflex actions independently of the brain.

Spine – The flexible bone column extending from the base of the skull to the tailbone. It is made up of 33 bones, known as vertebrae. The first 24 vertebrae are separated by discs known as intervertebral discs, and bound together by ligaments and muscles. Five vertebrae are fused together to form the sacrum and 4 vertebrae are fused together to form the coccyx. The spine is also referred to as the vertebral column, spinal column, or backbone.

Standardized Test – A systematic sample of performance obtained under prescribed conditions, scored according to definite rules, which allows professionals to compare your child's performance to every other child who takes the same test.

Stenosis – The narrowing or constriction of an opening, such as a blood vessel or heart valve.

Stent – A device made of expandable, metal mesh that is placed in a narrowed portion of a tubular organ to keep the tubular organ open.

Sterile – Inability to reproduce. Free from living micro organisms.

Sternum – The breastbone.

Steroid – A group of chemical substances, some of which are hormones that affect body processes such as the overcoming of inflammation. Steroids are naturally produced in the body and are also available as synthetically produced substances used as medication.

Stethoscope – An instrument for listening to sounds within the body.

Strabismus – A condition in which the visual axes of the eyes are not parallel and the eyes appear to be looking in different directions.

Streptococcal Infection ("Strep" Infection) – An infection, usually in the throat, resulting from the presence of streptococcus bacteria.

Streptokinase – A clot-dissolving drug used to treat heart attack patients.

Stress – Bodily or mental tension resulting from physical, chemical or emotional factors. Stress can refer to physical exertion as well as mental anxiety.

Stroke – A sudden disruption of blood flow to the brain, e.g. by a clot or a leak in a blood vessel.

Subarachnoid Hemorrhage – Bleeding from a blood vessel on the surface of the brain into the space between the pia mater and arachnoid membranes that cover the brain.

Sudden Death – Death that occurs unexpectedly and instantaneously or shortly after the onset of symptoms. The most common underlying reason for patients dying suddenly is cardiovascular disease, in particular, coronary heart disease.

Superior – Situated above or directed upward toward the head of an individual.

CPT © 2015 American Medical Association. All rights reserved.

Superior Vena Cava – The large vein that returns blood from the head and arms to the heart.

Surfactant – A substance formed in the lungs that helps keep the small air sacs or alveoli from collapsing and sticking together. A low level of surfactant in a premature baby contributes to respiratory distress syndrome (RDS).

Syncope – A temporary, insufficient blood supply to the brain which causes a loss of consciousness. Usually caused by a significant heart arrythmia.

Systolic Blood Pressure – The highest blood pressure measured in the arteries, which occurs when the heart muscle contracts.

Tachycardia – An abnormally fast heart rate.

Tachypnea – An abnormally fast breathing rate.

Tendon – The fibrous band of tissue that connects muscle to bone. It is mainly composed of collagen.

Testes – Male glands which secrete testosterone, which stimulates sperm production and development of male characteristics.

Testosterone – The hormone produced in the testes.

Tetany – Muscle twitching and cramps caused by a lack of calcium in the blood.

Thallium Stress Test – An x-ray study that follows the path of radioactive potassium carried by the blood into heart muscle. Damaged or dead muscle tissue can be defined, as can the extent of narrowing in an artery.

Thoracic Spine – The chest level region of the spine that is located between the cervical and lumbar vertebrae. It consists of 12 vertebrae which serve as attachment points for ribs.

Throat Culture – A test used to detect the possible presence of a bacterial infection in the throat.

Thrombolysis – The breaking up of a blood clot.

Thrombolytic Therapy – A drug that dissolves blood clots.

Thrombosis – A blood clot that forms inside the blood vessel or cavity of the heart.

Thrombus – A blood clot.

Thyroglobulin – A protein in the thyroid gland, a small amount of which circulates in the blood. Its level is followed after thyroid surgery to detect recurrence of thyroid cancer.

Thyroid Binding Globulin – A protein in the blood that binds with thyroxine (T4).

Thyroid Cancer – A malignant neoplasm of the thyroid gland.

Thyroidectomy – An operation removing all or part of the thyroid gland.

Thyroid Gland – An endocrine gland located in the anterior aspect of the neck below the larynx, that secretes the hormones thyroxin, triiodothyronine and calcitonin, which stimulate metabolism, body heat production, and bone growth.

Thyroiditis – Inflammation of the thyroid gland.

Thyroid Scan – An imaging test that uses radioactive iodine or technetium. The radioactive element is injected intravenously or taken orally and the amount of the element taken up by the thyroid is measured.

Thyroid Stimulating Hormone – A hormone produced by the pituitary that stimulates the thyroid gland.

Thyroxine (T4) – The primary hormone produced by the thyroid gland.

Tissue Plasminogen Activator (TPA) – A clot-dissolving drug used to treat heart attack patients.

Titration, Titrate – Adusting the concentration of a solution (such as an injectable drug) so that the smallest possible amount (or lowest concentration) of the active ingredient is used that will achieve the desired effect.

Tomography – An imaging technique that allows thin sections of tissue or organs to be evaluated.

Total Parenteral Nutrition (TPN) – Intravenous administration of nutritional solution that provides all the necessary nutrients –protein, sugar, fat, minerals, and vitamins.

Total Urine Protein – A kidney function test used to determine the amount of protein excreted by the kidyneys by collecting urine over a 12 or 24 hour period, and then measuring the amount of protein in the urine.

Tourette's Syndrome – An abnormal condition characterized by tics and other movements like eye blinks or facial twitches that cannot be controlled.

Toxic Goiter – An enlarged thyroid gland that produces too much thyroid hormone.

Trachea – The tubular respiratory system organ that connects the larynx and the main bronchi.

Transesophageal Echocardiography (TEE) – A diagnostic test performed using an endoscope inserted in the esophagus. The test analyzes sound waves bounced off the heart to assess heart function.

Trans Fat – Created when hydrogen is forced through an ordinary vegetable oil (hydrogenation), converting some polyunsaturates to monounsaturates, and some monounsaturates to saturates. Trans fat, like saturated fat, tends to raise LDL cholesterol levels and, unlike saturated fat, trans fat also lowers HDL cholesterol level at the same time.

Transient Ischemic Attack (TIA) – A temporary, stroke-like event that lasts for only a short time and is caused by a temporarily blocked blood vessel.

Transplantation – Replacing a defective organ with one from a donor.

Tricuspid Valve – The structure that controls blood flow from the heart's right atrium (upper chamber) into the right ventricle (lower chamber).

Triglycerides – The most common fatty substances found in the blood; normally stored as an energy source in fat tissue. High triglyceride levels tend to accompany high cholesterol levels and other risk factors for heart disease such as obesity.

Triiodothyronine (T3) – A hormone produced by the thyroid gland.

CPT © 2015 American Medical Association. All rights reserved.

Tunnel Vision – A reduced visual field in which the eyes only see straight ahead (no peripheral vision). It may be due to certain eye diseases, such as glaucoma.

Tympanometry – A test performed to diagnose conditions affecting the middle ear. The test uses air pressure to move the eardrum (tympanic membrane) back and forth, and then measures and graphs the movement.

Ultrasound – High-frequency sound waves. Ultrasound waves can be bounced off of tissues using special devices. The echoes are then converted into a picture called a sonogram. Ultrasound imaging, referred to as ultrasonography, allows the physician to view internal organs, soft tissues, and body cavities, without using invasive techniques.

Unilateral – Having, or relating to, one side.

Upper GI Series – An x-ray exam of the upper part of the digestive tract.

Urethritis – Inflammation or infection of the urethra.

Urokinase – An enzyme derived from human urine that dissolves blood clots.

Urticaria – A skin condition commonly known as hives.

Uvea – Part of the eye, the uvea collectively refers to the iris, the choroid of the eye, and the ciliary body.

Valvular Regurgitation – The backward flow of blood across a heart valve that does not close completely.

Valvuloplasty – The reshaping of a heart valve with surgical or catheter techniques.

Varicose Vein – Any vein that is abnormally dilated, usually from long-standing pressure within it.

Vascular – Pertaining to the blood vessels.

Vasodilators – Any medications that dilate (widen) the arteries.

Vasopressors – Any medications that elevate blood pressure.

Veins – Blood vessels that carry oxygen-depleted blood from various parts of the body back to the heart.

Ventricles (Right and Left) – The two lower chambers of the heart.

Ventricular Fibrillation – A condition in which the ventricles contract in a rapid, unsynchronized fashion. When fibrillation occurs, the ventricles cannot pump blood throughout the body.

Ventricular Tachycardia – An arrhythmia (abnormal heartbeat) in the ventricle, characterized by a very fast heartbeat

Vertebra – One of the 33 bones of the spinal column that surround and protect the spinal cord.

Vertigo – A feeling of dizziness or spinning.

Visual Acuity – The clarity or clearness of the vision; a measure of how well a person sees. The ability to distinguish details and shapes of objects; also called central vision.

Vitreous Humor – The vitreous humor is a clear, jelly-like substance that fills the middle of the eye.

Wolff-Parkinson-White Syndrome – A condition in which an extra electrical pathway connects the atria (two upper chambers) and the ventricles (two lower chambers). It may cause a rapid heartbeat.

X-ray – A form of radiation used to create a picture of internal body structures on film.

List of Nerves with Added Specificity

Codes 95900 and 95907-95913 involve the following nerves:

I. Upper Extremity/Cervical Plexus/Brachial Plexus Motor Nerves
- A. Axillary motor nerve to the deltoid
- B. Long thoracic motor nerve to the serratus anterior
- C. Median nerve
  1. Median motor nerve to the abductor pollicis brevis
  2. Median motor nerve, anterior interosseou branch, to the flexor pollicis longus
  3. Median motor nerve, anterior interosseous branch, to the pronator quadratus
  4. Median motor nerve to the first lumbrical
  5. Median motor nerve to the second lumbrical
- D. Musculocutaneous motor nerve to the biceps brachii
- E. Radial nerve
  1. Radial motor nerve to the extensor carpi ulnaris
  2. Radial motor nerve to the extensor digitorum communis
  3. Radial motor nerve to the extensor indicis proprius
  4. Radial motor nerve to the brachioradialis
- F. Suprascapular nerve
  1. Suprascapular motor nerve to the supraspinatus
  2. Suprascapular motor nerve to the infraspinatus
- G. Thoracodorsal motor nerve to the latissimus dorsi
- H. Ulnar nerve
  1. Ulnar motor nerve to the abductor digiti minimi
  2. Ulnar motor nerve to the palmar interosseous
  3. Ulnar motor nerve to the first dorsal interosseous
  4. Ulnar motor nerve to the flexor carpi ulnaris
- I. Other

II. Lower Extremity Motor Nerves
- A. Femoral motor nerve to the quadriceps
  1. Femoral motor nerve to vastus medialis
  2. Femoral motor nerve to vastus lateralis
  3. Femoral motor nerve to vastus intermedialis
  4. Femoral motor nerve to rectus femoris.
- B. Iloinguinal motor nerve
- C. Peroneal nerve
  1. Peroneal motor nerve to the extensor digitorum brevis
  2. Peroneal motor nerve to the peroneus brevis
  3. Peroneal motor nerve to the peroneus longus
  4. Peroneal motor nerve to the tibialis anterior
- D. Plantar motor nerve
- E. Sciatic nerve
- F. Tibial nerve
  1. Tibial motor nerve, inferior calcaneal branch, to the abductor digiti minimi
  2. Tibial motor nerve, medial plantar branch, to the abductor hallucis
  3. Tibial motor nerve, lateral plantar branch, to the flexor digiti minimi brevis
- G. Other

II. Cranial Nerves and Trunk
- A. Cranial nerve VII (facial motor nerve)
  1. Facial nerve to the frontalis
  2. Facial nerve to the nasalis
  3. Facial nerve to the orbicularis oculi
  4. Facial nerve to the orbicularis oris
- B. Cranial nerve XI (spinal accessory motor nerve)
- C. Cranial nerve XII (hypoglossal motor nerve)
- D. Intercostal motor nerve
- E. Phrenic motor nerve to the diaphragm
- F. Recurrent laryngeal nerve
- G. Other

IV. Nerve Roots
- A Cervical nerve root stimulation
  1. Cervical level 5 (CT)
  2. Cervical level 6 (C6)
  3. Cervical level 7 (C7)
  4. Cervical level 8 (C8)

CPT © 2015 American Medical Association. All rights reserved.

B. Thoracic nerve root stimulation
   1. Thoracic level 1 (T1)
   2. Thoracic level 2 (T2)
   3. Thoracic level 3 (T3)
   4. Thoracic level 4 (T4)
   5. Thoracic level 5 (T5)
   6. Thoracic level 6 (T6)
   7. Thoracic level 7 (T7)
   8. Thoracic level 8 (T8)
   9. Thoracic level 9 (T9)
   10. Thoracic level 10 (T10)
   11. Thoracic level 11 (T11)
   12. Thoracic level 12 (T12)
C. Lumbar nerve root stimulation
   1. Lumbar level 1 (L1)
   2. Lumbar level 2 (L2)
   3. Lumbar level 3 (L3)
   4. Lumbar level 4 (L4)
   5. Lumbar level 5 (L5)
D. Sacral nerve root stimulation
   1. Sacral level 1 (S1)
   2. Sacral level 2 (S2)
   3. Sacral level 3 (S3)
   4. Sacral level 4 (S4)

Code 95907-95913 involves the following nerves:

I. Upper Extremity Sensory and Mixed Nerves

A. Lateral antebrachial cutaneous sensory nerve
B. Medial antebrachial cutaneous sensory nerve
C. Medial brachial cutaneous sensory nerve
D. Median nerve
   1. Median sensory nerve to the 1st digit
   2. Median sensory nerve to the 2nd digit
   3. Median sensory nerve to the 3rd digit
   4. Median sensory nerve to the 4th digit
   5. Median palmar cutaneous sensory nerve
   6. Median palmar mixed nerve
E. Posterior antebrachial cutaneous sensory nerve
F. Radial sensory nerve

   1. Radial sensory nerve to the base of the thumb
   2. Radial sensory nerve to digit 1
G. Ulnar nerve
   1. Ulnar dorsal cutaneous sensory nerve
   2. Ulnar sensory nerve to the 4th digit
   3. Ulnar sensory nerve to the 5th digit
   4. Ulnar palmar mixed nerve
H. Intercostal sensory nerve
I. Other

II. Lower Extremity Sensory and Mixed Nerves

A. Lateral femoral cutaneous sensory nerve
B. Medial calcaneal sensory nerve
C. Medial femoral cutaneous sensory nerve
D. Peroneal nerve
   1. Deep peroneal sensory nerve
   2. Superficial peroneal sensory nerve, medial dorsal cutaneous branch
   3. Superficial peroneal sensory nerve, intermediate dorsal cutaneous branch
E. Posterior femoral cutaneous sensory nerve
F. Saphenous nerve
   1. Saphenous sensory nerve (distal technique)
   2. Saphenous sensory nerve (proximal technique)
G. Sural nerve
   1. Sural sensory nerve, lateral dorsal cutaneous branch
   2. Sural sensory nerve
H. Tibial sensory nerve (digital nerve to toe 1)
I. Tibial sensory nerve (medial plantar nerve)
J. Tibial sensory nerve (lateral plantar nerve)
K. Other

III. Head and Trunk Sensory Nerves

A. Dorsal nerve of the penis
B. Greater auricular nerve
C. Opthalmic branch of the trigeminal nerve
D. Pudendul sensory nerve
E. Suprascapular sensory nerves
F. Other

CPT © 2015 American Medical Association. All rights reserved.

2016 Procedural Code Changes

● New Code
▲ Revised Code

● 10035	● 50695	● 81272	▲ 99354
● 10036	● 50705	● 81273	▲ 99355
▲ 31632	● 50706	▲ 81275	● 99415
▲ 31633	● 54437	● 81276	● 99416
● 31652	● 54438	● 81311	▲ 6030F
● 31653	● 61645	● 81314	● 0381T
● 31654	● 61650	● 81412	● 0382T
● 33477	● 61651	● 81432	● 0383T
● 37252	● 64461	● 81433	● 0384T
● 37253	● 64462	● 81434	● 0385T
● 39401	● 64463	▲ 81435	● 0386T
● 39402	● 65785	▲ 81436	● 0387T
● 43210	● 69209	● 81437	● 0388T
● 47531	● 72081	● 81438	● 0389T
● 47532	● 72082	● 81442	● 0390T
● 47533	● 72083	● 81490	● 0391T
● 47534	● 72084	● 81493	● 0392T
● 47535	● 73501	● 81525	● 0393T
● 47536	● 73502	● 81528	● 0394T
● 47537	● 73503	● 81535	● 0395T
● 47538	● 73521	● 81536	● 0396T
● 47539	● 73522	● 81538	● 0397T
● 47540	● 73523	● 81540	● 0398T
● 47541	● 73551	● 81545	● 0399T
● 47542	● 73552	● 81595	● 0400T
● 47543	● 74712	● 88350	● 0401T
● 47544	● 74713	● 90620	● 0402T
● 49185	● 77767	● 90621	● 0403T
▲ 50387	● 77768	● 90625	● 0404T
● 50430	● 77770	● 90697	● 0405T
● 50431	● 77771	● 92537	● 0406T
● 50432	● 77772	● 92538	● 0407T
● 50433	▲ 78264	● 93050	
● 50434	● 78265	● 96931	
● 50435	● 78266	● 96932	
● 50606	● 80081	● 96933	
● 50693	● 81162	● 96934	
● 50694	● 81170	● 96935	
	▲ 81210	● 96936	
	● 81218	▲ 99174	
	● 81219	● 99177	

CPT © 2015 American Medical Association. All rights reserved.
© 2016 DecisionHealth

Deleted Code Crosswalk

Deleted Code	Crosswalked Code
21805	N/A
31620	31654
37202	61650, 61651
37250	37252
37251	37253
39400	39401
47136	N/A
47500	47532
47505	47531
47510	47533
47511	47534
47525	47536
47530	47535, 47536
47560	47541
47561	47543
47630	47544
50392	50432
50393	50433, 50693-50695
50394	50430, 50431
50398	50435
64412	64461, 64462, 64463
67112	67107, 67108, 67113
70373	70370
72010	72081-72084
72069	72081-72084
72090	72081-72084
73500	73501
73510	73502, 73503
73520	73521-73523
73530	73501-73503
73540	73521-73523

Deleted Code	Crosswalked Code
73550	73552
74305	47531
74320	47532
74327	47544
74475	50432
74480	50433, 50693-50695
75896	61650, 61651
75945	37252
75946	37253
75980	47533
75982	47534
77776	77761
77777	77762
77785	77767, 77770
77786	77768, 77771
77787	77768, 77772
82486	82542
82487	82542
82488	82542
82489	82542
82491	82542
82492	82542
82541	82542
82543	82542
82544	82542
83788	83789
88347	88346
90645	90647, 90648
90646	90647, 90648
90669	90670
90692	90690, 90691

Deleted Code	Crosswalked Code
90693	90690, 90691
90703	90702, 90714
90704	90707, 90710
90705	90707, 90710
90706	90707, 90710
90708	90707, 90710
90712	90713
90719	90702, 90714
90720	90697, 90698
90721	90697, 90698
90725	90625
90727	N/A
90735	90738
92543	92537, 92538
95973	95972
0099T	65785
0103T	N/A
0123T	N/A
0182T	0394T, 0395T
0223T	N/A
0224T	N/A
0225T	N/A
0233T	N/A
0240T	91010
0241T	91013
0243T	N/A
0244T	N/A
0262T	33477
0311T	93050

A

Abbe-Estlander Procedure
repair, 40525-40527, 40761

Abdomen, abdominal
abscess
  incision and drainage, 49020, 49040, 49405-49407
anesthesia, surgical
  lower, 00800-00882
  upper, 00700-00797
angiography, 74174-74175, 74185, 75726
aorta
  angiography, 75635
  aneurysm
    direct repair, 35081-35103
    endovascular repair, 34800-34826, 34841-34848
    radiological supervision, 75952
    prosthesis
      aorto-bi, 34831-34832
      aorto-uni, 34805
      bifurcated, 34802-34804
      extension, 34825-34826, 75953
      tube, 34800, 34830
biopsy, 49000, 49010, 49180
blood vessel
  ligation, 37617
  surgical anesthesia, 00770, 00880-00882
cannula
  insertion, 49419-49421, 49324
  removal, 49422
  revision, 49325
catheter
  insertion, 49419-49421, 49324
  removal, 49422
  revision, 49325
celiotomy
  exploratory, 49000
  for staging, 49220
colectomy
  laparoscopic, 44210-44212
  partial, 44147
  total, 44150-44158
computed tomography scan, 74150-74175, 74176-74178, 75635
cyst
  destruction, 49203-49205
  excision, 49203-49205
ectopic pregnancy, 59130
endometrioma
  destruction, 49203-49205
  excision, 49203-49205
excision
  infected graft, 35907
  skin, 11005-11006, 15830, 15847
  tumor, 22900, 49203-49205
exploration
  laparoscopic, 49320
  open, 49000-49010
  postoperative, 35840
  staging, 49220, 58960
  wound, 20102
fluid
  drainage, 49080-49081
hernia repair
  anesthesia, 00750-00756, 00830-00836
  laparoscopic, 49652-49653
    initial, 49654-49655
    recurrent, 49656-49657
  open, 49590
    initial, 49560-49561
    recurrent, 49565-49566
hysterectomy
  radical, 58210
  subtotal, 58180
  total, 58150-58152, 58200, 58240
hysterotomy, 59100
incision, 49000
  staging, 58960

Abdomen, abdominal — *continued*
infraumbilical panniculectomy, 15830
injection, 49400
laparoscopy, 49320-49329
laparotomy
  exploratory, 49000
  staging, 49220, 58960
magnetic resonance angiography (MRA), 74185
magnetic resonance imaging (MRI), 74181-74183
mass, 49180
pancreatitis, 48000
peritoneocentesis, 49080-49081
resection, 51597
repair
  blood vessel, 35221, 35251, 35281
  fistula, 35182, 35189
  hernia
    laparoscopic, 49652-49653
      initial, 49654-49655
      recurrent, 49656-49657
    open, 49590
      initial, 49560-49561
      recurrent, 49565-49566
  suture, 49900
shunt
  insertion, 49425
  ligation, 49428
  removal, 49429
  revision, 49426
tumor
  destruction, 49203-49205
  excision, 22900, 49203-49205
ultrasound, 76700-76705
wall
  debridement, 11005-11006
  reconstruction, 49905
  removal
    mesh, 11008
    prosthesis, 11008
  surgical anesthesia, 00700-00730, 00800-00802, 00820
  tumor, 22900
x-ray, 74000-74022

Abdominoplasty, 15830, 15847

Ablation
anal, 46615
bone, 20982-20983
cardiovascular, 93650-93657
cervix, 57513
cryosurgical, 19105, 50250, 50593
endometrial, 58353-58356, 58563
fibroadenoma, 19105
heart, 93650-93657
  arrhythmogenic focus, 33250-33251, 33261
leiomyomata, 0071T-0072T, 0336T, 0404T
lesion
  anal, 46615
  esophagus, 43229, 43270
  intracranial, MRI guided focused ultrasound, 0398T
  large intestine, 44401, 45320, 45346, 45388
  renal, 50520, 50541-50542, 50592-50593
  small intestine, 44368
liver, 47370-47371, 47380-47383
lung, 32998
polyp, esophagus, 43229
prostate, 55873
therapy
  endovenous, 36475-36479
cardiac tissue
  endoscopic, 33265-33266
  incisional, 33250-33261
  intracardiac catheter, 93650-93657
tongue, 41530
tumor
  bone, 20982-20983
  esophagus, 43229
  liver, 47370-47371, 47380-47383

Ablation — *continued*
tumor — *continued*
  pulmonary, 32998, 0340T
  rectal, 45190
turbinate mucosa, 30801-30802
uterine fibroids, 0071T-0072T, 0336T, 0404T
vein, 36475-36479

Abortion
incomplete, 01965, 59812
induced, 01966, 59840-59857
missed, 01965, 59820-59821
septic, 59830

Abrasion
arthroplasty, 29862, 29879
corneal, 65435
lesion(s), 15786-15793
tissue, 97602

Abscess
abdomen, 49020, 49040, 49405-49407
ankle, 27603, 27607
anus, 46040-46060
appendix, 44900, 44960
arm
  distal humerus, 24134
  elbow, 23930-23935
  forearm, 25028-25035, 25145
  olecranon, 24138
  radius, 24136
  shaft, 24134
  upper, 23930-23935
  wrist, 25028-25035, 25145
bladder, 51080
bone
  ankle, 27607, 28005
  clavicle, 23170
  elbow, 23935, 24134-24138
  face, 21025-21026
  femur, 27303, 27360
  fingers, 25035, 25145, 26034
  foot, 27607, 28005
  forearm, 25035, 25145, 26034
  hand, 25035, 25145, 26034
  hip, 26992, 27070-27071
  humerus, 23935, 24134-24138
  knee, 27303, 27360
  leg, 27607, 28005
  pelvis, 26992, 27070-27071
  scapula, 23172
  shoulder, 23035, 23174
  wrist, 25035, 25145, 26034
brain
  drainage, 61150-61151
  excision, 61514, 61522
  incision and drainage, 61320-61321
breast, 19020
dentoalveolar, 41800
ear, 69000-69020
eyelid, 67700
female reproductive organ, 56405, 56420, 57010, 58820
fingers, 26010-26011
foot, 28005
hip, 26990-26992, 27070-27071
kidney, 50020
leg
  lower, 27603, 27607
  upper, 27301, 27303, 27360
liver, 47010-47015, 47300
lung, 31645, 32200, 32551
lymph node, 38300-38305
male reproductive organ, 54700, 55100
mouth, 40800-40801, 41000-41009, 41015-41018
nose, 30000-30020
palate, 42000
peritoneal area, 49020
pharynx, 42700-42725
prostate, 52700, 55720-55725
rectum, 45000-45020
salivary gland, 42300-42320
shoulder, 23030-23035
skin, 10060-10061, 10160
soft tissue, 10030, 20005, 21501-20502

Abscess — *continued*
spine, 22010-22015
tongue, 41000-41009
wrist, 25028, 25035, 25145

Absorptiometry
dual photon, 78351
dual-energy x-ray, 77080-77086
single photon, 78350

Acetabulum
fracture, 27220-27228
osteotomy, 27146-27156
reconstruction, 27120-27122, 29915
replacement, 27130, 27137
tumor, 27076

Achilles tendon, 01472
lengthening, 27612
repair, 27650-27654
tenotomy, 27605-27606

Acid reflux
test, 78262, 91034-91038
treatment, 43257

Acne
abrasion, 15786-15787
chemical
  exfoliation, 17360
  peel, 15788-15793
cryotherapy, 17340
dermabrasion, 15780-15783
surgery, 10040, 10060-10061

Acromion
arthrocentesis, 20605-20606
arthrotomy, 23044, 23101
dislocation, 23540-23552
reconstruction, 23130, 23415-23420, 29826
x-ray, 73050

Actigraphy, 95803

Acute otitis externa, 4130F-4132F

ADAMTS-13, 85397

Adaptive Behavior
assessments, 0359T-0363T
treatment, 0364T-0374T

Adenoidectomy
primary, 42830-42831
secondary, 42835-42836
with tonsillectomy, 42820-42821

Adenoma
pancreas, 48120
thyroid, 60200, 78808

Adhesions
epidural, 2044F, 62263-62264
eye
  anterior chamber, 65860-65880
  vitreous, 67031
female reproductive organ
  fallopian tube, 58660, 58740
  intrauterine, 58559
  labia, 56441
  ovary, 58660, 58740
foreskin, 54162, 54450
intestines, 44005, 44180
intracranial, 62161
knee, 29884
labial, 56441
lung, 32124
shoulder, 29825
urethra, 53500

Administration, intracranial
pharmacologic agent, 61650-61651
for thrombolysis, 61645

Adrenal gland
angiography, 75731-75733
biopsy, 60540-60545
function test, 95922
imaging, 78075
removal, 60545, 60540-60545, 60650
venography, 75840-75842

Advance Care Planning, 99497-99498

Advancement
flexor tendon
  elbow, 24330-24331
  finger, 26350-26373

CPT © 2015 American Medical Association. All Rights Reserved.   © 2016 DecisionHealth

Angioplasty — *continued*
  balloon — *continued*
    percutaneous
      aortic, 35472
      brachiocephalic, 35475
      coronary, 92920-92921
      femoral-popliteal, 37224-37227
      iliac, 37220-37223
      intracranial, 61630
      pulmonary artery, 92997-92998
      renal, 35471
        radiological supervision, 75966-75968
      tibio-peroneal, 37228-37235
      visceral, 35471
        radiological supervision, 75966-75968
      venous, 35476
    peripheral artery
      radiological supervision, 75962-75964
  vein patch, 35879
Angioscopy
  non-coronary vessels, 35400
Ankle
  amputation, 27888-27889
  application
    cast, 29365
    splint, 29505
    strapping, 29540
  arthrocentesis, 20605-20606
  arthrodesis, 27870
  arthrography, 73615
  arthroplasty, 27700-27703
  arthroscopy, 01464, 29891-29899
  arthrotomy, 27610-27612, 27620-27626
  biopsy, 27613-27614, 27620
  disarticulation, 27889
  dislocation, 27840-27842, 27846-27848
  drainage, 27603-27604
  exploration, 27610, 27620
  fracture
    closed
      distal fibular, 27786-27788
      malleolus
        bimalleolar, 27808-27810
        medial, 27760-27762
        posterior, 27767-27768
        trimalleolar, 27816-27818
    open, 27766, 27769, 27792, 27814, 27822-27823, 27846-27848
      distal fibular, 27792
      malleolus
        bimalleolar, 27814
        medial, 27766
        posterior, 27769
        trimalleolar, 27822-27823
  fusion, 27870
  incision, 27607
    drainage, 27603-27604
  injection, 20605-20606, 27648
  lesion, 27630
  manipulation, 27860
  magnetic resonance imaging (MRI), 73721-73723
  manipulation, 27860
  removal, 28130
    foreign body, 27610, 27620, 27704
  repair
    ligament, 27695-27698
    tendon, 27612, 27650-27654, 27680-27687
  strapping, 29540
  surgical anesthesia, 01462-01486
  synovium, 27625-27626
  tendon, 27630, 27680-27686
  tenotomy, 27605-27606
  tumor, 27615-27619
  x-ray, 73600-73615

Annuloplasty, 0062T-0063T, 22526-22527
Anoplasty, 46700-46705
Anoscopy, 46600-46615, 0288T, 0377T
Antibiotic, 4042F-4043F, 4045F-4049F, 4120F-4124F
Anticonvulsant, 4191F, 4230F
Antihistamine, 4133F-4134F
Antigen
  allergen immunotherapy, 95144
  blood typing, 86902-86906, 86911
  carcinoembryonic, 82378
  detection, 87260-87899
  HLA typing, 86812-86817
  prostate specific (PSA), 3268F, 84152-84154
  tumor, 86294-86316
Antimicrobial, 4041F
  systemic therapy, 4131F-4132F
Anti-rheumatic, 4187F
Anus
  ablation, 46615
  biopsy, 46606
  crypt, 46210-46211
  dilation, 46604
  electromyography, 51784-51785
  endoscopy, 46600-46615
  exploration, 45990
  fissure, 46200, 46940-46942
  fistula, 0170T, 46270-46285, 46706-46712
  foreign body, 46030, 46608, 46754
  hemorrhage, 46614
  hemorrhoids
    destruction, 46930
    excision
      complete, 46250
      complex, 46260-46262
      ligature, 46221
      simple, 46255-46258
      thrombotic, 46320
    injection, 46500
    ligation, 46945-46946
    stapling, 46947
  imperforate, 46715-46742
  incision, 46070
    drainage, 46045-46050
  lesion
    destruction, 46900-46924
    excision, 45108, 46922
  manometry, 91122
  repair
    cloacal anomaly, 46744-46748
    high imperforate, 46730-46742
    low imperforate, 46715-46716
    sphincter, 46750-46751, 46760-46762
  seton, 46020
  sphincter
    chemodenervation, 46505
    electromyography, 51784-51785
    repair, 46750-46751, 46760-46762
  tag, 46220
Aorta, aortic
  abdominal
    aneurysm
      direct repair, 35081-35103
      endovascular repair, 34800-34826, 34841-34848
      radiological supervision, 75952
      prosthesis
        aorto-bi, 34831-34832
        aorto-uni, 34805
        bifurcated, 34802-34804
        extension, 34825-34826, 75953
        tube, 34800, 34830
    computed tomography (CT) angiography, 75635
    thoracoabdominal, 33877
    thromboendarterectomy, 35331
  anastomosis, 33606
  angiogram, 93567
  angioplasty, 35452, 35472
  aortography, 75600-75630

Aorta, aortic — *continued*
  atherectomy, 0236T
  balloon assist device, 33967-33974
  catheter introduction, 36160-36200
  circulation assist, 33967, 33970
  coarctation, 33840-33851
  duplex scan, 93978-93979
  insertion
    balloon, 33967
    graft, 33330-33335, 33860-33864, 33875
    shunt, 33755, 33762
  pulmonary artery
    reconstruction, 33778-33781
  repair
    anomaly, 33800-33853
    sinus, 33702-33720
    valve, 33400-33417
    wound, 33320-33322
  suspension, 33800
  thoracic
    aneurysm
      direct repair, 33860-33877
      endovascular repair, 33880-33884
  valve
    incision, 33420-33422
    repair, 33400-33417
    replacement, 33405-33413, 33430
  x-ray, 75600-75630
Apheresis, 0342T
Appendix
  incision and drainage, 44900
  removal, 44950-44970
Application
  caliper, 20660
  cast
    body
      halo, 29000
      Risser jacket, 29010-29015
      shoulder to hips, 29035-29046
    clubfoot, 29450
    elbow to finger, 29075
    figure of eight, 29049
    finger, 29086
    hand to forearm, 29085
    hip, 29305-29325
    knee to toes, 29405-29435
    rigid, 29445
    shoulder, 29055
      to hand, 29065
    thigh
      to ankle, 29365
      to toes, 29345-29358
    Velpeau, 29058
  compression system, 29581-29584
  external fixation device
    ankle, 27860
    knee, 27570
    multiplane, 20692
      unilateral, 20696-20697
    shoulder, 23700
    uniplane, 20690
  halo, 20661-20664, 21100
  head frame, 61800
  intervertebral device, 22851
  modality, 97010-97036
  pulmonary artery bands, 33620, 33690
  radioelement
    interstitial, 41019
      complex, 77778
      guidance, 76965
    intracavitary, 31643
      complex, 77763
      intermediate, 77762
      simple, 77761
    surface, 77789
  skin substitute, 15271-15278
  splint
    calf to foot, 29515
    finger, 29130-29131
    forearm to hand, 29125-29126
    shoulder to hand, 29105
    thigh to ankle, 29505
  topical fluoride, 99188

Arm
  amputation
    forearm, 25900-25915
    shoulder, 23900-23921
    upper, 24900-24940
    wrist, 25920-25931
  angiography, 73206
  application
    cast, 29065-29075
    splint, 29105-29126
  biopsy, 24065-24066
  bypass graft, 35903
  computed tomography (CT) scan 73200-73206
  decompression, 25020-25025
  drainage
    abscess, 23930, 25028
    bursa, 23931
    hematoma, 23930
  fasciotomy, 24495, 25020-25025
  lesion
    destruction, 17260-17266
    excision, 11400-11406
      malignant, 11600-11606
      tendon sheath, 25110
    Mohs, 17313-17314
    shaving, 11300-11303
  magnetic resonance imaging (MRI), 73218-73220, 73223
  muscle
    repair, 24330-24331, 24341
    transfer, 23395-23397, 24301
  nerve
    graft, 64892-64893, 64897-64898
    neuroplasty, 64708-64714
    suture, 64856-64857
  reconstruction, 25337
  removal
    cast, 29705
    foreign body, 24200-24201, 25248
  repair
    blood vessel, 35236, 35266
    muscle, 24341
      extensor, 25270-25274
      flexor, 25260-25265
      transfer, 24301, 24320
    tendon, 24341
      extensor, 25270-25274
      flexor, 25260-25265
      lengthening, 24305, 25280
      origin slide, 25315-25316
      sheath, 25275
      tenolysis, 25295
      tenoplasty, 24320
      tenotomy, 25290
      transfer, 24301, 25310-25312
  skin
    flap, 15572
      delay/sectioning, 15610
    graft
      acellular, 15170-15171, 15330-15331
      allograft, 15300-15301
      autograft
        dermal, 15130-15131
        epidermal, 15110-15111, 15150-15152
        split thickness, 15100-15101
      full-thickness, 15220-15221
      preparation, 15002-15003
      substitute, 15360-15361
      xenograft, 15400-15401
    repair, complex, 13120-13122
    tissue transfer, 14020-14021
  tendon, 25109
  tumor, 24075-24077
  x-ray, 73090-73092
Arteriovenous
  anastomosis, 36818-36820
  fistula, 4051F-4053F
    creation, 35686, 36825-36830
    repair, 76936
      aquired, 35188-35190
      congenital, 35180-35184

Arteriovenous – Autograft

Arteriovenous — *continued*
  fistula — *continued*
    repair — *continued*
      coronary, 33500-33501
      thrombectomy, 36831-36833
        percutaneous, 36870
    study, 90940
  malformation
    surgery
      arterial, 62294
      dural, 61690-61692
      infratentorial, 61684-61686
      intracranial, 61705-61708
      laminectomy, 63250-63252
      obliteration, 61613
      supratentorial, 61680-61682
  shunt
    needle/catheter introduction, 36145
    radiological supervision, 75790
Artery
  aortic pulmonary
    reconstruction, 33770-33781
  aortoiliofemoral, 35363
  basilar, 61698, 61702
  biopsy, 37609, 75970
  bypass graft
    axillary, 35516-35522, 35533, 35616-35623, 35650, 35654
    brachial, 35510, 35512, 35522-35525
    carotid, 33891, 35501-35510, 35526, 35601-35606, 35626, 35642
    celiac, 35531, 35631-35632
    coronary, 33503-33505
      anesthesia, 00566-00567
    femoral, 35521, 35533, 35540, 35558, 35565-35566, 35621, 35646-35647, 35651-35661, 35665-35666
    harvest
      composite, 35681-35683
      upper extremity, 35600
    iliac, 34900, 35531, 35537-35538, 35548-35549, 35563-35565, 35632-35634, 35637-35638, 35663-35665
    mammary, 4110F
    mesenteric, 35531, 35631, 35633
    popliteal, 35571, 35623, 35651, 35656, 35671
    radial, 35523
    renal, 35535, 35560, 35631-35636
    repair, 35700, 35883-35884
    splenic, 35536, 35636
    subclavian, 35506, 35511-35516, 35526, 35606-35616, 35626, 35645
    tibial, 35566-35571, 35585-35587
    ulnar, 35523
    vertebral, 35508, 35515, 35642-35645
  cannulization, 36810-36815, 36823
  catheterization
    abdominal, 36245-36248
    arteriovenous, 36145
    brachial, 36120, 36215-36218
    carotid, 36100
    coronary, 93454-93461
    extremity, 36140, 36245-36248
    femoral, 93510-93511
    pelvic, 36245-36248
    pulmonary, 36013-36015
    renal, 36251-36254
    thoracic, 36215-36218
    umbilical, 36660
    vertebral, 36100
  coronary
    bypass, 33510-33536
    repair, 33500-33508
    revascularization, 92937-92944

Artery — *continued*
  decompression, 61590-61591, 61595-61596
  embolectomy
    aortoiliac, 34151, 34201
    axillary, 34101
    brachial, 34101
    celiac, 34151
    carotid, 34001
    femoropopliteal, 34201
    innominate, 34001, 34051, 34101
    popliteal-tibio-peroneal, 34203
    pulmonary, 33910-33916
    radial, 34111
    renal, 34151
    ulnar, 34111
  exploration, 24495, 35701-35761
  ligation
    abdomen, 37617
    carotid, 37600-37606, 61610-61612
    chest, 37616
    coronary, 33502
    ethmoidal, 30915
    extremity, 37618
    fistula, 37607
    maxillary, 30920
    neck, 37615
    temporal, 37609
  pulmonary
    banding, 33620-33690
    balloon angioplasty, 92997-92998
    embolectomy, 33910-33915
    repair, 33690, 33925-33926
    shunt, 33750-33767
  sympathectomy, 64821-64822
  thrombectomy
    aortoiliac, 34151, 34201
    axillary, 34101
    brachial, 34101
    celiac, 34151
    carotid, 34001
    fistula, 36831-36833, 36870
    femoropopliteal, 34201
    graft, 35875-35876
    innominate, 34001, 34051, 34101
    mechanical, 37184-37186, 61645
    percutaneous transluminal, 37184-37186, 61645
    popliteal-tibio-peroneal, 34203
    radial, 34111
    renal, 34151
    ulnar, 34111
    venal caval, 50230
  thromboendarterectomy
    aorta, 35331, 35361-35363
    axillary, 35321
    carotid, 36301, 35390
    celiac, 35341
    femoral, 35302, 35355, 35363-35372
    iliac, 35351-35355, 35361-35363
    mesenteric, 35341
    peroneal, 35304-35306
    popliteal, 35303
    renal, 35341
    subclavian, 35301, 35311
    tibial, 35304-35306
    vertebral, 35301
  transection, 61611-61612
  x-ray, 75630
Arthrocentesis, 20600-20611
Arthrodesis
  ankle, 27870-27871, 29899
  elbow, 24800-24802
  foot, 28705-28760, 29907
  hand, 26841-26863
  hip, 27279-27286
  knee, 27580
  shoulder, 23800-23802
  spine, 0195T-0196T, 0309T, 22532-22812
  wrist, 25800-25830

Arthroplasty
  ankle, 27700
    total, 27702-27703
  disc
    removal, 22865, 0164T
    revision, 22862, 0165T
    total, 22857, 0163T
  elbow, 24360-24366, 24587
    revision, 24370-24371
  hand, 26530-26536
  hip, 29862
    partial, 27125
    total, 27130-27132
    revision, 27134-27138
  jaw, 21240-21243
  knee, 27437-27447, 29879
    revision, 27486-27487
    use of kinetic balance sensor, 0396T
  shoulder, 23470-23472
    revision, 23473-23474
  wrist, 25332, 25449
Arthroscopy
  ankle, 29891-29892, 29894-29899
  elbow
    diagnostic, 29830
    surgical, 29834-29838
  foot, 29904-29907
  hand, 29900-29902
  hip
    diagnostic, 29860
    surgical, 29861-29863, 29914-29916
  jaw, 29800-29804
  knee
    diagnostic, 29870
    repair, 29888-29889
    surgical, 29866-29868, 29871-29887
  shoulder
    diagnostic, 29805
    surgical, 29806-29828
  wrist
    diagnostic, 29840
    surgical, 29843-29847
Arthrotomy
  ankle, 27610-27612, 27620-27626
  biopsy, 23100-23101
  elbow, 24000-24006, 24100-24102
  foot, 28020-28024, 28050-28054
  hand, 26070-26110
  hip, 27030-27033, 27050-27054
  jaw, 21010
  knee, 27310, 27330-27335, 27403
  shoulder, 23040-23044, 23100-23107
  wrist, 25040, 25100-25107
Aspiration
  amniotic fluid, 59000-59001
  biopsy, 31629, 31633
  bladder, 51100-51102
  bone marrow, 01112, 38220
  brain, 61750-61751
  bursa, 20600-20611
  catheter, 31720-31725
  cyst
    breast, 19000-19001
    bone, 20615
    ganglion, 20612
    kidney, 50390
    spinal cord, 62268
    thyroid, 60300
  diagnostic, 62267
  inner ear, 69420-69421
  joint, 20600-20611
  liver, 47015
  lung, 32405
  lumbar, 62287
  pelvis, 49322
  puncture, 10160, 19000-19001
  stereotactic, 61750-61751, 63615
  therapeutic, tracheobronchial, 31645-31646
  thyroid, 60300
  with intubation
    duodenal, 43756-43757
    gastric, 43753-43755

Assays
  multianalyte (molecular), 81410-81471
    with algorithmic analysis, 81490-81599
  therapeutic drug, 80150-80299
Assessment
  adaptive behavior, 0359T-0363T
  emotional/behavioral, 96127
  endothelial function, 0337T
  interprofessional internet/telephone, 99446-99449
  myocardial mechanics, 0399T
  patient history/status/symptoms, 1000F-1494F
  visual field, 0378T-0379T
Atherectomy
  coronary, 92924-92925, 92933-92934
  open, percutaneous, 0234T-0238T, 37227, 33229, 37231, 37233, 37235
Atria
  ablation and reconstruction
    endoscopic, 33265-33266
    incisional, 33254-33259
Audiometry
  automated, 0208T-0212T
  Bekesy, 92560-92561
  comprehensive, 92556
  conditioning play, 92582
  evoked response, 92585-92586
  group testing, 92559
  pure tone, 92551-92553
  select picture, 92583
  speech, 92555-92556
  visual reinforcement, 92579
Auditory canal
  biopsy, 69105
  cerumen removal, 69209-69210
  decompression, 61591, 69960
  drainage, 69020
  foreign body, 69200-69205
  lesion, 69140-69155
  reconstruction, 69310-69320
Augmentation
  breast, 19324-19325
  esophageal sphincter, 0392T-0393T
  jaw, 21120-21127, 21208, 21270
  vertebral, 22513-22515
Autograft
  bone, 20936-20938
    head, 21120, 21123, 21182-21184, 21208, 21255
    forehead, 21138, 21180
    mandible, 21127, 21247
    midface, 21145-21147, 21151-21160, 21188
    orbit, 21172-21175, 21256
    temporomandibular joint, 21240
    lower extremity
      femur, 27130, 27357
      foot, 28102, 28106, 28305, 28307, 28446
      knee, 27416, 29866
      leg, 27637, 27724
      pelvis, 27065-27067, 27132-27137
    skull, 61559, 62146-62147
    upper extremity
      hand, 25135, 26205, 26215, 26255, 26261
      humerus, 24115, 24151, 24435
      radius, 24125, 24153, 25125, 25391, 25393, 25405, 25420-25426
      shoulder, 23145, 23155, 23221
  joint
    upper extremity, 26842, 26844, 26852, 26862-26863
  skin, 15100-15157
    harvest, 15040
  vocal cord, 31546

CPT © 2015 American Medical Association. All Rights Reserved.

© 2016 DecisionHealth

Autopsy
coroner's, 88045
forensic, 88040
gross only, 88000-88016
  with micro, 88020-88029
limited, 88036-88037
regional, 88036
single organ, 88037
Avulsion
nail plate, 11730-11740
nerve, 64732-64772
rotator cuff repair, 23420

B

Back, 2044F
biopsy, 21920-21925
pain, 1130F-1137F, 4240F-4248F
  imaging, 3330F-3331F
repair
  hernia, 49540
strapping, 29799
tumor
  excision, 21930
  radical resection, 21935
wound exploration, 20102
Bacteria
antibody, 86609
culture
  additional methods, 87077
  aerobic, 87040-87071
  anaerobic, 87073-87076
  blood, 87040
  other, 87070-87075
  screening, 87081
  stool, 87045-87046
  urine, 87086-87088
endotoxins, 87176
overgrowth breath test, 91065
Bactericidal titer, serum, 87197
Baker tube, 44021
Baker's cyst, 27345
Balanoplasty
plastic, 54440
prosthesis, 54408
Balloon
angioplasty
  open
    aortic, 35452
    brachiocephalic, 35458
    femoral-popliteal, 37224-37227
    iliac, 37220-37223
    renal, 35450
      radiological supervision, 75966-75968
    tibio-peroneal, 37228-37235
    visceral, 35450
      radiological supervision, 75966-75968
    venous, 35460
  percutaneous
    aortic, 35472
    brachiocephalic, 35475
    coronary, 92920-92921
    femoral-popliteal, 37224-37227
    iliac, 37220-37223
    intracranial, 61630
    pulmonary artery, 92997-92998
    renal, 35471
      radiological supervision, 75966-75968
    tibio-peroneal, 37228-37235
    visceral, 35471
      radiological supervision, 75966-75968
    venous, 35476
  peripheral artery
    radiological supervision, 75962-75964
assisted device
  aorta, 33967-33974

Banding
artery
  fistula, 37607
  pulmonary, 33620, 33690
Bankart procedure, 23455-23462
Bardenheuer operation, 37616
Bariatric surgery
laparoscopic
  gastric restrictive
    bypass, 43644-43645
    device, 43770-43774
open
  gastric restrictive
    bypass, 43846-43847
    gastroplasty, 43842-43843
    partial gastrectomy, 43845
    revision, 43848
    Bariumsubcutaneous port, 43886-43888
enema, 74270-74280
screen, 83015
Barr
bodies, 88130
procedure, 27690-27692
Bartholin's gland
abscess, 56420
cyst
  excision, 56740
  repair, 56440
excision, 56740
marsupialization, 56440
Bartonella
antibody, 86611
detection, 87470-87472
Basilar artery
aneurysm, 61698, 61702
Belsey IV procedure, 43325
Bender-Gestalt test, 96101-96103
Benign
lesion
  destruction, 17110-17111
  excision, 11400-11446
  paring, 11055-11057
tumor
  breast, 19120
  head
    contouring, 21029, 21181
    excision, 21030, 21040, 21046-21049, 61563-61564
  lower extremity 27065-27067, 27355-27358, 27635-27638, 28100-28108
  stomach, 43610
  rectum, 0184T, 46937
  upper extremity 23140-23156, 24110-24126, 25120-25136, 26200-26215
Bennett fracture, 26645-26665
Bernstein test, 91030
Beta
2 glycoprotein 1 antibody, 86146
2 microglobulin, 82232
blocker therapy, 4006F
glucosidase, 82963
hydroxydehydrogenase, 80406
hypophamine, 84588
Bethesda system, 88164-88167
Bicarbonate, 82374
Biceps tendon
insertion, 24342
Bichloride methylene, 82441
Bicuspid valve
incision, 33420-33422
repair, 33420-33427
replacement, 33430
Bifrontal craniotomy, 61557
anesthesia, 00211
Bile acids, 82239
blood, 82240
Bile duct
anastomosis, 47760, 47780-47785
  extrahepatic, 47760, 47780
  intrahepatic, 47785
biopsy, 47553

Bile duct — *continued*
drainage catheter
  exchange/conversion, 47535-47536
  placement, 47533-47534
  removal, 47538
cyst, 47715
destruction, 43265, 43278
dilation, 43277, 47542, 47555-47556, 74363
endoscopy 47550-47556
  retrograde catheterization, 43260-43265, 43273-43278
excision, 47711-47712, 47715
exploration, 47700, 47552
foreign body, 43275
imaging, 78223
incision, 43262, 47460
  and drainage, 47420-47425
reconstruction, 47800
repair, 47760, 47780-47785
stent
  placement, 43274
  removal, 43275-43276
stone
  destruction, 43265, 47544
  removal, 43264, 47420-47425, 47544, 47554
stricture, 74363
tumor
  destruction, 43278
  excision, 47711-47712
x-ray, intraoperative, 74300-74301
Biliary tree
access through to small bowel, 47541
biopsy, 47543
Bilirubin, 82247-82248, 82252, 88720
Billroth, 43631-43632, 43845
Bilobectomy, 32482, 32670
Binding globulin, 84270
Binet test, 96101-96103
Binocular microscopy, 92504
Biofeedback training, 90875-90876, 90901-90911
Bioimpedance, 93701-93702
Bioimplant, 15777
Biometry, 76516-76519, 92136
Biopsy
abdomen, 49000, 49180
ankle, 27613-27614, 27620
anus, 46606
arm, 24065-24066
artery, 37609
auditory canal, 69105
back, 21920-21925
biliary, 47553, 47543
bladder, 52204, 52224, 52250
bone, 20220-20251
bone marrow, 38221
brain, 61140, 61750-61751
  stem, 61575-61576
breast, 19081-19086, 19100-19101
bronchi, 31625, 31629, 31633, 31717
brush
  bronchi, 31717
  cystourethroscopy, 52204
  renal, 52007
  ureter, 52007
carpometacarpal joint, 26100
cervix, 57454-57455, 57460, 57500, 57520
  endoscopic, 57454-57455, 57460
  excision, 57500, 57520
chorionic villus, 59015
colon, 44025, 44100
  endoscopy, 44389, 45305, 45331, 45380, 45391-45392
  multiple, 44322
conjunctiva, 68100
cornea, 65410

Biopsy — *continued*
duodenum, 44010
ear, 69100-69105
elbow, 24065-24066, 24100-24101
embryo, 89290-89291
endometrium, 58100-58110, 58558
epididymis, 54800, 54865
esophagus, 43202
eye
  conjunctiva, 68100
  lid, 67810
  muscle, 67346
female
  genital organ, 56605-56606, 57100-57105, 57500
  reproductive organ, 58100-58110, 58900, 59015
flank, 21920-21925
gallbladder, 43261
gastrointestinal, 43202, 43239, 43605, 44100, 44361, 44377, 44389, 45305, 45331, 46606
gland
  adrenal, 60540-60545
  lacrimal, 68510
  salivary, 42405
heart, 93505
hip, 27040-27041
  joint, 27052
ileum, 44382
interphalangeal joint
  finger, 26110
  toe, 28050
intertarsal joint, 28050
intestines, 44020, 44100, 44361, 44377
joint
  acromioclavicular, 23101
  carpometacarpal, 26100
  glenohumeral, 23100
  hip, 27052
  interphalangeal, 26110, 28054
  intertarsal, 28050
  knee, 27330
  metacarpophalangeal, 26105
  metatarsophalangeal, 28052
  sacroiliac, 27050
  sternoclavicular, 23101
  tarsometatarsal, 28050
kidney
  endoscopic, 50555-50557, 50574-50576, 52354
  open, 50205
  percutaneous, 50200
knee, 27323-27324, 27330
  joint, 27330
lacrimal
  gland, 68510
  sac, 68525
larynx, 31510, 31576
leg
  lower, 27613-27614
  upper, 27323-27324
lip, 40490
liver, 47000-47001, 47100
lung, 31628, 31632, 32095-32100, 32400-32405
lymph node, 38500-38530
  injection, 38792
  laparoscopic, 38570-38572
  needle, 38505
  open, 38500, 38510-38530
male genital organ, 54100-54105, 54500-54505, 54800
mediastinum, 32405, 39401-39402
metacarpophalangeal joint, 26105
metatarsophalangeal joint, 28052
mouth, 40808, 41108
muscle, 20200-20206
nail unit, 11755
nasal, 30100, 31237
nasopharynx, 42804-42806
neck, 21550
nerve, 64795
ocular structure, 65410, 67346, 67810, 68100, 68510, 68525

© 2016 DecisionHealth

CPT © 2015 American Medical Association. All Rights Reserved.   © 2016 DecisionHealth

Biopsy – Blood

Blood — *continued*
　plasma exchange, 36514-36516
　platelet
　　aggregation, 85576
　　count, 85008
　　　automated, 85049
　　　manual, 85032
　pool imaging, 78472-78473,
　　　78481-78483, 78494-78496
　pressure, 2000F
　　analysis, 99090-99091
　　monitoring, 93660, 93784-
　　　93790, 93923, 95922
　　performance measure, 0001F,
　　　0501F, 2000F, 2010F,
　　　3074F-3080F
　　plan of care, 0513F
　　ventricular, 0086T
　　venous, 93770
　products
　　irradiation, 0520F, 86945
　　pooling, 86965
　　splitting, 86985
　　volume reduction, 86960
　red blood cell (RBC)
　　antibody, 86850-86870
　　　pretreatment, 86970-86972
　　count, 85032-85041
　　fragility
　　　mechanical, 85547
　　　osmotic, 85555-85557
　　hematocrit, 85014
　　morphology, 85007
　　platelet estimation, 85007
　　sedimentation rate
　　　automated, 85652
　　　manual, 85651
　　sequestration, 78140
　　sickling, 85660
　　survival test, 78130-78135
　　volume determination, 78120-
　　　78121
　sample, fetal, 59030
　stem cell
　　count, 86367
　　donor search, 38204
　　harvesting, 38205-38206
　　transplantation, 38240-38242
　　　concentration, 38215
　　　cryopreservation, 38207,
　　　　88240
　　　depletion
　　　　plasma, 38214
　　　　platelet, 38213
　　　　red blood cell, 38212
　　　　T-cell, 38210
　　　　tumor cell, 38211
　　　thawing, 38208-38209-
　　　　88241
　　　washing, 38209
　test
　　ascorbic acid, 82180
　　bone marrow, 3155F, 88237
　　catecholamines, 83283
　　clot assessment, 85396
　　chloride, 82435
　　cholesterol, 82465
　　complete, 85025-85027
　　creatinine, 82565
　　culture
　　　bacterial, 87040
　　　fungal, 87103
　　erythrocyte, 85032
　　gases
　　　CO22, 82803
　　　HCO3, 82803
　　　O2 saturation, 82805-82810
　　　pCO2, 82803
　　　pH, 82800-82803
　　　pO2, 82803
　　glucose, 82947-82948, 82962
　　helicobacter pylori, 83009
　　hematocrit, 85014
　　hemoglobin, 85018
　　iron
　　　stain, 85536
　　　stores, 3160F
　　Kt/V, 3082F-3084F

Blood — *continued*
　test — *continued*
　　leukocyte, 85032, 84048
　　　myeloperoxidase (MPO),
　　　　83876
　　lipoprotein, 3048F-3050F,
　　　83700-83704
　　lysis time, 85175
　　microhematocrit, 84013
　　myeloperoxidase (MPO), 83876
　　nuclear medicine
　　　plasma volume, 78110-78111
　　　platelet survival, 78190-78191
　　　red cell volume, 78120-78121
　　　whole blood volume, 78122
　　occult, 82270-82274
　　osmolality, 83930
　　panels
　　　electrolyte, 80051
　　　general health, 80050
　　　hepatic function, 80076
　　　hepatitis, 80074
　　　lipid, 3011F, 3278F, 80061
　　　metabolic, 80047-80048,
　　　　80053
　　　obstetric, 80055, 80081
　　　renal, 80069
　　phenylalanine (PKU), 84030
　　platelet, 85032, 85049
　　protein
　　　western blot, 84181-84182
　　red blood cell (RBC) 85041
　　reticulocyte, 85044-85046
　　smear, 85060, 88140
　　thromboplastin time, 85730
　　tissue, 88237
　　uric acid, 84550
　　volume determination, 78122
　　white blood (WBC), 85004-85009
　　　myeloperoxidase (MPO),
　　　　83876
　　xylose absorption, 84620
　　time, 85002, 85175, 85345-85348
　　transfusion, 36430, 86890-86891
　　　exchange, 36455
　　　　neonate/fetal, 36450
　　　push
　　　　infant, 36440
　　typing, 86900-86911, 86920-
　　　　86923, 3293F
　　urea nitrogen, 84520-84525
　　urine, 83491
　　viscosity, 85810
　　white blood cell
　　　alkaline phosphatase, 85540
　　　antibody, 86021
　　　count, 85032, 85048, 89055
　　　differential, 85004-85007, 85009
　　　histamine release test, 86343
　　　myeloperoxidase (MPO), 83876
　　　phagocystosis, 86344
　　　transfusion, 86950

Bloom syndrome, 88245

Blot test
　western
　　human immunodeficiency virus
　　　(HIV), 86689
　　protein, 84181-84182
　　tissue analysis, 88371-88372

Body
　acetone, 82009-82010
　Barr, 88130
　carotid, 60600-60605
　cast
　　halo, 29000
　　jacket
　　　Risser, 29010-29015
　　removal, 29700, 29710
　　repair, 29720
　　upper body, 29035
　　　and head, 29040
　　　and legs, 29044-29046
　ciliary
　　destruction
　　　cryotherapy, 66720
　　　cyclodialysis, 66740
　　　cyclophotocoagulation,
　　　　66710-66711

Body — *continued*
　ciliary — *continued*
　　destruction — *continued*
　　　diathermy, 66700
　　　endoscopic, 66711
　　　nonexcisional, 66770
　　　repair, 66680
　　fluid, 89060
　heinz, 85441-85445
　inclusion, 87207, 87210, 88106
　ketone, 82009-82010
　mass index, 3008F
　section
　　x-ray, 76100-76102
　vertebral
　　biopsy, 20250-20251
　　excision
　　　decompression, 63081-63103
　　　lesion, 63300-63308
　　　skull base surgery, 61597
　　fracture, 22305-22310
　　kyphectomy, 22818-22819

Boil
　incision and drainage, 10060-
　　10061, 56405

Bone
　ablation, tumor, 20982-20983
　abscess, excision, 21025-21026
　amputation
　　metatarsal, 28810
　　tarsal, 27888
　arthroplasty
　　ankle, 27700-27703
　　foot, 25443
　　lunate, 25444
　　wrist, 25443
　biopsy
　　deep, 20225, 20245
　　superficial, 20220, 20240
　　vertebral body, 20250-20251
　carpal
　　arthroplasty, 25443
　　cyst, 25130-25136
　　dislocation, 25690-25695
　　excision, 25145, 25210-25215
　　tumor, 25130-25136
　　fracture
　　　closed, 25622-25624,
　　　　25630-25635
　　　open, 25628, 25645
　　incision and drainage, 26034
　　insertion, 25430
　　osteoplasty, 25394
　　repair, 25431-25440
　　sequestrectomy, 25145
　　tumor, 25130-25136
　cheek
　　excision, 21030, 21034
　　fracture
　　　closed, 21355
　　　open, 21360-21366
　　graft, 15840-15845
　　reconstruction, 21270
　computed tomography (CT) scan
　　density, 77078-77079
　　facial, 70486-70488
　conduction hearing device
　　implantation, 69710
　　removal, 69711
　　repair, 69711
　　replacement, 69710
　coxa
　　application
　　　cast, 29305-29325
　　arthrocentesis, 20610-20611
　　arthrodesis, 27284-27286
　　arthrography, 73525
　　arthroplasty, 27125-27138
　　arthroscopy, 29860-29863
　　arthrotomy, 27030-27033
　　biopsy, 27040-27041, 27052
　　capsulectomy, 27036
　　　removal, 29710
　　craterization, 27070
　　denervation, 27035
　　dislocation treatment, 27250-
　　　27266

Bone — *continued*
　coxa — *continued*
　　drainage, 26992
　　incision
　　　abscess, 26990
　　　bursa, 26991
　　　hematoma, 26990
　　echography, 76885-76886
　　excision, 27070
　　　cyst, 27065-27067
　　　synovium, 27054, 29863
　　　tumor, 27047-27049, 27065-
　　　　27067, 27075-27076
　　exploration, 27033
　　fasciotomy, 27025-27027, 27057
　　fusion, 27284-27286
　　injection, 27093-27096
　　manipulation, 27275
　　osteotomy, 27146-27156
　　reconstruction, 27130
　　removal
　　　cast, 29710
　　　foreign body, 27033, 27086-
　　　　27087, 29861
　　　loose body, 29861
　　　prosthesis, 27090-27091
　　repair
　　　muscle, 27100-27105, 27111
　　　tendon, 27097
　　replacement, 27130-27132
　　resection
　　　radical, 27075-27079
　　strapping, 29520
　　tenotomy, 27000-27006
　　ultrasound, 76885-76886
　　x-ray, 73501-73503, 73521-
　　　73523
　craterization
　　calcaneus, 28120
　　clavicle, 23180
　　femur, 27070-27071, 27360
　　fibula, 27360, 27641
　　hip, 27070
　　humerus, 23184, 24140
　　ileum, 27070
　　metacarpal, 26230
　　metatarsal, 28122
　　olecranon process, 24147
　　phalanges, 26235-26236, 28124
　　pubis, 27070
　　radius, 24145, 25151
　　scapula, 23182
　　talus, 28120
　　tarsal, 28122
　　tibia, 27360, 27640
　　ulna, 24147, 25150
　cyst
　　drainage, 20615
　　excision
　　　facial, 21040, 21046-21049
　　　lower extremity, 27065-
　　　　27067, 27355-27358,
　　　　28100-28108
　　　upper extremity, 23140-
　　　　23156, 24110-24126,
　　　　25120-25136, 26200-
　　　　26215
　　injection, 20615
　debridement, 11044, 11047
　density, 78350-78351
　　appendicular skeleton, 77081
　　axial skeleton, 77078, 77080,
　　　77085
　　ultrasound, 76977
　　vertebral assessment, 77085-
　　　77086
　diaphysectomy, 28122
　dislocation
　　lunate, 25690, 25695
　　tarsal, 27840-27848
　　wrist, 25690, 25695
　dual energy x-ray absorptiometry,
　　3095F-3096F, 77080-77086
　excision
　　epyphyseal bar, 21050
　　exostosis, 69140
　　facial, 21026, 21030, 21032-
　　　21034

© 2016 DecisionHealth　　　　CPT © 2015 American Medical Association. All Rights Reserved.

Bone — continued
  excision — continued
    facial — continued
      cyst, 21040, 21046-21049
      tumor, 21034, 21040-21047
    mandible, 21025
    metatarsal, 28110-28114,
        28122, 28140
      tumor, 28104-28107, 28173
    sesamoid, 28315
      finger, 26185
      thumb, 26185
    tarsal
      tumor, 27615-27619
    temporal bone, 69535
    torus mandibularis, 21031
    wrist, 25145, 25210-25215
      cyst, 25130-25136
  exostosis, 69140
  facial
    abscess, 21025-21026
    foreign body, 41806
    fracture
      closed, 21310-21320
      open, 21325-21335
      x-ray, 70160
    graft, 21215
    osteotomy, 21198-21199
    reconstruction, 21275
      with implant, 21244-21246,
          21248-21249
    repair, 21208-21209
    torus mandibularis, 21031
    tumor
      excision, 21029-21030,
          21034, 21040-21047
      resection, 21015
    x-ray, 70100-70110, 70140-
        70150
  femur
    acetabuloplasty, 27122-27130
    amputation, 27590-27596
    arrest, 27475-27485, 27742
    arthroplasty, 27443, 27487
    biopsy, 20225-20245
    epiphysis, 27175-27187
    excision
      abscess, 27070, 27360
      cyst, 27065-27067
      ephiphyseal bar, 20150
    fixture device, 27495, 27506-
        27507
      external, 20663
      internal, 27244-27245,
          27358, 27511-27514,
          27519
    fracture
      closed, 27230-27232,
          27238-27240, 27267-
          27268, 27500-27503,
          27508, 27510, 27516-
          27517
      open, 27236, 27254,
          27269, 27506-27507,
          27511-27514, 27519
      percutaneous, 27235, 27509
    graft, 27170
    incision
      abscess, 27303
      fasciotomy, 27025-27027,
          27057
    nonunion repair, 27470-27472
    osteoplasty, 27465-27468
    osteotomy, 27151-27156,
        27161, 27448-27454
    repair, 27470-27472
    replacement, 27258-27259
    revision, 27138
    transfer, 27110-27111, 27140,
        27400
    tumor
      excision, 27078-27079
        benign, 27065-27067,
            27355-27358
      resection, 27365
    x-ray, 73551-73552
  fibula
    amputation, 27880-27888

Bone — continued
  fibula — continued
    arrest, 27477-27485, 27732-
        27742
    bone graft, 20955, 20962
    dislocation treatment, 27832
    excision, 27455-27457, 27641
      abscess, 27360, 27607
      epiphyseal bar 20150
      tumor, 27635-27638, 27646
    fracture
      closed, 27780-27781,
          27786-27788
      open, 27784, 27792, 27828
    nonunion repair, 27725-27726
    osteoplasty, 27715
    osteotomy, 27455-27457,
        27707-27709
    x-ray, 73590
  fixation
    caliper, 20660
    cranial tong, 20660
    halo, 20661-20663, 21100
      body cast, 29000
      cranial, 20661-20664
      femur, 20663
      maxillofacial, 21100
      pelvic, 20662
      removal, 20665
    interdental, 21110
    multiplane, 20692
      unilateral, 20696-20697
    pin, 20650
    removal, 20670-20680
    skeletal, 24566
    stereotactic frame, 20660
    uniplane, 20690
    wire, 20650
  foot
    metatarsal
      amputation, 28810
      anastomosis, 20972
      condyle
        excision, 28288
      craterization, 28122
      cyst
        excision, 28104-28107
      diaphysectomy, 28122
      excision
        complete, 28111-28114,
            28140
        condyle, 28288
        cyst, 28104-28107
        partial, 28110, 28112
        tumor, 28104-28107,
            28173
      fracture
        closed, 28470, 28475-
            28476
        open, 28485
      repair, 28322
        lengthening, 28306-28307
        osteotomy, 28306-28309
      saucerization, 28122
      tumor, 28104-28107, 28173
    navicular
      arthroplasty, 25443
      fracture
        closed, 25622, 25624
        open, 25628
      repair, 25440
    sesamoid
      excision, 28315
      fracture, 28530-28531
    tarsal
      fracture, 28456
  graft
    cranial, 61316, 61559, 62117,
        62146-62148
    craniofacial, 21436
    donor area, 20900-20902
    facial, 21121-21123, 21127,
        21138, 21145-21180,
        21182-21188, 21194,
        21210-21215, 21247,
        21256-21268, 21348,
        21366, 21395, 21408,
        21436

Bone — continued
  graft — continued
    facial — continued
      mandibular, 21127
      fascia, 15840
      muscle, 15841-15845
    femur, 27170
    harvesting, 20900-20902
    lower extremity, 20955-20973,
        27170, 27177, 27357,
        27472, 27637, 28102,
        28106-28107, 28305,
        28322, 29885
    malar, 21210
    mandible, 21215
    mandibular ramus, 21194
    maxilla, 21210
    microvascular anastomosis
        20955, 20962
    nasal, 21210
    nasomaxillary, 21348
    orbit, 21408
    osteocutaneous, 20969-20973
    other, 23145, 23485, 42210,
        63051
    reconstruction, 21275
      mandibular rami, 21194
      midface, 21145-21160
    skull, 61316, 62148
    spine
      allograft, 20930-20931
      autograft, 20936-20938
    upper extremity, 23155,
        23221, 24115, 24125,
        25125, 25135, 25431,
        25440, 25830, 26205,
        26215, 26546, 26551
    vascular pedicle, 25430
  healing
    electrical, 20974-20975
    ultrasound, 20979
  humerus
    amputation, 24900-24940
    arthrodesis, 23800-23802
    arthroplasty, 23470-23472
    biopsy, 24065-24066
    craterization, 23184, 24140,
    excision
      abscess, 23174, 24134
      cyst, 23150-23156, 24110-
          24116
      osteomyelitis, 24134, 24140
      tumor, 23220-23222,
          24075-24076
        benign, 23150-23156,
            24110-24116
        malignant, 24077
    diaphysectomy, 23184, 24140
    foreign body, 24200-24201
    fracture
      closed
        epicondylar, 24560-24566
        proximal, 23600-23605
        shaft, 24500-24505
        supracondylar, 24530-
            24538
        tuberosity, 23620-23625,
            23665
      open, 24587
        epicondylar, 24575-24586
        proximal, 23615-23616
        shaft, 24515-24516
        supracondylar, 24545-
            24546
        tuberosity, 23630, 23670
      condyle, 24576-24582
      epicondyle, 24560-24575
      greater tuberosity, 23620-
          23630
      shaft, 24500-24505,
          24515-24516
      supracondylar, 24530-24546
      transcondylar, 24530-24546
      with dislocation, 23665-
          23670
    incision/drainage
      abscess, 23930, 23935
      bursa, 23931

Bone — continued
  humerus — continued
    incision/drainage — continued
      glenohumeral joint, 23100,
          23105, 23107
      pinning, 23491, 24498
      prophylactic treatment, 23491,
          24498
    repair
      arrest, 24470
      malunion, 24430-24435
      nonunion, 24430-24435
      osteoplasty, 24420
      osteotomy, 24400-24410
      tendon, 24305-24320,
          24341-24342
      with graft, 24435
    resection
      head, 23195
      radical, 23220-23222
      tendon, 23440
      tumor, 24150-24151
    saucerization, 23184, 24140
    sequestrectomy, 23174, 24134
    tenodesis, 23430, 24340
    tenolysis, 24332
    transfer, 23395-23397, 24301
    x-ray, 73060
  hyoid, 21495
  infection, 20005
    elbow, 23935
    excision
      clavicle, 23180
      facial, 21026
      humerus, 23184
      mandible, 21025
      scapula, 23182
    femur, 27303
    finger, 26034
    hand, 26034
    hip, 26992
    humerus, 23935, 24134
    incision
      foot, 28005
      shoulder, 23035
      thorax, 21510
      pelvis, 26992
      radius, 24136, 24145
    sequestrectomy
      clavicle, 23170
      humeral head, 23174
      scapula, 23172
      skull, 61501
  imaging, nuclear medicine,
      78300-78320
  lesion (tumor)
    ablation, 20982-20983
    excision, 21025-21026, 21182-
        21184, 23140-23156,
        24110-24126, 25120-
        25136, 26200-26215,
        27065-27067, 28100-
        28108, 61500, 61563-
        61564
    head, 21025-21026,
        21034, 21040-21047
        21182-21184, 61500,
        61563-61564
    upper extremity, 23140-
        23156, 24110-24126,
        25120-25136, 26200-
        26215
    lower extremity, 27065-
        27067, 28100-28108
    resection, 23220-23222,
        27077, 27365, 27645-
        27647, 28171-28175,
        63101-63103
  marrow
    aspiration, 38220
    biopsy, 38221
    cytogenic testing, 3155F
    harvest, 38230-38232
    HPC transplantation, 38240-
        38242
    imaging (non-MRI), 78102-
        78104, 78300-78320
    magnetic resonance imaging
        (MRI), 77084

CPT © 2015 American Medical Association. All Rights Reserved.

Bone — *continued*
  marrow — *continued*
    smear, 85097
    therapy, intramuscular, 0263T-0265T
  metatarsal
    amputation, 28810
    anastomosis, 20972
    condyle, excision, 28288
    craterization, 28122
    cyst, 28104-28107
    diaphysectomy, 28122
    excision
      complete, 28111-28114, 28140
      condyle, 28288
      cyst, 28104-28107
      partial, 28110, 28112
      tumor, 28104-28107, 28173
    fracture
      closed, 28470, 28475-28476
      open, 28485
    repair, 28322
      lengthening, 28306-28307
      osteotomy, 28306-28309
    saucerization, 28122
    tumor, 28104-28107, 28173
  nasal
    fracture
      closed, 21310-21320
      open, 21325-21335
    x-ray, 70160
  navicular
    arthroplasty, 25443
    fracture
      closed, 25622, 25624
      open, 25628
    repair, 25440
  nuclear medicine, 3269F
    density study, 78350-78351
    imaging, 78300-78320
    single photon emission computed tomography (SPECT), 78320
  osteoporosis
    couseling, 4019F
    screening, 5015F
    therapy, 4005F
  osteoplasty, wrist, 25394
  osteotomy
    facial, 21198-21199, 21206
  plate, 21244
  protein, 83937
  reconstruction
    facial, 21244-21246, 21248-21249, 21275
  repair
    facial, 21208-21209
    foot
      metatarsal, 28306-28309, 28322
      navicular, 25440
    temporal
      electromagnetic device, 69711
    wrist, 25431-25440
  removal
    fixation device, 20670-20680
    foreign body
      facial, 41806
      tarsal, 27610, 27620
    temporal
      electromagnetic device, 69711
      tumor, 69970
  replacement
    cochlear, 69717-69718
    electromagnetic device, 69711
  scapula
    craterization, 23182
    excision, 23172, 23182, 23190
      cyst, 23140, 23145-23146
      tumor, 23140, 23145-23146
    fixation, 23400
    fracture treatment, 23570-23585
    incision, 23035
    ostectomy, 23190
    resection, 23210
    saucerization, 23172

Bone — *continued*
  scapula — *continued*
    scapulopexy, 23400
    sequestrectomy, 23172
    x-ray, 73010
  semilunar
    arthroplasty, 25444
    dislocation
      closed, 25690
      open, 25695
    sequestrectomy, wrist, 25145
  sesamoid
    excision, 28315
      finger, 28615
      thumb, 26185
    fracture
      foot, 26185
  single photon emission computed tomography (spect), 78320
  skull
    base surgery
      anterior cranial fossa
        bicoronal, 61586
        craniofacial, 61580-61583
        lesion, 61600-61601
        orbitocranial, 61584-61585
        transzygomatic, 61586
      carotid artery, 61610-61613
      defect, 61618-61619
      encephalocele, 62121
      middle cranial fossa
        infratemporal, 61590-61591
        lesion, 61605-61608
        midline, 61607-61608
      orbitocranial zygomatic approach, 61592
      posterior cranial fossa
        lesion, 61615-61616
        transcondylar, 61597
        transochlear, 61596
        transpetrosal, 61598
      transoral approach, 61575-61576
      transtemporal, 61595
    burr hole
      biopsy, 61140
      drainage, 61150-61151, 61154-61156
      exploration, 61250-61253
      injection, 61120
      insertion, 61210-61215
    decompression
      cranial nerves, 61458
      gasserian ganglion sensory root, 61450
      hypertension, 61322-61323
      medulla, 61343
      orbit, 61330
      posterior cranial fossa, 61345
      pseudotumor cerebri, 61340
      spinal cord, 61343
      subtemporal, 61340
    drill hole, 61105
    excision
      lesion, 61500
        anterior cranial fossa, 61600-61601
        infratemporal fossa, 61605-61606
        midline, 61607-61608
        posterior cranial fossa, 61615-61616
      osteomyelitis, 61501
      tumor, 61500
    exploration, 61332-61333
    fracture treatment, 62000-62010
    incision, 61550-61552
      hematoma evacuation, 61312-61315
    reconstruction
      defect, 62140-62141, 62145
      orbital rim, 21172-21180
    reduction, 62115-62117
    removal, 61333, 62142
    repair, 62100, 62120
    replacement, 62143
    x-ray, 70250-70260

Bone — *continued*
  spur, 69140
  stimulation, 20974-20979
  tarsal
    amputation, 27888
    arthroplasty, 27700-27703
    dislocation
      closed, 27840-27842
      open, 27846-27848
    foreign body, 27610-27620
    fracture, 28456
      bimalleolar, 27808-27814
      lateral, 27786-27814, 27792
      medial, 27760-27766, 27808-27814
      posterior, 27767-27769, 27808-27814
      trimalleolar, 27816-27823
    tumor, 27615-27619
    x-ray, 73600-73610, 73615
  temporal
    conduction hearing device, 69710-69711
    excision, 69535
    osseointegrated implant, 69714
    resection, 69535
    tumor, 69970
  tibia
    arthroscopy
      fracture treatment, 29855-29856
      repair, 29891-29892
    craterization, 27369, 27640
    diaphysectomy, 27360, 27649
    excision
      cyst, 27635-27638
      epiphyseal bar, 20150
      partial, 27640
      tumor, 27635-27638, 27645
    fracture treatment
      arthroscopic, 29855-29856
      closed, 27824-27825
      distal, 27824-27828
      intercondylar, 27538-27540
      malleolus, 27760-27766, 27808-27814
      open, 27535-27536, 27758-27759, 27826-27828
      plateau, 27530-27536
      shaft, 27752-27759
    osteotomy, 27455-27457, 27705, 27709-27712
    repair
      epiphysis, 27477-27485, 27730-27742
      pseudoarthrosis, 27727
      saucerization, 27360, 27640
    x-ray, 73590-73600
  wedge reversal, 21122
  wrist
    carpal
      arthroplasty, 25443
      cyst, 25130-25136
      dislocation, 25690-25695
      excision, 25145, 25210-25215
      tumor, 25130-25136
    fracture
      closed, 25622-25624, 25630-25635
      open, 25628, 25645
    incision and drainage, 26034
    insertion, 25430
    osteoplasty, 25394
    repair, 25431-25440
    sequestrectomy, 25145
    tumor, 25130-25136
  x-ray
    age study, 77072
    dual energy absorptiometry, 3095F-3096F, 77080-77086
    facial, 70100-70110, 70140-70150, 70160
    length study, 77073
    osseous survey, 77074-77077
    tarsal, 73600-73610, 73615

Bordetella
  antibody, 86615
  antigen detection, 87265
Borrelia, 86618-86619
Borrelia burgdorferi, 86617
Borreliosis (lyme), 86617-86618
Bost fusion, 25800-25810
Bottle type procedure, 55060
Botulinum toxin
  anal sphincter, 46505
  eccrine glands, 64650, 64653
  guidance
    electrical stimulation, 95873
    needle electromyography, 95874
  muscle
    extraocular, 67345
    extremity, 64642-64645
    facial, 64612
    neck, 64616
    trunk, 64646-64647
Boutonniere deformity, 26426-26428
Bowleg, 27455-27457
Brace leg cast, 29358
Brachial
  artery
    aneurysm, 35011-35013
    angiography, 75658
    bypass graft, 35510, 35512, 35522-35525
    catheterization, 36120
    embolectomy, 34101
    exploration, 24495
    exposure, 34834
    thrombectomy, 34101
    thromboendarterectomy, 35321
  plexus
    decompression, 64713
    injection, 64415-64416
    neuroplasty, 64713
    release, 64713
    repair, 64861
Brachiocephalic
  artery
    angioplasty, 35458
    atherectomy, 0237T
    catheterization, 36215-36218
Brachycephaly, 21175
Brachytherapy
  electronic, 0394T-0395T
  infusion/instillation, solution, 77750
  isodose plan, 77316-77318
  remote afterloading, high dose
    interstitial/intracavitary, 77770-77772
    skin surface, 77767-77768
  source application, 77761-77763
    interstitial, 77778
    intracavitary, 77761-77763
  supply placement, 19298, 57160, 58346, 92974
  surface application, low dose, 77789
Bradykinin, 82286
Brain
  abscess
    drainage, 61150-61151, 61320-61321
    excision, 61514, 61522
  adhesions, 62161
  angiography, 70496
  biopsy, 61140-61151, 61575-61576, 61750-61751
  catheter
    irrigation, 62194, 62225
    placement, 0169T
    replacement, 62160, 62194, 62225
  cisternography, 70015
  computer-assisted surgery, 61781-61782
  computed tomography (CT) scan, 0042T, 70450-70470, 70496, 78608
    performance measure, 3110F-3112F
  craniopharyngioma, 61545

Brain — *continued*
- cyst
  - drainage, 61150-61151, 62161-62162
  - excision, 61516, 61524, 62162
- death determination, 95824
- decompression
  - brainstem, 61575-61576
- electrode
  - insertion, 61531-61533, 61760, 61850-61870
  - removal, 61535, 61880
  - stimulation, 95961-95962
- excision
  - amygdala, 61566
  - choroid plexus, 61544
  - craniopharyngioma, 61545
  - cyst, 61516, 61524, 62162
  - epileptogenic focus, 61534, 61536
  - hemisphere, 61543
  - hippocampus, 61566
  - lesion, 61534, 61536, 61575-61576, 61600-61608, 61615-61616
  - lobe, 61323, 61539-61540
    - temporal, 61537-61538
  - meningioma, 61512, 61519
- exploration, 61304-61305
- foreign body, 61570, 62163
- hematoma
  - drainage, 61154
  - and incision, 61312-61315
- imaging, nuclear medicine, 78600-78607, 78610
- incision
  - corpus callosum, 61541
  - mesencephalic tract, 61480
  - subpial, 61567
- insertion
  - catheter, 61210
  - electrode, 61531-61533, 61760, 61850-61870
  - pulse generator, 61885-61886
  - reservoir, 61210-61215
- lesion
  - aspiration, 61750-61751
  - creation, 61720-61735, 61790-61791, 61796-61799
  - excision, 61534, 61536, 61575-61576, 61600-61608, 61615-61616
- lobe
  - excision
    - temporal, 61537-61538
    - other, 61323, 61539-61540
- magnetic resonance imaging (MRI), 70551-70559
- myelography, 70010
- nuclear medicine
  - blood flow, 78610
  - cerebrospinal fluid, 78630-78650
  - imaging, 78600-78607
  - vascular flow, 78610
- positron emission tomography (PET) scan, 78608-78609
- pulse generator
  - insertion, 61885-61886
  - removal, 61888
- radiation, 0520F, 77432
- radiosurgery, 61796-61799, 77371-77373, 77435
- removal
  - electrode, 61535, 61880
  - foreign body, 61570, 62163
  - pulse generator, 61888
  - shunt, 62256-62258
- repair procedure, 61618, 61571, 62010, 62145
- shunt
  - creation, 62180-62192, 62200-62223
  - removal, 62256-62258
  - replacement, 62160, 62194, 62225-62230, 62256-62258
  - reprogramming, 62252

Brain — *continued*
- stem
  - biopsy, 61575-61576
  - decompression, 61575-61576
  - evoked potentials, 92585-92586
  - lesion, 61575-61576
  - tractotomy, 61480
- stereotactic, 61800
  - aspiration, 61750-61751
  - biopsy, 61750-61751
  - catheter, 0169T
  - lesion, 61720-61735, 61790-61791
  - radiation, 0520F, 77432
  - radiosurgery, 61796-61799, 77371-77373, 77435
  - surgery navigation, 61781-61783
  - trigeminal tract, 61791
- stimulation
  - electrode, 95961-95962
- stroke, 1065F-1066F
- subpial
  - incision, 0169T
  - transection, 61567
- surface electrode, 95961-95962
- tractotomy
  - mesencephalon, 61480
- transection, subpial, 61567
- tumor
  - excision, 61510-61512, 61516-61521, 61524-61530, 61545, 61575-61576, 61600-61608, 61615-61616, 62164
- ventriculography, 78635
- X-ray, 70010-70015

Breast
- abscess, 19020
- aspiration
  - cyst, 19000-19001
- augmentation, 19324-19325
- biopsy, 19081-19086, 19100-19101
  - with placement localization device, 19081-19086
- capsules
  - excision, 19371
  - incision, 19370
  - removal, 19371
- catheter, 19296-19298, 20555, 41019
- cyst
  - aspiration, 19000-19001
  - excision, 19120-19126
- excision
  - biopsy, 19100-19101
  - capsules, 19371
  - cyst, 19120-19126
  - fistula, 19112
  - lesion, 19120-19126, 19301
  - mastectomy, 19300-19307
  - nipple, 19110
  - tumor, 19260-19272
- exploration, 19110, 19020
- fibroadenoma, 19105
- fistula, 19112
- implants
  - insertion, 19340-19342
  - preparation, 19396
  - removal, 19328-19330
  - supply, 19396
- incision
  - capsules, 19370
  - drainage, 19020
- injection, 19030
- lesion, 19120-19126, 19301
- magnetic resonance imaging (MRI), 0159T, 77058-77059
- mammoplasty
  - augmentation, 19324-19325
  - reduction, 19318
- mastectomy
  - excision 19300-19307
- mastopexy, 19316
- mammography, 77051-77052, 77055-77057
  - findings, 3014F, 5060F-5062F
  - performance measure, 3014F

Breast — *continued*
- oncoprotein, 83950
- periprosthetic
  - capsulectomy, 19371
  - capsulotomy, 19370
- placement
  - catheter, 19296-19298, 20555, 41019
  - metallic localization clip, 19281-19288
  - needle localization wire, 19281-19288
  - radiotherapy afterloading catheter, 19296-19298
- reconstruction, 19357-19369
  - augmentation, 19324-19325
  - flap
    - free, 19364
    - latissimus dorsi, 19361
    - myocutaneous, 19367-19369
  - mammoplasty, 19318-19325
  - nipple, 19350-19355
  - other, 19366
  - revision, 19380
  - tissue expander, 19357
- reduction, 19318
- removal
  - capsules, 19371
  - complete, 19303
  - implants, 19328-19330
  - partial, 19300-19302
  - radical, 19305-19307
  - subcutaneous, 19304
- repair, 19316
- revision, 19380
- tomosynthesis, 77061-77063
- tumor, 19260-19272
- ultrasound, 76641-76642
- x-ray, 76700, 77051-77052, 77055-77057

Breath
- inspiratory positive pressure breathing (IPPB)
  - continuous negative pressure breathing (CNPB), 94662
  - continuous positive airway pressure (CPAP), 94660
  - delivery room, 99465
- test
  - alcohol, 82075
  - heart transplant rejection detection, 0085T
  - helicobacter pylori, 78267-78268, 83013-83014
  - hydrogen, 91065

Bricker procedure, 50820
Brostow procedure, 23460-23462
Bronchial
- anastomosis, 32486
- biopsy, brush, 31717
- challenge, 95070-95071
Broncho-bronchial anastomosis, 32486
Bronchoalveolar lavage, 31624
Bronchography, 76499
- contrast injection, 31899
Bronchoplasty, 32501
- graft repair, 31770
- stenosis excision, 31775
Bronchopneumonia, 0012F, 86000, 86638
Bronchoplumonary lavage, 31624
Bronchoscopy
- aspiration
  - biopsy, 31629, 31633, 31652-31653
  - therapeutic, 31645-31646
- assessment, air leak, 31647, 31651
- biopsy
  - bronchial, 31625
  - lung, 31628, 31632
  - mediastinal/hilar lymph node, 31652-31653
  - needle aspiration, 31629, 31633
- brushings, 31623
- cell washing, 31622
- contrast injection, 31899

Bronchoscopy — *continued*
- diagnostic, 31622
- dilation, 31630-31631, 31636-31637
- foreign body, 31635
- fracture reduction, 31630
- insertion, valve, 31647, 31651
- lavage 31624
- occlusion, balloon, 31634, 31647, 31651
- placement
  - bronchial stent, 31636-31637
  - fiduciary markers, 31626
  - intracavitary catheter, 31643
  - tracheal stent, 31631
- removal, valve, 31648-31649
- stenosis relief, 31641
- stent
  - placement, 31631, 31636-31637
  - revision, 31638
- thermoplasty, 31660-31661
- tumor
  - destruction, 31641
  - excision, 31640
- ultrasound, 31654
- valve
  - insertion, 31647, 31651
  - removal, 31648-31649
Bronchospasm
- spirometry, 3023F-3027F, 94014-94016
Bronkodyl, 80198
Brow ptosis, 67900
Brucella, 86000
- antibody, 86622
Bruise
- ankle, 27603
- arm
  - lower, 25028
  - upper, 23930
- brain
  - drainage, 61154-61156
  - evacuation, 61312-61315
- drain, 61108
- ear, 69000, 69005
- elbow, 23930
- epididymis, 54700
- gums, 41800
- hip, 26990
- knee, 27301
- leg
  - lower, 27603
  - upper, 27301
- mouth, 40800-40801, 41005-41009, 41015-41018
- nose, 30000-30020
- pelvis, 26990
- scrotum, 54700
- shoulder, 23030
- skin, 10140, 10160
- subdural, 61108
- subungal, 11740
- testis, 54700
- tongue, 41000-41006, 41015
- vagina, 57022-57023
- wrist, 25028
Brunschwig operation, 58240
Brush
- biopsy, 31717
- border, 86308-86310
Bucca
- bone
  - excision, 21030, 21034
  - fracture
    - closed, 21355
    - open, 21360-21366
  - reconstruction, 21270
- graft
  - fascia, 15840
  - muscle, 15841-15845
Buccal mucosa, 40818
Bulbourethral gland, 53250
Bulla
- lung
  - excision-plication, 32141
  - endoscopic, 32655
  - puncture aspiration, 10160

CPT © 2015 American Medical Association. All Rights Reserved.   © 2016 DecisionHealth

Bunion
  repair, 28110, 28290-28299
Burgess amputation, 27889
Bunion surgery, 28110, 28290-28299
Burkitt herpesvirus, 86663-86665
Burn
  grafting procedures, 15050-15431
    allograft, 15300-15336
    tissue culture, 15100-15157
    xenograft, 15400-15431
  treatment, 16000-16036
    debridement, 01951-01953,
      15002-15005, 16020-
      16030
    dressings, 16020-16030
    escharotomy, 16035-16036
    initial, 16000
    preparation, 15002-15005
Burr hole, 0077T, 0169T, 61720-
  61751, 61850-61868
  biopsy, 61140
  catheterization, 61210
  drainage, 61150-61156
  exploration, 61250-61253
  implant, 61863-61868
  injection, 61120
  insertion, 61210
Bursa
  aspiration
    joint, 20600-20611
  excision
    elbow, 24105
    femur, 27062
    ischial, 27060
    knee, 27340
    wrist, 25115-25116
  incision and drainage
    ankle, 27604
    arm, lower, 25031
    elbow, 23931
    foot, 28001
    hip, 26991
    leg, lower, 27604
    palm, 26025-26030
    pelvis, 26991
    shoulder, 23031
    wrist, 25031
  injection, 20600-20611
Bursectomy
  elbow, 24105
  femur, 27062
  ischial, 27060
  knee, 27340
  wrist, 25115-25116
Bursocentesis, 20600-20611
Butyrylcholine esterase, 82480-82482
Bypass
  cardiopulmonary, 33926
    ablation, 33251, 33256,
      33259-33261
    lung transplant, 32852, 32854
    obliteration, 33814
    pericardiectomy, 33031
    pulmonary artery, 33910,
      33916, 33922, 33926
    replacement
      valve, 33405-33410,
        33430, 33465
    repair
      aortic arch, 33853
      atrial septal defect, 33641
      chamber, 33500
      coronary artery, 33504
      pulmonary artery, 33926
      sinus of valsalva, 33702-
        33720
      transposition, 33774-33777
      valve, 33496
    resection, 33120
    thoracic aorta, 33860-33877
    transmyocardial, 0167T
    wound, 33305, 33315, 33322,
      33335
    valve replacement, 33405-
      33410, 33430, 33465
    valvectomy, 33460
    valvotomy, 33422, 33474

Bypass — *continued*
  cardiopulmonary — *continued*
    valvuloplasty, 33400, 33403,
      33425-33427
    coronary artery, 33510-33536
    catheterization, 93454-93458
    gastric, 43644-43645, 43846-
      43847
  graft
    aortobi-iliac, 35538, 35638
    aortobifemoral, 35540, 35646
    aortofemoral, 35539, 35647
    aortoiliac, 35537, 35637
    axillary, 35516-35522, 35533,
      35616-35623, 35650,
      35654
    brachial, 35510, 35512,
      35522-35525
    carotid, 33891, 35501-35510,
      35526, 35601-35606,
      35626, 35642
    celiac, 35531, 35631
    composite graft, 35681
    computed tomography (CT)
      scan, 0146T-0149T
    coronary, 33510-33516,
      33533-33536, 93564
    duplex scan, 93925-93931,
      93978-93979
    excision, 35901-35907
    femoral, 35521, 35533, 35539-
      35558, 35566, 35621,
      35646-35647, 35654-
      35661, 35666, 35700
    harvest, 33508, 35500
    hepatorenal, 35535
    ilioceliac, 35632
    iliofemoral, 35565, 35665
    ilioiliac, 35563, 35663
    iliomesenteric, 35633
    iliorenal, 35634
    mammary, 4110F
    mesenteric, 35531, 35631, 35633
    peroneal, 35566-35571,
      35666-35671
    placement
      patch, 35685
    popliteal, 35556, 35571, 35623,
      35656, 35671, 35700
    renal, 35535-35536, 35560,
      35631-35636
    reoperation, 35700
    repair
      abdomen, 35907
      extremity, 35681-35683,
        35903
      neck, 35901
      secondary, 35870
      thorax, 35905
    revascularization, 35901,
      35903, 35905
    revision, 35879, 35881,
      35883-35884
    splenic, 35536, 35636
    subclavian, 35506, 35511-
      35516, 35526, 35606-
      35616, 35626, 35645
    thrombectomy, 35875-35876,
      37184-37186
    tibial, 35566-35571, 35623,
      35666-35671
    transcatheter, 37184-37186
    vertebral, 35508, 35515,
      35642-35645
  in-situ, 33548, 35583-35587
  revision, 35879-35884

C

C-13, 83013-83014
C-14, 78267-78268, 83013-83014
C-peptide, 80432, 84681
C-reactive protein, 86140-86141
Cadmium, 82300
**Caffeine halothane contracture test
  (CHCT)**, 89049
Calcaneal spur, 28119

Calcaneous
  craterization, 28120
  cyst
    excision, 28100-28103
  diaphysectomy, 28120
  excision
    bone, 28118-28122
    tumor, 27647, 28100-28103,
      28171
  fracture
    treatment, 28400-28420
  ostectomy, 28118-28119, 28300
  saucerization, 28120
  tumor
    excision, 27647, 28100-28103,
      28171
  x-ray, 73650
Calculus
  analysis, 82355-82370
  destruction
    biliary tract, 43265
    bladder, 51065, 52317-52318
    kidney, 50080-50081, 50590
    ureter, 52325, 52353
  removal
    biliary tract
      cholecystotomy, 47480
      choledochotomy, 47420-
        47425
      endoscopic, 43264, 47554
      transduodenal, 47460
    bladder, 51050, 52310-52318,
      52352
    kidney
      cystourethroscopy, 52352
      nephrolithotomy, 50060-
        50075
      nephrostolithotomy, 50080-
        50081
      nephrostomy, 50561
      nephrotomy, 50580
      pyelotomy, 50130
    pancreatic, 43264, 48020
    ureter, 52325, 52353
      cystourethroscopy, 52320-
        52325, 52352
      cystotomy, 51065
      ureterolithotomy, 50610-
        50630, 51060
      ureterostomy, 50961
      ureterotomy, 50980
    urethra, 52310-52315, 52352
Caldwell-Luc procedure, 21385,
  31030-31032
Caliper, 20660
Callander knee disarticulation, 27598
Calmette guerin bacillus vaccine,
  90585-90586
Caloric vestibular test, 92533
Calprotectin, 83993
Calycoplasty, 50405
Camey enterocystoplasty, 50825
Campbell procedure, 27422
Campylobacter, 86625
  pylori
    antibody, 86677
    antigen detection, 87338-87339
    stool, 87338
    test
      blood, 83009
      breath, 78267-78268,
        83013-83014
      urease, 83009, 83013-83014
Canal, auditory
  biopsy, 69105
  cerumen removal, 69209-69210
  decompression, 61591, 69960
  drainage, 69020
  foreign body
    removal, 69200-69205
  lesion
    excision, 69140-69155
  reconstruction, 69310-69320
  semicircular, fenestration, 69820,
    69840
Canalith, 95992

Canaloplasty, 69631, 69635
Candida
  antibody, 86628
  test, 86485
Cannulation
  arterial, 36620-36625
  arteriovenous, 36821
  dialysis, 36800-36815
  duct, 43273
  fallopian tube, 58565
  intraperitoneal
    delayed exit site creation, 49436
    insertion, 49324, 49419-49421
      extension, 49435
    removal, 49422
    revision, 49325
  renoportal, 37145
  sinus, 31000-31002, 31235
  thoracic duct, 38794
  vertebral, 22513-22515
Cannulization
  arteriovenous, 36145, 36810-
    36815
  declotting, 36593, 36860-36861
  extracorpeal circulation, 36823
  vas deferens, 55200
  vein, 36800
Canthocystostomy, 68745, 68750
Canthopexy, 21280, 21282
Canthoplasty, 67950
Canthorrhaphy, 67880-67882
Canthotomy, 67715
Canthus, 67950
Capsule
  arthrotomy
    elbow, 24006
  biopsy, 44100
  contraceptive procedures, 11975-
    11977
  endoscopy, 91110-91111
  excision
    breast, 19371
    elbow, 24006
    joint
      interphalangeal, 26525
      metacarpophalangeal, 25620
    lesion
      ankle, 27630
      foot, 28090-28092
      knee, 27347
      leg, 27630
      upper extremity, 26160
      wrist, 25320
  hymen, 58346
  incision
    joint
      interphalangeal, 26525
      metacarpophalangeal, 25620
    shoulder, 23020
  release
    ankle, 27612
    foot, 28260-28264
    joint
      interphalangeal, 28272,
        26525
      metacarpophalangeal, 26520
      metatarsophalangeal,
        28270, 28289
    knee, 27435
    wrist, 25085
  repair
    breast, 19370
    knee, 27405-27409
    shoulder, 23020, 23450-23466
    wrist, 25320
Capsulectomy, 19371
Capsulodesis, 26516-26518
Capsulorrhaphy, 23450-23466, 25320
Capsulotomy
  breast, 19370
  foot, 28260-28262
  hip, 27036
  joint
    interphalangeal, 28272
    metacarpophalangeal, 26520
    metatarsophalangeal, 28270

CPT © 2015 American Medical Association. All Rights Reserved.

© 2016 DecisionHealth

Care — *continued*
  therapy — *continued*
    orthotics training, 97760
    osteopathic manipulation, 98925-98929
    paraffin bath, 97018
    physical performance test, 97750
    prosthetic training, 97761
    sensory integration, 97533
    supervised procedure, 97010-97028
    traction, 97012, 97140
    ultrasound, 97035
    ultraviolet light, 97028
    vasopneumatic device, 97016
    wheelchair management, 97542
    whirlpool therapy, 97022
    work hardening, 97545-97546
    work reintegration, 97537

Carnitine, 82379
Carotene, 82380
Carotid
  aneurysm repair, 35001-35002, 61703-61710
  angiography, 3100F, 36222-36224, 36227
  artery
    aneurysm, 61710
    excision, 60605
    ligation, 37600-37606
    stent, 0075T-0076T
    transection, 61610-61612
  atheroma evaluation, 93895
  body
    lesion
      artery, 60605
      excision, 60600
  embolectomy, 34001
  excision
    artery, 60605
    lesion, 60600
  intima thickness, 93895
  ligation, 37600-37606, 61609-61612
  needle, stent or catheter
    introduction, 0075T-0076T, 36100, 37215-37216
  thromboendarterectomy, 35301, 35390

Carpal
  bone
    arthroplasty, 25443
    cyst, 25130-25136
    dislocation, 25690-25695
    excision, 25145, 25210-25215
      tumor, 25130-25136
    fracture
      closed, 25622-25624, 25630-25635
      open, 25628, 25645
    incision and drainage, 26034
    insertion, 25430
    osteoplasty, 25394
    repair, 25431-25440
    sequestrectomy, 25145
    tumor
      excision, 25130-25136
  incision and drainage, 25035
  ligament release, 29848
  tunnel
    injection, 20526
    neuroplasty, 64721

Carpectomy, 25210-25215
Carpometacarpal joint
  arthrodesis, 25800, 26841-26844
  arthroplasty, 25447
  arthrotomy, 26070, 26100
  biopsy, 26100
  dislocation treatment, 26641-26715, 26770-26785
  exploration, 26070
  fusion, 26841-26844
  removal
    foreign body, 26070
  repair, 25447
  synovectomy, 26130
  tendon transfer, 26480-26483

Cartilage, 4130F-4132F
  arytenoid, 31560-31561
  debridement, 29862, 29877
  excision, 23101, 27332-27333
  graft
    ear, 21235
    mandibular condyle, 21247
    nasal, 20912
    rib, 20910
      to chin, ear, face, nose, 21230
    septoplasty, 30520
    zygomatic arch, 21255
  shaving, 29862, 29877

Cartilaginous exostoses, 69140
Cast
  arm, 29065, 29075
  application, 29000-29086, 29305-29450
  body
    halo, 29000
    jacket
      Risser 29010-29015
    upper, 29035-29046
  brace
    leg, 29358
  clubfoot, 29450
  cranial, 20661-20664
  cylinder, 29365
  finger, 29086
    splint, 29130-29131
  femur, 20663
  hand, 29085
  hip, 29305-29325
  leg, 29345-29355, 29365, 29405-29450
    brace, 29358
    splint, 29505, 29515
  maxillofacial, 21100
  oral
    splint, 21085
  patellar tendon, 29435
  pelvic, 20662
  removal, 20665, 29700-29710
  repair, 29720
  shoulder, 29049-29058
  splint
    arm, 29105, 29125-29126
    finger, 29130-29131
    foot, 29590
    leg, 29505, 29515
    oral, 21085
  wedge, 29740-29750
  window, 29730
  wrist, 29085

Castration
  oophorectomy
    excisional, 58940-58943
    laparascopic, 58552, 58554, 58661
    vaginal, 58262-58263, 58291-58292
  orchiectomy
    laparoscopic, 54690
    partial, 54522
    radical, 54530-54535
    simple, 54520

Cataract, 4175F-4177
  assessment, 0014F, 3325F
  discission
    secondary membranous, 66820-66821
  removal
    extracapsular, 66982, 66984
    intracapsular, 66983
    secondary membranous, 66830

Catecholamines, 80424, 82382-82384
Cathepsin-D, 82387
Catheter
  aspiration, 31720-31725
  bladder
    insertion, 51701-51703
    irrigation, 51700
  brain, 0169T
  breast, 19296-19298, 20555, 41019
  bronchus, 31643

Catheter — *continued*
  central venous
    insertion, 36555-36558
    repair, 36575
    replacement, 36578-36582, 36584
    repositioning, 36597
  conversion
    biliary drainage, 47535-47536
    nephrostomy to nephroureteral, 50434
  declotting, 36593
  exchange
    biliary drainage, 47536
    cyst/abscess drainage, 49423
    nephrostomy, 50435
  intracardiac ablation, 93650-93657
  intracatheter, 36596, 99507
  intraperitoneal, insertion, 49419-49421
  introduction or selective
    placement, 36010-36015, 36200-36248
  pericatheter, 36595
  removal, 36589, 49422, 62355
  repair, 36575
  replacement, 36580-36581, 36584
  repositioning, 36597
  Swan-Ganz, 93503
  ureteral, insertion, 50433, 51045

Catheterization
  abdomen, 49421
    artery, 36245-36248
  aorta, 36160-36200
  artery
    abdomen, 36245-36248
    brachiocephalic, 36215-36218
    cerebral, 36215
    coronary, 93454-93461
    cutdown, 36625
    lower extremity, 36245-36248
    needle, 36100-36140
    percutaneous, 36620
    thoracic, 36215
    pelvic, 36245-36248
    pulmonary, 36013-36015
    renal, 36251-36254
    thoracic, 36215-36218
    umbilical, 36660
  bile duct, 47533-47534
  biliary ductal system, 74328, 74330
  bladder, 51701-51703, 51010, 51045
  brain, 0169T
    replacement, 62160, 62194, 62225
  bronchography, 31710
  cardiac, 36013, 93451-93533
    ablation, 93650-93657
    injection procedure, 93451-93461, 93563-93568
    pacemaker, 33210
  central, 36555-36566
  cystourethroscopy, 52005-52010
  fallopian, 58345, 74742
  jejenum, 44015
  kidney, 50432-50433
  legs, 36245-36248
  naso-tracheal, 31720
  pancreatic ductal system, 74329-74330
  peripheral, 36568-36571
  pleural cavity, 32550
  radioelement, 55875
  removal, 36595-36596, 37197
  salivary duct, 42660
  shunt
    arteriovenous, 36145
  skull, 61107
  spinal cord, 62350-62351
  tracheobronchi, 31725
  transthoracic, 33621
  umbilical, 36510, 36660
  ureter
    cystourethroscopy, 52005-52010, 52320-52330, 52353
    endoscopic, 50553, 50572, 50953, 50972, 52005
    injection, 50430-50431, 50684
    manometric, 50396, 50686

Catheterization — *continued*
  uterus, 58340
  vena cava, 36010
  vein
    central, 36555-36556, 36568-36569, 36580, 36584
    needle, 36000
    order
      first, 36011
      second, 36012
    organ, 36500
    portal, 36481
    umbilical, 36510
    ventricular, 61020-61026, 61210-61215
  with bronchial brush biopsy, 31717

Cauda equina
  decompression
    corpectomy, 63087-63091
    laminectomy, 63005-63011, 63017, 63047-63048
    transpedicular, 63055-63057
  exploration, 63005-63011, 63017

Cauterization
  anal fissure, 46940-46942
  cervix, 57510-57513, 57522
  everted punctum, 68705
  granulation tissue, 17250
  mucosa, inferior turbinate, 30801-30802
  nasal, 30901-30906
  nasopharyngeal, 42970
  punctum, everted, 68705
  skin
    lesion, 11055-11057, 17000-17004
    tags, 11200-11201

Cavernitides
  fibrous, 54110-54112, 54200-54205
Cavernosography, 54230
Cavernosometry, 54231
Cavus foot correction, 28309
Cecostomy
  evaluation, 49465
  injection
    contrast, 49465
      obstructive material removal, 49460
  insertion, 49442
  laparoscopic, 44188
  placement, 44300
  removal
    obstructive material, 49460
  replacement, 49450

Celiac
  artery
    aneurysm, 35121-35122
    embolectomy, 34151
    graft
      bypass, 35531, 35631-35632
    thrombectomy, 34151
    thromboendarterectomy, 35341
  plexus
    destruction, 64680
    injection, 64530, 64680

Celioscopy
  biopsy, removal, 69209
  drainage, 49323, 54690
Celiotomy, 49000, 49220
Cell
  blood
    CD4 and CD8, 86360
    count
      automated, 85049
      B-cells, 86355
      differential WBC, 85004-85007, 85009
      hematocrit, 85014
      hemoglobin, 85018
      hemogram
        automated, 85025-85027
        manual, 85032
      microhematocrit, 85013
      natural killer (NK) cells, 86357
      red blood cell (RBC), 85032-85041

Cell — *continued*
blood — *continued*
count — *continued*
reticulocyte, 85044-85046
smear, 85007-85008
stem cell, 86367
T-cell, 86359-86361
white blood cell, 85032,
85048, 89055
myeloperoxidase (MPO),
83876
enzyme activity, 82657
exchange, 36511-36513
sedimentation rate
automated, 85652
manual, 85651
count
blood
automated, 85049
B-cell, 86355
differential WBC, 85004-
85007, 85009
hematocrit, 85014
hemoglobin, 85018
hemogram
automated, 85025-85027
manual, 85032
microhematocrit, 85013
natural killer (NK) cells, 86357
red blood cell (RBC), 85032-
85041
reticulocyte, 85044-85046
smear, 85007-85008
stem cells, 86367
T-cells, 86359-86361
white blood cells, 85032,
85048, 89055
body fluid, 89050-89051
stem cell, 86367
enumeration, 86152-86153
fc receptor, 86243
islet
antibody, 86341
transplant, 0141T-0143T
stem
allograft, 65781
count, 86367
cryopreservation, 38207, 88240
depletion
plasma, 38214
platelet, 38213
red blood cell, 38212
T-cell, 38210
tumor, 38211
donor search, 38204
harvest, 38205-38206
thawing, 38208-38209, 88241
transplant
allogenic, 38240
infusions, 38242
autologous, 38241
concentration, 38215
washing, 38209
stimulating hormone, 80418,
80426, 83002
Cellobiase, 82963
Cellular inclusion, 87207, 87210, 88106
Central
catheter
insertion, 36555-36558,
36568-36569
repair, 36575
replacement, 36580-36585
removal, 36589
repositioning, 36597
shunt, 33764
Cephalic version, 01958, 59412
Cephalocele, 62120-62121
Cephalogram, 70350
Cerclage
cervix, 57700, 59320-59325, 59871
fracture
arm, 24515-24516
leg, 27244-27245, 27506-
27507, 27758-27759
femoral, 27244-27245
shaft, 27506-27507
tibial, 27758-27759

Cerebral
angiography, 36223-36224
angioplasty, 61630
artery
anastomosis, 61711
doppler velocimetry, 76821
death, 95824
epileptogenic focus
excision, 61536
hernia, 62120-62121
implant
neurostimulator electrodes,
61860
perfusion
analysis, 0042T
thermal probe implantation,
0077T
seizure focus monitoring, 95950-
95953, 95956
stent, 61635
thrombolysis, 37195
ventriculography, 78635
vessels
angioplasty, 61630
dilation, 61640-61642
occlusion, 61623
stent
placement, 61635
Cerebrose, 82760
Cerebrospinal
fluid, 86235
imaging, 78630-78647
leak, 63744
detection, 78650
repair
brain, 61618-61619, 62100
endoscopy, 31290-31291
skull base, 61618-61619
spinal cord, 63707-63709
shunt, 63740, 63746, 78650
creation, 62180-62192,
62200-62223
irrigation, 62194
removal, 62256-62258
replacement, 62160,
62194, 62225-62230
reprogramming, 62252
Ceruloplasmin, 82390
Cerumen, removal, 69209- 69210
Cervical
canal dilation, 57800
cap, 57170
dilator insertion, 59200
disc arthroplasty, 22856-22858,
0375T
removal, 0095T, 22864
revision, 22861, 0098T
discectomy, 63075-63076
discography, 72285 esophagus,
x-ray, 74210
injection
anesthetic agent, 64470-64480
interspace
laminotomy, 63020, 63035,
63040, 63043
laminectomy
arteriovenous malformation,
63250
cordotomy, 63194, 63196, 63198
decompression, 61343, 63001,
63015, 63045
facetectomy and
foraminotomy, 63048
intraspinal lesion, 63265, 63270
intraspinal neoplasm, 63275,
63280, 63285
myelotomy, 63170
section of ligaments, 63180-
63182
laminoplasty, 63050-63051
lymph node
biopsy, 38505-38520
excision, 38505-38520
lymphadenectomy, 38720-38724
penetration test, 89330
plexus, 64413
pregnancy, 59140
puncture, 61050-61055

Cervical — *continued*
rib
excision, 21615-21616
resection, 21705
spine
computed tomography (CT),
72125-72127
magnetic resonance imaging
(MRI), 72141-72142,
72156
myelography, 72240, 72270
x-ray, 72040-72052
smears
automated screening, 88174-
88175
Bethseda, 88164-88167
hormonal evaluation, 88155
physician interpretation, 88141
spine
excision, 22100, 22110
fracture, 23675-23680
stump
dilation and curettage, 57558
excision, 57540-57556
sympathectomy, 64802
tracheoplasty, 31750
vertebra
biopsy, 20251
excision, 22100, 22110
fracture treatment, 22326
osteotomy, 22210, 22220
resection, 63081-63082,
63300, 63304
Cervicectomy, 57530
Cervicoplasty, 15819
Cervicothoracic
ganglia, 64510
Cervix
amputation, 57530
biopsy
endoscopic, 57454-57455, 57460
excision, 57500, 57520
cautery, 57510-57513, 57522
cerclage, 57700, 59320-59325,
59871
colposcopy, 57420-57421, 57452-
57461
conization, 57461, 57520-57522
curettage, 57454, 57456, 57505
dilation, 57558, 57800
excision, 57540-57556
radical, 57531
total, 57530
exploration, 57452
insertion, 59200
oncoprotein, 83951
pregnancy, 59140
repair, 57720, 57700, 59320,
59325
Cesarean
care, 59610, 59515, 59618,
59622
delivery, 01961, 01968, 59514,
59618, 59620
hysterectomy, 01963, 01969,
59525
ligation, 58611
resuscitation, 99465
stabilization, 99464
Chalazion
excision, 67800-67801, 67805,
67808
Challenge
bronchial, 95070-95071
Chambers procedure, 28300
Change
catheter, 75984
dressing
burn, 15852, 16020-16030
fetal position, 59412
Cheek
graft, 15240-15241
lift, 15828
repair, 13131-13133
tissue transfer, 14040-14041
bone
excision, 21030, 21034

Cheek — *continued*
bone — *continued*
fracture
closed, 21355
open, 21360-21366
reconstruction, 21270
graft
fascia, 15840
muscle, 15841-15845
Cheilectomy, 28289
Cheiloplasty, 40650-40654
cleft lip, 40700-40761
Cheiloschisis, 30460-30462, 40700-
40761
Cheilotomy, 40806
Chemical
cauterization, 17250
exfoliation, 17360
lesion destruction, 40820, 42160,
46900, 54050
peel, 15788-15793
pleurodesis, 32560, 32650
Chemocauterization, 65435-65436
Chemodenervation
anal sphincter, 46505
bladder, 52887
eccrine glands, 64650-64653
electrical stimulation for guidance,
95873
larynx, 64617
muscle, 64612-64616, 64642-
64647, 67345
needle electromyography for
guidance, 95874
salivary glands, 64611
Chemonucleolysis, 62292
Chemosurgery
benign, 17110-17111
premalignant, 17000-17004
malignant, 17270, 17280
Chemotaxis, 86155
Chemotherapy administration, 0519F
catheter, 36640
brain, 61517, 96542
bladder, 51720
central nervous system, 61517,
96450
extracorporeal, 36823
filling, 96542
infusion
home, 99601-99602
intra-arterial infusion, 96373,
96379, 96420-96425
intralesional, 96405-96406
intramuscular, 96372, 96401-
96402
IV infusion, 96365-96368, 96379,
96413-96417
IV push, 96374-96376, 96409-
96411
kidney, 50391
pathology, 3317F-3318F
peritoneal, 96446
pleural cavity, 96440
pump, 95990-95991, 96521-
96522
subcutaneous, 96369-96372,
96401-96402
ureteral, 50391
Chest, 00520-00529
angiography, 71275, 71555
artery ligation, 37616
bioimpedance, 93701
biopsy, 00522, 21550, 32405,
39401-39402
cavity
endoscopy, 32601-32606,
32650-32665
graft, 35905
compression
delivery room, 99465
computed tomography (CT) scan,
71250-71275
cyst
excision, 32662, 39200

CPT © 2015 American Medical Association. All Rights Reserved.

Chest — *continued*
 excision
  cyst, 32662, 39200
  tumor, 19260-19272, 21555-21557, 32662, 39220
 exploration, 20101, 35820, 39000-39010
 funnel, 21740-21743
 incision
  drainage, 21501-21502, 21510, 39000-39010
  empyema, 32035-32036
 magnetic resonance imaging (MRI), 71550-71552
 removal, 39000-39010
 repair, 35211-35216
  graft, 35241-35246, 35271-35276
 strapping, 29200
 thoracostomy, 32551
 tumor
  ablation, 32998
  excision, 19260-19272, 21555-21557, 32662, 39220
 ultrasound, 76604
 wall
  closure, 32810
  fistula, 32906
  manipulation, 94667-94668
  mechanical oscillation, 94669
  reconstruction, 32820, 49904
  repair, 32810, 32905-32906
  resection, 32503-32504
  tumor
   ablation, 32998
   excision, 19260-19272
 x-ray, 3006F, 3319F-3320F, 0174T-0175T 71010-71035, 71090, 74022
Chevron procedure, 28296
Chicken pox vaccine, 90716
Chin
 cartilage graft, 21230
 genioplasty, 21120
  sliding, 21121-21123
 lift, 15828
 skin
  graft, 15240-15241
  pedicle, 15574
  repair, 13131-13133
  transfer, 14040-14041
Chinidin, 80194
Chiropractic treatment, 98940-98943
Chlamydia
 antibody, 86631-86632
 culture, 87110
 detection, 87270, 87320
Choramphenicol, 82415
Chloride, 82435-82438
 methylene, 82441
Chlorinated hydrocarbons, 82441
Chlorpromazine, 80342-80344
Choanal atresia, 30540-30545
Cholangiography
 injection, 47531-47532
 radiological supervision and interpretation, 74300-74301
 with
  bile duct exploration, 47700
  cholycystectomy, 47563, 47605, 47620
Cholangiopancreatography (ERCP), 43260-43265, 43273-43278
 with optical endomicroscopy, 0397T
Cholangiostomy, 47400
Cholecystectomy, 47600-47620
 laparoscopic, 47562-47564
Cholecystenterostomy, 47570, 47720-47741
Cholecystography, 74290
Cholecystotomy, 47480, 47490, 48001
Choledochoplasty, 47701, 47760, 47780-47785
Choledochoscopy, 47550

Choledochostomy, 47420-47425
Choledochus, 47715
Cholera, 90625
Cholesterol
 test, 80061, 82465, 83718-83721
Cholinesterase, 82480-82482
Cholylglycine, 82240
Chondroitin sulfate, 82485
Chondromalacia patellae, 27418
Chondrosteoma, 69140
Chopart procedure, 28800-28805
Chorionic
 gonadotropin
  stimulation panel, 80414-80415
  test, 84702-84704
 growth hormone, 83632
 meningitides, 86727
 tumor, 59100, 59870
 villus sampling, 59015
  test, 88235, 88267
  ultrasonic guidance, 76945
Choroid
 destruction, 67220-67225, 67299
 excision, 61544
Christmas factor, 85250
Chromaffinoma, 80424
Chromatin, 88130
Chromatography, 82542
Chromium, 82495
Chromogenic substrate, 85130
Chromosome analysis, 88230-88239, 88245-88269, 88280-88289
 myeloperoxidase, 83876
Chromotubation, 58350
Chronic
 care management, 99487-99490
 cystitis, 52260-52265
 erection, 54420-54430, 54435
Ciliary body
 destruction, 66700-66740
 lesion, 66770
 repair, 66680-66682
Cimino procedure, 36821
Cinefluorographies, 70371, 74230
Cineplasty, 24940
Cineradiography, 70371, 74230
Circulation
 assist, 33967, 33970
 carotid
  aneurysm surgery, 61697, 61700
 extracoporeal, 33946-33956, 36823
 vertebrobasilar
  aneurysm surgery, 61698, 61702
Circumcision, 54150-54161
 during hypospadias repair, 54322-54328
 repair, 54163
Cisternal puncture, 61050-61055
Cisternography, 70015, 78630
Citrate, 82507
Clagett procedure, 32810
Clavicle, 00450-00454
 dislocation, 23520-23552
 claviculectomy, 23120, 23125
 fracture
  closed, 23500-23505
  open, 23515
 osteotomy, 23480-23485
 prophylactic treatment, 23490
 sequestrectomy, 23170
 tumor
  excision, 23140-23146, 23180
  resection, 23200
 x-ray, 73000
Claw finger, 26499
Cleft
 cyst
  branchial, 42810-42815

Cleft — *continued*
 repair
  foot, 28360
  hand, 26580
  lip, 00102, 30460-30462, 40700-40761
  palate, 00172, 30460-30462, 42200-42225
Clitoroplasty, 56805
Clostridium
 difficile, 87324, 87803
Closure, 12001-13160
 amputation site
  ankle, 27888
  femur, 27594
  fibular, 27884
  finger, 26951
  forearm, 25907
  humerus, 24900
   secondary, 24925
  shoulder, 23921
  tibia, 27884
  wrist, 25922, 25929
 chest wall, 32810
 cranial, 61557-61559
 cystostomy, 51880
 distal segment, 44143, 44206
 enterostomy, 44227, 44620-44626
 eyelid, 67875
  wound, 67930-67935
 fistula
  anal, 46288
  bronchial, 32815
  bronchopleural, 32906
  esophageal, 43420-43425
  gastrocolic, 43880
  intestinal, 44650-44661
  lacrimal, 68770
  rectal, 45800-45825, 57300-57308
  renal, 50520-50526
  ureteral, 50920-50930
  urethral, 45820-45825, 53520, 57310-57311
  vaginal, 51900-51925, 57300-57330
 gastrostomy, 34870
 gland
  lacrimal, 68760-68761, 68770
 left atrial appendage, 0281T
 lip, 40510-40520
 oral or throat structure
  alveolar ridge, 42205-42210
  palate, 42106-42107
  pharyngeal wall, 42892-42894
  salivary, 00100, 42600
  tongue, 41112-41114
  tonsil, 42844-42845
  uvula, 42106-42107
  vestibule of mouth, 40830-40831
 septal defect
  atrial, 33615, 33647
  ventricular, 0166T-0167T, 93581
   direct, 33647
   multiple, 33675-33677
   single, 33681-33688
   tetralogy of Fallot, 33697
   transposition, 33776, 33780
 skin
  ulcer excision, 15922, 15934-15937, 15944-15946, 15952-15958
  wound, 12020, 12031-12057, 13160
 skin graft
  donor, 15200-15261, 15760
  recipient, 15300-15321, 15400-15421, 19367-19369
 spine, 63700-63702
 sternotomy, 21750
 tracheostomy, 31820-31825
 valve
  atrioventricular, 33600
  semilunar, 33602
  tunnel, 33722

Clot
 disorder, 85130, 85390
 factor, 85210-85293
 inhibitor, 85300-85305, 85307
 lysis time, 85175
 operation, 11765
 retraction, 85170
 test, 85303, 85306-85307
 thrombectomy
  by abdomen, 34151, 34401, 34451
  by arm, 34101, 34111, 34490
  by leg, 34201-34203, 34421-34451
  by neck, 34001, 34471
  by thoracic, 34051
  fistula, 36831-36833, 36870
  of graft, 35875-35876
  percutaneous transluminal mechanical
   arterial/bypass graft, 37184-37186
   coronary, 92973
   intracranial, 61645
  vena cava, 50230
 thromboendarterectomy
  aorta, 35331, 35361-35363
  axillary, 35321
  carotid, 36301, 35390
  celiac, 35341
  femoral, 35302, 35355, 35363-35372
  iliac, 35351-35355, 35361-35363
  mesenteric, 35341
  peroneal, 35304-35306
  popliteal, 35303
  renal, 35341
  subclavian, 35301, 35311
  tibial, 35304-35306
  vertebral, 35301
 time
  coagulation, 85345-85348
  lysis, 85175
Clubfoot
 cast, 29450
  wedge, 29750
Co-morbid, 1026F
Coagulation
 defect, 85390
  assay, 85130
 disorders, 34401-34490, 35875-35876, 50230
 factor
  I, 85384-85385
  II, 85210
  III
   inhibition, 85705
   inhibition test, 85347
   partial time, 85730-85732
  IV, 82331
  V, 85220
  VII, 85230
  VIII, 85240-85247
  IX, 85250
  X, 85260
  XI, 85270
  XII, 85280
  XIII, 85290-85290
 fibrinolysis, 85397
 hemorrhoid(s), 46930
 time, 85345-85348
Coagulin, 85347, 85705, 85730-85732
Coagulopathy, 85130, 85390
Cocaine, 80353
Coccidioides, 86635
Coccidioidomycosis, 86490
Coccygectomy, 15920-15922, 27080
Coccyx
 excision, 27080
 fracture treatment, 27200-27202
 pressure ulcer excision, 15920-15922
 tumor, 49215
 x-ray, 72220

Cochlear implant
  analysis, 92601-92604
  insertion, 69930
Codeine, 80323, 80361
Coffey operation, 58400, 58410
Cognitive, 3720F
  function, 96101-96120
  skills development, 97532
Cold
  agglutinine, 86156-86157
  pack, 97010
Colectomy
  partial, 44140, 44147, 44160
    laparoscopic, 44204-44208
      44213
    coloproctostomy, 44145-44146
    colostomy, 44141-44144,
      44206-44208
    ileocolostomy, 44205
    ilieostomy, 44144
  total
    laparoscopic, 44210-44212
    ileostomy, 44150-44158
    proctectomy, 45121
Collagen
  injection, 11950-11954
  links, 82523
Collar bone
  dislocation, 23520-23552
  claviculectomy, 23120, 23125
  fracture
    closed, 23500-23505
    open, 23515
  osteotomy, 23480-23485
  prophylactic treatment, 23490
  sequestrectomy, 23170
  tumor
    excision, 23140-23146, 23180
    resection, 23200
  x-ray, 73000
Collateral ligament
  reconstruction
    elbow, 24344, 24346
    wrist, hand or finger, 26541-
      26545, 29902
  repair
    ankle, 27695-27698
    elbow, 24343, 24345
    knee, 27405, 27409
    wrist, hand or finger, 26540
Collection
  blood, 36415-36416, 36591-36592
    allogenic, 38205
    autologous, 38206, 86890-
      86891
Colles' fracture, 25600-25605
Collis procedure, 43842-43843
Colon, 4180F
  biopsy, 44025, 44100
    endoscopy, 44389, 45305,
      45331, 45380, 45391-
      45392
    multiple, 44322
  closure
    diverticula, 44605
    fistula, 44650-44661
    plication, 44680
    stoma, 44620-44625
  colostomy, 44320
    revision, 44340-44346
  colotomy, 44322
  computed tomography (CT) scan,
    0066T-0067T
  dilation, 45386
  excision
    lesion, 44110-44111
    partial, 44140-44147, 44160,
      44204-44208
    total, 44150-44158, 44210-
      44215
  exploration, 44025, 44388,
    45378
  flexure, 44213
  hemorrhage, 44391, 45382
  hernia, 44050

Colon — *continued*
  incision, 44320-44322
    revision, 44340-44346
  interposition, 43108, 43113,
    43118, 43123, 43361
  lavage, 44701
  lysis, 44005
  motility study, 91117
  obstruction, 44025-44050
  reconstruction, 50810
  removal
    foreign body, 44025, 44390,
      45332, 45379
    polyp/tumor/lesion, 44392,
      44394, 45384-45385
  repair, 44050, 44055, 44605,
    44650-44661
  resection, 51597, 58240
  reservoir creation, 45397, 45400
  sigmoid
    ablation, 45346
    biopsy, 45331, 45342
    dilation, 45340
    exploration, 45330
    hemorrhage, 45334
    mucosal resection, 45349
    removal
      foreign body, 45332
      lesion/polyp/tumor, 45308-
        45309, 45315, 45333,
        45338, 45346
    stent, 45327, 45347
    ultrasound, 45341-45342
    volvulus, 45337
  stent, 45389
  stoma, 44320-44322, 44340-44346
    closure, 44620-44625
  tube
    insertion, 49442
    obstruction removal, 49460
    replacement, 49450
  ultrasound, 45391-45392
  virtual, 0066T-0067T
  x-ray, 74270-74280
Colonna procedure, 27120
Colonography
  computed tomography (CT) scan,
    0066T-0067T
Colonoscopy, 45378-45393, 45398
  ablation, 45388
  band ligation, 45398
  biopsy, 44389, 45380, 45392
  decompression, 45393
  dilation, 45386
  exploration, 44388, 45378
  hemorrhage, 44391, 45382
  injection, 45381
  mucosal resection, 45390
  performance measure, 3017F
  removal
    foreign body, 44390, 45379
    polyp, 44392, 44394, 45384-
      45385
  stent, 44402, 45389
  through stoma, 44388-44408
  ultrasound, 45391-45392
  virtual, 0066T-0067T
Color vision, 92283
Colorrhaphy, 44604
Colostomy
  abdominal, 50810, 57307
  colectomy, 44141-44144, 44146
  colorrhaphy, 44605
  enterostomy, 44320-44322
  establishment, 50810
  laparoscopy, 44188
    coloproctostomy, 44207-44208
    end, 44206
    rectal, 45395, 45563
      fistula, 45805, 45825
  maintenance visit, 99505
  perineal, 50810, 51597
  proctectomy, 45110, 45126
  revision
    complicated, 44345
    hernia, 44346
    simple, 44340

Colotomy, 44025
Colpectomy
  partial, 57106-57109, 58275-58280
  total, 57110-57112, 58275-58280
Colpourethrocystopexy, 58152,
  58267, 58293
Colpocentesis, 57020
Colpocleisis, 57120
Colphysterectomy, 58260, 58290
  enterocele, 58263, 58270,
    58280, 58292, 58294
  removal
    ovary, tube, 58262, 58291
    repair, 58263, 58292
  urethrocystopexy, 58267, 58293
  vaginectomy, 58275-58280,
Colpoperineorrhaphy, 57210
Colpopexy, 57280-57283, 57425
Colporrhaphy, 57200, 57240, 57250,
  57265-57267, 57289
Colposcopy
  cervix, 57420, 57452, 57456, 57461
    biopsy, 57421, 57454-57455,
      57460
  perineum, 99170
  uterus
    biopsy, 58110
  vagina, 57420
    biopsy, 57421
  vulva, 56820
    biopsy, 56821
Colpotomy, 57000, 57010
Column chromatography, 82542
Commissurotomy, 33476-33478
Communication
  device, 92605-92609
Compatability test, 86920, 86923
Complement, 86160-86162, 86171
Complete blood count (CBC)
  automated, 85049
  B-cell, 86355
  differential WBC, 85004-85007,
    85009
  hematocrit, 85014
  hemoglobin, 85018
  hemogram
    automated, 85025-85027
    manual, 85032
  microhematocrit, 85013
  natural killer (NK) cells, 86357
  red blood cell (RBC), 85032-85041
  reticulocyte, 85044-85046
  smear, 85007-85008
  stem cell, 86367
  T-cell, 86359-86361
  white blood cell, 85032, 85048,
    89055
Composite graft
  donor, 15760
  bypass, 35681-35683
Compression system, 29581-29584
Computed tomography,
  abdomen, 74150-74170
    and pelvis, 74176-74178
  bone density, 77078
  brain, 70450-70470
  chest, 71250-71270
  ear, 70480-70482
  extremity
    lower, 73700-73702
    upper, 73200-73202
  guidance
    ablation, 77013
    needle, 77012
    radiation therapy fields, 77014
    stereotactic localization, 77011
  head, 70450-70470
  limited, 76380
  maxillofacial, 70486-70488
  neck, 70490-70492
  orbit, 70480-70482
  pelvis, 72192-72194
  sella, 70480-70482
  spine
    cervical, 72125-72127

Computed tomography — *continued*
  spine — *continued*
    lumbar, 72131-72133
    thoracic, 72128-72130
  thorax, 71250-71270
  three dimensional, 76376-76377
Computer
  aided retinal images, 0380T
  analysis
    acoustic, 0068T-0070T
    data, 99090
  detection
    magnetic resonance imaging
      (MRI), 0159T
    mammography, 3014F,
      77051-77052
    radiograph
      chest, 0174T-0175T
    x-ray
      chest, 0152T
  navigation, 20985
  testing, 96103, 96120
Concentric procedure, 28296
Concha bullosa, 31240
Condyle
  femur
    arthroplasty, 27442-27443,
      27446-27447
    fracture treatment, 27508-
      27510, 27514
  foot
    metatarsal, 28288
    phalanges, 28126
  humerus
    fracture treatment, 24576-24582
  jaw
    fracture, 21465
    reconstruction, 21247
    removal, 21050
Condylectomy, 21050, 61596-61597
Condyloma, 54050-54065
Congenital
  arteriovenous
    excision
      spinal, 63250-63252
    injection
      spinal, 62294
    repair
      cranial, 61680-61692,
        61705-61708
      spinal, 63250-63252
  atresia
    exploration, bile ducts, 47700
    small intestine repair, 44126-
      44128
  AV fistula repair, 35180-35184
  cardiac anomaly
    diagnostic study, 93303-
      93304, 93315-93317
    treatment, 93530-93533,
      93580-93581
  defect repair
    esophagus, 43313-43314
  hip dislocation treatment, 27256-
    27259
  megacolon
    biopsy, 44322, 45100
    repair, 45120-45121
  kidney
    abnormality, 50070, 50135,
      50405
  laryngocele, 31300
  scapula elevation, 23400
  septal defect
    repair, 33813-33814
    ventricular, 33675-33688
      percutaneous, 93581
      transyocardial, 0166T-0167T
  vascular anomaly, 26115, 61710
Conization
  electrode, 57461, 57522
  laser, 57520
Conjunctiva
  biopsy, 68100
  drainage, 68020, 68745-68750
  expression, 68040

Conjunctiva — *continued*
- fistulization to nasal cavity, 68745-68750
- foreign body removal, 65205-65210
- graft, 65782, 68371
- incision and drainage, 68020
- injection, 68200
- lesion
  - destruction, 68135
  - excision, 68110-68130
- reconstruction
  - graft, 68335
  - partial, 68360
  - total, 68362
- repair
  - adhesion, 68330-68340
  - conjunctivoplasty, 68320-68335
  - wound, 65270-65273, 67930-67935
- resection, 67908
- stent, 68750

Construction
- artificial vagina, 57291-57292
- conduit
  - apical-aortic, 33404
  - ventricle to pulmonary artery, 33608, 33697
- finger, 26551-26556
- gastric tube, 43832
- intrapulmonary artery tunnel, 33505
- neobladder, 51596
- tracheoesophageal fistula, 31611

Consultation
- inpatient, 99251-99255
- medical physics, 77336-77370
- outpatient, 99241-99245
- pathology, 80500-80502, 88321-88334
- psychiatric, 90887
- x-ray, 76140

Contact lens
- fitting, 92071-92072
- modification, 92325
- prescription, 92310-92317
- replacement, 92326

Continuous
- negative pressure breathing (CNPB), 94662
- positive airway pressure (CPAP), 94660

Contouring, 11950-11954, 21029

Contraception
- fitting, 57170
- insertion, 58300
- removal, 11976, 58301

Contracture
- cast, finger, 29086
- release
  - elbow, 24149
  - palm, 26040-26045, 26121-26125
  - scar, 15002-15005
  - shoulder capsule, 23020
  - thumb, 26508
  - wrist, 25085

Contralateral ligament, 27405

Contrast
- bath, 97034
- injection
  - bronchography, 31899
  - catheter
    - cyst, 49424
    - hysterosalpingography, 58340-58345
    - sonohysterography, 58340
  - daryocystography, 68850
  - epidurography, 62310-62319
  - fluoroscopy, 36598
    - tube, 49440-49460
  - localization, 62310-62319
    - lysis, 62263-62264
  - radiological, 49465
  - shunt, 49427
  - urethrocystography, 51600-51610
- radiologic study
  - cholecystography, 74290
  - cisternography, 70015

Contrast — *continued*
- radiologic study — *continued*
  - computed tomography (CT)
    - aorta, 75635
    - abdomen, 74160-74175
    - cervical spine, 72126-72127
    - chest, 71275, 71551-71555
    - ear, 70481-70482
    - head, 70460-70470, 70496
    - lower extremity, 73701-73706
    - lumbar spine, 72132-72133
    - maxillofacial, 70487
    - neck, 70491-70492, 70498
    - orbit, 70481-70482
    - pelvis, 72191, 72193-72194
    - posterior fossa, 70481-70482
    - sella, 70481-70482
    - spinal canal, 72142, 72147, 72149-72159
    - thoracic spine, 72129-72130
    - thorax, 71260-71270
    - upper extremity, 73201-73206
  - magnetic resonance imaging (MRI)
    - abdomen, 74182-74185
    - brain, 70552-70553, 70558-70559
    - breast, 77058-77059
    - face, 70542-70543
    - head, 70545-70546
    - lower extremity, 73719-73720, 73722-73725
    - neck, 70542-70543, 70548-70549
    - orbit, 70542-70543
    - pelvis, 72196-72198
    - peritoneum, 74190
    - upper extremtiy, 73219-73220, 73222-73225

Contusion
- ankle, 27603
- arm
  - lower, 25028
  - upper, 23930
- brain
  - drainage, 61154-61156
  - evacuation, 61312-61315
- drain, 61108
- ear, 69000, 69005
- elbow, 23930
- epididymis, 54700
- gums, 41800
- hip, 26990
- knee, 27301
- leg
  - lower, 27603
  - upper, 27301
- mouth, 40800-40801, 41005-41009, 41015-41018
- nose, 30000-30020
- pelvis, 26990
- scrotum, 54700
- shoulder, 23030
- skin, 10140, 10160
- subdural, 61108
- subungal, 11740
- testis, 54700
- tongue, 41000-41006, 41015
- vagina, 57022-57023
- wrist, 25028

Conversion, catheter
- biliary drainage, 47535-47536
- nephrostomy to nephroureteral, 50434

Coombs test, 86880, 86885-86886

Copper, 82525

Coprobilinogen, 84577

Coproporphyrin, 84120

Coracoacromial ligament, 23415

Coracoid process, 23462

Cord
- spermatic
  - excision
    - hydrocele, 55500
    - lesion, 55520
    - vericocele, 55530-55540
  - laparoscopy, 55559
  - repair, 55530-55540

Cord — *continued*
- spinal
  - aspiration
    - cyst, 62268
    - diagnostic, 62267
    - stereotaxis, 63615
    - syrinx, 62268
  - biopsy, 62269, 63275-63290, 63615
  - creation
    - lesion, 63600
    - shunt, 63740-63741
  - decompression, 63001-63003, 63050-63051
  - destruction, lesion, 62280-62282
  - drainage, 62272
  - excision
    - lesion, 63265-63273, 63300-63308, 63615
    - neoplasm, 63275-63290
    - tumor, 63275-63290
  - exploration, 63001-63044
  - graft, 63710
  - implant, 63650-63655, 63685
  - incision, 63200
    - dentate ligament, 63180-63182
    - drainage
      - cyst, 63172-63173
      - tract, 63170, 63194-63199
  - injection
    - anesthetic, 62310-62319
    - blood, 62273
    - computed tomography (CT) scan, 62284
    - neurolytic agent, 62280-62282
    - other, 62310-62311
    - x-ray, 62284
  - irrigation
    - shunt, 63744
  - insertion, 63650-63655
  - puncture, 62270-62272
  - reconstruction, 63295
  - release, 63200
  - removal
    - catheter, 62355
    - electrode, 63660
    - pulse generator, 63688
    - pump, 62365
    - receiver, 63688
    - reservoir, 62365
    - shunt, 63746
  - repair, 63700-63709
  - replacement
    - shunt, 63744
  - section, 63180-63182, 63194-63199
  - stimulation, 63610
- vocal
  - injection, 31513, 31570-31571

Cordectomy, 31300

Cordocentesis, 59012

Cordotomy, 63194-63199

Corectomy
- iridectomy, 66600-66630

Coreoplasty, 66762

Cornea
- biopsy, 65410
- collagen crosslinking, 0402T
- curettage, 65435-65436
- destruction
  - lesion, 65450
- excision
  - epithelium, 65435-65436
  - lesion, 65400, 65420, 65426
  - pterygium, 65420
- hysteresis, 92145
- incision, 65772-65775
- laceration repair, 65275-65286
- lens prescription, 92310-92316
- measurement, 76514
- pachymetry, 76514
- prosthesis, 65770
- puncture, 65600
- removal
  - foreign body, 65220-65222

Cornea — *continued*
- repair, 65275, 65280-65286, 65772-65775
- reshape, 65760-65767
- scraping, 65430
- tattoo, 65600
- transplant, 65710-65757

Coronary
- angiography, 92975, 93454-93461
  - injection procedure, 93563-93568
- angioplasty
  - artery, 35471-35475, 92920-92921, 92997-92998
  - vein, 35476
- artery
  - bypass, 33510-33536
    - graft, 33503-33505, 33510-33516
    - anesthesia, 00567
    - arterial, 33533-33536, 33548, 4110F
    - arterial-venous, 33517-33523
    - beta blocker, 4115F
    - harvest, 35600
    - reoperation, 33530
    - venous, 33510-33516
  - computed tomography (CT) scan, 0146T-0149T
  - placement, 92974
  - repair, 33500-33508
  - stenting, 92928-92934
- atherectomy, 92924-92925, 92933-92934
- balloon angioplasty, 92920-92921
- chamber fistula repair, 33500-33501
- endarterectomy, 33572
- reconstruction, 33863-33864
- thrombolysis, 92975-92977
- vessel or graft ultrasound, 92978-92979

Coroner exam, 88045

Coronoidectomy, 21070

Corpectomy, 63101-63103

Corpora
- cavernosa
  - fistulization, 54435
  - injection, 54235
  - irrigation, 54220
  - plastic induration
    - exposure, 54205
    - graft, 54110-54112
    - injection, 54200
  - shunt
    - saphenous, 54420
    - spongiosum, 54430
  - x-ray, 74445
- cavernosography, 74445

Corpus
- callosum, 61541
- vertebrae
  - biopsy, 20250-20251
  - excision, 61597
    - decompression, 63081-63103
    - lesion, 63300-63308
  - fracture, 22305, 22310
  - kyphectomy, 22818-22819

Correction
- astigmatism, 65772-65775
- bunion, 28290-28299
- claw finger, 26499
- cleft palate, 00172, 30460-30462, 42200-42225
- eyelid disorder, 67820-67835, 67911-67912
- hammertoe, 28285
- intestinal malrotation, 44055
- inverted nipples, 19355
- male urinary incontinence, 53440
- osteotomy
  - metatarsal, 28306-28309, 28735
- osteotomy
  - toe, 28306-28312
- syndactyly, 26560-26562
- ureteropelvic junction, 50400-50405, 50540, 50544

CPT © 2015 American Medical Association. All Rights Reserved.   © 2016 DecisionHealth

Creation — *continued*
  stoma — *continued*
    kidney, 50395
    tympanic membrane, 69433-69436
    ureter, 50860
    vertebral cavity, 22513-22515
    window, 32659
Cricoid cartilage, 31587
Cricothyroid membrane, 31605
Cross
  finger flap, 15574
  match, 86920-86923
  tissue, 86812-86817, 86821-86822
Cruciate ligament
  repair, 27407-27409
    arthroscopic, 29888-29889
Cryo-
  ablation
    ciliary body, 66720
    fibroadenoma, 19105
    lesion
      kidney, 50250, 50593
  fibrinogen, 82585
  globulin, 82595
  preservation
    cells, 38207-38209, 88240-88241
    embryo, 89258
      thawing, 89352
    oocyte, 89337, 0357T
    ovarian tissue, 0058T
    sperm, 89259
      thawing, 89356
    storage, 38207, 88240
    testes, 89335
    tissue, 89354
  transplant
    heart, 33940
      lung, 33930
    intestine, 44132
    kidney, 50300-50320, 50547
    liver, 47133, 47140
    lung, 32850
      heart, 33930
    pancreas, 48550
  surgery
    labyrinthotomy, 69801-69802
    lesion
      anus, 46916, 46924
      benign, 17110-17111
      bladder, 52214-52240
      malignant, 17260-17286
      mouth, 40820
      penis, 54056, 54065
      premalignant, 17000-17004
      urethra, 52214-52240
      vagina, 57061-57065
      vulva, 56501-56515
    tumor
      rectal, 0184T, 45190
        benign, 46937
        malignant, 46938
  therapy
    ablation, 50593
    acne, 17340
    destruction
      ciliary body, 66720
    detachment
      retina, 67101, 67113, 67141
    lesion
      cornea, 65450
      retina, 67208, 67227
    retinopathy, 67229
    trichiasis, 67825
    tumor
      bronchial, 31641
Cryptectomy, 46210-46211
Cryptococcus
  antibody, 86641
  detection, 87327
Cryptorchism, 54550-54560
Cryptosporidium, 87272, 87328
Crystal identification, 89060

CT scan
  See computed tomography
Culture
  acid fast bacilli, 87116
  analysis
    chromosome, 88230, 88233, 88235, 88237
    myeloperoxidase (MPO), 83876
  bacteria, 87040-87077, 87081, 87086-87088
  chlamydia, 87110
  fungus, 87101-87103, 87106
  mold, 87107
  mycobacteria, 87116-87118
  mycoplasma, 87109
  oocytes, 89250-89251, 89272
  pathogen, 87084
  toxin, 87230
  tubercle bacilli, 87116
  typing, 87140-87158
  virus, 87252-87253
  yeast, 87106
Curettage
  anal fissure, 46940-46942
  and dilation, 59840
    cervical stump, 57558
    cervix, 57520-57522, 57558, 57800
    corpus uteri, 58120
    hysteroscopy, 58558
    injections, 59851
    postpartum, 59160
    suppositories, 59856
  bone, 21031-21032
    benign
      carpal, 25130-25136
      femur, 27355-27358
      foot, 28100-28108
    benign
      hand, 26200-26215
      head, 21030, 21040
      humerus, 24110-24116
      radius, 24120-24126
      shoulder, 23140-23156
      tibia, 27635-27638
      ulna, 25120-25126
    malignant, 21034
  cornea, 65435-65436
  endocervical, 57454-57456, 57505
  endometrial, 58356
  hydatidiform mole, 59870
  postpartum, 69160
  uterus, 58356, 59160
Curettement
  benign, 11055-11057, 17110
  malignant, 17270, 17280
  premalignant, 17004
Cutaneolipectomy, 15830-15839, 15876-15879
Cutaneous
  electrostimulation, 64550
  tag, 11200-11201
  tissue
    ablation
      breast, 19105
    biopsy, 11100-11101
    breast
      ablation, 19105
      excision, 19100-19101, 19110-19272, 19300-19307
      incision, 19000-19030
      metallic localization clip placement, 19281-19288
      needle localization, 19281-19288
      reconstruction, 19316-19396
      repair, 19316-19396
    burns, 16000-16030
      autograft, 15100-15101, 15120-15121
    escharotomy, 16035-16036
    preparation, 15002-15005
    xenograft, 15400-15401
    debridement, 11000-11006, 11010-11044

Cutaneous — *continued*
  tissue — *continued*
    destruction
      actinotherapy, 96900
      benign lesion, 17000-17004
      chemical exfoliation, 17360
      cryotherapy, 17340
      electrolysis epilation, 17380
      malignant lesion, 17260-17286
      photodynamic therapy, 96567-96571
      Mohs' micrographic surgery, 17311-17315
      photodynamic therapy, 96567-96571
      premalignant lesion, 17000-17004
    drainage
      acne, 10040
      abscess, 10060-10061, 10160
      bulla, 10160
      cyst, 10080-10081, 10160
      fluid, 10140
      hematoma, 10140-10160
      infection, 10180
      seroma, 10140
    excision
      benign, 11400-11471
      malignant, 11600-11646
    grafts
      allograft, 15300
      allogenic, 15300-15366
      autograft, 15040-15157
      preparation, 15002-15005
      replacement, 15170-15176
      xenograft, 15400-15431
    introduction, 11900-11977, 11981, 11983
    nails, 11720-11765
    paring, 11055-11057
    photography, 96904
    removal, 11982-11983
    repair, 15780-15879
      complex, 13100-13160
      flaps, 15740-15776
      grafts, 15050-15136, 15200-15321, 15420-15431
      intermediate, 12031-12057
      simple, 12001-12021
      skin, 15570-15738
      transfer, 14000-14350
    shaving, 11300-11313
    ulcers, 15920-15958
  vesicostomy, 51980
Cyanide, 82600
Cyanocobalamin, 82607-82608
Cyclodialysis, 66740
Cyclophotocoagulation, 66710-66711
Cyclosporine, 80158
Cyst
  ablation
    kidney, 50541
  anastomosis
    pancreas, 48520-48540
  aspiration
    bone, 20615
    brain, 61151, 61156
    breast, 19000-19001
    ganglion, 20612
    kidney, 50390
    ovarian, 49322
    pelvis, 50390
    skin, 10160
    spinal cord, 62268
    thyroid, 60300
  Baker's, 27345
  destruction
    ciliary, 66770
    iris, 66770
    intra-abdominal, 49203-49205
  dissection
    brain, 62161
  drainage
    abscess, 10060-10061

Cyst — *continued*
  drainage — *continued*
    brain, 61150
    conjunctiva, 68020
    gland
      lymph node, 49062, 49323
      salivary, 42409
      Skene's's, 53060
      sublingual, 42409
      thyroid, 60000
    gums, 41800
    injection, 49424, 76080
      kidney, 50390, 74470
    liver, 47010
    lung, 32200
    mouth, 40800-40801, 41000-41009, 41015-41018, 41800
    ovary, 58800-58805
    pilonidal, 10080-10081
    soft tissue, 10030
    spinal cord, 63172-63173
    wrist, 25111-25112
  echinococcosis, 86171, 86280
  excision
    ankle, 27630
    arm, 24120, 24125-24126
    biliary duct, 47715
    bladder, 51500
    bone, 28100-28103
    brain, 61516, 61524, 62162
    branchial cleft, 42810-42815
    breast, 19120
    carpal, 25130-25136
    cheek bone, 21030
    clavicle, 23140-23146
    digestive organ, 47715, 48120
    femur, 27065-27067, 27355-27358
    fibula, 27630, 27635-27638
    foot, 28090-28108
    gland
      Bartholin's, 56740
      lymph node, 38550-38555
      salivary, 00100, 42408
      seminal vesicle, 55680
      sublingual, 42408
      thyroid, 60200, 60280-60281
    hand, 26160, 26200-26215
    hip, 27065-27067
    humerus, 23150-23156, 24110-24116
    ileum, 27065-27067
    intra-abdominal, 49203-49205
    kidney, 50280-50290
    knee, 27345-27347
    lung, 32140
    mandible, 21040, 21046-21047
    maxilla, 21030, 21048-21049
    mediastinum, 32662, 39200
    Mullerian duct, 55680
    nose, 30124-30125
    ovary, 58925
    pancreas, 48120
    pericardium, 33050, 62661
    pilonidal, 11770-11772
    radial, 24120-24126, 25120-25126
    scapula, 23140-23146
    skin, 10040
    tibia, 27630, 27635-27638
    ulna, 24120-24126, 25120-25126
    vagina, 57135
    wrist, 25111-25112
    zygoma, 21030
  marsupialization
    liver, 47300
    pancreas, 48500
    salivary, 42409
  repair
    gland
      Bartholin's, 56740
      liver, 47300
Cystatin
  C, 82610
  kininogen, 85293

© 2016 DecisionHealth   CPT © 2015 American Medical Association. All Rights Reserved.

CPT © 2015 American Medical Association. All Rights Reserved.
© 2016 DecisionHealth

Destruction — *continued*
  tumor — *continued*
    prostate, 45320
    rectum, 0184T, 45190, 45320, 46937-46938
    skin, 96567
  ureter, 50957, 50976 52341-52342, 52344-52345, 52354
  urethra, 52214-52224, 52354, 52400, 53220, 53265, 53270, 53275
  uterus, 58356
Developmental testing, 96110-96111
Device
  evaluation
    defibrillator, 93260, 93282-93284, 93287
    interrogation, 93261, 93289-93292, 93295-93296
    leadless pacemaker system, 0389T-0391T
    pacemaker, 93279-93281, 93286, 93288
    transtelephonic, 93293
    recorder, 93285
    venous access, 36598
  insertion
    cochlear, 69930
    drug delivery, 62360-62362
    gastric restrictive, 43770
    iliac artery occlusion device, 34808
    intra-aortic balloon assist, 33967-33973
    intrauterine, 58300
    spinous process distraction, 0171T-0172T
    venous access, 36591-36592
      guidance, 77001
      port, 36560-36561, 36566, 36570-36571,
      pump, 36563-36565,
    ventricular assist, 33990-33991, 33975-33976, 33979
  intracardiac ischemic monitoring
    evaluation
      interrogation, 0306T
      programming, 0305T
    insertion, 0302T-0304T
    removal, 0307T
      with replacement, 0302T
  irrigation
    venous access, 96523
  removal
    gastric restrictive, 43772-43774, 43887-43888
    intra-aortic balloon assist, 33968, 33971, 33974
    intrauterine, 58301
    venous access, 36590, 36595-36596, 75901-75902
    ventricular assist, 33977-33978, 33980, 33992
  repositioning, 33993
  revision
    gastric restrictive, 43886, 43888
    venous access, 36576, 77001
      catheter, 36578
      complete, 36582-36583, 36585
Dexamethasone, 80420
Diabetes prevention program, 0403T
Diagnostic
  allergy test, 85004, 95004-95071
  amniocentesis, 59000
  arthroscopy, 29800, 29805, 29830, 29840, 29860, 29870, 29900
  aspiration, 62267
  colonography, 0067T
  colonoscopy, 44388, 45378
  endoscopy, 31231-31235, 43235, 43260, 44360, 44376, 44385, 47552
  infusion, 96365-96368
  injection, 20501
    intra-arterial, 96373, 96379

Diagnostic — *continued*
  injection — *continued*
    intramuscular, 96372
    intravenous, 96374-96379
    subcutaneous, 96372
  laryngoscopy, 31505, 31520-31526, 31575
  psychiatric interview, 90791-90792
  spinal tap, 62270
  thoracoscopy, 32601-32606
  ultrasound
    cardiac, 93662
    eyes, 76511-76514
    obstetrical, 76801-76828
    ophthalmic, 76510-76514
Dialysis
  cannula insertion, 36800-36815, 49421
  end stage renal disease (ESRD), 0505F-0507F, 90963-90970
  hemoperfusion, 90997
  peritoneal, 4055F
  procedures, 90935-90937, 90945-90947
  revision, 36832-36833
  shunt creation, 36145, 36831
  training, 90989-90993
Diaphragm
  repair, 39501-39545
  resection, 39560-39561
Diaphysectomy
  partial
    arm, 23184, 24140, 24145, 24147, 24150-24151
    clavicle, 23180
    foot, 28120-28124
    hand, 26230-26236
    leg, 27360, 27640-27641
    radial, 24145
    radius, 25151
    scapula, 23182
    ulna, 25150
Diathermy
  ciliary body, 66700
  retina
    detachment, 67101
      prophylaxis, 67141
    lesion, 67208
    modality, 97024
    retinopathy, 67227
Dibucaine number, 82638
Dichlorides, 82441
Digestive
  See Gastrointestinal
Digital
  artery sympathectomy, 64820
  nerve, 64455, 64632
  slit beam radiography, 77073
Digoxin, 4189F, 4220F, 80162-80163
Dihydrocodeinone, 82646
Dihydromophinone, 80361
Dihydrotestosterone, 80327-80328
Dilation
  ampulla, 53271
  anal sphincter, 45905
    anoscopy, 46604
    fissure, 46940-46942
  angioplasty
    artery, 75962-75968
    vein, 75978
  aqueous outflow canal, 66174-66175
  bile duct, 43277, 47542, 47555-47556, 74363
  bladder, 52260-52265
  bronchus, 31630, 31636-31638
  cerebral, 61640-61642
  cervix, 57558, 57800
  curettage
    abortion, 59840, 59851, 59856
    cervix, 58120
    canal, 57800
    conization, 57520-57522
    stump, 57558
  hysteroscopy, 58558

Dilation — *continued*
  curettage — *continued*
    postpartum, 59160
  esophagus, 43450-43453, 43213-43214, 43233
    endoscopy, 43249
    esophagoscopy, 43220-43226
    gastrotomy, 43510
  evacuation, 59841, 59851
  intestine, 44370
    colonoscopy, 45386
    proctosigmoidoscopy, 45303
    sigmoidoscopy, 45340
    stricturoplasty, 44615
  kidney, 50395, 52343, 52346
  lacrimal punctum, 68801
  larynx, 31528-31529
  nasolacrimal duct, 68816
  pancreatic duct, 43277
  rectum, 45303, 45910
  salivary duct, 42650-42660
  sinus ostium, 31295-31297
  stricture
    biliary duct, 47555-47556, 74363
    rectum, 45910
    ureter, 50706
  tracheal
    broncoscopy, 31630-31631, 31636-31638
    laryngoscopy, 31528-31529
  ureter, 50395, 53660-53665, 50706, 74485
    cystourethroscopy, 52260-52265, 52341-52346
    endoscopy, 50553, 50572, 50575, 50953, 50972
  urethra, 52601, 52647-52649, 53600-53665, 74485
    cystourethroscopy, 52281, 52285
    prostatectomy, 55801, 55821-55831
  vagina, 57400
Dimethadione, 80339-80341
Dioxide
  carbon, 82374
  silicon, 84285
Diptheria, 86648
  vaccine/toxoid, 90696-90702, 90714-90715, 90723
Dipropylacetic acid, 80164-80165
Disarticulation
  ankle, 27889
  hip, 27295
  knee, 27598
  shoulder, 23920-23921
  wrist, 25920-25924
Disc
  annuloplasty, 22526-22527
  arthroplasty, 0375T, 0163T, 22856-22858
    removal, 22864-22865, 0095T, 0164T
    revision, 22861-22862, 0098T, 0165T
  aspiration, 62267
  chemolysis, 62292
  discography, 72285, 72295
  excision
    decompression, 63075-63078
    herniated, 63020-63044, 63055-63066
  injection, 62292
  x-ray, 62290-62291
Discectomy
  arthrodesis, 22585, 22632
    cervical, 22554
    lumbar, 0195T-0196T, 22533-22534, 22558, 22630
    thoracic, 22532, 22534, 22556
  laminotomy
    cervical, 63020, 63035-63040, 63043
    lumbar, 63030-63035, 63042, 63044
  osteotomy, 22220-22226
  osteophytectomy, 63075-63078
  percutaneous, 62287

Discission, 66820-66821, 67030
Discography, 62290-62291
  cervical, 72285
  lumbar, 72295
  thoracic, 72285
Discolysis, 62292
Disease
  Durand-Nicolas-Favre, 86729
  Erb-Goldflam, 95857
  Heine-Medin, 86658, 90696-90698, 90713
  hydatid, 86171, 86280
  lyme, 86617-86618
  organ panel, 80050-80076
  Ormond, 50715
  Peyronie, 54110-54112, 54200-54205
  Posada-Wernicke, 86490
Dislocation
  closed treatment
    acromioclavicular, 23540-23545
    clavicle, 23540-23545
    hip
      post arthroplasty, 27265-27266
      spontaneous, 27256-27257
      traumatic, 27250-27252
    jaw, 21480-21485
    lower extremity
      ankle, 27830-27831, 27840-27842
      foot
        interphalangeal, 28660-28666
        metatarsophalangeal, 28630-28636
        talotarsal, 28570-28576
        tarsal, 28540-28546
        tarsometatarsal, 28600-28606
      knee, 27550-27552, 27560-27562
    pelvic ring, 27193-27194, 27216
    shoulder, 23650-23655, 23665, 23675
    sternoclavicular, 23520-23525
    upper extremity
      elbow, 24600-24605, 24620
      hand
        carpometacarpal, 26641-26650, 26670-26676
        interphalangeal, 26770-26776
        metacarpophalangeal, 26700-26706
      wrist
        intercarpal, 25660
        lunate, 25690
        radiocarpal, 25660
        radioulnar, 25520, 25671-25675
        trans-scaphoperilunar, 25680
    vertebra, 22305-22315
  open treatment
    acromioclavicular, 23550-23552
    clavicle, 23550-23552
    hip, 27253-27254, 27258-27259
    jaw, 21490
    lower extremity
      ankle, 27675-27676, 27832, 27846-27848
      foot
        interphalangeal, 28675
        metatarsophalangeal, 28645
        talotarsal, 28585
        tarsal, 28555
        tarsometatarsal, 28615
      knee, 27420-27424, 27556-27558, 27566, 27730
    pelvic ring, 27217-27218
    shoulder, 23660, 23670, 23680
    sternoclavicular, 23530-23532

Dislocation — *continued*
  open treatment — *continued*
    upper extremity
      elbow, 24586-24587, 24615, 24635
      hand
        carpometacarpal, 26665, 26685-26686
        interphalangeal, 26785
        metacarpophalangeal, 26715
      wrist
        intercarpal, 25670
        lunate, 25695
        radiocarpal, 25670
        radioulnar, 25525-25526, 25676
        trans-scaphoperilunar, 25685
      vertebra, 22318-22328

Dissection
  aortic repair, 34830-34832
    abdominal, 34800-34805, 34825-34826, 34841-34848, 75952-75953
    iliac, 34825-34826, 75953
    thoracic, 33880-33884, 75956-75958
  neck, 69155
    limited, 60252
    radical
      glossectomy, 41135, 41145, 41153-41155
      laryngectomy, 31365-31368
      lymphandectomy, 38724
      parotid, 42426
      pharyngolaryngectomy, 31390-31395
      thyroidectomy, 60254
      suprahyoid, 41153
  lymph nodes, 38542, 38550-38555
  neurovascular, 32503-32504, 38555, 42410-42420
  penis for hypospadias repair, 54328-54336, 54348-54352

Diuretic, 4190F, 4221F

Diverticulectomy, 43130-43135
  Meckel's, 44800

Diverticulum
  bladder, 51525, 52305
  Meckel's, 44800
  urethra, 53400-53405

Division, 28250
  isthmus, 50540
  scalenus, 21700-21705
  sternocleidomastoid, 21720-21725

DNA
  See deoxyribonucleic acid

Donor
  harvest, 01990
    conjunctival graft, 68371
    heart, 33940
      lung, 33930
    liver segment, 47140-47142
  search
    stem cell, 38204

Dopamine, 82382-82384

Doppler
  echocardiograph, 76827-76828, 93320-93352, 93662
  extracranial, 93875
  transcranial study, 93886-93923, 93965
  transesophageal, 93312-93318
  transthoracic, 93303-93308
  velocimetry, 76820-76821, 93571-93572
  scan
    artery, 76820-76821, 93922-93924, 93886-93893, 93965

Dosimetry, 77300-77331

Doxepin, 80335-80337

Drainage
  abscess
    abdominal, 49020-49062
    anus, 45005, 46045-46050
    appendix, 44900
    brain, 61150-61151
    ear, 69000-69020
    eyelid, 67700
    finger, 26010-26011
    forearm or wrist, 25028, 29843
    gastrointestinal, 43240, 43274
    hip, 26990
    image-guided, 10030, 49405-49407
    knee, 27301, 29871
    liver, 47010
    lower leg or ankle, 27603
    lung, 31645, 32200
    lymph node, 38300-38305
    neck, 21501-21502
    nose, 30000-30020
    oral structure
      dentoalveolar, 41800
      floor of mouth, 41000-41009, 41015-41018
      palate, 42000
      salivary, 42300-42320
      tongue, 41000-41009
      uvula, 42000
      vestibule of mouth, 40800-40801
    ovary, 55820-55822
    pelvic, 45000
    peritoneal, 49020, 49406-49407
    prostate, 52700, 55720-55725
    rectum, 45005-45020, 46040, 46060
    renal, 50020
    retroperitoneal, 49060, 49406-49407
    shoulder, 23030
    skin, 10060-10061
    soft tissue, 10030, 49405-49407
    spine, 22010-22015
    thigh, 27301
    thorax, 21501-21502
    throat structure, 42700-42725
    upper arm or elbow, 23930
    visceral, 49405
    x-ray, 75989
  amniotic fluid, 59000-59001
  bursa
    foot, 28001-28003
    forearm or wrist, 25031
    hip, 26991
    knee, 27301
    lower leg or ankle, 27604
    palm, 26025-26030
    shoulder, 23031
    thigh, 27301
    upper arm or elbow, 23931
  cyst
    bone, 20615
    brain, 61150-61151, 62161-62162
    breast, 19000-19001
    ganglion, 20612
    gland, 42409
    image-guided, 10030, 49405-49407
    liver, 47010-47011
    ovary, 58800-58805
    pilonidal, 10080-10081
    skin, 10080-10081
    soft tissue, 10030
  fluid
    brain, 61070
    cerebrospinal, 61000-61020, 61050, 61070, 62272
    cervical, 61050
    chest, 32554-32555
    cisternal, 61050
    fetal, 59074
    orbit, 67405, 67440
    pancreas, 48510
    paronychia, 10060-10061
    pericardium, 32659, 33010-33011
    skin, 10140, 10180

Drainage — *continued*
  fluid — *continued*
    urethra, 53080-53085
    ventricular, 61020
    hematoma
      brain, 61154-61156
        anesthesia, 00211
      image-guided, 10030, 49405-49407
      skin, 10040-10160
      soft tissue, 10030
      subungual, 11740
      vagina, 57022-57023
    implant, 66179-66185
    lymphocele, 10030, 49323, 49405-49407
    onychia, 10060-10061
    paracentesis
      abdominal, 49080-49081
      eye, 65800-65815
      pleural, 32556-32557
    tendon sheath
      digit or palm, 26020

Dressings, 15852, 16020-16030

Drill hole, 61105-61108
  electrode, 61850, 61863-61868

Drug
  alcohol, 80320-80322
  alkaloids, 80323
  amphetamines, 80324-80326
  anabolic steroids, 80327-80328
  analgesics, non-opioid, 80329-80331
  anticoagulant, 4075F, 4084F, 85300-85305, 85307
  antidepressants
    not otherwise specified, 80338
    serotonergic, 80332-80334
    tricyclic, 80335-80337
  antiepileptics, 80339-80341
  antipsychotics, 80342-80334
  assay/testing
    amikacin, 80150
    amitriptyline, 80335-80337
    benzodiazepine, 80346-80347
    caffeine, 80155
    carbamazepine, 80156-80157
    clozapine, 80159
    cyclosporine, 80158
    desipramine, 80335-80337
    digoxin, 80162-80163
    dipropylacetic acid, 80164-80165
    doxepin, 80335-80337
    ethosuximide, 80168
    everolimus, 80169
    gabapentin, 80171, 80355
    gentamicin, 80170
    gold, 80375
    haloperidol, 80173
    imipramine, 80335-80337
    lamotrigine, 80175
    levetiracetum, 80177
    lidocaine, 80176
    lithium, 80178
    mycophenolate, 80180
    nortriptyline, 80335-80337
    oxcarbazepine, 80183
    phenobarbital, 80184
    phenytoin, 80185-80186
    primidone, 80188
    procainamide, 80190-80192
    quinidine, 80194
    salicylate, 80329-80331
    sirolimus, 80195
    tacrolimus, 80197
    theophyline, 80198
    tiagabine, 80199
    tobramycin, 80200
    topiramate, 80201
    vancomycin, 80202
    zonisamide, 80203
  barbiturates, 80345
  buprenorphine, 80348
  cannabinoids
    natural, 80349
    synthetic, 80350-80352
  cocaine, 80353

Drug — *continued*
  delivery, 96365-96379
  analysis, 62367-62368
  implantation, 96522
    spinal, 62361-62362
  insertion
    intra-arterial, 36260
    intravenous, 36563
    ventricular, 61215
  removal
    intra-arterial, 36262
  repair
    intravenous, 36576
  replacement
    intravenous, 36583
  refilling, 95990-95991, 96521
    spinal, 95990-95991
    intra-arterial, 96522
    intravenous, 96522
  revision
    intra-arterial, 36261
  drug, not otherwise specified, 80375-80377
  fentanyl, 80354
  heroin metabolite, 80356
  instillation, 50391, 51720
  ketamine, 80357
  management
    psychiatric, 90863
  methadone, 80358
  methylenedioxyamphetamines, 80359
  methylphenidate, 80360
  muscle relaxants, 80369-80370
  opiate analogs, 80362-80364
  opiates, 80361
  opioids, 80362-80364
  oxycodone, 80365
  phencyclidine (PCP), 83992
  pregabalin, 80366
  propoxyphene, 80367
  screen, 80300-80304
  sedative hypnotics, 80368
  stereoisomer analysis, 80374
  stimulants, synthetic, 80371-tapentadol, 80372
  tramadol, 80373

Dual
  absorptiometry
    photon, 78351
    x-ray, 77080-77086

Duct
  bile
    anastomosis, 47760, 47780-47785
      extrahepatic, 47760, 47780
      intrahepatic, 47785
    biopsy, 47553
    cannulation, 43273
    catheter placement, 47533-47534
      conversion/exchange, 47535-47536
      removal, 47537
    cyst, 47715
    destruction, 43265
    dilation, 43270, 47555-47556
    endoscopic diagnosis and treatment, 43260-43265, 43273-43278, 47550-47556
    excision, 47711-47712, 47715
    exploration, 47700, 47552
    imaging, 78223
    incision, 43262, 47460
      and drainage, 47420-47425
    insertion/placement
      catheter, drainage, 47533-45734
        exchange/conversion, 47535-47536
        removal, 47537
      stent, 43274, 47538-47540, 47801
    reconstruction, 47800
    removal
      foreign body, 43275
      stent, 43275-43276

CPT © 2015 American Medical Association. All Rights Reserved.

© 2016 DecisionHealth

Duct — *continued*
bile — *continued*
removal — *continued*
stone, 43264, 47420-47425, 47544, 47554
repair, 47760, 47780-47785
stone
destruction, 43265, 47544
removal, 43264, 47420-47425, 47544, 47554
stricture treatment, 74363
tumor
excision, 47711-47712
x-ray
dilation, 74360
with contrast, 74300-74328, 74330
hepatic
anastomosis, 47465, 47802
exploration, 47400
incision and drainage, 47400
imaging
nuclear medicine, 78223
removal
calculus, 47400
repair, 47765, 47802
mammary
galactogram, 77053-77054
injection, 19030
nasolacrimal
probing, 68810-68816
x-ray, 70170
omphalomesenteric, 44800
pancreatic
cannulation, 43273
collection, 43260
destruction, 43265, 43278
dilation, 43277
incision, 43262
placement
stent, 73274
pressure, 43263
removal
calcali, 43264
debris, 43264
foreign body, 43275
stent, 43275-43276
sphincterotomy, 43262
x-ray, 74329-74330
parotid, 42300-42305, 42507-42510
salivary
biopsy, 42400, 42405
catheterization, 42660
dilation, 42650-42660
drainage, 42310-42320, 42409
excision
calculi, 42330-42340
cyst, 42408
injection, 42550
ligation, 42665
nuclear medicine, 78230-78232
repair
sialodochoplasty, 42500-42505
fistula, 42600
sialodochoplasty, 42500-42505
x-ray, 70380-70390
thoracic
cannulation, 38794
ligation, 38380-38382
suture, 38380-38382
Ductus
arteriosus, 33820-33824
percutaneous closure, 93582
deferens
anastomosis, 54900-54901
excision, 55250
incision, 55200, 55300
ligation 55450
repair, 55400
vasography, 74440
Duhamel procedure, 45120
Duodenostomy, 49441, 49451, 49460-49465
Duodenotomy, 44010

Duodenum
biopsy, 44010
exclusion, 48547
incision, 44010
intubation, 43756-43757
removal, 44010
study, 91022
x-ray, 74260
Duplex scan
artery, 93880-93882, 93925-93931
vein, 93970-93971, 93980-93981
Dupuytren's contracture, 26040-26045
injection, 20527
manipulation, 26341
Durand-Nicolas-Favre disease, 86729
Dwyer procedure, 28300
Dynamometry, 92260

E

Ear, 00120-00126
analysis, 62640
biopsy, 69100-69105
canal, 4130F-4132F
biopsy, 69105
decompression, 61591, 69960
drainage, 69020
foreign body
removal, 69200-69205
lesion
excision, 69140-69155
reconstruction, 69310-69320
canalith repositioning, 95992
cartilage, 4130F-4132F
graft, 21230-21235
collection, 36415-36416
computed tomography (CT) scan, 70480-70482
drainage, 69000-69005
drum
myringoplasty, 69620
myringotomy, 69420-69421
tympanic, 2035F, 69610
nerve, 69676
tympanometry, 92567
tympanolysis, 69450
tympanoplasty, 69631-69646
tympanostomy, 69433-69436
excision, 69110-69120, 69540, 69550-69554, 69905-69910
exploration, 69440, 69805-69806
function test, 92511-92520, 92531-92597
incision, 69000-69005, 69801-69806, 69820, 69840
insertion, 69820, 69840, 69930
lesion
destruction, 17280-17286
excision, 11440-11446, 11640-11646
shaving, 11310-11313
microscopy, 92504
pierce, 69090
protector attenuation, 92590-92595
reconstruction, 69300, 69631-69646
removal, ventilating tube, 69424
repair, 69666-69667
revision, 69662
skin
graft, 15115-15121, 15335-15336, 15365-15366, 15420-15421, 15760
transfer, 14060-14061, 15576
wax, removal, 62909-69210
wound
layer closure, 12051-12057
repair, 12011-12018, 13151-13153
Ebstein anomaly, 33468
Eccrine glands, 64650-64653, 64999
Echinococcosis, 86171, 86280

Echocardiography
doppler, 93320-93325
fetal, 76825-76828
intracardiac, 93662
performance measure, 3020F
transesophageal, 93312-93318, 93355
transthoracic, 93303-93317, 93350-93352
Echoencephalography, 76506
Echography
See ultrasound
ECMO, 33946-33966, 33969, 33984-33989
Ectopic
pregnancy treatment, 59120-59151
ureter repair, 50660, 52301
Ectropion repair, 67914-67917
Egg smear, 87177
Ehrlichia, 86666
Elastase, 82656
Elbow
advancement, 24330-24331
arthrectomy, 24155
arthrocentesis, 20605-20606
arthrodesis, 24800-24802
arthroplasty, 24360-24363, 25442
revision, 24370-24371
arthroscopy, 01732-01760, 29830-29838
arthrotomy, 24000-24006, 24100-24102
biopsy, 24065-24066, 24100-24101
epicondylitis, 24357-24359
excision, 24145-24147, 25240
abscess, 24138
bursa, 24105
cyst, 24120-24126
epiphyseal bar, 20150
tumor, 24075-24077, 24120-24126, 24150-24151
exploration, 24000, 24101
fracture and/or dislocation treatment, 24586-24640
closed, 24600-24605, 24620, 24640, 24670-24675
open, 24586-24587, 24615, 24635, 24685
incision, 23930-23935, 24000
injection, 24220
ligament, 24343-24346
magnetic resonance imaging (MRI), 73221
manipulation, 24300
muscle, 24301, 24341
removal
foreign body, 24000, 24101, 24200-24201
implant, 24160
resection, 24149-24151, 24155
strapping, 29260
tendon surgery, 24301-24359
tumor excision, 24075-24077
x-ray, 73070-73085
Electric
application, 64550
countershock, 92960-92961
stimulation
acupuncture, 97813-97814
bone, 20974-20975
cortical, 95961-95962
gastric
lapraroscopy, 0155T-0156T
laparotomy, 0157T-0158T
guidance, 95873
modality, 97014, 97032
Electro
analgesia, 64550
hydraulic, 52325
oculography (EOG), 92270
Electrocardiography (ECG) (EKG)
doppler, 93320-93325
monitoring, 93660, 93724, 99190-99192
external, 93224-93272

Electrocardiography (ECG) (EKG) — *continued*
monitoring — *continued*
interpretation and report, 0178T-0180T
stress test, 93015-93018
supervised, 93745
tracing, 93724
wearable, 93224-93272
patient demand, 93268-93272
recording
external, 0295T-0298T
rhythm
interpretation and report, 93040, 93042
tracing, 93041
routine
interpretation and report, 93000, 93010
tracing, 93005
signal averaged (SAECG), 93278
sleep study, 95806-95807
telephonic transmission, 93268-93272
transesophageal (TEE)
imaging, 93318
interpretation and report, 93314-93315, 93317
placement only, 93313, 93316
transthoracic
complete, 93303, 93306-93307
follow up, 93304, 93308
limited study, 93304, 93308
stress test, 93350-93352
Electrocautery, 17000-17286
Electroconvulsive therapy, 90870
Electrocorticogram, 95829
Electrode
cervical loop biopsy, 57460-57461, 57522
connection
cranial, 61885-61886
depth, 61760
implantation, 63650-63655, 64553-64565, 64568, 64575-64581
insertion
cardiac, 33202-33211, 33216-33217, 33224-33225, 33249
cortical, 61850-61870
depth, 61760
gastric stimulation, 43647, 43659
GERD test, 91034-91038
Eneurostimulator, 43647, 61863-61868, 63650, 64553-64565
removal, 64585
cardiac, 33234-33238, 33243-33244
cortical, 61880
gastric stimulation, 43648
neurostimulator, 43647, 61880, 63660, 64585
peripheral, 64585
spinal, 63660
repair
cardiac, 33218-33220
repositioning
cardiac, 33215, 33226, 33249
revision
cortical, 61880, 61886
peripheral, 64585
spinal, 63660
Electrodesiccation, 17000-17286, 54055
Electroejaculation, 55870
Electroencephalogram (EEG), 3650F, 95812-95827, 95830, 95950-95958
Electrogastrography, 91132-91133
Electrogram, 93615-93616
Electrolysis, 17380
Electromyography (EMG)
neuromuscular, 95860-95872, 95885-95887
sphincter, 51784-51785, 90911
surface, 96002-96004

Electron microscopy, 88348
Electronic analysis
neurostimulator pulse generator, 95970-95982
peripheral subcutaneous, 0285T
pump, 62367-62370, 95990-95991
Electrophoresis, 84165-84166, 86185, 86320-86327, 86334-86335
Electrophysiology procedure, 93600-93660
Electroretinography, 92275
Electrostimulation
See electric, stimulation
Electrosurgery, 17110-17111, 67825
Electroversion, 92960-92961
Elliot operation, 66130
Eloesser
procedure, 32035-32036, 32551
thoracoplasty, 32905-32906
Embolectomy, 34101
aortoiliac, 34151-34201
carotid, 34001
celiac, 34151
femoral, 34201
innominate, 34001-34101
peroneal, 34203
pulmonary, 33910-33916
radial, 34111
renal, 34151
tibial, 34203
Embolization
ureteral, 50705
vascular, 37241-37244
Embryo
biopsy, 89290-89291
cryopreservation, 89258
culture, 89250-89251
hatching, 89253
inoculation, 87250
monitoring, 59050-59051, 99500
storage, 89342
thawing, 89352
transfer, 58974-58976
preparation, 89255
Emission tomography
computerized
single photon (SPECT)
bone, 78320
brain, 78607
cerebrospinal, 78647
heart, 78464-78465
joint, 78320
kidney, 78710
liver, 78205
tumor, 78803
positron (PET)
brain, 78608-78609
heart, 78459
study, 78490-78492
Emmet operation, 59300
Empyema, 21501-21502
closure, 32810
thoracostomy, 32035-32036, 32551
Empyemectomy, 32540
Encephalitis, 86651-86654, 90738
Encephalocele, 62120-62121
Encephalon
abscess
drainage, 61150-61151, 61320-61321
excision, 61514, 61522
adhesions, 62161
amygdala
excision, 61566
angiography, 70496
biopsy, 61140-61151, 61575-61576, 61750-61751
catheter
irrigation, 62194, 62225
placement, 0169T
replacement, 62160, 62194, 62225
cisternography, 70015
choroid plexus
excision, 61544

Encephalon — continued
computer-assisted surgery, 61781-61783
computed tomography (CT) scan, 0042T, 70450-70470, 70496, 78608
corpus callosum
incision, 61541
coverings
tumor
excision, 61512, 61519
craniopharyngioma
excision, 61545
cyst
drainage, 61150-61151, 62161-62162
excision, 61516, 61524, 62162
death
determination, 95824
decompression
brainstem, 61575-61576
doppler
transcranial, 93886-93893
electrode
insertion, 61531-61533, 61760, 61850-61870
removal, 61535, 61880
stimulation, 95961-95962
epileptogenic focus
excision, 61534, 61536
excision
amygdala, 61566
choroid plexus, 61544
craniopharyngioma, 61545
cyst, 61516, 61524, 62162
epileptogenic focus, 61534, 61536
hemisphere, 61543
hippocampus, 61566
lesion, 61600-61608, 61615-61616
craniotomy, 61534, 61536
transoral, 61575-61576
lobe, 61323, 61539-61540
temporal, 61537-61538
meningioma, 61512, 61519
exploration, 61304-61305
foreign body
excision, 61570, 62163
hematoma
drainage, 61154
and incision, 61312-61315
anesthesia, 00211
hemisphere
excision, 61543
hippocampus
excision, 61566
imaging, nuclear medicine, 78600-78607, 78610
incision
corpus callosum, 61541
mesencephalic tract, 61480
subpial, 61567
insertion
catheter, 61210
electrode, 61531-61533, 61760, 61850-61870
pulse generator, 61885-61886
reservoir, 61210-61215
lesion, 61796-61799
aspiration, 61750-61751
creation, 61720-61735, 61790-61791
excision, 61534, 61536, 61575-61576, 61600-61608, 61615-61616
lobe
excision
temporal, 61537-61538
other, 61323, 61539-61540
magnetic resonance imaging (MRI), 70551-70559
meningioma
excision, 61512, 61519
mesencephalic tract
incision, 61480
myelography, 70010

Encephalon — continued
nuclear medicine
blood flow, 78610
cerebrospinal fluid, 78630-78650
imaging, 78600-78607
vascular flow, 78610
positron emission tomography (PET) scan, 78608-78609
pulse generator
insertion, 61885-61886
removal, 61888
radiation, 0520F, 77432
radiosurgery, 61796-61799, 77371-77373, 77435
removal
electrode, 61535, 61880
foreign body, 61570, 62163
pulse generator, 61888
shunt, 62256-62258
repair procedure, 61618, 61571, 62010, 62145
shunt
creation, 62180-62192, 62200-62223
removal, 62256-62258
replacement, 62160, 62194, 62225-62230, 62256-62258
reprogramming, 62252
skull
approach, 61595-61598
base
approach, 61580-61585, 61590-61592
stereotactic
aspiration, 61750-61751
biopsy, 61750-61751
catheter, 0169T
lesion, 61720-61735, 61790-61791, 61796-61799
radiation, 0520F, 77432
radiosurgery, 61796-61799, 77371-77373, 77435
surgery, 61781-61783
trigeminal tract, 61791
stimulation
electrode, 95961-95962
subpial
incision, 0169T
transection, 61567
surface electrode
stimulation, 95961-95962
tractotomy
mesencephalon, 61480
transection
subpial, 61567
trigeminal tract
stereotactic, 61791
tumor, lesion or cyst
excision, 61510-61512, 61516-61521, 61524-61530, 61545, 61575-61576, 61600-61608, 61615-61616, 62164
ventriculography
nuclear imaging, 78635
X-ray, 70010-70015
End-stage renal disease
See renal, end stage
Endarterectomy, 33572, 33916
Endocrine, 0141T-0143T, 86341
Endolymphatic sac, 69805-69806
Endometrial
ablation, 58353-58356, 58563
biopsy, 58100-58110, 58558
destruction, 58353-58356, 58563
sampling, 58100-58110, 58558
Endometrioma, 49203-49205
Endomyocardial
biopsy, 93505
Endoscopic retrograde cannulation of pancreatic duct (ERCP), 43260-43265, 43273-43278
Endoscopy
atria, 33265-33266

Endoscopy — continued
biliary, 43260-43265, 43273-43278, 47550-47556
bladder, 51715
brain, 62201
cardiac, 33265-33266, 33508
intracranial, 62160-62165
kidney, 50551-50580
large intestine, 45300-45398
nasal, 31231-31297, 0406T-0407T
ophthalmic, 66990
plantar fascia, 29893
small intestine, 44360-44379
stomal, 44380-44408
ureteral, 50951-50980
urethra, 51715
vascular, 33508, 37500-37501
wrist, 29848
Endosteal implant, 21248-21249
Endotracheal intubation, 31500
Endovascular
placement
graft, 34900
iliac artery occlusion device, 34808
repair
abdominal aortic aneurysm, 75952-75953
brachial, 34834
femoral, 34812-34813
iliac, 34820-34826, 34833
infrarenal, 34800-34805, 34825-34826, 34830-34832
transcatheter, 34806
visceral, 34841-34848
physician planning, 34839
descending thoracic aorta, 33880-33891, 75956-75958
therapy, 36475-36479, 61623
Enema, 74283
Entamoeba histolytica, 87336-87337
Enterectomy, 44120-44121, 44126-44128
harvest, 44132-44133
laparoscopy, 44202
Enterocele, 57556, 58280
Enterocystoplasty, 50825, 51960
Enterolysis, 44005, 44180
Enterorrhaphy, 44602-44603, 44615
Enterostomy, 44300, 44125, 44620-44626
Enterotomy, 44615, 45119
Enterovirus, 86658
Entropion repair, 67921-67924
Enucleation, 65101-65105
empyema, 32540
eye, 65101-65105
prostate, 52649
Enzyme
activity, 82657-82658
other, 87905
angiotensin converting (ACE), 4010F, 4188F, 4210F, 82164
myeloperoxidase (MPO), 83876
renin, 80408, 80416-80417, 84244
Eosinocyte, 89190
Epiandrosterone, 80327-80328
Epicondylitides, 24357-24359
Epidemic parotitis, 86735, 90707, 90710
Epididymectomy, 54860-54861
Epididymis
biopsy, 54800, 54865
drainage, 54700
excision, 54860-54861
lesion, 54830, 54840
spermatocele, 54840
exploration, 54865
repair, 54900-54901
X-ray, 74440
Epididymograms, 55300
Epididymography, 74440

CPT © 2015 American Medical Association. All Rights Reserved.

© 2016 DecisionHealth

Epidural, 2044F, 01996
  cervical, 62281, 62310, 62318,
    64479-64480
  craniotomy, 61535
  lumbar, 62282, 62311, 62319,
    64483-64484
  lysis, 62263-62264
  sacral, 62282, 62311, 62319,
    64483-64484
  thoracic, 62281, 62310, 62318,
    64479-64480
Epidurography, 72275
Epigastric, 49572, 49652-49653
Epiglottidectomy, 31420
Epikeratoplasty, 65767
Epilation, 17380
Epilepsy, 1205F, 4330F-4340F,
  5200F, 6070F
Epinephrine, 82383-82384
Epiphyseal
  arrest
    arm, 20150, 25450-25455
    leg, 20150, 27185, 27475-
      27485, 27730-27742
  bar excision, 20150
  separation treatment
    arm, 25600-25609
    leg, 27509, 27516-27519
Epiloectomy, 49255
Episotomy, 59300
Epispadias
  plastic repair, 54380-54390
Epistaxis, 30901-30906, 31238
Epley maneuver, 95992
Epstein-Barr virus, 86663-86665
Ergonovine provocation test, 93024
Erythrocyte
  antibody, 86850-86870
    pretreatment, 86970-86972
  count, 85032-85041
  fragility, 85547, 85555-85557
  hematocrit, 85014
  morphology, 85007
  platelet estimation, 85007
  sedimentation rate, 85651-85652
  sequestration, 78140
  sickling, 85660
  survival test, 78130-78135
  volume determination, 78120-
    78121
Erythropoietin, 4171F-4172F, 82668
Escharotomy, 16035-16036
Escherichia coli, 87335
Esophageal
  acid test, 91013, 91030
  biopsy, 3150F
  manipulation, 43450-43460
  motility study, 78258, 91010-
    91013
  polyp, 43229
  varices, 43205, 43400-43401
Esophagectomy, 43107-43124
Esophagoenterostomy, 43620
Esophagogastronomy, 43320
Esophagogastroduodenoscopy
  flexible, transoral, 43233, 43235-
    43255, 43257, 43259,
    43266, 43270
Esophagojejunostomy, 43340-43341
Esophagomyotomy, 32665, 43030,
  43279, 43330-43331
Esophagoplasty, 43300-43314
Esophagoscopy
  flexible
    transnasal, 43197-43198
    transoral, 43200-43232
  rigid, transoral, 43180-43196
Esophagostomy, 43351-43352
  closure, 43420-43425
Esophagotomy, 43020, 43045

Esophagus
  biopsy, 3150F, 43202, 43232
  dilation, 43213-43214, 43220-
    43226, 43233, 43248-
    43249, 43450-43453, 43510
  diverticulectomy, 43130-43135
  endoscopy, 43235-43259
  excision
    lesion, 43100-43101
  exploration, 43200
  lengthening, 43283-43338
  lesion ablation, 43229
  ligation, 43205, 43400, 43405
  neoplasm, 43229
  reconstruction, 43300-43314
  removal
    foreign bodies, 43020, 43045,
      43215, 74235
    polyp/tumor/lesion, 43216-
      43217, 43229
  repair, 43300-43425
  sphincter augmentation,
    0392T-0393T
  study
    motility, 78258, 91010-91013
    provocation, 91040
    reflux, 78262
  suture, 43405-43415
  test
    acid
      perfusion, 91013, 91030
      reflux, 91034-91038
    swallowing function, 3142F,
      74230
  transsection, 43401
  ultrasound, 43231-43232
  varix, 43205, 43400-43401
  x-ray, 74220
Estex operation, 58825
Estlander procedure, 40525
Estradiol, 50414, 82670
Estriol, 82677
Estrogen, 3315F-3316F, 82671-
  82672, 84233
Estrone, 82679
Ethanol, 80320-80322, 82075
Ethchlorvinol, 80320
Ethmoid, 21340
  sinus, 31200-31205, 31254-
    31255, 31290
Ethmoidectomy, 31200-31205,
  31254-31255, 61580-61581
Ethosuccimide, 80168
Etiocholanolone, 82696
Euglobulin lysis, 85360
Eustachian tube
  inflation, 69420-69421
Evaluation
  aldosterone suppression, 80408
  athletic training, 97005-97006
  auditory
    central function, 92620-92621
    otoacoustic emissions, 92588
    processing, 92506
    rehabilitation, 92626-92627
  body, 95833-95834
  carotid sinus baroreflex system,
    0272T-0273T
  condition, 1119F-1121F
  fetal and maternal ultrasound,
    76801-76812
  hearing aid, 92594-92595
  newborn, 99460-99463
    critical care, 99468-99469
  occupational therapy, 97003-
    97004
  ophthalmic, 92002-92019
  pediatric
    critical care, 99471-99476
    intensive care, 99478-99480
  physical therapy, 97001-97002
  programming
    intracardiac monitor, 0305T
  psychiatric, 90791-90792, 90885
  small intestine, 44385-44386

Evaluation — continued
  speech, 92521-92524
    prescription, 92605, 92607-
      92608
  sperm, 89329-89331
  swallowing, 3142F, 92610-92616
  voice, 92524
Evisceration, 45126, 58240, 65091-
  65093
Exenteration, 65110-65114
Evoked
  potential
    auditory, 92585-92586
    central motor, 95928-95929,
      95939
    somatosensory, 95925-95928
    visual, 95930
  otoacoustic emissions, 92558,
    92587-92588
Ewart procedure, 42226-42227
Excavatum, 21740-21743
Exchange
  catheter
    biliary drainage, 47536
    cyst/abscess drainage, 49423
    nephrostomy, 50435
  intraocular, 66986
  transfusion, 36450, 36455
  abscess
    arm, 24136-24138
    brain, 61514, 61522
    facial bone, 21025-21026
    leg, 27070-27071
    thigh, 27360
    pelvis, 27070-27071
  aorta, 33840-33851
  Bartholin's gland, 64740
  bone
    arm, 24110-24130, 24140-
      24147, 25120-25136,
      25150-25151, 25240
    epiphyseal bar, 20150
    facial, 21025-21026, 21031-
      21032
    foot, 28100-28116, 28120-
      28124
    hand, 26200-26236
    leg, 27635-27641
    rib, 21600, 21615-21616
    thigh, 27345-27347, 37355-
      27360
    pelvis, 27065-27071
    shoulder, 23140-23156,
      23180-23184
  bulbourethral gland, 53250
  bursa, 27340
    arm, 24105
    pelvis, 27060-27062
    wrist, 25115-25116
  cartilage, 23101, 27332-27333,
    27340-27345
  disc, 63020-63044
  duct, 19110-19112, 19120,
    42408, 42440-42450,
    44800, 53250, 53270,
    55680, 56740
  elbow, 24006
  electrode, 57522
  finger, 26596
  graft, 35901-35907
  hemorrhoid, 46230
  lacrimal, 68500-68505, 68520
  lesion
    brain, 61575-61576, 61600-
      61608, 61615-61616,
      61750-61751
    breast, 19120-19126
    cervix, 57500
    ear, 69145-69155
    esophagus, 43100-43101
    eye, 67840
      conjunctiva, 68110-68130
      cornia, 65400, 65420-
        65426
      sclera, 66130
    foot, 28080, 28090-28092
    hand, 26160

Exchange — continued
  lesion — continued
    intestine, 44110-44111
    kidney, 50290
    knee, 27347
    leg, 27630
    mediastinum, 39200
    mesentery, 44820
    mouth, 40810-40819, 41110-
      41114, 41116, 41825-
      41827, 42104-42107
    nasal, 30117-30118
    ovary, 58662
    pancreas, 48120
    pharynx, 42808, 42810-42815
    thigh, 27327-27328
    trachea, 31780-31781
    skin
      benign, 11400-11446
      malignant, 11600-11646
    spermatic cord, 55520-55540
    spinal, 63265-63273, 63300-
      63308, 63615
    testis, 54512, 54830
      spermatic cord, 55520-
        55540
    vertebrae, 22100-22116
    wrist, 25111-25112
  lung, 32141, 32655
  nerve, 64774-64786, 64788-
    64792
  organ
    bladder, 51500-51525, 51535
    cervix, 57540-57556
    rectal, 45130-45136
    urethral, 53230-53235, 53275
  plaque, 54110-54112
  polyp
    aural, 69540
    nasal, 30110-30115
    urethra, 53260-53265
  spinal, 61544, 63250-63252
  tendon
    arm, 25109-25110
    foot, 28090-28092, 28238
    hand, 26160-26180, 26390,
      26415
    leg, 27630
    thigh, 27327-27328
  tissue, 11450-11471
    anal, 46220
    ear, 69110-69140
    eye, 67961-67966
    foot, 28043-28045
    leg, 27618-27619
    Mohs' micrographic technique,
      17311-17315
    mouth, 40510-40527, 41115,
      41820-41823, 41828
    nasal, 30120-30130
    pelvis, 27047-27048
  tumor
    abdominal, 22900, 43610,
      49203-49215
      malignant, 43611
    arm, 24075-24076
      benign, 24110-24126,
        25120-25136
    aural, 69550-69554
    back, 21930
    bile duct, 47711-47712
    bladder, 51530
    brain, 61510, 61518-61521,
      61524-61530, 61535,
      62164-62165
    breast, 19120
    chest, 19260-19272
    cranium, 61500, 61563-61564
    endocrin, 60600-60605
    eye, 67800-67808
    facial, 21029-21030
      benign, 21029-21030,
        21040, 21046-21049
      malignant, 21034, 21044-
        21045
    foot, 28043-28045, 28100-
      28108
    gland, 60200, 68540-68550

Exchange — *continued*
  tumor — *continued*
    hand, 26115-26116, 26200-26215, 27065-27067
    heart, 33050-33120
    knee, 27327-27328
    larynx, 31540-31541
    leg, 27355-27358, 27618-27619, 27635-27638
    lung, 32661-32662
    mediastinum, 39200-39220
    Mohs' micrographic technique, 17311-17315
    mouth, 41822-41827, 42410-42426
    neck, 21555-21556
    pelvis, 27047-27048
     benign, 27065-27067
    penile, 45162
    pituitary, 61546-61548
    rectal, 0184T, 45160-45170
    shoulder, 23075-23076
     benign, 23140-23156
    spinal, 63275-63290
    testis, 55040
     spermatic cord, 55500-55540
    trachea, 31640, 31785-31786
    urethra, 53220
    uterus, 58140-58146
    vaginal, 57135
Exclusion, 44700, 48547
Exenteration, 45126, 58240, 65110-65114
Exostectomy, 28288, 28290
Exostoses, 69140
Expired gas, 0064T, 94680-94690, 64770, 95012
Exploration
  abdominal, 20102, 39000-39010, 43500, 49000-49002, 49010
  artery, 24495, 35701-35761
  arthrotomy
    ankle, 27610, 27620
    elbow, 24000, 24101
    foot, 28020-28024
    glenohumeral, 23040, 23107
    hand, 26070-26080
    hip, 27033
    knee, 27310, 27331
    sternoclavicular, 23040-23044, 23107
    wrist, 25040, 25101, 25248
  breast, 19020
  chest, 20101
  cranium, 61250-61253, 61304-61305, 61332-61333
  ear, 69440
  endocrine, 47400, 47480, 47610, 47700, 60500-60505, 60540-60545, 60650
  extremity, 20103
  eye, 37400, 67340
  gastrointestinal, 3130F-3141F, 43500, 44010, 44020, 44025
  heart, 33310-33315
  hemorrhage, 35800-35860, 47361-47362
  intestines, 44010
  kidney, 50010, 50045, 50120
  liver, 47361-47362
  neck, 20100
  nipple, 19110
  orbit, 61332-61333, 67400-67450
  penetrating wound, 20100-20103
  rectal, 45562-45563
  spinal cord, 22840, 63001-63017, 63040-63044
  spinal fusion, 22830
  testis, 54550-54560, 54865, 55110
  trachea, 31622
  uretal, 50600
  vaginal, 57000
  vascular, 35701-35860

External
  cephalic version, 59412
  ear
    abscess, 69000-69005
    auditory canal
     abscess, 69020
     biopsy, 69105
     excision
      exostosis, 69140
      lesion, 69140-69155
     reconstruction, 69310-69320
    biopsy, 69100
    drainage, 69000-69005
    excision, 69110-69120
    mastoidectomy cavity
     debridement, 69220-69222
    piercing, 69090
    repair, 69300
  fixation system
    adjustment, 20693
    application
     uniplane, 20690
     multiplane, 20692
      unilateral, 20696-20697
     facial, 21330, 21339, 21435, 21452, 21454
     hand, 26607
     hip, 27165, 27254
     leg, 27506, 27848, 29851
     wrist, 25332
    removal, 20694
Eye, 4177F, 5010F
  allergy test, 95060
  anesthesia, 00140-00148
  anterior chamber
    incision, 65800-65880
    injection, 66020-66030
    removal, 65900-65930
  assessment, 1055F
  biometry, 76516-76519, 92136
  biopsy
    conjunctiva, 68100
    cornea, 65410
    lid, 67810
    muscle, 67346
  choroid, 67220-67225
  ciliary
    destruction, 66700-66740
     lesion, 66770
    repair, 66680-66682
  computerized
    diagnostic imaging, 92132-92134
    topography, 92025
  cornea
    biopsy, 65410
    curettage, 65435-65436
    destruction
     lesion, 65450
    excision
     epithelium, 65435-65436
     lesion, 65400, 65420, 65426
     pterygium, 65420
    hysteresis, 92145
    implantation, intrastromal ring segments, 65785
    incision, 65772-65775
    laceration repair, 65275-65286
    lens prescription, 92310-92316
    measurement, 76514
    pachymetry, 76514
    prosthesis, 65770
    puncture, 65600
    reconstruction, 65780-65782
    removal
     epithelium, 65435-65436
     foreign body, 65220-65222
    repair, 65275, 65280-65286, 65772-65775
    reshape, 65760-65767
    scraping, 65430
    tattoo, 65600
    transplant, 65710-65757
  exam, 2019F-2027F, 92002-92019
  imaging, 92132-92134
  implant, 0100T
    modification, 65125
    insertion, 65130-65155

Eye — *continued*
  injection, 66020-66030
  iris
    destruction, 66761-66762
     cyst, 66770
    excision, 66600-66635
    incision, 66500-66505
    repair, 66680-66682
  lacrimal system
    biopsy, 68510, 68525
    dilation, 68801
    excision
     gland, 68500-68505
     tumor, 68540-68550
     sac, 68520
    incision, 68400-68440
    injection, 68850
    probing, 68810-68840
    removal
     foreign body, 68530
    repair, 68700-68705, 68760-68770
    fistulization, 68745-68750
  lens, 3073F, 4174F-4176F
    contact
     fitting, 92070, 92310-92313
     modification, 92325
     prescription, 92310-92317
     replacement, 92326
    incision, 66820-66825
    intraocular
     insertion, 66982-66990
     power calculation, 92136
    removal, 66830-66940
  lid
    biopsy, 67810
    blepharoplasty, 00103, 15820-15823
    drainage, 67700
    excision, 67800-67808, 67840-67850
    graft, 15115-15121, 15135-15136, 15155-15157, 15175-15176, 15260-15261, 15320-15321, 15335-15336, 15420-15421
    incision, 67700-67715
    reconstruction, 67950-67975
     wound, 67930-67935
    removal, 67938
    repair, 67900-67924
     lesion, 11310-11313, 11440-11446, 11640-11646, 17280-17286
     trichiasis, 67820-67835
     wound, 12011-12018, 12051-12057, 13151-13153, 67930-67935
    suture, 67875-67882
  muscles, 67311-67346
  orbit
    decompression, 67570
    excision, 67400-67450
    implant, 67550-67560
    injection, 67500-67515
  paracentesis, 65800-65815
  prosthesis, 21077, 92352-92353, 92371, 92358
  retina, 3072F
    destruction
     lesion, 67208-67218
     retinopathy, 67227-67229
    detachment
     prophylaxis, 67141-67145
     repair, 67101-67113
    imaging, 92134, 92227-92228
    membrane removal, 67042
    prosthetic implant, 0100T
    release, 67115
    removal, 67120-67121
  removal
    enucleation, 65101-65105
    evisceration, 65091-65093
    exenteration, 65110-65114
    foreign body, 65205-65265
    implant, 65175

Eye — *continued*
  repair
    laceration, 65270-65286
    wound, 65290
  sclera
    conjunctiva
     biopsy, 68100
     drainage, 68020, 68745-68750
     expression, 68040
     fistulization to nasal cavity, 68745-68750
     foreign body removal, 65205-65210
     graft, 65782, 68371
     incision and drainage, 68020
     injection, 68200
     lesion
      destruction, 68135
      excision, 68110-68130
     reconstruction
      graft, 68335
      partial, 68360
      total, 68362
     repair
      adhesion, 68330-68340
      conjunctivoplasty, 68320-68335
      wound, 65270-65273, 67930-67935
     resection, 67908
     stent, 68750
    excision
     lesion, 66130
    fistulization, 66150-66172
    reinforcement, 67255
    repair, 66220-66250
     wound, 65280-65286
    shunt, 66179-66185
  severing of adhesions, 65865-65880
  vitreous
    aspiration, 67015
    discission, 67030
    excision, 67036-67043
    incision
     strands, 67030-67031
    implantation, 67027
    injection
     fluid substitute, 67025
     pharmacological agent, 67028
    removal
     anterior approach, 67005
     subtotal, 67010
    severing strands, 67031
    subtotal removal, 67010
  x-ray, 70030

F

Face
  chemical peel, 15788-15789
  computed tomography (CT) scan, 70486-70488
  dermabrasion, 15780-15781
  destruction, 17000-17004, 17280-17286
  graft
    acellular, 15175-15176, 15335-15336
    allograft, 15320-15321
    autograft, 15115-15121
     dermal, 15135-15136
     epidermal, 15115-15121
     tissue cultured, 15155-15157
    full thickness, 15260-15261
    xenograft, 15420-15421
  excision
    lesion, 11310-11313, 11440-11446, 11640-11646
  lift, 15824-15828
  magnetic resonance imaging (MRI), 70540-70543
  repair
    wound, 12011-12018, 12051-12057
  tumor, 21015

CPT © 2015 American Medical Association. All Rights Reserved.
© 2016 DecisionHealth

Exchange — Face

Facial
asymmetries, 21247
bone, 00190-00192
contouring, 21029
excision
abscess, 21025-21026
cyst, 21040, 21046-21049
tumor, 21015, 21029-
21030, 21034,
21040-21049
fracture
closed
malar, 21355
mandibular, 21450-
21451, 21453
maxillary, 21421
nasal, 21310-21320
nasomaxillary, 21345
palatal, 21421
open
malar, 21360-21366
mandibular, 21454-21470
maxillary, 21422-21423
nasal, 21325-21335
nasomaxillary, 21346-
21348
palatal, 21422-21423
percutaneous, 21452
x-ray, 70160
graft
cheek, 15840-15845
craniofacial, 21436
malar, 21210
mandible, 21215
mandibular ramus, 21194
maxilla, 21210
nasal, 21210
nasomaxillary, 21348
osteoplasty, 21208-21209
osteotomy, 21198-21199, 21206
reconstruction, 21275
cheek, 21270
implant, 21244-21246,
21248-21249
mandibular rami, 21194
midface, 21145-21160
removal
foreign body, 41806
repair, 21208-21209
resection, 21015
torus mandibularis, 21031
x-ray, 70100-70110, 70140-
70150
nerve
anastomosis, 64866-64868
avulsion, 64742
decompression, 61590, 61596,
69720-69725, 69740-
69745, 69955
function studies, 92516
graft, 15840-15845
incision, 64742
injection, 64402
mobilization, 61590
paralysis, 15840-15845
suture, 64864-64865, 69740-
69745
transection, 64742
prosthesis, 21088
rhytidectomy, 15824-15828
Factor
blood coagulation
I, 85384-85385
II, 85210
III
inhibition, 85705
inhibition test, 85347
partial time, 85730-85732
IV, 82331
V, 85220
VII, 85230
VIII, 85240-85247
IX, 85250
X, 85260
XI, 85270
XII, 85280
XIII, 85290-85290
Fitzgerald, 85293

Factor — *continued*
Fletcher, 85292
inhibitor test, 85335
intrinsic, 83528, 86340
rheumatoid, 86430-86431
Falls, 0518F, 3288F
risk, 1100F-1101F
Fallopian tube
catheterization, 58345, 74742
excision, 58700-58720
laparoscopy, 58660-58679
ligation, 58600-58611
occlusion, 58615, 58565
pregnancy, 59120-59151
repair, 58740-58770
transfer, 58976
tumor
malignant, 58943-58952,
58957-58960
x-ray, 74742
Fanconi anemia, 88248
Farnsworth-Munsell color test, 92283
Fasanella-Servat procedure, 67908
Fascia
debridement, 11004-11006,
11011-11012
defect repair, 27656
graft
acromioclavicular, 23552
derma fat, 15770
facial nerve paralysis, 15840
hamstring, 27386
hip, 27100-27105
knee, 27381
lata, 20920-20922
metacarpophalangeal, 26541
pulley, 26502
sternoclavicular, 23532
plantar
division, 28250
removal, 28060-28062
Fasciectomy, 26121-26125, 28060-
28062
Fasciocutaneous flap
extremity, 15736-15738
neck, 15732
trunk, 15734
Fasciotomy
arm, 24495, 25020-25025
foot, 28008
hand, 26037-26045
hip, 27025
leg, 27305, 27496-27499, 27600-
27602, 27892-27894, 29893
pelvis, 27027, 27057
Fat measurement, 82705-82715
removal, 15876-15879
stain, 89125
Fatty acid, 0111T, 82725-82726
Fecal microbiota preparation, 44705
Femur
acetabuloplasty, 27122-27130,
29915
amputation, 01232, 27590-27596
anesthesia, 01220-01274, 01340-
01360
arrest, 27475-27485, 27742
artery, 01270-01274, 35363, 35540
aneurysm, 35141-35142
atherectomy, 37225, 37227
bypass, 35583-35585, 35883-
35884
graft, 35533, 35551-35558,
35566, 35621, 35646-
35647, 35651-35661,
35666, 35700, 35883-
35884
embolectomy, 34201
exploration, 35721
exposure, 34812-34813
thrombectomy, 34201
thromboendarterectomy,
35371-35372
arthroplasty, 27443, 27487
biopsy, 20225-20245
epiphysis, 27175-27187

Femur — *continued*
excision
abscess, 27070, 27360
cyst, 27065-27067
ephiphyseal bar, 20150
femoroplasty, 29914
fixture device, 27495, 27506-27507
external, 20663
internal, 27244-27245, 27358,
27511-27514, 27519
fracture
closed, 27230-27232, 27238-
27240, 27267-27268,
27500-27503, 27508,
27510, 27516-27517
open, 27236, 27254, 27269,
27506-27507, 27511-
27514, 27519
percutaneous, 27235, 27509
graft, 27170
incision
abscess, 27303
fasciotomy, 27025-27027, 27057
nerve, 01250
denervation, 27035
injection, 64447-64448
nonunion repair, 27470-27472
osteoplasty, 27465-27468
osteotomy, 27151-27156, 27161,
27448-27454
repair, 27470-27472
replacement, 27258-27259
revision, 27138
transfer, 27110-27111, 27140,
27400
tumor
excision, 27078-27079
benign, 27065-27067,
27355-27358
resection, 01234, 27365
vein, 01260, 34501
x-ray, 73551-73552
Fenestration
pericardium, 33015
procedure, 31610, 69820, 69840
Fern test, 87210, 89060
Ferric chloride, 81005
Ferritin, 82728
Fertility
control, 57170, 58300-58301
test, 89300-89322, 89329-
89331
Fertilization, 89251, 89280-89281
in vitro, 58321-58322
Fetal
amnioinfusion, 59070
cord occlusion, 59072
fluid drainage, 59074
magnetic resonance imaging,
74712-74713
monitoring, 59050-59051
shunt placement, 59076
test
blood
hemoglobin, 83030-83033,
85460-85461
scalp, 59030
contraction stress, 59020
echocardiography, 76825-76828
fibronectin, 82731
lung maturity, 83661-83664
non-stress, 59025, 76818
profile, 76818-76819
ultrasound, 76801-76817
velocimetry, 76820-76821
transfusion, 36460
Fibrillation, 33254-33256, 33265-
33266
Fibrin, 85384-85385
degradation, 85362-85380
lysis, 85390-85421
removal, 32150
stabilizing, 85290-85291
Fibrinadenoma, 19105, 19120-19126
Fibrinolysis, 85397

Fibrous
dysplasia, 21029, 21181-21184
penile, 54110-54112, 54200-54205
retroperitoneal, 50715
Fibula, 01390-01392
amputation, 27880-27888
arrest, 27477-27485, 27732-27742
bone graft, 20955, 20962
dislocation treatment, 27832
excision, 27455-27457, 27641
abscess, 27360, 27607
epiphyseal bar 20150
tumor, 27635-27638, 27646
fracture
closed, 27780-27781, 27786-
27788
open, 27784, 27792, 27828
nonunion repair, 27725-27726
osteoplasty, 27715
osteotomy, 27455-27457, 27707-
27709
x-ray, 73590
Filariasis, 86280
Fimbrioplasty, 58672, 58760
Finger
amputation, 26910-26952
arthrodesis, 26820-26863
arthroplasty, 26530-26536
biopsy, 26105-26110
decompression, 26035
drainage
abscess, 26010-26011
joint, 26075-26080
tendon sheath, 26020
excision, 26596
bone, 26185, 26235-26236
capsule, 26520-26525
lesion, 26160
tendon, 26170-26180
tumor, 26115-26116, 26260-
26262
benign, 26210-26215
malignant, 26117
exploration, 26075-26080
flap, 14350
fracture
closed, 25660, 26700-26705,
26720-26725, 26740-
26742, 26750-26755,
26770-26775
open, 26715, 26735, 26746,
26765, 26785
percutaneous, 26706, 26727,
26756, 26776
implant
rod, 26390, 26415
incision
abscess, 26034
fascia,
tendon, 26060
sheath, 26055
osteotomy, 26567-26568
release, 26055-26060, 26123-
26125, 26508
adhesions, 26440-26449
tenotomy, 26455-26460
removal
foreign body, 26075-26080
implant, 26320, 26392, 26416
tissue, 26135-26145
repair, 26499, 26580
joint, 25447, 26340
ligament, 26540
tendon, 26418-26434
lengthening, 26476, 26478
shortening, 26477, 26479
tenodesis, 26471-26474
transfer, 26497-26498, 26510,
26516-26518
web, 26560-26562, 26590
reconstruction
joint, 26548
ligament, 26541-26545
non-union, 26546
pollicization, 26550
transfer, 26551-26556
web, 26587
x-ray, 73140

Finney operation, 43810, 43850-43855
Fistula
  closure
    anal, 46288
    bronchial, 32815
    bronchopleural, 32906
    esophagus, 43420-43425
    intestinal, 43880, 44640-44661,
      45800-45825
    lacrimal, 68770
    middle ear, 69700
    salivary, 42600
    tracheal, 31820-31825
    urinary, 50520-50526, 50920-
      50930, 51920-51925
    vaginal, 51900, 57305-57330
  creation
    arteriovenous, 36825-36830
    conjunctiva, 68745-68750
    esophagus, 43351-43352
    intestinal, 44300-44346
    lacrimal, 68720
    pharynx, 42955
    sclera, 66150-66172
    tracheoesophageal, 31611
    tracheopharyngeal, 31755
    urinary, 54435
  ligation
    arteriovenous, 37607
  repair
    anal, 0170T, 46060, 46270-
      46285, 46706-46742
    arteriovenous, 33500-33501,
      35180-35890
    arteriovenous, 36831-36833,
      36870
    carotid-cavernous, 61710
    esophagus, 43360-43361
    middle ear, 69666-69667
    nasolabial, 42260
    oromaxillary, 30580
    oronasal, 30600
    tracheoesophageal, 43305,
      43312, 43314
    urinary, 53400
  x-ray, 86080
Fitting
  cervix
    cap, 57170
    diphragm, 57170
  eye
    contact lens, 92071-92072,
      92310-92313
    spectacles, 92340-92342,
      92354-92355
Fitzgerald factor, 85293
Fixation
  device
    external, 20650-20665
      chest, 21825
      hand, 26546, 26607
      head, 21100-21110, 21330,
        21339, 21340,
        21435, 21452, 21454
      hip, 26165
      leg, 27450, 27506, 27570,
        27848-27860, 29851
      multiplane, 20692
        unilateral, 20696-20697
      pelvis, 22848
      removal, 20694, 22850,
        22852-22855
      revision, 20693
      shoulder, 23700
      spine, 22840, 22842-
        22847, 22849
      uniplane, 20690
      wrist, 25332, 25431-25440
    internal, 20650, 20670-20680
      arm
        epicondylar, 24575,
          24579
        humerus, 24498, 24515-
          24516
        Monteggia, 24635
        radial, 24665-24666,
          25515, 25525-
          25526, 25574-25575

Fixation — continued
  device — continued
    internal — continued
      arm — continued
        supracondylar, 24545-
          24546
        ulnar, 24685, 25545,
          25574-25575
      foot, 28300
        calcaneal, 28415-28420
        interphalangeal, 28675
        metatarsal, 28485
        metatarsophalangeal,
          28645
        phalanx, 28505, 28525
        sesamoid, 28531
        talotarsal, 28585
        talus, 28445
        tarsal, 28465, 28555
        tarsometatarsal, 28615
      hand, 26390-26392,
        26415-26416
        carpometacarpal, 26665,
          26685, 26841-
          26842
        interphalangeal, 26785,
          26860-26863
        metacarpal, 26546, 26615
        metacarpophalangeal,
          26715, 26746,
          26850-26852
        phalanx, 26546, 26735,
          26765
      head, 21497
        craniofacial, 21431-21432,
          21435-21436
        malar, 21365
        mandibular, 21453, 21461-
          21462, 21470
        maxillary, 21421
        nasal, 21330
        nasoethmoid, 21340
        nasomaxillary, 21345-
          21346
        palatal, 21421
        temporomandibular, 21485
      hip, 27254
        acetabular wall, 27226-
          27228
        femoral, 27177-27178,
          27181, 27187,
          27236, 27269
        iliac, 27215
        ring, 27217-27218
        trochanteric, 27165,
          27244-27245, 27248
      leg, 27358
        ankle, 27814, 27823,
          27848-27860
        condylar, 27511-27514
        epiphyseal, 27519
        femur, 27450, 27507
        fibula, 27726, 27784,
          27792
        knee, 27540, 27556-
          27558, 27570,
          29851, 29885,
          29887, 29892
        malleolus, 27766, 27769
        patella, 27524
        tibia, 27535-27536, 27758-
          27759, 27826-
          27829, 27832,
          29855-29856
      mandibular, 21196
      shoulder, 23680
        clavicle, 23480-23490,
          23515
        humerus, 23491, 23615-
          23616
        scapular, 23585
        tuberosity, 23630, 23670
      spinal, 22318-22319,
        22841, 22851
      wrist, 25332
        carpal, 25431-25440,
          25629
        radial, 25607-25609

Fixation — continued
    kidney, 50400-50405
    latex, 86403-86406
    rectum, 45400-45402, 45540-
      45541, 45550
    test, 86171
    tongue, 41500
Flank
  biopsy, 21920-21925
  repair, 49540
  straping, 29220
  tumor
    excision, 21930
    radical resection, 21935
  wound exploration, 20102
Flap, 15757
  breast, 19364, 19367-19369
  closure, 15922, 15934-15937,
    15944-15946, 15952-
    15958
  fascia, 15758
  head, 15610-15630, 15731-15732
  island pedicle, 15740
  lower extremity, 15738
    foot, 14350, 15620
    leg, 15610
  muscle, 15842
  myocutaneous, 15756
  neurovascular pedicle, 15750
  omental, 49905-49906
  superficial musculoaponeurotic
    system (SMAS), 15829
  transfer, 15650
  trunk, 15600, 15734
  upper extremity, 15736
    arms, 15610
    hand, 14350, 15620
Flatfoot, 28735
Fletcher factor, 85292
Flow
  cytometry, 88182-88189
  volume loop, 94375
Fluid
  amniotic, 82106, 82143, 83661,
    83663-83664
  body, 89060
  cerebrospinal, 86325, 78630-
    78650
  skin, 10140
Fluorescein, 15860, 92287
  angiography, 92235
Fluorescent hybridization, 88364-
    88366
Fluoride, 82735
Fluoroscopy, 6045F, 76000-76010,
    76496
  chest, 71023, 71034
  larynx, 70370
  musculoskeletal, 0054T-0055T
  percutaneous, 75989
  pharynx, 70370
  spine, 77003
  stomach, 43752
  trachea, 31622-31624
  vascular, 36598, 77001-77002
Flurazepam, 80346-80347
Flush aortogram, 75722-75724
Foam stability, 83662
Folic acid, 82746-82747
Follitropin, 80418, 80426, 83001
Follow-up/Outcome documentation,
    5005F-5250F
Fontan procedure, 33615-33617
Foot, 01462-01486
  amputation, 28800-28825
  arthrodesis, 28705-28760
  arthroplasty, 25443
  biopsy, 28050-28054
  cast, 29345-29358, 29405-
    29445, 29505-29515
  clubfoot, 29450
    strapping, 29540-29580
  removal, 29700-29705
  wedging, 29740-29750
  window, 29730

Foot — continued
  computed tomography (CT) scan,
    73700-73706
  dislocation
    closed, 28540-28545, 28570-
      28575, 28600-28605,
      28630-28635, 28660-
      28665
    open, 28555, 28585, 28615,
      28645, 28675
  exam, 2028F
  excision, 28111-28124, 28130,
    28140-28150, 28288,
    28300-28315
    bunion, 28290-28299
    Tailor's, 28110
  fascia, 28060-28062
  foreign body, 28190-28193
  joint, 28070-28072, 28086-
    28092, 28160
  lesion, 28090-28092
  nerve, 28055
  neuroma, 28080, 64455,
    64782-64783
  tendon, 28086-28090
  tumor, 28043-28045, 28171-
    28175
    benign, 28100-28108
    malignant, 28046
  fracture, 28450-28455
    closed, 25622-25624 28400-
      28405, 28430-28435,
      28470-28475, 28490-
      28495, 28510-28551,
      28530
    open, 25628, 28415-28420,
      28445-28446, 28465,
      28485, 28505, 28525,
      28531
    percutaneous, 28406, 28436,
      28456, 28476, 28496
  incision, 28005
    bone, 28005
    drainage, 28001-28003,
      28020-28024
    exploration, 28020-28024
    fascia, 28008
    tendon, 28010-28011
  magnetic resonance angiography
    (MRA), 73725 magnetic
    resonance imaging (MRI),
    73706-73723
  nerve, 01470-01474
    destruction, 64632
    graft, 64890-64896
    suture, 64831-64834, 64837
  reconstruction, 28360
    tendon, 28238
    web, 28340-28345
  release, 28035, 28119, 28260,
    28289
  removal
    foreign body, 28020-28024,
      28190-28193
  repair, 28264, 28285-28286
    fascia, 28250
    joint, 28270-28272, 28289
    tendon, 28200-28234, 28240,
      28261-28262
    union, 25440, 28320-28322
    web, 28280
  replantation, 20838
  resection, 01482, 28046, 28126,
    28153, 28171-28175
  shock, 28890
  x-ray, 73620-73660
Forearm, 01810-01860
  amputation, 25900-25915
  angiography, 73206
  arrest, 25450-25455
  arthroplasty, 25441-25442,
    25444, 25446
  biopsy, 25065-25066
  cast, 01860, 29075
    splint, 29125-29126
  computed tomography (CT) scan,
    73200-73206
  decompression, 25020-25025

CPT © 2015 American Medical Association. All Rights Reserved.   © 2016 DecisionHealth

Forearm — *continued*
  dislocation
    closed, 25660, 25675, 25680, 25690
    open, 25670, 25676, 25685, 25695
    percutaneous, 25671
  excision, 25150-25151, 25210-25240
    abscess, 25145
    bursa, 25115-25116
    tendon, 25109-25110
    tumor, 25075-25076, 25170
      benign, 25120-25136
      malignant, 25077
  exploration, 25248, 35860
  fracture
    closed, 25500-25505, 25520, 25530-25535, 25560-25565, 25600-25605, 25622-25624, 25630-25635, 25650
    open, 25515, 25525-25526, 25545, 25574-25575, 25607-25609, 25628, 25645, 25652
    percutaneous, 25606, 25651
  graft, 35903
  incision and drainage, 25028-25040
  ligation, 37618
  magnetic resonance imaging (MRI), 73218-73220, 73223
  reconstruction, 25337-25394
  repair, 25315-25316, 25490-25492
    defect, 25425-25426
    tendon, 25260-25295
    union, 25400-25420
    vascular, 35236, 35266
  transplant, 20805
    tendon, 25310-25312
  ultrasound, 76881-76882
  x-ray, 73090-73092
Forehead
  lift, 15824
  reconstruction, 21159-21184, 21263
  reduction, 21137-21139
  skin
    flap, 15731
    repair, 13131-13133, 14040-14041, 15240-15241, 15574, 15620, 15731
Foreign body
  removal
    cardiac, 33310-33315
    ear, 69200-69205
    eye, 65205-65265, 65275
    intranasal, 30300-30320
    joint, 23040-23044, 23107
    lower extremity
      ankle, 27610, 29894
      foot, 28020-28024, 28190-28193, 29904
      hip, 27033, 27086-27087, 29861
      knee, 27310, 27372, 29874
      thigh, 27372
    lower gastrointestinal (GI) tract, 44020, 44025, 44363, 44390, 45307, 45332, 45379, 45915, 46608
    mediastinum, 39000-39010
    muscle, 20520-20525
    oral structure, 40804-40805, 41805-41806
    penile tissue, 54115
    peritoneal, 49402
    pharynx, 42809
    subcutaneous tissue, 10120-10121, 11010-11012
    thorax, 32150-32151, 32653, 32658
    throat, 31511, 31530-31531, 31577, 42809, 43020, 43045, 43215

Foreign body — *continued*
  removal — *continued*
    upper extremity
      elbow, 24000, 24101, 29834
      hand, 26070-26080
      shoulder, 23330-23333, 29819
      wrist, 25248
    upper gastrointestinal (GI) tract, 43020, 43045, 43215, 43247, 43275, 43500, 44010, 74235
    urinary organ, 50561, 50580, 50961, 50980, 52310-52315
    vagina, 57415
Forensic exam, 84061, 88040, 88125
Fowler-Stephens orchiopexy, 54650
Fracture
  arthroscopic treatment
    lower extremity, 29850-29856, 29892
    upper extremity, 29847
  blow-out
    orbital, 21385-21395
  closed treatment
    clavicle, 23500-23505
    head
      mandibular, 21450-21453
      maxillary, 21421, 21440
      nose, 21310-21320, 21337, 21345
      orbit, 21400-21401
    lower extremity
      acetabulum, 27220-27222
      ankle, 27760-27762, 27767-27768, 27808-27810, 27816-27818
      coccyx, 27200
      femur, 27230-27232, 27238-27246, 27267-27268, 27500-27503, 27508, 27510
      fibula, 27780-27781, 27786-27788
      foot, 28400-28405, 28430-28435, 28450-28455, 28470-28475, 28530
      knee, 27538
      patella, 27520
      pelvic ring, 27193-27194, 27216
      tibia, 27530-27532, 27750-27752, 27824-27825
      toe, 28490-28495, 28515
    rib, 21811-21813
    shoulder, 23570-23575, 23600-23605, 23620-23625, 23665, 23675
    sternum, 21820
    upper extremity
      elbow, 24620, 24650-24655, 24670-24675
      finger, 26720-26725, 26740-26742, 26750-26755
      hand, 26600-26607
      humerus, 24500-24505, 24530-24535, 24560-24565, 24576-24577
      radius, 25500-25505, 25520, 25560-25565, 25600-25605
      ulna, 25530-25535, 25560-25565, 25600-25605
      wrist, 25622-25624, 25630-25635, 25650, 25680
    vertebra, 22305-22315
  open treatment
    clavicle, 23515
    head
      cheek, 21356-21366
      hyoid, 21495
      mandibular, 21445, 21454-21470

Fracture — *continued*
  open treatment — *continued*
    head — *continued*
      maxillary, 21346-21348, 21422-21423, 21445
      nose, 21325-21336, 21338-21339, 21346-21348
      orbit, 21385-21395, 21406-21408
      sinus, 21343-21344
    larynx, 31584
    lower extremity
      acetabulum, 27226-27228
      ankle, 27766, 27769, 27814, 27822-27823
      coccyx, 27202
      femur, 27236, 27248, 27254, 27269, 27506-27507, 27511-27514, 27519
      fibula, 27784, 27792
      foot, 28415-28420, 28445-28446, 28465, 28485, 28531
      knee, 27540
      patella, 27524
      pelvis, 27215, 27215-27218
      pelvic ring, 27217-27218
      tibia, 27535-27536, 27758, 27759, 27826-27828
      toe, 28505, 28525
    rib, 21811-21813
    shoulder, 23585, 23615-23616, 23630, 23670, 23680
    sternum, 21825
    upper extremity
      elbow, 24586-24587, 24635, 24665-24666, 24685
      finger, 26735, 26746, 26765
      hand, 26615, 26665
      humerus, 24515-24516, 24545-24546, 24575, 24579
      radius, 25515, 25525-25526, 25574-25575, 25607-25609
      ulna, 25545, 25574-25575
      wrist, 25628, 25645, 25652, 25685
    vertebra, 22318-22328
  percutaneous treatment
    head
      cheek, 21355
      nose, 21340
    lower extremity
      femur, 27235, 27509
      foot, 28406, 28436, 28456, 28476
      pelvis, 27216
      tibia, 27756
      toe, 28496
    upper extremity
      finger, 26727, 26756
      hand, 26608, 26650
      humerus, 24538, 24566, 24582
      radius, 25606
      wrist, 25651
  treatment
    skull, 62000-62010
Fragile X, 88248
Fragility, 85547, 85555-85557
Francisella, 86000, 86668
Fredet-Ramstedt procedure, 43520
Frenulum
  incision, 40806, 41010, 41520
  removal, 40819, 41115
Frontal
  chest x-ray, 71010-71023
  craniotomy, 61556
    anesthesia, 00211
  sinus
    exploration, 31276
    fracture treatment, 21343-21344
  sinusotomy, 31070-31090

Frost suture, 67875
Fructose, 82757, 84375
  intolerance, 91065
Fulguration
  bladder, 51020, 52214, 52224-52240
  ureter, 50957, 50976, 52300-52301
  urethra, 52400, 53265
Function test
  pulmonary
    airway resistance, 94728
    capacity, 94150-94200, 94729
    continuous pressure, 94660-94662
    determination, 94726, 94727, 94770, 95012
    gas
      analysis, 0064T, 94680-94690, 94770
      collection, 94250
      diffusion, 94720-94725
      volume, 94726, 94727, 94750
    high altitude simulation test (HAST), 94452-94453
    inhalation, 94640-94645, 94664
    manipulation, 94667-94668
    recording, 94772-94777
    response, 94400-94450
    saturation, 82820, 94760-94762
    spirometry, 3023F-3027F, 94010-94070
    stress, 94620-94621
    surfactant, 94610
    ventilation, 94002-94005
    volume, 94375
    nasal, 92512
Fundoplasty, 43210, 43279-43280, 43325-43328
Fungus, 86671, 87101-87107, 87220
Furuncle, 10060-10061, 56405
Fusion, 32560
  lower extremity
    ankle, 27870-27871, 29899, 29907
    foot, 28705-28760
    hip, 27279-27286
    knee, 27580
  spine, 22532-22812
  upper extremity
    elbow, 24800-24802
    finger, 26843-26844
    hand, 26850-26863
    shoulder, 23800-23802
    thumb, 26820-26842
    wrist, 25800-25830

G

Gait training, 97116
Galactose
  blood, 82760
  galactogram, 77053-77054
    injection, 19030
  galactokinase
    blood, 82759
  galactose-1-phosphate
    uridyl transferase, 82775-82776
  uridyl transferase, 82775-82776
  urine, 82760
Galeazzi fracture/dislocation, 25525-25526
Gallbladder
  anastomosis
    with intestines, 47720-47741
  bile duct
    anastomosis, 47760, 47780-47785
      extrahepatic, 47760, 47780
      intrahepatic, 47785
    biopsy, 47553
    catheter placement, 47533-47534

Gallbladder — *continued*
  bile duct — *continued*
    catheter placement — *continued*
      conversion/exchange,
        47535-47536
      removal, 47537
    cyst, 47715
    destruction, 43265
    dilation, 43270, 47555-47556
    endoscopic diagnosis and
      treatment, 43260-43265,
      43273-43278, 47550-
      47556
    excision, 47711-47712, 47715
    exploration, 47700, 47552
    imaging, 78223
    incision, 43262, 47460
      and drainage, 47420-47425
    insertion
      catheter, drainage, 47533-
        45734
      exchange/conversion,
        47535-47536
      removal, 47537
      stent, 43274, 47538-47540,
        47801
    reconstruction, 47800
    removal
      foreign body, 43275
      stent, 43275-43276
      stone, 43264, 47420-
        47425, 47544, 47554
    repair, 47760, 47780-47785
    stone
      destruction, 43265, 47544
      removal, 43264, 47420-
        47425, 47544, 47554
    stricture treatment, 74363
    tumor
      excision, 47711-47712
    x-ray
      dilation, 74360
      with contrast, 74300-74328,
        74330
  biopsy, 43261
  calculi
    removal, 47480
  excision, 47562-47564, 47600-
    47620
  exploration, 47480
  imaging
    nuclear medicine, 78223
  incision, 47490
  incision and drainage, 47480
  nuclear medicine
    imaging, 78223
  repair
    with gastroenterostomy, 47741
    with intestines, 47720-47740
  x-ray
    with contrast, 74290
Gamete intrafallopian transfer (GIFT),
  58976
Gamma
  corten, 80420
  globulin, 82784-82787
  glutamyl transferase, 82977
  seminoprotein, 84152-84154
Gammulin Rh, 90384-90386
Ganglion
  cervicothoracicum
    anesthetic, 64510
  cyst
    aspiration, 20612
    drainage, 20612
    excision, wrist, 25111-25112
    injection, 20612
  excision
    wrist, 25111-25112
  gasserian
    decompression of sensory root,
      61450
    section, 61450
    stereotactic, 61790
  injection
    anesthetic, 64505, 64510
  pterygopalatinum
    anesthetic, 64505

Ganglion — *continued*
  sphenopalatine
    anesthetic, 64505
  stellate
    anesthetic, 64510
Gardner operation, 63700-63702
Gardnerella vaginalis detection,
  87510-87512
Gastric
  acid, analysis 82930
  electrodes
    neurostimulator
      implantation, 43647
      laparoscopic, open, 43881
      removal
        laparoscopic, 43648
        open, 43882
      replacement
        laparoscopic, 43647
        open, 43881
      revision
        laparoscopic, 43648
        open, 43882
  gastrectomy
    gastroduodenostomy, 43631
    partial, 43631-43635, 43845
    partial with gastrojejunostomy,
      43632
    total, 43621-43622
    total with
      esophagoenterostomy,
      43620
  gastroduodenostomy, 43810,
    43850-43855
  intubation, 43753-43755
  lavage, 43753
  tests
    manometry, 91020
  ulcer
    excision, 43610
    repair, 43501
    suture, 43840
Gastrin, 82938-82941
Gastrocnemius recession
  leg, lower, 27687
Gastroduodenostomy, 43810,
  43850-43855
Gastroenteritis, 4058F
Gastroenterology
  acid perfusion, 91030
  analysis, 43754-43755
  electrogastrography, 91132-91133
  function, 91037-91038
  hydrogen, 91065
  imaging, 91110-91111
  intubation, 43753-43755
  motility
    anorectal, 91122
    colon, 91117
    duodenal, 91022
    esophageal, 91010-91013
    gastric, 91020
  provocation, 91040
  reflux, 91034-91035
  sensation, 91120
Gastroenterostomy, 43644-43645,
  43842-43848
Gastrointestinal
  biopsy
    endoscopy, 43239
  breath hydrogen test, 91065
  dilation
    endoscopy, 43245
    esophagus, 43248
  endoscopy, 3130F-3142F, 00740
    ablation, 43270
    catheterization, 43241
    destruction, lesion, 43270
    dilation, 43245
    drainage, pseudocyst, 43240
    exploration, 43235
    foreign body removal, 43247
    hemorrhage, 43255
    inject varices, 43243
    injection, 43236
    lesion removal, 43251
    needle biopsy, 43238, 43242

Gastrointestinal — *continued*
  endoscopy — *continued*
    polyp removal, 43251
    radiation, thermal, 0520F, 43257
    stent placement, 43266
    suturing esophagogastric
      junction, 0008T
    thermal radiation, 0520F, 43257
    tube placement, 43246
    tumor removal, 43251
  esophagogastric fundoplasty,
    43210, 43280, 43325-43328
  esophagus tests
    acid
      perfusion, 91030
      reflux, 91034-91038
    balloon distention provocation
      study, 91040
    intubation with specimen
      collection, 43753-43757
    motility study, 91010-91013
  exploration, endoscopic, 43235
  gastroenterostomy
    for obesity, 43644-43645,
      43842-43848
  gastroesophageal reflux test,
    91034-91038
  gastrojejunostomy, 43860-43865
    conversion from gastrostomy
      tube, 49446
    contrast injection, 49465
    directed placement,
      endoscopic, 43246
    duodenal exclusion, 48547
    insertion, 49440
    obstructive material, removal,
      49460
    partial gastrectomy, 43632
    percutaneous placement,
      endoscopic, 43246
    percutaneous placement,
      nonendoscopic, 49440
    removal of obstructive material,
      49460
    replacement tube, 49542
    with, vagotomy, 43825
    without, vagotomy, 43820
  gastroplasty, morbid obesity,
    43842-43843
  gastrorrhaphy, 43840
  gastroschisis, 49605
  gastrostomy
    closure, 43870
    contrast injection, 49465
    conversion to gastro-
      jejunostomy tube, 49446
    laparoscopic, temporary, 43653
    neonatal, 43831
    pancreatic drain, with, 48001
    pyloroplasty, with, 43640
    temporary, laparoscopic, 43653
    temporary, neonatal, 43831
    tube change, 43760
    with, vagotomy, 43640
  gastrotomy, 43500-43501, 43510
  hemorrhage
    endoscopic control, 43255
  imaging
    intraluminal, 91110-91111
  injection
    submucosal, 43236
    varices, 43243
  lesion
    destruction, 43270
  ligation
    vein, 43244
  manometry, 91020
  needle biopsy
    endoscopy, 43238, 43242
  nuclear medicine
    blood loss study, 78278
    protein loss study, 78282
    shunt testing, 78291
  prophylaxis, 4017F
  reconstruction
    gastrointestinal tract, 43360-
      43361

Gastrointestinal — *continued*
  rectum
    manometry, 91122
    sensation, tone, and
      compliance test, 91120
    removal
      foreign body, 43247
      lesion, 43250
      polyp, 43250-43251
      tumor, 43250
    risk factor, 1008F
  stomach
    intubation with specimen prep,
      43754-43755
    stimulation of secretion, 43755
  tube
    placement, endoscopic, 43246
    replacement, 49450-49452
    repositioning, 43761
  ultrasound
    endoscopy, 43237-43238,
      43242, 43259, 76975
  upper gastrointestinal tract
    dilation, 83249
  x-ray
    contrast, 74246-74249
    guide
      dilator, 74360
      intubation, 74340
Gel diffusion, 86331
Genioplasty, 21120-21123
  augmentation, 21120-21123
  osteotomy, 21121-21123
Genitourinary sphincter, 53444-53449
Genomic sequencing, 81410-81471
Genotype analysis
  by nucleaic acid
    hepatitis C virus, 3218F,
      3265F-3266F, 87902
    HIV-1 protease/reverse
      transcriptase, 87901
    vanocomycin resistance, 87500
Gentamicin, 80170
Gentiobiase, 82963
GERD, 1118F, 91034-91038
German measles, 86762, 90707-
  90710
Gestational trophoblastic tumor,
  59870, 59100
Giardia
  antigen detection
    immunoassay technique, 87329
    immunofluorescence, 87269
  lamblia
    antibody, 86674
Gibbons stent, 52332
Gill operation, 63012
Gillies approach, 21356
Gingiva
  abscess
    incision and drainage, 41800
  alveolus
    excision, 41830
  cyst
    incision and drainage, 41800
  excision
    gingiva, 41820
    operculum, 41821
  gingivectomy, 41820
  gingivoplasty, 41872
  graft, mucosa, 41870
  hematoma
    incision and drainage, 41800
  lesion
    destruction, 41850
    excision, 41822-41828
  mucosa
    excision, 41828
  reconstruction
    alveolus, 41874
    gingiva, 41872
  removal
    foreign body, 41805
  tumor
    excision, 41825-41827

CPT © 2015 American Medical Association. All Rights Reserved.

© 2016 DecisionHealth

Gland

adrenal
  angiography, 75731-75733
  biopsy, 60540-60545
  function test, 95922
  imaging, 78075
  removal, 50545, 60540-60545, 60650
  venography, 75840-75842
Bartholin's
  abscess, drainage, 56420
  cyst
    excision, 56740
    repair, 56440
  excision, 56740
  marsupialization, 56440
bulbourethral, 53250
Cowper's, 53250
eccrine, 64650-64653, 64999
lacrimal
  gland
    biopsy, 68510
    drainage, 68400
    excision, 68500-68505
    tumor excision, 68540-68550
mammary
  ablation, 19105
  abscess, 19020
  aspiration
    cyst, 19000-19001
  augmentation, 19324-19325
  biopsy, 19100-19101
  capsules
    excision, 19371
    incision, 19370
    removal, 19371
  catheter, 19296-19298, 20555, 41019
  cryosurgery
    ablation, 19105
  cyst
    aspiration, 19000-19001
    excision, 19120-19126
  excision
    biopsy, 19100-19101
    capsules, 19371
    cyst, 19120-19126
    fistula, 19112
    lesion, 19120-19126, 19301
    mastectomy, 19300-19307
    nipple, 19110
    tumor, 19260-19272
  exploration, 19110, 19020
  fistula
    excision, 19112
  implants
    insertion, 19340-19342
    preparation, 19396
    removal, 19328-19330
    supply, 19396
  incision
    capsules, 19370
    drainage, 19020
  injection, 19030
  insertion
    implants, 19340-19342
  lesion
    excision, 19120-19126, 19301
  magnetic resonance imaging (MRI), 0159T, 77058-77059
  mammography, 77051-77052, 77055-77057
  performance measure, 3014F
  mammoplasty
    augmentation, 19324-19325
    reduction, 19318
  mastectomy
    excision 19300-19307
  mastopexy, 19316
  periprosthetic
    capsulectomy, 19371
    capsulotomy, 19370
  placement
    catheter, 19296-19298, 20555, 41019
    metallic localization clip, 19281-19288

Gland — *continued*
mammary — *continued*
  placement — *continued*
    needle localization wire, 19281-19288
    radiotherapy afterloading catheter, 19296-19298
  reconstruction, 19357-19369
    augmentation, 19324-19325
    flap
      free, 19364
      latissimus dorsi, 19361
      myocutaneous, 19367-19369
      mammoplasty, 19318-19325
      nipple, 19350-19355
      other, 19366
      revision, 19380
      tissue expander, 19357
    reduction, 19318
  removal
    capsules, 19371
    complete, 19303
    implants, 19328-19330
    partial, 19300-19302
    radical, 19305-19307
    subcutaneous, 19304
  revision, 19380
  repair, 19316
  tumor
    excision, 19260-19272
    ultrasound, 76641-76642
    x-ray, 76700, 77051-77052, 77055-77057
paraurethral, 53060
salivary
  biopsy
    needle, 42400
    incisional, 42405
  drainage
    abscess, 42310-42320
  excision
    cyst, 42408
  function study, 78232
  imaging, 78230
    with serial images, 78231
  incision, 42310-42320
  marsupialization
    cyst, 42409
  x-ray, 70380-70390
Skene's
  excision, 53260
  fulguration, 53260
  incision and drainage
    abscess, 53060
    cyst, 53060
sublingual, 42450
  excision
    calculus, 42330
  incision and drainage
    abscess, 42310-42320
  marsupialization
    cyst, 42409
submandibular
  excision, 42440, 42509
  incision
    calculus, 42330-42335
  ligation, 42510
thymus
  excision, 60520-60522
thyroid
  aspiration
    cyst, 60300
  biopsy
    percutaneous, 60100
  excision
    adenoma, 60200
    cervical, 60271
    complete, 60240
    cyst, 60200
    partial, 60210-60220
    remaining tissue, 60260
    substernal split, 60270
    total, 60220-60225, 60240, 60252-60254
    transthoracic, 60270
  incision and drainage, 60000

Gland — *continued*
thyroid — *continued*
  injection
    cyst, 60300
  nuclear medicine
    imaging, 78013-78018
      with flow, 78013
      with uptake, 78014
    metastases uptake, 78020
    uptake, 78012, 78014

Glaucoma
aqueous shunt, 66179-66180
  revision, 66184-66185
cryotherapy, 66720
cyclophotocoagulation, 66710-66711
diathermy, 66700
drainage implant, 0191T
  aqueous shunt, 66179-66185
fistulization, 66150
plan of care, 0517F
provocative test, 92140

Glenn procedure, 33766-33767

Glenohumeral joint
arthrotomy, 23040
biopsy, 23100
exploration, 23107
foreign body, 23107
loose body, 23107
synovectomy, 23105

Glenoid fossa, 21255

Globulin
antihuman, 86880-86886
binding
  corticosteroid, 84449
  sex hormone, 82470
  thyroxine, 84442
immune, 90378
  equine, 90287, 90296
  human
    intramuscular, 90281
      hepatitis B, 3216F, 90371
      rabies, 90375-90376
      respiratory syncytial, 90378
      Rho, 90384-90385
      tetanus, 90389
      vaccinia, 90393
      varicella-zoster, 90396
    intravenous, 90283
      botulism, 90288
      cytomegalovirus, 90291
      respiratory syncytial, 90379
      Rho, 90386
    subcutaneous, 90284
      rabies, 90375-90376

Glomus caroticum
artery, 60605
excision, 60600

Glossus
ablation, 41530
biopsy, 41100-41105
excision
  glossectomy, 41120-41155
  lesion, 41110-41114
  lingual frenum, 41115
fixation, 41500
frenoplasty, 41520
incision
  drainage, 41000-41009
  lingual frenum, 41010
repair
  wound, 41250-41252
  suture, 41510
  suspension, 41512

Glucagon, 82943
tolerance
  panel, 80422-80424
  test, 82946

Glucose
6-phosphate
  dehydrogenase, 82955-82960
blood test, 82947-82950, 82960
body fluid, 82945
continuous monitoring, 95250-95251

Glucose — *continued*
glucosidase, 82963
growth hormone supression, 80430
insulin
  supression, 80432
interstitial fluid
  continuous monitoring, 95250-95251
phosphate isomerase, 84087
tolerance
  panel, 80422-80424, 80434-80435
  test, 82951-82952

Glucuronide androstanediol, 82154

Glue
eye, 65286

Glutamate
dehydrogenase, 82965
transaminase
  alanine, 84460
  aspartic, 84450
  pyruvate, 84460

Glutamine, 82127-82131

Glutamyltransferase
gamma, 82977

Glutathione, 82978
reductase, 82979

Glycated protein, 82985

Glycohemoglobin, 83036

Glycosaminoglycan, 83864

Goeckerman treatment, 96910-96913

Gold, 80375

Goldwaite procedure, 27422

Gonadtropin
chorionic, 84702-84704
FSH, 83001
ICSH, 83002
LH, 83002
panel, 80426

Gonioscopy, 92020

Goniotomy, 65820

Goodenough Harris drawing test, 96101-96103

Graft
anal, 46753
aorta, 33840-33851, 33860-33877
artery
  coronary, 33503-33505
    anesthesia, 00567
  mammary, 4110F
bone
  anastomosis, microvascular, 20955-20962
  cranial, 61316, 61559, 62117, 62146-62148
  craniofacial, 21436
  donor area, 20900-20902
  facial, 21182-21184, 21436
    fascia, 15840
    forehead, 21138, 21172-21180
    genioplasty, 21121-21123
    malar, 21210, 21366
    mandibular, 21127, 21194, 21215, 21247
    maxillary, 21210
    midface, 21145-21160, 21188
    muscle, 15841-15845
    nasomaxillary, 21348
    orbit, 21256-21268, 21395, 21408
  femur, 27170
  harvesting, 20900-20902
  lower extremity, 20962
    calcaneous, 28102
    femoral, 27170, 27177, 27357, 27472
    fibula, 20955, 27637
    iliac crest, 20956
    knee, 29885
    metatarsal, 20957, 28322
    talus, 28102

CPT © 2015 American Medical Association. All Rights Reserved.
© 2016 DecisionHealth

Harvest — *continued*
  graft
    artery for bypass, 35600
    bone, 20900-20902
    cartilage, 20910-20912
    conjunctival, 68371
    fascia lata, 20920-20922
    tendon, 20924
    tissue, 20926
    vein for bypass, 33508, 35500, 35572
  intestines, 44132-44133
  kidney, 50300-50320, 50547
  liver, 47133, 47140-47142
  physiological support, 01990
  skin
    tissue culture, 15040
  stem cell, 38205-38206

Hauser procedure, 27420

Haygroves procedure, 27120

Head
  angiography, 70496, 70544-70546
  arthroplasty, 21240-21243
  augmentation, 21120
    mandibular body, 21125-21127
  brace, 20661, 21100
  computed tomography (CT) scan, 70450-70470, 70496
  dislocation
    temporomandibular, 21480-21490
  excision, 21015-21070
    abscess, 21025-21029
    condyle, 21050
    coronoid process, 21070
    meniscus, 21060
    torus, 21031-21032
    tumor
      benign, 21029-21030, 21040, 21046-21049
      malignant, 21015, 21034, 21044-21045
  fracture treatment, 21310-21497
  genioplasty, 21120-21123
  graft
    allograft, 21242
    autograft, 21240
    bone, 21210-21215
    cartilage, 21230-21235
    nerve, 64885-64886
  incision and drainage, 21010, 61316, 62148
  introduction, 21100-21116
    impression, 21076-21088
  lipectomy
    suction assisted, 15876
  magnetic resonance angiography (MRA), 70544-70546
  manipulation, 21073
  osteotomy, 21198-21206
  reconstruction
    benign tumor, 21181
    forehead, 21179-21180
    malar, 21270
    mandible, 21244-21249
    mandibular rami, 21193-21196
    mid-face, 21141-21160, 21188
    orbital, 21182-21184, 21256-21268
    superior-lateral orbital rim, 21172-21175
    zygomatic arch, 21255
  reduction
    facial bones, 21209
    forehead, 21137-21139
  rings, 20660
  removal, 21076-21116
  repair, 21120-21296
  revision, 21120-21296
  ultrasound, 76506, 76536
  x-ray, 70350

Hearing, 3230F
  aid
    bone conduction
      implantation, 69710
      removal, 69711
      repair, 69711
      replacement, 69710

Hearing — *continued*
  aid — *continued*
    check
      binaural, 92593
      monaural, 92592
    examination, 92590-92591
    services
      electroacoustic test, 92594-92595
    test, 92551-92597
    therapy, 92507-92508, 92601-92604

Heart
  ablation, 00537
    arrhythmogenic focus, 33250-33251, 33261
    atria, 33254-33256, 33265-33266
  aortic arch, 33852-33853
  arrhythmia, 93609
  arrhythmogenic focus, 33250-33251, 33261, 93650-93657
  assist, 92970-92971
  atria
    ablation, 33254-33256, 33265-33266
    endoscopy, 33265-33266
    reconstruction, 33254-33256, 33265-33266
  biopsy, 76932, 93505
  cardiopulmonary bypass, 32852, 32854
  catheterization
    angiography, 93454-93461
    biopsy, 93505
    dilution, 93561-93562
    flow directed, 93503
    injection, 93563-93568
    left heart, 93452-93453, 93458-93462
    pacemaker, 33210
    retrograde left and right, 93531
    right heart, 36013, 93451-93453, 93456-93457, 93460-93461
    transseptal left and right, 93532-93533
  closure, 33615
    valve, 33600-33602
    ventricle, 33675-33677, 33681-33688
  commissurotomy, 33476-33478
  computed tomography (CT) scan, 0144T-0151T
  defibrillator system, 93282-93284
    interrogation, 93261, 93289, 93292, 93295-93296
    peri-procedural, 93287
  electrode, 33202-33203
  electroversion, 92960-92961
  endoscopy
    atria, 33265-33266
  event recorder
    acoustic, 0068T-0070T, 33202-33203
    atria, 93602, 93615-93616
    bundle, 93600
    comprehensive, 93619-93622
    implantation, 33282
    mapping, 93609, 93613
    removal, 33284
    tachycardia, 93609
    ventricle, 93603
  excision
    donor, 33930, 33940
    tumor, 33120-33130
    valve, 33460
  exploration, 33310-33315
  failure assessment, 0001F
  fibrillation, 33254-33256, 33265-33266
  documentation, 1060F-1061F
  graft, 00566-00580
    allograft, 33933
  implantation
    artificial heart, 0051T
    assist, 33976, 33979
    event recorder, 33282

Heart — *continued*
  ligation, 37607
  magnetic resonance imaging (MRI) (CMRI), 75553-75564
  massage, 32160
  monitoring, 0086T
    evaluation, 93285, 93290-93291, 93297-93299
  nuclear medicine
    perfusion imaging, 78460-78465, 78478-78480
  output
    dilution, 93561-93562
    inert gas rebreathing, 93799
  pacemaker, 00530
    conversion, 33214
    evaluation, 93279-93281
      interrogation, 93288, 93294
      peri-procedural, 93286
      transtelephonic, 93293
    insertion, 33202-33213, 33216-33217, 33224-33225
    removal, 33233-33237
    replacement, 33206-33208
    catheter, 33210
    upgrade, 33214
  positron emission tomography (PET), 78459
    perfusion study, 78491-78492
  pulse generator, 33212-33213
  reconstruction, 34502
    atria, 33254-33256, 33265-33266
  rehabilitation, 93797-93798
  repair
    anomaly, 33608-33617
    aortic sinus, 33702-33722
    artificial heart, 0052T-0053T
    atrial septum, 33641, 33647
    atriventricular, 33660-33665, 33670
    cor triatriatum, 33732
    electrode, 33218
    fenestration, 93580
    infundibular, 33476-33478
    mitral valve, 33418-33430, 0345T
    myocardium, 33542
    outflow, 33476-33478
    postinfarction, 33542
    prosthetic, 33496
    septal defect, 0166T-0167T, 33608-33610, 33660, 33675-33688, 33813-33814, 93581
    sinus, 33645, 33702-33722
    system, 0052T-0053T
    tetralogy of Fallot, 33692-33697, 33924
    tricuspid valve, 33463-33468
    ventricle, 0166T-0167T, 33545, 33548, 33611-33612, 33619, 33647, 33681-33688, 33692-33697, 33722, 93581
    wound, 33300-33315
  resuscitation, 92950
  sounds, 0068T-0070T
  thrombectomy, 92973
  tissue ablation, 33250-33266
  transplantation, 00580, 33933, 33935, 33944-33945
  valve surgery, 33400-33478
  ventriculomyectomy, 33416
  vessels
    angioplasty, 92920-92921
    graft, 33330-33335
    thrombolysis, 92975-92977
    valvuloplasty, 92986-92990

Heavy metal
  quantitative, 83018
  screen, 83015

Heel
  collection, 36415-36416
  excision, 28120
    tumor, 27647, 28100-28103

Heel — *continued*
  fracture, 28400, 28405-28406, 28415-28420
  osteotomy, 28300
  spur, 28119
  x-ray, 73650

Heinz bodies, 85441-85445

Helicobacter pylori
  antibody, 86677
  antigen detection, 87338-87339
  blood test, 83009
  breath test, 78267-78268, 83013-83014
  stool, 87338
  urease activity, 83009, 83013-83014

Heller operation, 32665, 43279, 43330-43331

Helminth, 86682

Hemagglutination inhibition test, 86280

Hemangioma, 17106-17108, 96920-96922

Hemapheresis, 36511-36516

Hematoma
  drainage, 61108
    brain, 61154-61156
      anesthesia, 00211
    soft tissue, 10030
  evacuation
    brain, 61312-61315
      anesthesia, 00211
    subungual, 11740
  incision and drainage
    ankle, 27603
    arm, 23930, 25028
    brain, 61312-61315
    ear, 69000-69005
    elbow, 23930
    epididymis, 54700
    gums, 41800
    hip, 26990
    knee, 27301
    leg, 27301, 27603
    mouth, 40800-40801, 41005-41009, 41015-41018
    nasal septum, 30020
    neck, 21501-21502
    nose, 30000-30020
    pelvis, 26990
    scotum, 54700
    shoulder, 23030
    skin, 10140
    testis, 54700
    thorax, 21501-21502
    tongue, 41000-41006, 41015
    vagina, 57022-57023
    wrist, 25028
  puncture aspiration
    skin, 10160
  subdural, 61108
  subungual
    evacuation, 11740

Hematopoietic stem cell
  boost, 38243
  transplantation, 38240-38242

Hematopoietin, 82668

Hemiepiphyseal arrest, 24470

Hemipfacial microsomia, 21247

Hemilaminectomy, 63020-63044

Hemilaryngecomy, 31370-31382

Hemipelvectomy, 27290

Hemiphalangectomy, 28160

Hemispherectomy, 61543

Hemocytoblast
  allograft, 65781
  cell concentrate, 38215
  count, 86367
  cryopreservation, 38207, 88240
  donor search, 38204
  harvesting, 38205-38206
  plasma depletion, 38214
  platelet depletion, 38213
  red blood cell depletion, 38212
  T-cell depletion, 38210

Hemocytoblast – *continued*
thawing, 38208-38209
transplantation, 38240-38242
tumor cell depletion, 38211
washing, 38209
Hemodialysis, 4052F-4054F, 90935-90937
blood flow test, 90940
duplex scan, 93990
Hemodynamic monitoring, 0086T
Hemofiltration, 90945-90947
Hemoglobin, 3044F-3046F, 3279F-3281F
analysis
O2 affinity, 82820
carboxyhemoglobin, 82375-82376
chromotography, 83021
concentration, 85046
electrophoresis, 83020
F
chemical, 83030
quantitative, 83033
fetal, 83030-83033, 85460-85461
fractionation, 83020
glycosylated, 83036
methemoglobin, 83045-83050
non-automated, 83026
plan of care, 0514F
plasma, 83051
quantitation, 83020
carboxyhemoglobin, 88740
methemoglobin, 88741
sulfhemoglobin, 83060
thermolabile, 83065-83068
urine, 83069
Hemogram
automated, 85025-85027
manual, 85014-85018, 85032
Hemolysins, 85475
agglutinins, 86940-86941
Hemolytic complement, 86162
Hemoperfusion, 90997
Hemophil, 85210-85293
Haemophilus influenzae, 86684
vaccine, 90647-90648, 90748
Hemorrhage, control of
abdominal, 49002
cauterization
nose, 30901-30906
endoscopic
anal, 46614
chest cavity, 32654
colon, 44391, 43582
colon with sigmoid colon, 45334
esophagus, 43227
gastrointestinal, upper, 43255
intestines, small, 44366, 44378
nasal, 31238
rectum, 45317
liver, 47350
lung, 32110
nasal
cauterization, 30901-30906
nasopharynx, 42970-42972
oropharynx, 42960-42962
throat, 42960-42962
uterus
postpartum, 59160
vagina, 57180
Hemorrhoidectomy
complex, 46260-46262
external, 46250
ligature, 46221
simple, 46255, 46257-46258
Hemorrhoidopexy, 46947
Hemorrhoids
band ligation, 45350, 45398
destruction, 46930
incision, 46083
injection, 46500
ligation, 46945-46946, 0249T
stapling, 46947
suture, 46945-46946
Hemosiderin, 83070
Hemothorax, 32551

Heparin, 85520-85530
cofactor, 85300-85301
Hepatectomy
donor, 47133, 47140-47142
extensive, 47122
lobectomy, 47125-47130
Hepatic
abscess, 47010-47015, 47300
aneurysm, 35121-35122
duct
anastomosis, 47465, 47802
exploration, 47400
incision and drainage, 47400
nuclear medicine, 78223
removal
calculus, 47400
repair, 47765, 47802
graft, 35560
hemorrhage, 47350
portoenterostomy, 47802
transplant, 47135, 47143-47147
vein, 75810, 75885-75887
Hepaticodochotomy, 47400
Hepaticoenterostomy, 47802
Hepaticostomy, 47400
Hepaticotomy, 47400
Hepatitis, 3215F-3220F, 4150F-4159F
A
antibody, 86708-86709
vaccine, 90632-90634
B
antibody, 86704-86707
antigen
Be, 87350
surface, 87340-87341
vaccine, 90740-90748
virus, 87515-87517
C,
antibody, 86803-86804
detection, 87520-87522
delta agent, 86692
antigen, 87380
IgM, 86705, 86709
G, 87525-87527
Hepatobiliary imaging, 78226-78227
Hepatorrhaphy, 47300, 47350-47362
Hepatotomy, 47010
Hernia
repair
abdominal, 00750-00756, 00830-00836, 49560-49565, 49590
cerbral, 62120-62121
diaphragmic, 39540-39541
epigastic, 49570-49572
femoral, 49550-49557
incisional, 49561-49566
inguinal, 49491-49525
lumbar, 49540
lung, 32800
orchiopexy, 54640
paraesophageal, 43281-43282, 43332-43337
rectovaginal, 45560
spermatic cord, 55540
spigelian, 49590
umbilical, 49580-49587, 49600-49611
Herpes
simplex
antibody, 86694-86696
antigen detection
immunofluorescence, 87273-87374
nucleic acid, 87528-87530
identification
smear, 87207
stain, 87207
smear, 87207
virus
6, 87531-87533
gamma (4), 86663-86665
Herpetic vesicle, 54050-54065
Heteroantibody, 86308-86310
Heterograft, 15400-15421

Heterotropia, 67311-67345
Heyman procedure, 27179, 28264
Hib vaccination, 90647-90648
Hidradenitis
excision, 11450-11471
incision and drainage, 10060-10061
High altitude simulation test (HAST), 94452-94453
Hill procedure, 43325-43328
laparoscopic, 43280
Hinton positive, 86592-86593
Hip, 01200-01215
arthrocentesis, 20610-20611
arthrodesis, 27284-27286
arthrography, 73525
arthroplasty, 01214-01215, 27130-27132
arthroscopy, 01202, 29860-29863, 29914-29916
arthrotomy, 27030-27033
biopsy, 27040-27041, 27052
capsulectomy, 27036
capsulotomy, 27036
cast, 29305-29325
craterization, 27070
denervation, 27035
dislocation treatment, 27250-27266
echography, 76885-76886
drainage
abscess, 26990
bone, 26992
bursa, 26991
hematoma, 26990
excision, 27070
synovium, 27054, 29863
tumor, 27047-27049, 27065-27067, 27075-27076
exploration, 27033
fasciotomy, 27025-27027, 27057
fusion, 27284-27286
injection
radiological, 27093-27096
joint
arthroplasty, 27132, 27134-27138
biopsy, 27052
dislocation, 27250-27254, 27256-27259, 27265-27266
excision, 27054, 29863
manipulation, 27275
reconstruction, 27134-27138
release, 27036
replacement, 27132
manipulation, 27275
osteotomy, 27146-27156
prothesis
removal, 27090-27091
stem, 27125-27138
removal
cast, 29710
foreign body, 27033, 27086-27087, 29861
loose body, 29861
prothesis, 27090-27091
repair
labrum, 29916
muscle, 27100-27105, 27111
tendon, 27097
resection
radical, 27075-27079
saucerization, 27070
strapping, 29520
tenotomy, 27003-27006
total replacement, 27130-27132
ultrasound, 76885-76886
x-ray
bilateral, 73521-73523
unilateral, 73501-73503
Hippocampus, 61566
Histamine, 4185F-4186F, 83088, 86343
Histoplasma
antibody, 86698
antigen, 87385
test, 86510

HIV, 3292F
antibody, 86701-86703
antigen detection
-1, 87389-87390
-2, 87391
confirmation test, 86689
HLA typing, 86812-86817
Hoffman apparatus, 20690
Hofmeister operation, 43620-43622
Holten test, 82575
Home services
ADL, 99509
anticoagulant management, 99636-99664
apnea monitoring, 94774-94777
catheter care, 99507
counseling
family, 99510
individual, 99510
enema adminstration, 99511
established patient, 99347-99350
hemodialysis, 99512
home infusion, 99601-99602
injections
intramuscular, 99506
mechanical ventilation, 99504
new patient, 99341-99345
newborn care, 99502
postnatal assessment, 99501
prenatal monitoring, 99500
respiratory therapy, 99503
sleep studies, 95803-95811
stoma care, 99505
ventilation assistance, 94005
Homocystine, 82615, 83090
Homogenization, 87176
Homografts, 15271-15278
Homovanillic acid, 83150
Hormone
adrenocorticotropic (ACTH), 80400-80406, 80412, 80418, 82024
assay
ACTH, 82024
aldosterone, 82024
androstenedione, 82157
androsterone, 82160
angiotensin II, 82163
corticosterone, 82528
cortisol, 82533
dehydroepiandrosterone, 82626
dihydrotestosterone, 80327-80328
epiandrosterone, 80327-80328
estradiol, 82670
estriol, 82677
estrogen, 82671-82672
estone, 82679
follicle stimulating hormone, 83001
growth hormone, 83003
hydroxyprogesterone, 83498-83499
luteinizing hormone, 83002
somatotropin, 83003
testosterone, 84403
vasopressin, 84588
corticosteroid, 83491
corticotropic releasing, 80412
globulin, 84270
growth, 83003
human, 80418, 80428-80430, 86277
implantation
pellet, 11980
lactogen, 83632
luteinizing, 80418, 80426, 83002
parathormone, 83970
prolactin, 80418, 84146
somatostatin, 84307
thyroid stimulating, 3278F, 80418, 80438-80439, 84443
vasopressin, 84588
Hospital services
inpatient
discharge, 1110F-1111F, 99238-99239

CPT © 2015 American Medical Association. All Rights Reserved.   © 2016 DecisionHealth

Hospital services — *continued*
  inpatient — *continued*
    initial, 99221-99233
    newborn, 99477
    prolonged, 99356-99357
    subsequent, 99231-99233
  newborn
    transport, 99466-99467
    evaluation and management,
      99460-99463
    initial, 99477
  observation
    discharge, 1110F-1111F,
      99234-99236
    initial, 99218-99220
  same day admission
    discharge, 1110F-1111F,
      99234-99236
Hot pack treatment, 97010
Home/house visits, 99341-99350
HTLV, 86687-86689
Hubbard tank therapy, 97036
Hue test, 92283
Huggin operation, 54520
Huhner test, 89300
Human
  chorionic
    gonadotropin, 80414-80415,
      84702-84703
    somatomammotropin, 83632
  cytomegalovirus, 86644-86645,
    87271, 87332, 87495-87497
  growth hormone, 80418, 80428-
    80430
  herpes virus 4, 86663-86665
  immunodeficiency virus (HIV), 3292F
    antibody, 86701-86703
    antigen detection
      -1, 87389-87390
      -2, 87391
    confirmation test, 86689
  papillomavirus, 87623-87625
  T-cell leukemia, 86687-86689
Humerus
  amputation, 24900-24940
  arthrodesis, 23800-23802
  arthroplasty, 23470-23472
  biopsy, 24065-24066
  craterization, 23184, 24140,
  diaphysectomy, 23184, 24140
  excision
    abscess, 23174, 24134
    cyst, 23150-23156, 24110-
      24116
    osteomyelitis, 24134, 24140
    tumor, 23220-23222, 24075-
      24076
      benign, 23150-23156,
        24110-24116
      malignant, 24077
  fracture treatment
    closed
      humeral epicondylar, 24560-
        24566
      humeral shaft, 24500-
        24505
      humeral tuberosity, 23620-
        23625, 23665
      proximal humeral, 23600-
        23605
      supracondylar humeral,
        24530-24538
    open, 24587
      humeral epicondylar, 24575-
        24586
      humeral shaft, 24515-24516
      humeral tuberosity, 23630,
        23670
      proximal humeral, 23615-
        23616
      supracondylar humeral,
        24545-24546
    condyle, 24576-24582
    epicondyle, 24560-24575
    greater tuberosity, 23620-23630
    shaft, 24500-24505, 24515-
      24516

Humerus — *continued*
  fracture treatment — *continued*
    supracondylar, 24530-24546
    transcondylar, 24530-24546
    with dislocation, 23665-23670
  incision
    drainage
      abscess, 23930, 23935
      bursa, 23931
      glenohumeral joint, 23100,
        23105, 23107
    pinning, 23491, 24498
    prophylactic treatment, 23491,
      24498
  removal
    foreign body, 24200-24201
  repair
    arrest, 24470
    malunion, 24430-24435
    nonunion, 24430-24435
    osteoplasty, 24420
    osteotomy, 24400-24410
    tendon, 24305-24320, 24341-
      24342
    with graft, 24435
  resection
    head, 23195
    radical, 23220-23222
    tendon, 23440
    tumor, 24150-24151
  saucerization, 23184, 24140
  sequestrectomy, 23174, 24134
  tenodesis, 23430, 24340
  tenolysis, 24332
  transfer, 23395-23397, 24301
  x-ray, 73060
Hyaluron binding assay, 0087T
Hydatid disease, 86171, 86280
Hydatidiform mole, 59100, 59870
Hydration, 96360-96361
Hydrocarbon, 82441
Hydrocele
  aspiration, 55000
  excision
    spermatic cord, 55500
    tunica vaginalis, 55040-55041
  repair, 55060
Hydrochloric acid, 82930
Hydrocodone, 80361
Hydrogen ion, 83986
Hydrolase
  acetylcholine, 82013
  phosphoric monoester, 84061,
    84075, 84078, 84080
  triacylglycerol, 83690
Hydrotherapy, 97036
Hydrotubation, 58350
Hydroxycorticosteroid, 83491
Hydroxyindolacetic acid, 83497
Hydroxypregnenolone, 80406, 84143
Hydroxyprogesterone, 80402-80406,
  83498-83499
Hydroxyproline, 83500-83505
Hygroma, 38550-38555
Hymen
  excision, 56442, 56700
  ring, 56700
Hymenectomy, 56700
Hymenotomy, 56442
Hyoid
  fracture treatment, 21495
  muscle, 21685
**Hyperbaric oxygen pressurization/
  treatment**, 99183
Hypercycloidal x-ray, 76101-76102
Hyperhidrosis, 64650-64653
Hypertelorism
  orbit, 21260-21263
Hyperthermia
  therapy, 53850-53852
  treatment, 77600-77620
Hypnotherapy, 90880
Hypogastric plexus, 64517, 64681

Hypoglossal nerve, 64868
Hypophysectomy, 61546-61548,
  62165
Hypophysis, 61546-61548, 62165
Hypospadias
  repair, 54300, 54352
    complications, 54340-54348
    first stage, 54304, 54332
    one stage, 54322, 54336
    second stage, 54316
    third stage, 54318
    urethroplasty, 54324-54328
Hypothermia, 99184-99186
Hypoxia, 94450, 94452-94453
Hysterectomy
  abdominal
    radical, 58210
  after cesarean delivery, 01963,
    01969, 59525
    resection, 58951, 58953-58956
    supracervical, 58180
    total, 58100-58152, 58200,
      58956
  laparoscopic, 58541-58544
    radical, 58548
    total, 58570-58573
    vaginal, 58550, 58570-58570-
      58573
  vaginal, 01962, 58260-58270,
    58290-58294, 58550-58554
  with
    closure of vesicouterine fistula,
      51925
    colpectomy, 58275-58280
    colpo-urethrocystopexy,
    repair of enterocele, 58263,
      58292, 58294
Hysterolysis, 58559
Hysteroplasty, 58540
Hysterorrhaphy, 58520, 59350
Hysterosalpingography, 58340,
  58345, 74740
Hysteroscopy
  ablation, 58563
  biopsy, 58558
  diagnostic, 58555
  lysis, 58559
  placement, 58565
  removal, 58561-58562
  resection, 58560
Hysterotomy, 59100
  induced abortion, 59852, 59857
Hysterotrachelectomy, 57530

I

Icthyosis, 86592-86593
Identification
  oocyte, 89254
  sperm
    aspiration, 89257
    tissue, 89264
Ileal conduit, 50690
Ileoscopy, 44380-44386
Ileostomy, 44310, 45136
  continent (Kock procedure),
    44316
  laparoscopic, 44186-44187
  non-tube, 44187
  revision, 44312-44314
Ileum, 44382
Iliac
  artery
    aneurysm, 35131-35132,
      75954
    angioplasty, 37222
    atherectomy, 0238T
    embolectomy, 34151-34201
    exposure, 34820, 34833
    graft, 34900
      bypass, 35563, 35663
    occlusion device, 34808
    thrombectomy, 34151-34201

Iliac — *continued*
  artery — *continued*
    thromboendarterectomy,
      35351, 35361-35363
  crest
    anastomosis, 20970
Iliohypogastric nerve, 64425
Ilioinguinal nerve, 64425
Ilium
  excision, 27070
    tumor, 27065-27067
  fracture
    open treatment, 27215, 27218
Ilizarov procedure, 20692
Imaging
  capsule endoscopy, 0355T
  echography
    3D rendering, 76376-76377
    abdomen, 76700-76705
    arm, 76881-76882
    artery
      extracranial, 93880-93882
      intracranial, 93886-93893
      middle cerebral, 76821
      umbilical, 76820
    bladder, 51798
    breast, 76641-76642
    bronchi, endoscopic, 31654
    cardiac, 93303-93317, 93320-
      93321, 93350-93352,
      93662
    chest, 76604
    colon
      endoscopic, 45391-45392
      with sigmoid, 45341-45342
    drainage
      abscess, 75989
    esophagus
      endoscopic, 43231-43232
    eye
      arteries, 93875
      biometry, 76516-76519
      diagnostic, 76510-76513
      foreign body, 76529
      pachymetry, 76514
    fetus, 76818-76828
    follow-up, 76970
    gastrointestinal, 76975
      endoscopic, 43237-43238,
        43242, 43259
    guidance
      amniocentesis, 59001, 76946
      amniofusion, 59070
      arteriovenous fistula, 76936
      cardiac, 76932, 93662
      chorionic villus sampling,
        76945
      cryosurgery, 55873
      drainage, fetal fluid, 59074
      endometrial ablation, 58356
      fetal cordocentesis, 76941
      fetal transfusion, 76941
      heart biopsy, 76932
      needle biopsy, 43232,
        43238, 43242, 45342,
        45392, 76942
      occlusion, umbilical cord,
        59072
      ova retrieval, 76948
      percardiocentesis, 76930
      pseudoaneurysm, 76936
      radiation therapy, 0520F,
        77387
      radioelement, 76965
      shunt placement, fetal, 59076
      thoracentesis, 76942
      tissue ablation, 76940
      vascular access, 76937
    head, 76506, 76536
    heart
      fetal, 76825
    hips
      infant, 76885-76886
    hysterosonography, 76831
    intraoperative, 76998
    intravascular, noncoronary
      during procedure, 37252-
        37253

CPT © 2015 American Medical Association. All Rights Reserved.   © 2016 DecisionHealth

Imaging – Implantation

Implantation — *continued*
  brain
    chemotherapy, 0519F, 61517
    thermal perfusion probe, 0077T
    electrode, 61850-61870
  breast, 19340-19342
    preparation, 19396
    removal, 19328-19330
  cardiac event recorder, 33282
  carotid sinus baroeflex device,
    0266T-0268T
  drug delivery device, 11981,
    11983, 61517
  electrode (array)
    brain, 61850-61870
    cranial nerve, 64553, 64568
    epidural, 63650-63655
    gastric, 43647
    neuromuscular, 64565, 64580
    peripheral nerve, 64555, 64575
    sacral nerve, 64591, 64581
  eye
    anterior segment, 65920
    aqueous shunt to extraocular
      placement or replacement
      of pegs, 65125
    corneal ring segments, 65785
    posterior segment
      extraocular, 67120
      intraocular, 67121
    reservoir, 66179-66180
    vitreous drug delivery system,
      67027
  fallopian tube, 58565
  hearing aid hormone pellet
    bone conduction, 69710
  hip, 27125-27132
    revision, 27134-27138
  hormone pellet, 11980
  mesh
    debridement closure, 49568
    hernia repair, 49568
    vaginal repair, 57267
  nerve, 64553-64561, 64575-64581
  neurostimulators
    cranial
      pulse generator, 61885-
        61886
    gastric
      laparoscopic, 43647, 43659
      open, 43881
    subcutaneous, peripheral,
      0282T-0283T
  orbital, 67560, 67560
  ovum, 58976
  penile, 54400-54405
    removal, 54406, 54410-54417
    repair, 54408
  pulmonary valve, 33477
  pulse generator
    brain, 61885-61886
    spinal cord electrode array,
      63685
  receiver
    brain, 61885-61886
    spinal cord, 63685
  removal
    elbow, 24164
    radius, 24164
  reservoir vascular access device
    declotting, 36593
  retinal electrode array, 0100T
  spinal cord, 63650-63655
  subperiosteal, 21245-21246
  total replacement heart system,
    0051T
  tubouterine, 58752
  ureter, 50780-50785
  ventricular assist device
    extracorporeal, 33975-33976
    intracorporeal, 33979
    percutaneous, 33990-33991

Impression, maxillofacial
  prosthesis
    auricular, 21086
    facial, 21088
    mandibular, 21081
    nasal, 21087

Impression, maxillofacial — *continued*
  prosthesis — *continued*
    oburator, 21076
    definative, 21080
    interim, 21079
    orbital, 21077
    palatal, 21082-21083
    speech aid, 21084
  oral splint, 21085
In situ hybridization, 88272-88275,
  88364-88369, 88373-88374,
  88377
In vitro fertilization, 58321-58322
**In vivo nuclear magnetic resonance
  (NMR) spectroscopy**, 76390
Incision
  abdomen, 49000-49002, 58960,
    34151, 34401, 34451,
    34820, 34833
  abscess, 20005
  accessory nerve, 63191
  anal, 46020-46030, 46045-
    46050, 46070-46083
    fistula, 46270, 46280
    sphincter, 46080
  and drainage
    abdomen
      fluid, 49080-49081
      pancreatitis, 48000
    abscess
      abdomen, 49020, 49040
      anal, 46045-46050
      ankle, 27603
      appendix, 44900
      arm
        lower, 25028
        upper, 23930
      Bartholin's gland, 56420
      bladder, 51080
      brain, 61320-61321
      breast, 19020
      ear, 69000-69020
      elbow, 23930, 24000
      epididymis, 54700
      eyelid, 67700
      finger, 26010-26011
      gums, 41800
      hand, 26034
      hip, 26990
      kidney, 50020
      knee, 27301
      leg
        lower, 27603
        upper, 27301
      liver, 47010
      lung, 32200
      lymph node, 38300-38305
      mouth, 40800-40801, 41000-
        41009, 41015-41018
      nasal septum, 30020
      neck, 21501-21502
      nose, 30000-30200
      ovary, 58820-58822
      palate, 42000
      paraurethral gland, 53060
      parotid gland, 42300-42305
      pelvis, 26990, 45000
      perineum, 56405
      peritoneum, 49020, 49062
      prostate, 55720-55725
      rectum, 45005-45020,
        46040, 46050-46060
      retroperitoneal, 49060
      salivary gland, 42300-42320
      scrotum, 54700, 55100
      shoulder, 23030, 23035-
        23044
      Skene's gland, 53060
      skin, 10060-10061
      spine, 22010-22015
      subdiaphragmatic,
        percutaneous, 49040
      sublingual gland, 42310-
        42320
      submaxillary gland, 42310-
        42320
      subphrenic, percutaneous,
        49040

Incision — *continued*
  and drainage — *continued*
    abscess — *continued*
      testis, 54700
      thorax, 21501-21510
      throat, 42700-42725
      tongue, 41000-41009,
        41015
      tonsil, 42700-42725
      urethra, 53040
      uvula, 42000
      vagina, 57010
      vulva, 56405
      wrist, 25028, 25040
    ankle, 27603-27604, 27610
    appendix, 44900
    Bartholin's gland, 56420
    bile duct, 47420-47425, 47480
    bladder, 51040, 51080
    bulla, 10160
    bursa
      ankle, 27604
      arm
        lower, 25031
        upper, 25931
      elbow, 23931
      foot, 28001
      hand, 26025-26030
      hip, 26991
      knee, 27301
      leg
        lower, 27604
        upper, 27301
      palm, 26025-26030
      pelvis, 26991
      shoulder, 23031
      wrist, 25031
    carbuncle
      skin, 10060-10061
    carpals, 25035, 26034
    comedones
      skin, 10040
    conjunctiva, 68020-68040
    cyst
      conjunctiva, 68020
      gums, 41800
      liver, 47010
      lung, 32200
      mouth, 40800-40801,
        41000-41009, 41015-
        41018
      ovarian, 58800-58805
      Skene's gland, 53060
      skin, 10040, 10060-10061
        pilonidal, 10080-10081
        puncture aspiration, 10160
      spinal cord, 63172-63173
      thyroid gland, 60000
      tongue, 41000-41009, 60000
    ear, 69000-69020
    elbow
      abscess, 23930, 23935
      arthrotomy, 24000-24006
    femur, 27303
    fluid collection
      skin, 10140
    foot, 28001-28003, 28020-
      28024
    furuncle, 10060, 10061
    gallbladder, 47480
    gums, 41800
    hand, 26010-26030, 26070-
      26080
    hematoma
      ankle, 27603
      arm
        lower, 25028
        upper, 23930
      brain, 61312-61315
        anesthesia, 00211
      ear, external
        complicated, 69005
        simple, 69000
      elbow, 23930
      epididymis, 54700
      gums, 41800
      hip, 26990
      knee, 27301

Incision — *continued*
  and drainage — *continued*
    hematoma — *continued*
      leg
        lower, 27603
        upper, 27301
      lymph node, 38300-38305
      mouth, 40800-40801, 41000-
        41009, 41015-41018
      nasal septum, 30020
      neck, 21501-21502
      nose, 30000-30020
      pelvis, 26990
      scrotum, 54700
      shoulder, 23030, 23044
      skin, 10140, 10160
      skull, 61312-61315
      testis, 54700
      thorax, 21501-21502
      tongue, 41000-41009
      vagina, 57022-57023
      wrist, 25028
    hepatitic duct, 47400
    hip, 26990-26992, 27030
    humerus, 23935
    interphalangeal joint, 28024
    intertarsal joint, 28020
    kidney, 50020-50040, 50125
    knee, 27301, 27310
    lacrimal gland, 68400
    lacrimal sac, 68420
    leg
      lower, 27603-27604
      upper, 27301
    liver, 47010
    lung, 32036, 32200
    lymph node, 38300-38305
    mediastinum, 39000-39010
    metatarsophalangeal joint, 28022
    milia, multiple, 10040
    mouth, 40800-40801, 41000-
      41009, 41015-41018
    onychia, 10060-10061
    orbit, 67405, 67440
    ovary, 58800-58822
    palate, 42000
    paronychia, 10060-10061
    parotid gland, 42300-42305
    pelvic, 26990-26992
    penis, 54015
    pericardium, 33025
    peritoneum, 49020-49062
    phalanges, 26010-26020, 26080
    pilonidal cyst, 10080-10081
    prostate, 55720-55725
    pustules, 10040
    radius, 25035
    rectum, 45000-45020, 46040,
      46060
    scrotum, 55100
    seroma, 10140
    shoulder
      abscess, 23030
      arthrotomy, 23044
      bursa, 23031
      hematoma, 23030
    Skene's gland, 53060
    skin
      abscess, 10060-10061
      cyst, 10080-10081
      hematoma, 10140
      infection, 10180
    spine, 22010-22015
    submaxillary gland, 42310-42320
    tarsometatarsal joint, 28020
    tendon sheath, 26020
    testis, 54700
    thorax, 21510
    thyroid, 60000
    toe, 28024
    tongue, 41000-41009
    tonsil, 42700-42725
    ulna, 25035
    ureter, 50600
    urethra, 53040, 53080-53085
    uvula, 42000
    vagina, 57022-57023
    vulva, 56405

Influenza, 1030F
  A antigen detection
    immunofluorescence, 87276
    immunoassay technique, 87400
  B antigen detection
    immunofluorescence, 87275
    immunoassay technique, 87400
  vaccine, 90653-90668, 90672-
    90673, 90685-90688
  virus
    antibody, 86710
    by immunoassay
      with direct optical
        observation, 87804
Infraorbital nerve, 64734
Infrared light treatment, 97026
infratentorial craniectomy, 61520-
  61521
  anesthesia, 00211
Infusion
  amnion, 59072
  continuous, paraspinousl block,
    thoracic, 64463
  intraosseous, 36680
  intravenous, 96365-96338
  pump
    electronic analysis, 62367-
      62368
    insertion, 36260
    intra-arterial, 36261-36262
    intravenous
      insertion, 36563
      repair, 36576
      replacement, 36583
    maintenance, 95990-95991,
      96521-96522
    spinal cord, 62361-62362
    ventricular catheter, 61215
  radioelement, 77750
  subcutaneous, 96369-96371
  therapy, 62350-62351, 62360-
    62362
    arterial catherterization, 36640
    chemotherapy, 0519F, 96401-
      96542, 96545, 96549
    home infusion procedures,
      99601-99602
    intracranial, prolonged
      endovascular, 61650-
      61651
    pain, 0521F, 1116F, 62360-
      62362, 62367-62368
  thrombolysis
    cerebral, 37195
    coronary, 92975-92977
    other than coronary, 37211-
      37214
Ingestion challenge test, 95076, 95079
Inguinal hernia
  repair, 49491, 49495-49500, 49505
    incarcerated, 49492, 49496,
      49501, 49507, 49521
    laparoscopic, 49650-49651
    recurrent, 49520
    sliding, 49525
    strangulated, 49492
Ingrown nail, 11750-11755, 11765
Inhalation
  pentamidine, 94642
  provocation test, 95070-95071
  treatment, 94640
    aerosol, 94642
      continuous, 94644-94645
    evaluation, 94664
    home visit, 99503
Inhibin A, 86336
Inhibition
  fertilization
    capsules, 11975-11977
    fitting, 57170
    intrautirine device (IUD),
      58300-58301
  test, 86280
Inhibitor
  alpha 1, 82103-82104
  alpha 2, 85410
  aromatase, 4179F

Inhibitory concentration, 87186
Initial consultation, 99251-99255
Injection
  abdomen, 49400
  angiography, 75746
  ankle, 27648
  antigen (allergen), 95115-95125
  aorta (aortography), 93567
  aponeurosis, 20550
  bladder, 51600-51610
  brain canal, 61070
  bronchography, 31899
  bursa, 20600-20611
  cardiac catheterization, 93563-
    93568
  chemotherapy, 0519F, 96401-
    96542, 96545, 96549
  cholangiography, percutaneous,
    47531-47532
  cistern, 61055
  contrast, 49465
    catheter, 36598, 49424
  corpora cavernosa, 54235
  cyst
    bone, 20615
    kidney, 50390
    pelvis, 50390
    thyroid, 60300
  diagnostic, 96372-96379
  Dupuytren's cord, 20527
  elbow, 24220
  esophageal varices, 43243
  esophagus
    sclerosing agent, 43204
    submucosal, 43201
  extremity, 36002
  eye
    air, 66020
    medication or other, 66030
  eyelid, 68200
  ganglion, 64505, 64510
    cyst, 20612
  gastric
    secretion stimulant, 43755
    varices, 43243
  heart vessels, 93563-93568
  hemorrhoids, 46500
  hip, 27093-27095
  insect venom, 95130-95134
  intervertebral disc, 62290-62292
  intra-amniotic, 59852
  intra-arterial, 96373, 96379
    thrombolytic, 37184-37186,
      61645
  intradermal, 11920-11922
  intralesional, 11900-11901
  intramuscular, 96372
    therapeutic, 99506
  intravenous, 96374-96379
    diagnostic, 37187-37188
    infusion, 96360-96368
    vascular flow check, graft, 15860
  intravenous push, 96374-96376
  joint, 20600-20611
  kidney
    drugs, 50391
    radiologic, 50430-50431
  knee, 27370
  lacrimal gland, 68850
  larynx, 64617
  left heart, 93565
  lesion, 11900-11901
  ligament, 20550
  liver, 47015
  mammary ductogram/
    galactogram, 19030
  muscle chemodenervation
    cervical spinal, 64615
    extremity, 64642-64645
    facial, 64612, 64615
    larynx, 64617
    neck, 64616
    trigeminal, 64615
    trunk, 64646-64647
  nerve
    anesthetic, 01991-01992,
      64400-64530
    neurolytic agent, 64600-
      64640, 64680-64681

Injection — *continued*
  orbit
    retrobulbar
      alcohol, 67505
      medication, 67500
    Tenon's capsule, 67515
  palmar fascial cord, 20527
  pancreatography, 48400
  paraspinous, thoracic, 64461-64462
  parathyroid, 78808
  paravertebral facet joint/nerve,
    64470-64476, 0213T-0218T
  penis
    erection, 54235
    Peyronie disease, 54200
    Peyronie disease with surgical
      exposure of plaque, 54205
    radiology, 54230
    vasoactive drugs, 54231
  platelet rich plasma, 0232T
  prophylactic, 96365-96379
  radioactive tracer, 38792
  radiologic, 19030, 78808
  rectum, 45520
  right heart, 93566
  sacroiliac joint, 27096
  salivary duct, 42660
  salivary gland, 42550
  sclerosing agent
    esophagus, 43204
    intravenous, 36470-36471
  sentinel node identification, 38792
  shoulder, 23350
  shunt, 49427
  sinus tract, 20500-20501
  spider veins, 36468
  spinal
    artery, 62294
    cord
      anesthetic, 62310-62319
      blood, 62273
      neurolytic agent, 62280-
        62282
      other, 62310-62311
      radiological, 62284
  steroids, 52283
  subcutaneous, 96372
    infusion, 96369
    silicone, 11950-11954
    therapeutic, 90782
  temporomandibular joint, 21116
  tendon, 20550-20551
  therapeutic, 96365-96379
    extremity pseudoaneurysm,
      36002
    lung, 32960
    thyroid, 60300
    turbinate, 30200
  trachea, 31612
  transforaminal epidural,
    0228T-0231T
  transtracheal, 31899
  trigger point(s)
    one or two muscles, 20552
    three or more muscles, 20553
  turbinate, 30200
  ureter
    drugs, 50391
    radiologic, 50684
  venography, 36005
  ventricle
    dye, 61120
    medication or other, 61026
  vitreous, 67028
    fluid substitute, 67025
  vocal cords, 31513, 31570-31571
  wrist
    carpal tunnel, therapeutic, 20526
    radiologic, 25246
Inner ear
  canalith repositioning, 95992
  cochlear device, 69930
  computed tomography (CT) scan,
    70480-70482
  endolymphatic sac, 69805-69806
  labyrinth
    excision, 69905-69910
    incision, 69801-69802

Inner ear — *continued*
  semicurcular canal
    incision, 69840
    insertion, 69820
Innominate
  artery
    angioplasty, 35458
    atherectomy, 0237T
    catheter, 36215-36218
  tumor, 27077
INR test review, 99363-99364
Insemination, 58321-58322, 89268
Insertion
  abdomen
    catheter, 49324, 49419-
      49421, 49435
    artery, 36245-36248
    shunt, 49425-49426
  aorta
    catheter, 36200
    graft, 33330-33335
    needle, 36160
  artery
    abdominal
      catheter, 36245-36248
    brachiocephalic, 36215-36218
    extremity
      catheter, 36245-36248
    iliac
      occlusion device, 34808
    pelvic
      catheter, 36245-36248
    pulmonary
      catheter, 36013-36015
    thoracic
      catheter, 36215-36218
    to vein
      cannula, 36810-36815
      shunt, 36145
  bile duct
    catheter, 47533-47534
    stent, 43274, 47538-47540,
      47801
  bladder
    catheter, 51045, 51701-51703
      indwelling, 50605
    radioactive material, 51020,
      52250
    stent, 51045
  bone
    cochlear stimulator, 69714-
      69718
    needle, 36680
    pin, 20650
    vascular pedicle, 25430
    wire, 20650
  brain
    catheter, 0169T, 61210, 61770
    electrode, 61531-61533,
      61760, 61850-61870
    cerebrum, 61760
    cortical, 61850-61860, 61870
    subcortical, 61863-61868,
      61870
    subdural, 61531-61533
    probe, 61770
    pulse generator, 61885-61886
    reservoir, 61210-61215
  breast
    catheter, 0169T, 19296-19298,
      20555, 41019
    implant, 19340-19342
  bronchus
    catheter, 31643, 31717
    valve, 31647, 31651
  cardiac
    catheter, 33621, 93503
  cervix
    dilator, 59200
    laminaria, 59200
    prostaglandin, 59200
  colon
    tube, 49442
  duodenum
    tube, 49441
  ear
    cochlear device, 69930
    tube, 69433-69436

Influenza – Insertion

Insertion — *continued*
  esophagus
    stent, 43212
    tamponade, 43460
    tube, 43510
  eye
    aqueous
      drainage device, 66183
      shunt, 66179-66180
    conjunctival stent, 68750
    lacrimal duct
      implant, 0356T
      stent, 68815
    lens, 66982-66985
    muscle, 65135-65155
    ocular telescope prosthesis, 0308T
    orbit, 67550
    retinal electrode, 0100T
    scleral implant, 65130
  gastrointestinal
    catheter, 43241
    guide wire, 43226, 43248
    stent, 43266, 44370, 44379, 44384, 44402, 45327, 45347, 45389
    tube, 43241
  hand
    graft, 26392
    vascular pedicle, 25430
  heart
    electrode, 93620-93622
      epicardial, 33202-33203
      pacing, 33224-33225
      transvenous, 33210-33211, 33216-33217
    pacemaker, 33206-33208
    generator, 33212-33213, 33221
    permanent leadless, ventricular, 0387T
    right, catheter, 36013
    ventricular assist device, 33975
  vessel
    graft, 33330-33335
  intracardiac monitoring system, 0302T-0304T
  intra-aortic
    balloon, 33967, 33973
  intra-arterial
    infusion pump, 36260
    needle, 36100-36140
  intravenous
    infusion pump, 36563
    needle, 36000
  jejunum
    catheter, 44015
    tube, 44372, 49441
  kidney
    catheter, 50432-50433
    guide, 50395
  larynx
    keel, 31580
    obturator, 31527
  left atrial monitor, 0293T-0294T
  liver shunt, 37182
  knee prosthesis, 27438, 27445
  nerve
    electrode, 64553-64581
    neurostimulator, 64590
  nose
    catheter, 31720
    prosthesis, 30220
  palate
    prosthesis, 42281
  pancreatic stent, 43274
  pelvic mesh, 57267
  penile prosthesis, 54400-54405
  peritoneum, catheter, tunneled, 49324, 49419-49421
  pleural cavity catheter, 32550
  prostate
    catheter, 55875
    needle, 55875-55876
    radioactive substance, 55860
  skin
    drug delivery implant, 11981, 11983

Insertion — *continued*
  skin — *continued*
    expander, 11960-11971
    reservoir, 49419
  skull catheter, 61107
  sphenoid electrode, 95830
  spine
    catheter, 62350-62351
    distraction device, 0171T-0172T
    electrode, 63650-63655
    infusion pump, 62361-62362
    instrument, 22849
      anterior, 22845-22847
      fixation, 22841
        pelvic, 22848
      posterior
        nonsegmental, 22840
        segmental, 22842-22844
      process, 0171T-0172T, 22841
      prosthetic device, 22851
    pulse generator, 63685
    reservoir, 62360
  stomach
    electrode, 0155T, 0157T, 43647, 43881
    gastrostomy tube, 43246, 43653
  suprapubic catheter, 51010
  testicular prosthesis, 54660
  thoracic duct cannula, 38794
  trachea
    bronchial
      catheter, 31725
    catheter, 31700
    endotrachea tube, 31500
    naso
      catheter, 31720
      needle wire, 31730
    tube, 31730
  ureter
    catheter, 50433
    guide, 50395
      wire, 52334
    stent, 50605, 50693-50695, 50947, 52332
  urethra
    catheter, 51701-51703
    prosthesis, 53444-53445
    stent, 0084T, 52282
  uterus
    capsule, 58346
    intrauterine device (IUD), 58300
    oviduct, 58350
    tandem, 57155
  vagina
    interloading apparatus, 57156
    ovoid, 57155
    packing, 57180
    pessary, 57160
  vein
    access device, 36560-36566, 36570-36571
    cannula, 36800
    catheter, 36011-36012, 36400-36410, 36420-36425, 36500-36510, 36555-36558, 36568-36569
    central, 36555-36558
      peripheral (PICC), 36568-36569
    selective, 36011-36012
    sampling, 36500
    umbilical, 36510
    venipuncture, 36400-36410, 36420-36425
  portal catheter, 36481
  shunt, 49425-49426
  vena cava
    catheter, 36010
    filter, 37191

Instillation
  bladder, 51720
  kidney, 50391
  ureter, 50391

Instrumentation
  spinal
    insertion, 22840-22848, 22851
    reinsertion, 22849
    removal, 22850, 22852-22955

Insufflation, 69420-69421
Insulin, 80422, 80432-80435
  antibody, 86337
  blood, 83525
  C peptide, 80432, 84681
  free, 83527
  like growth factor, 84305
Insurance
  basic life/disablilty
    evaluation services, 99450
    examination, 99450-99456
Integumentary system, 00300, 00400-00410
  biopsy, 11100-11101
  breast
    ablation, 19105
    excision, 19100-19101, 19110-19272, 19300-19307
    incision, 19000-19030
    metallic localization clip placement, 19281-19288
    needle localization, 19281-19288
    reconstruction, 19316-19396
    repair, 19316-19396
  burns, 16000-16030
    autograft, 15100-15101, 15120-15121
    escharotomy, 16035-16036
    preparation, 15002-15005
    xenograft, 15400-15401
  debridement, 11000-11006, 11010-11044
  destruction
    actinotherapy, 96900
    chemical exfoliation, 17360
    cryotherapy, 17340
    electrolysis epilation, 17380
    lesion
      benign, 17000-17004
      malignant, 17260-17286
      photodynamic therapy, 96567-96571
      premalignant, 17000-17004
    Mohs' micrographic surgery, 17311-17315
    photodynamic therapy, 96567-96571
  excision
    benign, 11400-11471
    malignant, 11600-11646
  grafts
    allograft, 15300
    allogenic, 15300-15366
    autograft, 15040-15157
    preparation, 15002-15005
    replacement, 15170-15176
    xenograft, 15400-15431
  incision
    drainage
      acne, 10040
      abscess, 10060-10061, 10160
      bulla, 10160
      cyst, 10080-10081, 10160
      fluid, 10140
      hematoma, 10140-10160
      infection, 10180
      seroma, 10140
    introduction, 11900-11977, 11981, 11983
  nails, 11720-11765
  paring, 11055-11057
  photography, 96904
  removal, 11200-11201, 11982-11983
  repair, 15780-15879
    complex, 13100-13160
    flaps, 15740-15776
    grafts, 15050-15136, 15200-15321, 15420-15431
    intermediate, 12031-12057
    simple, 12001-12021
    skin, 15570-15738
    transfer, 14000-14350
  shaving, 11300-11313
  ulcers, 15920-15958
Intelligence test, 96101-96103

Intercarpal joint, 25447, 25660
  arthrodesis, 25820-25825
Intercostal nerve, 64620
  injection, 64420-64421, 64620
Interdental
  fixation, 21110, 21453, 21462, 21497
  wire, 21431
Interferometry, 92136
Internal
  ear
    cochlear device, 69930
    computed tomography (CT) scan, 70480-70482
    endolymphatic sac, 69805-69806
    labyrinth
      excision, 69905-69910
      incision, 69801-69802
    semicurcular canal
      incision, 69840
      insertion, 69820
  fixation, 20650, 20670-20680
  arm
    humerus, 24498, 24515-24516
      epicondylar, 24575, 24579
      Monteggia, 24635
      supracondylar, 24545-24546
      radial, 24665-24666, 25515, 25525-25526, 25574-25575
      ulnar, 24685, 25545, 25574-25575
    foot, 28300
      calcaneal, 28415-28420
      interphalangeal, 28675
      metatarsal, 28485
      metatarsophalangeal, 28645
      phalanx, 28505, 28525
      sesamoid, 28531
      talotarsal, 28585
      talus, 28445
      tarsal, 28465, 28555
      tarsometatarsal, 28615
    hand, 26390-26392, 26415-26416
      carpometacarpal, 26665, 26685, 26841-26842
      interphalangeal, 26785, 26860-26863
      metacarpal, 26546, 26615
      metacarpophalangeal, 26715, 26746, 26850-26852
      phalanx, 26546, 26735, 26765
    head, 21497
      craniofacial, 21431-21432, 21435-21436
      malar, 21365
      mandibular, 21453, 21461-21462, 21470
      maxillary, 21421
      nasal, 21330
      nasoethmoid, 21340
      nasomaxillary, 21345-21346
      palatal, 21421
      temporomandibular, 21485
    hip, 27254
      acetabular wall, 27226-27228
      femoral, 27177-27178, 27181, 27187, 27236, 27269
      iliac, 27215
      ring, 27217-27218
      trochanteric, 27165, 27244-27245, 27248
    leg, 27358
      ankle, 27814, 27823, 27848-27860
      femur, 27450, 27507
        condylar, 27511-27514
        epiphyseal, 27519
      fibula, 27726, 27784, 27792

CPT © 2015 American Medical Association. All Rights Reserved.

Internal — *continued*
  fixation — *continued*
    leg — *continued*
      knee, 27540, 27556-27558,
        27570, 29851, 29885,
        29887, 29892
      malleolus, 27766, 27769
      patella, 27524
      tibia, 27535-27536, 27758-
        27759, 27826-27829,
        27832, 29855-29856
    mandibular, 21196
    shoulder, 23680
      clavicle, 23480-23490,
        23515
      humerus, 23491, 23615-
        23616
        tuberosity, 23630, 23670
      scapular, 23585
    spinal, 22318-22319, 22841,
      22851
    wrist, 25332
      carpal, 25431-25440, 25629
      radial, 25607-25609
  prosthesis
    breast, 19328-19330, 19340-
      19342, 19396

Internet
  assessment/management,
    interprofessional, 99446-
    99449

Interphalangeal joint
  biopsy, 26110, 28054

Intersex
  state, 56805, 57335
  surgery, 55970, 55980

Interstitial
  cell stimulator, 80418, 80426,
    83002
  cystitis, 52260-52265
  fluid pressure, 20950

Intertarsal joint
  arthrotomy, 28020
  biopsy, 28050
  excision, 28070

Interthoracoscapular amputation,
  23900

Intertrochanteric fracture, 24238,
  27244

Intervetebral
  chemonucleolysis, 62292
  disc
    annuloplasty, 22526-22527
    arthroplasty, 0098T,
      0163T-0165T, 22856-
      22858
      lumbar, 0163T, 22857-
      22862, 22865
    discography, 72285, 72295
    excision, 63075-63078
      herniated, 63020-63044,
      63055-63066
    x-ray, 62290-62291

Intestine
  allotransplantation, 44135-44136
  anastomosis, 47760-47785,
    50800, 50810, 50820-
    50825, 51590, 51960
  biopsy, 44010, 44025, 44100,
    44322
  cecostomy, 44188, 44322
    tube, 44300
  cholecystoenterostomy, 47720-
    47741
  closure
    enterostomy, 44227, 44620-
      44626
    fistula, 44640-44661
  colectomy
    partial, 44140-44147
      laparoscopy, 44204-44208
      mobilization, 44139, 44213
    total, 44150-44160
      laparoscopy, 44210-44212
  colostomy, 44188, 44320-44346
  correction, 44055
  enterectomy, 44132-44133

Intestine — *continued*
  enteroenterostomy, 44130
  enterolysis, 44005
    laparoscopy, 44180
  enterostomy, 44300
  excision
    lesion, 44110-44111
  exploration, 44010, 44025
  hepaticoenterostomy, 47802
  ileostomy, 44187, 44310-44316,
    45136
  imaging, 78290
  introduction, 44500
  invagination, 74283
  jujenostomy, 44015, 44310, 44373,
    49441, 49451-49452
    laparoscopy, 44186-44187
  large
    colonoscopy, 45378-45393,
      45398
      ablation, 44401, 45388
      biopsy, 44389, 45380,
        45391-45392
      removal
        foreign body, 44390,
          45379
        lesion, 44392, 44394,
          45384-45385
      ultrasound, 45391-45392
    colostomy, 45395
    computed tomography (CT)
      scan, 0066T-0067T
    creation, 45397
    enterostomy, 45119
    lavage, 44701
    suture, 44604-44605
    x-ray, 74270-74280
  peptide, 84586
  plication, 44680
  reduction, 44050
  removal
    allograft, 44137
    foreign body, 44010, 44025
  sigmoid
    biopsy, 45331
    proctosigmoidoscopy, 45300-
      45303, 45317, 45321
      ablation, 45320
      biopsy, 45305
      placement, 45327
      removal
        foreign body, 45307
        lesion, 45308-45315
    sigmoidoscopy, 45330-45350
      ablation, 45346
      band ligation, 45350
      biopsy, 45331
      mucosal resection, 45349
      placement, stent, 45347
      removal
        foreign body, 45332
        lesion, 45333, 45338
      ultrasound, 45341-45342
  small
    endoscopy, 00810, 44360,
      44366, 44376, 44378
      ablation, 44369
      biopsy, 44361, 44377
      evaluation, 44385-44386
      placement, 44370-44372,
        44379
      removal
        foreign body, 44363
        lesion, 44364-44365
    enterectomy, 44120-44128
      laparoscopy, 44202-44203
    enterocele, 57268, 57270
    enterotomy, 44020-44021
    exclusion, 44700
    ileoileostomy, 43845
    ileoscopy, 44380-44386
    specimen collection, 43756-
      43757
    suture, 44602-44603
    x-ray, 74250-74251
  strictureoplasty, 44615
  transplantation
    preparation, 44715-44721

Intima media thickness (IMT), 0126T
Intimectomy, 33572, 33916
Intra-
  abdominal voiding, 51797
  arterial injection, 37184-37186,
    61645, 96373, 96379
  capsular extraction, 66920, 66930
  osseous infusion, 36680

Intracardiac echocardiogram, 93662
Intracranial
  adhesions, 62161
  anastomosis, 61711
  aneurysm, 61697-61710
  angioplasty, 61630
  arterial perfusion, 61624
  biopsy, 61140
  electrode, 61880
  lesion, 61750-61751
  malformation, 61680-61692
  neoplasm
    craniopharyngioma, 61545
    mengioma, 61512, 61519
  neuroendoscopy, 62160-62165
  occlusion, 61623-61626
  stent, 61635
  stereotactic, 61781-61783
  vasospasm, 61640-61642

Intramuscular injection, 96372,
  96379, 99506
Intraocular, 3284F-3285F, 3325F
  lens, 66982-66986
  radiation, 0190T
Intratracheal intubation, 31500
Intrauterine
  adhesions, 58559
  contraceptive device (IUD), 58300-
    58301
Intravascular
  pressure study, 93982
  stent, 0075T-0076T, 37215-37216
  ultrasound, 37252-37253
Intravenous
  infusion, 96360-96361
  injection, 15860
    thrombolytic, 37187-37188
  pyelogram, 74400-74415
  radiopharmaceutical, 78808
  therapy, 96365-96368
Intravesical instillation, 51720
Intravitreal injection, 67028
Intrisic factor, 83528, 86340
Introduction
  breast, 19281-19288
  capsules, 11975-11977
  drug delivery, 11981, 11983
  tissue expander, 11960-11971
  tube, long gastrointestinal, 44500,
    74340
Intubation
  duodenal, 43756-43757
  endotracheal, 31500
  gastric, 43753-43755
Invagination, 44050, 74283
Inversion, 19355
Ionization, 89230, 97033
Iridectomy
  corneal/corneoscleral section,
    66600
  laser, 66761
  peripheral, 66625
  sclerotomy, 66160
  thermocauterization, 66155
  transfixion, 66605
  trephination, 66150
Iridodialysis, 66680
Iridoplasty, 66762
Iridotomy
  excision
    optical, 66635
    peripheral, 66625
    corneal/corneoscleral section,
      66600
    cyclectomy, 66605

Iridotomy — *continued*
  incision
    stab, 66500
    transfixion, 66505
  laser, 66761
  optical, 66635
  peripherally, 66625
  sector, 66630
Iris
  destruction, 66761-66762, 66770
  excision, 66600-66635
  incision, 66500-66505
  repair, 66680-66682
Iron, 83540
  binding capacity, 83550
  plan of care, 0516F
  stain, 85536, 88313
    hematoxylin, 88312
Irradiation, 0520F, 86945
Irrigation
  bladder, 51700
  brain, 62194, 62225
  corpora cavernosa, 54220
  penis, 54220
  sinus tract
    maxillary, 31000
    sphenoid, 31002
  spinal cord, 63744
  vagina, 57150
  venous access device, 96523
Irving sterilization, 58600-58611,
  58670
Ischial
  bursa, 27060
  tumor, 27078-27079
Ischiectomy, 15941
Island pedicle flaps, 15740
Islet cell
  antibody, 86341
  transplantation, 0141T-0143T
Isocitrate dehydrogenase, 83570
Isolation, 89260-89261
Isomerase, phosphohexose, 84087
Isopropanol, 80320
Isthmusectomy, 60210, 60225
Ivy bleeding time, 85002

J

Jaboulay operation, 43810, 43850-
  43855
Janeway procedure, 43832
Jannetta procedure, 61458
Japanese
  encephalitis, 90738
  river fever, 86000
Jatene type, 33770-33781
Jaw
  augmentation, mandible
    bone graft, 21127
    prosthetic, 21125
  fracture/dislocation treatment
    mandible, closed, 21440,
      21450-21451, 21453
    mandible, open, 21445,
      21454-21470
    maxilla, closed, 21421, 21440
    maxilla, open, 21422-21423,
      21445
    temporomandibular joint,
      closed, 21480-21485
    temporomandibular joint, open,
      21490
  interdental fixation/wiring, 21110,
    20670-20680, 21453,
    21462, 21470, 21497
  manipulation, 21073
  muscle reduction, 21295-21296
  osteomyelitis
    mandible, 21025
    arthroplasty, 21240-21243
  percutaneous treatment, 21452

Jaw — continued
reconstruction
mandible, 21244-21249
maxilla, 21245-21246, 21248-21249
temporomandibular joint
arthrocentesis, 20605-20606
arthrography, 70328-70332
arthroplasty, 21240-21243
arthroscopy, 29800-29804
arthrotomy, 21010
condylectomy, 21050
injection, 21116, 70332
magnetic resonance imaging (MRI), 70336
manipulation, 21073
meniscectomy, 21060
x-ray, 70328-70332
tumor excision
benign
mandible, 21040, 21046-21047
maxilla, 21030, 21048-21049
malignant
mandible, 21044-21045
maxilla, 21034
x-ray, 70100-70110, 70328-70332, 70355

Jejunostomy
catheter, 44015
contrast injection, 49465
laparoscopic, 44186-44187
non-tube, 44310
obstructive material, 49460
tube
placement, 49441
replacement, 49451
with pancreatic drain, 48001

Jejunum, 43496, 44186

Johannsen procedure, 53400

Joint
acromioclavicular
arthrography, 23350, 73040
arthroplasty, 23470-23472
arthrotomy, 23044
dislocation, 23550-23552
ankle
arthrocentesis, 20605-20606
arthrodesis, 27870
arthrography, 27648, 73615
arthroplasty, 27700-27703
arthroscopy, 29891-29899
arthrotomy, 27610-27612, 27620-27626
biopsy, 27613-27614, 27620
dislocation/fracture treatment, 27840-27848
injection, 27648
manipulation, 27860
x-ray, 73600-73610
antiinflammatory, 4016F
arthrodesis
spinal deformity, 22800-22812
spinal fusion, 22830
aspiration, 20600-20611
carpometacarpal
arthrodesis, 25800-25810, 26841-26844
arthrography, 25246, 73115
arthroplasty, 25443, 25447
arthrotomy, 26070, 26100
biopsy, 26100
dislocation, 26670-26676, 26685-26686
prosthesis, 25250-25251
elbow
arthrectomy, 24155
arthrocentesis, 20605-20606
arthrodesis, 24800-24802
arthrography, 24220, 73085
arthroplasty, 24360-24366
arthroscopy, 29830-29838
arthrotomy, 24000-24006, 24100-24102
biopsy, 24065-24066, 24101

Joint — continued
elbow — continued
dislocation/fracture treatment, 24600-24615, 24620-24635, 24586-24587, 24640
injection, 24220
manipulation, 24300
x-ray, 73070-73080
fibulotalar
arthrodesis, 29899
glenohumeral
arthrocentesis, 20610-20611
arthrodesis, 23800-23802
arthrography, 23350, 73040
arthroplasty, 23470-23472
arthroscopy, 29805-29828
arthrotomy, 23100-23107
biopsy, 23100-23106
dislocation/fracture treatment, 23650-23680
injection, 23350
manipulation, 23700
x-ray, 73020-73030
hip, 01200-01215
arthrocentesis, 20610-20611
arthrodesis, 27284-27286
arthrography, 27093-27095, 73525
arthroplasty, 27125, 27130-27138
arthroscopy, 29860-29863
arthrotomy, 27030-27033, 27052-27054
biopsy, 27052
dislocation/fracture treatment, 27250-27266
injection, 27093-27096
manipulation, 27275
prosthesis, 27090-27091
x-ray
bilateral, 73521-73523
unilateral, 73501-73503
injection, 20600-20611
intercarpal
arthrodesis, 25800-25825
arthrography, 25246, 73115
arthroplasty, 25443, 25447
dislocation, 25660, 25670
repair, 25447
interphalangeal
arthrodesis, 26860-26863, 28755, 28760
arthroplasty, 26535-26536
arthrotomy, 26080, 28024, 28054
biopsy, 26110, 28054
dislocation, 26340, 26770, 26776, 26785, 28660-28666, 28675
excision, 26140, 26525, 28160
fracture, 26740, 26742, 26746
fusion, 26860-26863, 28755, 28760
incision, 26525
repair, 26545, 26548
intertarsal
arthrotomy, 28020, 28050
biopsy, 28050
excision, 28070
intervertebral
arthrodesis
cervical, 22548, 22554, 22590-22600
lumbar, 22533-22534, 22558, 22585, 22612-22614, 22630-22632
thoracic, 22532, 22534, 22556, 22610
arthroplasty, 0095T-0098T, 0163T-0165T, 0375T, 22856-22865
dislocation, 22305-22328
prosthesis, 22851
knee, 01380-01382
arthrocentesis, 20610-20611
arthrodesis, 27580
arthrography, 27370, 73580

Joint — continued
knee — continued
arthroplasty, 27437-27447, 27486-27487
arthroscopy, 01400-01404, 29870-29887
arthrotomy, 27310, 27330-27335, 27403
biopsy, 27323-27324, 27330-27331
dislocation/fracture treatment, 01420, 27520-27524, 27550-27566, 29850-29851
injection, 27370
manipulation, 27570
prosthesis, 27438, 27445
x-ray, 73560-73565
magnetic resonance imaging (MRI)
lower extremity joint, 73721-73723
upper extremity joint, 73221-73223
metacarpohalangeal
arthrodesis, 26850-26852
arthrography, 25246, 73115
arthroplasty 26530-26531
arthroscopy, 01382, 29900-29902
arthrotomy, 26075, 26105
biopsy, 26105
capsulodesis, 26516-26518
dislocation, 26340, 26700-26706, 26715
excision, 26135, 26520
fracture, 26740, 26742, 26746
fusion, 26516-26518, 26850-26852
repair, 26540-26542
metatarsophalangeal
arthrodesis, 28750
arthrotomy, 28022, 28052
biopsy, 28052
dislocation, 28630-28636, 28645
excision, 28072
fusion, 28750
repair, 28270, 28289
midcarpal midioccipital, 25040
nuclear imaging, 78300-78320
pubis symphysis, 01160-01170
arthrodesis, 27282
radiocarpal
arthrodesis, 25800-25825
arthrography, 25246, 73115
arthroplasty, 25441, 25443, 25447
arthrotomy, 25040
dislocation, 25660, 25670
radioulnar
arthrodesis, 25830
arthrography, 25246, 73115
arthroplasty, 25447, 25441-25442
dislocation, 25520-25526, 25671, 25675-25676
sacroiliac, 01160-01170
arthrodesis, 27279-27280
arthrography, 27096
arthrotomy, 27050
biopsy, 27050
dislocation, 27218
x-ray, 72200-72202, 73542
sternoclavicular
arthrotomy, 23044, 23101, 23106
dislocation, 23520-23532
stress application, 77071
survey, 77077
talotarsal
dislocation, 28570-28576, 28585
magnetic resonance imaging (MRI), 73721-73723
stabilization, 0335T
talus
arthrodesis, 28705-28725, 29907

Joint — continued
talus — continued
dislocation, 28546, 28570-28576, 28585
tarsal
arthrodesis, 28122, 28730-28735, 28737, 28740
excision, 28104-28107, 28116, 28122, 28171
dislocation, 28540-28546, 28555
fracture, 28450, 28455-28456, 28465
repair, 28304-28305, 28320
tarsometatarsal
arthrodesis, 28730-28735, 28740
arthrotomy, 28020, 28050
biopsy, 28050
dislocation, 28600-28606, 28615
excision, 28070
magnetic resonance imaging (MRI), 73721-73723
temporomandibular joint
arthrocentesis, 20605-20606
arthrography, 21116, 70328-70332
arthroplasty, 21240-21243
arthroscopy, 29800-29804
arthrotomy, 21010
condylectomy, 21050
dislocation, 21480-21485, 21490
injection, 21116, 70332
manipulation, 21073
meniscectomy, 21060
magnetic resonance imaging (MRI), 70336
x-ray, 70328-70332
tibiofibular
arthrodesis, 27871
dislocation, 27830-27832
tibiotalar
arthrodesis, 29899

Jones procedure, 28760

Joplin procedure, 28294

Jugal bone
excision, 21030, 21034
fracture
closed, 21355
open, 21360-21366
reconstruction, 21270

Jugular vein, 62190, 75860

K

K wire fixation, 41500
Kala Azar smear, 87207
Kallidin, 82286
Kallikrein, 84152-84153
Kasai procedure, 47701
Kedani fever, 86000
Keel, 31580
Kelikian procedure, 28280
Keller procedure, 28292
Keratectomy, 65400
Keratomileusis, 65760
Keratophakia, 65765
Keratoplasty, 65710-65757
Keratoprosthesis, 65770
Keratosteroids, 83586-83593
Keratotomy, 65771
Ketone bodies, 82009-82010
Kidner procedure, 28238
Kidney
ablation, 50250, 50541-50542, 50592-50593
cryosurgical, 50250
cryotherapy, 50593
laparoscopic, 50541-50542
radiofrequency, 50592
abscess, 50020
aspiration, 50390

CPT © 2015 American Medical Association. All Rights Reserved.   © 2016 DecisionHealth

Kidney — *continued*
biopsy
endoluminal, 50606
endoscopic, 50555-50557, 50574-50576, 52354
open, 50205
percutaneous, 50200
calculus removal/destruction
endoscopic, 50561, 50580
lithotripsy, 50590, 52353
open incisional, 50060-50065, 50075, 50130
catheterization, 50432-50433, 50572
cyst study, 74470
dilation, 50395, 50553, 52343, 52346
endoscopy, 50551-50580
tumor resection, 50562
with biopsy, 50555-50557, 50574, 50576, 52354
with ureteral catheterization, 50553, 50572
excision
cyst, 50280-50290
donor, 50300-50320, 50547
laparoscopic, 50543, 50547, 50545-50548
partial, 50240, 50543
radical, 50230, 50545
recipient, 50340
tumor, 52355
with ureters, 50220-50236, 50546, 50548
exploration, 50010, 50045, 50120, 52351
foreign body removal, 50561, 50580
nephrostomy tube, 50389
function study, 78725
incision, 50010, 50045
drainage, 50040, 50125
injection
cyst, 50390
for nephrostogram/ureterogram, 50430-50431
therapeutic agent, 50391
laparoscopy, 50541-50549
lithotripsy, 50590, 52353, 52356
manometry, 50396
nuclear imaging, 78700-78710
removal
foreign body, 50561-50580
suture, 50500, 50520-50526, 50540
transplantation, 50300-50380
backbench preparation, 50323-50329
tube, 50389, 50398
ultrasound, 76770-76776
ureteral stent, 50382-50387
Kinase, 82550-82552
Kineplasty, 24940
Kinetic therapy, 97530
Kininase, 82164
Kininogen, 85293
Kleihauer Betke test, 85460
Kloramfenikol, 82405
Knee, 01320-01444
arthrocentesis, 20610-20611
arthrodesis, 27580
arthrography, 73580
arthroplasty, 01402, 27440-27447, 27486-27487
arthroscopy, 01382, 01400-01404, 29870-29887
arthrotomy, 27310, 27330-27335, 27403
Baker's cyst, 27345
biopsy, 27323-27324, 27330-27331
chondromalacia, 27418
disarticulation, 01404, 27598
dislocation/fracture treatment, 01420, 27520-27524, 27550-27566, 29850-29851

Knee — *continued*
excision
bursa, 27340
cap, 27350
cartilage, 27332-27333
cyst, 27345-27347
lesion, 27347
synovium, 27334-27335
tumor, 27327-27329, 27365
exploration, 27310, 27331
foreign body removal, 27310
deep, 27372
loose body, 27331
prosthesis, 27488
fusion, 27580
incision
capsule, 27435
drainage, 27301-27303, 27310
fasiotomy, 27305, 27496-27499
injection, 27370
magnetic resonance imaging (MRI), 73721-73723
manipulation, 27570
meniscectomy, 27332-27333
osteochondral graft, 27412-27416, 29866-29867
prosthesis, 27438, 27445, 27488
reconstruction, 27445
cap, 27424, 27437-27438
ligament, 27427-27429
patella, 27437-27438
release, 27425
removal, 27310, 27331, 27372, 27488
repair, 27403-27409
cap, 27420-27424
tendon, 27380-27381
replacement, 27447
kinetic balance sensor use, 0396T
strapping, 29530
transplantation
chonodrocytes, 27412
graft, 27412, 27415, 29866-29867
meniscus, 29868
x-ray, 73560-73565, 73580
Kock
formation, 50825
procedure, 44316
Kraske procedure, 45116
Kroenlein procedure, 67420
Krukenberg procedure, 25915
Kuhlmann test, 96101-96103
Kyphectomy, 22818-22819
Kyphoplasty, 22513-22515

L

Labial adhesion, 56441
Labyrinth
excision, 69905-69910, 61596
incision, 69801
Laceration
repair
conjunctiva, 65270-65273
cornea, 65275-65286
diaphragm, 39501
esophagogastric, 43502
mouth, 40830-40831
palate, 42180-42182
tongue, 41250-41252
Lacrimal
duct
dilation, 68816
exploration, 68810-68811, 68815, 68840
removal, 68530
repair, 68700
x-ray, 70170
foreign body removal, 68530
gland
biopsy, 68510
closure, 68770
drainage, 68400
excision, 68500-68505
tumor, 68540-68550

Lacrimal— *continued*
gland— *continued*
fistulization, 68720
nuclear medicine, 78660
removal, 68530
repair, 68770
x-ray, 68850, 70170
punctum
closure, 68760-68761
dilation, 68801
incision, 68440
repair, 68705
sac
biopsy, 68525
drainage, 68420
excision, 68520
fistulization, 68720
Lactase deficiency test, 91065
Lactate, 83605
Lactic
acid, 83605
dehydrogenase, 83615-83625
duct, 19110, 19112
Lactoferrin, 83630-83631
Lactogen, 83632
hormone, 80418, 84146
Lactose, 83633
Ladd procedure, 44055
Lagopthalmos, 67912
Laki Lorand factor, 85290-85291
Lamblia intestinalis, 86674
Lamellar keratoplasty, 65710
Laminectomy, 63191
catheter, 62351
cervical, 61343, 63180-63182
cordotomy, 63194, 63196, 63198
decompression, 63045, 63048, 0274T
exploration, 63001, 63015
drainage, 63172-63173
interspace preparation, 22630-22632
lesion, 63265-3273
lumbar, 63005, 63012, 63017
decompression, 63047-63048, 0275T
release, 63200
malformation, 63250-63252
myelotomy, 63170
neoplasm, 63275-63290
rhizotomy, 63185-63190
sacral, 63011
thoracic, 63003, 63016
cordotomy, 63195, 63197, 63199
decompression, 63046, 63048, 0274T
Laminoplasty, 63050-63051
Language
evaluation, 92523
therapy, 92507-92508
Laparoscopy, 0143T
abdominal, 49320-49329, 49650-49657
adrenal, 50545, 60650
appendiceal, 44970-44979
biliary tract, 47562-47579
bladder, 51990-51999
espohageal, 43279-43289
fallopian tube, 59150-59151
gastric, 0155T-0156T, 43644-43659, 43770-43774, 43848, 43886-43888
intestinal, 44180-44238,
liver, 47370-47379
lymphatic, 38570-38589
ovary/oviducts, 49322, 58660-58679
prostate, 55866
renal, 50541-50549
rectal, 45395-45499
spermatic cord, 55550
spleen, 38120-38219, 44213
testicular, 54690-54699
ureteral, 50945-50949
uterus, 58541-58554, 58570-58578
vagina, 57425

Laparotomy
biopsy, 49000
bleeding, 49002
electrode
implantation, 0157T, 43881
removal, 0158T, 43882
exploration, 35840, 47015, 49000-49002
staging, 49220, 58960
Lapidus procedure, 28297
Laroyenne operation, 57010
Larynx, 00320-00326
aspiration, 31515
biopsy, 31510, 31535-31536, 31576
electromyography, 95865
excision
lesion, 31512, 31545-31546, 31578
tumor, 31300, 31540-31541
laryngeal
reinnervation, 31590
study, 92520
testing, 92614-92617
laryngectomy
partial, 31370-31382
subtotal, 31367-31368
total, 31360-31365
laryngocele, 31300
laryngoscopy
direct, 31515-31571
flexible fiberoptic, 31575-31579
indirect, 31505-31513
laryngopharyngectomy, 31390-31395
laryngoplasty, 31580-31588
laryngoscopy, 31505-31579
laryngotomy, 31300-31320
nerve, 31590-31595
removal, 31511-31512, 31530-31531, 31545-31546, 31577-31578
section, 31595
vocal cords, 31513, 31570-31571
x-ray, 70370-70371
Laser
revascularization
transmyocardial, 33141-33141
surgery
anal, 46614, 46917, 46924
arms, 17260-17266
bladder, 52214-52346
cervix, 57513-57520
choroid, 67220
ears, 17280-17286
esophagus, 43227
eye
chamber, 65855-65860
iris, 66761
lens, 66821
vitreous, 67031, 67043
face, 17280-17286
feet, 17270-17276
genitalia, 17270-17276
penis, 54057, 54065
vagina, 57061-57065
vulva, 56501-56515
hands, 17270-17276
intestines, 44366, 44378, 44391, 45317-45320, 45334, 45382
lacrimal punctum, 68760
legs, 17260-17266
lips, 17280-17286
mouth, 40820
myocardium, 33140-33141
neck, 17270-17276
nose, 17280-17286, 30117-30118
prostate, 52647-52649
rectum, 45190
scalp, 17270-17276
skin, 17000-17111, 17260-17286
trachea, 31641
trunk, 17260-17266

Laser — *continued*
  treatment
    skin, 17000-17286, 96920-96922

Lateral epicondylitis, 24357-24359

Latex fixation, 86403-86406

Lavage
  bladder, 51700
  colonic, 44701
  lung, 31624, 32997
  peritoneal, 49084
  sinuses, 31000-31002

Lead, 83655

Leadbetter procedure, 53431

Lecithin sphingomyelin ratio, 83661

Lecithinase C, 86812-86817, 86821-86822

Lee and White test, 85345

LEEP procedure, 57460

LeFort procedure
  I, 21141-21147, 21421-21423, 21155, 21160
  II, 21150-21151, 21345-21348
  III, 21154-21160, 21431-21436

Leg
  amputation
    lower, 27598, 27880-27886
    upper, 27590-27596
  application
    brace, 29358
    cast, 29305-29325, 29445-29450
      lower, 29405-29435, 49450
      upper, 29345-29355, 29365, 29450
    walker, 29440
  halo, 20663
  splint
    lower, 29515
    upper, 29505
  strapping, 29580
  biopsy
    lower, 27613-27614
    upper, 27323-27324
  computed tomography (CT) scan, 73700-73706, 75635
  destruction
    lower, 17260-17266
  excision
    lesion, 11400-11406, 11600-11606
      lower, 27630
    nerve
      lower, 27325-27326
    skin, 15833
    tumor
      lower, 27615-27619
      upper, 27327-27329
  exploration, 20103, 35860
  graft, 35286
    bypass, 01500-01502, 35903
    nerve, 64892-64893, 64897-64898
    skin, 15100-15111, 15130-15313, 15150-15152
    vein, 35256
  incision
    drainage
      abscess
        lower, 27603, 27607
        upper, 27301
      bursa
        lower, 27604
        upper, 27301
      fascia, 27600-27602, 27892-27894
        lower, 27600-27602, 27892-27894
        upper, 27305, 27496-27499, 27892-27894
  ligation, 37618
  magnetic resonance imaging (MRI), 73718-73720
  neuroplasty, 01470-01474, 64708-64714
  removal, 27372, 29705

Leg — *continued*
  repair
    fascia, 01470-01474, 27656
    muscle, 01470-01474, 27385-27386, 27400, 27430
    skin, 13120-13122, 14020-14021
    tendon, 01470-01474, 27658-27692
      lower, 27658-27692
      upper, 27306-27307, 27390-27392
    vessel, 01500-01522, 35226, 35256, 35286
  shaving, 11300-11303
  suture
    muscle, 27385-27386
    nerve, 64856-64857
    tendon, 27658-27665
  ultrasound, 76881-76881
  x-ray, 73592

Legionella, 86713
  antigen, 87540-87542
  micdadei, 87277
  pneumophila, 87278

Leiomyomata
  embolization, 37243
  removal, 58140, 58545-58546, 58561

Leishmania, 86717

Lens
  contact
    fitting, 92070, 92310-92313
    modification, 92325
    prescription, 92310-92317
    replacement, 92326
  incision, 66820-66825
  intraocular, 3325F
    insertion, 66982-66990
    power calculation, 92136
  removal, 66830-66940

Leptomeningioma, 61512, 61519

Leptospira, 86720

Leriche operation, 64809

Lesion
  ablation
    anal, 46615
    esophagus, 43229, 43270
    intracranial, MRI guided focused ultrasound, 0398T
    kidney, 50250, 50542
    large intestine, 44401, 45320, 45346, 45388
    renal, 50542
    small intestine, 44369
    upper gastrointestinal (GI) tract, 43270
  abrasion, 15786-15787
  analysis, skin, digital, 0400T-0401T
  biopsy
    nasopharynx, 42804-42806
    skin, 11100-11101
    ureteral, 52354
  chemotherapy, 0519F, 67220-67225, 96405-96406
  creation
    alcohol, 61790-61791
    brain, 61720-61735, 61790-61791, 61796-61799
    spinal cord, 63600
  cutting
    skin, 11055-11057
  destruction
    anus, 46900-46924
    bladder, 51030
    choroid, 67220-67225, 67299
    ciliary body, 66770
    colon, 44401, 45388
    conjunctiva, 68135
    cornea, 65450
    dentoalveolar structures, 41850
    eyelid, 67850
    intranasal, 30117-30118
    iris, 66770
    macular drusen, 67299

Lesion — *continued*
  destruction — *continued*
    oral structure, 40820, 41850, 42160
    ovary, 58662
    pelvis, 58662
    penis, 54050-54065
    pharynx, 42808
    retina, 67208-67218, 67299
    skin, 96567
      benign, 17110-17111
      malignant, 17260-17286
      premalignant, 17000-17004
      vascular proliferative, 17106-17108
    spinal, 63620-63621
    vagina, 57061-57065
    vulva, 56501-56515
  excision
    ankle, 27630
    arm, 25110
    auditory canal, 69145-69155
    brain, 61575-61576, 61600-61608, 61615-61616
    breast, 19120-19126
    colon, 44110-44111
    conjunctiva, 68110-68130
    cornea, 65400, 65420-65426
    dentoalveolar structures, 41822-41827
    ear, 69540
    epididymis, 54830
    esophagus, 43100-43101, 43216-43217
    foot, 28080, 28090
    hand, 26160
    intranasal, 30117-30118
    intraspinal, 63265-63273, 63300-63308
    knee, 27347
    leg, 27630
    lower extremity capsule, 25110, 26160, 27347, 27630, 28090-28092
    mandible, 21046-21047
    maxilla, 21048-21049
    mesentery, 44820
    mouth, 40812-40816, 41116, 42104-42107, 42160
    ovary, 58662
    pancreas, 48120
    pelvis, 58662
    pharynx, 42808
    sclera, 66130
    skin
      benign, 11400-11446
      hidradenitis, 11450-11471
      malignant, 11600-11646
    skull, 61500
    spermatic cord, 55520
    testis, 54512
    toe, 28092
    tongue, 41110-41114
    vertebra, 22110-22116
    vocal cord, 31545-31546
    wrist, 25110
  fulguration, 52224, 52354, 53265, 58662
  injection
    skin, 11900-11901
  paring/cutting
    hyperkeratotic, 11055-11057
  placement, localization device
    breast, 19281-19288
    soft tissue, 10035-10036
  radiosurgery, 63620-63621
  removal
    anus, 46610-46612
    esophagus, 43216-43217
    intestine, 44364-44365, 44392, 44394, 45308-45315, 45333, 45338, 45384-45385
    larynx, 31512, 31578
    orbit, 61333, 67412
    skin tags, 11200-11201
    upper gastrointestinal (GI) tract, 43250-43251

Lesion — *continued*
  resection
    brain, 61600-61608, 61615-61616
    palate, 42120
  shaving
    skin, 11300-11313
    cranial, 77371-77372, 77432

Leu 2, 86360

Leucine aminopeptidase, 83670

Leukemia
  lymphoma virus I, 86687, 86689
  lymphoma virus II, 86688
  myeloperoxidase (MPO), 83876
  oncoprotein, 83951

Leukoagglutinins, 86021

Levarternol, 82383-82384

Leveen shunt, 49425-49426
  test, 78291

Levulose, 82757, 84375

Lid
  biopsy, 67810
  blepharoplasty, 00103, 15820-15823
  drainage, 67700
  excision, 67800-67808, 67840-67850
  graft, 15115-15121, 15135-15136, 15155-15157, 15175-15176, 15260-15261, 15320-15321, 15335-15336, 15420-15421
  incision, 67700-67715
  reconstruction, 67950-67975
    wound, 67930-67935
  removal, 67938
  repair, 67900-67924
    lesion, 11310-11313, 11440-11446, 11640-11646, 17280-17286
    trichiasis, 67820-67835
    wound, 12011-12018, 12051-12057, 13151-13153, 67930-67935
  suture, 67875-67882

Lidocaine, 80176

Ligament
  injection, 20550
  reconstruction
    elbow, 24344, 24346, 24362
    hand, finger, 26541-26545
    knee, 27427-27429
  release
    coroacromial, 23130, 23415
    wrist, 29848
  repair
    ankle, 27695-27698
    canthal, 21340
    elbow, 24343, 24345
    hand, finger, 26540
    knee, 27405-27409, 27556-27558, 29888-29889

Ligation
  artery, 37607
    abdomen, 37617
    carotid, 37600-37606, 61610-61612
    chest, 37616
    coronary, 33502
    ethmoidal, 30915
    extremity, 37618
    maxillary, 30920
    neck, 37615
    temporal, 37609
  duct
    salivary, 42665
    submandibular, 42510
    thoracic, 38380-38382
  esophagus, 43405
  fallopian tube(s), 58600-58611
  hemorrhoids, 46945-46946, 0249T
  shunt, 33924, 49428
  varices
    esophageal, 43205, 43244, 43400

Laser – Ligation

CPT © 2015 American Medical Association. All Rights Reserved.   © 2016 DecisionHealth

Ligation — *continued*
varices — *continued*
gastric, 43244
vas deferens, 55450
vein
femoral, 37650
iliac, 37660
jugular, 37565
perforator, 37500, 37760
saphenous, 37700-37735, 37780
spermatic, 55530-55550
varicose, 37785
vena cava, 37619
Ligature strangulation, 11200-11201
Light
chemotherapy, 0519F, 36522, 96570-96571, 96910-96913
density, 77083
scattering, 83883
sensitivity, 85056
therapy, 0168T, 36522, 96567, 96900
Lingual
bone, 21495, 21685
frenectomy, 41115
nerve, 64740
tonsil, 42870
Linton procedure, 37760
Lip
biopsy, 40490
excision, 40510-40527
lesion
destruction, 17280-17286
excision, 11440-11446, 11640-11646
shaving, 11310-11313
repair, 12011-12018, 12051-12057, 13151-13153, 40650-40654
cleft, 00102, 40700-40761
resection, 40530
shaving, 40500
Lipase, 83690
Lipectomy, 15830-15839
aspiration, 15876-15879
Lipids, 3278F, 82705-82710
Lipoprotein, 83695-83721
Liposuction, 15876-15879
Listeria monocytogenes, 86723
Lithium, 80178
Litholapaxy, 52317-52318
Lithotripsy, 00872-00873, 43265, 50080-50081, 50590, 52353
Liver
aspiration, 47015
assist system oversight, 0405T
biopsy, 47000-47001, 47100
drainage, 47010
elastography, 91200
hemorrhage management, 47350-47362
imaging, 78201-78216
injection, 47015
marsupialization, 47300
nuclear medicine, 78201-78220
resection, 47120-47130
transplant, 47135
donor, 47133, 47140-47142
backbench, 47143-47147
tumor ablation, 47370-47371, 47380-47383
Lobectomy
brain, 61323, 61537-61540
gland
parotid, 42410-42415
thyroid, 60210-60225
liver, 47120-47130, 47141-47142
lung, 32480-32486, 32663
Loopogram, 74425
Loose body
ankle, 27620, 29894
elbow, 24101, 29834
foot, 28020-28024
hand, 26070-26080
hip, 27033, 29861
knee, 27331, 29874

Loose body — *continued*
shoulder, 23107, 29819
wrist, 25101
Lord procedure, 45905
Louis Bar syndrome, 88248
Low
birth weight, 99478-99480
density lipoprotein, 3048F-3050F, 83700-83704, 83721
frequency ultrasound, 97610
vision aid, 92354-92355
Lumbar
arthrodesis, 22533-22534, 22558, 22612, 22630
arthroplasty, 0163T-0165T, 22857-22865
augmentation, 22514-22515
biopsy, 20251-20251
neoplasm, 63277, 63282, 63287-63290
computed tomography (CT) scan, 72131-72133
corpectomy, 63087-63091, 63102-63103
lesion, 63287-63303, 63306-63307
destruction, 64622-64623
excision, 22102, 22114
fracture, 22305, 22325, 22328, 22510-22515
hernia, 49540
incision
drainage, 22015
injection, 64520
aspiration, 62287
catheter, 64449
discography, 62290, 62292
epidural, 2044F, 62282, 62311, 62319, 64483-64484
facet joint, 64475-64476
vertebroplasty, 22511-22512
laminectomy, 63005, 63017, 63047-63048
Gill type, 63012
lesion, 63267, 63272
malformation, 63252
myleotomy, 63170
neoplasm, 63277, 63282, 63287-63290
release, 63200
laminotomy, 63030-63035, 63042, 63044
magnetic resonance imaging (MRI), 72148-72149, 72158
manipulation, 22505
neuroplasty, 64714
osteotomy, 22207, 22214, 22224
plastic repair, 22511-22512
puncture, 62270
resection, 63087-63091, 63102-63103, 63303, 63307
shunt
replacement, 63744
removal, 63746
spinal tap, 62270
suture, 64862
sympathectomy, 64809-64818
transpedicular approach, 63056-63057
Lumen dilation, 74360
Lumpectomy, 19301-19302
Lunate, 25444, 25690-25695
Lung
ablation, 32998
biopsy
bronchoscopy, 31628, 31632
brush, 31717
needle, 32400, 32405
thoracoscopy, 32604-32609
thoracotomy, 32096-32098
bronchoscopy, 31622-31661
closure, 32815, 32906
decortication, 32220-32225, 32320, 32651-32652
drainage
abscess, 31645-31646, 32200
empyema, 32035-32036

Lung — *continued*
excision
bulla, 32141, 32655
cyst, 32661-32662
empyema, 32540
pleura, 32310-32320, 32656
stenosis, 31775
tumor, 32503-32504, 32661-32662
expiratory volume, 3040F-3042F
hemorrhage, 32110, 32654
lavage, 31624, 32997
lysis, 32124, 32652, 32940
pneumocentesis, 32405
pneumogram, 94772
pneumothorax, 32215, 32560, 32960
puncture, 32405
removal
apical tumor, 32503-32504
cyst, 32140
extrapleural, 32445
one lobe, 32480, 32663
one segment, 32484, 32669
sleeve lobectomy, 32486
sleeve pneumonectomy, 32488
total pneumonectomy, 32440-32445, 32671
two lobes, 32482, 32670
volume reduction, 32491, 32672
wedge, 32505-32507, 32666-32668
repair
bronchus, 32501
hernia, 32800
tear, 32110
resection, 32141, 32491, 32505-32507
bronchus, 32486
pericardial sac, 32659
tumor, 32503-32504
stent, 31636-31638, 31730
sympathectomy, 32664
thoracoplasty, 32905-32906
thoracoscopy
diagnostic, 32601-32609
surgical, 32650-32674
Heller type, 32665
transplant, 00580, 32851-32854
donor, 32850, 32855-32856
tube, 32551
ultrasound, 31654
volume reduction, 32491
Lupus, 85705
Luteinizing
hormone, 80418, 80426, 83002
release factor, 83727
Luteotropin, 80418, 84146
placental, 83632
Lyme disease, 86617-86618
Lymph, 00320-00322
channels, 38308
duct, 38790
thoracic, 38380-38382
node(s)
biopsy, 38500-38530, 58943
injection, 38792
laparoscopic, 38570-38572
needle, 38505
open, 38500, 38510-38530
prostate, 55812-55815, 55842-55845, 55862
cannulation, 38794
dissection, 38542, 38724
drainage
abscess, 38300-38305
cyst, 49062, 49323
excision, 19305-19307, 38500-38530
hygroma, 38550-38555
open, 38500, 38510-38530
injection, 38790-38792
lymphadenectomy
abdominal, 38747
axillary, 19302, 38740-38745
cervical, 38720-38724
gastric, 38747

Lymph — *continued*
node(s) — *continued*
lymphadenectomy — *continued*
inguinofemoral
bilateral, 54130, 56632, 56637
complete, 56631, 56640
superficial, 38760-38765
unilateral, 56631, 56634
mediastinal, 19272, 21632, 32674
para-aortic, 58951, 58954, 58958-58960
pelvic, 38770, 58954, 58958-58960
bilateral, 51575, 54135, 55815, 55845, 55865
complete, 51585, 51595, 56640
laparoscopy, 38571-38572
limited, 38562, 55812, 55842, 55862, 58951
total, 57109, 57112, 57531, 58210, 58548
portal, 38747
regional, 50230, 32674
retroperitoneal, 38564, 38780
sentinel node, 38792
suprahyoid, 38700
thoracic, 38746
lymphadenitis, 38300-38305
lymphangiotomy, 38308
lymphoblast, 86353
lymphocyte, 86805-86806, 86821-86822
choriomeningitis, 86727
thymus dependent, 86359-86361
lymphocytotoxicity, 86805-86806
lymphogranuloma venereum, 86729
lymphoma virus, 86663-86665
nuclear medicine, 78195
sampling, 38570, 38572, 58200
vessels
incision, 38308
lymphangiography, 38790
abdomen, 75805-75807
extremity, 75801-75803
nuclear medicine, 78195
Lymphocele
drainage, 10030
Lynch procedure, 31075
Lysergic acid, 80299
Lysis
adhesions
intestine, 44005
knee, 29884
labia, 56441
ovary, 58660, 58740
nose, 30560
penile, 54162, 54450
shoulder, 29825
spine, 62263-62264
ureter, 50715-50725
urethra, 53500
uterus, 58559
artery, 35701-35761
euglobulin, 85360
Lysozyme, 85549

M

Macrodactylia, 26590
Magnesium, 83735
Magnetic resonance
angiography (MRA)
abdomen, 74185
chest, 71555
head, 70544-70546
lower extremity, 73725
neck, 70547-70549
pelvis, 72198

Magnetic resonance — *continued*
　angiography (MRA) — *continued*
　　spine, 72159
　　upper extremity, 73225
　guidance, 77021-77022
　imaging (MRI), 3319F-3320F
　　abdomen, 74181-74183
　　ankle, 73721-73723
　　arm, 73218-73220
　　bone marrow, 77084
　　brain, 70551-70555, 70557-70559
　　breast, 0159T, 77058-77059
　　chest, 71550-71552
　　elbow, 73221-73223
　　face, 70540-70543
　　fetal, 74712-74713
　　finger joint, 73221-73223
　　foot, 73718-73720
　　foot joint, 73721-73723
　　hand, 73218-73220
　　heart, 75557-75564
　　intraoperative, 70557-70559
　　lower extremity, 73718-73723
　　　foot, 73718-73720
　　　foot joint, 73721-73723
　　　knee, 73721-73723
　　　leg, 73718-73720
　　　pelvis, 72195-72197
　　　toe joint, 73721-73723
　　knee, 73721-73723
　　leg, 73718-73720
　　neck, 70540-70543
　　orbit, 70540-70543
　　pelvis, 72195-72197
　　spine, 72141-72158
　　temporomandibular joint, 70336
　　toe joint, 73721-72723
　　unlisted, 76498
　　upper extremity, 73218-73223
　　　arm, 73218-73220
　　　elbow, 73221-73223
　　　finger joint, 73221-73223
　　　hand, 73218-73220
　　　wrist, 73221-73223
　spectroscopy, 76390
　three dimensional rendering, 76376-76377

Magnetoencephalography (MEG), 95965-95967

Magnuson procedure, 23450

MAGPI operation, 54322

Malar
　augmentation, 21270
　excision, 21030, 21034
　fracture treatment, 21355, 21360-21366
　graft, 21210
　reconstruction, 21270

Malaria
　antibody, 86750
　smear, 87207

Malate dehydrogenase, 83775

Maldescent, 54550-54560

Malformation
　arteriovenous
　　cranial, 61680-61692, 61705-61708
　　spinal, 62294, 63250-63252

Malleolus
　bimalleolar, 27808-27810, 27814
　lateral, 27786-27788
　medial, 27760-27762, 27766
　trimalleolar, 27816-27818, 27822-27823

Mallet finger, 26432

Maltose, 82951-82952

Malunion
　repair
　　femur, 27470-27472
　　metatarsal, 28322
　　tarsal, 28320

Mammary
　ablation, 19105
　abscess, 19020
　angiography, 75756

Mammary — *continued*
　aspiration
　　cyst, 19000-19001
　augmentation, 19324-19325
　biopsy, 19100-19101
　capsules
　　excision, 19371
　　incision, 19370
　　removal, 19371
　catheter, 19296-19298, 20555, 41019
　cryosurgery
　　ablation, 19105
　cyst
　　aspiration, 19000-19001
　　excision, 19120-19126
　ductogram, 19030, 77053-77054
　excision
　　biopsy, 19100-19101
　　capsules, 19371
　　cyst, 19120-19126
　　fistula, 19112
　　lesion, 19120-19126, 19301
　　mastectomy, 19300-19307
　　nipple, 19110
　　tumor, 19260-19272
　exploration, 19110, 19020
　fistula
　　excision, 19112
　graft, 4110F
　implants
　　insertion, 19340-19342
　　preparation, 19396
　　removal, 19328-19330
　　supply, 19396
　incision
　　capsules, 19370
　　drainage, 19020
　injection, 19030
　insertion
　　implants, 19340-19342
　lesion
　　excision, 19120-19126, 19301
　magnetic resonance imaging (MRI), 0159T, 77058-77059
　mammillaplasty, 19350-19355
　mammogram, 3341F-3350F
　　findings, 5060F-5062F
　mammography
　　bilateral, 77056
　　　with computer-aided detection, 77051
　　magnetic resonance
　　　bilateral, 77059
　　　unilateral, 77058
　　screening
　　　bilateral, 77057
　　　　with computer-aided detection, 77052
　　　unilateral, 77055
　　　　with computer-aided detection, 77051
　mammoplasty, 19318-19325
　　augmentation, 19324-19325
　　reduction, 19318
　mastectomy
　　excision 19300-19307
　mastopexy, 19316
　periprosthetic
　　capsulectomy, 19371
　　capsulotomy, 19370
　placement
　　catheter, 19296-19298, 20555, 41019
　　metallic localization clip, 19281-19288
　　needle localization wire, 19281-19288
　　radiotherapy afterloading catheter, 19296-19298
　reconstruction, 19357-19369
　　augmentation, 19324-19325
　　flap
　　　free, 19364
　　　latissimus dorsi, 19361
　　　myocutaneous, 19367-19369

Mammary — *continued*
　reconstruction — *continued*
　　mammoplasty, 19318-19325
　　nipple, 19350-19355
　　other, 19366
　　revision, 19380
　　tissue expander, 19357
　reduction, 19318
　removal
　　capsules, 19371
　　complete, 19303
　　implants, 19328-19330
　　partial, 19300-19302
　　radical, 19305-19307
　　subcutaneous, 19304
　revision, 19380
　repair, 19316
　stimulating hormone, 80418, 84146
　tumor
　　excision, 19260-19272
　ultrasound, 76641-76642
　x-ray, 76700, 77051-77057

Mandible
　augmentation, 21125-21127
　bone graft, 21215
　excision
　　abscess, 21025
　　condyle, 21050
　　cyst, 21040, 21046-21047
　　foreign body, 41806
　　torus mandibularis, 21031
　　tumor, 21040-21047
　fracture treatment
　　closed, 21450-21451, 21453
　　open, 21454-21470
　　percutaneous, 21452
　graft, 21215
　osteotomy, 21198-21199
　prosthesis, 21081
　reconstruction, 21244-21249
　　rami, 21193-21196
　removal, 41806
　x-ray, 70100-70110

Manganese, 83785

Manipulation
　chest wall, 94667-94668
　chiropractic, 98940-98943
　Dupuytren's contracture, 26341
　foreskin, 54450
　fracture/dislocation
　　acetabulum, 01173, 27222
　　acromioclavicular, 23545
　　ankle, 27810, 27818, 27860
　　carpometacarpal, 26670-26676
　　clavicle, 23505
　　elbow, 24300, 24640
　　femur, 27232, 27240, 27502, 27510, 27517
　　fibula, 27781, 27788
　　finger, 26725-26727, 26742, 26755, 26770-26776
　　hand, 26670-26676
　　hip, 27222, 27257
　　humerus, 23605, 23625, 24505, 24535, 24565, 24577
　　intercarpal, 25660
　　interphalangeal joint, 26340, 26742, 26770-26776
　　malar, 21355
　　mandibular, 21451
　　metacarpal, 26605-26607
　　metacarpophalangeal, 26340, 26700-26706, 26742
　　metatarsal, 28475-28476
　　nose, 21315-21320
　　orbit, 21401
　　radius, 24655, 25505, 25565
　　radiocarpal, 25660
　　radioulnar, 25675
　　scapula, 23575
　　shoulder, 23650-23655, 23665, 23700
　　sternoclavicular, 23525, 23675
　　talus, 28435-28436
　　tarsus, 28455-28456
　　thumb, 26641-26650
　　tibia, 27532, 27752, 27762

Manipulation — *continued*
　fracture/dislocation — *continued*
　　ulna, 25535
　　vertebra, 22315
　　wrist, 25259, 25624, 25635, 25660, 25675, 25680, 25690
　globe, 92018-92019
　knee, 27570
　osteopathic, 98925-98929
　palmar fasical cord, 26341
　spine, 22505
　temporomandibular joint, 21073

Manometric study
　anus, 91122
　pressure
　　kidney, 50396
　　ureter, 50686
　rectum, 91122

Manometry
　rectal, 90911

Mantoux test, 86580

Manual therapy, 97140

Mapping
　motor function, 0310T
　sentinel node, 38900

Maquet procedure, 27418

Marrow
　aspiration, 38220
　biopsy, 38221
　cytogenic testing, 3155F
　harvest, 38221, 38230
　HPC transplantation, 38240-38242
　imaging (non-MRI), 78102-78104, 78300-78320
　magnetic resonance imaging (MRI), 77084
　smear, 85097

Marshall-Marchetti-Kranz procedure, 51840-51841, 58152, 58267, 58293

Marsupialization
　cyst
　　Bartholin's Gland, 56440
　　liver, 47300
　　pancreatic, 48500
　　sublingual, 42409
　diverticulum
　　urethra, 53240
　skin, 10040

Mass spectrometry, 83789

Massage, 97124
　cardiac, 32160

Masseter, 21295-21296

Mastectomy
　complete, 19303
　gynecomastia, 19300
　halsted, 19303-19306
　partial, 19301-19302
　radical, 19305-19306
　　modified, 19307
　simple, 19303
　subcutaneous, 19304

Mastoid(s)
　debridement, 69220-69222
　excision, 69601-69603
　　complete, 69502
　　radical, 69505, 69511, 69530
　　simple, 69501
　mastoidectomy
　　complete, 69502
　　　revision, 69601
　　osseointegrated implant
　　　implantation, 69715
　　　replacement, 69718
　　radical, 69511
　　　modified, 69505, 69602
　　　revision, 69602-69603
　　　with petrous apicectomy, 69530
　　revision
　　　complete, 69601
　　　modified radical, 69602
　　　radical, 69603
　　　with tympanoplasty, 69604
　　　with apicectomy, 69605

Mastoid(s) — *continued*
mastoidectomy — *continued*
with labyrinthectomy, 69910
with tympanoplasty
complete, 69645-69646
radical, 69645-69646
with intact, reconstructed
wall, 69643-69644
with ossicular chain
reconstruction, 69642,
69644, 69646
without ossicular chain
reconstruction, 69641,
69643, 69645
mastoidotomy, 69635-69637
mastopexy, 19316
mastotomy, 19020
obliteration, 69670
polytomography, 76101-76102
repair, 69601-69605
fistula, 69700
x-ray, 70120-70130
Maternity care, 59000-59899
abortion
evacuation, 59870
incomplete, 59812
induced, 59840-59857
missed, 59820-59821
multifetal reduction, 59866
septic, 59830
amniocentesis, 59000-59001
cordocentesis, 59012
curettage, 59160
delivery, 59425-59430
cesarean, 59510-59525
attempted vaginal, 59618-
59622
external cephalic version, 59412
placenta, 59414
vaginal, 59400-59410
previous cesarean, 59610-
59614
dilator, 59200
ectopic pregnancy, 59120-59151
excision
hysterectomy, 59135
hysterotomy, 59100
oophorectomy, 59120, 59151
salpingectomy, 59120, 59151
monitoring, 59050-59051
repair, 59300-59350
removal, 59871
resection, 59136
sampling
chorionic villus, 59015
fetal scalp blood, 59030
stabilization, 99464
stress test, 59020-59025
ultrasound, 59070-59076
Maxilla(ry)
antrostomy, 31256-31267
bone graft, 21210
computed tomography (CT) scan,
70486-70488
excision
cyst, 21030
sinus, 31225-31230
tumor, 21030, 21034, 21048-
21049
torus palatinus, 21032
exploration, 31020-31032, 31233
fracture treatment, 21345-21347
closed, 21345, 21421
open, 21346-21348, 21422-
21423
incision, 31020-31032, 31256-
31267
irrigation, 31000
ligation, 30920
maxillectomy, 31225-31230
maxillofacial
fixation, 21100
impression, 21076-21089
osteotomy, 21206
reconstruction, 21245-21246,
21248-21249
surgery, 61581
Maximal sterile barrier (MSB), 6030F

Maydl procedure, 45563, 50810
Mayo
hernia repair, 49580-49587
procedure, 28292
Maze procedure, 33254-33256,
33265-33266
McBride procedure, 28292
McCannell procedure, 66682
McKissock procedure, 19318
Measles, 86765, 87283, 90707-90710
german, 86762
Measurement
lung volumes, 94013
gastrointestinal transit, 91112
ocular blood flow, 0198T
spirometric forced expiratory
flows, 94011-94012
Meatoplasty, 69310
Meatotomy
in cystourethroscopy, 52281
prostate, 52601, 52647-52648
ureteral, 52290-52305
urethral, 53020
infant, 53025
Meckel's diverticulum
excision, 44800
Median nerve, 64721
compression, 64721
repair, 64835
Mediastinum
biopsy, 32405, 39401-39402
drainage/exploration, 39000-39010
excision
cyst, 32662, 39200
tumor, 32662, 39220
mediastinoscopy,39401-39402
mediastinotomy, 39000-39010
removal foreign body, 39000-39010
Medical
conference, 99366-99368
evaluation, disability, 99455-99456
genetic counseling, 96040
testimony, 99075
Meibomian cyst, 67800-67808
Melanoma, 0015F
Membrane
mucosa
biopsy, 57100-57105
destruction, 30801-30802,
96567
excision, 40810-40818, 41828,
44369
graft, 41870
imaging, 78290
urethra, 53450
tympanic
incision, 69420-69421
reconstruction, 69620
repair, 69450, 69610
stoma, 69433-69436
Meningioma, 61512, 61519
Meningitis, 86727
Meningocele, 63700-63702
Meningococcal, 90733-90734
Meningococcus, 86741
Meniscus
excision
knee, 27332-27333
temporomandibular joint, 21060
repair, 27403
transplantation, 29868
Mental nerve incision, 64736
Meprobamate, 80369-80370
Mercury, 83015, 83825
Mesencephalon, 61480
Mesentery
aneurysm, 35121-35122
embolectomy, 34151
excision, 44820
graft, 35531, 35631
repair, 44850
Mesh
insertion, 49568
pelvic floor, 57267

Mesh — *continued*
removal, 11008
repair, 49568
Metabisulfite test, 85660
Metacarpal
amputation, 26910
excision
cyst, 26200-26205
diaphysis, 26230
tumor, 26200-26205, 26250-
26255
fracture treatment, 26600-26615
repair, 26546, 26565, 26568
Metacarpophalangeal joint
arthrodesis, 26850-26852
arthroplasty, 26530-26531
arthroscopy, 29900-29902
biopsy, 26105
dislocation treatment, 26700-26715
excision
capsule, 26520, 26560
synovectomy, 26135
exploration, 26075
fracture treatment, 26740-26746
fusion, 26850-26852
capsule, 26516-26518
incision
capsule, 26520
exploration, 26075
removal, foreign body, 26075
repair, 26540-26542
synovectomy, 26135
Metadrenaline, 83535
Metals, 83015-83018
Metatarsal
amputation, 28810
anastomosis, 20972
excision, 28110-28114, 28140
condyle, 28288
cyst, 28104-28107
diaphysis, 28122
tumor, 28104-28107, 28173
fracture treatment, 28470-28485
repair, 28306-28309, 28322
Metatarsophalangeal joint
arthrotomy, 28052
exploration, 28022
removal, foreign body, 28022
biopsy, 28052
capsulotomy, 28270
cheilectomy, 28289
dislocation treatment, 28630-28645
exploration, 28022
fusion
great toe, 28750
removal, foreign body, 28022
repair, 28289
synovectomy, 28072
Methadone, 80358
Methamphetamine, 80324-80326
Methanol, 80320
Methemalbumin, 83857
Methemoglobin, 83045-83050
Methenamine silver, 88312
Methopyrapone, 80436
Methsuximide, 80339-80341
Methyl alcohol, 80320
Methylene bichloride, 82441
Methylfluoprednisolone, 80420
Methylmorphine, 80323, 82468
Metroplasty, 58540
Metyrapone, 80436
Microalbumin, 3060F-3062F, 82043-
82044
Microbiology, 87003-87999
Microdissection, 88380-88381
Microfluorometries, 88182-88189
Microglobulin, 82232
Micrographic surgery, 17311-17315
Microopthalmia, 21256
Micropigmentation, 11920-11922

Microscop(ic)(y), 69990
electron, 88348
evaluation, 96902
exam, 92504
Microsomal antibody, 86376
Microsomia, 21247
Microsurgery, 69990
Microvascular anastomosis
bone graft, 20955, 20962
flap
free, 15756-15758
osteocutaneous, 20969-20973
Midcarpal joint, 25040
Middle
cerebral artery, 76821
ear
computed tomography (CT)
scan, 70480-70482
excision, 69540, 69550-69554
exploration, 69440
reconstruction, 69631-69646
removal, 69424
repair, 69662, 69666-69667
Midface, 21141-21160, 21188
Migration inhibitory factor (MIF), 86378
Milia, 10040
Miller procedure, 28737
Miiller-abbot intubation, 44500, 74340
Minerva cast, 29035, 29710
Minimum concentration, 87186-87187
**Minnesota multiphasic personality
inventory (MMPI),** 96101-96103
Miscarriage
incomplete, 59812
missed, 59820-59821
septic, 59830
Mitchell procedure, 28296
Mitogen blastogenesis, 86353
Mitral valve, 33418-33430, 0345T
MMR vaccine, 90707
Mobilization
splenic flexure, 44139, 44213
stapes, 69650
Moderate sedation, 99143-99150
Modified radical mastectomy, 19307
Mohs' micrographic surgery, 17311-
17315
Molar pregnancy, 59100, 59870
Mold, 87101
Molecular
assays, multianalyte, 81410-81471
diagnostics, 81200-81599
pathology
ABL1, 81170
APC, 81201-81203
ASPA, 81200
BCKDHB, 81205
BCR/ABL1, 81206-81208
BLM, 81209
BRAF, 81210, 81162
BRCA1, 81214-81215
BRCA2, 81216-81217
BRCA1, BRCA2, 81211-81213
CALR, 81219
CEBPA, 81218
CFTR, 81220-81224
Chimerism analysis, 81267-
81268
Comparative analysis, STR
markers, 81265-81266
CYP2C9, 81227
CYP2C19, 81225
CYP2D6, 81226
Cytogenomic constitutional
microarray, 81228-81229
DMD, 81161
F2, 81240
F5, 81241
FANCC, 81242
FLT3, 81245-81246
FMR1, 81243-81244
G6PC, 81250
GBA, 81251
GJB2, 81252-81253

© 2016 DecisionHealth

CPT © 2015 American Medical Association. All Rights Reserved.

CPT © 2015 American Medical Association. All Rights Reserved.
© 2016 DecisionHealth

Nuclear — *continued*
  medicine — *continued*
    dacryocystography, 78660
    diagnostic imaging, 78012, 78999
    endocrine system
      adrenal, 78075
      parathyroid, 78070-78072
      thyroid, 78012-78020
      unlisted procedure, 78099
    esophageal motility, 78258
    gastric
      emptying, 78264-78266
      mucosa, 78261
    gastroesophageal reflux, 78262
    gastrointestinal system, 78201-78299
      blood loss, 78278
      intestine, 78290
      liver, 78201-78216
      protein loss, 78282
      salivary gland, 78230-78232
      unlisted procedure, 78299
      urea breath test, 78267-78268
      vitamin B12, 78270-78272
    genitourinary system, 78700-78799
      bladder, residual, 78730
      kidney, 78700-78725
      testicle, 78761
      ureteral reflux, 78740
    hematopoietic/lymphatic system, 78102-78199
      bone marrow, 3155F, 78102-78104
      lymphatics, 78195
      plasma volume, 78110-78111
      platelet survival, 78190-78191
      red cell, 78120-78121, 78130-78140
      spleen, 78185
      whole blood, 78122
    hepatobiliary system, 78226-78227
    inflammatory process localization, 78805-78807
    intestine imaging, 78290
    joint imaging, 78300-78320
    kidney, 78700-78725
      function study, 78725
      morphology imaging, 78700-78709
      tomographic (SPECT), 78710
      vascular flow, 78701-78709
    liver, 78201-78216
    lymphatics imaging, 78195
    musculoskeletal system, 78300-78399
      bone, 78300-78351
      joint, 78300-78320
    myocardial
      imaging, 78459, 78466-78469, 78491-78492
      perfusion, 78460-78465, 78478-78480
    nervous system, 78600-78699
      brain imaging, 78600-78610
      cerebrospinal fluid, 78630-78650
    dacryocystography, 78660
    parathyroid, 78070-78072
    plasma volume, 78110-78111
    platelet survival, 78190-78191
    positron emission tomography (PET), 78811-78816
      limited area, 78811, 78814
      skull base to mid thigh, 78812, 78815
      whole body, 78813, 78816
      with concurrent computed tomography (CT), 78814-78816
    red blood cell, 78120-78121, 78130-78140
      sequestration, 78140

Nuclear — *continued*
  medicine — *continued*
    red blood cell — *continued*
      survival study, 78130-78135
      volume, 78120-78121
    respiratory system, 78579-78598
      pulmonary perfusion, 78580-78598
      quantitative differential, 78597-78598
      unlisted procedure, 78599
      ventilation imaging, 78579, 78582, 78598
    salivary gland, 78230-78232
    spleen, 78185
      with liver, 78215-78216
    testicles, 78761
    therapeutic (radiopharmaceutical), 79005-79999
      interstitial colloid, 79300
      intra-arterial, 79445
      intra-articular, 79440
      intracavitary, 79200
      intravenous, 79101, 79403
      monoclonal antibody, 79403
      oral, 79005
    thyroid, 78012-78020
      carcinoma metastases, 78015-78020
      imaging, 78013-78014
      uptake, 78012, 78014
    tumor localization, 78800-78804
    urea breath test, 78267-78268
    ureteral reflux study, 78740
    venous thrombosis, 78456-78458
    whole blood, 78122
  three dimensional rendering, 76376-76377
Nucleases (DNA), 86225-86226
  endonuclease, 86215
  probe
    molecular, 88271-88275, 88291
Nucleic acid probe
  amplified probe detection
    bartonella, 87471
    borrelia burgdorferi, 87476
    candida, 78481
    chlamydia, 87486, 87491
    cytomegalovirus, 87496
    enterovirus, 87498, 87500
    gardnerella vaginalis, 87511
    hepatitis, 3215F-3220F, 87516, 87521, 87526
    herpes simplex, 87529
    herpes virus 6, 87532
    human immunodeficiency virus (HIV), 87535, 87538
    legionella, 87541
    multiple organisms, 87801
    mycobacteria, 87551, 87556, 87561
    mycoplasma pneumoniae, 87581
    neisseria gonorrheae, 87591
    not otherwise specified, 87798, 87801
    staphylococcus, 87640-87641
    streptococcus, 87651, 87653
  direct probe detection
    bartonella, 87470
    borrelia burgdorferi, 87475
    candida, 87480
    chlamydia, 87485, 87490
    cytomegalovirus, 87495
    gardnerella vaginalis, 87510
    hepatitis, 3215F-3220F, 87515, 87520, 87525
    herpes simplex, 87528
    herpes virus 6, 87531
    human immunodeficiency virus (HIV), 87534, 87537
    legionella, 87540
    multiple organisms, 87800
    mycobacteria, 87550, 87555, 87560
    mycoplasma pneumoniae, 87580

Nucleic acid probe — *continued*
  direct probe detection — *continued*
    neisseria gonorrheae, 87590
    not otherwise specified, 87797
    streptococcus group A, 87650
    trichomonas vaginalis, 87660
  genotype analysis
    hepatitis B, 87912
    hepatitis C, 87902
    human immunodeficiency virus (HIV)-1, 87901, 87906
  in situ hybridization, 88364-88369, 88373-88374, 88377
  phenotype analysis
    human immunodeficiency virus (HIV)-1, 87903-87904
  quantification
    bartonella, 87472
    borrelia burgdorferi, 87477
    candida, 87482
    chlamydia, 87487, 87492
    cytomegalovirus, 87497
    bardnerella vaginalis, 87512
    hepatitis, 3215F-3220F, 87517, 87522, 87527
    herpes simplex, 87530
    herpes virus 6, 87533
    human immunodeficiency virus (HIV), 87536, 87539
    legionella, 87542
    mycobacteria, 87552, 87557, 87562
    mycoplasma pneumoniae, 87582
    neisseria gonorrheae, 87592
    not otherwise specified, 87799
    streptococcus group A, 87652
Nucleolysis, 62292
Nucleotidase, 83915
Nursemaid elbow, 24640
Nuss procedure, 21742-21743
Nutrition, 97802-97804
Nystagmus test, 92531-92532, 92534, 92541-92542, 92544

O

O₂ saturation, 82805-82810
Ober-Yount procedure, 27025
Obliteration
  mastoid, 69670
  vagina, 57110-57112, 57120
Observation, 99234-99236
Obstetrical care
  abortion
    incomplete, 59812
    induced, 59840-59857
    missed, 59820-59821
    septic, 59830
    spontaneous, 59812
    therapeutic, 59840-59857
  amniocentesis, 59000-59001
  amnioinfusion, 59070
  antepartum, 59000-59076, 59425-59426
    amniocentesis, 59000-59001
    amnioinfusion, 59070
    care only, 59425-59426
    chorionic villus sampling, 59015
    cordocentesis, 59012
    fetal
      blood sampling, 59030
      fluid drainage, 59074
      monitoring, 59050-59051
      shunt, 95076
      stress test, 59020-59025
    umbilical cord occlusion, 59072
  cesarean-section, 59510-59525, 59618-59622
    delivery only, 59514-59515, 59620-59622
    with hysterectomy, 59525
    with routine care, 59510, 59618
  cerclage
    abdominal, 59325
    suture removal, 59871
    vaginal, 59320

Obstetrical care — *continued*
  cervical dilator, 59200
  chorionic villus sampling, 59015
  cordocentesis, 59012
  curettage
    postpartum, 59160
  delivery, 59400-59622
    cesarean, 59510-59515, 59618-59622
    placenta, 59414
    vaginal, 59400-59410, 59610-59614
    following previous C-section, 59610-59622
  ectopic pregnancy, 59120-59151
    abdominal, 59130
    cervical, 59140
    interstitial, 59135-59136
    laparoscopic treatment, 59150-59151
    tubal/ovarian, 59120-59121
  evacuation
    ectopic pregnancy, 59140
    hydatidiform mole, 59870
  fetal
    blood sampling, 59030
    fluid drainage, 59074
    monitoring, 59050-59051
    paracentesis, 59074
    shunt placement, 95076
    stress test, 59020-59025
    thoracocentesis, 59074
    vesicocentesis, 59074
  hydatidiform mole
    evacuation, 59870
    excision, 59100
  hysterorrhaphy, 59350
  laminaria insertion, 59200
  multifetal reduction, 59866
  postpartum
    care only, 59430
    curettage, 59160
  prostaglandin insertion, 59200
  umbilical cord occlusion, 59072
Obstruction
  arterial
    permanent, 61624-61625
    temporary, 61623
  colonic
    reduction, 44050
    removal, 44025
  fallopian tube
    band, clip, ring, 58615
    implant, 58565
  removal
    venous access device, 36595-36596
  umbilical cord, 59072
  vein
    penile, 37790
  venous access device
    removal, 36595-36596
Obturator
  nerve, 64763-64766
  prosthesis, 21076
    auricular, 21086
    definitive, 21080
    facial, 21088
    interim, 21079
    larynx, 31527
    mandibular, 21081
    nasal, 21087
    oral, 21085
    orbital, 21077
    palatal, 21082-21083
    speech, 21084
Occipital nerve
  injection, 64405
  incision, 64744
Occlusion
  arterial
    permanent, 61624-61625
    temporary, 61623
  bronchus, 31634
  fallopian tube
    band, clip, ring, 58615
    implant, 58565
  umbilical cord, 59072

Nuclear – Occlusion

Occlusion — *continued*
  vascular, 37241-37244
  vein, penile, 37790
  venous access device
    removal, 36595-36596
Occult blood, 82270-82272
  immunoassay, 82274
Occupational therapy, 97003-97004
Ocular
  implant
    insertion, 65130-65140, 67550
    modification, 65125
    reinsertion, 65150-65155
    removal, 65175, 67560
  muscle
    biopsy, 67346
    chemodenervation, 67345
    scar tissue release, 67343
    strabismus repair, 67311-
      67318, 67331-67340
    transposition, 67320
  orbital
    aspiration, 67415
    biopsy, 61332
      fine needle aspiration,
        67415
      with exploration, 67400,
        67450
    computed tomography (CT)
      scan, 70480-70482
    decompression, 61330, 67414,
      67445
    exploration, 61332, 67400,
      64750
      with biopsy, 61332, 67400,
        67450
      with lesion removal, 61333
    floor blow out, 21385-21395
      combined approach, 21387
      periorbital approach, 21386,
        21390-21395
      transantral approach, 21385
    fracture treament
      closed, 21400-21401
      open, blowout, 21385-21395
      open, except blowout,
        21406-21408
    hypertelorism treatment,
      21260-21263
    implant
      insertion, 67550
      removal, 67560
      revision, 67560
    incision and drainage, 67405,
      67440
    injection, 67500-67515
      medication, 67500, 67515
      retrobulbar, 67500-67505
    magnetic resonance imaging
      (MRI), 70540-70543
    osteotomy
      for repositioning, 21267-
        21268
      hypertelorism, 21260-21263
      periorbital, 21260-21263
      reconstruction, 21256
      repositioning, 21267-21268
      with forehead advancement,
        21263
    prosthesis, 21077
    reconstruction, 21256
      orbitocraniofacial, 21275
      rim with forehead, 21172-
        21180
      rims, 21182-21184
      secondary, 21275
      walls, 21182-21184
    repositioning, 21267-21268
    rim, 21182-21184
    rim and forehead, 21172-21180
    transplant, 67560
    wall, 21182-21184
  photoscreening, 99174
  prosthesis
    custom preparation, 21077
    intraocular lens, 66982-66985
    keratoprosthesis, 65770
    service, aphakia, 92358

Odontoid
  dislocation/fracture
    treatment, 22318-22319
  process, excision, 22548
Oestradiol, 80414, 82670
Olecranon (process)
  arthrocentesis, bursa, 20605-
    20606
  craterization/saucerization, 24147
  diaphysectomy, 24147
  excision
    abscess, 24138
    cyst/benign tumor, 24120-24126
    osteomyelitis, 24138
    partial, 24147
  fracture treatment
    closed, 24670-24675
    open, 24685
  sequestrectomy, 24138
Oligoclonal bands, 83916
Omentectomy, 49255
  malignancy
    abdominal hysterectomy,
      58953-58956
    oophorectomy, 58943
      bilateral salpingo-
        oophorectomy, 58950-
        58956
    resection
      ovarian, 58950-58952
      peritoneal, 58950-58958
      tubal, 58950-58958
    staging/restaging, 58960
    tumor debulking, 58957-58958
    total, 58956
Omentum
  excision, 49255, 58950-58958
  flap, 49904-49906
  suspension, 49326
Omphalectomy, 49250
Omphalocele
  first stage, 49610
  large, 49605-49606
  second stage, 49611
  small, 49600
Omphalomesenteric duct, 44800
Oncoprotein
  des gamma carboxy prothrombin
    (DCP), 83951
  HER-2/neu, 83950
Online management service
  nonphysician, 98969
  physician, 99444
Onychia
  drainage, 10060-10061
  excision, 11750-11752
Oocyte
  biopsy, 89290-89291
  culture, 89250-89251, 89272
  fertilization, 89280-89281
  identification, 89254
  insemination, 89268
  retrieval, 58970
  storage, 89346
  thawing, 89356
Oophorectomy
  bilateral, 58940-58956
  ectopic pregnancy, 59120
  hysterectomy
    radical, 58210
      laparoscopic, 58548
    supracervical, 58180
      laparoscopic, 58542, 58544
    total, 58150-58152, 58200,
      58240
      laparoscopic, 58571, 58573
    vaginal, 58262-58263, 58291-
      58292
      laparoscopic, 58552, 58554
  partial/total, 58661, 58940-58940
  unilateral, 58940-58943
Operating microscope, 69990
Operation
  Bardenheurer, 37616
  Blalock-Hanlon, 33735
  Blalock-Taussig, 33750

Operation — *continued*
  Brunschwig, 58240
  Burch, 58152
  Chopart, 28800
  Coffey, 58400, 58410
  Cotte, 58400-58410
  D'Ombrain, 65426
  Damus-Kaye-Stansel, 33606
  Dana, 63185-63190
  Dandy, 62200-62201
  Douglas, 41510
  Doyle, 64435
  Duhamel, 45112
  Dunn, 28715
  Durham-Caldwell, 24301
  Elliot, 66130
  Emmet, 59300
  Estes, 58825
  Estlander, 32905, 40525
  Fasanella-Servat, 67908
  Finney, 43810, 43850-43855
  Foley, 50400-50405
  Fontan, 33615-33617
  Gardner, 63700-63702
  Ghormley, 27284-27286
  Gill, 63102
  Gill-Stein, 25820
  Gol-Vernet, 50120
  Green, 23400
  Grice, 29907
  Gritti-Stokes, 27598
  Guyon, 27888
  Hegar, 57250
  Heller, 32665, 43279, 43330-
    43331
  Hofmeister, 43620-43622
  Huggin, 54520
  Hutch, 50780-50785
  Jaboulay, 43810, 43850-43855
  Janeway, 43832
  Jannetta, 61458
  Jones, 28760
  Kessler, 25447
  Kroenlein, 67420
  Laroyenne, 57010
  Leriche, 64809
  Lynch, 31075
  Marshall-Marchetti-Krants, 58152,
    58267, 58293
  Miller, 28737
  Norman Miller, 57335
  Norwood, 33619
  Pereyra, 58267, 58293
  Sauve-Kapandjii, 25830
  Schauta, 58285
  Sofield, 24410
  Stallard, 68745-68750
  Steindler, 24330-24331
  Strassman, 58540
  Trendelenburg, 37785
  Trepine, 31070
  Urban, 19306
Operculectomy, 41821
Opthalmic membrane test, 95060
Ophthalmology services, 92002-
  92499
  anterior segment photography,
    92286
    with fluorescein angiography,
      92287
  biometry, 92136
  color vision exam, 92283
  contact lens, 92310-92326
    fitting, for disease, 92070
    modification, 92325
    prescription, 92310-92317
    replacement, 92326
  dark adaptation, 92284
  diagnostic imaging
    scanner, 92132-92134
  electromyography, 92265
  electro-oculography, 92270
  electroretinography, 92275
  established patient, 92012-92014
  examination
    color vision, 92283
    complete, 92018
    dark adaptation, 92284

Ophthalmology services — *continued*
  examination — *continued*
    established patient, 92012-
      92014
    limited, 92019
    new patient, 92002-92004
    sensorimotor, 92060
    under general anesthesia,
      92018-92019
    slit lamp, 92018
    visual field, 92081-92083
  fundus photography, 92250
  glaucoma, provocative test, 92140
  goniophotography, 92285
  gonioscopy, 92020
  interferometry, 92136
  needle electromyography, 92265
  new patient, 92002-92004
  ocular photography, 92285
    anterior segment, 92286-92287
  oculoelectromyography, 92265
  ophthalmoscopy, 92225-92260
    extended, 92225-92226
    fluorescein angiography,
      92235, 92287
    fluorescein angioscopy, 92230
    fundus photography, 92250
    indocyanine-green angiography,
      92240
    ophthalmodynamometry, 92260
  orthoptic/pleoptic training, 92065
  photoscreening, 99174
  provacative test
    glaucoma, 92140
  refractive state, 92015
  screening
    computerized, 99172, 99174
    photoscreening, 99174
    visual acuity, 99172-99173
    visual function, 99172, 99174
  sensorimotor exam, 92060
  serial tonometry, 92100
  slit lamp photography, 92285
  spectacles, 92340-92371
    fitting, 92340-92355
    prosthesis for aphakia, 92358,
      92371
    repair, 92370-92371
  stereophotography, 92285
  tonography, 92120-92130
  tonometry, 92100
  topography
    computerized, 92025
  ultrasound, 76511-76529
  visual acuity screen, 99172-99173
  visual field exam
    intermediate, 92082
    limited, 92081
    extended, 92083
  visual function, 99172
Ophthalmoscopy, 92225-92260
  extended, 92225-92226
  fluorescein
    angiography, 92235, 92287
    angioscopy, 92230
  fundus photography, 92250
  indocyanine-green angiography,
    92240
  ophthalmodynamometry, 92260
Opiates, 80361-80364
Optic nerve
  decompression, 31294, 67570
Optokinetic nystagmus test, 92534,
  92544
Oral
  lactose tolerance test, 82951-82952
  mucosa, 40818
  splint, 21085
Orbit(al)
  aspiration, 67415
  biopsy, 61332
    fine needle aspiration, 67415
    exploration, 67400, 67450
  computed tomography (CT) scan,
    70480-70482
  decompression, 61330, 67414,
    67445
    orbit wall, 31292-31293

Orbit(al) — *continued*
excision
　lesion, 67412, 67420
　tumor, 61333
exploration
　biopsy, 61332, 67400, 67450
　lesion removal, 61333
floor blow out, 21385-21395
　combined approach, 21387
　periorbital approach, 21386, 21390-21395
　transantral approach, 21385
fracture treament
　closed, 21400-21401
　open, blowout, 21385-21395
　open, except blowout, 21406-21408
hypertelorism treatment, 21260-21263
implant
　insertion, 67550
　removal, 67560
　revision, 67560
incision and drainage, 67405, 67440
injection, 67500-67515
　medication, 67500, 67515
　retrobulbar, 67500-67505
magnetic resonance imaging (MRI), 70540-70543
osteotomy
　for repositioning, 21267-21268
　hypertelorism, 21260-21263
　periorbital, 21260-21263
　reconstruction, 21256
　repositioning, 21267-21268
　with forehead advancement, 21263
prosthesis, 21077
reconstruction, 21256
　orbitocraniofacial, 21275
　rim with forehead, 21172-21180
　rims, 21182-21184
　secondary, 21275
　walls, 21182-21184
removal
　foreign body, 67413, 67430
　implant, 67560
repostitioning, 21267-21268
rim, 21182-21184
rim and forehead, 21172-21180
sella turcica, 70482
transplant, 67560
wall, 21182-21184
x-ray, 70190-70200

Orbitotomy, 67400-67450
biopsy, 67400, 67450
bone flap, 67420-67450
decompression, 67414, 67445
drainage, 67405, 67440
exploration, 67400, 67450
foreign body removal, 67413, 67430
lesion removal, 67412, 67420
without bone flap, 67400-67414

Orchidectomy
laparoscopic, 54690
partial, 54522
radical, 54530-54535
simple, 54520
tumor, 54530-54535

Orchiectomy, 54520-54535
laparoscopic, 54690
partial, 54522
radical, 54530-54535
simple, 54520

Orchiopexy
abdominal, 54650
inguinal, 54640
laparoscopic, 54692

Orchioplasty
fixation, 54620
prosthesis, 54660
suture, injury, 54670
torsion reduction, 54600
transplantation, 54680

Organ
grafting
　eye, 65780-65782

Organ — *continued*
grafting — *continued*
eye — *continued*
　conjunctiva, 65782
　cornea, 65710, 65730-65757
　heart, 33933, 33944-33945
　lung, 33935
　intestine, 44132-44136, 44715-44721
　liver, 47135, 47143-47147
　lung, 32850-32856, 33933
　pancreas, 0141T-0143T, 48160, 48550-48556
　renal, 50300-50380
　skin, 15002-15431
　testis, 54680
panel, 80050
　hepatic, 80074-80076
　renal function, 80069

Organic acid
qualitative, 83919
single, 83921
total, 83918

Ormond disease, 50715

Orogastric tube, 43752

Oropharynx, 42800

Orthodentic cephalogram, 70350

Orthomyxoviridus,
antibody, 86710
immunoassay, 87804

Orthopantogram, 70355

Orthopedic
cast
　arm, 29065, 29075
　body
　　halo, 29000
　　upper, 29035-29046
　clubfoot, 29450
　cranial, 20661-20664
　cylinder, 29365
　finger, 29086
　femur, 20663
　hand, 29085
　hip, 29305-29325
　leg, 29345-29355, 29365, 29405-29450
　maxillofacial, 21100
　patellar tendon, 29435
　pelvic, 20662
　shoulder, 29049-29058
　wedge, 29740-29750
　window, 29730
　wrist, 29085
surgery, 20985

Orthoptic training, 92065

Orthoroentgenogram, 77073

Orthosis, 97760-97762

Os calcis fracture, 28400-28420

Osmolality, 83930-83935

Osseous Survey, 77074-77076

Ossicles
excision, 69660-69661
mobilization, 69650
reconstruction
　mastoidectomy, 69642, 69644, 69646
　mastoidotomy, 69636, 69637
　replacement prostheis, 69633, 69637
　without mastoidectomy, 69632-69633
release, 69650
stapes
　excision, 69660-69661
　mobilization, 69650
　revision, 69662

Ostectomy
metacarpal, 26250-26255
metatarsal, 28288
phalanx
　distal, 26262
　middle, 26260
scapula, 23190
sternum, 21620
ulcer
　coccyx, 15920

Ostectomy — *continued*
ulcer — *continued*
　ischial, 15941, 15945-15946
　sacral, 15933, 15935, 15937
　trochanteric, 15951, 15953, 15956

Osteoarthritis, 0005F, 1006F-1007F, 2004F

Osteocalcin, 83937

Osteochondroma, 69140

Osteocutaneous flap, 20969-20973

Osteoma, 31075

Osteomyelitis
clavicle, 23170, 23180
elbow, 23935
face, 21026
femur, 27303
finger, 26034
foot, 28005
hand, 26034
hip, 26992
humerus, 23174, 23184, 23935, 24134
incision
　superficial, 2000
　deep, 2005
knee, 27303
olecranon process, 24138, 24147
mandible, 21025
pelvis, 26992
radius, 24136, 21415
scapula, 23172, 23182
shoulder, 23035
skull, 61501
thorax, 21510

Osteopathic manipulation, 98925-98929

Osteoperosis, 4005F

Osteoplasty
carpals, 25394
face, 21208-21209
femur
　lengthening, 27466-27468
　neck, 27179
　shortening, 27465, 27468
fibula, 27715
humerus, 24420
metacarpal, 26568
phalanx, 26568
radius, 25390-25391
　ulna, 25392-25393
tibia, 27715
ulna, 25390-25391
　radius, 25392-25393
vertebra
　lumbar, 22511-22512, 22514-22515
　thoracic, 22510, 22512, 22513, 22515

Osteotomy
calcaneus, 28300
chin, 21121-21123
clavicle, 23480-23485
femur
　epiphysis, 27181
　greater trochanter, 27140
　iliac, 27151-27156
　intertrochanteric, 27165
　neck, 27161
　shaft, 27448-27450, 27454
　subtrochanteric, 27165
　supracondylar, 27448-27450
fibula, 27707
　and tibia, 27709
finger, 26567
graft, 21267-21268
hip, 27146-27151
humerus, 24400
　shaft, 24410
mandible
　extraoral, 21047
　intraoral, 21046
　segmental, 21198-21199
maxilla
　extraoral, 21049
　intraoral, 21048
　segmental, 21206

Osteotomy — *continued*
metacarpal, 26565
metatarsal
　first, 28306-28307
　other than first, 28308
　multiple, 28309
orbital
　hypertelorism, 21260-21263
　periorbital, 21260-21263
　repositioning, 21267-21268
　reconstruction, 21256
pelvis, 27158
phalanx
　any toe, 28312
　finger, 26567
　first toe, proximal, 28310
radius
　distal, 25350
　middle/proximal, 25355
　multiple, 25370
　with ulna, 25365, 25375
skull
　anterior cranial fossa, 61582-61583
　supraorbital ridge, 61584-61585
　zygoma, 61592
spine
　anterior, 22220-22226
　posterior, 22206-22216
talus, 28302
tarsal bone, except talus/calcaneous, 28304-28305
tibia, 27705
　and fibula, 27709
　multiple, 27712
　proximal, 27455-27457
ulna, 25360
　multiple, 25370
　with radius, 25365, 25375
vertebra
　anterior, 22220-22226
　cervical, 22210, 22216-22220, 22226
　lumbar, 22207-22208, 22214-22216, 22224-22226
　posterior, 22206-22216
　thoracic, 22206, 22208, 22212, 22216, 22222, 22226

Otolaryngology exam, 92502

Otoplasty, 69300

Otorhinolaryngology services, 92502-92700
audiology function tests, 92551-92597
diagnostic analysis
　brain stem implant, 92640
　cochlear implant, 92601-92604
evaluation
　auditory rehab status, 92626-92627
　central auditory function, 92620-92621
　electroacoustic, 92594-92595
　non-speech-generating device, 92605
　speech-generating device, 92607-92608
　speech, language, voice, 92521-92524
　swallowing function, 3142F, 92610
　voice prosthetic device, 92597
facial nerve function, 92516
flexible fiberoptic endoscopy, 92612-92617
laryngeal function, 92520
nasal function study, 92512
swallowing function, 3142F, 92610
therapeutic, 92606, 92609
vestibular function tests, 92531-92548

Outpatient services
consultation, 99201-99215
education, 4003F, 4014F, 4058F
established patient, 99211-99215
new patient, 99201-99205
office visit, 99201-99215
prolonged services, 99354-99355

Orbit(al) — Outpatient services

Output, cardiac
  dilution, 93561-93562
Ova smear, 87177
Oval window
  fistula repair, 69666
Ovariolysis, 58740
Ovary(ian)
  abscess, 58820-58822
  adhesions, 58660, 58740
  biopsy, 58900
  cyst
    excision, 58925
    incision, 58800-58805
  excision
    bilateral/unilateral, 58940-
      58943, 58950-58956
    ectopic pregnancy, 59120
    hysterectomy
      radical, 58210, 58548
      supracervical, 58180,
        58542, 58544
      total, 58150-58152, 58200,
        58240, 58571, 58573
      vaginal, 58262-58263,
        58291-58292, 58552,
        58554
      partial/total, 58661, 58940-
        58940
      radical hysterectomy, 58210,
        58548
  transposition, 58825
  vein syndrome, 50722
  wedge resection, 58920
Oviduct
  adhesions, 58660, 58740
  anastomosis, 58750
  chromotubation, 58350
  excision
    bilateral, 58700-58720,
      58950-58956
    ectopic pregnancy, 59120
    hysterectomy
      radical, 58210, 58548
      supracervical, 58180,
        58542, 58544
      total, 58150-58152, 58200,
        58240, 58571, 58573
      vaginal, 58262-58263,
        58291-58292, 58552,
        58554
      partial/total, 58661, 58700-
        58720
    with radical hysterectomy,
      58210, 58548
  fulguration, 58670
  ligation, 58600-58611
  occlusion, 58615, 58671
  stoma, 58770
  transection, 58600-58611
  x-ray, 74740
Ovocyte
  biopsy, 89290-89291
  culture, 89250-89251, 89272
  fertilization, 89280-89281
  identification, 89254
  insemination, 89268
  retrieval, 58970
  storage, 89346
  thawing, 89356
Ovulation test, 84830
Ovum, 58976
Oxalate, 83945
Oxidase, 82390
Oxidoreductase, 82943
  measurement, 84588
  tolerance, 80422-80424, 82946
Oximetry, 94760-94762
Oxoisomerase, 84087
Oxosteroid, 83586-83593
Oxygen saturation, 82805-82810
Oxygenation
  extracorporeal, 33946-33966,
    33969, 33984-33989
Oxyproline, 83500-83505
Oxytocin stress test, 59020

P

Pacemaker
  evaluation, 93279-93281
    device, leadless system,
      0389T-0391T
    interrogation, 93288, 93294
    peri-procedural, 93286
    transtelephonic, 93293
  insertion, 00530, 33206-33208
    electrode, 33210-33211, 33216-
      33217, 33224-33225
    pulse generator only, 33212-
      33213, 33221
  removal, 33233-33237
    thoracotomy, 33236-33237
  repair, 33218-33220
  replacement
    catheter, 33210
    electrode, 33210-33211
    insertion, 33206-33208
    pulse generator, 33226-33229
  repositioning, 33215, 33226
  revise pocket, 33222
  upgrade, 33214
Pachymetry, 76514
Packing
  nasal hemorrhage, 30901-30906
Pain, 1125F-1126F, 2040F
  management, 0521F, 1116F
    epidural/intrathecal, 2044F,
      62350-62351, 62360-
      62362, 99601-99602
Palate
  biopsy, 42100
  destruction, 42160
  excision, 42145
    lesion, 42104-42120
  fracture
    closed treatment, 21421
    open treatment, 21422-21423
  incision and drainage, 42000
  palatoplasty, 42200-42225
  prosthesis
    augmentation, 21082
    impression, 42280
    insertion, 42281
    lift, 21083
  reconstruction, 42226-42227
  repair
    cleft, 00172, 42200-42225
    laceration, 42180-42182
    vomer flap, 42235
Palm
  excision
    tendon, 26170
      sheath, 26145
  fasciectomy, 26121-26125
  fasciotomy, 26040-26045
  incision and drainage
    bursa, 26025-26030
    tendon sheath, 26020
Palsy, 15840-15845
Pancreas
  anastomosis, 48548
    cyst, 48520-48540
  biopsy, 48100
    needle, 48102
  collection, 43260
  cannulation, 43273
  debridement
    peripancreatic tissue, 48105
  destruction
    calculi, 43265
    tumor, 43278
  dilation, 43277
  drainage, 48510
  elastase 1 (PE1), 82656
  excision
    ampulla of vater, 48148
    duct, 48148
    lesion, 48120
    partial, 48140-48146, 48150,
      48154, 48160
    peripancreatic tissue, 48105
    total, 48155-48160

Pancreas — *continued*
  islet cell, 0141T-0143T
  pancreateceomy
    donor, 48550
    partial, 48140-48146, 48150-
      48154, 48160
    total, 48155-48160
    with transplantation, 48160
  pancreaticojejunostomy, 48548
  pancreatography
    injection procedure, 48400
    intraoperative, 74300-74301
  pancreatorrhaphy, 48545
  pancreatotomy, 48000-48001
  pancreozymin-secretin test, 82938
  placement
    drainage, 48000-48001
    stent, 43274
  pseudocyst
    drainage, open, 48510
  removal
    allograft, 48556
    calculi (stone), 43264, 48020
    foreign body, 43275
    stent, 43275-43276
  repair
    cyst, 48500
  resection, 48105
  sphincter, 43262-43263
  suture, 48545
  transplantation, 48160, 48550,
    48554-48556
    allograft preparation, 48550-
      48552
    islet cell, 0141T-0143T
  x-ray with contrast, 74300-74301
    guide catheter, 74329-74330
    injection procedure, 48400
Panel
  electrolyte, 80051
  general health, 80050
  hepatic function, 80076
  hepatitis, 80074
  lipid, 3011F, 3278F, 80061
  metabolic, 80047-80048, 80053
  obstetric, 80055, 80081
  renal, 80069
Panniculectomy, 15830-15839,
  15876-15879
Pap smears, 88141
  preservative fluid, 88142-88143
    thin layer prep, 88174-88175
  slide, 88150-88155
    Bethesda system, 88164-88167
  smear, 88147-88148
Papillectomy, 46220, 46230
Papilloma
  anus, 46900-46924
  penis, 54050-54065
Para-tyrosine, 84510
Paracentesis
  abdomen, 49082-49083
  eye
    aqueous removal, 65800
    blood removal, 65815
    vitreous removal, 65810
    membrane, 65810
  thorax, 32554-32555
Paracervical nerve
  injection, 64435
Paraffin bath therapy, 97018
Parainfluenza virus, 87279
Paralysis
  facial nerve, 15840-15845
  infantile, 86658, 90696-90698,
    90713
Parasites
  blood, 87206-87209
  examination, 87169
  smear, 87177
  tissue, 87220
  worms, helminth, 86682
Parathyrine, 83970
Parathyroid
  autotransplant, 60512
  excision, 60500-60502

Parathyroid — *continued*
  exploration, 60500-60505
  hormone, 83970
  imaging, 78070-78072
  parathyroidectomy, 60500-60505
Paraurethral gland, 53060
Paravertebral nerve
  destruction, 64622-64627
  injection, 0213T-0218T
    anesthetic, 64470-64484
    neurolytic, 64622-64627
Parietal
  cell vagotomy, 43641
  craniotomy, 61556
    anesthesia, 00211
Paring
  skin lesions
    benign hyperkeratotic, 11055-
      11057
    1 lesion, 11055
    2-4 lesions, 11056
    4 lesions or more, 11057
Paronychia, 10060-10061
Parotid
  abscess, 42300-42305
  excision
    calculi, 42330, 42340
    partial, 42410-42415
    total, 42420-42426
    tumor, 42410-42426
  reconstruction
    duct, 42507-42510
Parkinsons, 1400F, 4324F-4328F,
  4400F, 6080F-6090F
Parotitides, 86735
  immunization, 90707, 90710
Pars abdominalis aortae
  aneurysm, 34800-34805, 34825-
    34832, 34841-34848,
    35081-35103, 75952-75953
  computed tomography (CT)
    angiography, 75635
  repair, 33877, 34800-34805,
    34830-34832, 34841-
    34848, 35081-35103, 75952
  thromboendarterectomy, 35331
Partial
  arthroplasty
    hip, 27125
  decortication, 32225, 32651
  diaphysectomy
    arm, 23184, 24140, 24145,
      24147, 24150-24151
    clavicle, 23180
    foot, 28120-28124
    hand, 26230-26236
    leg, 27360, 27640-27641
    radial, 24145
    radius, 25151
    scapula, 23182
    ulna, 25150
  excision
    bladder, 55150-55165
    breast, 19300-19302
    colectomy
      partial, 44140, 44147, 44160
        laparoscopic, 44204-
          44208 44213
      coloproctostomy, 44145-
        44146
      colostomy, 44141-44144,
        44206-44208
      ileocolostomy, 44205
      ilieostomy, 44144
    esophagus, 43116-43124
    kidney, 50240, 50543
    larynx, 31370-31382
    liver, 47120
    metatarsal, 28110-28112
    olecranon process, 24147
    oviduct, 58661, 58700-58720
    pancreas, 48140-48146,
      48150-48154, 48160
    parotid, 42410-42415
    penis, 54120
    pharynx, 42890
    prostate, 55801, 55821-55831

CPT © 2015 American Medical Association. All Rights Reserved.
© 2016 decisionHealth

Partial — *continued*
  excision — *continued*
    radius, 25145
    rectum, 45111, 45113-45116, 45123
    spleen, 38101, 38115
    stomach, 43631-43635, 43845
    testis, 54522
    thyroid, 60210-60220
    tibia, 27370, 27640
    tongue, 41120-41135
    ovary, 58661, 58940-58943
    ulna, 25145-25151, 25240
    ureter, 50220-50230, 50546
    uterus, 58180
    vagina, 57106-57109
    vulva, 56620, 56630-56632
  reconstruction
    conjunctiva, 68360
  repair
    pulmonary vein, 33724
  replacement
    ossicular prosthesis (PORP), 69633, 69637
  resection
    uterus, 59136
Particle agglutination, 86403-86406
Parvovirus, 86747
Patella, 01390-01392
  chondromalacia, 27418
  dislocation, 27560-27566
  excision, 27424
    bursa, 27340
  fracture, 27520-27524
  patellar tendon bearing (PTB) cast, 29435
  patellectomy, 27424
  reconstruction, 27437-27438
    arthroplasty, 27437-27438, 27447
    dislocating, 27420-27424
  repair
    chondromalacia, 27418
    instability, 27420-27424
  tendon
    suture, 27380-27381
    transplant, 27396-27397
Paternity testing, 86910-86911
Patey's operation, 19303-19306
Pathology
  consultation
    clinical, 80500-80502
    surgical, 88321-88325
      intraoperative, 88329-88334
  decalcification procedure, 88311
  electron microscopy, 88348
  gross and/or micro exam
    level I, 88300
    level II, 88302
    level III, 88304
    level IV, 88305
    level V, 88307
    level VI, 88309
  histochemistry, 88313-88314
  immunocytochemistry, 88341-88344
  immunofluorescence, single antibody stain, 88346, 88350
  immunohistochemistry, 88341-88344
  malignancy, 3317F-3318F
  morphometry
    nerve, 88356
    skeletal muscle, 88355
    tumor, 88358-88361
  nerve testing, 88362
  staining, 88312-88319
  tissue hybridization, 88364-88366
Patient care management, 0500F-0557F, 0575F, 0580F-0584F
Pectoral cavity
  exploration, 32601-32606
  graft, 35905
  surgery, 32650-32665
Pectus
  reconstructive repair, 21740-21742
  thoracoscopy, 21743

Pediatric
  critical care
    evaluation and management, 99471-99476
    transport, 99466-99467
  intensive care
    low birth weight, 99478-99480
Pedicle
  fixation
    insertion, 22842-22844
  flap
    formation, 15570-15576
    island, 15740
    neurovascular, 15750
    transfer, 15650
Pelvi-ureteroplasty, 50400-50405, 50540, 50544
Pelvic, 01120-01190
  angiography, 72191
  biopsy, 27040-27041
  brace application, 20662
  computed tomography (CT) scan, 72191-72194, 74176-74178
  cyst
    aspiration, 50390
    injection, 50390
  destruction
    lesion, 58662
  endoscopy
    destruction of lesion, 58662
    lysis of adhesions, 58660
    oviduct surgery, 58670-58671
  examination, 57410
  excision, 27047-27049
  exclusion
    small intestine, 44700
  exenteration, 45126, 51597, 58240
  fixation, 22848
  halo, 20662
  incision and drainage
    abscess, 26990, 45000
    bone, 26992
    bursa, 26991
    hematoma, 26990
  lymphadenectomy, 58210, 58958
  lysis, 58660
  magnetic resonance angiography (MRA), 72198
  magnetic resonance imaging (MRI), 72195-72197
  osteotomy, 27158
  pelvimetry, 74710
  pelviolithotomy, 50130
  pemberton osteotomy, 27158
  removal
    foreign body, 27086-27087
  repair
    osteotomy, 27158
    tendon, 27098
  ring
    dislocation, 27193-27194, 27216-27218
    fracture, closed treatment, 27193-27194
  ultrasound, 76856-76857
  x-ray, 72170-72190
    manometry, 74710
Penetrating keratoplasty, 65750-65755
Penis, 00920-00938
  amputation
    partial, 54120
    radical, 54130-54135
    total, 54125
  biopsy, 54100-54105
  circumcision
    newborn, 54150, 54160
    repair, 54163
  destruction
    lesion
      cryosurgery, 54056
      electrodesiccation, 54055
      excision, surgical, 54060
      extensive, 54065
      laser surgery, 54057
      penile plaque, 54110-54112
      simple, 54050-54060

Penis — *continued*
  excision
    frenulum, 54164
    partial, 54120
    plaque, 54110-54112
    prepuce, 54150-54161, 54163
    total, 54125-54135
  incision
    drainage, 54015
    prepuce, 54000-54001
  induration, 54200
  injection
    erection, 54235
    Peyronie disease, 54200
    plaque, surgical exposure, 54205
    vasoactive drugs, 54231
    x-ray, 54230
  insertion
    inflatable prosthesis, 54401-54405
    noninflatable prosthesis, 54400
  irrigation, 54220
  lysis
    adhesions, 54162
  occlusion, 37790
  penectomy
    partial, 54120
    radical, 54130-54135
    total, 54125
  plaque
    excision, 54110-54112
  plethysmography, 54240
  prepuce
    excision, 54150-54161, 54163
    incision, 54000-54001
    stretch, 54450
  prosthesis
    inflatable, 54401-54405
      removal, 54406, 54410-54417
      repair, 54408
      replacement, 54410-54411, 54416-54417
    noninflatable, 54400
      removal, 54415-54417
      replacement, 54416-54417
  reconstruction
    angulation, 54360
    chordee, 54300-54304, 54328
    complications, 54340-54348
    epispadias, 54380-54390
    hypospadias, 54328-54352
    injury, 54440
  removal
    foreign body, 54115
    prosthesis, 54406, 54410-54417
  repair
    corporeal tears, 54437
    fistulization, 54435
    inflatable prosthesis, 54408
    priapism with shunt, 54420-54430
  replacement
    inflatable prosthesis, 54410-54411, 54416-54417
    semi-rigid prosthesis, 54416-54417
  replantation of amputation, 54438
  revascularization, 37788
  test
    erection, 54250
    nocturnal penile tumescence, 54250
    rigidity, 54250
  venous studies, 93980-93981
Pentagastrin test, 43755
Peptidase
  P, 82164
  S, 83670
Peptide
  C, 80432, 84681
  vasoactive intestinal, 84586
Percutaneous
  abdominal paracentesis, 49080-49081
  allergy test, 95004, 95017-95018

Percutaneous — *continued*
  arthrectomy, 37225, 37227, 37229, 37231, 37233, 37235, 0234T-0238T
  aspiration, 62267
  biopsy
    bile duct, 47552-47556
    cholecystostomy, 47490
    kidney, 50200
    spinal cord, 62269
    thyroid, 60100
  catheter, 36620
  discectomy, 62287
  drainage, 75989
  electric nerve stimulation, 64550
  fixation
    ankle, 27842
    femur, 27235, 27509
    finger, 26432, 26727, 26756, 26776
    foot, 28436, 28476, 28546, 28576, 28606, 28636, 28666
    forearm, 25671
    hand, 26608, 26650
    humerus, 24538, 24566, 24582
    radius, 25525, 25606
    tibia, 27756
    toe fixation, 28496
    wrist, 25651
  fluoroscopy, 75989
  fracture treatment
    cheek, 21355
    facial, 21452
    femur, 27235, 27509
    finger, 26706, 26727, 26756, 26776
    foot, 28406, 28436, 28456, 28476, 28496
    forearm, 25606, 25651
    hand
      carpometacarpal, 26650, 26676
      metacarpal, 26608
      metacarpophalangeal, 26706
    nose, 21330, 21340, 21345-21347
    pelvis, 01130, 27216
    radius, 25606
    tarsal, 28456
    tibia, 27756
    toe, 28496
  gastrostomy, 43246, 49440
  implant, 64561
  lysis, 62263-62264
  nephrostomy, 52334
  transcatheter
    closure
      atrial septal defect, 93580
      interatrial communication, 93580
      patent ductus arteriosus, 93582
      ventricular septal defect, 93581
    septal reduction therapy, 93583
  transluminal angioplasty
    artery
      aortic, 35472
      brachiocephalic, 35475
      coronary, 92920-92921
      femoral-popliteal, 37224-37227
      iliac, 37220-37223
      pulmonary, 92997-92998
      renal, 35471
      tibioperoneal, 37228-37235
      visceral, 35471
    venous, 35476
  valvuloplasty
    aortic, 92986
    mitral, 92987
    pulmonary, 92990
  venipuncture, 36400-36410
Pereyra procedure, 51845, 57289, 58267

Partial – Pereyra procedure

Performance measures
  assessment
    clinical, 2000F-2060F
    patient history/status,
      1000F-1494F
    symptoms, 1000F-1494F,
      1500F-1505F
  composite measures,
    0001F-0015F
  follow-up, 5005F-5250F
  documentation
    plan of care, 0500F-0575F
    safety measures, 6005F-6110F
    results, 3006F-3763F
    screening, 3006F-3763F
  nonmeasure codes, 9001F-9007F
  outcomes, 5005F-5250F
  patient care management,
    0500F-0575F
  physical examination, 2000F-2060F
  therapy/intervention, 4000F-4563F
  structural measures, 7010F-7025F
Performance test
  cognitive, 96125
  physical, 97750
  psychological, 96101-96103
Perfusion
  brain, 0042T
  intracranial arterial thrombolysis,
    61624
  myocardial, 78460-78465,
    78478-78480
    imaging, 78466-78469
  positron emission tomography
    (PET), 78491-78492
  pulmonary, imaging, 78580-78598
Pericardium
  excision, 32659, 33030-33031
    cyst, 32661, 33050
    tumor, 32661, 33050
  incision, 33020
    drainage, 33025
    tube, 33015
  pericardial sac, 32659, 33025
  pericardiectomy
    complete, 33030-33031
    subtotal, 33030-33031
  pericardiocentesis, 33010-33011,
    76930
  pericardiostomy, 33015
  pericardiotomy, 33020
  puncture aspiration, 33010-33011
  removal, 32658
  window, 32659, 33025
Peridural, 62281-62282, 62310-
    62319, 64479-64484
Perineum, 00904
  biopsy, 56605-56606
  colposcopy, 99170
  incision and drainage, 56405
  debridement, 11004, 11006
  perineoplasty, 56810
  perineorrhaphy, 57250
  prostatectomy, 55801, 55810-
    55815
  prosthesis, 53442
  repair, 56810
  x-ray with contrast, 74775
Periorbital region
  osteotomy, 21260-21263
  osteotomy with graft, 21267-21268
Peripheral
  artery disease, 93668
  nerve, 64856-64859
Periprosthetic capsulectomy, 19371
Peristaltic pump
  electronic analysis, 62367-
    62368 insertion, 36260
  intra-arterial, 36261-36262
  intravenous
    insertion, 36563
    repair, 36576
    replacement, 36583
  maintenance, 95990-95991,
    96521-96522
  spinal cord, 62361-62362
  ventricular catheter, 61215

Peritoneocentesis, 49082-49083
Peritoneum
  abscess, 49020
  biopsy, 49000, 49320-49321
  catheter, 49418-49422
  chemotherapy, 0519F, 96446
  dialysis, 90945-90947
  injection
    contrast, 49424
    shunt, 49427
  lavage, 49084
  ligation
    shunt, 49428
  pneumoperitoneum, 49400
  removal
    cannula/catheter, 49422
    foreign body, 49402
    shunt, 49429
  tumor, 58950-58958
  x-ray, 74190
Persistent
  truncus arteriosus, 33786
  omphalomesenteric duct, 44800
Personality test, 96101-96103
Pessary, 57160
Pesticides, 82441
PET (Positron emission tomography),
    3319F-3320F
  limited, 78811
    computed tomography (CT),
      78814
  skull base to mid-thigh, 78812
    computed tomography (CT),
      78815
  whole body, 78813
    computed tomography (CT),
      78816
Petrous temporal, 69530
Peyronie disease
  injection, 54200
  surgical exposure, 54205
    with graft, 54110-54112
pH
  exhaled breath condensate, 83987
  other fluid, 83986
  urine, 83986
Phacoemulsification
  extracapsular cataract, 66982,
    66984
  secondary membranous cataract,
    66850
Phagocytosis, 86344
Phalanx
  finger
    amputation, 26910-26952
    arthrodesis, 26820-26863
    arthroplasty, 26535-26536
    biopsy, 11755, 26110
    decompression, 26035
    diaphysectomy, 26235-26236
    excision
      capsule, 26525
      cyst, 26210-26215
      lesion, 26160
      radical, 26260-26262
      ring, 26596
      sesamoid, 26185
      tendon, 26180, 26415
      tumor, 26115-26117,
        26210-26215
    exploration, 26080
    fracture
      articular
        closed treatment, 26740
        open treatment, 26746
        with manipulation, 26742
      distal
        closed treatment, 26750
        open treatment, 26756
        percutaneous fixation,
          26756
      shaft fracture, 26720-26727
        open treatment, 26735
    incision, 26034, 26055-26060,
      26080

Phalanx — *continued*
  finger — *continued*
    incision — *continued*
      drainage
        abscess, 26010-26011
        tendon sheath, 26020
    manipulation, 26340
    open treatment, 26735
    osteotomy, 26567
    pollicization, 26550
    release, 26508
    removal, 26080
      implant, 26320
      rod, 26416
    repair, 26418, 26426-26434
      claw finger, 26499
      joint, 26540
      lengthening, 26478, 26568
      macrodactyly, 26590
      nonunion, 26546
      osteotomy, 26567
      polydactyly, 26587
      shortening, 26477, 26479
      syndactyly, 26560-26562
      volar plate, 26548
    synovectomy, 26135-26145
    tenolysis, 26440-26449
    tenotomy, 26455-26460
    transfer, 26497-26498, 26551-
      26556
  toe
    amputation, 28810-28825
    arthrodesis, 28750-28760
    biopsy, 11755, 28052-28054
    diaphysectomy, 28124
    excision, 28110-28114, 28124,
      28150, 28160
      capsule, 28270-28272
      condyle, 28126
      cyst, 28108
      fascia, 28008
      lesion, 28092
      neuroma, 28080
      tumor, 28108, 28175
    fracture
      great, 28490
        open treatment, 28505
        with manipulation,
          28495-28496
        percutaneous fixation,
          28496
        without manipulation,
          28490
      open treatment, 28525
        with manipulation, 28515
        without manipulation, 28510
    incision, 28010-28011, 28234
      drainage, 28020-28024
    release, 28289
    removal
      foreign body, 28020-28024
    repair, 28286, 28312-28315
      bunion, 28289-28299
      hammertoe, 28285
      macrodactyly, 28340-28341
      osteotomy, 28310-28312
      polydactyly, 28344
      syndactyly, 28280, 28345
    replantation, 20816-20822
    resection, 28126, 28153, 28175
    synovectomy, 28072
Pharmacotherapy, 4063F
Pharynx
  biopsy, 42800-42806
  cineradiography, 70371, 74230
  creation, 42955
  excision, 42145
    lesion, 42808
    partial, 42890
    resection, 42892-42894
    with larynx, 31390-31395
  hemorrhage, 42960-42962,
    42970-42972
  pharyngectomy, 42890
  pharyngolaryngectomy, 31390-
    31395
  pharyngoplasty, 42950
  pharyngorrhaphy, 42900

Pharynx — *continued*
  pharyngostomy, 42955
  pharyngotomy, 42955
  reconstruction, 42950
  removal, 42809
  repair, 42953
  tonsil, 42820-42821, 42830-42836
  video study, 70371, 74230
  x-ray, 70370, 74210
Phencyclidine, 83992
Phenobarbital, 80345
  assay, 80184
Phenothiazine, 80342-80344
Phenotype
  analysis
    HIV-1 drug resistance, 87903-
      87904
  prediction, 87900
Phenylaline, 84030
Phenylketones, 84035
Phenytoin, 80185-80186
Pheochromocytoma, 80424
Pheresis, 36511-36516
Phlebectomy, 37765-37766
Phlebography
  adrenal, 75840-75842
  arm, 75820-75822
  epidural, 2044F, 75872
  hepatic portal, 75885-75887
  injection, 36005
  jugular, 75860
  leg, 75820-75822
  liver, 75889-75891
  neck, 75860
  nuclear medicine, 78445, 78457-
    78458
  orbit, 75880
  renal, 75831-75833
  sagittal sinus, 75870
  sampling, 75893
  vena cava, 75825-75827
Phleborrhaphy, 37620-37660
Phlebotomy, 99195
Phoria, 67345
  repair, 67311-67340
Phosphatase
  acid, 84060
    blood, 84066
  alkaline, 84075, 84080
    blood, 84078
  forensic examination, 84061
Phosphate, 84207
Phosphatidyl
  choline, 86812-86817, 86821-
    86822
  glycerol, 84081
Phosphidylglycerol, 84081
Phosphocreatine, 82550-82552
Phosphogluconate-6
  dehydrogenase, 84085
Phosphoglyceride, 84081
Phosphohexose isomerase, 84087
Phosphohydrolases
  acid, 84060
    blood, 84066
  alkaline, 84075, 84080
    blood, 84078
  forensic examination, 84061
Phosphokinase, 82550-82552
Phospholipid
  antibody, 86147
  cofactor antibody, 86849
  neutralization, 85597-85598
Phosphorus, 3278F, 84100
  urine, 84105
Photo patch, 95052
Photochemotherapy, 0519F, 96910-
    96913
  endoscopic, 96570-96571
  extracorporeal, 36522
Photocoagulation
  iridoplasty, 66762

CPT © 2015 American Medical Association. All Rights Reserved.   © 2016 DecisionHealth

Photocoagulation — *continued*
  lesion
    cornea, 65450
    retina, 67210, 67228 -67229
  retinal detachment
    prophylaxis, 67145
    repair, 67105
  vitrectomy
    endolaser panretinal, 67040
    focal endolaser, 67040
Photodensity, 77083
Photodynamic therapy, 96567
Photography
  eye, 92225-92226
  skin, 96904
Photopheresis, 0168T, 96900
  extracorporeal, 36522
Photoscreen, 99174
Photosensitivity testing, 95056
Phrenic nerve
  avulsion, 64746
  incision, 64746
  injection, 64410
  transection, 64746
Physical examination measures, 2000F-2060F
Physical/occupational therapy, 4018F
  activities
    daily living, 97535, 99509
      therapeutic, 97530
  acquatic, 97113
  check-out, 97762
  cognitive skills development, 97532
  community reintegration, 97537
  contrast baths, 97034
  diathermy treatment, 97024
  direct, 97032-97039
  electric stimulation
    attended, 97032
    unattended, 97014
  evaluation, 97001-97002
  exercises, 4240F-4242F, 97110
  group, 97150
  hot or cold pack, 97010
  hydrotherapy (Hubbard tank), 97036
  infrared light treatment, 97026
  iontophoresis, 97033
  kinetic, 97530
  manual, 97140
  massage, 97124
  microwave, 97024
  neuromuscular re-education, 97112
  osteopathic manipulation, 98925-98929
  paraffin bath, 97018
  physical performance test, 97750
  sensory integration, 97533
  supervised procedure, 97010-97028
  traction, 97012, 97140
  training
    athletic, 97005-97006
    gait, 97116
    orthotics, 97760
    prosthetics, 97761
  ultrasound, 97035
  ultraviolet light, 97028
  vasopneumatic device, 97016
  wheelchair management, 97542
  whirlpool, 97022
  work
    hardening, 97545-97546
    reintegration, 95537
  work hardening, 97545-97546
Physician services
  advanced life support, 99288
  care plan oversight, 99339-99340, 99374-99380
  domiciliary facility, 99339-99340
  home health agency care, 99374
  home or rest home care, 99339-99340
  hospice, 99377-99378
  nursing facility, 99379-99380
  case management, 99366-99368
  online, 99444

Physician services — *continued*
  prolonged
    direct patient contact, 99354-99357
    inpatient, 99356-99357
    outpatient/office, 99354-99355
    without direct patient contact, 99358-99359
  standby, 99360
  supervision, 99339-99340, 99374-99380
  team conference, 99367
  telephone, 99441-99443
Piercing, 69090
Piles
  destruction, 46930
  incision, 46083
  injection, 46500
  ligation, 46945-46946
  stapling, 46947
  suture, 46945-46946
Pilonidal cyst
  excision, 11770-11772
  incision and drainage, 10080-10081
Pin
  insertion, 20650
  prophylactic treatment
    femur, 27187
    humerus, 24498
    shouler, 23490-23491
  removal, 20650
Pinch graft, 15050
Pinna
  biopsy, 69100
  computed tomography (CT) scan, 70480-70482
  destruction, 17280-17286
  drainage, 69000-69005
  excision, 69110-69110
    lesion
      benign, 11440-11446
      malignant, 11640-11646
  flap
    formation, 15576
    delay, 15630
  graft, 21235
    acellular, 15175-15176
    allograft, 15320-15321
      acellular, 15335-15336
    autograft
      dermal, 15135-15136
      epidermal, 15115-15116, 15155-15157
      split thickness, 15120-15121
    full thickness, 15260-15261
    preparation, 15004-15005
    substitute, 15365-15366
    xenograft, 15420-15421
  piercing, 69090
  reconstruction, 69300
  repair
    wound
      complex, 13151-13153
      layer closure, 12051-12057
      simple, 12011-12018
    shaving, 11310-11313
    transfer, 14060-14061
Pinworms, 87172
Pirogoff procedure, 27888
Pituitary
  epidermoid tumor, 61545
  gland
    excision, 61546-61548, 62165
  hormone
    growth, 83003, 80418, 80428-80430, 86277
    lactogenic, 80418, 84146
Placement
  access through biliary tree, 47541
  amniotic membrane, 65778-65779
  catheter
    aneurysm, 34806, 93982
    brain, 0169T
    breast, 19296-19298, 20555, 41019
    bronchus, 31643

Placement — *continued*
  catheter — *continued*
    guidance, 75989
    head, 41019
    heart, 93503
    neck, 41019
    pelvis, 55920
    prostate, 55875
  clip
    breast, 19281-19288
    soft tissue, 10035-10036
  device
    dosimeter, 49327, 49412, 55876
    gastric restrictive, 43770
    interstitial, 55876
    intracoronary, 92974
  drain
    pancreas, 48001
  filter, 37191
  intrafacet implant, 0219T-0222T
  marker
    fiducial, 49327, 49412, 55876
  needle
    bone, 36680
    breast, 19281-19288
    genitalia, 55920
    head, 41019
    muscle, 20555
    neck, 41019
    pelvis, 55920
    prostate, 55875-55876
    soft tissue, 10035-10036, 20555
  prosthesis
    endovascular, 33883-33886
    guidance, 75958-75959
  sensor, 34806
  stent
    bronchial, 31636-31637
    colonic, 44402, 45327, 45347, 45389
    coronary artery, 92928-92934
    intracranial, 61635
    intravascular
      carotid artery, 37215-37218
      extracranial, 0075T-0076T
      innominate artery, 37217-37218
      intracoronary, 92928-92929, 92933-92934, 92937-92938, 92941, 92943-92944
      intracranial, 61635
      lower extremity artery, 37221, 37223, 37226, 37230, 37231, 37234, 37235
      other artery, 37236-37237
      ureter, 50693-50695
      vein, 37238-37239
  tube
    cecostomy, 44300, 49442
    duodenostomy, 49441
    enterostomy, 44300
    gastostomy, 43246, 49440
    jujenostomy, 44372, 49441
    nasogastric, 43752
    orogastric, 43752
    ureteral, 50947
  wire
    breast 19281-19286
    soft tissue, 10035-100036
Placenta, 59414
  alpha microglobulin, 84112
  villi, 59015
Plagiocephaly, 21175
Planing, 30120
Plantar
  digital nerve, 64726, 64632
  pressure measurement, 96001, 96004
Plasma
  frozen preparation, 86927
  protein-A, pregnancy associated (PAPP-A), 84163
  thromboplastin
    antecedent, 85270
    component, 85250
  volume determination, 78110-78111

Plasmin, 85400
  antiactivator, 85410
Plasminogen, 4077F, 85420-85421
Plasmodium, 86750
Plate
  bone, 21244
Platelet
  aggregation, 85576
  antibody, 86022-86023
  assay, 85055
  blood, 85025
  cofactor, 85210-85293
  count, 85032, 85049
  neutralization, 85597
  survival test, 78190-78191
Platysmal flap, 15825
Pleoptic training, 92065
Plethysmography
  extremities, 93922-93923
    veins, 93965
  lung, 94726
  penis, 54240
  total body, 94726
Pleura
  biopsy, 32098, 32400
  decortication, 32320
  excision
    empyema, 32540
    endoscopic, 32656
    parietal, 32310-32320
  pleurectomy
    endoscopic, 32656
    parietal, 32310-32320
  pleurodesis
    chemical, 32560
    endoscopic, 32650
  removal
    foreign body, 32653
  repair, 32215
  thoracotomy, 32098-32100
Pleural
  cavity
    aspiration, 32554-32555
    catheterization, 32250
    chemotherapy administration, 0519F, 96440
    fusion, 32560
    incision
      abscess, 21501-21502
      empyema, 32035-32036
      pneumothroax, 32551
      puncture and drainage, 32554-32555
    scarification, 32215
    thoracostomy, 32035-32036
  endoscopy
    diagnostic, 32601-32606
    surgical, 21743, 32650-32665
  tap, 32554-32555
Plexus
  brachial
    decompression, 64713
    injection, 64415-64416
    neuroplasty, 64713
    repair, 64861
  celiac
    destruction, 64680
    injection, 64530, 64680
  cervical, 64413
  choroid, 61544
  lumbar
    decompression, 64714
    injection, 64449
    neuroplasty, 64714
    repair, 64862
Plication, 51845
Pneumocentesis, 32405
Pneumocisternogram, 70015, 78630
Pneumococcal vaccine, 90670, 90732
Pneumocystis carinii, 87281
Pneumogastric nerve
  abdominal, 64760
  incision, 43640-43641
  injection, 64408
  selective, 43652, 64755
  truncal, 43651

CPT © 2015 American Medical Association. All Rights Reserved.

© 2016 DecisionHealth

Probe — *continued*
nucleic acid — *continued*
amplified detection — *continued*
not otherwise specified,
87798, 87801
staphylococcus, 87640-87641
streptococcus, 87651, 87653
direct detection
bartonella, 87470
borrelia burgdorferi, 87475
candida, 87480
chlamydia, 87485, 87490
cytomegalovirus, 87495
gardnerella vaginalis, 87510
hepatitis, 87515, 87520,
87525
herpes simplex, 87528
herpes virus 6, 87531
human immunodeficiency
virus (HIV), 87534,
87537
legionella, 87540
multiple organisms, 87800
mycobacteria, 87550,
87555, 87560
mycoplasma pneumoniae,
87580
neisseria gonorrheae, 87590
not otherwise specified,
87797
streptococcus group A, 87650
trichomonas Vaginalis, 87660
genotype analysis
hepatitis C, 3265F-3266F,
87902
human immunodeficiency
virus (HIV)-1, 87901
other, 87905
parathyroid, 78808
phenotype analysis
human immunodeficiency
virus (HIV)-1, 87903-
87904
quantification
bartonella, 87472
borrelia burgdorferi, 87477
candida, 87482
chlamydia, 87487, 87492
cytomegalovirus, 87497
bardnerella vaginalis, 87512
hepatitis, 87517, 87522,
87527
herpes simplex, 87530
herpes virus 6, 87533
human immunodeficiency
virus (HIV), 87536,
87539
legionella, 87542
mycobacteria, 87552,
87557, 87562
mycoplasma pneumoniae,
87582
neisseria gonorrheae, 87592
not otherwise specified,
87799
streptococcus group A, 87652
Procainamide, 80190-80192
Procalcitonin (PCT), 0194T
Procidentia
excision, 45130-45135
repair, 45900
Procoagulant activity
inhibition, 85705
test, 85347
partial time, 85730-85732
Proconvertin, 85230
Proctectasis, 45303, 45910
Proctectomy
partial
open, 45111, 45113-45116,
45123
total
colectomy, 44155-44158, 44212
laparoscopic, 45395-45397
open, 45110, 45112-45120,
45123
colon, 45121

Proctocele, 45560
Proctopexy
laparoscopic, 45400-45402
open, 45540-45541
Proctoplasty, 45500-45505
Proctorrhaphy, 45800-45825
prolapse, 45540-45541
Proctoscopy
ablation, 46615
biopsy, 46606
exploration, 46600-46601
removal, 46608-46612
Proctosigmoidoscopy
ablation, 45320
biopsy, 45305
destruction, 45320
dilation, 45303
exploration, 45300
hemorrhage control, 45317
removal
foreign body, 45307
polyp or lesion, 45308-45315
tumor, 45315
stent, 45327
volvulus repair, 45321
Proetz therapy, 30210
Profibrinolysin, 85420-85421
Progenitor cell
allograft, 65781
count, 86367
cryopreservation, 38207, 88240
depletion
plasma, 38214
platelet, 38213
red blood cell, 38212
T-cell, 38210
tumor, 38211
donor search, 38204
harvest, 38205-38206
thawing, 38208-38209, 88241
transplant
allogenic, 38240
infusions, 38242
autologous, 38241
concentration, 38215
Progesterone, 84144
receptors, 84234
Proinsulin, 84206
Projective test, 96101-96103
Prokallikrien plasma, 85292
Prolactin, 80418, 80440, 80146
Prolapse
excision, 45130-45135
repair, 45900
Prolastin, 82103-82104
Prolonged services, 99354-99357,
99360
without direct patient contact,
99358-99359
Prophylactic treatment
femur, 27495
neck, 27187
humerus, 24498
radius, 25490, 25492
shoulder
clavicle, 23490
humerus, 23491
tibia, 27745
ulna, 25491-25492
Prophylaxis
retina detachment, 67141, 67145
Prostaglandin, 84150
insertion, 59200
Prostate, 3268F-3274F, 4163F-4164F
ablation, 55873
antigen, 84152-84154
biopsy, 55700-55706, 55812,
55842
brachytherapy, 55875-55876
coagulation, 52647
destruction
cryosurgery, 55873
microwave thermotherapy,
53850
radio frequency, 53852

Prostate — *continued*
drainage
abscess, 52700
electroejaculation, 55870
enucleation, 52649
excision
partial, 55801, 55821-55831
perineal, 55801-55815
radical, 55810-55815, 55840-
55845
retropubic, 55831-55845
suprapubic, 55821
transurethral, 52402, 52601
exploration
exposure, 55860
nodes, 55862-55865
incision
drainage, 55720-55725
exposure, 55860
transurethral, 52450
insertion
catheter, 55875
needle, 55875
radioactive substance, 55860
placement
catheter, 55875
dosimeter, 55876
fiducial marker, 55876
interstitial device, 55876
needle, 55875
prostatectomy, 52601
laparoscopic, 55866
perineal
partial, 55801
radical, 55810-55815
retropubic
partial, 55831
radical, 55840-55845, 55866
suprapubic, partial, 55821
prostate specific antigen (PSA),
3268F, 84152-84154
prostatotomy, 55720-55725
radiotherapy, 4165F, 4200F-4201F
stent, 0084T
thermotherapy, 53850-53852
ultrasound, 76872-76873
vaporization, 52648
Prosthesis
auricular, 21806
breast
insertion, 19340-19342
removal, 19328-19330
supply, 19396
check-out, 97762
cornea, 65770
endovascular
thoracic aorta, 33883-33886
facial, 21088
hernia, 49568
hip, 27090-27091
intestines, 44700
knee, 27438, 27445
lens
insertion, 66982-66985
manual or mechanical
technique, 66982-66984
not associated with concurrent
cataract removal, 66985
mandibular body
augmentation, 21125
resection, 21081
nasal, 21087
septum, 30220
obturator, 01180-01190, 21076
definitive, 21080
interim, 21079
ocular, 21077, 65770, 66982-
66985, 92358
loan, 92358
orbital, 21077
partial or total, 69633, 69637
orthotic
checkout, 97762
training, 97761
ossicle reconstruction, 69633
palate, 42280-42281
augmentation, 21082
lift, 21083

Prosthesis — *continued*
penile
insertion, 54400-54405
removal, 54406, 54410-54417
repair, 54408
replacement, 54410-54411,
54416-54417
perineum, 53442
skull plate
removal, 62142
replacement, 62143
spectacle
fitting, 92352-92353
repair, 92371
speech aid, 21084
spinal, 22851
synthetic, 69633, 69637
temporomandibular joint, 21243
testicular, 54660
training, 97761
urethral sphincter
insertion, 53444-53445
removal, 53446-53447
repair, 53449
replacement, 53448
vagina, 57267
wrist, 25250-25251
Protease F, 85400
Protein
A plasma (PAPP-A), 84163
blotting, 84181-84182
tissue, 88371
C
activator, 85337
antigen, 85302
assay, 85303
reactive, 86140-86141
resistance, 85307
electropheresis, 84165-84166
glycated, 82985
myelin basic, 83873
osteocalcin, 83937
other fluids, 84166
prealbumin, 84134
S
assay, 85306
total, 85305
serum, 84155, 84165
total, 84155-84160
urine, 84156
Prothrombase, 85260
Prothrombin, 85210
time, 85610-85611
Prothrombokinase, 85230
Proton treatment delivery
complex, 77525
intermediate, 77523
simple, 77520-77522
Protoporphyrin, 84202-84203
Protozoa, 86753
Provocation
test, 92140
tonography, 92130
Prower factor, 85260
Pseudocyst, 48510
Psoriasis treatment, 96910-96922
Psychiatric services
biofeedback training, 90875-90876
consultation with family, 90887
drug management, 90863
electroconvulsive therapy, 90870
environmental intervention, 90882
evaluation of records or reports,
90885
family, 90846-90849, 99510
group, 90853
hypnotherapy, 90880
individual, 90832-90838
home visit, 99510
interactive complexity, 90785
interview and evaluation, 90791-
90792
narcosynthesis analysis, 90865
pharmacologic management, 90863
psychoanalysis, 90845

CPT © 2015 American Medical Association. All Rights Reserved.   © 2016 DecisionHealth

Radiation — *continued*
  X-ray — *continued*
    intestines, small, 74250-74251
    jaw, 70355
    joint, 77071
    knee, 73560-73564, 73580
    larynx, 70370
    leg, 73592
    mandible, 70100-70110
    mastoids, 70120-70130
    nasal bone, 70160
    neck, 70360
    orbit, 70190-70200
    pelvis, 72170-72190
      manometry, 74710
    peritoneum, 74190
    pharynx, 70370, 74210
    ribs, 71100-71111
    sacroiliac joint, 72200-72202,
      73542
    sacrum, 72220
    salivary gland, 70380
    scapula, 73010
    sella turcica, 70240
    shoulder, 73020-73030,
      73050
    sinus tract, 76080
    skull, 70250-70260
    specimen, 76098
    spine
      cervical, 72020-72052
      complete, 72081-72084
      lumbosacral, 72100-72120
      thoracic, 72020, 72070-72074
      thoracolumbar junction, 72080
    sternum, 71120-71130
    teeth, 70300-70320
    tibia, 73590
    toe, 73660
    with contrast
      ankle, 72615
      aorta, 75600-75630,
        75952-75953
      bile duct, 74300-74301
      bladder, 74430, 74450-
        74455
      brain, 70010-70015
      bronchus, 76499
      central venous access
        device, 36598
      colon, 74270-74270
      corpora cavernosa, 74445
      elbow, 73085
      epididymis, 74440
      gallbladder, 74290
      gastrointestinal tract,
        74246-74249
      hip, 73525
      iliofemoral artery, 75630
      intervertebral disc, 72285-
        72295
      joint, 77071
      kidney cyst, 74470
      lacriminal duct, 70170
      lymph vessel, 75801-75807
      mammary duct, 77053-
        77054
      nasolacriminal duct, 70170
      oviduct, 74740
      pancreas, 74300-74301
      pancreatic duct, 74329-
        74330
      perineum, 74775
      peritoneum, 74190
      salivary gland, 70390
      seminal vesicles, 74440
      shoulder, 73040
      spine, 72240-72270
      tempomandibular joint,
        70328-70332
      ureter, 74485
      urethra, 74450-74455
      urinary tract, 74400-74425
      uterus, 74740
      vas deferens, 74440
      wrist, 73100-73110

Radical
  dissection
    auditory canal, 69155
    glossectomy, 41135, 41145,
      41153-41155
    laryngotomy, 31365-31368
    lymphadenectomy, 38724
    pharyngolaryngectomy, 31390-
      31395
    salivary gland, 42426
    thyroidectomy, 60254
  excision
    hysterectomy, 58210, 58548
    mastectomy, 19305-19307
    mastoidectomy, 69511
      modified, 69505, 69602
      revision, 69602-69603
      petrous apicectomy, 69530
      tympanoplasty, 69645-
        69646
    nephrectomy, 50230, 50545
    oophorectomy, 58210
      laparoscopic, 58548
    orchiectomy, 54530-54535
    penectomy, 54130-54135
    prostatectomy, 55810-55815,
      55840-55845
    salpingectomy, 58210
    styloidectomy, 25230
    tonsilectomy, 42842-42845
    trachelectomy, 57531
    vulvectomy, 00906, 56630-
      56640
  resection
    abdomen, 51597
    acetabulum, 27076
    ankle, 27615
    arm, 25077
    back, 21935
    calcaneus, 27647
    clavicle, 23200
    coxa, 27075-27079
    elbow, 24149
    face, 21015
    fibula, 27646
    finger, 26117, 26260-26262
    flank, 21935
    foot, 28046
    forearm, 25077
    hand, 26115
    hip, 27049, 27075-27079
    humerus, 23220-23222
    innominate, 27077
    ischial, 27078-27079
    knee, 27329
    leg, 27329, 27615
    metacarpal, 26250-26255
    metatarsal, 28173
    mouth, 41150, 41155
    ovary, 58950-58956
    pelvis, 27049
    peritoneum, 58952-58956
    radius, 25170
    scalp, 21015
    scapula, 23210
    shoulder, 23077, 23220-23222
    sternum, 21630-21632
    talus, 27647
    tarsal, 28171
    tibia, 27645
    toe, 28175
    tonsil, 42842-42845
    ulna, 25170
    wrist, 25077

Radio cobalt B12, 78270-78272
Radioactive
  colloid therapy, 79300
  substance, 55860
Radiocarpal joint
  arthrotomy, 25040
  dislocation treatment, 25660
Radiocinematography
  esophagus, 74230
  evaluation, 70371, 74230
  pharynx, 70371, 74230

Radioelement
  application
    interstitial, 77778
    intracavitary, 77761-77763
    remote afterloading, 77767-77772
    surface, 77789
    ultrasound guidance, 79695
  catheter placement
    breast, 19296-19298
    bronchus, 31643
    muscle/soft tissue, 20555
    prostate, 55875
  handling, 77790
  infusion, 77750
  needle placement
    muscle/soft tissue, 20555
    prostate, 55875-55876

Radioimmunosorbent test, 82784-
  82787

Radioisotope
  brachytherapy, 77750-77790
    dose, 77316-77318
  scan
    adrenal imaging, 78075
    bladder
      residual study, 78730
    bone, 78300-78351
      density, 78350
      marrow imaging, 78102-
        78104
    brain imaging, 78600-78610
      positron emission
        tomography (PET),
        78608-78609
      static view, 78600-78606
      tomographic (SPECT),
        78607
      vascular flow, 78610
    cardiac blood pool imaging,
      78472-78473, 78481-
      78483, 78494-78496
      first pass technique, 78481-
        78483
      gated equilibrium, 78472-
        78473, 78494-
        78496
    cardiovascular system, 78414-
      78499
      cardiac blood pool imaging,
        78472-78473, 78481-
        78483, 78494-78496
      myocardial imaging, 78459,
        78466-78469, 78491-
        78492
      perfusion, 78460-78465,
        78478-78480
      shunt detection, 78428
      venous thrombosis, 4070F,
        78456-78457
    cerebrospinal fluid flow, 78630-
      78650
      cisternography, 78630
      shunt evaluation, 78645
      tomographic (SPECT),
        78647
      ventriculography, 78635
    dacryocystography, 78660
    diagnostic imaging, 78012-
      78999
    endocrine system
      adrenal, 78075
      parathyroid, 78070-78072
      thyroid, 78012-78020
      unlisted procedure, 78099
    gastric
      emptying, 78264-78266
      mucosa, 78261
    gastroesophageal reflux, 78262
    gastrointestinal system, 78201-
      78299
      blood loss, 78278
      intestine, 78290
      liver, 78207-78220
      protein loss, 78282
      salivary gland, 78230-
        78232
      unlisted procedure, 78299

Radioisotope — *continued*
  scan — *continued*
    gastrointestinal system — *continued*
      urea breath test, 78267-
        78268
      vitamin B12, 78270-78272
    genitourinary system, 78700-
      78799
      bladder, residual, 78730
      kidney, 78700-78725
      testicle, 78761
      ureteral reflux, 78740
    hematopoietic/lymphatic
      system, 78102-78199
      bone marrow, 78102-78104
      lymphatics, 78195
      plasma volume, 78110-
        78111
      platelet survival, 78190-
        78191
      red cell, 78120-78121,
        78130-78140
      spleen, 78185
      whole blood, 78122
    inflammatory process
      localization, 78805-78807
    intestine imaging, 78290
    joint imaging, 78300-78320
    kidney, 78700-78725
      function study, 78725
      morphology imaging, 78700-
        78709
      tomographic (SPECT), 78710
      vascular flow, 78701-78709
    liver, 78207-78220
      function study, 78220
      imaging, 78201-78261
    lymphatics imaging, 78195
    musculoskeletal system,
      78300-78399
      bone, 78300-78351
      joint, 78300-78320
    myocardial
      imaging, 78459, 78466-
        78469, 78491-78492
      perfusion, 78460-78465,
        78478-78480
    nervous system, 78600-78699
      brain imaging, 78600-
        78610
      cerebrospinal fluid, 78630-
        78650
      dacryocystography, 78660
    parathyroid, 78070-78072
    plasma volume, 78110-78111
    platelet survival, 78190-78191
    positron emission tomography
      (PET), 78811-78816
      limited area, 78811, 78814
      skull base to mid thigh,
        78812, 78815
      whole body, 78813, 78816
      with concurrent computed
        tomography (CT),
        78814-78816
    red blood cell, 78120-78121,
      78130-78140
      sequestration, 78140
      survival study, 78130-
        78135
      volume, 78120-78121
    respiratory system, 78580-
      78599
      pulmonary perfusion,
        78580-78585, 78588
      quantitative differential,
        78596
      unlisted procedure, 78599
      ventilation imaging, 78586-
        78587, 78591-78594
    salivary gland, 78230-78232
    spleen, 78185
      with liver, 78215-78216
    testicles, 78761
    therapeutic
      (radiopharmaceutical),
      79005-79999
      interstitial colloid, 79300

Radiation – Radioisotope

CPT © 2015 American Medical Association. All Rights Reserved.
© 2016 DecisionHealth

Reduction — *continued*
  skull
    enlarged cranium, 62115-62117
    facial bone, 21209
Reflectance confocal microscopy, 96931-96936
Reflex test, 95907-95913, 95933
Reflux study, 78262
  gastroesophageal, 91034-91038
Refraction, 92015
Rehabilitation
  auditory, 92630-92633
    status evaluation, 92626-92627
  cardiac, 93797-93798
  peripheral artery disease, 93668
Reimplantation
  artery, 35691-35697
    carotid-subclavian, 35695
    pulmonary, 33788
    subclavian-carotid, 35694
    vertebral-carotid, 35691
    vertebral-subclavian, 35693
    visceral, 35697
  kidney, 50380
  ovary, 58825
  ureter, 50780-50785, 51565
Reinforcement, soft tissue, 15777
Reinnervation, 31590
Reinsch test, 83015
Reinsertion
  drug delivery implant, 11983
  spinal fixation device, 22849
Relative density, 84315
Release
  carpal tunnel, 64721
  contraction
    elbow, 24149
    hip flexor muscle, 27036
    knee muscle, 27422
  hormone, 84307
  nerve, 64702-64727
  retinal material, 67115
  spinal cord, 63200
  stapes, 69650
  tarsal tunnel, 28035
  tendon, 24332, 25295
Removal
  balloon assist device
    intra-aortic, 33968, 33971, 33974
  blood component, 36511-36516
    plasma, 36514
      reinfusion, 36515-36516
    platelets, 36513
    red blood cell, 36512
    white blood cell, 36411
  breast, 19300-19307
  bronchial valve, 31648-31649
  calculus
    bile duct, 43264, 47420-47425, 47544, 47554
    bladder, 51050, 52310-52318, 52352
    gallbladder, 47480
    hepatic duct, 47400
    kidney, 50060-50081, 50130, 50561, 50580, 52352
    lacrimal, 68530
    pancreas, 48020
    pancreatic duct, 43264
    salivary gland, 42330-42340
    ureter, 50610-50630, 50961, 50980, 51060-51065, 52320-52330, 52352
    urethra, 52310-52315, 52352
  cast, 29700-29710
  cataract, 66982-66984
  catheter
    central venous, 36589
    fractured, 37197
    peritoneal, 49422
    spinal, 62355
  cervical cerclage, 59871
  cerumen, 69209-69210
  contraceptive capsules, 11976
  cranial tongs, 20665

Removal — *continued*
  dacryolith, 68530
  defibrillator, 33241-33244
  drug delivery implant, 11982-11983
  ear wax, 69209-69210
  electrode
    brain, 61535, 61880
    heart, 33238
    nerve, 64585
    spinal, 63660
    stomach, 0156T, 0158T, 43648, 43882
  device
    cardiac event recorder, 33284
    carotid sinus baroreflex, 0269T-0271T
    central venous catheter, 36589
    contraceptive capsules, 11976
    cranial tongs, 20665
    defibrillator, 33241-33244
    drug delivery implant, 11982-11983
    electrodes, neurostimulator, 0156T, 0158T, 43648, 43882, 61880, 63660, 64585
    external fixation, 20694
    fixation, 20670-20680
    fractured catheter, 37197
    gastric restriction, 43772-43774
    halo, 20665
    hearing aid, 69711
    infusion pump, 36262, 36590, 62365
    intervertebral disc, artificial, 0095T, 22864
    intra-aortic balloon assist, 33968, 33971, 33974
    peritoneal catheter, 49422
    ocular implant, 65175
    pacemaker, 33233-33237
    pulse generator/receiver, 61888, 63688, 64595
    sling, 53442, 57287
    spinal catheter, 62355
    spinal instrumentation, 22850, 22852-22855
    stent, 43275-43276, 50382-50387, 52310-52315
    subcutaneous port, 43887-43888
    tube, 50389, 69424
    venous access device, 36590
    ventricular assist, 33977-33978, 33980
  eye, 65091-65114
    implant, 65175
    foreign body, 65205-65265
  fallopian tube
    bilateral, 58700-58720, 58950-58956
    ectopic pregnancy, 59120
    partial/total, 58661, 58700-58720
    with radical hysterectomy, 58210, 58548
    with supracervical hysterectomy, 58180, 58542, 58544
    with total hysterectomy, 58150-58152, 58200, 58240, 58571, 58573
    with vaginal hysterectomy, 58262-58263, 58291-58292, 58552, 58554
  fat, 15876-15879
  fecal impaction, 45915
  fibrin deposit, 32150
  foreign body
    anus, 46608
    ankle, 27610, 27620
    arm, 24200-24201, 25248
    ear canal, 69200-69205
    bile duct, 43275
    bladder, 52310-52315
    brain, 61570, 62163
    bronchi, 31635

Removal — *continued*
  foreign body — *continued*
    colon, 44025, 44390, 45332, 45379
    conjunctivus, 65210
    cornea, 65220-65222
    duodenum, 44010
    elbow, 24000, 24101, 24200-24201
    esophagus, 43020, 43045, 43215, 74235
    eye, 65205-65265
    eyelid, 67938
    finger, 26075-26080
    foot, 28190-28193
    gastrointestinal, 43247
    gums, 41805
    hand, 26070
    hip, 27033, 27086-27087
    intertarsal joint, 28020
    intestines, 44020, 44363
    kidney, 50561, 50580
    knee, 27310, 27331, 27372
    lacrimal, 68530
    larynx, 31511, 31530-31531, 31577
    leg, 27372
    lung, 32151
    mandible, 41806
    mediastinum, 39000-39010
    metatarsophalangeal joint, 28022
    mouth, 40804-40805
    muscle, 20520-20525
    nose, 30300-30320
    orbit, 67413, 67430
    pancreatic duct, 43275
    pelvis, 27086-27087
    penis, 54115
    pericardium, 32658, 33020
    peritoneum, 49402
    pharynx, 42809
    pleura, 32150-32151, 32653
    rectum, 45307, 45915
    scrotum, 55120
    shoulder, 23040-23044, 23330-23333
    skin, 11010-11012
    stomach, 43500
    subcutaneous tissue, 10120-10121, 11010-11012
    tarsometatarsal joint, 28020
    tendon sheath, 20520-20525
    toe, 28022-28024
    ureter, 50961, 50980
    urethra, 52310-52315
    uterus, 58562
    vagina, 57415
    wrist, 25040, 25101, 25248
  gastric restriction device, 43772-43774
  graft
    intestine, 44137
  hair, 17380
  halo, 20665
  hearing aid, 69711
  hematoma, brain, 61312-61315
    anesthesia, 00211
  implant
    mammary, 19328-19330
    ocular, 65175, 65920
    orbital, 67560
    infusion pump
      intra-arterial, 36262
      intravenous, 36590
      spinal cord, 62365
    intervertebral disc, artificial
      cervical, 0095T, 22864
      lumbar, 22865, 0164T
    intra-aortic balloon, 33968, 33971, 33974
  intestine
    allograft, 44137
  lacrimal
    calculus, 68530
    gland, 68500-68505
    sac, 68520
  laryngocele, 31300

Removal — *continued*
  leiomyomata, 58561
    intramural, 58545-58546
  lens, 66840-66852, 66920-66940
  loose body, joint
    ankle, 27620
    carpometacarpal, 26070
    elbow, 24101
    interphalangeal, 28024
    intertarsal, 28020
    knee, 27331
    metatarsophalangeal, 28022
    tarsometatarsal, 28020
    wrist, 25101
  lung
    apical tumor, 32503-32504
    cyst, 32140
    extrapleural, 32445
    one lobe, 32480, 32663
    one segment, 32484, 32669
    sleeve lobectomy, 32486
    sleeve pneumonectomy, 32488
    total pneumonectomy, 32440-32445, 32671
    two lobes, 32482, 32670
    volume reduction, 32491, 32672
    wedge, 32505-32507, 32666-32668
  lymph nodes
    abdominal, 38747
    inguinofemoral, 38760-38765
    pelvic, 38770
    retroperitoneal, 38746, 38780
  mastoid cell, 69670
  mesh, 11008
  nails, 11750-11752
  neurostimulator
    electrodes, 0156T, 0158T, 43648, 43882, 61880, 63660, 64585
    pulse generator/receiver, 61888, 63688, 64595
  ovary(ies)
    bilateral/unilateral, 58940-58943, 58950-58956
    ectopic pregnancy, 59120
    laparoscopic, 58542, 58544, 58548, 58552, 58554, 58571, 58573
    partial/total, 58661, 58940-58940
    radical hysterectomy, 58210, 58548
    supracervical hysterectomy, 58180, 58542, 58544
    total hysterectomy, 58150-58152, 58200, 58240, 58571, 58573
    vaginal hysterectomy, 58262-58263, 58291-58292, 58552, 58554
  pacemaker, 33233-33237
  permanent leadless, ventricular, 0388T
  polyp
    anal, 46610-46612
    colon, 44392, 45333, 45385
    esophagus, 43217, 43250
    gastrointestinal, 43250-43251
    rectum, 45315
    sphenoid sinus, 31051
  prosthesis
    abdominal, 11008, 49606
    hip, 27090-27091
    knee, 27488
    penis, 54406, 54410-54417
    perineal, 53442
    shoulder, 23334-23335
    skull, 62142
    urethral sphincter, 53446-53447
    wrist, 25250-25251
  pulse generator/receiver
    cranial, 61888
    gastric, 64595
    peripheral, 64595
    spinal, 63688

Removal – Repair

CPT © 2015 American Medical Association. All Rights Reserved.   © 2016 DecisionHealth

Repair — *continued*
- heart
  - anomaly, 33600-33619
  - atria, 33265-33266, 33640, 33647, 33660-33665, 33670
  - blood vessel, 33320-33322
  - cor triatriatum, 33732
  - coronary artery, 33500-33507
  - electrode, 33218-33220
  - infundibular, 33476-33478
  - myocardium, 33542
  - outflow, 33414, 33478
  - pulmonary
    - artery, 33502-33506, 33924
    - valve, 33470-33474
    - septal defect, 33545, 33608-33610, 33641, 33647, 33681-33688, 33692-33697
  - replacement system, 0052T-0053T
  - sinus
    - aortic, 33702-33722
    - valsalva, 33702-33722
    - venosus, 33645
  - tetralogy of fallot, 33692-33697
  - valve
    - aortic, 33400-33403
    - atrioventricular, 33660-33670
    - mitral, 33420-33427
    - prosthetic, 33496, 33670, 33852-33853
    - pulmonary, 33470-33474
    - tricuspid, 33460-33464
  - ventricle, 33545, 33611-33612, 33619
  - ventricular tunnel, 33722
  - wound, 33300-33305
- hepatic duct, 47765, 47802
- hernia
  - diaphragmatic, 39540-39541
  - epigastric, 49570-49572
  - femoral, 49550-49557
  - incisional, 49654-49657
  - inguinal, 49491-49525, 49650-49651
  - lumbar, 49540
  - lung, 32800
  - paracolostomy, 44346
  - paraesophageal, 43281-43282, 43332-43337
  - umbilical, 49580-49587, 49652-49653, 51500
  - ventral, 49560-49566
- hip
  - acetabuloplasty, 27120-27122, 29915
  - arthroplasty, 27125-27132
  - muscle, 27100-27111
  - osteotomy, 27140-27156
- intestine
  - enterolysis, 44180
  - stricturoplasty, 44615
  - suture, 44602-44605, 44620-44661
- jacket, 29720
- jejunum, 43496
- kidney
  - pyeloplasty, 50400-50405, 50544
  - suture, 50500-50526
  - symphysiotomy, 50540
- knee
  - ligament, 27405-27409
  - meniscus, 27403
  - tendon, 27380-27381
  - union, 27470-27472
- larynx, 31580-31590
- leg
  - lower, 27726
    - fascia, 27656
    - ligament, 29888-29889
    - tendon
      - achilles, 27650-27654
      - extensor, 27664-27665, 27680

Repair — *continued*
- leg — *continued*
  - lower — *continued*
    - tendon — *continued*
      - flexor, 27658-27659, 27680
      - lengthening, 27685-27686
      - peroneal, 27675-27676
      - union, 27720-27726
  - upper
    - muscle, 27385-27386
    - tendon
      - lengthening, 27393-27395
      - tenotomy, 27390-27392
      - union, 27470-27472
- lip, 40650-40654, 42260
  - cleft, 40700-40761
- liver, 47300, 47350-47361
- lung, 32940
  - hernia, 32800
  - tear, 32110
- maxilla, 21206
- mesentery, 44850
- mouth, 40830-40845
  - floor, 41250-41252
- neck
  - division, 21700-21725
  - suspension, 21685
- nose 40700-40761, 42260
  - artresia, 30540-30545
  - cerebrospinal fluid leak, 31290-31291
  - fistula, 30580-30600
  - rhinoplasty, 30400-30462
  - septum, 30630
  - vestible, 30465
- palate, 42235-42260
  - cleft, 42200-42225
  - lengthening, 42226-42227
  - wound, 42180-42182
- pancreas, 48500-48511
  - wound, 48545-48547
- pelvis, 27158
- penis
  - corporeal tears, 54437
  - hypospadias, 54300-54352
  - prosthesis, 54408
  - wound, 54440
- perineum, 56810
- pharynx, 42953
- rectum, 0170T
  - imperforate anus, 46740-46742
  - proctoplasty, 45500-45505
  - rectocele, 45560
  - suture, 45800-45825
  - wound, 45562-45563
- scapula, 23400
- scrotum, 55175-55180
- shoulder
  - capsulorrhaphy, 23450-23466
  - cuff, 23410-23412, 23420
  - deformity, 23400
  - ligament, 23415
  - muscle, 23395-23397
  - tendon, 23405-23406, 23430-23440
- skin
  - hidradenitis, 11450-11471
  - wound
    - complex, 13100-13153
    - simple, 12001-12018
- skull
  - cerebrospinal fluid leak, 62100
  - cranioplasty, 62140-62141, 62145-62148
  - elevation, 62000-62010
  - ecephalocele, 62120
- spine
  - annuloplasty, 22526-22527
  - augmentation, 22513-22515
  - fluid leak, 63707-63709
  - hernia, 49540
  - meningocele, 63700-63706
  - osteotomy, 22206-22226
  - vertebroplasty, 22510-22515
- spleen, 38115
- spica, 29720

Repair — *continued*
- stomach
  - cardioplasty, 43320
  - fundoplasty, 43210, 43280, 43325-43328
  - pyloroplasty, 43800
  - suture, 43502, 43840 43870-43880
- testis, 54600-54680
- tongue, 41250-41252, 41500
- toe
  - capsule, 28270-28272
  - sesamoid, 28315
  - syndactyly, 28280
  - tendon, 28232-28234
- trachea, 31755
  - fistula, 43300-43314
  - suture, 31800-31825
  - tracheoplasty, 31750-31760
- tunica vaginalis, 55060
- ureter
  - fascia, 50728
  - lysis, 50715-50725
  - suture, 50900-5930
  - ureteroplasty, 50700
- urethra
  - sphincter, 57220
  - suture, 45820-45825, 53502-53520
  - urethrocele, 57230
  - urethromeatoplasty, 53450-53460
  - urethroplasty, 53400-53431
- uterus, 51920-51928, 58400-58410, 58520, 59350
- vagina, 59300
  - clitoroplasty, 56805
  - defect, 57284-57285, 57423
  - enterocele, 57268-57270
  - imperforate anus, 46705-46706
  - introitus, 56800
  - perineoplasty, 56810
  - sphincter, 57220
  - suture, 51900, 57200-57210, 57240-57265, 57289, 57300-57330
  - urethrocele, 57230
  - vaginoplasty, 57335
- vas deferens, 55400
- vein, 33730, 34501, 34520, 34510, 35460, 35476, 75978
- vessel, 33320-33322
- vulva, 59300
- wrist
  - capsulorrhaphy, 25320
  - muscle, 25260-25274
  - tendon, 25260-25274
    - lengthening, 25280
    - sheath, 25275
    - slide, 25315-25316
    - tenodesis, 25300-25301
    - tenotomy, 25290
    - tenolysis, 25295
    - transplant, 25310-25312

Replacement
- aortic valve, 33361-33369, 33405-33413
- band, 43773
- catheter
  - pacemaker, 33210
  - venous, 36578-36585
  - ventricular, 62160-62161
- carotid sinus baroreflex device, 0266T-0268T
- defibrillator, 33262-33264, 33249
- electrode
  - cardiac, 33210-33211
  - gastric neurostimulator, 43647, 43881
  - gastric stimulation, 0155T, 0157T
  - pacing, 33216-33217, 33224
- hearing aid, 69710, 69717-69718
- heart
  - system, 0052T-0053T
  - valve
    - aortic, 33405-33413
    - mitral, 33430
    - pulmonary, 33475

Replacement — *continued*
- infusion pump, 62361-62362
- reservoir, 63260
- neurostimulator pulse generator/ receiver
  - cranial, 61885-61886, 63685
  - gastric, 64590
- pacemaker, 33206-33208
  - permanent leadless, ventricular, 0387T
  - pulse generator, 33227-33229
- prosthetic
  - disc, 0375T, 0163T, 22856-22862
  - elbow, 24361, 24363
  - hip, 27130-27132, 27134-27138, 27236, 27258-27259
  - jaw, 21243
  - knee, 27447
  - ossicle, 69633, 69637
  - penis, 54410-54417
  - proximal humerus, 23222, 23472, 23616
  - radial head, 24666
  - shoulder, 23472
  - skull, 62143
  - sphincter, 53448
  - wrist, 25441-25446
- skin, 15271-15278
- shunt
  - cerebrospinal fluid, 62160, 62194, 62225-62230
  - lumbosubarachnoid, 63744
- stent
  - ureteral, 50382, 50385, 50387
- tube, 43760, 49450-49452
- valve, aortic, 33361-33369, 33405-33413

Replantation
- arm, 20802-20805
- finger, 20816-20827
- foot, 20838
- hand, 20808
- penis, 54438

Repositioning
- catheter
  - central venous, 36597
  - electrode, 93620-93622
  - epidural, 62350-62351
- defibrillator, 33215
- digit, 26551-26556
- filter, 37192
- gastric feeding tube, 43761
- lens, 66825
- orbital, 21267-21268
- pacemaker, 33215
  - electrode, 33226, 33249
- valve, 33468
- ventricular assist device, 33993

Reprogramming, 62252
Reptilase test, 85635
Resection
- ankle
  - talus, 27647
  - tissue, 27615
- arm
  - lower, 25170
    - tissue, 25077
    - ulna, 25240, 25830
  - upper, 24150-24153
    - capsule, 24149
    - humerus, 23220-23222
    - tissue, 24077
- back, 21935
- bladder, 52234-52240
  - diverticulum, 52305
  - neck, 52400-52402, 52500, 52640
  - sphincter, 52277
  - tissue, 52630
  - ureterocele, 52300-52301
- bronchus, 32486, 32501
- cardiac, 33025
  - atrium, 33732
  - external, 33130
  - infundibular, 33676, 33684
  - intracardiac, 33120
  - myocardium, 33542-33545

Resection — *continued*
- cardiac — *continued*
  - valve, 33415
  - vena cava, 37799
  - ventricle, 33476
- chest, 19260-19272
- cranium, 61600-61608, 61615-61616
- diaphragm, 39560-39561
- ear, 69535
- elbow
  - capsule, 24149
  - tissue, 24077
- eye, 67311-67316
  - lid, 67903-67904, 67908
- face, 21015
- fallopian tube, 58957-58958
- flank, 21935
- foot
  - metatarsal, 28173
  - phalanx, 28175
    - base, 28126
    - condyle, 28153
    - tissue, 28340
  - tarsal, 28171
  - tissue, 28046
- hand
  - metacarpal, 26250
  - phalanx, 26260-26262
  - tissue, 26117
- hip
  - ilium, 27075-27076
  - innominate, 27077
  - ischial, 27078-27079
  - tissue, 27049
- intestine, 43860-43865, 44661
  - large, 44144, 44625-44626
    - laparascopy, 44227
    - sigmoid, 45402
  - small, 44120-44128, 44625-44626
    - laparascopy, 44202-44203, 44227
- kidney, 50562, 52355
- knee, 27365
  - tissue, 27329
- leg
  - lower
    - fibula, 27646
    - talus, 27647
    - tibia, 27645
    - tissue, 27615
  - upper
    - femur, 27122, 27365
    - tissue, 27329
- lip, 40530
- liver, 47120-47130
- lung
  - apical tumor, 32503
  - emphysematous, 32491, 32672
  - wedge, 32505-32507, 32666-32668
- mandible, 21045, 41150
- mouth, 41150-41155
- nose
  - concha bullosa, 31240
  - submucous, 30140, 30520
- ovary, 58950-58958
  - wedge, 58920
- palate, 42120
- pancreas, 48105
- pericardium, 32659, 33025-33031
  - cyst/tumor, 32661, 33050
- peritoneum, 58957-58958
- pharynx, 42892-42894
- prostate
  - transurethral, 00914, 52601, 52648-52649
- rectum, 45111, 45190
- rib
  - cervical, 21705
  - chest wall tumor, 19260-19272
  - empyema, 32035
  - extrapleural, 32900
  - kidney, 50220-50230
- shoulder, 23077, 23220-23222
  - clavicle, 23200
  - humeral head, 23195

Resection — *continued*
- shoulder — *continued*
  - scapula, 23210
  - sternum, 21630-21632
  - thorax, 21557
  - thymus, 32673, 60520-60522
  - tonsil, 42842-42845
  - ureter, 52355
  - uterus, 52300-52301
  - vertebra, 22818-22819, 63308
    - C1-C3, 61597
    - cervical, 63081-63082, 63300, 63304
    - lumbar, 63087-63091, 63102-63103, 63303, 63307
    - sacral, 63090-63091, 63303, 63307
    - thoracic, 63085-63101, 63103, 63301-63302, 63305-63306

Respiratory
- pattern recording, 94772
- syncytial virus, 86756
  - direct fluorescence, 87280
  - direct optical, 87807
  - immunoassay technique, 87420

Results documentation, 3006F-3725F

Reticulocyte, 85044-85045

Retina
- destruction, 67299
  - lesion, 67208-67218
  - retinopathy, 67227-67229
- detachment
  - prophylaxis, 67141-67145
  - repair, 67101-67113
- membrane removal, 67042
- prosthetic implant, 0100T
- release, 67115
- removal, 67120-67121

Retinacular, 27425

Retinopathy, 67227-67229

Retraction, 85170

Retrieval, 37193, 37197

Retrocaval ureter, 50725

Retrograde
- cholangiopancreatography, 43260-43265, 43274-43278
  - with optical endomicroscopy, 0397T
- urethrocystography, 51610
- urography, 74420

Retroperitoneal
- abscess drainage, 49060
- biopsy, 49010, 49180
- duplex scan, 93975-93976
- excision
  - cyst, 49203-49205
  - tumor, 58952-58953, 58958
- fibrosis, 50715
- lymph node procedure, 38564, 38570, 38780
- ultrasound, 76770-76775

Retropubic prostatectomy, 55831
- radical, 55840-55845, 55866

Revascularization
- artery
  - coronary, 92937-92944
  - femoral/popliteal, 37224-37227
  - iliac, 37220-37223
  - tibial/peroneal, 37228-37235
- penis, 37788
- transmyocardial, 33140-33141
- upper extremity, 36838

Reverse
- triidothyronine, 84482
- vasectomy, 55400

Revision
- anastomosis
  - intestinal, 43850-43865, urinary, 50727-50728
- arthroplasty
  - ankle, 27703
  - disc, 22861-22862, 0098T, 0165T
  - hip, 27134-27138
  - knee, 27486-27487
  - wrist, 25449

Revision — *continued*
- breast reconstruction, 19380
- bypass, 35879-35884
- carotid sinus baroreflex device, 0269T-0271T
- catheter
  - abdomen, 49325
  - colostomy, 44340-44346
  - fenestration, 69840
  - fistula, 36832-36833
  - fixation, 20693
- gastric restrictive procedure, 43848
  - device component, 43771
  - port, 43886
- graft, 57295-57296
- ileostomy, 44312-44314
- mastoidectomy, 69601-69605
- neurostimulator
  - cranial, 61880, 61888
  - gastric, 0156T-0158T, 0165T, 43648, 43882, 64595
  - peripheral, 64585, 64595
  - spinal, 63600, 63688
- pocket, 33222-33223
- pump, 36261
- ring, 56700
- scar
  - arm, 24925, 25907
  - leg, 27594, 27884
  - shoulder, 23921
  - tracheostomy, 31830
  - wrist, 25922, 25929
- sling, 53442, 57287
- stapedectomy, 69662
- stent/shunt/tube
  - eye, 66185
  - gastrostomy, 44373
  - trachea, 31638
  - transvenous intrahepatic portosystemic shunt (TIPS), 37183
- tracheostoma, 31613-31614
- typanoplasty, 69631-69633

Rheumatoid factor, 86430-86431

Rhinectomy, 30150, 30160

Rhinomanometry, 92512

Rhinophototherapy, 0168T

Rhinophyma, 30120

Rhinoplasty, 30400-30462

Rhinotomy, 30118, 30320

Rhizotomy, 63185-63190

Rho variant, 86905

Rhytidectomy, 15824-15829

Rib
- biopsy, 20220-20240
- cartilage harvest, 20936, 21230
- excision, 21600, 21615-21616
  - chest wall tumor, 19260-19272
  - ostectomy, 21502
- fracture treatment, 21811-21813
- resection, 00470-00474
  - cervical, 21705
  - empyema, 32035
  - extrapleural, 32900
  - lung tumor, 32503-32504
  - nephrectomy, 50220-50230
- x-ray, 71100-71111

Riboflavin, 84252

Richardson procedure, 53460

Rickettsia, 86757

Risser jacket, 29010-29015, 29710

Rocky mountain spotted fever, 86000

Ropes test, 83872

Rorschach test, 96101

Ross
- assessment, 96125
- procedure, 33413

Rotator cuff
- reconstruction, 23420
- repair, 23410-23412, 29827

Rotavirus
- antibody, 86759
- detection, 87425
- vaccine, 90680-90681

Roux-en-Y
- anatomosis, 47780-47785, 48540
- cholecystoenterostomy, 47740-47741
- gastroenterostomy, 43644, 43846, 47741
- reconstruction, 43621, 43633

Rubella, 86762
- vaccine, 90707-90710

Rubeola, 86765, 87283

Russell viper venom, 85612-85613

S

Sac, 69805-69806

Saccomanno technique, 88108

Sacral nerve
- neurostimulator electrode implants, incisional, 64581
  - percutaneous, 64561
- removal, 64585-64595
- replacement, 64590
- revision, 64585-64595

Sacroiliac joint
- anesthesia, 01160, 01170
- arthrodesis, 27279-27280
- arthrotomy, 27050
- biopsy, 27050
- dislocation treatment, 27218
- fracture, 27216-27218
- injection, 27096
- x-ray, 72200-72202, 73542

Sacrum
- excision
  - tumor, 49215
- fracture treatment, 27216-27218
- x-ray, 72220

Safety measures documentation, 6005F-6110F

Sahli test, 43754-43755

Salicylate, 80329-80331

Salivary duct
- catheterization, 42660
- dilation, 42650-42660
- injection, 42550
- ligation, 42665
- repair
  - sialodochoplasty, 42500-42505
  - fistula, 42600

Salivary gland, 00100
- biopsy
  - needle, 42400
  - incisional, 42405
- chemodenervation, 64610
- drainage
  - abscess, 42310-42320
    - parotid, 42300-42305
  - cyst, 42409
- excision
  - cyst, 42408
  - stone, 42330-42340
- function study, 78232
- imaging, 78230
  - with serial images, 78231
- incision, 42310-42320
- marsupialization
  - cyst, 42409
- virus, 86644-86645
  - direct fluorescence, 87271
  - enzyme, 87332
  - nucleic acid, 87495-87497
- x-ray, 70380-70390
  - injection, 42550

Salmonella, 86768

Salpingectomy
- complete, total, 58700-58720
  - laparoscopic, 58661
- for ectopic pregnancy, 59120, 59151
- for malignancy, 58950-58956
- partial, 58700-58720
  - laparoscopic, 58661
- with abdominal hysterectomy
  - radical, 58210
  - total, 58200, 58240

CPT © 2015 American Medical Association. All Rights Reserved.

© 2016 DecisionHealth

Salpingectomy — *continued*
  with supracervical hysterectomy,
    58180
    laparoscopic, 58542, 58544
  with vaginal hysterectomy, 58260-
    58263, 58291-58292
Salpingo-oophorectomy
  complete, 58720
  for ectopic pregnancy, 59120,
    59151
  for malignancy, 58950-58956
  laparoscopic
    partial, 58661
    total, 58661
  partial, 58720
  with abdominal hysterectomy
    radical, 58210
    total, 58200, 58240
  with supracervical hysterectomy,
    58180
    laparoscopic, 58542, 58544
  with vaginal hysterectomy, 58260–
    58263, 58291-58292
Salpingolysis, 58740
Salpingoneostomy, 58673, 58770
Salpingoplasty, 58750-58752
Salpingostomy, 58673, 58770
Sang-Park procedure, 33735-33737
Sao Paulo typhus, 86000
Saucerization
  calcaneus, 28120
  clavicle, 23180
  femur, 27070, 27360
  fibula, 27360, 27641
  hip, 27070
  humerus, 23184, 24140
  ilium, 27070
  metacarpal, 26230
  metatarsal, 28122
  olecranon process, 24147
  phalanx
    toe, 26235-26236
    finger, 28124
  pubis, 27070
  radius, 24145, 25151
  scapula, 23182
  talus, 28120
  tarsal, 28122
  tibia, 27360, 27640
  ulna, 24147, 25150
Scabies, 87220
Scalenotomy, 21700-21705
Scalp
  adjacent tissue transfer, 14020-
    14021
  blood sampling, 59030
  excision
    skin lesion, 11420-11426,
      11620-11626
    recipeint grafting site, 15004
  formation
    pedicle, 15572
  graft
    allogenic dermal substitute,
      15365-15366
    allograft, 15320-15321,
      15335-15336
    autograft, 15115-15116, 15135-
      15136, 15115-15157
    full thickness, 15220-15221
    xenograft, 15420-15421
  repair
    laceration, 12001-12007,
      12031-12037, 13120-
      13122
  resection
    tumor, 21015
  shaving
    skin lesion, 11305-11308
Scan, CT
  abdomen, 74150-74170
    and pelvis, 74176-74178
  bone density, 77078
  brain, 70450-70470
  chest, 71250-71270
  ear, 70480-70482

Scan, CT — *continued*
  extremity
    lower, 73700-73702
    upper, 73200-73202
  guidance
    ablation, 77013
    needle, 77012
    radiation therapy fields, 77014
    stereotactic localization, 77011
  head, 70450-70470
  limited, 76380
  maxillofacial, 70486-70488
  neck, 70490-70492
  orbit, 70480-70482
  pelvis, 72192-72194
  sella, 70480-70482
  spine
    cervical, 72125-72127
    lumbar, 72131-72133
    thoracic, 72128-72130
  thorax, 71250-71270
  three dimensional, 76376-76377
Scanogram
  bone length studies, 77073
Scaphoid fracture, 25622-25628
Scapula, 00450-00454
  craterization, 23182
  excision, 23172, 23182, 23190
    cyst, 23140, 23145-23146
    tumor, 23140, 23145-23146
  fixation, 23400
  fracture treatment, 23570-23585
  incision, 23035
  ostectomy, 23190
  resection, 23210
  saucerization, 23172
  scapulopexy, 23400
  sequestrectomy, 23172
  x-ray, 73010
Scapulopexy, 23400
Scarification
  pleural, 32215
Schede procedure, 32905-32906
Schilling test, 78270
Schlicter test, 87197
Schuchard procedure, 21206
Sciatic nerve
  decompression, 64712
  excision
    lesion, 64786
    neuroma, 64786
  graft, 64897-64901
  injection, 64445-64446
  neuroplasty, 64712
  neurorrhaphy, 64858
  release, 64712
  repair, 64858
  suture, 64858
Scintigraphy, 78607
Sclera
  excision, 66160
    lesion, 66130
  fistulization for glaucoma
    iridectomy, 66150-66155
    sclerectomy, 66160
    thermocauterization, 66155
    trabeculectomy ab externa,
      66170-66172
    trephination, 66150
  reinforcement
    with graft, 67255
    without graft, 67255
  removal, foreign body, 65235
  repair
    laceration, 65280-65286
    reinforcement, 67250-67255
    staphyloma, 66220-66225
    wound, 68250, 65280-65286
  shunt, 66179-66185
Sclerotherapy
  fluid collection, 49185
  hemorrhoids, 46500
  perirectal, 45520
  varices
    esophageal, 43205, 43243
    venous, 36468-36471

Screening
  alcohol abuse, 99408-99409
  audiologic function test
    pure tone, air only, 92551
  Bekesy audio, 92560
  cervical cancer, 3015F
  colorectal neoplasm, 82270
  cytopathology, vaginal/cervical
    smears
    automated, 88147-88148,
      88174-88175
    manual, 88142-88143, 88150-
      88154, 88164, 88167
  cytopathology, other source
    smears, 88160-88162
  depression, 3351F-3354F, 3725F
  developmental, 96110
  documentation, 3006F-3725F
  drug, 80300-80304
  drug abuse, 99408-99409
  dyspnea, 3450F-3452F
  evoked otoacoustic emissions,
    92558
  Group B Streptococcus, 3294F
  mammography, 3014F, 77052,
    77057
  ocular, intrument-based, 99174,
    99177
  tobacco use, 4004F
  TB, 3455F
  visual field
    suprathreshold, 92082
  visual function, 99172
Scribner cannulization, 36810
Scrotum
  duplex scan, 93975-93976
  excision, 55150
  exploration, 55110
  incision and drainage
    abscess, 54700, 55100
    hematoma, 54700
  removal, 55120
  repair, 55175-55180
    hypospadias (Cecil repair), 54318
  resection, 55150
  scrotoplasty, 55175-55180
  ultrasound, 76870
Scrub typhus, 86000
Section
  cranium
    mesencephalic tract, 61480
    nerve, 61460
      trigeminal, 61450
    spine access, 63191
  spine
    accessory nerve, 63191
    cord, 63194-63199
    ligament, 63180-63182
    nerve root, 63185-63190
  vestibular nerve, 69915, 69950
Sedation
  conscious (moderate)
    same physician, 99143-99145
    different physician, 99148-
      99150
Seddon-Brookes procedure, 24320
Sedimentation rate
  automated, 85652
  manual, 86551
Segmentectomy
  breast, 19301-19302
  liver
    partial, 47120
    trisegmentectomy, 47122
  lung, 32484, 32669
Selective cellular enhancement, 88112
Selenium, 84255
Sella turcica, 70240, 70480-70482
Semen
  analysis, 89300-89322
  sperm
    analysis, 89331
    antibodies, 89325
    storage, 89343
    thawing
      cryopreserved, 89353
      with sperm isolation, 89260-89261

Semenogelase, 84152-84153
Semicircular canal, 69820-69840
Seminal vesicle
  excision, 55650
    cyst, 55680
    Mullerian duct, 55680
  incision, 55600-55605
  vesiculography, 74440
  x-ray, 74440
Seminin, 84152-84153
Semiquantitative, 81005
Semont maneuver, 95992
Sengstaken tamponade, 43460
Senning procedure, 33774-33777
Sensitivity study
  agar, 87181
  disc, 87184
  enzyme, 87185
  human immunodifficiency virus
    (HIV)-1, 87904
  macrobroth, 87188
  minimum inhibitory concentration
    (MIC), 87186
  microtiter, 87186
  multiple chemical (MCS), 87187
  mycobacteria, 87190
Sensor, 34806
Sensorimotor exam, 92060
Sensory nerve
  common, 64834
  graft, 64890-64891, 64895-64896
Sentinel node, 38792, 38900
Separation, 21431-21436
Septal defect, 33813-33814
  ventricle, 0166T-0167T
    closure, 33675-33688
    percutaneous, 93581
Septectomy
  atrial, 33735-33737
    balloon, 92992
    blade method, 92993
  nasal, 30520
Septic, 59830
Septoplasty, 30520
Septostomy
  atrial
    closed heart, 33735
    open heart, 33736-33737
Septum
  drainage, 30020
  fracture, 21336-21337
  repair, 30630
  resection, 30520
Sequestrectomy
  arm
    humerus, 24134
    radius, 24136, 25145
    ulna, 24138, 25145
  elbow, 24138
  shoulder
    clavicle, 23170
    humeral head, 23174
    scapula, 23172
  skull, 61501
  wrist, 25145
Seruakigraphy, 75625
Serologic test, 86592-86593
Seroma, 10140
Serotonin measurement testing, 84260
Serum, 3278F
  albumin, 82040
  antibody, 86975-86978
  creatine kinase, 82550
  glutamate
    oxaloacetic transaminase
      (SGOT), 84450
    pyruvate transaminase (SGPT),
      84460
  immune globulin, 90281-90284
Sesamoid bone
  excision, 28315
    digit, 26185
  fracture, 28530-28531

CPT © 2015 American Medical Association. All Rights Reserved.   © 2016 DecisionHealth

Skin — *continued*
graft — *continued*
free, 15757
full thickness, 15200-15261
pinch, 15050
punch, 15775-15776
recipient site preparation, 15002-15005
xenograft, 15271-15278
implant
device, 11981-11983
hormone, 11980
incision
acne, 10040
drainage
abscess, 10060-10061
cyst, 10080-10081
hematoma, 10140
infection, 10180
escharotomy, 16035-16036
removal
foreign body, 10120-10121
injection
agent, 15860
collagen, 11950-11954
lesion, 11900-11901
insertion
drug delivery, 11981
tissue expander, 11960, 11970
introduction
pigment, 11920-11922
lipectomy, 15876-15879
mohs micrographic procedure, 17311-17315
moles, 1050F
paring, 11055-11057
photography, 96904
planing, 30120
removal
acne, 10040
contraceptive, 11976
drug delivery, 11982-11983
foreign body, 10120-10121, 11010-11012
prosthetic, 11008
skin tag, 11200-11201
sutures, 15850-15851
tissue expander, 11971
repair
complex, 13100-13153
layer closure
wound, 12031-12057
secondary closure, 13160
superficial
wound, 12001-12018
rhytidectomy, 15824-15829
shaving
arm, 11300-11303
face, 11310-11313
feet, 11305-11308
genitalia, 11305-11308
hand, 11305-11308
leg, 11300-11303
scalp, 11305-11308
trunk, 11300-11303
substitute, 15271-15278
treatment
wound, 12020-12021

Skull
anesthesia, 00190-00192
base surgery
anterior cranial fossa
bicoronal, 61586
craniofacial, 61580-61583
lesion, 61600-61601
orbitocranial, 61584-61585
transzygomatic, 61586
carotid artery, 61610-61613
defect, 61618-61619
encephalocele, 62121
middle cranial fossa
infratemporal, 61590-61591
lesion, 61605-61608
midline, 61607-61608
orbitocranial zygomatic
approach, 61592

Skull — *continued*
base surgery
posterior cranial fossa
lesion, 61615-61616
transcondylar, 61597
transochlear, 61596
transpetrosal, 61598
transoral approach, 61575-61576
transtemporal, 61595
burr hole
biopsy, 61140
drainage, 61150-61151, 61154-61156
exploration, 61250-61253
injection, 61120
insertion, 61210-61215
decompression
cranial nerves, 61458
gasserian ganglion sensory
root, 61450
hypertension, 61322-61323
medulla, 61343
orbit, 61330
posterior cranial fossa, 61345
pseudotumor cerebri, 61340
spinal cord, 61343
subtemporal, 61340
drill hole, 61105
excision
hematoma evacuation, 61312-61315
anesthesia, 00211
lesion, 61500
anterior cranial fossa, 61600-61601
infratemporal fossa, 61605-61606
midline, 61607-61608
posterior cranial fossa, 61615-61616
osteomyelitis, 61501
tumor, 61500
exploration, 61332-61333
fracture treatment, 62000-62010
incision, 61550-61552
hematoma evacuation, 61312-61315
insertion, 61107
puncture
cervical, 61050
cervical, with medication
injection, 61055
fluid, 61020, 61070
subdural, 61000-61001
reconstruction
defect, 62140-62141, 62145
orbital rim, 21172-21180
reduction, 62115-62117
removal, 61333, 62142
repair, 62100, 62120
replacement, 62143
x-ray, 70250-70260

Sleep studies
actigraphy, 95803
attended, 95807
polysomnography
1-3 parameters, 95808
4 or more additional
parameters, 95810-95811
unattended, 95806, 95800-95801
wakefulness testing, 95805

Sling operation, 57287
stress incontinence
female, 57288
laparoscopic, 51992
urinary incontinence
male, 53440-53442

Small increment sensitivity index
(SISI) test, 92564

Smears
cervical
automated, 88147-88174
rescreening, 88148, 88175
manual, 88142
rescreening, 88143
other source, 88160-88162

Smears — *continued*
stain
cornea, 65430
fluorescent, 87206
giesma, 87205
ova, 87177, 87209
parasites, 87207-87209
wet mount, 87210
vaginal
automated, 88147-88174
rescreening, 88148, 88175
manual, 88142
rescreening, 88143

Smith fracture, 25600-25605
Smoking cessation, 4000F-40001F, 99406-99407
Soave, 45120
Sodium
glycinate, 80198
other source, 84302
serum, 84295
urine, 84300
Sofield procedure, 24410
Solar plexus
destruction, 64680
injection, 64530, 64680
Somatomammotropin, 83632
Somatomedin, 84305
Somatosensory testing
head, 95927
lower limbs, 95926
trunk, 95927
upper limbs, 95925
Somatostatin, 84307
Somatotropin, 83003
Somnography, 95808-95811
Somophyllin T, 80198
Sonography
abdomen, 76700-76705
arm, 76881-76882
arteries
extracranial, 93880-93882
intracranial, 93886-93893
breast, 76641-76642
cardiac, 93303-93307, 93320-93321, 93350-93352, 93662
chest, 76604
eyes, 76510-76529
head, 76536
hip
infant, 76885-76886
intraoperative, 76998
kidney, transplanted, 76776
leg, 76881-76882
neck, 76536
pelvis, 76856-76857
prostate, 76872-76873
retroperitoneal, 76770-76775
scrotum, 76870
spine, 76800
transvaginal, 76817, 76830
uterus
pregnant, 76801-76828
vagina, 76817, 76830
Sonohysterography, 76831
catheterization, 58340
Specific gravity testing, 84315
Specimen
collection, 43754-43757
concentration, 87015
handling, 99000-99001
SPECT
bone, 78320
cerebrospinal fluid, 78647
heart
multiple, 78465
kidney, 78710
localization
abscess, 78807
tumor, 78803
liver, 78205
Spectacle services
fitting
low vision aid, 92354-92355
prosthesis, 92352-92353

Spectacle services — *continued*
fitting — *continued*
spectacles, 92340-92342
repair, 92370-92371
Spectrometry, 83789
Spectrophotometry, 84311
Spectroscopy, 0064T
atomic absorption, 82190
bioimpedance, 93702
coronary vessel graft, 0205T
lower extremity wounds, 0287T
magnetic resonance, 76390
Speech
evaluation, 92521-92523
cine, 70371
video, 70371
prosthesis, 21084
evaluation, 92597, 92607-92608
modification, 92609
programming, 92609
therapy, 92507-92508
Sperm
analysis
antibodies, 89325
hyaluron binding assay, 0087T
identification, 89257, 89261
isolation, 89260-89261
motility, 89300-89322
penetration test, 89329-89330
cryopreservation, 89259, 89353
evaluation, 89329-89331
storage, 89343
washing, 58323
Spermatic
cord
excision
hydrocele, 55500
lesion, 55520
varicocele, 55530-55540
repair, 55530-55540
vein
excision, 55530-55540
ligation, 55550
Spermatocystectomy, 54840
Sphenoid sinus
biopsy, 31050-31051
excision, 31287-31288
incision, 31287-31288
injection, 64505
irrigation, 31002
repair, 31291
sinusotomy, 31050-31051
x-ray, 70210-70220
Sphenopalatine ganglion, 64505
Sphincter
anal
dilation, 45905
incision, 46080
repair, 46750-46751, 46760-46762
bile duct, 47460
bladder, 51845
oddi, 43263
pyloric
incision, 43520
reconstruction, 43800
urethral
prosthesis, 53444-53449
Spica cast
hip, 29305-29325
repair, 29720
shoulder, 29055
Spinal
cord
aspiration
cyst, 62268
diagnostic, 62267
syrinx, 62268
biopsy, 63275-63290
needle, 62269
decompression, 63001-63003, 63050-63051
destruction
lesion, 62280-62282
excision
lesion, 63265-63273, 63300-63308

CPT © 2015 American Medical Association. All Rights Reserved.

© 2016 DecisionHealth

Stimulation — *continued*
  gonadotropin panel
    releasing hormone, 80426
  growth hormone panel, 80430
  lymphocyte, 86353
  magnetic, 90867-90868
  nerve
    peripheral, 95925-95927
    repetitive, 95937
  neurostimulation
    application, 64550
  peripheral vein renin panel, 80417
  programmed
    with pacing after IV drug
      infusion, 93623
  renal vein renin panel, 80416
  spinal cord, 63610
  subcortical, 95961-95962
  thyroid uptake, 78012, 78014
  thyrotropin releasing hormone
    panel
    one hour, 80438
    two hour, 80439
  transcranial
    magnetic, 90867–90869, 95939
    motor, 95928-95929
Stimulus evoked response, 51792
Stoma
  bladder, 51980
  kidney, 50551-50561
  stomach, 43830-43831
  ureter, 50860, 50951-50961
Stomach
  anastomosis
    duodenal, 43810, 43850-43855
    jejunum, 43820-43825,
      43860-43865
  biopsy, 43605
  creation
    stoma, 43653, 43830-43831
  excision
    partial, 43631-43635, 43845
    total, 43620-43622
    tumor, 43610-43611
  exploration, 43500
  gastric bypass, 43644-43645,
    43845
    revision, 43848
  gastric restrictive procedures
    laparoscopic, 43770-43774
    open, 43842-43848
  implantation
    electrodes, 0155T, 0157T,
      43647, 43881
  incision
    pyloric sphincter, 43520
  intubation, 43753-43755
  nuclear medicine
    blood loss study, 78278
    gastric emptying study, 78264-
      78266
    imaging, 78261
    protein loss study, 78282
    reflux study, 78262
    vitamin B-12 absorption,
      78270-78272
  reconstruction
    Roux-en-Y, 43644, 43846
  removal
    electrode, 0156T, 058T, 43882
    foreign body, 43500
  repair
    fistula, 43880
    fundoplasty, 43210, 43280,
      43325-43328
    laceration, 43501-43502
    stoma, 43870
    ulcer, 43501
  replacement
    electrodes, 0155T, 0157T,
      43647, 43881
  specimen collection, 43754-
    43757
  stimulation
    secretion, 43755
  suture
    fistula, 93880
    stoma, 43870

Stomach — *continued*
  suture — *continued*
    ulcer, 43840
    wound, 43840
Stomatoplasty, 40830-40831
Stone
  lithopaxy, 52317-52318
  lithotripsy
    biliary duct, 43265
    pancreatic duct, 43265
    ureter, 52353
  removal
    anesthesia, 00918
    biliary duct, 43264, 47400-
      47480, 47554
    bladder, 51045-51065,
    kidney, 50060-50081, 50130,
      50561, 50580
    ureter, 50610-50630, 50961,
      50980, 52320-52325,
      53252
    pancreatic duct, 43264
    pancreas, 48020
  qualitative analysis, 82355
  quanitative analysis, 82360
  spectroscopy
    infrared, 82365
  x-ray
    defraction, 82370
    salivary gland, 70380
Storage
  embryo, 89342
  oocyte, 89346
  reproductive tissue, 89344
  sperm, 89343
Strabismus
  chemodenervation, 67345
  previous surgery, 67331
  release
    scar tissue, 67343
  repair
    extraocular muscles, 67340
    horizontal muscle, 67311-67312
    posterior technique, 67334-
      67335
    superior oblique muscle, 67318
    sutures, 67335
    vertical muscle, 67314-67316
  transposition, 67320
Strapping
  ankle, 29540
  back, 29799
  elbow, 29260
  finger, 29280
  foot, 29540
  hand, 29280
  hip, 29520
  knee, 29530
  shoulder, 29240
  thorax, 29200
  toes, 29550
  Unna boot, 29580
  wrist, 29260
Strassman procedure, 58540
Strayer procedure, 27687
Streptococcus
  group A
    antigen, 87430
      nucleic acid, 87650-87652
    observation, 87880
  group B, 87802
  pneumoniae vaccine, 90732
Streptokinase, 86590
Stress test
  cardiovascular, 93015-93024
  multiple uptake gated acqusition
    (MUGA), 78472-78473
  myocardial perfusion imaging,
    78460-78465
  pulmonary, 94620-94621
Stricture
  anoplasty, 46700-46705
  dilation
    biliary duct, 47555-47556,
      74363
    intrarenal, 52346

Stricture — *continued*
  dilation — *continued*
    rectal, 45910
    ureter, 50700, 52341
    ureteropelvic, 52342, 52345
    urethra, 52281, 53600-53621
  division
    rectum, 45150
  electrocautery
    intrarenal, 52346
    ureteral, 52341, 52345
    ureteropelvic, 52342, 52345
  incision
    hypospadias, 54343-54348
    intrarenal, 52346
    ureteral, 52341, 52345
    ureteropelvic, 52342, 52345
  injection
    urethral, 52283
  laser
    intrarenal, 52346
    ureteral, 52341, 52344
    ureteropelvic, 52342, 52345
  repair
    urethra, 53400-53405
  urethroplasty, 53400-53405
Strictureplasty, 44615
Stroboscopy, 31579
Stuart Prower factor, 85260
Sturmdorf procedure, 57520
Styloid process
  excision, 25230
  fracture treatment
    ulna, 25600-25605, 25650-
      25652
Stypven time, 85612-85613
Subacromial bursa, 20610-20611
Subclavian artery
  aneurysm, 35001-35002, 35021-
    35022
  angioplasty, 35458
  embolectomy, 34001-34101
  graft, 35506, 35511-35516,
    35526, 35606-35616,
    35626, 35645
  thrombectomy, 34001-34101
  thromboendarterectomy, 35301,
    35311
  transposition, 33889
Subcutaneous
  injection, 11950-11954
    therapy, 90782
  mastectomy, 19304
  tissue, 15830-15839, 15847
    debridement, 11004-11047
Subdiaphragmatic abscess, 49040
Subdural
  electrode
    insertion, 61531-61533
    removal, 61535
  hematoma, 61108
  puncture, 61105-61108
  tap, 61000-61001
Sublingual gland, 42450
  excision, 42330
  incision and drainage, 42310-
    42320
  marsupialization, 42409
Subluxation, 24640
Submandibular gland
  excision, 42440, 42508-42509
  incision, 42330-42335
  ligation, 42510
Submaxillary
  excision, 42440
  incision, 42330-42335
    drainage, 42310-42320
Submucous resection, 30520
Subperiosteal implant
  mandible, 21245-21246
  maxilla, 21245-21246
Subphrenic abscess, 49040
Subtrochanteric fracture, 27238-
  27245

Sudiferous gland
  axillary, 11450-11451
  inguinal, 11462-11463
  perianal, 11470-11471
  umbilical, 11470-11471
Sugar, 84375-84379
  water test, 85555-85557
Sulfate
  chondroitin, 82485
  dehydroepiandrosenesulfate
    (DHA), 82626
Sumatran mite fever, 86000
Superficial musculoaponeurotic
  system (SMAS) flap, 15829
Supernumerary digit, 26587
Supression test, 80400-80439
Suprahyoid, 38700
Supraorbital
  avulsion, 64732
  destruction, 64600
  reconstruction, 21179-21180
  transection, 64732
Supracapsular nerve, 64418
Supracellar cyst, 61545
Surface
  CD4, 86360
  radiotherapy, 77789
Suspension
  aorta, 33800
  hyoid, 21685
  kidney, 50400-50405
  testis, 54620-54640
  tongue, 41512
  urethra, 51840-51841, 57289
  uterus, 58400-58410
  vagina
    abdominal, 57280
    extraperitoneal, 57282
    intraperitoneal, 57283
    laparoscopic, 57425
  vesical neck, 51845
Suture
  abdomen, 49900
  aorta, 33320-33322
  artery
    abdomen, 37617
    carotid, 37605-37606
    chest, 37616
    extremity, 37618
    neck, 37615
    temporal, 37609
  bile duct, 47900
  bladder, 51860-51865
  cervix, 57720
  colon
    diverticulum, 44604-44605
    plication, 44680
    stoma, 44620-44625
    ulcer, 44604-44605
    wound, 44604-44605
  esophagus, 43410-43415
  eyelid
    intermarginal adhesions,
      67880-67882
    temporary closure, 67875
    wound, 67930-67935
  fistula
    arteriovenous, 37607
  gastroesophageal, 43405
  hemorrhoids, 46945-46946
  intestine
    large, 44604-44605
    small, 44602-44603, 44680
    stoma, 44620-44625
  iris and ciliary body, 66682
  kidney, 50500
  leg
    muscle, 27385-27386
    tendon, 27658-27665
  liver, 47350-47361
  mesentery, 44850
  nerve, 69740-69745, 64831-64876
  pancreas, 48545
  pharynx, 42900
  rectum, 45540-45541
  removal, 15850-15851

Tenotomy — *continued*
- hip — *continued*
  - adductor, 27000-27003
  - iliopsoas, 27005
  - leg, 27306-27307, 27390-27392
  - toe, 28010, 28232, 28234, 28240

TENS, 64550, 97014, 97032

Terman-Merrill test, 96101-96103

Test
- acid reflux, 78262, 91034-91038
- adrenal gland, 95922
- allergy
  - food, 95076, 95079
  - inhalation, 95070-95071
  - intracutaneous, 95017-95028
  - patch, 95044-95052
  - percutaneous, 95004, 95017-95018
  - photo, 95052-95056
  - ophthalmic, 95060
- amines, 82120
- Bender-Getsalt, 96101-96103
- Bernstein, 91030
- Binet, 96101-96103
- blood
  - ascorbic acid, 82180
  - bone marrow, 3155F, 88237
  - catecholamines, 83283
  - clot assessment, 85396
  - chloride, 82435
  - cholesterol, 82465
  - complete, 85025-85027
  - creatinine, 82565
  - culture
    - bacterial, 87040
    - fungal, 87103
  - erythrocyte, 85032
  - gases
    - CO22, 82803
    - HCO3, 82803
    - O2 saturation, 82805-82810
    - pCO2, 82803
    - pH, 82800-82803
    - pO2, 82803
  - glucose, 82947-82948, 82962
  - helicobacter pylori, 83009
  - hematocrit, 85014
  - hemoglobin, 85018
  - iron
    - stain, 85536
    - stores, 3160F
  - Kt/V, 3082F-3084F
  - leukocyte, 85032, 84048
    - myeloperoxidase (MPO), 83876
  - lipoprotein, 3048F-3050F, 83700-83704
  - lysis time, 85175
  - microhematocrit, 84013
  - nuclear medicine
    - plasma volume, 78110-78111
    - platelet survival, 78190-78191
    - red cell volume, 78120-78121
    - whole blood volume, 78122
  - occult, 82270-82274
  - osmolality, 83930
  - panels
    - electrolyte, 80051
    - general health, 80050
    - hepatic function, 80076
    - hepatitis, 80074
    - lipid, 3011F, 3278F, 80061
    - metabolic, 80047-80048, 80053
    - obstetric, 80055, 80081
    - renal, 80069
  - phenylalanine (PKU), 84030
  - platelet, 85032, 85049
  - protein
    - western blot, 84181-84182
  - red blood cell (RBC) 85041
  - reticulocyte, 85044-85046
  - smear, 85060, 88140
  - thromboplastin time, 85730
  - tissue, 88237

Test — *continued*
- blood — *continued*
  - uric acid, 84550
  - volume determination, 78122
  - WBC, 85004-85009
  - western blot
    - human immunodeficiency virus (HIV), 86689
    - protein, 84181-84182
    - tissue analysis, 88371-88372
  - xylose absorption, 84620
- breath
  - alcohol, 82075
  - heart transplant rejection detection, 0085T
  - helicobacter pylori, 78267-78268, 83013-83014
  - hydrogen, 91065
- caffeine halothane contracture (CHCT), 89049
- caloric vestibular, 92533
- candida, 86485
- cholesterol, 80061, 82465, 83718-83721
- cholinesterase inhibitor, 95857
- compatability, 86920, 86923
- Coombs, 86880, 86885-86886
- D-xylose absorption, 84620
- dark room, 92140
- defibrillator, 93640-93644
- developmental, 96110-96111
- ear function, 92511-92520, 92531-92597
- ergonovine provocation, 93024
- esophagus acid, 91013, 91030
- Farnsworth-Munsell color, 92283
- Fern, 87210, 89060
- fertility, 89300-89322, 89329-89331
- fetal
  - blood
    - hemoglobin, 83030-83033, 85460-85461
    - scalp, 59030
  - contraction stress, 59020
  - echocardiography, 76825-76828
  - fibronectin, 82731
  - lung maturity, 83661-83664
  - non-stress, 59025, 76818
  - profile, 76818-76819
  - ultrasound, 76801-76817
  - velocimetry, 76820-76821
- function
  - nasal, 92512
  - neurological
    - autonomic nervous system, 95921-95924, 95943
    - aphasia, 96105
    - cognitive, 96116
    - developmental, 96110-96111
    - neuropsychological, 96118-96120
  - pulmonary
    - capacity, 94200-94240
    - continuous pressure, 94660-94662
    - determination, 94350-94370, 95012
    - gas
      - analysis, 0064T, 94680-94690, 94770
      - collection, 94250
      - diffusion, 94720-94725
      - volume, 94260, 94750
    - high altitude simulation test (HAST), 94452-94453
    - inhalation, 94640-94645, 94664
    - manipulation, 94667-94668
    - perfusion, 78596
    - recording, 94772-94777
    - response, 94400-94450
    - saturation, 82820, 94760-94762
    - spirometry, 94010-94070
    - stress, 94620-94621
    - surfactant, 94610
    - ventilation, 94002-94005
    - volume, 94375

Test — *continued*
- GERD, 91034-91038
- glass, 81020
- glucagon tolerance, 82946
- gonadotropin, 84702-84704
- Goodenough Harris drawing test, 96101-96103
- guaiac, 82270-82272
- Gunning-Lieben, 82009-82010
- Guthrie, 84030
- Hamster penetration, 89329
- hemagglutination inhibition, 86280
- high altitude simulation (HAST), 94452-94453
- histoplasma, 86510
- Holten, 82575
- human immunodeficiency, 86689
- hue, 92283
- Huhner, 89300
- impedance, 92567
- infection, 86403-86406
- ingestion challenge, 95076, 95079
- inhalation provocation, 95070-95071
- inhibition, 86280
- intelligence, 96101-96103
- Kleihauer Betke, 85460
- Kuhlmann, 96101-96103
- lactase deficiency, 91065
- lactose tolerance, 82951-82953
- larynx, 92614-92617
- Lee and White, 85345
- Leveen shunt, 78291
- Mantoux, 86580
- Metabisulfite, 85660
- monitoring, 4189F-4191F
- monospot, 86308
- Mosenthal, 81002
- mucous membrane, 95060-95065
- multiple sleep latency (MSLT), 95805
- muscle
  - eye, 92260-92265
  - manual, 95831-95834
- myasthenia gravis, 95857
- Nagel, 92283
- nerve, 88362
- neurofunctional, 96020
- neuromuscluar junction, 95937
- neurophysiologic
  - autonomic, 95921-95923
  - intraoperative, 95940-95941
- neuropsychology, 96118-96125
- neutralization, 86382
- nitroblue tetrazolium, 83684
- nocturnal penile, 54250
- Nystagmus, 92531-92532, 92534, 92541-92542, 92544
- opthalmic membrane, 95060
- optokinetic nystagmus, 92534, 92544
- ovulation, 84830
- oxytocin stress, 59020
- pacemaker
  - antitachycardia, 93724
- pain, 1125F-1126F, 1130F-1137F, 2040F, 3330F-3331F
- pancreozymin-secretin, 82938
- paternity, 86910-86911
- penetration, 89330
- penile, 54250
- pentagastrin, 43755
- performance
  - cognitive, 96125
  - physical, 97750
  - psychological, 96101-96103
- personality, 96101-96103
- photosensitivity, 95056
- physical performance, 97750
- positional nystagmus, 92532-92542
- pregnancy, 84702-84704
- projective, 96101-96103
- psychological, 96101-96103, 96125
- quantitative sensory
  - cooling, 0108T
  - heat-pain, 0109T
  - other, 0110T
  - touch pressure, 0106T
  - vibration, 0107T

Test — *continued*
- quick, 85610-85611
- radioimmunosorbent, 82784-82787
- rapid
  - infection, 86308, 86403-86406
  - plasma reagent, 86592-86593
- Rapoport, 52005
- reflex, 95907-95913, 95933
- Reinsch, 83015
- reptilase, 85635
- Ropes, 83872
- Rorschach, 96101
- Sahli, 43754-43755
- Schilling, 78270
- Schlicter, 87197
- serologic, 86592-86593
- serotonin, 84260
- six minute walk, 94620
- skin
  - immunologic
    - candida, 86485
    - coccidiodomycosis, 86490
    - histoplasmosis, 86510
    - other, 86486
    - tuberculosis, 17999
- small increment sensitivity index (SISI), 82564
- somatosensory, 95925-95927
- specific gravity, 84315
- Stenger, 92565, 92577
- stress, 78473, 93015-93018, 93024
- supression, 80400-80439
- sweat, 82435
- syphilis, 86592-86593
- Terman Merrill, 96101-96103
- tissue factor, 85347
- tolerance
  - glucagon, 82946
  - glucose, 82951-82952
  - heparine-protamine, 85530
  - insulin, 80434-80435
  - maltose, 82951-82952
- torsion swing, 92546
- tracking, 92545
- tuberculosis, 86480, 86580
- urea, 78267-78268
- urodynamic
  - bladder capacity, 51798
  - cystometrogram, 51725-51726
  - electromyographic study, 51785
  - residual urine, 51798
  - stimulus evoked response, 51792
  - urethra pressure profile, 51772
  - uroflowmetry, 51736-51741
  - voiding pressure studies
    - bladder, 51795
    - intra-abdominal, 51797
    - rectal, 51797
- VanDen Bergh, 82247-82248
- villus sampling, 88235, 88267
- vitamin test
  - A, 84590
  - B, 82607-82608, 84207, 84252, 84425
    - absorption study, 78270-78272
  - C, 82180
  - D, 82306-82307, 82652
  - E, 84446
  - K, 84597
- WADA, 95958
- wakefullness, 95805
- water test, 85555-85557
- Wintrobe, 85651-85652
- xylose absorption, 84620

Testis, 00920-00938
- biopsy, 54500-54505
- cryopreservation, 89335
- excision, 54690
  - lesion, 54512
  - partial, 54522
  - radical, 54530-54535
  - simple, 54520
- incision, 54700
- insertion, 54660
- nuclear medicine, 78761

Testis — *continued*
repair, 54600-54670
transplant, 54680
undescended, 54550-54560
Testosterone, 84402-84403
binding, 84270
response, 80414-80415
Tetanus, 86280
antibody, 86774
immunoglobulin, 90389
vaccine, 90714-90715
Tetrachloride, 82441
Tetralogy of Fallot, 33692-33697, 33924
Thal-Nissen procedure, 43325
Thawing
blood, 86930-86932
cell, 38208-38209
expansion, 88241
embryo, 89352
oocytes, 89356
sperm, 89353
tissue, 89354
Theleplasty, 19350
Theophylline, 80198
Thermocauterization, 67922
cornea, 65450
Thermocoagulation, 17000-17286, 46930
Thermoplasty, 31660-31661
Thermotherapy, 53850-53852
Thiamine, 84425
Thiersch
operation, 15050
procedure, 46753
Thiocyanate, 84430
Thompson procedure, 27430
Thoracentesis, 32554-32555
Thoracoplasty, 32905-32906
Thoracoscopy
bilobectomy, 32670
decortication, 32651-32652
diagnostic, 32601
biopsies, 32604-32609
esophagomyotomy, 32665
excision, cyst/tumor/mass
mediastinal, 32662
pericardial, 32661
hemorrhage control, 32654
lobectomy, 32663
lymphadenectomy, 32674
pericardial window, 32659
pleurodesis, 32650
pleurectomy, 32656
removal
clot, 32658
foreign body, 32653, 32658
lung, 32671
single segment, 32669
two lobes, 32670
resection
plication, 32655, 32672
thymus, 32673
wedge, 32666-32668
segmentectomy, 32669
sympathectomy, 32664
Thoracostomy, 32035-32036, 32551
Thoracotomy
biopsy
lung, 32096-32097
pleura, 32098
cardiac massage, 32160
exploration, 32100
hemorrhage control, 32110
pneumolysis, 32124
postoperative, 32120
removal
cyst, 32140
electrodes
defibrillator, 33243
permanent transvenous, 33238
foreign body, 32150-32151
pacemaker, 33236-33237

Thoracotomy — *continued*
repair, lung tear, 32110
revascularization, transmyocardial, 33140-33141
resection
bullae, 32141
wedge, 32505-32507
Thorax
angiography, 71275
artery, 36215-36218
bioimpedance, 93701
biopsy, 21550
cavity
exploration, 32601-32606
graft, 35905
surgery, 32650-32665
computed tomography (CT) scan, 71250-71275
duct
cannulation, 38794
ligation, 38380-38382
suture, 38380-38382
empyema, 32035-32036
excision, 21555-21558
incision, 32035-32036
deep, 21510
drainage, 21501-21502
resection, 21557
strapping, 29200
target delineation, 32701
Throat
biopsy, 42800-42806
hemorrhage, 42960-42962
incision and drainage, 42700-42725
reconstruction, 42950
removal, 42809
repair
pharyngoesophageal, 42953
wound, 42900
suture, 42900
Thrombectomy
artery
aortoiliac, 34201
axillary, 34101
brachial, 34101
carotid, 34001
celiac, 34151
coronary, 92973
femoral, 34201
innominate, 34001-34101
mesentary, 34151
peroneal, 34203
popliteal, 34203
radial, 34111
renal, 34151
subclavian, 34001-34101
tibial, 34203
ulnar, 34111
arteriovenous fistula
graft, 36870
bypass graft, 35875-35876
dialysis, 36831
vein
axillary, 34490
femoropopliteal, 34421-34451
iliac, 34401-34451
subclavian, 34471-34490
vena cava, 34401-34451
Thrombin
inhibitor, 85300-85301
time, 85670-85675
Thrombocyte
aggregation, 85576
antibody, 86022-86023
count, 85008
automated, 85049
manual, 85032
Thromboembolism, 4044F
Thromboendarterectomy
artery
aorta, 35331
aortoiliofemoral, 35363
axillary, 35321
brachial, 35321
carotid, 35301, 35390
celiac, 35341
femoral, 35302, 35371-35372

Thromboendarterectomy — *continued*
artery — *continued*
iliac, 35351, 35361-35363
iliofemoral, 35355, 35363
innominate, 35311
mesentaric, 35341
peroneal, 35305-35306
popliteal, 35303
renal, 35341
subclavian, 35301, 35311
tibial, 35305-35306
tibioperoneal trunk, 35304
vertebral, 35301
Thrombokinase, 85260
Thrombolysis
catheter exchange, 37213-37214
cerebral, 37195
coronary vessels, 92975-92977
other than coronary, 37211-37214
Thrombomodulin, 85337
Thromboplastin
factor
christmas, 85250
clotting, 85210-85293
inhibition, 85705
test, 85347
partial time, 85730-85732
plasma, 85250
antecedent, 85270
Thumb
amputation, 26910-26952
arthrodesis, 26841-26842
dislocation treatment
open, 26665
with fracture, 26645-26650
fracture treatment
open, 26665
with dislocation, 26645-26650
fusion, 26820
opponenplasty, 26490-26496
reconstruction, 26550
opponenplasty, 26490-26496
repair, 26508
sesamoidectomy, 26185
transfer
muscle, 26494
tendon, 26510
Thymectomy
sternal split, 60520-60521
transcervical, 60520
transthoracic, 60520-60521
Thymotaxin, 82232
Thymus gland, 32673, 60520-60522
Thyrocalcitonin, 80410, 82308
Thyroglobulin, 86800, 84432
Thyroglossal duct, 60280-60281
Thyroid, 00320-00322
gland
aspiration, 60300
biopsy, 60100
excision
adenoma, 60200
cervical, 60271
complete, 60240
cyst, 60200
partial, 60210-60220
remaining tissue, 60260
substernal split, 60270
total, 60220-60225, 60240, 60252-60254
transthoracic, 60270
incision and drainage, 60000
injection, 60300
nuclear medicine
imaging, 78012-78018
imaging with flow, 78013
imaging with uptake, 78014
metastases uptake, 78020
uptake, 78012, 78014
hormone binding, 84479
hormone stimulation, 84443
immune globulins, 84445
pituitary evaluation, 80418
thyrotropin, 80438-80439
uptake, 84479
nuclear medicine
imaging, 78013-78018
flow, 78013-78014

Thyroid — *continued*
nuclear medicine — *continued*
imaging — *continued*
metastases, 78015-78018
uptake, 78020
uptake, 78012, 78014
metastases, 78020
Thyroidectomy
partial, 60210-60225
secondary, 60260
sternal split, 60270
tissue, 60260
total
cervical, 60271
for malignancy, 60252-6254
transthoracic, 60270
Thyrolingual cyst
excision, 60200
incision and drainage, 60280-60281
Thyrotomy, 31300
Thyrotropin releasing hormone, 80438-80439
Thyroxine
binding gobulin, 84442
free, 84439
neonatal, 84437
total, 84436
true, 84439
Tibia, 01390-01392
artery
bypass
graft, 35566-35571, 35623, 35666-35671
in situ, 35585-35587
embolectomy, 34203
thromboendarterectomy, 35305-35306
arthroscopy
fracture treatment, 29855-29856
repair, 29891-29892
craterization, 27369, 27640
diaphysectomy, 27360, 27649
excision
cyst, 27635-27638
epiphyseal bar, 20150
partial, 27640
tumor, 27635-27638, 27645
fracture treatment
arthroscopic, 29855-29856
closed, 27824-27825
distal, 27824-27828
intercondylar, 27538-27540
malleolus, 27760-27766, 27808-27814
open, 27535-27536, 27758-27759, 27826-27828
plateau, 27530-27536
shaft, 27752-27759
nerve, 64840
osteotomy, 27455-27457, 27705, 27709-27712
repair
epiphysis, 27477-27485, 27730-27742
nerve, 64840
pseudoarthrosis, 27727
saucerization, 27360, 27640
x-ray, 73590-73600
Tibiofibular joint
arthrodesis, 27871
dislocation treatment, 27830-27832
disruption
open treatment, 27829
fusion, 27871
x-ray, 73590-73600
Time
bleeding, 85002
prothrombin, 85610-85611
thrombin, 85670-85675
thromboplastin, 85730-85732
Tinnitus, 92625
Tissue
crystal identification, 89060

CPT © 2015 American Medical Association. All Rights Reserved.
© 2016 decisionHealth

Tissue — *continued*
  culture
    antitoxin, 87230
    chromosome analysis, 88230-88239
    graft, 15150-15157, 15340-15366
    harvest, 15040
    homogenization, 87176
    non-neoplastic disorder, 88230, 88237
    skin grafts, 15100-15101, 15120-15121
    toxin, 87230
  enzyme activity, 82657
  examination
    ecoparasites, 87220
    fungi, 87220
  expander
    breast reconstruction, 19357
    insertion, 11950
    removal, 11971
    replacement, 11970
  factor, 85705
    test, 85347
    time, 85730-85732
  graft, 20926
  granulation, 17250
  granulation
  homogenization, 87176
  hybridization, 88364-88369, 88373-88374, 88377
  skin harvest, 15040
  transfer
    adjacent, 14000-14350, 67961
    facial muscle, 15845
    finger flap, 14350
    toe flap, 14350
  typing, 86805-86849
    human leukocyte antigens (HLA), 86812-86817
    antibody to, 86828-86835
    crossmatch, 86825-86826
    lymphocyte culture, 86821-86822
    lymphocytotoxicity, 86805-86806
    serum screening, PRA, 86807-86808
TLC, 84375
TMS, 90867-90869
Tobramycin, 80200
Tocolysis, 59412
Tocopherol, 84446
Toe
  amputation, 28810-28825
  arthrocentesis, 20600-20604
  capsulotomy, 28270-28272
  excision, 28092
  fasciotomy, 28008
  flap, 14350
  fracture treatment
    closed, 28490-28496, 28510-28515
    open, 28505, 28525
  magnetic resonance imaging (MRI), 73722-73723
  reconstruction
    angle deformity, 28313
    extra digit, 26587
    hammertoe, 28285-28286
    macrodactyly, 28340-28341
    polydactyly, 28344
    syndactyly, 28345
    webbed, 28345
  repair
    bunion, 28290-28299
    extra digit, 26587
    macrodactyly, 26590
    muscle, 28340
    tendon, 28232-28234, 28240
    webbed, 28280
  repositioning
    to hand, 26551-26556
  strapping, 29550
  tenotomy, 28010-28011, 28232-28234
  x-ray, 73660

Tolerance test
  glucagon, 82946
  glucose, 82951-82952
  heparine-protamine, 85530
  insulin, 80434-80435
  maltose, 82951-82952
Tomography
  computed (CT) scan
    3D rendering, 76376-76377
    ablation, 76362, 77013
    abdomen, 74150-74170
    arm, 73200-73202
    bone density study, 77078
    brain, 70450-70470
    ear, 70480-70482
    face, 70486-70488
    follow-up study, 76380
    head, 70450-70470
    heart, 75571-75573
    leg, 73700-73702
    maxilla, 70486-70488
    neck, 70490-70492
    needle placement, 77012
    orbit, 70480-70482
    pelvis, 72192-72194
    radiation therapy, 77014
    sella turcica, 70480-70482
    spine, 72125-72133
    thorax, 71250-71270
  optical coherence
    breast, 0351T-0354T
    intravascular, 0291T-0292T
Tomosynthesis, 77061-77063
Tompkins metroplasty, 58540
Tongue
  ablation, 41530
  biopsy, 41100-41105
  excision
    complete, 41140-41155
    frenum, 41115
    lesion, 41110-41114
    partial, 41120-41135
    with mouth resection, 41150-41153
    with neck resection, 41135, 41145, 41153-41155
  fixation, 41500
  incision, 41010
    drainage
      abscess, 41000-41006, 41015
      cyst, 41000-41006, 41015
      hematoma, 41000-41006, 41005
  reconstruction, 41520
  repair
    laceration, 41250-41252
    suture, 41510
  suture, 41510
  suspension, 41512
Tonometry, 92100
Tonsil
  destruction
    lingual, 42870
  excision
    lingual, 42870
    radical, 42842-42845
    tag, 42860
    with adenoids, 42820-42821
Tonsillectomy
  and adnoidectomy, 42820
  primary, 42825-42831
  radical
    resection, 42842-42845
  secondary, 42825-42826, 42835-42836
Topiramate, 80201
Torek procedure, 54640, 54650, 54692
Torkildsen procedure, 62180
TORP (total ossicular replacement prosthesis), 69633, 69637
Torsion swing test, 92546
Torula, 86641, 87327
Torus mandibularis, 21031

Total
  claviculectomy, 23125
  colectomy, 44150-44158, 44210-44212
  dacryoadenectomy, 68500
  esophagectomy, 43107-43113, 43124
  glossectomy, 41140-41145
  hepatectomy, 47125-47130
  hysterectomy
    abdominal, 58150-58200
    bilateral, 58953-58956
    cesarean, 59525
    ectopic pregnancy, 59135
    laparoscopy, 58570-58573
    lobectomy, 60220-60225
    oophorectomy, 58940-58943
    pancreatectomy, 48155-48160
    thymectomy, 60520-60522
    thyroidectomy, 60240-60254
    ureterectomy, 50234-50236
Touroff operation, 37615
Toxicology screening, 80300-80304
Toxin assay, 87230
  assay, 87230
Toxoplasma, 86777-86778
Trabeculectomy, 66170-66172
Trabeculoplasty, 65855
Trabeculotomy, 65850
Trachea, 00320-00326
  aspiration, 31720-31725
    puncture, 31612
  dilation, 31630-31631, 31636-31638
  endoscopy
    fracture treatment, 31630
    through tracheostomy, 31615
  excision
    stenosis, 31780-31781
    tumor, 31785-31786
  fistula closure, 31820
    with plastic repair, 31825
  fracture treatment, 31630
  incision
    emergency, 31603-31605
    planned, 31600-31601
    with flaps, 31610
  injection, 31612
  introduction, 31730
  placement
    stent, 31631
    tube, 31500
  puncture aspiration, 31612
  reconstruction
    carina, 31766
    cervical, 31750
    fistula, 31755
    intrathoracic, 31760
  repair
    stenosis, 31780-31781
    stoma, 31613-31614
  revision, 31830
  stent, 31631
  stoma
    repair, 31820-31825
    revision, 31830
    suture, 31800-31805
  tracheostomy
    emergency, 31603-31605
    planned, 31600-31601
    with flaps, 31610
  tube, 31500
Trachelectomy, 57530-57531
Trachelorrhaphy, 57720
Tracheobronchoscopy, 31615
Tracheostoma, 31613-31614
Tracheostomy
  closure, 31820
    with plastic repair, 31825
  emergency, 31603-31605
  planned, 31600-31601
  revision, 31830
  tracheobronchoscopy, 31615
    with flaps, 31610
Tracheotomy, 31502
Tracking test, 92545

Traction therapy
  manual, 97140
  mechanical, 97012
Tractotomy, 61480
Training
  biofeedback, 90901-90911
  integration
    sensory, 97533
  management
    home, 97535, 99509
    wheelchair, 97542
  orthoptic, 92065
  orthotics, 97760
  prosthetics, 97761
  reintegration
    community, 97537
    work, 97537
  self care, 97535, 98960-98962, 99509
  skills, cognitive, 97532
TRAM flap, 19367-19369
Trans-scaphoperilunar, 25680-25685
Transaminase
  oxalacetic, 84450
  pyruvic, 84460
Transcortin, 84449
Transcranial
  doppler study, 93886-93893
  stimulation
    magnetic, 90867-90869
    motor, 95928-95929, 95939
Transection
  artery
    carotid, 61610-61612
    pulmonary, 33922
  brain, 61567
  kidney
    blood vessel, 50100
  nerve, 64732-64772
Transesophageal, 93312-93318, 93355
Transfer
  bone
    lower extremity, 27140, 27468
    upper extremity, 23462
  digit, 26551-26556, 28760
  muscle
    facial, 15845
    trunk, 27100-27111
    upper extremity, 23395-23397, 24301
  pedicle
    nerve, 64905-64907
    skin, 15570-15576, 15650
  tendon
    lower extremity
      adductor, 27098
      foot, 27690-27692
      hamstring, 27400
    upper extremity
      elbow, 24301
        to shoulder, 24320
      forearm, 25310-25312, 25316
      hand, 26480-26498, 26510
      upper arm, 24301
      wrist, 25310-25312, 25316-25320, 25337
  tissue, 14000-14300, 67961-67975
Transferase
  asparate amino, 84450
  glutamic oxaloacetic, 84450
Transferrin, 84466
Transformation, 86353
Transfusion
  blood, 36430
    autologous, 86890-86891
    exchange, 36450-36455
    fetal, 36460
    push, infant, 36440
  blood parts
    exchange, 36511-36516
  leukocyte, 86950
  push
    infant, 36440
  white blood cell, 86950

Transluminal
angioplasty
aortic, 35452
arterial, 75962-75968
brachiocephalic, 35458
iliac, 37220-37223
femoral, 37224-37227
popliteal, 37224-37227
renal, 35450
tibioperoneal, 37228-37235
venous, 35460
visceral, 35450
atherectomy
aorta, 0236T
brachiocephalic, 0237T
coronary, 92924-92925,
92933-92934
femoral, 37225, 37227
iliac, 0238T
popliteal, 37225, 37227
renal, 0234T-0235T
tibioperoneal, 35495
visceral, 0234T-0235T
Transmyocardial revascularization,
33140-33141
Transosteal plate, 21244
Transpeptidase, 82977
Transplant
bone marrow—derived HPCs,
38240-38242
cartilage
knee, 27412-27415, 29866-
29867
chondrocytes
knee, 27412
conjunctiva, 65782
cornea
endothelial, 65756-65757
for aphakia, 65750
lamellar, 65710
penetrating, 65730-65755
eye
amniotic membrane, 65780
conjunctiva, 65782
stem cell, 65781
hair
punch graft, 15775-15776
strip, 15220-15221
harvest, 01990
heart, 00580, 33945
heart-lung, 00580, 33935
intestines
cadaver, 44135
living donor, 44136
islet cell, 0141T-0143T, 48160
kidney
allotransplantation, 50360
autotransplantation, 50380
liver, orthotopic, 47135
lung
double, 32853-32854
single, 32851-32852
meniscus
knee, 29868
muscle
anus, 46760
pancreas, 48554
islet cell, 0141T-0143T
parathyroid, 60512
renal
allotransplantation, 50360
autotransplantation, 50380
stem cells, 38240-38242
tendon
carpometacarpal, 26480-26483
hamstring, 27396-27397
palmar, 26485-26489
tibial, 27690-27692
wrist, 25310-25312
ureter, 50860
Transposition
artery
carotid, 33889, 35691, 35694-
35695
subclavian, 33889, 35693-
35695
vertebral, 35691-35693

Transposition — continued
muscle, eye, 67320
nerve
cranial, 64716
peripheral, 64856
ovary, 58825
repair, great arteries, 33770-33781
valve, venous, 34510
Transthoracic echocardiography,
93304-93318, 93350-93352
Transthyretin, 84134
Transureteroureterostomy, 50770
Transurethral procedure, 00910-00918
prostate
incision, 52450
thermotherapy, 53850-53852
Trapezium, 25445
Treacher-Collins syndrome, 21150-
21151
Treatment
plan, 5050F
report, 5020F
Trendelenburg operation, 37785
Trephine procedure, 31070
Treponema pallidum
antibody, 86781
antigen detection, 87285
Triacylglycerol, 84478
hydrolase, 83690
Trichiasis
epilation, 67820-67825
incision, lid margin, 67830-67835
Trichina, 86784
trichogram, 96902
Trichonosis vaginalis
antigen detection
nucleic acid, 87660-87661
observation, 87808
Trichrome stain, 88313
Tricuspid valve
excision, 33460
repair, 33463-33465
replacement, 33465
repositioning, 33468
Tridymite, 84285
Trigeminal
ganglia, 61450
stereotactic, 61790
nerve
destruction, 64600-64610
injection
anesthetic, 64400
neurolytic, 64600-64610
tract, 61791
Trigger
finger repair, 26055
point, 20552-20553
Triglyceridase, 83690
Triglycerides, 84478
Trigonocephaly, 21175
Triiodothyronine
free, 84481
reverse, 84482
total, 84480
true, 84480
Triolean hydrolase, 83690
Trioxopurine, 84550, 84560
Tripcellim, 84485
feces, 84488-84490
Trisegmentomy, 47122
Trocar biopsy, 38221
Trochanteric fracture, 27246-27248
Trophoblastic tumor, 59100, 59870
Troponin
qualitative, 84512
quantitative, 84484
Truncal vagotomy, 43640
Truncus
arteriosus, 33786
brachiocephalic
angioplasty, 35458
atherectomy, 0237T
catheter, 36215-36218

Trypanosomiases, 86171, 86280
Trypsin
duodenum, 84485
feces, 84488-84490
inhibitor, 82103-82104
Tsutsugamushi disease, 86000
Tubal
embryo transfer, 58974-58976
ligation
laparoscopic, 58670
with cesarean section, 58611
occlusion, 58615, 58671
pregnancy
excision
fallopian tube, 59120
laparoscopic, 59150-59151
postpartum curettage, 59160
surgical treatment
abdominal, 59130
cervical, 59140
ovarian, 59121
tubal, 59121
uterine, 59135-59136
Tube
Baker's, 44021
change
colon, 49450
duodenostomy, 49451
gastro-jejunostomy, 49452
gastrostomy, 43760, 49446
jejunostomy, 49451
tracheostomy, 31502
eustachian
inflation, 69420-69421
fallopian
catheterization, 58345, 74742
excision, 58700-58720
laparoscopy, 58660-58679
ligation, 58600-58611
occlusion, 58615, 58565
pregnancy, 59120-59151
repair, 58740-58770
transfer, 58976
tumor
malignant, 58943-58952,
58957-58960
x-ray, 74742
placement
cecostomy, 44300, 49442
duodenostomy, 49441
endoscopic
bile duct, 43274
jejunostomy, 49441
nasobiliary, 43274
nasopancreatic, 43274
pancreatic duct, 43274
enterostomy, 44300
gastrostomy, 43246, 49440
nasogastric, 43752
orogastric, 43752
Tubed pedicle flap, 15570-15576
Tubercle bacilli, 87116
Tubercleplasty, 27418
Tuberculosis
antigen response test, 86480-
86481
culture, 87116
skin test, 86580
vaccine, 90585-90586
Tumor, 3260F, 3268F, 3323F
ablation
bone, 20982-20983
duodenum, 43270
esophagus, 43229, 43270
intestine, 44369
kidney, 50592-50593
liver, 47370-47371, 47380-
47383
pancreas, 43278
pulmonary, 32998
rectum, 45320, 45346
renal, 50592-50593
stomach, 43270
chemosurgery
skin, 17311-17315
cryosurgery
bladder, 52234-52240

Tumor — continued
cryosurgery — continued
liver, 47371, 47381
rectum, 46937-46938
destruction
abdomen, 49203-49205
bile duct, 43278
central nervous system, 61624-
61626
colon, 44401, 45320, 45346,
45388
intestine, 44369
pancreatic duct, 43278
rectum, 45190, 45320, 46937-
46938
retroperitoneum, 49203-49205
urethra, 53220
excision
abdomen, 22900, 49203-
49205
acetabulum, 27076
ankle, 27618-27619
arm, 24075-24077, 25075-
25077
back, 21930
bile duct, 47711-47712
bladder, 51530, 52355
brain, 61510-61512, 61518-
61521, 61526-61530,
61545, 62164
breast, 19120-19126
bronchus, 31640
calcaneus, 27647, 28100-28103
carotid, 60600-60605
carpal, 25130-25136
clavicle, 23140-23146, 23200
chest wall, 19260-19272
coccyx, 49215
dentoalveolar, 41825-41827
ear, 69550-69554
elbow, 24075-24077
femur, 27355-27358
facial bone, 21029-21030,
21034
flank, 21930
fibula, 27635-27638
finger, 26115-26117
foot, 28043-28045
gums, 41825-41827
hand, 26115-26117
hip, 27047-27049, 27075-
27076
humerus, 23220-23222,
24110-24116
proximal, 23150-23156
ilium, 27065-27067
intracardiac, 33120
ischium, 27078-27079
innominate, 27077
kidney, 50562, 52355
knee, 27327-27329, 27365
lacrimal duct, 68540-68550
larynx, 31300, 31540-31541,
31578
leg, 27327-27329, 27615-
27619
mandible, 21040-21047
maxilla, 21030, 21034, 21048-
21049
maxillary torus palatinus,
21032
mediastinum, 32662, 39220
meningioma, 61512, 61519
metacarpal, 26200-26205
metatarsal, 28104-28107
neck, 21555-21556
olecranon, 24120-24126
parotid gland, 42410-42426
pelvis, 27047-27048
pericardial, 32661, 33050
phalanx, 26210-26215, 28108
pituitary gland, 61546-61548,
62145
presacral, 49215
pubis, 27065-27067
radius, 24120-24130, 25120-
25126
rectum, 45160-45170

CPT © 2015 American Medical Association. All Rights Reserved. | © 2016 DecisionHealth

Tumor — *continued*
　excision — *continued*
　　retroperitoneum, 49203-49205, 60545
　　sacrococcygeal, 49215
　　sacrum, 49215
　　salivary, 42410-42426
　　scapula, 23140-23146, 23210
　　shoulder, 23075-23077
　　skull, 61500
　　spinal cord, 63275-63290
　　stomach, 43610-43611
　　talus, 28100-28103
　　tarsal, 28104-28107
　　testis, 54530-54535
　　thigh, 27327-27328
　　thorax, 21555-21556
　　thyroid, 60200
　　tibia, 27635-27638
　　torus mandibularis, 21031
　　trachea, 31785-31786
　　ulna, 25120-25126
　　ureter, 52355
　　urethra, 53220
　　uterus, 58140-58146
　　vagina, 57135
　　vertebra, 22100-22116
　　wrist, 25075-25077, 25135-25136
　　zygoma, 21030, 21034
　exenteration, 51597
　extrahepatic, 47711
　immunoassay
　　antigen screening, 86294, 86316
　　CA 125, 86304
　　CA 15-3, 86300
　　CA 19-9, 86301,
　localization, 78800-78804
　orchiectomy, 54530-54535
　removal
　　anus, 46610-46612
　　colon, 44392-44394
　　duodenum, 44392-44394
　　esophagus, 43216-43217, 43250-43251
　　face, 21029
　　intestine, 44364-44365
　　rectum, 45308-45315, 45333, 45338
　　stomach, 43250-43251
　　temporal bone, 69970
　resection
　　ankle, 27615
　　back, 21935
　　bladder, 52234-52240
　　calcaneus, 27647, 28100-28103
　　cardiac, 33130
　　clavicle, 23200
　　elbow, 24077
　　fallopian tube, 58950, 58952-58958
　　femur, 27365
　　fibula, 27646
　　flank, 21935
　　foot, 28046
　　forearm, 25077
　　hand, 26117
　　head, 21015
　　hip, 27049, 27075-27079
　　humerus, 24150-24151
　　　proximal, 23220-23222
　　kidney, 50562, 52355
　　knee, 27329
　　leg, 27615
　　lung, 32503-32504
　　mandible, 21045
　　metacarpal, 26250-26255
　　metatarsal, 28173
　　neck, 21557
　　ovary, 58950-58958
　　pelvis, 27049, 27075-27079
　　peritoneum, 58950-58958
　　phalanx, 26260-26262, 28175
　　radius, 24152-24153, 25170
　　scalp, 21015
　　scapula, 23210

Tumor — *continued*
　resection — *continued*
　　shoulder, 23077
　　talus, 27647
　　tarsal, 28171
　　thigh, 27329
　　thorax, 21557
　　tibia, 27645
　　ulna, 25170
　　ureter, 52355
　　urethra, 52234-52240
　　uterus, 58950-58958
　　wrist, 25077
Tunica vaginalis
　hydrocele
　　aspiration, 55000
　　excision, 55040-55041
　　repair, 55060
Turbinate
　excision, 30130-30140
　fracture treatment, 30930
　injection, 30200
　mucosa, 30801-30802
　resection
　　submucous, 30140
Turcica
　computed tomography (CT) scan, 70480-70482
　x-ray, 70240
Tylenol, 80329-80331
Tympanic
　membrane, 2035F
　　incision, 69420-69421
　　reconstruction, 69620
　　repair, 68450, 69610
　　stoma, 69433-69436
　nerve, 69676
　tympanolysis, 69450
　tympanometry, 92567
　tympanoplasty, 69631-69644
　tympanostomy, 69433-69436
　tympanotomy, 69420-69421
Typhoid vaccine
　oral, 90690
　polysaccharide, 90691
Typhus, 86000
Typing
　blood
　　ABO only, 86900
　　antigen screening, 86902-86904
　　crossmatch, 86920-86923
　　paternity testing, 86910-86911
　　RBC antigens, other, 86905
　　Rh (D), 86901
　　Rh phenotype, 86906
　HLA, 86812-86817
　tissue, 86912-86817, 86821-86822
Tyrosine, 84510
Tzank smear, 88160-88161

U

UFR, 51736-51741
Ulcer
　anal, 46200, 46940-46942
　decubitus, 15920-15998
　excision
　　decubitus, 15920-15998
　　stomach, 43610
　　pressure, 15920-15998
　pinch graft, 15050
Ulna
　artery
　　aneurysm, 35045
　　embolectomy, 34111
　　sympathectomy, 64822
　　thrombectomy, 34111
　arthrodesis, 25830
　arthroplasty, 25442
　centralization, 25335
　craterization, 24147, 25150-25151
　diaphysectomy, 24147, 25150-25151

Ulna — *continued*
　excision
　　abscess, 24138
　　complete, 25240
　　cyst, 24125-24126, 25120-25126
　　epiphyseal bar, 20150
　　olecranon, 24147
　　partial, 25145-25151, 25240
　　tumor, 24125-24126, 25120-25126, 25170
　fracture treatment
　　closed, 25530-25535
　　olecranon, 24670-24675
　　open, 24685, 25545
　　shaft, 25530-25545
　　styloid, 24620, 25651-25652
　　with dislocation, 24620-24635
　　with radius, 25560-25575
　incision and drainage, 25035
　nerve, 64718-64719, 64836-64838
　osteoplasty, 25390-25393
　prophylactic treatment, 25491-25492
　reconstruction, 25337
　repair
　　epiphyseal arrest, 25450-25455
　　malunion, 25400, 25415
　　nonunion, 25400, 25415
　　osteotomy, 25360, 25370-25375
　　with radius, 25365
　sequestrectomy, 24138, 25145
Ultrasound, 3319F-3320F
　3D rendering, 76376-76377
　abdomen, 76700-76705
　arm, 76881-76882
　artery
　　extracranial, 93880-93882
　　intracranial, 93886-93893
　　middle cerebral, 76821
　　umbilical, 76820
　bladder, 51798
　breast, 76641-76642
　bronchi, endoscopic, 31654
　cardiac, 93303-93317, 93320-93321, 93350-93352, 93662
　chest, 76604, 76645
　colon
　　endoscopic, 45391-45392
　　with sigmoid, 45341-45342
　drainage
　　abscess, 75989
　elastography, 0346T
　esophagus
　　endoscopic, 43231-43232
　eye
　　arteries, 93875
　　biometry, 76516-76519
　　diagnostic, 76510-76513
　　foreign body, 76529
　　pachymetry, 76514
　fetus, 76818-76828
　follow-up, 76970
　gastrointestinal, 76975
　　endoscopic, 43237-43238, 43242, 43259
　guidance
　　amniocentesis, 59001, 76946
　　amniofusion, 59070
　　arteriovenous fistula, 76936
　　cardiac, 76932, 93662
　　chorionic villus sampling, 76945
　　cryosurgery, 55873
　　drainage, fetal fluid, 59074
　　endometrial ablation, 58356
　　fetal cordocentesis, 76941
　　fetal transfusion, 76941
　　heart biopsy, 76932
　　needle biopsy, 43232, 43238, 43242, 45342, 45392, 76942
　　occlusion, umbilical cord, 59072
　　ova retrieval, 76948
　　percardiocentesis, 76930
　　pseudoaneurysm, 76936

Ultrasound — *continued*
　guidance — *continued*
　　radiation therapy, 0520F, 77387
　　radioelement, 76965
　　shunt placement, fetal, 59076
　　thoracentesis, 76942
　　tissue ablation, 76940
　　vascular access, 76937
　head, 76506, 76536
　heart
　　fetal, 76825
　hips
　　infant, 76885-76886
　hysterosonography, 76831
　intraoperative, 76998
　intravascular, noncoronary
　　during procedure, 37250-37253
　kidney, 76770-76776
　leg, 76881-76882
　neck, 76536
　needle
　　placement, 20555
　pelvis, 76856-76857
　physical therapy, 97035
　placement
　　catheter, 20555
　　needle, 20555
　　therapy fields, 77387
　prostate, 76872-76873
　rectal, 76872-76873
　retroperitoneal, 76770-76775
　scrotum, 76870
　sonohysterography, 76831
　spine, 76800
　stimulation
　　bone healing, 20979
　transvaginal, 76817, 86830
　umbilical artery, 76820
　uterus
　　pregnant, 76801-76828
　　tumor ablation, 0071T-0072T
　vagina, 76817, 76830
　wound assessment
　　noncontact, nonthermal, 97610
Ultraviolet light therapy
　actinotherapy, 96900
　dermatoses, 96913
　psoralens, 96912
Umbilicus
　catheterization
　　artery, 36660
　　vein, 36510
　excision, 49250
　hernia, 49580-49587
　occlusion
　　cord, 59072
　omphalocele, 49600-49611
　ultrasound
　　artery, 76820
Unna boot, 29700
　strapping, 29580
UPP (urethra pressure profile), 51772
Urachal cyst, 51500
Urea
　breath test, 78267-78268, 83014
　nitrogen test
　　clearance, 84545
　　quantitative, 84520
　　semiquantitative, 84525
　　urine, 84540
Urecholine supersensitivity, 51725-51726
Ureter
　biopsy
　　brush, 52007
　　　with cystourethroscopy, 52204
　　cystourethroscopy, 52007, 52354
　　endoluminal, 50606
　　endoscopic, 50955-50957, 50974-50976
　catheterization, 52005
　　endoscopic, 50953, 50972, 52005
　continent diversion, 50825
　destruction, 50957, 50976
　lesion, 52354

© 2016 DecisionHealth　　　　CPT © 2015 American Medical Association. All Rights Reserved.

Ureter — *continued*
dilation, 50706, 52341-52342, 52344-52345
  endoscopic, 50553, 50572, 50953, 50972
embolization/occlusion, 50705
excision, 52355
exploration, 50600
  endoscopic, 52351
incision and drainage, 50600
injection
  drugs, 50391
  implant material, 52327
  radiologic, 50684, 50690
insertion/placement
  catheter, 50433
  guide wire, 52334
  stent, 50693-50695
    endoscopic, 50947, 52332-52334
lithotripsy, 52353, 52356
lysis, 50715-50725
manipulation, 52330
manometric study, 50686
meatotomy, 52290
reconstruction, 50700, 50840
  bladder, 50780-50785
  colon, 50810-50815
  intestine, 50800, 50820-50825
  kidney, 50740-50750
  ureter, 50760-50770
reflux study, 78740
reimplantation, 51565
removal
  anastomosis, 50830
  calculus, 50610-50630, 51060-51065
    endoscopic, 50961, 50980, 52320-52325, 52352
  foreign body, 50961, 50980
  stent, 50382-50387
repair
  anastomosis, 50740-50825
  continent diversion, 50825
  deligation, 50940
  fistula, 50920-50930
  ureterocele, 51535, 52300-52301
  urinary undiversion, 50830
  wound, 50900
replacement
  stent, 50382, 50387
  with intestine, 50840
resection, 52355
revision, 50727-50728
splint, 50400-50405
stent
  change, 50688
  insertion/placement, 50605, 50693-50695
stoma, 50860
suture
  deligation, 50940
  fistula, 50920-50930
  wound, 50900
x-ray, dilation, 74485
Ureterectomy
partial, 50220, 50546
total, 50548, 50660
with bladder cuff, 50650
Ureterocalycostomy, 50750
Ureterocele
excision, 51535
fulguration
  ectopic, 52301
  orthotopic, 52300
incision, 51535
repair, 51535
resection
  ectopic, 52301
  orthotopic, 52300
Ureterocolon conduit, 50815
Ureteroenterostomy, 50800
revision, 50830
Ureterography
injection, 50430-50431, 50684
radiologic, 74425

Ureteroileal conduit, 50820-50830
cystectomy, 51590
Ureterolithotomy, 50610-50630
laparoscopic, 50945
transvesical, 51060
Ureterolysis
ovarian vein syndrome, 50722
retrocaval ureter, 50725
retroperitoneal fibrosis, 50715
Ureteroneocystostomy, 50780-50785, 50830, 51565
laparoscopic, 50947-50948
Ureteroplasty, 50700
Ureteropyelography, 50951, 52005
injection, 50684, 50690
Ureteropyelostomy, 50740
Ureteroscopy
biopsy, 52354
destruction, 52354
diagnostic, 52351
dilation
  renal, 52346
  ureter, 52344-52345
excision, 52355
lithotripsy, 52353, 52356
removal, 52352
Ureterosigmoidostomy, 50810, 50830
Ureterostomy, 50860, 50951
injection, 50684
manometric studies, 50686
tube, change, 50688
Ureterotomy, 50600
stent, 50605
Ureteroureterostomy, 50760-50770, 50830
Urethra
biofeedback training, 90911
biopsy, 52204, 52354, 53200
catheterization, endoscopic, 52010
destruction, 52214-52224
  endoscopic, 52354, 52400
  polyp, 53260
  prolapse, 53275
  tumor, 53255, 53220
dilation, 52260-52265, 53600-53621
  female, 53665
  stenosis, 52281
  stricture, 52281, 53600-53621
  suppository, 53660-53661
drainage, 53080-53085
electomyography, 51784-51785
evacuation, 52001
excision
  diverticulum, 53230-53235
  lesion, 53260
  polyp, 53260
  prolapse, 53275
  tumor, 52355, 53220
  total, 53210-53215
injection
  implant material, 51715
  steroids, 52283
incision, 53000-53010
  drainage
    paraurethral gland, 53060
    Skene's gland, 53060
  ejaculatory duct, 52402
  meatus, 53020-53025
insertion
  prosthesis, 53444
  stent, 0084T, 52282
lithotripsy, 52353
marsupialization, 53240
pressure profile, 51772
prosthesis, 53444
radiotracer, 52250
reconstruction, 53410-53440, 53445
  complications, 54340-54348
  meatus, 53450-53460
  sphincter, 53445
  with bladder, 51800-51820
removal
  calculus, 52310-52315, 52352

Urethra — *continued*
removal — *continued*
  foreign body, 52310-52315
  prosthesis, 53446-53447
  sling, 53442
  stent, 52310-52315
repair
  diverticulum, 53240, 53400-53405
  ejaculatory duct, 52402
  fistula, 45820-45825, 53400-53405, 53520
  hypospadias, 54308-54336
  prolapse, 53275
  prosthesis, 53449
  sphincter, 57220
  stricture, 53400-53405
  ureterocele, 57230
  wound, 53502-53515
sphincter, 90911
  electromyography, 51784-51785
  prosthesis, 53444
    removal, 53446-53447
    repair, 53449
    replacement, 53448
  reconstruction, 53445
suture
  bladder, 51840-51841
  fistula, 45820-45825, 53520
  wound, 53502-53515
x-ray, 74450-74455
Urethrectomy
female, 53210
male, 53215
Urethrocele, 53275
Urethrocystography
contrast and/or chain, 51605
radiologic, 74450-74455
retrograde, 51610
voiding, 51600
Urethrocystopexy, 51840-51841
Urethromeatoplasty, 53450-53460
Urethropexy, 51840-51841
Urethroplasty
first stage, 53400
one stage
  hypospadias, 54322-54328
reconstruction
  female, 53430
  male, 53410
    membranous urethra, 53410-53425
  prostatic urethra, 53410-53425
repair
  cloacal anomaly, 46746-46748
second stage, 53405
  hypospadias, 54308-54316
third stage
  hypospadias, 54318
Urethrorrhaphy, 53502-53515
Urethroscopy, 52000
biopsy, 52204, 52354, 53200
catheter, 52010
destruction, 52354, 52400
evacuation, 52001
excision, 52355
exploration 52351
incision, 52402
injection, 51715
lithotripsy, 52353
removal, 52352
resection, 52402
vasectomy, 52402
Urethrostomy, 53000-53010
Urethrotomy, 53000-53010
direct
  with cystourethroscopy, 52276
internal, 52601, 52647-52648
  female, 52270
  male, 52275
Uric acid
blood, 84550
other source, 84560
urine, 84560

Uridyltransferase
galactose-1-phosphate, 82775-82776
Urinalysis
automated, 81001, 81003
glass test, 81020
microalbumin, 82043-82044
microscopic, 81015
non-automated, 81002
pregnancy test, 81025
qualitative, 81005
routine, 81002
screening, 81007
volume measurement, 81050
Urinary
bladder
  abscess
    incision and drainage, 51080
  anastomosis, 51960
  aspiration, 51100-51102
  biopsy, 52204, 52224, 52250
  catheterization, 51045, 51701-51703
  change tube, 51705-51710
  cyst
    excision, 51500
  destruction
    lesion, 51030
    52214-52224, 52354
  dilation, 52260-52265, 52341-52342, 52344-52345
  diverticulum, 51525, 52305
  endoscopy, 52000
    biopsy, 52204, 52354
    catheterization, 52005, 52010
    destruction, 52214-52224, 52400
    dilation, 52260-52265
    diverticulum, 52305
    evacuation
      clot, 52001
    excision
      tumor, 52234-52240, 52355
    exploration, 52351
    injection, 52283
    lithotripsy, 52353
    neck, 51715
    radiotracer, 52250
    removal
      calculus, 52310-52315, 52352
      foreign body, 52310-52315
    surgery
      sphincter, 52277
      ureter, 52290-52300
    tumor
      excision, 52234-52240, 52355
    urethral syndrome, 52285
    urethrotomy, 52270-52276
  excision
    cyst, 51500
    neck, 51520
    partial, 51550-51565
    total, 51570, 51580, 51590-51597
    with nodes, 51575, 51585, 51595
    tumor, 51530, 52234-52240, 52355
    transurethral, 52640
  incision
    catheter, 51045
    destruction, 51020-51030
    drainage, 51040
    radiotracer, 51020
  incision and drainage, 51040
  injection, 51600-51610
  insertion
    stent, 51045, 52334
  instillation, 51720
  irrigation, 51700
  laparoscopy, 51999
  lesion
    destruction, 51030

CPT © 2015 American Medical Association. All Rights Reserved.

Urinary — *continued*
　bladder — *continued*
　　neck, 51715, 51520
　　nuclear medicine, 78730
　　radiotracer, 51020, 52250
　　reconstruction
　　　intestines, 51960
　　　urethra, 51800-51820
　　removal, 51550-51597
　　　calculus, 51050, 52310-52315
　　　foreign body, 52310-52315
　　　stent, 52310-52315
　　repair, 51800, 51845-51865
　　　diverticulum, 52305
　　　extrophy, 51940
　　　fistula, 44660-44661, 45800-45805, 51880-51925
　　　neck, 51845
　　　wound, 51860-51865
　　resection, 52500
　　sphincter surgery, 52277
　　stoma, 51980
　　stone removal, 52317-52318
　　study, 51795, 51798, 78730
　　suspension, 51990
　　suture
　　　fistula, 44660-44661, 45800-45805, 51880-51925
　　　wound, 51860-51865
　　tumor
　　　excision, 51530
　　urethrocystography, 74450-74455
　　urethrotomy, 52270-52276
　　urinary incontinence, 0509F, 1090F-1091F, 51990-51992
　　voiding, 51795
　　x-ray, 74430
　　　contrast, 74450-74455
　catheter, 51700
　sphincter
　　insertion, 53444-53445
　　removal, 53446-53447
　　repair, 53448-53449
　tract
　　x-ray, 74400-74425

Urine
　albumin, 82042-82044
　blood, 83491
　colony count, 87086
　test, 81001
　　pregnancy, 81025

Urobilinogen
　feces, 84577
　urine, 84578-84583

Urodynamic tests
　bladder capacity, 51798
　cystometrogram, 51725-51726
　electromyographic study, 51785
　residual urine, 51798
　stimulus evoked response, 51792
　urethra pressure profile, 51772
　uroflowmetry, 51736-51741
　voiding pressure studies
　　bladder, 51795
　　intra-abdominal, 51797
　　rectal, 51797

Uroflowmetry, 51736-51741

Urography
　antegrade, 74425
　infusion, 74410-74415
　intravenous, 74400
　retrograde, 74420

Uroporphyrin, 84120

Uterus
　ablation
　　endometrium, 58353-58356, 58363
　　fibroids/leiomyomata
　　　focused ultrasound, 0071T-0072T
　　　radiofrequency, 0336T, 0404T

Uterus — *continued*
　biopsy
　　endometrium, 58100-58110, 59015
　　endoscopic, 58558, 59015
　brachytherapy, 58346
　catheterization, 58340
　chorionic villus, 59015
　chromotubation, 58350
　curettage, 58356
　　postpartum, 59160
　dilation and curettage, 58120
　　postpartum, 59160
　ectopic pregnancy, 59135-59136
　embolization, 37243
　exploration, 58555
　excision
　　fibroid tumor, 58140-58146, 58545-58546
　　hydatidiform mole, 59100
　　laparoscopic, 58541-58544, 58550-58554
　　lesion, 58545-58546, 59100
　　partial, 58180
　　radical, 58210, 58285, 58548
　　total
　　　abdominal, 58150-58152, 58200
　　　laparoscopy, 58570-58573
　　　bilateral, 58953-58956
　　　vaginal
　　　　250g or less, 58260-58270
　　　　251g or more, 58290-58294
　　　　laparoscopy, 58550-58554
　　　　vaginectomy, 58275-58280
　hemorrhage control, 59160
　hydrotubation, 58350
　hysterosalpingography, 74740
　hysteroscopy, 58555-58560
　incision, 59100
　insertion, 58300
　　hyman capsule, 58346
　　tandem, 57155
　lysis, 58559
　placement, 58565
　reconstruction, 58540
　removal
　　endometrial, 58563
　　foreign body, 58562
　　intrauterine device (IUD), 58301
　　leimyomata, 58561
　　lesion, 58210, 58285, 58548
　repair
　　fistula, 51920-51925
　　rupture, 58520, 59350
　　suspension, 58400-58410
　sonohysterography, 76831
　suture, 59350
　x-ray, 74740

UV light therapy
　actinotherapy, 96900
　for dermatoses, 96913
　psoralens, 96912

Uvula
　biopsy, 42100
　destruction, 42145
　excision, 42140-42145
　tumor, 42104-42107
　incision and drainage
　　abscess, 42000

Uvulectomy, 42140

V

V flap, 54322
Vaccines/Toxoids
　adenovirus, 90476-90477
　anthrax, 90581
　bacillus Calmette-Guerin, 90585-90586
　chicken pox, 90716
　cholera, 90625
　diphtheria, 90696-90702, 90714-90715, 90723
　haemophilus influenze b, 90647-90648

Vaccines — *continued*
　hepatitis
　　A, 90632-90364
　　A and B, 90636
　　B, 90739-90748
　human papilloma virus, 90649-90651
　influenza virus, 90630, 90653-90668, 90672-90673, 90685-90688
　Japanese encephalitis, 90738
　measles, 90707-90710
　meningococcal
　　conjugate, 90644, 90734
　　polysaccharide, 90733
　　recombinant, 90620-90621
　mumps, 90707, 90710
　pertussis, 90696-90700, 90715, 90723
　pneumococcal
　　conjugate, 90670
　　polysaccharide, 90732
　poliovirus, 90696-90698, 90713
　rabies, 90675-90676
　rotavirus, 90680-90681
　rubella, 90707-90710
　tetanus, 90714-90715
　typhoid, 90690-90691
　varicella virus, 90716
　yellow fever, 90717
　zoster (shingles), 90736

Vagina, 00940-00952
　amines test, 82120
　biopsy
　　colposcopy, 57421
　　endocervical, 57454
　　extensive, 57105
　　simple, 57100
　brachytherapy, 57155
　closure, 27120
　colpocentesis, 57020
　colpocleisis, 57120
　colposcopy, 57420-57421, 57455-57456, 57461
　construction
　　with graft, 57292
　　without graft, 57291
　destruction, 57061-57065
　dilation, 57400
　excision
　　complete, 57110-57112
　　cyst, 57135
　　partial, 57106-57109
　　septum, 57130
　　total, 57110, 58275-58280
　　tumor, 57135
　exploration
　　endocervical, 57452
　　incision, 57000
　fixation, 57282
　hemorrhage control, 57180
　hysterectomy, 58290, 58550-58554
　incision and drainage, 57020
　　abscess, 57010
　　hematoma, 57022-57023
　insertion
　　ovoid, brachytherapy, 57155
　　packing, 57180
　　pessary, 57160
　　prosthesis, 57267
　irrigation, 57150
　removal
　　foreign body, 57415
　　prosthetic graft, 57295-57296
　　sling, 57287
　repair
　　cystocele, 57240, 57260-57265
　　enterocele, 57265
　　fistula, 51900, 57300-57330
　　incontinence, 57284-57285, 57288
　　obstetric, 59300
　　paravaginal defect, 57284-57285, 57423
　　prolapse, 57284-57285, 57288
　　rectocele, 57250-57265

Vagina — *continued*
　repair — *continued*
　　urethral sphincter, 57220
　　wound, 57200-57210
　revision
　　prosthetic graft, 57295-57296
　　sling, 57287
　suspension, 57280-57283
　　laparoscopic, 57425
　suture
　　cystocele, 57240, 57260
　　enterocele, 57265
　　fistula, 51900, 57300-57330
　　rectocele, 57250-57260
　　wound, 57200-57210
　ultrasound, 76830
　x-ray, 74775

Vaginal
　delivery, 01960, 01967, 59409
　　antepartum care, 59400
　　cesarean, 59618-59622
　　　previous, 59610-59612
　　　attempted, 59618-59622
　　external, 59412
　　placenta, 59414
　　postpartum care, 59410, 59614
　　routine care
　hysterectomy, 58552-58554
　resuscitation, 99465
　sialidase, 87905
　stabilization, 99464
　suppository, 59855-59857

Vaginectomy
　partial, 57106-57109, 58275-58280
　total, 57110-57112, 58275-58280

Vaginoplasty, 57335

Vaginorrhaphy, 57200, 57240, 57250, 57265-57267, 57289

Vaginoscopy
　biopsy, 57454
　exploration, 57452

Vaginotomy, 57000, 57010

Vagotomy
　abdominal, 64760
　highly selective, 43641, 64755
　parietal cell, 43641, 64755
　reconstruction, 43635
　revision
　　gastroduodenostomy, 43855
　　gastrojejunostomy, 43865, selective, 43640
　　truncal, 43640

Vagus nerve
　avulsion/transection
　　abdominal, 64760
　　selective, 64755
　injection, 64408

Valproic acid, 80164-80165

Valsalva sinus, 33645

Valve
　aortic
　　incision, 33420-33422
　　repair, 33420-33427
　　replacement, 33405-33413, 33430
　　　transcatheter, 33361-33369
　　valvuloplasty, 33400-33403
　artrioventricular, 33420-33427, 33430
　bicuspid
　　incision, 33420-33422
　　repair, 33420-33427
　　replacement, 33430
　cardiopulmonary, 33405-33410, 33430, 33465
　mitral, 33420-33427, 33430
　tricuspid
　　excision, 33460
　　repair, 33463-33465
　　replacement, 33465
　　repositioning, 33468

Valvectomy, 33460

Valvotomy
　mitral valve, 33420-33422
　pulmonary valve, 33470-33474
　reoperation, 33530

Urinary – Valvotomy

Valvuloplasty
aortic, 33400-33403
  percutaneous, 92986
femoral vein, 34501
mitral, 33425-33427
  percutaneous, 92987
prosthetic, 33496
pulmonary valve
  percutaneous, 92990
reoperation, 33530
tricuspid valve, 33463-33465

Van Den Bergh test, 82247-82248

Vancomycin, 87500
therapeutic assay, 80202

Vanillylmandelic acid, 84585

Varicella-Zoster
antibody, 86787
antigen detection
  direct fluorescence, 87290

Varices
esophageal
  ligation, 43205, 43400
  repair, 43401
  transection, 43401

Varicocele, 55530-55540

Varicose vein
ablation, 36475-36479
removal, 37720, 37730, 37765-37785
tissue, 37735-37760

Vas deferens
anastomosis, 54900-54901
excision, 55250
incision, 55200, 55300
ligation, 55450
suture, 55400
x-ray, 74440

Vasectomy, 55250
laser, 52647-52648
resection, 52601, 52648
reversal, 55400
transurethral, 52402

Vasoactive
drug, 54231
peptide, 84586

Vasogram, 74440

Vasopneumatic device, 97016

Vasopressin, 84588

Vasotomy, 52000, 55300
transurethral, 52402

Vasovasorrhaphy, 55400

Vasovasotomy, 55400

Vein, 00532
ablation, 36475-36479
anastomosis
  caval, 37160
  hepatic, 37182-37183
  portocaval, 37140
  saphenopopliteal, 34530
  splenorenal, 37180-37181
angioplasty, 35460, 35879-35881, 75978
biopsy, 75970
cannulization, 36800-36815
  external, 36860-36861
catheterization
  insertion, 36555-36558
    peripheral, 36568-36569
  organ, 36500
  portal, 36481
  removal, 36589
  repair, 36575
  replacement, 36578-36581, 36584
division, 37718-37722
excision, 55530-55540
guidance
  fluoroscopic, 77001
  ultrasound, 76937
harvest, 35500, 35572
  arm, 35500
  endoscopic, 35508
  leg, 35572
injection, 36468-36471
insertion, 75940

Vein — *continued*
interruption
  femoral, 37650
  iliac, 37660
  vena cava, 37620
ligation
  cluster, 37785
  esophagus, 43205
  jugular, 37565
  perforation, 37760
  saphenous, 37700-37735, 37780
  secondary, 37785
  spermatic, 55550
nuclear medicine, 78456-78458
placement, 75940
removal
  cluster, 37785
  saphenous, 37720, 37730-37735, 37780
  varicose, 37720, 37730, 37765-37766
repair
  aneurysm, 36834
  angioplasty, 75978
  femoral, 34501
  graft, 34520
  pulmonary, 33730
splenoportography, 75810
stripping, 37718-37735
study, 93965-93971
thrombectomy, 37187-37188
  axillary, 34490
  femoropopliteal, 34421-34451
  iliac, 34401-34451
  other, 35875-35876
  subclavian, 34471-34490
  vena cava, 34401-34451
transposition, 34510
venography
  adrenal, 75840-75842
  arm, 75820-75822
  hepatic portal, 75810
  jugular, 75860
  leg, 75820-75822
  liver, 75889-75891
  neck, 75860
  orbit, 75880
  renal, 75831-75833
  sampling, 75893
  sinus, 75870
  skull, 75870-75872
  vena cava, 75825-75827

Velpeau cast, 29058

Vena cava
catheterization, 36010
filter, 37191-37193
ligation, 37619
reconstruction, 34502
  resection, 37799
thrombectomy, 50230

Venipuncture
cutdown, 36420-36425
percutaneous, 36400-36410
routine, 36415

Venography
adrenal, 75840-75842
arm, 75820-75822
epidural, 2044F, 75872
hepatic portal, 75885-75887
injection, 75860
jugular, 75860
leg, 75820-75822
liver, 75889-75891
neck, 75860
orbit, 75880
renal, 75831-75833
sagittal sinus, 75870
vena cava, 75825-75827
venous sampling, 75893

Venorrhaphy
femoral, 37650
iliac, 37660
vena cava, 37620

Venous
access device
  collection
    blood, 36591-36592
    declotting, 36593-36596
    fluoroscopic guidance, 77001
  insertion
    central, 36560-36566
    peripheral, 36570-36571
  blood pressure, 93770

Venovenostomy, 37140-37160, 37182-37183
sapheopopliteal, 34530

Ventilation
assist, 94002-94005, 99504
delivery room, 99465
tube
  insertion, 69433
  removal, 69424

Ventricular puncture, 61020-61026, 61105-61120

Ventriculocisternostomy, 62180, 62200-62201

Ventriculography
anesthesia
  brain, 00214
  cardiac, 01920
nuclear imaging, 78635

Ventriculomyectomy, 33416

Vermilionectomy, 40500

Verruca, 17110-17111

Vertebra
aneurysm, 35005, 61698, 61702
angiography, 36225-36226
arthrodesis
  anterior, 22548-22585, 22808-22812
  exploration, 22830
  extracavitary, 22532-22534
  posterior, 22590-22804
  spinal deformity, 22800-22812
augmentation, 22513-22515
biopsy, 20250-20251
catheterization, 36100
corpectomy, 63081-63103, 63300-63308
decompression, 61597
distraction device, 0171T-0172T
excision, 61597
  decompression, 63081-63103
  lesion, 63300-63308
  segment, 22103, 22116
  tumor
    cervical, 22100, 22110
    lumbar, 22102, 22114
    thoracic, 22101, 22112
fracture treatment, 22305-22310
  bracing, 22315
  cervical, 22326, 23675-23680
  lumbar, 22325
  segment, 22328
  thoracic, 22327
graft, 35508, 35515, 35642-35645
kyphectomy, 22818-22819
osteoplasty
  lumbar, 22511-22512
  thoracic, 22510, 22512
osteotomy
  anterior, 22216, 22226
  cervical, 22210, 22220
  lumbar, 22214, 22224
  thoracic, 22212, 22222
thromboendarterectomy, 35301

Vesication, 10160, 32141, 32655

Vesicle, 74440

Vesico-psoas hitch, 50785

Vesicostomy, 51980

Vesicourethropexy, 51840-51841

Vesicovaginal, 51900, 57320-57330

Vesiculectomy, 55650

Vesiculogram, 55300, 74440

Vesiculotomy, 55600-55605

Vessel
ablation, 36475-36479

Vessel — *continued*
anastomosis
  artery, 33606, 61711
  vein, 34530, 37140-37183
aneurysm
  arteriovenous, 36834
  axillary-brachial, 35011-35013
  carotid, 61697-61710
  celiac, 35121-35122
  femoral, 35141-35142
  hepatic, 35121-35122
  iliac, 35131-35132, 75954
  mesenteric, 35121-35122
  popliteal, 35151-35152
  radial, 35045
  renal, 35121-35122
  splenic, 35111-35112
  subclavian, 35001-35002, 35021-35022
  ulnar, 35045
  vertebral, 35005
  vein, 36834
angiography, 36221-36227, 36251-36254, 75658-75774
angioplasty
  artery, 35450-35458, 37228-37235, 75962-75968
  vein, 35460, 75978
angioscopy, 35400
aortic pulmonary
  reconstruction, 33770-33781
aortoiliofemoral, 35363
atherectomy, 37229, 37231, 37233, 37235, 92924-92925, 92933-92934, 0234T-0238T
basilar, 61698, 61702
biopsy, 37609, 75970
bypass graft
  axillary, 35516-35522, 35533, 35616-35623, 35650, 35654
  brachial, 35510, 35512, 35522-35525
  carotid, 33891, 35501-35510, 35526, 35601-35606, 35626, 35642
  celiac, 35531, 35631
  coronary, 33503-33505
    anesthesia, 00567
  femoral, 35521, 35533, 35540, 35558, 35565-35566, 35621, 35646-35647, 35651-35661, 35665-35666
  harvest
    multiple locations, 35682-35683
    prosthetic, 35681-35683
  iliac, 34900, 35538, 35563-35565, 35637-35638, 35663-35665
  mesenteric, 35531, 35631
  popliteal, 35571, 35623, 35651, 35656, 35671
  radial, 35523
  renal, 35535, 35560, 35631-35636
  repair, 34520, 35700, 35883-35884
  splenic, 35536, 35636
  subclavian, 35506, 35511-35516, 35526, 35606-35616, 35626, 35645
  ulnar, 35523
  vertebral, 35508, 35515, 35642-35645
cannulization, 36810-36815, 36800, 36823
catheterization
  artery
    abdominal, 36245-36248
    arteriovenous, 36145
    brachial, 36120, 36215-36218, 93458-93461
    carotid, 36100
    coronary, 93454-93461
    extremity, 36140, 36245-36248

CPT © 2015 American Medical Association. All Rights Reserved.

Vessel — *continued*
  catheterization — *continued*
    artery — *continued*
      pelvic, 36245-36248
      pulmonary, 36013-36015
      thoracic, 36215-36218
      umbilical, 36660
      vertebral, 36100
    vein
      central insertion, 36555-36558
      declotting, 36860-36861
      organ blood, 36500
      peripheral insertion, 36568-36569
      portal, 36481
      removal, 36589
      repair, 36575
      replacement, 36578-36581, 36584
      umbilical, 36510
  coronary
    bypass, 33510-33536
    repair, 33500-33508
  decompression, 61590-61591, 61595-61596
  division, saphenous, 37718-37722
  embolectomy, 34001-34101, 34111, 34151-34201, 34203
  endoscopy, 37500
  excision, 55530-55540, 63250-63252
  exploration
    artery
      brachial, 24495
      carotid, 35701
      femoral, 35721
      popliteal, 35741
      other, 35761
    vein
      abdomen, 35840
      chest, 35820
      extremity, 35860
      neck, 35800
  extremity, 93965-93971
  femoral, 34501
  harvest
    artery, 35600
    vein, 35500, 35508, 35572
  hepatic, 75810
  imaging
    nuclear medicine, 78456-78458
  injection, 36468-36471
  insertion, 75940
  interrupt, 37620, 37650, 37660
  kidney, 50100
  ligation
    artery
      abdomen, 37617
      carotid, 37600-37606, 61610-61612
      chest, 37616
      coronary, 33502
      ethmoidal, 30915
      extremity, 37618
      fistula, 37607
      maxillary, 30920
      neck, 37615
      temporal, 37609
    vein
      clusters, 37785
      esophagus, 43205
      jugular, 37565
      perforation, 37760
      saphenous, 37700-37735, 37780
      secondary, 37785
      spermatic, 55550
  non-pulmonary
    embolectomy, 34001-34203
    thrombectomy, 34001-34203
  nuclear medicine
    imaging, 78456-78458
  pulmonary
    balloon angioplasty, 92997-92998
    embolectomy, 33910-33915
    repair, 33690, 33730, 33925-33926

Vessel — *continued*
  pulmonary — *continued*
    shunt, 33750-33767
  removal
    clusters, 37785
    saphenous, 37720, 37730-37735, 37780
    varicose vein, 37720, 37730, 37765-37785
  repair
    abdomen
      aneurysm, 34800-34805, 34825-34832, 34841, 34848, 35081-35103, 75952-75953
      composite graft, 35681-35683
      other graft, 35281
      vein graft, 35251
    aneurysm, 61705-61708
    arteriovenous
      malformation, 61680-61692, 61705-61710, 63250-63252
    chest
      composite graft, 35681-35683
      other graft, 35271-35276
      vein graft, 35241-35246
    direct, 35201-35226
    finger, 35207
    graft defect, 35870
    hand, 35207
    lower extremity, 35226
      composite graft, 35681-35683
      other graft, 35281
      vein graft, 35251
    neck
      composite graft, 35681-35683
      other graft, 35261
      vein graft, 35231
    upper extremity, 35206
      composite graft, 35681-35683
      other graft, 35266
      vein graft, 35236
  shunt, 36818, 36821, 36835
    revision, 36832
    with graft, 35686, 36825-36830
  splenoportography, 75810
  stripping, 37718-37735
  suture, 33320-3322
  sympathectomy, 64821-64822
  thrombectomy
    by abdomen, 34151
    by arm, 34101, 34111
    by leg, 34201-34203
    by neck, 34001
    by thoracic, 34051
    fistula, 36831-36833, 36870
    iliac, 34401-34451
    of graft, 35875
    other, 35875-35876
    percutaneous transluminal mechanical
      arterial/bypass graft, 37184-37186
      coronary, 92973
      intracranial, 61645
    subclavian, 34471-34490
    vena cava, 34401-34451
  thromboendaterectomy
    aorta, 35331, 35361-35363
    axillary, 35321
    carotid, 36301, 35390
    celiac, 35341
    femoral, 35302, 35355, 35363-35372
    femoropopliteal, 34421-34451
    iliac, 35351-35355, 35361-35363
    mesenteric, 35341
    peroneal, 35304-35306
    popliteal, 35303
    renal, 35341

Vessel — *continued*
  thromboendaterectomy — *continued*
    subclavian, 35301, 35311
    tibial, 35304-35306
    vertebral, 35301
  transection, 61611-61612
  valve transposition, 34510
  varicosity, 37785, 37735-37760
  venography
    adrenal, 75840-75842
    arm, 75820-75822
    hepatic, 75885-75887
    jugular, 75860
    leg, 75820-75822
    liver, 75889-75891
    neck, 75860
    orbit, 75880
    renal, 75831-75833
    sampling, 75893
    sinus, 75870
    skull, 75870-75872
    vena cava, 75825-75827
    x-ray, 75630

Vestibular
  function test
    caloric, 92533, 92537-92538
    electrodes, 92547
    nystagmus
      otokinetic, 92534, 92544
      positional, 92532, 92542
      spontaneous, 92431, 92541
    posturography, 92548
    sinusoidal rotational testing, 92546
    torsion swing test, 92546
    tracking test, 92545
  nerve, 69915, 69950

Vestibule of mouth
  destruction, 40808-40820
  incision, 40800-40806
  removal, 40804
  repair, 40830-40845

Vestibuloplasty, 40840-40845

Video
  esophagus, 74230
  pharynx, 70371, 74230
  speech, 70371
  swallowing, 74230

Villus, 59015

Villusectomy
  elbow, 24102
  excision
    carpometacarpal joint, 26130
    finger joint, 26135-26140
    hip joint, 27054
    interphalangeal joint, 26140
    knee joint, 27334-27335
    metacarpophalangeal joint, 26135
    palm, 25105, 25118-25119
  incision
    glenohumeral joint, 23105
    sternoclavicular joint, 23106
  wrist, 25105, 25115-25116, 25118-25119

Viral antibodies, 86280

Virtual colonoscopy, 0066T-0067T

Virus
  cytomegalovirus, 86644-86645
    direct fluorescence, 87271
    immunoassay, 87332
    nucleic acid, 87495-87497
  Epstein-Barr, 86663-86665
  human immunodeficiency, 86689, 86701-86703, 87901, 87906
    antigen detection, 87389-87391
  identification, 87254
  influenza, 86710, 87501-87503, 87804
  isolation, 87250-87255
  JC, 86711
  respiratory, 87631-87633
    syncytial, 86756
      direct fluorescence, 87280
      immunoassay, 87420
      observation, 87807

Visceral larval migrans, 86280

Visit, 0525F-0526F

Visual
  acuity screen, 99172-99173
  evoked potential, 0333T
  field exam, 92081-92083
  function screen, 99172
  reinforcement, 92579

Visualization, 50690

Vital capacity measurement, 94150

Vitamin test, 84591
  A, 84590
  B, 82607-82608, 84207, 84252, 84425
    absorption study, 78270-78272
  C, 82180
  D, 82306-82307, 82652
  E, 84446
  K, 84597

Vitelline duct, 44800

Vitrectomy
  anterior approach, 67005
  implantation, 67027
  pars plana approach, 67036-67043
  photocoagulation, 67039
  replacement, 67027
  retinal detatchment, 67108, 67113

Vitreous
  aspiration, 67015
  discission, 67030
  excision, 67036-67043
  incision, 67030-67031
  implantation, 67027
  injection
    fluid substitute, 67025
    pharmacological agent, 67028
  removal
    anterior approach, 67005
    subtotal, 67010
  severing strands, 67031
  subtotal removal, 67010

Vocal cords, 31513
  therapeutic, 31570-31571

Voice button, 31611

Voiding pressure studies
  abdominal, 51797
  bladder, 51795
  rectum, 51797

Volatiles, 84600

Volkman contracture, 25315-25316

Volume reduction
  blood products, 86960
  lung, 32491

Vulva
  biopsy
    colposcopy, 56821
    perineum, 56605-56606
  destruction, 56501-56515
  incision and drainage, 56405
  repair, 59300

Vulvectomy
  complete, 56625, 56633-56640
  partial, 56620, 56620-56632
  radical, 56630-56640
  simple, 56620-56625

W

WADA activation test, 95958

WAIS, 96101-96102

Waldius procedure, **27445**

Wall
  debridement, 11005-11006
  excision, 22900
  reconstruction, 49905
  removal, 11008

Warfarin, 4012F

Warming, 4250F

Warts, 17110-17111

Washing, 58323

Wassmund procedure, 21206

Waterson procedure, 33755

Watson-Jones procedure, 27695-27698

Wedge
excision, 21122
resection, 58920
West Nile virus, 86788-86789
Western Blot
human immunodeficiency virus
(HIV), 86689
protein, 84181-84182
Wheelchair management, 97542
Wheeler procedure, 66820
Whipple procedure, 48150
Whirlpool therapy, 97022
White blood cell
alkaline phosphatase, 85540
antibody, 86021
count, 85032, 85048, 89055
differential, 85004-85007, 85009
histamine release, 86343
myeloperoxidase, 83876
phagocytosis, 86344
transfusion, 86950
Whitman
astragalectomy, 97022
procedure, 27120
Wick catheter, 20950
Window
orbit, 67420-67450
oval, 69666
pericardial, 32659, 33025
round, 69667
technic, 33015
Winiwarter operation, 47720-47740
Winter procedure, 54435
Wintrobe test, 85651-85652
Wire
humerus, 24498
interdental, 21497
skeletal, 20650
Witzel operation, 43500, 43520,
43830-43832
Work hardening, 97545-97546
Worm, 86682
Wound
allograft, 15271-15278
care, 97597, 97610
debridement
non-selective, 97602
selective, 97597-97598
exploration, 20100-20103
incision and drainage, 10180
negative pressure therapy, 97605-
97608
repair
complex, 13100-13160
dehiscence, 12020-12021,
13160
intermediate, 12031-12057
simple, 12001-12021
vaginal, 57200-57210
suture
bladder, 51860-51865
kidney, 50500
trachea, 31800-31805
urethra, 53502-53515
Wrist, 01810-01860
arthrocentesis, 20605-20606
arthrodesis, 25800-25810
arthrography, 73115
arthroplasty, 25332, 25443-25449
arthroscopy, 01829-01832,
29840-29848
biopsy, 25065-25066, 25100-
25101
cast, 29085
decompression, 25020-25025
disarticulation, 25920-25924
dislocation treatment, 25660-25675
excision
bursa, 25115-25116
carpal, 25210-25215
cartilage, 25107
ganglion cyst, 25111-25112
lesion, 25110
synovium, 25101, 25115-25119
tendon, 25109

Wrist — *continued*
excision — *continued*
tendon sheath, 25115-25116
tumor, 25075-25077
exploration, 25040, 25101
fasciotomy, 01810, 25020-25025
fracture treatment, 25622-25635,
25680-25685
incision
drainage
abscess, 25028
cyst, 25130-25136
hematoma, 25028
tendon sheath, 25000-25001
injection
carpal tunnel, 20526
x-ray, 25246
magentic resonance imaging
(MRI), 73221
reconstruction, 25320, 25335,
25394, 25430
removal
foreign body, 25040, 25101,
25248
implant, 25449
loose body, 25101
prothesis, 25250-25251
repair
bone, 25431, 25440
muscle, 01810, 25260, 25270
tendon sheath, 25275
strapping, 29260
tenodesis, 25300-25301
tenotomy, 25290
x-ray, 73100-73115

X

X-ray, 3319F-3320F
abdominal, 74000-74022, 75726
abscess, 76080
acromioclavicular joint, 73050
adrenal, 75731-75733
ankle, 73600-73610
aorta, 75600-75630, 75952-75953
arm, 73090-73092
auditory meatus, 70134
bile duct dilation, 74360
bone
age study, 77072
dual energy absorptiometry,
3095F-3096F, 77080-
77086
length study, 77073
osseous survey, 77074-77077
ultrasound, 76977
breast, 77055-77057
computer-aided detection,
77051-77052
calcaneous, 73650
chest, 3006F, 71010-71035
clavicle, 73000
coccyx, 72220
consultation, 76140
duodenum, 74260
elbow, 73070-73080
esophagus, 74220
eye, 70030
facial bones, 70140-70150
fallopian tube, 74742
femur, 73551-73552
fibula, 73590
finger, 73140
foot, 73620-73630
gastrointestinal tract, upper,
74240-74249
hand, 73120-73130
head, 70350
heel, 73650
hip
bilateral, 73521-73523
unilateral, 73501-73503
humerus, 73060
intestines, small, 774250-74251
jaw, 70355
joint, 77071
knee, 73560-73564, 73580
larynx, 70370

X-ray — *continued*
leg, 73592
mandible, 70100-70110
mastoids, 70120-70130
nasal bone, 70160
neck, 70360
orbit, 70190-70200
pelvis, 72170-72190
manometry, 74710
peritoneum, 74190
pharynx, 70370, 74210
ribs, 71100-71111
sacroiliac joint, 72200-72202,
73542
sacrum, 72220
salivary gland, 70380
scapula, 73010
sella turcica, 70240
shoulder, 73020-73030, 73050
sinus tract, 76080
skull, 70250-70260
specimen, 76098
spine
cervical, 72020-72052
complete, 72081-72084
lumbosacral, 72100-72120
thoracic, 72020, 72070-72074
thoracolumbar junction, 72080
sternum, 71120-71130
teeth, 70300-70320
tibia, 73590
toe, 73660
with contrast
ankle, 72615
aorta, 75600-75630, 75952-
75953
bile duct, 74300-74301
bladder, 74430, 74450-74455
brain, 70010-70015
bronchus, 76499
central venous access device,
36598
colon, 74270-74270
corpora cavernosa, 74445
elbow, 73085
epididymis, 74440
gallbladder, 74290
gastrointestinal tract, 74246-
74249
hip, 73525
iliofemoral artery, 75630
intervertebral disc, 72285-72295
joint, 77071
kidney cyst, 74470
lacriminal duct, 70170
lymph vessel, 75801-75807
mammary duct, 77053-77054
nasolacriminal duct, 70170
oviduct, 74740
pancreas, 74300-74301
pancreatic duct, 74329-74330
perineum, 74775
peritoneum, 74190
salivary gland, 70390
seminal vesicles, 74440
shoulder, 73040
spine, 72240-72270
tempomandibular joint, 70328-
70332
ureter, 74485
urethra, 74450-74455
urinary tract, 74400-74425
uterus, 74740
vas deferens, 74440
wrist, 73100-73110
Xenoantibody, 86308-86310
Xenograft, 15271-15278
Xylose absorption test
blood, 84620
urine, 84620

Y

Yeast culture, 87106
Yellow fever vaccine, 90717
Yersinia antibody, 86793

Z

Ziegler procedure, 66820
Zinc
blood, 84630
urine, 84630
Zygoma
fracture treatment, 21355-21366

CPT © 2015 American Medical Association. All Rights Reserved.   © 2016 DecisionHealth

Evaluation and Management Services

In addition to the information presented in the Introduction, several other items unique to this section are defined or identified here.

Classification of Evaluation and Management (E/M) Services

The E/M section is divided into broad categories such as office visits, hospital visits, and consultations. Most of the categories are further divided into two or more subcategories of E/M services. For example, there are two subcategories of office visits (new patient and established patient) and there are two subcategories of hospital visits (initial and subsequent). The subcategories of E/M services are further classified into levels of E/M services that are identified by specific codes. This classification is important because the nature of work varies by type of service, place of service, and the patient's status.

The basic format of the levels of E/M services is the same for most categories. First, a unique code number is listed. Second, the place and/or type of service is specified, eg, office consultation. Third, the content of the service is defined, eg, comprehensive history and comprehensive examination. (See "Levels of E/M Services," next page, for details on the content of E/M services.) Fourth, the nature of the presenting problem(s) usually associated with a given level is described. Fifth, the time typically required to provide the service is specified.

Definitions of Commonly Used Terms

Certain key words and phrases are used throughout the E/M section. The following definitions are intended to reduce the potential for differing interpretations and to increase the consistency of reporting by physicians in differing specialties. E/M services may also be reported by other qualified health care professionals who are authorized to perform such services within the scope of their practice.

New and Established Patient

Solely for the purposes of distinguishing between new and established patients, **professional services** are those face-to-face services rendered by physicians and other qualified health care professionals who may report evaluation and management services reported by a specific CPT code(s). A new patient is one who has not received any professional services from the physician/qualified health care professional or another physician/qualified health care professional of the **exact** same specialty **and subspecialty** who belongs to the same group practice, within the past three years.

An established patient is one who has received professional services from the physician/qualified health care professional or another physician/qualified health care professional of the **exact** same specialty **and subspecialty** who belongs to the same group practice, within the past three years. See Decision Tree.

In the instance where a physician/qualified health care professional is on call for or covering for another physician/qualified health care professional, the patient's encounter will be classified as it would have been by the physician/qualified health care professional who is not available. When advanced practice nurses and physician assistants are working with physicians they are considered as working in the exact same specialty and exact same subspecialties as the physician.

No distinction is made between new and established patients in the emergency department. E/M services in the emergency department category may be reported for any new or established patient who presents for treatment in the emergency department.

The decision tree on the next page is provided to aid in determining whether to report the E/M service provided as a new or an established patient encounter.

Coding tip
Instructions for Use of the CPT Codebook

When advanced practice nurses and physician assistants are working with physicians they are considered as working in the exact same specialty and exact same subspecialties as the physician. A "physician or other qualified health care professional" is an individual who is qualified by education, training, licensure/regulation (when applicable), and facility privileging (when applicable) who performs a professional service within his or her scope of practice and independently reports that professional services. These professionals are distinct from "clinical staff." A clinical staff member is a person who works under the supervision of a physician or other qualified health care professional, and who is allowed by law, regulation and facility policy to perform or assist in the performance of a specific professional service, but does not individually report that professional service. Other policies may also affect who may report specific services.

CPT Coding Guidelines, Introduction, Instructions for Use of the CPT Codebook

Chief Complaint

A chief complaint is a concise statement describing the symptom, problem, condition, diagnosis, or other factor that is the reason for the encounter, usually stated in the patient's words.

Concurrent Care and Transfer of Care

Concurrent care is the provision of similar services (eg, hospital visits) to the same patient by more than one physician or other qualified health care professional on the same day. When concurrent care is provided, no special reporting is required. Transfer of care is the process whereby a physician or other qualified health care professional who is providing management for some or all of a patient's problems relinquishes this responsibility to another physician or other qualified health care professional who explicitly agrees to accept this responsibility and who, from the initial encounter, is not providing consultative services. The physician or other qualified health care professional transferring care is then no longer providing care for these problems though he or she may continue providing care for other conditions when appropriate. Consultation codes should not be reported by the physician or other qualified health care professional who has agreed to accept transfer of care before an initial evaluation but are appropriate to report if the decision to accept transfer of care cannot be made until after the initial consultation evaluation, regardless of site of service.

Counseling

Counseling is a discussion with a patient and/or family concerning one or more of the following areas:

- Diagnostic results, impressions, and/or recommended diagnostic studies
- Prognosis
- Risks and benefits of management (treatment) options
- Instructions for management (treatment) and/or follow-up
- Importance of compliance with chosen management (treatment) options
- Risk factor reduction
- Patient and family education

(For psychotherapy, see 90832-90834, 90836-90840)

Family History

A review of medical events in the patient's family that includes significant information about:

- The health status or cause of death of parents, siblings, and children
- Specific diseases related to problems identified in the Chief Complaint or History of the Present Illness, and/or System Review
- Diseases of family members that may be hereditary or place the patient at risk

History of Present Illness

A chronological description of the development of the patient's present illness from the first sign and/or symptom to the present. This includes a description of location, quality, severity, timing, context, modifying factors, and associated signs and symptoms significantly related to the presenting problem(s).

● New   ▲ Revised   ✖ Deleted   ⊙ Moderate Sedation   ✚ Add-on Codes   ⊘ High Risk Denial   Ⓐ Age Edit   ♀ Female   ♂ Male   **AMA** *CPT® Assistant*   **MUE** Medically Unlikely Edit   ⊘ Modifier 51 Exempt   ⊖ Modifier 63 Exempt   ✖ Unlisted   **Modifiers:** *See Inside Back Cover*   Ⓜ Maternity   A2-Z3 ASC Payment Indicators   A-Y OPPS Status Indicators

© 2016 DecisionHealth   CPT © 2015 American Medical Association. All Rights Reserved.   **115**

Levels of E/M Services

Within each category or subcategory of E/M service, there are three to five levels of E/M services available for reporting purposes. Levels of E/M services are **not** interchangeable among the different categories or subcategories of service. For example, the first level of E/M services in the subcategory of office visit, new patient, does not have the same definition as the first level of E/M services in the subcategory of office visit, established patient.

The levels of E/M services include examinations, evaluations, treatments, conferences with or concerning patients, preventive pediatric and adult health supervision, and similar medical services, such as the determination of the need and/or location for appropriate care. Medical screening includes the history, examination, and medical decision-making required to determine the need and/or location for appropriate care and treatment of the patient (eg, office and other outpatient setting, emergency department, nursing facility). The levels of E/M services encompass the wide variations in skill, effort, time, responsibility, and medical knowledge required for the prevention or diagnosis and treatment of illness or injury and the promotion of optimal health. Each level of E/M services may be used by all physicians or other qualified health care professionals.

The descriptors for the levels of E/M services recognize seven components, six of which are used in defining the levels of E/M services. These components are:

- History
- Examination
- Medical decision making
- Counseling
- Coordination of care
- Nature of presenting problem
- Time

The first three of these components (history, examination, and medical decision making) are considered the **key** components in selecting a level of E/M services. (See "Determine the Extent of History Obtained.")

The next three components (counseling, coordination of care, and the nature of the presenting problem) are considered **contributory** factors in the majority of encounters. Although the first two of these contributory factors are important E/M services, it is not required that these services be provided at every patient encounter.

Coordination of care with other physicians, other health care professionals, or agencies without a patient encounter on that day is reported using the case management codes.

The final component, time, is discussed in detail on the next page.

Any specifically identifiable procedure (ie, identified with a specific CPT code) performed on or subsequent to the date of initial or subsequent E/M services should be reported separately.

The actual performance and/or interpretation of diagnostic tests/studies ordered during a patient encounter are not included in the levels of E/M services. Physician performance of diagnostic tests/studies for which specific CPT codes are available may be reported separately, in addition to the appropriate E/M code. The physician's interpretation of the results of diagnostic tests/studies (ie, professional component) with preparation of a separate distinctly identifiable signed written report may also be reported separately, using the appropriate CPT code with modifier 26 appended.

The physician or other health care professional may need to indicate that on the day a procedure or service identified by a CPT code was performed, the patient's condition required a significant separately identifiable E/M service above and beyond other services provided or beyond the usual preservice and postservice care associated with the procedure that was performed. The E/M service may be caused or prompted by the symptoms or condition for which the procedure and/or service was provided. This circumstance may be reported by adding modifier 25 to the appropriate level of E/M service. As such, different diagnoses are not required for reporting of the procedure and the E/M services on the same date.

DecisionTree for New vs Established Patients

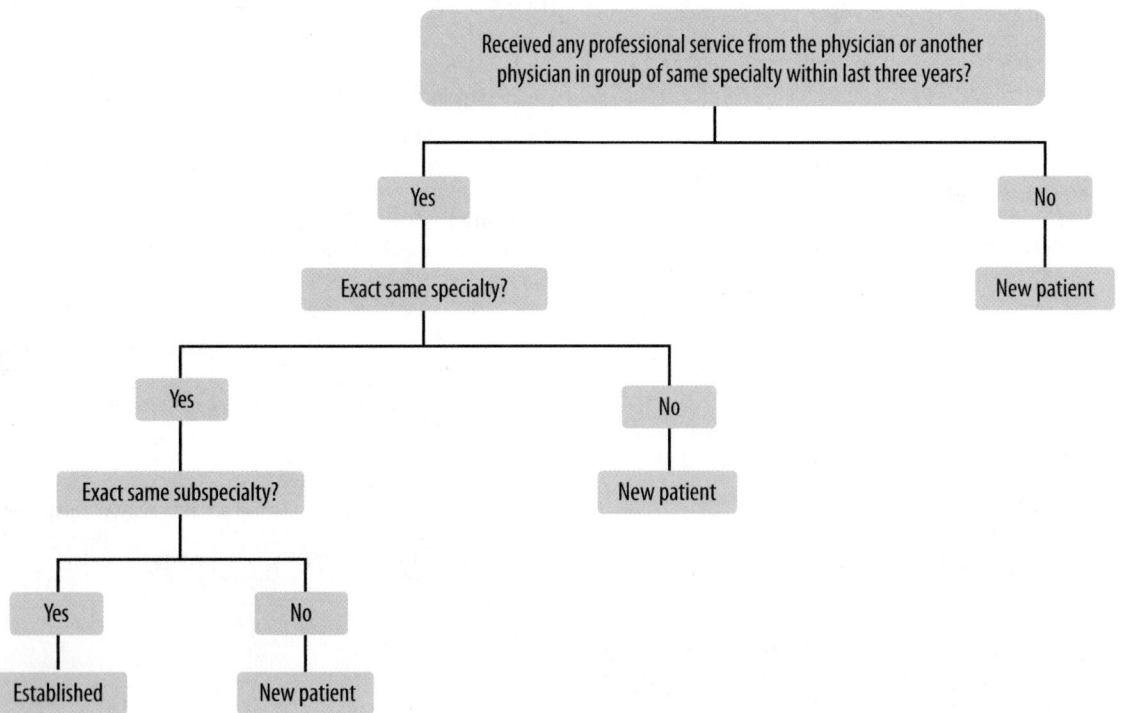

● New   ▲ Revised   ✖ Deleted   ⊙ Moderate Sedation   ✚ Add-on Codes   ⊖ High Risk Denial   Ⓐ Age Edit   ♀ Female   ♂ Male   **AMA** *CPT® Assistant*   **MUE** Medically Unlikely Edit

⊘ Modifier 51 Exempt   ⊖ Modifier 63 Exempt   ☒ Unlisted   **Modifiers:** *See Inside Back Cover*   Ⓜ Maternity   **A2–Z3** ASC Payment Indicators   **A–Y** OPPS Status Indicators

116   CPT © 2015 American Medical Association. All Rights Reserved.   © 2016 DecisionHealth

Nature of Presenting Problem

A presenting problem is a disease, condition, illness, injury, symptom, sign, finding, complaint, or other reason for encounter, with or without a diagnosis being established at the time of the encounter. The E/M codes recognize five types of presenting problems that are defined as follows:

Minimal: A problem that may not require the presence of the physician or other qualified health care professional, but service is provided under the physician's or other qualified health care professional's supervision.

Self-limited or minor: A problem that runs a definite and prescribed course, is transient in nature, and is not likely to permanently alter health status OR has a good prognosis with management/compliance.

Low severity: A problem where the risk of morbidity without treatment is low; there is little to no risk of mortality without treatment; full recovery without functional impairment is expected.

Moderate severity: A problem where the risk of morbidity without treatment is moderate; there is moderate risk of mortality without treatment; uncertain prognosis OR increased probability of prolonged functional impairment.

High severity: A problem where the risk of morbidity without treatment is high to extreme; there is a moderate to high risk of mortality without treatment OR high probability of severe, prolonged functional impairment.

Past History

A review of the patient's past experiences with illnesses, injuries, and treatments that includes significant information about:

- Prior major illnesses and injuries
- Prior operations
- Prior hospitalizations
- Current medications
- Allergies (eg, drug, food)
- Age appropriate immunization status
- Age appropriate feeding/dietary status

Social History

An age appropriate review of past and current activities that includes significant information about:

- Marital status and/or living arrangements
- Current employment
- Occupational history
- Military history
- Use of drugs, alcohol, and tobacco
- Level of education
- Sexual history
- Other relevant social factors

System Review (Review of Systems)

An inventory of body systems obtained through a series of questions seeking to identify signs and/or symptoms that the patient may be experiencing or has experienced. For the purposes of the CPT codebook the following elements of a system review have been identified:

- Constitutional symptoms (fever, weight loss, etc)
- Eyes
- Ears, nose, mouth, throat
- Cardiovascular
- Respiratory
- Gastrointestinal
- Genitourinary
- Musculoskeletal
- Integumentary (skin and/or breast)
- Neurological
- Psychiatric
- Endocrine
- Hematologic/lymphatic
- Allergic/immunologic

The review of systems helps define the problem, clarify the differential diagnosis, identify needed testing, or serves as baseline data on other systems that might be affected by any possible management options.

Time

The inclusion of time in the definitions of levels of E/M services has been implicit in prior editions of the CPT codebook. The inclusion of time as an explicit factor beginning in *CPT 1992* is done to assist in selecting the most appropriate level of E/M services. It should be recognized that the specific times expressed in the visit code descriptors are averages and, therefore, represent a range of times that may be higher or lower depending on actual clinical circumstances.

Time is **not** a descriptive component for the emergency department levels of E/M services because emergency department services are typically provided on a variable intensity basis, often involving multiple encounters with several patients over an extended period of time. Therefore, it is often difficult to provide accurate estimates of the time spent face-to-face with the patient.

Studies to establish levels of E/M services employed surveys of practicing physicians to obtain data on the amount of time and work associated with typical E/M services. Since "work" is not easily quantifiable, the codes must rely on other objective, verifiable measures that correlate with physicians' estimates of their "work." It has been demonstrated that estimations of intraservice time (as explained on the next page), both within and across specialties, is a variable that is predictive of the "work" of E/M services. This same research has shown there is a strong relationship between intraservice time and total time for E/M services. Intraservice time, rather than total time, was chosen for inclusion with the codes because of its relative ease of measurement and because of its direct correlation with measurements of the total amount of time and work associated with typical E/M services.

Intraservice times are defined as **face-to-face** time for office and other outpatient visits and as **unit/floor** time for hospital and other inpatient visits. This distinction is necessary because most of the work of typical office visits takes place during the face-to-face time with the patient, while most of the work of typical hospital visits takes place during the time spent on the patient's floor or unit. When prolonged time occurs in either the office or the inpatient areas, the appropriate add-on code should be reported.

Face-to-face time (office and other outpatient visits and office consultations): For coding purposes, face-to-face time for these services is defined as only that time spent face-to-face with the patient and/or family. This includes the time spent performing such tasks as obtaining a history, examination, and counseling the patient.

Time is also spent doing work before or after the face-to-face time with the patient, performing such tasks as reviewing records and tests, arranging for further services, and communicating further with other professionals and the patient through written reports and telephone contact.

This **non-face-to-face** time for office services-also called pre- and postencounter time-is not included in the time component described in the E/M codes. However, the pre- and post-non-face-to-face work associated with an encounter was included in calculating the total work of typical services in physician surveys.

Thus, the face-to-face time associated with the services described by any E/M code is a valid proxy for the total work done before, during, and after the visit.

Unit/floor time (hospital observation services, inpatient hospital care, initial inpatient hospital consultations, nursing facility): For reporting purposes, intraservice time for these services is defined as unit/floor time, which includes the time present on the patient's hospital unit and at the bedside rendering services for that patient. This includes the time to establish and/or review the patient's chart, examine the patient, write notes, and communicate with other professionals and the patient's family.

In the hospital, pre- and post-time includes time spent off the patient's floor performing such tasks as reviewing pathology and radiology findings in another part of the hospital.

This pre- and postvisit time is not included in the time component described in these codes. However, the pre- and postwork performed during the time spent off the floor or unit was included in calculating the total work of typical services in physician surveys.

Thus, the unit/floor time associated with the services described by any code is a valid proxy for the total work done before, during, and after the visit.

Unlisted Service

An E/M service may be provided that is not listed in this section of the CPT codebook. When reporting such a service, the appropriate unlisted code may be used to indicate the service, identifying it by "Special Report," as discussed in the following paragraph. The "Unlisted Services" and accompanying codes for the E/M section are as follows:

99429   **Unlisted preventive** medicine service

99499   **Unlisted evaluation and management** service

Special Report

An unlisted service or one that is unusual, variable, or new may require a special report demonstrating the medical appropriateness of the service. Pertinent information should include an adequate definition or description of the nature, extent, and need for the procedure and the time, effort, and equipment necessary to provide the service. Additional items that may be included are complexity of symptoms, final diagnosis, pertinent physical findings, diagnostic and therapeutic procedures, concurrent problems, and follow-up care.

Instructions for Selecting a Level of E/M Service

Review the Reporting Instructions for the Selected Category or Subcategory

Most of the categories and many of the subcategories of service have special guidelines or instructions unique to that category or subcategory. Where these are indicated, eg, "Inpatient Hospital Care," special instructions will be presented preceding the levels of E/M services.

Review the Level of E/M Service Descriptors and Examples in the Selected Category or Subcategory

The descriptors for the levels of E/M services recognize seven components, six of which are used in defining the levels of E/M services. These components are:

- History
- Examination
- Medical decision making
- Counseling
- Coordination of care
- Nature of presenting problem
- Time

The first three of these components (ie, history, examination, and medical decision making) should be considered the **key** components in selecting the level of E/M services. An exception to this rule is in the case of visits that consist predominantly of counseling or coordination of care (see numbered paragraph 3, next page).

The nature of the presenting problem and time are provided in some levels to assist the physician in determining the appropriate level of E/M service.

Determine the Extent of History Obtained

The extent of the history is dependent upon clinical judgment and on the nature of the presenting problem(s). The levels of E/M services recognize four types of history that are defined as follows:

Problem focused: Chief complaint; brief history of present illness or problem.

Expanded problem focused: Chief complaint; brief history of present illness; problem pertinent system review.

Detailed: Chief complaint; extended history of present illness; problem pertinent system review extended to include a review of a limited number of additional systems; **pertinent** past, family, and/or social history **directly related to the patient's problems**.

Comprehensive: Chief complaint; extended history of present illness; review of systems that is directly related to the problem(s) identified in the history of the present illness plus a review of all additional body systems; **complete** past, family, and social history.

The comprehensive history obtained as part of the preventive medicine E/M service is not problem-oriented and does not involve a chief complaint or present illness. It does, however, include a comprehensive system review and comprehensive or interval past, family, and social history as well as a comprehensive assessment/history of pertinent risk factors.

Determine the Extent of Examination Performed

The extent of the examination performed is dependent on clinical judgment and on the nature of the presenting problem(s). The levels of E/M services recognize four types of examination that are defined as follows:

Problem focused: A limited examination of the affected body area or organ system.

Expanded problem focused: A limited examination of the affected body area or organ system and other symptomatic or related organ system(s).

Detailed: An extended examination of the affected body area(s) and other symptomatic or related organ system(s).

Comprehensive: A general multisystem examination or a complete examination of a single organ system. **Note:** The comprehensive examination performed as part of the preventive medicine E/M service is multisystem, but its extent is based on age and risk factors identified.

For the purposes of these CPT definitions, the following body areas are recognized:

- Head, including the face
- Neck
- Chest, including breasts and axilla
- Abdomen
- Genitalia, groin, buttocks
- Back
- Each extremity

For the purposes of these CPT definitions, the following organ systems are recognized:

- Eyes
- Ears, nose, mouth, and throat
- Cardiovascular
- Respiratory
- Gastrointestinal
- Genitourinary
- Musculoskeletal
- Skin
- Neurologic
- Psychiatric
- Hematologic/lymphatic/immunologic

● New   ▲ Revised   ✖ Deleted   ⊙ Moderate Sedation   ✚ Add-on Codes   ⊘ High Risk Denial   Ⓐ Age Edit   ♀ Female   ♂ Male   **AMA** *CPT® Assistant*   ***MUE*** Medically Unlikely Edit
     ⊘ Modifier 51 Exempt   ⊖ Modifier 63 Exempt   ✗ Unlisted   **Modifiers:** *See Inside Back Cover*   Ⓜ Maternity   **A̲2̲–Z̲3̲** ASC Payment Indicators   **A̲–Y̲** OPPS Status Indicators

118   CPT © 2015 American Medical Association. All Rights Reserved.   © 2016 DecisionHealth

Determine the Complexity of Medical Decision Making

Medical decision making refers to the complexity of establishing a diagnosis and/or selecting a management option as measured by:

The number of possible diagnoses and/or the number of management options that must be considered

- The amount and/or complexity of medical records, diagnostic tests, and/or other information that must be obtained, reviewed, and analyzed

- The risk of significant complications, morbidity, and/or mortality, as well as comorbidities, associated with the patient's presenting problem(s), the diagnostic procedure(s), and/or the possible management options

- Four types of medical decision making are recognized: straightforward, low complexity, moderate complexity, and high complexity. To qualify for a given type of decision making, two of the three elements in Table 1 must be met or exceeded.

- Comorbidities/underlying diseases, in and of themselves, are not considered in selecting a level of E/M services *unless* their presence significantly increases the complexity of the medical decision making.

Select the Appropriate Level of E/M Services Based on the Following

1. For the following categories/subcategories, **all of the key components**, ie, history, examination, and medical decision making, must meet or exceed the stated requirements to qualify for a particular level of E/M service: office, new patient; hospital observation services; initial hospital care; office consultations; initial inpatient consultations; emergency department services; initial nursing facility care; domiciliary care, new patient; and home, new patient.

2. For the following categories/subcategories, **two of the three key components** (ie, history, examination, and medical decision making) must meet or exceed the stated requirements to qualify for a particular level of E/M services: office, established patient; subsequent hospital care; subsequent nursing facility care; domiciliary care, established patient; and home, established patient.

3. When counseling and/or coordination of care dominates (more than 50%) the encounter with the patient and/or family (face-to-face time in the office or other outpatient setting or floor/unit time in the hospital or nursing facility), then **time** shall be considered the key or controlling factor to qualify for a particular level of E/M services. This includes time spent with parties who have assumed responsibility for the care of the patient or decision making whether or not they are family members (eg, foster parents, person acting in loco parentis, legal guardian). The extent of counseling and/or coordination of care must be documented in the medical record.

Table 1

Complexity of Medical Decision Making

Number of Diagnoses or Management Options	Amount and/or Complexity of Data to be Reviewed	Risk of Complications and/or Morbidity or Mortality	Type of Decision Making
minimal	minimal or none	minimal	straightforward
limited	limited	low	low complexity
multiple	moderate	moderate	moderate complexity
extensive	extensive	high	high complexity

Office/Outpatient Visits

The following codes are used to report evaluation and management services provided in the office or in an outpatient or other ambulatory facility. A patient is considered an outpatient until inpatient admission to a health care facility occurs.

To report services provided to a patient who is admitted to a hospital or nursing facility in the course of an encounter in the office or other ambulatory facility, see the notes for initial hospital inpatient care or initial nursing facility care.

For services provided in the emergency department, see 99281-99285.

For observation care, see 99217-99226.

For observation or inpatient care services (including admission and discharge services), see 99234-99236.

Determination of Patient Status as New or Established Patient

Solely for the purposes of distinguishing between new and established patients, **professional services** are those face-to-face services rendered by physicians and other qualified health care professionals who may report evaluation and management services reported by a specific CPT code(s). A new patient is one who has not received any professional services from the physician/qualified health care professional or another physician/qualified health care professional of the **exact** same specialty and subspecialty who belongs to the same group practice, within the past three years.

An established patient is one who has received professional services from the physician/qualified health care professional or another physician/qualified health care professional of the exact same specialty and subspecialty who belongs to the same group practice, within the past three years.

In the instance where a physician/qualified health care professional is on call for or covering for another physician/qualified health care professional, the patient's encounter will be classified as it would have been by the physician/qualified health care professional who is not available. When advanced practice nurses and physician assistants are working with physicians they are considered as working in the **exact** same specialty and exact same **subspecialties** as the physician.

CPT Coding Guidelines, Evaluation and Management, Definitions of Commonly Used Terms, New and Established Patient

New Office/Outpatient Visits

99201 Office or other outpatient visit for the evaluation and management of a new patient, which requires these 3 key components:

- A problem focused history;
- A problem focused examination;
- Straightforward medical decision making.

Counseling and/or coordination of care with other physicians, other qualified health care professionals, or agencies are provided consistent with the nature of the problem(s) and the patient's and/or family's needs. Usually, the presenting problem(s) are self limited or minor. Typically, 10 minutes are spent face-to-face with the patient and/or family. ▣

RVU		Global Days	Modifiers				
Mod	Non-Fac Total	Fac Total		51	50	62	80	MUE
	1.24	0.76	XXX	0	0	0	0	1

AMA: Apr 05: 1, Apr 07: 11, Apr 12: 10, Aug 01: 2, Aug 06: 12, Aug 09: 5, Aug 13: 13, 14, Aug 14: 3, Dec 05: 10, Dec 09: 9, Fall 93: 9, Fall 95: 9, Feb 00: 3, 9, 11, Feb 06: 14, Jan 11: 3, Jan 12: 5, Jan 13: 9, Jan 15: 12, Jul 10: 10, Jul 98: 9, Jun 05: 11, Jun 06: 1, Jun 13: 3, Jun 99: 8, Mar 05: 11, Mar 09: 3, Mar 12: 4, 8, May 05: 1, May 06: 1, Nov 08: 10, Nov 14: 14, Oct 04: 11, Oct 06: 15, Oct 14: 3, Sep 07: 1, Sep 98: 5, Spring 92: 13, 24, Spring 93: 34, Spring 95: 1, Summer 92: 1, 24, Summer 93: 2, Summer 95: 4, Winter 91: 11

Pub 100-04, 32, 12.1

99202 Office or other outpatient visit for the evaluation and management of a new patient, which requires these 3 key components:

- An expanded problem focused history;
- An expanded problem focused examination;
- Straightforward medical decision making.

Counseling and/or coordination of care with other physicians, other qualified health care professionals, or agencies are provided consistent with the nature of the problem(s) and the patient's and/or family's needs. Usually, the presenting problem(s) are of low to moderate severity. Typically, 20 minutes are spent face-to-face with the patient and/or family. ▣

RVU		Global Days	Modifiers				
Mod	Non-Fac Total	Fac Total		51	50	62	80	MUE
	2.11	1.42	XXX	0	0	0	0	1

AMA: Apr 02: 14, Apr 05: 1, 3, Apr 07: 11, Aug 01: 2, Aug 09: 5, Aug 13: 13, 14, Dec 05: 10, Dec 09: 9, Fall 93: 9, Fall 95: 9, Feb 00: 11, Jan 11: 3, Jan 13: 9, Jan 15: 12, Jul 98: 9, Jun 05: 11, Jun 06: 1, Jun 13: 3, Mar 09: 3, Mar 12: 4, 8, May 06: 1, Oct 04: 10, Oct 06: 15, Sep 07: 1, Sep 98: 5, Spring 92: 13, 24, Spring 93: 34, Spring 95: 1, Summer 92: 1, 24, Summer 93: 2, Summer 95: 4, Winter 91: 11

Pub 100-04, 32, 12.1

99203 Office or other outpatient visit for the evaluation and management of a new patient, which requires these 3 key components:

- A detailed history;
- A detailed examination;
- Medical decision making of low complexity.

Counseling and/or coordination of care with other physicians, other qualified health care professionals, or agencies are provided consistent with the nature of the problem(s) and the patient's and/or family's needs. Usually, the presenting problem(s) are of moderate severity. Typically, 30 minutes are spent face-to-face with the patient and/or family. ▣

RVU		Global Days	Modifiers				
Mod	Non-Fac Total	Fac Total		51	50	62	80	MUE
	3.05	2.17	XXX	0	0	0	0	1

AMA: Apr 02: 14, Apr 05: 1, 3, Apr 07: 11, Aug 01: 2, Aug 09: 5, Aug 13: 13, 14, Dec 05: 10, Dec 09: 9, Fall 93: 9, Fall 95: 9, Feb 00: 11, Feb 05: 9, Jan 11: 3, Jan 13: 9, Jan 15: 12, Jul 98: 9, Jun 05: 11, Jun 06: 1, Jun 13: 3, Mar 09: 3, Mar 12: 4, 8, May 06: 1, Oct 04: 10, Oct 06: 15, Sep 07: 1, Sep 98: 5, Spring 92: 14, 24, Spring 93: 34, Spring 95: 1, Summer 92: 1, 24, Summer 93: 2, Summer 95: 4, Winter 91: 11

Pub 100-04, 32, 12.1

99204 Office or other outpatient visit for the evaluation and management of a new patient, which requires these 3 key components:

- A comprehensive history;
- A comprehensive examination;
- Medical decision making of moderate complexity.

● New   ▲ Revised   ✖ Deleted   ⊙ Moderate Sedation   ✚ Add-on Codes   ⊘ High Risk Denial   ⓐ Age Edit   ♀ Female   ♂ Male   **AMA** *CPT® Assistant*   **MUE** Medically Unlikely Edit
⊘ Modifier 51 Exempt   ⊖ Modifier 63 Exempt   ✗ Unlisted   **Modifiers:** *See Inside Back Cover*   Ⓜ Maternity   A2–Z3 ASC Payment Indicators   A–Y OPPS Status Indicators

120 | CPT © 2014 American Medical Association. All Rights Reserved. | © 2016 DecisionHealth

Counseling and/or coordination of care with other physicians, other qualified health care professionals, or agencies are provided consistent with the nature of the problem(s) and the patient's and/or family's needs. Usually, the presenting problem(s) are of moderate to high severity. Typically, 45 minutes are spent face-to-face with the patient and/or family. **B**

RVU			Global Days	Modifiers				
Mod	Non-Fac Total	Fac Total		51	50	62	80	MUE
	4.64	3.67	XXX	0	0	0	0	1

AMA: Apr 02: 14, Apr 05: 1, 3, Apr 07: 11, Aug 01: 2, Aug 09: 5, Aug 13: 13, 14, Dec 05: 10, Dec 09: 9, Fall 93: 9, Fall 95: 9, Feb 00: 11, Jan 11: 3, Jan 13: 9, Jan 15: 12, Jul 98: 9, Jun 05: 11, Jun 06: 1, Jun 13: 3, Mar 09: 3, Mar 12: 4, 8, May 02: 1, May 06: 1, Oct 04: 10, Oct 06: 15, Sep 07: 1, Sep 98: 5, Spring 92: 14, 24, Spring 93: 34, Spring 95: 1, Summer 92: 1, 24, Summer 93: 2, Summer 95: 4, Winter 91: 11

Pub 100-04, 32, 12.1

99205 Office or other outpatient visit for the evaluation and management of a new patient, which requires these 3 key components:

- A comprehensive history;
- A comprehensive examination;
- Medical decision making of high complexity.

Counseling and/or coordination of care with other physicians, other qualified health care professionals, or agencies are provided consistent with the nature of the problem(s) and the patient's and/or family's needs. Usually, the presenting problem(s) are of moderate to high severity. Typically, 60 minutes are spent face-to-face with the patient and/or family. **B**

RVU			Global Days	Modifiers				
Mod	Non-Fac Total	Fac Total		51	50	62	80	MUE
	5.82	4.77	XXX	0	0	0	0	1

AMA: Apr 02: 2, Apr 05: 1, 3, Apr 07: 11, Aug 01: 2, Aug 09: 5, Aug 13: 13, 14, Dec 05: 10, Dec 09: 9, Fall 93: 9, Fall 95: 9, Feb 00: 11, Jan 11: 3, Jan 12: 3, Jan 13: 9, Jan 15: 12, Jul 10: 4, Jul 98: 9, Jun 05: 11, Jun 06: 1, Jun 13: 3, Mar 09: 3, Mar 12: 4, 8, May 02: 1, May 06: 1, Oct 04: 10, Oct 06: 15, Sep 07: 1, Sep 98: 5, Spring 92: 14, 24, Spring 93: 34, Spring 95: 1, Summer 92: 1, 24, Summer 93: 2, Summer 95: 4, Winter 91: 11

Pub 100-04, 32, 12.1

Established Office/Outpatient Visits

99211 Office or other outpatient visit for the evaluation and management of an established patient, that may not require the presence of a physician or other qualified health care professional. Usually, the presenting problem(s) are minimal. Typically, 5 minutes are spent performing or supervising these services. B

RVU			Global Days	Modifiers				
Mod	Non-Fac Total	Fac Total		51	50	62	80	MUE
	0.56	0.26	XXX	0	0	0	0	1

AMA: Apr 05: 1, 3, Apr 07: 11, Apr 10: 10, Apr 12: 10, Aug 01: 2, Aug 08: 13, Aug 09: 5, Aug 13: 13, 14, Dec 05: 10, Dec 07: 9, Fall 93: 9, Fall 95: 9, Feb 00: 11, Feb 05: 15, Feb 06: 14, Feb 97: 9, Jan 02: 2, Jan 11: 3, Jan 12: 3, Jan 13: 9, Jan 15: 12, Jul 06: 19, Jul 07: 1, Jul 98: 9, Jun 05: 11, Jun 06: 1, Jun 13: 3, Mar 05: 11, Mar 08: 3, Mar 09: 3, Mar 12: 4, 8, Mar 13: 13, Mar 14: 14, May 05: 1, May 06: 1, May 97: 4, Nov 05: 1, Nov 06: 21, Nov 13: 3, Oct 04: 10, Oct 06: 15, Oct 96: 10, Oct 99: 9, Sep 07: 1, Sep 98: 5, Spring 92: 14, 24, Spring 93: 34, Spring 95: 1, Summer 92: 1, 24, Summer 93: 2, Summer 95: 4, Winter 91: 11

Pub 100-04, 13, 70.2; 100-04, 32, 12.1, 130.1

99212 Office or other outpatient visit for the evaluation and management of an established patient, which requires at least 2 of these 3 key components:

- A problem focused history;
- A problem focused examination;
- Straightforward medical decision making.

Counseling and/or coordination of care with other physicians, other qualified health care professionals, or agencies are provided consistent with the nature of the problem(s) and the patient's and/or family's needs. Usually, the presenting problem(s) are self limited or minor. Typically, 10 minutes are spent face-to-face with the patient and/or family. **B**

RVU			Global Days	Modifiers				
Mod	Non-Fac Total	Fac Total		51	50	62	80	MUE
	1.23	0.72	XXX	0	0	0	0	2

AMA: Apr 04: 14, Apr 05: 1, 3, Apr 07: 11, Apr 12: 17, Aug 01: 2, Aug 09: 5, Aug 13: 13, 14, Dec 05: 10, Fall 93: 9, Fall 95: 9, Feb 00: 11, Feb 10: 13, Feb 14: 11, Jan 02: 2, Jan 11: 3, Jan 13: 9, Jan 15: 12, Jul 07: 1, Jul 10: 4, Jul 98: 9, Jun 00: 11, Jun 05: 11, Jun 06: 1, 11, Jun 11: 3, Jun 13: 3, Mar 08: 3, Mar 09: 3, Mar 12: 4, 8, Mar 13: 13, May 02: 3, May 06: 1, Oct 04: 10, Oct 06: 15, Sep 06: 8, Sep 07: 1, Sep 10: 4, Sep 98: 5, Spring 92: 14, 24, Spring 93: 34, Spring 95: 1, Summer 92: 1, 24, Summer 93: 2, Summer 95: 4, Winter 91: 11

Pub 100-04, 13, 70.2; 100-04, 32, 12.1, 130.1

99213 Office or other outpatient visit for the evaluation and management of an established patient, which requires at least 2 of these 3 key components:

- An expanded problem focused history;
- An expanded problem focused examination;
- Medical decision making of low complexity.

Counseling and coordination of care with other physicians, other qualified health care professionals, or agencies are provided consistent with the nature of the problem(s) and the patient's and/or family's needs. Usually, the presenting problem(s) are of low to moderate severity. Typically, 15 minutes are spent face-to-face with the patient and/or family. **B**

RVU			Global Days	Modifiers				
Mod	Non-Fac Total	Fac Total		51	50	62	80	MUE
	2.05	1.44	XXX	0	0	0	0	2

AMA: Apr 04: 14, Apr 05: 1, 3, Apr 07: 11, Aug 01: 2, Aug 09: 5, Aug 13: 13, 14, Dec 05: 10, Fall 93: 9, Fall 95: 9, Jan 11: 3, Jan 13: 9, Jan 15: 12, Jan 97: 10, Jul 07: 1, Jul 98: 9, Jun 05: 11, Jun 06: 1, 11, Jun 11: 3, Jun 13: 3, Mar 05: 11, Mar 08: 3, Mar 09: 3, Mar 12: 4, 8, Mar 13: 13, May 02: 3, May 06: 1, Oct 03: 5, Oct 04: 10, Oct 06: 15, Sep 06: 8, Sep 07: 1, Sep 10: 4, Sep 98: 5, Spring 92: 14, 24, Spring 93: 34, Spring 95: 1, Summer 92: 1, 24, Summer 93: 2, Summer 95: 4, Winter 91: 11

Pub 100-04, 13, 70.2; 100-04, 32, 12.1, 130.1

● New   ▲ Revised   ✖ Deleted   ⊙ Moderate Sedation   ✚ Add-on Codes   ⊘ High Risk Denial   Ⓐ Age Edit   ♀ Female   ♂ Male   **AMA** *CPT® Assistant*   **MUE** Medically Unlikely Edit
⊘ Modifier 51 Exempt   ⊖ Modifier 63 Exempt   ✗ Unlisted   **Modifiers:** *See Inside Back Cover*   Ⓜ Maternity   A2-Z3 ASC Payment Indicators   A-Y OPPS Status Indicators

99214 Office or other outpatient visit for the evaluation and management of an established patient, which requires at least 2 of these 3 key components:

- A detailed history;

- A detailed examination;

- Medical decision making of moderate complexity. Counseling and/or coordination of care with other physicians, other qualified health care professionals, or agencies are provided consistent with the nature of the problem(s) and the patient's and/or family's needs. Usually, the presenting problem(s) are of moderate to high severity. Typically, 25 minutes are spent face-to-face with the patient and/or family.   **B**

RVU			Global Days	Modifiers				
Mod	Non-Fac Total	Fac Total		51	50	62	80	MUE
	3.02	2.21	XXX	0	0	0	0	2

AMA: Apr 04: 14, Apr 05: 1, 3, Apr 07: 11, Aug 01: 2, Aug 09: 5, Aug 13: 13, 14, Dec 05: 10, Fall 93: 9, Fall 95: 9, Jan 02: 2, Jan 11: 3, Jan 13: 9, Jan 15: 12, Jul 07: 1, Jul 98: 9, Jun 05: 11, Jun 06: 1, 11, Jun 11: 3, Jun 13: 3, Mar 08: 3, Mar 09: 3, Mar 12: 4, 8, Mar 13: 13, May 02: 1, 2, May 06: 1, May 97: 4, Oct 03: 5, Oct 04: 10, Oct 06: 15, Sep 06: 8, Sep 07: 1, Sep 10: 4, Sep 98: 5, Spring 92: 15, 24, Spring 93: 34, Spring 95: 1, Summer 92: 1, 24, Summer 93: 2, Summer 95: 4, Winter 91: 11

Pub 100-04, 13, 70.2; 100-04, 32, 12.1, 130.1

99215 Office or other outpatient visit for the evaluation and management of an established patient, which requires at least 2 of these 3 key components:

- A comprehensive history;

- A comprehensive examination;

- Medical decision making of high complexity. Counseling and/or coordination of care with other physicians, other qualified health care professionals, or agencies are provided consistent with the nature of the problem(s) and the patient's and/or family's needs. Usually, the presenting problem(s) are of moderate to high severity. Typically, 40 minutes are spent face-to-face with the patient and/or family.   **B**

RVU			Global Days	Modifiers				
Mod	Non-Fac Total	Fac Total		51	50	62	80	MUE
	4.07	3.12	XXX	0	0	0	0	1

AMA: Apr 04: 14, Apr 05: 1, 3, Apr 07: 11, Apr 12: 10, Aug 01: 2, Aug 09: 5, Aug 13: 13, 14, Aug 14: 3, Dec 05: 10, Fall 93: 9, Fall 95: 9, Jan 02: 2, Jan 11: 3, Jan 12: 3, Jan 13: 9, Jan 15: 12, Jan 97: 10, Jul 07: 1, Jul 10: 4, Jul 98: 9, Jun 05: 11, Jun 06: 1, 11, Jun 11: 3, Jun 13: 3, Mar 05: 11, Mar 08: 3, Mar 09: 3, Mar 12: 4, 8, Mar 13: 13, May 02: 1, 3, May 06: 1, Nov 13: 3, Nov 14: 14, Oct 04: 10, Oct 06: 15, Oct 14: 3, Sep 06: 8, Sep 07: 1, Sep 10: 4, Sep 98: 5, Spring 92: 15, 24, Spring 93: 34, Spring 95: 1, Summer 92: 1, 24, Summer 93: 2, Summer 95: 4, Winter 91: 11

Pub 100-04, 13, 70.2; 100-04, 32, 12.1, 130.1

Hospital Observation Visits

The following codes are used to report evaluation and management services provided to patients designated/admitted as "observation status" in a hospital. It is not necessary that the patient be located in an observation area designated by the hospital.

If such an area does exist in a hospital (as a separate unit in the hospital, in the emergency department, etc.), these codes are to be utilized if the patient is placed in such an area.

For definitions of key components and commonly used terms, please see *Evaluation and Management Services Guidelines.*

Hospital Observation Discharge Services

Observation care discharge of a patient from "observation status" includes final examination of the patient, discussion of the hospital stay, instructions for continuing care, and preparation of discharge records. For observation or inpatient hospital care including admission and discharge on the same date, see codes 99234-99236 as appropriate.

99217 Observation care discharge day management

(This code is to be utilized to report all services provided to a patient on discharge from "observation status" if the discharge is on other than the initial date of "observation status."

To report services to a patient designated as "observation status" or "inpatient status" and discharged on the same date, use the codes for Observation or Inpatient Care Services [including Admission and Discharge Services, 99234-99236 as appropriate.])   **B**

RVU			Global Days	Modifiers				
Mod	Non-Fac Total	Fac Total		51	50	62	80	MUE
	2.05	2.05	XXX	0	0	0	0	1

AMA: Dec 06: 14, Jan 13: 9, Jul 12: 10, 11, 14, Jun 11: 3, Jun 13: 3, Mar 98: 1, May 05: 1, May 98: 3, Nov 05: 10, Nov 14: 14, Nov 97: 2, Sep 00: 3, Sep 06: 8, Sep 10: 4, Sep 98: 5

Pub 100-02, 15, 30; 100-04, 32, 130.1

Initial Observation Care

New or Established Patient

The following codes are used to report the encounter(s) by the supervising physician or other qualified health care professional for patient designated as "observation status." This refers to the initiation of observation status, supervision of the care plan for observation and performance of periodic reassessments. For observation encounters by other physicians, see office or other outpatient consultation codes, 99241-99245 or subsequent observation care codes (99224-99226) as appropriate.

To report services provided to a patient who is admitted to the hospital after receiving hospital observation care services on the same date, see the notes for initial hospital inpatient care. For observation care services on other than the initial or discharge date, see subsequent observation services codes (99224-99226). For a patient admitted to the hospital on a date subsequent to the date of observation status, the hospital admission would be reported with the appropriate initial hospital Care code, 99221-99223. For a patient admitted and discharged from observation of inpatient status on the same date, the services should be reported with codes 99234-99236, as appropriate. Do not report observation discharge, 99217, in conjunction with a hospital admission.

When "observation status" is initiated in the course of an encounter in another site of service (e.g., hospital emergency department, physician's office, nursing facility), all evaluation and management services provided by the supervising physician should include the services related to initiating "observation status" are considered part of the initial observation care when performed on the same date. The observation care level of service reported by the supervising physician or other qualified health care professional should include the services related to initiating "observation status" provided in the other sites of service as well as in the observation setting.

Evaluation and management services on the same date provided in sites that are related to initiating "observation status" should not be reported separately.

These codes may not be utilized for post-operative recovery if the procedure is considered part of the surgical "package." These codes apply to all evaluation and management services that are provided on the same date of initiating "observation status."

● New   ▲ Revised   ✖ Deleted   ⊙ Moderate Sedation   ✚ Add-on Codes   ⊘ High Risk Denial   ⓐ Age Edit   ♀ Female   ♂ Male   **AMA** *CPT® Assistant*   **MUE** Medically Unlikely Edit
⊘ Modifier 51 Exempt   ⊖ Modifier 63 Exempt   ✗ Unlisted   **Modifiers:** *See Inside Back Cover*   Ⓜ Maternity   **A2-Z3** ASC Payment Indicators   **A-Y** OPPS Status Indicators

122   CPT © 2014 American Medical Association. All Rights Reserved.   © 2016 DecisionHealth

99218 Initial observation care, per day, for the evaluation and management of a patient which requires these 3 key components:

- A detailed or comprehensive history;

- A detailed or comprehensive examination;

- and Medical decision making that is straightforward or of low complexity.

Counseling and/or coordination of care with other physicians, other qualified health care professionals, or agencies are provided consistent with the nature of the problem(s) and the patient's and/or family's needs. Usually, the problem(s) requiring admission to "observation status" are of low severity. Typically, 30 minutes are spent at the bedside and on the patient's hospital floor or unit.**B**

RVU			Global Days	Modifiers				
Mod	Non-Fac Total	Fac Total		51	50	62	80	MUE
	2.81	2.81	XXX	0	0	0	0	1

AMA: Aug 04: 11, Aug 13: 13, Dec 06: 14, Fall 95: 9, Jan 03: 10, Jan 13: 9, Jul 12: 11, 14, Jul 15: 4, Jun 11: 3, Jun 13: 3, Mar 15: 3, Mar 98: 1, May 05: 1, Nov 05: 10, Nov 97: 2, Oct 10: 6, Sep 00: 3, Sep 06: 8, Sep 10: 4, Sep 98: 5, Spring 93: 34

Pub 100-04, 32, 130.1

99219 Initial observation care, per day, for the evaluation and management of a patient, which requires these 3 key components:

- A comprehensive history;

- A comprehensive examination;

- and Medical decision making of moderate complexity.

Counseling and/or coordination of care with other physicians, other qualified health care professionals, or agencies are provided consistent with the nature of the problem(s) and the patient's and/or family's needs. Usually, the problem(s) requiring admission to "observation status" are of moderate severity. Typically, 50 minutes are spent at the bedside and on the patient's hospital floor or unit.　　　　　　　　　　　**B**

RVU			Global Days	Modifiers				
Mod	Non-Fac Total	Fac Total		51	50	62	80	MUE
	3.81	3.81	XXX	0	0	0	0	1
	3.81	3.81	XXX	0	0	0	0	1

AMA: Aug 04: 11, Aug 13: 13, Dec 06: 14, Fall 95: 16, Jan 03: 10, Jan 13: 9, Jul 12: 11, 14, Jun 11: 3, Jun 13: 3, Mar 98: 1, Nov 05: 10, Nov 97: 2, Oct 10: 6, Sep 00: 3, Sep 06: 8, Sep 10: 4, Sep 98: 5, Spring 93: 34

Pub 100-04, 32, 130.1

99220 Initial observation care, per day, for the evaluation and management of a patient, which requires these 3 key components:

- A comprehensive history;

- A comprehensive examination;

- and Medical decision making of high complexity.

Counseling and/or coordination of care with other physicians, other qualified health care professionals, or agencies are provided consistent with the nature of the problem(s) and the patient's and/or family's needs. Usually, the problem(s) requiring admission to "observation status" are of high severity. Typically, 70 minutes are spent at the bedside and on the patient's hospital floor or unit.**B**

RVU			Global Days	Modifiers				
Mod	Non-Fac Total	Fac Total		51	50	62	80	MUE
	5.22	5.22	XXX	0	0	0	0	1

AMA: Aug 04: 11, Aug 13: 13, Dec 06: 14, Fall 95: 16, Jan 03: 10, Jan 13: 9, Jul 12: 11, Jun 11: 3, Jun 13: 3, Mar 98: 1, Nov 05: 10, Nov 14: 14, Nov 97: 2, Oct 10: 6, Sep 00: 3, Sep 06: 8, Sep 10: 4, Sep 98: 5, Spring 93: 34

Pub 100-04, 32, 130.1

Hospital Inpatient Visits

The following codes are used to report evaluation and management services provided to hospital inpatients. Hospital inpatient services include those services provided to patients in a "partial hospital" setting. These codes are to be used to report these partial hospitalization services. For definitions of key components and commonly used terms, see Evaluation and Management Services Guidelines.

For Hospital Observation Services, see 99218-99220, 99224-99226. For a patient admitted and discharged from observation or inpatient status on the same date, the service should be reported with codes 99234-99236, as appropriate.

Significance of the Time Factor in Selecting an Evaluation and Management Code

The inclusion of time as an explicit factor beginning in CPT 1992 was done to assist physicians in selecting the most appropriate level of E/M service. It should be recognized that the specific times expressed in the visit code descriptors are averages and, therefore, represent a range of times that may be higher or lower depending on actual clinical circumstances.

Intraservice times are defined as face-to-face times for office and other outpatient visits and as unit/floor time for hospital and other in inpatients visits. This distinction is necessary because more of the work of typical office visits take place during the face-to-face time with the patient, while most of the work of typical hospital visits takes place during the time spent on the patient's floor or unit.

Unit/floor time in hospital observation services, inpatient hospital care and initial hospital inpatient consultations, and nursing facility:

Intraservice time for these services is defined as unit/floor time, which includes the time that the physician is present on the patient's hospital unit and at the bedside rendering services. This includes the time in which the physician establishes and/or reviews the patient's chart, examines the patient, writes notes, and communicates with other professionals and the patient's family.

Pre- and post-time in the hospital includes the time spent off the patient's floor performing tasks such as reviewing pathology and radiology findings in another part of the hospital. Pre- and post-visit time is not included in the time component described in these codes. However, the pre- and post-work performed during the time spent off the floor or unit was included in calculating the total work of typical services in physician surveys. Thus, the unit/floor time associated with the services described by any code is a valid proxy for the total work done before, during and after the visit.

● New　　▲ Revised　　✖ Deleted　　⊙ Moderate Sedation　　✚ Add-on Codes　　⊘ High Risk Denial　　Ⓐ Age Edit　　♀ Female　　♂ Male　　**AMA** *CPT® Assistant*　　***MUE*** Medically Unlikely Edit
⊘ Modifier 51 Exempt　　⊖ Modifier 63 Exempt　　✖ Unlisted　　**Modifiers:** *See Inside Back Cover*　　Ⓜ Maternity　　**A2–Z3** ASC Payment Indicators　　**A–Y** OPPS Status Indicators

© 2016 DecisionHealth　　　　CPT © 2014 American Medical Association. All Rights Reserved.　　　　**123**

Evaluation and Management (E/M) Services

99221 – 99223

Initial Hospital Care

New or Established Patient

The following codes are used to report the first hospital inpatient encounter with the patient by the admitting physician. For initial inpatient encounters by physicians other than the admitting physician, see initial inpatient consultation codes, 99251-99255 or subsequent hospital care codes, 99231-99233. For admission services for the neonate (28 days of age or less) requiring intensive observation, frequent interventions, and other intensive care services, see 99477.

When the patient is admitted to the hospital as an inpatient in the course of an encounter in another site of service (e.g., hospital emergency department, observation status in a hospital, physician's office, nursing facility), all evaluation and management services provided by that physician in conjunction with that admission are considered to be part of the initial hospital care when performed on the same date as the admission. The inpatient care level of service reported by the admitting physician should include the services related to the admission he/she provided in the other sites of service as well as in the inpatient setting.

Evaluation and management services on the same date provided in sites that are related to the admission "observation status" should not be reported separately. For a patient admitted and discharge from observation or inpatient status on the same date, the services should be reported with codes 99234-99236, as appropriate.

99221 Initial hospital care, per day, for the evaluation and management of a patient, which requires these 3 key components:

- A detailed or comprehensive history;
- A detailed or comprehensive examination;
- and Medical decision making that is straightforward or of low complexity.

Counseling and/or coordination of care with other physicians, other qualified health care professionals, or agencies are provided consistent with the nature of the problem(s) and the patient's and/or family's needs. Usually, the problem(s) requiring admission are of low severity. Typically, 30 minutes are spent at the bedside and on the patient's hospital floor or unit. **B**

RVU			Global Days	Modifiers				
Mod	Non-Fac Total	Fac Total		51	50	62	80	MUE
	2.86	2.86	XXX	0	0	0	0	1

AMA: Apr 03: 26, Apr 04: 14, Aug 04: 11, Aug 13: 13, Fall 92: 1, Fall 95: 9, Feb 14: 11, Jan 02: 2, 3, Jan 13: 9, Jul 07: 12, Jul 12: 12, Jul 96: 11, Jun 13: 3, Mar 98: 1, May 05: 1, May 14: 4, Nov 14: 14, Nov 97: 2, Sep 06: 8, Sep 96: 10, Sep 98: 5, Spring 92: 14, 24, Spring 93: 34, Spring 95: 1, Summer 92: 10, 24, Winter 91: 11

99222 Initial hospital care, per day, for the evaluation and management of a patient, which requires these 3 key components:

- A comprehensive history;
- A comprehensive examination;
- and Medical decision making of moderate complexity.

Counseling and/or coordination of care with other physicians, other qualified health care professionals, or agencies are provided consistent with the nature of the problem(s) and the patient's and/or family's needs. Usually, the problem(s) requiring admission are of moderate severity. Typically, 50 minutes are spent at the bedside and on the patient's hospital floor or unit. **B**

RVU			Global Days	Modifiers				
Mod	Non-Fac Total	Fac Total		51	50	62	80	MUE
	3.86	3.86	XXX	0	0	0	0	1

AMA: Apr 03: 26, Apr 04: 14, Aug 04: 11, Aug 13: 13, Fall 92: 1, Fall 95: 9, Jan 02: 2, 3, Jan 13: 9, Jul 07: 12, Jul 12: 12, Jul 96: 11, Jun 13: 3, Mar 15: 3, Mar 98: 1, Nov 97: 2, Sep 06: 8, Sep 96: 10, Sep 98: 5, Spring 92: 14, 24, Spring 93: 34, Spring 95: 1, Summer 92: 10, 24, Winter 91: 11

99223 Initial hospital care, per day, for the evaluation and management of a patient, which requires these 3 key components:

- A comprehensive history;
- A comprehensive examination;
- and Medical decision making of high complexity.

Counseling and/or coordination of care with other physicians, other qualified health care professionals, or agencies are provided consistent with the nature of the problem(s) and the patient's and/or family's needs. Usually, the problem(s) requiring admission are of high severity. Typically, 70 minutes are spent at the bedside and on the patient's hospital floor or unit. **B**

RVU			Global Days	Modifiers				
Mod	Non-Fac Total	Fac Total		51	50	62	80	MUE
	5.70	5.70	XXX	0	0	0	0	1

AMA: Apr 03: 26, Apr 04: 14, Aug 04: 11, Aug 13: 13, Fall 92: 1, Fall 95: 9, Jan 02: 2, 3, Jan 13: 9, Jul 07: 12, Jul 12: 12, Jul 96: 11, Jun 13: 3, Mar 98: 1, May 14: 4, Nov 14: 14, Nov 97: 2, Sep 06: 8, Sep 96: 10, Sep 98: 5, Spring 92: 14, 24, Spring 93: 34, Spring 95: 1, Summer 92: 10, 24, Winter 91: 11

Subsequent Observation Care

All levels of subsequent observation care include reviewing the medical record and reviewing the results of diagnostic studies and changes in the patient's status (ie, changes in history, physical condition, and response to management) since the last assessment.

● New ▲ Revised ✖ Deleted ⊙ Moderate Sedation ✚ Add-on Codes ⊘ High Risk Denial Ⓐ Age Edit ♀ Female ♂ Male **AMA** CPT® Assistant **MUE** Medically Unlikely Edit
⊘ Modifier 51 Exempt ⊖ Modifier 63 Exempt ✗ Unlisted **Modifiers:** See Inside Back Cover Ⓜ Maternity A2–Z3 ASC Payment Indicators A–Y OPPS Status Indicators

124 CPT © 2014 American Medical Association. All Rights Reserved. © 2016 DecisionHealth

99224 **Subsequent observation care, per day, for the evaluation and management of a patient, which requires at least 2 of these 3 key components:**

- Problem focused interval history;
- Problem focused examination;
- Medical decision making that is straightforward or of low complexity.

Counseling and/or coordination of care with other physicians, other qualified health care professionals, or agencies are provided consistent with the nature of the problem(s) and the patient's and/or family's needs. Usually, the patient is stable, recovering, or improving. Typically, 15 minutes are spent at the bedside and on the patient's hospital floor or unit.   **B**

Coding tip: Subsequent observation care codes (99224-99226) are listed out of numeric order in CPT. Refer to codes 99218-99220 for initial observation care services.

RVU			Global Days	Modifiers				
Mod	Non-Fac Total	Fac Total		51	50	62	80	MUE
	1.12	1.12	XXX	0	0	0	0	1

AMA: Aug 11: 11, Aug 13: 13, Jul 12: 10, 11, Jun 11: 3, Jun 13: 3, Nov 14: 14

99225 **Subsequent observation care, per day, for the evaluation and management of a patient, which requires at least 2 of these 3 key components:**

- An expanded problem focused interval history;
- An expanded problem focused examination;
- Medical decision making of moderate complexity.

Counseling and/or coordination of care with other physicians, other qualified health care professionals, or agencies are provided consistent with the nature of the problem(s) and the patient's and/or family's needs. Usually, the patient is responding inadequately to therapy or has developed a minor complication. Typically, 25 minutes are spent at the bedside and on the patient's hospital floor or unit.   **B**

Coding tip: Subsequent observation care codes (99224-99226) are listed out of numeric order in CPT. Refer to codes 99218-99220 for initial observation care services.

RVU			Global Days	Modifiers				
Mod	Non-Fac Total	Fac Total		51	50	62	80	MUE
	2.05	2.05	XXX	0	0	0	0	1

AMA: Aug 11: 11, Aug 13: 13, Jan 13: 9, Jul 12: 10, 11, Jun 11: 3, Jun 13: 3

99226 **Subsequent observation care, per day, for the evaluation and management of a patient, which requires at least 2 of these 3 key components:**

- A detailed interval history;
- A detailed examination;
- Medical decision making of high complexity.

Counseling and/or coordination of care with other physicians, other qualified health care professionals, or agencies are provided consistent with the nature of the problem(s) and the patient's and/or family's needs. Usually, the patient is unstable or has developed a significant complication or a significant new problem. Typically, 35 minutes are spent at the bedside and on the patient's hospital floor or unit.   **B**

Coding tip: Subsequent observation care codes (99224-99226) are listed out of numeric order in CPT. Refer to codes 99218-99220 for initial observation care services.

RVU			Global Days	Modifiers				
Mod	Non-Fac Total	Fac Total		51	50	62	80	MUE
	2.95	2.95	XXX	0	0	0	0	1

AMA: Aug 11: 11, Aug 13: 13, Jan 13: 9, Jul 12: 10, 11, Jun 11: 3, Jun 13: 3, Nov 14: 14

Subsequent Hospital Inpatient Visits

All levels of subsequent care include reviewing the medical record and reviewing the results of diagnostic studies and changes in the patient's status (ie, changes in history, physical condition, and response to management) since the last assessment.

99231 **Subsequent hospital care, per day, for the evaluation and management of a patient, which requires at least 2 of these 3 key components:**

- A problem focused interval history;
- A problem focused examination;
- Medical decision making that is straightforward or of low complexity.

Counseling and/or coordination of care with other physicians, other qualified health care professionals, or agencies are provided consistent with the nature of the problem(s) and the patient's and/or family's needs. Usually, the patient is stable, recovering or improving. Typically, 15 minutes are spent at the bedside and on the patient's hospital floor or unit.   **B**

RVU			Global Days	Modifiers				
Mod	Non-Fac Total	Fac Total		51	50	62	80	MUE
	1.11	1.11	XXX	0	0	0	0	1

AMA: Apr 04: 14, Aug 01: 2, Aug 04: 11, Aug 13: 14, Dec 09: 9, Fall 92: 1, Fall 95: 16, Jan 02: 2, 3, Jan 13: 9, Jan 99: 10, Jul 06: 4, Jul 07: 1, Jul 12: 12, Jun 11: 3, Jun 13: 3, Mar 05: 11, Mar 07: 9, Mar 09: 3, May 05: 1, May 06: 1, 16, May 14: 4, Nov 14: 14, Nov 97: 2, Nov 99: 5, Sep 13: 18, Sep 98: 5, Spring 92: 14, 24, Spring 93: 34, Spring 95: 1, Summer 92: 10, 24, Winter 91: 11

99232 **Subsequent hospital care, per day, for the evaluation and management of a patient, which requires at least 2 of these 3 key components:**

- An expanded problem focused interval history;
- An expanded problem focused examination;
- Medical decision making of moderate complexity.

Counseling and/or coordination of care with other physicians, other qualified health care professionals, or agencies are provided consistent with the nature of the problem(s) and the patient's and/or family's needs. Usually, the patient is responding inadequately to therapy or has developed a minor complication. Typically, 25 minutes are spent at the bedside and on the patient's hospital floor or unit.   **B**

RVU			Global Days	Modifiers				
Mod	Non-Fac Total	Fac Total		51	50	62	80	MUE
	2.03	2.03	XXX	0	0	0	0	1

AMA: Apr 04: 14, Aug 01: 2, Aug 04: 11, Aug 13: 14, Dec 09: 9, Fall 92: 1, Fall 95: 16, Jan 00: 11, Jan 13: 9, Jan 99: 10, Jul 06: 4, Jul 07: 1, Jul 12: 12, Jun 11: 3, Jun 13: 3, Mar 07: 9, Mar 09: 3, May 06: 1, 16, Nov 97: 2, Nov 99: 5, Sep 98: 5, Spring 92: 14, 24, Spring 93: 34, Spring 95: 1, Summer 92: 10, 24, Winter 91: 11

● New   ▲ Revised   ✖ Deleted   ⊙ Moderate Sedation   ➕ Add-on Codes   ⊘ High Risk Denial   Ⓐ Age Edit   ♀ Female   ♂ Male   **AMA** *CPT® Assistant*   **MUE** Medically Unlikely Edit
⊘ Modifier 51 Exempt   ⊖ Modifier 63 Exempt   ⚿ Unlisted   **Modifiers:** *See Inside Back Cover*   Ⓜ Maternity   A2–Z3 ASC Payment Indicators   A–Y OPPS Status Indicators

© 2016 DecisionHealth   CPT © 2014 American Medical Association. All Rights Reserved.   **125**

Evaluation and Management (E/M) Services

99233 – 99236

99233 Subsequent hospital care, per day, for the evaluation and management of a patient, which requires at least 2 of these 3 key components:

- A detailed interval history;

- A detailed examination;

- Medical decision making of high complexity.

Counseling and/or coordination of care with other physicians, other qualified health care professionals, or agencies are provided consistent with the nature of the problem(s) and the patient's and/or family's needs. Usually, the patient is unstable or has developed a significant complication or a significant new problem. Typically, 35 minutes are spent at the bedside and on the patient's hospital floor or unit.   **B**

RVU			Global Days	Modifiers				
Mod	*Non-Fac Total*	*Fac Total*		51	50	62	80	MUE
	2.93	2.93	XXX	0	0	0	0	1

AMA: Apr 04: 14, Aug 01: 2, Aug 04: 11, Aug 13: 13, 14, Dec 09: 9, Fall 92: 1, Fall 95: 16, Jan 13: 9, Jan 99: 10, Jul 06: 4, Jul 07: 1, Jul 12: 12, Jun 11: 3, Jun 13: 3, Mar 07: 9, Mar 09: 3, May 06: 1, 16, May 14: 4, Nov 14: 14, Nov 97: 2, Nov 99: 5, Sep 98: 5, Spring 92: 14, 24, Spring 93: 34, Spring 95: 1, Summer 92: 10, 24, Winter 91: 11

Observation/Inpatient Visits, Same Day

The following codes are used to report observation or inpatient hospital care services provided to patients admitted and discharged on the same date of service. When a patient is admitted to the hospital from observations status on the same date, report only the initial hospital care code. The initial hospital care code reported by the admitting physician should include the services related to the observation status services he/she provided on the same date of inpatient admission.

When "observation status" is initiated in the course of an encounter in another site of service (e.g., hospital emergency department, physician's office, nursing facility), all evaluation and management services provided by the supervising physician in conjunction with initiating "observation status" are considered part of the initial observation care when performed on the same date. The observation care level of service should include the services related to initiating "observations status" provided in the other sites of service as well as in the observation setting when provided by the same individual.

For patients admitted to observation or inpatient care and discharges on a different date, see codes 99218-99220, 99224-99226, 99217, or 99221-99223 and 99238, 99326.

99234 Observation or inpatient hospital care, for the evaluation and management of a patient including admission and discharge on the same date, which requires these 3 key components:

- A detailed or comprehensive history;

- A detailed or comprehensive examination;

- Medical decision making that is straightforward or of low complexity.

Counseling and/or coordination of care with other physicians, other qualified health care professionals, or agencies are provided consistent with the nature of the problem(s) and the patient's and/or family's needs. Usually the presenting problem(s) requiring admission are of low severity. Typically, 40 minutes are spent at the bedside and on the patient's hospital floor or unit.   **B**

RVU			Global Days	Modifiers				
Mod	*Non-Fac Total*	*Fac Total*		51	50	62	80	MUE
	3.76	3.76	XXX	0	0	0	0	1

AMA: Dec 06: 14, Jan 00: 11, Jan 02: 2, Jan 03: 10, Jul 12: 14, Jun 02: 10, Jun 11: 3, Jun 13: 3, Mar 98: 2, May 05: 1, May 98: 1, Nov 05: 10, Nov 97: 2, Sep 00: 3, Sep 06: 8, Sep 10: 4, Sep 98: 5

99235 Observation or inpatient hospital care, for the evaluation and management of a patient including admission and discharge on the same date, which requires these 3 key components:

- A comprehensive history;

- A comprehensive examination; and

- Medical decision making of moderate complexity.

Counseling and/or coordination of care with other physicians, other qualified health care professionals, or agencies are provided consistent with the nature of the problem(s) and the patient's and/or family's needs. Usually the presenting problem(s) requiring admission are of moderate severity. Typically, 50 minutes are spent at the bedside and on the patient's hospital floor or unit. **B**

RVU			Global Days	Modifiers				
Mod	*Non-Fac Total*	*Fac Total*		51	50	62	80	MUE
	4.76	4.76	XXX	0	0	0	0	1

AMA: Dec 06: 14, Jan 00: 11, Jan 02: 2, Jan 03: 10, Jul 12: 14, Jun 02: 10, Jun 11: 3, Jun 13: 3, Mar 98: 2, May 98: 1, Nov 05: 10, Nov 97: 2, Sep 00: 3, Sep 06: 8, Sep 10: 4, Sep 98: 5

99236 Observation or inpatient hospital care, for the evaluation and management of a patient including admission and discharge on the same date, which requires these 3 key components:

- A comprehensive history;

- A comprehensive examination; and

- Medical decision making of high complexity.

Counseling and/or coordination of care with other physicians, other qualified health care professionals, or agencies are provided consistent with the nature of the problem(s) and the patient's and/or family's needs. Usually the presenting problem(s) requiring admission are of high severity. Typically, 55 minutes are spent at the bedside and on the patient's hospital floor or unit. **B**

RVU			Global Days	Modifiers				
Mod	*Non-Fac Total*	*Fac Total*		51	50	62	80	MUE
	6.13	6.13	XXX	0	0	0	0	1

AMA: Dec 06: 14, Jan 00: 11, Jan 02: 2, Jan 03: 10, Jul 12: 14, Jun 02: 10, Jun 11: 3, Jun 13: 3, Mar 98: 2, May 98: 1, Nov 05: 10, Nov 97: 2, Sep 00: 3, Sep 06: 8, Sep 10: 4, Sep 98: 5

● New   ▲ Revised   ✖ Deleted   ⊙ Moderate Sedation   ✚ Add-on Codes   ⊘ High Risk Denial   Ⓐ Age Edit   ♀ Female   ♂ Male   **AMA** *CPT® Assistant*   ***MUE*** Medically Unlikely Edit
⊘ Modifier 51 Exempt   ⊖ Modifier 63 Exempt   ✻ Unlisted   **Modifiers:** *See Inside Back Cover*   Ⓜ Maternity   A 2–Z 3 ASC Payment Indicators   A –Y OPPS Status Indicators

126   CPT © 2014 American Medical Association. All Rights Reserved.   © 2016 DecisionHealth

Hospital Discharge Visits

The hospital discharge day management codes are to be used to report the total duration of time spent by a physician for final hospital discharge of a patient. The codes include, as appropriate, final examination of the patient, discussion of the hospital stay, even if the time spent by the physician on that date is not continuous, instructions for continuing care to all relevant caregivers, and preparation of discharge records, prescriptions and referral forms.

For a patient admitted and discharged from observation or inpatient status on the same date, the services should be reported with codes 99234-99236.

99238 Hospital discharge day management; 30 minutes or less B

RVU			Global Days	Modifiers				
Mod	Non-Fac Total	Fac Total		51	50	62	80	MUE
	2.04	2.04	XXX	0	0	0	0	1

AMA: Aug 04: 11, Aug 13: 13, Dec 09: 9, Fall 92: 1, Jan 02: 2, Jan 99: 10, Jul 11: 16, Jul 12: 10, 12, Jun 13: 3, Mar 98: 3, 11, May 05: 1, May 98: 2, Nov 09: 10, Nov 97: 4, Sep 06: 8, Spring 93: 4

Pub 100-02, 15, 30; 100-04, 13, 70.2

99239 Hospital discharge day management; more than 30 minutes B

RVU			Global Days	Modifiers				
Mod	Non-Fac Total	Fac Total		51	50	62	80	MUE
	3.02	3.02	XXX	0	0	0	0	1

AMA: Aug 04: 11, Aug 13: 13, Dec 09: 9, Jan 02: 2, Jan 99: 10, Jul 11: 16, Jul 12: 12, Jun 13: 3, Mar 98: 3, 11, May 98: 2, Nov 09: 10, Nov 97: 4, Sep 06: 8

Pub 100-02, 15, 30

Consultation Visits

A consultation is a type of evaluation and management service provided by a physician at the request of another physician or appropriate source to either recommend care for a specific condition or problem or to determine whether to accept responsibility for ongoing management of the patient's entire care or for the care of a specific condition or problem.

A physician consultant may initiate diagnostic and/or therapeutic services at the same or subsequent visit.

A "consultation" initiated by a patient and/or family, and not requested by a physician or other appropriate source (e.g., physician assistant, nurse practitioner, doctor of chiropractic, physical therapist, occupational therapist, speech-language pathologist, psychologist, social worker, lawyer, or insurance company), is not reported using the consultation codes, but may be reported using the office visit, home service, or domiciliary/rest home care codes.

The written or verbal request for consult may be made by a physician or other appropriate source and documented in the patient's medical record by either the consulting or requesting physician or appropriate source. The consultant's opinion and any services that were ordered or performed must also be documented in the patient's medical record and communicated by written report to the requesting physician or other appropriate source.

If a consultation is mandated (e.g., by a third-party payer), modifier 32 should also be reported.

Any specifically identifiable procedure (i.e., identified with a specific CPT code) performed on or subsequent to the date of the initial consultation should be reported separately.

If subsequent to the completion of a consultation the consultant assumes responsibility for management of a portion or all of the patient's condition(s), the appropriate Evaluation and Management services code for the site of service should be reported. In the hospital or nursing facility setting, the consulting physician should use the appropriate inpatient consultation code for the initial encounter and then subsequent hospital or nursing facility setting, the consulting physician should use the appropriate inpatient consultation code for the initial encounter and then subsequent hospital or nursing facility care codes. In the office setting, the consultant should use the appropriate office or other outpatient consultation codes and then the established patient office or other outpatient services codes.

To report services provided to a patient who is admitted to a hospital or nursing facility in the course of an encounter in the office or other ambulatory facility, see the notes for Initial Hospital Inpatient Care or Initial Nursing Facility Care.

For definitions of key components and commonly used terms, see Evaluation and Management Services Guidelines.

Office or Other Outpatient Consultations

New or Established Patient

The following set of codes are used to report consultations provided in the office or in an outpatient or other ambulatory facility, including hospital observation services, home services, domiciliary, rest home, or emergency department (see the preceding consultation information). Follow-up visits in the consultant's office or other outpatient facility that are initiated by the physician consultant or patient are reported using the appropriate codes for established patients, office visits, 99211-99215, domiciliary, rest home, 99334-99337, or home, 99347-99350. If an additional request for an opinion or advice regarding the same or a new problem is received from another physician or other appropriate source and documented in the medical record, the office consultation codes may be used again. Services that constitute transfer of care (ie, are provided for the management of the patient's entire care or for the care of a specific condition or problem) are reported with the appropriate new or established patient care codes for office or other outpatient visits, domiciliary, rest home services, or home services.

Definition of Transfer of Care

Transfer of care is the process whereby a physician who is providing management for some or all of a patient's problems relinquishes this responsibility to another physician who explicitly agrees to accept this responsibility and who, from the initial encounter, is not providing consultative serves. The physician transferring care is then no longer providing care for these problems though he or she may continue providing care for other conditions when appropriate. Consultation codes should not be reported by the physician who has agreed to accept transfer of care before an initial evaluation but are appropriate to report if the decision to accept transfer of care cannot be made until after the initial consultation evaluation, regardless of site of service.

99241 Office consultation for a new or established patient, which requires these 3 key components:

- A problem focused history;
- A problem focused examination; and
- Straightforward medical decision making.

Counseling and/or coordination of care with other physicians, other qualified health care professionals, or agencies are provided consistent with the nature of the problem(s) and the patient's and/or family's needs. Usually, the presenting problem(s) are self limited or minor. Typically, 15 minutes are spent face-to-face with the patient and/or family. ⊘ E

RVU			Global Days	Modifiers				
Mod	Non-Fac Total	Fac Total		51	50	62	80	MUE
	1.34	0.92	XXX	9	9	9	9	

AMA: Apr 00: 10, Apr 07: 11, Apr 12: 10, Aug 01: 3, Aug 09: 9, Aug 14: 3, Dec 05: 10, Jan 02: 2, Jan 06: 46, Jan 07: 28, Jan 10: 3, Jan 13: 9, Jan 15: 12, Jul 02: 2, Jul 07: 1, Jul 10: 4, Jun 06: 1, Jun 11: 3, Jun 13: 3, Jun 99: 10, May 05: 1, May 06: 1, 16, May 08: 13, Nov 08: 10, Nov 14: 14, Oct 97: 1, Sep 02: 11, Sep 06: 8, Sep 14: 13, Sep 98: 5, Spring 92: 4, 23, 24, Spring 93: 4, Spring 95: 1, Summer 92: 12, Winter 91: 11

Pub 100-02, 15, 30; 100-04, 32, 130.1

© 2016 DecisionHealth CPT © 2014 American Medical Association. All Rights Reserved.

Evaluation and Management (E/M) Services

99242 – 99251

99242 Office consultation for a new or established patient, which requires these 3 key components:

- An expanded problem focused history;
- An expanded problem focused examination; and
- Straightforward medical decision making.

Counseling and/or coordination of care with other physicians, other qualified health care professionals, or agencies are provided consistent with the nature of the problem(s) and the patient's and/or family's needs. Usually, the presenting problem(s) are of low severity. Typically, 30 minutes are spent face-to-face with the patient and/or family. ⊗🅴

RVU			Global Days	Modifiers				
Mod	Non-Fac Total	Fac Total		51	50	62	80	MUE
	2.52	1.93	XXX	9	9	9	9	

AMA: Apr 07: 11, Aug 01: 3, Dec 05: 10, Jan 02: 2, Jan 10: 3, Jan 13: 9, Jan 15: 12, Jul 02: 2, Jul 07: 1, Jun 06: 1, Jun 11: 3, Jun 13: 3, May 06: 1, 16, Oct 97: 1, Sep 02: 11, Sep 06: 8, Sep 14: 13, Sep 98: 5, Spring 92: 4, 23, 24, Spring 93: 2, 34, Spring 95: 1, Summer 92: 12, Winter 91: 11

Pub 100-02, 15, 30; 100-04, 32, 130.1

99243 Office consultation for a new or established patient, which requires these 3 key components:

- A detailed history;
- A detailed examination; and
- Medical decision making of low complexity.

Counseling and/or coordination of care with other physicians, other qualified health care professionals, or agencies are provided consistent with the nature of the problem(s) and the patient's and/or family's needs. Usually, the presenting problem(s) are of moderate severity. Typically, 40 minutes are spent face-to-face with the patient and/or family. ⊗🅴

RVU			Global Days	Modifiers				
Mod	Non-Fac Total	Fac Total		51	50	62	80	MUE
	3.45	2.70	XXX	9	9	9	9	

AMA: Apr 07: 11, Aug 01: 3, Dec 05: 10, Jan 02: 2, Jan 10: 3, Jan 13: 9, Jan 15: 12, Jul 02: 2, Jul 07: 1, Jun 06: 1, Jun 11: 3, Jun 13: 3, May 06: 1, 16, Oct 03: 5, Oct 97: 1, Sep 02: 11, Sep 06: 8, Sep 14: 13, Sep 98: 5, Spring 92: 4, 23, 24, Spring 93: 2, 34, Spring 95: 1, Summer 92: 12, Winter 91: 11

Pub 100-02, 15, 30; 100-04, 32, 130.1

99244 Office consultation for a new or established patient, which requires these 3 key components:

- A comprehensive history;
- A comprehensive examination; and
- Medical decision making of moderate complexity.

Counseling and/or coordination of care with other physicians, other qualified health care professionals, or agencies are provided consistent with the nature of the problem(s) and the patient's and/or family's needs. Usually, the presenting problem(s) are of moderate to high severity. Typically, 60 minutes are spent face-to-face with the patient and/or family. ⊗🅴

RVU			Global Days	Modifiers				
Mod	Non-Fac Total	Fac Total		51	50	62	80	MUE
	5.16	4.34	XXX	9	9	9	9	

AMA: Apr 07: 11, Aug 01: 3, Aug 13: 12, Dec 05: 10, Jan 02: 2, Jan 10: 3, Jan 13: 9, Jan 15: 12, Jul 02: 2, Jul 07: 1, Jun 06: 1, Jun 11: 3, Jun 13: 3, May 06: 1, 16, Oct 03: 5, Oct 97: 1, Sep 02: 11, Sep 06: 8, Sep 14: 13, Sep 98: 5, Spring 92: 3, 23, 24, Spring 93: 2, 34, Spring 95: 1, Summer 92: 12, Winter 91: 11

Pub 100-02, 15, 30; 100-04, 32, 130.1

99245 Office consultation for a new or established patient, which requires these 3 key components:

- A comprehensive history;
- A comprehensive examination; and
- Medical decision making of high complexity.

Counseling and/or coordination of care with other physicians, other qualified health care professionals, or agencies are provided consistent with the nature of the problem(s) and the patient's and/or family's needs. Usually, the presenting problem(s) are of moderate to high severity. Typically, 80 minutes are spent face-to-face with the patient and/or family. ⊗🅴

RVU			Global Days	Modifiers				
Mod	Non-Fac Total	Fac Total		51	50	62	80	MUE
	6.29	5.37	XXX	9	9	9	9	

AMA: Apr 07: 11, Apr 12: 10, Aug 01: 2, Aug 14: 3, Dec 05: 10, Jan 02: 2, Jan 10: 3, Jan 13: 9, Jan 15: 12, Jul 02: 2, Jul 07: 1, Jul 10: 4, Jun 06: 1, Jun 11: 3, Jun 13: 3, May 06: 1, 16, Oct 97: 1, Sep 02: 11, Sep 06: 8, Sep 14: 13, Sep 98: 5, Spring 92: 4, 23, 24, Spring 93: 2, 34, Spring 95: 1, Summer 92: 12, Winter 91: 11

Pub 100-02, 15, 30; 100-04, 32, 130.1

Inpatient Consultation Visits

New or Established Patient

The following codes are used to report physician or other qualified healthcare professional consultations provided to hospital inpatients, residents of nursing facilities, or patients in a partial hospital setting. Only one consultation should be reported by a consultant per admission. Subsequent services during the same admission are reported using subsequent hospital care codes (99231-99233) or subsequent nursing facility care codes (99307-99310), including services to complete the initial consultation, monitor progress, revise recommendations, or address a new problem. Use subsequent hospital care codes (99231-99233) or subsequent nursing facility care codes (99307-99310) to report transfer of care services (see Concurrent Care and Transfer of Care definitions).

When an inpatient consultation is performed on a date that a patient is admitted to a hospital or nursing facility, all evaluation and management services provided by the consultant related to the admission are reported with the inpatient consultation service code (99251-99255). If a patient is admitted after an outpatient consultation (office, emergency department, etc), and the patient is not seen on the unit on the date of admission, only report the outpatient consultation code (99241-99245). If the patient is seen by the consultant on the unit on the date of admission, report all evaluation and management services provided by the consultant related to the admission with either the inpatient consultant code (99251-99255) or with the initial inpatient admission service code (99221-99223). Do not report both an outpatient consultation and inpatient consultation for service related to the same inpatient stay. When transfer of care services are provided on a date subsequent to the outpatient consultation, use the subsequent hospital care (99231-99233) or subsequent nursing facility care codes (99307-99310).

99251 Inpatient consultation for a new or established patient, which requires these 3 key components:

- A problem focused history;
- A problem focused examination; and
- Straightforward medical decision making.

● New   ▲ Revised   ✖ Deleted   ⊙ Moderate Sedation   ✚ Add-on Codes   ⊘ High Risk Denial   Ⓐ Age Edit   ♀ Female   ♂ Male   **AMA** *CPT® Assistant*   **MUE** Medically Unlikely Edit
⊘ Modifier 51 Exempt   ⊖ Modifier 63 Exempt   🅇 Unlisted   **Modifiers:** *See Inside Back Cover*   Ⓜ Maternity   🄰2–🅉3 ASC Payment Indicators   🄰–🅈 OPPS Status Indicators

128   CPT © 2014 American Medical Association. All Rights Reserved.   © 2016 DecisionHealth

Counseling and/or coordination of care with other physicians, other qualified health care professionals, or agencies are provided consistent with the nature of the problem(s) and the patient's and/or family's needs. Usually, the presenting problem(s) are self limited or minor. Typically, 20 minutes are spent at the bedside and on the patient's hospital floor or unit. ⊝E

RVU			Global Days	Modifiers				
Mod	Non-Fac Total	Fac Total		51	50	62	80	MUE
	1.38	1.38	XXX	9	9	9	9	

AMA: Aug 01: 3, Jan 10: 3, Jan 13: 9, Jul 06: 19, Jul 07: 1, Jun 06: 1, Jun 13: 3, May 05: 1, May 06: 1, 16, Oct 97: 1, Sep 02: 11, Sep 98: 5, Spring 92: 16, 23, 24, Spring 93: 34, Spring 95: 1, Summer 92: 12, Winter 91: 11

Pub 100-02, 15, 30

99252 **Inpatient consultation for a new or established patient, which requires these 3 key components:**

- An expanded problem focused history;
- An expanded problem focused examination; and
- Straightforward medical decision making.

Counseling and/or coordination of care with other physicians, other qualified health care professionals, or agencies are provided consistent with the nature of the problem(s) and the patient's and/or family's needs. Usually, the presenting problem(s) are of low severity. Typically, 40 minutes are spent at the bedside and on the patient's hospital floor or unit. ⊝E

RVU			Global Days	Modifiers				
Mod	Non-Fac Total	Fac Total		51	50	62	80	MUE
	2.11	2.11	XXX	9	9	9	9	

AMA: Aug 01: 4, Jan 10: 3, Jan 13: 9, Jul 06: 19, Jul 07: 1, Jun 06: 1, Jun 13: 3, May 06: 1, 16, Oct 97: 1, Sep 02: 11, Sep 98: 5, Spring 92: 16, 23, 24, Spring 95: 1, Summer 92: 12, Summer 93: 34, Winter 91: 11

Pub 100-02, 15, 30

99253 **Inpatient consultation for a new or established patient, which requires these 3 key components:**

- A detailed history;
- A detailed examination; and
- Medical decision making of low complexity.

Counseling and/or coordination of care with other physicians, other qualified health care professionals, or agencies are provided consistent with the nature of the problem(s) and the patient's and/or family's needs. Usually, the presenting problem(s) are of moderate severity. Typically, 55 minutes are spent at the bedside and on the patient's hospital floor or unit. ⊝E

RVU			Global Days	Modifiers				
Mod	Non-Fac Total	Fac Total		51	50	62	80	MUE
	3.24	3.24	XXX	9	9	9	9	

AMA: Aug 01: 4, Jan 10: 3, Jan 13: 9, Jul 06: 19, Jul 07: 1, Jun 06: 1, Jun 13: 3, May 06: 1, 16, Oct 97: 1, Sep 02: 11, Sep 98: 5, Spring 92: 16, 23, 24, Spring 95: 1, Summer 92: 12, Summer 93: 34, Winter 91: 11

Pub 100-02, 15, 30

99254 **Inpatient consultation for a new or established patient, which requires these 3 key components:**

- A comprehensive history;
- A comprehensive examination; and
- Medical decision making of moderate complexity.

Counseling and/or coordination of care with other physicians, other qualified health care professionals, or agencies are provided consistent with the nature of the problem(s) and the patient's and/or family's needs. Usually, the presenting problem(s) are of moderate to high severity. Typically, 80 minutes are spent at the bedside and on the patient's hospital floor or unit. ⊝E

RVU			Global Days	Modifiers				
Mod	Non-Fac Total	Fac Total		51	50	62	80	MUE
	4.72	4.72	XXX	9	9	9	9	

AMA: Aug 01: 4, Jan 10: 3, Jan 13: 9, Jul 06: 19, Jul 07: 1, Jun 06: 1, Jun 13: 3, May 06: 1, 16, Oct 97: 1, Sep 02: 11, Sep 98: 5, Spring 92: 16, 23, 24, Spring 95: 1, Summer 92: 12, Summer 93: 34, Winter 91: 11

Pub 100-02, 15, 30

99255 **Inpatient consultation for a new or established patient, which requires these 3 key components:**

- A comprehensive history;
- A comprehensive examination; and
- Medical decision making of high complexity.

Counseling and/or coordination of care with other physicians, other qualified health care professionals, or agencies are provided consistent with the nature of the problem(s) and the patient's and/or family's needs. Usually, the presenting problem(s) are of moderate to high severity. Typically, 110 minutes are spent at the bedside and on the patient's hospital floor or unit. ⊝E

RVU			Global Days	Modifiers				
Mod	Non-Fac Total	Fac Total		51	50	62	80	MUE
	5.68	5.68	XXX	9	9	9	9	

AMA: Aug 01: 4, Jan 10: 3, Jan 13: 9, Jul 06: 19, Jul 07: 1, Jun 06: 1, Jun 13: 3, May 06: 1, 16, Nov 14: 14, Oct 97: 1, Sep 02: 11, Sep 98: 5, Spring 92: 16, 23, 24, Spring 95: 1, Summer 92: 12, Summer 93: 34, Winter 91: 11

Pub 100-02, 15, 30

Emergency Department Visits

New or Established Patient

The following codes are used to report evaluation and management services provided in the emergency department. No distinction is made between new and established patients in the emergency department.

An emergency department is defined as an organized hospital-based facility for the provision of unscheduled episodic services to patients who present for immediate medical attention. The facility must be available 24 hours a day.

For critical care services provided in the emergency department, see Critical Care notes and 99291, 99292.

For evaluation and management services provided to a patient in an observation area of a hospital, see 99217-99220.

For observation or inpatient care services services (including admission and discharge services), see 99234-99236.

Time as a Factor in the Emergency Department Setting

Time is not a descriptive component for the emergency department levels of E/M services because emergency department services are typically provided on a variable intensity basis, often involving multiple encounters with several patients over an extended period of time. Therefore, it is often difficult for physicians to provide accurate estimates of the time spent face-to-face with the patient.

● New   ▲ Revised   ✖ Deleted   ⊙ Moderate Sedation   ✚ Add-on Codes   ⊘ High Risk Denial   Ⓐ Age Edit   ♀ Female   ♂ Male   **AMA** *CPT® Assistant*   ***MUE*** Medically Unlikely Edit

⊘ Modifier 51 Exempt   ⊖ Modifier 63 Exempt   ☒ Unlisted   **Modifiers:** *See Inside Back Cover*   Ⓜ Maternity   A2–Z3 ASC Payment Indicators   A–Y OPPS Status Indicators

© 2016 DecisionHealth   CPT © 2014 American Medical Association. All Rights Reserved.   **129**

Evaluation and Management (E/M) Services

99281 – 99285

99281 **Emergency department visit for the evaluation and management of a patient, which requires these 3 key components:**

- A problem focused history;
- A problem focused examination; and
- Straightforward medical decision making.

Counseling and/or coordination of care with other physicians, other qualified health care professionals, or agencies are provided consistent with the nature of the problem(s) and the patient's and/or family's needs. Usually, the presenting problem(s) are self limited or minor.   **J2**

RVU			Global Days	Modifiers				
Mod	Non-Fac Total	Fac Total		51	50	62	80	MUE
	0.60	0.60	XXX	0	0	0	0	1

AMA: Apr 02: 14, Dec 06: 14, Dec 07: 13, Feb 00: 11, Feb 06: 14, Feb 96: 3, Jan 00: 11, Jan 13: 9, Jan 15: 12, Jul 02: 2, Jun 13: 3, Nov 05: 10, Nov 14: 14, Sep 00: 3, Sep 98: 5, Spring 92: 24, Spring 93: 34, Spring 95: 1, Summer 92: 18, Winter 91: 11

Pub 100-04, 13, 70.2

99282 **Emergency department visit for the evaluation and management of a patient, which requires these 3 key components:**

- An expanded problem focused history;
- An expanded problem focused examination; and
- Medical decision making of low complexity.

Counseling and/or coordination of care with other physicians, other qualified health care professionals, or agencies are provided consistent with the nature of the problem(s) and the patient's and/or family's needs. Usually, the presenting problem(s) are of low to moderate severity.   **J2**

RVU			Global Days	Modifiers				
Mod	Non-Fac Total	Fac Total		51	50	62	80	MUE
	1.17	1.17	XXX	0	0	0	0	1

AMA: Apr 02: 14, Dec 06: 14, Dec 07: 13, Feb 00: 11, Feb 06: 14, Feb 96: 3, Jan 00: 11, Jan 13: 9, Jan 15: 12, Jul 02: 2, Jun 13: 3, Nov 05: 10, Sep 00: 3, Sep 98: 5, Spring 92: 24, Spring 93: 34, Spring 95: 1, Summer 92: 18, Summer 95: 1, Winter 91: 11

Pub 100-04, 13, 70.2

99283 **Emergency department visit for the evaluation and management of a patient, which requires these 3 key components:**

- An expanded problem focused history;
- An expanded problem focused examination; and
- Medical decision making of moderate complexity.

Counseling and/or coordination of care with other physicians, other qualified health care professionals, or agencies are provided consistent with the nature of the problem(s) and the patient's and/or family's needs. Usually, the presenting problem(s) are of moderate severity.   **J2**

RVU			Global Days	Modifiers				
Mod	Non-Fac Total	Fac Total		51	50	62	80	MUE
	1.75	1.75	XXX	0	0	0	0	1

AMA: Apr 02: 14, Dec 06: 14, Dec 07: 13, Feb 00: 11, Feb 06: 14, Feb 96: 3, Jan 00: 11, Jan 13: 9, Jan 15: 12, Jul 02: 2, Jun 13: 3, Nov 05: 10, Sep 00: 3, Sep 98: 5, Spring 92: 24, Spring 93: 34, Spring 95: 1, Summer 92: 18, Summer 95: 1, Winter 91: 11

Pub 100-04, 13, 70.2

99284 **Emergency department visit for the evaluation and management of a patient, which requires these 3 key components:**

- A detailed history;
- A detailed examination; and
- Medical decision making of moderate complexity.

Counseling and/or coordination of care with other physicians, other qualified health care professionals, or agencies are provided consistent with the nature of the problem(s) and the patient's and/or family's needs. Usually, the presenting problem(s) are of high severity, and require urgent evaluation by the physician, or other qualified health care professionals but do not pose an immediate significant threat to life or physiologic function.   **J2**

RVU			Global Days	Modifiers				
Mod	Non-Fac Total	Fac Total		51	50	62	80	MUE
	3.32	3.32	XXX	0	0	0	0	1

AMA: Apr 02: 14, Dec 06: 14, Dec 07: 13, Feb 00: 11, Feb 06: 14, Feb 96: 3, Jan 00: 11, Jan 13: 9, Jan 15: 12, Jul 02: 2, Jun 13: 3, Nov 05: 10, Sep 00: 3, Sep 98: 5, Spring 92: 24, Spring 93: 34, Spring 95: 1, Summer 92: 18, Summer 95: 1, Winter 91: 11

Pub 100-04, 13, 70.2

99285 **Emergency department visit for the evaluation and management of a patient, which requires these 3 key components within the constraints imposed by the urgency of the patient's clinical condition and/or mental status:**

- A comprehensive history;
- A comprehensive examination; and
- Medical decision making of high complexity.

Counseling and/or coordination of care with other physicians, other qualified health care professionals, or agencies are provided consistent with the nature of the problem(s) and the patient's and/or family's needs. Usually, the presenting problem(s) are of high severity and pose an immediate significant threat to life or physiologic function.   **J2**

RVU			Global Days	Modifiers				
Mod	Non-Fac Total	Fac Total		51	50	62	80	MUE
	4.90	4.90	XXX	0	0	0	0	1

AMA: Apr 02: 14, Aug 98: 8, Dec 06: 14, Dec 07: 13, Feb 00: 11, Feb 06: 14, Feb 96: 3, Jan 00: 11, Jan 13: 9, Jan 15: 12, Jul 02: 2, Jun 13: 3, Mar 05: 11, Nov 05: 10, Nov 14: 14, Nov 99: 23, Sep 00: 3, Sep 02: 11, Sep 98: 5, Spring 92: 24, Spring 93: 34, Spring 95: 1, Summer 92: 18, Summer 95: 1, Winter 91: 11

Pub 100-04, 13, 70.2

Emergency Department Classification of New vs Established Patient

No distinction is made between new and established patients in the emergency department. E/M services in the emergency department category may be reported for any new or established patient who presents for treatment in the emergency department.

● New   ▲ Revised   ✖ Deleted   ⊙ Moderate Sedation   ✚ Add-on Codes   ⊘ High Risk Denial   Ⓐ Age Edit   ♀ Female   ♂ Male   **AMA** *CPT® Assistant*   *MUE* Medically Unlikely Edit
⊘ Modifier 51 Exempt   ⊖ Modifier 63 Exempt   ✂ Unlisted   **Modifiers:** *See Inside Back Cover*   Ⓜ Maternity   **A2–Z3** ASC Payment Indicators   **A–Y** OPPS Status Indicators

Other Emergency Department Services

In directed emergency care, advanced life support, the physician or other qualified healthcare professional is located in a hospital emergency or critical care department, and is in two-way voice communication with ambulance or rescue personnel outside the hospital. The physician directs the performance of necessary medical procedures, including but not limited to: telemetry of cardiac rhythm; cardiac and/or pulmonary resuscitation; endotracheal or esophageal obturator airway intubation; administration of intravenous fluids and/or administration of intramuscular, intratracheal, or subcutaneous drugs; and/or electrical conversion of arrhythmia.

99288 **Physician or other qualified health care professional direction of emergency medical systems (EMS) emergency care, advanced life support** ⊘B

RVU			Global Days	Modifiers				
Mod	Non-Fac Total	Fac Total		51	50	62	80	MUE
	0.00	0.00	XXX	9	9	9	9	0

AMA: May 05: 1, May 13: 6, Nov 07: 5, Summer 92: 18

Critical Care

Critical care is the direct delivery by a physician or other qualified health care professional of medical care for a critically ill or critically injured patient. A critical illness or injury acutely impairs one of more vital organ systems such that there is a high probability of imminent or life threatening deterioration in the patient's condition. Critical care involves high complexity decision making to assess, manipulate, and support vital system function(s) to treat single or multiple vital organ system failure and/or to prevent further life threatening deterioration of the patient's condition. Examples of vital organ system failure include, but are not limited to: central nervous system failure, circulatory failure, shock, renal, hepatic, metabolic, and/or respiratory failure.

Although critical care typically requires interpretation of multiple physiologic parameters and/or application of advanced technology(s), critical care may be provided in life threatening situations when these elements are not present. Critical care may be provided on multiple days, even if no changes are made in the treatment rendered to the patient, provided that the patient's condition continues to require the level of physician attention described above.

Providing medical care to a critically ill, injured, or post-operative patient qualifies as a critical care service only if both the illness or injury and the treatment being provided meet the above requirements. Critical care is usually but not always, given in a critical care area, such as the coronary care unit, intensive care unit, or the emergency care facility.

Inpatient critical care services provided to infants 29 days through 71 months of age are reported with pediatric critical care codes 99471-99476. The pediatric critical care codes are reported as long as the infant/young child qualifies for critical care services during the hospital stay through 71 months of age. Inpatient critical care services provided to neonates (28 days of age or younger) are reported with the neonatal critical care codes 99468 and 99469. The neonatal critical care codes are reported as long as the neonate qualifies for critical care services during the hospital stay through the 28th postnatal day. The reporting of pediatric and neonatal critical care services is not based on time or the type of unit (eg, pediatric or neonatal critical care unit) and it is not dependent upon the type of provider delivering the care. To report critical care services provided in the outpatient setting (eg, emergency department or office), of neonates and pediatric patients up through 71 months of age, see the critical care codes 99291, 99292. If the same physician provides critical care services for a neonatal or pediatric patient in both the outpatient and inpatient settings on the same day, report only the appropriate neonatal or pediatric critical care code 99468-99472 for all critical care services provided on that day. Also report 99291-99292 for neonatal or pediatric critical care services provided by the physician providing critical care at one facility but transferring the patient to another facility. Critical care services provided by a second physician or a different specialty not reporting a per day neonatal or pediatric critical care code can be reported with codes 99291-99292. For additional instructions on reporting these services, see the Neonatal and Pediatric Critical Care section and codes 99468-99476.

Services for a patient who is not critically ill but happens to be in a critical care unit are reported using other appropriate E/M codes.

Critical care and other E/M services may be provided to the same patient on the same date by the same individual.

For reporting by professionals, the following services are included in reporting critical care when performed during the critical period by the physician(s) providing critical care: the interpretation of cardiac output measurements (93561, 93562), chest X-rays (71010, 71015, 71020), pulse oximetry (94760, 94761, 94762), blood gases, and information data stored in computers (eg, ECGs, blood pressures, hematologic data [99090]; gastric intubation (43752, 43753); temporary transcutaneous pacing (92953); ventilator management (94002-94004, 94660, 94662); and vascular access procedures (36000, 36410, 36415, 36591, 36600). Any services performed that are not included in this listing should be reported separately. Facilities may report the above services separately.

Codes 99291, 99292 should be reported for the attendance during the transport of critically ill or critically injured patients older than 24 months of age to or from a facility or hospital. For physician transport service of critically ill or critically injured pediatric patients 24 months of age or younger see 99466, 99467.

The critical care codes 99291 and 99292 are used to report the total duration of time spent providing critical care services to a critically ill or critically injured patient, even if the time spent by the physician on that date is not continuous. For any given period of time spent providing critical care services, the individual must devote his or her full attention to the patient and, therefore, cannot provide services to any other patient during the same time period.

Time spent with the individual patient should be recorded in the patient's record. The time that can be reported as critical care is the time spent engaged in work directly related to the individual patient's care whether that time was spent at the immediate bedside or elsewhere on the floor or unit. For example, time spent on the unit or at the nursing station on the floor reviewing test results or imaging studies, discussing the critically ill patient's care with other medical staff or documenting critical care services in the medical record would be reported as critical care, even though it does not occur at the beside, Also, when the patient is unable or lacks capacity to participate in discussions, time spent on the floor or unit with family members or surrogate decision makers obtaining a medical history, reviewing the patient's condition or prognosis, or discussing treatment or limitation(s) of treatment may be reported as critical care, provided that the conversation bears directly on the management of the patient.

Time spent in activities that occur outside of the unit or off the floor (eg, telephone calls whether taken at home, in the office, or elsewhere in the hospital) may not be reported as critical care since the individual is not immediately available to the patient. Time spent in activities that do not directly contribute to the treatment of the patient may not be reported as critical care, even if they are performed in the critical care unit (eg, participation in administrative meetings or telephone calls to discuss other patients). Time spent performing separately reportable procedures or services should not be included in the time reported as critical care time. No individual may report remote real-time interactive video-conferenced critical care services (0188T, 0189T) for the period in which any other physician or other qualified healthcare professional reports 99291, 99292.

Code 99291 is used to report the first 30-74 minutes of critical care on a given date. It should be used only once per date even if the time spent by the individual is not continuous on that date. Critical care of less than 30 minutes total duration on a given date should be reported with the appropriate E/M code. Code 99292 is used to report additional block(s) of time of up to 30 minutes each beyond the first 74 minutes. (See the following table.)

The following examples illustrate the correct reporting of critical care services:

● New   ▲ Revised   ✖ Deleted   ⊙ Moderate Sedation   ✚ Add-on Codes   ⊘ High Risk Denial   Ⓐ Age Edit   ♀ Female   ♂ Male   **AMA** *CPT® Assistant*   **MUE** Medically Unlikely Edit
🚫 Modifier 51 Exempt   ⊖ Modifier 63 Exempt   🚫 Unlisted   **Modifiers:** *See Inside Back Cover*   Ⓜ Maternity   A2-Z3 ASC Payment Indicators   A-Y OPPS Status Indicators

© 2016 DecisionHealth   CPT © 2014 American Medical Association. All Rights Reserved.   **131**

Total Duration of Critical Care	Codes
Less than 30 minutes	Other E/M code(s)
30 minutes -74 minutes (30 minutes-1 hour, 14 minutes)	99291 x 1
75 minutes -104 minutes (1 hour, 15 minutes – 1 hour, 44 minutes	99291 x 1 + 99292 x 1
105 minutes -134 minutes (1 hour, 45 minutes – 2 hours, 14 minutes)	99291 x 1 + 99292 x 2
135 minutes -164 minutes (2 hours, 15 minutes – 2 hours, 44 minutes)	99291 x 1 + 99292 x 3
165 minutes -194 minutes (2 hours, 45 minutes – 3 hours, 15 minutes)	99291 x 1 + 99292 x 4
195 minutes or longer (3 hours, 14 minutes or longer)	99291 x 1 + 99292 as appropriate (see illustrated reporting examples above)

99291 Critical care, evaluation and management of the critically ill or critically injured patient; first 30-74 minutes

RVU			Global Days	Modifiers				
Mod	Non-Fac Total	Fac Total		51	50	62	80	MUE
	7.74	6.31	XXX	0	0	0	0	1

AMA: Apr 00: 6, Apr 97: 3, Aug 04: 7, 10, Aug 11: 10, Aug 14: 5, Dec 00: 15, Dec 06: 13, Dec 98: 6, Feb 03: 15, Feb 13: 17, Feb 15: 10, Jan 09: 5, Jan 96: 7, Jul 02: 2, Jul 05: 15, Jul 06: 4, Jul 09: 10, Jul 12: 13, Mar 09: 3, May 05: 1, May 13: 6, May 14: 4, Nov 05: 10, Nov 07: 5, Nov 99: 3, Oct 03: 2, Oct 04: 14, Oct 14: 14, Sep 00: 1, Sep 11: 3, Summer 92: 18, Summer 93: 1, Summer 95: 1

+ 99292 Critical care, evaluation and management of the critically ill or critically injured patient; each additional 30 minutes (List separately in addition to code for primary service)

RVU			Global Days	Modifiers				
Mod	Non-Fac Total	Fac Total		51	50	62	80	MUE
	3.46	3.16	ZZZ	0	0	0	0	

AMA: Apr 00: 6, Apr 97: 3, Aug 04: 10, Aug 11: 10, Aug 14: 5, Dec 00: 15, Dec 06: 13, Dec 98: 6, Feb 03: 15, Feb 13: 17, Feb 15: 10, Jan 09: 5, Jan 96: 7, Jul 05: 15, Jul 06: 4, Mar 09: 3, May 13: 6, May 14: 4, Nov 05: 10, Nov 07: 5, Nov 99: 3, Oct 03: 2, Oct 04: 14, Oct 14: 14, Sep 00: 1, Sep 11: 3, Summer 92: 18, Summer 93: 1, Summer 95: 1

Services that are Included in Critical Care

For professional reporting, the following services are included in critical care when performed during the critical period by the physician(s) providing critical care: the interpretation of cardiac output measurements (93561, 93562), chest X-rays (71010, 71015, 71020), pulse oximetry (94760, 94761, 94762), blood gases, and information data stored in computers (eg, ECGs, blood pressures, hematologic data (99090), gastric intubation (43752, 43753), temporary transcutaneous pacing (92953), ventilator management (94002-94004, 94660, 94662), and vascular access procedures (36000, 36410, 36415, 36591, 36600). Any services performed that are not listed above should be reported separately. Facilities may report the above services separately.

Nursing Facility Visits

The following codes are used to report evaluation and management services to patients in nursing facilities (formerly known as skilled nursing facilities [SNF's], intermediate care facilities [ICF's], or long term care facilities [LTCF's]).

The codes are also used to report of evaluation and management services provided to a patient in a psychiatric residential treatment center (a facility or distinct part of a facility for psychiatric care, which provides a 24-hour therapeutically planned and professionally staffed group living and learning environment). If procedures such as medical psychotherapy are provided in addition to evaluation and management services, these should be reported in addition to the evaluation and management services provided.

Nursing facilities that provide convalescent, rehabilitative, or long term care are required to conduct comprehensive, accurate, standardized, and reproducible assessments of each resident's functional capacity using a Resident Assessment Instrument (RAI). All RAIs include the Minimum Data Set (MDS), Resident Assessment Protocols (RAPs), and utilization guidelines. The MDS is the primary screening and assessment tool; the RAPs trigger the identification of potential problems and provide guidelines for follow-up assessments.

Physicians have a central role in assuring that all residents receive thorough assessments and that medical plans of care are instituted or revised to enhance or maintain the residents' physical and psychosocial functioning. This role includes providing input in the development of the MDS and a multi-disciplinary plan of care, as required by regulations pertaining to the care of nursing facility residents. Initial assessments in a nursing facility are only provided by physicians.

Two major subcategories of nursing facility services are recognized: Initial Nursing Facility Care and Subsequent Nursing Facility Care. Both subcategories apply to new or established patients.

For definitions of key components and commonly used terms, please see Evaluation and Management Guidelines.

(For care plan oversight services provided to nursing facility residents, see 99379-99380).

Initial Nursing Facility Visits
New or Established Patient

When the patient is admitted to the nursing facility in the course of an encounter in another site of service (e.g., office, hospital emergency department), all evaluation and management services provided by that physician in conjunction with that admission are considered part of the initial nursing facility care when performed on the same date as the admission or readmission. The nursing facility care level of service reported by the admitting physician should include the services related to the admission he/she provided in the other sites of services as well as in the nursing facility setting.

Hospital discharge or observation discharge services performed on the same date of nursing facility admission or readmission may be reported separately. For a patient discharged from inpatient status on the same date of nursing facility admission or readmission, the hospital discharge services should be reported with codes 99238, 99239 as appropriate. For a patient discharged from observation status on the same date of nursing facility admission or readmission, the observation care discharge services should be reported with code 99217. For a patient admitted and discharged from observation or inpatient status on the same date, see codes 99234-99236. (For nursing facility care discharge, see 99315, 99316.)

Significance of Time as a Factor in Selection of an E/M Code

The inclusion of time as an explicit factor beginning in CPT 1992 is done to assist physicians in selecting the most appropriate level of E/M services. It should be recognized that the specific times expressed in the visit code descriptors are averages and, therefore, represent a range of times that may be higher or lower depending on actual clinical circumstances.

Intraservice times are defined as face-to-face time for office and other outpatient visits and unit/floor time for hospital and other inpatient visits. This distinction is necessary because most of the work of typical office visits takes place during the face-to-face time with the patient, while most of the work of typical hospital visits takes place during the time spent on the patient's floor or unit.

Unit/Floor Time Nursing Facility Care

For reporting purposes, intraservice time for these services is defined as unit/floor time, which includes the time that the physician is present on the patient's hospital unit and at the bedside rendering services for that patient. This includes the time in which the physician establishes and/or reviews the patient's chart, examines the patients, writes notes, and communicates with other professionals and the patient's family.

In the nursing facility, pre- and post-time includes time spent off the patient's floor performing such tasks as reviewing pathology and radiology findings in another part of the hospital.

The pre- and post-visit time is not included in the time component described in these codes. However, the pre- and post-work performed during the time spent off the floor or unit was included in calculating the total work of typical services in the physician surveys.

Thus, the unit/floor time associated with the services described by any code is a valid proxy for the work done before, during, and after the visit.

● New   ▲ Revised   ✖ Deleted   ⊙ Moderate Sedation   ✚ Add-on Codes   ⊘ High Risk Denial   Ⓐ Age Edit   ♀ Female   ♂ Male   **AMA** *CPT® Assistant*   **MUE** Medically Unlikely Edit   ⊘ Modifier 51 Exempt   ⊖ Modifier 63 Exempt   ⚡ Unlisted   **Modifiers:** *See Inside Back Cover*   Ⓜ Maternity   A2–Z3 ASC Payment Indicators   A–Y OPPS Status Indicators

132   CPT © 2014 American Medical Association. All Rights Reserved.   © 2016 DecisionHealth

99304 **Initial nursing facility care, per day, for the evaluation and management of a patient, which requires these 3 key components:**

- A detailed or comprehensive history;
- A detailed or comprehensive examination; and
- Medical decision making that is straightforward or of low complexity.

Counseling and/or coordination of care with other physicians, other qualified health care professionals, or agencies are provided consistent with the nature of the problem(s) and the patient's and/or family's needs. Usually, the problem(s) requiring admission are of low severity. Typically, 25 minutes are spent at the bedside and on the patient's facility floor or unit. **B**

RVU			Global Days	Modifiers				
Mod	*Non-Fac Total*	*Fac Total*		*51*	*50*	*62*	*80*	*MUE*
	2.58	2.58	XXX	0	0	0	0	1

AMA: Jan 11: 3, Jan 12: 3, Jan 13: 9, Jul 10: 4, Jul 12: 12, Jun 11: 3, Jun 13: 3, Nov 14: 14

99305 **Initial nursing facility care, per day, for the evaluation and management of a patient, which requires these 3 key components:**

- A comprehensive history;
- A comprehensive examination; and
- Medical decision making of moderate complexity.

Counseling and/or coordination of care with other physicians, other qualified health care professionals, or agencies are provided consistent with the nature of the problem(s) and the patient's and/or family's needs. Usually, the problem(s) requiring admission are of moderate severity. Typically, 35 minutes are spent at the bedside and on the patient's facility floor or unit. **B**

RVU			Global Days	Modifiers				
Mod	*Non-Fac Total*	*Fac Total*		*51*	*50*	*62*	*80*	*MUE*
	3.67	3.67	XXX	0	0	0	0	1

AMA: Jan 11: 3, Jan 13: 9, Jul 12: 12, Jun 11: 3, Jun 13: 3

99306 **Initial nursing facility care, per day, for the evaluation and management of a patient, which requires these 3 key components:**

- A comprehensive history;
- A comprehensive examination; and
- Medical decision making of high complexity.

Counseling and/or coordination of care with other physicians, other qualified health care professionals, or agencies are provided consistent with the nature of the problem(s) and the patient's and/or family's needs. Usually, the problem(s) requiring admission are of high severity. Typically, 45 minutes are spent at the bedside and on the patient's facility floor or unit. **B**

RVU			Global Days	Modifiers				
Mod	*Non-Fac Total*	*Fac Total*		*51*	*50*	*62*	*80*	*MUE*
	4.68	4.68	XXX	0	0	0	0	1

AMA: Jan 11: 3, Jan 12: 3, Jan 13: 9, Jul 12: 12, Jun 11: 3, Jun 13: 3

Subsequent Nursing Facility Visits

All levels of subsequent nursing facility care include reviewing the medical record and reviewing the results of diagnostic studies and changes in the patient's status (ie, changes in history, physical condition, and response to management) since the last assessment by the physician or other qualified health care professional.

99307 **Subsequent nursing facility care, per day, for the evaluation and management of a patient, which requires at least 2 of these 3 key components:**

- A problem focused interval history;
- A problem focused examination;
- Straightforward medical decision making.

Counseling and/or coordination of care with other physicians, other qualified health care professionals, or agencies are provided consistent with the nature of the problem(s) and the patient's and/or family's needs. Usually, the patient is stable, recovering, or improving. Typically, 10 minutes are spent at the bedside and on the patient's facility floor or unit. **B**

RVU			Global Days	Modifiers				
Mod	*Non-Fac Total*	*Fac Total*		*51*	*50*	*62*	*80*	*MUE*
	1.26	1.26	XXX	0	0	0	0	1

AMA: Jan 11: 3, Jan 12: 3, Jan 13: 9, Jul 07: 1, Jul 09: 3, 8, Jul 12: 12, Jun 06: 1, 19, Jun 13: 3, Mar 07: 9, May 06: 1, 16

99308 **Subsequent nursing facility care, per day, for the evaluation and management of a patient, which requires at least 2 of these 3 key components:**

- An expanded problem focused interval history;
- An expanded problem focused examination;
- Medical decision making of low complexity.

Counseling and/or coordination of care with other physicians, other qualified health care professionals, or agencies are provided consistent with the nature of the problem(s) and the patient's and/or family's needs. Usually, the patient is responding inadequately to therapy or has developed a minor complication. Typically, 15 minutes are spent at the bedside and on the patient's facility floor or unit. **B**

RVU			Global Days	Modifiers				
Mod	*Non-Fac Total*	*Fac Total*		*51*	*50*	*62*	*80*	*MUE*
	1.94	1.94	XXX	0	0	0	0	1

AMA: Jan 11: 3, Jan 13: 9, Jul 07: 1, Jul 09: 3, 8, Jul 12: 12, Jun 06: 1, 19, Jun 13: 3, Mar 07: 9, May 06: 1, 16

99309 **Subsequent nursing facility care, per day, for the evaluation and management of a patient, which requires at least 2 of these 3 key components:**

- A detailed interval history;
- A detailed examination;
- Medical decision making of moderate complexity.

Counseling and/or coordination of care with other physicians, other qualified health care professionals, or agencies are provided consistent with the nature of the problem(s) and the patient's and/or family's needs. Usually, the patient has developed a significant complication or a significant new problem. Typically, 25 minutes are spent at the bedside and on the patient's facility floor or unit. **B**

RVU			Global Days	Modifiers				
Mod	*Non-Fac Total*	*Fac Total*		*51*	*50*	*62*	*80*	*MUE*
	2.56	2.56	XXX	0	0	0	0	1

● New ▲ Revised ✖ Deleted ⊙ Moderate Sedation ➕ Add-on Codes ⊘ High Risk Denial Ⓐ Age Edit ♀ Female ♂ Male **AMA** *CPT® Assistant* **MUE** Medically Unlikely Edit

⊘ Modifier 51 Exempt ⊖ Modifier 63 Exempt ✖ Unlisted **Modifiers:** *See Inside Back Cover* Ⓜ Maternity A2–Z3 ASC Payment Indicators A–Y OPPS Status Indicators

© 2016 DecisionHealth CPT © 2014 American Medical Association. All Rights Reserved. **133**

AMA: Jan 11: 3, Jan 13: 9, Jul 07: 1, Jul 09: 3, 8, Jul 12: 12, Jun 06: 1, 19, Jun 13: 3, Mar 07: 9, May 06: 1, 16

99310 **Subsequent nursing facility care, per day, for the evaluation and management of a patient, which requires at least 2 of these 3 key components:**

- A comprehensive interval history;

- A comprehensive examination;

- Medical decision making of high complexity.

Counseling and/or coordination of care with other physicians, other qualified health care professionals, or agencies are provided consistent with the nature of the problem(s) and the patient's and/or family's needs. The patient may be unstable or may have developed a significant new problem requiring immediate physician attention. Typically, 35 minutes are spent at the bedside and on the patient's facility floor or unit.   B

RVU			Global Days	Modifiers				
Mod	Non-Fac Total	Fac Total		51	50	62	80	MUE
	3.82	3.82	XXX	0	0	0	0	1

AMA: Jan 11: 3, Jan 12: 3, Jan 13: 9, Jul 07: 1, Jul 09: 3, 8, Jul 10: 4, Jul 12: 12, Jun 06: 1, 19, Jun 13: 3, Mar 07: 9, May 06: 1, 16

Other Nursing Facility Services

The nursing facility discharge day management codes are to be used to report the total duration of time spent by a physician or other qualified health care professional for the final nursing facility discharge of a patient. The codes include, as appropriate, final examination of the patient, discussion of the nursing facility stay, even if the time spent on that date is not continuous. Instructions are given for continuing care to all relevant caregivers, and preparation of discharge records, prescriptions and referral forms.

99315 **Nursing facility discharge day management; 30 minutes or less**   B

RVU			Global Days	Modifiers				
Mod	Non-Fac Total	Fac Total		51	50	62	80	MUE
	2.05	2.05	XXX	0	0	0	0	1

AMA: Jan 11: 3, Jan 12: 3, Jan 13: 9, Jul 09: 3, Jul 12: 12, Jun 13: 3, May 02: 19, May 05: 1, Nov 02: 11, Nov 97: 5, 6, Sep 98: 5

99316 **Nursing facility discharge day management; more than 30 minutes**   B

RVU			Global Days	Modifiers				
Mod	Non-Fac Total	Fac Total		51	50	62	80	MUE
	2.98	2.98	XXX	0	0	0	0	1

AMA: Jan 11: 3, Jan 13: 9, Jul 09: 3, Jul 12: 12, Jun 13: 3, May 02: 19, Nov 02: 11, Nov 97: 5, 6, Sep 98: 5

Other Nursing Facility Services

99318 **Evaluation and management of a patient involving an annual nursing facility assessment, which requires these 3 key components:**

- A detailed interval history;

- A comprehensive examination; and

- Medical decision making that is of low to moderate complexity.

Counseling and/or coordination of care with other physicians, other qualified health care professionals, or agencies are provided consistent with the nature of the problem(s) and the patient's and/or family's needs. Usually, the patient is stable, recovering, or improving. Typically, 30 minutes are spent at the bedside and on the patient's facility floor or unit.   B

RVU			Global Days	Modifiers				
Mod	Non-Fac Total	Fac Total		51	50	62	80	MUE
	2.70	2.70	XXX	0	0	0	0	1

AMA: Jan 11: 3, Jan 12: 3, Jan 13: 9, Jun 13: 3, Nov 14: 14

Domiciliary, Rest Homes (e.g., Boarding Home), or Custodial Care Services

The following codes are used to report evaluation and management services in a facility which provides room, board and other personal assistance services, generally on a long-term basis. They also are used to report evaluation and management services in an assisted living facility.

The facility's services do not include a medical component.

For definitions of key components and commonly used terms, please see Evaluation and Management Services Guidelines.

New Assisted Living Facility/Rest Home Visits

99324 **Domiciliary or rest home visit for the evaluation and management of a new patient, which requires these 3 key components:**

- A problem focused history;
- A problem focused examination; and
- Straightforward medical decision making.

Counseling and/or coordination of care with other physicians, other qualified health care professionals, or agencies are provided consistent with the nature of the problem(s) and the patient's and/or family's needs. Usually, the presenting problem(s) are of low severity. Typically, 20 minutes are spent with the patient and/or family or caregiver.   B

RVU			Global Days	Modifiers				
Mod	Non-Fac Total	Fac Total		51	50	62	80	MUE
	1.56	1.56	XXX	0	0	0	0	1

AMA: Apr 12: 10, Aug 09: 5, Jan 06: 1, Jan 11: 3, Jan 12: 3, Jan 13: 9, Jul 09: 8, Jun 06: 1, Jun 13: 3, Nov 14: 14, Oct 14: 3

99325 **Domiciliary or rest home visit for the evaluation and management of a new patient, which requires these 3 key components:**

- An expanded problem focused history;
- An expanded problem focused examination; and
- Medical decision making of low complexity.

Counseling and/or coordination of care with other physicians, other qualified health care professionals, or agencies are provided consistent with the nature of the problem(s) and the patient's and/or family's needs. Usually, the presenting problem(s) are of moderate severity. Typically, 30 minutes are spent with the patient and/or family or caregiver.   B

RVU			Global Days	Modifiers				
Mod	Non-Fac Total	Fac Total		51	50	62	80	MUE
	2.27	2.27	XXX	0	0	0	0	1

AMA: Aug 09: 5, Jan 06: 1, Jan 11: 3, Jan 13: 9, Jul 09: 8, Jun 06: 1, Jun 13: 3

● New   ▲ Revised   ✖ Deleted   ⊙ Moderate Sedation   ✚ Add-on Codes   ⊗ High Risk Denial   Ⓐ Age Edit   ♀ Female   ♂ Male   **AMA** CPT® Assistant   **MUE** Medically Unlikely Edit

⊘ Modifier 51 Exempt   ⊖ Modifier 63 Exempt   ⊠ Unlisted   **Modifiers:** See Inside Back Cover   Ⓜ Maternity   A2–Z3 ASC Payment Indicators   A–Y OPPS Status Indicators

134   CPT © 2014 American Medical Association. All Rights Reserved.   © 2016 DecisionHealth

99326 Domiciliary or rest home visit for the evaluation and management of a new patient, which requires these 3 key components:

- A detailed history;
- A detailed examination; and
- Medical decision making of moderate complexity.

Counseling and/or coordination of care with other physicians, other qualified health care professionals, or agencies are provided consistent with the nature of the problem(s) and the patient's and/or family's needs. Usually, the presenting problem(s) are of moderate to high severity. Typically, 45 minutes are spent with the patient and/or family or caregiver. **B**

RVU			Global Days	Modifiers				
Mod	Non-Fac Total	Fac Total		51	50	62	80	MUE
	3.92	3.92	XXX	0	0	0	0	1

AMA: Aug 09: 5, Jan 06: 1, Jan 11: 3, Jan 13: 9, Jul 09: 8, Jun 06: 1, Jun 13: 3

99327 Domiciliary or rest home visit for the evaluation and management of a new patient, which requires these 3 key components:

- A comprehensive history;
- A comprehensive examination; and
- Medical decision making of moderate complexity.

Counseling and/or coordination of care with other physicians, other qualified health care professionals, or agencies are provided consistent with the nature of the problem(s) and the patient's and/or family's needs. Usually, the presenting problem(s) are of high severity. Typically, 60 minutes are spent with the patient and/or family or caregiver. **B**

RVU			Global Days	Modifiers				
Mod	Non-Fac Total	Fac Total		51	50	62	80	MUE
	5.22	5.22	XXX	0	0	0	0	1

AMA: Aug 09: 5, Jan 06: 1, Jan 11: 3, Jan 13: 9, Jul 09: 8, Jun 06: 1, Jun 13: 3

99328 Domiciliary or rest home visit for the evaluation and management of a new patient, which requires these 3 key components:

- A comprehensive history;
- A comprehensive examination; and
- Medical decision making of high complexity.

Counseling and/or coordination of care with other physicians, other qualified health care professionals, or agencies are provided consistent with the nature of the problem(s) and the patient's and/or family's needs. Usually, the patient is unstable or has developed a significant new problem requiring immediate physician attention. Typically, 75 minutes are spent with the patient and/or family or caregiver. **B**

RVU			Global Days	Modifiers				
Mod	Non-Fac Total	Fac Total		51	50	62	80	MUE
	6.10	6.10	XXX	0	0	0	0	1

AMA: Aug 09: 5, Jan 06: 1, Jan 11: 3, Jan 12: 3, Jan 13: 9, Jul 09: 8, Jun 06: 1, Jun 13: 3

Established Patient Services

99334 Domiciliary or rest home visit for the evaluation and management of an established patient, which requires at least 2 of these 3 key components:

- A problem focused interval history;
- A problem focused examination;
- Straightforward medical decision making.

Counseling and/or coordination of care with other physicians, other qualified health care professionals, or agencies are provided consistent with the nature of the problem(s) and the patient's and/or family's needs. Usually, the presenting problem(s) are self-limited or minor. Typically, 15 minutes are spent with the patient and/or family or caregiver. **B**

RVU			Global Days	Modifiers				
Mod	Non-Fac Total	Fac Total		51	50	62	80	MUE
	1.70	1.70	XXX	0	0	0	0	1

AMA: Aug 09: 5, Jan 06: 1, Jan 11: 3, Jan 12: 3, Jan 13: 9, Jul 07: 1, Jul 09: 8, Jun 06: 1, Jun 13: 3, Nov 13: 3

99335 Domiciliary or rest home visit for the evaluation and management of an established patient, which requires at least 2 of these 3 key components:

- An expanded problem focused interval history;
- An expanded problem focused examination;
- Medical decision making of low complexity.

Counseling and/or coordination of care with other physicians, other qualified health care professionals, or agencies are provided consistent with the nature of the problem(s) and the patient's and/or family's needs. Usually, the presenting problem(s) are of low to moderate severity. Typically, 25 minutes are spent with the patient and/or family or caregiver. **B**

RVU			Global Days	Modifiers				
Mod	Non-Fac Total	Fac Total		51	50	62	80	MUE
	2.67	2.67	XXX	0	0	0	0	1

AMA: Aug 09: 5, Jan 06: 1, Jan 11: 3, Jan 13: 9, Jul 07: 1, Jul 09: 8, Jun 06: 1, Jun 13: 3

99336 Domiciliary or rest home visit for the evaluation and management of an established patient, which requires at least 2 of these 3 key components:

- A detailed interval history;
- A detailed examination;
- Medical decision making of moderate complexity.

Counseling and/or coordination of care with other physicians, other qualified health care professionals, or agencies are provided consistent with the nature of the problem(s) and the patient's and/or family's needs. Usually, the presenting problem(s) are of moderate to high severity. Typically, 40 minutes are spent with the patient and/or family or caregiver. **B**

RVU			Global Days	Modifiers				
Mod	Non-Fac Total	Fac Total		51	50	62	80	MUE
	3.79	3.79	XXX	0	0	0	0	1

AMA: Aug 09: 5, Jan 06: 1, Jan 11: 3, Jan 13: 9, Jul 07: 1, Jul 09: 8, Jun 06: 1, Jun 13: 3

● New　▲ Revised　✖ Deleted　⊙ Moderate Sedation　✚ Add-on Codes　⊗ High Risk Denial　Ⓐ Age Edit　♀ Female　♂ Male　**AMA** CPT® Assistant　**MUE** Medically Unlikely Edit　⊘ Modifier 51 Exempt　⊖ Modifier 63 Exempt　Ⓧ Unlisted　**Modifiers:** See Inside Back Cover　Ⓜ Maternity　Ⓐ2–Z3 ASC Payment Indicators　Ⓐ–Y OPPS Status Indicators

© 2016 DecisionHealth　　CPT © 2014 American Medical Association. All Rights Reserved.　　**135**

Evaluation and Management (E/M) Services

99337 – 99342

99337 Domiciliary or rest home visit for the evaluation and management of an established patient, which requires at least 2 of these 3 key components:

- A comprehensive interval history;
- A comprehensive examination;
- Medical decision making of moderate to high complexity.

Counseling and/or coordination of care with other physicians, other qualified health care professionals, or agencies are provided consistent with the nature of the problem(s) and the patient's and/or family's needs. Usually, the presenting problem(s) are of moderate to high severity. The patient may be unstable or may have developed a significant new problem requiring immediate physician attention. Typically, 60 minutes are spent with the patient and/or family or caregiver. **B**

RVU			Global Days	Modifiers				
Mod	Non-Fac Total	Fac Total		51	50	62	80	MUE
	5.41	5.41	XXX	0	0	0	0	1

AMA: Apr 12: 10, Aug 09: 5, Jan 06: 1, Jan 11: 3, Jan 12: 3, Jan 13: 9, Jul 07: 1, Jul 09: 8, Jun 06: 1, Jun 13: 3, Nov 13: 3, Nov 14: 14, Oct 14: 3

Domiciliary, Rest Homes (e.g., Boarding Home), or Custodial Care Services

99339 Individual physician supervision of a patient (patient not present) in home, domiciliary or rest home (eg, assisted living facility) requiring complex and multidisciplinary care modalities involving regular physician development and/or revision of care plans, review of subsequent reports of patient status, review of related laboratory and other studies, communication (including telephone calls) for purposes of assessment or care decisions with health care professional(s), family member(s), surrogate decision maker(s) (eg, legal guardian) and/or key caregiver(s) involved in patient's care, integration of new information into the medical treatment plan and/or adjustment of medical therapy, within a calendar month; 15-29 minutes ⊙**B**

RVU			Global Days	Modifiers				
Mod	Non-Fac Total	Fac Total		51	50	62	80	MUE
	2.18	2.18	XXX	9	9	9	9	

AMA: Apr 13: 3, Dec 06: 4, Jan 06: 1, Jan 12: 3, Jul 09: 5, 10, Jun 13: 3, Mar 07: 11, Nov 13: 3, Oct 14: 3, Sep 08: 3, Sep 13: 15

99340 Individual physician supervision of a patient (patient not present) in home, domiciliary or rest home (eg, assisted living facility) requiring complex and multidisciplinary care modalities involving regular physician development and/or revision of care plans, review of subsequent reports of patient status, review of related laboratory and other studies, communication (including telephone calls) for purposes of assessment or care decisions with health care professional(s), family member(s), surrogate decision maker(s) (eg, legal guardian) and/or key caregiver(s) involved in patient's care, integration of new information into the medical treatment plan and/or adjustment of medical therapy, within a calendar month; 30 minutes or more ⊙**B**

RVU			Global Days	Modifiers				
Mod	Non-Fac Total	Fac Total		51	50	62	80	MUE
	3.06	3.06	XXX	9	9	9	9	

AMA: Apr 13: 3, Dec 06: 4, Jan 06: 1, Jan 12: 3, Jul 09: 5, 10, Jun 13: 3, Mar 07: 11, Nov 13: 3, Oct 14: 3, Sep 08: 3, Sep 13: 15

Home Services

The following codes are used to report evaluation and management services provided in a private residence.

For definitions of key components and commonly used terms, please see Evaluation and Management Services Guidelines.

New Home Visits

99341 Home visit for the evaluation and management of a new patient, which requires these 3 key components:

- A problem focused history;
- A problem focused examination; and
- Straightforward medical decision making.

Counseling and/or coordination of care with other physicians, other qualified health care professionals, or agencies are provided consistent with the nature of the problem(s) and the patient's and/or family's needs. Usually, the presenting problem(s) are of low severity. Typically, 20 minutes are spent face-to-face with the patient and/or family. **B**

RVU			Global Days	Modifiers				
Mod	Non-Fac Total	Fac Total		51	50	62	80	MUE
	1.56	1.56	XXX	0	0	0	0	1

AMA: Apr 12: 10, Aug 09: 5, Jan 06: 1, Jan 11: 3, Jan 12: 3, Jan 13: 9, Jul 09: 8, Jun 13: 3, Jun 97: 6, May 05: 1, Nov 14: 14, Nov 97: 6, 8, Oct 03: 7, Oct 14: 3, Oct 98: 6, Spring 92: 24, Spring 93: 34, Spring 95: 1, Summer 92: 12, Winter 91: 11

99342 Home visit for the evaluation and management of a new patient, which requires these 3 key components:

- An expanded problem focused history;
- An expanded problem focused examination; and
- Medical decision making of low complexity.

● New ▲ Revised ✖ Deleted ⊙ Moderate Sedation ✚ Add-on Codes ⊘ High Risk Denial Ⓐ Age Edit ♀ Female ♂ Male **AMA** CPT® Assistant **MUE** Medically Unlikely Edit ⃠ Modifier 51 Exempt ⊖ Modifier 63 Exempt ✗ Unlisted **Modifiers:** See Inside Back Cover Ⓜ Maternity Ⓐ2–Z3 ASC Payment Indicators Ⓐ–Ⓨ OPPS Status Indicators

Counseling and/or coordination of care with other physicians, other qualified health care professionals, or agencies are provided consistent with the nature of the problem(s) and the patient's and/or family's needs. Usually, the presenting problem(s) are of moderate severity. Typically, 30 minutes are spent face-to-face with the patient and/or family. **B**

RVU			Global Days	Modifiers				
Mod	Non-Fac Total	Fac Total		51	50	62	80	MUE
	2.24	2.24	XXX	0	0	0	0	1

AMA: Aug 09: 5, Jan 06: 1, Jan 11: 3, Jan 13: 9, Jul 09: 8, Jun 13: 3, Jun 97: 6, Nov 97: 6, 8, Oct 98: 6, Spring 92: 24, Spring 93: 34, Spring 95: 1, Summer 92: 12, Winter 91: 11

99343 Home visit for the evaluation and management of a new patient, which requires these 3 key components:

- A detailed history;
- A detailed examination; and
- Medical decision making of moderate complexity.

Counseling and/or coordination of care with other physicians, other qualified health care professionals, or agencies are provided consistent with the nature of the problem(s) and the patient's and/or family's needs. Usually, the presenting problem(s) are of moderate to high severity. Typically, 45 minutes are spent face-to-face with the patient and/or family. **B**

RVU			Global Days	Modifiers				
Mod	Non-Fac Total	Fac Total		51	50	62	80	MUE
	3.66	3.66	XXX	0	0	0	0	1

AMA: Aug 09: 5, Jan 06: 1, Jan 11: 3, Jan 13: 9, Jul 09: 8, Jun 13: 3, Jun 97: 6, Nov 97: 6, 8, Oct 98: 6, Spring 92: 24, Spring 93: 34, Spring 95: 1, Summer 92: 12, Winter 91: 11

99344 Home visit for the evaluation and management of a new patient, which requires these 3 key components:

- A comprehensive history;
- A comprehensive examination; and
- Medical decision making of moderate complexity.

Counseling and/or coordination of care with other physicians, other qualified health care professionals, or agencies are provided consistent with the nature of the problem(s) and the patient's and/or family's needs. Usually, the presenting problem(s) are of high severity. Typically, 60 minutes are spent face-to-face with the patient and/or family. **B**

RVU			Global Days	Modifiers				
Mod	Non-Fac Total	Fac Total		51	50	62	80	MUE
	5.12	5.12	XXX	0	0	0	0	1

AMA: Aug 09: 5, Jan 06: 1, Jan 11: 3, Jan 13: 9, Jul 09: 8, Jun 13: 3, Nov 97: 6, 8, Oct 98: 6

99345 Home visit for the evaluation and management of a new patient, which requires these 3 key components:

- A comprehensive history;
- A comprehensive examination; and
- Medical decision making of high complexity.

Counseling and/or coordination of care with other physicians, other qualified health care professionals, or agencies are provided consistent with the nature of the problem(s) and the patient's and/or family's needs. Usually, the patient is unstable or has developed a significant new problem requiring immediate physician attention. Typically, 75 minutes are spent face-to-face with the patient and/or family. **B**

RVU			Global Days	Modifiers				
Mod	Non-Fac Total	Fac Total		51	50	62	80	MUE
	6.21	6.21	XXX	0	0	0	0	1

AMA: Aug 09: 5, Jan 06: 1, Jan 11: 3, Jan 12: 3, Jan 13: 9, Jul 09: 8, Jun 13: 3, Nov 97: 6, 8, Oct 98: 6

Established Patient Services

99347 Home visit for the evaluation and management of an established patient, which requires at least 2 of these 3 key components:

- A problem focused interval history;
- A problem focused examination;
- Straightforward medical decision making.

Counseling and/or coordination of care with other physicians, other qualified health care professionals, or agencies are provided consistent with the nature of the problem(s) and the patient's and/or family's needs. Usually, the presenting problem(s) are self limited or minor. Typically, 15 minutes are spent face-to-face with the patient and/or family. **B**

RVU			Global Days	Modifiers				
Mod	Non-Fac Total	Fac Total		51	50	62	80	MUE
	1.57	1.57	XXX	0	0	0	0	1

AMA: Aug 09: 5, Jan 06: 1, Jan 11: 3, Jan 12: 3, Jan 13: 9, Jul 07: 1, Jul 09: 8, Jun 13: 3, May 05: 1, Nov 13: 3, Nov 97: 6, 8, Oct 98: 6

99348 Home visit for the evaluation and management of an established patient, which requires at least 2 of these 3 key components:

- An expanded problem focused interval history;
- An expanded problem focused examination;
- Medical decision making of low complexity.

Counseling and/or coordination of care with other physicians, other qualified health care professionals, or agencies are provided consistent with the nature of the problem(s) and the patient's and/or family's needs. Usually, the presenting problem(s) are of low to moderate severity. Typically, 25 minutes are spent face-to-face with the patient and/or family. **B**

RVU			Global Days	Modifiers				
Mod	Non-Fac Total	Fac Total		51	50	62	80	MUE
	2.38	2.38	XXX	0	0	0	0	1

AMA: Aug 09: 5, Jan 06: 1, Jan 11: 3, Jan 13: 9, Jul 07: 1, Jul 09: 8, Jun 13: 3, Nov 97: 6, 8, Oct 98: 6

99349 Home visit for the evaluation and management of an established patient, which requires at least 2 of these 3 key components:

- A detailed interval history;
- A detailed examination;
- Medical decision making of moderate complexity.

Counseling and/or coordination of care with other physicians, other qualified health care professionals, or agencies are provided consistent with the nature of the problem(s) and the patient's and/or family's needs. Usually, the presenting problem(s) are moderate to high severity. Typically, 40 minutes are spent face-to-face with the patient and/or family. **B**

RVU			Global Days	Modifiers				
Mod	Non-Fac Total	Fac Total		51	50	62	80	MUE
	3.61	3.61	XXX	0	0	0	0	1

AMA: Aug 09: 5, Jan 06: 1, Jan 13: 9, Jul 07: 1, Jul 09: 8, Jun 13: 3, Nov 97: 6, 8, Oct 98: 6

99350 **Home visit for the evaluation and management of an established patient, which requires at least 2 of these 3 key components:**

- A comprehensive interval history;
- A comprehensive examination;
- Medical decision making of moderate to high complexity.

Counseling and/or coordination of care with other physicians, other qualified health care professionals, or agencies are provided consistent with the nature of the problem(s) and the patient's and/or family's needs. Usually, the presenting problem(s) are of moderate to high severity. The patient may be unstable or may have developed a significant new problem requiring immediate physician attention. Typically, 60 minutes are spent face-to-face with the patient and/or family. **B**

RVU			Global Days	Modifiers				
Mod	Non-Fac Total	Fac Total		51	50	62	80	MUE
	5.00	5.00	XXX	0	0	0	0	1

AMA: Apr 12: 10, Aug 09: 5, Jan 06: 1, Jan 12: 3, Jan 13: 9, Jul 07: 1, Jul 09: 8, Jun 13: 3, Nov 13: 3, Nov 14: 14, Nov 97: 6, 8, Oct 03: 7, Oct 14: 3, Oct 98: 6

Prolonged Services

Prolonged Physician Service With Direct (Face-To-Face) Patient Contact

Codes 99354-99357 are used when a physician or other qualified health care professional provides prolonged service involving direct patient contact that is beyond the usual service in either the inpatient or outpatient setting. Direct patient contact is face-to-face and includes additional non-face-to-face services on the patient's floor or unit in the hospital or nursing facility during the same session. This service is reported in addition to the designated evaluation and management services at any level and any other services provided at the same session as evaluation and management services. Appropriate codes should be selected for supplies provided or procedures performed in the care of the patient during this period.

Codes 99354-99355 are used to report the total duration of face-to-face time spent by a physician or other qualified health care professional on a given date providing prolonged service in the office or other outpatient setting, even if the time spent by the physician or other qualified health care professional on that date is not continuous. Codes 99356-99357 are used to report the total duration of time spent by a physician or other qualified health care professional at the bedside and on the patient's floor or unit, in the hospital or nursing facility on a given date providing prolonged service to a patient, even if the time spent by the physician or other qualified health care professional on that date is not continuous.

Code 99354 or 99356 is used to report the first hour of prolonged service on a given date, depending on the place of service.

Either code should be used only once per date, even if the time spent by the physician or other qualified health care professional is not continuous

on that date. Prolonged service of less than 30 minutes total duration on a given date is not separately reported because the work involved is included in the total work of the evaluation and management codes.

Code 99355 or 99357 is used to report each additional 30 minutes beyond the first hour, depending on the place of service. Either code may also be used to report the final 15-30 minutes of prolonged service on a given date. Prolonged service of less than 15 minutes beyond the first hour or less than 15 minutes beyond the final 30 minutes is not reported separately.

The use of the time based add-on codes requires that the primary evaluation and management service have a typical or specified time published in the CPT codebook.

The following examples illustrate the correct reporting of prolonged physician or other qualified health care professional service with direct patient contact in the office setting:

Total Duration of Prolonged Services	Code(s)
Less than 30 minutes (less than 30 minutes)	Not reported separately
30 minutes -74 minutes (30 minutes – 1 hour, 14 minutes)	99354 x 1
75 minutes – 104 minutes (1 hour, 15 minutes – 1 hour, 44 minutes)	99354 x 1 + 99355 x 1
105 minutes or more (1 hour, 45 minutes or more)	99354 x 1 + 99355 x 2 or more for each additional 30 minutes

Reporting a Service of Less than 30 Minutes
Prolonged service of less than 30 minutes total duration on a given date is not separately reported because the work involved is included in the total work of the E/M codes.

+▲99354 **Prolonged evaluation and management or psychotherapy service(s) (beyond the typical service time of the primary procedure) in the office or other outpatient setting requiring direct patient contact beyond the usual service; first hour (List separately in addition to code for office or other outpatient Evaluation and Management or psychotherapy service)** **N**

RVU			Global Days	Modifiers				
Mod	Non-Fac Total	Fac Total		51	50	62	80	MUE
	2.82	2.62	ZZZ	0	0	0	0	1

AMA: Apr 12: 10, Apr 14: 6, Aug 12: 3, 4, 5, Jul 01: 2, Jul 09: 8, Jun 08: 12, Jun 13: 3, Jun 14: 14, May 05: 1, May 13: 12, May 97: 3, Nov 05: 10, Oct 13: 11, Sep 00: 2, Sep 08: 3, Sep 98: 5, Spring 94: 30, 32

+▲99355 **Prolonged evaluation and management or psychotherapy service(s) (beyond the typical service time of the primary procedure) in the office or other outpatient setting requiring direct patient contact beyond the usual service; each additional 30 minutes (List separately in addition to code for prolonged service)** **N**

RVU			Global Days	Modifiers				
Mod	Non-Fac Total	Fac Total		51	50	62	80	MUE
	2.74	2.54	ZZZ	0	0	0	0	

AMA: Apr 12: 10, Apr 14: 6, Aug 12: 3, 4, 5, Jul 01: 2, Jul 09: 8, Jun 08: 12, Jun 13: 3, Jun 14: 14, May 13: 12, May 97: 3, Nov 05: 10, Oct 13: 11, Sep 00: 2, Sep 08: 3, Sep 98: 5, Spring 94: 30, 32

● New   ▲ Revised   ✖ Deleted   ⊙ Moderate Sedation   ✚ Add-on Codes   ⊗ High Risk Denial   Ⓐ Age Edit   ♀ Female   ♂ Male   **AMA** CPT® Assistant   **MUE** Medically Unlikely Edit
⊘ Modifier 51 Exempt   ⊖ Modifier 63 Exempt   𝕏 Unlisted   **Modifiers:** See Inside Back Cover   Ⓜ Maternity   Ⓐ2–Ⓩ3 ASC Payment Indicators   Ⓐ–Ⓨ OPPS Status Indicators

138   CPT © 2014 American Medical Association. All Rights Reserved.   © 2016 DecisionHealth

+ 99356 Prolonged service in the inpatient or observation setting, requiring unit/floor time beyond the usual service; first hour (List separately in addition to code for inpatient Evaluation and Management service)   C

RVU		Global Days	Modifiers				
Mod	Non-Fac Total	Fac Total		51	50	62	80	MUE
	2.58	2.58	ZZZ	0	0	0	0	1

AMA: Apr 14: 6, Apr 97: 3, Aug 11: 11, Aug 12: 3, 4, 5, Jul 01: 2, Jul 09: 8, Jul 12: 11, Jun 08: 12, Jun 11: 3, Jun 13: 3, Jun 14: 14, May 13: 12, May 97: 3, Nov 05: 10, Oct 13: 11, Sep 00: 2, Sep 08: 3, Sep 98: 5, Spring 94: 30, 32

+ 99357 Prolonged service in the inpatient or observation setting, requiring unit/floor time beyond the usual service; each additional 30 minutes (List separately in addition to code for prolonged service)   C

RVU		Global Days	Modifiers				
Mod	Non-Fac Total	Fac Total		51	50	62	80	MUE
	2.57	2.57	ZZZ	0	0	0	0	

AMA: Apr 14: 6, Apr 97: 3, Aug 11: 11, Aug 12: 3, 4, 5, Jul 01: 2, Jul 09: 8, Jul 12: 11, Jun 08: 12, Jun 11: 3, Jun 13: 3, Jun 14: 14, May 13: 12, May 97: 3, Nov 05: 10, Oct 13: 11, Sep 00: 2, Sep 08: 3, Sep 98: 5, Spring 94: 34

Prolonged Physician Service Without Direct (Face-To-Face) Patient Contact

Codes 99358 and 99359 are used when a prolonged service is provided that is neither face-to-face time in the office or outpatient setting, nor additional unit/floor time in the hospital or nursing facility setting during the same session of an evaluation and management service and is beyond the usual physician or other qualified health care professional service time.

This service is to be reported in relation to other physician or other qualified health care professional services, including evaluation and management services at any level. This prolonged service may be reported on a different date than the primary service to which it is related. For example, extensive record review may relate to a previous evaluation and management service performed earlier and commences upon receipt of past records. However, it must relate to a service or patient where direct (face-to-face) patient care has occurred or will occur and relate to ongoing patient management. A typical time for the primary service need not be established within CPT code set.

Codes 99358 and 99359 are used to report the total duration of non-face-to-face time spent by a physician or other qualified health care professional on a given date providing prolonged service, even if the time spent by the physician or other qualified health care professional on that date is not continuous. Code 99358 is used to report the first hour of prolonged service on a given date regardless of the place of service. It should be used only once per date.

Prolonged service of less than 30 minutes total duration on a given date is not separately reported.

Code 99359 is used to report each additional 30 minutes beyond the first hour regardless of the place of service. It may also be used to report the final 15 to 30 minutes of prolonged service on a given date.

Prolonged service of less than 15 minutes beyond the first hour or less than 15 minutes beyond the final 30 minutes is not reported separately.

Do not report 99358-99359 for time spent in medical team conferences, on-line medical evaluations, care plan oversight services, anticoagulation management, or other non-face-to-face services that have more specific codes and no upper time limit in the CPT code set. Codes 99358-99359 may be reported when related to other non-face-to-face services codes that have a published maximum time (eg, telephone services)

99358 Prolonged evaluation and management service before and/or after direct patient care; first hour   ⊘N

RVU		Global Days	Modifiers				
Mod	Non-Fac Total	Fac Total		51	50	62	80	MUE
	3.06	3.06	XXX	9	9	9	9	

AMA: Apr 13: 3, Aug 12: 3, 4, 5, Jun 08: 12, Nov 05: 10, Nov 13: 3, Nov 98: 3, Oct 13: 11, Oct 14: 3, Sep 00: 3, Sep 08: 3, Spring 94: 34

+ 99359 Prolonged evaluation and management service before and/or after direct patient care; each additional 30 minutes (List separately in addition to code for prolonged service)   ⊘N

RVU		Global Days	Modifiers				
Mod	Non-Fac Total	Fac Total		51	50	62	80	MUE
	1.48	1.48	ZZZ	9	9	9	9	

AMA: Apr 13: 3, Aug 12: 3, 4, 5, Jun 08: 12, Nov 05: 10, Nov 13: 3, Oct 13: 11, Oct 14: 3, Sep 00: 3, Sep 08: 3, Spring 94: 34

Physician Standby Services

Code 99360 is used to report physician or other qualified healthcare professional standby service that is requested by another physician and that involves prolonged physician attendance without direct (face-to-face) patient contact. The individual may not be providing care or services to other patients during this period. This code is not used to report time spent proctoring another physician. It is also not used if the period of standby ends with the performance of a procedure subject to a surgical package by the individual who was on standby. Code 99360 is used to report the total duration of time spent by a physician on a given date on standby. Standby service of less than 30 minutes total duration on a given date is not reported separately. Second and subsequent periods of standby beyond the first 30 minutes may be reported only if a full 30 minutes of standby was provided for each unit of service reported.

99360 Standby service, requiring prolonged attendance, each 30 minutes (eg, operative standby, standby for frozen section, for cesarean/high risk delivery, for monitoring EEG)   ⊘B

RVU		Global Days	Modifiers				
Mod	Non-Fac Total	Fac Total		51	50	62	80	MUE
	1.73	1.73	XXX	9	9	9	9	

AMA: Apr 14: 5, 11, Apr 97: 10, Aug 00: 3, Aug 97: 18, Feb 11: 3, Mar 08: 14, May 05: 1, May 13: 8, Nov 05: 10, Nov 06: 23, Nov 97: 8, Nov 99: 5, 6, Sep 00: 3, Spring 94: 32

Case Management Services

Case management is a process in which a physician or another qualified health care professional is responsible for direct care of a patient and additionally for coordinating, managing access to, initiating, and/or supervising other health care services needed by the patient.

Anticoagulant Management

Anticoagulation services are intended to describe the outpatient management of warfarin therapy, including ordering, review, and interpretation of International Normalized Ratio (INR) testing, communication with the patient, and dosage adjustments as appropriate.

When reporting these services, the work of anticoagulant management may not be used as a basis for reporting an evaluation and management (E/M) service or care plan oversight time during the reporting period. Do not report these services with 98966-98969, 99441-99444 when telephone or on-line services address anticoagulation with warfarin management. If a significant, separately identifiable E/M service is performed, report the appropriate E/M service code using modifier 25.

These services are outpatient services only. When anticoagulation therapy is initiated or continued in the inpatient or observation setting, a new period begins after discharge and is reported with 99364. Do not report 99363-99364 with 99217-99239, 99291-99292, 99304-99318, 99471-99480 or other code(s) for physician review, interpretation, and patient

● New   ▲ Revised   ✖ Deleted   ⊙ Moderate Sedation   ✚ Add-on Codes   ⊘ High Risk Denial   ⊛ Age Edit   ♀ Female   ♂ Male   **AMA** CPT® Assistant   **MUE** Medically Unlikely Edit
⊘ Modifier 51 Exempt   ⊖ Modifier 63 Exempt   ⊠ Unlisted   **Modifiers:** See Inside Back Cover   M Maternity   A2-Z3 ASC Payment Indicators   A-Y OPPS Status Indicators

© 2016 DecisionHealth   CPT © 2014 American Medical Association. All Rights Reserved.   **139**

Evaluation and Management (E/M) Services

99363 – 99368

management of home INR testing for a patient with mechanical heart valve(s).

Any period less than 60 continuous outpatient days is not reported. If less than the specified minimum number of services per period are performed, do not report the anticoagulant management services (99363-99364).

99363 **Anticoagulant management for an outpatient taking warfarin, physician review and interpretation of International Normalized Ratio (INR) testing, patient instructions, dosage adjustment (as needed), and ordering of additional tests; initial 90 days of therapy (must include a minimum of 8 INR measurements)** ⊙Ⓑ

RVU			Global Days	Modifiers				
Mod	Non-Fac Total	Fac Total		51	50	62	80	MUE
	3.59	2.38	XXX	9	9	9	9	

AMA: Apr 13: 3, Jul 09: 5, Nov 13: 3, Oct 14: 3, Sep 07: 1

99364 **Anticoagulant management for an outpatient taking warfarin, physician review and interpretation of International Normalized Ratio (INR) testing, patient instructions, dosage adjustment (as needed), and ordering of additional tests; each subsequent 90 days of therapy (must include a minimum of 3 INR measurements)** ⊙Ⓑ

RVU			Global Days	Modifiers				
Mod	Non-Fac Total	Fac Total		51	50	62	80	MUE
	1.22	0.91	XXX	9	9	9	9	

AMA: Apr 13: 3, Jul 09: 5, Nov 13: 3, Oct 14: 3, Sep 07: 1

Medical Team Conferences

Medical team conferences include face-to-face participation by a minimum of three qualified health care professionals from different specialties or disciplines (each of whom provide direct care to the patient), with or without the presence of the patient, family members(s), community agencies, surrogate decision maker(s) (eg, legal guardian), and/or caregiver(s). The participants are actively involved in the development, revision, coordination, and implementation of health care services needed by the patient. Reporting participants shall have performed face-to-face evaluations or treatments of the patient, independent of any team conference, within the previous 60 day.

Physicians or other qualified healthcare professionals may report their time spent in a team conference with the patient and/or family present using evaluation and management (E/M) codes (and time as the key controlling factor for code selection when counseling and/or coordination of care dominates the service). These introductory guidelines do not apply to services reported using E/M codes (see E/M services guidelines). However, the individual must be directly involved with the patient, providing face-to-face services outside of the conference visit with other providers or agencies.

Reporting participants shall document their participation in the team conference as well as their contributed information and subsequent treatment recommendations.

No more than one individual from the same specialty may report 99366-99368 at the same encounter.

Individuals should not report 99366-99368 when their participation in the medical team conference is part of a facility or organizational service contractually provided by the organization or facility provider.

The team conference starts at the beginning of the review of an individual patient and ends at the conclusion of the review. Time related to record keeping and report generation is not reported. The reporting participant shall be present for all time reported. The time reported is not limited to the time that the participant is communicating to the other team members or patient and/or family. Time reported for medical team conferences may not be used in the determination of time for other services such as care plan oversight (99374-99380), home, domiciliary, or rest home care plan oversight (99339-99340), prolonged services

(99354-99359), psychotherapy, or any E/M service. For team conferences where the patient is present for any part of the duration of the conference, nonphysician qualified health care professionals report the team conference face-to-face code 99366.

Medical Team Conference Services, Face to Face

99366 **Medical team conference with interdisciplinary team of health care professionals, face-to-face with patient and/or family, 30 minutes or more, participation by nonphysician qualified health care professional** ⊙Ⓝ

RVU			Global Days	Modifiers				
Mod	Non-Fac Total	Fac Total		51	50	62	80	MUE
	1.21	1.18	XXX	9	9	9	9	0

AMA: Apr 13: 3, Jun 14: 3, Oct 14: 3

Medical Team Conference Services, Non-Face to Face

99367 **Medical team conference with interdisciplinary team of health care professionals, patient and/or family not present, 30 minutes or more; participation by physician** ⊙Ⓝ

RVU			Global Days	Modifiers				
Mod	Non-Fac Total	Fac Total		51	50	62	80	MUE
	1.59	1.59	XXX	9	9	9	9	0

AMA: Apr 13: 3, Jun 14: 3

99368 **Medical team conference with interdisciplinary team of health care professionals, patient and/or family not present, 30 minutes or more; participation by nonphysician qualified health care professional** ⊙Ⓝ

RVU			Global Days	Modifiers				
Mod	Non-Fac Total	Fac Total		51	50	62	80	MUE
	1.04	1.04	XXX	9	9	9	9	0

AMA: Apr 13: 3, Jun 14: 3, Oct 14: 3

Care Plan Oversight Services

Care plan oversight services are reported separately from codes for office/outpatient, hospital, home, nursing facility or domiciliary, or non-face-to-face services. The complexity and approximate time of the care plan oversight services provided within a 30-day period determine code selection. Only one individual may report services for a given period of time, to reflect the sole or predominant supervisory role with a particular patient. These codes should not be reported for supervision of patients in nursing facilities or under the care of home health agencies unless they require recurrent supervision of therapy.

The work involved in providing very low intensity or infrequent supervision services is included in the pre- and post-encounter work for home, office/outpatient and nursing facility or domiciliary visit codes.

● New   ▲ Revised   ✖ Deleted   ⊙ Moderate Sedation   ✚ Add-on Codes   ⊘ High Risk Denial   Ⓐ Age Edit   ♀ Female   ♂ Male   **AMA** *CPT® Assistant*   **MUE** Medically Unlikely Edit
⊘ Modifier 51 Exempt   ⊖ Modifier 63 Exempt   ✗ Unlisted   **Modifiers:** *See Inside Back Cover*   Ⓜ Maternity   Ⓐ2–Ⓩ3 ASC Payment Indicators   Ⓐ–Ⓨ OPPS Status Indicators

140   CPT © 2014 American Medical Association. All Rights Reserved.   © 2016 DecisionHealth

99374 Supervision of a patient under care of home health agency (patient not present) in home, domiciliary or equivalent environment (eg, Alzheimer's facility) requiring complex and multidisciplinary care modalities involving regular development and/or revision of care plans by that individual, review of subsequent reports of patient status, review of related laboratory and other studies, communication (including telephone calls) for purposes of assessment or care decisions with health care professional(s), family member(s), surrogate decision maker(s) (eg, legal guardian) and/or key caregiver(s) involved in patient's care, integration of new information into the medical treatment plan and/or adjustment of medical therapy, within a calendar month; 15-29 minutes ⊘B

RVU			Global Days	Modifiers				
Mod	Non-Fac Total	Fac Total		51	50	62	80	MUE
	1.98	1.59	XXX	9	9	9	9	

AMA: Apr 13: 3, Dec 06: 4, Feb 14: 11, Jul 09: 5, 10, Jul 13: 11, Mar 07: 11, Mar 08: 6, May 05: 1, Nov 13: 3, Nov 97: 8, 9, Oct 14: 3, Sep 08: 3, Sep 13: 15, Summer 94: 9

99375 Supervision of a patient under care of home health agency (patient not present) in home, domiciliary or equivalent environment (eg, Alzheimer's facility) requiring complex and multidisciplinary care modalities involving regular development and/or revision of care plans by that individual, review of subsequent reports of patient status, review of related laboratory and other studies, communication (including telephone calls) for purposes of assessment or care decisions with health care professional(s), family member(s), surrogate decision maker(s) (eg, legal guardian) and/or key caregiver(s) involved in patient's care, integration of new information into the medical treatment plan and/or adjustment of medical therapy, within a calendar month; 30 minutes or more ⊘E

RVU			Global Days	Modifiers				
Mod	Non-Fac Total	Fac Total		51	50	62	80	MUE
	2.95	2.49	XXX	9	9	9	9	

AMA: Apr 13: 3, Dec 06: 4, Jul 09: 5, 10, Jul 13: 11, Mar 07: 11, Mar 08: 6, Nov 97: 8, 9, Sep 08: 3, Sep 13: 15, Summer 94: 9

99377 Supervision of a hospice patient (patient not present) requiring complex and multidisciplinary care modalities involving regular development and/or revision of care plans by that individual, review of subsequent reports of patient status, review of related laboratory and other studies, communication (including telephone calls) for purposes of assessment or care decisions with health care professional(s), family member(s), surrogate decision maker(s) (eg, legal guardian) and/or key caregiver(s) involved in patient's care, integration of new information into the medical treatment plan and/or adjustment of medical therapy, within a calendar month; 15-29 minutes ⊘B

RVU			Global Days	Modifiers				
Mod	Non-Fac Total	Fac Total		51	50	62	80	MUE
	1.98	1.59	XXX	9	9	9	9	

AMA: Apr 13: 3, Dec 06: 4, Jul 09: 5, 10, Jul 13: 11, Mar 07: 11, Nov 97: 8, 9, Sep 08: 3, Sep 13: 15

99378 Supervision of a hospice patient (patient not present) requiring complex and multidisciplinary care modalities involving regular development and/or revision of care plans by that individual, review of subsequent reports of patient status, review of related laboratory and other studies, communication (including telephone calls) for purposes of assessment or care decisions with health care professional(s), family member(s), surrogate decision maker(s) (eg, legal guardian) and/or key caregiver(s) involved in patient's care, integration of new information into the medical treatment plan and/or adjustment of medical therapy, within a calendar month; 30 minutes or more ⊘E

RVU			Global Days	Modifiers				
Mod	Non-Fac Total	Fac Total		51	50	62	80	MUE
	2.95	2.49	XXX	9	9	9	9	

AMA: Apr 13: 3, Dec 06: 4, Jul 09: 5, 10, Jul 13: 11, Mar 07: 11, Mar 08: 6, Nov 97: 8, 9, Sep 08: 3, Sep 13: 15

99379 Supervision of a nursing facility patient (patient not present) requiring complex and multidisciplinary care modalities involving regular development and/or revision of care plans by that individual, review of subsequent reports of patient status, review of related laboratory and other studies, communication (including telephone calls) for purposes of assessment or care decisions with health care professional(s), family member(s), surrogate decision maker(s) (eg, legal guardian) and/or key caregiver(s) involved in patient's care, integration of new information into the medical treatment plan and/or adjustment of medical therapy, within a calendar month; 15-29 minutes ⊘B

RVU			Global Days	Modifiers				
Mod	Non-Fac Total	Fac Total		51	50	62	80	MUE
	1.98	1.59	XXX	9	9	9	9	

AMA: Apr 13: 3, Dec 06: 4, Jul 09: 5, Jul 13: 11, Mar 08: 6, Sep 08: 3, Sep 13: 15

● New　▲ Revised　✖ Deleted　⊙ Moderate Sedation　✚ Add-on Codes　⊘ High Risk Denial　Ⓐ Age Edit　♀ Female　♂ Male　**AMA** CPT® Assistant　**MUE** Medically Unlikely Edit
⊘ Modifier 51 Exempt　⊖ Modifier 63 Exempt　✖ Unlisted　**Modifiers:** See Inside Back Cover　Ⓜ Maternity　A2–Z3 ASC Payment Indicators　A–Y OPPS Status Indicators

Evaluation and Management (E/M) Services

99380 – 99384

99380 **Supervision of a nursing facility patient (patient not present) requiring complex and multidisciplinary care modalities involving regular development and/or revision of care plans by that individual, review of subsequent reports of patient status, review of related laboratory and other studies, communication (including telephone calls) for purposes of assessment or care decisions with health care professional(s), family member(s), surrogate decision maker(s) (eg, legal guardian) and/or key caregiver(s) involved in patient's care, integration of new information into the medical treatment plan and/or adjustment of medical therapy, within a calendar month; 30 minutes or more** ⊙B

RVU		Global Days	Modifiers				
Mod	Non-Fac Total	Fac Total		51	50	62	80	MUE
	2.95	2.49	XXX	9	9	9	9	

AMA: Apr 13: 3, Dec 06: 4, Jul 09: 5, Jul 13: 11, Mar 08: 6, Nov 13: 3, Nov 97: 8, 9, Oct 14: 3, Sep 08: 3, Sep 13: 15

Preventive Medicine Services

The following codes are used to report the preventive medicine evaluation and management of infants, children, adolescents, and adults.

The extent and focus of the services will largely depend on the age of the patient.

If an abnormality is encountered or a preexisting problem is addressed in the process of performing this preventive medicine evaluation and management service, and if the problem or abnormality is significant enough to require additional work to perform the key components of a problem-oriented E/M service, then the appropriate Office/Outpatient code 99201-99215 should also be reported. Modifier 25 should be added to the Office/Outpatient code to indicate that a significant, separately identifiable evaluation and management service was provided by the same physician on the same day as the preventive medicine service. The appropriate preventive medicine service is additionally reported.

An insignificant or trivial problem/abnormality that is encountered in the process of performing the preventive medicine evaluation and management service and which does not require additional work and the performance of the key components of a problem-oriented E/M service should not be reported.

The "comprehensive" nature of the Preventive Medicine Services codes 99381-99397 reflects an age and gender appropriate history/exam and is not synonymous with the "comprehensive" examination required in Evaluation and Management codes 99201-99350.

Codes 99381-99397 include counseling/anticipatory guidance/risk factor reduction interventions which are provided at the time of the initial or period comprehensive preventive medicine examination. (Refer to codes 99401-99412 for reporting those counseling/anticipatory guidance/risk factor reduction interventions that are provided at an encounter separate from the preventive medicine examination.)

Vaccine/toxoids products, immunization administrations, ancillary studies involving laboratory, radiology, other procedures, or screening tests (eg, vision, hearing, developmental) identified with a specific CPT code are reported separately. For immunization administration and vaccine risk/benefit counseling, see 90460, 90461, 90471-90474. For vaccine/toxoids products, see 90476-90749.

New Patient Services

99381 **Initial comprehensive preventive medicine evaluation and management of an individual including an age and gender appropriate history, examination, counseling/anticipatory guidance/ risk factor reduction interventions, and the ordering of laboratory/diagnostic procedures, new patient; infant (age younger than 1 year)** ⊙ⒶE

RVU			Global Days	Modifiers				
Mod	Non-Fac Total	Fac Total		51	50	62	80	MUE
	3.11	2.16	XXX	9	9	9	9	

AMA: Aug 05: 15, Aug 09: 5, Aug 97: 1, Dec 14: 18, Jan 13: 9, Jul 09: 7, Jul 98: 9, Mar 09: 3, May 02: 1, May 05: 1, Nov 98: 3, 4, Oct 06: 15, Sep 98: 5, Spring 93: 14, 34, Spring 95: 1, Winter 91: 11

99382 **Initial comprehensive preventive medicine evaluation and management of an individual including an age and gender appropriate history, examination, counseling/anticipatory guidance/ risk factor reduction interventions, and the ordering of laboratory/diagnostic procedures, new patient; early childhood (age 1 through 4 years)** ⊙ⒶE

RVU			Global Days	Modifiers				
Mod	Non-Fac Total	Fac Total		51	50	62	80	MUE
	3.25	2.30	XXX	9	9	9	9	

AMA: Aug 05: 15, Aug 09: 5, Aug 97: 1, Dec 14: 18, Jan 13: 9, Jul 09: 5, Jul 98: 9, May 02: 1, Nov 98: 3, 4, Oct 06: 15, Sep 98: 5, Spring 93: 14, 34, Spring 95: 1, Winter 91: 11

99383 **Initial comprehensive preventive medicine evaluation and management of an individual including an age and gender appropriate history, examination, counseling/anticipatory guidance/ risk factor reduction interventions, and the ordering of laboratory/diagnostic procedures, new patient; late childhood (age 5 through 11 years)** ⊙ⒶE

RVU			Global Days	Modifiers				
Mod	Non-Fac Total	Fac Total		51	50	62	80	MUE
	3.38	2.45	XXX	9	9	9	9	

AMA: Aug 05: 15, Aug 09: 5, Aug 97: 1, Dec 14: 18, Jan 13: 9, Jul 09: 7, Jul 98: 9, May 02: 1, Nov 98: 3, 4, Oct 06: 15, Sep 98: 5, Spring 93: 14, 34, Spring 95: 1, Winter 91: 11

99384 **Initial comprehensive preventive medicine evaluation and management of an individual including an age and gender appropriate history, examination, counseling/anticipatory guidance/ risk factor reduction interventions, and the ordering of laboratory/diagnostic procedures, new patient; adolescent (age 12 through 17 years)** ⊙ⒶE

RVU			Global Days	Modifiers				
Mod	Non-Fac Total	Fac Total		51	50	62	80	MUE
	3.82	2.89	XXX	9	9	9	9	

AMA: Aug 05: 15, Aug 09: 5, Aug 97: 1, Dec 14: 18, Jan 13: 9, Jan 15: 12, Jul 09: 7, Jul 98: 9, May 02: 1, Nov 98: 3, 4, Oct 06: 15, Sep 98: 5, Spring 93: 14, 34, Spring 95: 1, Winter 91: 11

● New   ▲ Revised   ✖ Deleted   ⊙ Moderate Sedation   ✚ Add-on Codes   ⊘ High Risk Denial   Ⓐ Age Edit   ♀ Female   ♂ Male   **AMA** *CPT® Assistant*   **MUE** Medically Unlikely Edit
◌ Modifier 51 Exempt   ⊖ Modifier 63 Exempt   ✗ Unlisted   **Modifiers:** *See Inside Back Cover*   Ⓜ Maternity   A2–Z3 ASC Payment Indicators   A–Y OPPS Status Indicators

142   CPT © 2014 American Medical Association. All Rights Reserved.   © 2016 DecisionHealth

99385 Initial comprehensive preventive medicine evaluation and management of an individual including an age and gender appropriate history, examination, counseling/anticipatory guidance/ risk factor reduction interventions, and the ordering of laboratory/diagnostic procedures, new patient; 18-39 years ⊘Ⓐ🄴

RVU			Global Days	Modifiers				
Mod	Non-Fac Total	Fac Total		51	50	62	80	MUE
	3.70	2.77	XXX	9	9	9	9	

AMA: Aug 05: 15, Aug 09: 5, Aug 97: 7, Dec 14: 18, Jan 13: 9, Jan 15: 12, Jul 09: 5, Jul 98: 9, May 02: 1, Nov 98: 3, 4, Oct 06: 15, Sep 98: 5, Spring 93: 14, 34, Spring 95: 1, Winter 91: 11

99386 Initial comprehensive preventive medicine evaluation and management of an individual including an age and gender appropriate history, examination, counseling/anticipatory guidance/ risk factor reduction interventions, and the ordering of laboratory/diagnostic procedures, new patient; 40-64 years ⊘Ⓐ🄴

RVU			Global Days	Modifiers				
Mod	Non-Fac Total	Fac Total		51	50	62	80	MUE
	4.30	3.36	XXX	9	9	9	9	

AMA: Aug 05: 15, Aug 09: 5, Aug 97: 1, Dec 14: 18, Jan 13: 9, Jan 15: 12, Jul 09: 7, Jul 98: 9, May 02: 1, Nov 98: 3, 4, Oct 06: 15, Sep 98: 5, Spring 93: 14, 34, Spring 95: 1, Winter 91: 11

99387 Initial comprehensive preventive medicine evaluation and management of an individual including an age and gender appropriate history, examination, counseling/anticipatory guidance/ risk factor reduction interventions, and the ordering of laboratory/diagnostic procedures, new patient; 65 years and older ⊘Ⓐ🄴

RVU			Global Days	Modifiers				
Mod	Non-Fac Total	Fac Total		51	50	62	80	MUE
	4.66	3.61	XXX	9	9	9	9	

AMA: Aug 05: 15, Aug 09: 5, Aug 97: 1, Dec 14: 18, Jan 13: 9, Jul 09: 7, Jul 98: 9, May 02: 1, Nov 98: 3, 4, Oct 06: 15, Sep 98: 5, Spring 93: 14, 34, Spring 95: 1, Winter 91: 11

Established Patient Services

99391 Periodic comprehensive preventive medicine reevaluation and management of an individual including an age and gender appropriate history, examination, counseling/anticipatory guidance/ risk factor reduction interventions, and the ordering of laboratory/diagnostic procedures, established patient; infant (age younger than 1 year) ⊘Ⓐ🄴

RVU			Global Days	Modifiers				
Mod	Non-Fac Total	Fac Total		51	50	62	80	MUE
	2.79	1.97	XXX	9	9	9	9	

AMA: Aug 05: 15, Aug 09: 5, Aug 97: 1, Dec 14: 18, Jan 13: 9, Jul 09: 7, Jul 98: 9, Mar 09: 3, May 02: 1, May 05: 1, Nov 98: 3, 4, Oct 06: 15, Sep 98: 5, Spring 93: 14, 34, Spring 95: 1, Winter 91: 11

99392 Periodic comprehensive preventive medicine reevaluation and management of an individual including an age and gender appropriate history, examination, counseling/anticipatory guidance/ risk factor reduction interventions, and the ordering of laboratory/diagnostic procedures, established patient; early childhood (age 1 through 4 years) ⊘Ⓐ🄴

RVU			Global Days	Modifiers				
Mod	Non-Fac Total	Fac Total		51	50	62	80	MUE
	2.98	2.16	XXX	9	9	9	9	

AMA: Aug 05: 15, Aug 97: 1, Dec 14: 18, Jan 13: 9, Jul 09: 7, Jul 98: 9, May 02: 1, Nov 98: 3, 4, Oct 06: 15, Sep 98: 5, Spring 93: 14, 34, Spring 95: 1, Winter 91: 11

99393 Periodic comprehensive preventive medicine reevaluation and management of an individual including an age and gender appropriate history, examination, counseling/anticipatory guidance/ risk factor reduction interventions, and the ordering of laboratory/diagnostic procedures, established patient; late childhood (age 5 through 11 years) ⊘Ⓐ🄴

RVU			Global Days	Modifiers				
Mod	Non-Fac Total	Fac Total		51	50	62	80	MUE
	2.97	2.16	XXX	9	9	9	9	

AMA: Aug 05: 15, Aug 97: 1, Dec 14: 18, Jan 13: 9, Jul 09: 7, Jul 98: 9, May 02: 1, Nov 98: 3, 4, Oct 06: 15, Sep 98: 5, Spring 93: 14, 34, Spring 95: 1, Winter 91: 11

99394 Periodic comprehensive preventive medicine reevaluation and management of an individual including an age and gender appropriate history, examination, counseling/anticipatory guidance/ risk factor reduction interventions, and the ordering of laboratory/diagnostic procedures, established patient; adolescent (age 12 through 17 years) ⊘Ⓐ🄴

RVU			Global Days	Modifiers				
Mod	Non-Fac Total	Fac Total		51	50	62	80	MUE
	3.26	2.45	XXX	9	9	9	9	

AMA: Aug 05: 15, Aug 97: 1, Dec 14: 18, Jan 13: 9, Jan 15: 12, Jul 09: 7, Jul 98: 9, May 02: 1, Nov 98: 3, 4, Oct 06: 15, Sep 98: 5, Spring 93: 14, 34, Spring 95: 1, Winter 91: 11

99395 Periodic comprehensive preventive medicine reevaluation and management of an individual including an age and gender appropriate history, examination, counseling/anticipatory guidance/ risk factor reduction interventions, and the ordering of laboratory/diagnostic procedures, established patient; 18-39 years ⊘Ⓐ🄴

RVU			Global Days	Modifiers				
Mod	Non-Fac Total	Fac Total		51	50	62	80	MUE
	3.33	2.52	XXX	9	9	9	9	

AMA: Aug 05: 15, Aug 97: 1, Dec 14: 18, Jan 13: 9, Jan 15: 12, Jul 09: 7, Jul 98: 9, Mar 08: 3, May 02: 1, Nov 98: 3, 4, Oct 06: 15, Sep 98: 5, Spring 93: 14, 34, Spring 95: 1, Winter 91: 11

Evaluation and Management (E/M) Services

99396 – 99407

99396 Periodic comprehensive preventive medicine reevaluation and management of an individual including an age and gender appropriate history, examination, counseling/anticipatory guidance/ risk factor reduction interventions, and the ordering of laboratory/diagnostic procedures, established patient; 40-64 years ⊘Ⓐ🄴

RVU			Global Days	Modifiers				
Mod	Non-Fac Total	Fac Total		51	50	62	80	MUE
	3.55	2.74	XXX	9	9	9	9	

AMA: Aug 05: 15, Aug 97: 1, Dec 14: 18, Jan 13: 9, Jan 15: 12, Jul 09: 7, Jul 98: 9, Mar 12: 4, May 02: 1, Nov 98: 3, 4, Oct 06: 15, Sep 98: 5, Spring 93: 14, 34, Spring 95: 1, Winter 91: 11

99397 Periodic comprehensive preventive medicine reevaluation and management of an individual including an age and gender appropriate history, examination, counseling/anticipatory guidance/ risk factor reduction interventions, and the ordering of laboratory/diagnostic procedures, established patient; 65 years and older ⊘Ⓐ🄴

RVU			Global Days	Modifiers				
Mod	Non-Fac Total	Fac Total		51	50	62	80	MUE
	3.83	2.89	XXX	9	9	9	9	

AMA: Aug 05: 15, Aug 97: 1, Dec 14: 18, Jan 13: 9, Jul 09: 7, Jul 98: 9, May 02: 1, Nov 98: 3, 4, Oct 06: 15, Sep 98: 5, Spring 93: 14, 34, Spring 95: 1, Winter 91: 11

Counseling Risk Factor Reduction and Behavior Change Intervention

New or Established Patient

These codes are used to report services provided face-to-face by a physician or other qualified health care professional for the purpose of promoting health and preventing illness or injury. They are distinct from evaluation and management (E/M) services that may be reported separately when performed. Risk factor reduction services are used for persons without a specific illness for which the counseling might otherwise be used as part of treatment.

Preventive medicine counseling and risk factor reduction interventions will vary with age and should address such issues are family problems, diet and exercise, substance use, sexual practices, injury prevention, dental health, and diagnostic and laboratory test results available at the time of the encounter.

Behavior change interventions are for persons who have a behavior that is often considered an illness itself, such as tobacco use and addiction, substance abuse/misuse, or obesity. Behavior change services may be reported when performed as part of the treatment of condition(s) related to or potentially exacerbated by the behavior or when performed to change the harmful behavior that has not yet resulted in illness. Any E/M services reported on the same day must be distinct, and time spent providing these services may not be used as a basis for the E/M code selection. Behavior change services involve specific validated interventions of assessing readiness for change and barriers to change, advising a change in behavior, assisting by providing specific suggested actions and motivational counseling, and arranging for services and follow-up.

For counseling groups of patients with symptoms or established illness, use 99078.

Health and Behavior Assessment/Intervention services (96150-96155) should not be reported on the same day as codes 99401-99412.

Preventative Medicine, Individual Counseling

99401 Preventive medicine counseling and/or risk factor reduction intervention(s) provided to an individual (separate procedure); approximately 15 minutes ⊘🄴

RVU			Global Days	Modifiers				
Mod	Non-Fac Total	Fac Total		51	50	62	80	MUE
	1.02	0.69	XXX	9	9	9	9	

AMA: Aug 07: 9, Aug 14: 5, Aug 97: 1, Dec 10: 3, Jan 13: 9, Jan 98: 12, May 05: 1, Oct 10: 3

99402 Preventive medicine counseling and/or risk factor reduction intervention(s) provided to an individual (separate procedure); approximately 30 minutes ⊘🄴

RVU			Global Days	Modifiers				
Mod	Non-Fac Total	Fac Total		51	50	62	80	MUE
	1.74	1.42	XXX	9	9	9	9	

AMA: Aug 97: 1, Dec 10: 3, Jan 13: 9, Jan 98: 12, May 05: 1, Oct 10: 3

99403 Preventive medicine counseling and/or risk factor reduction intervention(s) provided to an individual (separate procedure); approximately 45 minutes ⊘🄴

RVU			Global Days	Modifiers				
Mod	Non-Fac Total	Fac Total		51	50	62	80	MUE
	2.44	2.11	XXX	9	9	9	9	

AMA: Aug 97: 1, Dec 10: 3, Jan 13: 9, Jan 98: 12, May 05: 1, Oct 10: 3

99404 Preventive medicine counseling and/or risk factor reduction intervention(s) provided to an individual (separate procedure); approximately 60 minutes ⊘🄴

RVU			Global Days	Modifiers				
Mod	Non-Fac Total	Fac Total		51	50	62	80	MUE
	3.14	2.82	XXX	9	9	9	9	

AMA: Aug 14: 5, Aug 97: 1, Dec 10: 3, Jan 13: 9, Jan 98: 12, May 05: 1, Oct 10: 3

Behavioral Change Interventions, Individual

99406 Smoking and tobacco use cessation counseling visit; intermediate, greater than 3 minutes up to 10 minutes Ⓢ

RVU			Global Days	Modifiers				
Mod	Non-Fac Total	Fac Total		51	50	62	80	MUE
	0.40	0.35	XXX	0	0	0	0	1

AMA: Dec 10: 3, Jan 08: 1, Jan 13: 9, Oct 10: 3, Sep 09: 11

Pub 100-04, 12, 190.3; 100-04, 18, 150.3, 150.4; 100-04, 32, 12.1, 12.3

99407 Smoking and tobacco use cessation counseling visit; intensive, greater than 10 minutes Ⓢ

RVU			Global Days	Modifiers				
Mod	Non-Fac Total	Fac Total		51	50	62	80	MUE
	0.78	0.73	XXX	0	0	0	0	1

AMA: Dec 10: 3, Jan 08: 1, Jan 13: 9, Oct 10: 3, Sep 09: 11

Pub 100-04, 12, 190.3; 100-04, 18, 150.3, 150.4; 100-04, 32, 12.1, 12.3

● New   ▲ Revised   ✖ Deleted   ⊙ Moderate Sedation   ✚ Add-on Codes   ⊘ High Risk Denial   Ⓐ Age Edit   ♀ Female   ♂ Male   **AMA** *CPT® Assistant*   **MUE** Medically Unlikely Edit
⊘ Modifier 51 Exempt   ⊖ Modifier 63 Exempt   🅇 Unlisted   **Modifiers:** *See Inside Back Cover*   Ⓜ Maternity   A2–Z3 ASC Payment Indicators   A–Y OPPS Status Indicators

CPT © 2014 American Medical Association. All Rights Reserved.   © 2016 DecisionHealth

99408 Alcohol and/or substance (other than tobacco) abuse structured screening (eg, AUDIT, DAST), and brief intervention (SBI) services; 15 to 30 minutes ⊘🄴

RVU			Global Days	Modifiers				
Mod	Non-Fac Total	Fac Total		51	50	62	80	MUE
	0.99	0.94	XXX	9	9	9	9	

AMA: Dec 10: 3, Jan 13: 9, Oct 10: 3

99409 Alcohol and/or substance (other than tobacco) abuse structured screening (eg, AUDIT, DAST), and brief intervention (SBI) services; greater than 30 minutes ⊘🄴

RVU			Global Days	Modifiers				
Mod	Non-Fac Total	Fac Total		51	50	62	80	MUE
	1.93	1.88	XXX	9	9	9	9	

AMA: Dec 10: 3, Jan 13: 9, Oct 10: 3

Preventative Medicine Group Counseling

99411 Preventive medicine counseling and/or risk factor reduction intervention(s) provided to individuals in a group setting (separate procedure); approximately 30 minutes ⊘🄴

RVU			Global Days	Modifiers				
Mod	Non-Fac Total	Fac Total		51	50	62	80	MUE
	0.46	0.22	XXX	9	9	9	9	

AMA: Aug 97: 1, Dec 10: 3, Jan 13: 9, Jan 98: 12, May 05: 1, Oct 10: 3, Sep 98: 5

99412 Preventive medicine counseling and/or risk factor reduction intervention(s) provided to individuals in a group setting (separate procedure); approximately 60 minutes ⊘🄴

RVU			Global Days	Modifiers				
Mod	Non-Fac Total	Fac Total		51	50	62	80	MUE
	0.60	0.36	XXX	9	9	9	9	

AMA: Aug 07: 9, Aug 97: 1, Dec 10: 3, Jan 13: 9, Jan 98: 12, May 05: 1, Oct 10: 3, Sep 98: 5

+● 99415 Prolonged clinical staff service (the service beyond the typical service time) during an evaluation and management service in the office or outpatient setting, direct patient contact with physician supervision; first hour (List separately in addition to code for outpatient Evaluation and Management service) 🄽

RVU			Global Days	Modifiers				
Mod	Non-Fac Total	Fac Total		51	50	62	80	MUE
	0.25	0.25	XXX	0	0	0	0	1

+● 99416 Prolonged clinical staff service (the service beyond the typical service time) during an evaluation and management service in the office or outpatient setting, direct patient contact with physician supervision; each additional 30 minutes (List separately in addition to code for prolonged service) 🄽

RVU			Global Days	Modifiers				
Mod	Non-Fac Total	Fac Total		51	50	62	80	MUE
	0.02	0.02	XXX	0	0	0	0	

Other Preventative Care Visits

99420 Administration and interpretation of health risk assessment instrument (eg, health hazard appraisal) ⊘🄴

RVU			Global Days	Modifiers				
Mod	Non-Fac Total	Fac Total		51	50	62	80	MUE
	0.31	0.31	XXX	9	9	9	9	

AMA: Dec 10: 3, Jan 13: 9, May 05: 1, Oct 10: 3

99429 Unlisted preventive medicine service ⊘🆇🄴

RVU			Global Days	Modifiers				
Mod	Non-Fac Total	Fac Total		51	50	62	80	MUE
	0.00	0.00	XXX	9	9	9	9	

AMA: Dec 10: 3, Jan 13: 9, May 05: 1, Oct 10: 3, Sep 98: 5

Non-Face-to-Face Physician Services

Telephone Services

Telephone services are non-face-to-face evaluation and management (E/M) services provided to a patient using the telephone by a physician or other qualified healthcare professional who may report evaluation and management services. These codes are used to report episodes of care initiated by an established patient or guardian of an established patient. If the telephone service ends with a decision to see the patient within 24 hours or next available urgent visit appointment, the code is not reported; rather the encounter is considered part of the preservice work of the subsequent E/M service, procedure, and visit. Likewise, if the telephone call referes to an E/M service performed and reported by the physician within the previous seven days (either requested or unsolicited patient follow-up) or within the postoperative period of the previously completed procedure, then the service(s) are considered part of that pervious E/M service or procedure.

99441 Telephone evaluation and management service by a physician or other qualified health care professional who may report evaluation and management services provided to an established patient, parent, or guardian not originating from a related E/M service provided within the previous 7 days nor leading to an E/M service or procedure within the next 24 hours or soonest available appointment; 5-10 minutes of medical discussion ⊘🄴

RVU			Global Days	Modifiers				
Mod	Non-Fac Total	Fac Total		51	50	62	80	MUE
	0.39	0.36	XXX	9	9	9	9	

AMA: Apr 13: 3, Mar 08: 6, Nov 13: 3, Oct 13: 11, Oct 14: 3

99442 Telephone evaluation and management service by a physician or other qualified health care professional who may report evaluation and management services provided to an established patient, parent, or guardian not originating from a related E/M service provided within the previous 7 days nor leading to an E/M service or procedure within the next 24 hours or soonest available appointment; 11-20 minutes of medical discussion ⊘🄴

RVU			Global Days	Modifiers				
Mod	Non-Fac Total	Fac Total		51	50	62	80	MUE
	0.76	0.72	XXX	9	9	9	9	

AMA: Apr 13: 3, Mar 08: 6, Oct 13: 11

● New ▲ Revised ✖ Deleted ⊙ Moderate Sedation ✚ Add-on Codes ⊘ High Risk Denial ⒶAge Edit ♀ Female ♂ Male **AMA** *CPT® Assistant* **MUE** Medically Unlikely Edit
🚫 Modifier 51 Exempt ⊖ Modifier 63 Exempt 🅇 Unlisted **Modifiers:** *See Inside Back Cover* Ⓜ Maternity 🄰2–🅉3 ASC Payment Indicators 🄰–🆈 OPPS Status Indicators

© 2016 DecisionHealth   CPT © 2014 American Medical Association. All Rights Reserved.   **145**

Evaluation and Management (E/M) Services

99443 – 99450

99443 Telephone evaluation and management service by a physician or other qualified health care professional who may report evaluation and management services provided to an established patient, parent, or guardian not originating from a related E/M service provided within the previous 7 days nor leading to an E/M service or procedure within the next 24 hours or soonest available appointment; 21-30 minutes of medical discussion ⊗🄴

RVU			Global Days	Modifiers				
Mod	Non-Fac Total	Fac Total		51	50	62	80	MUE
	1.12	1.08	XXX	9	9	9	9	

AMA: Apr 13: 3, Mar 08: 6, Nov 13: 3, Oct 13: 11, Oct 14: 3

On-Line Medical Evaluation

An on-line electronic medical evaluation is a non-face-to-face evaluation and management (E/M) service by a physician to a patient using Internet resources in response to a patient's on-line inquiry. Reportable services involve the physician's personal timely response to the patient's inquiry and must involve permanent storage (electronic or hard copy) of the encounter. This service is reported only once for the same episode of care during a seven-day period, although multiple physicians could report their exchange with the same patient. If the on-line medical evaluation refers to an E/M service previously performed and reported by the physician within the previous seven days (either physician requested or unsolicited patient follow-up) or within the postoperative period of the previously completed procedure, then the service(s) are considered covered by the previous E/M service or procedure. A reportable service encompasses the sum of communication (eg, related telephone calls, prescription provision, laboratory orders) pertaining to the on-line patient encounter.

(For an on-line medical evaluation provided by a qualified nonphysician health care professional, use 98969.)

99444 Online evaluation and management service provided by a physician or other qualified health care professional who may report evaluation and management services provided to an established patient or guardian, not originating from a related E/M service provided within the previous 7 days, using the Internet or similar electronic communications network ⊗🄴

RVU			Global Days	Modifiers				
Mod	Non-Fac Total	Fac Total		51	50	62	80	MUE
	0.00	0.00	XXX	9	9	9	9	

AMA: Apr 13: 3, Nov 12: 13, Nov 13: 3, Oct 13: 11, Oct 14: 3

99446 Interprofessional telephone/Internet assessment and management service provided by a consultative physician including a verbal and written report to the patient's treating/requesting physician or other qualified health care professional; 5-10 minutes of medical consultative discussion and review ⊗🄴

RVU			Global Days	Modifiers				
Mod	Non-Fac Total	Fac Total		51	50	62	80	MUE
	0.00	0.00	XXX	9	9	9	9	1

AMA: Jun 14: 14

99447 Interprofessional telephone/Internet assessment and management service provided by a consultative physician including a verbal and written report to the patient's treating/requesting physician or other qualified health care professional; 11-20 minutes of medical consultative discussion and review ⊗🄴

RVU			Global Days	Modifiers				
Mod	Non-Fac Total	Fac Total		51	50	62	80	MUE
	0.00	0.00	XXX	9	9	9	9	1

AMA: Jun 14: 14

99448 Interprofessional telephone/Internet assessment and management service provided by a consultative physician including a verbal and written report to the patient's treating/requesting physician or other qualified health care professional; 21-30 minutes of medical consultative discussion and review ⊗🄴

RVU			Global Days	Modifiers				
Mod	Non-Fac Total	Fac Total		51	50	62	80	MUE
	0.00	0.00	XXX	9	9	9	9	1

AMA: Jun 14: 14

99449 Interprofessional telephone/Internet assessment and management service provided by a consultative physician including a verbal and written report to the patient's treating/requesting physician or other qualified health care professional; 31 minutes or more of medical consultative discussion and review ⊗🄴

RVU			Global Days	Modifiers				
Mod	Non-Fac Total	Fac Total		51	50	62	80	MUE
	0.00	0.00	XXX	9	9	9	9	1

AMA: Jun 14: 14

Special Evaluation and Management Services

The following codes are used to report evaluations performed to establish baseline information prior to life or disability insurance certificates being issued. This service is performed in the office or other setting, and applies to both new and established patients. When using these codes, no active management of the problem(s) is undertaken during the encounter.

If other evaluation and management services and/or procedures are performed on the same date, the appropriate E/M or procedure code(s) should be reported in addition to these codes.

Basic Life and/or Disability Evaluation Services

99450 Basic life and/or disability examination that includes:

    - Measurement of height, weight, and blood pressure;
    - Completion of a medical history following a life insurance pro forma;
    - Collection of blood sample and/or urinalysis complying with "chain of custody" protocols; and
    - Completion of necessary documentation/certificates. ⊗🄴

RVU			Global Days	Modifiers				
Mod	Non-Fac Total	Fac Total		51	50	62	80	MUE
	0.00	0.00	XXX	9	9	9	9	

AMA: May 05: 1, Sep 98: 5, Summer 95: 14

● New   ▲ Revised   ✖ Deleted   ⊙ Moderate Sedation   ✚ Add-on Codes   ⊗ High Risk Denial   Ⓐ Age Edit   ♀ Female   ♂ Male   **AMA** CPT® Assistant   **MUE** Medically Unlikely Edit
Ⓢ Modifier 51 Exempt   ⊖ Modifier 63 Exempt   ☒ Unlisted   **Modifiers:** See Inside Back Cover   Ⓜ Maternity   A2–Z3 ASC Payment Indicators   A–Y OPPS Status Indicators

146   CPT © 2014 American Medical Association. All Rights Reserved.   © 2016 DecisionHealth

Work-Related or Medical Disability Visits

99455 **Work related or medical disability examination by the treating physician that includes:**

- Completion of a medical history commensurate with the patient's condition;
- Performance of an examination commensurate with the patient's condition;
- Formulation of a diagnosis, assessment of capabilities and stability, and calculation of impairment;
- Development of future medical treatment plan; and
- Completion of necessary documentation/ certificates and report. ⊙🅑

RVU			Global Days	Modifiers				
Mod	Non-Fac Total	Fac Total		51	50	62	80	MUE
	0.00	0.00	XXX	0	0	0	0	1

AMA: Aug 13: 13, May 05: 1, Sep 98: 5, Summer 95: 14

99456 **Work related or medical disability examination by other than the treating physician that includes:**

- Completion of a medical history commensurate with the patient's condition;
- Performance of an examination commensurate with the patient's condition;
- Formulation of a diagnosis, assessment of capabilities and stability, and calculation of impairment;
- Development of future medical treatment plan; and
- Completion of necessary documentation/ certificates and report. ⊙🅑

RVU			Global Days	Modifiers				
Mod	Non-Fac Total	Fac Total		51	50	62	80	MUE
	0.00	0.00	XXX	0	0	0	0	1

AMA: Aug 13: 13, Sep 98: 5, Summer 95: 14

Newborn Care Services

The following codes are used to report the services provided to newborns (birth through the first 28 days) in several different settings. Use of the normal newborn codes is limited to the initial care of the newborn in the first days after birth prior to home discharge.

Evaluation and Management (E/M) services for the newborn include maternal and/or fetal and newborn history, newborn physical examination(s), ordering of diagnostic tests and treatments, meeting with the family, and documentation in the medical record.

When delivery room attendance services (99464) or delivery room resuscitation services (99465) are required, report these in addition to normal newborn services Evaluation and Management codes.

For E/M services provided to newborns who are other than normal, see codes for hospital inpatient services (99221-99233) and neonatal intensive and critical care services (99466-99469, 99477-99480). When normal newborn services are provided by the individual on the same date that the newborn later becomes ill and receives additional intensive or critical care services, report the appropriate E/M code with modifier 25 for these services in addition to the normal newborn code.

Procedures (eg, 54150, newborn circumcision) are not included with the normal newborn codes, and when performed, should be reported in addition to the newborn services.

When newborns are seen in follow-up after the date of discharge in the office or outpatient setting, see 99201-99215, 99381, 99391 as appropriate.

99460 **Initial hospital or birthing center care, per day, for evaluation and management of normal newborn infant** ⊙🅐🆅

RVU			Global Days	Modifiers				
Mod	Non-Fac Total	Fac Total		51	50	62	80	MUE
	2.72	2.72	XXX	0	0	0	0	1

99461 **Initial care, per day, for evaluation and management of normal newborn infant seen in other than hospital or birthing center** 🅐🅜

RVU			Global Days	Modifiers				
Mod	Non-Fac Total	Fac Total		51	50	62	80	MUE
	2.79	1.86	XXX	0	0	0	0	1

99462 **Subsequent hospital care, per day, for evaluation and management of normal newborn** ⊙🅐🅒

RVU			Global Days	Modifiers				
Mod	Non-Fac Total	Fac Total		51	50	62	80	MUE
	1.18	1.18	XXX	0	0	0	0	1

99463 **Initial hospital or birthing center care, per day, for evaluation and management of normal newborn infant admitted and discharged on the same date** ⊙🅐🆅

RVU			Global Days	Modifiers				
Mod	Non-Fac Total	Fac Total		51	50	62	80	MUE
	3.36	3.36	XXX	0	0	0	0	1

Delivery/Birthing Room Attendance and Resuscitation Services

99464 **Attendance at delivery (when requested by the delivering physician or other qualified health care professional) and initial stabilization of newborn** ⊙🅐🅝

RVU			Global Days	Modifiers				
Mod	Non-Fac Total	Fac Total		51	50	62	80	MUE
	2.02	2.02	XXX	0	0	0	0	1

99465 **Delivery/birthing room resuscitation, provision of positive pressure ventilation and/or chest compressions in the presence of acute inadequate ventilation and/or cardiac output** ⊙🅐🆂

RVU			Global Days	Modifiers				
Mod	Non-Fac Total	Fac Total		51	50	62	80	MUE
	4.31	4.31	XXX	0	0	0	0	1

Inpatient Neonatal Intensive Care Services and Pediatric and Neonatal Critical Care Services

Pediatric Critical Care Patient Transport

The following codes (99466, 99467) are used to report the physical attendance and direct face-to-face care by a physician during the interfacility transport of a critically ill or critically injured pediatric patient 24 months of age or younger. Codes 99485 and 99486 are used to report the control physician's non face-to-face supervision of interfacility transport of a critically ill or critically injured pediatric patient 24 months of age or younger. For the purpose of reporting codes 99466 and 99467, face-to-face care begins when the physician assumes primary responsibility of the pediatric patient at the referring hospital/facility, and ends when the receiving hospital/facility accepts the responsibility for the pediatric patient's care. Only the time the physician spends in direct face-to-face contact with the patient during the transport should be reported. Pediatric patient transport services involving less than 30 minutes of face-to-face physician care should not be reported using codes 99466, 99467. Procedure(s) or service(s) performed by other members of the transporting team may not be reported by the supervising physician.

● New   ▲ Revised   ✖ Deleted   ⊙ Moderate Sedation   ✚ Add-on Codes   ⊘ High Risk Denial   Ⓐ Age Edit   ♀ Female   ♂ Male   **AMA** *CPT® Assistant*   **MUE** Medically Unlikely Edit

⊙ Modifier 51 Exempt   ⊖ Modifier 63 Exempt   🆇 Unlisted   **Modifiers:** *See Inside Back Cover*   🅜 Maternity   🄰2–🅉3 ASC Payment Indicators   🄰–🆈 OPPS Status Indicators

Codes 99485, 99486 are used to report control physician's non-face-to-face supervision of interfacility pediatric critical care transport, which includes all two-way communication between the control physician and the specialized transport team prior to transport, at the referring facility and during transport of the patient back to the receiving facility. The "control" physician is the physician directing transport services. These codes do not include pre-transport communication between the control physician and the referring facility before or following patient transport. These codes are only reported for patients 24 months of age or younger who are critically ill or critically injured. The control physician provides treatment advice to a specialized transport team who are present and delivering the hands-on patient care. The control physician does not report any services provided by the specialized transport team. The control physician's non-face-to-face time begins with the first contact by the control physician with the specialized transport team and ends when the patient's care is handed over to the receiving facility team. Refer to 99466 and 99467 for face-to-face transport care of the critically ill/injured patient. Time spent with the individual patient's transport team and reviewing data submissions should be recorded. Code 99485 is used to report the first 16-45 minutes of direction on a given date and should only be used once even if time spent by the physician is discontinuous. Do not report services of 15 minutes or less or any time when another physician is reporting 99466, 99467. Do not report 99485 or 99486 in conjunction with 99466, 99467 when performed by the same physician.

For the definition of the critically injured pediatric patient, see the Neonatal and Pediatric Critical Care Services section.

The non-face-to-face direction of emergency care to a patient's transporting staff by a physician located in a hospital or other facility by two-way communication is not considered direct face-to-face care and should not be reported with 99466, 99467. Physician-directed non-face-to-face emergency care through outside voice communication to transporting staff personnel is reported with 99288 or 99485, 99486 based upon the age and clinical condition of the patient.

Emergency department services (99281-99285), initial hospital care (99221-99223), critical care (99291, 99292), initial date neonatal intensive (99477) or critical care (99468) are only reported after the patient has been admitted to the emergency department, the inpatient floor, or the critical care unit of the receiving facility. If inpatient critical care services are reported in the referring facility prior to transfer to the receiving hospital, use the critical care codes (99291, 99292).

The following services are included when performed during the pediatric patient transport by the physician providing critical care and may not be reported separately: routine monitoring evaluations (e.g., heart rate, respiratory rate, blood pressure, and pulse oximetry), the interpretation of cardiac output measurements (93562), ches X-rays (71010, 71015, 71020), pulse oximetry (94760, 94761, 94762), blood gases and information data stored in computers (e.g., ECGs, blood pressures, hematologic data (99090), gastric intubation (43752, 43753), temporary transcutaneous pacing (92953), ventilatory management (94002, 94003, 94660, 94662), and vascular access procedures (36000, 36400, 36405, 36406, 36415, 36591, 36600). Any services performed which are not listed above should be reported separately.

Services provided by the specialized transport team during non-face-to-face transport supervision are not reported by the control physician.

Code 99466 is used to report the first 30 to 74 minutes of direct face-to-face time with the transport pediatric patient and should be reported only once on a given date. Code 99467 is used to report each additional 30 minutes provided on a given date. Face-to-face services of less than 30 minutes should not be reported with these codes.

Code 99485 is used to report the first 30 minutes of non-face-to-face supervision of an interfacility transport of a critically ill or critically injured pediatric patient and should be reported only once per date of service. Only the communication time spent by the supervising physician with the specialty transport team members during an interfacility transport should be reported. Code 99486 is used to report each additional 30 minutes beyond the initial 30 minutes. Non-face-to-face interfacility transport of 15 minutes or less is not reported.

(For total body and selective head cooling of neonates, see 99481, 99482)

99466   **Critical care face-to-face services, during an interfacility transport of critically ill or critically injured pediatric patient, 24 months of age or younger; first 30-74 minutes of hands-on care during transport** ⊗Ⓐℕ

RVU		Global Days	Modifiers				
Mod	Non-Fac Total	Fac Total		51	50	62	80	MUE
	6.49	6.49	XXX	0	0	0	0	1

AMA: May 13: 6, May 14: 4, Sep 11: 3

✚ **99467**   **Critical care face-to-face services, during an interfacility transport of critically ill or critically injured pediatric patient, 24 months of age or younger; each additional 30 minutes (List separately in addition to code for primary service)** ⊗Ⓐℕ

RVU		Global Days	Modifiers				
Mod	Non-Fac Total	Fac Total		51	50	62	80	MUE
	3.28	3.28	ZZZ	0	0	0	0	

AMA: May 13: 6, May 14: 4, Sep 11: 3

99468   **Initial inpatient neonatal critical care, per day, for the evaluation and management of a critically ill neonate, 28 days of age or younger** ⊗Ⓐ©

RVU		Global Days	Modifiers				
Mod	Non-Fac Total	Fac Total		51	50	62	80	MUE
	26.63	26.63	XXX	0	0	0	0	1

AMA: Feb 15: 10, May 14: 4, Nov 11: 5

99469   **Subsequent inpatient neonatal critical care, per day, for the evaluation and management of a critically ill neonate, 28 days of age or younger** ⊗Ⓐ©

RVU		Global Days	Modifiers				
Mod	Non-Fac Total	Fac Total		51	50	62	80	MUE
	11.22	11.22	XXX	0	0	0	0	1

AMA: Feb 15: 10, May 14: 4, Nov 11: 5

99471   **Initial inpatient pediatric critical care, per day, for the evaluation and management of a critically ill infant or young child, 29 days through 24 months of age** ⊗Ⓐ©

RVU		Global Days	Modifiers				
Mod	Non-Fac Total	Fac Total		51	50	62	80	MUE
	24.76	24.76	XXX	0	0	0	0	1

AMA: Feb 15: 10, Nov 11: 5

99472   **Subsequent inpatient pediatric critical care, per day, for the evaluation and management of a critically ill infant or young child, 29 days through 24 months of age** ⊗Ⓐ©

RVU		Global Days	Modifiers				
Mod	Non-Fac Total	Fac Total		51	50	62	80	MUE
	11.56	11.56	XXX	0	0	0	0	1

AMA: Feb 15: 10, Nov 11: 5

99475   **Initial inpatient pediatric critical care, per day, for the evaluation and management of a critically ill infant or young child, 2 through 5 years of age** Ⓐ©

RVU		Global Days	Modifiers				
Mod	Non-Fac Total	Fac Total		51	50	62	80	MUE
	16.28	16.28	XXX	0	0	0	0	1

AMA: Feb 15: 10

● New   ▲ Revised   ✖ Deleted   ⊙ Moderate Sedation   ✚ Add-on Codes   ⊗ High Risk Denial   Ⓐ Age Edit   ♀ Female   ♂ Male   **AMA** CPT® Assistant   **MUE** Medically Unlikely Edit
⊖ Modifier 51 Exempt   ⊖ Modifier 63 Exempt   🄴 Unlisted   **Modifiers:** See Inside Back Cover   Ⓜ Maternity   🄰2–🅉3 ASC Payment Indicators   🄰–🅈 OPPS Status Indicators

CPT © 2014 American Medical Association. All Rights Reserved.   © 2016 DecisionHealth

99476 Subsequent inpatient pediatric critical care, per day, for the evaluation and management of a critically ill infant or young child, 2 through 5 years of age Ⓐ🅲

RVU			Global Days	Modifiers				
Mod	Non-Fac Total	Fac Total		51	50	62	80	MUE
	9.78	9.78	XXX	0	0	0	0	1

AMA: Feb 15: 10

Initial and Continuing Intensive Care Services

Code 99477 represents the initial day of inpatient care for a child who is not critically ill but requires intensive observation, frequent interventions, and other intensive care services. Codes 99478-99480 are used to report subsequent day services provided by a physician directing the continuing intensive care of the low birth weight (LBW 1500-2500 grams) present body weight infant, very low birth weight (VLBW less than 1500 grams) present body weight infant, or normal (2501-5000 grams) present body weight newborn who does not meet the definition of critically ill but continues to require intensive observation, frequent interventions, and other intensive care services. These services are for infants and neonates who are not critically ill but continue to require intensive cardiac and respiratory monitoring, continuous and/or frequent vital sign monitoring, heat maintenance, enteral and/or parenteral nutritional adjustments, laboratory and oxygen monitoring, and constant observation by the health care team under direct supervision of the physician or other qualified health care professional. Codes 99477-99480 may be reported by a single individual and only once per day, per patient in a given facility. If readmitted to the intensive care unit during the same hospital stay, report 99478-99480 for the first day of intensive care and for each successive day that the child requires intensive care services. These codes include the same procedures that are outlined in the Neonatal and Pediatric Critical Care Services section and these services should not be separately reported.

The initial day neonatal intensive care code (99477) can be used in addition to 99464 or 99465 as appropriate, when the physician or other qualified health care professional is present for the delivery (99464) or resuscitation (99465) is required. In this situation, report 99477 with modifier 25. Other procedures performed as a necessary part of the resuscitation (e.g., endotracheal intubation [31500]) are also reported separately when performed as part of the pre-admission delivery room care. In order to report these procedures separately, they must be performed as a necessary component of the resuscitation and not simply as a convenience before admission to the neonatal intensive care unit. The same procedures are included as bundled services with the neonatal intensive care codes as those listed for the neonatal (99468, 99469) and pediatric (99471-99476) critical care codes.

When the neonate or infant improves after the initial day and no longer requires intensive care services and is transferred to a lower level of care, the transferring individual does not report a per day intensive care service. Subsequent hospital care (99231-99233) or subsequent normal newborn care (99460, 99462) is reported as appropriate based upon the condition of the neonate or infant. If the transfer to a lower level of care occurs on the same day as initial intensive care services were provided by the transferring individual, 99477 may be reported. When the neonate or infant is transferred after the initial day within the same facility to the care of another individual in a different group, both individuals report subsequent hospital care (99231-99233) services. The receiving individual reports subsequent hospital care (99231-99233) or subsequent normal newborn care (99462).

When the neonate or infant becomes critically ill on a day when initial or subsequent intensive care services (99477 -99480) have been reported by one individual and is transferred to a critical care level of care provided by a different individual from a different group, the transferring individual reports either the time-based critical care services performed (99291, 99292) for the time spent providing critical care to the patient or the initial or subsequent intensive care (99477-99480) service, but not both. The receiving individual reports initial or subsequent inpatient neonatal or pediatric critical care (99468-99476) based upon the patient's age and whether this is the first or subsequent admission to critical care for the same hospital stay.

When the neonate or infant becomes critically ill on a day when initial or subsequent intensive care services (99477-99480) have been performed by the same individual or group, report only initial or subsequent inpatient neonatal or pediatric critical care (99468-99476) based upon the patient's age and whether this is the first or subsequent admission to critical care for the same hospital stay.

For the subsequent care of the sick neonate younger than 28 days of age but more than 5000 grams who does not require intensive or critical care services, use codes 99231-99233.

99477 Initial hospital care, per day, for the evaluation and management of the neonate, 28 days of age or younger, who requires intensive observation, frequent interventions, and other intensive care services ⊗Ⓐ🅲

RVU			Global Days	Modifiers				
Mod	Non-Fac Total	Fac Total		51	50	62	80	MUE
	10.08	10.08	XXX	0	0	0	0	1

AMA: Jan 08: 8, Jul 08: 10, Mar 09: 3, May 14: 4, Nov 11: 5

99478 Subsequent intensive care, per day, for the evaluation and management of the recovering very low birth weight infant (present body weight less than 1500 grams) ⊗Ⓐ🅲

RVU			Global Days	Modifiers				
Mod	Non-Fac Total	Fac Total		51	50	62	80	MUE
	3.86	3.86	XXX	0	0	0	0	1

99479 Subsequent intensive care, per day, for the evaluation and management of the recovering low birth weight infant (present body weight of 1500-2500 grams) ⊗Ⓐ🅲

RVU			Global Days	Modifiers				
Mod	Non-Fac Total	Fac Total		51	50	62	80	MUE
	3.51	3.51	XXX	0	0	0	0	1

99480 Subsequent intensive care, per day, for the evaluation and management of the recovering infant (present body weight of 2501-5000 grams) ⊗Ⓐ🅲

RVU			Global Days	Modifiers				
Mod	Non-Fac Total	Fac Total		51	50	62	80	MUE
	3.37	3.37	XXX	0	0	0	0	1

AMA: Jul 15: 4, May 14: 4

Coordination of Complex Chronic Care

Complex chronic care coordination services are patient-centered management and support services provided by physicians, other qualified health care professionals, and clinical staff to an individual who resides at home or in a domiciliary, rest home, or assisted living facility. These services typically involve clinical staff implementing a care plan directed by the physician or other qualified health care professional. These services address the coordination of care by multiple disciplines and community service agencies. The reporting individual provides or oversees the management and/or coordination of services, as needed, for all medical conditions, psychosocial needs, and activities of daily living.

Patients who require complex chronic care coordination services may be identified by algorithms that utilize reported conditions and services (e.g., predictive modeling risk score or repeat admissions or emergency department use) or by clinician judgment. Typical patients have 1 or more chronic continuous or episodic health conditions expected to last at least 12 months, or until the death of the patient, that place the patient at significant risk of death, acute exacerbation/decompensation, or functional decline. Because of the complex nature of their diseases and morbidities, these patients commonly require the coordination of a number of specialties and services. Patients may have medical and psychiatric behavioral co-morbidities (e.g., dementia and chronic obstructive pulmonary disease or substance abuse and diabetes) that complicate their care. Social support weaknesses or access to care difficulties may cause a need for these services. Medical, functional, and/or psychosocial problems that require medical decision making of moderate

● New   ▲ Revised   ✖ Deleted   ⊙ Moderate Sedation   ✚ Add-on Codes   ⊗ High Risk Denial   Ⓐ Age Edit   ♀ Female   ♂ Male   **AMA** CPT® Assistant   **MUE** Medically Unlikely Edit
⊘ Modifier 51 Exempt   ⊖ Modifier 63 Exempt   🅇 Unlisted   **Modifiers:** See Inside Back Cover   Ⓜ Maternity   🅰2-🅩3 ASC Payment Indicators   🅰–Ⓨ OPPS Status Indicators

Evaluation and Management (E/M) Services

99486 – 99487

or high complexity and extensive clinical staff support are expected. Medical decision making as defined in the Evaluation and Management (E/M) guidelines is not only applied to the face-to-face services but is determined by the nature of the problems addressed by the reporting individual during the month. A plan of care should be documented and shared with the patient and/or caregiver.

Codes 99487, 99489, 99490 are reported only once per calendar month and include all non-face-to-face complex chronic care coordination services and none or 1 face-to-face office or other outpatient, home, or domiciliary visit. Codes 99487, 99489, 99490 may only be reported by the single physician or other qualified health care professional who assumes the care coordination role with a particular patient for the calendar month.

Code selection is as follows:

Code 99487 is reported when, during the calendar month, there is no face-to-face visit with the physician or other qualified health care professional and at least 60-89 minutes of clinical staff time is spent in care coordination activities. To report one or more face-to-face visits, performed in the same calendar month, use the appropriate E/M code.

The face-to-face and non-face-to-face time spent by the clinical staff in communicating with the patient and/or family, caregivers, other professionals and agencies; revising, documenting and implementing the care plan; or teaching self-management is used in determining the complex chronic care coordination clinical staff time for the month. Note: Do not count any clinical staff time on the date of the first visit or on a day when the physician or qualified health care professional reports an E/M service (office or other outpatient services 99201-99205, 99211-99215; domiciliary; rest home services 99327-99337; home services 99341-99350).

Code 99490 is used when at least 20 minutes of clinical staff time is spend on care management activities during the calendar month.

Care coordination activities performed by clinical staff may include:

- communication (with patient, family members, guardian or caretaker, surrogate decision makers, and/or other professionals) regarding aspects of care;
- communication with home health agencies and other community services utilized by the patient;
- collection of health outcomes data and registry documentation;
- patient and/or family/caretaker education to support self-management, independent living, and activities of daily living;
- assessment and support for treatment regimen adherence and medication management;
- identification of available community and health resources;
- facilitating access to care and services needed by the patient and/or family;
- development and maintenance of a comprehensive care plan.

Additional E/M services beyond the first visit may be reported separately by the same physician or other qualified health care professional during the same calendar month. Complex care coordination services include care plan oversight services (99339, 99340, 99374-99378), prolonged services without direct patient contact (99358, 99359), anticoagulant management (99363, 99364), medical team conferences (99366-99368), education and training (98960-98962, 99071, 99078), telephone services (98966-98968, 99441-99443), on-line medical evaluation (98969, 99444), preparation of special reports (99080), analysis of data (99090, 99091), transitional care management services (99495, 99496), medication therapy management services (99605-99607), and if performed, these services may not be reported separately during the month for which 99487-99489 are reported. All other services may be reported. Do not report 99487, 99489, 99490 if reporting ESRD services (90951-90970) during the same month. If the complex chronic care coordination services are performed within the postoperative period of a reported surgery, the same individual may not report 99487, 99489, 99490.

Complex chronic care coordination can be reported in any calendar month during which the clinical staff time requirements are met. If care coordination resumes after a discharge during a new month, start a new period or report transitional care management services (99495, 99496) as appropriate. If discharge occurs in the same month, continue the reporting period or report transitional care management services. Do not report 99487, 99489, 99490 for any post-discharge complex chronic care

coordination services for any days within 30 days of discharge, if reporting 99495, 99496.

99485   **Supervision by a control physician of interfacility transport care of the critically ill or critically injured pediatric patient, 24 months of age or younger, includes two-way communication with transport team before transport, at the referring facility and during the transport, including data interpretation and report; first 30 minutes**   ⊘🅱

Coding tip: Pediatric interfacility transport care codes 99485-99486 are listed out of numeric order in CPT. Refer to codes 99466-99467 for additional pediatric interfacility transport services.

RVU			Global Days	Modifiers				
Mod	Non-Fac Total	Fac Total		51	50	62	80	MUE
	2.16	2.16	XXX	9	9	9	9	1

AMA: May 13: 6, May 14: 4

✚ 99486   **Supervision by a control physician of interfacility transport care of the critically ill or critically injured pediatric patient, 24 months of age or younger, includes two-way communication with transport team before transport, at the referring facility and during the transport, including data interpretation and report; each additional 30 minutes (List separately in addition to code for primary procedure)**   ⊘🅱

Coding tip: Pediatric interfacility transport care codes 99485-99486 are listed out of numeric order in CPT. Refer to codes 99466-99467 for additional pediatric interfacility transport services.

RVU			Global Days	Modifiers				
Mod	Non-Fac Total	Fac Total		51	50	62	80	MUE
	1.88	1.88	XXX	9	9	9	9	

AMA: May 13: 6, May 14: 4

99487   **Complex chronic care management services, with the following required elements: multiple (two or more) chronic conditions expected to last at least 12 months, or until the death of the patient, chronic conditions place the patient at significant risk of death, acute exacerbation/decompensation, or functional decline, establishment or substantial revision of a comprehensive care plan, moderate or high complexity medical decision making; 60 minutes of clinical staff time directed by a physician or other qualified health care professional, per calendar month.**   ⊘ℕ

RVU			Global Days	Modifiers				
Mod	Non-Fac Total	Fac Total		51	50	62	80	MUE
	0.00	0.00	XXX	0	0	0	0	1

AMA: Apr 13: 3, Feb 14: 3, Jun 14: 3, 5, Nov 13: 3, Oct 14: 3, Sep 13: 15

● New   ▲ Revised   ✖ Deleted   ⊙ Moderate Sedation   ✚ Add-on Codes   ⊘ High Risk Denial   Ⓐ Age Edit   ♀ Female   ♂ Male   **AMA** CPT® Assistant   **MUE** Medically Unlikely Edit

⊘ Modifier 51 Exempt   ⊖ Modifier 63 Exempt   ✗ Unlisted   **Modifiers:** See Inside Back Cover   Ⓜ Maternity   🄰2–🅉3 ASC Payment Indicators   🄰–🅈 OPPS Status Indicators

150   CPT © 2014 American Medical Association. All Rights Reserved.   © 2016 DecisionHealth

+ 99489 **Complex chronic care management services, with the following required elements: multiple (two or more) chronic conditions expected to last at least 12 months, or until the death of the patient, chronic conditions place the patient at significant risk of death, acute exacerbation/decompensation, or functional decline, establishment or substantial revision of a comprehensive care plan, moderate or high complexity medical decision making; 60 minutes of clinical staff time directed by a physician or other qualified health care professional, per calendar month.; each additional 30 minutes of clinical staff time directed by a physician or other qualified health care professional, per calendar month (List separately in addition to code for primary procedure)** ⊙N

RVU			Global Days	Modifiers				
Mod	Non-Fac Total	Fac Total		51	50	62	80	MUE
	0.00	0.00	ZZZ	0	0	0	0	

AMA: Apr 13: 3, Jun 14: 5, Nov 13: 3, Oct 14: 3, Sep 13: 15

99490 **Chronic care management services, at least 20 minutes of clinical staff time directed by a physician or other qualified health care professional, per calendar month, with the following required elements: multiple (two or more) chronic conditions expected to last at least 12 months, or until the death of the patient; chronic conditions place the patient at significant risk of death, acute exacerbation/decompensation, or functional decline; comprehensive care plan established, implemented, revised, or monitored.** V

RVU			Global Days	Modifiers				
Mod	Non-Fac Total	Fac Total		51	50	62	80	MUE
	1.14	0.88	XXX	0	0	0	9	1

AMA: Feb 15: 3, Oct 14: 3

Transitional Care Management Services

Codes 99495 and 99496 are used to report transitional care management services (TCM). These services are for a new or established patient whose medical and/or psychosocial problems require moderate or high complexity medical decision making during transitions in care from an inpatient hospital setting (including acute hospital, rehabilitation hospital, long-term acute care hospital), partial hospital, observation status in a hospital, or skilled nursing facility/nursing facility, to the patient's community setting (home, domiciliary, rest home, or assisted living). TCM commences upon the date of discharge and continues for the next 29 days.

TCM is comprised of one face-to-face visit within the specified time frames, in combination with non- face-to-face services that may be performed by the physician or other qualified health care professional and/or licensed clinical staff under his or her direction.

Non-face-to-face services provided by clinical staff, under the direction of the physician or other qualified health care professional, may include:

- communication (with patient, family members, guardian or caretaker, surrogate decision makers, and/or other professionals) regarding aspects of care;
- communication with home health agencies and other community services utilized by the patient;
- patient and/or family/caretaker education to support self-management, independent living, and activities of daily living;
- assessment and support for treatment regimen adherence and medication management;
- identification of available community and health resources;
- facilitating access to care and services needed by the patient and/or family.

Non-face-to-face services provided by the physician or other qualified health care provider may include:

- obtaining and reviewing the discharge information (e.g., discharge summary, as available, or continuity of care documents);
- reviewing need for or follow-up on pending diagnostic tests and treatments;
- interaction with other qualified health care professionals who will assume or reassume care of the patient's system-specific problems;
- education of patient, family, guardian, and/or caregiver;
- establishment or reestablishment of referrals and arranging for needed community resources;
- assistance in scheduling any required follow-up with community providers and services.

TCM requires a face-to-face visit, initial patient contact, and medication reconciliation within specified time frames. The first face-to-face visit is part of the TCM service and not reported separately. Additional E/M services provided on subsequent dates after the first face-to-face visit may be reported separately. TCM requires an interactive contact with the patient or caregiver, as appropriate, within two business days of discharge. The contact may be direct (face-to-face), telephonic, or by electronic means. Medication reconciliation and management must occur no later than the date of the face-to-face visit.

These services address any needed coordination of care performed by multiple disciplines and community service agencies. The reporting individual provides or oversees the management and/or coordination of services, as needed, for all medical conditions, psychosocial needs, and activities of daily living support by providing first contact and continuous access.

Medical decision making and the date of the first face-to-face visit are used to select and report the appropriate TCM code. For 99496, the face-to-face visit must occur within 7 calendar days of the date of discharge, and medical decision making must be of high complexity. For 99495, the face-to-face visit must occur within 14 calendar days of the date of discharge, and medical decision making must be of at least moderate complexity.

Type of Medical Decision Making	Face-to-face visit within 7 days	Face-to-face visit within 8-14 days
Moderate Complexity	99495	99495
High Complexity	99496	99495

Medical decision making is defined by the Evaluation and Management Services Guidelines. The medical decision making over the service period reported is used to define the medical decision making of TCM. Documentation includes the timing of the initial post-discharge communication with the patient or caregivers, date of the face-to-face visit, and the complexity of medical decision making.

Only one individual may report these services and only once per patient within 30 days of discharge. Another TCM may not be reported by the same individual or group for any subsequent discharges) within the 30 days. The same individual may report hospital or observation discharge services and TCM. However, the discharge service may not constitute the required face-to-face visit. The same individual should not report TCM services provided in the postoperative period of a service that the individual reported.

A physician or other qualified health care professional who reports codes 99495, 99496 may not report care plan oversight services (99339, 99340, 99374-99380), prolonged services without direct patient contact (99358, 99359), anticoagulant management (99363, 99364), medical team conferences (99366-99368), education and training (98960-98962,99071,99078), telephone services (98966-98968, 99441-99443), end stage renal disease services (90951-90970), online medical evaluation services (98969, 99444), preparation of special reports (99080), analysis of data (99090, 99091), complex chronic care coordination services (99487-99489), or medication therapy management services (99605-99607) during the time period covered by the transitional care management services codes.

● New   ▲ Revised   ✖ Deleted   ⊙ Moderate Sedation   ✚ Add-on Codes   ⊘ High Risk Denial   ⊛ Age Edit   ♀ Female   ♂ Male   **AMA** *CPT® Assistant*   **MUE** Medically Unlikely Edit
⊙ Modifier 51 Exempt   ⊖ Modifier 63 Exempt   ✗ Unlisted   **Modifiers:** *See Inside Back Cover*   Ⓜ Maternity   A2–Z3 ASC Payment Indicators   A–Y OPPS Status Indicators

© 2016 DecisionHealth   CPT © 2014 American Medical Association. All Rights Reserved.   **151**

99495 Transitional Care Management Services with the following required elements: Communication (direct contact, telephone, electronic) with the patient and/or caregiver within 2 business days of discharge Medical decision making of at least moderate complexity during the service period Face-to-face visit, within 14 calendar days of discharge ⓥ

RVU			Global Days	Modifiers				
Mod	Non-Fac Total	Fac Total		51	50	62	80	MUE
	4.60	3.11	XXX	0	0	0	0	1

AMA: Apr 13: 3, Aug 13: 13, Dec 13: 11, Jul 13: 11, Mar 14: 13, Nov 13: 3, Oct 14: 3, Sep 13: 15

Pub 100-04, 12, 190.3

99496 Transitional Care Management Services with the following required elements: Communication (direct contact, telephone, electronic) with the patient and/or caregiver within 2 business days of discharge Medical decision making of high complexity during the service period Face-to-face visit, within 7 calendar days of discharge ⓥ

RVU			Global Days	Modifiers				
Mod	Non-Fac Total	Fac Total		51	50	62	80	MUE
	6.49	4.50	XXX	0	0	0	0	1

AMA: Apr 13: 3, Aug 13: 13, Jul 13: 11, Mar 14: 13, Nov 13: 3, Oct 14: 3, Sep 13: 15

Pub 100-04, 12, 190.3

Advance Care Planning

An advance directive is a document appointing an agent and/or recording the wishes of a patient pertaining to his/her medical treatment at a future time should he/she lack decisional capacity at that time. Face-to-face services between a physician or other qualified health care professional and a patient, family member, or surrogate for counseling and discussing advance directives, with or without completing relevant legal forms, are reported using codes 99497, 99498. NOTE: No active management of the problem(s) is performed during the time period reported by these codes. You may report 99497, 99498 separately if these services are performed on the same day as another EM service.

99497 Advance care planning including the explanation and discussion of advance directives such as standard forms (with completion of such forms, when performed), by the physician or other qualified health care professional; first 30 minutes, face-to-face with the patient, family member(s), and/or surrogate ⓠ1

RVU			Global Days	Modifiers				
Mod	Non-Fac Total	Fac Total		51	50	62	80	MUE
	2.40	2.22	XXX	0	0	0	0	

AMA: Dec 14: 11

+ 99498 Advance care planning including the explanation and discussion of advance directives such as standard forms (with completion of such forms, when performed), by the physician or other qualified health care professional; each additional 30 minutes (List separately in addition to code for primary procedure) ⓝ

RVU			Global Days	Modifiers				
Mod	Non-Fac Total	Fac Total		51	50	62	80	MUE
	2.09	2.08	ZZZ	0	0	0	0	

AMA: Dec 14: 11

Other Evaluation and Management Services

99499 Unlisted evaluation and management service ⊘ⓧⒷ

RVU			Global Days	Modifiers				
Mod	Non-Fac Total	Fac Total		51	50	62	80	MUE
	0.00	0.00	XXX	0	0	0	0	

AMA: Apr 12: 10, Apr 96: 11, Jan 06: 46, Jan 07: 30, Jul 12: 10, 11, Mar 05: 11, May 05: 1, May 11: 7, Nov 12: 13, Oct 14: 9, Sep 06: 8

CPT © 2014 American Medical Association. All Rights Reserved.   © 2016 DecisionHealth

Anesthesia Services

The anesthesia services in the *Procedural Coding Expert* identify services provided by an anesthesiologist or another practitioner, such as a certified registered nurse anesthetist (CRNA) or anesthesia assistant (AA). The CRNA may perform anesthesia services with or without supervision of an anesthesiologist where the AA must always have supervision of an anesthesiologist.

Anesthesia services under the codes in this section are provided as a package. Included in this package are the following services:

- The preoperative evaluation
  - Sufficient history
  - Physical examination
  - Assessment of risk of adverse reactions to anesthesia
  - Alternative anesthesia approaches
  - Any patient questions answered
- Standard preparation
  - Transporting, positioning, and prepping the patient
  - Placement of intravenous lines for medication and fluid administration
  - Placement of endotracheal/orotracheal tube for ventilation
  - Placement of devices for cardiac monitoring
  - Placement of airway/nasogastric/orogastric tube(s)
- Monitoring of anesthesia during procedure
  - Physiological parameters (e.g., heart rate, blood pressure, oxygen saturation levels)
- Administration of anesthesia
  - Local
  - Regional
  - Epidural
  - General
  - Moderate conscious sedation
  - Monitored anesthesia care (MAC)
- Administration of other medication, blood, and other fluids
- Interpretation of laboratory tests performed intraoperatively
  - pH
  - pO2
  - pCO2
  - bicarbonate
  - hematology
  - blood chemistry
- Post-anesthesia recovery care until release of the patient to the surgeon or other practitioner

Note: Procedures performed that are not listed above, such as Swan-Ganz catheterization (to see blood movement through the heart and monitor heart function), or unusual postoperative pain and/or ventilator management that is unrelated to the procedure, may be reported separately in addition to the anesthesia code.

Anesthesia Coding Guidance

A. Reporting

Only one anesthesia code is reported with the exception of an add-on code. Both the primary anesthesia code and an add-on anesthesia code are reported, when appropriate (see C. Anesthesia Qualifying Circumstances for examples of add-on codes).

B. Time Units

Time is the most significant element when reporting anesthesia services. Each anesthesia service has a basic unit value. In addition to this basic unit value (which is determined by the ASA (American Society of Anesthesiologists) or CMS (Centers for Medicare and Medicaid Services)), the anesthesiologist, or other practitioner providing the anesthesia services, documents the time. Reimbursement for anesthesia services increases as time increases. Time begins when the practitioner starts to prepare the patient for anesthesia and continues until the patient is released to the care of the surgeon or other practitioner and the anesthesiologist is no longer personally in attendance. An exception to this rule is when it is medically necessary for the patient to be monitored continuously during an interval period, which may be included when calculating the anesthesia time.

C. Anesthesia Qualifying Circumstances

For those instances with special or extreme circumstances (e.g., age younger than one year/older than 70) or some type of impairment, the following code(s) should be reported in addition to the anesthesia code:

+ 99100   **Anesthesia for patient of extreme age, younger than one year and older than 70 years (List separately in addition to code for primary anesthesia procedure)**

     (For procedure performed on infants younger than 1 year of age at time of surgery, see anesthesia codes 00326, 00561, 00834, 00836)

+ 99116   **Anesthesia complicated by utilization of total body hypothermia (List separately in addition to code for primary anesthesia procedure)**

+ 99135   **Anesthesia complicated by utilization of controlled hypotension (List separately in addition to code for primary anesthesia procedure)**

+ 99140   **Anesthesia complicated by emergency conditions (specify) (List separately in addition to code for primary anesthesia procedure)**

Note: An emergency condition is a situation when delay in patient treatment would lead to a considerable increase in the threat to life or body part. Additional payment may be made on the qualifying circumstances codes; check with the payer to determine guidelines.

D. Modifiers

1. Anesthesia Modifiers

When appropriate, the following modifiers may be used with the anesthesia codes:

22   **Increased Procedural Services.** This modifier is used when the service performed involves substantially more work and time than is normally required for the procedure and documentation notes the reason for the additional work.

23   **Unusual Anesthesia.** This modifier is used when the anesthesia service performed would not normally require that it be carried out under general anesthesia (e.g., unruly child).

Note: Modifier 47 Anesthesia by Surgeon, should not be reported by an anesthesiologist or other practitioner administering anesthesia if not performing the procedure.

● New   ▲ Revised   Deleted   ⊙ Moderate Sedation   ✚ Add-on Codes   ⊘ High Risk Denial   Ⓐ Age Edit   ♀ Female   ♂ Male   **AMA** *CPT® Assistant*   **MUE** Medically Unlikely Edit
⊘ Modifier 51 Exempt   ⊖ Modifier 63 Exempt   ✗ Unlisted   **Modifiers:** *See Inside Back Cover*   Ⓜ Maternity   A2–Z3 ASC Payment Indicators   A–Y OPPS Status Indicators

© 2016 DecisionHealth   CPT © 2014 American Medical Association. All Rights Reserved.   **153**

2. HCPCS Level II Anesthesia Modifiers

HCPCS Level II modifiers are available specifically for anesthesia services to identify who performed the procedure, if medical direction was given, or for other special circumstances:

AA   Anesthesia services performed personally by anesthesiologist

AD   Medical supervision by a physician; more than four concurrent anesthesia procedures

G8   Monitored anesthesia care (MAC) for deep complex, complicated, or markedly invasive surgical procedure

G9   Monitored anesthesia care (MAC) for patient who has history of severe cardiopulmonary condition

GF   Nonphysician (e.g. nurse practitioner (NP), certified registered nurse anesthetist (CRNA), certified registered nurse (CRN), clinical nurse specialist (CNS), physician assistant (PA) services in a critical access hospital.

QK   Medical direction of two, three, or four concurrent anesthesia procedures involving qualified individuals

QS   Monitored anesthesia care service

QX   CRNA service: with medical direction by a physician

QY   Medical direction of one certified registered nurse anesthetist (CRNA) by an anesthesiologist

QZ   CRNA service: without medical direction by a physician

Check with payers to determine the use of HCPCS Level II Modifiers.

3. Anesthesia Physical Status Modifiers

All anesthesia procedures require the use of a physical (P) status modifier. These P status modifiers identify the health condition of the patient (e.g., healthy, with systemic disease, or brain dead). The following is a list of the P status modifiers:

- P1 – A normal healthy patient
- P2 – A patient with mild systemic disease
- P3 – A patient with severe systemic disease
- P4 – A patient with severe systemic disease that is a constant threat to life
- P5 – A moribund patient who is not expected to survive without the operation
- P6 – A declared brain-dead patient whose organs are being removed for donor purposes

E. Moderate (Conscious) Sedation

CPT codes 99143-99150 report conscious sedation services, but are not found within the Anesthesia Services section of the *Procedural Coding Expert*. These codes are listed in the Medicine Procedures/Services section, under Conscious Sedation.

F. Monitored Anesthesia Care (MAC)

MAC uses sedatives, hypnotics, analgesics, and other anesthetic agents, with a dosage that is low enough for patients to remain responsive and breathe without assistance. It is often used to supplement local and regional anesthesia, particularly during simple procedures and minor surgery.

A

nesthesia Services

Head Anesthesia Procedures

00100   **Anesthesia for procedures on salivary glands, including biopsy** Ⓝ

Base Units	Global Days	Modifiers 51	50	62	80
5	XXX	9	9	9	9

AMA: Feb 97: 4, Nov 99: 6, Feb 06: 9, Mar 06: 15, Nov 07: 8, Oct 11: 3, Jul 12: 13, Aug 14: 6

00102   **Anesthesia for procedures involving plastic repair of cleft lip** Ⓝ

Base Units	Global Days	Modifiers 51	50	62	80
6	XXX	9	9	9	9

AMA: Nov 99: 6

00103   **Anesthesia for reconstructive procedures of eyelid (eg, blepharoplasty, ptosis surgery)** Ⓝ

Base Units	Global Days	Modifiers 51	50	62	80
5	XXX	9	9	9	9

AMA: Nov 99: 6

00104   **Anesthesia for electroconvulsive therapy** Ⓝ

Base Units	Global Days	Modifiers 51	50	62	80
4	XXX	9	9	9	9

00120   **Anesthesia for procedures on external, middle, and inner ear including biopsy; not otherwise specified** Ⓝ

Base Units	Global Days	Modifiers 51	50	62	80
5	XXX	9	9	9	9

00124   **Anesthesia for procedures on external, middle, and inner ear including biopsy; otoscopy** Ⓝ

Base Units	Global Days	Modifiers 51	50	62	80
4	XXX	9	9	9	9

AMA: Nov 99: 7

00126   **Anesthesia for procedures on external, middle, and inner ear including biopsy; tympanotomy** Ⓝ

Base Units	Global Days	Modifiers 51	50	62	80
4	XXX	9	9	9	9

00140   **Anesthesia for procedures on eye; not otherwise specified** Ⓝ

Base Units	Global Days	Modifiers 51	50	62	80
5	XXX	9	9	9	9

00142   **Anesthesia for procedures on eye; lens surgery** Ⓝ

Base Units	Global Days	Modifiers 51	50	62	80
4	XXX	9	9	9	9

00144   **Anesthesia for procedures on eye; corneal transplant** Ⓝ

Base Units	Global Days	Modifiers 51	50	62	80
6	XXX	9	9	9	9

● New   ▲ Revised   ✖ Deleted   ⊙ Moderate Sedation   ✚ Add-on Codes   ⊘ High Risk Denial   Ⓐ Age Edit   ♀ Female   ♂ Male   **AMA** *CPT® Assistant*   *MUE* Medically Unlikely Edit

⊘ Modifier 51 Exempt   ⊖ Modifier 63 Exempt   ✖ Unlisted   **Modifiers:** *See Inside Back Cover*   Ⓜ Maternity   Ⓐ2–Ⓩ3 ASC Payment Indicators   Ⓐ–Ⓨ OPPS Status Indicators

154   CPT © 2014 American Medical Association. All Rights Reserved.   © 2016 DecisionHealth

00145 Anesthesia for procedures on eye; vitreoretinal surgery N

Base Units	Global Days	Modifiers 51	50	62	80
6	XXX	9	9	9	9

00147 Anesthesia for procedures on eye; iridectomy N

Base Units	Global Days	Modifiers 51	50	62	80
4	XXX	9	9	9	9

00148 Anesthesia for procedures on eye; ophthalmoscopy N

Base Units	Global Days	Modifiers 51	50	62	80
4	XXX	9	9	9	9

00160 Anesthesia for procedures on nose and accessory sinuses; not otherwise specified N

Base Units	Global Days	Modifiers 51	50	62	80
5	XXX	9	9	9	9

00162 Anesthesia for procedures on nose and accessory sinuses; radical surgery N

Base Units	Global Days	Modifiers 51	50	62	80
7	XXX	9	9	9	9

00164 Anesthesia for procedures on nose and accessory sinuses; biopsy, soft tissue N

Base Units	Global Days	Modifiers 51	50	62	80
4	XXX	9	9	9	9

00170 Anesthesia for intraoral procedures, including biopsy; not otherwise specified N

Base Units	Global Days	Modifiers 51	50	62	80
5	XXX	9	9	9	9

00172 Anesthesia for intraoral procedures, including biopsy; repair of cleft palate N

Base Units	Global Days	Modifiers 51	50	62	80
6	XXX	9	9	9	9

00174 Anesthesia for intraoral procedures, including biopsy; excision of retropharyngeal tumor N

Base Units	Global Days	Modifiers 51	50	62	80
6	XXX	9	9	9	9

00176 Anesthesia for intraoral procedures, including biopsy; radical surgery C

Base Units	Global Days	Modifiers 51	50	62	80
7	XXX	9	9	9	9

00190 Anesthesia for procedures on facial bones or skull; not otherwise specified N

Base Units	Global Days	Modifiers 51	50	62	80
5	XXX	9	9	9	9

00192 Anesthesia for procedures on facial bones or skull; radical surgery (including prognathism) C

Base Units	Global Days	Modifiers 51	50	62	80
7	XXX	9	9	9	9

00210 Anesthesia for intracranial procedures; not otherwise specified N

Base Units	Global Days	Modifiers 51	50	62	80
11	XXX	9	9	9	9

00211 Anesthesia for intracranial procedures; craniotomy or craniectomy for evacuation of hematoma C

Base Units	Global Days	Modifiers 51	50	62	80
10	XXX	9	9	9	9

00212 Anesthesia for intracranial procedures; subdural taps N

Base Units	Global Days	Modifiers 51	50	62	80
5	XXX	9	9	9	9

00214 Anesthesia for intracranial procedures; burr holes, including ventriculography C

Base Units	Global Days	Modifiers 51	50	62	80
9	XXX	9	9	9	9

AMA: Nov 99: 7

00215 Anesthesia for intracranial procedures; cranioplasty or elevation of depressed skull fracture, extradural (simple or compound) C

Base Units	Global Days	Modifiers 51	50	62	80
9	XXX	9	9	9	9

00216 Anesthesia for intracranial procedures; vascular procedures N

Base Units	Global Days	Modifiers 51	50	62	80
15	XXX	9	9	9	9

00218 Anesthesia for intracranial procedures; procedures in sitting position N

Base Units	Global Days	Modifiers 51	50	62	80
13	XXX	9	9	9	9

00220 Anesthesia for intracranial procedures; cerebrospinal fluid shunting procedures N

Base Units	Global Days	Modifiers 51	50	62	80
10	XXX	9	9	9	9

00222 Anesthesia for intracranial procedures; electrocoagulation of intracranial nerve N

Base Units	Global Days	Modifiers 51	50	62	80
6	XXX	9	9	9	9

AMA: Jul 12: 13

Neck Anesthesia Procedures

00300 Anesthesia for all procedures on the integumentary system, muscles and nerves of head, neck, and posterior trunk, not otherwise specified N

Base Units	Global Days	Modifiers 51	50	62	80
5	XXX	9	9	9	9

AMA: Nov 99: 7, Mar 06: 15, Oct 11: 3, Jul 12: 13

● New   ▲ Revised   Deleted   ⊙ Moderate Sedation   ✚ Add-on Codes   ⊘ High Risk Denial   Ⓐ Age Edit   ♀ Female   ♂ Male   **AMA** CPT® Assistant   **MUE** Medically Unlikely Edit
⦸ Modifier 51 Exempt   ⊖ Modifier 63 Exempt   ☒ Unlisted   **Modifiers:** See Inside Back Cover   Ⓜ Maternity   A2–Z3 ASC Payment Indicators   A–Y OPPS Status Indicators

00320 Anesthesia for all procedures on esophagus, thyroid, larynx, trachea and lymphatic system of neck; not otherwise specified, age 1 year or older Ⓐ Ⓝ

Base Units	Global Days	Modifiers			
		51	50	62	80
6	XXX	9	9	9	9

00322 Anesthesia for all procedures on esophagus, thyroid, larynx, trachea and lymphatic system of neck; needle biopsy of thyroid Ⓝ

Base Units	Global Days	Modifiers			
		51	50	62	80
3	XXX	9	9	9	9

00326 Anesthesia for all procedures on the larynx and trachea in children younger than 1 year of age Ⓢ Ⓐ Ⓝ

Base Units	Global Days	Modifiers			
		51	50	62	80
7	XXX	9	9	9	9

00350 Anesthesia for procedures on major vessels of neck; not otherwise specified Ⓝ

Base Units	Global Days	Modifiers			
		51	50	62	80
10	XXX	9	9	9	9

00352 Anesthesia for procedures on major vessels of neck; simple ligation Ⓝ

Base Units	Global Days	Modifiers			
		51	50	62	80
5	XXX	9	9	9	9

AMA: Nov 07: 8, Jul 12: 13

Chest Wall, Thorax, Shoulder Girdle Anesthesia Procedures

00400 Anesthesia for procedures on the integumentary system on the extremities, anterior trunk and perineum; not otherwise specified Ⓝ

Base Units	Global Days	Modifiers			
		51	50	62	80
3	XXX	9	9	9	9

AMA: Mar 06: 15, Nov 07: 8, Oct 11: 3, Jul 12: 13

00402 Anesthesia for procedures on the integumentary system on the extremities, anterior trunk and perineum; reconstructive procedures on breast (eg, reduction or augmentation mammoplasty, muscle flaps) Ⓝ

Base Units	Global Days	Modifiers			
		51	50	62	80
5	XXX	9	9	9	9

00404 Anesthesia for procedures on the integumentary system on the extremities, anterior trunk and perineum; radical or modified radical procedures on breast Ⓝ

Base Units	Global Days	Modifiers			
		51	50	62	80
5	XXX	9	9	9	9

00406 Anesthesia for procedures on the integumentary system on the extremities, anterior trunk and perineum; radical or modified radical procedures on breast with internal mammary node dissection Ⓝ

Base Units	Global Days	Modifiers			
		51	50	62	80
13	XXX	9	9	9	9

00410 Anesthesia for procedures on the integumentary system on the extremities, anterior trunk and perineum; electrical conversion of arrhythmias Ⓝ

Base Units	Global Days	Modifiers			
		51	50	62	80
4	XXX	9	9	9	9

00450 Anesthesia for procedures on clavicle and scapula; not otherwise specified Ⓝ

Base Units	Global Days	Modifiers			
		51	50	62	80
5	XXX	9	9	9	9

00454 Anesthesia for procedures on clavicle and scapula; biopsy of clavicle Ⓝ

Base Units	Global Days	Modifiers			
		51	50	62	80
3	XXX	9	9	9	9

00470 Anesthesia for partial rib resection; not otherwise specified Ⓝ

Base Units	Global Days	Modifiers			
		51	50	62	80
6	XXX	9	9	9	9

00472 Anesthesia for partial rib resection; thoracoplasty (any type) Ⓝ

Base Units	Global Days	Modifiers			
		51	50	62	80
10	XXX	9	9	9	9

00474 Anesthesia for partial rib resection; radical procedures (eg, pectus excavatum) Ⓒ

Base Units	Global Days	Modifiers			
		51	50	62	80
13	XXX	9	9	9	9

AMA: Nov 07: 8, Jul 12: 13

Intrathorax Anesthesia Procedures

00500 Anesthesia for all procedures on esophagus Ⓝ

Base Units	Global Days	Modifiers			
		51	50	62	80
15	XXX	9	9	9	9

AMA: Mar 06: 15, Nov 07: 8, Oct 11: 3, Jul 12: 13

00520 Anesthesia for closed chest procedures; (including bronchoscopy) not otherwise specified Ⓝ

Base Units	Global Days	Modifiers			
		51	50	62	80
6	XXX	9	9	9	9

AMA: Nov 99: 7

00522 Anesthesia for closed chest procedures; needle biopsy of pleura Ⓝ

Base Units	Global Days	Modifiers			
		51	50	62	80
4	XXX	9	9	9	9

● New   ▲ Revised   ✖ Deleted   ⊙ Moderate Sedation   ✚ Add-on Codes   ⊖ High Risk Denial   Ⓐ Age Edit   ♀ Female   ♂ Male   **AMA** *CPT® Assistant*   **MUE** Medically Unlikely Edit
⊘ Modifier 51 Exempt   ⊖ Modifier 63 Exempt   Ⓧ Unlisted   **Modifiers:** *See Inside Back Cover*   Ⓜ Maternity   Ⓐ②–Ⓩ③ ASC Payment Indicators   Ⓐ–Ⓨ OPPS Status Indicators

156

CPT © 2014 American Medical Association. All Rights Reserved.   © 2016 DecisionHealth

00524 Anesthesia for closed chest procedures; pneumocentesis Ⓒ

Base Units	Global Days	Modifiers			
		51	50	62	80
4	XXX	9	9	9	9

00528 Anesthesia for closed chest procedures; mediastinoscopy and diagnostic thoracoscopy not utilizing 1 lung ventilation Ⓝ

Base Units	Global Days	Modifiers			
		51	50	62	80
8	XXX	9	9	9	9

AMA: Nov 99: 7

00529 Anesthesia for closed chest procedures; mediastinoscopy and diagnostic thoracoscopy utilizing 1 lung ventilation Ⓝ

Base Units	Global Days	Modifiers			
		51	50	62	80
11	XXX	9	9	9	9

AMA: Jun 04: 3

00530 Anesthesia for permanent transvenous pacemaker insertion Ⓝ

Base Units	Global Days	Modifiers			
		51	50	62	80
4	XXX	9	9	9	9

00532 Anesthesia for access to central venous circulation Ⓝ

Base Units	Global Days	Modifiers			
		51	50	62	80
4	XXX	9	9	9	9

00534 Anesthesia for transvenous insertion or replacement of pacing cardioverter-defibrillator Ⓝ

Base Units	Global Days	Modifiers			
		51	50	62	80
7	XXX	9	9	9	9

00537 Anesthesia for cardiac electrophysiologic procedures including radiofrequency ablation Ⓝ

Base Units	Global Days	Modifiers			
		51	50	62	80
7	XXX	9	9	9	9

00539 Anesthesia for tracheobronchial reconstruction Ⓝ

Base Units	Global Days	Modifiers			
		51	50	62	80
18	XXX	9	9	9	9

00540 Anesthesia for thoracotomy procedures involving lungs, pleura, diaphragm, and mediastinum (including surgical thoracoscopy); not otherwise specified Ⓒ

Base Units	Global Days	Modifiers			
		51	50	62	80
12	XXX	9	9	9	9

00541 Anesthesia for thoracotomy procedures involving lungs, pleura, diaphragm, and mediastinum (including surgical thoracoscopy); utilizing 1 lung ventilation Ⓝ

Base Units	Global Days	Modifiers			
		51	50	62	80
15	XXX	9	9	9	9

00542 Anesthesia for thoracotomy procedures involving lungs, pleura, diaphragm, and mediastinum (including surgical thoracoscopy); decortication Ⓒ

Base Units	Global Days	Modifiers			
		51	50	62	80
15	XXX	9	9	9	9

00546 Anesthesia for thoracotomy procedures involving lungs, pleura, diaphragm, and mediastinum (including surgical thoracoscopy); pulmonary resection with thoracoplasty Ⓒ

Base Units	Global Days	Modifiers			
		51	50	62	80
15	XXX	9	9	9	9

00548 Anesthesia for thoracotomy procedures involving lungs, pleura, diaphragm, and mediastinum (including surgical thoracoscopy); intrathoracic procedures on the trachea and bronchi Ⓝ

Base Units	Global Days	Modifiers			
		51	50	62	80
17	XXX	9	9	9	9

AMA: Nov 97: 10

00550 Anesthesia for sternal debridement Ⓝ

Base Units	Global Days	Modifiers			
		51	50	62	80
10	XXX	9	9	9	9

00560 Anesthesia for procedures on heart, pericardial sac, and great vessels of chest; without pump oxygenator Ⓒ

Base Units	Global Days	Modifiers			
		51	50	62	80
15	XXX	9	9	9	9

00561 Anesthesia for procedures on heart, pericardial sac, and great vessels of chest; with pump oxygenator, younger than 1 year of age ⊘ⒶⒸ

Base Units	Global Days	Modifiers			
		51	50	62	80
25	XXX	9	9	9	9

00562 Anesthesia for procedures on heart, pericardial sac, and great vessels of chest; with pump oxygenator, age 1 year or older, for all noncoronary bypass procedures (eg, valve procedures) or for re-operation for coronary bypass more than 1 month after original operation Ⓒ

Base Units	Global Days	Modifiers			
		51	50	62	80
20	XXX	9	9	9	9

00563 Anesthesia for procedures on heart, pericardial sac, and great vessels of chest; with pump oxygenator with hypothermic circulatory arrest Ⓝ

Base Units	Global Days	Modifiers			
		51	50	62	80
25	XXX	9	9	9	9

00566 Anesthesia for direct coronary artery bypass grafting; without pump oxygenator Ⓝ

Base Units	Global Days	Modifiers			
		51	50	62	80
25	XXX	9	9	9	9

● New   ▲ Revised   Deleted   ⊙ Moderate Sedation   ✚ Add-on Codes   ⊘ High Risk Denial   Ⓐ Age Edit   ♀ Female   ♂ Male   **AMA** *CPT® Assistant*   **MUE** Medically Unlikely Edit
⊘ Modifier 51 Exempt   ⊖ Modifier 63 Exempt   Ⓧ Unlisted   **Modifiers:** *See Inside Back Cover*   Ⓜ Maternity   Ⓐ2–Ⓩ3 ASC Payment Indicators   Ⓐ–Ⓨ OPPS Status Indicators

Anesthesia Services

00567 – 00756

00567 Anesthesia for direct coronary artery bypass grafting; with pump oxygenator   C

Base Units	Global Days	Modifiers			
		51	50	62	80
18	XXX	9	9	9	9

00580 Anesthesia for heart transplant or heart/lung transplant   C

Base Units	Global Days	Modifiers			
		51	50	62	80
20	XXX	9	9	9	9

AMA: Nov 07: 8, Jul 12: 13

Spine/Spinal Cord Anesthesia Procedures

00600 Anesthesia for procedures on cervical spine and cord; not otherwise specified   N

Base Units	Global Days	Modifiers			
		51	50	62	80
10	XXX	9	9	9	9

AMA: Mar 06: 15, May 07: 9, Nov 07: 8, Oct 11: 3, Jul 12: 13

00604 Anesthesia for procedures on cervical spine and cord; procedures with patient in the sitting position   C

Base Units	Global Days	Modifiers			
		51	50	62	80
13	XXX	9	9	9	9

00620 Anesthesia for procedures on thoracic spine and cord, not otherwise specified   N

Base Units	Global Days	Modifiers			
		51	50	62	80
10	XXX	9	9	9	9

AMA: Mar 07: 9

00625 Anesthesia for procedures on the thoracic spine and cord, via an anterior transthoracic approach; not utilizing 1 lung ventilation   N

Base Units	Global Days	Modifiers			
		51	50	62	80
13	XXX	9	9	9	9

AMA: Mar 07: 9

00626 Anesthesia for procedures on the thoracic spine and cord, via an anterior transthoracic approach; utilizing 1 lung ventilation   N

Base Units	Global Days	Modifiers			
		51	50	62	80
15	XXX	9	9	9	9

AMA: Mar 07: 9

00630 Anesthesia for procedures in lumbar region; not otherwise specified   N

Base Units	Global Days	Modifiers			
		51	50	62	80
8	XXX	9	9	9	9

00632 Anesthesia for procedures in lumbar region; lumbar sympathectomy   C

Base Units	Global Days	Modifiers			
		51	50	62	80
7	XXX	9	9	9	9

00635 Anesthesia for procedures in lumbar region; diagnostic or therapeutic lumbar puncture   N

Base Units	Global Days	Modifiers			
		51	50	62	80
4	XXX	9	9	9	9

00640 Anesthesia for manipulation of the spine or for closed procedures on the cervical, thoracic or lumbar spine   N

Base Units	Global Days	Modifiers			
		51	50	62	80
3	XXX	9	9	9	9

00670 Anesthesia for extensive spine and spinal cord procedures (eg, spinal instrumentation or vascular procedures)   C

Base Units	Global Days	Modifiers			
		51	50	62	80
13	XXX	9	9	9	9

AMA: Nov 07: 8, Jul 12: 13

Abdominal Anesthesia Procedures

00700 Anesthesia for procedures on upper anterior abdominal wall; not otherwise specified   N

Base Units	Global Days	Modifiers			
		51	50	62	80
4	XXX	9	9	9	9

AMA: Mar 06: 15, Nov 07: 8, Oct 11: 3, Jul 12: 13

00702 Anesthesia for procedures on upper anterior abdominal wall; percutaneous liver biopsy   N

Base Units	Global Days	Modifiers			
		51	50	62	80
4	XXX	9	9	9	9

00730 Anesthesia for procedures on upper posterior abdominal wall   N

Base Units	Global Days	Modifiers			
		51	50	62	80
5	XXX	9	9	9	9

00740 Anesthesia for upper gastrointestinal endoscopic procedures, endoscope introduced proximal to duodenum   N

Base Units	Global Days	Modifiers			
		51	50	62	80
5	XXX	9	9	9	9

AMA: Nov 99: 7

00750 Anesthesia for hernia repairs in upper abdomen; not otherwise specified   N

Base Units	Global Days	Modifiers			
		51	50	62	80
4	XXX	9	9	9	9

00752 Anesthesia for hernia repairs in upper abdomen; lumbar and ventral (incisional) hernias and/or wound dehiscence   N

Base Units	Global Days	Modifiers			
		51	50	62	80
6	XXX	9	9	9	9

00754 Anesthesia for hernia repairs in upper abdomen; omphalocele   N

Base Units	Global Days	Modifiers			
		51	50	62	80
7	XXX	9	9	9	9

00756 Anesthesia for hernia repairs in upper abdomen; transabdominal repair of diaphragmatic hernia   N

Base Units	Global Days	Modifiers			
		51	50	62	80
7	XXX	9	9	9	9

● New   ▲ Revised   ✖ Deleted   ⊙ Moderate Sedation   ✚ Add-on Codes   ⊘ High Risk Denial   Ⓐ Age Edit   ♀ Female   ♂ Male   **AMA** *CPT® Assistant*   *MUE* Medically Unlikely Edit
⊘ Modifier 51 Exempt   ⊖ Modifier 63 Exempt   ✗ Unlisted   **Modifiers:** *See Inside Back Cover*   Ⓜ Maternity   A2–Z3 ASC Payment Indicators   A–Y OPPS Status Indicators

158   CPT © 2014 American Medical Association. All Rights Reserved.   © 2016 DecisionHealth

00770 Anesthesia for all procedures on major abdominal blood vessels   N

Base Units	Global Days	Modifiers 51	50	62	80
15	XXX	9	9	9	9

00790 Anesthesia for intraperitoneal procedures in upper abdomen including laparoscopy; not otherwise specified   N

Base Units	Global Days	Modifiers 51	50	62	80
7	XXX	9	9	9	9

00792 Anesthesia for intraperitoneal procedures in upper abdomen including laparoscopy; partial hepatectomy or management of liver hemorrhage (excluding liver biopsy)   C

Base Units	Global Days	Modifiers 51	50	62	80
13	XXX	9	9	9	9

00794 Anesthesia for intraperitoneal procedures in upper abdomen including laparoscopy; pancreatectomy, partial or total (eg, Whipple procedure)   C

Base Units	Global Days	Modifiers 51	50	62	80
8	XXX	9	9	9	9

00796 Anesthesia for intraperitoneal procedures in upper abdomen including laparoscopy; liver transplant (recipient)   C

Base Units	Global Days	Modifiers 51	50	62	80
30	XXX	9	9	9	9

00797 Anesthesia for intraperitoneal procedures in upper abdomen including laparoscopy; gastric restrictive procedure for morbid obesity   N

Base Units	Global Days	Modifiers 51	50	62	80
11	XXX	9	9	9	9

AMA: Nov 07: 8, Jul 12: 13

00800 Anesthesia for procedures on lower anterior abdominal wall; not otherwise specified   N

Base Units	Global Days	Modifiers 51	50	62	80
4	XXX	9	9	9	9

AMA: Mar 06: 15, Nov 07: 8, Oct 11: 3, Jul 12: 13

00802 Anesthesia for procedures on lower anterior abdominal wall; panniculectomy   C

Base Units	Global Days	Modifiers 51	50	62	80
5	XXX	9	9	9	9

00810 Anesthesia for lower intestinal endoscopic procedures, endoscope introduced distal to duodenum   N

Base Units	Global Days	Modifiers 51	50	62	80
5	XXX	9	9	9	9

AMA: Nov 99: 7

Pub 100-04, 18, 1.2, 60.1.1

00820 Anesthesia for procedures on lower posterior abdominal wall   N

Base Units	Global Days	Modifiers 51	50	62	80
5	XXX	9	9	9	9

00830 Anesthesia for hernia repairs in lower abdomen; not otherwise specified   N

Base Units	Global Days	Modifiers 51	50	62	80
4	XXX	9	9	9	9

00832 Anesthesia for hernia repairs in lower abdomen; ventral and incisional hernias   N

Base Units	Global Days	Modifiers 51	50	62	80
6	XXX	9	9	9	9

00834 Anesthesia for hernia repairs in the lower abdomen not otherwise specified, younger than 1 year of age   ⊘ⒶN

Base Units	Global Days	Modifiers 51	50	62	80
5	XXX	9	9	9	9

00836 Anesthesia for hernia repairs in the lower abdomen not otherwise specified, infants younger than 37 weeks gestational age at birth and younger than 50 weeks gestational age at time of surgery   ⊘ⒶN

Base Units	Global Days	Modifiers 51	50	62	80
6	XXX	9	9	9	9

00840 Anesthesia for intraperitoneal procedures in lower abdomen including laparoscopy; not otherwise specified   N

Base Units	Global Days	Modifiers 51	50	62	80
6	XXX	9	9	9	9

00842 Anesthesia for intraperitoneal procedures in lower abdomen including laparoscopy; amniocentesis   ♀N

Base Units	Global Days	Modifiers 51	50	62	80
4	XXX	9	9	9	9

00844 Anesthesia for intraperitoneal procedures in lower abdomen including laparoscopy; abdominoperineal resection   C

Base Units	Global Days	Modifiers 51	50	62	80
7	XXX	9	9	9	9

00846 Anesthesia for intraperitoneal procedures in lower abdomen including laparoscopy; radical hysterectomy   ♀C

Base Units	Global Days	Modifiers 51	50	62	80
8	XXX	9	9	9	9

00848 Anesthesia for intraperitoneal procedures in lower abdomen including laparoscopy; pelvic exenteration   C

Base Units	Global Days	Modifiers 51	50	62	80
8	XXX	9	9	9	9

● New   ▲ Revised   Deleted   ⊙ Moderate Sedation   ✚ Add-on Codes   ⊘ High Risk Denial   Ⓐ Age Edit   ♀ Female   ♂ Male   **AMA** *CPT® Assistant*   *MUE* Medically Unlikely Edit

⊘ Modifier 51 Exempt   ⊖ Modifier 63 Exempt   ✗ Unlisted   **Modifiers:** *See Inside Back Cover*   Ⓜ Maternity   A2–Z3 ASC Payment Indicators   A–Y OPPS Status Indicators

Anesthesia Services

00851 – 00918

00851 Anesthesia for intraperitoneal procedures in lower abdomen including laparoscopy; tubal ligation/transection ⚥Ⓝ

Base Units	Global Days	Modifiers			
		51	50	62	80
6	XXX	9	9	9	9

AMA: Oct 14: 14

00860 Anesthesia for extraperitoneal procedures in lower abdomen, including urinary tract; not otherwise specified Ⓝ

Base Units	Global Days	Modifiers			
		51	50	62	80
6	XXX	9	9	9	9

00862 Anesthesia for extraperitoneal procedures in lower abdomen, including urinary tract; renal procedures, including upper one-third of ureter, or donor nephrectomy Ⓝ

Base Units	Global Days	Modifiers			
		51	50	62	80
7	XXX	9	9	9	9

00864 Anesthesia for extraperitoneal procedures in lower abdomen, including urinary tract; total cystectomy Ⓒ

Base Units	Global Days	Modifiers			
		51	50	62	80
8	XXX	9	9	9	9

00865 Anesthesia for extraperitoneal procedures in lower abdomen, including urinary tract; radical prostatectomy (suprapubic, retropubic) ♂Ⓒ

Base Units	Global Days	Modifiers			
		51	50	62	80
7	XXX	9	9	9	9

00866 Anesthesia for extraperitoneal procedures in lower abdomen, including urinary tract; adrenalectomy Ⓒ

Base Units	Global Days	Modifiers			
		51	50	62	80
10	XXX	9	9	9	9

00868 Anesthesia for extraperitoneal procedures in lower abdomen, including urinary tract; renal transplant (recipient) Ⓒ

Base Units	Global Days	Modifiers			
		51	50	62	80
10	XXX	9	9	9	9

00870 Anesthesia for extraperitoneal procedures in lower abdomen, including urinary tract; cystolithotomy Ⓝ

Base Units	Global Days	Modifiers			
		51	50	62	80
5	XXX	9	9	9	9

00872 Anesthesia for lithotripsy, extracorporeal shock wave; with water bath Ⓝ

Base Units	Global Days	Modifiers			
		51	50	62	80
7	XXX	9	9	9	9

00873 Anesthesia for lithotripsy, extracorporeal shock wave; without water bath Ⓝ

Base Units	Global Days	Modifiers			
		51	50	62	80
5	XXX	9	9	9	9

00880 Anesthesia for procedures on major lower abdominal vessels; not otherwise specified Ⓝ

Base Units	Global Days	Modifiers			
		51	50	62	80
15	XXX	9	9	9	9

00882 Anesthesia for procedures on major lower abdominal vessels; inferior vena cava ligation Ⓒ

Base Units	Global Days	Modifiers			
		51	50	62	80
10	XXX	9	9	9	9

Perineal Anesthesia Procedures

00902 Anesthesia for; anorectal procedure Ⓝ

Base Units	Global Days	Modifiers			
		51	50	62	80
5	XXX	9	9	9	9

AMA: Mar 06: 15, Oct 11: 3, Jul 12: 13

00904 Anesthesia for; radical perineal procedure Ⓒ

Base Units	Global Days	Modifiers			
		51	50	62	80
7	XXX	9	9	9	9

00906 Anesthesia for; vulvectomy ♀Ⓝ

Base Units	Global Days	Modifiers			
		51	50	62	80
4	XXX	9	9	9	9

00908 Anesthesia for; perineal prostatectomy ♂Ⓒ

Base Units	Global Days	Modifiers			
		51	50	62	80
6	XXX	9	9	9	9

00910 Anesthesia for transurethral procedures (including urethrocystoscopy); not otherwise specified Ⓝ

Base Units	Global Days	Modifiers			
		51	50	62	80
3	XXX	9	9	9	9

00912 Anesthesia for transurethral procedures (including urethrocystoscopy); transurethral resection of bladder tumor(s) Ⓝ

Base Units	Global Days	Modifiers			
		51	50	62	80
5	XXX	9	9	9	9

00914 Anesthesia for transurethral procedures (including urethrocystoscopy); transurethral resection of prostate ♂Ⓝ

Base Units	Global Days	Modifiers			
		51	50	62	80
5	XXX	9	9	9	9

00916 Anesthesia for transurethral procedures (including urethrocystoscopy); post-transurethral resection bleeding Ⓝ

Base Units	Global Days	Modifiers			
		51	50	62	80
5	XXX	9	9	9	9

00918 Anesthesia for transurethral procedures (including urethrocystoscopy); with fragmentation, manipulation and/or removal of ureteral calculus Ⓝ

Base Units	Global Days	Modifiers			
		51	50	62	80
5	XXX	9	9	9	9

AMA: Nov 99: 8, Apr 09: 8

● New ▲ Revised ✖ Deleted ⊙ Moderate Sedation ➕ Add-on Codes ⊘ High Risk Denial Ⓐ Age Edit ♀ Female ♂ Male **AMA** *CPT® Assistant* **MUE** Medically Unlikely Edit
⊘ Modifier 51 Exempt ⊖ Modifier 63 Exempt ✗ Unlisted **Modifiers:** *See Inside Back Cover* Ⓜ Maternity A2–Z3 ASC Payment Indicators A–Y OPPS Status Indicators

00920 Anesthesia for procedures on male genitalia (including open urethral procedures); not otherwise specified ♂Ⓝ

Base Units	Global Days	Modifiers			
		51	50	62	80
3	XXX	9	9	9	9

AMA: Sep 12: 16

00921 Anesthesia for procedures on male genitalia (including open urethral procedures); vasectomy, unilateral or bilateral ∞♂Ⓝ

Base Units	Global Days	Modifiers			
		51	50	62	80
3	XXX	9	9	9	9

00922 Anesthesia for procedures on male genitalia (including open urethral procedures); seminal vesicles ♂Ⓝ

Base Units	Global Days	Modifiers			
		51	50	62	80
6	XXX	9	9	9	9

00924 Anesthesia for procedures on male genitalia (including open urethral procedures); undescended testis, unilateral or bilateral ♂Ⓝ

Base Units	Global Days	Modifiers			
		51	50	62	80
4	XXX	9	9	9	9

00926 Anesthesia for procedures on male genitalia (including open urethral procedures); radical orchiectomy, inguinal ♂Ⓝ

Base Units	Global Days	Modifiers			
		51	50	62	80
4	XXX	9	9	9	9

00928 Anesthesia for procedures on male genitalia (including open urethral procedures); radical orchiectomy, abdominal ♂Ⓝ

Base Units	Global Days	Modifiers			
		51	50	62	80
6	XXX	9	9	9	9

00930 Anesthesia for procedures on male genitalia (including open urethral procedures); orchiopexy, unilateral or bilateral ♂Ⓝ

Base Units	Global Days	Modifiers			
		51	50	62	80
4	XXX	9	9	9	9

00932 Anesthesia for procedures on male genitalia (including open urethral procedures); complete amputation of penis ♂Ⓒ

Base Units	Global Days	Modifiers			
		51	50	62	80
4	XXX	9	9	9	9

00934 Anesthesia for procedures on male genitalia (including open urethral procedures); radical amputation of penis with bilateral inguinal lymphadenectomy ♂Ⓒ

Base Units	Global Days	Modifiers			
		51	50	62	80
6	XXX	9	9	9	9

00936 Anesthesia for procedures on male genitalia (including open urethral procedures); radical amputation of penis with bilateral inguinal and iliac lymphadenectomy ♂Ⓒ

Base Units	Global Days	Modifiers			
		51	50	62	80
8	XXX	9	9	9	9

00938 Anesthesia for procedures on male genitalia (including open urethral procedures); insertion of penile prosthesis (perineal approach) ♂Ⓝ

Base Units	Global Days	Modifiers			
		51	50	62	80
4	XXX	9	9	9	9

00940 Anesthesia for vaginal procedures (including biopsy of labia, vagina, cervix or endometrium); not otherwise specified ♀Ⓝ

Base Units	Global Days	Modifiers			
		51	50	62	80
3	XXX	9	9	9	9

00942 Anesthesia for vaginal procedures (including biopsy of labia, vagina, cervix or endometrium); colpotomy, vaginectomy, colporrhaphy, and open urethral procedures ♀Ⓝ

Base Units	Global Days	Modifiers			
		51	50	62	80
4	XXX	9	9	9	9

00944 Anesthesia for vaginal procedures (including biopsy of labia, vagina, cervix or endometrium); vaginal hysterectomy ♀Ⓒ

Base Units	Global Days	Modifiers			
		51	50	62	80
6	XXX	9	9	9	9

00948 Anesthesia for vaginal procedures (including biopsy of labia, vagina, cervix or endometrium); cervical cerclage ♀Ⓝ

Base Units	Global Days	Modifiers			
		51	50	62	80
4	XXX	9	9	9	9

00950 Anesthesia for vaginal procedures (including biopsy of labia, vagina, cervix or endometrium); culdoscopy ♀Ⓝ

Base Units	Global Days	Modifiers			
		51	50	62	80
5	XXX	9	9	9	9

00952 Anesthesia for vaginal procedures (including biopsy of labia, vagina, cervix or endometrium); hysteroscopy and/or hysterosalpingography ♀Ⓝ

Base Units	Global Days	Modifiers			
		51	50	62	80
4	XXX	9	9	9	9

AMA: Nov 99: 8, Jul 12: 13

Pelvic Anesthesia Procedures

01112 Anesthesia for bone marrow aspiration and/or biopsy, anterior or posterior iliac crest Ⓝ

Base Units	Global Days	Modifiers			
		51	50	62	80
5	XXX	9	9	9	9

AMA: Mar 06: 15, Oct 11: 3, Jul 12: 13

● New   ▲ Revised   Deleted   ⊙ Moderate Sedation   ✚ Add-on Codes   ⊘ High Risk Denial   Ⓐ Age Edit   ♀ Female   ♂ Male   **AMA** *CPT® Assistant*   **MUE** Medically Unlikely Edit

⊘ Modifier 51 Exempt   ⊖ Modifier 63 Exempt   Ⓧ Unlisted   **Modifiers:** *See Inside Back Cover*   Ⓜ Maternity   A2–Z3 ASC Payment Indicators   A–Y OPPS Status Indicators

Anesthesia Services

01120 – 01270

01120 Anesthesia for procedures on bony pelvis   N

Base Units	Global Days	Modifiers			
		51	50	62	80
6	XXX	9	9	9	9

01130 Anesthesia for body cast application or revision N

Base Units	Global Days	Modifiers			
		51	50	62	80
3	XXX	9	9	9	9

01140 Anesthesia for interpelviabdominal (hindquarter) amputation   C

Base Units	Global Days	Modifiers			
		51	50	62	80
15	XXX	9	9	9	9

01150 Anesthesia for radical procedures for tumor of pelvis, except hindquarter amputation   C

Base Units	Global Days	Modifiers			
		51	50	62	80
10	XXX	9	9	9	9

01160 Anesthesia for closed procedures involving symphysis pubis or sacroiliac joint   N

Base Units	Global Days	Modifiers			
		51	50	62	80
4	XXX	9	9	9	9

01170 Anesthesia for open procedures involving symphysis pubis or sacroiliac joint   N

Base Units	Global Days	Modifiers			
		51	50	62	80
8	XXX	9	9	9	9

01173 Anesthesia for open repair of fracture disruption of pelvis or column fracture involving acetabulum   N

Base Units	Global Days	Modifiers			
		51	50	62	80
12	XXX	9	9	9	9

AMA: Jun 04: 3, 4

01180 Anesthesia for obturator neurectomy; extrapelvic   N

Base Units	Global Days	Modifiers			
		51	50	62	80
3	XXX	9	9	9	9

01190 Anesthesia for obturator neurectomy; intrapelvic   N

Base Units	Global Days	Modifiers			
		51	50	62	80
4	XXX	9	9	9	9

AMA: Nov 07: 8, Jul 12: 13

Upper Leg Anesthesia Procedures

01200 Anesthesia for all closed procedures involving hip joint   N

Base Units	Global Days	Modifiers			
		51	50	62	80
4	XXX	9	9	9	9

AMA: Mar 06: 15, Nov 07: 8, Jul 12: 13

01202 Anesthesia for arthroscopic procedures of hip joint   N

Base Units	Global Days	Modifiers			
		51	50	62	80
4	XXX	9	9	9	9

01210 Anesthesia for open procedures involving hip joint; not otherwise specified   N

Base Units	Global Days	Modifiers			
		51	50	62	80
6	XXX	9	9	9	9

01212 Anesthesia for open procedures involving hip joint; hip disarticulation   C

Base Units	Global Days	Modifiers			
		51	50	62	80
10	XXX	9	9	9	9

01214 Anesthesia for open procedures involving hip joint; total hip arthroplasty   C

Base Units	Global Days	Modifiers			
		51	50	62	80
8	XXX	9	9	9	9

01215 Anesthesia for open procedures involving hip joint; revision of total hip arthroplasty   N

Base Units	Global Days	Modifiers			
		51	50	62	80
10	XXX	9	9	9	9

01220 Anesthesia for all closed procedures involving upper two-thirds of femur   N

Base Units	Global Days	Modifiers			
		51	50	62	80
4	XXX	9	9	9	9

01230 Anesthesia for open procedures involving upper two-thirds of femur; not otherwise specified   N

Base Units	Global Days	Modifiers			
		51	50	62	80
6	XXX	9	9	9	9

01232 Anesthesia for open procedures involving upper two-thirds of femur; amputation   C

Base Units	Global Days	Modifiers			
		51	50	62	80
5	XXX	9	9	9	9

01234 Anesthesia for open procedures involving upper two-thirds of femur; radical resection   C

Base Units	Global Days	Modifiers			
		51	50	62	80
8	XXX	9	9	9	9

01250 Anesthesia for all procedures on nerves, muscles, tendons, fascia, and bursae of upper leg   N

Base Units	Global Days	Modifiers			
		51	50	62	80
4	XXX	9	9	9	9

01260 Anesthesia for all procedures involving veins of upper leg, including exploration   N

Base Units	Global Days	Modifiers			
		51	50	62	80
3	XXX	9	9	9	9

01270 Anesthesia for procedures involving arteries of upper leg, including bypass graft; not otherwise specified   N

Base Units	Global Days	Modifiers			
		51	50	62	80
8	XXX	9	9	9	9

● New   ▲ Revised   ✖ Deleted   ⊙ Moderate Sedation   ✚ Add-on Codes   ⊘ High Risk Denial   Ⓐ Age Edit   ♀ Female   ♂ Male   **AMA** *CPT® Assistant*   **MUE** Medically Unlikely Edit

⊘ Modifier 51 Exempt   ⊖ Modifier 63 Exempt   ✗ Unlisted   **Modifiers:** *See Inside Back Cover*   Ⓜ Maternity   A2–Z3 ASC Payment Indicators   A–Y OPPS Status Indicators

162   CPT © 2014 American Medical Association. All Rights Reserved.   © 2016 DecisionHealth

01272 Anesthesia for procedures involving arteries of upper leg, including bypass graft; femoral artery ligation   **C**

Base Units	Global Days	Modifiers			
		51	50	62	80
4	XXX	9	9	9	9

01274 Anesthesia for procedures involving arteries of upper leg, including bypass graft; femoral artery embolectomy   **C**

Base Units	Global Days	Modifiers			
		51	50	62	80
6	XXX	9	9	9	9

AMA: Nov 07: 8, Jul 12: 13

Knee/Knee Region Anesthesia Procedures

01320 Anesthesia for all procedures on nerves, muscles, tendons, fascia, and bursae of knee and/or popliteal area   **N**

Base Units	Global Days	Modifiers			
		51	50	62	80
4	XXX	9	9	9	9

AMA: Mar 06: 15, Nov 07: 8, Oct 11: 3, Jul 12: 13

01340 Anesthesia for all closed procedures on lower one-third of femur   **N**

Base Units	Global Days	Modifiers			
		51	50	62	80
4	XXX	9	9	9	9

01360 Anesthesia for all open procedures on lower one-third of femur   **N**

Base Units	Global Days	Modifiers			
		51	50	62	80
5	XXX	9	9	9	9

01380 Anesthesia for all closed procedures on knee joint   **N**

Base Units	Global Days	Modifiers			
		51	50	62	80
3	XXX	9	9	9	9

01382 Anesthesia for diagnostic arthroscopic procedures of knee joint   **N**

Base Units	Global Days	Modifiers			
		51	50	62	80
3	XXX	9	9	9	9

01390 Anesthesia for all closed procedures on upper ends of tibia, fibula, and/or patella   **N**

Base Units	Global Days	Modifiers			
		51	50	62	80
3	XXX	9	9	9	9

01392 Anesthesia for all open procedures on upper ends of tibia, fibula, and/or patella   **N**

Base Units	Global Days	Modifiers			
		51	50	62	80
4	XXX	9	9	9	9

01400 Anesthesia for open or surgical arthroscopic procedures on knee joint; not otherwise specified   **N**

Base Units	Global Days	Modifiers			
		51	50	62	80
4	XXX	9	9	9	9

01402 Anesthesia for open or surgical arthroscopic procedures on knee joint; total knee arthroplasty   **C**

Base Units	Global Days	Modifiers			
		51	50	62	80
7	XXX	9	9	9	9

01404 Anesthesia for open or surgical arthroscopic procedures on knee joint; disarticulation at knee   **C**

Base Units	Global Days	Modifiers			
		51	50	62	80
5	XXX	9	9	9	9

01420 Anesthesia for all cast applications, removal, or repair involving knee joint   **N**

Base Units	Global Days	Modifiers			
		51	50	62	80
3	XXX	9	9	9	9

01430 Anesthesia for procedures on veins of knee and popliteal area; not otherwise specified   **N**

Base Units	Global Days	Modifiers			
		51	50	62	80
3	XXX	9	9	9	9

01432 Anesthesia for procedures on veins of knee and popliteal area; arteriovenous fistula   **N**

Base Units	Global Days	Modifiers			
		51	50	62	80
6	XXX	9	9	9	9

01440 Anesthesia for procedures on arteries of knee and popliteal area; not otherwise specified   **N**

Base Units	Global Days	Modifiers			
		51	50	62	80
8	XXX	9	9	9	9

01442 Anesthesia for procedures on arteries of knee and popliteal area; popliteal thromboendarterectomy, with or without patch graft   **C**

Base Units	Global Days	Modifiers			
		51	50	62	80
8	XXX	9	9	9	9

01444 Anesthesia for procedures on arteries of knee and popliteal area; popliteal excision and graft or repair for occlusion or aneurysm   **C**

Base Units	Global Days	Modifiers			
		51	50	62	80
8	XXX	9	9	9	9

AMA: Nov 07: 8, Jul 12: 13

Lower Leg/Ankle/Foot Anesthesia Procedures

01462 Anesthesia for all closed procedures on lower leg, ankle, and foot   **N**

Base Units	Global Days	Modifiers			
		51	50	62	80
3	XXX	9	9	9	9

AMA: Mar 06: 15, Nov 07: 8, Oct 11: 3, Jul 12: 13

01464 Anesthesia for arthroscopic procedures of ankle and/or foot   **N**

Base Units	Global Days	Modifiers			
		51	50	62	80
3	XXX	9	9	9	9

● New   ▲ Revised   Deleted   ⊙ Moderate Sedation   ✚ Add-on Codes   ⊘ High Risk Denial   ⊛ Age Edit   ♀ Female   ♂ Male   **AMA** *CPT® Assistant*   **MUE** Medically Unlikely Edit
⊘ Modifier 51 Exempt   ⊖ Modifier 63 Exempt   ✗ Unlisted   **Modifiers:** *See Inside Back Cover*   Ⓜ Maternity   **A2**–**Z3** ASC Payment Indicators   **A**–**Y** OPPS Status Indicators

© 2016 DecisionHealth   CPT © 2014 American Medical Association. All Rights Reserved.   **163**

01470 Anesthesia for procedures on nerves, muscles, tendons, and fascia of lower leg, ankle, and foot; not otherwise specified   N

Base Units	Global Days	Modifiers 51	50	62	80
3	XXX	9	9	9	9

01472 Anesthesia for procedures on nerves, muscles, tendons, and fascia of lower leg, ankle, and foot; repair of ruptured Achilles tendon, with or without graft   N

Base Units	Global Days	Modifiers 51	50	62	80
5	XXX	9	9	9	9

01474 Anesthesia for procedures on nerves, muscles, tendons, and fascia of lower leg, ankle, and foot; gastrocnemius recession (eg, Strayer procedure) N

Base Units	Global Days	Modifiers 51	50	62	80
5	XXX	9	9	9	9

01480 Anesthesia for open procedures on bones of lower leg, ankle, and foot; not otherwise specified   N

Base Units	Global Days	Modifiers 51	50	62	80
3	XXX	9	9	9	9

01482 Anesthesia for open procedures on bones of lower leg, ankle, and foot; radical resection (including below knee amputation)   N

Base Units	Global Days	Modifiers 51	50	62	80
4	XXX	9	9	9	9

01484 Anesthesia for open procedures on bones of lower leg, ankle, and foot; osteotomy or osteoplasty of tibia and/or fibula   N

Base Units	Global Days	Modifiers 51	50	62	80
4	XXX	9	9	9	9

01486 Anesthesia for open procedures on bones of lower leg, ankle, and foot; total ankle replacement   C

Base Units	Global Days	Modifiers 51	50	62	80
7	XXX	9	9	9	9

01490 Anesthesia for lower leg cast application, removal, or repair   N

Base Units	Global Days	Modifiers 51	50	62	80
3	XXX	9	9	9	9

01500 Anesthesia for procedures on arteries of lower leg, including bypass graft; not otherwise specified   N

Base Units	Global Days	Modifiers 51	50	62	80
8	XXX	9	9	9	9

01502 Anesthesia for procedures on arteries of lower leg, including bypass graft; embolectomy, direct or with catheter   C

Base Units	Global Days	Modifiers 51	50	62	80
6	XXX	9	9	9	9

01520 Anesthesia for procedures on veins of lower leg; not otherwise specified   N

Base Units	Global Days	Modifiers 51	50	62	80
3	XXX	9	9	9	9

01522 Anesthesia for procedures on veins of lower leg; venous thrombectomy, direct or with catheter   N

Base Units	Global Days	Modifiers 51	50	62	80
5	XXX	9	9	9	9

AMA: Nov 07: 8, Jul 12: 13

Shoulder/Axilla Anesthesia Procedures

01610 Anesthesia for all procedures on nerves, muscles, tendons, fascia, and bursae of shoulder and axilla   N

Base Units	Global Days	Modifiers 51	50	62	80
5	XXX	9	9	9	9

AMA: Mar 06: 15, Nov 07: 8, Oct 11: 3, Jul 12: 13

01620 Anesthesia for all closed procedures on humeral head and neck, sternoclavicular joint, acromioclavicular joint, and shoulder joint   N

Base Units	Global Days	Modifiers 51	50	62	80
4	XXX	9	9	9	9

01622 Anesthesia for diagnostic arthroscopic procedures of shoulder joint   N

Base Units	Global Days	Modifiers 51	50	62	80
4	XXX	9	9	9	9

01630 Anesthesia for open or surgical arthroscopic procedures on humeral head and neck, sternoclavicular joint, acromioclavicular joint, and shoulder joint; not otherwise specified   N

Base Units	Global Days	Modifiers 51	50	62	80
5	XXX	9	9	9	9

01634 Anesthesia for open or surgical arthroscopic procedures on humeral head and neck, sternoclavicular joint, acromioclavicular joint, and shoulder joint; shoulder disarticulation   C

Base Units	Global Days	Modifiers 51	50	62	80
9	XXX	9	9	9	9

01636 Anesthesia for open or surgical arthroscopic procedures on humeral head and neck, sternoclavicular joint, acromioclavicular joint, and shoulder joint; interthoracoscapular (forequarter) amputation   C

Base Units	Global Days	Modifiers 51	50	62	80
15	XXX	9	9	9	9

01638 Anesthesia for open or surgical arthroscopic procedures on humeral head and neck, sternoclavicular joint, acromioclavicular joint, and shoulder joint; total shoulder replacement   C

Base Units	Global Days	Modifiers 51	50	62	80
10	XXX	9	9	9	9

● New   ▲ Revised   ✖ Deleted   ⊙ Moderate Sedation   ➕ Add-on Codes   ⊘ High Risk Denial   Ⓐ Age Edit   ♀ Female   ♂ Male   **AMA** CPT® Assistant   **MUE** Medically Unlikely Edit
⊘ Modifier 51 Exempt   ⊖ Modifier 63 Exempt   ✗ Unlisted   **Modifiers:** See Inside Back Cover   Ⓜ Maternity   A2–Z3 ASC Payment Indicators   A–Y OPPS Status Indicators

CPT © 2014 American Medical Association. All Rights Reserved.   © 2016 DecisionHealth

01650 Anesthesia for procedures on arteries of shoulder and axilla; not otherwise specified N

Base Units	Global Days	Modifiers 51	50	62	80
6	XXX	9	9	9	9

01652 Anesthesia for procedures on arteries of shoulder and axilla; axillary-brachial aneurysm C

Base Units	Global Days	Modifiers 51	50	62	80
10	XXX	9	9	9	9

01654 Anesthesia for procedures on arteries of shoulder and axilla; bypass graft C

Base Units	Global Days	Modifiers 51	50	62	80
8	XXX	9	9	9	9

01656 Anesthesia for procedures on arteries of shoulder and axilla; axillary-femoral bypass graft C

Base Units	Global Days	Modifiers 51	50	62	80
10	XXX	9	9	9	9

01670 Anesthesia for all procedures on veins of shoulder and axilla N

Base Units	Global Days	Modifiers 51	50	62	80
4	XXX	9	9	9	9

01680 Anesthesia for shoulder cast application, removal or repair; not otherwise specified N

Base Units	Global Days	Modifiers 51	50	62	80
3	XXX	9	9	9	9

01682 Anesthesia for shoulder cast application, removal or repair; shoulder spica ⊙N

Base Units	Global Days	Modifiers 51	50	62	80
4	XXX	9	9	9	9

AMA: Nov 07: 8, Jul 12: 13

Upper Arm/Elbow Anesthesia Procedures

01710 Anesthesia for procedures on nerves, muscles, tendons, fascia, and bursae of upper arm and elbow; not otherwise specified N

Base Units	Global Days	Modifiers 51	50	62	80
3	XXX	9	9	9	9

AMA: Mar 06: 15, Nov 07: 8, Oct 11: 3, Jul 12: 13

01712 Anesthesia for procedures on nerves, muscles, tendons, fascia, and bursae of upper arm and elbow; tenotomy, elbow to shoulder, open N

Base Units	Global Days	Modifiers 51	50	62	80
5	XXX	9	9	9	9

01714 Anesthesia for procedures on nerves, muscles, tendons, fascia, and bursae of upper arm and elbow; tenoplasty, elbow to shoulder N

Base Units	Global Days	Modifiers 51	50	62	80
5	XXX	9	9	9	9

01716 Anesthesia for procedures on nerves, muscles, tendons, fascia, and bursae of upper arm and elbow; tenodesis, rupture of long tendon of biceps N

Base Units	Global Days	Modifiers 51	50	62	80
5	XXX	9	9	9	9

01730 Anesthesia for all closed procedures on humerus and elbow N

Base Units	Global Days	Modifiers 51	50	62	80
3	XXX	9	9	9	9

01732 Anesthesia for diagnostic arthroscopic procedures of elbow joint N

Base Units	Global Days	Modifiers 51	50	62	80
3	XXX	9	9	9	9

01740 Anesthesia for open or surgical arthroscopic procedures of the elbow; not otherwise specified N

Base Units	Global Days	Modifiers 51	50	62	80
4	XXX	9	9	9	9

01742 Anesthesia for open or surgical arthroscopic procedures of the elbow; osteotomy of humerus N

Base Units	Global Days	Modifiers 51	50	62	80
5	XXX	9	9	9	9

01744 Anesthesia for open or surgical arthroscopic procedures of the elbow; repair of nonunion or malunion of humerus N

Base Units	Global Days	Modifiers 51	50	62	80
5	XXX	9	9	9	9

01756 Anesthesia for open or surgical arthroscopic procedures of the elbow; radical procedures C

Base Units	Global Days	Modifiers 51	50	62	80
6	XXX	9	9	9	9

01758 Anesthesia for open or surgical arthroscopic procedures of the elbow; excision of cyst or tumor of humerus N

Base Units	Global Days	Modifiers 51	50	62	80
5	XXX	9	9	9	9

01760 Anesthesia for open or surgical arthroscopic procedures of the elbow; total elbow replacement N

Base Units	Global Days	Modifiers 51	50	62	80
7	XXX	9	9	9	9

01770 Anesthesia for procedures on arteries of upper arm and elbow; not otherwise specified N

Base Units	Global Days	Modifiers 51	50	62	80
6	XXX	9	9	9	9

01772 Anesthesia for procedures on arteries of upper arm and elbow; embolectomy N

Base Units	Global Days	Modifiers 51	50	62	80
6	XXX	9	9	9	9

● New ▲ Revised   Deleted   ⊙ Moderate Sedation   ✚ Add-on Codes   ⊘ High Risk Denial   Ⓐ Age Edit   ♀ Female   ♂ Male   **AMA** CPT® Assistant   **MUE** Medically Unlikely Edit
⊘ Modifier 51 Exempt   ⊖ Modifier 63 Exempt   ☒ Unlisted   **Modifiers:** See Inside Back Cover   Ⓜ Maternity   A2–Z3 ASC Payment Indicators   A–Y OPPS Status Indicators

© 2016 DecisionHealth   CPT © 2014 American Medical Association. All Rights Reserved.   **165**

Anesthesia Services

01780 – 01930

01780 Anesthesia for procedures on veins of upper arm and elbow; not otherwise specified ⓝ

Base Units	Global Days	Modifiers 51	50	62	80
3	XXX	9	9	9	9

01782 Anesthesia for procedures on veins of upper arm and elbow; phleborrhaphy ⓝ

Base Units	Global Days	Modifiers 51	50	62	80
4	XXX	9	9	9	9

AMA: Nov 07: 8, Jul 12: 13

Forearm/Wrist/Hand Anesthesia Procedures

01810 Anesthesia for all procedures on nerves, muscles, tendons, fascia, and bursae of forearm, wrist, and hand ⓝ

Base Units	Global Days	Modifiers 51	50	62	80
3	XXX	9	9	9	9

AMA: Mar 06: 15, Nov 07: 8, Oct 11: 3, Jul 12: 13

01820 Anesthesia for all closed procedures on radius, ulna, wrist, or hand bones ⓝ

Base Units	Global Days	Modifiers 51	50	62	80
3	XXX	9	9	9	9

01829 Anesthesia for diagnostic arthroscopic procedures on the wrist ⓝ

Base Units	Global Days	Modifiers 51	50	62	80
3	XXX	9	9	9	9

01830 Anesthesia for open or surgical arthroscopic/endoscopic procedures on distal radius, distal ulna, wrist, or hand joints; not otherwise specified ⓝ

Base Units	Global Days	Modifiers 51	50	62	80
3	XXX	9	9	9	9

01832 Anesthesia for open or surgical arthroscopic/endoscopic procedures on distal radius, distal ulna, wrist, or hand joints; total wrist replacement ⓝ

Base Units	Global Days	Modifiers 51	50	62	80
6	XXX	9	9	9	9

01840 Anesthesia for procedures on arteries of forearm, wrist, and hand; not otherwise specified ⓝ

Base Units	Global Days	Modifiers 51	50	62	80
6	XXX	9	9	9	9

01842 Anesthesia for procedures on arteries of forearm, wrist, and hand; embolectomy ⓝ

Base Units	Global Days	Modifiers 51	50	62	80
6	XXX	9	9	9	9

01844 Anesthesia for vascular shunt, or shunt revision, any type (eg, dialysis) ⓝ

Base Units	Global Days	Modifiers 51	50	62	80
6	XXX	9	9	9	9

01850 Anesthesia for procedures on veins of forearm, wrist, and hand; not otherwise specified ⓝ

Base Units	Global Days	Modifiers 51	50	62	80
3	XXX	9	9	9	9

01852 Anesthesia for procedures on veins of forearm, wrist, and hand; phleborrhaphy ⓝ

Base Units	Global Days	Modifiers 51	50	62	80
4	XXX	9	9	9	9

01860 Anesthesia for forearm, wrist, or hand cast application, removal, or repair ⓝ

Base Units	Global Days	Modifiers 51	50	62	80
3	XXX	9	9	9	9

AMA: Nov 07: 8, Jul 12: 13

Radiological Anesthesia Procedures

01916 Anesthesia for diagnostic arteriography/venography ⓝ

Base Units	Global Days	Modifiers 51	50	62	80
5	XXX	9	9	9	9

AMA: Nov 07: 8, Oct 11: 3, Jul 12: 13

01920 Anesthesia for cardiac catheterization including coronary angiography and ventriculography (not to include Swan-Ganz catheter) ⓝ

Base Units	Global Days	Modifiers 51	50	62	80
7	XXX	9	9	9	9

01922 Anesthesia for non-invasive imaging or radiation therapy ⓝ

Base Units	Global Days	Modifiers 51	50	62	80
7	XXX	9	9	9	9

01924 Anesthesia for therapeutic interventional radiological procedures involving the arterial system; not otherwise specified ⓝ

Base Units	Global Days	Modifiers 51	50	62	80
5	XXX	9	9	9	9

01925 Anesthesia for therapeutic interventional radiological procedures involving the arterial system; carotid or coronary ⓝ

Base Units	Global Days	Modifiers 51	50	62	80
7	XXX	9	9	9	9

01926 Anesthesia for therapeutic interventional radiological procedures involving the arterial system; intracranial, intracardiac, or aortic ⓝ

Base Units	Global Days	Modifiers 51	50	62	80
8	XXX	9	9	9	9

01930 Anesthesia for therapeutic interventional radiological procedures involving the venous/lymphatic system (not to include access to the central circulation); not otherwise specified ⓝ

Base Units	Global Days	Modifiers 51	50	62	80
5	XXX	9	9	9	9

● New   ▲ Revised   ✖ Deleted   ⊙ Moderate Sedation   ✚ Add-on Codes   ⊗ High Risk Denial   Ⓐ Age Edit   ♀ Female   ♂ Male   **AMA** *CPT® Assistant*   **MUE** Medically Unlikely Edit
⊘ Modifier 51 Exempt   ⊖ Modifier 63 Exempt   Ⓧ Unlisted   **Modifiers:** *See Inside Back Cover*   Ⓜ Maternity   Ⓐ2–Ⓩ3 ASC Payment Indicators   Ⓐ–Ⓨ OPPS Status Indicators

01931 Anesthesia for therapeutic interventional radiological procedures involving the venous/lymphatic system (not to include access to the central circulation); intrahepatic or portal circulation (eg, transvenous intrahepatic portosystemic shunt[s] [TIPS])   N

Base Units	Global Days	Modifiers 51	50	62	80
7	XXX	9	9	9	9

AMA: Apr 08: 3

01932 Anesthesia for therapeutic interventional radiological procedures involving the venous/lymphatic system (not to include access to the central circulation); intrathoracic or jugular   N

Base Units	Global Days	Modifiers 51	50	62	80
6	XXX	9	9	9	9

01933 Anesthesia for therapeutic interventional radiological procedures involving the venous/lymphatic system (not to include access to the central circulation); intracranial   N

Base Units	Global Days	Modifiers 51	50	62	80
7	XXX	9	9	9	9

01935 Anesthesia for percutaneous image guided procedures on the spine and spinal cord; diagnostic   N

Base Units	Global Days	Modifiers 51	50	62	80
5	XXX	9	9	9	9

AMA: Apr 08: 3

01936 Anesthesia for percutaneous image guided procedures on the spine and spinal cord; therapeutic   N

Base Units	Global Days	Modifiers 51	50	62	80
5	XXX	9	9	9	9

AMA: Apr 08: 3, Jul 12: 13

Burn Excision/Debridement Anesthesia Procedures

01951 Anesthesia for second- and third-degree burn excision or debridement with or without skin grafting, any site, for total body surface area (TBSA) treated during anesthesia and surgery; less than 4% total body surface area   N

Base Units	Global Days	Modifiers 51	50	62	80
3	XXX	9	9	9	9

AMA: Mar 06: 15, Oct 11: 3, Jul 12: 13

01952 Anesthesia for second- and third-degree burn excision or debridement with or without skin grafting, any site, for total body surface area (TBSA) treated during anesthesia and surgery; between 4% and 9% of total body surface area   N

Base Units	Global Days	Modifiers 51	50	62	80
5	XXX	9	9	9	9

+ 01953 Anesthesia for second- and third-degree burn excision or debridement with or without skin grafting, any site, for total body surface area (TBSA) treated during anesthesia and surgery; each additional 9% total body surface area or part thereof (List separately in addition to code for primary procedure)   N

Base Units	Global Days	Modifiers 51	50	62	80
1	XXX	9	9	9	9

AMA: Jun 11: 13, Jul 12: 13

Obstetrical Anesthesia Procedures

01958 Anesthesia for external cephalic version procedure   N

Base Units	Global Days	Modifiers 51	50	62	80
5	XXX	9	9	9	9

AMA: Jun 04: 5, 6, Oct 11: 3, Jul 12: 13

01960 Anesthesia for vaginal delivery only   ♀ M N

Base Units	Global Days	Modifiers 51	50	62	80
5	XXX	9	9	9	9

AMA: Dec 01: 3

01961 Anesthesia for cesarean delivery only   ♀ M N

Base Units	Global Days	Modifiers 51	50	62	80
7	XXX	9	9	9	9

01962 Anesthesia for urgent hysterectomy following delivery   ♀ N

Base Units	Global Days	Modifiers 51	50	62	80
8	XXX	9	9	9	9

01963 Anesthesia for cesarean hysterectomy without any labor analgesia/anesthesia care   ♀ N

Base Units	Global Days	Modifiers 51	50	62	80
8	XXX	9	9	9	9

01965 Anesthesia for incomplete or missed abortion procedures   ♀ N

Base Units	Global Days	Modifiers 51	50	62	80
4	XXX	9	9	9	9

01966 Anesthesia for induced abortion procedures   ⊙ ♀ N

Base Units	Global Days	Modifiers 51	50	62	80
4	XXX	9	9	9	9

01967 Neuraxial labor analgesia/anesthesia for planned vaginal delivery (this includes any repeat subarachnoid needle placement and drug injection and/or any necessary replacement of an epidural catheter during labor)   ♀ M N

Base Units	Global Days	Modifiers 51	50	62	80
5	XXX	9	9	9	9

AMA: Dec 01: 3, Oct 14: 14

● New   ▲ Revised   Deleted   ⊙ Moderate Sedation   ✚ Add-on Codes   ⊘ High Risk Denial   Ⓐ Age Edit   ♀ Female   ♂ Male   **AMA** *CPT® Assistant*   *MUE* Medically Unlikely Edit
⊘ Modifier 51 Exempt   ⊖ Modifier 63 Exempt   ✗ Unlisted   **Modifiers:** *See Inside Back Cover*   M Maternity   A2–Z3 ASC Payment Indicators   A–Y OPPS Status Indicators

Anesthesia Services

01968 – 01999

+ **01968** Anesthesia for cesarean delivery following neuraxial labor analgesia/anesthesia (List separately in addition to code for primary procedure performed) ♀N

Base Units	Global Days	Modifiers			
		51	50	62	80
2	XXX	9	9	9	9

AMA: Dec 01: 3, Jun 11: 13, Oct 14: 14

+ **01969** Anesthesia for cesarean hysterectomy following neuraxial labor analgesia/anesthesia (List separately in addition to code for primary procedure performed) ♀N

Base Units	Global Days	Modifiers			
		51	50	62	80
5	XXX	9	9	9	9

AMA: Dec 01: 3, Jun 11: 13, Jul 12: 13

Other Anesthesia Procedures

01990 Physiological support for harvesting of organ(s) from brain-dead patient ©C

Base Units	Global Days	Modifiers			
		51	50	62	80
7	XXX	9	9	9	9

AMA: Mar 06: 15, Nov 07: 8, Oct 11: 3, Jul 12: 13

01991 Anesthesia for diagnostic or therapeutic nerve blocks and injections (when block or injection is performed by a different physician or other qualified health care professional); other than the prone position N

Base Units	Global Days	Modifiers			
		51	50	62	80
3	XXX	9	9	9	9

Pub 100-04, 12, 50

01992 Anesthesia for diagnostic or therapeutic nerve blocks and injections (when block or injection is performed by a different physician or other qualified health care professional); prone position N

Base Units	Global Days	Modifiers			
		51	50	62	80
5	XXX	9	9	9	9

Coding Guidance

In the postoperative period, patients treated with epidural or subarachnoid continuous drug administration may require daily hospital adjustment/ management of the catheter, dosage, etc. This service may be reported by the anesthesia practitioner with CPT code 01996. The management of postoperative pain by the surgeon who performed the procedure, including epidural or subarachnoid drug administration, is included in the global period services associated with the operative procedure. If the only surgery performed is placement of an epidural or subarachnoid catheter for continuous drug administration, CPT code 01996 may be reported on subsequent days by the managing physician.

01996 Daily hospital management of epidural or subarachnoid continuous drug administration N

Base Units	Global Days	Modifiers			
		51	50	62	80
3	XXX	9	9	9	9

AMA: Feb 97: 5, Nov 97: 10, May 99: 6, Jul 12: 5, Oct 12: 14, May 15: 10

Pub 100-04, 12, 50

01999 Unlisted anesthesia procedure(s) ⊘xN

Base Units	Global Days	Modifiers			
		51	50	62	80
0	XXX	9	9	9	9

AMA: Feb 97: 4, Feb 06: 9, Mar 06: 15, Jan 07: 30, Nov 07: 8, Oct 11: 3, Jul 12: 13, Aug 14: 6, 14, May 15: 10

● New   ▲ Revised   ✖ Deleted   ⊙ Moderate Sedation   ✛ Add-on Codes   ⊘ High Risk Denial   Ⓐ Age Edit   ♀ Female   ♂ Male   **AMA** *CPT® Assistant*   *MUE* Medically Unlikely Edit
⊘ Modifier 51 Exempt   ⊖ Modifier 63 Exempt   ✗ Unlisted   **Modifiers:** *See Inside Back Cover*   Ⓜ Maternity   A2–Z3 ASC Payment Indicators   A–Y OPPS Status Indicators

168   CPT © 2014 American Medical Association. All Rights Reserved.   © 2016 DecisionHealth

Surgical Procedures

The Surgery Section of CPT (10021-69990) is the largest section, containing codes for surgical procedures performed using a variety of techniques. Surgical procedures classified in this section are organized into subsections based on anatomic areas and type of procedure.

Coding procedures within the surgical section requires an understanding of the surgery guidelines, the surgical package, and appropriate modifier usage.

Surgical Package

In CPT, the global surgical package includes the pre-operative, intra-operative, and post-operative surgical services. The pre-procedure and post-procedure work are inclusive components of each procedure as standard medical/surgical practice; so it is inappropriate to report services separately that are integral to that procedure.

Note that Medicare has established a definition of the global surgical package that is quite similar to the CPT surgical package except that Medicare defines the global period for each code (0, 10, or 90 days) while CPT does not. Also unlike CPT, Medicare includes treatment of complications that do not require additional trips to the operating room as part of the surgical package. Both the CPT and Medicare packages include one E/M service subsequent to the decision for surgery and prior to the procedure. According to both CPT and Medicare, the encounter where the decision for surgery is made is not included in the surgical package and should be reported separately with the appropriate Evaluation and Management code.

Included in the CPT surgical package are certain pre-operative services, the surgical procedure with all integral components, and all uncomplicated follow-up care. In addition to the procedure itself, CPT surgical codes always include:

- Local infiltration of an anesthetic, digital (metacarpal, metatarsal) nerve blocks, or other application of topical anesthesia
- One related Evaluation and Management service subsequent to the decision for surgery, on the date immediately prior to or on the same date of the procedure
- Immediate postoperative care, including dictating operative notes, talking with family and other physicians or other qualified health care professionals
- Writing orders
- Postanesthesia recovery evaluation of the patient
- Typical postoperative follow-up care, which is usually a part of the surgical service

Services integral to a procedure are based on the standards of medical/surgical practice. For example, surgical lysis is considered part of a surgical procedure so different methods of surgical destruction are not reported separately.

Some of these integral services have specific CPT codes for reporting that same service when not performed as an integral part of another procedure. Other integral services do not have specific CPT codes, such as wound irrigation, which is integral to treating all wounds and as such does not have a CPT code. Examples of services integral to most procedures include:

- Cleansing, shaving, and prepping of skin
- Draping and positioning of patient
- Insertion of intravenous access for medication administration
- Insertion of urinary catheter
- Sedative administration by the physician performing the procedure
- Local, topical, or regional anesthesia administered by the physician performing the procedure
- Surgical approach including identification of anatomical landmarks, incision, evaluation of the surgical field, debridement of traumatized tissue, lysis of adhesions, and isolation of structures limiting access to the surgical field such as bone, blood vessels, nerves, and muscles—including stimulation for identification or monitoring
- Surgical cultures
- Wound irrigation
- Insertion and removal of drains, suction devices, and pumps into the same site
- Surgical closure and dressings
- Application, management, and removal of postoperative dressings and analgesic devices (peri-incisional)
- Application of TENS unit
- Institution of patient controlled anesthesia
- Preoperative, intraoperative, and postoperative documentation, including photographs, drawings, dictation, or transcription as necessary to document the services provided
- Surgical supplies (except where CMS policy permits separate payment)

Postoperative follow-up care, which is usually a part of the surgical service, is included in all surgical procedure codes. For diagnostic procedures such as endoscopy or arthroscopy, follow-up care only includes care that is related to recovery from the diagnostic procedure itself. Follow-up care for therapeutic surgical procedures includes only care that is related to the condition for which the procedure was performed.

Codes designated as "separate procedures" are not reported in addition to the code for the total procedure. If a designated separate procedure is distinct, unrelated to, and/or performed independently from another procedure, it may be reported by itself or in addition to other procedures/services with the modifier 59.

General/Integumentary System Surgical Procedures 10021-19499

Integumentary procedures are those performed on the skin, subcutaneous tissue, accessory structures, and the breast.

Excisions are specified by the method of removal and by the type of lesion:

- excision of benign or malignant lesions, or pressure ulcers
- debridement of exzematous skin, fractures, or necrotizing soft tissue
- paring of hyperkeratotic lesions
- shaving of epidermal lesion

Wound repairs are coded by the level of complexity. Grafts, flaps, and tissue transfers are organized by the specific type, site, and size.

Mohs' micrographic surgical technique for removing complex and ill-defined lesions for examination with the margins is also reported in the integumentary system.

Breast procedures cover biopsies and removal of breast lesions or structures, as well as mastectomy and repair and reconstruction procedures.

● New   ▲ Revised   Deleted   ⊙ Moderate Sedation   ✚ Add-on Codes   ⊘ High Risk Denial   ⊕ Age Edit   ♀ Female   ♂ Male   **AMA** *CPT® Assistant*   **MUE** Medically Unlikely Edit
⊘ Modifier 51 Exempt   ⊖ Modifier 63 Exempt   ✗ Unlisted   **Modifiers:** *See Inside Back Cover*   Ⓜ Maternity   A2–Z3 ASC Payment Indicators   A–Y OPPS Status Indicators

© 2016 DecisionHealth   CPT © 2015 American Medical Association. All Rights Reserved.   **169**

Fine Needle Aspiration

Coding Guidance

Fine needle aspiration (FNA) codes are not generally reported with another biopsy procedure done on the same lesion, unless the initial FNA specimen is inadequate for diagnosis. If the specimen is adequate, an additional one is not necessary. When the FNA sample is inadequate and another type of biopsy, such as open needle, is subsequently done, the additional biopsy procedure may also be reported with a modifier.

10021 Fine needle aspiration; without imaging guidance

P 3 T

RVU			Global Days	Modifiers				
Mod	Non-Fac Total	Fac Total		51	50	62	80	MUE
	3.50	2.00	XXX	0	0	0	0	4

AMA: Aug 02: 10, Mar 05: 11

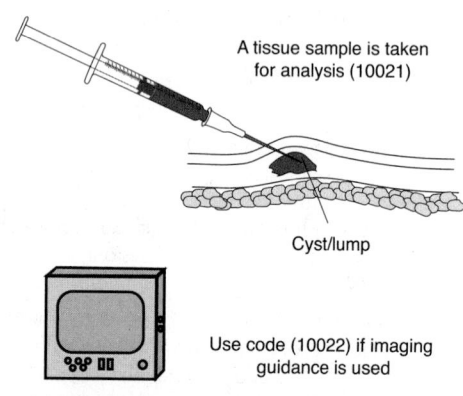

Fine needle aspiration

A tissue sample is taken for analysis (10021)

Cyst/lump

Use code (10022) if imaging guidance is used

10022 Fine needle aspiration; with imaging guidance

P 3 T

RVU			Global Days	Modifiers				
Mod	Non-Fac Total	Fac Total		51	50	62	80	MUE
	3.99	1.88	XXX	0	0	0	0	4

AMA: Nov 02: 1, Jun 07: 10

⊙ 10030 Image-guided fluid collection drainage by catheter (eg, abscess, hematoma, seroma, lymphocele, cyst), soft tissue (eg, extremity, abdominal wall, neck), percutaneous

P 2 T

RVU			Global Days	Modifiers				
Mod	Non-Fac Total	Fac Total		51	50	62	80	MUE
	22.15	4.88	XXX	2	9	0	0	2

AMA: May 14: 3, 9

● 10035 Placement of soft tissue localization device(s) (eg, clip, metallic pellet, wire/needle, radioactive seeds), percutaneous, including imaging guidance; first lesion

N I T

RVU			Global Days	Modifiers				
Mod	Non-Fac Total	Fac Total		51	50	62	80	MUE
	15.18	2.50	000	2	1	0	0	1

✚● 10036 Placement of soft tissue localization device(s) (eg, clip, metallic pellet, wire/needle, radioactive seeds), percutaneous, including imaging guidance; each additional lesion (List separately in addition to code for primary procedure)

N I N

RVU			Global Days	Modifiers				
Mod	Non-Fac Total	Fac Total		51	50	62	80	MUE
	13.19	1.26	ZZZ	2	0	0	0	

Skin Procedures

Incision and/or Drainage Procedures

10040 Acne surgery (eg, marsupialization, opening or removal of multiple milia, comedones, cysts, pustules)

N I Q I

RVU			Global Days	Modifiers				
Mod	Non-Fac Total	Fac Total		51	50	62	80	MUE
	2.89	2.52	010	2	0	0	1	1

AMA: Fall 92: 10, Feb 08: 8

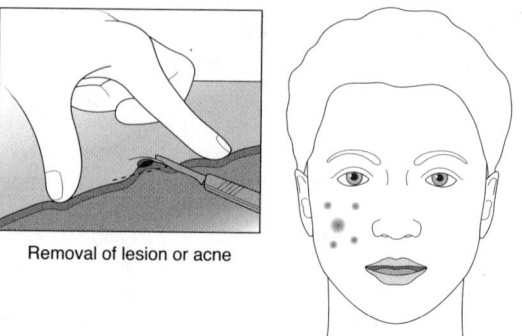

Acne surgery

Removal of lesion or acne

The physician creates a small incision over the acne site or lesion and removes the overlying skin. The lesion is either drained and cleansed to facilitate healing or removed.

Coding Guidance

Incision and drainage services, as related to the integumentary system, generally involve cutaneous or subcutaneous drainage of cysts, pustules, infections, hematomas, abscesses, seromas or fluid collections. When excision, destruction, repair, or removal of a lesion involves drainage for access to the surgical site, the incision and drainage done at the same session and site is not coded.

10060 Incision and drainage of abscess (eg, carbuncle, suppurative hidradenitis, cutaneous or subcutaneous abscess, cyst, furuncle, or paronychia); simple or single

P 2 T

RVU			Global Days	Modifiers				
Mod	Non-Fac Total	Fac Total		51	50	62	80	MUE
	3.32	2.77	010	2	0	0	1	1

AMA: Sep 12: 10

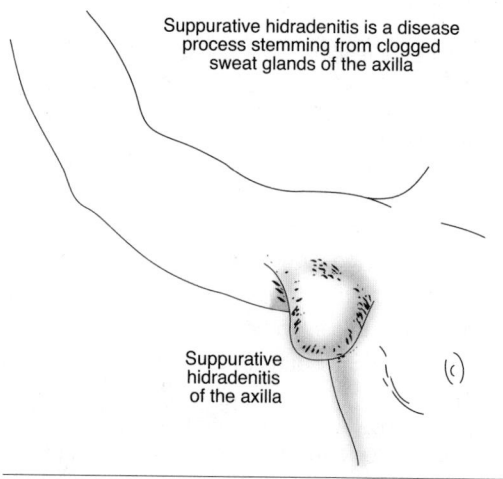

Incision and drainage of abscess

Suppurative hidradenitis is a disease process stemming from clogged sweat glands of the axilla

Suppurative hidradenitis of the axilla

● New   ▲ Revised   ✖ Deleted   ⊙ Moderate Sedation   ✚ Add-on Codes   ⊘ High Risk Denial   Ⓐ Age Edit   ♀ Female   ♂ Male   **AMA** *CPT® Assistant*   **MUE** Medically Unlikely Edit
⊘ Modifier 51 Exempt   ⊖ Modifier 63 Exempt   Ⓧ Unlisted   **Modifiers:** *See Inside Back Cover*   Ⓜ Maternity   **A 2**–**Z 3** ASC Payment Indicators   **A**–**Y** OPPS Status Indicators

CPT © 2015 American Medical Association. All Rights Reserved.   © 2016 DecisionHealth

10061 Incision and drainage of abscess (eg, carbuncle, suppurative hidradenitis, cutaneous or subcutaneous abscess, cyst, furuncle, or paronychia); complicated or multiple `P 3 T`

RVU		Global Days	Modifiers				
Mod	Non-Fac Total	Fac Total		51	50	62	80	MUE
	5.85	5.12	010	2	0	0	1	1

AMA: Sep 12: 10

10080 Incision and drainage of pilonidal cyst; simple `P 2 T`

RVU		Global Days	Modifiers				
Mod	Non-Fac Total	Fac Total		51	50	62	80	MUE
	5.07	2.94	010	2	0	0	1	1

AMA: Fall 92: 13, Dec 06: 15, May 07: 5

Incision and drainage of pilonidal cyst

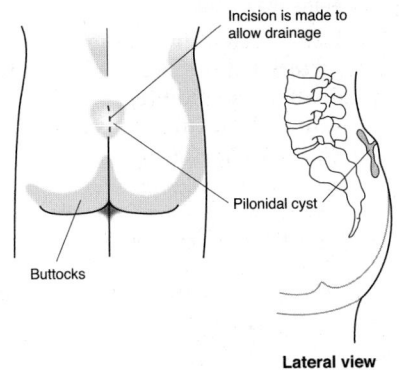

Incision is made to allow drainage

Pilonidal cyst

Buttocks

Lateral view

10081 Incision and drainage of pilonidal cyst; complicated `P 3 T`

RVU		Global Days	Modifiers				
Mod	Non-Fac Total	Fac Total		51	50	62	80	MUE
	7.60	4.85	010	2	0	0	1	1

AMA: Fall 92: 13, Dec 06: 15, May 07: 5

10120 Incision and removal of foreign body, subcutaneous tissues; simple `P 3 T`

Coding tip: For removal of foreign body from the vagina, see 57415

Documentation Finder: The level of difficulty in removing the foreign body or bodies from the sub-q tissues is decided upon by the provider

RVU		Global Days	Modifiers				
Mod	Non-Fac Total	Fac Total		51	50	62	80	MUE
	4.30	2.95	010	2	0	0	1	3

AMA: Sep 12: 10, Apr 13: 10, Dec 13: 16

Incision and removal of foreign body, subcutaneous tissues

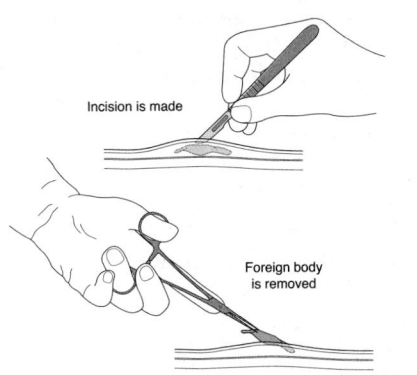

Incision is made

Foreign body is removed

10121 Incision and removal of foreign body, subcutaneous tissues; complicated `A 2 T`

Coding tip: For removal of foreign body from the vagina, see 57415

RVU		Global Days	Modifiers				
Mod	Non-Fac Total	Fac Total		51	50	62	80	MUE
	7.81	5.34	010	2	0	0	1	2

AMA: Spring 91: 7, Dec 06: 15, Sep 12: 10, Dec 13: 16

Coding Guidance

When excision, destruction, repair, or removal of a lesion involves drainage for access to the site, the incision and drainage done at the same session or site is not coded.

10140 Incision and drainage of hematoma, seroma or fluid collection `P 3 T`

RVU		Global Days	Modifiers				
Mod	Non-Fac Total	Fac Total		51	50	62	80	MUE
	4.61	3.38	010	2	0	0	1	2

AMA: Nov 14: 5

10160 Puncture aspiration of abscess, hematoma, bulla, or cyst `P 3 T`

RVU		Global Days	Modifiers				
Mod	Non-Fac Total	Fac Total		51	50	62	80	MUE
	3.71	2.75	010	2	0	0	1	3

Coding Guidance

Complex incision and drainage of a postoperative wound infection is never reported for the same patient encounter as the procedure causing the postoperative infection. It may be separately reportable with a subsequent procedure depending upon the circumstances. If it is performed to gain access to an anatomic region for another procedure, CPT code 10180 is not separately reportable. However, if the procedure described by CPT code 10180 is performed at an anatomic site unrelated to another procedure, it may be reported separately with the procedure using the appropriate modifier to identify a distinct procedural service. When drainage of a complex postoperative empyema is required to accomplish another primary procedure, the incision and drainage is included in the main procedure, even when it was necessitated by the complication of a prior surgery.

10180 Incision and drainage, complex, postoperative wound infection `A 2 T`

Documentation Finder: The procedure note should describe a prior surgical site, which is now infected with subdermal debris and the fluid that must be removed.

RVU		Global Days	Modifiers				
Mod	Non-Fac Total	Fac Total		51	50	62	80	MUE
	7.02	5.14	010	2	0	0	1	2

AMA: Nov 14: 5

● New ▲ Revised Deleted ⊙ Moderate Sedation ✚ Add-on Codes ⊘ High Risk Denial Ⓐ Age Edit ♀ Female ♂ Male **AMA** CPT® Assistant **MUE** Medically Unlikely Edit
⊘ Modifier 51 Exempt ⊖ Modifier 63 Exempt ☒ Unlisted **Modifiers:** See Inside Back Cover Ⓜ Maternity `A 2`–`Z 3` ASC Payment Indicators `A`–`Y` OPPS Status Indicators

Surgical Procedures

11000 – 11011

Excisional Debridement Procedures

Coding Guidance

If lesion removal, incision, or repair requires debridement of non-viable tissue surrounding a lesion, incision, or injury in order to complete the procedure, the debridement is not separately reportable.

11000 Debridement of extensive eczematous or infected skin; up to 10% of body surface `P 3 T`

Mod	RVU Non-Fac Total	Fac Total	Global Days	Modifiers 51	50	62	80	MUE
	1.55	0.82	000	2	0	0	1	1

AMA: May 99: 10, Oct 12: 3

Debridement of extensive eczematous or infected skin

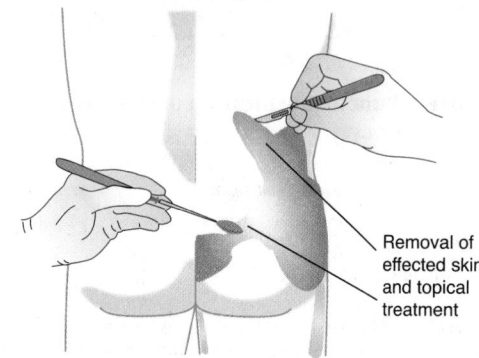

Removal of effected skin and topical treatment

Up to 10% of body surface (11000);
each additional 10% of the body surface (11001)

+ 11001 Debridement of extensive eczematous or infected skin; each additional 10% of the body surface, or part thereof (List separately in addition to code for primary procedure) `N I N`

Mod	RVU Non-Fac Total	Fac Total	Global Days	Modifiers 51	50	62	80	MUE
	0.61	0.41	ZZZ	0	0	0	1	1

AMA: May 99: 10, Oct 12: 3

11004 Debridement of skin, subcutaneous tissue, muscle and fascia for necrotizing soft tissue infection; external genitalia and perineum `C`

Mod	RVU Non-Fac Total	Fac Total	Global Days	Modifiers 51	50	62	80	MUE
	16.79	16.79	000	2	0	0	1	1

AMA: Jan 12: 6, Oct 12: 3, Oct 13: 15

11005 Debridement of skin, subcutaneous tissue, muscle and fascia for necrotizing soft tissue infection; abdominal wall, with or without fascial closure `C`

Mod	RVU Non-Fac Total	Fac Total	Global Days	Modifiers 51	50	62	80	MUE
	22.74	22.74	000	0	0	0	0	1

AMA: Jan 12: 6, Oct 12: 3, Oct 13: 15

11006 Debridement of skin, subcutaneous tissue, muscle and fascia for necrotizing soft tissue infection; external genitalia, perineum and abdominal wall, with or without fascial closure `C`

Mod	RVU Non-Fac Total	Fac Total	Global Days	Modifiers 51	50	62	80	MUE
	20.37	20.37	000	2	0	0	1	1

AMA: Jan 12: 6, Oct 12: 3, Oct 13: 15

+ 11008 Removal of prosthetic material or mesh, abdominal wall for infection (eg, for chronic or recurrent mesh infection or necrotizing soft tissue infection) (List separately in addition to code for primary procedure) `⊘ C`

Mod	RVU Non-Fac Total	Fac Total	Global Days	Modifiers 51	50	62	80	MUE
	8.00	8.00	ZZZ	0	0	0	0	1

AMA: Jan 12: 6, Oct 12: 3

11010 Debridement including removal of foreign material at the site of an open fracture and/or an open dislocation (eg, excisional debridement); skin and subcutaneous tissues `A 2 T`

Documentation Finder: The medical record may detail various types, shapes, and sizes of devitalized and loose tissue, as well as contamination and/or foreign matter in and around the open fracture wound (or open dislocation wound). Excisional debridement is carried out in preparation for the fracture or dislocation treatment.

Mod	RVU Non-Fac Total	Fac Total	Global Days	Modifiers 51	50	62	80	MUE
	14.02	8.05	010	2	2	0	1	2

AMA: Mar 97: 2, Apr 97: 10, Aug 97: 6, Oct 03: 10, May 11: 3, Oct 12: 13

Debridement including removal of foreign material associated with open fracture(s)/dislocation(s)

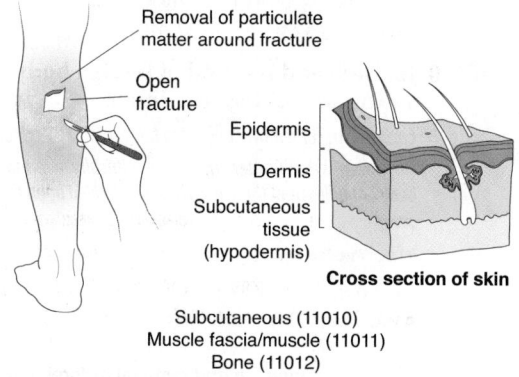

Removal of particulate matter around fracture

Open fracture

Epidermis
Dermis
Subcutaneous tissue (hypodermis)

Cross section of skin

Subcutaneous (11010)
Muscle fascia/muscle (11011)
Bone (11012)

11011 Debridement including removal of foreign material at the site of an open fracture and/or an open dislocation (eg, excisional debridement); skin, subcutaneous tissue, muscle fascia, and muscle `A 2 T`

Mod	RVU Non-Fac Total	Fac Total	Global Days	Modifiers 51	50	62	80	MUE
	15.24	8.64	000	2	2	0	1	2

AMA: Mar 97: 2, Apr 97: 10, Aug 97: 6, May 11: 3, Oct 12: 13

● New   ▲ Revised   ✖ Deleted   ⊙ Moderate Sedation   ✚ Add-on Codes   ⊘ High Risk Denial   Ⓐ Age Edit   ♀ Female   ♂ Male   **AMA** *CPT® Assistant*   *MUE* Medically Unlikely Edit

⊘ Modifier 51 Exempt   ⊖ Modifier 63 Exempt   ✗ Unlisted   **Modifiers:** *See Inside Back Cover*   Ⓜ Maternity   `A 2`–`Z 3` ASC Payment Indicators   `A`–`Y` OPPS Status Indicators

CPT © 2015 American Medical Association. All Rights Reserved.   © 2016 DecisionHealth

11012 Debridement including removal of foreign material at the site of an open fracture and/or an open dislocation (eg, excisional debridement); skin, subcutaneous tissue, muscle fascia, muscle, and bone   A 2 T

RVU			Global Days	Modifiers				
Mod	Non-Fac Total	Fac Total		51	50	62	80	MUE
	20.46	12.37	000	2	2	0	1	2

AMA: Mar 97: 2, Apr 97: 10, Aug 97: 6, Oct 03: 10, May 11: 3, Oct 12: 13

11042 Debridement, subcutaneous tissue (includes epidermis and dermis, if performed); first 20 sq cm or less   A 2 T

Coding tip: Debridement, subcutaneous tissue, each additional 20 sq cm - 11045

Coding tip: Do not report together with 53448, 54411, 54417, 97602

RVU			Global Days	Modifiers				
Mod	Non-Fac Total	Fac Total		51	50	62	80	MUE
	3.31	1.77	000	2	0	0	1	1

AMA: Winter 92: 10, May 96: 6, Feb 97: 7, Aug 97: 6, Jun 05: 1, 10, Oct 07: 15, May 11: 3, Sep 11: 11, Jan 12: 6, Nov 10: 9, Mar 12: 3, Oct 12: 13, Feb 13: 16, Sep 13: 17, Oct 13: 15, Nov 14: 5

Debridement

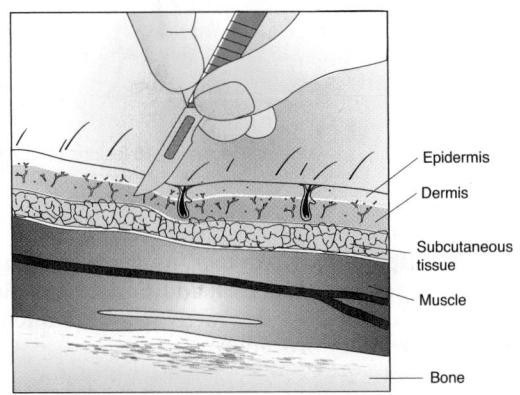

Subcutaneous tissue (11042, 11045); subcutaneous tissue, muscle and/or fascia (11043, 11046); subcutaneous tissue, muscle and/or fascia, bone (11044, 11047)

11043 Debridement, muscle and/or fascia (includes epidermis, dermis, and subcutaneous tissue, if performed); first 20 sq cm or less   A 2 T

Coding tip: Do not report together with 53448, 54411, 54417, 97602

Coding tip: Debridement, muscle/fascia, each additional 20 sq cm - 11046

RVU			Global Days	Modifiers				
Mod	Non-Fac Total	Fac Total		51	50	62	80	MUE
	6.49	4.48	000	2	0	0	1	1

AMA: May 96: 6, Feb 97: 7, Apr 97: 11, Aug 97: 6, Dec 99: 10, Jun 05: 1, 10, Oct 07: 15, May 11: 3, Sep 11: 11, Jan 12: 6, Nov 10: 9, Mar 12: 3, Oct 12: 13, Feb 13: 16, Nov 14: 5

11044 Debridement, bone (includes epidermis, dermis, subcutaneous tissue, muscle and/or fascia, if performed); first 20 sq cm or less   A 2 T

Coding tip: Debridement, bone, each additional 20 sq cm - 11047

RVU			Global Days	Modifiers				
Mod	Non-Fac Total	Fac Total		51	50	62	80	MUE
	8.98	6.68	000	2	0	0	1	1

AMA: Fall 93: 21, Mar 96: 10, May 96: 6, Feb 97: 7, Apr 97: 11, Aug 97: 6, Jun 05: 1, 10, Oct 07: 15, May 11: 3, Sep 11: 11, Jan 12: 6, Nov 10: 9, Mar 12: 3, Oct 12: 13, Feb 13: 16, Nov 14: 5

+ 11045 Debridement, subcutaneous tissue (includes epidermis and dermis, if performed); each additional 20 sq cm, or part thereof (List separately in addition to code for primary procedure)   N 1 N

Coding tip: Code 11045 is listed out of numerical order in CPT. Related debridement services - 11042 (subcutaneous tissue); 11043 and 11046 (muscle and fascia); 11044 and 11047 (bone)

RVU			Global Days	Modifiers				
Mod	Non-Fac Total	Fac Total		51	50	62	80	MUE
	1.16	0.75	ZZZ	0	0	0	0	12

AMA: May 11: 3, Sep 11: 11, Jan 12: 6, Mar 12: 3, Oct 12: 13, Nov 14: 5

+ 11046 Debridement, muscle and/or fascia (includes epidermis, dermis, and subcutaneous tissue, if performed); each additional 20 sq cm, or part thereof (List separately in addition to code for primary procedure)   N 1 N

Coding tip: Code 11046 is listed out of numerical order in CPT. Related debridement services - 11043 (muscle and fascia); 11042 and 11045 (subcutaneous tissue); 11044 and 11047 (bone)

RVU			Global Days	Modifiers				
Mod	Non-Fac Total	Fac Total		51	50	62	80	MUE
	2.09	1.62	ZZZ	0	0	0	0	10

AMA: May 11: 3, Sep 11: 11, Jan 12: 6, Mar 12: 3, Oct 12: 13, Feb 13: 16, Nov 14: 5

+ 11047 Debridement, bone (includes epidermis, dermis, subcutaneous tissue, muscle and/or fascia, if performed); each additional 20 sq cm, or part thereof (List separately in addition to code for primary procedure)   N 1 N

Coding tip: Debridement, bone, initial 20 sq cm or less - 11044

RVU			Global Days	Modifiers				
Mod	Non-Fac Total	Fac Total		51	50	62	80	MUE
	3.55	2.88	ZZZ	0	0	0	0	10

AMA: May 11: 3, Sep 11: 11, Jan 12: 6, Mar 12: 3, Oct 12: 13, Nov 14: 5

Paring/Cutting Procedures

11055 Paring or cutting of benign hyperkeratotic lesion (eg, corn or callus); single lesion   N 1 Q 1

RVU			Global Days	Modifiers				
Mod	Non-Fac Total	Fac Total		51	50	62	80	MUE
	1.35	0.46	000	2	0	0	1	1

AMA: Nov 97: 11, Jan 99: 11

Pub 100-04, 32, 80.8

Paring or cutting of benign hyperkeratotic lesion (eg, corn or callus); single lesion

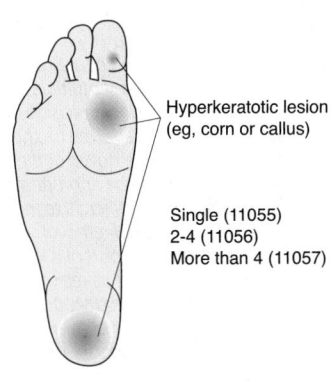

Hyperkeratotic lesion (eg, corn or callus)

Single (11055)
2-4 (11056)
More than 4 (11057)

A benign skin lesion is sliced away.

● New   ▲ Revised   Deleted   ⊙ Moderate Sedation   ✚ Add-on Codes   ⊘ High Risk Denial   Ⓐ Age Edit   ♀ Female   ♂ Male   **AMA** *CPT® Assistant*   **MUE** Medically Unlikely Edit
⊘ Modifier 51 Exempt   ⊖ Modifier 63 Exempt   Ⓧ Unlisted   **Modifiers:** *See Inside Back Cover*   Ⓜ Maternity   A 2 – Z 3 ASC Payment Indicators   A – Y OPPS Status Indicators

Surgical Procedures

11012 – 11055

Surgical Procedures

11056 – 11301

11056 Paring or cutting of benign hyperkeratotic lesion (eg, corn or callus); 2 to 4 lesions   N I Q I

RVU		Global Days	Modifiers				
Mod	Non-Fac Total	Fac Total		51	50	62	80	MUE
	1.65	0.65	000	2	0	0	1	1

AMA: Nov 97: 11, Jan 99: 11, Sep 10: 9

Pub 100-04, 32, 80.8

11057 Paring or cutting of benign hyperkeratotic lesion (eg, corn or callus); more than 4 lesions   P 3 T

RVU		Global Days	Modifiers				
Mod	Non-Fac Total	Fac Total		51	50	62	80	MUE
	1.86	0.85	000	2	0	0	1	1

AMA: Nov 97: 11, Jan 99: 11, May 99: 10

Pub 100-04, 32, 80.8

Biopsy Procedures

Coding Guidance

Biopsy is usually a partial removal of a lesion specifically for obtaining a specimen. If a specimen is obtained as part of a complete lesion removal, it is included in the overall procedure and should not be reported separately. It should be reported only when a biopsy is obtained on a separate date at a separate session from a definitive procedure.

11100 Biopsy of skin, subcutaneous tissue and/or mucous membrane (including simple closure), unless otherwise listed; single lesion   P 3 T

RVU		Global Days	Modifiers				
Mod	Non-Fac Total	Fac Total		51	50	62	80	MUE
	2.93	1.40	000	2	0	0	1	1

AMA: Fall 94: 20, Mar 97: 12, Jun 97: 12, Apr 00: 7, Nov 02: 6, Jul 04: 5, Oct 04: 4, Nov 06: 1, Feb 08: 1, Feb 13: 16, Mar 13: 6

+ 11101 Biopsy of skin, subcutaneous tissue and/or mucous membrane (including simple closure), unless otherwise listed; each separate/additional lesion (List separately in addition to code for primary procedure)   N I N

RVU		Global Days	Modifiers				
Mod	Non-Fac Total	Fac Total		51	50	62	80	MUE
	0.93	0.72	ZZZ	0	0	0	1	6

AMA: Fall 94: 20, Apr 00: 6, 7, Nov 02: 6, Jul 04: 5, Oct 04: 4, Nov 06: 1, Feb 08: 1, Feb 13: 16, Mar 13: 6

Skin Tag Removal Procedures

Coding Guidance

Only one type of removal is reported per lesion, whether destruction, paring, debridement, shaving, excision, or curettement. Multiple codes describing destruction of one single lesion are not reported. When an initial attempt at lesion removal using a less invasive method must be followed using a more invasive type of lesion removal, only the more complex procedure should be reported. If a removal procedure is begun by one method but is converted to another method to complete the procedure, only the code describing the completed procedure may be reported. If multiple lesions are included in a single removal procedure, such as a single excision of skin containing three nevi, only one removal code may be reported for the procedure. If multiple, separate lesions of the same site are removed at the same session using the same or different methods, it may be appropriate to report additional codes with anatomic modifiers or modifier 59 to indicate the different site or lesion treated. Biopsy is usually a partial removal specifically for obtaining a specimen. If a specimen is obtained as part of a lesion removal, it is included in the overall procedure and should not be reported separately. Only when a biopsy is obtained on a separate date at a separate session from a definitive procedure should it be reported. The site of the lesion removal may require some kind of closure. Strip closure, bandaging, tissue glue, or simple repairs (12001-12021) are included in the initial excision. Intermediate and complex repairs are reported separately. When debridement of non-viable tissue around

a lesion or wound is performed in order to accomplish the primary removal, destruction, repair, incision, or closure, it is considered to be a necessary part of the whole procedure and should not be reported separately.

11200 Removal of skin tags, multiple fibrocutaneous tags, any area; up to and including 15 lesions   N I Q I

RVU		Global Days	Modifiers				
Mod	Non-Fac Total	Fac Total		51	50	62	80	MUE
	2.49	2.09	010	2	0	0	1	1

AMA: Winter 90: 3, Nov 97: 11, 12, Nov 02: 11, Aug 09: 7, Jun 11: 13

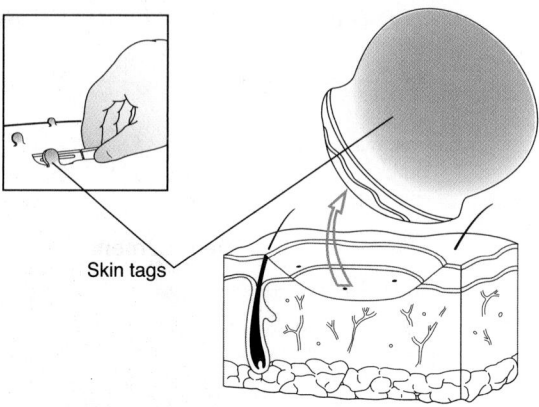

Removal of skin tags multiple fibrocutaneous tags, any area

Skin tags

Up to and including 15 lesions (11200); each additional 10 lesions (11201)

+ 11201 Removal of skin tags, multiple fibrocutaneous tags, any area; each additional 10 lesions, or part thereof (List separately in addition to code for primary procedure)   ⊘ N I N

RVU		Global Days	Modifiers				
Mod	Non-Fac Total	Fac Total		51	50	62	80	MUE
	0.54	0.48	ZZZ	0	0	0	1	0

AMA: Winter 90: 3, Nov 97: 11, 12, Nov 02: 11, Jun 11: 13

Shaving - Epidermal/Dermal Skin Lesions

11300 Shaving of epidermal or dermal lesion, single lesion, trunk, arms or legs; lesion diameter 0.5 cm or less   N I Q I

Coding tip: See anatomical site codes for destruction of lesions in specific areas

Coding tip: See also paring or cutting of hyperkeratotic lesions, corns, calluses - 11055-11057

Coding tip: For removal or other type destruction of skin or fibrocutaneous tags, see 11200-11201

RVU		Global Days	Modifiers				
Mod	Non-Fac Total	Fac Total		51	50	62	80	MUE
	2.75	1.01	000	2	9	0	0	5

AMA: Feb 00: 11, Nov 02: 11, Feb 08: 1

11301 Shaving of epidermal or dermal lesion, single lesion, trunk, arms or legs; lesion diameter 0.6 to 1.0 cm   N I Q I

RVU		Global Days	Modifiers				
Mod	Non-Fac Total	Fac Total		51	50	62	80	MUE
	3.38	1.54	000	2	9	0	0	6

AMA: Feb 00: 11, Feb 08: 1

● New   ▲ Revised   ✖ Deleted   ⊙ Moderate Sedation   ✚ Add-on Codes   ⊘ High Risk Denial   Ⓐ Age Edit   ♀ Female   ♂ Male   **AMA** *CPT® Assistant*   **MUE** Medically Unlikely Edit

⊘ Modifier 51 Exempt   ⊖ Modifier 63 Exempt   ⊠ Unlisted   **Modifiers:** *See Inside Back Cover*   Ⓜ Maternity   A2–Z3 ASC Payment Indicators   A–Y OPPS Status Indicators

174   CPT © 2015 American Medical Association. All Rights Reserved.   © 2016 DecisionHealth

Surgical Procedures

11302   Shaving of epidermal or dermal lesion, single lesion, trunk, arms or legs; lesion diameter 1.1 to 2.0 cm   N I Q I

RVU			Global Days	Modifiers				
Mod	Non-Fac Total	Fac Total		51	50	62	80	MUE
	3.99	1.81	000	2	9	0	0	4

AMA: Feb 00: 11, Feb 08: 1

11303   Shaving of epidermal or dermal lesion, single lesion, trunk, arms or legs; lesion diameter over 2.0 cm   N I Q I

RVU			Global Days	Modifiers				
Mod	Non-Fac Total	Fac Total		51	50	62	80	MUE
	4.41	2.15	000	2	9	0	0	3

AMA: Feb 00: 11, Feb 08: 1

11305   Shaving of epidermal or dermal lesion, single lesion, scalp, neck, hands, feet, genitalia; lesion diameter 0.5 cm or less   N I Q I

Coding tip: See also paring or cutting of hyperkeratotic lesions, corns, calluses - 11055-11057

Coding tip: See anatomical site codes for destruction of lesions in specific areas

Coding tip: For removal or other type destruction of skin or fibrocutaneous tags, see 11200-11201

RVU			Global Days	Modifiers				
Mod	Non-Fac Total	Fac Total		51	50	62	80	MUE
	2.81	1.13	000	2	9	0	0	4

AMA: Feb 00: 11, Feb 08: 1

Shaving of epidermal/dermal lesion

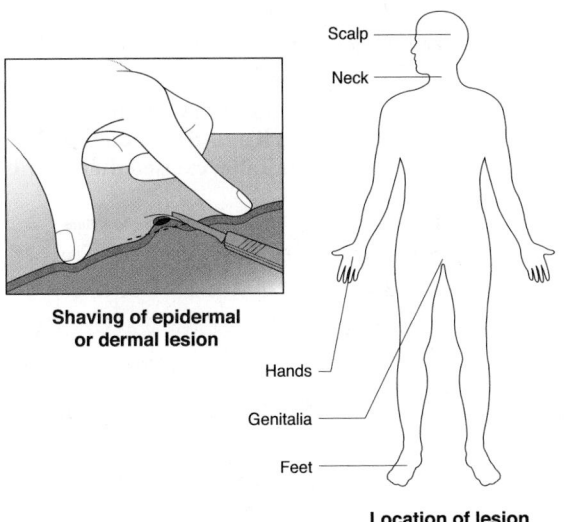

Shaving of epidermal or dermal lesion

Scalp
Neck
Hands
Genitalia
Feet

Location of lesion

11306   Shaving of epidermal or dermal lesion, single lesion, scalp, neck, hands, feet, genitalia; lesion diameter 0.6 to 1.0 cm   N I Q I

RVU			Global Days	Modifiers				
Mod	Non-Fac Total	Fac Total		51	50	62	80	MUE
	3.45	1.50	000	2	9	0	0	4

AMA: Feb 00: 11, Feb 08: 1

11307   Shaving of epidermal or dermal lesion, single lesion, scalp, neck, hands, feet, genitalia; lesion diameter 1.1 to 2.0 cm   P 3 T

RVU			Global Days	Modifiers				
Mod	Non-Fac Total	Fac Total		51	50	62	80	MUE
	4.06	1.92	000	2	9	0	0	3

AMA: Feb 00: 11, Feb 08: 1

11308   Shaving of epidermal or dermal lesion, single lesion, scalp, neck, hands, feet, genitalia; lesion diameter over 2.0 cm   N I Q I

RVU			Global Days	Modifiers				
Mod	Non-Fac Total	Fac Total		51	50	62	80	MUE
	4.27	2.12	000	2	9	0	0	4

AMA: Feb 00: 11, Feb 08: 1

11310   Shaving of epidermal or dermal lesion, single lesion, face, ears, eyelids, nose, lips, mucous membrane; lesion diameter 0.5 cm or less   P 3 T

Coding tip: See anatomical site codes for destruction of lesions in specific areas

Coding tip: For removal or other type destruction of skin or fibrocutaneous tags, see 11200-11201

Coding tip: See also paring or cutting of hyperkeratotic lesions, corns, calluses - 11055-11057

RVU			Global Days	Modifiers				
Mod	Non-Fac Total	Fac Total		51	50	62	80	MUE
	3.22	1.36	000	2	9	0	0	4

AMA: Feb 00: 11, Feb 08: 1, Feb 13: 16, Mar 13: 6

Shaving of epidermal/dermal lesion

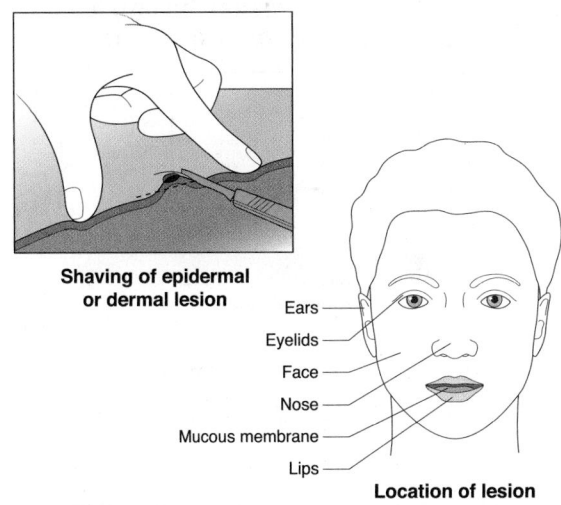

Shaving of epidermal or dermal lesion

Ears
Eyelids
Face
Nose
Mucous membrane
Lips

Location of lesion

11311   Shaving of epidermal or dermal lesion, single lesion, face, ears, eyelids, nose, lips, mucous membrane; lesion diameter 0.6 to 1.0 cm   P 3 T

RVU			Global Days	Modifiers				
Mod	Non-Fac Total	Fac Total		51	50	62	80	MUE
	3.17	1.90	000	2	9	0	0	4

AMA: Feb 00: 11, Feb 08: 1, Feb 13: 16, Mar 13: 6

● New   ▲ Revised   Deleted   ⊙ Moderate Sedation   ✚ Add-on Codes   ⊘ High Risk Denial   Ⓐ Age Edit   ♀ Female   ♂ Male   **AMA** CPT® Assistant   **MUE** Medically Unlikely Edit
⊘ Modifier 51 Exempt   ⊖ Modifier 63 Exempt   ✗ Unlisted   **Modifiers:** See Inside Back Cover   Ⓜ Maternity   A 2 – Z 3 ASC Payment Indicators   A – Y OPPS Status Indicators

© 2016 DecisionHealth   CPT © 2015 American Medical Association. All Rights Reserved.   **175**

11312 Shaving of epidermal or dermal lesion, single lesion, face, ears, eyelids, nose, lips, mucous membrane; lesion diameter 1.1 to 2.0 cm   P 3 T

RVU			Global Days	Modifiers				
Mod	Non-Fac Total	Fac Total		51	50	62	80	MUE
	4.54	2.25	000	2	9	0	0	3

AMA: Feb 00: 11, Feb 08: 1, Feb 13: 16, Mar 13: 6

11313 Shaving of epidermal or dermal lesion, single lesion, face, ears, eyelids, nose, lips, mucous membrane; lesion diameter over 2.0 cm   ⊘ P 3 T

RVU			Global Days	Modifiers				
Mod	Non-Fac Total	Fac Total		51	50	62	80	MUE
	5.27	2.90	000	2	9	0	0	3

AMA: Feb 00: 11, Feb 08: 1, Feb 13: 16, Mar 13: 6

Excisional Benign Skin Lesion Procedures

Coding Guidance

Excision of benign lesions with excised diameter of 0.5 cm or less includes simple, intermediate, or complex repairs which should not be reported separately.

11400 Excision, benign lesion including margins, except skin tag (unless listed elsewhere), trunk, arms or legs; excised diameter 0.5 cm or less   P 3 T

RVU			Global Days	Modifiers				
Mod	Non-Fac Total	Fac Total		51	50	62	80	MUE
	3.50	2.30	010	2	0	0	1	3

AMA: Summer 92: 22, Fall 93: 7, Fall 95: 3, May 96: 11, Aug 00: 5, Nov 02: 5, 7, Aug 06: 10, Jul 08: 5, Apr 10: 3, Jul 10: 10, Jan 11: 9, May 12: 13, Apr 14: 10, Mar 14: 4, 12

Excision, benign lesion
(trunk, arms or legs)

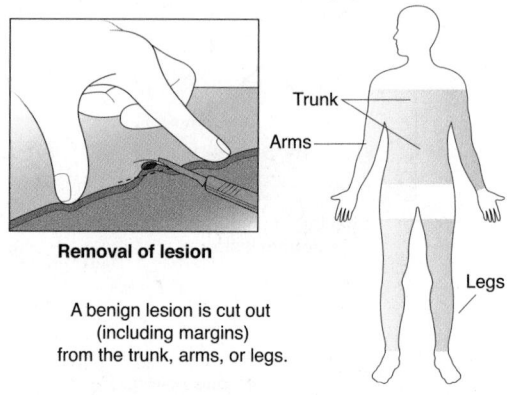

Removal of lesion

A benign lesion is cut out
(including margins)
from the trunk, arms, or legs.

11401 Excision, benign lesion including margins, except skin tag (unless listed elsewhere), trunk, arms or legs; excised diameter 0.6 to 1.0 cm   P 3 T

RVU			Global Days	Modifiers				
Mod	Non-Fac Total	Fac Total		51	50	62	80	MUE
	4.21	2.97	010	2	0	0	1	3

AMA: Summer 92: 22, Fall 93: 7, Fall 95: 3, May 96: 11, Nov 02: 5, 7, Jul 10: 10, Jan 11: 9, May 12: 13, Mar 14: 4, 12

11402 Excision, benign lesion including margins, except skin tag (unless listed elsewhere), trunk, arms or legs; excised diameter 1.1 to 2.0 cm   P 3 T

RVU			Global Days	Modifiers				
Mod	Non-Fac Total	Fac Total		51	50	62	80	MUE
	4.69	3.27	010	2	0	0	1	3

AMA: Summer 92: 22, Fall 93: 7, Fall 95: 3, May 96: 11, Nov 02: 5, 7, Jul 10: 10, Jan 11: 9, May 12: 13, Mar 14: 4, 12

11403 Excision, benign lesion including margins, except skin tag (unless listed elsewhere), trunk, arms or legs; excised diameter 2.1 to 3.0 cm   P 3 T

RVU			Global Days	Modifiers				
Mod	Non-Fac Total	Fac Total		51	50	62	80	MUE
	5.42	4.22	010	2	0	0	1	2

AMA: Summer 92: 22, Fall 93: 7, Fall 95: 3, May 96: 11, Nov 02: 5, 7, Jul 10: 10, Jan 11: 9, May 12: 13, Mar 14: 4, 12

11404 Excision, benign lesion including margins, except skin tag (unless listed elsewhere), trunk, arms or legs; excised diameter 3.1 to 4.0 cm   A 2 T

RVU			Global Days	Modifiers				
Mod	Non-Fac Total	Fac Total		51	50	62	80	MUE
	6.17	4.66	010	2	0	0	1	2

AMA: Summer 92: 22, Fall 93: 7, Fall 95: 3, May 96: 11, Nov 02: 5, 7, Jul 10: 10, Jan 11: 9, May 12: 13, Mar 14: 4, 12

11406 Excision, benign lesion including margins, except skin tag (unless listed elsewhere), trunk, arms or legs; excised diameter over 4.0 cm   A 2 T

RVU			Global Days	Modifiers				
Mod	Non-Fac Total	Fac Total		51	50	62	80	MUE
	8.92	7.09	010	2	0	0	1	2

AMA: Summer 92: 22, Fall 93: 7, Fall 95: 3, May 96: 11, Nov 02: 5, 7, Apr 14: 10, Jul 10: 10, May 12: 13, Jan 11: 9, Mar 14: 4, 12

11420 Excision, benign lesion including margins, except skin tag (unless listed elsewhere), scalp, neck, hands, feet, genitalia; excised diameter 0.5 cm or less   P 3 T

RVU			Global Days	Modifiers				
Mod	Non-Fac Total	Fac Total		51	50	62	80	MUE
	3.46	2.32	010	2	0	0	1	3

AMA: Summer 92: 22, Fall 95: 3, Jul 08: 5, Jul 10: 10, Mar 14: 4, 12, May 12: 13, Jan 13: 15

Excision, benign lesion

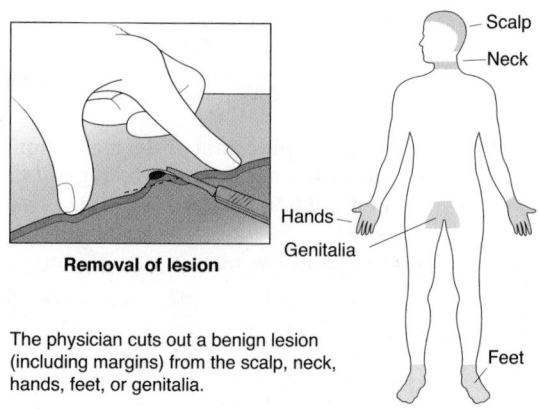

Removal of lesion

The physician cuts out a benign lesion
(including margins) from the scalp, neck,
hands, feet, or genitalia.

● New   ▲ Revised   ✖ Deleted   ⊙ Moderate Sedation   ✚ Add-on Codes   ⊘ High Risk Denial   Ⓐ Age Edit   ♀ Female   ♂ Male   **AMA** *CPT® Assistant*   *MUE* Medically Unlikely Edit

⊘ Modifier 51 Exempt   ⊖ Modifier 63 Exempt   ✗ Unlisted   **Modifiers:** *See Inside Back Cover*   Ⓜ Maternity   A 2 – Z 3 ASC Payment Indicators   A – Y OPPS Status Indicators

CPT © 2015 American Medical Association. All Rights Reserved.   © 2016 DecisionHealth

11421 Excision, benign lesion including margins, except skin tag (unless listed elsewhere), scalp, neck, hands, feet, genitalia; excised diameter 0.6 to 1.0 cm   P 3 T

RVU			Global Days	Modifiers				
Mod	Non-Fac Total	Fac Total		51	50	62	80	MUE
	4.43	3.15	010	2	0	0	1	3

AMA: Summer 92: 22, Fall 95: 3, May 96: 11, Jul 10: 10, May 12: 13, Jan 13: 15, Mar 14: 4, 12

11422 Excision, benign lesion including margins, except skin tag (unless listed elsewhere), scalp, neck, hands, feet, genitalia; excised diameter 1.1 to 2.0 cm   P 3 T

RVU			Global Days	Modifiers				
Mod	Non-Fac Total	Fac Total		51	50	62	80	MUE
	4.96	3.88	010	2	0	0	1	3

AMA: Summer 92: 22, Fall 95: 3, May 96: 11, Aug 00: 5, Jul 10: 10, Mar 12: 4, May 12: 13, Jan 13: 15, Mar 14: 4, 12

11423 Excision, benign lesion including margins, except skin tag (unless listed elsewhere), scalp, neck, hands, feet, genitalia; excised diameter 2.1 to 3.0 cm   P 3 T

RVU			Global Days	Modifiers				
Mod	Non-Fac Total	Fac Total		51	50	62	80	MUE
	5.72	4.50	010	2	0	0	1	2

AMA: Summer 92: 22, Fall 95: 3, May 96: 11, Jul 10: 10, May 12: 13, Jan 13: 15, Mar 14: 4, 12

11424 Excision, benign lesion including margins, except skin tag (unless listed elsewhere), scalp, neck, hands, feet, genitalia; excised diameter 3.1 to 4.0 cm   A 2 T

RVU			Global Days	Modifiers				
Mod	Non-Fac Total	Fac Total		51	50	62	80	MUE
	6.62	5.16	010	2	0	0	1	2

AMA: Summer 92: 22, Fall 95: 3, May 96: 11, Jul 10: 10, May 12: 13, Jan 13: 15, Mar 14: 4, 12

11426 Excision, benign lesion including margins, except skin tag (unless listed elsewhere), scalp, neck, hands, feet, genitalia; excised diameter over 4.0 cm   A 2 T

RVU			Global Days	Modifiers				
Mod	Non-Fac Total	Fac Total		51	50	62	80	MUE
	9.51	7.92	010	2	0	0	1	2

AMA: Summer 92: 22, Fall 95: 3, May 96: 11, Jul 10: 10, May 12: 13, Jan 13: 15, Mar 14: 4, 12

11440 Excision, other benign lesion including margins, except skin tag (unless listed elsewhere), face, ears, eyelids, nose, lips, mucous membrane; excised diameter 0.5 cm or less   P 3 T

RVU			Global Days	Modifiers				
Mod	Non-Fac Total	Fac Total		51	50	62	80	MUE
	3.81	2.95	010	2	0	0	1	4

AMA: Summer 92: 22, Fall 95: 3, May 96: 11, Jul 08: 5, Jul 10: 10, May 12: 13, Mar 14: 4, 12

Excision, other benign lesion including margins, except skin tag

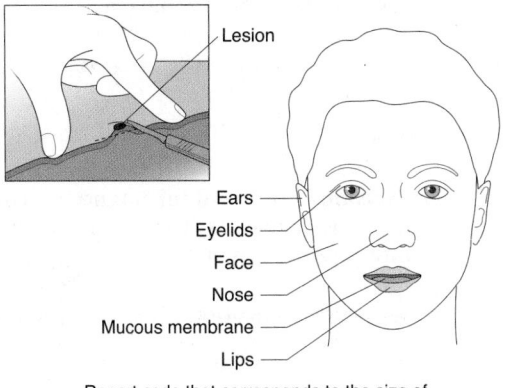

Report code that corresponds to the size of lesion plus margins for total excised diameter

11441 Excision, other benign lesion including margins, except skin tag (unless listed elsewhere), face, ears, eyelids, nose, lips, mucous membrane; excised diameter 0.6 to 1.0 cm   P 3 T

RVU			Global Days	Modifiers				
Mod	Non-Fac Total	Fac Total		51	50	62	80	MUE
	4.75	3.76	010	2	0	0	1	3

AMA: Summer 92: 22, Fall 95: 3, May 96: 11, Jul 10: 10, May 12: 13, Mar 14: 4, 12

11442 Excision, other benign lesion including margins, except skin tag (unless listed elsewhere), face, ears, eyelids, nose, lips, mucous membrane; excised diameter 1.1 to 2.0 cm   P 3 T

RVU			Global Days	Modifiers				
Mod	Non-Fac Total	Fac Total		51	50	62	80	MUE
	5.34	4.18	010	2	0	0	1	3

AMA: Summer 92: 22, Fall 95: 3, May 96: 11, Aug 00: 5, Jun 08: 14, Jul 10: 10, May 12: 13, Mar 14: 4, 12

11443 Excision, other benign lesion including margins, except skin tag (unless listed elsewhere), face, ears, eyelids, nose, lips, mucous membrane; excised diameter 2.1 to 3.0 cm   P 3 T

RVU			Global Days	Modifiers				
Mod	Non-Fac Total	Fac Total		51	50	62	80	MUE
	6.37	5.11	010	2	0	0	1	2

AMA: Summer 92: 22, Fall 95: 3, May 96: 11, Jul 10: 10, May 12: 13, Mar 14: 4, 12

11421 – 11443

● New   ▲ Revised   Deleted   ⊙ Moderate Sedation   ✚ Add-on Codes   ⊘ High Risk Denial   Ⓐ Age Edit   ♀ Female   ♂ Male   **AMA** *CPT® Assistant*   **MUE** Medically Unlikely Edit

⊘ Modifier 51 Exempt   ⊖ Modifier 63 Exempt   ✗ Unlisted   **Modifiers**: *See Inside Back Cover*   Ⓜ Maternity   A 2 – Z 3 ASC Payment Indicators   A – Y OPPS Status Indicators

11444 Excision, other benign lesion including margins, except skin tag (unless listed elsewhere), face, ears, eyelids, nose, lips, mucous membrane; excised diameter 3.1 to 4.0 cm   A 2 T

RVU			Global Days	Modifiers				
Mod	Non-Fac Total	Fac Total		51	50	62	80	MUE
	8.00	6.52	010	2	0	0	1	2

AMA: Summer 92: 22, Fall 95: 3, May 96: 11, Jul 10: 10, May 12: 13, Mar 14: 4, 12

11446 Excision, other benign lesion including margins, except skin tag (unless listed elsewhere), face, ears, eyelids, nose, lips, mucous membrane; excised diameter over 4.0 cm   A 2 T

RVU			Global Days	Modifiers				
Mod	Non-Fac Total	Fac Total		51	50	62	80	MUE
	11.14	9.37	010	2	0	0	1	2

AMA: Summer 92: 22, Fall 95: 3, May 96: 11, Aug 06: 10, Jul 08: 5, Apr 10: 3, Jul 10: 10, May 12: 13, Mar 14: 4, 12

11450 Excision of skin and subcutaneous tissue for hidradenitis, axillary; with simple or intermediate repair   A 2 T

RVU			Global Days	Modifiers				
Mod	Non-Fac Total	Fac Total		51	50	62	80	MUE
	10.84	7.25	090	2	1	0	1	1

AMA: May 12: 13

11451 Excision of skin and subcutaneous tissue for hidradenitis, axillary; with complex repair   A 2 T

RVU			Global Days	Modifiers				
Mod	Non-Fac Total	Fac Total		51	50	62	80	MUE
	13.87	9.37	090	2	1	0	0	1

AMA: May 12: 13

11462 Excision of skin and subcutaneous tissue for hidradenitis, inguinal; with simple or intermediate repair   A 2 T

RVU			Global Days	Modifiers				
Mod	Non-Fac Total	Fac Total		51	50	62	80	MUE
	10.59	6.92	090	2	1	0	0	1

AMA: May 12: 13

11463 Excision of skin and subcutaneous tissue for hidradenitis, inguinal; with complex repair   A 2 T

RVU			Global Days	Modifiers				
Mod	Non-Fac Total	Fac Total		51	50	62	80	MUE
	14.04	9.41	090	2	1	0	0	1

AMA: May 12: 13

11470 Excision of skin and subcutaneous tissue for hidradenitis, perianal, perineal, or umbilical; with simple or intermediate repair   A 2 T

RVU			Global Days	Modifiers				
Mod	Non-Fac Total	Fac Total		51	50	62	80	MUE
	11.78	8.11	090	2	0	0	1	3

AMA: May 12: 13

11471 Excision of skin and subcutaneous tissue for hidradenitis, perianal, perineal, or umbilical; with complex repair   A 2 T

RVU			Global Days	Modifiers				
Mod	Non-Fac Total	Fac Total		51	50	62	80	MUE
	14.59	10.08	090	2	0	0	0	2

AMA: May 12: 13

Excisional Malignant Skin Lesion Procedures

11600 Excision, malignant lesion including margins, trunk, arms, or legs; excised diameter 0.5 cm or less   P 3 T

RVU			Global Days	Modifiers				
Mod	Non-Fac Total	Fac Total		51	50	62	80	MUE
	5.43	3.41	010	2	0	0	1	2

AMA: Fall 95: 3, May 96: 11, Nov 02: 5, Oct 04: 4, Feb 08: 8, Feb 10: 3, Apr 10: 3, May 12: 13, Jul 12: 12, Mar 14: 4, 12

Excision, malignant lesion including margins, trunk, arms, or legs

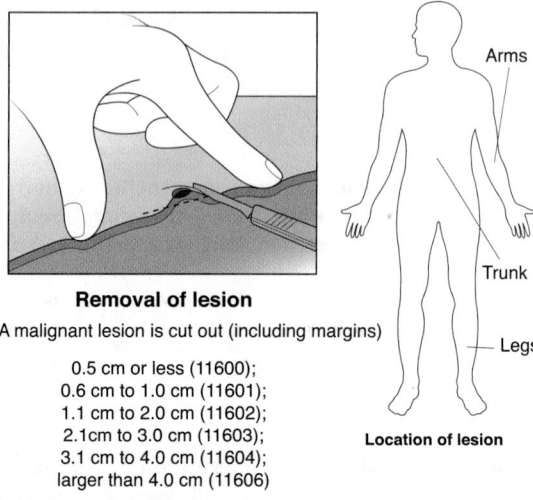

Removal of lesion

A malignant lesion is cut out (including margins)

0.5 cm or less (11600);
0.6 cm to 1.0 cm (11601);
1.1 cm to 2.0 cm (11602);
2.1cm to 3.0 cm (11603);
3.1 cm to 4.0 cm (11604);
larger than 4.0 cm (11606)

Arms

Trunk

Legs

Location of lesion

11601 Excision, malignant lesion including margins, trunk, arms, or legs; excised diameter 0.6 to 1.0 cm   P 3 T

RVU			Global Days	Modifiers				
Mod	Non-Fac Total	Fac Total		51	50	62	80	MUE
	6.46	4.27	010	2	0	0	1	2

AMA: Fall 95: 3, May 96: 11, Nov 02: 5, Feb 10: 3, Mar 12: 7, May 12: 13, Jul 12: 12, Mar 14: 4, 12

11602 Excision, malignant lesion including margins, trunk, arms, or legs; excised diameter 1.1 to 2.0 cm   P 3 T

RVU			Global Days	Modifiers				
Mod	Non-Fac Total	Fac Total		51	50	62	80	MUE
	7.02	4.69	010	2	0	0	1	3

AMA: Fall 95: 3, May 96: 11, Nov 02: 5, Feb 08: 8, Feb 10: 3, Apr 10: 3, Mar 12: 4, May 12: 13, Jul 12: 12, Mar 14: 4, 12

11603 Excision, malignant lesion including margins, trunk, arms, or legs; excised diameter 2.1 to 3.0 cm   P 3 T

RVU			Global Days	Modifiers				
Mod	Non-Fac Total	Fac Total		51	50	62	80	MUE
	8.04	5.63	010	2	0	0	1	2

AMA: Fall 95: 3, May 96: 11, Nov 02: 5, Feb 08: 8, Feb 10: 3, May 12: 13, Jul 12: 12, Mar 14: 4, 12

● New   ▲ Revised   ✖ Deleted   ⊙ Moderate Sedation   ✚ Add-on Codes   ⊘ High Risk Denial   Ⓐ Age Edit   ♀ Female   ♂ Male   **AMA** *CPT® Assistant*   **MUE** Medically Unlikely Edit
⊘ Modifier 51 Exempt   ⊖ Modifier 63 Exempt   ⊠ Unlisted   **Modifiers:** *See Inside Back Cover*   Ⓜ Maternity   A 2 – Z 3 ASC Payment Indicators   A – Y OPPS Status Indicators

CPT © 2015 American Medical Association. All Rights Reserved.   © 2016 DecisionHealth

11604 Excision, malignant lesion including margins, trunk, arms, or legs; excised diameter 3.1 to 4.0 cm `A 2 T`

RVU		Global Days	Modifiers				
Mod	*Non-Fac Total* *Fac Total*		51	50	62	80	*MUE*
	8.95 6.20	010	2	0	0	1	2

AMA: Fall 95: 3, May 96: 11, Nov 02: 5, Feb 08: 8, Feb 10: 3, May 12: 13, Jul 12: 12, Mar 14: 4, 12

11606 Excision, malignant lesion including margins, trunk, arms, or legs; excised diameter over 4.0 cm `A 2 T`

RVU		Global Days	Modifiers				
Mod	*Non-Fac Total* *Fac Total*		51	50	62	80	*MUE*
	12.85 9.25	010	2	0	0	1	2

AMA: Fall 91: 6, Fall 95: 3, May 96: 11, Nov 02: 5, Feb 08: 8, Feb 10: 3, May 12: 13, Jul 12: 12, Mar 14: 4, 12

11620 Excision, malignant lesion including margins, scalp, neck, hands, feet, genitalia; excised diameter 0.5 cm or less `P 3 T`

RVU		Global Days	Modifiers				
Mod	*Non-Fac Total* *Fac Total*		51	50	62	80	*MUE*
	5.49 3.46	010	2	0	0	1	2

AMA: Fall 95: 3, Nov 02: 5, Oct 04: 4, Feb 08: 8, Feb 10: 3, May 12: 13, Jul 12: 12, Mar 14: 4, 12

Excision, malignant lesion
(scalp, neck, hands, feet, genitalia)

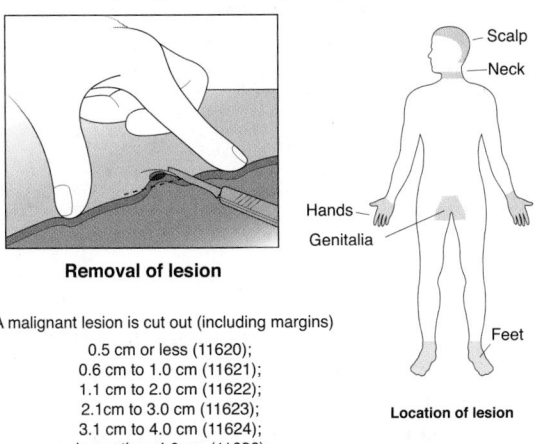

Removal of lesion

A malignant lesion is cut out (including margins)

    0.5 cm or less (11620);
    0.6 cm to 1.0 cm (11621);
    1.1 cm to 2.0 cm (11622);
    2.1cm to 3.0 cm (11623);
    3.1 cm to 4.0 cm (11624);
    larger than 4.0 cm (11626)

Location of lesion

11621 Excision, malignant lesion including margins, scalp, neck, hands, feet, genitalia; excised diameter 0.6 to 1.0 cm `P 3 T`

RVU		Global Days	Modifiers				
Mod	*Non-Fac Total* *Fac Total*		51	50	62	80	*MUE*
	6.51 4.31	010	2	0	0	1	2

AMA: Fall 95: 3, May 96: 11, Nov 02: 5, Feb 08: 8, Feb 10: 3, May 12: 13, Mar 14: 4, 12

11622 Excision, malignant lesion including margins, scalp, neck, hands, feet, genitalia; excised diameter 1.1 to 2.0 cm `P 3 T`

RVU		Global Days	Modifiers				
Mod	*Non-Fac Total* *Fac Total*		51	50	62	80	*MUE*
	7.27 4.94	010	2	0	0	1	2

AMA: Fall 95: 3, May 96: 11, Nov 02: 5, Feb 08: 8, Feb 10: 3, May 12: 13, Mar 14: 4, 12

11623 Excision, malignant lesion including margins, scalp, neck, hands, feet, genitalia; excised diameter 2.1 to 3.0 cm `P 3 T`

RVU		Global Days	Modifiers				
Mod	*Non-Fac Total* *Fac Total*		51	50	62	80	*MUE*
	8.55 6.11	010	2	0	0	1	2

AMA: Fall 95: 3, May 96: 11, Nov 02: 5, Feb 08: 8, Feb 10: 3, May 12: 13, Mar 14: 4, 12

11624 Excision, malignant lesion including margins, scalp, neck, hands, feet, genitalia; excised diameter 3.1 to 4.0 cm `A 2 T`

RVU		Global Days	Modifiers				
Mod	*Non-Fac Total* *Fac Total*		51	50	62	80	*MUE*
	9.64 6.92	010	2	0	0	1	2

AMA: Fall 95: 3, May 96: 11, Nov 02: 5, Feb 08: 8, Feb 10: 3, May 12: 13, Mar 14: 4, 12

11626 Excision, malignant lesion including margins, scalp, neck, hands, feet, genitalia; excised diameter over 4.0 cm `A 2 T`

RVU		Global Days	Modifiers				
Mod	*Non-Fac Total* *Fac Total*		51	50	62	80	*MUE*
	11.66 8.52	010	2	0	0	1	2

AMA: Fall 95: 3, May 96: 11, Nov 02: 5, Feb 08: 8, Feb 10: 3, May 12: 13, Mar 14: 4, 12

11640 Excision, malignant lesion including margins, face, ears, eyelids, nose, lips; excised diameter 0.5 cm or less `P 3 T`

RVU		Global Days	Modifiers				
Mod	*Non-Fac Total* *Fac Total*		51	50	62	80	*MUE*
	5.67 3.59	010	2	0	0	1	2

AMA: Fall 95: 3, May 96: 11, Nov 02: 5, Oct 04: 4, Feb 08: 8, Feb 10: 3, May 12: 13, Mar 14: 4, 12

Excision, malignant lesion

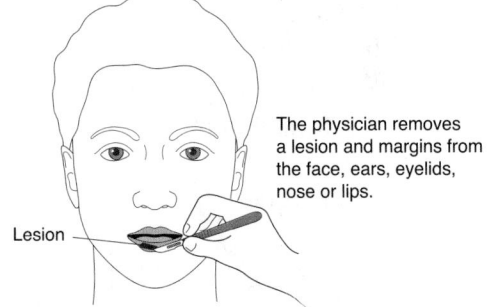

The physician removes a lesion and margins from the face, ears, eyelids, nose or lips.

Lesion

0.5 cm or less (11640); 0.6 cm to 1.0 cm (11641); 1.1 cm to 2.0 cm (11642); 2.1cm to 3.0 cm (11643); 3.1 cm to 4.0 cm (11644); larger than 4.0 cm (11646)

11641 Excision, malignant lesion including margins, face, ears, eyelids, nose, lips; excised diameter 0.6 to 1.0 cm `P 3 T`

RVU		Global Days	Modifiers				
Mod	*Non-Fac Total* *Fac Total*		51	50	62	80	*MUE*
	6.74 4.49	010	2	0	0	1	2

AMA: Fall 95: 3, May 96: 11, Feb 08: 8, Feb 10: 3, May 12: 13, Mar 14: 4, 12

● New   ▲ Revised   Deleted   ⊙ Moderate Sedation   ✚ Add-on Codes   ⊘ High Risk Denial   Ⓐ Age Edit   ♀ Female   ♂ Male   **AMA** *CPT® Assistant*   *MUE* Medically Unlikely Edit
⊘ Modifier 51 Exempt   ⊖ Modifier 63 Exempt   ⌧ Unlisted   **Modifiers:** *See Inside Back Cover*   Ⓜ Maternity   `A 2`–`Z 3` ASC Payment Indicators   `A`–`Y` OPPS Status Indicators

Surgical Procedures

11604 – 11641

11642 Excision, malignant lesion including margins, face, ears, eyelids, nose, lips; excised diameter 1.1 to 2.0 cm   P 3 T

RVU			Global Days	Modifiers				
Mod	Non-Fac Total	Fac Total		51	50	62	80	MUE
	7.71	5.31	010	2	0	0	1	3

AMA: Fall 95: 3, May 96: 11, Feb 08: 8, Feb 10: 3, May 12: 13, Mar 14: 4, 12

11643 Excision, malignant lesion including margins, face, ears, eyelids, nose, lips; excised diameter 2.1 to 3.0 cm   P 3 T

RVU			Global Days	Modifiers				
Mod	Non-Fac Total	Fac Total		51	50	62	80	MUE
	9.10	6.64	010	2	0	0	1	2

AMA: Fall 95: 3, May 96: 11, Feb 08: 8, Feb 10: 3, May 12: 13, Mar 14: 4, 12

11644 Excision, malignant lesion including margins, face, ears, eyelids, nose, lips; excised diameter 3.1 to 4.0 cm   A 2 T

RVU			Global Days	Modifiers				
Mod	Non-Fac Total	Fac Total		51	50	62	80	MUE
	11.25	8.24	010	2	0	0	1	2

AMA: Fall 95: 3, May 96: 11, Feb 08: 8, Feb 10: 3, May 12: 13, Mar 14: 4, 12

11646 Excision, malignant lesion including margins, face, ears, eyelids, nose, lips; excised diameter over 4.0 cm   A 2 T

RVU			Global Days	Modifiers				
Mod	Non-Fac Total	Fac Total		51	50	62	80	MUE
	14.74	11.47	010	2	0	0	1	2

AMA: Fall 95: 3, May 96: 11, Feb 08: 8, Feb 10: 3, Apr 10: 3, May 12: 13, Mar 14: 4, 12

Nail Procedures

11719 Trimming of nondystrophic nails, any number   N I Q I

RVU			Global Days	Modifiers				
Mod	Non-Fac Total	Fac Total		51	50	62	80	MUE
	0.40	0.22	000	2	0	0	1	1

AMA: Nov 97: 12, Dec 02: 4
Pub 100-04, 32, 80.8

Trimming of nondystrophic nails

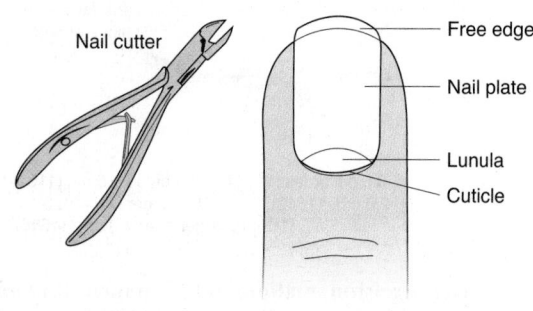

Nail cutter
Free edge
Nail plate
Lunula
Cuticle

Healthy, nondystrophic fingernails/toenails are trimmed and inspected for potential problems.

11720 Debridement of nail(s) by any method(s); 1 to 5   N I Q I

RVU			Global Days	Modifiers				
Mod	Non-Fac Total	Fac Total		51	50	62	80	MUE
	0.91	0.42	000	0	0	0	1	1

AMA: Nov 96: 3, Dec 02: 4
Pub 100-04, 32, 80.8

11721 Debridement of nail(s) by any method(s); 6 or more   N I Q I

RVU			Global Days	Modifiers				
Mod	Non-Fac Total	Fac Total		51	50	62	80	MUE
	1.27	0.71	000	0	0	0	1	1

AMA: Nov 96: 3, Dec 02: 4
Pub 100-04, 32, 80.8

11730 Avulsion of nail plate, partial or complete, simple; single   N I Q I

RVU			Global Days	Modifiers				
Mod	Non-Fac Total	Fac Total		51	50	62	80	MUE
	2.81	1.46	000	2	0	0	1	1

AMA: Mar 96: 10, Dec 02: 4, Dec 03: 11

Avulsion of nail plate

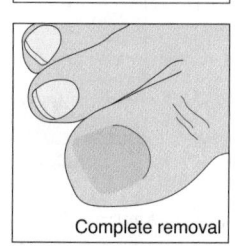

After

Before

Partial removal

Complete removal

+ 11732 Avulsion of nail plate, partial or complete, simple; each additional nail plate (List separately in addition to code for primary procedure)   N I N

RVU			Global Days	Modifiers				
Mod	Non-Fac Total	Fac Total		51	50	62	80	MUE
	1.01	0.58	ZZZ	0	0	0	1	9

AMA: Dec 02: 4

11740 Evacuation of subungual hematoma   N I Q I

Coding tip: For avulsion of nail plate, see 11730-11732

RVU			Global Days	Modifiers				
Mod	Non-Fac Total	Fac Total		51	50	62	80	MUE
	1.41	0.94	000	2	0	0	1	3

AMA: Dec 02: 4

● New   ▲ Revised   ✖ Deleted   ⊙ Moderate Sedation   ✚ Add-on Codes   ⊗ High Risk Denial   Ⓐ Age Edit   ♀ Female   ♂ Male   **AMA** *CPT® Assistant*   **MUE** Medically Unlikely Edit
⊘ Modifier 51 Exempt   ⊖ Modifier 63 Exempt   ✗ Unlisted   **Modifiers:** *See Inside Back Cover*   Ⓜ Maternity   A2–Z3 ASC Payment Indicators   A–Y OPPS Status Indicators

180   CPT © 2015 American Medical Association. All Rights Reserved.   © 2016 DecisionHealth

11750 Excision of nail and nail matrix, partial or complete (eg, ingrown or deformed nail), for permanent removal P 3 T

RVU			Global Days	Modifiers				
Mod	Non-Fac Total	Fac Total		51	50	62	80	MUE
	5.10	4.00	010	2	0	0	1	6

AMA: Dec 02: 4

11752 Excision of nail and nail matrix, partial or complete (eg, ingrown or deformed nail), for permanent removal; with amputation of tuft of distal phalanx P 3 T

RVU			Global Days	Modifiers				
Mod	Non-Fac Total	Fac Total		51	50	62	80	MUE
	9.20	7.50	010	2	0	0	1	3

AMA: Dec 02: 4

11755 Biopsy of nail unit (eg, plate, bed, matrix, hyponychium, proximal and lateral nail folds) (separate procedure) P 3 T

Coding tip: Report only when tissue sample removal is performed alone, not when done in conjunction with another type of procedure on the nail unit

RVU			Global Days	Modifiers				
Mod	Non-Fac Total	Fac Total		51	50	62	80	MUE
	3.78	2.23	000	2	0	0	0	4

AMA: Mar 96: 11, Dec 02: 4, Oct 04: 14

Biopsy of nail unit

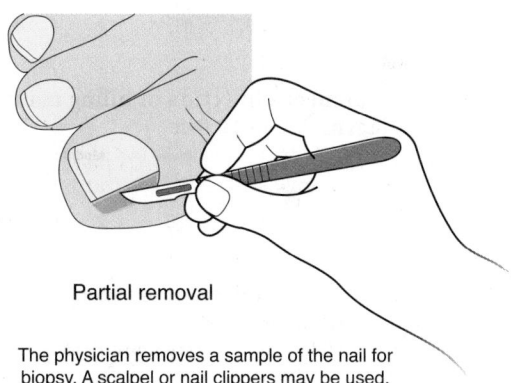

Partial removal

The physician removes a sample of the nail for biopsy. A scalpel or nail clippers may be used.

11760 Repair of nail bed G 2 T

Coding tip: Removal of all or a portion of the nail plate is included

Coding tip: Local or digital block anesthesia is included

Coding tip: Add simple/intermediate/complex repair codes when a soft tissue laceration on the pulp or back of the finger is also repaired

RVU			Global Days	Modifiers				
Mod	Non-Fac Total	Fac Total		51	50	62	80	MUE
	5.54	3.37	010	2	0	0	1	4

AMA: Dec 02: 4

11762 Reconstruction of nail bed with graft P 3 T

Coding tip: Local or digital block anesthesia is included

Coding tip: Split-thickness graft acquisition is generally from the bed of the great toe and requires avulsion of the donor nail plate

RVU			Global Days	Modifiers				
Mod	Non-Fac Total	Fac Total		51	50	62	80	MUE
	7.99	5.29	010	2	0	0	1	2

AMA: Dec 02: 4

11765 Wedge excision of skin of nail fold (eg, for ingrown toenail) N I Q I

Coding tip: Local or digital block anesthesia is included

RVU			Global Days	Modifiers				
Mod	Non-Fac Total	Fac Total		51	50	62	80	MUE
	4.74	2.69	010	2	0	0	1	4

AMA: Dec 02: 4

Excisional Pilonidal Cyst Procedures

Coding Guidance

During an excision procedure of pilonidal cysts and/or sinuses it may be necessary to first incise and drain one or more of the cysts. It is inappropriate to report CPT codes 10080 or 10081 separately for the incision and drainage procedure.

11770 Excision of pilonidal cyst or sinus; simple A 2 T

RVU			Global Days	Modifiers				
Mod	Non-Fac Total	Fac Total		51	50	62	80	MUE
	7.89	5.32	010	2	0	0	1	1

Excision of pilonidal cyst or sinus

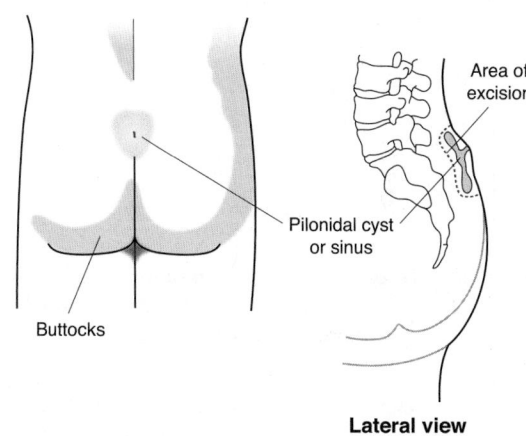

Area of excision

Pilonidal cyst or sinus

Buttocks

Lateral view

11771 Excision of pilonidal cyst or sinus; extensive A 2 T

RVU			Global Days	Modifiers				
Mod	Non-Fac Total	Fac Total		51	50	62	80	MUE
	16.34	12.50	090	2	0	0	1	1

11772 Excision of pilonidal cyst or sinus; complicated A 2 T

RVU			Global Days	Modifiers				
Mod	Non-Fac Total	Fac Total		51	50	62	80	MUE
	19.81	16.55	090	2	0	0	1	1

● New   ▲ Revised   Deleted   ⊙ Moderate Sedation   ✚ Add-on Codes   ⊗ High Risk Denial   Ⓐ Age Edit   ♀ Female   ♂ Male   **AMA** *CPT® Assistant*   **MUE** Medically Unlikely Edit
⊘ Modifier 51 Exempt   ⊖ Modifier 63 Exempt   ⊠ Unlisted   **Modifiers:** *See Inside Back Cover*   Ⓜ Maternity   A 2–Z 3 ASC Payment Indicators   A –Y OPPS Status Indicators

© 2016 DecisionHealth   CPT © 2015 American Medical Association. All Rights Reserved.   **181**

Surgical Procedures

11900 – 11970

Introduction/Removal Skin Procedures

Coding Guidance

Codes 11900-11901 describe intralesional injections of non-chemotherapeutic agents. Nonspecific lesion injection codes should not be used to report the administration of local anesthesia for another definitive procedure. Codes 11900 and 11901 are not reported together, unless separate groups of lesions are injected with different agents, in which case, a modifier should be attached.

11900 Injection, intralesional; up to and including 7 lesions N I Q I

RVU			Global Days	Modifiers				
Mod	Non-Fac Total	Fac Total		51	50	62	80	MUE
	1.57	0.90	000	2	0	0	1	1

AMA: Sep 96: 5, May 98: 10, Nov 99: 8, Feb 00: 11, Sep 04: 12, Nov 13: 14

Intralesional injection

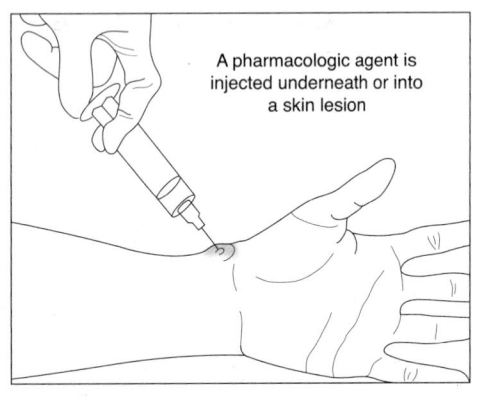

A pharmacologic agent is injected underneath or into a skin lesion

11901 Injection, intralesional; more than 7 lesions N I Q I

RVU			Global Days	Modifiers				
Mod	Non-Fac Total	Fac Total		51	50	62	80	MUE
	1.98	1.40	000	2	0	0	1	1

AMA: Sep 96: 5, May 98: 10, Nov 99: 8, Feb 00: 11, Sep 04: 12

11920 Tattooing, intradermal introduction of insoluble opaque pigments to correct color defects of skin, including micropigmentation; 6.0 sq cm or less P 3 T

RVU			Global Days	Modifiers				
Mod	Non-Fac Total	Fac Total		51	50	62	80	MUE
	4.87	3.29	000	2	0	0	0	1

Pub 100-04, 13, 70.2

Tattooing

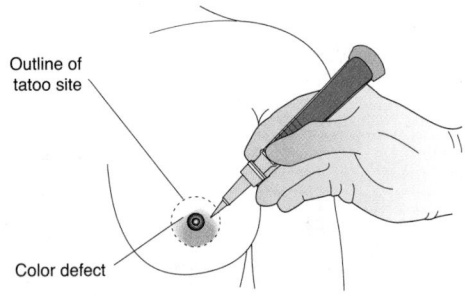

Outline of tatoo site

Color defect

For 6.0 sq. cm or less (11920); 6.1 to 20.0 sq cm (11921); each additional 20.0 sq cm, or part thereof (11922)

11921 Tattooing, intradermal introduction of insoluble opaque pigments to correct color defects of skin, including micropigmentation; 6.1 to 20.0 sq cm P 3 T

RVU			Global Days	Modifiers				
Mod	Non-Fac Total	Fac Total		51	50	62	80	MUE
	5.68	3.90	000	2	0	0	0	1

Pub 100-04, 13, 70.2

+ 11922 Tattooing, intradermal introduction of insoluble opaque pigments to correct color defects of skin, including micropigmentation; each additional 20.0 sq cm, or part thereof (List separately in addition to code for primary procedure) N I N

RVU			Global Days	Modifiers				
Mod	Non-Fac Total	Fac Total		51	50	62	80	MUE
	1.76	0.86	ZZZ	0	0	0	0	1

Pub 100-04, 13, 70.2

11950 Subcutaneous injection of filling material (eg, collagen); 1 cc or less ⊗ P 3 T

RVU			Global Days	Modifiers				
Mod	Non-Fac Total	Fac Total		51	50	62	80	MUE
	2.09	1.47	000	2	0	0	0	1

AMA: Jun 12: 15

11951 Subcutaneous injection of filling material (eg, collagen); 1.1 to 5.0 cc P 3 T

RVU			Global Days	Modifiers				
Mod	Non-Fac Total	Fac Total		51	50	62	80	MUE
	2.77	2.07	000	2	0	0	0	1

AMA: Jun 12: 15

11952 Subcutaneous injection of filling material (eg, collagen); 5.1 to 10.0 cc ⊗ P 3 T

RVU			Global Days	Modifiers				
Mod	Non-Fac Total	Fac Total		51	50	62	80	MUE
	3.72	2.78	000	2	0	0	0	1

AMA: Jun 12: 15

11954 Subcutaneous injection of filling material (eg, collagen); over 10.0 cc ⊗ P 3 T

RVU			Global Days	Modifiers				
Mod	Non-Fac Total	Fac Total		51	50	62	80	MUE
	4.52	3.32	000	2	0	0	0	1

AMA: Jun 12: 15

11960 Insertion of tissue expander(s) for other than breast, including subsequent expansion A 2 T

RVU			Global Days	Modifiers				
Mod	Non-Fac Total	Fac Total		51	50	62	80	MUE
	27.27	27.27	090	2	0	0	1	2

AMA: Winter 91: 2

11970 Replacement of tissue expander with permanent prosthesis A 2 J I

RVU			Global Days	Modifiers				
Mod	Non-Fac Total	Fac Total		51	50	62	80	MUE
	17.66	17.66	090	2	1	0	1	2

AMA: Aug 05: 1, Jan 13: 15

● New ▲ Revised ✖ Deleted ⊙ Moderate Sedation ✚ Add-on Codes ⊗ High Risk Denial Ⓐ Age Edit ♀ Female ♂ Male **AMA** *CPT® Assistant* **MUE** Medically Unlikely Edit
⊗ Modifier 51 Exempt ⊖ Modifier 63 Exempt ⊠ Unlisted **Modifiers:** *See Inside Back Cover* Ⓜ Maternity A2–Z3 ASC Payment Indicators A–Y OPPS Status Indicators

CPT © 2015 American Medical Association. All Rights Reserved.   © 2016 DecisionHealth

11971   Removal of tissue expander(s) without insertion of prosthesis   A 2 Q 2

RVU			Global Days	Modifiers				
Mod	Non-Fac Total	Fac Total		51	50	62	80	MUE
	13.49	9.22	090	2	1	0	0	2

AMA: Jun 05: 11

11976   Removal, implantable contraceptive capsules   ⊘♀ P 3 Q 2

RVU			Global Days	Modifiers				
Mod	Non-Fac Total	Fac Total		51	50	62	80	MUE
	4.05	2.69	000	2	0	0	0	1

11980   Subcutaneous hormone pellet implantation (implantation of estradiol and/or testosterone pellets beneath the skin)   N I Q I

Coding tip: See also insertion of implantable contraceptive capsules - 11981

RVU			Global Days	Modifiers				
Mod	Non-Fac Total	Fac Total		51	50	62	80	MUE
	2.66	1.61	000	2	0	0	1	1

AMA: Nov 99: 8

11981   Insertion, non-biodegradable drug delivery implant   N I Q I

Coding tip: See also implantation of hormone pellets - 11980

RVU			Global Days	Modifiers				
Mod	Non-Fac Total	Fac Total		51	50	62	80	MUE
	4.00	2.38	XXX	2	0	0	0	1

AMA: Apr 11: 12

Non-biodegradable drug delivery implant

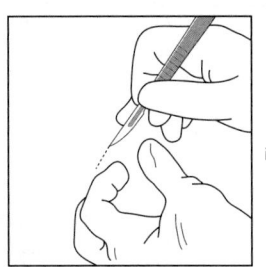

Small incision is made in the appropriate location

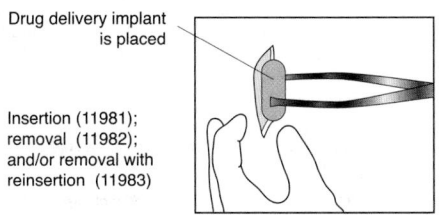

Drug delivery implant is placed

Insertion (11981); removal (11982); and/or removal with reinsertion (11983)

11982   Removal, non-biodegradable drug delivery implant   N I Q I

RVU			Global Days	Modifiers				
Mod	Non-Fac Total	Fac Total		51	50	62	80	MUE
	4.54	2.89	XXX	2	0	0	0	1

11983   Removal with reinsertion, non-biodegradable drug delivery implant   N I Q I

Coding tip: See also implantation of hormone pellets - 11980

RVU			Global Days	Modifiers				
Mod	Non-Fac Total	Fac Total		51	50	62	80	MUE
	6.31	4.99	XXX	2	0	0	0	1

Laceration Repair/Reconstructive Skin Procedures

Coding Guidance

Wound closures using topical dermal adhesive, tape, or adhesive strips alone are not separately reportable. These types of wound closures are included in an E&M service when there is no inclusive operative procedure performed.

12001   Simple repair of superficial wounds of scalp, neck, axillae, external genitalia, trunk and/or extremities (including hands and feet); 2.5 cm or less   N I Q I

RVU			Global Days	Modifiers				
Mod	Non-Fac Total	Fac Total		51	50	62	80	MUE
	2.52	1.27	000	2	0	0	1	1

AMA: Jun 96: 7, Feb 98: 11, Jan 00: 11, Feb 00: 10, Apr 00: 8, Jul 00: 10, Jan 02: 10, Feb 07: 10, Feb 08: 8, Mar 12: 5

12002   Simple repair of superficial wounds of scalp, neck, axillae, external genitalia, trunk and/or extremities (including hands and feet); 2.6 cm to 7.5 cm   N I Q I

RVU			Global Days	Modifiers				
Mod	Non-Fac Total	Fac Total		51	50	62	80	MUE
	3.07	1.67	000	2	0	0	1	1

AMA: Feb 00: 10, Jan 02: 10, Feb 08: 8, Oct 14: 14

12004   Simple repair of superficial wounds of scalp, neck, axillae, external genitalia, trunk and/or extremities (including hands and feet); 7.6 cm to 12.5 cm   N I Q I

RVU			Global Days	Modifiers				
Mod	Non-Fac Total	Fac Total		51	50	62	80	MUE
	3.62	2.09	000	2	0	0	1	1

AMA: Feb 00: 10, Jan 02: 10, Feb 08: 8

12005   Simple repair of superficial wounds of scalp, neck, axillae, external genitalia, trunk and/or extremities (including hands and feet); 12.6 cm to 20.0 cm   A 2 Q I

RVU			Global Days	Modifiers				
Mod	Non-Fac Total	Fac Total		51	50	62	80	MUE
	4.57	2.72	000	2	0	0	1	1

AMA: Feb 00: 10, Jan 02: 10, Feb 08: 8

12006   Simple repair of superficial wounds of scalp, neck, axillae, external genitalia, trunk and/or extremities (including hands and feet); 20.1 cm to 30.0 cm   A 2 Q 2

RVU			Global Days	Modifiers				
Mod	Non-Fac Total	Fac Total		51	50	62	80	MUE
	5.42	3.35	000	2	0	0	1	1

AMA: Feb 98: 11, Feb 00: 10, Jan 02: 10, Feb 08: 8

12007   Simple repair of superficial wounds of scalp, neck, axillae, external genitalia, trunk and/or extremities (including hands and feet); over 30.0 cm   A 2 T

RVU			Global Days	Modifiers				
Mod	Non-Fac Total	Fac Total		51	50	62	80	MUE
	6.34	4.23	000	2	0	1	1	1

AMA: Feb 00: 10, Jan 02: 10, Feb 08: 8

● New   ▲ Revised   Deleted   ⊙ Moderate Sedation   ✚ Add-on Codes   ⊘ High Risk Denial   Ⓐ Age Edit   ♀ Female   ♂ Male   **AMA** *CPT® Assistant*   **MUE** Medically Unlikely Edit
⊘ Modifier 51 Exempt   ⊖ Modifier 63 Exempt   ✗ Unlisted   **Modifiers:** *See Inside Back Cover*   Ⓜ Maternity   A 2 – Z 3 ASC Payment Indicators   A – Y OPPS Status Indicators

© 2016 DecisionHealth   CPT © 2015 American Medical Association. All Rights Reserved.   **183**

Surgical Procedures

12011 – 12031

12011 Simple repair of superficial wounds of face, ears, eyelids, nose, lips and/or mucous membranes; 2.5 cm or less   N I Q I

Mod	Non-Fac Total	Fac Total	Global Days	51	50	62	80	MUE
	3.09	1.58	000	2	0	0	1	1

RVU / Modifiers

AMA: Feb 00: 10, May 00: 8, Jan 02: 10, Feb 08: 8, May 14: 5

Simple repair of superficial wounds of face, ears, eyelids, nose, lips and/or mucous membranes

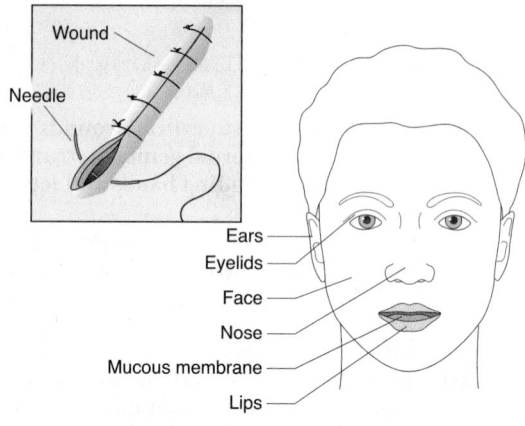

Report according to total length repaired.
Single layer stitching is used to repair the wound.

12013 Simple repair of superficial wounds of face, ears, eyelids, nose, lips and/or mucous membranes; 2.6 cm to 5.0 cm   N I Q I

Mod	Non-Fac Total	Fac Total	Global Days	51	50	62	80	MUE
	3.23	1.66	000	2	0	0	1	1

AMA: Feb 00: 10, Jan 02: 10, Feb 08: 8

12014 Simple repair of superficial wounds of face, ears, eyelids, nose, lips and/or mucous membranes; 5.1 cm to 7.5 cm   N I Q I

Mod	Non-Fac Total	Fac Total	Global Days	51	50	62	80	MUE
	3.78	2.14	000	2	0	0	1	1

AMA: Feb 00: 10, Jan 02: 10, Feb 08: 8

12015 Simple repair of superficial wounds of face, ears, eyelids, nose, lips and/or mucous membranes; 7.6 cm to 12.5 cm   G 2 Q I

Mod	Non-Fac Total	Fac Total	Global Days	51	50	62	80	MUE
	4.58	2.70	000	2	0	0	1	1

AMA: Feb 00: 10, Jan 02: 10, Feb 08: 8

12016 Simple repair of superficial wounds of face, ears, eyelids, nose, lips and/or mucous membranes; 12.6 cm to 20.0 cm   A 2 Q I

Mod	Non-Fac Total	Fac Total	Global Days	51	50	62	80	MUE
	5.81	3.68	000	2	0	0	1	1

AMA: Feb 00: 10, Jan 02: 10, Feb 08: 8

12017 Simple repair of superficial wounds of face, ears, eyelids, nose, lips and/or mucous membranes; 20.1 cm to 30.0 cm   A 2 Q I

Mod	Non-Fac Total	Fac Total	Global Days	51	50	62	80	MUE
	4.41	4.41	000	2	0	0	0	1

AMA: Feb 00: 10, Jan 02: 10, Feb 08: 8

12018 Simple repair of superficial wounds of face, ears, eyelids, nose, lips and/or mucous membranes; over 30.0 cm   A 2 Q I

Mod	Non-Fac Total	Fac Total	Global Days	51	50	62	80	MUE
	5.00	5.00	000	2	0	0	2	1

AMA: Feb 00: 10, Jan 02: 10, Feb 07: 10, Feb 08: 8, May 14: 5

12020 Treatment of superficial wound dehiscence; simple closure   A 2 T

Mod	Non-Fac Total	Fac Total	Global Days	51	50	62	80	MUE
	8.25	5.60	010	2	0	0	1	2

AMA: Feb 00: 10, Jan 02: 10, Feb 08: 8

Treatment of superficial dehiscence

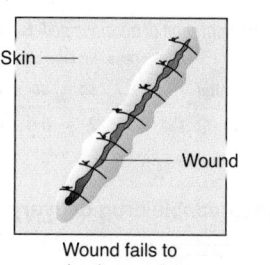

Wound fails to heal properly

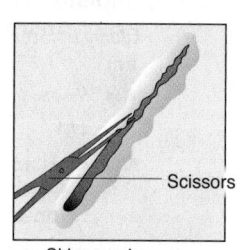

Skin margins may be trimmed

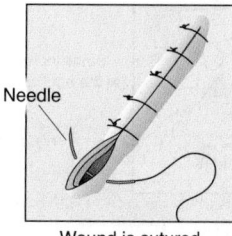

Wound is sutured if not infected

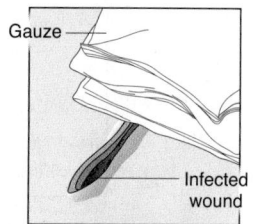

Wound is left open and packed with gauze strips if infected

12021 Treatment of superficial wound dehiscence; with packing   A 2 T

Mod	Non-Fac Total	Fac Total	Global Days	51	50	62	80	MUE
	4.75	4.06	010	2	0	0	1	3

AMA: Feb 00: 10, Jan 02: 10, Feb 08: 8

12031 Repair, intermediate, wounds of scalp, axillae, trunk and/or extremities (excluding hands and feet); 2.5 cm or less   P 2 T

Coding tip: Add excision of benign lesion - 11400-11446 or malignant lesion - 11600-11646

Mod	Non-Fac Total	Fac Total	Global Days	51	50	62	80	MUE
	6.72	4.41	010	2	0	0	1	1

AMA: Sep 97: 11, Feb 00: 10, Apr 00: 8, Jan 02: 10, Aug 06: 1, Feb 07: 10, Apr 10: 3

● New   ▲ Revised   ✖ Deleted   ⊙ Moderate Sedation   ✚ Add-on Codes   ⊘ High Risk Denial   Ⓐ Age Edit   ♀ Female   ♂ Male   **AMA** *CPT® Assistant*   **MUE** Medically Unlikely Edit
⊘ Modifier 51 Exempt   ⊖ Modifier 63 Exempt   ⊠ Unlisted   **Modifiers:** *See Inside Back Cover*   Ⓜ Maternity   A 2 – Z 3 ASC Payment Indicators   A – Y OPPS Status Indicators

184   CPT © 2015 American Medical Association. All Rights Reserved.   © 2016 DecisionHealth

12032 Repair, intermediate, wounds of scalp, axillae, trunk and/or extremities (excluding hands and feet); 2.6 cm to 7.5 cm P 2 T

RVU			Global Days	Modifiers				
Mod	Non-Fac Total	Fac Total		51	50	62	80	MUE
	8.60	5.61	010	2	0	0	1	1

AMA: May 96: 6, Jun 96: 8, Feb 00: 10, Jan 02: 10, Feb 07: 10

12034 Repair, intermediate, wounds of scalp, axillae, trunk and/or extremities (excluding hands and feet); 7.6 cm to 12.5 cm A 2 T

RVU			Global Days	Modifiers				
Mod	Non-Fac Total	Fac Total		51	50	62	80	MUE
	8.85	5.95	010	2	0	0	1	1

AMA: Fall 91: 6, Feb 00: 10, Jan 02: 10, Feb 07: 10

12035 Repair, intermediate, wounds of scalp, axillae, trunk and/or extremities (excluding hands and feet); 12.6 cm to 20.0 cm A 2 T

RVU			Global Days	Modifiers				
Mod	Non-Fac Total	Fac Total		51	50	62	80	MUE
	10.88	6.92	010	2	0	0	1	1

AMA: Feb 00: 10, Jan 02: 10, Feb 07: 10

12036 Repair, intermediate, wounds of scalp, axillae, trunk and/or extremities (excluding hands and feet); 20.1 cm to 30.0 cm A 2 T

RVU			Global Days	Modifiers				
Mod	Non-Fac Total	Fac Total		51	50	62	80	MUE
	12.02	8.07	010	2	0	0	1	1

AMA: Feb 00: 10, Jan 02: 10, Feb 07: 10

12037 Repair, intermediate, wounds of scalp, axillae, trunk and/or extremities (excluding hands and feet); over 30.0 cm A 2 T

RVU			Global Days	Modifiers				
Mod	Non-Fac Total	Fac Total		51	50	62	80	MUE
	13.64	9.46	010	2	0	1	0	1

AMA: Feb 00: 10, Jan 02: 10, Feb 07: 10

12041 Repair, intermediate, wounds of neck, hands, feet and/or external genitalia; 2.5 cm or less P 2 Q 2

Coding tip: *Add excision of benign lesion - 11400-11446; malignant lesion - 11600-11646*

RVU			Global Days	Modifiers				
Mod	Non-Fac Total	Fac Total		51	50	62	80	MUE
	6.72	4.33	010	2	0	0	1	1

AMA: Sep 97: 11, Feb 00: 10, Apr 00: 8, Jan 02: 10, Feb 07: 10, Jan 13: 15

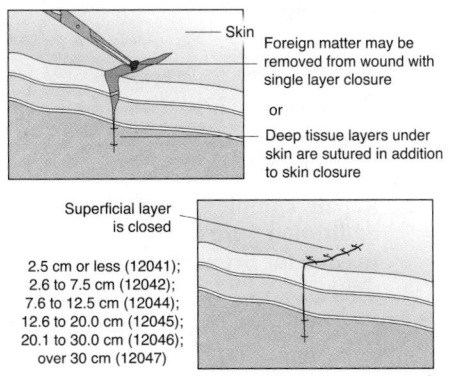

Repair, intermediate, wounds of neck, hands, feet and/or external genitalia

Skin — Foreign matter may be removed from wound with single layer closure

or

Deep tissue layers under skin are sutured in addition to skin closure

Superficial layer is closed

2.5 cm or less (12041);
2.6 to 7.5 cm (12042);
7.6 to 12.5 cm (12044);
12.6 to 20.0 cm (12045);
20.1 to 30.0 cm (12046);
over 30 cm (12047)

12042 Repair, intermediate, wounds of neck, hands, feet and/or external genitalia; 2.6 cm to 7.5 cm P 2 T

RVU			Global Days	Modifiers				
Mod	Non-Fac Total	Fac Total		51	50	62	80	MUE
	8.20	5.77	010	2	0	0	1	1

AMA: Feb 00: 10, Apr 00: 9, Jan 02: 10, Feb 07: 10, Jan 13: 15

12044 Repair, intermediate, wounds of neck, hands, feet and/or external genitalia; 7.6 cm to 12.5 cm A 2 T

RVU			Global Days	Modifiers				
Mod	Non-Fac Total	Fac Total		51	50	62	80	MUE
	10.20	6.18	010	2	0	0	1	1

AMA: Feb 00: 10, Jan 02: 10, Feb 07: 10, Jan 13: 15

12045 Repair, intermediate, wounds of neck, hands, feet and/or external genitalia; 12.6 cm to 20.0 cm A 2 T

RVU			Global Days	Modifiers				
Mod	Non-Fac Total	Fac Total		51	50	62	80	MUE
	11.45	7.77	010	2	0	0	1	1

AMA: Feb 00: 10, Jan 02: 10, Feb 07: 10, Jan 13: 15

12046 Repair, intermediate, wounds of neck, hands, feet and/or external genitalia; 20.1 cm to 30.0 cm A 2 T

RVU			Global Days	Modifiers				
Mod	Non-Fac Total	Fac Total		51	50	62	80	MUE
	13.60	8.95	010	2	0	0	0	1

AMA: Feb 00: 10, Jan 02: 10, Feb 07: 10, Jan 13: 15

12047 Repair, intermediate, wounds of neck, hands, feet and/or external genitalia; over 30.0 cm A 2 T

RVU			Global Days	Modifiers				
Mod	Non-Fac Total	Fac Total		51	50	62	80	MUE
	14.79	9.97	010	2	0	1	2	1

AMA: Feb 00: 10, Jan 02: 10, Feb 07: 10, Jan 13: 15

12051 Repair, intermediate, wounds of face, ears, eyelids, nose, lips and/or mucous membranes; 2.5 cm or less P 2 T

Coding tip: *Add excision of benign lesion - 11400-11446; malignant lesion - 11600-11646*

RVU			Global Days	Modifiers				
Mod	Non-Fac Total	Fac Total		51	50	62	80	MUE
	7.34	4.95	010	2	0	0	1	1

AMA: Sep 97: 11, Feb 00: 10, Apr 00: 8, Jan 02: 10, Feb 07: 10, May 14: 5

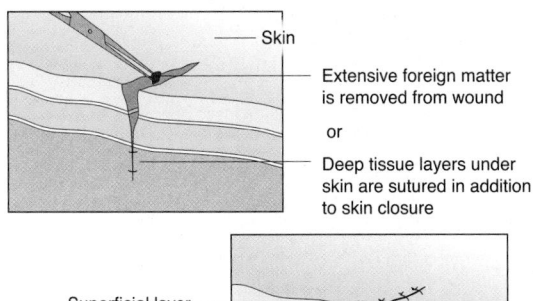

Layered closure of wounds

Extensive cleaning or removal of foreign matter is done with single layer closure

Skin

Extensive foreign matter is removed from wound

or

Deep tissue layers under skin are sutured in addition to skin closure

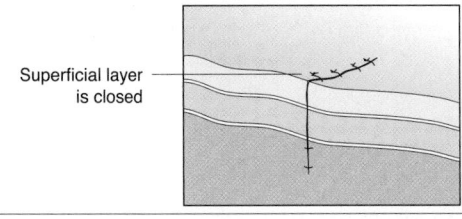

Superficial layer is closed

● New ▲ Revised Deleted ⊙ Moderate Sedation ✚ Add-on Codes ⊘ High Risk Denial Ⓐ Age Edit ♀ Female ♂ Male **AMA** *CPT® Assistant* **MUE** Medically Unlikely Edit
⊘ Modifier 51 Exempt ⊖ Modifier 63 Exempt Ⓧ Unlisted **Modifiers:** *See Inside Back Cover* Ⓜ Maternity A2–Z3 ASC Payment Indicators A–Y OPPS Status Indicators

© 2016 DecisionHealth · CPT © 2015 American Medical Association. All Rights Reserved.

12052 Repair, intermediate, wounds of face, ears, eyelids, nose, lips and/or mucous membranes; 2.6 cm to 5.0 cm   `P 2 T`

RVU		Global Days	Modifiers				
Mod	Non-Fac Total	Fac Total		51	50	62	80	MUE
	8.36	5.87	010	2	0	0	1	1

AMA: Feb 00: 10, Aug 00: 9, Jan 02: 10, Feb 07: 10, Jul 08: 5

12053 Repair, intermediate, wounds of face, ears, eyelids, nose, lips and/or mucous membranes; 5.1 cm to 7.5 cm   `P 2 T`

RVU		Global Days	Modifiers				
Mod	Non-Fac Total	Fac Total		51	50	62	80	MUE
	9.81	6.27	010	2	0	0	1	1

AMA: Feb 00: 10, Jan 02: 10, Feb 07: 10

12054 Repair, intermediate, wounds of face, ears, eyelids, nose, lips and/or mucous membranes; 7.6 cm to 12.5 cm   `A 2 Q 2`

RVU		Global Days	Modifiers				
Mod	Non-Fac Total	Fac Total		51	50	62	80	MUE
	10.25	6.42	010	2	0	0	1	1

AMA: Feb 00: 10, Jan 02: 10, Feb 07: 10

12055 Repair, intermediate, wounds of face, ears, eyelids, nose, lips and/or mucous membranes; 12.6 cm to 20.0 cm   `A 2 T`

RVU		Global Days	Modifiers				
Mod	Non-Fac Total	Fac Total		51	50	62	80	MUE
	13.32	8.82	010	2	0	0	1	1

AMA: Feb 00: 10, Jan 02: 10, Feb 07: 10

12056 Repair, intermediate, wounds of face, ears, eyelids, nose, lips and/or mucous membranes; 20.1 cm to 30.0 cm   `A 2 Q 2`

RVU		Global Days	Modifiers				
Mod	Non-Fac Total	Fac Total		51	50	62	80	MUE
	15.69	10.99	010	2	0	0	0	1

AMA: Feb 00: 10, Jan 02: 10, Feb 07: 10

12057 Repair, intermediate, wounds of face, ears, eyelids, nose, lips and/or mucous membranes; over 30.0 cm   `A 2 T`

RVU		Global Days	Modifiers				
Mod	Non-Fac Total	Fac Total		51	50	62	80	MUE
	16.09	11.78	010	2	0	1	2	1

AMA: Feb 00: 10, Jan 02: 10, Feb 07: 10, Apr 10: 3, May 14: 5

13100 Repair, complex, trunk; 1.1 cm to 2.5 cm   `A 2 T`

RVU		Global Days	Modifiers				
Mod	Non-Fac Total	Fac Total		51	50	62	80	MUE
	9.51	5.95	010	2	0	0	1	1

AMA: Sep 97: 11, Dec 98: 5, Nov 99: 9, 10, Feb 00: 10, Apr 00: 8, Apr 10: 3, Feb 10: 3, May 11: 4, Jan 12: 8, Dec 12: 6

Complex repair

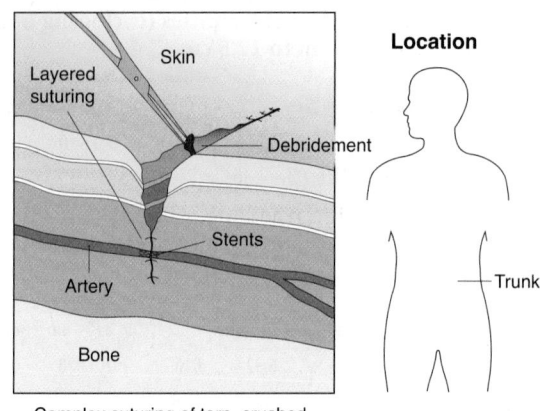

Complex suturing of torn, crushed, or deeply lacerated tissue

13101 Repair, complex, trunk; 2.6 cm to 7.5 cm   `A 2 T`

RVU		Global Days	Modifiers				
Mod	Non-Fac Total	Fac Total		51	50	62	80	MUE
	11.25	7.32	010	2	0	0	1	1

AMA: Dec 98: 5, Nov 99: 9, 10, Feb 00: 10, Apr 00: 9, Feb 10: 3, May 11: 4, Jan 12: 8, Dec 12: 6

+ 13102 Repair, complex, trunk; each additional 5 cm or less (List separately in addition to code for primary procedure)   `N I N`

RVU		Global Days	Modifiers				
Mod	Non-Fac Total	Fac Total		51	50	62	80	MUE
	3.48	2.16	ZZZ	0	0	0	1	9

AMA: Nov 99: 9, 10, Feb 00: 10, Apr 00: 9, Feb 10: 3, May 11: 4, Jan 12: 8, Dec 12: 6

13120 Repair, complex, scalp, arms, and/or legs; 1.1 cm to 2.5 cm   `A 2 T`

RVU		Global Days	Modifiers				
Mod	Non-Fac Total	Fac Total		51	50	62	80	MUE
	9.96	6.82	010	2	0	0	1	1

AMA: Sep 97: 11, Apr 99: 11, Nov 99: 9, 10, Feb 00: 10, Apr 00: 8, Feb 10: 3, May 11: 4, Jan 12: 8, Dec 12: 6

13121 Repair, complex, scalp, arms, and/or legs; 2.6 cm to 7.5 cm   `A 2 T`

RVU		Global Days	Modifiers				
Mod	Non-Fac Total	Fac Total		51	50	62	80	MUE
	12.14	7.73	010	2	0	0	1	1

AMA: Dec 98: 5, Nov 99: 9, 10, Feb 00: 10, Apr 10: 3, Feb 10: 3, May 11: 4, Jan 12: 8, Dec 12: 6

+ 13122 Repair, complex, scalp, arms, and/or legs; each additional 5 cm or less (List separately in addition to code for primary procedure)   `N I N`

RVU		Global Days	Modifiers				
Mod	Non-Fac Total	Fac Total		51	50	62	80	MUE
	3.80	2.48	ZZZ	0	0	0	1	9

● New   ▲ Revised   ✖ Deleted   ⊙ Moderate Sedation   ✚ Add-on Codes   ⊘ High Risk Denial   Ⓐ Age Edit   ♀ Female   ♂ Male   **AMA** *CPT® Assistant*   **MUE** Medically Unlikely Edit
⊘ Modifier 51 Exempt   ⊖ Modifier 63 Exempt   ⊠ Unlisted   **Modifiers:** *See Inside Back Cover*   Ⓜ Maternity   `A 2`–`Z 3` ASC Payment Indicators   `A`–`Y` OPPS Status Indicators

186   CPT © 2015 American Medical Association. All Rights Reserved.   © 2016 DecisionHealth

AMA: Nov 99: 10, Feb 10: 3, May 11: 4, Jan 12: 8, Dec 12: 6

13131 Repair, complex, forehead, cheeks, chin, mouth, neck, axillae, genitalia, hands and/or feet; 1.1 cm to 2.5 cm   A2T

RVU			Global Days	Modifiers				
Mod	Non-Fac Total	Fac Total		51	50	62	80	MUE
	10.96	7.22	010	2	0	0	1	1

AMA: Fall 93: 7, Sep 97: 11, Dec 98: 5, Nov 99: 10, Feb 00: 10, Apr 00: 8, Feb 10: 3, May 11: 4, Jan 12: 8, Dec 12: 6, Jan 13: 15

Complex repair

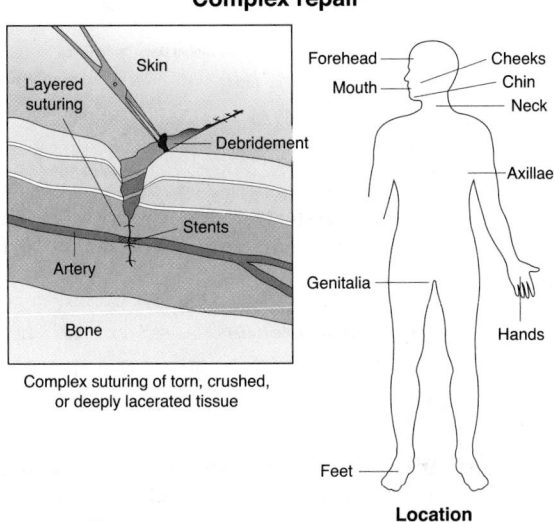

Complex suturing of torn, crushed, or deeply lacerated tissue

Location

13132 Repair, complex, forehead, cheeks, chin, mouth, neck, axillae, genitalia, hands and/or feet; 2.6 cm to 7.5 cm   A2T

RVU			Global Days	Modifiers				
Mod	Non-Fac Total	Fac Total		51	50	62	80	MUE
	13.55	9.10	010	2	0	0	1	1

AMA: Fall 93: 7, Dec 98: 5, Nov 99: 10, Dec 99: 10, Feb 00: 10, Apr 00: 9, Aug 00: 9, Feb 10: 3, May 11: 4, Jan 12: 8, Dec 12: 6, Jan 13: 15, Oct 14: 14

+ 13133 Repair, complex, forehead, cheeks, chin, mouth, neck, axillae, genitalia, hands and/or feet; each additional 5 cm or less (List separately in addition to code for primary procedure)   N1N

RVU			Global Days	Modifiers				
Mod	Non-Fac Total	Fac Total		51	50	62	80	MUE
	5.09	3.81	ZZZ	0	0	0	1	7

AMA: Fall 93: 7, Feb 00: 10, Apr 00: 9, Feb 10: 3, May 11: 4, Jan 12: 8, Dec 12: 6, Jan 13: 15

13151 Repair, complex, eyelids, nose, ears and/or lips; 1.1 cm to 2.5 cm   A2T

RVU			Global Days	Modifiers				
Mod	Non-Fac Total	Fac Total		51	50	62	80	MUE
	12.02	8.31	010	2	0	0	1	1

AMA: Dec 98: 5, Nov 99: 10, Feb 00: 10, Feb 10: 3, May 11: 4, Jan 12: 8, Dec 12: 6, Mar 14: 12, May 14: 3, 5

13152 Repair, complex, eyelids, nose, ears and/or lips; 2.6 cm to 7.5 cm   A2T

RVU			Global Days	Modifiers				
Mod	Non-Fac Total	Fac Total		51	50	62	80	MUE
	14.44	10.09	010	2	0	0	1	1

AMA: Dec 98: 5, Nov 99: 10, Feb 00: 10, Feb 10: 3, May 11: 4, Jan 12: 8, Dec 12: 6, May 14: 3, Oct 14: 14

+ 13153 Repair, complex, eyelids, nose, ears and/or lips; each additional 5 cm or less (List separately in addition to code for primary procedure)   N1N

RVU			Global Days	Modifiers				
Mod	Non-Fac Total	Fac Total		51	50	62	80	MUE
	5.54	4.11	ZZZ	0	0	0	1	2

AMA: Nov 99: 10, Feb 00: 10, Feb 10: 3, Apr 10: 3, May 11: 4, Jan 12: 8, Dec 12: 6, May 14: 3, 5

13160 Secondary closure of surgical wound or dehiscence, extensive or complicated   A2T

RVU			Global Days	Modifiers				
Mod	Non-Fac Total	Fac Total		51	50	62	80	MUE
	23.27	23.27	090	2	0	0	1	2

AMA: Sep 97: 11, Dec 98: 5, Apr 00: 8, May 11: 4, Dec 12: 6

Adjacent Tissue Transfer/Rearrangement Procedures

Coding Guidance

Codes 14000-14350 involve excision, including the lesion, with repair by adjacent tissue transfer or rearrangement. Separate excision codes (11400-11646) and repair codes (12001-13160) should not be used when these codes are reported. Debridement necessary to perform a tissue transfer procedure is also included in the procedure. Debridement codes (11000, 11042-11047, 97597, 97598) should not be reported with adjacent tissue transfer for the same lesion/injury. Skin grafting used in conjunction with these procedures may be reported separately. When traumatic wounds are closed and coincidentally result in repair by a W- or Z-plasty type closure technique, the code for the most appropriate level of more simple wound closure should be used instead of a tissue transfer code. Any tissue samples or cultures obtained as specimens from an adjacent tissue transfer procedure are included in the closure code.

14000 Adjacent tissue transfer or rearrangement, trunk; defect 10 sq cm or less   A2T

RVU			Global Days	Modifiers				
Mod	Non-Fac Total	Fac Total		51	50	62	80	MUE
	17.80	14.53	090	2	0	0	1	2

AMA: Sep 96: 11, Jul 99: 3, Jul 00: 10, Jan 06: 47, Dec 06: 15, Jul 08: 5, Mar 10: 4, Apr 10: 3, Jan 12: 8, May 12: 13, Nov 12: 13, Dec 12: 6, Apr 14: 10, Feb 15: 10

14001 Adjacent tissue transfer or rearrangement, trunk; defect 10.1 sq cm to 30.0 sq cm   A2T

RVU			Global Days	Modifiers				
Mod	Non-Fac Total	Fac Total		51	50	62	80	MUE
	22.88	18.92	090	2	0	0	1	2

AMA: Aug 96: 8, Jul 99: 3, Jan 06: 47, Dec 06: 15, Jul 08: 5, Mar 10: 4, Jan 12: 8, May 12: 13, Nov 12: 13, Dec 12: 6, Apr 14: 10, Feb 15: 10

● New   ▲ Revised   Deleted   ⊙ Moderate Sedation   ✚ Add-on Codes   ⊘ High Risk Denial   Ⓐ Age Edit   ♀ Female   ♂ Male   **AMA** *CPT® Assistant*   **MUE** Medically Unlikely Edit
⊘ Modifier 51 Exempt   ⊖ Modifier 63 Exempt   ✗ Unlisted   **Modifiers:** *See Inside Back Cover*   Ⓜ Maternity   A2–Z3 ASC Payment Indicators   A–Y OPPS Status Indicators

Surgical Procedures

14020 – 14350

14020 Adjacent tissue transfer or rearrangement, scalp, arms and/or legs; defect 10 sq cm or less   A 2 T

RVU			Global Days	Modifiers				
Mod	Non-Fac Total	Fac Total		51	50	62	80	MUE
	19.91	16.42	090	2	0	0	1	4

AMA: Jul 99: 3, Jan 06: 47, Dec 06: 15, Jul 08: 5, Mar 10: 4, Jan 12: 8, May 12: 13, Nov 12: 13, Dec 12: 6

Adjacent tissue transfer or rearrangement scalp, arms and/or legs

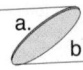
a. b.   Skin incision is reflected back

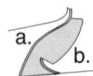
a. b.   Two additional incisions intersect

a. b.   The flaps are transposed

Code 14020 for defects that are 10.0 sq. cm or less.
Code 14021 for defects that are 10.1 sq. cm to 30.0 sq. cm.

14021 Adjacent tissue transfer or rearrangement, scalp, arms and/or legs; defect 10.1 sq cm to 30.0 sq cm   A 2 T

RVU			Global Days	Modifiers				
Mod	Non-Fac Total	Fac Total		51	50	62	80	MUE
	24.90	20.78	090	2	0	0	1	3

AMA: Jul 99: 3, Jan 06: 47, Dec 06: 15, Jul 08: 5, Mar 10: 4, Jan 12: 8, May 12: 13, Nov 12: 13, Dec 12: 6

14040 Adjacent tissue transfer or rearrangement, forehead, cheeks, chin, mouth, neck, axillae, genitalia, hands and/or feet; defect 10 sq cm or less   A 2 T

RVU			Global Days	Modifiers				
Mod	Non-Fac Total	Fac Total		51	50	62	80	MUE
	21.78	18.28	090	2	0	0	1	4

AMA: Jul 99: 3, Jul 00: 10, Jan 06: 47, Dec 06: 15, Jul 08: 5, Mar 10: 4, Jan 12: 8, May 12: 13, Nov 12: 13, Dec 12: 6

Adjacent tissue transfer or rearrangement forehead, cheeks, chin, mouth, neck, axillae, genitalia, hands and/or feet

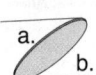
a. b.   Skin incision is reflected back

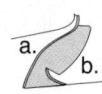
a. b.   Two additional incisions intersect

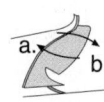
a. b.   The flaps are transposed

Code 14040 for defects that are 10.0 sq. cm or less; code 14041 for defects that are 10.1 sq cm to 30.0 sq. cm.

14041 Adjacent tissue transfer or rearrangement, forehead, cheeks, chin, mouth, neck, axillae, genitalia, hands and/or feet; defect 10.1 sq cm to 30.0 sq cm   A 2 T

RVU			Global Days	Modifiers				
Mod	Non-Fac Total	Fac Total		51	50	62	80	MUE
	26.95	22.49	090	2	0	0	1	3

AMA: Jul 99: 3, Jan 06: 47, Dec 06: 15, Jul 08: 5, Mar 10: 4, Jan 12: 8, May 12: 13, Nov 12: 13, Dec 12: 6

14060 Adjacent tissue transfer or rearrangement, eyelids, nose, ears and/or lips; defect 10 sq cm or less   A 2 T

RVU			Global Days	Modifiers				
Mod	Non-Fac Total	Fac Total		51	50	62	80	MUE
	22.21	19.46	090	2	0	0	1	4

AMA: Fall 93: 7, Jul 99: 3, Jan 06: 47, Dec 06: 15, Jul 08: 5, Mar 10: 4, Jan 12: 8, May 12: 13, Aug 12: 13, Nov 12: 13, Dec 12: 6

14061 Adjacent tissue transfer or rearrangement, eyelids, nose, ears and/or lips; defect 10.1 sq cm to 30.0 sq cm   A 2 T

RVU			Global Days	Modifiers				
Mod	Non-Fac Total	Fac Total		51	50	62	80	MUE
	28.99	24.07	090	2	0	0	1	2

AMA: Jul 99: 3, Jan 06: 47, Dec 06: 15, Jul 08: 5, Mar 10: 4, Jan 12: 8, May 12: 13, Nov 12: 13, Dec 12: 6

14301 Adjacent tissue transfer or rearrangement, any area; defect 30.1 sq cm to 60.0 sq cm   G 2 T

RVU			Global Days	Modifiers				
Mod	Non-Fac Total	Fac Total		51	50	62	80	MUE
	30.88	25.57	090	2	0	0	2	2

AMA: May 12: 13, Nov 12: 13, Dec 12: 6

+ 14302 Adjacent tissue transfer or rearrangement, any area; each additional 30.0 sq cm, or part thereof (List separately in addition to code for primary procedure)   N 1 N

RVU			Global Days	Modifiers				
Mod	Non-Fac Total	Fac Total		51	50	62	80	MUE
	6.42	6.42	ZZZ	0	0	0	2	8

AMA: May 12: 13, Nov 12: 13, Dec 12: 6

14350 Filleted finger or toe flap, including preparation of recipient site   A 2 T

RVU			Global Days	Modifiers				
Mod	Non-Fac Total	Fac Total		51	50	62	80	MUE
	20.01	20.01	090	2	0	0	0	2

AMA: Jan 06: 47, Jul 08: 5, Mar 10: 4, May 12: 13, Dec 12: 6

CPT © 2015 American Medical Association. All Rights Reserved.   © 2016 DecisionHealth

Skin Preparation and Grafting Procedures

Coding Guidance

When a graft is applied after incisional or excisional preparation of the wound recipient site, the surgical preparation is reported separately. These services do not describe simple wound debridement prior to skin grafting, which is included in the skin graft code.

15002 Surgical preparation or creation of recipient site by excision of open wounds, burn eschar, or scar (including subcutaneous tissues), or incisional release of scar contracture, trunk, arms, legs; first 100 sq cm or 1% of body area of infants and children ▨2▨

RVU			Global Days	Modifiers				
Mod	Non-Fac Total	Fac Total		51	50	62	80	MUE
	9.96	6.58	000	0	0	0	0	1

AMA: Jan 12: 6, Oct 12: 13, Dec 12: 6, Feb 13: 16, Mar 14: 12

Surgical preparation or creation of recipient site by excision of open wounds, burn eschar, or scar: trunk, arms, legs

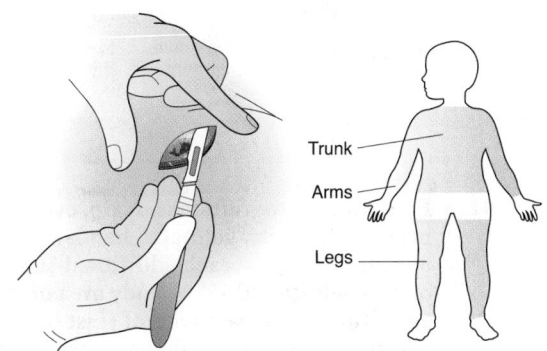

First 100 sq cm or 1 body area of infant/child (15002); each additional 1% of body area of infant/child (15003)

+ **15003** Surgical preparation or creation of recipient site by excision of open wounds, burn eschar, or scar (including subcutaneous tissues), or incisional release of scar contracture, trunk, arms, legs; each additional 100 sq cm, or part thereof, or each additional 1% of body area of infants and children (List separately in addition to code for primary procedure) ▧▨▧

Documentation Finder: Add-on codes, such as 15003, describe additional intraoperative procedures or services associated with the primary procedure(s); documentation must support this service was performed by same physician on same date and at same surgical session as primary procedure(s).

RVU			Global Days	Modifiers				
Mod	Non-Fac Total	Fac Total		51	50	62	80	MUE
	2.17	1.32	ZZZ	0	0	0	0	60

AMA: Jan 12: 6, Oct 12: 13, Feb 13: 16, Mar 14: 12

15004 Surgical preparation or creation of recipient site by excision of open wounds, burn eschar, or scar (including subcutaneous tissues), or incisional release of scar contracture, face, scalp, eyelids, mouth, neck, ears, orbits, genitalia, hands, feet and/or multiple digits; first 100 sq cm or 1% of body area of infants and children ▨2▨

RVU			Global Days	Modifiers				
Mod	Non-Fac Total	Fac Total		51	50	62	80	MUE
	11.48	7.83	000	0	0	0	0	1

AMA: Jan 12: 6, Oct 12: 13, Feb 13: 16, Mar 14: 12

Surgical preparation or creation of recipient site by excision of open wounds, burn eschar, or scar

(Face, scalp, eyelids, mouth, neck, ears, orbits, genitalia, hands and feet)

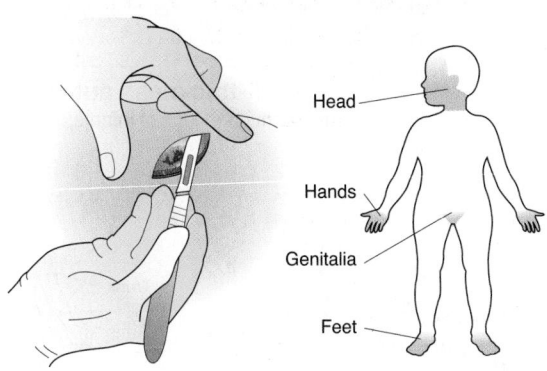

First 100 sq cm or 1% body area of infant/child (15002); each additional 100 sq cm or 1% of body area of infant/child (15003)

+ **15005** Surgical preparation or creation of recipient site by excision of open wounds, burn eschar, or scar (including subcutaneous tissues), or incisional release of scar contracture, face, scalp, eyelids, mouth, neck, ears, orbits, genitalia, hands, feet and/or multiple digits; each additional 100 sq cm, or part thereof, or each additional 1% of body area of infants and children (List separately in addition to code for primary procedure) ▧▨▧

RVU			Global Days	Modifiers				
Mod	Non-Fac Total	Fac Total		51	50	62	80	MUE
	3.58	2.64	ZZZ	0	0	0	0	19

AMA: Jan 12: 6, Oct 12: 13, Feb 13: 16, Mar 14: 12

Autograft Procedures

Coding Guidance

Codes for skin grafts and skin substitutes are classified by size, location of recipient area defect, and type of graft or skin substitute. Generally, there are two or three codes including a primary code and one or two add-on codes for each site and type of skin graft or skin substitute. Only one primary code is assigned with one unit of service, and add-on codes are used for coverage of an additional area. Only one type of skin graft/substitute may be applied to a given area, making the primary codes mutually exclusive of each other. When multiple areas are grafted using different kinds of grafts, the separate sites should be identified using modifier 59 or anatomic modifiers.

15040 Harvest of skin for tissue cultured skin autograft, 100 sq cm or less ▨2▨

RVU			Global Days	Modifiers				
Mod	Non-Fac Total	Fac Total		51	50	62	80	MUE
	7.31	3.70	000	0	0	0	1	1

AMA: Aug 06: 10, Oct 06: 1, Feb 08: 3, Apr 10: 3, Jan 12: 6

● New   ▲ Revised   Deleted   ⊙ Moderate Sedation   ✚ Add-on Codes   ⊘ High Risk Denial   Ⓐ Age Edit   ♀ Female   ♂ Male   **AMA** *CPT® Assistant*   **MUE** Medically Unlikely Edit
⃠ Modifier 51 Exempt   ⊖ Modifier 63 Exempt   ✗ Unlisted   **Modifiers:** *See Inside Back Cover*   Ⓜ Maternity   A2–Z3 ASC Payment Indicators   A–Y OPPS Status Indicators

© 2016 DecisionHealth   CPT © 2015 American Medical Association. All Rights Reserved.   **189**

Surgical Procedures

15002 – 15040

15050 Pinch graft, single or multiple, to cover small ulcer, tip of digit, or other minimal open area (except on face), up to defect size 2 cm diameter   A2 T

	RVU		Global Days	Modifiers				
Mod	Non-Fac Total	Fac Total		51	50	62	80	MUE
	16.04	12.77	090	2	0	0	1	1

AMA: Apr 97: 4, Sep 97: 2, Nov 98: 6, Jan 12: 6

15100 Split-thickness autograft, trunk, arms, legs; first 100 sq cm or less, or 1% of body area of infants and children (except 15050)   A2 T

	RVU		Global Days	Modifiers				
Mod	Non-Fac Total	Fac Total		51	50	62	80	MUE
	24.64	20.73	090	2	0	0	1	1

AMA: Fall 93: 7, Apr 97: 4, Aug 97: 6, Sep 97: 3, Nov 98: 6, Sep 02: 3, Oct 06: 1, Feb 08: 3, Mar 11: 9, Jan 12: 6, Oct 12: 3

Split-thickness autograft
(trunk, arms and legs of infants and children)

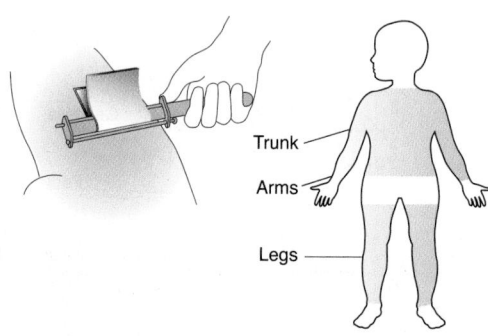

First 1% of body area of infants and children (15100); each additional 1% of body area of infants and children (15101)

+ 15101 Split-thickness autograft, trunk, arms, legs; each additional 100 sq cm, or each additional 1% of body area of infants and children, or part thereof (List separately in addition to code for primary procedure)   N I N

	RVU		Global Days	Modifiers				
Mod	Non-Fac Total	Fac Total		51	50	62	80	MUE
	5.33	3.23	ZZZ	0	0	0	1	40

AMA: Apr 97: 4, Nov 98: 6, Sep 02: 3, Feb 08: 3, Mar 11: 9, Jan 12: 6, Oct 12: 3

15110 Epidermal autograft, trunk, arms, legs; first 100 sq cm or less, or 1% of body area of infants and children   A2 T

	RVU		Global Days	Modifiers				
Mod	Non-Fac Total	Fac Total		51	50	62	80	MUE
	22.92	20.02	090	2	0	0	1	1

AMA: Feb 08: 3, Mar 11: 9, Jan 12: 6, Oct 12: 3

+ 15111 Epidermal autograft, trunk, arms, legs; each additional 100 sq cm, or each additional 1% of body area of infants and children, or part thereof (List separately in addition to code for primary procedure)   N I N

	RVU		Global Days	Modifiers				
Mod	Non-Fac Total	Fac Total		51	50	62	80	MUE
	3.33	3.01	ZZZ	0	0	0	1	5

AMA: Feb 08: 3, Mar 11: 9, Jan 12: 6, Oct 12: 3

15115 Epidermal autograft, face, scalp, eyelids, mouth, neck, ears, orbits, genitalia, hands, feet, and/or multiple digits; first 100 sq cm or less, or 1% of body area of infants and children   A2 T

	RVU		Global Days	Modifiers				
Mod	Non-Fac Total	Fac Total		51	50	62	80	MUE
	23.58	20.63	090	2	0	0	1	1

AMA: Feb 08: 3, Mar 11: 9, Jan 12: 6, Oct 12: 3

Epidermal autograft

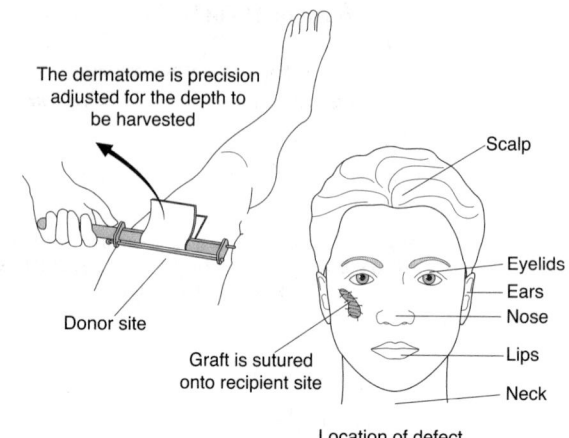

The dermatome is precision adjusted for the depth to be harvested

Donor site

Graft is sutured onto recipient site

Scalp
Eyelids
Ears
Nose
Lips
Neck

Location of defect

+ 15116 Epidermal autograft, face, scalp, eyelids, mouth, neck, ears, orbits, genitalia, hands, feet, and/or multiple digits; each additional 100 sq cm, or each additional 1% of body area of infants and children, or part thereof (List separately in addition to code for primary procedure)   N I N

	RVU		Global Days	Modifiers				
Mod	Non-Fac Total	Fac Total		51	50	62	80	MUE
	4.40	3.98	ZZZ	0	0	1	1	2

AMA: Feb 08: 3, Mar 11: 9, Jan 12: 6, Oct 12: 3

15120 Split-thickness autograft, face, scalp, eyelids, mouth, neck, ears, orbits, genitalia, hands, feet, and/or multiple digits; first 100 sq cm or less, or 1% of body area of infants and children (except 15050)   A2 T

	RVU		Global Days	Modifiers				
Mod	Non-Fac Total	Fac Total		51	50	62	80	MUE
	24.44	20.23	090	2	0	0	1	1

AMA: Apr 97: 4, Aug 97: 6, Sep 97: 3, Nov 98: 6, Jan 99: 4, Sep 02: 3, Feb 08: 3, Jul 08: 5, Mar 11: 9, Jan 12: 6, Oct 12: 3

+ 15121 Split-thickness autograft, face, scalp, eyelids, mouth, neck, ears, orbits, genitalia, hands, feet, and/or multiple digits; each additional 100 sq cm, or each additional 1% of body area of infants and children, or part thereof (List separately in addition to code for primary procedure)   N I N

	RVU		Global Days	Modifiers				
Mod	Non-Fac Total	Fac Total		51	50	62	80	MUE
	5.97	3.86	ZZZ	0	0	1	1	8

AMA: Apr 97: 4, Aug 97: 6, Sep 97: 3, Nov 98: 6, Jan 99: 4, Sep 02: 3, Feb 08: 3, Mar 11: 9, Jan 12: 6, Oct 12: 3

● New   ▲ Revised   ✖ Deleted   ⊙ Moderate Sedation   ✚ Add-on Codes   ⊘ High Risk Denial   Ⓐ Age Edit   ♀ Female   ♂ Male   **AMA** CPT® Assistant   **MUE** Medically Unlikely Edit
⊘ Modifier 51 Exempt   ⊖ Modifier 63 Exempt   ✖ Unlisted   **Modifiers:** See Inside Back Cover   Ⓜ Maternity   A2–Z3 ASC Payment Indicators   A–Y OPPS Status Indicators

CPT © 2015 American Medical Association. All Rights Reserved.   © 2016 DecisionHealth

15130 Dermal autograft, trunk, arms, legs; first 100 sq cm or less, or 1% of body area of infants and children `A2 T`

RVU			Global Days	Modifiers				
Mod	Non-Fac Total	Fac Total		51	50	62	80	MUE
	19.25	16.27	090	2	0	0	1	1

AMA: Feb 08: 3, Mar 11: 9, Jan 12: 6, Oct 12: 3

+ 15131 Dermal autograft, trunk, arms, legs; each additional 100 sq cm, or each additional 1% of body area of infants and children, or part thereof (List separately in addition to code for primary procedure) `N N`

RVU			Global Days	Modifiers				
Mod	Non-Fac Total	Fac Total		51	50	62	80	MUE
	2.88	2.65	ZZZ	0	0	1	1	2

AMA: Feb 08: 3, Mar 11: 9, Jan 12: 6, Oct 12: 3

15135 Dermal autograft, face, scalp, eyelids, mouth, neck, ears, orbits, genitalia, hands, feet, and/or multiple digits; first 100 sq cm or less, or 1% of body area of infants and children `A2 T`

RVU			Global Days	Modifiers				
Mod	Non-Fac Total	Fac Total		51	50	62	80	MUE
	24.15	21.23	090	2	0	0	1	1

AMA: Feb 08: 3, Mar 11: 9, Jan 12: 6, Oct 12: 3

+ 15136 Dermal autograft, face, scalp, eyelids, mouth, neck, ears, orbits, genitalia, hands, feet, and/or multiple digits; each additional 100 sq cm, or each additional 1% of body area of infants and children, or part thereof (List separately in addition to code for primary procedure) `N N`

RVU			Global Days	Modifiers				
Mod	Non-Fac Total	Fac Total		51	50	62	80	MUE
	2.74	2.56	ZZZ	0	0	1	1	1

AMA: Mar 11: 9, Jan 12: 6, Oct 12: 3

15150 Tissue cultured skin autograft, trunk, arms, legs; first 25 sq cm or less `A2 T`

RVU			Global Days	Modifiers				
Mod	Non-Fac Total	Fac Total		51	50	62	80	MUE
	20.00	18.34	090	2	0	0	1	1

AMA: Oct 06: 1, Feb 08: 3, Mar 11: 9, Jan 12: 6, Oct 12: 3

+ 15151 Tissue cultured skin autograft, trunk, arms, legs; additional 1 sq cm to 75 sq cm (List separately in addition to code for primary procedure) `N N`

RVU			Global Days	Modifiers				
Mod	Non-Fac Total	Fac Total		51	50	62	80	MUE
	3.52	3.25	ZZZ	0	0	0	1	1

AMA: Oct 06: 1, Feb 08: 3, Mar 11: 9, Jan 12: 6, Oct 12: 3

+ 15152 Tissue cultured skin autograft, trunk, arms, legs; each additional 100 sq cm, or each additional 1% of body area of infants and children, or part thereof (List separately in addition to code for primary procedure) `⊘N N`

RVU			Global Days	Modifiers				
Mod	Non-Fac Total	Fac Total		51	50	62	80	MUE
	4.31	4.05	ZZZ	0	0	0	1	2

AMA: Oct 06: 1, Feb 08: 3, Mar 11: 9, Jan 12: 6, Oct 12: 3

15155 Tissue cultured skin autograft, face, scalp, eyelids, mouth, neck, ears, orbits, genitalia, hands, feet, and/or multiple digits; first 25 sq cm or less `A2 T`

RVU			Global Days	Modifiers				
Mod	Non-Fac Total	Fac Total		51	50	62	80	MUE
	20.65	19.13	090	2	0	0	1	1

AMA: Oct 06: 1, Feb 08: 3, Mar 11: 9, Jan 12: 6, Oct 12: 3

+ 15156 Tissue cultured skin autograft, face, scalp, eyelids, mouth, neck, ears, orbits, genitalia, hands, feet, and/or multiple digits; additional 1 sq cm to 75 sq cm (List separately in addition to code for primary procedure) `N N`

RVU			Global Days	Modifiers				
Mod	Non-Fac Total	Fac Total		51	50	62	80	MUE
	4.55	4.32	ZZZ	0	0	1	1	1

AMA: Oct 06: 1, Feb 08: 3, Mar 11: 9, Jan 12: 6, Oct 12: 3

+ 15157 Tissue cultured skin autograft, face, scalp, eyelids, mouth, neck, ears, orbits, genitalia, hands, feet, and/or multiple digits; each additional 100 sq cm, or each additional 1% of body area of infants and children, or part thereof (List separately in addition to code for primary procedure) `⊘N N`

RVU			Global Days	Modifiers				
Mod	Non-Fac Total	Fac Total		51	50	62	80	MUE
	5.00	4.67	ZZZ	0	0	1	1	1

AMA: Oct 06: 1, Feb 08: 3, Apr 10: 3, Mar 11: 9, Jan 12: 6, Oct 12: 3

15200 Full thickness graft, free, including direct closure of donor site, trunk; 20 sq cm or less `A2 T`

RVU			Global Days	Modifiers				
Mod	Non-Fac Total	Fac Total		51	50	62	80	MUE
	23.81	19.46	090	2	0	0	1	1

AMA: Aug 96: 11, Aug 97: 6, Sep 97: 3, Feb 08: 3, Mar 08: 14, Jan 12: 6, Oct 12: 3

Full thickness graft

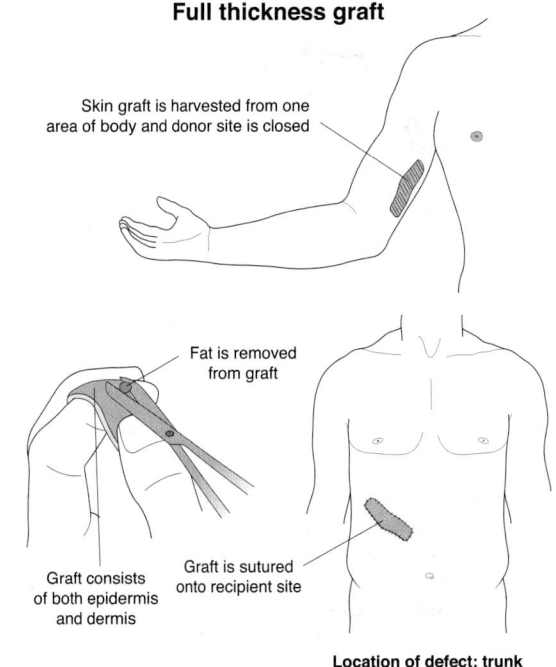

Skin graft is harvested from one area of body and donor site is closed

Fat is removed from graft

Graft consists of both epidermis and dermis

Graft is sutured onto recipient site

Location of defect: trunk

● New   ▲ Revised   Deleted   ⊙ Moderate Sedation   ✚ Add-on Codes   ⊘ High Risk Denial   Ⓐ Age Edit   ♀ Female   ♂ Male   **AMA** CPT® Assistant   **MUE** Medically Unlikely Edit
⊘ Modifier 51 Exempt   ⊖ Modifier 63 Exempt   ✗ Unlisted   **Modifiers:** See Inside Back Cover   Ⓜ Maternity   A2–Z3 ASC Payment Indicators   A–Y OPPS Status Indicators

+ 15201 Full thickness graft, free, including direct closure of donor site, trunk; each additional 20 sq cm, or part thereof (List separately in addition to code for primary procedure) N I N

RVU			Global Days	Modifiers				
Mod	Non-Fac Total	Fac Total		51	50	62	80	MUE
	4.24	2.29	ZZZ	0	0	0	1	9

AMA: Apr 97: 4, Aug 97: 6, Sep 97: 3, Feb 08: 3, Mar 08: 14, Jan 12: 6, Oct 12: 3

15220 Full thickness graft, free, including direct closure of donor site, scalp, arms, and/or legs; 20 sq cm or less A 2 T

RVU			Global Days	Modifiers				
Mod	Non-Fac Total	Fac Total		51	50	62	80	MUE
	22.06	17.79	090	2	0	0	1	1

AMA: Apr 97: 4, Aug 97: 6, Sep 97: 3, Aug 98: 9, Feb 08: 3, Mar 08: 14, Jan 12: 6, Oct 12: 3

+ 15221 Full thickness graft, free, including direct closure of donor site, scalp, arms, and/or legs; each additional 20 sq cm, or part thereof (List separately in addition to code for primary procedure) N I N

RVU			Global Days	Modifiers				
Mod	Non-Fac Total	Fac Total		51	50	62	80	MUE
	3.91	2.07	ZZZ	0	0	0	1	9

AMA: Apr 97: 4, Aug 97: 6, Sep 97: 3, Aug 98: 9, Feb 08: 3, Mar 08: 14, Jan 12: 6, Oct 12: 3

15240 Full thickness graft, free, including direct closure of donor site, forehead, cheeks, chin, mouth, neck, axillae, genitalia, hands, and/or feet; 20 sq cm or less A 2 T

RVU			Global Days	Modifiers				
Mod	Non-Fac Total	Fac Total		51	50	62	80	MUE
	26.75	23.20	090	2	0	0	1	1

AMA: Apr 97: 4, Aug 97: 6, Sep 97: 3, Nov 00: 10, Feb 08: 3, Mar 08: 14, Jan 12: 6, Oct 12: 3

+ 15241 Full thickness graft, free, including direct closure of donor site, forehead, cheeks, chin, mouth, neck, axillae, genitalia, hands, and/or feet; each additional 20 sq cm, or part thereof (List separately in addition to code for primary procedure) N I N

RVU			Global Days	Modifiers				
Mod	Non-Fac Total	Fac Total		51	50	62	80	MUE
	5.30	3.24	ZZZ	0	0	0	1	9

AMA: Apr 97: 4, Aug 97: 6, Sep 97: 3, Feb 08: 3, Mar 08: 14, Jan 12: 6, Oct 12: 3

Coding Guidance

A full-thickness graft is included as part of the total service for 67911, correction of lid retraction. Do not report code 15260 in addition to 67911.

15260 Full thickness graft, free, including direct closure of donor site, nose, ears, eyelids, and/or lips; 20 sq cm or less A 2 T

RVU			Global Days	Modifiers				
Mod	Non-Fac Total	Fac Total		51	50	62	80	MUE
	28.93	24.83	090	2	0	0	1	1

AMA: Fall 91: 7, Fall 93: 7, Apr 97: 4, Aug 97: 6, Sep 97: 3, Jul 99: 3, Feb 08: 3, Mar 08: 14, Jan 12: 6, Oct 12: 3

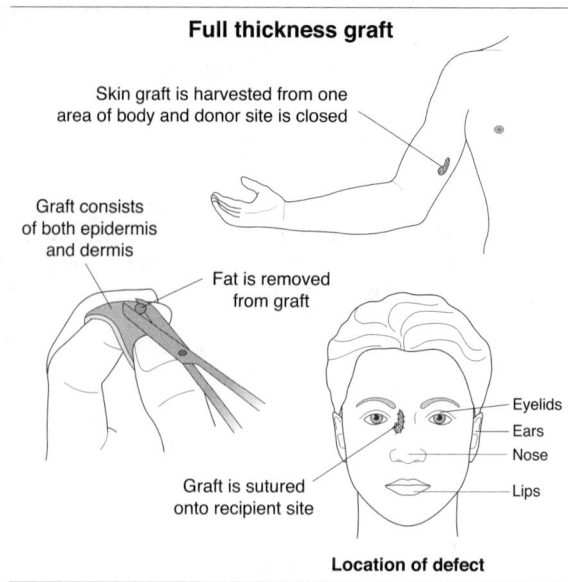

Full thickness graft

Skin graft is harvested from one area of body and donor site is closed

Graft consists of both epidermis and dermis

Fat is removed from graft

Graft is sutured onto recipient site

Eyelids
Ears
Nose
Lips

Location of defect

+ 15261 Full thickness graft, free, including direct closure of donor site, nose, ears, eyelids, and/or lips; each additional 20 sq cm, or part thereof (List separately in addition to code for primary procedure) N I N

RVU			Global Days	Modifiers				
Mod	Non-Fac Total	Fac Total		51	50	62	80	MUE
	6.17	4.08	ZZZ	0	0	0	1	6

AMA: Fall 91: 7, Apr 97: 4, Aug 97: 6, Sep 97: 3, Feb 08: 3, Mar 08: 14, Apr 10: 3, Jan 12: 6, Oct 12: 3

Skin Replacement Graft Procedures

Coding Guidance

Simple debridement of a skin wound (11000, 11040-11042) prior to a graft/skin substitute is included in the skin graft/substitute procedure (CPT codes 15050-15278) and should not be reported as a separate code on a claim. If the recipient site requires excision of open wounds, burn eschar, or scar or release of scar contracture, 15002-15005 may be reported. The supply of the graft may be reported separately with 99070 or a HCPCS Level II code(s) - C9363, (Medicare outpatient hospital - OPPS only), and Q4100-Q4130.

15271 Application of skin substitute graft to trunk, arms, legs, total wound surface area up to 100 sq cm; first 25 sq cm or less wound surface area G 2 T

RVU			Global Days	Modifiers				
Mod	Non-Fac Total	Fac Total		51	50	62	80	MUE
	4.00	2.44	000	2	0	0	1	1

AMA: Jan 12: 6, Oct 12: 3, Jun 14: 14

+ 15272 Application of skin substitute graft to trunk, arms, legs, total wound surface area up to 100 sq cm; each additional 25 sq cm wound surface area, or part thereof (List separately in addition to code for primary procedure) N I N

RVU			Global Days	Modifiers				
Mod	Non-Fac Total	Fac Total		51	50	62	80	MUE
	0.77	0.50	ZZZ	0	0	0	1	3

AMA: Jan 12: 6, Oct 12: 3, Oct 13: 15, Jun 14: 14

● New   ▲ Revised   ✖ Deleted   ⊙ Moderate Sedation   ✚ Add-on Codes   ⊘ High Risk Denial   Ⓐ Age Edit   ♀ Female   ♂ Male   **AMA** *CPT® Assistant*   **MUE** Medically Unlikely Edit
⊘ Modifier 51 Exempt   ⊖ Modifier 63 Exempt   🗷 Unlisted   **Modifiers:** *See Inside Back Cover*   Ⓜ Maternity   A 2 – Z 3 ASC Payment Indicators   A – Y OPPS Status Indicators

CPT © 2015 American Medical Association. All Rights Reserved.   © 2016 DecisionHealth

15273 Application of skin substitute graft to trunk, arms, legs, total wound surface area greater than or equal to 100 sq cm; first 100 sq cm wound surface area, or 1% of body area of infants and children   `G2T`

RVU			Global Days	Modifiers				
Mod	Non-Fac Total	Fac Total		51	50	62	80	MUE
	8.45	5.82	000	2	0	0	1	1

AMA: Jan 12: 6, Oct 12: 3, Oct 13: 15, Nov 13: 14, Jun 14: 14

Application of skin substitute graft

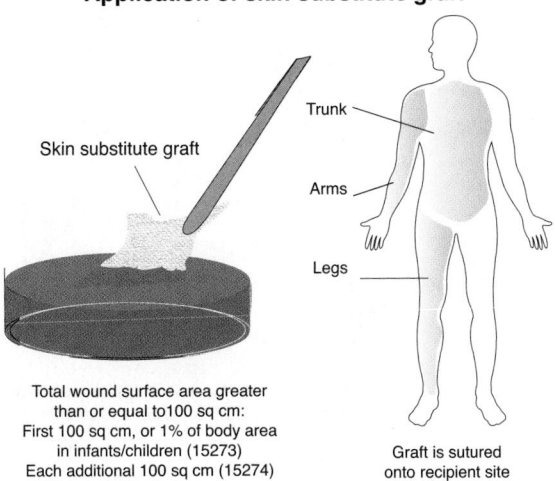

Skin substitute graft

Trunk

Arms

Legs

Total wound surface area greater than or equal to100 sq cm: First 100 sq cm, or 1% of body area in infants/children (15273) Each additional 100 sq cm (15274)

Graft is sutured onto recipient site

+ 15274 Application of skin substitute graft to trunk, arms, legs, total wound surface area greater than or equal to 100 sq cm; each additional 100 sq cm wound surface area, or part thereof, or each additional 1% of body area of infants and children, or part thereof (List separately in addition to code for primary procedure)   `NIN`

RVU			Global Days	Modifiers				
Mod	Non-Fac Total	Fac Total		51	50	62	80	MUE
	2.04	1.33	ZZZ	0	0	0		1

AMA: Jan 12: 6, Oct 12: 3, Oct 13: 15, Nov 13: 14, Jun 14: 14

15275 Application of skin substitute graft to face, scalp, eyelids, mouth, neck, ears, orbits, genitalia, hands, feet, and/or multiple digits, total wound surface area up to 100 sq cm; first 25 sq cm or less wound surface area   `G2T`

RVU			Global Days	Modifiers				
Mod	Non-Fac Total	Fac Total		51	50	62	80	MUE
	4.23	2.75	000	2	0	0	1	1

AMA: Jan 12: 6, Oct 12: 3, Oct 13: 15, Jun 14: 14

+ 15276 Application of skin substitute graft to face, scalp, eyelids, mouth, neck, ears, orbits, genitalia, hands, feet, and/or multiple digits, total wound surface area up to 100 sq cm; each additional 25 sq cm wound surface area, or part thereof (List separately in addition to code for primary procedure)   `NIN`

RVU			Global Days	Modifiers				
Mod	Non-Fac Total	Fac Total		51	50	62	80	MUE
	0.99	0.73	ZZZ	0	0	0	1	3

AMA: Jan 12: 6, Oct 12: 3, Oct 13: 15, Jun 14: 14

15277 Application of skin substitute graft to face, scalp, eyelids, mouth, neck, ears, orbits, genitalia, hands, feet, and/or multiple digits, total wound surface area greater than or equal to 100 sq cm; first 100 sq cm wound surface area, or 1% of body area of infants and children   `G2T`

RVU			Global Days	Modifiers				
Mod	Non-Fac Total	Fac Total		51	50	62	80	MUE
	9.20	6.50	000	2	0	1	1	1

AMA: Jan 12: 6, Oct 12: 3, Oct 13: 15, Nov 13: 14, Jun 14: 14

+ 15278 Application of skin substitute graft to face, scalp, eyelids, mouth, neck, ears, orbits, genitalia, hands, feet, and/or multiple digits, total wound surface area greater than or equal to 100 sq cm; each additional 100 sq cm wound surface area, or part thereof, or each additional 1% of body area of infants and children, or part thereof (List separately in addition to code for primary procedure)   `NIN`

RVU			Global Days	Modifiers				
Mod	Non-Fac Total	Fac Total		51	50	62	80	MUE
	2.44	1.66	ZZZ	0	0	1	1	

AMA: Jan 12: 6, Oct 12: 3, Oct 13: 15, Nov 13: 14, Jun 14: 14

Skin Flap Procedures

15570 Formation of direct or tubed pedicle, with or without transfer; trunk   `A2T`

RVU			Global Days	Modifiers				
Mod	Non-Fac Total	Fac Total		51	50	62	80	MUE
	26.29	21.36	090	2	0	0	1	2

AMA: Nov 02: 7, Apr 10: 3, Mar 10: 4, Dec 12: 6

Formation of direct or tubed pedicle with or without transfer

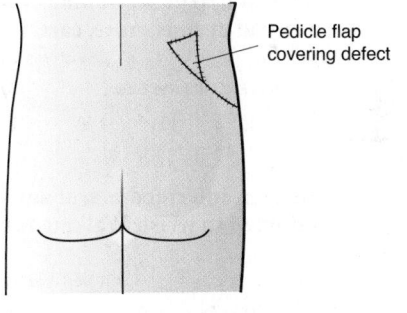

Pedicle flap covering defect

15572 Formation of direct or tubed pedicle, with or without transfer; scalp, arms, or legs   `A2T`

RVU			Global Days	Modifiers				
Mod	Non-Fac Total	Fac Total		51	50	62	80	MUE
	25.50	21.64	090	2	0	0	1	2

AMA: Mar 10: 4, Dec 12: 6

● New   ▲ Revised   Deleted   ⊙ Moderate Sedation   ✚ Add-on Codes   ⊗ High Risk Denial   Ⓐ Age Edit   ♀ Female   ♂ Male   **AMA** CPT® Assistant   **MUE** Medically Unlikely Edit
⊘ Modifier 51 Exempt   ⊖ Modifier 63 Exempt   ⊠ Unlisted   **Modifiers:** See Inside Back Cover   Ⓜ Maternity   `A2`–`Z3` ASC Payment Indicators   `A`–`Y` OPPS Status Indicators

Surgical Procedures

15273 – 15572

15574 Formation of direct or tubed pedicle, with or without transfer; forehead, cheeks, chin, mouth, neck, axillae, genitalia, hands or feet A 2 T

	RVU		Global Days	Modifiers				
Mod	Non-Fac Total	Fac Total		51	50	62	80	MUE
	26.21	22.22	090	2	0	0	1	2

AMA: Mar 10: 4, Dec 12: 6

15576 Formation of direct or tubed pedicle, with or without transfer; eyelids, nose, ears, lips, or intraoral A 2 T

	RVU		Global Days	Modifiers				
Mod	Non-Fac Total	Fac Total		51	50	62	80	MUE
	23.10	19.41	090	2	0	0	1	2

AMA: Mar 10: 4, Dec 12: 6

15600 Delay of flap or sectioning of flap (division and inset); at trunk A 2 T

	RVU		Global Days	Modifiers				
Mod	Non-Fac Total	Fac Total		51	50	62	80	MUE
	9.26	5.98	090	2	0	0	0	2

AMA: Nov 99: 10, Mar 10: 4, Dec 12: 6

15610 Delay of flap or sectioning of flap (division and inset); at scalp, arms, or legs A 2 T

	RVU		Global Days	Modifiers				
Mod	Non-Fac Total	Fac Total		51	50	62	80	MUE
	10.19	6.98	090	2	0	0	0	2

AMA: Mar 10: 4, Dec 12: 6

15620 Delay of flap or sectioning of flap (division and inset); at forehead, cheeks, chin, neck, axillae, genitalia, hands, or feet A 2 T

	RVU		Global Days	Modifiers				
Mod	Non-Fac Total	Fac Total		51	50	62	80	MUE
	12.61	9.45	090	2	0	0	1	2

AMA: Mar 10: 4, Dec 12: 6

15630 Delay of flap or sectioning of flap (division and inset); at eyelids, nose, ears, or lips A 2 T

	RVU		Global Days	Modifiers				
Mod	Non-Fac Total	Fac Total		51	50	62	80	MUE
	13.12	10.00	090	2	0	0	1	2

AMA: Mar 10: 4, Dec 12: 6

15650 Transfer, intermediate, of any pedicle flap (eg, abdomen to wrist, Walking tube), any location A 2 T

	RVU		Global Days	Modifiers				
Mod	Non-Fac Total	Fac Total		51	50	62	80	MUE
	14.39	11.02	090	2	0	0	0	1

AMA: Mar 10: 4, Dec 12: 6

15731 Forehead flap with preservation of vascular pedicle (eg, axial pattern flap, paramedian forehead flap) A 2 T

	RVU		Global Days	Modifiers				
Mod	Non-Fac Total	Fac Total		51	50	62	80	MUE
	32.41	29.20	090	2	0	0	0	1

AMA: Dec 12: 6

15732 Muscle, myocutaneous, or fasciocutaneous flap; head and neck (eg, temporalis, masseter muscle, sternocleidomastoid, levator scapulae) A 2 T

	RVU		Global Days	Modifiers				
Mod	Non-Fac Total	Fac Total		51	50	62	80	MUE
	36.94	32.32	090	2	0	1	1	3

AMA: Dec 12: 6

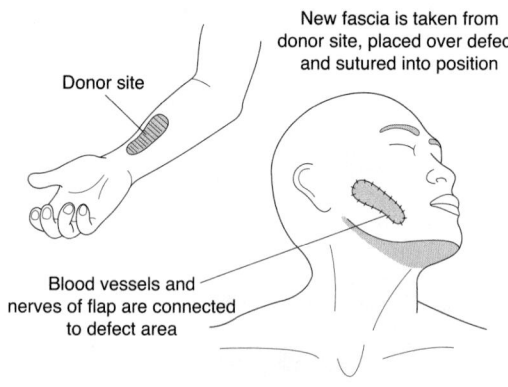

Myocutaneous muscle or fasciocutaneous flap

New fascia is taken from donor site, placed over defect, and sutured into position

Donor site

Blood vessels and nerves of flap are connected to defect area

Donor sites: Head/neck (15732); trunk (15734); upper extremities (15736); lower extremities (15738)

15734 Muscle, myocutaneous, or fasciocutaneous flap; trunk A 2 T

	RVU		Global Days	Modifiers				
Mod	Non-Fac Total	Fac Total		51	50	62	80	MUE
	43.31	38.24	090	2	0	1	2	4

AMA: Dec 12: 6, Apr 14: 10, Oct 13: 15

15736 Muscle, myocutaneous, or fasciocutaneous flap; upper extremity A 2 T

	RVU		Global Days	Modifiers				
Mod	Non-Fac Total	Fac Total		51	50	62	80	MUE
	38.13	33.12	090	2	0	1	1	2

AMA: Dec 12: 6, Mar 13: 13

15738 Muscle, myocutaneous, or fasciocutaneous flap; lower extremity A 2 T

	RVU		Global Days	Modifiers				
Mod	Non-Fac Total	Fac Total		51	50	62	80	MUE
	40.42	35.72	090	2	0	1	2	4

AMA: Sep 03: 15, Apr 10: 3, Dec 12: 6

Other Flap/Grafting Procedures

15740 Flap; island pedicle requiring identification and dissection of an anatomically named axial vessel A 2 T

	RVU		Global Days	Modifiers				
Mod	Non-Fac Total	Fac Total		51	50	62	80	MUE
	29.21	24.73	090	2	0	0	1	3

AMA: Mar 04: 11, Sep 04: 12, Oct 04: 15, Apr 10: 3, Dec 12: 6

15750 Flap; neurovascular pedicle A 2 T

	RVU		Global Days	Modifiers				
Mod	Non-Fac Total	Fac Total		51	50	62	80	MUE
	26.63	26.63	090	2	0	0	2	2

● New   ▲ Revised   ✖ Deleted   ⊙ Moderate Sedation   ✚ Add-on Codes   ⊘ High Risk Denial   Ⓐ Age Edit   ♀ Female   ♂ Male   **AMA** *CPT® Assistant*   **MUE** Medically Unlikely Edit
⊘ Modifier 51 Exempt   ⊖ Modifier 63 Exempt   ✗ Unlisted   **Modifiers:** *See Inside Back Cover*   Ⓜ Maternity   A 2 – Z 3 ASC Payment Indicators   A – Y OPPS Status Indicators

CPT © 2015 American Medical Association. All Rights Reserved.   © 2016 DecisionHealth

15756 **Free muscle or myocutaneous flap with microvascular anastomosis** `C`

RVU			Global Days	Modifiers				
Mod	Non-Fac Total	Fac Total		51	50	62	80	MUE
	67.50	67.50	090	2	0	2	2	2

AMA: Apr 97: 5, Nov 97: 12, Nov 98: 6

Free muscle or myocutaneous flap with microvascular anastomosis

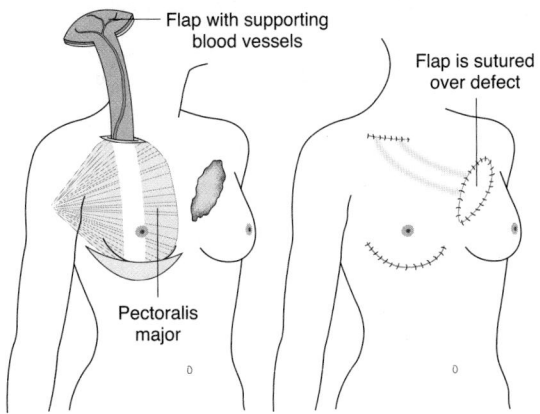

Flap with supporting blood vessels

Flap is sutured over defect

Pectoralis major

A free muscle or myocutaneous flap is implanted into a defect area.

15757 **Free skin flap with microvascular anastomosis** `C`

RVU			Global Days	Modifiers				
Mod	Non-Fac Total	Fac Total		51	50	62	80	MUE
	66.52	66.52	090	2	0	2	2	2

AMA: Apr 97: 5, Nov 98: 6

15758 **Free fascial flap with microvascular anastomosis** `C`

RVU			Global Days	Modifiers				
Mod	Non-Fac Total	Fac Total		51	50	62	80	MUE
	66.62	66.62	090	2	0	2	2	2

AMA: Apr 97: 5, Nov 98: 6

15760 **Graft; composite (eg, full thickness of external ear or nasal ala), including primary closure, donor area** `A 2 T`

RVU			Global Days	Modifiers				
Mod	Non-Fac Total	Fac Total		51	50	62	80	MUE
	24.49	20.54	090	2	0	0	1	2

AMA: Sep 97: 3

15770 **Graft; derma-fat-fascia** `A 2 T`

RVU			Global Days	Modifiers				
Mod	Non-Fac Total	Fac Total		51	50	62	80	MUE
	19.45	19.45	090	2	0	1	2	2

AMA: Sep 97: 3, Apr 10: 3

15775 **Punch graft for hair transplant; 1 to 15 punch grafts** `A 2 T`

RVU			Global Days	Modifiers				
Mod	Non-Fac Total	Fac Total		51	50	62	80	MUE
	8.56	6.43	000	2	0	0	0	1

AMA: Sep 97: 3

15776 **Punch graft for hair transplant; more than 15 punch grafts** `A 2 T`

RVU			Global Days	Modifiers				
Mod	Non-Fac Total	Fac Total		51	50	62	80	MUE
	14.28	10.38	000	2	0	0	0	1

AMA: Sep 97: 3

+ **15777** **Implantation of biologic implant (eg, acellular dermal matrix) for soft tissue reinforcement (ie, breast, trunk) (List separately in addition to code for primary procedure)** `N I N`

RVU			Global Days	Modifiers				
Mod	Non-Fac Total	Fac Total		51	50	62	80	MUE
	6.22	6.22	ZZZ	0	1	0	1	1

AMA: Jan 12: 10, Oct 13: 15

Other Skin Procedures

15780 **Dermabrasion; total face (eg, for acne scarring, fine wrinkling, rhytids, general keratosis)** `P 3 T`

RVU			Global Days	Modifiers				
Mod	Non-Fac Total	Fac Total		51	50	62	80	MUE
	23.90	18.14	090	2	0	0	0	1

AMA: Apr 03: 27

Dermabrasion

Abrasive tip

Acellular dermis
Epidermis
Dermis
Subcutaneous tissue

Total face (15780); segmental, face (15781); regional, other than face (15782); superficial, any site (15783)

15781 **Dermabrasion; segmental, face** `P 2 T`

RVU			Global Days	Modifiers				
Mod	Non-Fac Total	Fac Total		51	50	62	80	MUE
	15.92	12.54	090	2	0	0	1	1

15782 **Dermabrasion; regional, other than face** `⊘P 3 T`

RVU			Global Days	Modifiers				
Mod	Non-Fac Total	Fac Total		51	50	62	80	MUE
	18.32	12.96	090	2	0	0	0	1

15783 **Dermabrasion; superficial, any site (eg, tattoo removal)** `⊘P 2 T`

RVU			Global Days	Modifiers				
Mod	Non-Fac Total	Fac Total		51	50	62	80	MUE
	13.14	10.27	090	2	0	0	0	1

AMA: Apr 03: 27

● New ▲ Revised Deleted ⊙ Moderate Sedation ✚ Add-on Codes ⊘ High Risk Denial Ⓐ Age Edit ♀ Female ♂ Male **AMA** *CPT® Assistant* ***MUE*** Medically Unlikely Edit
⊘ Modifier 51 Exempt ⊖ Modifier 63 Exempt ✗ Unlisted **Modifiers:** *See Inside Back Cover* Ⓜ Maternity A 2 – Z 3 ASC Payment Indicators A – Y OPPS Status Indicators

© 2016 DecisionHealth | CPT © 2015 American Medical Association. All Rights Reserved. | **195**

Surgical Procedures

15756 – 15783

15786 Abrasion; single lesion (eg, keratosis, scar) N I Q I

RVU			Global Days	Modifiers				
Mod	Non-Fac Total	Fac Total		51	50	62	80	MUE
	6.94	3.89	010	2	0	0	1	1

+ 15787 Abrasion; each additional 4 lesions or less (List separately in addition to code for primary procedure) N I N

RVU			Global Days	Modifiers				
Mod	Non-Fac Total	Fac Total		51	50	62	80	MUE
	1.39	0.50	ZZZ	0	0	0	1	2

15788 Chemical peel, facial; epidermal N I Q I

RVU			Global Days	Modifiers				
Mod	Non-Fac Total	Fac Total		51	50	62	80	MUE
	13.11	7.08	090	2	0	0	1	1

15789 Chemical peel, facial; dermal P 2 T

RVU			Global Days	Modifiers				
Mod	Non-Fac Total	Fac Total		51	50	62	80	MUE
	15.67	11.91	090	2	0	0	1	1

15792 Chemical peel, nonfacial; epidermal N I Q I

RVU			Global Days	Modifiers				
Mod	Non-Fac Total	Fac Total		51	50	62	80	MUE
	12.60	7.55	090	2	0	0	0	1

15793 Chemical peel, nonfacial; dermal N I Q I

RVU			Global Days	Modifiers				
Mod	Non-Fac Total	Fac Total		51	50	62	80	MUE
	14.03	10.55	090	2	0	0	0	1

15819 Cervicoplasty ⊘ G 2 T

RVU			Global Days	Modifiers				
Mod	Non-Fac Total	Fac Total		51	50	62	80	MUE
	21.26	21.26	090	2	0	0	0	1

15820 Blepharoplasty, lower eyelid ⊘ A 2 T

RVU			Global Days	Modifiers				
Mod	Non-Fac Total	Fac Total		51	50	62	80	MUE
	16.01	14.45	090	2	1	0	0	1

AMA: Feb 04: 11, May 04: 12, Feb 05: 16

15821 Blepharoplasty, lower eyelid; with extensive herniated fat pad ⊘ A 2 T

RVU			Global Days	Modifiers				
Mod	Non-Fac Total	Fac Total		51	50	62	80	MUE
	17.28	15.53	090	2	1	0	0	1

AMA: Feb 04: 11, May 04: 12, Feb 05: 16

15822 Blepharoplasty, upper eyelid A 2 T

RVU			Global Days	Modifiers				
Mod	Non-Fac Total	Fac Total		51	50	62	80	MUE
	12.67	11.15	090	2	1	0	1	1

AMA: Feb 04: 11, May 04: 12, Feb 05: 16

Blepharoplasty, upper eyelid

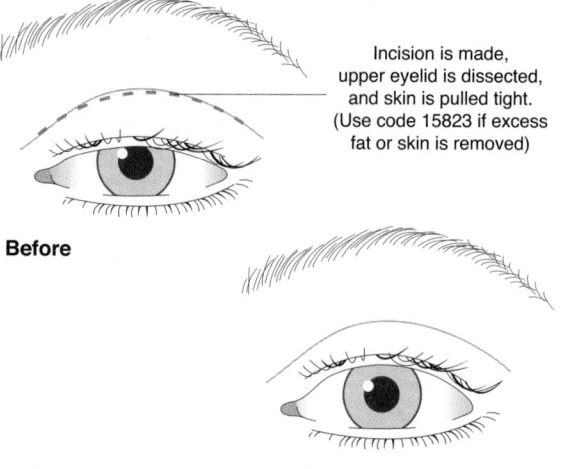

Incision is made, upper eyelid is dissected, and skin is pulled tight. (Use code 15823 if excess fat or skin is removed)

Before

After

15823 Blepharoplasty, upper eyelid; with excessive skin weighting down lid A 2 T

RVU			Global Days	Modifiers				
Mod	Non-Fac Total	Fac Total		51	50	62	80	MUE
	17.25	15.48	090	2	1	0	1	1

AMA: Sep 00: 7, Feb 04: 11, May 04: 12, Feb 05: 16, Aug 11: 8

15824 Rhytidectomy; forehead ⊘ A 2 T

RVU			Global Days	Modifiers				
Mod	Non-Fac Total	Fac Total		51	50	62	80	MUE
	0.00	0.00	000	2	1	0	0	1

15825 Rhytidectomy; neck with platysmal tightening (platysmal flap, P-flap) ⊘ A 2 T

RVU			Global Days	Modifiers				
Mod	Non-Fac Total	Fac Total		51	50	62	80	MUE
	0.00	0.00	000	2	1	0	0	1

15826 Rhytidectomy; glabellar frown lines ⊘ A 2 T

RVU			Global Days	Modifiers				
Mod	Non-Fac Total	Fac Total		51	50	62	80	MUE
	0.00	0.00	000	2	1	0	0	1

15828 Rhytidectomy; cheek, chin, and neck ⊘ A 2 T

RVU			Global Days	Modifiers				
Mod	Non-Fac Total	Fac Total		51	50	62	80	MUE
	0.00	0.00	000	2	1	0	0	1

15829 Rhytidectomy; superficial musculoaponeurotic system (SMAS) flap ⊘ A 2 T

RVU			Global Days	Modifiers				
Mod	Non-Fac Total	Fac Total		51	50	62	80	MUE
	0.00	0.00	000	2	1	0	0	1

● New   ▲ Revised   ✖ Deleted   ⊙ Moderate Sedation   ✚ Add-on Codes   ⊘ High Risk Denial   Ⓐ Age Edit   ♀ Female   ♂ Male   **AMA** CPT® Assistant   **MUE** Medically Unlikely Edit
⊝ Modifier 51 Exempt   ⊖ Modifier 63 Exempt   ✗ Unlisted   **Modifiers:** See Inside Back Cover   Ⓜ Maternity   A 2 – Z 3 ASC Payment Indicators   A – Y OPPS Status Indicators

Coding Guidance

A panniculectomy (removal of excess skin and subcutaneous tissue) at the incision site of an open procedure, such as hernia repair, is not separately reportable. However, when an abdominoplasty is also done that requires a significant amount of work more than a panniculectomy, both 15830 and 15847 for the abdominplasty may be reported.

15830 Excision, excessive skin and subcutaneous tissue (includes lipectomy); abdomen, infraumbilical panniculectomy [A 2 T]

RVU			Global Days	Modifiers				
Mod	Non-Fac Total	Fac Total		51	50	62	80	MUE
	33.99	33.99	090	2	0	1	2	1

15832 Excision, excessive skin and subcutaneous tissue (includes lipectomy); thigh ⊘[A 2 T]

RVU			Global Days	Modifiers				
Mod	Non-Fac Total	Fac Total		51	50	62	80	MUE
	26.63	26.63	090	2	1	1	2	1

15833 Excision, excessive skin and subcutaneous tissue (includes lipectomy); leg ⊘[A 2 T]

RVU			Global Days	Modifiers				
Mod	Non-Fac Total	Fac Total		51	50	62	80	MUE
	24.99	24.99	090	2	1	0	0	1

15834 Excision, excessive skin and subcutaneous tissue (includes lipectomy); hip ⊘[A 2 T]

RVU			Global Days	Modifiers				
Mod	Non-Fac Total	Fac Total		51	50	62	80	MUE
	25.78	25.78	090	2	1	0	0	1

15835 Excision, excessive skin and subcutaneous tissue (includes lipectomy); buttock ⊘[A 2 T]

RVU			Global Days	Modifiers				
Mod	Non-Fac Total	Fac Total		51	50	62	80	MUE
	26.93	26.93	090	2	0	0	0	1

15836 Excision, excessive skin and subcutaneous tissue (includes lipectomy); arm ⊘[A 2 T]

RVU			Global Days	Modifiers				
Mod	Non-Fac Total	Fac Total		51	50	62	80	MUE
	22.06	22.06	090	2	1	0	0	1

15837 Excision, excessive skin and subcutaneous tissue (includes lipectomy); forearm or hand [G 2 T]

RVU			Global Days	Modifiers				
Mod	Non-Fac Total	Fac Total		51	50	62	80	MUE
	23.13	19.38	090	2	0	0	0	2

15838 Excision, excessive skin and subcutaneous tissue (includes lipectomy); submental fat pad [G 2 T]

RVU			Global Days	Modifiers				
Mod	Non-Fac Total	Fac Total		51	50	62	80	MUE
	16.51	16.51	090	2	0	0	0	1

15839 Excision, excessive skin and subcutaneous tissue (includes lipectomy); other area [A 2 T]

RVU			Global Days	Modifiers				
Mod	Non-Fac Total	Fac Total		51	50	62	80	MUE
	25.35	21.31	090	2	0	0	0	2

15840 Graft for facial nerve paralysis; free fascia graft (including obtaining fascia) [A 2 T]

RVU			Global Days	Modifiers				
Mod	Non-Fac Total	Fac Total		51	50	62	80	MUE
	29.17	29.17	090	2	0	0	1	1

Graft for facial nerve paralysis

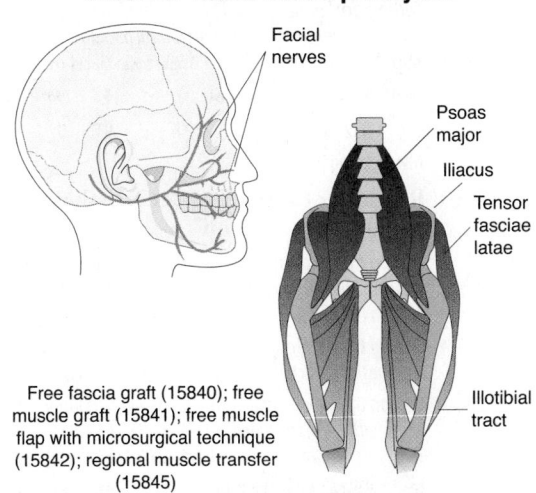

Facial nerves
Psoas major
Iliacus
Tensor fasciae latae
Illotibial tract

Free fascia graft (15840); free muscle graft (15841); free muscle flap with microsurgical technique (15842); regional muscle transfer (15845)

15841 Graft for facial nerve paralysis; free muscle graft (including obtaining graft) [A 2 T]

RVU			Global Days	Modifiers				
Mod	Non-Fac Total	Fac Total		51	50	62	80	MUE
	46.80	46.80	090	2	0	1	2	2

15842 Graft for facial nerve paralysis; free muscle flap by microsurgical technique [G 2 T]

RVU			Global Days	Modifiers				
Mod	Non-Fac Total	Fac Total		51	50	62	80	MUE
	76.54	76.54	090	2	0	1	2	2

15845 Graft for facial nerve paralysis; regional muscle transfer [A 2 T]

RVU			Global Days	Modifiers				
Mod	Non-Fac Total	Fac Total		51	50	62	80	MUE
	28.86	28.86	090	2	0	0	2	2

+ 15847 Excision, excessive skin and subcutaneous tissue (includes lipectomy), abdomen (eg, abdominoplasty) (includes umbilical transposition and fascial plication) (List separately in addition to code for primary procedure) [N 1 N]

RVU			Global Days	Modifiers				
Mod	Non-Fac Total	Fac Total		51	50	62	80	MUE
	0.00	0.00	YYY	0	0	1	2	1

Coding Guidance

Codes for suture removal or dressing change under anesthesia (15850-15852) should not be reported when a patient requires anesthesia for a related procedure, such as a return to the operating room for treatment of complications where an incision is reopened necessitating removal of sutures and redressing.

● New ▲ Revised Deleted ⊙ Moderate Sedation ✚ Add-on Codes ⊘ High Risk Denial Ⓐ Age Edit ♀ Female ♂ Male **AMA** *CPT® Assistant* **MUE** Medically Unlikely Edit
⊗ Modifier 51 Exempt ⊖ Modifier 63 Exempt ⊠ Unlisted **Modifiers:** *See Inside Back Cover* Ⓜ Maternity [A 2]–[Z 3] ASC Payment Indicators [A]–[Y] OPPS Status Indicators

15850 Removal of sutures under anesthesia (other than local), same surgeon ⊘G2T

Coding tip: Suture removal by a physician other than the operating surgeon who initially placed the sutures (not under anesthesia) is reported with an E/M code

Coding tip: Re-dressing of wounds, wound irrigation, or irrigation of tubes/catheters is included

Coding tip: Suture removal by the operating surgeon (not under anesthesia) is part of the global surgical package

RVU			Global Days	Modifiers				
Mod	Non-Fac Total	Fac Total		51	50	62	80	MUE
	2.52	1.19	XXX	9	9	9	9	

AMA: Spring 93: 34, Nov 97: 22

15851 Removal of sutures under anesthesia (other than local), other surgeon P3T

Coding tip: Suture removal by a physician other than the operating surgeon who initially placed the sutures (not under anesthesia) is reported with an E/M code

Coding tip: Suture removal by the operating surgeon (not under anesthesia) is part of the global surgical package

Coding tip: Re-dressing of wounds, wound irrigation, or irrigation of tubes/catheters is included

RVU			Global Days	Modifiers				
Mod	Non-Fac Total	Fac Total		51	50	62	80	MUE
	2.80	1.31	000	2	0	0	1	1

AMA: Spring 93: 34, Nov 97: 22

15852 Dressing change (for other than burns) under anesthesia (other than local) N1Q1

Coding tip: Report when surgical dressing change without suture removal is done under anesthesia

RVU			Global Days	Modifiers				
Mod	Non-Fac Total	Fac Total		51	50	62	80	MUE
	1.35	1.35	000	2	0	0	1	1

15860 Intravenous injection of agent (eg, fluorescein) to test vascular flow in flap or graft N1Q1

RVU			Global Days	Modifiers				
Mod	Non-Fac Total	Fac Total		51	50	62	80	MUE
	3.21	3.21	000	2	0	0	0	1

Intravenous injection of agent to test vascular flow in flap or graft

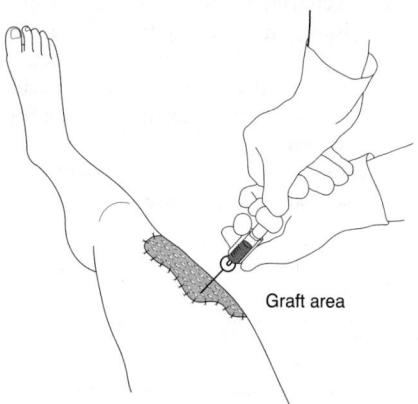

Graft area

The physician injects a dye agent (e.g., fluorescein) to test vascular flow in a flap or graft area. The agent is injected intravenously.

15876 Suction assisted lipectomy; head and neck ⊘A2T

RVU			Global Days	Modifiers				
Mod	Non-Fac Total	Fac Total		51	50	62	80	MUE
	0.00	0.00	000	2	0	0	0	1

15877 Suction assisted lipectomy; trunk ⊘A2T

RVU			Global Days	Modifiers				
Mod	Non-Fac Total	Fac Total		51	50	62	80	MUE
	0.00	0.00	000	2	0	0	0	1

AMA: Oct 99: 10, Feb 05: 14

15878 Suction assisted lipectomy; upper extremity ⊘A2T

RVU			Global Days	Modifiers				
Mod	Non-Fac Total	Fac Total		51	50	62	80	MUE
	0.00	0.00	000	2	1	0	0	1

15879 Suction assisted lipectomy; lower extremity ⊘A2T

RVU			Global Days	Modifiers				
Mod	Non-Fac Total	Fac Total		51	50	62	80	MUE
	0.00	0.00	000	2	1	0	0	1

Excisional Decubitus Ulcer Procedures

15920 Excision, coccygeal pressure ulcer, with coccygectomy; with primary suture A2T

RVU			Global Days	Modifiers				
Mod	Non-Fac Total	Fac Total		51	50	62	80	MUE
	17.48	17.48	090	2	0	0	0	1

15922 Excision, coccygeal pressure ulcer, with coccygectomy; with flap closure A2T

RVU			Global Days	Modifiers				
Mod	Non-Fac Total	Fac Total		51	50	62	80	MUE
	22.65	22.65	090	2	0	1	2	1

15931 Excision, sacral pressure ulcer, with primary suture A2T

RVU			Global Days	Modifiers				
Mod	Non-Fac Total	Fac Total		51	50	62	80	MUE
	19.79	19.79	090	2	0	0	1	1

15933 Excision, sacral pressure ulcer, with primary suture; with ostectomy A2T

RVU			Global Days	Modifiers				
Mod	Non-Fac Total	Fac Total		51	50	62	80	MUE
	24.51	24.51	090	2	0	0	0	1

● New ▲ Revised ✖ Deleted ⊙ Moderate Sedation ✚ Add-on Codes ⊘ High Risk Denial Ⓐ Age Edit ♀ Female ♂ Male **AMA** CPT® Assistant **MUE** Medically Unlikely Edit
Ⓢ Modifier 51 Exempt ⊖ Modifier 63 Exempt ⊠ Unlisted **Modifiers:** See Inside Back Cover Ⓜ Maternity A2–Z3 ASC Payment Indicators A–Y OPPS Status Indicators

CPT © 2015 American Medical Association. All Rights Reserved. © 2016 DecisionHealth

15934 Excision, sacral pressure ulcer, with skin flap closure A2T

Mod	RVU Non-Fac Total	Fac Total	Global Days	51	50	62	80	MUE
	26.79	26.79	090	2	0	0	1	1

Excision of sacral pressure ulcer

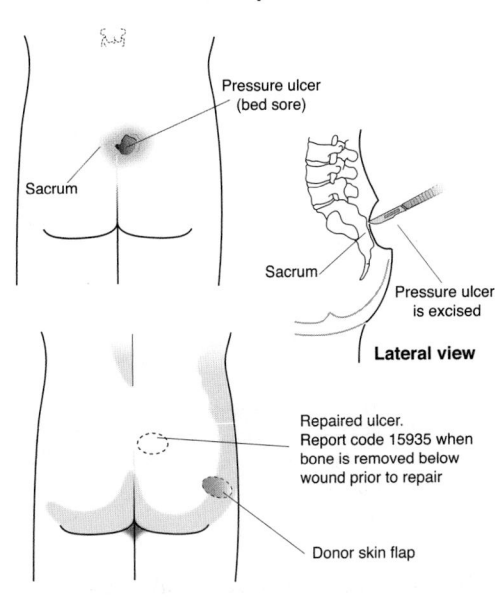

Pressure ulcer (bed sore)
Sacrum
Sacrum
Pressure ulcer is excised
Lateral view
Repaired ulcer. Report code 15935 when bone is removed below wound prior to repair
Donor skin flap

15935 Excision, sacral pressure ulcer, with skin flap closure; with ostectomy A2T

Mod	RVU Non-Fac Total	Fac Total	Global Days	51	50	62	80	MUE
	31.57	31.57	090	2	0	1	2	1

15936 Excision, sacral pressure ulcer, in preparation for muscle or myocutaneous flap or skin graft closure A2T

Mod	RVU Non-Fac Total	Fac Total	Global Days	51	50	62	80	MUE
	25.73	25.73	090	2	0	1	1	1

AMA: Nov 98: 6, 7

15937 Excision, sacral pressure ulcer, in preparation for muscle or myocutaneous flap or skin graft closure; with ostectomy A2T

Mod	RVU Non-Fac Total	Fac Total	Global Days	51	50	62	80	MUE
	29.91	29.91	090	2	0	1	1	1

15940 Excision, ischial pressure ulcer, with primary suture A2T

Mod	RVU Non-Fac Total	Fac Total	Global Days	51	50	62	80	MUE
	20.25	20.25	090	2	0	0	1	2

15941 Excision, ischial pressure ulcer, with primary suture; with ostectomy (ischiectomy) A2T

Mod	RVU Non-Fac Total	Fac Total	Global Days	51	50	62	80	MUE
	25.97	25.97	090	2	0	0	0	2

15944 Excision, ischial pressure ulcer, with skin flap closure A2T

Mod	RVU Non-Fac Total	Fac Total	Global Days	51	50	62	80	MUE
	25.58	25.58	090	2	0	0	0	2

15945 Excision, ischial pressure ulcer, with skin flap closure; with ostectomy A2T

Mod	RVU Non-Fac Total	Fac Total	Global Days	51	50	62	80	MUE
	28.18	28.18	090	2	0	0	0	2

15946 Excision, ischial pressure ulcer, with ostectomy, in preparation for muscle or myocutaneous flap or skin graft closure A2T

Mod	RVU Non-Fac Total	Fac Total	Global Days	51	50	62	80	MUE
	47.45	47.45	090	2	0	1	1	2

AMA: Nov 98: 6, 7, Jun 02: 10, Jan 03: 23

15950 Excision, trochanteric pressure ulcer, with primary suture A2T

Mod	RVU Non-Fac Total	Fac Total	Global Days	51	50	62	80	MUE
	17.03	17.03	090	2	0	0	1	2

15951 Excision, trochanteric pressure ulcer, with primary suture; with ostectomy A2T

Mod	RVU Non-Fac Total	Fac Total	Global Days	51	50	62	80	MUE
	25.47	25.47	090	2	0	1	0	2

15952 Excision, trochanteric pressure ulcer, with skin flap closure A2T

Mod	RVU Non-Fac Total	Fac Total	Global Days	51	50	62	80	MUE
	25.99	25.99	090	2	0	1	2	2

15953 Excision, trochanteric pressure ulcer, with skin flap closure; with ostectomy A2T

Mod	RVU Non-Fac Total	Fac Total	Global Days	51	50	62	80	MUE
	28.84	28.84	090	2	0	1	1	2

15956 Excision, trochanteric pressure ulcer, in preparation for muscle or myocutaneous flap or skin graft closure A2T

Mod	RVU Non-Fac Total	Fac Total	Global Days	51	50	62	80	MUE
	33.28	33.28	090	2	0	1	1	2

AMA: Nov 98: 6, 7

15958 Excision, trochanteric pressure ulcer, in preparation for muscle or myocutaneous flap or skin graft closure; with ostectomy A2T

Mod	RVU Non-Fac Total	Fac Total	Global Days	51	50	62	80	MUE
	33.93	33.93	090	2	0	1	1	2

AMA: Nov 98: 6, 7

15999 Unlisted procedure, excision pressure ulcer xT

Mod	RVU Non-Fac Total	Fac Total	Global Days	51	50	62	80	MUE
	0.00	0.00	YYY	2	0	1	0	

● New ▲ Revised Deleted ⊙ Moderate Sedation ✚ Add-on Codes ⊘ High Risk Denial Ⓐ Age Edit ♀ Female ♂ Male **AMA** *CPT® Assistant* **MUE** Medically Unlikely Edit
⊘ Modifier 51 Exempt ⊖ Modifier 63 Exempt ☒ Unlisted **Modifiers:** *See Inside Back Cover* Ⓜ Maternity A2–Z3 ASC Payment Indicators A–Y OPPS Status Indicators

Burn Treatment

16000 Initial treatment, first degree burn, when no more than local treatment is required `N` `I` `Q` `I`

RVU		Global Days	Modifiers				
Mod	Non-Fac Total	Fac Total		51	50	62	80	MUE
	1.95	1.32	000	2	0	0	1	1

AMA: Aug 97: 6, Oct 12: 3

Pub 100-04, 13, 70.2

Initial first degree burn treatment

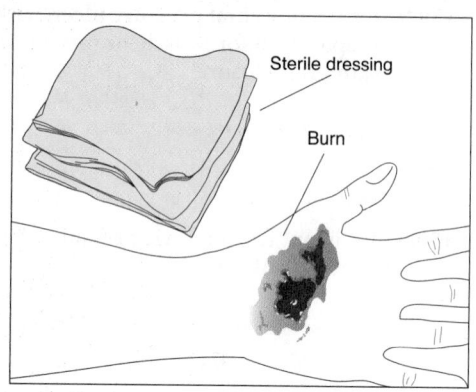

Sterile dressing

Burn

Cream and a sterile dressing is applied as needed.

16020 Dressings and/or debridement of partial-thickness burns, initial or subsequent; small (less than 5% total body surface area) `N` `I` `Q` `I`

RVU		Global Days	Modifiers				
Mod	Non-Fac Total	Fac Total		51	50	62	80	MUE
	2.31	1.55	000	2	0	0	1	1

AMA: Aug 97: 6, Oct 12: 3

Pub 100-04, 13, 70.2

16025 Dressings and/or debridement of partial-thickness burns, initial or subsequent; medium (eg, whole face or whole extremity, or 5% to 10% total body surface area) `A` `2` `T`

RVU		Global Days	Modifiers				
Mod	Non-Fac Total	Fac Total		51	50	62	80	MUE
	4.20	3.20	000	2	0	0	1	1

AMA: Aug 97: 6, Jun 08: 14, Oct 12: 3

Pub 100-04, 13, 70.2

16030 Dressings and/or debridement of partial-thickness burns, initial or subsequent; large (eg, more than 1 extremity, or greater than 10% total body surface area) `A` `2` `T`

RVU		Global Days	Modifiers				
Mod	Non-Fac Total	Fac Total		51	50	62	80	MUE
	5.29	3.86	000	2	0	0	1	1

AMA: Aug 97: 6, Jun 08: 14, Oct 12: 3

Pub 100-04, 13, 70.2

16035 Escharotomy; initial incision `G` `2` `T`

RVU		Global Days	Modifiers				
Mod	Non-Fac Total	Fac Total		51	50	62	80	MUE
	5.61	5.61	000	2	0	0	1	1

AMA: Aug 97: 6, Oct 12: 3

Escharotomy

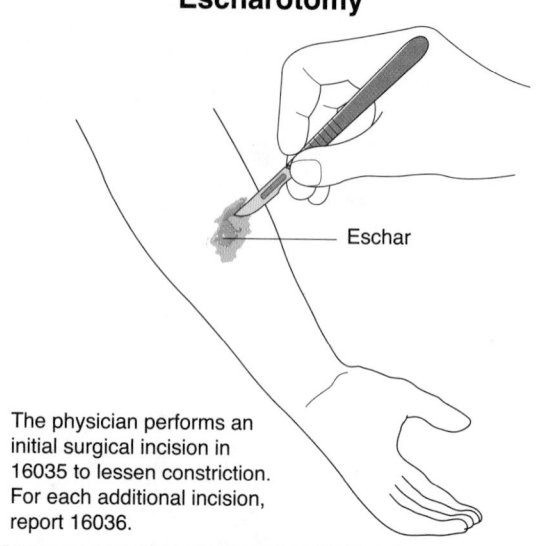

Eschar

The physician performs an initial surgical incision in 16035 to lessen constriction. For each additional incision, report 16036.

+ 16036 Escharotomy; each additional incision (List separately in addition to code for primary procedure) `C`

RVU		Global Days	Modifiers				
Mod	Non-Fac Total	Fac Total		51	50	62	80	MUE
	2.34	2.34	ZZZ	0	0	0	1	8

AMA: Oct 12: 3

Skin Lesion Destruction Procedures

Coding Guidance

Only one type of removal is reported per given lesion, whether destruction, paring, debridement, shaving, excision, or curettement. Multiple codes describing destruction of one single lesion are not reported. If multiple, separate lesions are removed at the same session using different methods, a modifier should be used to indicate the different site or lesion treated, or different method used. When an initial attempt at lesion removal using a less invasive method must be followed by a more invasive type of lesion removal, only the more complex procedure should be reported. Lesions removed by any method usually require some kind of closure. Strip closure, bandaging, tissue glueing, or simple repairs (12001-12021) are included in the initial excision. Intermediate and complex repairs are reported separately. When debridement of non-viable tissue around a lesion or wound is performed in order to accomplish the primary removal, destruction, repair, incision, or closure, it is a necessary part of the whole procedure and should not be reported separately.

● New ▲ Revised ✖ Deleted ⊙ Moderate Sedation ✚ Add-on Codes ⊘ High Risk Denial Ⓐ Age Edit ♀ Female ♂ Male **AMA** *CPT® Assistant* **MUE** Medically Unlikely Edit
⊘ Modifier 51 Exempt ⊖ Modifier 63 Exempt ✗ Unlisted **Modifiers:** *See Inside Back Cover* Ⓜ Maternity `A2`–`Z3` ASC Payment Indicators `A`–`Y` OPPS Status Indicators

CPT © 2015 American Medical Association. All Rights Reserved.   © 2016 DecisionHealth

17000 Destruction (eg, laser surgery, electrosurgery, cryosurgery, chemosurgery, surgical curettement), premalignant lesions (eg, actinic keratoses); first lesion N I Q I

RVU		Global Days	Modifiers				
Mod	Non-Fac Total	Fac Total		51	50	62	80	MUE
	1.89	1.52	010	2	0	0	1	1

AMA: Winter 90: 3, Nov 97: 12, Jun 99: 10, May 06: 19, Feb 07: 10, Aug 09: 7, Mar 10: 10, Mar 12: 7, May 12: 13

Destruction of lesions

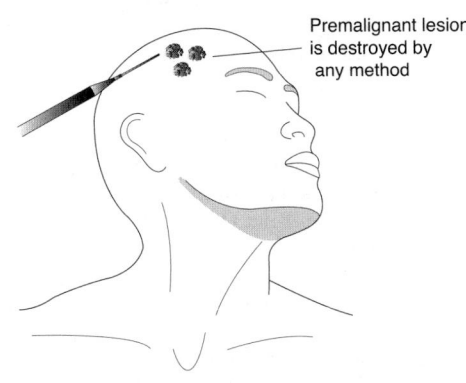

Premalignant lesion is destroyed by any method

First lesion (17000); each additional lesion up to 14 (17003); 15 or more lesions (17004)

+ 17003 Destruction (eg, laser surgery, electrosurgery, cryosurgery, chemosurgery, surgical curettement), premalignant lesions (eg, actinic keratoses); second through 14 lesions, each (List separately in addition to code for first lesion) N I N

RVU		Global Days	Modifiers				
Mod	Non-Fac Total	Fac Total		51	50	62	80	MUE
	0.16	0.07	ZZZ	0	0	0	1	13

AMA: Nov 97: 12, Jun 99: 10, May 06: 19, Feb 07: 10, Aug 09: 7, Mar 10: 10

⊘ 17004 Destruction (eg, laser surgery, electrosurgery, cryosurgery, chemosurgery, surgical curettement), premalignant lesions (eg, actinic keratoses), 15 or more lesions P 3 T

RVU		Global Days	Modifiers				
Mod	Non-Fac Total	Fac Total		51	50	62	80	MUE
	4.26	2.86	010	0	0	0	1	1

AMA: Nov 97: 12, Nov 98: 7, Jun 99: 10, Mar 03: 21, Feb 07: 10, Aug 09: 7, Mar 10: 10

17106 Destruction of cutaneous vascular proliferative lesions (eg, laser technique); less than 10 sq cm P 3 T

RVU		Global Days	Modifiers				
Mod	Non-Fac Total	Fac Total		51	50	62	80	MUE
	9.71	7.91	090	2	0	0	1	1

AMA: Winter 90: 3, Apr 07: 11, Jun 08: 14, Aug 09: 7

Destruction of cutaneous vascular proliferative lesions

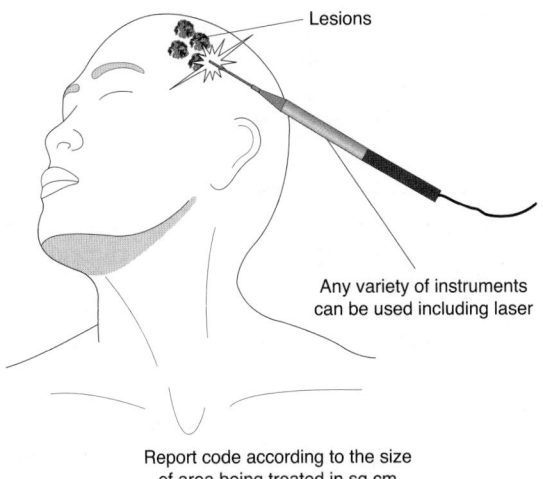

Lesions

Any variety of instruments can be used including laser

Report code according to the size of area being treated in sq cm

17107 Destruction of cutaneous vascular proliferative lesions (eg, laser technique); 10.0 to 50.0 sq cm P 2 T

RVU		Global Days	Modifiers				
Mod	Non-Fac Total	Fac Total		51	50	62	80	MUE
	12.35	9.97	090	2	0	0	1	1

AMA: Winter 90: 3, Apr 07: 11, Jun 08: 14, Aug 09: 7

17108 Destruction of cutaneous vascular proliferative lesions (eg, laser technique); over 50.0 sq cm P 3 T

RVU		Global Days	Modifiers				
Mod	Non-Fac Total	Fac Total		51	50	62	80	MUE
	18.21	15.13	090	2	0	0	0	1

AMA: Winter 90: 3, Apr 07: 11, Jun 08: 14, Aug 09: 7

17110 Destruction (eg, laser surgery, electrosurgery, cryosurgery, chemosurgery, surgical curettement), of benign lesions other than skin tags or cutaneous vascular proliferative lesions; up to 14 lesions N I Q I

Coding tip: For destruction of premalignant lesions - 17000-17003; malignant lesions - 17260-17286

RVU		Global Days	Modifiers				
Mod	Non-Fac Total	Fac Total		51	50	62	80	MUE
	3.14	2.00	010	2	0	0	1	1

AMA: Nov 97: 13, Feb 07: 10, Apr 07: 11, Nov 08: 10, Aug 09: 7

● New ▲ Revised Deleted ⊙ Moderate Sedation ✛ Add-on Codes ⊘ High Risk Denial Ⓐ Age Edit ♀ Female ♂ Male **AMA** *CPT® Assistant* **MUE** Medically Unlikely Edit
⊘ Modifier 51 Exempt ⊖ Modifier 63 Exempt ✗ Unlisted **Modifiers:** *See Inside Back Cover* Ⓜ Maternity A 2 – Z 3 ASC Payment Indicators A – Y OPPS Status Indicators

© 2016 DecisionHealth | CPT © 2015 American Medical Association. All Rights Reserved. | **201**

Surgical Procedures

17111 – 17270

17111 Destruction (eg, laser surgery, electrosurgery, cryosurgery, chemosurgery, surgical curettement), of benign lesions other than skin tags or cutaneous vascular proliferative lesions; 15 or more lesions   N I Q I

Coding tip: For destruction of premalignant lesions - 17004; malignant lesions - 17260-17286

RVU			Global Days	Modifiers				
Mod	Non-Fac Total	Fac Total		51	50	62	80	MUE
	3.72	2.46	010	2	0	0	1	1

AMA: Nov 97: 13, Feb 07: 10, Apr 07: 11, Nov 08: 10, Aug 09: 7

17250 Chemical cauterization of granulation tissue (proud flesh, sinus or fistula)   N I Q I

RVU			Global Days	Modifiers				
Mod	Non-Fac Total	Fac Total		51	50	62	80	MUE
	2.25	1.06	000	2	0	0	1	4

AMA: May 12: 13, Dec 12: 15

17260 Destruction, malignant lesion (eg, laser surgery, electrosurgery, cryosurgery, chemosurgery, surgical curettement), trunk, arms or legs; lesion diameter 0.5 cm or less   N I Q I

Coding tip: For destruction of premalignant lesions, these codes are for quantity, not size of lesion - 17000-17004; benign lesions, these codes are for quantity, not size of lesion - 17110-17111

RVU			Global Days	Modifiers				
Mod	Non-Fac Total	Fac Total		51	50	62	80	MUE
	2.69	2.02	010	2	0	0	1	7

AMA: May 12: 13

Destruction of a malignant lesion

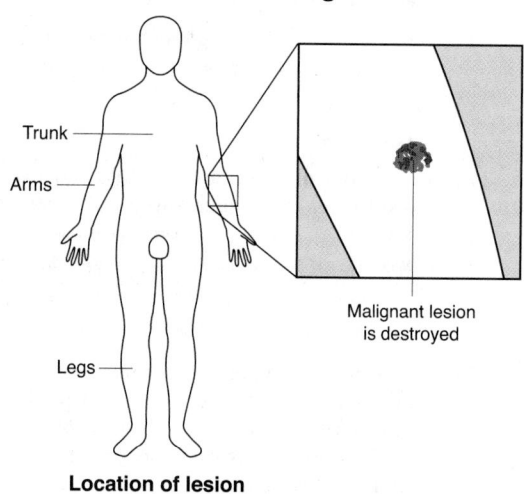

Trunk

Arms

Legs

Malignant lesion is destroyed

Location of lesion

17261 Destruction, malignant lesion (eg, laser surgery, electrosurgery, cryosurgery, chemosurgery, surgical curettement), trunk, arms or legs; lesion diameter 0.6 to 1.0 cm   N I Q I

RVU			Global Days	Modifiers				
Mod	Non-Fac Total	Fac Total		51	50	62	80	MUE
	4.07	2.63	010	2	0	0	1	7

17262 Destruction, malignant lesion (eg, laser surgery, electrosurgery, cryosurgery, chemosurgery, surgical curettement), trunk, arms or legs; lesion diameter 1.1 to 2.0 cm   N I Q I

RVU			Global Days	Modifiers				
Mod	Non-Fac Total	Fac Total		51	50	62	80	MUE
	4.96	3.35	010	2	0	0	1	6

17263 Destruction, malignant lesion (eg, laser surgery, electrosurgery, cryosurgery, chemosurgery, surgical curettement), trunk, arms or legs; lesion diameter 2.1 to 3.0 cm   N I Q I

RVU			Global Days	Modifiers				
Mod	Non-Fac Total	Fac Total		51	50	62	80	MUE
	5.42	3.72	010	2	0	0	1	5

17264 Destruction, malignant lesion (eg, laser surgery, electrosurgery, cryosurgery, chemosurgery, surgical curettement), trunk, arms or legs; lesion diameter 3.1 to 4.0 cm   P 2 T

RVU			Global Days	Modifiers				
Mod	Non-Fac Total	Fac Total		51	50	62	80	MUE
	5.82	3.97	010	2	0	0	1	3

17266 Destruction, malignant lesion (eg, laser surgery, electrosurgery, cryosurgery, chemosurgery, surgical curettement), trunk, arms or legs; lesion diameter over 4.0 cm   P 3 T

RVU			Global Days	Modifiers				
Mod	Non-Fac Total	Fac Total		51	50	62	80	MUE
	6.59	4.65	010	2	0	0	1	2

17270 Destruction, malignant lesion (eg, laser surgery, electrosurgery, cryosurgery, chemosurgery, surgical curettement), scalp, neck, hands, feet, genitalia; lesion diameter 0.5 cm or less   P 3 T

Coding tip: For destruction of premalignant lesions, these codes are for quantity, not size of lesion - 17000-17004; benign lesions, these codes are for quantity, not size of lesion - 17110-17111

RVU			Global Days	Modifiers				
Mod	Non-Fac Total	Fac Total		51	50	62	80	MUE
	4.26	2.87	010	2	0	0	1	6

Destruction of a malignant lesion

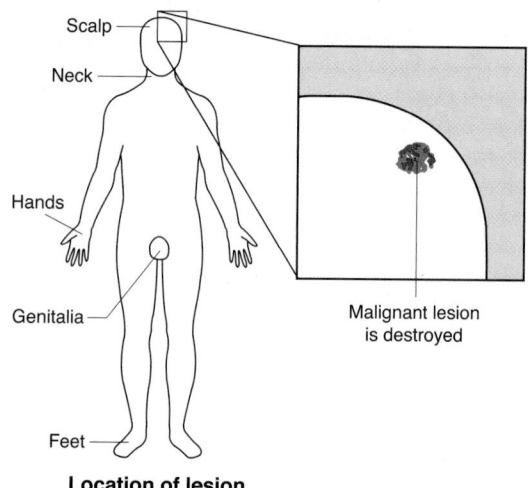

Scalp

Neck

Hands

Genitalia

Feet

Malignant lesion is destroyed

Location of lesion

● New   ▲ Revised   ✖ Deleted   ⊙ Moderate Sedation   ✚ Add-on Codes   ⊘ High Risk Denial   Ⓐ Age Edit   ♀ Female   ♂ Male   **AMA** *CPT® Assistant*   **MUE** Medically Unlikely Edit
⊘ Modifier 51 Exempt   ⊖ Modifier 63 Exempt   ✗ Unlisted   **Modifiers:** *See Inside Back Cover*   Ⓜ Maternity   A2–Z3 ASC Payment Indicators   A–Y OPPS Status Indicators

202   CPT © 2015 American Medical Association. All Rights Reserved.   © 2016 DecisionHealth

17271 Destruction, malignant lesion (eg, laser surgery, electrosurgery, cryosurgery, chemosurgery, surgical curettement), scalp, neck, hands, feet, genitalia; lesion diameter 0.6 to 1.0 cm   P 3 T

RVU			Global Days	Modifiers				
Mod	Non-Fac Total	Fac Total		51	50	62	80	MUE
	4.62	3.18	010	2	0	0	1	4

17272 Destruction, malignant lesion (eg, laser surgery, electrosurgery, cryosurgery, chemosurgery, surgical curettement), scalp, neck, hands, feet, genitalia; lesion diameter 1.1 to 2.0 cm   N1 Q1

RVU			Global Days	Modifiers				
Mod	Non-Fac Total	Fac Total		51	50	62	80	MUE
	5.28	3.69	010	2	0	0	1	5

17273 Destruction, malignant lesion (eg, laser surgery, electrosurgery, cryosurgery, chemosurgery, surgical curettement), scalp, neck, hands, feet, genitalia; lesion diameter 2.1 to 3.0 cm   P 3 T

RVU			Global Days	Modifiers				
Mod	Non-Fac Total	Fac Total		51	50	62	80	MUE
	5.89	4.16	010	2	0	0	1	4

17274 Destruction, malignant lesion (eg, laser surgery, electrosurgery, cryosurgery, chemosurgery, surgical curettement), scalp, neck, hands, feet, genitalia; lesion diameter 3.1 to 4.0 cm   P 3 T

RVU			Global Days	Modifiers				
Mod	Non-Fac Total	Fac Total		51	50	62	80	MUE
	6.96	5.08	010	2	0	0	1	4

17276 Destruction, malignant lesion (eg, laser surgery, electrosurgery, cryosurgery, chemosurgery, surgical curettement), scalp, neck, hands, feet, genitalia; lesion diameter over 4.0 cm   P 3 T

RVU			Global Days	Modifiers				
Mod	Non-Fac Total	Fac Total		51	50	62	80	MUE
	8.07	6.10	010	2	0	0	1	3

17280 Destruction, malignant lesion (eg, laser surgery, electrosurgery, cryosurgery, chemosurgery, surgical curettement), face, ears, eyelids, nose, lips, mucous membrane; lesion diameter 0.5 cm or less   N1 Q1

Coding tip: For destruction of premalignant lesions, these codes are for quantity, not size of lesion - 17000-17004; benign lesions, these codes are for quantity, not size of lesion - 17110-17111

RVU			Global Days	Modifiers				
Mod	Non-Fac Total	Fac Total		51	50	62	80	MUE
	3.99	2.61	010	2	0	0	1	6

17281 Destruction, malignant lesion (eg, laser surgery, electrosurgery, cryosurgery, chemosurgery, surgical curettement), face, ears, eyelids, nose, lips, mucous membrane; lesion diameter 0.6 to 1.0 cm   P 3 T

RVU			Global Days	Modifiers				
Mod	Non-Fac Total	Fac Total		51	50	62	80	MUE
	5.04	3.59	010	2	0	0	1	6

17282 Destruction, malignant lesion (eg, laser surgery, electrosurgery, cryosurgery, chemosurgery, surgical curettement), face, ears, eyelids, nose, lips, mucous membrane; lesion diameter 1.1 to 2.0 cm   P 3 T

RVU			Global Days	Modifiers				
Mod	Non-Fac Total	Fac Total		51	50	62	80	MUE
	5.80	4.16	010	2	0	0	1	5

17283 Destruction, malignant lesion (eg, laser surgery, electrosurgery, cryosurgery, chemosurgery, surgical curettement), face, ears, eyelids, nose, lips, mucous membrane; lesion diameter 2.1 to 3.0 cm   P 2 T

RVU			Global Days	Modifiers				
Mod	Non-Fac Total	Fac Total		51	50	62	80	MUE
	6.94	5.18	010	2	0	0	1	4

17284 Destruction, malignant lesion (eg, laser surgery, electrosurgery, cryosurgery, chemosurgery, surgical curettement), face, ears, eyelids, nose, lips, mucous membrane; lesion diameter 3.1 to 4.0 cm   P 2 T

RVU			Global Days	Modifiers				
Mod	Non-Fac Total	Fac Total		51	50	62	80	MUE
	7.94	6.04	010	2	0	0	1	3

17286 Destruction, malignant lesion (eg, laser surgery, electrosurgery, cryosurgery, chemosurgery, surgical curettement), face, ears, eyelids, nose, lips, mucous membrane; lesion diameter over 4.0 cm   P 2 T

RVU			Global Days	Modifiers				
Mod	Non-Fac Total	Fac Total		51	50	62	80	MUE
	10.19	8.10	010	2	0	0	1	3

Mohs Micrographic Procedures

Coding Guidance

Mohs micrographic surgery is performed to remove a complex or ill-defined cutaneous malignancy. A single physician performs both the surgery and pathologic examination of the specimen(s). Mohs' micrographic surgery includes by definition the biopsy, surgical excision of the lesion and its margins, and the surgical pathology services. It is inappropriate to report either the surgery or the pathology services as separate portions of the procedure. An exception may be made for the biopsy and pathological exam of a suspected skin malignancy if the biopsy is performed to determine the medical necessity of performing a more extensive procedure. This circumstance requires the use of modifier 58 staged procedure or modifier 59 distinct procedural service appended to the appropriate biopsy code(s) (11100, 11101) and frozen section pathology code (88331)Necessary repairs, grafts and flaps following Mohs' micrographic surgery may be coded separately.

17311 Mohs micrographic technique, including removal of all gross tumor, surgical excision of tissue specimens, mapping, color coding of specimens, microscopic examination of specimens by the surgeon, and histopathologic preparation including routine stain(s) (eg, hematoxylin and eosin, toluidine blue), head, neck, hands, feet, genitalia, or any location with surgery directly involving muscle, cartilage, bone, tendon, major nerves, or vessels; first stage, up to 5 tissue blocks   P 2 T

RVU			Global Days	Modifiers				
Mod	Non-Fac Total	Fac Total		51	50	62	80	MUE
	18.80	10.94	000	2	0	0	1	4

AMA: Feb 14: 10, Oct 14: 14

● New   ▲ Revised   Deleted   ⊙ Moderate Sedation   ✛ Add-on Codes   ⊘ High Risk Denial   Ⓐ Age Edit   ♀ Female   ♂ Male   **AMA** *CPT® Assistant*   **MUE** Medically Unlikely Edit
⊘ Modifier 51 Exempt   ⊖ Modifier 63 Exempt   ✗ Unlisted   **Modifiers:** *See Inside Back Cover*   Ⓜ Maternity   A2–Z3 ASC Payment Indicators   A–Y OPPS Status Indicators

Surgical Procedures

17312 – 17999

✚ **17312** Mohs micrographic technique, including removal of all gross tumor, surgical excision of tissue specimens, mapping, color coding of specimens, microscopic examination of specimens by the surgeon, and histopathologic preparation including routine stain(s) (eg, hematoxylin and eosin, toluidine blue), head, neck, hands, feet, genitalia, or any location with surgery directly involving muscle, cartilage, bone, tendon, major nerves, or vessels; each additional stage after the first stage, up to 5 tissue blocks (List separately in addition to code for primary procedure) **N I N**

RVU		Global Days	Modifiers				
Mod	Non-Fac Total	Fac Total		51	50	62	80	MUE
	11.02	5.82	ZZZ	0	0	0	1	6

17313 Mohs micrographic technique, including removal of all gross tumor, surgical excision of tissue specimens, mapping, color coding of specimens, microscopic examination of specimens by the surgeon, and histopathologic preparation including routine stain(s) (eg, hematoxylin and eosin, toluidine blue), of the trunk, arms, or legs; first stage, up to 5 tissue blocks **P 2 T**

RVU		Global Days	Modifiers				
Mod	Non-Fac Total	Fac Total		51	50	62	80	MUE
	17.57	9.80	000	2	0	0	1	3

Mohs micrographic technique

A tumor is removed one layer at a time. Each layer is viewed under a microscope to track the tumor's removal down to the roots. If cancer cells are found, the location is noted and another layer is removed where the cancer cells remain.

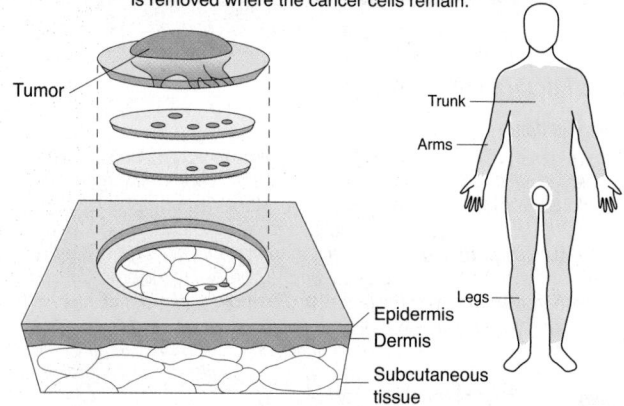

Code 17313 for first stage, up to five tissue blocks; code 17314 each additional stage, up to five tissue blocks; and code 17315 for incremental blocks after first five blocks

✚ **17314** Mohs micrographic technique, including removal of all gross tumor, surgical excision of tissue specimens, mapping, color coding of specimens, microscopic examination of specimens by the surgeon, and histopathologic preparation including routine stain(s) (eg, hematoxylin and eosin, toluidine blue), of the trunk, arms, or legs; each additional stage after the first stage, up to 5 tissue blocks (List separately in addition to code for primary procedure) **N I N**

RVU		Global Days	Modifiers				
Mod	Non-Fac Total	Fac Total		51	50	62	80	MUE
	10.58	5.39	ZZZ	0	0	0	1	4

✚ **17315** Mohs micrographic technique, including removal of all gross tumor, surgical excision of tissue specimens, mapping, color coding of specimens, microscopic examination of specimens by the surgeon, and histopathologic preparation including routine stain(s) (eg, hematoxylin and eosin, toluidine blue), each additional block after the first 5 tissue blocks, any stage (List separately in addition to code for primary procedure) **N I N**

RVU		Global Days	Modifiers				
Mod	Non-Fac Total	Fac Total		51	50	62	80	MUE
	2.27	1.53	ZZZ	0	0	0	1	15

AMA: May 12: 13, Feb 14: 10, Oct 14: 14

Other Integumentary Procedures

17340 Cryotherapy (CO2 slush, liquid N2) for acne **N I Q I**

Coding tip: For surgical procedures to treat acne (comedones/cysts/milia/ pustules) - 10040; or abscess - 10060-10061

RVU		Global Days	Modifiers				
Mod	Non-Fac Total	Fac Total		51	50	62	80	MUE
	1.46	1.40	010	2	0	0	1	1

AMA: May 12: 13

17360 Chemical exfoliation for acne (eg, acne paste, acid) **N I Q I**

Coding tip: For surgical procedures to treat acne (comedones/cysts/milia/ pustules) - 10040; or abscess - 10060-10061

RVU		Global Days	Modifiers				
Mod	Non-Fac Total	Fac Total		51	50	62	80	MUE
	3.67	2.83	010	2	0	0	1	1

17380 Electrolysis epilation, each 30 minutes ⊘ **R 2 T**

RVU		Global Days	Modifiers				
Mod	Non-Fac Total	Fac Total		51	50	62	80	MUE
	0.00	0.00	000	2	0	0	0	1

17999 Unlisted procedure, skin, mucous membrane and subcutaneous tissue ⊘ ✗ **O I**

RVU		Global Days	Modifiers				
Mod	Non-Fac Total	Fac Total		51	50	62	80	MUE
	0.00	0.00	YYY	2	0	1	0	

AMA: Dec 98: 9, May 99: 11, Jun 05: 11, Nov 08: 10, Mar 11: 9, May 12: 13, Oct 13: 15

Breast Procedures

Incisional Breast Procedures

Coding Guidance

Excision of lesions occur automatically in the course of performing a mastectomy. Breast lesion excisions are not reported together with the mastectomy code. A biopsy or lesion excision to procure tissue for an undetermined diagnosis may be separately reported in cases when the decision to proceed with a mastectomy depends upon the establishment of a malignant diagnosis from the pathology results. Modifier 58 can be utilized in these situations to denote that the biopsy or lesion excision and mastectomy are staged procedures. Lymph node and muscle tissue excision frequently done with mastectomies have been included in CPT coding for mastectomy and should not be separately reported. Biopsy of a sentinel lymph node may be separately reported when it is done before performing breast tissue excision or mastectomy. Biopsy or excision of the contralateral lymph nodes that is deemed necessary after breast lesion detection can be reported separately (38500-38530).

● New   ▲ Revised   ✖ Deleted   ⊙ Moderate Sedation   ✚ Add-on Codes   ⊘ High Risk Denial   Ⓐ Age Edit   ♀ Female   ♂ Male   **AMA** CPT® Assistant   **MUE** Medically Unlikely Edit
⊘ Modifier 51 Exempt   ⊖ Modifier 63 Exempt   ✗ Unlisted   **Modifiers:** See Inside Back Cover   Ⓜ Maternity   **A 2 – Z 3** ASC Payment Indicators   **A – Y** OPPS Status Indicators

CPT © 2015 American Medical Association. All Rights Reserved.   © 2016 DecisionHealth

19000   Puncture aspiration of cyst of breast   P 3 T

RVU			Global Days	Modifiers				
Mod	Non-Fac Total	Fac Total		51	50	62	80	MUE
	3.21	1.26	000	2	0	0	1	2

AMA: Fall 94: 18, Apr 05: 6, Nov 08: 10, Dec 13: 17

+ 19001   Puncture aspiration of cyst of breast; each additional cyst (List separately in addition to code for primary procedure)   N 1 N

RVU			Global Days	Modifiers				
Mod	Non-Fac Total	Fac Total		51	50	62	80	MUE
	0.77	0.63	ZZZ	0	0	0	1	5

AMA: Fall 94: 18, Apr 05: 6, Dec 13: 17

19020   Mastotomy with exploration or drainage of abscess, deep   A 2 T

RVU			Global Days	Modifiers				
Mod	Non-Fac Total	Fac Total		51	50	62	80	MUE
	13.45	8.78	090	2	1	0	1	2

AMA: Apr 05: 6, Dec 14: 16

Mastotomy
With exploration or drainage of abscess

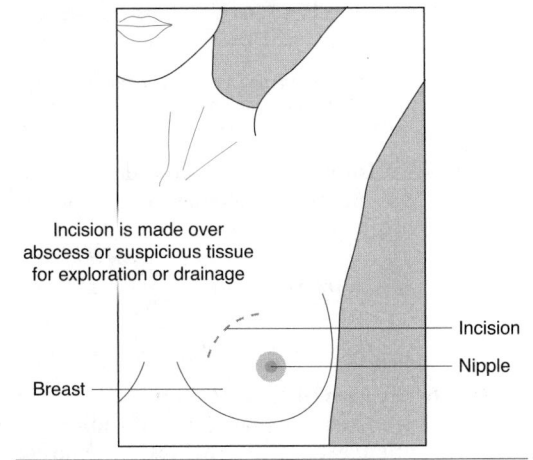

Incision is made over abscess or suspicious tissue for exploration or drainage

Incision

Nipple

Breast

19030   Injection procedure only for mammary ductogram or galactogram   N 1 N

RVU			Global Days	Modifiers				
Mod	Non-Fac Total	Fac Total		51	50	62	80	MUE
	4.67	2.24	000	2	1	0	1	1

AMA: Jul 04: 8, Apr 05: 6

19081   Biopsy, breast, with placement of breast localization device(s) (eg, clip, metallic pellet), when performed, and imaging of the biopsy specimen, when performed, percutaneous; first lesion, including stereotactic guidance   G 2 T

RVU			Global Days	Modifiers				
Mod	Non-Fac Total	Fac Total		51	50	62	80	MUE
	19.67	4.89	000	2	1	0	0	1

AMA: Mar 15: 5, May 14: 3, Jun 14: 14, May 15: 8

Biopsy, breast, with placement of breast localization device(s), percutaneous, including stereotactic guidance
First lesion (19081), each additional lesion (19082)

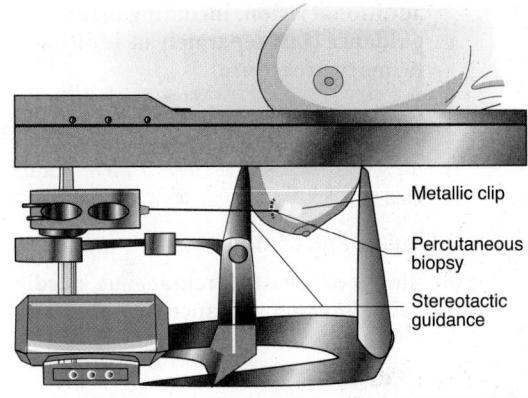

Metallic clip

Percutaneous biopsy

Stereotactic guidance

+ 19082   Biopsy, breast, with placement of breast localization device(s) (eg, clip, metallic pellet), when performed, and imaging of the biopsy specimen, when performed, percutaneous; each additional lesion, including stereotactic guidance (List separately in addition to code for primary procedure)   N 1 N

RVU			Global Days	Modifiers				
Mod	Non-Fac Total	Fac Total		51	50	62	80	MUE
	16.25	2.45	ZZZ	0	0	0	0	2

AMA: Mar 15: 5, May 14: 3, Jun 14: 14, May 15: 8

19083   Biopsy, breast, with placement of breast localization device(s) (eg, clip, metallic pellet), when performed, and imaging of the biopsy specimen, when performed, percutaneous; first lesion, including ultrasound guidance   G 2 T

RVU			Global Days	Modifiers				
Mod	Non-Fac Total	Fac Total		51	50	62	80	MUE
	19.03	4.60	000	2	1	0	0	1

AMA: Mar 15: 5, May 14: 3, Jun 14: 14, May 15: 8

+ 19084   Biopsy, breast, with placement of breast localization device(s) (eg, clip, metallic pellet), when performed, and imaging of the biopsy specimen, when performed, percutaneous; each additional lesion, including ultrasound guidance (List separately in addition to code for primary procedure)   N 1 N

RVU			Global Days	Modifiers				
Mod	Non-Fac Total	Fac Total		51	50	62	80	MUE
	15.63	2.29	ZZZ	0	0	0	0	2

AMA: Mar 15: 5, May 14: 3, Jun 14: 14, May 15: 8

● New   ▲ Revised   Deleted   ⊙ Moderate Sedation   ✚ Add-on Codes   ⊘ High Risk Denial   Ⓐ Age Edit   ♀ Female   ♂ Male   **AMA** CPT® Assistant   **MUE** Medically Unlikely Edit
⊘ Modifier 51 Exempt   ⊖ Modifier 63 Exempt   ✗ Unlisted   **Modifiers:** See Inside Back Cover   Ⓜ Maternity   A 2 – Z 3 ASC Payment Indicators   A – Y OPPS Status Indicators

19085
Biopsy, breast, with placement of breast localization device(s) (eg, clip, metallic pellet), when performed, and imaging of the biopsy specimen, when performed, percutaneous; first lesion, including magnetic resonance guidance G2T

RVU			Global Days	Modifiers				
Mod	Non-Fac Total	Fac Total		51	50	62	80	MUE
	29.21	5.39	000	2	1	0	0	1

AMA: Mar 15: 5, May 14: 3, Jun 14: 14, May 15: 8

+ 19086
Biopsy, breast, with placement of breast localization device(s) (eg, clip, metallic pellet), when performed, and imaging of the biopsy specimen, when performed, percutaneous; each additional lesion, including magnetic resonance guidance (List separately in addition to code for primary procedure) NIN

RVU			Global Days	Modifiers				
Mod	Non-Fac Total	Fac Total		51	50	62	80	MUE
	23.13	2.67	ZZZ	0	0	0	0	2

AMA: Mar 15: 5, May 14: 3, Jun 14: 14, May 15: 8

Excisional Breast Procedures

19100
Biopsy of breast; percutaneous, needle core, not using imaging guidance (separate procedure) A2T

RVU			Global Days	Modifiers				
Mod	Non-Fac Total	Fac Total		51	50	62	80	MUE
	4.28	2.02	000	2	1	0	1	4

AMA: Spring 93: 35, Fall 94: 18, Apr 96: 8, Mar 97: 4, Nov 97: 24, Nov 98: 7, Jan 01: 10, May 02: 18, Apr 05: 6, Dec 06: 10, Nov 08: 10, May 14: 3

19101
Biopsy of breast; open, incisional A2T

RVU			Global Days	Modifiers				
Mod	Non-Fac Total	Fac Total		51	50	62	80	MUE
	9.73	6.37	010	2	1	0	1	3

AMA: Spring 93: 35, Fall 94: 19, Nov 97: 24, Jan 01: 8, May 02: 18, Apr 05: 6, May 14: 3

19105
Ablation, cryosurgical, of fibroadenoma, including ultrasound guidance, each fibroadenoma P3T

RVU			Global Days	Modifiers				
Mod	Non-Fac Total	Fac Total		51	50	62	80	MUE
	60.59	5.60	000	2	1	0	1	2

19110
Nipple exploration, with or without excision of a solitary lactiferous duct or a papilloma lactiferous duct A2T

RVU			Global Days	Modifiers				
Mod	Non-Fac Total	Fac Total		51	50	62	80	MUE
	13.85	9.85	090	2	1	0	1	1

AMA: Apr 05: 6

19112
Excision of lactiferous duct fistula A2T

RVU			Global Days	Modifiers				
Mod	Non-Fac Total	Fac Total		51	50	62	80	MUE
	12.98	8.93	090	2	1	0	0	2

AMA: Apr 05: 6

19120
Excision of cyst, fibroadenoma, or other benign or malignant tumor, aberrant breast tissue, duct lesion, nipple or areolar lesion (except 19300), open, male or female, 1 or more lesions A2T

RVU			Global Days	Modifiers				
Mod	Non-Fac Total	Fac Total		51	50	62	80	MUE
	14.14	11.92	090	2	1	0	1	1

AMA: Feb 96: 9, Nov 97: 14, Jan 01: 8, May 01: 10, Apr 05: 6, 13, Mar 15: 5, Mar 14: 13

Excision of cyst, fibroadenoma, or other benign or malignant tumor, aberrant breast tissue

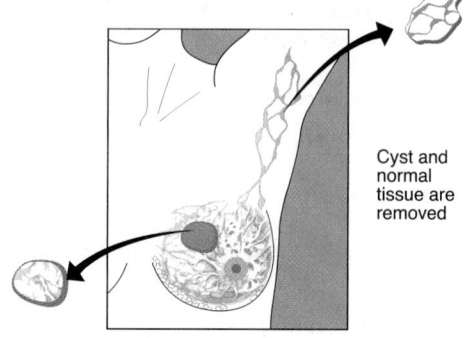

Cyst and normal tissue are removed

The physician excises one or more tumors, cysts, lesions, or fibroadenomas from the tissue of the breast.

19125
Excision of breast lesion identified by preoperative placement of radiological marker, open; single lesion A2T

RVU			Global Days	Modifiers				
Mod	Non-Fac Total	Fac Total		51	50	62	80	MUE
	15.68	13.24	090	2	1	1	1	1

AMA: Fall 94: 18, Mar 98: 10, Jan 01: 8, Apr 05: 6, Mar 09: 10, Mar 15: 5

+ 19126
Excision of breast lesion identified by preoperative placement of radiological marker, open; each additional lesion separately identified by a preoperative radiological marker (List separately in addition to code for primary procedure) NIN

RVU			Global Days	Modifiers				
Mod	Non-Fac Total	Fac Total		51	50	62	80	MUE
	4.70	4.70	ZZZ	0	0	1	1	3

AMA: Fall 94: 18, Mar 98: 10, Jan 01: 8, Apr 05: 6

19260   Excision of chest wall tumor including ribs   🅣

Mod	RVU Non-Fac Total	Fac Total	Global Days	Modifiers 51	50	62	80	MUE
	34.84	34.84	090	2	0	1	2	2

AMA: Apr 05: 6, 7, Apr 10: 3

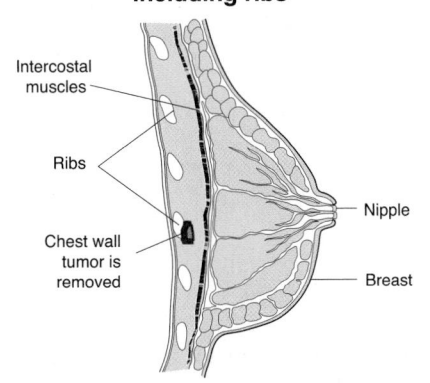

Excision of chest wall tumor including ribs

Intercostal muscles

Ribs

Chest wall tumor is removed

Nipple

Breast

Tumor and adjacent ribs (19260), with plastic reconstruction (19271), with mediastinal lymphadenectomy (19272)

19271   Excision of chest wall tumor involving ribs, with plastic reconstruction; without mediastinal lymphadenectomy   🅒

Mod	RVU Non-Fac Total	Fac Total	Global Days	Modifiers 51	50	62	80	MUE
	47.19	47.19	090	2	0	1	2	1

AMA: Apr 05: 6, 7

19272   Excision of chest wall tumor involving ribs, with plastic reconstruction; with mediastinal lymphadenectomy   🅒

Mod	RVU Non-Fac Total	Fac Total	Global Days	Modifiers 51	50	62	80	MUE
	51.52	51.52	090	2	0	1	2	1

AMA: Apr 05: 6, 7

19281   Placement of breast localization device(s) (eg, clip, metallic pellet, wire/needle, radioactive seeds), percutaneous; first lesion, including mammographic guidance   NIQI

Mod	RVU Non-Fac Total	Fac Total	Global Days	Modifiers 51	50	62	80	MUE
	6.78	2.92	000	2	1	0	0	1

AMA: May 14: 3, Jun 14: 14, May 15: 8

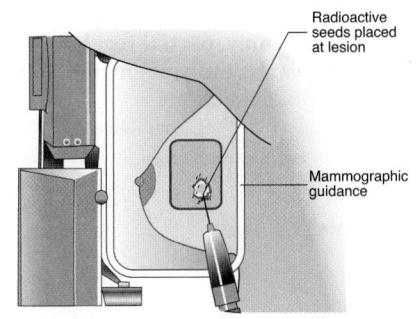

Placement of breast localization device(s), percutaneous, including mammographic guidance
First lesion (19281), each additional lesion (19282)

Radioactive seeds placed at lesion

Mammographic guidance

+ 19282   Placement of breast localization device(s) (eg, clip, metallic pellet, wire/needle, radioactive seeds), percutaneous; each additional lesion, including mammographic guidance (List separately in addition to code for primary procedure)   NIN

Mod	RVU Non-Fac Total	Fac Total	Global Days	Modifiers 51	50	62	80	MUE
	4.75	1.47	ZZZ	0	0	0	0	2

AMA: May 14: 3, Jun 14: 14, May 15: 8

19283   Placement of breast localization device(s) (eg, clip, metallic pellet, wire/needle, radioactive seeds), percutaneous; first lesion, including stereotactic guidance   NIQI

Mod	RVU Non-Fac Total	Fac Total	Global Days	Modifiers 51	50	62	80	MUE
	7.64	2.95	000	2	1	0	0	1

AMA: May 14: 3, May 15: 8

+ 19284   Placement of breast localization device(s) (eg, clip, metallic pellet, wire/needle, radioactive seeds), percutaneous; each additional lesion, including stereotactic guidance (List separately in addition to code for primary procedure)   NIN

Mod	RVU Non-Fac Total	Fac Total	Global Days	Modifiers 51	50	62	80	MUE
	5.76	1.49	ZZZ	0	0	0	0	2

AMA: May 14: 3, May 15: 8

19285   Placement of breast localization device(s) (eg, clip, metallic pellet, wire/needle, radioactive seeds), percutaneous; first lesion, including ultrasound guidance   NIQI

Mod	RVU Non-Fac Total	Fac Total	Global Days	Modifiers 51	50	62	80	MUE
	14.59	2.50	000	2	1	0	0	1

AMA: May 14: 3, May 15: 8

+ 19286   Placement of breast localization device(s) (eg, clip, metallic pellet, wire/needle, radioactive seeds), percutaneous; each additional lesion, including ultrasound guidance (List separately in addition to code for primary procedure)   NIN

Mod	RVU Non-Fac Total	Fac Total	Global Days	Modifiers 51	50	62	80	MUE
	12.81	1.25	ZZZ	0	0	0	0	2

AMA: May 14: 3, May 15: 8

19287   Placement of breast localization device(s) (eg clip, metallic pellet, wire/needle, radioactive seeds), percutaneous; first lesion, including magnetic resonance guidance   NIQI

Mod	RVU Non-Fac Total	Fac Total	Global Days	Modifiers 51	50	62	80	MUE
	24.39	3.76	000	2	1	0	0	1

AMA: May 14: 3

● New   ▲ Revised   Deleted   ⊙ Moderate Sedation   + Add-on Codes   ⊘ High Risk Denial   Ⓐ Age Edit   ♀ Female   ♂ Male   **AMA** *CPT® Assistant*   ***MUE*** Medically Unlikely Edit
⊘ Modifier 51 Exempt   ⊖ Modifier 63 Exempt   🅧 Unlisted   **Modifiers:** *See Inside Back Cover*   Ⓜ Maternity   A2–Z3 ASC Payment Indicators   A–Y OPPS Status Indicators

© 2016 DecisionHealth   CPT © 2015 American Medical Association. All Rights Reserved.

+ 19288 Placement of breast localization device(s) (eg clip, metallic pellet, wire/needle, radioactive seeds), percutaneous; each additional lesion, including magnetic resonance guidance (List separately in addition to code for primary procedure) N I N

	RVU			Global Days	Modifiers				
Mod	Non-Fac Total	Fac Total			51	50	62	80	MUE
	19.66	1.87	ZZZ		0	0	0	0	2

AMA: May 14: 3

19296 Placement of radiotherapy afterloading expandable catheter (single or multichannel) into the breast for interstitial radioelement application following partial mastectomy, includes imaging guidance; on date separate from partial mastectomy J 8 J 1

	RVU			Global Days	Modifiers				
Mod	Non-Fac Total	Fac Total			51	50	62	80	MUE
	112.31	6.11	000		2	1	0	0	1

AMA: Apr 05: 6, 8, Nov 05: 15, Apr 09: 3, Dec 09: 9, Mar 10: 10

+ 19297 Placement of radiotherapy afterloading expandable catheter (single or multichannel) into the breast for interstitial radioelement application following partial mastectomy, includes imaging guidance; concurrent with partial mastectomy (List separately in addition to code for primary procedure) N I N

	RVU			Global Days	Modifiers				
Mod	Non-Fac Total	Fac Total			51	50	62	80	MUE
	2.75	2.75	ZZZ		0	0	0	0	2

AMA: Apr 05: 6, 8, Nov 05: 15, Apr 09: 3, Mar 10: 10

⊙ 19298 Placement of radiotherapy afterloading brachytherapy catheters (multiple tube and button type) into the breast for interstitial radioelement application following (at the time of or subsequent to) partial mastectomy, includes imaging guidance J 8 J 1

	RVU			Global Days	Modifiers				
Mod	Non-Fac Total	Fac Total			51	50	62	80	MUE
	29.49	9.40	000		2	1	0	0	1

AMA: Apr 05: 6, 7, 9, 16, Nov 05: 15, Apr 09: 3, Mar 10: 10

Placement of radiotherapy afterloading brachytherapy catheters

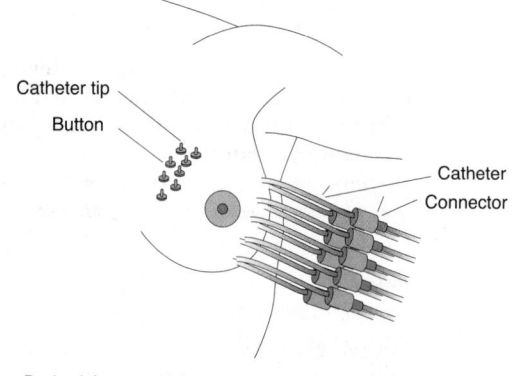

During/after a partial mastectomy, tubes are positioned into remaining cancerous tissue with needles.

Mastectomies

Coding Guidance

Mastectomy codes describe removal of breast tissue including all lesions within the breast tissue. Breast biopsy and excision codes (10021-10022, 19100-19126) generally are not separately reportable unless performed at a site unrelated to the mastectomy. An exception is a diagnostic biopsy or breast lesion excision procedure performed for the purpose of pathological examination to determine the necessity of a more definitive procedure. In this case, the breast biopsy/excision and mastectomy codes are separately reportable. Modifier 58 may be used to indicate a staged procedure. However, if a diagnosis was established preoperatively, the biopsy/excision procedure is not reported separately. An excision procedure for the purpose of obtaining additional pathologic material is not reported separately. For mastectomy codes described as with lymphadenectomy and/or removal of muscle tissues, lymph node excision of the specified lymph node chains on the same side (ipsilateral) are not separately reportable. Lymph node excisions on the opposite side (contralateral) may be reported separately with the appropriate anatomical modifiers (LT, RT). Sentinel lymph node biopsy is separately reportable when performed prior to a mastectomy without lymphadenectomy. Sentinel lymph node biopsy is not separately reportable with a mastectomy procedure that includes lymphadenectomy in the anatomic area of the sentinel lymph node biopsy.

19300 Mastectomy for gynecomastia ♂ A 2 T

	RVU			Global Days	Modifiers				
Mod	Non-Fac Total	Fac Total			51	50	62	80	MUE
	14.98	11.90	090		2	1	0	1	1

AMA: Feb 07: 4, Mar 14: 13

19301 Mastectomy, partial (eg, lumpectomy, tylectomy, quadrantectomy, segmentectomy) A 2 T

	RVU			Global Days	Modifiers				
Mod	Non-Fac Total	Fac Total			51	50	62	80	MUE
	18.86	18.86	090		2	1	0	0	1

AMA: Feb 07: 4, Dec 07: 8, Sep 08: 5, Mar 10: 10, Mar 15: 5, Nov 13: 14

Partial Mastectomy

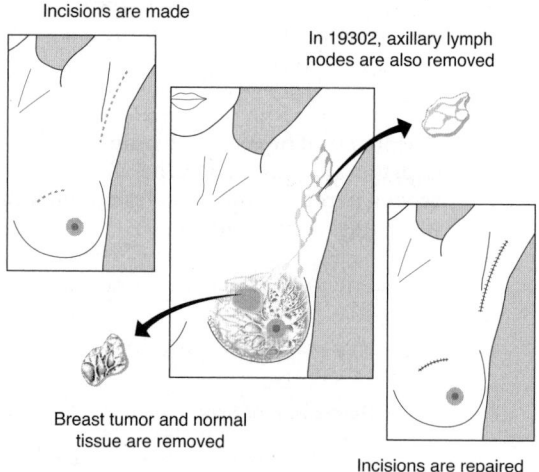

Incisions are made

In 19302, axillary lymph nodes are also removed

Breast tumor and normal tissue are removed

Incisions are repaired

19302 Mastectomy, partial (eg, lumpectomy, tylectomy, quadrantectomy, segmentectomy); with axillary lymphadenectomy A 2 T

	RVU			Global Days	Modifiers				
Mod	Non-Fac Total	Fac Total			51	50	62	80	MUE
	25.94	25.94	090		2	1	1	2	1

AMA: Feb 07: 4, Dec 07: 8, Sep 08: 5, Mar 10: 10, Mar 15: 5

● New   ▲ Revised   ✖ Deleted   ⊙ Moderate Sedation   ✚ Add-on Codes   ⊘ High Risk Denial   Ⓐ Age Edit   ♀ Female   ♂ Male   **AMA** *CPT® Assistant*   **MUE** Medically Unlikely Edit
⊘ Modifier 51 Exempt   ⊖ Modifier 63 Exempt   ✗ Unlisted   **Modifiers:** *See Inside Back Cover*   Ⓜ Maternity   A 2 - Z 3 ASC Payment Indicators   A - Y OPPS Status Indicators

CPT © 2015 American Medical Association. All Rights Reserved.

© 2016 DecisionHealth

19303 Mastectomy, simple, complete   A2 T

Mod	Non-Fac Total	Fac Total	Global Days	51	50	62	80	MUE
	29.17	29.17	090	2	1	1	2	1

AMA: Feb 07: 4, Mar 15: 5

19304 Mastectomy, subcutaneous   A2 T

Mod	Non-Fac Total	Fac Total	Global Days	51	50	62	80	MUE
	16.53	16.53	090	2	1	1	2	1

AMA: Feb 07: 4, Dec 07: 7, 8

19305 Mastectomy, radical, including pectoral muscles, axillary lymph nodes   C

Mod	Non-Fac Total	Fac Total	Global Days	51	50	62	80	MUE
	32.56	32.56	090	2	1	1	2	1

AMA: Feb 07: 4, Sep 08: 5

19306 Mastectomy, radical, including pectoral muscles, axillary and internal mammary lymph nodes (Urban type operation)   C

Mod	Non-Fac Total	Fac Total	Global Days	51	50	62	80	MUE
	34.62	34.62	090	2	1	1	2	1

AMA: Feb 07: 4, Sep 08: 5

19307 Mastectomy, modified radical, including axillary lymph nodes, with or without pectoralis minor muscle, but excluding pectoralis major muscle   T

Mod	Non-Fac Total	Fac Total	Global Days	51	50	62	80	MUE
	34.53	34.53	090	2	1	1	2	1

AMA: Feb 07: 4, Sep 08: 5, Mar 15: 5

Breast Repair/Reconstruction Procedures

19316 Mastopexy   A2 T

Mod	Non-Fac Total	Fac Total	Global Days	51	50	62	80	MUE
	22.25	22.25	090	2	1	1	2	1

AMA: Jan 03: 7, Apr 05: 6, Feb 12: 11

19318 Reduction mammaplasty   A2 T

Mod	Non-Fac Total	Fac Total	Global Days	51	50	62	80	MUE
	31.97	31.97	090	2	1	1	2	1

AMA: Jan 03: 7, Apr 05: 6, Apr 14: 10

19324 Mammaplasty, augmentation; without prosthetic implant   A2 T

Mod	Non-Fac Total	Fac Total	Global Days	51	50	62	80	MUE
	14.10	14.10	090	2	1	0	0	1

AMA: Apr 05: 6

19325 Mammaplasty, augmentation; with prosthetic implant   J8 J1

Mod	Non-Fac Total	Fac Total	Global Days	51	50	62	80	MUE
	18.56	18.56	090	2	1	0	0	1

AMA: Apr 05: 6

19328 Removal of intact mammary implant   A2 Q2

Mod	Non-Fac Total	Fac Total	Global Days	51	50	62	80	MUE
	14.38	14.38	090	2	1	0	1	1

AMA: Apr 05: 6

19330 Removal of mammary implant material   A2 Q2

Mod	Non-Fac Total	Fac Total	Global Days	51	50	62	80	MUE
	18.40	18.40	090	2	1	0	1	1

AMA: Nov 01: 11, Apr 05: 6

Coding Guidance

Breast reconstruction codes that include the insertion of a prosthetic implant should not be reported with codes that separately describe the insertion of a breast prosthesis.

19340 Immediate insertion of breast prosthesis following mastopexy, mastectomy or in reconstruction   A2 T

Mod	Non-Fac Total	Fac Total	Global Days	51	50	62	80	MUE
	29.14	29.14	090	2	1	1	1	1

AMA: Aug 96: 8, Apr 05: 6, Aug 05: 1, Mar 10: 9

19342 Delayed insertion of breast prosthesis following mastopexy, mastectomy or in reconstruction   J8 J1

Mod	Non-Fac Total	Fac Total	Global Days	51	50	62	80	MUE
	26.78	26.78	090	2	1	1	0	1

AMA: Aug 96: 8, Apr 05: 6, Aug 05: 1, Jan 13: 15

19350 Nipple/areola reconstruction   A2 T

Mod	Non-Fac Total	Fac Total	Global Days	51	50	62	80	MUE
	23.78	19.54	090	2	1	0	1	1

AMA: Aug 96: 11, Apr 05: 6, Jan 13: 15

19355 Correction of inverted nipples   ⊘ A2 T

Mod	Non-Fac Total	Fac Total	Global Days	51	50	62	80	MUE
	20.14	16.50	090	2	1	0	0	1

AMA: Apr 05: 6

19357 Breast reconstruction, immediate or delayed, with tissue expander, including subsequent expansion   J8 J1

Mod	Non-Fac Total	Fac Total	Global Days	51	50	62	80	MUE
	43.68	43.68	090	2	1	1	2	1

AMA: Winter 91: 2, Apr 05: 6, Aug 05: 1, Mar 10: 9, Oct 13: 15, Feb 15: 10

19361 Breast reconstruction with latissimus dorsi flap, without prosthetic implant   C

Mod	Non-Fac Total	Fac Total	Global Days	51	50	62	80	MUE
	45.69	45.69	090	2	1	1	2	1

AMA: Apr 05: 6, Aug 05: 1, Mar 10: 9, Feb 15: 10

19364 Breast reconstruction with free flap   C

Mod	Non-Fac Total	Fac Total	Global Days	51	50	62	80	MUE
	80.13	80.13	090	2	1	1	2	1

AMA: Aug 96: 8, Nov 98: 7, Apr 05: 6, Aug 05: 1, Dec 11: 14, Jun 10: 8, Jul 12: 12, Mar 13: 13, Apr 14: 10, Feb 15: 10

● New   ▲ Revised   Deleted   ⊙ Moderate Sedation   ✚ Add-on Codes   ⊘ High Risk Denial   Ⓐ Age Edit   ♀ Female   ♂ Male   **AMA** *CPT® Assistant*   **MUE** Medically Unlikely Edit
⊘ Modifier 51 Exempt   ⊖ Modifier 63 Exempt   ✗ Unlisted   **Modifiers:** *See Inside Back Cover*   Ⓜ Maternity   A2–Z3 ASC Payment Indicators   A–Y OPPS Status Indicators

Surgical Procedures

19366 – 19499

19366 Breast reconstruction with other technique `A 2 T`

Mod	Non-Fac Total	Fac Total	Global Days	51	50	62	80	MUE
	40.73	40.73	090	2	1	1	2	1

AMA: Aug 96: 8, Nov 98: 7, Apr 05: 6, Apr 14: 10, Dec 11: 14, Feb 15: 10

19367 Breast reconstruction with transverse rectus abdominis myocutaneous flap (TRAM), single pedicle, including closure of donor site `C`

Mod	Non-Fac Total	Fac Total	Global Days	51	50	62	80	MUE
	51.95	51.95	090	2	1	1	2	1

AMA: Nov 98: 7, Apr 05: 6, Aug 05: 1, Feb 15: 10

19368 Breast reconstruction with transverse rectus abdominis myocutaneous flap (TRAM), single pedicle, including closure of donor site; with microvascular anastomosis (supercharging) `C`

Mod	Non-Fac Total	Fac Total	Global Days	51	50	62	80	MUE
	64.06	64.06	090	2	1	1	2	1

AMA: Nov 98: 7, Apr 05: 6, Aug 05: 1, Feb 15: 10

19369 Breast reconstruction with transverse rectus abdominis myocutaneous flap (TRAM), double pedicle, including closure of donor site `C`

Mod	Non-Fac Total	Fac Total	Global Days	51	50	62	80	MUE
	59.29	59.29	090	2	1	1	2	1

AMA: Oct 00: 3, Apr 05: 6, Aug 05: 1, Feb 15: 10

19370 Open periprosthetic capsulotomy, breast `A 2 T`

Mod	Non-Fac Total	Fac Total	Global Days	51	50	62	80	MUE
	19.92	19.92	090	2	1	0	1	1

AMA: Aug 96: 8, Apr 05: 6

19371 Periprosthetic capsulectomy, breast `A 2 T`

Mod	Non-Fac Total	Fac Total	Global Days	51	50	62	80	MUE
	22.76	22.76	090	2	1	0	1	1

AMA: Aug 96: 8, Nov 01: 11, Apr 05: 6, Jan 13: 15

19380 Revision of reconstructed breast `A 2 T`

Mod	Non-Fac Total	Fac Total	Global Days	51	50	62	80	MUE
	22.44	22.44	090	2	1	0	1	1

AMA: Apr 05: 6

19396 Preparation of moulage for custom breast implant `G 2 T`

Mod	Non-Fac Total	Fac Total	Global Days	51	50	62	80	MUE
	7.97	4.07	000	2	1	0	0	1

AMA: Jan 03: 7, Apr 05: 6

Other Breast Procedures

19499 Unlisted procedure, breast `⊗ x T`

Mod	Non-Fac Total	Fac Total	Global Days	51	50	62	80	MUE
	0.00	0.00	YYY	2	1	1	0	

AMA: Apr 05: 6, Dec 09: 9, Nov 13: 14, Dec 14: 16

● New   ▲ Revised   ✖ Deleted   ⊙ Moderate Sedation   ✚ Add-on Codes   ⊘ High Risk Denial   Ⓐ Age Edit   ♀ Female   ♂ Male   **AMA** *CPT® Assistant*   **MUE** Medically Unlikely Edit
⊘ Modifier 51 Exempt   ⊖ Modifier 63 Exempt   ✗ Unlisted   **Modifiers:** *See Inside Back Cover*   Ⓜ Maternity   `A 2`–`Z 3` ASC Payment Indicators   `A`–`Y` OPPS Status Indicators

CPT © 2015 American Medical Association. All Rights Reserved.
© 2016 DecisionHealth

Musculoskeletal Procedures

Musculoskeletal Surgical Procedures 20005-29999

Musculoskeletal codes include those performed on bones, joints, muscles, fascia and other related soft tissue, tendons, ligaments, and traumatic wound exploration. The codes are organized first by body site, e.g., hand and fingers, shoulder, pelvis and hip joint, then by type of procedure, e.g., excision, incision, introduction/removal, manipulation, repair/reconstruction, fracture/dislocation, osteotomy, arthrodesis.

Fractures/dislocations must be coded by the type of treatment—closed, open, or percutaneous fixation—used for reduction and fixation or stabilization. The type of fracture itself has no coding relevancy.

Skeletal traction applies a distraction or pulling force to a limb through a screw, wire, pin, or clamp device penetrated into the bone.

External fixation is the application of bone pins that are attached to an external mechanical device for healing/stabilizing.

Spinal procedures are organized by the type, e.g., excision, osteotomy, fracture/dislocation, arthrodesis, spinal instrumentation, the level or number of segments, e.g., thoracic, lumbar, and by the approach, e.g., lateral extracavitary, anterior, posterolateral.

Basic Musculoskeletal Procedures

Musculoskeletal Incisional Procedures

20005 **Incision and drainage of soft tissue abscess, subfascial (ie, involves the soft tissue below the deep fascia)** `G2 T`

Coding tip: Report debridement separately when gross contamination requires prolonged cleansing or removal of extensive amounts of devitalized tissue

Coding tip: For debridement of soft tissue associated with other conditions - 11042-11043, 11045-11046

Coding tip: For debridement of soft tissue associated with open fractures or dislocations - 11010-11011

RVU		Global Days	Modifiers				
Mod	*Non-Fac Total*	*Fac Total*		51	50	62	80	MUE
	8.84	6.72	010	2	0	0	1	4

Traumatic Wound Exploration Procedures

20100 **Exploration of penetrating wound (separate procedure); neck** `T`

RVU		Global Days	Modifiers				
Mod	*Non-Fac Total*	*Fac Total*		51	50	62	80	MUE
	17.59	17.59	010	2	1	0	2	2

AMA: Jun 96: 7, Aug 96: 10, Sep 06: 13

Exploration of penetrating wound

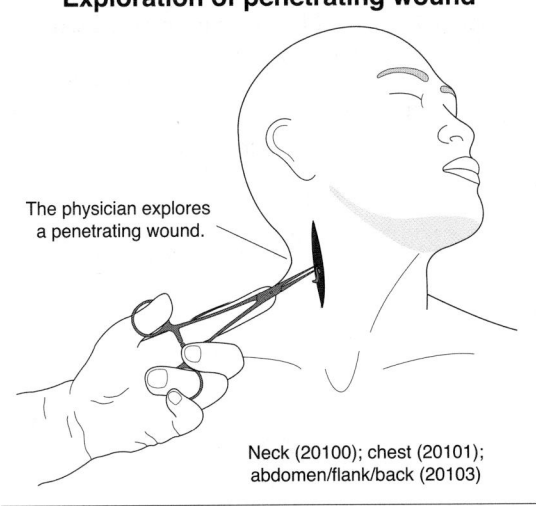

The physician explores a penetrating wound.

Neck (20100); chest (20101); abdomen/flank/back (20103)

20101 **Exploration of penetrating wound (separate procedure); chest** `T`

RVU		Global Days	Modifiers				
Mod	*Non-Fac Total*	*Fac Total*		51	50	62	80	MUE
	12.79	6.04	010	2	0	0	1	2

AMA: Jun 96: 7, Sep 06: 13

20102 **Exploration of penetrating wound (separate procedure); abdomen/flank/back** `T`

RVU		Global Days	Modifiers				
Mod	*Non-Fac Total*	*Fac Total*		51	50	62	80	MUE
	14.04	7.39	010	2	0	0	1	3

AMA: Jun 96: 7, Sep 06: 13

20103 **Exploration of penetrating wound (separate procedure); extremity** `G2 T`

RVU		Global Days	Modifiers				
Mod	*Non-Fac Total*	*Fac Total*		51	50	62	80	MUE
	16.73	10.08	010	2	0	0	0	4

AMA: Jun 96: 7, Aug 96: 10, Sep 06: 13

Excisional/Biopsy Procedures

20150 **Excision of epiphyseal bar, with or without autogenous soft tissue graft obtained through same fascial incision** `G2 T`

RVU		Global Days	Modifiers				
Mod	*Non-Fac Total*	*Fac Total*		51	50	62	80	MUE
	26.14	26.14	090	2	1	1	2	2

Excision of epiphyseal bar

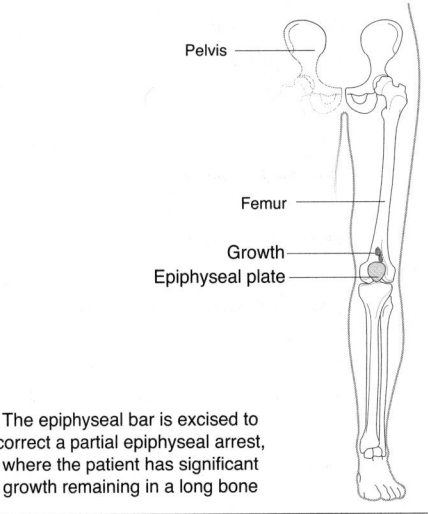

Pelvis

Femur

Growth
Epiphyseal plate

The epiphyseal bar is excised to correct a partial epiphyseal arrest, where the patient has significant growth remaining in a long bone

20200 **Biopsy, muscle; superficial** `A2 T`

Coding tip: Code 99000 for specimen transfer from office setting to an outside laboratory

RVU		Global Days	Modifiers				
Mod	*Non-Fac Total*	*Fac Total*		51	50	62	80	MUE
	5.91	2.77	000	2	0	0	1	2

● New   ▲ Revised   Deleted   ☉ Moderate Sedation   ✚ Add-on Codes   ⊘ High Risk Denial   Ⓐ Age Edit   ♀ Female   ♂ Male   **AMA** *CPT® Assistant*   **MUE** Medically Unlikely Edit
⊘ Modifier 51 Exempt   ⊖ Modifier 63 Exempt   ☒ Unlisted   **Modifiers:** *See Inside Back Cover*   Ⓜ Maternity   A2–Z3 ASC Payment Indicators   A–Y OPPS Status Indicators

Surgical Procedures

20205 – 20525

20205 Biopsy, muscle; deep `A2 T`

Coding tip: Code 99001 for specimen transfer from a facility to an outside laboratory

Coding tip: For excision of foreign body in muscle, deep - 20525

RVU			Global Days	Modifiers				
Mod	Non-Fac Total	Fac Total		51	50	62	80	MUE
	8.26	4.51	000	2	0	0	1	4

20206 Biopsy, muscle, percutaneous needle `A2 T`

Coding tip: Report an additional code for radiological needle guidance - ultrasound 76942, fluoroscopy 77002, CT 77012, MRI 77021

RVU			Global Days	Modifiers				
Mod	Non-Fac Total	Fac Total		51	50	62	80	MUE
	6.70	1.71	000	2	0	0	1	3

Coding Guidance

Use 88307 for the surgical pathology evaluation of bone matrix structure. Do not report code 38221 for bone marrow biopsy together with code 20220 for bone biopsy. When it is necessary to evaluate both bone matrix structure and bone marrow, only one code can be reported: either 38221 or 20220. If two separate biopsies are required at separate sites, both codes may be reported using modifier 59 on one code. If only one specimen is submitted for pathological evaluation, only one interpretation code may be reported, whether or not the report includes a morphological evaluation of both bone structure and bone marrow.

20220 Biopsy, bone, trocar, or needle; superficial (eg, ilium, sternum, spinous process, ribs) `A2 T`

RVU			Global Days	Modifiers				
Mod	Non-Fac Total	Fac Total		51	50	62	80	MUE
	4.78	2.10	000	2	0	0	1	4

AMA: Winter 92: 17, Jul 98: 4

20225 Biopsy, bone, trocar, or needle; deep (eg, vertebral body, femur) `A2 T`

Coding tip: Code 99000 for specimen transfer from a facility to an outside laboratory

RVU			Global Days	Modifiers				
Mod	Non-Fac Total	Fac Total		51	50	62	80	MUE
	14.92	3.14	000	2	0	0	1	4

AMA: Winter 92: 17, Jul 98: 4, Jun 12: 10, Jan 15: 8

20240 Biopsy, bone, open; superficial (eg, ilium, sternum, spinous process, ribs, trochanter of femur) `A2 T`

RVU			Global Days	Modifiers				
Mod	Non-Fac Total	Fac Total		51	50	62	80	MUE
	4.48	4.48	010	2	0	0	1	4

AMA: Winter 92: 17, Jul 98: 4, Aug 04: 11, Aug 05: 13

Open bone biopsy

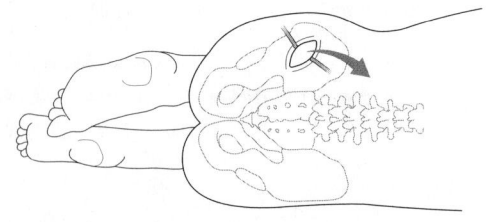

A sample of bone is obtained through an incision

20245 Biopsy, bone, open; deep (eg, humerus, ischium, femur) `A2 T`

Coding tip: Code 99001 for specimen transfer from a facility to an outside laboratory

RVU			Global Days	Modifiers				
Mod	Non-Fac Total	Fac Total		51	50	62	80	MUE
	14.88	14.88	010	2	0	0	1	4

AMA: Winter 92: 17, Jul 98: 4

20250 Biopsy, vertebral body, open; thoracic `A2 T`

RVU			Global Days	Modifiers				
Mod	Non-Fac Total	Fac Total		51	50	62	80	MUE
	11.33	11.33	010	2	0	0	1	3

AMA: Winter 92: 17, Jul 98: 4

20251 Biopsy, vertebral body, open; lumbar or cervical `A2 T`

Coding tip: Code 99001 for specimen transfer from a facility to an outside laboratory

RVU			Global Days	Modifiers				
Mod	Non-Fac Total	Fac Total		51	50	62	80	MUE
	12.23	12.23	010	2	0	0	2	3

AMA: Winter 92: 17, Jul 98: 4

Introduction/Injection/Removal

20500 Injection of sinus tract; therapeutic (separate procedure) `P3 T`

Coding tip: Therapeutic injection code 20500 should not be used to report administration of local anesthesia for a procedure.

RVU			Global Days	Modifiers				
Mod	Non-Fac Total	Fac Total		51	50	62	80	MUE
	2.96	2.42	010	2	0	0	1	2

20501 Injection of sinus tract; diagnostic (sinogram) `N I N`

Coding tip: Report the radiological portion of the diagnostic examination with 76080

RVU			Global Days	Modifiers				
Mod	Non-Fac Total	Fac Total		51	50	62	80	MUE
	3.35	1.10	000	2	0	0	1	2

20520 Removal of foreign body in muscle or tendon sheath; simple `P3 T`

RVU			Global Days	Modifiers				
Mod	Non-Fac Total	Fac Total		51	50	62	80	MUE
	5.80	4.21	010	2	0	0	1	4

20525 Removal of foreign body in muscle or tendon sheath; deep or complicated `A2 T`

RVU			Global Days	Modifiers				
Mod	Non-Fac Total	Fac Total		51	50	62	80	MUE
	13.77	7.18	010	2	0	0	1	4

● New   ▲ Revised   ✖ Deleted   ⊙ Moderate Sedation   ✛ Add-on Codes   ⊘ High Risk Denial   Ⓐ Age Edit   ♀ Female   ♂ Male   **AMA** *CPT® Assistant*   **MUE** Medically Unlikely Edit
⊘ Modifier 51 Exempt   ⊖ Modifier 63 Exempt   ⓍUnlisted   **Modifiers:** *See Inside Back Cover*   Ⓜ Maternity   `A2`–`Z3` ASC Payment Indicators   `A`–`Y` OPPS Status Indicators

212   CPT © 2015 American Medical Association. All Rights Reserved.   © 2016 DecisionHealth

20526 Injection, therapeutic (eg, local anesthetic, corticosteroid), carpal tunnel P 3 T

Coding tip: Therapeutic injection codes 20526 should not be used to report administration of local anesthesia for a separately reportable procedure.

Coding tip: Injection into tendon - 20550-20551; trigger points - 20552-20553

RVU			Global Days	Modifiers				
Mod	Non-Fac Total	Fac Total		51	50	62	80	MUE
	2.21	1.66	000	2	1	0	1	1

AMA: Mar 02: 7

20527 Injection, enzyme (eg, collagenase), palmar fascial cord (ie, Dupuytren's contracture) P 3 T

RVU			Global Days	Modifiers				
Mod	Non-Fac Total	Fac Total		51	50	62	80	MUE
	2.42	1.93	000	2	1	0	1	2

AMA: Jul 12: 8, 14

Coding Guidance

Therapeutic injection codes 20550-20553 should not be used to report administration of local anesthesia for a separately reportable procedure.

20550 Injection(s); single tendon sheath, or ligament, aponeurosis (eg, plantar "fascia") P 3 T

RVU			Global Days	Modifiers				
Mod	Non-Fac Total	Fac Total		51	50	62	80	MUE
	1.68	1.20	000	2	1	0	1	5

AMA: Jan 96: 7, Jun 98: 10, Mar 02: 7, Aug 03: 14, Sep 03: 13, Dec 03: 11, Jan 09: 6, Jul 12: 14, Oct 14: 9

Injections

Plantar fascia

Achilles tendon

Aponeurosis

A therapeutic agent is injected into a single tendon sheath, ligament or aponeurosis

A therapeutic agent is injected into a tendon origin or insertion point

20551 Injection(s); single tendon origin/insertion P 3 T

Coding tip: Report an additional code with injection procedures that require radiological needle guidance - ultrasound 76942; fluoroscopy 77002; CT 77012; MRI 77021

RVU			Global Days	Modifiers				
Mod	Non-Fac Total	Fac Total		51	50	62	80	MUE
	1.73	1.23	000	2	0	0	1	5

AMA: Mar 02: 7, Sep 03: 13, Oct 14: 9

20552 Injection(s); single or multiple trigger point(s), 1 or 2 muscle(s) P 3 T

RVU			Global Days	Modifiers				
Mod	Non-Fac Total	Fac Total		51	50	62	80	MUE
	1.57	1.09	000	2	0	0	1	1

AMA: Mar 02: 7, May 03: 19, Sep 03: 11, Feb 10: 9, Jul 11: 16, Feb 11: 5, Apr 12: 19, Oct 14: 9

Injection

An anesthetic or therapeutic solution is injected into one or more trigger points in one or more muscles

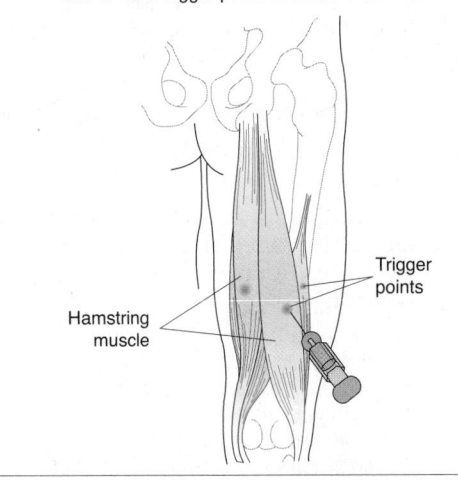

Trigger points

Hamstring muscle

20553 Injection(s); single or multiple trigger point(s), 3 or more muscles P 3 T

RVU			Global Days	Modifiers				
Mod	Non-Fac Total	Fac Total		51	50	62	80	MUE
	1.81	1.24	000	2	0	0	1	1

AMA: Mar 02: 7, May 03: 19, Sep 03: 11, Jun 08: 8, Feb 10: 9, Jul 11: 16, Feb 11: 5, Oct 14: 9

20555 Placement of needles or catheters into muscle and/or soft tissue for subsequent interstitial radioelement application (at the time of or subsequent to the procedure) R 2 T

Coding tip: Report an additional code when correct placement of the needles or catheters requires radiological guidance - ultrasound 76942; fluoroscopy 77002; CT 77012; MRI 77021

RVU			Global Days	Modifiers				
Mod	Non-Fac Total	Fac Total		51	50	62	80	MUE
	9.43	9.43	000	2	0	0	0	1

AMA: Feb 08: 8

● New ▲ Revised Deleted ⊙ Moderate Sedation ✛ Add-on Codes ⊘ High Risk Denial Ⓐ Age Edit ♀ Female ♂ Male **AMA** *CPT® Assistant* **MUE** Medically Unlikely Edit
⊘ Modifier 51 Exempt ⊖ Modifier 63 Exempt ✗ Unlisted **Modifiers:** *See Inside Back Cover* Ⓜ Maternity A 2 – Z 3 ASC Payment Indicators A – Y OPPS Status Indicators

Coding Guidance

Therapeutic injection/aspiration codes 20600-20610 should not be used to report administration of local anesthesia for a separately reportable procedure.

20600 Arthrocentesis, aspiration and/or injection, small joint or bursa (eg, fingers, toes); without ultrasound guidance `P 3 T`

Coding tip: Report an additional code for radiological needle guidance - ultrasound 76942, fluoroscopy 77002, CT 77012, MRI 77021

Documentation Finder: The procedure note or medical record documentation may detail the patient's condition as arthralgia, tenosynovitis, and chronic pain syndrome, among other types of inflammatory conditions and pain syndromes. If a drug is injected, the provider should document the name of the drug and the amount.

RVU			Global Days	Modifiers				
Mod	Non-Fac Total	Fac Total		51	50	62	80	MUE
	1.36	1.02	000	2	1	0	1	6

AMA: Dec 07: 10, Feb 15: 6

20604 Arthrocentesis, aspiration and/or injection, small joint or bursa (eg, fingers, toes); with ultrasound guidance, with permanent recording and reporting `P 3 T`

Documentation Finder: The procedure note or medical record documentation may detail the patient's condition as arthralgia, tenosynovitis, and chronic pain syndrome, among other types of inflammatory conditions and pain syndromes. If a drug is injected, the provider should document the name of the drug and the amount. Operative note should include a radiological report.

RVU			Global Days	Modifiers				
Mod	Non-Fac Total	Fac Total		51	50	62	80	MUE
	2.06	1.32	000	2	1	0	1	4

AMA: Feb 15: 6, Jul 15: 10

Arthrocentesis, aspiration and/or injection, small joint or bursa (eg, fingers, toes).

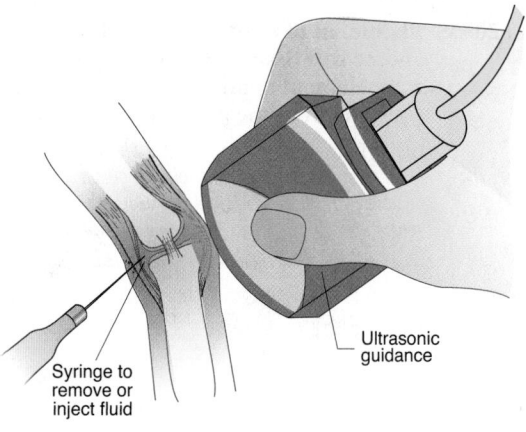

Syringe to remove or inject fluid

Ultrasonic guidance

20605 Arthrocentesis, aspiration and/or injection, intermediate joint or bursa (eg, temporomandibular, acromioclavicular, wrist, elbow or ankle, olecranon bursa); without ultrasound guidance `P 3 T`

Documentation Finder: The procedure note or medical record documentation may detail the patient's condition as arthralgia, tenosynovitis, and chronic pain syndrome, among other types of inflammatory conditions and pain syndromes. If a drug is injected, the provider should document the name of the drug and the amount.

RVU			Global Days	Modifiers				
Mod	Non-Fac Total	Fac Total		51	50	62	80	MUE
	1.43	1.07	000	2	1	0	1	4

AMA: Dec 07: 10, Feb 15: 6

20606 Arthrocentesis, aspiration and/or injection, intermediate joint or bursa (eg, temporomandibular, acromioclavicular, wrist, elbow or ankle, olecranon bursa); with ultrasound guidance, with permanent recording and reporting `P 3 T`

Documentation Finder: The procedure note or medical record documentation may detail the patient's condition as arthralgia, tenosynovitis, and chronic pain syndrome, among other types of inflammatory conditions and pain syndromes. If a drug is injected, the provider should document the name of the drug and the amount. Operative note should include a radiological report.

RVU			Global Days	Modifiers				
Mod	Non-Fac Total	Fac Total		51	50	62	80	MUE
	2.28	1.52	000	2	1	0	1	4

AMA: Feb 15: 6, Jul 15: 10

20610 Arthrocentesis, aspiration and/or injection, major joint or bursa (eg, shoulder, hip, knee, subacromial bursa); without ultrasound guidance `P 3 T`

Documentation Finder: The procedure note or medical record documentation may detail the patient's condition as arthralgia, tenosynovitis, and chronic pain syndrome, among other types of inflammatory conditions and pain syndromes. If a drug is injected, the provider should document the name of the drug and the amount.

RVU			Global Days	Modifiers				
Mod	Non-Fac Total	Fac Total		51	50	62	80	MUE
	1.72	1.33	000	2	1	0	1	4

AMA: Spring 92: 8, Mar 01: 10, Apr 04: 15, Jul 06: 1, Dec 07: 10, Jul 08: 9, Mar 12: 6, Jun 12: 14, Aug 15: 6, Dec 14: 18, Feb 15: 6

20611 Arthrocentesis, aspiration and/or injection, major joint or bursa (eg, shoulder, hip, knee, subacromial bursa); with ultrasound guidance, with permanent recording and reporting `P 3 T`

Documentation Finder: The procedure note or medical record documentation may detail the patient's condition as arthralgia, tenosynovitis, and chronic pain syndrome, among other types of inflammatory conditions and pain syndromes. If a drug is injected, the provider should document the name of the drug and the amount. Operative note should include a radiological report.

RVU			Global Days	Modifiers				
Mod	Non-Fac Total	Fac Total		51	50	62	80	MUE
	2.61	1.77	000	2	1	0	1	4

AMA: Feb 15: 6, Aug 15: 6, Jul 15: 10

CPT © 2015 American Medical Association. All Rights Reserved.   © 2016 DecisionHealth

20612 Aspiration and/or injection of ganglion cyst(s) any location P 3 T

RVU			Global Days	Modifiers				
Mod	Non-Fac Total	Fac Total		51	50	62	80	MUE
	1.73	1.21	000	2	0	0	1	2

20615 Aspiration and injection for treatment of bone cyst P 3 T

Coding tip: *Add radiologic guidance for needle placement for aspiration or injection of cyst - ultrasound 76942; fluoroscopy 77002; CT 77012; MRI 77021*

RVU			Global Days	Modifiers				
Mod	Non-Fac Total	Fac Total		51	50	62	80	MUE
	6.98	4.70	010	2	0	0	1	1

20650 Insertion of wire or pin with application of skeletal traction, including removal (separate procedure) A 2 T

RVU			Global Days	Modifiers				
Mod	Non-Fac Total	Fac Total		51	50	62	80	MUE
	5.96	4.53	010	2	0	1	1	4

20660 Application of cranial tongs, caliper, or stereotactic frame, including removal (separate procedure) ⊗ Q 2

RVU			Global Days	Modifiers				
Mod	Non-Fac Total	Fac Total		51	50	62	80	MUE
	7.14	7.14	000	2	0	0	1	1

AMA: Jun 96: 10, Nov 97: 14, Jan 06: 46, Dec 06: 10, Feb 08: 8, Jul 08: 10, Nov 09: 6, Apr 12: 11, Aug 12: 14

20661 Application of halo, including removal; cranial C

RVU			Global Days	Modifiers				
Mod	Non-Fac Total	Fac Total		51	50	62	80	MUE
	14.76	14.76	090	2	0	0	1	1

AMA: Nov 97: 14, Aug 12: 14

Application of halo

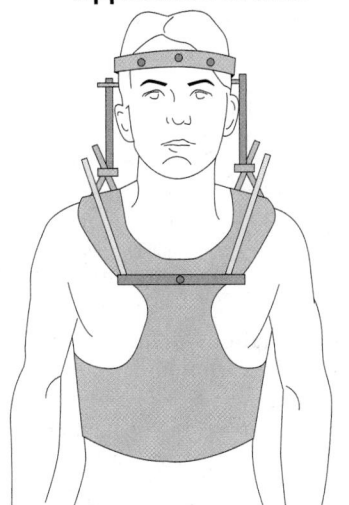

A halo is applied for stabilization of the spine. Code 20661 for a cranial halo; 20662 for a pelvic halo; and 20663 for a femoral halo

20662 Application of halo, including removal; pelvic ⊗ R 2 T

RVU			Global Days	Modifiers				
Mod	Non-Fac Total	Fac Total		51	50	62	80	MUE
	12.39	12.39	090	2	0	0	0	1

20663 Application of halo, including removal; femoral ⊗ R 2 T

RVU			Global Days	Modifiers				
Mod	Non-Fac Total	Fac Total		51	50	62	80	MUE
	13.54	13.54	090	2	1	0	0	1

20664 Application of halo, including removal, cranial, 6 or more pins placed, for thin skull osteology (eg, pediatric patients, hydrocephalus, osteogenesis imperfecta) C

RVU			Global Days	Modifiers				
Mod	Non-Fac Total	Fac Total		51	50	62	80	MUE
	25.56	25.56	090	2	0	0	1	1

AMA: Nov 97: 14, Aug 12: 5, Aug 13: 12

20665 Removal of tongs or halo applied by another individual G 2 Q 1

RVU			Global Days	Modifiers				
Mod	Non-Fac Total	Fac Total		51	50	62	80	MUE
	3.00	2.59	010	2	0	0	0	1

AMA: Apr 12: 12

Coding Guidance

When a buried wire, pin, rod, or other deep or superficial implant requires surgical removal, and the procedure is done separately, it may be reported. When the service is necessary for accomplishing another procedure in the same area, the implant removal may not be reported separately.

20670 Removal of implant; superficial (eg, buried wire, pin or rod) (separate procedure) A 2 Q 2

RVU			Global Days	Modifiers				
Mod	Non-Fac Total	Fac Total		51	50	62	80	MUE
	10.89	4.25	010	2	0	0	1	3

AMA: Dec 07: 7, 8, Jun 09: 7, Apr 12: 17

Removal of implant

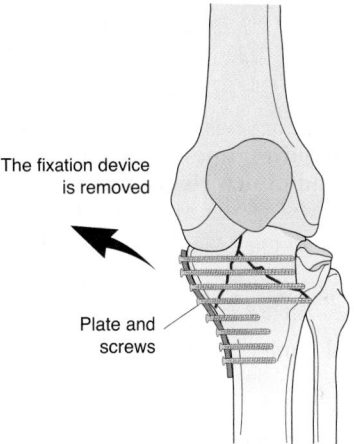

The fixation device is removed

Plate and screws

In 20670, a superficial implant is removed, such as a wire, pin or rod. After creating an incision at the site of the implant, the implant is unscrewed, or pulled out. Use code, 20680 if the implant is deep.

● New   ▲ Revised   Deleted   ⊙ Moderate Sedation   ✚ Add-on Codes   ⊘ High Risk Denial   Ⓐ Age Edit   ♀ Female   ♂ Male   **AMA** *CPT® Assistant*   ***MUE*** Medically Unlikely Edit
⊘ Modifier 51 Exempt   ⊖ Modifier 63 Exempt   ✖ Unlisted   **Modifiers:** *See Inside Back Cover*   Ⓜ Maternity   A 2 – Z 3 ASC Payment Indicators   A – Y OPPS Status Indicators

20680 Removal of implant; deep (eg, buried wire, pin, screw, metal band, nail, rod or plate) `A2 Q2`

Mod	RVU Non-Fac Total	Fac Total	Global Days	Modifiers 51	50	62	80	MUE
	17.75	12.23	090	2	0	0	0	3

AMA: Spring 92: 11, Jun 09: 7, Sep 12: 16, Mar 14: 4

20690 Application of a uniplane (pins or wires in 1 plane), unilateral, external fixation system `A2 J1`

Mod	RVU Non-Fac Total	Fac Total	Global Days	Modifiers 51	50	62	80	MUE
	17.20	17.20	090	2	0	0	1	2

AMA: Winter 90: 4, Winter 92: 11, Fall 93: 21, Oct 99: 5, Jan 04: 27, Jun 05: 12, Oct 07: 7, Jan 08: 4, Feb 08: 9, Jun 09: 7

Insertion of a uniplane/multiplane external fixation device

Use code 20693 if external fixation device is adjusted or revised and code 20694 if device is removed

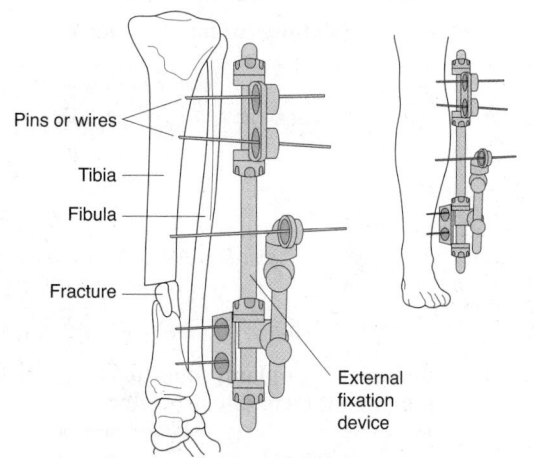

20692 Application of a multiplane (pins or wires in more than 1 plane), unilateral, external fixation system (eg, Ilizarov, Monticelli type) `A2 J1`

Mod	RVU Non-Fac Total	Fac Total	Global Days	Modifiers 51	50	62	80	MUE
	32.30	32.30	090	2	0	1	2	2

AMA: Winter 90: 4, Fall 93: 21, Oct 99: 5, Jul 00: 11, Feb 08: 9, Jun 09: 7

20693 Adjustment or revision of external fixation system requiring anesthesia (eg, new pin[s] or wire[s] and/or new ring[s] or bar[s]) `A2 T`

Mod	RVU Non-Fac Total	Fac Total	Global Days	Modifiers 51	50	62	80	MUE
	12.80	12.80	090	2	0	0	1	2

AMA: Fall 93: 21, Oct 99: 5, Jul 00: 11, Jun 09: 7

20694 Removal, under anesthesia, of external fixation system `A2 Q2`

Mod	RVU Non-Fac Total	Fac Total	Global Days	Modifiers 51	50	62	80	MUE
	12.14	9.70	090	2	0	0	1	2

AMA: Winter 92: 10, Fall 93: 21, Oct 99: 5, Jul 00: 11

20696 Application of multiplane (pins or wires in more than 1 plane), unilateral, external fixation with stereotactic computer-assisted adjustment (eg, spatial frame), including imaging; initial and subsequent alignment(s), assessment(s), and computation(s) of adjustment schedule(s) `J8 J1`

Mod	RVU Non-Fac Total	Fac Total	Global Days	Modifiers 51	50	62	80	MUE
	34.73	34.73	090	2	0	1	2	2

⊘ **20697** Application of multiplane (pins or wires in more than 1 plane), unilateral, external fixation with stereotactic computer-assisted adjustment (eg, spatial frame), including imaging; exchange (ie, removal and replacement) of strut, each ⊘ `P2 T`

Mod	RVU Non-Fac Total	Fac Total	Global Days	Modifiers 51	50	62	80	MUE
	56.67	56.67	000	0	0	1	2	4

Amputation Reattachment Procedures

20802 Replantation, arm (includes surgical neck of humerus through elbow joint), complete amputation `C`

Mod	RVU Non-Fac Total	Fac Total	Global Days	Modifiers 51	50	62	80	MUE
	69.36	69.36	090	2	1	1	2	1

Replantation of arm

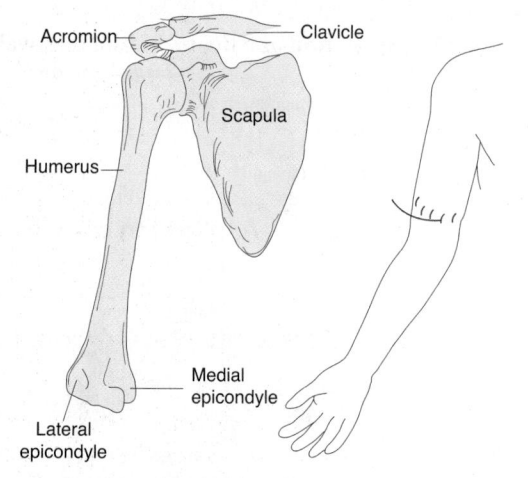

A replantation of an arm is performed, which has been completely amputated.

20805 Replantation, forearm (includes radius and ulna to radial carpal joint), complete amputation ⊘ `C`

Mod	RVU Non-Fac Total	Fac Total	Global Days	Modifiers 51	50	62	80	MUE
	95.86	95.86	090	2	1	1	2	1

20808 Replantation, hand (includes hand through metacarpophalangeal joints), complete amputation ⊘ `C`

Mod	RVU Non-Fac Total	Fac Total	Global Days	Modifiers 51	50	62	80	MUE
	116.77	116.77	090	2	1	1	2	1

● New   ▲ Revised   ✖ Deleted   ⊙ Moderate Sedation   ✚ Add-on Codes   ⊘ High Risk Denial   Ⓐ Age Edit   ♀ Female   ♂ Male   **AMA** CPT® Assistant   **MUE** Medically Unlikely Edit
⊘ Modifier 51 Exempt   ⊖ Modifier 63 Exempt   ✗ Unlisted   **Modifiers:** See Inside Back Cover   Ⓜ Maternity   `A2`–`Z3` ASC Payment Indicators   `A`–`Y` OPPS Status Indicators

216   CPT © 2015 American Medical Association. All Rights Reserved.   © 2016 DecisionHealth

Surgical Procedures   20680 — 20808

20816 Replantation, digit, excluding thumb (includes metacarpophalangeal joint to insertion of flexor sublimis tendon), complete amputation   C

RVU			Global Days	Modifiers				
Mod	Non-Fac Total	Fac Total		51	50	62	80	MUE
	60.04	60.04	090	2	0	1	2	3

AMA: Oct 96: 11

20822 Replantation, digit, excluding thumb (includes distal tip to sublimis tendon insertion), complete amputation   G2T

RVU			Global Days	Modifiers				
Mod	Non-Fac Total	Fac Total		51	50	62	80	MUE
	52.20	52.20	090	2	0	1	2	3

20824 Replantation, thumb (includes carpometacarpal joint to MP joint), complete amputation   C

RVU			Global Days	Modifiers				
Mod	Non-Fac Total	Fac Total		51	50	62	80	MUE
	59.42	59.42	090	2	1	1	2	1

20827 Replantation, thumb (includes distal tip to MP joint), complete amputation   C

RVU			Global Days	Modifiers				
Mod	Non-Fac Total	Fac Total		51	50	62	80	MUE
	53.00	53.00	090	2	1	1	2	1

20838 Replantation, foot, complete amputation   ⊙C

RVU			Global Days	Modifiers				
Mod	Non-Fac Total	Fac Total		51	50	62	80	MUE
	70.07	70.07	090	2	1	1	2	1

Grafting/Implantation

20900 Bone graft, any donor area; minor or small (eg, dowel or button)   A2T

RVU			Global Days	Modifiers				
Mod	Non-Fac Total	Fac Total		51	50	62	80	MUE
	11.94	5.47	000	2	0	1	2	2

AMA: Dec 00: 15, Jul 11: 18

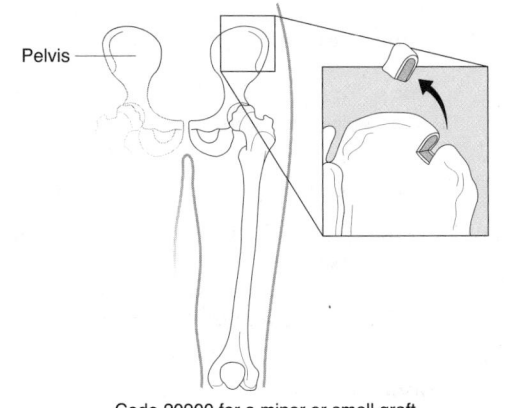

Bone graft from any donor area

Pelvis

Code 20900 for a minor or small graft.
Code 20902 for a large or major graft.

20902 Bone graft, any donor area; major or large   A2J1

RVU			Global Days	Modifiers				
Mod	Non-Fac Total	Fac Total		51	50	62	80	MUE
	8.25	8.25	000	2	0	1	2	2

AMA: Dec 00: 15, Jul 11: 18

20910 Cartilage graft; costochondral   A2T

RVU			Global Days	Modifiers				
Mod	Non-Fac Total	Fac Total		51	50	62	80	MUE
	11.82	11.82	090	2	0	0	0	1

AMA: Jan 13: 15

20912 Cartilage graft; nasal septum   A2T

RVU			Global Days	Modifiers				
Mod	Non-Fac Total	Fac Total		51	50	62	80	MUE
	13.89	13.89	090	2	0	0	0	1

20920 Fascia lata graft; by stripper   A2T

RVU			Global Days	Modifiers				
Mod	Non-Fac Total	Fac Total		51	50	62	80	MUE
	11.31	11.31	090	2	0	1	1	1

AMA: Aug 99: 5, Jan 05: 8

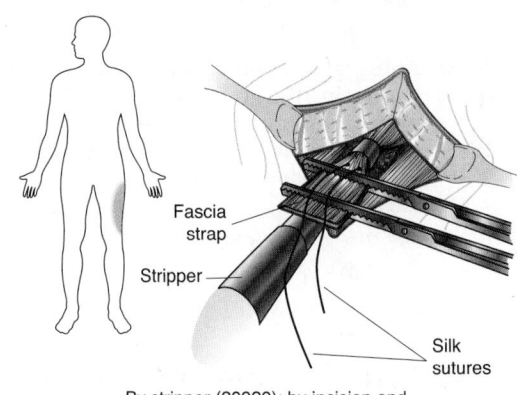

Fascia lata graft

Fascia strap

Stripper

Silk sutures

By stripper (20920); by incision and
area exposure, complex or sheet (20922)

20922 Fascia lata graft; by incision and area exposure, complex or sheet   A2T

RVU			Global Days	Modifiers				
Mod	Non-Fac Total	Fac Total		51	50	62	80	MUE
	17.98	14.82	090	2	0	1	2	1

AMA: Jan 05: 8

20924 Tendon graft, from a distance (eg, palmaris, toe extensor, plantaris)   A2T

RVU			Global Days	Modifiers				
Mod	Non-Fac Total	Fac Total		51	50	62	80	MUE
	14.51	14.51	090	2	0	1	2	2

Coding Guidance

Code 20926 is a general tissue grafting code for use when the primary procedure does not already include grafting in its description or when there is no other grafting code that more accurately describes the service done. Code 20926 should not be used with procedure codes where grafting is included or with other grafting codes.

● New   ▲ Revised   Deleted   ⊙ Moderate Sedation   ✚ Add-on Codes   ⊘ High Risk Denial   Ⓐ Age Edit   ♀ Female   ♂ Male   **AMA** *CPT® Assistant*   **MUE** Medically Unlikely Edit
⊘ Modifier 51 Exempt   ⊖ Modifier 63 Exempt   ✗ Unlisted   **Modifiers:** *See Inside Back Cover*   Ⓜ Maternity   A2–Z3 ASC Payment Indicators   A–Y OPPS Status Indicators

20926 Tissue grafts, other (eg, paratenon, fat, dermis)

`A2 T`

RVU			Global Days	Modifiers				
Mod	Non-Fac Total	Fac Total		51	50	62	80	MUE
	12.24	12.24	090	2	0	0	1	2

AMA: Summer 91: 12, Aug 99: 5, Nov 99: 10, May 06: 16, Jun 12: 15

+ 20930 Allograft, morselized, or placement of osteopromotive material, for spine surgery only (List separately in addition to code for primary procedure)

`⊘ N I N`

RVU			Global Days	Modifiers				
Mod	Non-Fac Total	Fac Total		51	50	62	80	MUE
	0.00	0.00	XXX	9	9	9	9	

AMA: Feb 96: 6, Mar 96: 4, Sep 97: 8, Nov 99: 10, Feb 02: 6, Jan 04: 27, Dec 07: 1, Feb 08: 8, Jul 11: 18, Dec 11: 15, Nov 10: 8, Apr 12: 14, Jun 12: 11, Jul 13: 3

+ 20931 Allograft, structural, for spine surgery only (List separately in addition to code for primary procedure)

`N I N`

RVU			Global Days	Modifiers				
Mod	Non-Fac Total	Fac Total		51	50	62	80	MUE
	3.30	3.30	ZZZ	0	0	1	1	1

AMA: Feb 96: 6, Feb 02: 6, Feb 05: 15, Feb 08: 8, Jul 11: 18, Sep 11: 12, Dec 11: 15, Nov 10: 8, Apr 12: 14, Jun 12: 11, Jul 13: 3

+ 20936 Autograft for spine surgery only (includes harvesting the graft); local (eg, ribs, spinous process, or laminar fragments) obtained from same incision (List separately in addition to code for primary procedure)

`⊘ N`

RVU			Global Days	Modifiers				
Mod	Non-Fac Total	Fac Total		51	50	62	80	MUE
	0.00	0.00	XXX	9	9	9	9	

AMA: Feb 96: 6, Sep 97: 8, Feb 02: 6, Feb 08: 8, Dec 11: 15, Apr 12: 14, Jun 12: 11, Jul 13: 3

+ 20937 Autograft for spine surgery only (includes harvesting the graft); morselized (through separate skin or fascial incision) (List separately in addition to code for primary procedure)

`N`

RVU			Global Days	Modifiers				
Mod	Non-Fac Total	Fac Total		51	50	62	80	MUE
	4.79	4.79	ZZZ	0	0	1	2	1

AMA: Feb 96: 6, Sep 97: 8, Dec 99: 2, Feb 02: 6, Feb 08: 8, Dec 11: 15, Apr 12: 11, Jun 12: 11, Jul 13: 3

+ 20938 Autograft for spine surgery only (includes harvesting the graft); structural, bicortical or tricortical (through separate skin or fascial incision) (List separately in addition to code for primary procedure)

`N`

RVU			Global Days	Modifiers				
Mod	Non-Fac Total	Fac Total		51	50	62	80	MUE
	5.30	5.30	ZZZ	0	0	1	2	1

AMA: Feb 96: 6, Mar 96: 5, Sep 97: 8, Feb 02: 6, Feb 08: 8, Jul 11: 18, Dec 11: 15, Apr 12: 12, May 12: 11, Jun 12: 11, Jul 13: 3

Other General Musculoskeletal Procedures

20950 Monitoring of interstitial fluid pressure (includes insertion of device, eg, wick catheter technique, needle manometer technique) in detection of muscle compartment syndrome

`G2 T`

Coding tip: During the postoperative period following some procedures monitoring of interstitial fluid pressure is routinely performed (e.g., distal lower extremity procedures). Code 20950 should not be reported separately for routine postoperative monitoring.

RVU			Global Days	Modifiers				
Mod	Non-Fac Total	Fac Total		51	50	62	80	MUE
	7.22	2.64	000	2	0	0	0	2

AMA: Sep 07: 10

Monitoring of interstitial fluid pressure

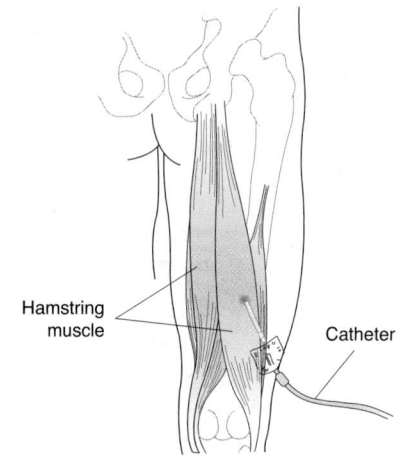

Hamstring muscle

Catheter

An interstitial fluid pressure monitoring device is inserted into a muscle compartment.

20955 Bone graft with microvascular anastomosis; fibula

`C`

RVU			Global Days	Modifiers				
Mod	Non-Fac Total	Fac Total		51	50	62	80	MUE
	72.79	72.79	090	2	0	1	2	1

AMA: Apr 97: 4

20956 Bone graft with microvascular anastomosis; iliac crest

`C`

RVU			Global Days	Modifiers				
Mod	Non-Fac Total	Fac Total		51	50	62	80	MUE
	77.03	77.03	090	2	0	1	2	1

AMA: Apr 97: 4

20957 Bone graft with microvascular anastomosis; metatarsal

`C`

RVU			Global Days	Modifiers				
Mod	Non-Fac Total	Fac Total		51	50	62	80	MUE
	71.07	71.07	090	2	0	1	2	1

AMA: Apr 97: 4

20962 Bone graft with microvascular anastomosis; other than fibula, iliac crest, or metatarsal

`C`

RVU			Global Days	Modifiers				
Mod	Non-Fac Total	Fac Total		51	50	62	80	MUE
	61.23	61.23	090	2	0	1	2	1

AMA: Apr 97: 4

● New   ▲ Revised   ✖ Deleted   ⊙ Moderate Sedation   ✚ Add-on Codes   ⊘ High Risk Denial   ⓐ Age Edit   ♀ Female   ♂ Male   **AMA** CPT® Assistant   **MUE** Medically Unlikely Edit

⊘ Modifier 51 Exempt   ⊖ Modifier 63 Exempt   ⓧ Unlisted   **Modifiers:** See Inside Back Cover   Ⓜ Maternity   `A2`–`Z3` ASC Payment Indicators   `A`–`Y` OPPS Status Indicators

20969 Free osteocutaneous flap with microvascular anastomosis; other than iliac crest, metatarsal, or great toe   C

RVU			Global Days	Modifiers				
Mod	Non-Fac Total	Fac Total		51	50	62	80	MUE
	80.33	80.33	090	2	0	1	2	2

AMA: Apr 97: 4

Free osteocutaneous flap with microvascular anastomosis

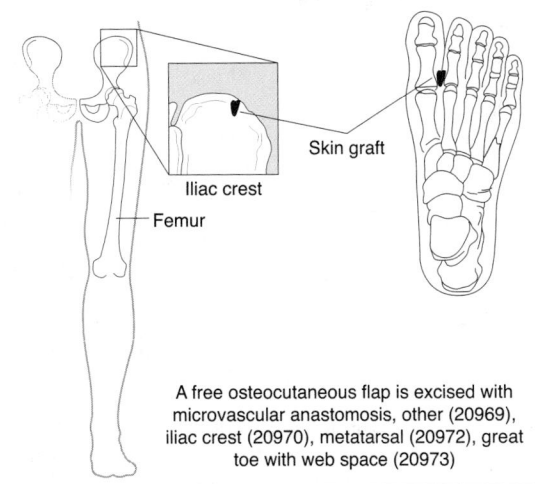

Skin graft
Iliac crest
Femur

A free osteocutaneous flap is excised with microvascular anastomosis, other (20969), iliac crest (20970), metatarsal (20972), great toe with web space (20973)

20970 Free osteocutaneous flap with microvascular anastomosis; iliac crest   C

RVU			Global Days	Modifiers				
Mod	Non-Fac Total	Fac Total		51	50	62	80	MUE
	84.92	84.92	090	2	0	1	2	1

AMA: Apr 97: 4

20972 Free osteocutaneous flap with microvascular anastomosis; metatarsal   G2J1

RVU			Global Days	Modifiers				
Mod	Non-Fac Total	Fac Total		51	50	62	80	MUE
	67.99	67.99	090	2	0	0	2	2

AMA: Apr 97: 4

20973 Free osteocutaneous flap with microvascular anastomosis; great toe with web space   R2J1

RVU			Global Days	Modifiers				
Mod	Non-Fac Total	Fac Total		51	50	62	80	MUE
	76.26	76.26	090	2	1	1	2	1

AMA: Apr 97: 4

⊘ **20974** Electrical stimulation to aid bone healing; noninvasive (nonoperative)   A

RVU			Global Days	Modifiers				
Mod	Non-Fac Total	Fac Total		51	50	62	80	MUE
	2.19	1.45	000	0	0	0	1	1

AMA: Sep 96: 11, Nov 00: 8

⊘ **20975** Electrical stimulation to aid bone healing; invasive (operative)   N1N

RVU			Global Days	Modifiers				
Mod	Non-Fac Total	Fac Total		51	50	62	80	MUE
	5.09	5.09	000	0	0	1	2	1

AMA: Nov 00: 8

20979 Low intensity ultrasound stimulation to aid bone healing, noninvasive (nonoperative)   N1Q1

RVU			Global Days	Modifiers				
Mod	Non-Fac Total	Fac Total		51	50	62	80	MUE
	1.49	0.93	000	0	0	0	1	1

AMA: Nov 99: 10, Nov 00: 8
Pub 100-04, 32, 110.3

⊙ **20982** Ablation therapy for reduction or eradication of 1 or more bone tumors (eg, metastasis) including adjacent soft tissue when involved by tumor extension, percutaneous, including imaging guidance when performed; radiofrequency   G2T

Documentation Finder: Cryoablation is sometimes referred to as percutaneous ablation, cryosurgery or cryotherapy.

RVU			Global Days	Modifiers				
Mod	Non-Fac Total	Fac Total		51	50	62	80	MUE
	85.83	11.03	000	2	1	0	1	1

AMA: Jul 15: 8

⊙ **20983** Ablation therapy for reduction or eradication of 1 or more bone tumors (eg, metastasis) including adjacent soft tissue when involved by tumor extension, percutaneous, including imaging guidance when performed; cryoablation   G2T

RVU			Global Days	Modifiers				
Mod	Non-Fac Total	Fac Total		51	50	62	80	MUE
	207.53	11.81	000	2	1	0	1	1

AMA: Jul 15: 8

Ablation therapy for bone tumors (eg, metastasis)
including adjacent soft tissue, percutaneous, and imaging guidance when performed; cryoablation

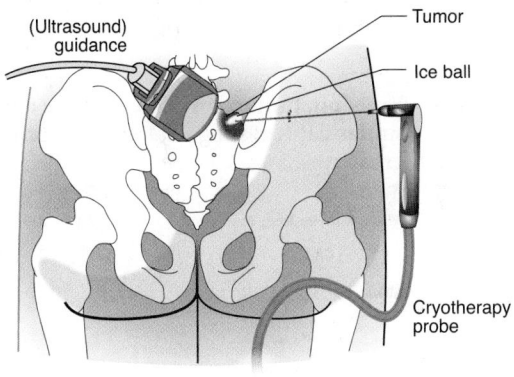

(Ultrasound) guidance
Tumor
Ice ball
Cryotherapy probe

+ **20985** Computer-assisted surgical navigational procedure for musculoskeletal procedures, image-less (List separately in addition to code for primary procedure)   N1N

RVU			Global Days	Modifiers				
Mod	Non-Fac Total	Fac Total		51	50	62	80	MUE
	4.27	4.27	ZZZ	0	0	0	0	2

AMA: Jul 11: 12

● New   ▲ Revised   Deleted   ⊙ Moderate Sedation   ✚ Add-on Codes   ⊘ High Risk Denial   Ⓐ Age Edit   ♀ Female   ♂ Male   **AMA** *CPT® Assistant*   **MUE** Medically Unlikely Edit
⊘ Modifier 51 Exempt   ⊖ Modifier 63 Exempt   Ⓧ Unlisted   **Modifiers:** *See Inside Back Cover*   Ⓜ Maternity   A2–Z3 ASC Payment Indicators   A–Y OPPS Status Indicators

Surgical Procedures

20999 – 21030

20999 Unlisted procedure, musculoskeletal system, general ⊗xT

RVU			Global Days	Modifiers				
Mod	Non-Fac Total	Fac Total		51	50	62	80	MUE
	0.00	0.00	YYY	2	0	1	0	

AMA: Sep 03: 13, Jul 15: 8

Musculoskeletal Head/Skull/Face Procedures

Head/Skull/Face Incisional Procedures

21010 Arthrotomy, temporomandibular joint A2JT

RVU			Global Days	Modifiers				
Mod	Non-Fac Total	Fac Total		51	50	62	80	MUE
	21.46	21.46	090	2	1	0	0	1

Head/Skull/Face Excisional Procedures

21011 Excision, tumor, soft tissue of face or scalp, subcutaneous; less than 2 cm P3T

RVU			Global Days	Modifiers				
Mod	Non-Fac Total	Fac Total		51	50	62	80	MUE
	10.00	7.49	090	2	0	0	2	4

AMA: Apr 10: 3, Feb 10: 3

21012 Excision, tumor, soft tissue of face or scalp, subcutaneous; 2 cm or greater R2T

RVU			Global Days	Modifiers				
Mod	Non-Fac Total	Fac Total		51	50	62	80	MUE
	9.78	9.78	090	2	0	0	2	3

AMA: Apr 10: 3, Feb 10: 3

21013 Excision, tumor, soft tissue of face and scalp, subfascial (eg, subgaleal, intramuscular); less than 2 cm P3T

RVU			Global Days	Modifiers				
Mod	Non-Fac Total	Fac Total		51	50	62	80	MUE
	14.94	11.62	090	2	0	0	2	4

AMA: Apr 10: 3, Feb 10: 3

21014 Excision, tumor, soft tissue of face and scalp, subfascial (eg, subgaleal, intramuscular); 2 cm or greater R2T

RVU			Global Days	Modifiers				
Mod	Non-Fac Total	Fac Total		51	50	62	80	MUE
	15.08	15.08	090	2	0	0	2	3

AMA: Apr 10: 3, Feb 10: 3

21015 Radical resection of tumor (eg, sarcoma), soft tissue of face or scalp; less than 2 cm G2T

RVU			Global Days	Modifiers				
Mod	Non-Fac Total	Fac Total		51	50	62	80	MUE
	20.58	20.58	090	2	0	0	1	1

AMA: Apr 10: 3, Feb 10: 3

Radical resection of tumor

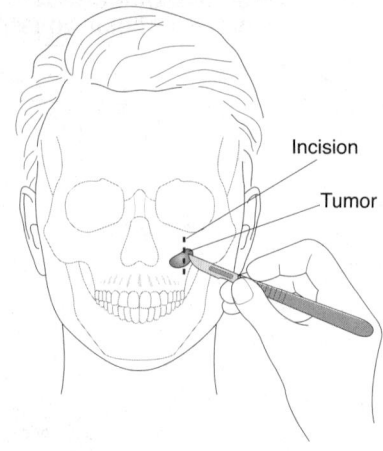

Both the tumor and its surrounding tissues are excised.
Less than (21015), or greater than (21016) 2 Cm.

21016 Radical resection of tumor (eg, sarcoma), soft tissue of face or scalp; 2 cm or greater G2T

RVU			Global Days	Modifiers				
Mod	Non-Fac Total	Fac Total		51	50	62	80	MUE
	29.70	29.70	090	2	0	0	2	2

AMA: Feb 10: 3, Apr 10: 3

21025 Excision of bone (eg, for osteomyelitis or bone abscess); mandible A2JT

RVU			Global Days	Modifiers				
Mod	Non-Fac Total	Fac Total		51	50	62	80	MUE
	25.97	21.98	090	2	0	0	1	2

AMA: Oct 11: 10

21026 Excision of bone (eg, for osteomyelitis or bone abscess); facial bone(s) A2T

RVU			Global Days	Modifiers				
Mod	Non-Fac Total	Fac Total		51	50	62	80	MUE
	17.98	14.57	090	2	0	0	1	2

21029 Removal by contouring of benign tumor of facial bone (eg, fibrous dysplasia) A2T

RVU			Global Days	Modifiers				
Mod	Non-Fac Total	Fac Total		51	50	62	80	MUE
	22.25	18.57	090	2	0	0	0	1

21030 Excision of benign tumor or cyst of maxilla or zygoma by enucleation and curettage P3T

RVU			Global Days	Modifiers				
Mod	Non-Fac Total	Fac Total		51	50	62	80	MUE
	15.10	12.22	090	2	1	0	1	1

AMA: Nov 03: 9

● New ▲ Revised ✖ Deleted ⊙ Moderate Sedation ✚ Add-on Codes ⊘ High Risk Denial Ⓐ Age Edit ♀ Female ♂ Male **AMA** CPT® Assistant **MUE** Medically Unlikely Edit
⊘ Modifier 51 Exempt ⊖ Modifier 63 Exempt ✖ Unlisted **Modifiers:** See Inside Back Cover Ⓜ Maternity A2–Z3 ASC Payment Indicators A–Y OPPS Status Indicators

220   CPT © 2015 American Medical Association. All Rights Reserved.   © 2016 DecisionHealth

21031 Excision of torus mandibularis ⊙ P 3 T

RVU			Global Days	Modifiers				
Mod	Non-Fac Total	Fac Total		51	50	62	80	MUE
	11.48	8.64	090	2	1	0	1	2

21032 Excision of maxillary torus palatinus P 3 T

RVU			Global Days	Modifiers				
Mod	Non-Fac Total	Fac Total		51	50	62	80	MUE
	11.67	8.55	090	2	0	0	1	1

21034 Excision of malignant tumor of maxilla or zygoma A 2 J 1

RVU			Global Days	Modifiers				
Mod	Non-Fac Total	Fac Total		51	50	62	80	MUE
	38.13	33.66	090	2	0	1	2	1

AMA: Nov 03: 9

21040 Excision of benign tumor or cyst of mandible, by enucleation and/or curettage A 2 T

RVU			Global Days	Modifiers				
Mod	Non-Fac Total	Fac Total		51	50	62	80	MUE
	15.22	12.24	090	2	0	0	1	2

AMA: Nov 03: 9

21044 Excision of malignant tumor of mandible A 2 J 1

RVU			Global Days	Modifiers				
Mod	Non-Fac Total	Fac Total		51	50	62	80	MUE
	25.47	25.47	090	2	0	1	2	1

21045 Excision of malignant tumor of mandible; radical resection C

RVU			Global Days	Modifiers				
Mod	Non-Fac Total	Fac Total		51	50	62	80	MUE
	35.75	35.75	090	2	0	1	2	1

21046 Excision of benign tumor or cyst of mandible; requiring intra-oral osteotomy (eg, locally aggressive or destructive lesion[s]) A 2 J 1

RVU			Global Days	Modifiers				
Mod	Non-Fac Total	Fac Total		51	50	62	80	MUE
	32.70	32.70	090	2	0	1	0	2

AMA: Nov 03: 9

21047 Excision of benign tumor or cyst of mandible; requiring extra-oral osteotomy and partial mandibulectomy (eg, locally aggressive or destructive lesion[s]) A 2 J 1

RVU			Global Days	Modifiers				
Mod	Non-Fac Total	Fac Total		51	50	62	80	MUE
	38.57	38.57	090	2	0	1	2	2

AMA: Nov 03: 9

21048 Excision of benign tumor or cyst of maxilla; requiring intra-oral osteotomy (eg, locally aggressive or destructive lesion[s]) R 2 J 1

RVU			Global Days	Modifiers				
Mod	Non-Fac Total	Fac Total		51	50	62	80	MUE
	33.52	33.52	090	2	0	1	0	2

AMA: Nov 03: 9

21049 Excision of benign tumor or cyst of maxilla; requiring extra-oral osteotomy and partial maxillectomy (eg, locally aggressive or destructive lesion[s]) J 1

RVU			Global Days	Modifiers				
Mod	Non-Fac Total	Fac Total		51	50	62	80	MUE
	35.16	35.16	090	2	0	1	2	1

AMA: Nov 03: 9

21050 Condylectomy, temporomandibular joint (separate procedure) A 2 J 1

RVU			Global Days	Modifiers				
Mod	Non-Fac Total	Fac Total		51	50	62	80	MUE
	24.46	24.46	090	2	1	0	0	1

21060 Meniscectomy, partial or complete, temporomandibular joint (separate procedure) ⊙ A 2 J 1

RVU			Global Days	Modifiers				
Mod	Non-Fac Total	Fac Total		51	50	62	80	MUE
	23.16	23.16	090	2	1	1	2	1

21070 Coronoidectomy (separate procedure) A 2 J 1

RVU			Global Days	Modifiers				
Mod	Non-Fac Total	Fac Total		51	50	62	80	MUE
	17.68	17.68	090	2	1	0	0	1

Manipulation Procedures

21073 Manipulation of temporomandibular joint(s) (TMJ), therapeutic, requiring an anesthesia service (ie, general or monitored anesthesia care) P 3 T

RVU			Global Days	Modifiers				
Mod	Non-Fac Total	Fac Total		51	50	62	80	MUE
	11.23	7.39	090	2	1	0	0	1

AMA: Feb 08: 9

Head Prostheses Impression and Preparation

21076 Impression and custom preparation; surgical obturator prosthesis P 2 T

RVU			Global Days	Modifiers				
Mod	Non-Fac Total	Fac Total		51	50	62	80	MUE
	29.24	24.57	010	2	0	0	0	1

21077 Impression and custom preparation; orbital prosthesis P 3 J 1

RVU			Global Days	Modifiers				
Mod	Non-Fac Total	Fac Total		51	50	62	80	MUE
	73.31	61.68	090	2	1	0	0	1

21079 Impression and custom preparation; interim obturator prosthesis P 3 J 1

RVU			Global Days	Modifiers				
Mod	Non-Fac Total	Fac Total		51	50	62	80	MUE
	49.36	41.08	090	2	0	0	1	1

AMA: Winter 90: 5, Sep 06: 13, Dec 06: 10

21080 Impression and custom preparation; definitive obturator prosthesis P 3 J 1

RVU			Global Days	Modifiers				
Mod	Non-Fac Total	Fac Total		51	50	62	80	MUE
	55.39	45.72	090	2	0	0	1	1

AMA: Winter 90: 5, Sep 06: 13, Dec 06: 10

● New   ▲ Revised   Deleted   ⊙ Moderate Sedation   ✚ Add-on Codes   ⊘ High Risk Denial   ⒶAge Edit   ♀ Female   ♂ Male   **AMA** CPT® Assistant   **MUE** Medically Unlikely Edit
⊘ Modifier 51 Exempt   ⊖ Modifier 63 Exempt   ✗ Unlisted   **Modifiers:** See Inside Back Cover   Ⓜ Maternity   A 2 – Z 3 ASC Payment Indicators   A – Y OPPS Status Indicators
© 2016 DecisionHealth   CPT © 2015 American Medical Association. All Rights Reserved.   **221**

Surgical Procedures

21081   Impression and custom preparation; mandibular resection prosthesis P 3 J I

RVU			Global Days	Modifiers				
Mod	Non-Fac Total	Fac Total		51	50	62	80	MUE
	51.15	42.06	090	2	0	0	0	1

AMA: Winter 90: 5, Sep 06: 13, Dec 06: 10

21082   Impression and custom preparation; palatal augmentation prosthesis P 3 J I

RVU			Global Days	Modifiers				
Mod	Non-Fac Total	Fac Total		51	50	62	80	MUE
	48.34	39.46	090	2	0	0	0	1

AMA: Winter 90: 5, Sep 06: 13, Dec 06: 10

21083   Impression and custom preparation; palatal lift prosthesis P 3 J I

RVU			Global Days	Modifiers				
Mod	Non-Fac Total	Fac Total		51	50	62	80	MUE
	46.03	36.59	090	2	0	0	0	1

AMA: Winter 90: 5, Sep 06: 13, Dec 06: 10

21084   Impression and custom preparation; speech aid prosthesis P 3 J I

RVU			Global Days	Modifiers				
Mod	Non-Fac Total	Fac Total		51	50	62	80	MUE
	52.95	42.48	090	2	0	0	0	1

AMA: Winter 90: 5, Sep 06: 13, Dec 06: 10

21085   Impression and custom preparation; oral surgical splint P 2 T

RVU			Global Days	Modifiers				
Mod	Non-Fac Total	Fac Total		51	50	62	80	MUE
	22.16	16.65	010	2	0	0	0	1

AMA: Winter 90: 5, Sep 06: 13, Dec 06: 10

21086   Impression and custom preparation; auricular prosthesis P 3 J I

RVU			Global Days	Modifiers				
Mod	Non-Fac Total	Fac Total		51	50	62	80	MUE
	54.53	45.71	090	2	1	0	0	1

AMA: Winter 90: 5, Sep 06: 13, Dec 06: 10

21087   Impression and custom preparation; nasal prosthesis P 3 J I

RVU			Global Days	Modifiers				
Mod	Non-Fac Total	Fac Total		51	50	62	80	MUE
	54.44	45.61	090	2	0	0	0	1

AMA: Winter 90: 5, Sep 06: 13, Dec 06: 10

21088   Impression and custom preparation; facial prosthesis R 2 J I

RVU			Global Days	Modifiers				
Mod	Non-Fac Total	Fac Total		51	50	62	80	MUE
	0.00	0.00	090	0	0	0	0	1

AMA: Winter 90: 5, Sep 06: 13, Dec 06: 10

21089   Unlisted maxillofacial prosthetic procedure ⊘ x T

RVU			Global Days	Modifiers				
Mod	Non-Fac Total	Fac Total		51	50	62	80	MUE
	0.00	0.00	YYY	0	0		1	1

AMA: Winter 90: 5, Sep 06: 13, Dec 06: 10

Head Introduction/Removal Procedures

21100   Application of halo type appliance for maxillofacial fixation, includes removal (separate procedure) A 2 J I

RVU			Global Days	Modifiers				
Mod	Non-Fac Total	Fac Total		51	50	62	80	MUE
	29.78	14.56	090	2	0	0	0	1

21110   Application of interdental fixation device for conditions other than fracture or dislocation, includes removal P 2 Q 2

RVU			Global Days	Modifiers				
Mod	Non-Fac Total	Fac Total		51	50	62	80	MUE
	23.42	19.66	090	2	0	0	1	2

AMA: Mar 97: 10, Dec 13: 16

21116   Injection procedure for temporomandibular joint arthrography N I N

RVU			Global Days	Modifiers				
Mod	Non-Fac Total	Fac Total		51	50	62	80	MUE
	4.16	1.27	000	2	1	0	1	1

AMA: Aug 15: 6

Head Repair/Revision/Reconstruction Procedures

21120   Genioplasty; augmentation (autograft, allograft, prosthetic material) A 2 J I

RVU			Global Days	Modifiers				
Mod	Non-Fac Total	Fac Total		51	50	62	80	MUE
	19.07	15.13	090	2	0	1	1	1

Genioplasty

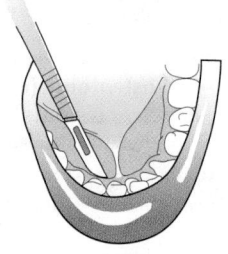 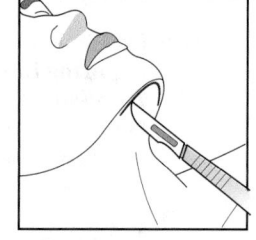

Incision inside mouth   Incision under chin

For augmentation (21120); for sliding osteo, single (21121); for sliding osteotomies, 2 or more (21122); for sliding, augmentation (21123)

21121   Genioplasty; sliding osteotomy, single piece ⊘ A 2 T

RVU			Global Days	Modifiers				
Mod	Non-Fac Total	Fac Total		51	50	62	80	MUE
	23.63	19.75	090	2	0	0	2	1

21122   Genioplasty; sliding osteotomies, 2 or more osteotomies (eg, wedge excision or bone wedge reversal for asymmetrical chin) A 2 T

RVU			Global Days	Modifiers				
Mod	Non-Fac Total	Fac Total		51	50	62	80	MUE
	19.04	19.04	090	2	0	0	2	1

● New   ▲ Revised   ✖ Deleted   ⊙ Moderate Sedation   ✚ Add-on Codes   ⊘ High Risk Denial   ⓐ Age Edit   ♀ Female   ♂ Male   **AMA** *CPT® Assistant*   **MUE** Medically Unlikely Edit
⊘ Modifier 51 Exempt   ⊖ Modifier 63 Exempt   x̶ Unlisted   **Modifiers:** *See Inside Back Cover*   Ⓜ Maternity   A2–Z3 ASC Payment Indicators   A–Y OPPS Status Indicators

21123 Genioplasty; sliding, augmentation with interpositional bone grafts (includes obtaining autografts)　A2 T

RVU			Global Days	Modifiers				
Mod	Non-Fac Total	Fac Total		51	50	62	80	MUE
	27.43	27.43	090	2	0	1	2	1

21125 Augmentation, mandibular body or angle; prosthetic material　A2 T

RVU			Global Days	Modifiers				
Mod	Non-Fac Total	Fac Total		51	50	62	80	MUE
	87.87	22.83	090	2	0	0	2	2

21127 Augmentation, mandibular body or angle; with bone graft, onlay or interpositional (includes obtaining autograft)　⊗A2 J1

RVU			Global Days	Modifiers				
Mod	Non-Fac Total	Fac Total		51	50	62	80	MUE
	128.02	26.14	090	2	0	1	2	2

21137 Reduction forehead; contouring only　G2 T

RVU			Global Days	Modifiers				
Mod	Non-Fac Total	Fac Total		51	50	62	80	MUE
	22.03	22.03	090	2	0	0	2	1

21138 Reduction forehead; contouring and application of prosthetic material or bone graft (includes obtaining autograft)　G2 J1

RVU			Global Days	Modifiers				
Mod	Non-Fac Total	Fac Total		51	50	62	80	MUE
	25.76	25.76	090	2	0	1	2	1

21139 Reduction forehead; contouring and setback of anterior frontal sinus wall　G2 J1

RVU			Global Days	Modifiers				
Mod	Non-Fac Total	Fac Total		51	50	62	80	MUE
	27.49	27.49	090	2	0	1	2	1

21141 Reconstruction midface, LeFort I; single piece, segment movement in any direction (eg, for Long Face Syndrome), without bone graft　C

RVU			Global Days	Modifiers				
Mod	Non-Fac Total	Fac Total		51	50	62	80	MUE
	39.14	39.14	090	2	0	1	2	1

21142 Reconstruction midface, LeFort I; 2 pieces, segment movement in any direction, without bone graft　C

RVU			Global Days	Modifiers				
Mod	Non-Fac Total	Fac Total		51	50	62	80	MUE
	41.09	41.09	090	2	0	1	2	1

21143 Reconstruction midface, LeFort I; 3 or more pieces, segment movement in any direction, without bone graft　C

RVU			Global Days	Modifiers				
Mod	Non-Fac Total	Fac Total		51	50	62	80	MUE
	41.29	41.29	090	2	0	1	2	1

21145 Reconstruction midface, LeFort I; single piece, segment movement in any direction, requiring bone grafts (includes obtaining autografts)　C

RVU			Global Days	Modifiers				
Mod	Non-Fac Total	Fac Total		51	50	62	80	MUE
	45.98	45.98	090	2	0	0	2	1

Reconstruction midface; LeFort I
(Segment movement in any direction requiring bone grafts, includes obtaining autograft)

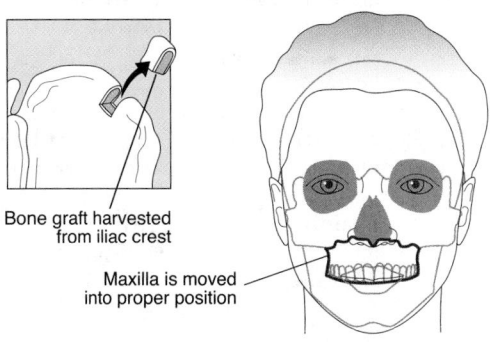

Bone graft harvested from iliac crest

Maxilla is moved into proper position

For single piece (21145); for 2 pieces (21146); and for 3 or more pieces (21147)

21146 Reconstruction midface, LeFort I; 2 pieces, segment movement in any direction, requiring bone grafts (includes obtaining autografts) (eg, ungrafted unilateral alveolar cleft)　C

RVU			Global Days	Modifiers				
Mod	Non-Fac Total	Fac Total		51	50	62	80	MUE
	44.86	44.86	090	2	0	1	2	1

21147 Reconstruction midface, LeFort I; 3 or more pieces, segment movement in any direction, requiring bone grafts (includes obtaining autografts) (eg, ungrafted bilateral alveolar cleft or multiple osteotomies)　⊗C

RVU			Global Days	Modifiers				
Mod	Non-Fac Total	Fac Total		51	50	62	80	MUE
	50.99	50.99	090	2	0	0	2	1

21150 Reconstruction midface, LeFort II; anterior intrusion (eg, Treacher-Collins Syndrome)　G2 J1

RVU			Global Days	Modifiers				
Mod	Non-Fac Total	Fac Total		51	50	62	80	MUE
	48.71	48.71	090	2	0	0	2	1

21151 Reconstruction midface, LeFort II; any direction, requiring bone grafts (includes obtaining autografts)　C

RVU			Global Days	Modifiers				
Mod	Non-Fac Total	Fac Total		51	50	62	80	MUE
	59.12	59.12	090	2	0	0	2	1

21154 Reconstruction midface, LeFort III (extracranial), any type, requiring bone grafts (includes obtaining autografts); without LeFort I　C

RVU			Global Days	Modifiers				
Mod	Non-Fac Total	Fac Total		51	50	62	80	MUE
	60.72	60.72	090	2	0	1	2	1

● New　▲ Revised　Deleted　⊙ Moderate Sedation　✚ Add-on Codes　⊗ High Risk Denial　Ⓐ Age Edit　♀ Female　♂ Male　**AMA** *CPT® Assistant*　**MUE** Medically Unlikely Edit
⊘ Modifier 51 Exempt　⊖ Modifier 63 Exempt　🅇 Unlisted　**Modifiers**: *See Inside Back Cover*　Ⓜ Maternity　A2–Z3 ASC Payment Indicators　A–Y OPPS Status Indicators

© 2016 DecisionHealth　　　CPT © 2015 American Medical Association. All Rights Reserved.　　　**223**

21155 Reconstruction midface, LeFort III (extracranial), any type, requiring bone grafts (includes obtaining autografts); with LeFort I ◨

RVU			Global Days	Modifiers				
Mod	Non-Fac Total	Fac Total		51	50	62	80	MUE
	62.63	62.63	090	2	0	0	2	1

21159 Reconstruction midface, LeFort III (extra and intracranial) with forehead advancement (eg, mono bloc), requiring bone grafts (includes obtaining autografts); without LeFort I ◨

RVU			Global Days	Modifiers				
Mod	Non-Fac Total	Fac Total		51	50	62	80	MUE
	72.45	72.45	090	2	0	1	2	1

21160 Reconstruction midface, LeFort III (extra and intracranial) with forehead advancement (eg, mono bloc), requiring bone grafts (includes obtaining autografts); with LeFort I ◨

RVU			Global Days	Modifiers				
Mod	Non-Fac Total	Fac Total		51	50	62	80	MUE
	92.94	92.94	090	2	0	0	2	1

21172 Reconstruction superior-lateral orbital rim and lower forehead, advancement or alteration, with or without grafts (includes obtaining autografts) ⊘ J I

RVU			Global Days	Modifiers				
Mod	Non-Fac Total	Fac Total		51	50	62	80	MUE
	52.39	52.39	090	2	0	1	2	1

21175 Reconstruction, bifrontal, superior-lateral orbital rims and lower forehead, advancement or alteration (eg, plagiocephaly, trigonocephaly, brachycephaly), with or without grafts (includes obtaining autografts) J I

RVU			Global Days	Modifiers				
Mod	Non-Fac Total	Fac Total		51	50	62	80	MUE
	62.76	62.76	090	2	0	0	2	1

21179 Reconstruction, entire or majority of forehead and/or supraorbital rims; with grafts (allograft or prosthetic material) ◨

RVU			Global Days	Modifiers				
Mod	Non-Fac Total	Fac Total		51	50	62	80	MUE
	41.96	41.96	090	2	0	0	2	1

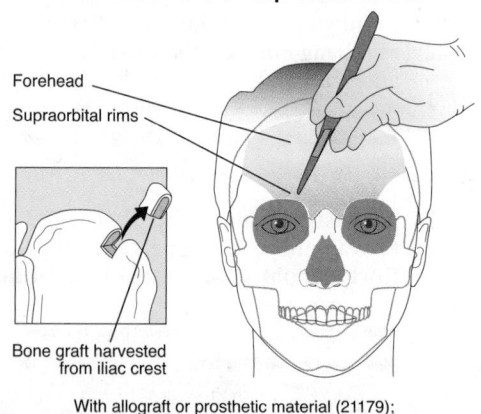

Reconstruction, entire or majority of forehead and/or supraorbital rims

Forehead

Supraorbital rims

Bone graft harvested from iliac crest

With allograft or prosthetic material (21179); and with autograft (21180)

21180 Reconstruction, entire or majority of forehead and/or supraorbital rims; with autograft (includes obtaining grafts) ◨

RVU			Global Days	Modifiers				
Mod	Non-Fac Total	Fac Total		51	50	62	80	MUE
	44.64	44.64	090	2	0	1	2	1

21181 Reconstruction by contouring of benign tumor of cranial bones (eg, fibrous dysplasia), extracranial A2 J I

RVU			Global Days	Modifiers				
Mod	Non-Fac Total	Fac Total		51	50	62	80	MUE
	21.54	21.54	090	2	0	0	0	1

21182 Reconstruction of orbital walls, rims, forehead, nasoethmoid complex following intra- and extracranial excision of benign tumor of cranial bone (eg, fibrous dysplasia), with multiple autografts (includes obtaining grafts); total area of bone grafting less than 40 sq cm ◨

RVU			Global Days	Modifiers				
Mod	Non-Fac Total	Fac Total		51	50	62	80	MUE
	56.16	56.16	090	2	0	1	2	1

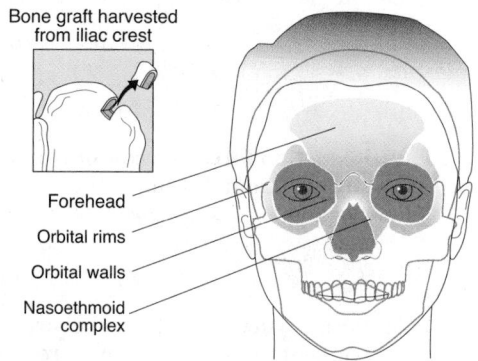

Reconstruction of orbital walls, rims, forehead, nasoethmoid complex

Bone graft harvested from iliac crest

Forehead

Orbital rims

Orbital walls

Nasoethmoid complex

For area of bone grafting less than 40 sq cm (21182); for area of bone grafting 40 to 80 sq cm (21183); and for area of bone grafting greater than 80 sq cm 21184

21183 Reconstruction of orbital walls, rims, forehead, nasoethmoid complex following intra- and extracranial excision of benign tumor of cranial bone (eg, fibrous dysplasia), with multiple autografts (includes obtaining grafts); total area of bone grafting greater than 40 sq cm but less than 80 sq cm ⊘ ◨

RVU			Global Days	Modifiers				
Mod	Non-Fac Total	Fac Total		51	50	62	80	MUE
	67.52	67.52	090	2	0	1	2	1

21184 Reconstruction of orbital walls, rims, forehead, nasoethmoid complex following intra- and extracranial excision of benign tumor of cranial bone (eg, fibrous dysplasia), with multiple autografts (includes obtaining grafts); total area of bone grafting greater than 80 sq cm ◨

RVU			Global Days	Modifiers				
Mod	Non-Fac Total	Fac Total		51	50	62	80	MUE
	61.77	61.77	090	2	0	0	2	1

● New   ▲ Revised   ✖ Deleted   ⊙ Moderate Sedation   ✚ Add-on Codes   ⊘ High Risk Denial   Ⓐ Age Edit   ♀ Female   ♂ Male   **AMA** *CPT® Assistant*   **MUE** Medically Unlikely Edit

⊘ Modifier 51 Exempt   ⊖ Modifier 63 Exempt   ⊠ Unlisted   **Modifiers:** *See Inside Back Cover*   Ⓜ Maternity   A2–Z3 ASC Payment Indicators   A–Y OPPS Status Indicators

CPT © 2015 American Medical Association. All Rights Reserved.   © 2016 DecisionHealth

21188 Reconstruction midface, osteotomies (other than LeFort type) and bone grafts (includes obtaining autografts)   C

RVU			Global Days	Modifiers				
Mod	Non-Fac Total	Fac Total		51	50	62	80	MUE
	46.84	46.84	090	2	0	0	2	1

21193 Reconstruction of mandibular rami, horizontal, vertical, C, or L osteotomy; without bone graft   J I

RVU			Global Days	Modifiers				
Mod	Non-Fac Total	Fac Total		51	50	62	80	MUE
	35.42	35.42	090	2	2	1	2	1

AMA: Apr 96: 11

21194 Reconstruction of mandibular rami, horizontal, vertical, C, or L osteotomy; with bone graft (includes obtaining graft)   C

RVU			Global Days	Modifiers				
Mod	Non-Fac Total	Fac Total		51	50	62	80	MUE
	41.73	41.73	090	2	2	0	2	1

AMA: Apr 96: 11

21195 Reconstruction of mandibular rami and/or body, sagittal split; without internal rigid fixation   J I

RVU			Global Days	Modifiers				
Mod	Non-Fac Total	Fac Total		51	50	62	80	MUE
	38.92	38.92	090	2	2	0	2	1

AMA: Apr 96: 11

21196 Reconstruction of mandibular rami and/or body, sagittal split; with internal rigid fixation   C

RVU			Global Days	Modifiers				
Mod	Non-Fac Total	Fac Total		51	50	62	80	MUE
	43.35	43.35	090	2	2	1	2	1

AMA: Apr 96: 11, Mar 97: 11

21198 Osteotomy, mandible, segmental   G2 T

RVU			Global Days	Modifiers				
Mod	Non-Fac Total	Fac Total		51	50	62	80	MUE
	34.21	34.21	090	2	0	1	2	1

AMA: Dec 13: 16

Osteotomy, mandible

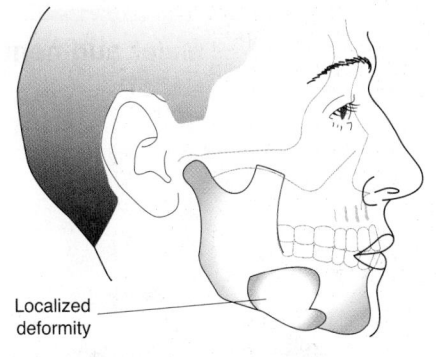

Localized deformity

Segmental (21198); and segmental
with genioglossus advancement (21199)

21199 Osteotomy, mandible, segmental; with genioglossus advancement   G2 J I

RVU			Global Days	Modifiers				
Mod	Non-Fac Total	Fac Total		51	50	62	80	MUE
	31.25	31.25	090	2	0	1	2	1

21206 Osteotomy, maxilla, segmental (eg, Wassmund or Schuchard)   A2 J I

RVU			Global Days	Modifiers				
Mod	Non-Fac Total	Fac Total		51	50	62	80	MUE
	34.37	34.37	090	2	0	1	2	1

21208 Osteoplasty, facial bones; augmentation (autograft, allograft, or prosthetic implant)   A2 J I

RVU			Global Days	Modifiers				
Mod	Non-Fac Total	Fac Total		51	50	62	80	MUE
	54.85	24.40	090	2	0	0	0	1

21209 Osteoplasty, facial bones; reduction   A2 J I

RVU			Global Days	Modifiers				
Mod	Non-Fac Total	Fac Total		51	50	62	80	MUE
	23.44	17.90	090	2	0	0	2	1

21210 Graft, bone; nasal, maxillary or malar areas (includes obtaining graft)   A2 J I

RVU			Global Days	Modifiers				
Mod	Non-Fac Total	Fac Total		51	50	62	80	MUE
	66.41	25.34	090	2	0	0	1	2

Graft, bone;
nasal, maxillary or malar areas
(includes obtaining graft)

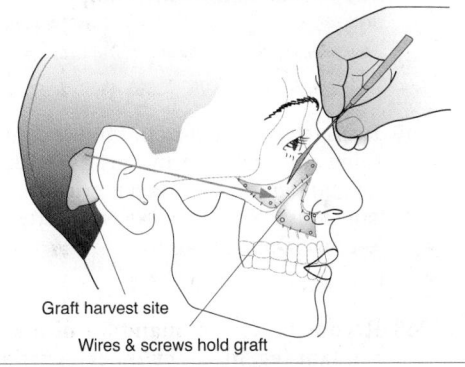

Graft harvest site

Wires & screws hold graft

21215 Graft, bone; mandible (includes obtaining graft)   A2 J I

RVU			Global Days	Modifiers				
Mod	Non-Fac Total	Fac Total		51	50	62	80	MUE
	118.10	26.36	090	2	0	1	1	2

21230 Graft; rib cartilage, autogenous, to face, chin, nose or ear (includes obtaining graft)   A2 J I

RVU			Global Days	Modifiers				
Mod	Non-Fac Total	Fac Total		51	50	62	80	MUE
	20.61	20.61	090	2	0	0	0	2

21235 Graft; ear cartilage, autogenous, to nose or ear (includes obtaining graft)   A2 T

RVU			Global Days	Modifiers				
Mod	Non-Fac Total	Fac Total		51	50	62	80	MUE
	20.98	16.46	090	2	0	0	1	2

● New   ▲ Revised   Deleted   ⊙ Moderate Sedation   ✚ Add-on Codes   ⊘ High Risk Denial   Ⓐ Age Edit   ♀ Female   ♂ Male   **AMA** CPT® Assistant   **MUE** Medically Unlikely Edit
⃠ Modifier 51 Exempt   ⊖ Modifier 63 Exempt   ✗ Unlisted   **Modifiers:** See Inside Back Cover   Ⓜ Maternity   A2 – Z3 ASC Payment Indicators   A – Y OPPS Status Indicators

© 2016 DecisionHealth   CPT © 2015 American Medical Association. All Rights Reserved.   **225**

Surgical Procedures

21240 – 21270

21240 Arthroplasty, temporomandibular joint, with or without autograft (includes obtaining graft) A2 J1

RVU			Global Days	Modifiers				
Mod	Non-Fac Total	Fac Total		51	50	62	80	MUE
	32.77	32.77	090	2	1	1	2	1

21242 Arthroplasty, temporomandibular joint, with allograft A2 J1

RVU			Global Days	Modifiers				
Mod	Non-Fac Total	Fac Total		51	50	62	80	MUE
	30.04	30.04	090	2	1	1	2	1

21243 Arthroplasty, temporomandibular joint, with prosthetic joint replacement J8 J1

RVU			Global Days	Modifiers				
Mod	Non-Fac Total	Fac Total		51	50	62	80	MUE
	49.69	49.69	090	2	1	1	2	1

21244 Reconstruction of mandible, extraoral, with transosteal bone plate (eg, mandibular staple bone plate) A2 J1

RVU			Global Days	Modifiers				
Mod	Non-Fac Total	Fac Total		51	50	62	80	MUE
	31.18	31.18	090	2	0	1	2	1

21245 Reconstruction of mandible or maxilla, subperiosteal implant; partial A2 J1

RVU			Global Days	Modifiers				
Mod	Non-Fac Total	Fac Total		51	50	62	80	MUE
	32.05	25.68	090	2	0	0	2	2

21246 Reconstruction of mandible or maxilla, subperiosteal implant; complete ⊘ A2 J1

RVU			Global Days	Modifiers				
Mod	Non-Fac Total	Fac Total		51	50	62	80	MUE
	25.29	25.29	090	2	0	0	2	2

21247 Reconstruction of mandibular condyle with bone and cartilage autografts (includes obtaining grafts) (eg, for hemifacial microsomia) ⊘ C

RVU			Global Days	Modifiers				
Mod	Non-Fac Total	Fac Total		51	50	62	80	MUE
	45.10	45.10	090	2	1	1	2	1

21248 Reconstruction of mandible or maxilla, endosteal implant (eg, blade, cylinder); partial ⊘ A2 J1

RVU			Global Days	Modifiers				
Mod	Non-Fac Total	Fac Total		51	50	62	80	MUE
	32.36	26.52	090	2	0	0	1	2

21249 Reconstruction of mandible or maxilla, endosteal implant (eg, blade, cylinder); complete ⊘ A2 J1

RVU			Global Days	Modifiers				
Mod	Non-Fac Total	Fac Total		51	50	62	80	MUE
	44.31	37.68	090	2	0	0	0	2

21255 Reconstruction of zygomatic arch and glenoid fossa with bone and cartilage (includes obtaining autografts) C

RVU			Global Days	Modifiers				
Mod	Non-Fac Total	Fac Total		51	50	62	80	MUE
	40.47	40.47	090	2	1	1	2	1

21256 Reconstruction of orbit with osteotomies (extracranial) and with bone grafts (includes obtaining autografts) (eg, micro-ophthalmia) J1

RVU			Global Days	Modifiers				
Mod	Non-Fac Total	Fac Total		51	50	62	80	MUE
	34.77	34.77	090	2	1	1	2	1

21260 Periorbital osteotomies for orbital hypertelorism, with bone grafts; extracranial approach G2 J1

RVU			Global Days	Modifiers				
Mod	Non-Fac Total	Fac Total		51	50	62	80	MUE
	40.55	40.55	090	2	0	1	2	1

21261 Periorbital osteotomies for orbital hypertelorism, with bone grafts; combined intra- and extracranial approach J1

RVU			Global Days	Modifiers				
Mod	Non-Fac Total	Fac Total		51	50	62	80	MUE
	60.90	60.90	090	2	0	1	2	1

21263 Periorbital osteotomies for orbital hypertelorism, with bone grafts; with forehead advancement J1

RVU			Global Days	Modifiers				
Mod	Non-Fac Total	Fac Total		51	50	62	80	MUE
	56.26	56.26	090	2	0	1	2	1

21267 Orbital repositioning, periorbital osteotomies, unilateral, with bone grafts; extracranial approach A2 J1

RVU			Global Days	Modifiers				
Mod	Non-Fac Total	Fac Total		51	50	62	80	MUE
	45.22	45.22	090	2	1	1	2	1

21268 Orbital repositioning, periorbital osteotomies, unilateral, with bone grafts; combined intra- and extracranial approach C

RVU			Global Days	Modifiers				
Mod	Non-Fac Total	Fac Total		51	50	62	80	MUE
	50.27	50.27	090	2	1	1	2	1

21270 Malar augmentation, prosthetic material A2 J1

RVU			Global Days	Modifiers				
Mod	Non-Fac Total	Fac Total		51	50	62	80	MUE
	27.69	20.81	090	2	1	1	2	1

Malar augmentation

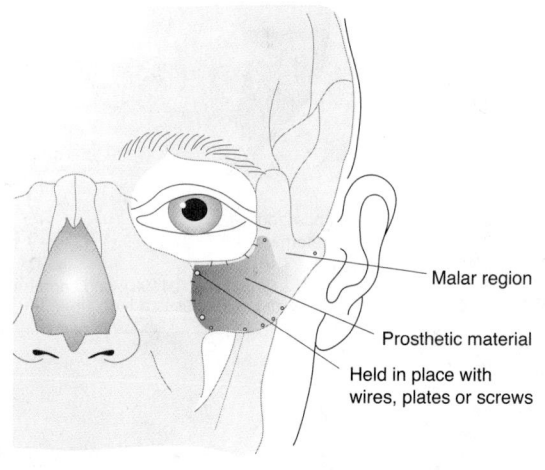

Malar region
Prosthetic material
Held in place with wires, plates or screws

● New ▲ Revised ✖ Deleted ⊙ Moderate Sedation ✚ Add-on Codes ⊘ High Risk Denial Ⓐ Age Edit ♀ Female ♂ Male **AMA** CPT® Assistant **MUE** Medically Unlikely Edit
⊘ Modifier 51 Exempt ⊖ Modifier 63 Exempt ✗ Unlisted **Modifiers:** See Inside Back Cover Ⓜ Maternity A2–Z3 ASC Payment Indicators A–Y OPPS Status Indicators

21275 Secondary revision of orbitocraniofacial reconstruction A 2 J 1

RVU			Global Days	Modifiers				
Mod	Non-Fac Total	Fac Total		51	50	62	80	MUE
	24.36	24.36	090	2	0	1	2	1

21280 Medial canthopexy (separate procedure) A 2 J 1

RVU			Global Days	Modifiers				
Mod	Non-Fac Total	Fac Total		51	50	62	80	MUE
	16.28	16.28	090	2	1	0	0	1

21282 Lateral canthopexy A 2 T

RVU			Global Days	Modifiers				
Mod	Non-Fac Total	Fac Total		51	50	62	80	MUE
	10.94	10.94	090	2	1	0	1	1

21295 Reduction of masseter muscle and bone (eg, for treatment of benign masseteric hypertrophy); extraoral approach A 2 T

RVU			Global Days	Modifiers				
Mod	Non-Fac Total	Fac Total		51	50	62	80	MUE
	5.17	5.17	090	2	1	0	0	1

21296 Reduction of masseter muscle and bone (eg, for treatment of benign masseteric hypertrophy); intraoral approach A 2 T

RVU			Global Days	Modifiers				
Mod	Non-Fac Total	Fac Total		51	50	62	80	MUE
	12.49	12.49	090	2	1	0	0	1

21299 Unlisted craniofacial and maxillofacial procedure ⊗ x T

RVU			Global Days	Modifiers				
Mod	Non-Fac Total	Fac Total		51	50	62	80	MUE
	0.00	0.00	YYY	2	0	1	0	

Head Fracture/Dislocation Procedures

21310 Closed treatment of nasal bone fracture without manipulation A 2 T

RVU			Global Days	Modifiers				
Mod	Non-Fac Total	Fac Total		51	50	62	80	MUE
	3.75	0.78	000	2	0	0	1	1

21315 Closed treatment of nasal bone fracture; without stabilization A 2 T

RVU			Global Days	Modifiers				
Mod	Non-Fac Total	Fac Total		51	50	62	80	MUE
	7.95	4.38	010	2	0	0	1	1

21320 Closed treatment of nasal bone fracture; with stabilization A 2 T

RVU			Global Days	Modifiers				
Mod	Non-Fac Total	Fac Total		51	50	62	80	MUE
	7.38	3.91	010	2	0	0	1	1

21325 Open treatment of nasal fracture; uncomplicated A 2 T

RVU			Global Days	Modifiers				
Mod	Non-Fac Total	Fac Total		51	50	62	80	MUE
	13.72	13.72	090	2	0	0	0	1

21330 Open treatment of nasal fracture; complicated, with internal and/or external skeletal fixation A 2 T

RVU			Global Days	Modifiers				
Mod	Non-Fac Total	Fac Total		51	50	62	80	MUE
	16.41	16.41	090	2	0	0	0	1

21335 Open treatment of nasal fracture; with concomitant open treatment of fractured septum A 2 T

RVU			Global Days	Modifiers				
Mod	Non-Fac Total	Fac Total		51	50	62	80	MUE
	21.04	21.04	090	2	0	0	1	1

21336 Open treatment of nasal septal fracture, with or without stabilization A 2 T

RVU			Global Days	Modifiers				
Mod	Non-Fac Total	Fac Total		51	50	62	80	MUE
	18.64	18.64	090	2	0	0	0	1

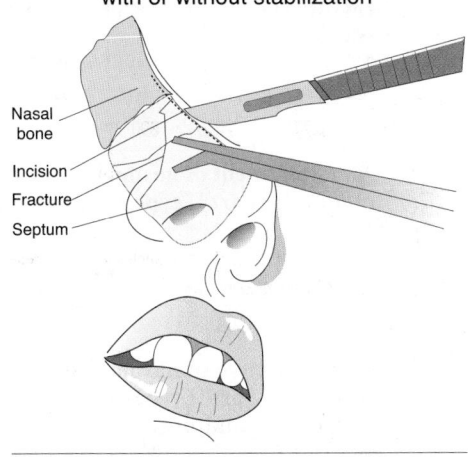

Open treatment of nasal septal fracture
with or without stabilization

Nasal bone
Incision
Fracture
Septum

21337 Closed treatment of nasal septal fracture, with or without stabilization A 2 T

RVU			Global Days	Modifiers				
Mod	Non-Fac Total	Fac Total		51	50	62	80	MUE
	11.65	8.53	090	2	0	0	0	1

21338 Open treatment of nasoethmoid fracture; without external fixation ⊗ A 2 J 1

RVU			Global Days	Modifiers				
Mod	Non-Fac Total	Fac Total		51	50	62	80	MUE
	20.96	20.96	090	2	0	0	0	1

21339 Open treatment of nasoethmoid fracture; with external fixation A 2 T

RVU			Global Days	Modifiers				
Mod	Non-Fac Total	Fac Total		51	50	62	80	MUE
	22.25	22.25	090	2	0	1	2	1

21340 Percutaneous treatment of nasoethmoid complex fracture, with splint, wire or headcap fixation, including repair of canthal ligaments and/or the nasolacrimal apparatus A 2 J 1

RVU			Global Days	Modifiers				
Mod	Non-Fac Total	Fac Total		51	50	62	80	MUE
	21.83	21.83	090	2	0	0	0	1

● New   ▲ Revised   Deleted   ⊙ Moderate Sedation   ✛ Add-on Codes   ⊗ High Risk Denial   Ⓐ Age Edit   ♀ Female   ♂ Male   **AMA** CPT® Assistant   **MUE** Medically Unlikely Edit
⊘ Modifier 51 Exempt   ⊖ Modifier 63 Exempt   x Unlisted   **Modifiers**: See Inside Back Cover   Ⓜ Maternity   A 2–Z 3 ASC Payment Indicators   A–Y OPPS Status Indicators

© 2016 DecisionHealth   CPT © 2015 American Medical Association. All Rights Reserved.   **227**

21343 Open treatment of depressed frontal sinus fracture C

RVU			Global Days	Modifiers				
Mod	Non-Fac Total	Fac Total		51	50	62	80	MUE
	35.11	35.11	090	2	0	1	2	1

21344 Open treatment of complicated (eg, comminuted or involving posterior wall) frontal sinus fracture, via coronal or multiple approaches C

RVU			Global Days	Modifiers				
Mod	Non-Fac Total	Fac Total		51	50	62	80	MUE
	40.36	40.36	090	2	0	2	2	1

21345 Closed treatment of nasomaxillary complex fracture (LeFort II type), with interdental wire fixation or fixation of denture or splint A2 T

RVU			Global Days	Modifiers				
Mod	Non-Fac Total	Fac Total		51	50	62	80	MUE
	23.46	18.98	090	2	0	0	0	1

21346 Open treatment of nasomaxillary complex fracture (LeFort II type); with wiring and/or local fixation J1

RVU			Global Days	Modifiers				
Mod	Non-Fac Total	Fac Total		51	50	62	80	MUE
	26.27	26.27	090	2	0	1	1	1

21347 Open treatment of nasomaxillary complex fracture (LeFort II type); requiring multiple open approaches C

RVU			Global Days	Modifiers				
Mod	Non-Fac Total	Fac Total		51	50	62	80	MUE
	33.18	33.18	090	2	0	1	2	1

21348 Open treatment of nasomaxillary complex fracture (LeFort II type); with bone grafting (includes obtaining graft) C

RVU			Global Days	Modifiers				
Mod	Non-Fac Total	Fac Total		51	50	62	80	MUE
	35.21	35.21	090	2	0	2	2	1

21355 Percutaneous treatment of fracture of malar area, including zygomatic arch and malar tripod, with manipulation A2 J1

RVU			Global Days	Modifiers				
Mod	Non-Fac Total	Fac Total		51	50	62	80	MUE
	12.34	9.26	010	2	1	0	0	1

21356 Open treatment of depressed zygomatic arch fracture (eg, Gillies approach) A2 T

RVU			Global Days	Modifiers				
Mod	Non-Fac Total	Fac Total		51	50	62	80	MUE
	14.52	11.00	010	2	1	0	0	1

21360 Open treatment of depressed malar fracture, including zygomatic arch and malar tripod G2 J1

RVU			Global Days	Modifiers				
Mod	Non-Fac Total	Fac Total		51	50	62	80	MUE
	15.63	15.63	090	2	1	0	2	1

21365 Open treatment of complicated (eg, comminuted or involving cranial nerve foramina) fracture(s) of malar area, including zygomatic arch and malar tripod; with internal fixation and multiple surgical approaches J1

RVU			Global Days	Modifiers				
Mod	Non-Fac Total	Fac Total		51	50	62	80	MUE
	32.35	32.35	090	2	1	1	2	1

21366 Open treatment of complicated (eg, comminuted or involving cranial nerve foramina) fracture(s) of malar area, including zygomatic arch and malar tripod; with bone grafting (includes obtaining graft) C

RVU			Global Days	Modifiers				
Mod	Non-Fac Total	Fac Total		51	50	62	80	MUE
	33.41	33.41	090	2	1	2	2	1

21385 Open treatment of orbital floor blowout fracture; transantral approach (Caldwell-Luc type operation) J1

RVU			Global Days	Modifiers				
Mod	Non-Fac Total	Fac Total		51	50	62	80	MUE
	19.71	19.71	090	2	1	1	2	1

21386 Open treatment of orbital floor blowout fracture; periorbital approach J1

RVU			Global Days	Modifiers				
Mod	Non-Fac Total	Fac Total		51	50	62	80	MUE
	20.23	20.23	090	2	1	0	2	1

21387 Open treatment of orbital floor blowout fracture; combined approach J1

RVU			Global Days	Modifiers				
Mod	Non-Fac Total	Fac Total		51	50	62	80	MUE
	20.59	20.59	090	2	1	0	2	1

21390 Open treatment of orbital floor blowout fracture; periorbital approach, with alloplastic or other implant G2 J1

RVU			Global Days	Modifiers				
Mod	Non-Fac Total	Fac Total		51	50	62	80	MUE
	22.99	22.99	090	2	1	1	2	1

Open treatment of orbital floor blowout fracture; periorbital approach with alloplastic or other implant

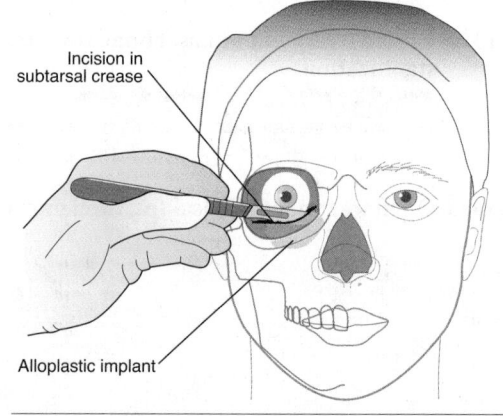

Incision in subtarsal crease

Alloplastic implant

● New ▲ Revised ✖ Deleted ⊙ Moderate Sedation ✚ Add-on Codes ⊘ High Risk Denial Ⓐ Age Edit ♀ Female ♂ Male **AMA** *CPT® Assistant* **MUE** Medically Unlikely Edit
⊘ Modifier 51 Exempt ⊖ Modifier 63 Exempt ✗ Unlisted **Modifiers:** *See Inside Back Cover* Ⓜ Maternity A2–Z3 ASC Payment Indicators A–Y OPPS Status Indicators

21395 Open treatment of orbital floor blowout fracture; periorbital approach with bone graft (includes obtaining graft) `J 1`

RVU			Global Days	Modifiers				
Mod	Non-Fac Total	Fac Total		51	50	62	80	MUE
	29.20	29.20	090	2	1	1	2	1

21400 Closed treatment of fracture of orbit, except blowout; without manipulation `A 2 T`

RVU			Global Days	Modifiers				
Mod	Non-Fac Total	Fac Total		51	50	62	80	MUE
	5.53	4.50	090	2	1	0	0	1

21401 Closed treatment of fracture of orbit, except blowout; with manipulation `A 2 T`

Coding tip: Add modifier 77 for re-reduction of the fracture by another physician

RVU			Global Days	Modifiers				
Mod	Non-Fac Total	Fac Total		51	50	62	80	MUE
	12.72	8.27	090	2	1	0	2	1

21406 Open treatment of fracture of orbit, except blowout; without implant `G 2 J 1`

RVU			Global Days	Modifiers				
Mod	Non-Fac Total	Fac Total		51	50	62	80	MUE
	15.01	15.01	090	2	1	1	2	1

21407 Open treatment of fracture of orbit, except blowout; with implant `G 2 J 1`

RVU			Global Days	Modifiers				
Mod	Non-Fac Total	Fac Total		51	50	62	80	MUE
	18.71	18.71	090	2	1	1	2	1

21408 Open treatment of fracture of orbit, except blowout; with bone grafting (includes obtaining graft) `⊙ J 1`

RVU			Global Days	Modifiers				
Mod	Non-Fac Total	Fac Total		51	50	62	80	MUE
	25.52	25.52	090	2	1	2	2	1

21421 Closed treatment of palatal or maxillary fracture (LeFort I type), with interdental wire fixation or fixation of denture or splint `A 2 J 1`

RVU			Global Days	Modifiers				
Mod	Non-Fac Total	Fac Total		51	50	62	80	MUE
	21.93	18.51	090	2	0	0	0	1

21422 Open treatment of palatal or maxillary fracture (LeFort I type) `C`

RVU			Global Days	Modifiers				
Mod	Non-Fac Total	Fac Total		51	50	62	80	MUE
	19.61	19.61	090	2	0	1	2	1

21423 Open treatment of palatal or maxillary fracture (LeFort I type); complicated (comminuted or involving cranial nerve foramina), multiple approaches `C`

RVU			Global Days	Modifiers				
Mod	Non-Fac Total	Fac Total		51	50	62	80	MUE
	23.90	23.90	090	2	0	2	2	1

21431 Closed treatment of craniofacial separation (LeFort III type) using interdental wire fixation of denture or splint `C`

RVU			Global Days	Modifiers				
Mod	Non-Fac Total	Fac Total		51	50	62	80	MUE
	21.53	21.53	090	2	0	0	2	1

21432 Open treatment of craniofacial separation (LeFort III type); with wiring and/or internal fixation `C`

RVU			Global Days	Modifiers				
Mod	Non-Fac Total	Fac Total		51	50	62	80	MUE
	18.98	18.98	090	2	0	0	2	1

21433 Open treatment of craniofacial separation (LeFort III type); complicated (eg, comminuted or involving cranial nerve foramina), multiple surgical approaches `C`

RVU			Global Days	Modifiers				
Mod	Non-Fac Total	Fac Total		51	50	62	80	MUE
	50.57	50.57	090	2	0	1	2	1

21435 Open treatment of craniofacial separation (LeFort III type); complicated, utilizing internal and/or external fixation techniques (eg, head cap, halo device, and/or intermaxillary fixation) `C`

RVU			Global Days	Modifiers				
Mod	Non-Fac Total	Fac Total		51	50	62	80	MUE
	36.52	36.52	090	2	0	0	2	1

21436 Open treatment of craniofacial separation (LeFort III type); complicated, multiple surgical approaches, internal fixation, with bone grafting (includes obtaining graft) `C`

RVU			Global Days	Modifiers				
Mod	Non-Fac Total	Fac Total		51	50	62	80	MUE
	60.69	60.69	090	2	0	2	2	1

21440 Closed treatment of mandibular or maxillary alveolar ridge fracture (separate procedure) `P 3 T`

RVU			Global Days	Modifiers				
Mod	Non-Fac Total	Fac Total		51	50	62	80	MUE
	16.80	13.65	090	2	0	0	0	2

Closed treatment of mandibular or maxillary alveolar ridge fracture
(separate procedure)

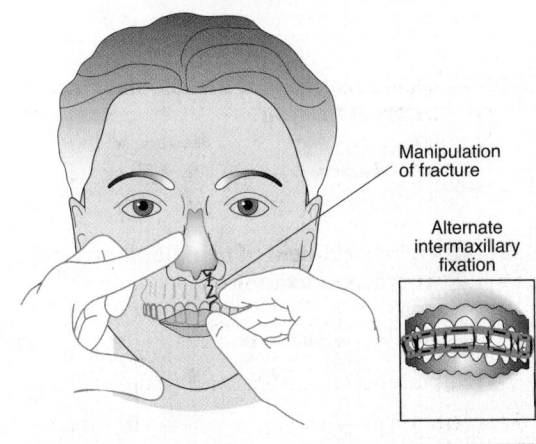

Manipulation of fracture

Alternate intermaxillary fixation

● New ▲ Revised Deleted ⊙ Moderate Sedation ✚ Add-on Codes ⊘ High Risk Denial Ⓐ Age Edit ♀ Female ♂ Male **AMA** *CPT® Assistant* **MUE** Medically Unlikely Edit
⊘ Modifier 51 Exempt ⊖ Modifier 63 Exempt Ⓧ Unlisted **Modifiers:** *See Inside Back Cover* Ⓜ Maternity `A 2`–`Z 3` ASC Payment Indicators `A`–`Y` OPPS Status Indicators

Surgical Procedures

21445 – 21499

21445 Open treatment of mandibular or maxillary alveolar ridge fracture (separate procedure) A 2 J 1

RVU			Global Days	Modifiers				
Mod	Non-Fac Total	Fac Total		51	50	62	80	MUE
	22.46	18.30	090	2	0	0	2	2

21450 Closed treatment of mandibular fracture; without manipulation A 2 T

RVU			Global Days	Modifiers				
Mod	Non-Fac Total	Fac Total		51	50	62	80	MUE
	17.83	14.34	090	2	0	0	0	1

21451 Closed treatment of mandibular fracture; with manipulation A 2 T

RVU			Global Days	Modifiers				
Mod	Non-Fac Total	Fac Total		51	50	62	80	MUE
	22.21	18.65	090	2	0	0	0	1

21452 Percutaneous treatment of mandibular fracture, with external fixation A 2 T

RVU			Global Days	Modifiers				
Mod	Non-Fac Total	Fac Total		51	50	62	80	MUE
	17.28	10.18	090	2	0	0	0	1

21453 Closed treatment of mandibular fracture with interdental fixation A 2 J 1

RVU			Global Days	Modifiers				
Mod	Non-Fac Total	Fac Total		51	50	62	80	MUE
	26.66	22.88	090	2	0	0	0	1

AMA: Dec 07: 7, 8

Closed treatment of mandibular fracture, with interdental fixation

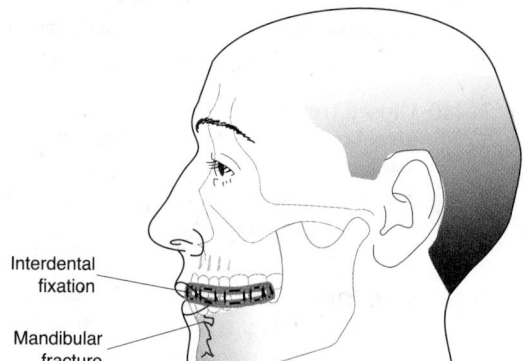

Interdental fixation

Mandibular fracture

21454 Open treatment of mandibular fracture with external fixation A 2 J 1

RVU			Global Days	Modifiers				
Mod	Non-Fac Total	Fac Total		51	50	62	80	MUE
	17.37	17.37	090	2	0	1	0	1

21461 Open treatment of mandibular fracture; without interdental fixation A 2 J 1

RVU			Global Days	Modifiers				
Mod	Non-Fac Total	Fac Total		51	50	62	80	MUE
	62.39	27.48	090	2	0	1	1	1

21462 Open treatment of mandibular fracture; with interdental fixation A 2 J 1

RVU			Global Days	Modifiers				
Mod	Non-Fac Total	Fac Total		51	50	62	80	MUE
	66.11	30.57	090	2	0	1	2	1

21465 Open treatment of mandibular condylar fracture A 2 J 1

RVU			Global Days	Modifiers				
Mod	Non-Fac Total	Fac Total		51	50	62	80	MUE
	28.05	28.05	090	2	1	1	2	1

21470 Open treatment of complicated mandibular fracture by multiple surgical approaches including internal fixation, interdental fixation, and/or wiring of dentures or splints J 1

RVU			Global Days	Modifiers				
Mod	Non-Fac Total	Fac Total		51	50	62	80	MUE
	35.16	35.16	090	2	0	1	2	1

AMA: Nov 02: 10

21480 Closed treatment of temporomandibular dislocation; initial or subsequent A 2 T

RVU			Global Days	Modifiers				
Mod	Non-Fac Total	Fac Total		51	50	62	80	MUE
	2.84	0.92	000	2	1	0	1	1

21485 Closed treatment of temporomandibular dislocation; complicated (eg, recurrent requiring intermaxillary fixation or splinting), initial or subsequent A 2 T

RVU			Global Days	Modifiers				
Mod	Non-Fac Total	Fac Total		51	50	62	80	MUE
	20.43	17.10	090	2	1	0	0	1

21490 Open treatment of temporomandibular dislocation A 2 J 1

RVU			Global Days	Modifiers				
Mod	Non-Fac Total	Fac Total		51	50	62	80	MUE
	26.71	26.71	090	2	1	1	2	1

21495 Open treatment of hyoid fracture G 2 T

RVU			Global Days	Modifiers				
Mod	Non-Fac Total	Fac Total		51	50	62	80	MUE
	20.42	20.42	090	2	0	0	2	1

Coding Guidance

Interdental wiring necessary for fracture treatment, reconstructive facial surgery, or arthoplasty, is included in the service. Code 21497 may be reported with other head and neck procedure codes as a separate, distinct service, using modifier 59.

21497 Interdental wiring, for condition other than fracture ⊙ A 2 T

RVU			Global Days	Modifiers				
Mod	Non-Fac Total	Fac Total		51	50	62	80	MUE
	21.49	17.87	090	2	0	0	0	1

AMA: Mar 97: 10

Other Head Procedures

21499 Unlisted musculoskeletal procedure, head x T

RVU			Global Days	Modifiers				
Mod	Non-Fac Total	Fac Total		51	50	62	80	MUE
	0.00	0.00	YYY	2	0	1	0	

● New   ▲ Revised   ✖ Deleted   ⊙ Moderate Sedation   ✚ Add-on Codes   ⊗ High Risk Denial   Ⓐ Age Edit   ♀ Female   ♂ Male   **AMA** *CPT® Assistant*   **MUE** Medically Unlikely Edit
⊘ Modifier 51 Exempt   ⊖ Modifier 63 Exempt   ✗ Unlisted   **Modifiers:** *See Inside Back Cover*   Ⓜ Maternity   A 2 – Z 3 ASC Payment Indicators   A – Y OPPS Status Indicators

CPT © 2015 American Medical Association. All Rights Reserved.   © 2016 DecisionHealth

Musculoskeletal Neck/Thorax Procedures

Neck/Thorax Incisional Procedures

21501 Incision and drainage, deep abscess or hematoma, soft tissues of neck or thorax `A2` `T`

RVU			Global Days	Modifiers				
Mod	Non-Fac Total	Fac Total		51	50	62	80	MUE
	13.02	9.28	090	2	0	0	1	3

AMA: Dec 14: 16

21502 Incision and drainage, deep abscess or hematoma, soft tissues of neck or thorax; with partial rib ostectomy `A2` `T`

RVU			Global Days	Modifiers				
Mod	Non-Fac Total	Fac Total		51	50	62	80	MUE
	15.38	15.38	090	2	0	0	2	1

21510 Incision, deep, with opening of bone cortex (eg, for osteomyelitis or bone abscess), thorax `C`

RVU			Global Days	Modifiers				
Mod	Non-Fac Total	Fac Total		51	50	62	80	MUE
	13.01	13.01	090	2	0	0	0	1

Neck/Thorax Excisional Procedures

21550 Biopsy, soft tissue of neck or thorax `G2` `T`

Coding tip: Biopsy is usually included as a component of a more complex procedure

Coding tip: Report this procedure separately only when performed alone, or distinct from other procedures on the same day

Coding tip: Code 99000 for specimen transfer from office setting to an outside laboratory

RVU			Global Days	Modifiers				
Mod	Non-Fac Total	Fac Total		51	50	62	80	MUE
	7.52	4.56	010	2	0	0	1	3

Biopsy, soft tissue of neck or thorax

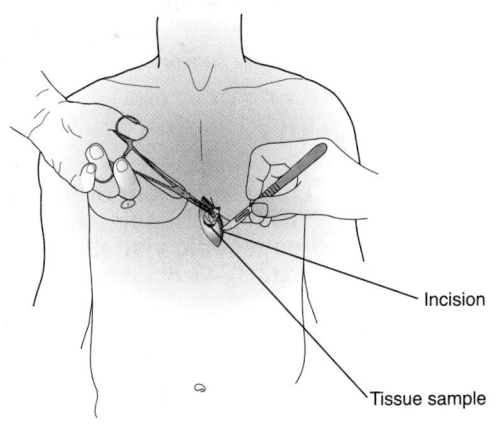

Incision

Tissue sample

21552 Excision, tumor, soft tissue of neck or anterior thorax, subcutaneous; 3 cm or greater `G2` `T`

Coding tip: Code 21552 is listed out of numerical order in CPT. Related soft tissue tumor excision procedures - 21555 (subcutaneous tissue); 21554 and 21556 (subfascial).

RVU			Global Days	Modifiers				
Mod	Non-Fac Total	Fac Total		51	50	62	80	MUE
	12.91	12.91	090	2	0	0	2	4

21554 Excision, tumor, soft tissue of neck or anterior thorax, subfascial (eg, intramuscular); 5 cm or greater `G2` `T`

Coding tip: Code 21554 is listed out of numerical order in CPT. Related soft tissue tumor excision procedures - 21555 and 21552 (subcutaneous tissue); 21556 (subfascial).

RVU			Global Days	Modifiers				
Mod	Non-Fac Total	Fac Total		51	50	62	80	MUE
	21.18	21.18	090	2	0	0	2	2

21555 Excision, tumor, soft tissue of neck or anterior thorax, subcutaneous; less than 3 cm `G2` `T`

Coding tip: Related soft tissue tumor excision - 21552

RVU			Global Days	Modifiers				
Mod	Non-Fac Total	Fac Total		51	50	62	80	MUE
	11.91	8.84	090	2	0	0	1	4

AMA: Oct 02: 11

21556 Excision, tumor, soft tissue of neck or anterior thorax, subfascial (eg, intramuscular); less than 5 cm `G2` `T`

Coding tip: Related soft tissue tumor excision - 21554

RVU			Global Days	Modifiers				
Mod	Non-Fac Total	Fac Total		51	50	62	80	MUE
	15.34	15.34	090	2	0	0	1	3

21557 Radical resection of tumor (eg, sarcoma), soft tissue of neck or anterior thorax; less than 5 cm `G2` `T`

RVU			Global Days	Modifiers				
Mod	Non-Fac Total	Fac Total		51	50	62	80	MUE
	27.79	27.79	090	2	0	1	2	1

AMA: Apr 10: 11

21558 Radical resection of tumor (eg, sarcoma), soft tissue of neck or anterior thorax; 5 cm or greater `G2` `T`

RVU			Global Days	Modifiers				
Mod	Non-Fac Total	Fac Total		51	50	62	80	MUE
	39.11	39.11	090	2	0	1	2	1

21600 Excision of rib, partial `A2` `T`

RVU			Global Days	Modifiers				
Mod	Non-Fac Total	Fac Total		51	50	62	80	MUE
	16.10	16.10	090	2	0	1	2	5

AMA: Jul 12: 12, Mar 13: 13

21610 Costotransversectomy (separate procedure) `A2` `T`

RVU			Global Days	Modifiers				
Mod	Non-Fac Total	Fac Total		51	50	62	80	MUE
	34.88	34.88	090	2	0	0	2	1

21615 Excision first and/or cervical rib `C`

RVU			Global Days	Modifiers				
Mod	Non-Fac Total	Fac Total		51	50	62	80	MUE
	17.83	17.83	090	2	1	1	2	1

AMA: Mar 14: 13

21616 Excision first and/or cervical rib; with sympathectomy `C`

RVU			Global Days	Modifiers				
Mod	Non-Fac Total	Fac Total		51	50	62	80	MUE
	21.79	21.79	090	2	1	0	2	1

● New ▲ Revised Deleted ⊙ Moderate Sedation ✚ Add-on Codes ⊘ High Risk Denial Ⓐ Age Edit ♀ Female ♂ Male **AMA** *CPT® Assistant* **MUE** Medically Unlikely Edit
⊘ Modifier 51 Exempt ⊖ Modifier 63 Exempt ✗ Unlisted **Modifiers:** *See Inside Back Cover* Ⓜ Maternity `A2`–`Z3` ASC Payment Indicators `A`–`Y` OPPS Status Indicators

21620 Ostectomy of sternum, partial   C

	RVU		Global Days	Modifiers				
Mod	Non-Fac Total	Fac Total		51	50	62	80	MUE
	14.58	14.58	090	2	0	1	2	1

21627 Sternal debridement   C

	RVU		Global Days	Modifiers				
Mod	Non-Fac Total	Fac Total		51	50	62	80	MUE
	15.56	15.56	090	2	0	0	2	1

AMA: May 11: 3

21630 Radical resection of sternum   C

	RVU		Global Days	Modifiers				
Mod	Non-Fac Total	Fac Total		51	50	62	80	MUE
	34.98	34.98	090	2	0	1	2	1

21632 Radical resection of sternum; with mediastinal lymphadenectomy   C

	RVU		Global Days	Modifiers				
Mod	Non-Fac Total	Fac Total		51	50	62	80	MUE
	35.17	35.17	090	2	0	1	2	1

Neck/Thorax Repair/Revision/Reconstruction Procedures

21685 Hyoid myotomy and suspension   G2 T

	RVU		Global Days	Modifiers				
Mod	Non-Fac Total	Fac Total		51	50	62	80	MUE
	29.05	29.05	090	2	0	1	2	1

AMA: Aug 04: 11

21700 Division of scalenus anticus; without resection of cervical rib   ⊘ A2 T

	RVU		Global Days	Modifiers				
Mod	Non-Fac Total	Fac Total		51	50	62	80	MUE
	10.80	10.80	090	2	1	0	2	1

21705 Division of scalenus anticus; with resection of cervical rib   C

	RVU		Global Days	Modifiers				
Mod	Non-Fac Total	Fac Total		51	50	62	80	MUE
	16.01	16.01	090	2	1	0	2	1

AMA: Mar 14: 13

21720 Division of sternocleidomastoid for torticollis, open operation; without cast application   A2 T

	RVU		Global Days	Modifiers				
Mod	Non-Fac Total	Fac Total		51	50	62	80	MUE
	13.12	13.12	090	2	0	0	2	1

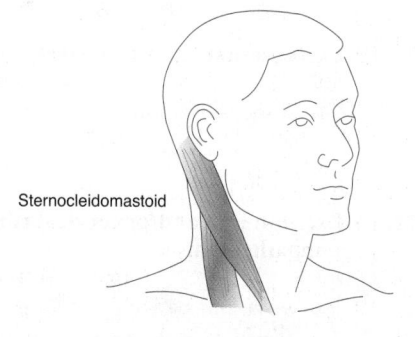

Division of sternocleidomastoid

Sternocleidomastoid

Transection of spinal accessory
and cervical nerves for torticollis.

21725 Division of sternocleidomastoid for torticollis, open operation; with cast application   A2 T

	RVU		Global Days	Modifiers				
Mod	Non-Fac Total	Fac Total		51	50	62	80	MUE
	15.34	15.34	090	2	0	1	2	1

21740 Reconstructive repair of pectus excavatum or carinatum; open   C

	RVU		Global Days	Modifiers				
Mod	Non-Fac Total	Fac Total		51	50	62	80	MUE
	29.73	29.73	090	2	0	1	2	1

21742 Reconstructive repair of pectus excavatum or carinatum; minimally invasive approach (Nuss procedure), without thoracoscopy   T

	RVU		Global Days	Modifiers				
Mod	Non-Fac Total	Fac Total		51	50	62	80	MUE
	0.00	0.00	090	2	0	1	2	1

21743 Reconstructive repair of pectus excavatum or carinatum; minimally invasive approach (Nuss procedure), with thoracoscopy   T

	RVU		Global Days	Modifiers				
Mod	Non-Fac Total	Fac Total		51	50	62	80	MUE
	0.00	0.00	090	2	0	1	2	1

21750 Closure of median sternotomy separation with or without debridement (separate procedure)   C

	RVU		Global Days	Modifiers				
Mod	Non-Fac Total	Fac Total		51	50	62	80	MUE
	19.81	19.81	090	2	0	1	2	1

AMA: May 11: 3

✖ 21805 Open treatment of rib fracture without fixation, each

21811 Open treatment of rib fracture(s) with internal fixation, includes thoracoscopic visualization when performed, unilateral; 1-3 ribs   T

	RVU		Global Days	Modifiers				
Mod	Non-Fac Total	Fac Total		51	50	62	80	MUE
	17.75	17.75	000	2	1	0	2	1

AMA: Aug 15: 3

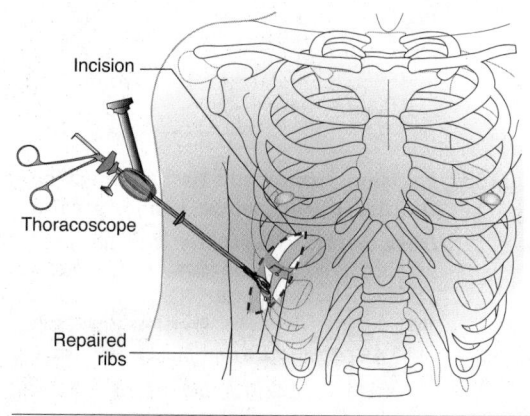

**Open treatment of rib fracture(s)
with internal fixation, includes
thoracoscopic visualization, unilateral;**
1-3 ribs (21811), 4-6 ribs (21812), 7 or more ribs (21813)

Incision

Thoracoscope

Repaired
ribs

● New   ▲ Revised   ✖ Deleted   ⊙ Moderate Sedation   ✚ Add-on Codes   ⊘ High Risk Denial   Ⓐ Age Edit   ♀ Female   ♂ Male   **AMA** *CPT® Assistant*   **MUE** Medically Unlikely Edit

⊘ Modifier 51 Exempt   ⊖ Modifier 63 Exempt   🗵 Unlisted   **Modifiers:** *See Inside Back Cover*   Ⓜ Maternity   A2–Z3 ASC Payment Indicators   A–Y OPPS Status Indicators

CPT © 2015 American Medical Association. All Rights Reserved.   © 2016 DecisionHealth

21812 Open treatment of rib fracture(s) with internal fixation, includes thoracoscopic visualization when performed, unilateral; 4-6 ribs   **T**

RVU			Global Days	Modifiers				
Mod	Non-Fac Total	Fac Total		51	50	62	80	MUE
	21.29	21.29	000	2	1	0	2	1

AMA: Aug 15: 3

21813 Open treatment of rib fracture(s) with internal fixation, includes thoracoscopic visualization when performed, unilateral; 7 or more ribs   **T**

RVU			Global Days	Modifiers				
Mod	Non-Fac Total	Fac Total		51	50	62	80	MUE
	27.84	27.84	000	2	1	0	2	1

AMA: Aug 15: 3

Coding Guidance
Sternal fracture repair is not reported for median sternotomy performed to accomplish cardiothoracic procedures; the necessary sternal repair is part of the primary procedure.

21820 Closed treatment of sternum fracture   **A2 T**

RVU			Global Days	Modifiers				
Mod	Non-Fac Total	Fac Total		51	50	62	80	MUE
	4.01	4.11	090	2	0	0	1	1

21825 Open treatment of sternum fracture with or without skeletal fixation   **C**

RVU			Global Days	Modifiers				
Mod	Non-Fac Total	Fac Total		51	50	62	80	MUE
	15.67	15.67	090	2	0	1	2	1

Other Neck/Thorax Procedures

21899 Unlisted procedure, neck or thorax   **x T**

RVU			Global Days	Modifiers				
Mod	Non-Fac Total	Fac Total		51	50	62	80	MUE
	0.00	0.00	YYY	2	0	1	0	

AMA: Aug 15: 3

Back/Trunk Musculoskeletal Procedures

Back/Trunk Excisional Procedures

21920 Biopsy, soft tissue of back or flank; superficial   **P3 T**

Coding tip: Code 99000 for specimen transfer from office setting to an outside laboratory

RVU			Global Days	Modifiers				
Mod	Non-Fac Total	Fac Total		51	50	62	80	MUE
	7.36	4.63	010	2	0	0	1	3

21925 Biopsy, soft tissue of back or flank; deep   **A2 T**

RVU			Global Days	Modifiers				
Mod	Non-Fac Total	Fac Total		51	50	62	80	MUE
	12.67	10.13	090	2	0	0	1	3

21930 Excision, tumor, soft tissue of back or flank, subcutaneous; less than 3 cm   **G2 T**

RVU			Global Days	Modifiers				
Mod	Non-Fac Total	Fac Total		51	50	62	80	MUE
	13.57	10.55	090	2	0	0	1	5

21931 Excision, tumor, soft tissue of back or flank, subcutaneous; 3 cm or greater   **G2 T**

RVU			Global Days	Modifiers				
Mod	Non-Fac Total	Fac Total		51	50	62	80	MUE
	13.59	13.59	090	2	0	0	2	3

21932 Excision, tumor, soft tissue of back or flank, subfascial (eg, intramuscular); less than 5 cm   **G2 T**

RVU			Global Days	Modifiers				
Mod	Non-Fac Total	Fac Total		51	50	62	80	MUE
	19.15	19.15	090	2	0	0	2	4

21933 Excision, tumor, soft tissue of back or flank, subfascial (eg, intramuscular); 5 cm or greater   **G2 T**

RVU			Global Days	Modifiers				
Mod	Non-Fac Total	Fac Total		51	50	62	80	MUE
	21.33	21.33	090	2	0	0	2	3

21935 Radical resection of tumor (eg, sarcoma), soft tissue of back or flank; less than 5 cm   **G2 T**

RVU			Global Days	Modifiers				
Mod	Non-Fac Total	Fac Total		51	50	62	80	MUE
	29.75	29.75	090	2	0	1	1	1

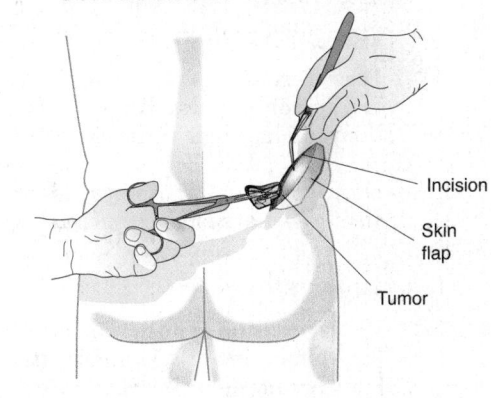

Radical resection of tumor, soft tissue of back or flank

Incision
Skin flap
Tumor

Less than 5 cm (21935); 5 cm or greater (21936)

21936 Radical resection of tumor (eg, sarcoma), soft tissue of back or flank; 5 cm or greater   **G2 T**

RVU			Global Days	Modifiers				
Mod	Non-Fac Total	Fac Total		51	50	62	80	MUE
	40.95	40.95	090	2	0	1	2	1

Spinal Column/Vertebral Procedures

Spinal Column/Vertebral Incisional Procedures

22010 Incision and drainage, open, of deep abscess (subfascial), posterior spine; cervical, thoracic, or cervicothoracic   **C**

RVU			Global Days	Modifiers				
Mod	Non-Fac Total	Fac Total		51	50	62	80	MUE
	27.73	27.73	090	2	0	0	0	2

● New   ▲ Revised   Deleted   ⊙ Moderate Sedation   ✚ Add-on Codes   ⊘ High Risk Denial   Ⓐ Age Edit   ♀ Female   ♂ Male   **AMA** *CPT® Assistant*   **MUE** Medically Unlikely Edit
⊘ Modifier 51 Exempt   ⊖ Modifier 63 Exempt   **x** Unlisted   **Modifiers:** *See Inside Back Cover*   Ⓜ Maternity   **A2–Z3** ASC Payment Indicators   **A–Y** OPPS Status Indicators

© 2016 DecisionHealth   CPT © 2015 American Medical Association. All Rights Reserved.   **233**

22015 Incision and drainage, open, of deep abscess (subfascial), posterior spine; lumbar, sacral, or lumbosacral ☐C

	RVU		Global Days	Modifiers				
Mod	Non-Fac Total	Fac Total		51	50	62	80	MUE
	27.14	27.14	090	2	0	0	1	2

Spinal Column/Vertebral Excisional Procedures

Coding Guidance
Codes 22100-22116 for partial excision of vertebral components are distinct services and should not be reported together with laminotomy or laminectomy procedures unless those separate services are performed as defined in the code description.

22100 Partial excision of posterior vertebral component (eg, spinous process, lamina or facet) for intrinsic bony lesion, single vertebral segment; cervical ☐T

	RVU		Global Days	Modifiers				
Mod	Non-Fac Total	Fac Total		51	50	62	80	MUE
	25.45	25.45	090	2	0	1	2	1

AMA: Jul 13: 3

22101 Partial excision of posterior vertebral component (eg, spinous process, lamina or facet) for intrinsic bony lesion, single vertebral segment; thoracic ☐T

	RVU		Global Days	Modifiers				
Mod	Non-Fac Total	Fac Total		51	50	62	80	MUE
	24.81	24.81	090	2	0	1	2	1

AMA: Jul 13: 3

22102 Partial excision of posterior vertebral component (eg, spinous process, lamina or facet) for intrinsic bony lesion, single vertebral segment; lumbar G2T

	RVU		Global Days	Modifiers				
Mod	Non-Fac Total	Fac Total		51	50	62	80	MUE
	22.77	22.77	090	2	0	1	2	1

AMA: Jul 13: 3

+ **22103 Partial excision of posterior vertebral component (eg, spinous process, lamina or facet) for intrinsic bony lesion, single vertebral segment; each additional segment (List separately in addition to code for primary procedure)** N1N

	RVU		Global Days	Modifiers				
Mod	Non-Fac Total	Fac Total		51	50	62	80	MUE
	4.04	4.04	ZZZ	0	0	1	2	3

AMA: Feb 96: 6

22110 Partial excision of vertebral body, for intrinsic bony lesion, without decompression of spinal cord or nerve root(s), single vertebral segment; cervical ☐C

	RVU		Global Days	Modifiers				
Mod	Non-Fac Total	Fac Total		51	50	62	80	MUE
	30.35	30.35	090	2	0	1	2	1

AMA: Jul 13: 3

22112 Partial excision of vertebral body, for intrinsic bony lesion, without decompression of spinal cord or nerve root(s), single vertebral segment; thoracic ☐C

	RVU		Global Days	Modifiers				
Mod	Non-Fac Total	Fac Total		51	50	62	80	MUE
	28.72	28.72	090	2	0	1	2	1

AMA: Jul 13: 3

22114 Partial excision of vertebral body, for intrinsic bony lesion, without decompression of spinal cord or nerve root(s), single vertebral segment; lumbar ☐C

	RVU		Global Days	Modifiers				
Mod	Non-Fac Total	Fac Total		51	50	62	80	MUE
	28.84	28.84	090	2	0	1	2	1

AMA: Jul 13: 3

+ **22116 Partial excision of vertebral body, for intrinsic bony lesion, without decompression of spinal cord or nerve root(s), single vertebral segment; each additional vertebral segment (List separately in addition to code for primary procedure)** ☐C

	RVU		Global Days	Modifiers				
Mod	Non-Fac Total	Fac Total		51	50	62	80	MUE
	4.04	4.04	ZZZ	0	0	1	2	3

AMA: Feb 96: 6

Spinal Osteotomy Procedures

22206 Osteotomy of spine, posterior or posterolateral approach, 3 columns, 1 vertebral segment (eg, pedicle/vertebral body subtraction); thoracic ☐C

	RVU		Global Days	Modifiers				
Mod	Non-Fac Total	Fac Total		51	50	62	80	MUE
	70.89	70.89	090	2	0	1	2	1

AMA: Feb 08: 9, Jul 13: 3

22207 Osteotomy of spine, posterior or posterolateral approach, 3 columns, 1 vertebral segment (eg, pedicle/vertebral body subtraction); lumbar ☐C

	RVU		Global Days	Modifiers				
Mod	Non-Fac Total	Fac Total		51	50	62	80	MUE
	69.47	69.47	090	2	0	1	2	1

AMA: Feb 08: 9, Jul 13: 3

+ **22208 Osteotomy of spine, posterior or posterolateral approach, 3 columns, 1 vertebral segment (eg, pedicle/vertebral body subtraction); each additional vertebral segment (List separately in addition to code for primary procedure)** ☐C

	RVU		Global Days	Modifiers				
Mod	Non-Fac Total	Fac Total		51	50	62	80	MUE
	16.53	16.53	ZZZ	0	0	1	2	6

AMA: Feb 08: 9

22210 Osteotomy of spine, posterior or posterolateral approach, 1 vertebral segment; cervical ☐C

	RVU		Global Days	Modifiers				
Mod	Non-Fac Total	Fac Total		51	50	62	80	MUE
	51.85	51.85	090	2	0	1	2	1

AMA: Jul 13: 3

● New ▲ Revised ✖ Deleted ⊙ Moderate Sedation ✛ Add-on Codes ⊘ High Risk Denial Ⓐ Age Edit ♀ Female ♂ Male **AMA** *CPT® Assistant* **MUE** Medically Unlikely Edit
⊘ Modifier 51 Exempt ⊖ Modifier 63 Exempt 🅇 Unlisted **Modifiers:** *See Inside Back Cover* Ⓜ Maternity A2–Z3 ASC Payment Indicators A–Y OPPS Status Indicators

CPT © 2015 American Medical Association. All Rights Reserved. © 2016 DecisionHealth

22212 Osteotomy of spine, posterior or posterolateral approach, 1 vertebral segment; thoracic C

RVU			Global Days	Modifiers				
Mod	Non-Fac Total	Fac Total		51	50	62	80	MUE
	42.87	42.87	090	2	0	1	2	1

AMA: Dec 07: 1, Jul 13: 3

22214 Osteotomy of spine, posterior or posterolateral approach, 1 vertebral segment; lumbar C

RVU			Global Days	Modifiers				
Mod	Non-Fac Total	Fac Total		51	50	62	80	MUE
	42.91	42.91	090	2	0	1	2	1

AMA: Dec 07: 1, Jul 13: 3, Dec 14: 16

+ 22216 Osteotomy of spine, posterior or posterolateral approach, 1 vertebral segment; each additional vertebral segment (List separately in addition to primary procedure) C

RVU			Global Days	Modifiers				
Mod	Non-Fac Total	Fac Total		51	50	62	80	MUE
	10.39	10.39	ZZZ	0	0	1	2	6

AMA: Dec 07: 1

22220 Osteotomy of spine, including discectomy, anterior approach, single vertebral segment; cervical C

RVU			Global Days	Modifiers				
Mod	Non-Fac Total	Fac Total		51	50	62	80	MUE
	46.37	46.37	090	2	0	1	2	1

AMA: Feb 02: 4, Jul 13: 3

22222 Osteotomy of spine, including discectomy, anterior approach, single vertebral segment; thoracic C

RVU			Global Days	Modifiers				
Mod	Non-Fac Total	Fac Total		51	50	62	80	MUE
	45.23	45.23	090	2	0	1	2	1

AMA: Feb 02: 4

22224 Osteotomy of spine, including discectomy, anterior approach, single vertebral segment; lumbar C

RVU			Global Days	Modifiers				
Mod	Non-Fac Total	Fac Total		51	50	62	80	MUE
	45.71	45.71	090	2	0	1	2	1

AMA: Feb 02: 4, Jul 13: 3

+ 22226 Osteotomy of spine, including discectomy, anterior approach, single vertebral segment; each additional vertebral segment (List separately in addition to code for primary procedure) C

RVU			Global Days	Modifiers				
Mod	Non-Fac Total	Fac Total		51	50	62	80	MUE
	10.33	10.33	ZZZ	0	0	1	2	4

AMA: Feb 96: 6, Feb 02: 4

Spinal Fracture/Dislocation Procedures

22305 Closed treatment of vertebral process fracture(s) A2T

RVU			Global Days	Modifiers				
Mod	Non-Fac Total	Fac Total		51	50	62	80	MUE
	5.49	4.99	090	2	0	0	1	1

AMA: Jul 13: 3

22310 Closed treatment of vertebral body fracture(s), without manipulation, requiring and including casting or bracing A2T

RVU			Global Days	Modifiers				
Mod	Non-Fac Total	Fac Total		51	50	62	80	MUE
	8.87	8.18	090	2	0	0	1	1

AMA: Jun 12: 10, Jul 13: 3, Jul 14: 8

22315 Closed treatment of vertebral fracture(s) and/or dislocation(s) requiring casting or bracing, with and including casting and/or bracing by manipulation or traction A2T

RVU			Global Days	Modifiers				
Mod	Non-Fac Total	Fac Total		51	50	62	80	MUE
	25.49	22.34	090	2	0	0	1	1

AMA: Apr 12: 11, Jun 12: 10, Jul 13: 3

22318 Open treatment and/or reduction of odontoid fracture(s) and or dislocation(s) (including os odontoideum), anterior approach, including placement of internal fixation; without grafting C

RVU			Global Days	Modifiers				
Mod	Non-Fac Total	Fac Total		51	50	62	80	MUE
	47.91	47.91	090	2	0	2	2	1

AMA: Nov 99: 11, Apr 12: 13, Jul 13: 3

22319 Open treatment and/or reduction of odontoid fracture(s) and or dislocation(s) (including os odontoideum), anterior approach, including placement of internal fixation; with grafting C

RVU			Global Days	Modifiers				
Mod	Non-Fac Total	Fac Total		51	50	62	80	MUE
	53.54	53.54	090	2	0	2	2	1

AMA: Nov 99: 11, Apr 12: 16, Jul 13: 3

22325 Open treatment and/or reduction of vertebral fracture(s) and/or dislocation(s), posterior approach, 1 fractured vertebra or dislocated segment; lumbar C

RVU			Global Days	Modifiers				
Mod	Non-Fac Total	Fac Total		51	50	62	80	MUE
	41.47	41.47	090	2	0	1	2	1

AMA: Sep 97: 8, Jun 12: 10, Jul 13: 3

Open treatment and/or reduction of vertebral fracture(s) and/or dislocation

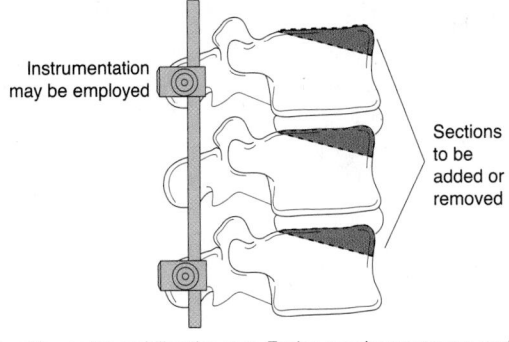

Instrumentation may be employed

Sections to be added or removed

A rod is used to stabilize the area. Fusion may be necessary, and is achieved via grafting (separately reportable) or internal fixation. The incision is closed. Code 22325 for a lumbar procedure; 22326 for cervical; 22327 for a thoracic site; and 22328 for each additional fractured or dislocated vertebra or segment in addition to the primary procedure.

● New   ▲ Revised   Deleted   ⊙ Moderate Sedation   ✚ Add-on Codes   ⊘ High Risk Denial   Ⓐ Age Edit   ♀ Female   ♂ Male   **AMA** *CPT® Assistant*   **MUE** Medically Unlikely Edit
⊘ Modifier 51 Exempt   ⊖ Modifier 63 Exempt   Ⓧ Unlisted   **Modifiers:** *See Inside Back Cover*   Ⓜ Maternity   A2-Z3 ASC Payment Indicators   A-Y OPPS Status Indicators

© 2016 DecisionHealth   CPT © 2015 American Medical Association. All Rights Reserved.   **235**

Surgical Procedures

22326 – 22512

22326 Open treatment and/or reduction of vertebral fracture(s) and/or dislocation(s), posterior approach, 1 fractured vertebra or dislocated segment; cervical   C

RVU			Global Days	Modifiers				
Mod	Non-Fac Total	Fac Total		51	50	62	80	MUE
	43.34	43.34	090	2	0	1	2	1

AMA: Sep 97: 8, Jul 13: 3

22327 Open treatment and/or reduction of vertebral fracture(s) and/or dislocation(s), posterior approach, 1 fractured vertebra or dislocated segment; thoracic   C

RVU			Global Days	Modifiers				
Mod	Non-Fac Total	Fac Total		51	50	62	80	MUE
	43.73	43.73	090	2	0	1	2	1

AMA: Sep 97: 8, Jun 12: 10, Jul 13: 3

+ 22328 Open treatment and/or reduction of vertebral fracture(s) and/or dislocation(s), posterior approach, 1 fractured vertebra or dislocated segment; each additional fractured vertebra or dislocated segment (List separately in addition to code for primary procedure)   C

RVU			Global Days	Modifiers				
Mod	Non-Fac Total	Fac Total		51	50	62	80	MUE
	8.02	8.02	ZZZ	0	0	1	2	6

AMA: Feb 96: 6

Spinal Manipulation

Coding Guidance
Do not report the separate manipulation under anesthesia code when the service is necessary to accomplish fracture reduction or assess range of motion as part of another related procedure.

22505 Manipulation of spine requiring anesthesia, any region   ⊘A 2 T

RVU			Global Days	Modifiers				
Mod	Non-Fac Total	Fac Total		51	50	62	80	MUE
	3.70	3.70	010	2	0	0	1	1

AMA: Mar 97: 11, Jan 99: 11

Vertabroplasty/Vertebral Augmentation, Percutaneous

⊙ 22510 Percutaneous vertebroplasty (bone biopsy included when performed), 1 vertebral body, unilateral or bilateral injection, inclusive of all imaging guidance; cervicothoracic   G 2 T

Documentation Finder: *The operative report may indicate a preoperative diagnosis of any number of vertebra-related disorders, injuries or diseases including but not limited to traumatic vertebral fracture (rarely), pathologic vertebral fracture, vertebral defect due to disease, osteoporosis, and bone cyst, among other diagnoses.*

RVU			Global Days	Modifiers				
Mod	Non-Fac Total	Fac Total		51	50	62	80	MUE
	50.35	13.10	010	2	0	0	1	1

Percutaneous vertebroplasty, 1 vertebral body, unilateral or bilateral injection,
cervicothoracic (22510), lumbosacral (22511), each additional cervicothoracic or lumbosacral vertebral body (22512)

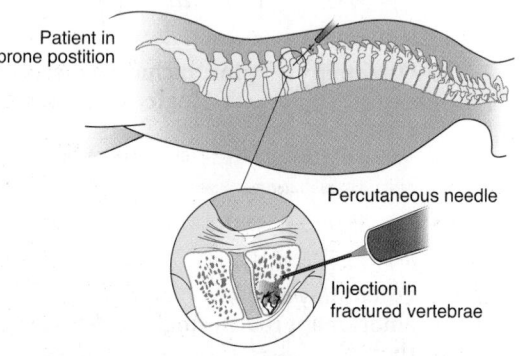

Patient in prone postition

Percutaneous needle

Injection in fractured vertebrae

⊙ 22511 Percutaneous vertebroplasty (bone biopsy included when performed), 1 vertebral body, unilateral or bilateral injection, inclusive of all imaging guidance; lumbosacral   G 2 T

RVU			Global Days	Modifiers				
Mod	Non-Fac Total	Fac Total		51	50	62	80	MUE
	49.85	12.30	010	2	0	0	1	1

AMA: Jan 15: 8, Apr 15: 8

⊙+22512 Percutaneous vertebroplasty (bone biopsy included when performed), 1 vertebral body, unilateral or bilateral injection, inclusive of all imaging guidance; each additional cervicothoracic or lumbosacral vertebral body (List separately in addition to code for primary procedure)   N I N

RVU			Global Days	Modifiers				
Mod	Non-Fac Total	Fac Total		51	50	62	80	MUE
	27.94	6.09	ZZZ	0	0	0	1	5

AMA: Jan 15: 8

● New   ▲ Revised   ✖ Deleted   ⊙ Moderate Sedation   ✚ Add-on Codes   ⊘ High Risk Denial   Ⓐ Age Edit   ♀ Female   ♂ Male   **AMA** *CPT® Assistant*   **MUE** Medically Unlikely Edit
⊘ Modifier 51 Exempt   ⊖ Modifier 63 Exempt   ✗ Unlisted   **Modifiers:** *See Inside Back Cover*   Ⓜ Maternity   A 2 – Z 3 ASC Payment Indicators   A – Y OPPS Status Indicators

CPT © 2015 American Medical Association. All Rights Reserved.   © 2016 DecisionHealth

22513 Percutaneous vertebral augmentation, including cavity creation (fracture reduction and bone biopsy included when performed) using mechanical device (eg, kyphoplasty), 1 vertebral body, unilateral or bilateral cannulation, inclusive of all imaging guidance; thoracic **G2 J1**

Documentation Finder: This procedure may be described in the operative report as a kyphoplasty. The operative report may describe a preoperative diagnosis of pathologic fracture, compression fracture, progressive osteoporosis or other bone-eroding disease processes.

RVU			Global Days	Modifiers				
Mod	Non-Fac Total	Fac Total		51	50	62	80	MUE
	209.45	15.65	010	2	0	0	1	1

22514 Percutaneous vertebral augmentation, including cavity creation (fracture reduction and bone biopsy included when performed) using mechanical device (eg, kyphoplasty), 1 vertebral body, unilateral or bilateral cannulation, inclusive of all imaging guidance; lumbar **G2 J1**

Documentation Finder: This procedure may be described in the operative report as a kyphoplasty. The operative report may describe a preoperative diagnosis of pathologic fracture, compression fracture, progressive osteoporosis or other bone-eroding disease processes.

RVU			Global Days	Modifiers				
Mod	Non-Fac Total	Fac Total		51	50	62	80	MUE
	209.22	14.59	010	2	0	0	1	1

+22515 Percutaneous vertebral augmentation, including cavity creation (fracture reduction and bone biopsy included when performed) using mechanical device (eg, kyphoplasty), 1 vertebral body, unilateral or bilateral cannulation, inclusive of all imaging guidance; each additional thoracic or lumbar vertebral body (List separately in addition to code for primary procedure) **N1 N**

Documentation Finder: This procedure may be described in the operative report as a kyphoplasty. The operative report may describe a preoperative diagnosis of pathologic fracture, compression fracture, progressive osteoporosis or other bone-eroding disease processes.

RVU			Global Days	Modifiers				
Mod	Non-Fac Total	Fac Total		51	50	62	80	MUE
	126.77	6.61	ZZZ	0	0	0	1	5

22526 Percutaneous intradiscal electrothermal annuloplasty, unilateral or bilateral including fluoroscopic guidance; single level **E**

RVU			Global Days	Modifiers				
Mod	Non-Fac Total	Fac Total		51	50	62	80	MUE
	67.90	10.12	010	9	9	9	9	

AMA: Sep 07: 10, Nov 10: 3, Jan 11: 8, Jan 15: 8
Pub 100-04, 32, 220.2

+22527 Percutaneous intradiscal electrothermal annuloplasty, unilateral or bilateral including fluoroscopic guidance; 1 or more additional levels (List separately in addition to code for primary procedure) **E**

RVU			Global Days	Modifiers				
Mod	Non-Fac Total	Fac Total		51	50	62	80	MUE
	56.34	4.60	ZZZ	9	9	9	9	

AMA: Sep 07: 10, Nov 10: 3, Jan 11: 8, Jan 15: 8
Pub 100-04, 32, 220.2

Spinal Arthrodesis

22532 Arthrodesis, lateral extracavitary technique, including minimal discectomy to prepare interspace (other than for decompression); thoracic **C**

RVU			Global Days	Modifiers				
Mod	Non-Fac Total	Fac Total		51	50	62	80	MUE
	51.51	51.51	090	2	0	2	2	1

AMA: Apr 12: 16, Jul 13: 3

Arthrodesis

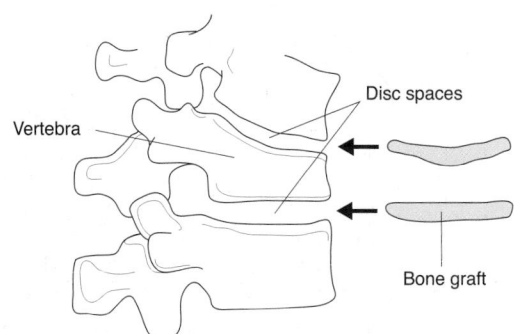

Vertebra — Disc spaces — Bone graft

A bone graft is used to fuse two vertebrae together. Code 22532 for thoracic vertebra; use 22533 for lumbar vertebra. Add 22534 for each additional vertebral segment that is fused.

22533 Arthrodesis, lateral extracavitary technique, including minimal discectomy to prepare interspace (other than for decompression); lumbar **C**

RVU			Global Days	Modifiers				
Mod	Non-Fac Total	Fac Total		51	50	62	80	MUE
	47.83	47.83	090	2	0	2	2	1

AMA: Apr 12: 16, Jul 13: 3

+22534 Arthrodesis, lateral extracavitary technique, including minimal discectomy to prepare interspace (other than for decompression); thoracic or lumbar, each additional vertebral segment (List separately in addition to code for primary procedure) **C**

RVU			Global Days	Modifiers				
Mod	Non-Fac Total	Fac Total		51	50	62	80	MUE
	10.27	10.27	ZZZ	0	0	2	2	3

22548 Arthrodesis, anterior transoral or extraoral technique, clivus-C1-C2 (atlas-axis), with or without excision of odontoid process **C**

RVU			Global Days	Modifiers				
Mod	Non-Fac Total	Fac Total		51	50	62	80	MUE
	58.11	58.11	090	2	0	2	2	1

AMA: Spring 93: 36, Feb 96: 7, Sep 97: 8, Sep 00: 10, Feb 02: 4, Apr 12: 16, Jul 13: 3

● New ▲ Revised Deleted ⊙ Moderate Sedation + Add-on Codes ⊖ High Risk Denial Ⓐ Age Edit ♀ Female ♂ Male **AMA** CPT® Assistant **MUE** Medically Unlikely Edit ⊘ Modifier 51 Exempt ⊖ Modifier 63 Exempt ⊠ Unlisted **Modifiers:** See Inside Back Cover Ⓜ Maternity A2-Z3 ASC Payment Indicators A-Y OPPS Status Indicators

© 2016 DecisionHealth   CPT © 2015 American Medical Association. All Rights Reserved.   **237**

22551 Arthrodesis, anterior interbody, including disc space preparation, discectomy, osteophytectomy and decompression of spinal cord and/or nerve roots; cervical below C2   J 8 J I

	RVU		Global Days	Modifiers				
Mod	Non-Fac Total	Fac Total		51	50	62	80	MUE
	49.87	49.87	090	2	0	2	2	1

AMA: Apr 12: 16, Jul 13: 3, Jan 15: 13

Arthrodesis; anterior interbody, cervical below C-2

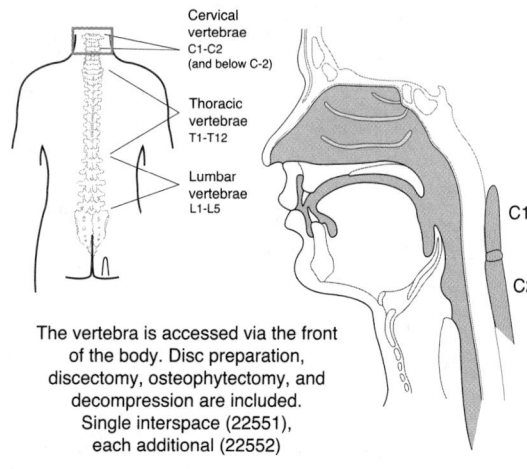

Cervical vertebrae C1-C2 (and below C-2)

Thoracic vertebrae T1-T12

Lumbar vertebrae L1-L5

C1

C2

The vertebra is accessed via the front of the body. Disc preparation, discectomy, osteophytectomy, and decompression are included. Single interspace (22551), each additional (22552)

+ 22552 Arthrodesis, anterior interbody, including disc space preparation, discectomy, osteophytectomy and decompression of spinal cord and/or nerve roots; cervical below C2, each additional interspace (List separately in addition to code for separate procedure)   N

	RVU		Global Days	Modifiers				
Mod	Non-Fac Total	Fac Total		51	50	62	80	MUE
	11.35	11.35	ZZZ	0	0	2	2	5

AMA: Apr 12: 16, Jul 13: 3

22554 Arthrodesis, anterior interbody technique, including minimal discectomy to prepare interspace (other than for decompression); cervical below C2   J 8 J I

	RVU		Global Days	Modifiers				
Mod	Non-Fac Total	Fac Total		51	50	62	80	MUE
	36.26	36.26	090	2	0	2	2	1

AMA: Spring 93: 36, Sep 97: 8, Sep 00: 10, Jan 01: 12, Feb 02: 4, Apr 12: 16, Jul 13: 3, Apr 15: 7

22556 Arthrodesis, anterior interbody technique, including minimal discectomy to prepare interspace (other than for decompression); thoracic   C

	RVU		Global Days	Modifiers				
Mod	Non-Fac Total	Fac Total		51	50	62	80	MUE
	48.53	48.53	090	2	0	2	2	1

AMA: Spring 93: 36, Jul 96: 7, Sep 97: 8, Sep 00: 10, Feb 02: 4, Apr 12: 16, Jul 13: 3

22558 Arthrodesis, anterior interbody technique, including minimal discectomy to prepare interspace (other than for decompression); lumbar   C

	RVU		Global Days	Modifiers				
Mod	Non-Fac Total	Fac Total		51	50	62	80	MUE
	44.78	44.78	090	2	0	2	2	1

AMA: Spring 93: 36, Mar 96: 6, Jul 96: 7, Sep 97: 8, Sep 00: 10, Feb 02: 4, Oct 09: 9, Apr 12: 16, Jul 13: 3, Mar 15: 9

+ 22585 Arthrodesis, anterior interbody technique, including minimal discectomy to prepare interspace (other than for decompression); each additional interspace (List separately in addition to code for primary procedure)   C

	RVU		Global Days	Modifiers				
Mod	Non-Fac Total	Fac Total		51	50	62	80	MUE
	9.44	9.44	ZZZ	0	0	2	2	7

AMA: Spring 93: 36, Feb 96: 6, Mar 96: 6, Sep 97: 8, Sep 00: 10, Feb 02: 4, Apr 08: 11

22586 Arthrodesis, pre-sacral interbody technique, including disc space preparation, discectomy, with posterior instrumentation, with image guidance, includes bone graft when performed, L5-S1 interspace   C

	RVU		Global Days	Modifiers				
Mod	Non-Fac Total	Fac Total		51	50	62	80	MUE
	52.58	52.58	090	2	0	2	2	1

22590 Arthrodesis, posterior technique, craniocervical (occiput-C2)   C

	RVU		Global Days	Modifiers				
Mod	Non-Fac Total	Fac Total		51	50	62	80	MUE
	46.14	46.14	090	2	0	2	2	1

AMA: Spring 93: 36, Sep 97: 8, Apr 12: 16, Jul 13: 3

22595 Arthrodesis, posterior technique, atlas-axis (C1-C2)   C

	RVU		Global Days	Modifiers				
Mod	Non-Fac Total	Fac Total		51	50	62	80	MUE
	44.00	44.00	090	2	0	2	2	1

AMA: Spring 93: 36, Sep 97: 8, Apr 12: 12, Jul 13: 3

22600 Arthrodesis, posterior or posterolateral technique, single level; cervical below C2 segment   C

	RVU		Global Days	Modifiers				
Mod	Non-Fac Total	Fac Total		51	50	62	80	MUE
	37.46	37.46	090	2	0	2	2	1

AMA: Spring 93: 36, Sep 97: 8, Nov 10: 8, Apr 12: 16, Jun 12: 11, Jul 13: 3

22610 Arthrodesis, posterior or posterolateral technique, single level; thoracic (with lateral transverse technique, when performed)   C

	RVU		Global Days	Modifiers				
Mod	Non-Fac Total	Fac Total		51	50	62	80	MUE
	36.63	36.63	090	2	0	2	2	1

AMA: Spring 93: 36, Sep 97: 8, Nov 10: 8, Apr 12: 16, Jun 12: 10, Jul 13: 3

● New ▲ Revised ✖ Deleted ⊙ Moderate Sedation ✚ Add-on Codes ⊘ High Risk Denial ⓐ Age Edit ♀ Female ♂ Male **AMA** CPT® Assistant **MUE** Medically Unlikely Edit ⊘ Modifier 51 Exempt ⊖ Modifier 63 Exempt ✗ Unlisted **Modifiers:** See Inside Back Cover Ⓜ Maternity A 2–Z 3 ASC Payment Indicators A –Y OPPS Status Indicators

238   CPT © 2015 American Medical Association. All Rights Reserved.   © 2016 DecisionHealth

22612 Arthrodesis, posterior or posterolateral technique, single level; lumbar (with lateral transverse technique, when performed)   G2 J-1

RVU			Global Days	Modifiers				
Mod	Non-Fac Total	Fac Total		51	50	62	80	MUE
	46.12	46.12	090	2	0	2	2	1

AMA: Spring 93: 36, Mar 96: 7, Sep 97: 8, 11, Apr 08: 11, Jul 08: 7, Oct 09: 9, Dec 11: 14, Nov 10: 8, Apr 12: 16, Jun 12: 10, Jan 12: 3, Jul 13: 3, Dec 13: 14

+ 22614 Arthrodesis, posterior or posterolateral technique, single level; each additional vertebral segment (List separately in addition to code for primary procedure)   N1 N

RVU			Global Days	Modifiers				
Mod	Non-Fac Total	Fac Total		51	50	62	80	MUE
	11.20	11.20	ZZZ	0	0	2	2	13

AMA: Feb 96: 6, Mar 96: 7, Nov 10: 8, Jun 12: 11, Jul 13: 3

22630 Arthrodesis, posterior interbody technique, including laminectomy and/or discectomy to prepare interspace (other than for decompression), single interspace; lumbar   C

RVU			Global Days	Modifiers				
Mod	Non-Fac Total	Fac Total		51	50	62	80	MUE
	45.51	45.51	090	2	0	2	2	1

AMA: Spring 93: 36, Sep 97: 8, Nov 99: 11, Dec 99: 2, Jan 01: 12, Oct 09: 9, Nov 11: 10, Dec 11: 14, Jan 12: 3, Apr 12: 16, Jun 12: 11, Jul 13: 3

+ 22632 Arthrodesis, posterior interbody technique, including laminectomy and/or discectomy to prepare interspace (other than for decompression), single interspace; each additional interspace (List separately in addition to code for primary procedure)   C

RVU			Global Days	Modifiers				
Mod	Non-Fac Total	Fac Total		51	50	62	80	MUE
	9.14	9.14	ZZZ	0	0	2	2	4

AMA: Feb 96: 6, Sep 97: 8, Dec 99: 2, Jun 12: 11, Jul 13: 3

22633 Arthrodesis, combined posterior or posterolateral technique with posterior interbody technique including laminectomy and/or discectomy sufficient to prepare interspace (other than for decompression), single interspace and segment; lumbar   C

RVU			Global Days	Modifiers				
Mod	Non-Fac Total	Fac Total		51	50	62	80	MUE
	53.69	53.69	090	2	0	2	2	1

AMA: Dec 11: 14, Jan 12: 3, Jun 12: 10, Jul 13: 3

+ 22634 Arthrodesis, combined posterior or posterolateral technique with posterior interbody technique including laminectomy and/or discectomy sufficient to prepare interspace (other than for decompression), single interspace and segment; each additional interspace and segment (List separately in addition to code for primary procedure)   C

RVU			Global Days	Modifiers				
Mod	Non-Fac Total	Fac Total		51	50	62	80	MUE
	14.09	14.09	ZZZ	0	0	2	2	4

AMA: Dec 11: 14, Jan 12: 3, Jun 12: 10, Jul 13: 3

22800 Arthrodesis, posterior, for spinal deformity, with or without cast; up to 6 vertebral segments   C

RVU			Global Days	Modifiers				
Mod	Non-Fac Total	Fac Total		51	50	62	80	MUE
	39.07	39.07	090	2	0	1	2	1

AMA: Apr 12: 16, Jul 13: 3

22802 Arthrodesis, posterior, for spinal deformity, with or without cast; 7 to 12 vertebral segments   C

RVU			Global Days	Modifiers				
Mod	Non-Fac Total	Fac Total		51	50	62	80	MUE
	60.86	60.86	090	2	0	1	2	1

AMA: Mar 96: 10, Apr 12: 16, Jul 13: 3

22804 Arthrodesis, posterior, for spinal deformity, with or without cast; 13 or more vertebral segments   C

RVU			Global Days	Modifiers				
Mod	Non-Fac Total	Fac Total		51	50	62	80	MUE
	70.48	70.48	090	2	0	1	2	1

AMA: Apr 12: 16, Jul 13: 3

22808 Arthrodesis, anterior, for spinal deformity, with or without cast; 2 to 3 vertebral segments   C

RVU			Global Days	Modifiers				
Mod	Non-Fac Total	Fac Total		51	50	62	80	MUE
	53.42	53.42	090	2	0	1	2	1

AMA: Feb 02: 4, Apr 12: 16, Jul 13: 3

22810 Arthrodesis, anterior, for spinal deformity, with or without cast; 4 to 7 vertebral segments   C

RVU			Global Days	Modifiers				
Mod	Non-Fac Total	Fac Total		51	50	62	80	MUE
	58.89	58.89	090	2	0	1	2	1

AMA: Mar 96: 10, Sep 97: 8, Feb 02: 4, Apr 12: 16, Jul 13: 3

22812 Arthrodesis, anterior, for spinal deformity, with or without cast; 8 or more vertebral segments   C

RVU			Global Days	Modifiers				
Mod	Non-Fac Total	Fac Total		51	50	62	80	MUE
	70.67	70.67	090	2	0	1	2	1

AMA: Feb 02: 4, Apr 12: 16, Jul 13: 3

22818 Kyphectomy, circumferential exposure of spine and resection of vertebral segment(s) (including body and posterior elements); single or 2 segments   C

RVU			Global Days	Modifiers				
Mod	Non-Fac Total	Fac Total		51	50	62	80	MUE
	63.21	63.21	090	2	0	2	2	1

AMA: Nov 97: 14

● New   ▲ Revised   Deleted   ⊙ Moderate Sedation   ✚ Add-on Codes   ⊘ High Risk Denial   Ⓐ Age Edit   ♀ Female   ♂ Male   **AMA** *CPT® Assistant*   **MUE** Medically Unlikely Edit
⊘ Modifier 51 Exempt   ⊖ Modifier 63 Exempt   ⊠ Unlisted   **Modifiers:** *See Inside Back Cover*   Ⓜ Maternity   A2-Z3 ASC Payment Indicators   A-Y OPPS Status Indicators

© 2016 DecisionHealth   CPT © 2015 American Medical Association. All Rights Reserved.

22819 Kyphectomy, circumferential exposure of spine and resection of vertebral segment(s) (including body and posterior elements); 3 or more segments   🄲

RVU			Global Days	Modifiers				
Mod	Non-Fac Total	Fac Total		51	50	62	80	MUE
	81.44	81.44	090	2	0	2	2	1

AMA: Nov 97: 14

Kyphectomy, circumferential exposure of spine and resection of vertebral segment

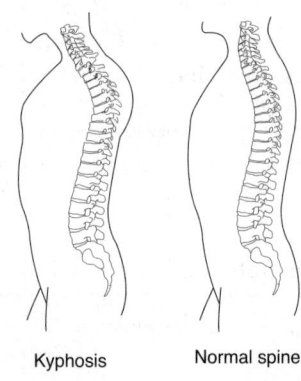

A condition is fixed in which the spine bulges out, causing a hump in the patients' back. Damaged and deformed vertebrae are removed, and the physician uses bone grafts and metal rods and wires to correct the deformity.

Kyphosis   Normal spine

Coding Guidance

Do not report exploration of spinal fusion with other procedures involving the spine, unless performed at a different anatomic site.

22830 Exploration of spinal fusion   🄲

RVU			Global Days	Modifiers				
Mod	Non-Fac Total	Fac Total		51	50	62	80	MUE
	23.49	23.49	090	2	0	1	2	1

AMA: Sep 97: 11, Mar 10: 9

Segmental/Nonsegmental Spinal Instrumentation

✚ **22840** Posterior non-segmental instrumentation (eg, Harrington rod technique, pedicle fixation across 1 interspace, atlantoaxial transarticular screw fixation, sublaminar wiring at C1, facet screw fixation) (List separately in addition to code for primary procedure)   🄲

RVU			Global Days	Modifiers				
Mod	Non-Fac Total	Fac Total		51	50	62	80	MUE
	21.66	21.66	ZZZ	0	0	1	2	1

AMA: Feb 96: 6, Jul 96: 10, Sep 97: 8, Nov 99: 12, Feb 02: 6, Dec 11: 15, Nov 10: 8, Jan 11: 9, Apr 12: 12, Jun 12: 11, Jul 13: 3, Dec 13: 17, Oct 14: 15

✚ **22841** Internal spinal fixation by wiring of spinous processes (List separately in addition to code for primary procedure)   ⊘🄲

RVU			Global Days	Modifiers				
Mod	Non-Fac Total	Fac Total		51	50	62	80	MUE
	0.00	0.00	XXX	9	9	9	9	

AMA: Feb 96: 6, Sep 97: 8, Feb 02: 6, Jun 12: 11, Jul 13: 3

✚ **22842** Posterior segmental instrumentation (eg, pedicle fixation, dual rods with multiple hooks and sublaminar wires); 3 to 6 vertebral segments (List separately in addition to code for primary procedure)   🄲

RVU			Global Days	Modifiers				
Mod	Non-Fac Total	Fac Total		51	50	62	80	MUE
	21.76	21.76	ZZZ	0	0	2	2	1

AMA: Feb 96: 6, Mar 96: 7, Sep 97: 8, Feb 02: 6, Dec 11: 15, Jun 12: 11, Jul 13: 3

✚ **22843** Posterior segmental instrumentation (eg, pedicle fixation, dual rods with multiple hooks and sublaminar wires); 7 to 12 vertebral segments (List separately in addition to code for primary procedure)   🄲

RVU			Global Days	Modifiers				
Mod	Non-Fac Total	Fac Total		51	50	62	80	MUE
	23.48	23.48	ZZZ	0	0	2	2	1

AMA: Feb 96: 6, Sep 97: 8, Feb 02: 6, Dec 11: 15, Jun 12: 11, Jul 13: 3

✚ **22844** Posterior segmental instrumentation (eg, pedicle fixation, dual rods with multiple hooks and sublaminar wires); 13 or more vertebral segments (List separately in addition to code for primary procedure)   🄲

RVU			Global Days	Modifiers				
Mod	Non-Fac Total	Fac Total		51	50	62	80	MUE
	28.42	28.42	ZZZ	0	0	2	2	1

AMA: Feb 96: 6, Sep 97: 8, Feb 02: 6, Dec 11: 15, Jun 12: 11, Jul 13: 3

✚ **22845** Anterior instrumentation; 2 to 3 vertebral segments (List separately in addition to code for primary procedure)   🄲

RVU			Global Days	Modifiers				
Mod	Non-Fac Total	Fac Total		51	50	62	80	MUE
	20.78	20.78	ZZZ	0	0	2	2	1

AMA: Feb 96: 6, Mar 96: 10, Jul 96: 7, 10, Sep 97: 8, Feb 02: 6, Jun 12: 11, Jul 13: 3, Nov 14: 14, Jan 15: 13, Mar 15: 9, Apr 15: 7

✚ **22846** Anterior instrumentation; 4 to 7 vertebral segments (List separately in addition to code for primary procedure)   🄲

RVU			Global Days	Modifiers				
Mod	Non-Fac Total	Fac Total		51	50	62	80	MUE
	21.55	21.55	ZZZ	0	0	2	2	1

AMA: Feb 96: 6, Sep 97: 8, Feb 02: 6, Jun 12: 11, Jul 13: 3

✚ **22847** Anterior instrumentation; 8 or more vertebral segments (List separately in addition to code for primary procedure)   🄲

RVU			Global Days	Modifiers				
Mod	Non-Fac Total	Fac Total		51	50	62	80	MUE
	23.68	23.68	ZZZ	0	0	2	2	1

AMA: Feb 96: 6, Sep 97: 8, Feb 02: 6, Jun 12: 11, Jul 13: 3

● New   ▲ Revised   ✖ Deleted   ⊙ Moderate Sedation   ✚ Add-on Codes   ⊖ High Risk Denial   Ⓐ Age Edit   ♀ Female   ♂ Male   **AMA** *CPT® Assistant*   *MUE* Medically Unlikely Edit

⊘ Modifier 51 Exempt   ⊖ Modifier 63 Exempt   ⓧ Unlisted   **Modifiers:** *See Inside Back Cover*   Ⓜ Maternity   A2–Z3 ASC Payment Indicators   A–Y OPPS Status Indicators

CPT © 2015 American Medical Association. All Rights Reserved.   © 2016 DecisionHealth

+ 22848 Pelvic fixation (attachment of caudal end of instrumentation to pelvic bony structures) other than sacrum (List separately in addition to code for primary procedure) C

RVU			Global Days	Modifiers				
Mod	Non-Fac Total	Fac Total		51	50	62	80	MUE
	10.34	10.34	ZZZ	0	0	2	2	1

AMA: Feb 96: 6, Sep 97: 8, Feb 02: 6, Jun 12: 11, Jul 13: 3

22849 Reinsertion of spinal fixation device C

RVU			Global Days	Modifiers				
Mod	Non-Fac Total	Fac Total		51	50	62	80	MUE
	37.68	37.68	090	2	0	1	2	1

AMA: Feb 96: 6, Sep 97: 8, Feb 02: 6, Nov 02: 3, Oct 11: 10, Jun 12: 11, Jul 13: 3

Reinsertion of spinal fixation device

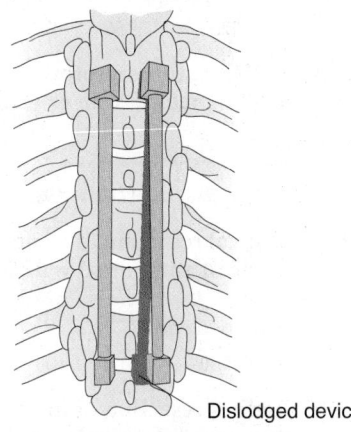

Dislodged device

This procedure is performed to reattach a device to the spine that has become dislodged.

22850 Removal of posterior nonsegmental instrumentation (eg, Harrington rod) C

RVU			Global Days	Modifiers				
Mod	Non-Fac Total	Fac Total		51	50	62	80	MUE
	20.95	20.95	090	2	0	1	2	1

AMA: Feb 96: 6, Sep 97: 8, Feb 02: 6, Jun 12: 11, Jul 13: 3

+ 22851 Application of intervertebral biomechanical device(s) (eg, synthetic cage(s), methylmethacrylate) to vertebral defect or interspace (List separately in addition to code for primary procedure) N

RVU			Global Days	Modifiers				
Mod	Non-Fac Total	Fac Total		51	50	62	80	MUE
	11.57	11.57	ZZZ	0	0	2	2	5

AMA: Feb 96: 6, Sep 97: 8, Nov 99: 12, Dec 99: 2, May 00: 11, Mar 01: 2, Feb 02: 6, Feb 05: 14, 15, Oct 11: 10, Dec 11: 15, Nov 10: 8, Jun 12: 11, Jul 13: 3, Nov 14: 14, Jan 15: 13, Mar 15: 9, Apr 15: 7

22852 Removal of posterior segmental instrumentation C

RVU			Global Days	Modifiers				
Mod	Non-Fac Total	Fac Total		51	50	62	80	MUE
	20.09	20.09	090	2	0	1	2	1

AMA: Feb 96: 6, Sep 97: 8, Feb 02: 6, May 06: 16, Jun 12: 11

22855 Removal of anterior instrumentation C

RVU			Global Days	Modifiers				
Mod	Non-Fac Total	Fac Total		51	50	62	80	MUE
	32.02	32.02	090	2	0	1	2	1

AMA: Feb 96: 6, Sep 97: 8, Feb 02: 6, Nov 02: 2, Jun 12: 11

Removal of anterior instrumentation

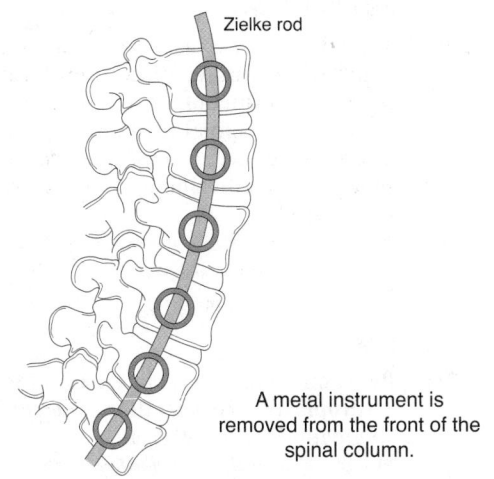

Zielke rod

A metal instrument is removed from the front of the spinal column.

22856 Total disc arthroplasty (artificial disc), anterior approach, including discectomy with end plate preparation (includes osteophytectomy for nerve root or spinal cord decompression and microdissection); single interspace, cervical J1

Documentation Finder: The operative report may describe underlying preoperative diagnoses including, but not limited to, vertebral degenerative disease, degenerative disc disease, disc herniation with or without myelopathy, traumatic or pathological fracture, or other disease processes such as neoplasm. Congenital defects also may be listed.

RVU			Global Days	Modifiers				
Mod	Non-Fac Total	Fac Total		51	50	62	80	MUE
	47.13	47.13	090	2	0	2	2	1

AMA: Apr 15: 7

Total disc arthroplasty (artificial disc), anterior approach, including discectomy with end plate preparation; second level,
Cervical (22856), additional cervical treatment (22858)

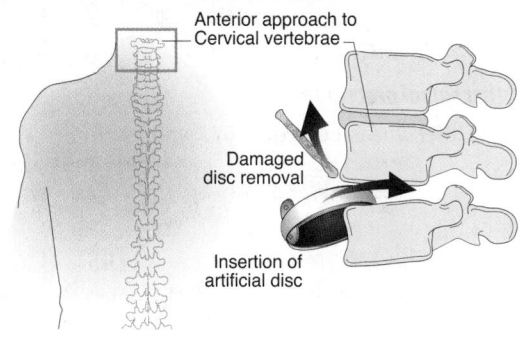

Anterior approach to Cervical vertebrae

Damaged disc removal

Insertion of artificial disc

● New　▲ Revised　Deleted　⊙ Moderate Sedation　✚ Add-on Codes　⊘ High Risk Denial　Ⓐ Age Edit　♀ Female　♂ Male　**AMA** CPT® Assistant　**MUE** Medically Unlikely Edit
⊘ Modifier 51 Exempt　⊖ Modifier 63 Exempt　✗ Unlisted　**Modifiers:** See Inside Back Cover　Ⓜ Maternity　A2-Z3 ASC Payment Indicators　A-Y OPPS Status Indicators

Surgical Procedures

22857   Total disc arthroplasty (artificial disc), anterior approach, including discectomy to prepare interspace (other than for decompression), single interspace, lumbar   ⊗**C**

	RVU		Global Days	Modifiers				
Mod	Non-Fac Total	Fac Total		51	50	62	80	MUE
	57.34	57.34	090	2	0	2	2	1

Pub 100-04, 32, 170.2

+ 22858   Total disc arthroplasty (artificial disc), anterior approach, including discectomy with end plate preparation (includes osteophytectomy for nerve root or spinal cord decompression and microdissection); second level, cervical (List separately in addition to code for primary procedure)   **C**

	RVU		Global Days	Modifiers				
Mod	Non-Fac Total	Fac Total		51	50	62	80	MUE
	14.76	14.76	ZZZ	0	0	2	2	1

AMA: Apr 15: 7

22861   Revision including replacement of total disc arthroplasty (artificial disc), anterior approach, single interspace; cervical   **C**

	RVU		Global Days	Modifiers				
Mod	Non-Fac Total	Fac Total		51	50	62	80	MUE
	58.36	58.36	090	2	0	2	2	1

22862   Revision including replacement of total disc arthroplasty (artificial disc), anterior approach, single interspace; lumbar   ⊗**C**

	RVU		Global Days	Modifiers				
Mod	Non-Fac Total	Fac Total		51	50	62	80	MUE
	58.06	58.06	090	2	0	2	2	1

AMA: Jun 07: 1

22864   Removal of total disc arthroplasty (artificial disc), anterior approach, single interspace; cervical   **C**

	RVU		Global Days	Modifiers				
Mod	Non-Fac Total	Fac Total		51	50	62	80	MUE
	60.49	60.49	090	2	0	2	2	1

22865   Removal of total disc arthroplasty (artificial disc), anterior approach, single interspace; lumbar   **C**

	RVU		Global Days	Modifiers				
Mod	Non-Fac Total	Fac Total		51	50	62	80	MUE
	59.64	59.64	090	2	0	2	2	1

AMA: Jun 07: 1

Other spinal procedures

22899   Unlisted procedure, spine   ✗**T**

	RVU		Global Days	Modifiers				
Mod	Non-Fac Total	Fac Total		51	50	62	80	MUE
	0.00	0.00	YYY	2	0	1	2	

AMA: May 00: 11, Sep 00: 10, Jul 06: 19, Feb 10: 13, Jan 12: 14, Nov 10: 4, Sep 12: 16, Dec 12: 13, Dec 13: 14, 17, Oct 14: 15, Jan 15: 8

Abdominal Musculoskeletal Procedures

22900   Excision, tumor, soft tissue of abdominal wall, subfascial (eg, intramuscular); less than 5 cm **G2T**

	RVU		Global Days	Modifiers				
Mod	Non-Fac Total	Fac Total		51	50	62	80	MUE
	16.32	16.32	090	2	0	1	2	3

22901   Excision, tumor, soft tissue of abdominal wall, subfascial (eg, intramuscular); 5 cm or greater   **G2T**

	RVU		Global Days	Modifiers				
Mod	Non-Fac Total	Fac Total		51	50	62	80	MUE
	19.22	19.22	090	2	0	1	2	2

22902   Excision, tumor, soft tissue of abdominal wall, subcutaneous; less than 3 cm   **G2T**

	RVU		Global Days	Modifiers				
Mod	Non-Fac Total	Fac Total		51	50	62	80	MUE
	12.59	9.56	090	2	0	1	2	4

22903   Excision, tumor, soft tissue of abdominal wall, subcutaneous; 3 cm or greater   **G2T**

	RVU		Global Days	Modifiers				
Mod	Non-Fac Total	Fac Total		51	50	62	80	MUE
	12.69	12.69	090	2	0	1	2	3

22904   Radical resection of tumor (eg, sarcoma), soft tissue of abdominal wall; less than 5 cm   **G2T**

	RVU		Global Days	Modifiers				
Mod	Non-Fac Total	Fac Total		51	50	62	80	MUE
	30.40	30.40	090	2	0	1	2	1

22905   Radical resection of tumor (eg, sarcoma), soft tissue of abdominal wall; 5 cm or greater   **G2T**

	RVU		Global Days	Modifiers				
Mod	Non-Fac Total	Fac Total		51	50	62	80	MUE
	38.54	38.54	090	2	0	1	2	1

22999   Unlisted procedure, abdomen, musculoskeletal system   ✗**T**

	RVU		Global Days	Modifiers				
Mod	Non-Fac Total	Fac Total		51	50	62	80	MUE
	0.00	0.00	YYY	2	0	1	0	

Musculoskeletal Shoulder Procedures

Incisional Shoulder Procedures

23000   Removal of subdeltoid calcareous deposits, open   **A2T**

	RVU		Global Days	Modifiers				
Mod	Non-Fac Total	Fac Total		51	50	62	80	MUE
	16.76	10.67	090	2	1	1	2	1

● New   ▲ Revised   ✖ Deleted   ⊙ Moderate Sedation   ✚ Add-on Codes   ⊗ High Risk Denial   ⑧ Age Edit   ♀ Female   ♂ Male   **AMA** *CPT® Assistant*   **MUE** Medically Unlikely Edit

⊘ Modifier 51 Exempt   ⊖ Modifier 63 Exempt   ✗ Unlisted   **Modifiers:** *See Inside Back Cover*   Ⓜ Maternity   **A2–Z3** ASC Payment Indicators   **A–Y** OPPS Status Indicators

242   CPT © 2015 American Medical Association. All Rights Reserved.   © 2016 DecisionHealth

23020 Capsular contracture release (eg, Sever type procedure)   A 2 T

RVU			Global Days	Modifiers				
Mod	Non-Fac Total	Fac Total		51	50	62	80	MUE
	19.74	19.74	090	2	1	0	2	1

Capsular contracture release

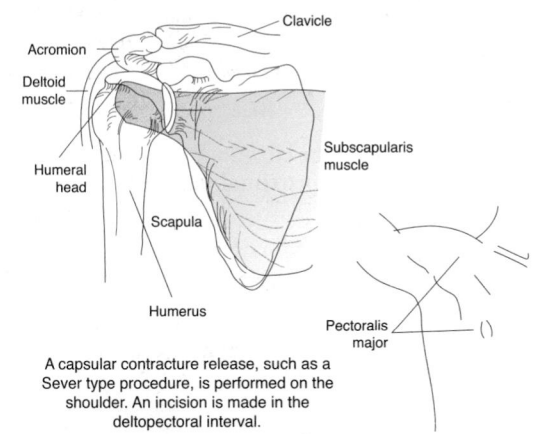

A capsular contracture release, such as a Sever type procedure, is performed on the shoulder. An incision is made in the deltopectoral interval.

23030 Incision and drainage, shoulder area; deep abscess or hematoma   A 2 T

RVU			Global Days	Modifiers				
Mod	Non-Fac Total	Fac Total		51	50	62	80	MUE
	12.68	7.39	010	2	0	0	1	2

23031 Incision and drainage, shoulder area; infected bursa   A 2 T

RVU			Global Days	Modifiers				
Mod	Non-Fac Total	Fac Total		51	50	62	80	MUE
	12.21	6.32	010	2	1	0	1	1

23035 Incision, bone cortex (eg, osteomyelitis or bone abscess), shoulder area   A 2 T

RVU			Global Days	Modifiers				
Mod	Non-Fac Total	Fac Total		51	50	62	80	MUE
	19.51	19.51	090	2	1	0	2	1

23040 Arthrotomy, glenohumeral joint, including exploration, drainage, or removal of foreign body   A 2 T

RVU			Global Days	Modifiers				
Mod	Non-Fac Total	Fac Total		51	50	62	80	MUE
	20.76	20.76	090	2	1	1	2	1

AMA: Nov 98: 8

23044 Arthrotomy, acromioclavicular, sternoclavicular joint, including exploration, drainage, or removal of foreign body   A 2 T

RVU			Global Days	Modifiers				
Mod	Non-Fac Total	Fac Total		51	50	62	80	MUE
	16.36	16.36	090	2	1	1	1	1

AMA: Nov 98: 8

Excisional Shoulder Procedures

23065 Biopsy, soft tissue of shoulder area; superficial   P 3 T

Coding tip: Code 99000 for specimen transfer from office setting to an outside laboratory

RVU			Global Days	Modifiers				
Mod	Non-Fac Total	Fac Total		51	50	62	80	MUE
	6.19	4.82	010	2	1	0	1	2

23066 Biopsy, soft tissue of shoulder area; deep   A 2 T

RVU			Global Days	Modifiers				
Mod	Non-Fac Total	Fac Total		51	50	62	80	MUE
	15.90	10.25	090	2	1	0	1	2

23071 Excision, tumor, soft tissue of shoulder area, subcutaneous; 3 cm or greater   G 2 T

Coding tip: Code 23071 is listed out of numerical order in CPT. Related soft tissue tumor excision procedures - 23075 (subcutaneous tissue); 23076 and 23073 (subfascial)

RVU			Global Days	Modifiers				
Mod	Non-Fac Total	Fac Total		51	50	62	80	MUE
	12.12	12.12	090	2	1	0	2	2

23073 Excision, tumor, soft tissue of shoulder area, subfascial (eg, intramuscular); 5 cm or greater   G 2 T

Coding tip: Code 23073 is listed out of numerical order in CPT. Related soft tissue tumor excision procedures - 23075 and 23071 (subcutaneous tissue); 23076 (subfascial)

RVU			Global Days	Modifiers				
Mod	Non-Fac Total	Fac Total		51	50	62	80	MUE
	20.03	20.03	090	2	1	0	2	2

23075 Excision, tumor, soft tissue of shoulder area, subcutaneous; less than 3 cm   G 2 T

Coding tip: Related soft tissue tumor excision codes - 23071, 23073, and 23076

RVU			Global Days	Modifiers				
Mod	Non-Fac Total	Fac Total		51	50	62	80	MUE
	13.39	9.40	090	2	1	0	1	3

AMA: Summer 92: 22, Nov 98: 8

23076 Excision, tumor, soft tissue of shoulder area, subfascial (eg, intramuscular); less than 5 cm   G 2 T

Coding tip: Related soft tissue tumor excision codes - 23071, 23073, and 23075

RVU			Global Days	Modifiers				
Mod	Non-Fac Total	Fac Total		51	50	62	80	MUE
	15.60	15.60	090	2	1	0	1	2

AMA: Summer 92: 22, Oct 09: 7

23077 Radical resection of tumor (eg, sarcoma), soft tissue of shoulder area; less than 5 cm   G 2 T

RVU			Global Days	Modifiers				
Mod	Non-Fac Total	Fac Total		51	50	62	80	MUE
	33.22	33.22	090	2	1	1	2	1

23078 Radical resection of tumor (eg, sarcoma), soft tissue of shoulder area; 5 cm or greater   G 2 T

RVU			Global Days	Modifiers				
Mod	Non-Fac Total	Fac Total		51	50	62	80	MUE
	41.64	41.64	090	2	1	1	2	1

● New   ▲ Revised   Deleted   ⊙ Moderate Sedation   ✚ Add-on Codes   ⊘ High Risk Denial   Ⓐ Age Edit   ♀ Female   ♂ Male   **AMA** *CPT® Assistant*   **MUE** Medically Unlikely Edit
⊘ Modifier 51 Exempt   ⊖ Modifier 63 Exempt   ✗ Unlisted   **Modifiers:** *See Inside Back Cover*   Ⓜ Maternity   A2-Z3 ASC Payment Indicators   A -Y OPPS Status Indicators

© 2016 DecisionHealth   CPT © 2015 American Medical Association. All Rights Reserved.   **243**

23100 Arthrotomy, glenohumeral joint, including biopsy A 2 T

Mod	Non-Fac Total	Fac Total	Global Days	51	50	62	80	MUE
	14.37	14.37	090	2	1	1	2	1

AMA: Nov 98: 8

23101 Arthrotomy, acromioclavicular joint or sternoclavicular joint, including biopsy and/or excision of torn cartilage A 2 T

Mod	Non-Fac Total	Fac Total	Global Days	51	50	62	80	MUE
	13.09	13.09	090	2	1	1	1	2

AMA: Nov 98: 8

23105 Arthrotomy; glenohumeral joint, with synovectomy, with or without biopsy A 2 T

Mod	Non-Fac Total	Fac Total	Global Days	51	50	62	80	MUE
	18.33	18.33	090	2	1	1	2	1

AMA: Nov 98: 8

23106 Arthrotomy; sternoclavicular joint, with synovectomy, with or without biopsy A 2 T

Mod	Non-Fac Total	Fac Total	Global Days	51	50	62	80	MUE
	14.19	14.19	090	2	1	1	1	1

23107 Arthrotomy, glenohumeral joint, with joint exploration, with or without removal of loose or foreign body A 2 T

Mod	Non-Fac Total	Fac Total	Global Days	51	50	62	80	MUE
	18.98	18.98	090	2	1	1	2	1

23120 Claviculectomy; partial A 2 T

Mod	Non-Fac Total	Fac Total	Global Days	51	50	62	80	MUE
	16.77	16.77	090	2	1	1	2	1

AMA: Sep 12: 16

23125 Claviculectomy; total A 2 T

Mod	Non-Fac Total	Fac Total	Global Days	51	50	62	80	MUE
	20.49	20.49	090	2	1	1	2	1

23130 Acromioplasty or acromionectomy, partial, with or without coracoacromial ligament release A 2 T

Mod	Non-Fac Total	Fac Total	Global Days	51	50	62	80	MUE
	17.60	17.60	090	2	1	1	1	1

AMA: Aug 01: 11, Mar 15: 7, Feb 15: 10

23140 Excision or curettage of bone cyst or benign tumor of clavicle or scapula A 2 T

Mod	Non-Fac Total	Fac Total	Global Days	51	50	62	80	MUE
	15.35	15.35	090	2	1	0	1	1

23145 Excision or curettage of bone cyst or benign tumor of clavicle or scapula; with autograft (includes obtaining graft) A 2 T

Mod	Non-Fac Total	Fac Total	Global Days	51	50	62	80	MUE
	20.08	20.08	090	2	1	1	2	1

23146 Excision or curettage of bone cyst or benign tumor of clavicle or scapula; with allograft A 2 J 1

Mod	Non-Fac Total	Fac Total	Global Days	51	50	62	80	MUE
	17.89	17.89	090	2	1	0	0	1

23150 Excision or curettage of bone cyst or benign tumor of proximal humerus A 2 T

Mod	Non-Fac Total	Fac Total	Global Days	51	50	62	80	MUE
	18.87	18.87	090	2	1	1	2	1

23155 Excision or curettage of bone cyst or benign tumor of proximal humerus; with autograft (includes obtaining graft) A 2 T

Mod	Non-Fac Total	Fac Total	Global Days	51	50	62	80	MUE
	22.93	22.93	090	2	1	1	2	1

23156 Excision or curettage of bone cyst or benign tumor of proximal humerus; with allograft A 2 J 1

Mod	Non-Fac Total	Fac Total	Global Days	51	50	62	80	MUE
	19.51	19.51	090	2	1	0	2	1

23170 Sequestrectomy (eg, for osteomyelitis or bone abscess), clavicle A 2 T

Mod	Non-Fac Total	Fac Total	Global Days	51	50	62	80	MUE
	16.08	16.08	090	2	1	0	1	1

23172 Sequestrectomy (eg, for osteomyelitis or bone abscess), scapula A 2 T

Mod	Non-Fac Total	Fac Total	Global Days	51	50	62	80	MUE
	16.36	16.36	090	2	1	0	2	1

23174 Sequestrectomy (eg, for osteomyelitis or bone abscess), humeral head to surgical neck A 2 T

Mod	Non-Fac Total	Fac Total	Global Days	51	50	62	80	MUE
	21.66	21.66	090	2	1	1	2	1

● New   ▲ Revised   ✖ Deleted   ⊙ Moderate Sedation   ✚ Add-on Codes   ⊘ High Risk Denial   Ⓐ Age Edit   ♀ Female   ♂ Male   **AMA** *CPT® Assistant*   **MUE** Medically Unlikely Edit
⊘ Modifier 51 Exempt   ⊖ Modifier 63 Exempt   ✗ Unlisted   **Modifiers:** *See Inside Back Cover*   Ⓜ Maternity   A 2–Z 3 ASC Payment Indicators   A – Y OPPS Status Indicators

244   CPT © 2015 American Medical Association. All Rights Reserved.   © 2016 DecisionHealth

23180 Partial excision (craterization, saucerization, or diaphysectomy) bone (eg, osteomyelitis), clavicle `A2T`

RVU			Global Days	Modifiers				
Mod	Non-Fac Total	Fac Total		51	50	62	80	MUE
	19.15	19.15	090	2	1	1	1	1

AMA: Nov 98: 9

Partial excision clavicle bone

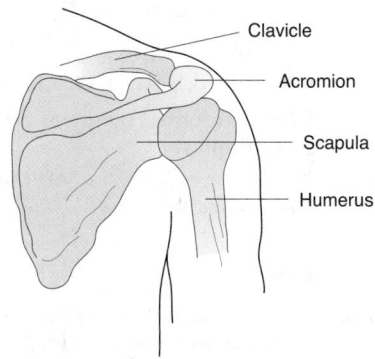

An incision is made in the top of the shoulder area, down to the bone. Part of the collar bone is then removed due to infection or disease. The incision is then closed. Code 23180 for partial excision. Code 23182 partial excision of scapula. Use 23184 for partial excision of proximal humerus.

23182 Partial excision (craterization, saucerization, or diaphysectomy) bone (eg, osteomyelitis), scapula `A2T`

RVU			Global Days	Modifiers				
Mod	Non-Fac Total	Fac Total		51	50	62	80	MUE
	18.63	18.63	090	2	1	0	2	1

AMA: Nov 98: 9

23184 Partial excision (craterization, saucerization, or diaphysectomy) bone (eg, osteomyelitis), proximal humerus `A2T`

RVU			Global Days	Modifiers				
Mod	Non-Fac Total	Fac Total		51	50	62	80	MUE
	21.19	21.19	090	2	1	1	2	1

AMA: Nov 98: 9

23190 Ostectomy of scapula, partial (eg, superior medial angle) `A2T`

RVU			Global Days	Modifiers				
Mod	Non-Fac Total	Fac Total		51	50	62	80	MUE
	16.34	16.34	090	2	1	1	2	1

23195 Resection, humeral head `A2 J I`

RVU			Global Days	Modifiers				
Mod	Non-Fac Total	Fac Total		51	50	62	80	MUE
	21.76	21.76	090	2	1	1	2	1

23200 Radical resection of tumor; clavicle `C`

RVU			Global Days	Modifiers				
Mod	Non-Fac Total	Fac Total		51	50	62	80	MUE
	43.12	43.12	090	2	1	1	2	1

23210 Radical resection of tumor; scapula `C`

RVU			Global Days	Modifiers				
Mod	Non-Fac Total	Fac Total		51	50	62	80	MUE
	51.43	51.43	090	2	1	1	2	1

23220 Radical resection of tumor, proximal humerus `C`

RVU			Global Days	Modifiers				
Mod	Non-Fac Total	Fac Total		51	50	62	80	MUE
	56.16	56.16	090	2	1	1	2	1

AMA: Nov 98: 8

Shoulder Introduction/Removal Procedures

23330 Removal of foreign body, shoulder; subcutaneous `A2T`

RVU			Global Days	Modifiers				
Mod	Non-Fac Total	Fac Total		51	50	62	80	MUE
	6.79	4.32	010	2	1	0	0	2

AMA: Aug 99: 3, Mar 14: 4

23333 Removal of foreign body, shoulder; deep (subfascial or intramuscular) `G2T`

RVU			Global Days	Modifiers				
Mod	Non-Fac Total	Fac Total		51	50	62	80	MUE
	13.09	13.09	090	2	1	0	0	1

AMA: Mar 14: 4

23334 Removal of prosthesis, includes debridement and synovectomy when performed; humeral or glenoid component `G2T`

RVU			Global Days	Modifiers				
Mod	Non-Fac Total	Fac Total		51	50	62	80	MUE
	31.19	31.19	090	2	1	1	1	1

AMA: Mar 14: 4

Removal of prosthesis, includes debridement and synovectomy when performed; humeral *or* glenoid component (23334), humeral *and* glenoid components (23335)

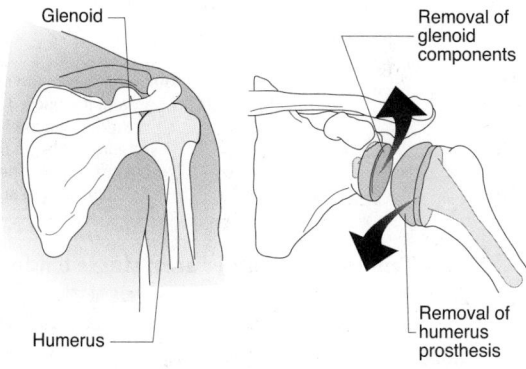

23335 Removal of prosthesis, includes debridement and synovectomy when performed; humeral and glenoid components (eg, total shoulder) `C`

RVU			Global Days	Modifiers				
Mod	Non-Fac Total	Fac Total		51	50	62	80	MUE
	37.11	37.11	090	2	1	1	1	1

AMA: Mar 14: 4

● New ▲ Revised Deleted ⊙ Moderate Sedation ✚ Add-on Codes ⊗ High Risk Denial Ⓐ Age Edit ♀ Female ♂ Male **AMA** *CPT® Assistant* *MUE* Medically Unlikely Edit
⊘ Modifier 51 Exempt ⊖ Modifier 63 Exempt 🗶 Unlisted **Modifiers:** *See Inside Back Cover* Ⓜ Maternity A2–Z3 ASC Payment Indicators A–Y OPPS Status Indicators

© 2016 DecisionHealth CPT © 2015 American Medical Association. All Rights Reserved. **245**

Surgical Procedures

23350 – 23455

23350 **Injection procedure for shoulder arthrography or enhanced CT/MRI shoulder arthrography** N I N

Coding tip: When contrast is injected with fluoroscopic guidance for enhanced CT/MRI imaging, report additional codes for fluoroscopic needle guidance and for the enhanced CT/MRI imaging

RVU			Global Days	Modifiers				
Mod	Non-Fac Total	Fac Total		51	50	62	80	MUE
	3.70	1.47	000	2	1	0	1	1

AMA: Jul 01: 3, Aug 15: 6

Shoulder Repair/Revision/Reconstruction Procedures

23395 **Muscle transfer, any type, shoulder or upper arm; single** A 2 J I

RVU			Global Days	Modifiers				
Mod	Non-Fac Total	Fac Total		51	50	62	80	MUE
	37.04	37.04	090	2	0	1	2	1

23397 **Muscle transfer, any type, shoulder or upper arm; multiple** A 2 T

RVU			Global Days	Modifiers				
Mod	Non-Fac Total	Fac Total		51	50	62	80	MUE
	33.01	33.01	090	2	0	1	2	1

23400 **Scapulopexy (eg, Sprengels deformity or for paralysis)** A 2 J I

RVU			Global Days	Modifiers				
Mod	Non-Fac Total	Fac Total		51	50	62	80	MUE
	28.11	28.11	090	2	1	1	2	1

Scapulopexy

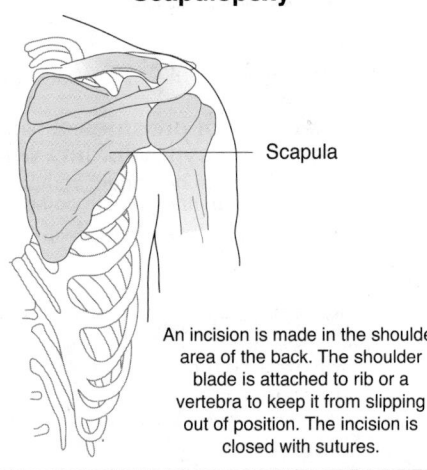

An incision is made in the shoulder area of the back. The shoulder blade is attached to rib or a vertebra to keep it from slipping out of position. The incision is closed with sutures.

Scapula

23405 **Tenotomy, shoulder area; single tendon** A 2 T

RVU			Global Days	Modifiers				
Mod	Non-Fac Total	Fac Total		51	50	62	80	MUE
	17.95	17.95	090	2	0	1	2	2

AMA: Nov 98: 8

23406 **Tenotomy, shoulder area; multiple tendons through same incision** A 2 T

RVU			Global Days	Modifiers				
Mod	Non-Fac Total	Fac Total		51	50	62	80	MUE
	22.09	22.09	090	2	0	0	2	1

AMA: Nov 98: 8

23410 **Repair of ruptured musculotendinous cuff (eg, rotator cuff) open; acute** A 2 J I

RVU			Global Days	Modifiers				
Mod	Non-Fac Total	Fac Total		51	50	62	80	MUE
	23.68	23.68	090	2	1	1	2	1

AMA: Aug 01: 11, Feb 02: 11

23412 **Repair of ruptured musculotendinous cuff (eg, rotator cuff) open; chronic** A 2 J I

RVU			Global Days	Modifiers				
Mod	Non-Fac Total	Fac Total		51	50	62	80	MUE
	24.53	24.53	090	2	1	1	2	1

AMA: Feb 02: 11, Sep 12: 16, Feb 15: 10, Jun 15: 10

23415 **Coracoacromial ligament release, with or without acromioplasty** A 2 T

RVU			Global Days	Modifiers				
Mod	Non-Fac Total	Fac Total		51	50	62	80	MUE
	20.12	20.12	090	2	1	1	1	1

AMA: Mar 15: 7

23420 **Reconstruction of complete shoulder (rotator) cuff avulsion, chronic (includes acromioplasty)** A 2 J I

RVU			Global Days	Modifiers				
Mod	Non-Fac Total	Fac Total		51	50	62	80	MUE
	27.92	27.92	090	2	1	1	2	1

AMA: Feb 02: 11, Oct 05: 23

23430 **Tenodesis of long tendon of biceps** A 2 J I

RVU			Global Days	Modifiers				
Mod	Non-Fac Total	Fac Total		51	50	62	80	MUE
	21.44	21.44	090	2	1	1	2	1

23440 **Resection or transplantation of long tendon of biceps** A 2 T

RVU			Global Days	Modifiers				
Mod	Non-Fac Total	Fac Total		51	50	62	80	MUE
	21.73	21.73	090	2	1	1	2	1

23450 **Capsulorrhaphy, anterior; Putti-Platt procedure or Magnuson type operation** A 2 T

RVU			Global Days	Modifiers				
Mod	Non-Fac Total	Fac Total		51	50	62	80	MUE
	27.27	27.27	090	2	1	1	2	1

23455 **Capsulorrhaphy, anterior; with labral repair (eg, Bankart procedure)** A 2 J I

RVU			Global Days	Modifiers				
Mod	Non-Fac Total	Fac Total		51	50	62	80	MUE
	28.84	28.84	090	2	1	1	2	1

AMA: Nov 98: 8

● New ▲ Revised ✖ Deleted ⊙ Moderate Sedation ✚ Add-on Codes ⊗ High Risk Denial Ⓐ Age Edit ♀ Female ♂ Male **AMA** *CPT® Assistant* **MUE** Medically Unlikely Edit
⊘ Modifier 51 Exempt ⊖ Modifier 63 Exempt ✗ Unlisted **Modifiers:** *See Inside Back Cover* Ⓜ Maternity A 2 – Z 3 ASC Payment Indicators A – Y OPPS Status Indicators

CPT © 2015 American Medical Association. All Rights Reserved. © 2016 DecisionHealth

23460 Capsulorrhaphy, anterior, any type; with bone block

A2 T

Mod	Non-Fac Total	Fac Total	Global Days	Modifiers				
				51	50	62	80	MUE
	31.56	31.56	090	2	1	1	2	1

Capsulorrhaphy with bone block

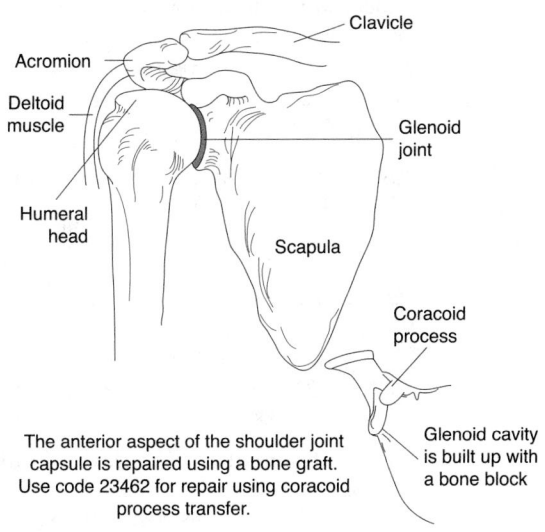

Clavicle
Acromion
Deltoid muscle
Glenoid joint
Humeral head
Scapula
Coracoid process
Glenoid cavity is built up with a bone block

The anterior aspect of the shoulder joint capsule is repaired using a bone graft. Use code 23462 for repair using coracoid process transfer.

23462 Capsulorrhaphy, anterior, any type; with coracoid process transfer

A2 J1

Mod	Non-Fac Total	Fac Total	Global Days	Modifiers				
				51	50	62	80	MUE
	30.61	30.61	090	2	1	1	2	1

23465 Capsulorrhaphy, glenohumeral joint, posterior, with or without bone block

G2 J1

Mod	Non-Fac Total	Fac Total	Global Days	Modifiers				
				51	50	62	80	MUE
	32.00	32.00	090	2	1	1	2	1

AMA: Nov 98: 8

23466 Capsulorrhaphy, glenohumeral joint, any type multi-directional instability

A2 J1

Mod	Non-Fac Total	Fac Total	Global Days	Modifiers				
				51	50	62	80	MUE
	32.18	32.18	090	2	1	1	2	1

AMA: Nov 98: 8

23470 Arthroplasty, glenohumeral joint; hemiarthroplasty

J1

Mod	Non-Fac Total	Fac Total	Global Days	Modifiers				
				51	50	62	80	MUE
	34.74	34.74	090	2	1	1	2	1

AMA: Nov 98: 8, Mar 14: 4

23472 Arthroplasty, glenohumeral joint; total shoulder (glenoid and proximal humeral replacement (eg, total shoulder))

C

Mod	Non-Fac Total	Fac Total	Global Days	Modifiers				
				51	50	62	80	MUE
	42.03	42.03	090	2	1	1	2	1

AMA: Jun 96: 10, Nov 98: 8, Mar 13: 12, Mar 14: 4

23473 Revision of total shoulder arthroplasty, including allograft when performed; humeral or glenoid component

J1

Mod	Non-Fac Total	Fac Total	Global Days	Modifiers				
				51	50	62	80	MUE
	46.68	46.68	090	2	1	1	2	1

AMA: Mar 13: 12, Feb 13: 11, Mar 14: 4

Revision of total shoulder arthroplasty, including allograft when performed;
humeral *or* glenoid component (23473),
humeral *and* glenoid components (23474)

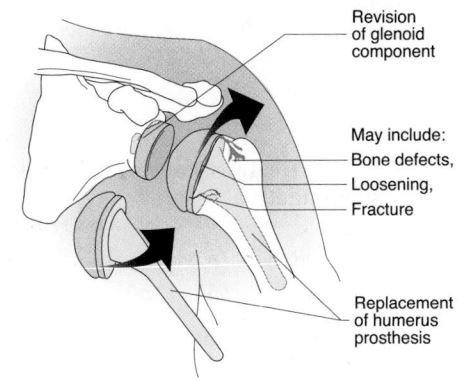

Revision of glenoid component
May include:
Bone defects,
Loosening,
Fracture
Replacement of humerus prosthesis

23474 Revision of total shoulder arthroplasty, including allograft when performed; humeral and glenoid component

C

Mod	Non-Fac Total	Fac Total	Global Days	Modifiers				
				51	50	62	80	MUE
	50.45	50.45	090	2	1	1	2	1

AMA: Mar 13: 12, Feb 13: 11, Mar 14: 4

23480 Osteotomy, clavicle, with or without internal fixation

A2 T

Mod	Non-Fac Total	Fac Total	Global Days	Modifiers				
				51	50	62	80	MUE
	23.74	23.74	090	2	1	1	1	1

23485 Osteotomy, clavicle, with or without internal fixation; with bone graft for nonunion or malunion (includes obtaining graft and/or necessary fixation)

G2 J1

Mod	Non-Fac Total	Fac Total	Global Days	Modifiers				
				51	50	62	80	MUE
	27.54	27.54	090	2	1	1	2	1

23490 Prophylactic treatment (nailing, pinning, plating or wiring) with or without methylmethacrylate; clavicle

A2 J1

Mod	Non-Fac Total	Fac Total	Global Days	Modifiers				
				51	50	62	80	MUE
	24.32	24.32	090	2	1	0	2	1

23491 Prophylactic treatment (nailing, pinning, plating or wiring) with or without methylmethacrylate; proximal humerus

G2 J1

Mod	Non-Fac Total	Fac Total	Global Days	Modifiers				
				51	50	62	80	MUE
	29.30	29.30	090	2	1	1	2	1

AMA: Nov 98: 8

● New ▲ Revised Deleted ⊙ Moderate Sedation ✚ Add-on Codes ⊘ High Risk Denial Ⓐ Age Edit ♀ Female ♂ Male **AMA** *CPT® Assistant* *MUE* Medically Unlikely Edit
⊘ Modifier 51 Exempt ⊖ Modifier 63 Exempt ✗ Unlisted **Modifiers:** *See Inside Back Cover* Ⓜ Maternity A2 –Z3 ASC Payment Indicators A –Y OPPS Status Indicators

Surgical Procedures

23500 – 23570

Shoulder Fracture/Dislocation Procedures

Coding Guidance

Open treatment of fractures or dislocations includes the application of casts, straps, or splints; do not report their application separately. The physician who treated the fracture or dislocation with an initial cast, splint, or strap and assumed the follow-up care cannot report the casting/splinting/strapping codes, as they are inclusive in the fracture/dislocation care codes. The physician who treated the fracture or dislocation with a cast, splint, or strap as an initial service minus any other definitive care and expects to do only the initial casting, may report an E&M service code (if significant and separately identifiable), the casting/strapping/splinting application code, and a supply code (Q4001-Q4051) for the cast/splint/strap used. According to OPPS rules, a hospital that treats the fracture or dislocation with a cast, splint, or strap as an initial service minus any other definitive care, reports the casting/strapping/splinting application code, while payment for the supply of the cast/splint/strap is included. When closed fracture reduction is followed by open reduction for the same patient encounter, only the open reduction service can be reported. Use codes 11010-11012 for debridement of tissue with open fractures or dislocations.

23500 Closed treatment of clavicular fracture; without manipulation   A 2 T

RVU			Global Days	Modifiers				
Mod	Non-Fac Total	Fac Total		51	50	62	80	MUE
	6.29	6.39	090	2	1	0	1	1

23505 Closed treatment of clavicular fracture; with manipulation   A 2 T

Coding tip: Add modifier 77 for re-reduction of the fracture by another physician

RVU			Global Days	Modifiers				
Mod	Non-Fac Total	Fac Total		51	50	62	80	MUE
	10.15	9.59	090	2	1	0	1	1

23515 Open treatment of clavicular fracture, includes internal fixation, when performed   A 2 J T

RVU			Global Days	Modifiers				
Mod	Non-Fac Total	Fac Total		51	50	62	80	MUE
	20.75	20.75	090	2	1	1	2	1

AMA: Jan 08: 4

23520 Closed treatment of sternoclavicular dislocation; without manipulation   A 2 T

Coding tip: Closed treatment of sternum fracture - 21820

Coding tip: Closed treatment of acromioclavicular dislocation - 23540

RVU			Global Days	Modifiers				
Mod	Non-Fac Total	Fac Total		51	50	62	80	MUE
	6.41	6.51	090	2	1	0	0	1

23525 Closed treatment of sternoclavicular dislocation; with manipulation   A 2 T

Coding tip: Add modifier 77 for re-reduction of the dislocation by another physician

Coding tip: Closed treatment of acromioclavicular dislocation with manipulation - 23545

RVU			Global Days	Modifiers				
Mod	Non-Fac Total	Fac Total		51	50	62	80	MUE
	10.79	9.98	090	2	1	0	0	1

23530 Open treatment of sternoclavicular dislocation, acute or chronic   A 2 T

RVU			Global Days	Modifiers				
Mod	Non-Fac Total	Fac Total		51	50	62	80	MUE
	15.85	15.85	090	2	1	0	2	1

23532 Open treatment of sternoclavicular dislocation, acute or chronic; with fascial graft (includes obtaining graft)   A 2 J T

RVU			Global Days	Modifiers				
Mod	Non-Fac Total	Fac Total		51	50	62	80	MUE
	17.94	17.94	090	2	1	0	2	1

23540 Closed treatment of acromioclavicular dislocation; without manipulation   A 2 T

Coding tip: Closed treatment of sternoclavicular dislocation - 23520

RVU			Global Days	Modifiers				
Mod	Non-Fac Total	Fac Total		51	50	62	80	MUE
	6.49	6.60	090	2	1	0	1	1

23545 Closed treatment of acromioclavicular dislocation; with manipulation   A 2 T

Coding tip: Closed treatment of sternoclavicular dislocation with manipulation - 23525

Coding tip: Add modifier 77 for re-reduction of the fracture by another physician

RVU			Global Days	Modifiers				
Mod	Non-Fac Total	Fac Total		51	50	62	80	MUE
	9.69	8.81	090	2	1	0	0	1

23550 Open treatment of acromioclavicular dislocation, acute or chronic   A 2 J T

RVU			Global Days	Modifiers				
Mod	Non-Fac Total	Fac Total		51	50	62	80	MUE
	16.16	16.16	090	2	1	1	2	1

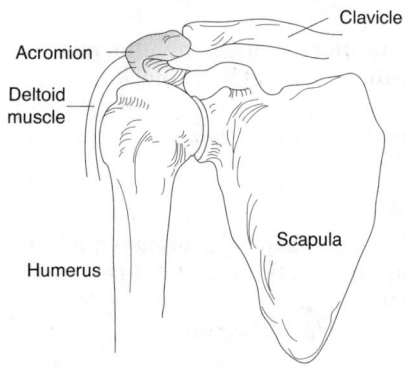

Open treatment of acromioclavicular dislocation

The physician makes an incision over a dislocation of the collar bone where it meets the top bone of the shoulder. The joint is stabilized using a screw tendon transfer (23550) or fascial graft (23552).

23552 Open treatment of acromioclavicular dislocation, acute or chronic; with fascial graft (includes obtaining graft)   G 2 J T

RVU			Global Days	Modifiers				
Mod	Non-Fac Total	Fac Total		51	50	62	80	MUE
	18.85	18.85	090	2	1	1	2	1

23570 Closed treatment of scapular fracture; without manipulation   A 2 T

RVU			Global Days	Modifiers				
Mod	Non-Fac Total	Fac Total		51	50	62	80	MUE
	6.65	6.86	090	2	1	0	1	1

● New   ▲ Revised   ✖ Deleted   ⊙ Moderate Sedation   ✚ Add-on Codes   ⊘ High Risk Denial   Ⓐ Age Edit   ♀ Female   ♂ Male   **AMA** *CPT® Assistant*   **MUE** Medically Unlikely Edit
⊗ Modifier 51 Exempt   ⊖ Modifier 63 Exempt   ✗ Unlisted   **Modifiers:** *See Inside Back Cover*   Ⓜ Maternity   A 2–Z 3 ASC Payment Indicators   A –Y OPPS Status Indicators

CPT © 2015 American Medical Association. All Rights Reserved.   © 2016 DecisionHealth

23575 Closed treatment of scapular fracture; with manipulation, with or without skeletal traction (with or without shoulder joint involvement) A 2 T

Coding tip: Skeletal traction requires the use of a wire, pin, screw, or clamp attached through the bone, which is included in the initial placement - code separately only when a subsequent traction device is placed

Coding tip: Removal of the initial traction device is included - code separately only when a subsequent traction device is removed

RVU			Global Days	Modifiers				
Mod	Non-Fac Total	Fac Total		51	50	62	80	MUE
	11.45	10.74	090	2	1	0	0	1

23585 Open treatment of scapular fracture (body, glenoid or acromion) includes internal fixation, when performed A 2 J I

RVU			Global Days	Modifiers				
Mod	Non-Fac Total	Fac Total		51	50	62	80	MUE
	28.31	28.31	090	2	1	1	2	1

AMA: Oct 04: 10

23600 Closed treatment of proximal humeral (surgical or anatomical neck) fracture; without manipulation P 2 T

Coding tip: Closed treatment of humeral shaft fracture - 24500

Coding tip: Closed treatment of greater humeral tuberosity fracture - 23620

RVU			Global Days	Modifiers				
Mod	Non-Fac Total	Fac Total		51	50	62	80	MUE
	9.37	8.84	090	2	1	0	1	1

23605 Closed treatment of proximal humeral (surgical or anatomical neck) fracture; with manipulation, with or without skeletal traction A 2 T

Coding tip: Closed treatment of greater humeral tuberosity fracture with manipulation - 23625

Coding tip: Skeletal traction requires the use of a wire, pin, screw, or clamp attached through the bone, which is included in the initial placement - code separately only when a subsequent traction device is placed

Coding tip: Removal of the initial traction device is included - code separately only when a subsequent traction device is removed

Coding tip: Closed treatment of humeral shaft fracture with manipulation - 24505

Coding tip: Add modifier 77 for re-reduction of the fracture by another physician

RVU			Global Days	Modifiers				
Mod	Non-Fac Total	Fac Total		51	50	62	80	MUE
	13.35	12.26	090	2	1	0	1	1

23615 Open treatment of proximal humeral (surgical or anatomical neck) fracture, includes internal fixation, when performed, includes repair of tuberosity(s), when performed G 2 J I

RVU			Global Days	Modifiers				
Mod	Non-Fac Total	Fac Total		51	50	62	80	MUE
	25.53	25.53	090	2	1	1	2	1

AMA: Jan 08: 4

23616 Open treatment of proximal humeral (surgical or anatomical neck) fracture, includes internal fixation, when performed, includes repair of tuberosity(s), when performed; with proximal humeral prosthetic replacement J 8 J I

RVU			Global Days	Modifiers				
Mod	Non-Fac Total	Fac Total		51	50	62	80	MUE
	35.87	35.87	090	2	1	2	2	1

23620 Closed treatment of greater humeral tuberosity fracture; without manipulation P 2 T

Coding tip: Closed treatment of humeral shaft fracture - 24500

Coding tip: Closed treatment of proximal humeral (neck) fracture - 23600

RVU			Global Days	Modifiers				
Mod	Non-Fac Total	Fac Total		51	50	62	80	MUE
	7.71	7.35	090	2	1	0	1	1

AMA: Nov 98: 8

Closed treatment of greater humeral tuberosity fracture

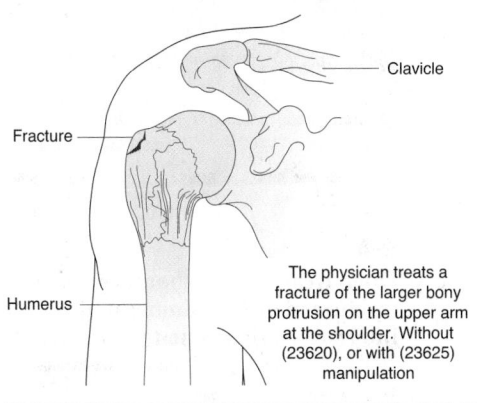

Clavicle

Fracture

Humerus

The physician treats a fracture of the larger bony protrusion on the upper arm at the shoulder. Without (23620), or with (23625) manipulation

23625 Closed treatment of greater humeral tuberosity fracture; with manipulation A 2 T

Coding tip: Closed treatment of proximal humeral (neck) fracture with manipulation - 23605

Coding tip: Add modifier 77 for re-reduction of the fracture by another physician

Coding tip: Closed treatment of humeral shaft fracture with manipulation - 24505

RVU			Global Days	Modifiers				
Mod	Non-Fac Total	Fac Total		51	50	62	80	MUE
	10.91	10.17	090	2	1	0	1	1

23630 Open treatment of greater humeral tuberosity fracture, includes internal fixation, when performed A 2 J I

RVU			Global Days	Modifiers				
Mod	Non-Fac Total	Fac Total		51	50	62	80	MUE
	22.55	22.55	090	2	1	1	2	1

AMA: Nov 98: 8

23650 Closed treatment of shoulder dislocation, with manipulation; without anesthesia A 2 T

Coding tip: Add modifier 77 for re-reduction of the dislocation by another physician

RVU			Global Days	Modifiers				
Mod	Non-Fac Total	Fac Total		51	50	62	80	MUE
	8.91	8.18	090	2	1	0	1	1

● New ▲ Revised Deleted ⊙ Moderate Sedation ✚ Add-on Codes ⊘ High Risk Denial Ⓐ Age Edit ♀ Female ♂ Male **AMA** *CPT® Assistant* **MUE** Medically Unlikely Edit
⊘ Modifier 51 Exempt ⊖ Modifier 63 Exempt ☒ Unlisted **Modifiers:** *See Inside Back Cover* Ⓜ Maternity A 2 – Z 3 ASC Payment Indicators A – Y OPPS Status Indicators

© 2016 DecisionHealth | CPT © 2015 American Medical Association. All Rights Reserved. | **249**

Surgical Procedures

23575 – 23650

23655 **Closed treatment of shoulder dislocation, with manipulation; requiring anesthesia** `A2 T`

Coding tip: Add modifier 77 for re-reduction of the dislocation by another physician

RVU			Global Days	Modifiers				
Mod	Non-Fac Total	Fac Total		51	50	62	80	MUE
	11.57	11.57	090	2	1	0	1	1

23660 **Open treatment of acute shoulder dislocation** `A2 T`

RVU			Global Days	Modifiers				
Mod	Non-Fac Total	Fac Total		51	50	62	80	MUE
	16.72	16.72	090	2	1	1	2	1

AMA: Feb 96: 5

23665 **Closed treatment of shoulder dislocation, with fracture of greater humeral tuberosity, with manipulation** `A2 T`

Coding tip: Closed treatment of humeral fracture without concomitant dislocation - 23600-23605, 23620-23625

Coding tip: Closed treatment of shoulder dislocation without concomitant humeral fracture - 23650-23655

Coding tip: Closed treatment of shoulder dislocation with proximal humeral neck fracture - 23675

Coding tip: Add modifier 77 for re-reduction by another physician

RVU			Global Days	Modifiers				
Mod	Non-Fac Total	Fac Total		51	50	62	80	MUE
	12.23	11.41	090	2	1	0	1	1

AMA: Nov 98: 8

23670 **Open treatment of shoulder dislocation, with fracture of greater humeral tuberosity, includes internal fixation, when performed** `A2 J I`

RVU			Global Days	Modifiers				
Mod	Non-Fac Total	Fac Total		51	50	62	80	MUE
	25.25	25.25	090	2	1	1	2	1

AMA: Nov 98: 8

23675 **Closed treatment of shoulder dislocation, with surgical or anatomical neck fracture, with manipulation** `A2 T`

Coding tip: Closed treatment of humeral fracture without concomitant dislocation - 23600-23605, 23620-23625

Coding tip: Closed treatment of shoulder dislocation without concomitant humeral fracture - 23650-23655

Coding tip: Add modifier 77 for re-reduction by another physician

Coding tip: Closed treatment of shoulder dislocation with greater humeral tuberosity fracture - 23665

RVU			Global Days	Modifiers				
Mod	Non-Fac Total	Fac Total		51	50	62	80	MUE
	15.85	14.46	090	2	1	0	1	1

23680 **Open treatment of shoulder dislocation, with surgical or anatomical neck fracture, includes internal fixation, when performed** `G2 J I`

RVU			Global Days	Modifiers				
Mod	Non-Fac Total	Fac Total		51	50	62	80	MUE
	26.79	26.79	090	2	1	1	2	1

Shoulder Manipulation

23700 **Manipulation under anesthesia, shoulder joint, including application of fixation apparatus (dislocation excluded)** `A2 T`

Coding tip: Do not report 23700 if general anesthesia is not used

RVU			Global Days	Modifiers				
Mod	Non-Fac Total	Fac Total		51	50	62	80	MUE
	5.66	5.66	010	2	1	0	1	1

AMA: Jan 99: 10, Apr 05: 14, May 09: 8, Jun 15: 10

Shoulder Arthrodesis

23800 **Arthrodesis, glenohumeral joint** `G2 J I`

RVU			Global Days	Modifiers				
Mod	Non-Fac Total	Fac Total		51	50	62	80	MUE
	29.69	29.69	090	2	1	1	2	1

AMA: Nov 98: 8

23802 **Arthrodesis, glenohumeral joint; with autogenous graft (includes obtaining graft)** `G2 J I`

RVU			Global Days	Modifiers				
Mod	Non-Fac Total	Fac Total		51	50	62	80	MUE
	36.67	36.67	090	2	1	1	2	1

Shoulder Amputation

23900 **Interthoracoscapular amputation (forequarter)** `C`

RVU			Global Days	Modifiers				
Mod	Non-Fac Total	Fac Total		51	50	62	80	MUE
	40.27	40.27	090	2	0	0	2	1

23920 **Disarticulation of shoulder** `C`

RVU			Global Days	Modifiers				
Mod	Non-Fac Total	Fac Total		51	50	62	80	MUE
	32.54	32.54	090	2	1	1	2	1

23921 **Disarticulation of shoulder; secondary closure or scar revision** `A2 T`

RVU			Global Days	Modifiers				
Mod	Non-Fac Total	Fac Total		51	50	62	80	MUE
	13.51	13.51	090	2	1	0	1	1

Other Shoulder Procedures

23929 **Unlisted procedure, shoulder** `x T`

RVU			Global Days	Modifiers				
Mod	Non-Fac Total	Fac Total		51	50	62	80	MUE
	0.00	0.00	YYY	2	0	1	2	

Musculoskeletal Upper Arm/Elbow Procedures

Upper Arm/Elbow Incisional Procedures

23930 **Incision and drainage, upper arm or elbow area; deep abscess or hematoma** `A2 T`

RVU			Global Days	Modifiers				
Mod	Non-Fac Total	Fac Total		51	50	62	80	MUE
	10.10	6.21	010	2	1	0	1	2

23931 **Incision and drainage, upper arm or elbow area; bursa** `A2 T`

RVU			Global Days	Modifiers				
Mod	Non-Fac Total	Fac Total		51	50	62	80	MUE
	8.21	4.59	010	2	1	0	1	2

AMA: Nov 98: 8

● New   ▲ Revised   ✖ Deleted   ⊙ Moderate Sedation   ✚ Add-on Codes   ⊘ High Risk Denial   Ⓐ Age Edit   ♀ Female   ♂ Male   **AMA** CPT® Assistant   **MUE** Medically Unlikely Edit
⊘ Modifier 51 Exempt   ⊖ Modifier 63 Exempt   ✗ Unlisted   **Modifiers:** See Inside Back Cover   Ⓜ Maternity   `A2`–`Z3` ASC Payment Indicators   `A`–`Y` OPPS Status Indicators

CPT © 2015 American Medical Association. All Rights Reserved.   © 2016 DecisionHealth

23935 Incision, deep, with opening of bone cortex (eg, for osteomyelitis or bone abscess), humerus or elbow `A 2 T`

RVU			Global Days	Modifiers				
Mod	Non-Fac Total	Fac Total		51	50	62	80	MUE
	14.60	14.60	090	2	1	0	0	2

24000 Arthrotomy, elbow, including exploration, drainage, or removal of foreign body `A 2 T`

RVU			Global Days	Modifiers				
Mod	Non-Fac Total	Fac Total		51	50	62	80	MUE
	13.75	13.75	090	2	1	1	0	1

AMA: Nov 98: 8, 9

24006 Arthrotomy of the elbow, with capsular excision for capsular release (separate procedure) `A 2 T`

RVU			Global Days	Modifiers				
Mod	Non-Fac Total	Fac Total		51	50	62	80	MUE
	20.40	20.40	090	2	1	2	2	1

Upper Arm/Elbow Excisional Procedures

24065 Biopsy, soft tissue of upper arm or elbow area; superficial `P 3 T`

Coding tip: Code 99000 for specimen transfer from office setting to an outside laboratory

RVU			Global Days	Modifiers				
Mod	Non-Fac Total	Fac Total		51	50	62	80	MUE
	7.32	4.83	010	2	1	0	1	2

24066 Biopsy, soft tissue of upper arm or elbow area; deep (subfascial or intramuscular) `A 2 T`

RVU			Global Days	Modifiers				
Mod	Non-Fac Total	Fac Total		51	50	62	80	MUE
	17.87	11.97	090	2	1	0	1	2

24071 Excision, tumor, soft tissue of upper arm or elbow area, subcutaneous; 3 cm or greater `G 2 T`

Coding tip: Code 24071 is listed out of numerical order in CPT. Related soft tissue tumor excision procedures - 24075 (subcutaneous); 24076 and 24073 (subfascial)

RVU			Global Days	Modifiers				
Mod	Non-Fac Total	Fac Total		51	50	62	80	MUE
	11.72	11.72	090	2	1	0	2	3

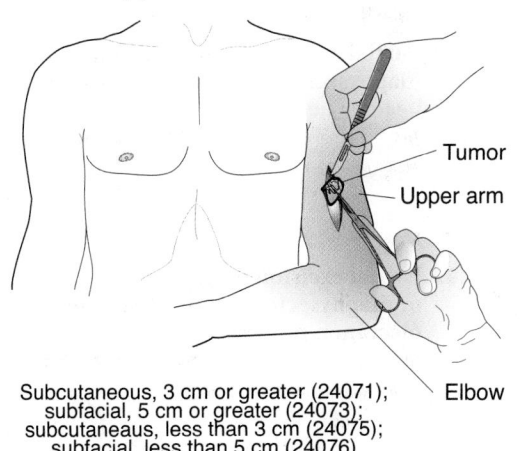

Excision, tumor, soft tissue of upper arm or elbow area

Tumor
Upper arm
Elbow

Subcutaneous, 3 cm or greater (24071); subfacial, 5 cm or greater (24073); subcutaneaus, less than 3 cm (24075); subfacial, less than 5 cm (24076)

24073 Excision, tumor, soft tissue of upper arm or elbow area, subfascial (eg, intramuscular); 5 cm or greater `G 2 T`

Coding tip: Code 24073 is listed out of numerical order in CPT. Related soft tissue tumor excision procedures - 24071 and 24075 (subcutaneous); 24076 (subfascial)

RVU			Global Days	Modifiers				
Mod	Non-Fac Total	Fac Total		51	50	62	80	MUE
	20.02	20.02	090	2	1	0	2	3

24075 Excision, tumor, soft tissue of upper arm or elbow area, subcutaneous; less than 3 cm `G 2 T`

Coding tip: Related soft tissue tumor excision codes - 24071, 24073, 24076

RVU			Global Days	Modifiers				
Mod	Non-Fac Total	Fac Total		51	50	62	80	MUE
	14.06	9.52	090	2	1	0	1	5

24076 Excision, tumor, soft tissue of upper arm or elbow area, subfascial (eg, intramuscular); less than 5 cm `G 2 T`

Coding tip: Related soft tissue tumor excision codes - 24071, 24073, 24075

RVU			Global Days	Modifiers				
Mod	Non-Fac Total	Fac Total		51	50	62	80	MUE
	15.70	15.70	090	2	1	0	1	4

24077 Radical resection of tumor (eg, sarcoma), soft tissue of upper arm or elbow area; less than 5 cm `G 2 T`

RVU			Global Days	Modifiers				
Mod	Non-Fac Total	Fac Total		51	50	62	80	MUE
	30.03	30.03	090	2	1	1	1	1

24079 Radical resection of tumor (eg, sarcoma), soft tissue of upper arm or elbow area; 5 cm or greater `G 2 T`

RVU			Global Days	Modifiers				
Mod	Non-Fac Total	Fac Total		51	50	62	80	MUE
	38.34	38.34	090	2	1	1	2	1

24100 Arthrotomy, elbow; with synovial biopsy only `A 2 T`

RVU			Global Days	Modifiers				
Mod	Non-Fac Total	Fac Total		51	50	62	80	MUE
	12.06	12.06	090	2	1	1	2	1

24101 Arthrotomy, elbow; with joint exploration, with or without biopsy, with or without removal of loose or foreign body `A 2 T`

RVU			Global Days	Modifiers				
Mod	Non-Fac Total	Fac Total		51	50	62	80	MUE
	14.43	14.43	090	2	1	0	2	1

24102 Arthrotomy, elbow; with synovectomy `A 2 T`

RVU			Global Days	Modifiers				
Mod	Non-Fac Total	Fac Total		51	50	62	80	MUE
	17.79	17.79	090	2	1	1	2	1

● New ▲ Revised Deleted ⊙ Moderate Sedation ✚ Add-on Codes ⊘ High Risk Denial Ⓐ Age Edit ♀ Female ♂ Male **AMA** *CPT® Assistant* **MUE** Medically Unlikely Edit
⊘ Modifier 51 Exempt ⊖ Modifier 63 Exempt ✘ Unlisted **Modifiers:** *See Inside Back Cover* Ⓜ Maternity `A 2`–`Z 3` ASC Payment Indicators `A`–`Y` OPPS Status Indicators

© 2016 DecisionHealth   CPT © 2015 American Medical Association. All Rights Reserved.   **251**

24105 Excision, olecranon bursa `A 2 T`

Mod	RVU Non-Fac Total	Fac Total	Global Days	Modifiers 51	50	62	80	MUE
	10.11	10.11	090	2	1	0	1	1

24110 Excision or curettage of bone cyst or benign tumor, humerus `A 2 T`

Mod	RVU Non-Fac Total	Fac Total	Global Days	Modifiers 51	50	62	80	MUE
	16.74	16.74	090	2	1	1	1	1

24115 Excision or curettage of bone cyst or benign tumor, humerus; with autograft (includes obtaining graft) `A 2 T`

Mod	RVU Non-Fac Total	Fac Total	Global Days	Modifiers 51	50	62	80	MUE
	21.33	21.33	090	2	1	1	2	1

24116 Excision or curettage of bone cyst or benign tumor, humerus; with allograft `A 2 T`

Mod	RVU Non-Fac Total	Fac Total	Global Days	Modifiers 51	50	62	80	MUE
	24.94	24.94	090	2	1	0	2	1

24120 Excision or curettage of bone cyst or benign tumor of head or neck of radius or olecranon process `A 2 T`

Mod	RVU Non-Fac Total	Fac Total	Global Days	Modifiers 51	50	62	80	MUE
	15.26	15.26	090	2	1	0	0	1

24125 Excision or curettage of bone cyst or benign tumor of head or neck of radius or olecranon process; with autograft (includes obtaining graft) `A 2 T`

Mod	RVU Non-Fac Total	Fac Total	Global Days	Modifiers 51	50	62	80	MUE
	17.69	17.69	090	2	1	1	2	1

24126 Excision or curettage of bone cyst or benign tumor of head or neck of radius or olecranon process; with allograft `A 2 T`

Mod	RVU Non-Fac Total	Fac Total	Global Days	Modifiers 51	50	62	80	MUE
	18.74	18.74	090	2	1	0	2	1

24130 Excision, radial head `A 2 T`

Mod	RVU Non-Fac Total	Fac Total	Global Days	Modifiers 51	50	62	80	MUE
	14.70	14.70	090	2	1	1	1	1

24134 Sequestrectomy (eg, for osteomyelitis or bone abscess), shaft or distal humerus `A 2 J 1`

Mod	RVU Non-Fac Total	Fac Total	Global Days	Modifiers 51	50	62	80	MUE
	21.57	21.57	090	2	1	0	2	1

Sequestrectomy

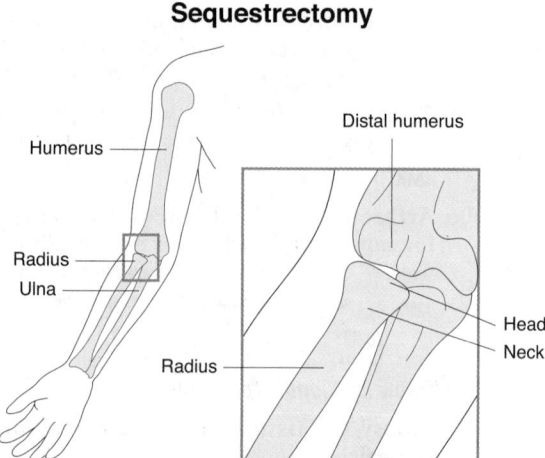

Dead bone tissue, walled-off (sequestered) within sound bone tissue, is removed; shaft or distal humerus (24134), radial head or neck (24136), olecranon process (24138), at the elbow.

24136 Sequestrectomy (eg, for osteomyelitis or bone abscess), radial head or neck `A 2 T`

Mod	RVU Non-Fac Total	Fac Total	Global Days	Modifiers 51	50	62	80	MUE
	18.28	18.28	090	2	1	0	1	1

24138 Sequestrectomy (eg, for osteomyelitis or bone abscess), olecranon process `A 2 T`

Mod	RVU Non-Fac Total	Fac Total	Global Days	Modifiers 51	50	62	80	MUE
	19.39	19.39	090	2	1	0	2	1

24140 Partial excision (craterization, saucerization, or diaphysectomy) bone (eg, osteomyelitis), humerus `A 2 T`

Mod	RVU Non-Fac Total	Fac Total	Global Days	Modifiers 51	50	62	80	MUE
	20.22	20.22	090	2	1	0	2	1

AMA: Nov 98: 9

24145 Partial excision (craterization, saucerization, or diaphysectomy) bone (eg, osteomyelitis), radial head or neck `A 2 T`

Mod	RVU Non-Fac Total	Fac Total	Global Days	Modifiers 51	50	62	80	MUE
	17.09	17.09	090	2	1	1	1	1

AMA: Nov 98: 9

24147 Partial excision (craterization, saucerization, or diaphysectomy) bone (eg, osteomyelitis), olecranon process `A 2 T`

Mod	RVU Non-Fac Total	Fac Total	Global Days	Modifiers 51	50	62	80	MUE
	17.95	17.95	090	2	1	1	1	1

AMA: Nov 98: 9

● New   ▲ Revised   ✖ Deleted   ⊙ Moderate Sedation   ➕ Add-on Codes   ⊗ High Risk Denial   Ⓐ Age Edit   ♀ Female   ♂ Male   **AMA** CPT® Assistant   **MUE** Medically Unlikely Edit
⊘ Modifier 51 Exempt   ⊖ Modifier 63 Exempt   ✖ Unlisted   **Modifiers:** See Inside Back Cover   Ⓜ Maternity   `A 2`–`Z 3` ASC Payment Indicators   `A`–`Y` OPPS Status Indicators

24149 Radical resection of capsule, soft tissue, and heterotopic bone, elbow, with contracture release (separate procedure) G2T

RVU			Global Days	Modifiers				
Mod	Non-Fac Total	Fac Total		51	50	62	80	MUE
	34.01	34.01	090	2	1	1	2	1

AMA: Nov 96: 4

24150 Radical resection of tumor, shaft or distal humerus T

RVU			Global Days	Modifiers				
Mod	Non-Fac Total	Fac Total		51	50	62	80	MUE
	45.17	45.17	090	2	1	1	2	1

24152 Radical resection of tumor, radial head or neck G2T

RVU			Global Days	Modifiers				
Mod	Non-Fac Total	Fac Total		51	50	62	80	MUE
	38.69	38.69	090	2	1	1	2	1

24155 Resection of elbow joint (arthrectomy) A2T

RVU			Global Days	Modifiers				
Mod	Non-Fac Total	Fac Total		51	50	62	80	MUE
	24.40	24.40	090	2	1	1	2	1

Upper Arm/Elbow Introduction/Removal Procedures

24160 Removal of prosthesis, includes debridement and synovectomy when performed; humeral and ulnar components A2Q2

RVU			Global Days	Modifiers				
Mod	Non-Fac Total	Fac Total		51	50	62	80	MUE
	36.70	36.70	090	2	1	1	1	1

AMA: Feb 13: 11, Mar 14: 4

24164 Removal of prosthesis, includes debridement and synovectomy when performed; radial head A2Q2

RVU			Global Days	Modifiers				
Mod	Non-Fac Total	Fac Total		51	50	62	80	MUE
	21.13	21.13	090	2	1	1	1	1

AMA: Mar 14: 4

24200 Removal of foreign body, upper arm or elbow area; subcutaneous P3T

RVU			Global Days	Modifiers				
Mod	Non-Fac Total	Fac Total		51	50	62	80	MUE
	5.90	4.01	010	2	1	0	0	3

AMA: Mar 14: 4

24201 Removal of foreign body, upper arm or elbow area; deep (subfascial or intramuscular) A2T

RVU			Global Days	Modifiers				
Mod	Non-Fac Total	Fac Total		51	50	62	80	MUE
	15.61	10.40	090	2	1	0	1	3

AMA: Nov 98: 8, Mar 14: 4

24220 Injection procedure for elbow arthrography N1N

RVU			Global Days	Modifiers				
Mod	Non-Fac Total	Fac Total		51	50	62	80	MUE
	4.56	1.99	000	2	1	0	0	1

AMA: Aug 15: 6

Upper Arm/Elbow Repair/Revision/Reconstruction Procedures

24300 Manipulation, elbow, under anesthesia G2T

RVU			Global Days	Modifiers				
Mod	Non-Fac Total	Fac Total		51	50	62	80	MUE
	12.02	12.02	090	2	1	0	1	1

24301 Muscle or tendon transfer, any type, upper arm or elbow, single (excluding 24320-24331) A2T

RVU			Global Days	Modifiers				
Mod	Non-Fac Total	Fac Total		51	50	62	80	MUE
	21.63	21.63	090	2	0	1	2	2

Coding Guidance

Neuroplasty of the ulnar nerve (64718) is included in the tendon lengthening described by 24305 and is not separately reportable. If the surgeon also performs an ulnar nerve transposition at the elbow, in addition to the tendon lengthening, then 64718 can be reported with modifier 59.

24305 Tendon lengthening, upper arm or elbow, each tendon A2T

RVU			Global Days	Modifiers				
Mod	Non-Fac Total	Fac Total		51	50	62	80	MUE
	16.68	16.68	090	2	0	0	0	4

AMA: Nov 98: 8

Tendon lengthening, upper arm or elbow, each tendon

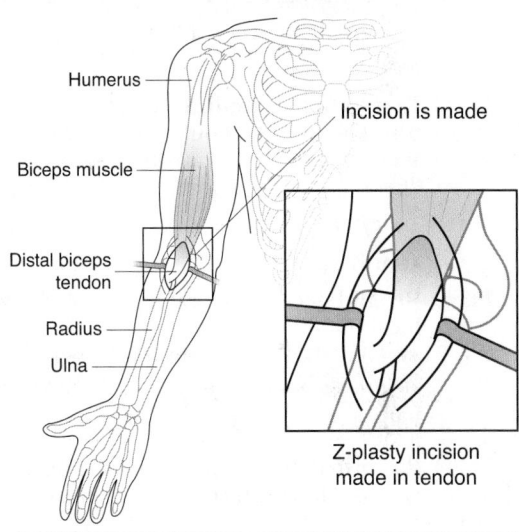

Humerus

Biceps muscle

Distal biceps tendon

Radius

Ulna

Incision is made

Z-plasty incision made in tendon

24310 Tenotomy, open, elbow to shoulder, each tendon A2T

RVU			Global Days	Modifiers				
Mod	Non-Fac Total	Fac Total		51	50	62	80	MUE
	13.58	13.58	090	2	0	0	0	3

AMA: Nov 98: 8

24320 Tenoplasty, with muscle transfer, with or without free graft, elbow to shoulder, single (Seddon-Brookes type procedure) A2T

RVU			Global Days	Modifiers				
Mod	Non-Fac Total	Fac Total		51	50	62	80	MUE
	22.59	22.59	090	2	0	1	2	2

● New ▲ Revised Deleted ⊙ Moderate Sedation ✚ Add-on Codes ⊘ High Risk Denial Ⓐ Age Edit ♀ Female ♂ Male **AMA** *CPT® Assistant* **MUE** Medically Unlikely Edit
⊘ Modifier 51 Exempt ⊖ Modifier 63 Exempt ✗ Unlisted **Modifiers:** *See Inside Back Cover* Ⓜ Maternity A2–Z3 ASC Payment Indicators A–Y OPPS Status Indicators

© 2016 DecisionHealth   CPT © 2015 American Medical Association. All Rights Reserved.   **253**

Surgical Procedures

24330 – 24366

24330 Flexor-plasty, elbow (eg, Steindler type advancement) `A 2 T`

Mod	Non-Fac Total	Fac Total	Global Days	51	50	62	80	MUE
	20.75	20.75	090	2	1	0	2	1

24331 Flexor-plasty, elbow (eg, Steindler type advancement); with extensor advancement `A 2 T`

Mod	Non-Fac Total	Fac Total	Global Days	51	50	62	80	MUE
	22.74	22.74	090	2	1	0	2	1

24332 Tenolysis, triceps `G 2 T`

Mod	Non-Fac Total	Fac Total	Global Days	51	50	62	80	MUE
	17.64	17.64	090	2	1	0	1	1

24340 Tenodesis of biceps tendon at elbow (separate procedure) `A 2 J 1`

Mod	Non-Fac Total	Fac Total	Global Days	51	50	62	80	MUE
	17.59	17.59	090	2	1	1	2	1

24341 Repair, tendon or muscle, upper arm or elbow, each tendon or muscle, primary or secondary (excludes rotator cuff) `A 2 T`

Mod	Non-Fac Total	Fac Total	Global Days	51	50	62	80	MUE
	21.52	21.52	090	2	1	1	2	2

AMA: Nov 96: 4

24342 Reinsertion of ruptured biceps or triceps tendon, distal, with or without tendon graft `A 2 T`

Mod	Non-Fac Total	Fac Total	Global Days	51	50	62	80	MUE
	22.36	22.36	090	2	1	1	2	2

AMA: Nov 96: 4

24343 Repair lateral collateral ligament, elbow, with local tissue `G 2 T`

Mod	Non-Fac Total	Fac Total	Global Days	51	50	62	80	MUE
	20.35	20.35	090	2	1	1	2	1

24344 Reconstruction lateral collateral ligament, elbow, with tendon graft (includes harvesting of graft) `G 2 J 1`

Mod	Non-Fac Total	Fac Total	Global Days	51	50	62	80	MUE
	31.69	31.69	090	2	1	1	2	1

24345 Repair medial collateral ligament, elbow, with local tissue `A 2 T`

Mod	Non-Fac Total	Fac Total	Global Days	51	50	62	80	MUE
	20.28	20.28	090	2	1	1	2	1

24346 Reconstruction medial collateral ligament, elbow, with tendon graft (includes harvesting of graft) `G 2 J 1`

Mod	Non-Fac Total	Fac Total	Global Days	51	50	62	80	MUE
	31.64	31.64	090	2	1	1	2	1

24357 Tenotomy, elbow, lateral or medial (eg, epicondylitis, tennis elbow, golfer's elbow); percutaneous `G 2 T`

Mod	Non-Fac Total	Fac Total	Global Days	51	50	62	80	MUE
	12.32	12.32	090	2	1	0	0	2

AMA: Jan 08: 4

24358 Tenotomy, elbow, lateral or medial (eg, epicondylitis, tennis elbow, golfer's elbow); debridement, soft tissue and/or bone, open `G 2 T`

Mod	Non-Fac Total	Fac Total	Global Days	51	50	62	80	MUE
	15.07	15.07	090	2	1	0	0	2

AMA: Jan 08: 4

24359 Tenotomy, elbow, lateral or medial (eg, epicondylitis, tennis elbow, golfer's elbow); debridement, soft tissue and/or bone, open with tendon repair or reattachment `G 2 T`

Mod	Non-Fac Total	Fac Total	Global Days	51	50	62	80	MUE
	19.05	19.05	090	2	1	0	0	2

AMA: Jan 08: 4

24360 Arthroplasty, elbow; with membrane (eg, fascial) `A 2 J 1`

Mod	Non-Fac Total	Fac Total	Global Days	51	50	62	80	MUE
	25.60	25.60	090	2	1	1	2	1

AMA: Nov 98: 8

24361 Arthroplasty, elbow; with distal humeral prosthetic replacement `J 8 J 1`

Mod	Non-Fac Total	Fac Total	Global Days	51	50	62	80	MUE
	28.87	28.87	090	2	1	1	2	1

24362 Arthroplasty, elbow; with implant and fascia lata ligament reconstruction `J 8 J 1`

Mod	Non-Fac Total	Fac Total	Global Days	51	50	62	80	MUE
	30.68	30.68	090	2	1	0	2	1

24363 Arthroplasty, elbow; with distal humerus and proximal ulnar prosthetic replacement (eg, total elbow) `J 8 J 1`

Mod	Non-Fac Total	Fac Total	Global Days	51	50	62	80	MUE
	42.16	42.16	090	2	1	0	2	1

AMA: Feb 13: 11

24365 Arthroplasty, radial head `G 2 J 1`

Mod	Non-Fac Total	Fac Total	Global Days	51	50	62	80	MUE
	18.34	18.34	090	2	1	1	2	1

24366 Arthroplasty, radial head; with implant `J 8 J 1`

Mod	Non-Fac Total	Fac Total	Global Days	51	50	62	80	MUE
	19.62	19.62	090	2	1	1	2	1

● New ▲ Revised ✖ Deleted ⊙ Moderate Sedation ✚ Add-on Codes ⊘ High Risk Denial Ⓐ Age Edit ♀ Female ♂ Male **AMA** *CPT® Assistant* **MUE** Medically Unlikely Edit

⊘ Modifier 51 Exempt ⊖ Modifier 63 Exempt ✗ Unlisted **Modifiers:** *See Inside Back Cover* Ⓜ Maternity `A 2`–`Z 3` ASC Payment Indicators `A`–`Y` OPPS Status Indicators

254   CPT © 2015 American Medical Association. All Rights Reserved.   © 2016 DecisionHealth

24370 Revision of total elbow arthroplasty, including allograft when performed; humeral or ulnar component `J 8 J 1`

RVU			Global Days	Modifiers				
Mod	Non-Fac Total	Fac Total		51	50	62	80	MUE
	45.03	45.03	090	2	1	0	2	1

AMA: Feb 13: 11, Mar 14: 4

24371 Revision of total elbow arthroplasty, including allograft when performed; humeral and ulnar component `J 8 J 1`

RVU			Global Days	Modifiers				
Mod	Non-Fac Total	Fac Total		51	50	62	80	MUE
	51.58	51.58	090	2	1	0	2	1

AMA: Feb 13: 11, Mar 14: 4

24400 Osteotomy, humerus, with or without internal fixation `A 2 J 1`

RVU			Global Days	Modifiers				
Mod	Non-Fac Total	Fac Total		51	50	62	80	MUE
	23.54	23.54	090	2	1	1	2	1

AMA: Mar 14: 4

24410 Multiple osteotomies with realignment on intramedullary rod, humeral shaft (Sofield type procedure) `J 8 J 1`

RVU			Global Days	Modifiers				
Mod	Non-Fac Total	Fac Total		51	50	62	80	MUE
	30.60	30.60	090	2	1	1	2	1

24420 Osteoplasty, humerus (eg, shortening or lengthening) (excluding 64876) `A 2 T`

RVU			Global Days	Modifiers				
Mod	Non-Fac Total	Fac Total		51	50	62	80	MUE
	28.26	28.26	090	2	1	1	2	1

24430 Repair of nonunion or malunion, humerus; without graft (eg, compression technique) `G 2 J 1`

RVU			Global Days	Modifiers				
Mod	Non-Fac Total	Fac Total		51	50	62	80	MUE
	30.51	30.51	090	2	1	1	2	1

24435 Repair of nonunion or malunion, humerus; with iliac or other autograft (includes obtaining graft) `J 8 J 1`

RVU			Global Days	Modifiers				
Mod	Non-Fac Total	Fac Total		51	50	62	80	MUE
	31.09	31.09	090	2	1	1	2	1

24470 Hemiepiphyseal arrest (eg, cubitus varus or valgus, distal humerus) `A 2 T`

RVU			Global Days	Modifiers				
Mod	Non-Fac Total	Fac Total		51	50	62	80	MUE
	16.28	16.28	090	2	1	0	2	1

24495 Decompression fasciotomy, forearm, with brachial artery exploration `A 2 T`

RVU			Global Days	Modifiers				
Mod	Non-Fac Total	Fac Total		51	50	62	80	MUE
	18.85	18.85	090	2	1	0	0	1

24498 Prophylactic treatment (nailing, pinning, plating or wiring), with or without methylmethacrylate, humeral shaft `G 2 J 1`

RVU			Global Days	Modifiers				
Mod	Non-Fac Total	Fac Total		51	50	62	80	MUE
	25.00	25.00	090	2	1	1	2	1

AMA: Nov 98: 8

Upper Arm/Elbow Fracture/Dislocation Procedures

Coding Guidance

Open treatment of fractures or dislocations includes the application of casts, straps, or splints. Do not report their application separately. The physician who treated the fracture or dislocation with an initial cast, splint, or strap and assumed the follow-up care cannot report the casting/splinting/strapping codes, as they are inclusive in the fracture/dislocation care codes. The physician who treated the fracture or dislocation with a cast, splint, or strap as an initial service minus any other definitive care and expects to do only the initial casting, may report an E&M service code (if significant and separately identifiable), the casting/strapping/splinting application code, and a supply code (Q4001-Q4051) for the cast/splint/strap used. According to OPPS rules, a hospital that treats the fracture or dislocation with a cast, splint, or strap as an initial service minus any other definitive care, reports the casting/strapping/splinting application code, while payment for the supply of the cast/splint/strap is included. When closed fracture reduction is followed by open reduction for the same patient encounter, only the open reduction service can be reported. Use codes 11010-11012 for debridement of tissue with open fractures or dislocations.

24500 Closed treatment of humeral shaft fracture; without manipulation `A 2 T`

Coding tip: Closed treatment of greater humeral tuberosity fracture - 23620

Coding tip: Closed treatment of proximal humeral (neck) fracture - 23600

RVU			Global Days	Modifiers				
Mod	Non-Fac Total	Fac Total		51	50	62	80	MUE
	10.27	9.37	090	2	1	0	1	1

Closed treatment of humeral shaft fracture

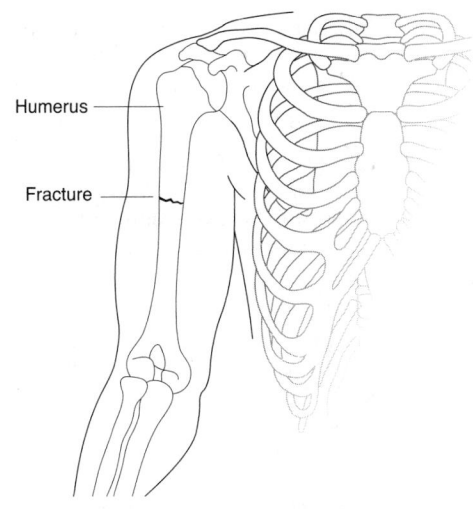

Humerus

Fracture

Without manipulation (24500); with manipulation, with or without skeletal traction (24505)

● New   ▲ Revised   Deleted   ⊙ Moderate Sedation   ✚ Add-on Codes   ⊘ High Risk Denial   Ⓐ Age Edit   ♀ Female   ♂ Male   **AMA** *CPT® Assistant*   **MUE** Medically Unlikely Edit
⊘ Modifier 51 Exempt   ⊖ Modifier 63 Exempt   ✗ Unlisted   **Modifiers:** *See Inside Back Cover*   Ⓜ Maternity   `A 2`–`Z 3` ASC Payment Indicators   `A`–`Y` OPPS Status Indicators

24505 Closed treatment of humeral shaft fracture; with manipulation, with or without skeletal traction
A 2 T

Coding tip: Removal of the initial traction device is included - code separately only when a subsequent traction device is removed

Coding tip: Add modifier 77 for re-reduction of the fracture by another physician

Coding tip: Closed treatment of greater humeral tuberosity fracture with manipulation - 23625

Coding tip: Closed treatment of proximal humeral (neck) fracture with manipulation - 23605

Coding tip: Skeletal traction requires the use of a wire, pin, screw, or clamp attached through the bone, which is included in the initial placement - code separately only when a subsequent traction device is placed

RVU			Global Days	Modifiers				
Mod	Non-Fac Total	Fac Total		51	50	62	80	MUE
	14.36	13.03	090	2	1	0	1	1

24515 Open treatment of humeral shaft fracture with plate/screws, with or without cerclage
G 2 J 1

RVU			Global Days	Modifiers				
Mod	Non-Fac Total	Fac Total		51	50	62	80	MUE
	25.27	25.27	090	2	1	1	2	1

24516 Treatment of humeral shaft fracture, with insertion of intramedullary implant, with or without cerclage and/or locking screws
G 2 J 1

RVU			Global Days	Modifiers				
Mod	Non-Fac Total	Fac Total		51	50	62	80	MUE
	24.83	24.83	090	2	1	2	2	1

AMA: Feb 96: 4, Jun 09: 7

24530 Closed treatment of supracondylar or transcondylar humeral fracture, with or without intercondylar extension; without manipulation
A 2 T

Coding tip: Closed treatment of humeral condylar fracture - 24576

Coding tip: Closed treatment of humeral epicondylar fracture - 24560

RVU			Global Days	Modifiers				
Mod	Non-Fac Total	Fac Total		51	50	62	80	MUE
	10.93	9.92	090	2	1	0	1	1

24535 Closed treatment of supracondylar or transcondylar humeral fracture, with or without intercondylar extension; with manipulation, with or without skin or skeletal traction
A 2 T

Coding tip: Removal of the initial traction device is included - code separately only when a subsequent traction device is removed

Coding tip: Skeletal traction requires the use of a wire, pin, screw, or clamp attached through the bone, which is included in the initial placement - code separately only when a subsequent traction device is placed

Coding tip: Closed treatment of humeral epicondylar fracture with manipulation - 24565

Coding tip: Closed treatment of humeral condylar fracture with manipulation - 24577

Coding tip: Add modifier 77 for re-reduction of the fracture by another physician

RVU			Global Days	Modifiers				
Mod	Non-Fac Total	Fac Total		51	50	62	80	MUE
	17.69	16.36	090	2	1	0	1	1

24538 Percutaneous skeletal fixation of supracondylar or transcondylar humeral fracture, with or without intercondylar extension
A 2 T

RVU			Global Days	Modifiers				
Mod	Non-Fac Total	Fac Total		51	50	62	80	MUE
	21.47	21.47	090	2	1	0	1	1

AMA: Winter 92: 10

24545 Open treatment of humeral supracondylar or transcondylar fracture, includes internal fixation, when performed; without intercondylar extension
J 8 J 1

RVU			Global Days	Modifiers				
Mod	Non-Fac Total	Fac Total		51	50	62	80	MUE
	26.81	26.81	090	2	1	1	2	1

24546 Open treatment of humeral supracondylar or transcondylar fracture, includes internal fixation, when performed; with intercondylar extension
J 8 J 1

RVU			Global Days	Modifiers				
Mod	Non-Fac Total	Fac Total		51	50	62	80	MUE
	30.01	30.01	090	2	1	2	2	1

24560 Closed treatment of humeral epicondylar fracture, medial or lateral; without manipulation
A 2 T

Coding tip: Closed treatment of humeral condylar fracture - 24576

Coding tip: Closed treatment of humeral supracondylar/transcondylar fracture - 24530

RVU			Global Days	Modifiers				
Mod	Non-Fac Total	Fac Total		51	50	62	80	MUE
	9.19	8.24	090	2	1	0	1	1

24565 Closed treatment of humeral epicondylar fracture, medial or lateral; with manipulation
A 2 T

Coding tip: Add modifier 77 for re-reduction of the fracture by another physician

Coding tip: Closed treatment of humeral supracondylar/transcondylar fracture with manipulation - 24535

Coding tip: Closed treatment of humeral condylar fracture with manipulation - 24577

RVU			Global Days	Modifiers				
Mod	Non-Fac Total	Fac Total		51	50	62	80	MUE
	15.18	13.97	090	2	1	0	1	1

24566 Percutaneous skeletal fixation of humeral epicondylar fracture, medial or lateral, with manipulation
A 2 T

RVU			Global Days	Modifiers				
Mod	Non-Fac Total	Fac Total		51	50	62	80	MUE
	20.71	20.71	090	2	1	0	1	1

24575 Open treatment of humeral epicondylar fracture, medial or lateral, includes internal fixation, when performed
G 2 J 1

RVU			Global Days	Modifiers				
Mod	Non-Fac Total	Fac Total		51	50	62	80	MUE
	21.10	21.10	090	2	1	1	2	1

● New   ▲ Revised   ✖ Deleted   ⊙ Moderate Sedation   ✚ Add-on Codes   ⊘ High Risk Denial   Ⓐ Age Edit   ♀ Female   ♂ Male   **AMA** *CPT® Assistant*   **MUE** Medically Unlikely Edit
⊘ Modifier 51 Exempt   ⊖ Modifier 63 Exempt   ✗ Unlisted   **Modifiers:** *See Inside Back Cover*   Ⓜ Maternity   A2–Z3 ASC Payment Indicators   A–Y OPPS Status Indicators

256   CPT © 2015 American Medical Association. All Rights Reserved.   © 2016 DecisionHealth

24576 Closed treatment of humeral condylar fracture, medial or lateral; without manipulation `A 2 T`

Coding tip: Closed treatment of humeral supracondylar/transcondylar fracture - 24530

Coding tip: Closed treatment of humeral epicondylar fracture - 24560

RVU			Global Days	Modifiers				
Mod	Non-Fac Total	Fac Total		51	50	62	80	MUE
	9.75	8.78	090	2	1	0	1	1

Closed treatment of humeral condylar fracture, medial or lateral

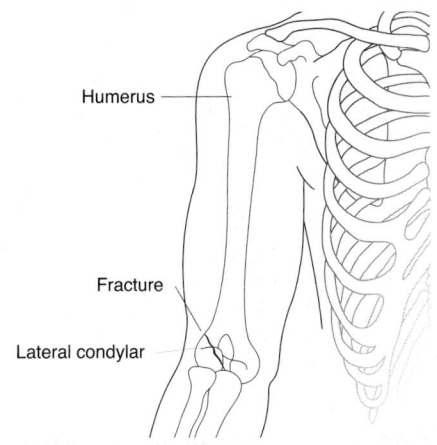

Humerus

Fracture

Lateral condylar

Without manipulation (24576); with manipulation, (24577)

24577 Closed treatment of humeral condylar fracture, medial or lateral; with manipulation `A 2 T`

Coding tip: Closed treatment of humeral supracondylar/transcondylar fracture with manipulation - 24535

Coding tip: Add modifier 77 for re-reduction of the fracture by another physician

Coding tip: Closed treatment of humeral epicondylar fracture with manipulation - 24565

RVU			Global Days	Modifiers				
Mod	Non-Fac Total	Fac Total		51	50	62	80	MUE
	15.63	14.34	090	2	1	0	1	1

24579 Open treatment of humeral condylar fracture, medial or lateral, includes internal fixation, when performed `G 2 J I`

RVU			Global Days	Modifiers				
Mod	Non-Fac Total	Fac Total		51	50	62	80	MUE
	24.13	24.13	090	2	1	1	2	1

24582 Percutaneous skeletal fixation of humeral condylar fracture, medial or lateral, with manipulation `A 2 T`

RVU			Global Days	Modifiers				
Mod	Non-Fac Total	Fac Total		51	50	62	80	MUE
	23.24	23.24	090	2	1	0	1	1

24586 Open treatment of periarticular fracture and/or dislocation of the elbow (fracture distal humerus and proximal ulna and/or proximal radius) `G 2 J I`

RVU			Global Days	Modifiers				
Mod	Non-Fac Total	Fac Total		51	50	62	80	MUE
	31.31	31.31	090	2	1	1	2	1

24587 Open treatment of periarticular fracture and/or dislocation of the elbow (fracture distal humerus and proximal ulna and/or proximal radius); with implant arthroplasty `J 8 J I`

RVU			Global Days	Modifiers				
Mod	Non-Fac Total	Fac Total		51	50	62	80	MUE
	31.25	31.25	090	2	1	1	2	1

24600 Treatment of closed elbow dislocation; without anesthesia `A 2 T`

RVU			Global Days	Modifiers				
Mod	Non-Fac Total	Fac Total		51	50	62	80	MUE
	10.41	9.56	090	2	1	0	1	1

24605 Treatment of closed elbow dislocation; requiring anesthesia `A 2 T`

RVU			Global Days	Modifiers				
Mod	Non-Fac Total	Fac Total		51	50	62	80	MUE
	13.55	13.55	090	2	1	0	1	1

24615 Open treatment of acute or chronic elbow dislocation `A 2 J I`

RVU			Global Days	Modifiers				
Mod	Non-Fac Total	Fac Total		51	50	62	80	MUE
	20.58	20.58	090	2	1	1	2	1

24620 Closed treatment of Monteggia type of fracture dislocation at elbow (fracture proximal end of ulna with dislocation of radial head), with manipulation `A 2 T`

RVU			Global Days	Modifiers				
Mod	Non-Fac Total	Fac Total		51	50	62	80	MUE
	15.88	15.88	090	2	1	0	0	1

24635 Open treatment of Monteggia type of fracture dislocation at elbow (fracture proximal end of ulna with dislocation of radial head), includes internal fixation, when performed `A 2 J I`

RVU			Global Days	Modifiers				
Mod	Non-Fac Total	Fac Total		51	50	62	80	MUE
	19.42	19.42	090	2	1	1	2	1

24640 Closed treatment of radial head subluxation in child, nursemaid elbow, with manipulation `⊗ Ⓐ P 3 T`

Coding tip: Add modifier 77 for re-reduction of subluxation by another physician

RVU			Global Days	Modifiers				
Mod	Non-Fac Total	Fac Total		51	50	62	80	MUE
	3.86	2.65	010	2	1	0	0	1

24650 Closed treatment of radial head or neck fracture; without manipulation `P 2 T`

RVU			Global Days	Modifiers				
Mod	Non-Fac Total	Fac Total		51	50	62	80	MUE
	7.49	6.89	090	2	1	0	1	1

24655 Closed treatment of radial head or neck fracture; with manipulation `A 2 T`

Coding tip: Add modifier 77 for re-reduction of the fracture by another physician

RVU			Global Days	Modifiers				
Mod	Non-Fac Total	Fac Total		51	50	62	80	MUE
	12.47	11.38	090	2	1	0	1	1

● New   ▲ Revised   Deleted   ⊙ Moderate Sedation   ✚ Add-on Codes   ⊗ High Risk Denial   Ⓐ Age Edit   ♀ Female   ♂ Male   **AMA** *CPT® Assistant*   ***MUE*** Medically Unlikely Edit
⊘ Modifier 51 Exempt   ⊖ Modifier 63 Exempt   ✗ Unlisted   **Modifiers:** *See Inside Back Cover*   Ⓜ Maternity   A 2 – Z 3 ASC Payment Indicators   A – Y OPPS Status Indicators

Surgical Procedures

24665 Open treatment of radial head or neck fracture, includes internal fixation or radial head excision, when performed   A2 J I

Mod	Non-Fac Total	Fac Total	Global Days	51	50	62	80	MUE
	18.78	18.78	090	2	1	1	2	1

24666 Open treatment of radial head or neck fracture, includes internal fixation or radial head excision, when performed; with radial head prosthetic replacement   G2 J I

Mod	Non-Fac Total	Fac Total	Global Days	51	50	62	80	MUE
	21.15	21.15	090	2	1	1	2	1

24670 Closed treatment of ulnar fracture, proximal end (eg, olecranon or coronoid process[es]); without manipulation   A2 T

Mod	Non-Fac Total	Fac Total	Global Days	51	50	62	80	MUE
	8.35	7.55	090	2	1	0	1	1

24675 Closed treatment of ulnar fracture, proximal end (eg, olecranon or coronoid process[es]); with manipulation   A2 T

Coding tip: Add modifier 77 for re-reduction of the fracture by another physician

Coding tip: Closed treatment of proximal ulnar fracture with radial head dislocation - 24620

Mod	Non-Fac Total	Fac Total	Global Days	51	50	62	80	MUE
	13.02	11.90	090	2	1	0	1	1

24685 Open treatment of ulnar fracture, proximal end (eg, olecranon or coronoid process[es]), includes internal fixation, when performed   A2 J I

Mod	Non-Fac Total	Fac Total	Global Days	51	50	62	80	MUE
	18.86	18.86	090	2	1	1	2	1

Upper Arm/Elbow Arthrodesis

24800 Arthrodesis, elbow joint; local   A2 J I

Mod	Non-Fac Total	Fac Total	Global Days	51	50	62	80	MUE
	23.98	23.98	090	2	1	1	2	1

24802 Arthrodesis, elbow joint; with autogenous graft (includes obtaining graft)   G2 J I

Mod	Non-Fac Total	Fac Total	Global Days	51	50	62	80	MUE
	28.32	28.32	090	2	1	0	2	1

Upper Arm/Elbow Amputation

24900 Amputation, arm through humerus; with primary closure   C

Mod	Non-Fac Total	Fac Total	Global Days	51	50	62	80	MUE
	21.14	21.14	090	2	1	1	2	1

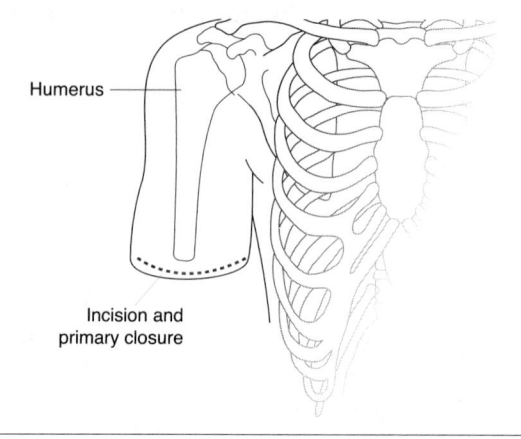

Amputation, arm through humerus; with primary closure

Humerus

Incision and primary closure

24920 Amputation, arm through humerus; open, circular (guillotine)   C

Mod	Non-Fac Total	Fac Total	Global Days	51	50	62	80	MUE
	21.13	21.13	090	2	1	1	2	1

24925 Amputation, arm through humerus; secondary closure or scar revision   A2 T

Mod	Non-Fac Total	Fac Total	Global Days	51	50	62	80	MUE
	15.79	15.79	090	2	1	0	2	1

24930 Amputation, arm through humerus; re-amputation   C

Mod	Non-Fac Total	Fac Total	Global Days	51	50	62	80	MUE
	22.22	22.22	090	2	1	0	2	1

24931 Amputation, arm through humerus; with implant   C

Mod	Non-Fac Total	Fac Total	Global Days	51	50	62	80	MUE
	23.06	23.06	090	2	1	0	2	1

24935 Stump elongation, upper extremity   J I

Mod	Non-Fac Total	Fac Total	Global Days	51	50	62	80	MUE
	32.07	32.07	090	2	1	0	0	1

24940 Cineplasty, upper extremity, complete procedure   ⊗ C

Mod	Non-Fac Total	Fac Total	Global Days	51	50	62	80	MUE
	0.00	0.00	090	2	1	0	2	1

● New   ▲ Revised   ✖ Deleted   ⊙ Moderate Sedation   ✚ Add-on Codes   ⊗ High Risk Denial   Ⓐ Age Edit   ♀ Female   ♂ Male   **AMA** *CPT® Assistant*   **MUE** Medically Unlikely Edit
⊘ Modifier 51 Exempt   ⊖ Modifier 63 Exempt   ✗ Unlisted   **Modifiers:** *See Inside Back Cover*   Ⓜ Maternity   A2–Z3 ASC Payment Indicators   A–Y OPPS Status Indicators

258   CPT © 2015 American Medical Association. All Rights Reserved.   © 2016 DecisionHealth

Other Upper Arm/Elbow Procedures

24999 Unlisted procedure, humerus or elbow ☒T

RVU			Global Days	Modifiers				
Mod	Non-Fac Total	Fac Total		51	50	62	80	MUE
	0.00	0.00	YYY	2	1	1	0	

Forearm/Wrist Procedures

Forearm/Wrist Incisional Procedures

25000 Incision, extensor tendon sheath, wrist (eg, deQuervains disease) A2T

RVU			Global Days	Modifiers				
Mod	Non-Fac Total	Fac Total		51	50	62	80	MUE
	9.72	9.72	090	2	1	0	1	2

AMA: Nov 98: 8

25001 Incision, flexor tendon sheath, wrist (eg, flexor carpi radialis) G2T

RVU			Global Days	Modifiers				
Mod	Non-Fac Total	Fac Total		51	50	62	80	MUE
	9.85	9.85	090	2	1	0	1	1

25020 Decompression fasciotomy, forearm and/or wrist, flexor OR extensor compartment; without debridement of nonviable muscle and/or nerve A2T

RVU			Global Days	Modifiers				
Mod	Non-Fac Total	Fac Total		51	50	62	80	MUE
	16.64	16.64	090	2	1	0	1	1

25023 Decompression fasciotomy, forearm and/or wrist, flexor OR extensor compartment; with debridement of nonviable muscle and/or nerve A2T

RVU			Global Days	Modifiers				
Mod	Non-Fac Total	Fac Total		51	50	62	80	MUE
	31.81	31.81	090	2	1	0	0	1

25024 Decompression fasciotomy, forearm and/or wrist, flexor AND extensor compartment; without debridement of nonviable muscle and/or nerve A2T

RVU			Global Days	Modifiers				
Mod	Non-Fac Total	Fac Total		51	50	62	80	MUE
	22.39	22.39	090	2	1	0	1	1

25025 Decompression fasciotomy, forearm and/or wrist, flexor AND extensor compartment; with debridement of nonviable muscle and/or nerve A2T

RVU			Global Days	Modifiers				
Mod	Non-Fac Total	Fac Total		51	50	62	80	MUE
	34.97	34.97	090	2	1	0	0	1

25028 Incision and drainage, forearm and/or wrist; deep abscess or hematoma A2T

RVU			Global Days	Modifiers				
Mod	Non-Fac Total	Fac Total		51	50	62	80	MUE
	15.09	15.09	090	2	1	0	1	4

25031 Incision and drainage, forearm and/or wrist; bursa A2T

RVU			Global Days	Modifiers				
Mod	Non-Fac Total	Fac Total		51	50	62	80	MUE
	10.31	10.31	090	2	1	0	0	2

AMA: Nov 98: 9

25035 Incision, deep, bone cortex, forearm and/or wrist (eg, osteomyelitis or bone abscess) A2T

RVU			Global Days	Modifiers				
Mod	Non-Fac Total	Fac Total		51	50	62	80	MUE
	16.71	16.71	090	2	1	0	1	2

25040 Arthrotomy, radiocarpal or midcarpal joint, with exploration, drainage, or removal of foreign body A2T

RVU			Global Days	Modifiers				
Mod	Non-Fac Total	Fac Total		51	50	62	80	MUE
	16.25	16.25	090	2	1	0	0	1

Forearm/Wrist Excisional Procedures

25065 Biopsy, soft tissue of forearm and/or wrist; superficial P3T

Coding tip: Code 99000 for specimen transfer from office setting to an outside laboratory

RVU			Global Days	Modifiers				
Mod	Non-Fac Total	Fac Total		51	50	62	80	MUE
	7.25	4.70	010	2	1	0	1	3

Biopsy, soft tissue of forearm and/or wrist

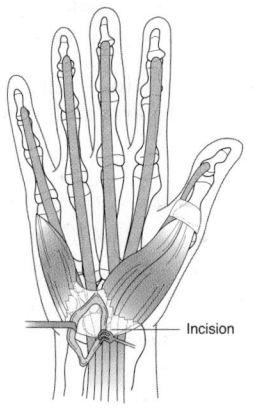

Superficial (25065), deep, subfascial or intramuscular (25066)

25066 Biopsy, soft tissue of forearm and/or wrist; deep (subfascial or intramuscular) A2T

RVU			Global Days	Modifiers				
Mod	Non-Fac Total	Fac Total		51	50	62	80	MUE
	10.29	10.29	090	2	1	0	1	2

AMA: Nov 98: 8, Apr 10: 3

25071 Excision, tumor, soft tissue of forearm and/or wrist area, subcutaneous; 3 cm or greater G2T

Coding tip: Code 25071 is listed out of numerical order in CPT. Related soft tissue tumor excision procedures - 25075 (subcutaneous tissue); 25076, 25073 (subfascial).

RVU			Global Days	Modifiers				
Mod	Non-Fac Total	Fac Total		51	50	62	80	MUE
	12.30	12.30	090	2	1	0	2	3

● New ▲ Revised Deleted ⊙ Moderate Sedation ✚ Add-on Codes ⊘ High Risk Denial Ⓐ Age Edit ♀ Female ♂ Male **AMA** *CPT® Assistant* **MUE** Medically Unlikely Edit
⊘ Modifier 51 Exempt ⊖ Modifier 63 Exempt ☒ Unlisted **Modifiers:** *See Inside Back Cover* Ⓜ Maternity A2–Z3 ASC Payment Indicators A–Y OPPS Status Indicators

25073 Excision, tumor, soft tissue of forearm and/or wrist area, subfascial (eg, intramuscular); 3 cm or greater   G2T

Coding tip: Code 25073 is listed out of numerical order in CPT. Related soft tissue tumor excision procedures - 25071, 25075 (subcutaneous tissue); 25076 (subfascial)

RVU			Global Days	Modifiers				
Mod	Non-Fac Total	Fac Total		51	50	62	80	MUE
	15.37	15.37	090	2	1	0	2	3

25075 Excision, tumor, soft tissue of forearm and/or wrist area, subcutaneous; less than 3 cm   G2T

Coding tip: Related soft tissue tumor excision codes - 25071, 25073, and 25076

RVU			Global Days	Modifiers				
Mod	Non-Fac Total	Fac Total		51	50	62	80	MUE
	13.70	9.12	090	2	1	0	1	6

25076 Excision, tumor, soft tissue of forearm and/or wrist area, subfascial (eg, intramuscular); less than 3 cm   G2T

Coding tip: Related soft tissue tumor excision codes - 25071, 25073, and 25075

RVU			Global Days	Modifiers				
Mod	Non-Fac Total	Fac Total		51	50	62	80	MUE
	14.95	14.95	090	2	1	0	1	5

25077 Radical resection of tumor (eg, sarcoma), soft tissue of forearm and/or wrist area; less than 3 cm   G2T

RVU			Global Days	Modifiers				
Mod	Non-Fac Total	Fac Total		51	50	62	80	MUE
	25.64	25.64	090	2	1	0	1	1

25078 Radical resection of tumor (eg, sarcoma), soft tissue of forearm and/or wrist area; 3 cm or greater   G2T

RVU			Global Days	Modifiers				
Mod	Non-Fac Total	Fac Total		51	50	62	80	MUE
	33.74	33.74	090	2	1	0	2	1

25085 Capsulotomy, wrist (eg, contracture)   A2T

RVU			Global Days	Modifiers				
Mod	Non-Fac Total	Fac Total		51	50	62	80	MUE
	12.96	12.96	090	2	1	0	2	1

25100 Arthrotomy, wrist joint; with biopsy   A2T

RVU			Global Days	Modifiers				
Mod	Non-Fac Total	Fac Total		51	50	62	80	MUE
	9.91	9.91	090	2	1	0	0	1

25101 Arthrotomy, wrist joint; with joint exploration, with or without biopsy, with or without removal of loose or foreign body   A2T

RVU			Global Days	Modifiers				
Mod	Non-Fac Total	Fac Total		51	50	62	80	MUE
	11.61	11.61	090	2	1	0	0	1

25105 Arthrotomy, wrist joint; with synovectomy   A2T

RVU			Global Days	Modifiers				
Mod	Non-Fac Total	Fac Total		51	50	62	80	MUE
	13.95	13.95	090	2	1	1	0	1

25107 Arthrotomy, distal radioulnar joint including repair of triangular cartilage, complex   A2T

RVU			Global Days	Modifiers				
Mod	Non-Fac Total	Fac Total		51	50	62	80	MUE
	17.78	17.78	090	2	1	1	2	1

25109 Excision of tendon, forearm and/or wrist, flexor or extensor, each   G2T

RVU			Global Days	Modifiers				
Mod	Non-Fac Total	Fac Total		51	50	62	80	MUE
	15.59	15.59	090	2	1	0	1	4

25110 Excision, lesion of tendon sheath, forearm and/or wrist   A2T

RVU			Global Days	Modifiers				
Mod	Non-Fac Total	Fac Total		51	50	62	80	MUE
	9.86	9.86	090	2	1	0	1	3

25111 Excision of ganglion, wrist (dorsal or volar); primary   A2T

RVU			Global Days	Modifiers				
Mod	Non-Fac Total	Fac Total		51	50	62	80	MUE
	9.23	9.23	090	2	1	0	1	1

25112 Excision of ganglion, wrist (dorsal or volar); recurrent   A2T

RVU			Global Days	Modifiers				
Mod	Non-Fac Total	Fac Total		51	50	62	80	MUE
	11.16	11.16	090	2	1	0	1	1

25115 Radical excision of bursa, synovia of wrist, or forearm tendon sheaths (eg, tenosynovitis, fungus, Tbc, or other granulomas, rheumatoid arthritis); flexors   A2T

RVU			Global Days	Modifiers				
Mod	Non-Fac Total	Fac Total		51	50	62	80	MUE
	21.97	21.97	090	2	1	0	1	1

AMA: Jun 12: 15

Radical excision of bursa, synovia of wrist or forearm tendon sheaths

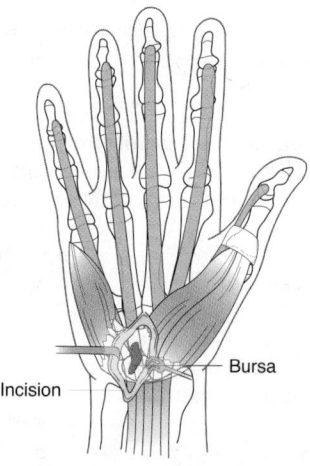

Incision — Bursa

Flexor tendons (25115), extensor tendons, with or without transposition of dorsal retinaculum (25116)

● New   ▲ Revised   ✖ Deleted   ⊙ Moderate Sedation   ✚ Add-on Codes   ⊘ High Risk Denial   Ⓐ Age Edit   ♀ Female   ♂ Male   **AMA** *CPT® Assistant*   **MUE** Medically Unlikely Edit
⊘ Modifier 51 Exempt   ⊖ Modifier 63 Exempt   ✗ Unlisted   **Modifiers:** *See Inside Back Cover*   Ⓜ Maternity   A2–Z3 ASC Payment Indicators   A–Y OPPS Status Indicators

CPT © 2015 American Medical Association. All Rights Reserved.   © 2016 DecisionHealth

25116 Radical excision of bursa, synovia of wrist, or forearm tendon sheaths (eg, tenosynovitis, fungus, Tbc, or other granulomas, rheumatoid arthritis); extensors, with or without transposition of dorsal retinaculum **A2 T**

RVU		Global Days	Modifiers				
Mod	Non-Fac Total	Fac Total		51	50	62	80	MUE
	17.33	17.33	090	2	1	1	0	1

25118 Synovectomy, extensor tendon sheath, wrist, single compartment **A2 T**

RVU		Global Days	Modifiers				
Mod	Non-Fac Total	Fac Total		51	50	62	80	MUE
	11.03	11.03	090	2	1	0	1	5

AMA: Apr 12: 17, Jun 15: 10

25119 Synovectomy, extensor tendon sheath, wrist, single compartment; with resection of distal ulna **A2 T**

RVU		Global Days	Modifiers				
Mod	Non-Fac Total	Fac Total		51	50	62	80	MUE
	14.29	14.29	090	2	1	1	2	1

25120 Excision or curettage of bone cyst or benign tumor of radius or ulna (excluding head or neck of radius and olecranon process) **A2 T**

RVU		Global Days	Modifiers				
Mod	Non-Fac Total	Fac Total		51	50	62	80	MUE
	14.36	14.36	090	2	1	1	0	1

25125 Excision or curettage of bone cyst or benign tumor of radius or ulna (excluding head or neck of radius and olecranon process); with autograft (includes obtaining graft) **A2 T**

RVU		Global Days	Modifiers				
Mod	Non-Fac Total	Fac Total		51	50	62	80	MUE
	16.67	16.67	090	2	1	0	0	1

25126 Excision or curettage of bone cyst or benign tumor of radius or ulna (excluding head or neck of radius and olecranon process); with allograft **A2 T**

RVU		Global Days	Modifiers				
Mod	Non-Fac Total	Fac Total		51	50	62	80	MUE
	17.11	17.11	090	2	1	0	2	1

25130 Excision or curettage of bone cyst or benign tumor of carpal bones **A2 T**

RVU		Global Days	Modifiers				
Mod	Non-Fac Total	Fac Total		51	50	62	80	MUE
	12.90	12.90	090	2	1	0	0	1

25135 Excision or curettage of bone cyst or benign tumor of carpal bones; with autograft (includes obtaining graft) **A2 T**

RVU		Global Days	Modifiers				
Mod	Non-Fac Total	Fac Total		51	50	62	80	MUE
	15.95	15.95	090	2	1	1	2	1

25136 Excision or curettage of bone cyst or benign tumor of carpal bones; with allograft **A2 T**

RVU		Global Days	Modifiers				
Mod	Non-Fac Total	Fac Total		51	50	62	80	MUE
	14.18	14.18	090	2	1	1	2	1

25145 Sequestrectomy (eg, for osteomyelitis or bone abscess), forearm and/or wrist **A2 T**

RVU		Global Days	Modifiers				
Mod	Non-Fac Total	Fac Total		51	50	62	80	MUE
	14.92	14.92	090	2	1	0	2	1

25150 Partial excision (craterization, saucerization, or diaphysectomy) of bone (eg, for osteomyelitis); ulna **A2 T**

RVU		Global Days	Modifiers				
Mod	Non-Fac Total	Fac Total		51	50	62	80	MUE
	16.38	16.38	090	2	1	1	1	1

25151 Partial excision (craterization, saucerization, or diaphysectomy) of bone (eg, for osteomyelitis); radius **A2 T**

RVU		Global Days	Modifiers				
Mod	Non-Fac Total	Fac Total		51	50	62	80	MUE
	16.79	16.79	090	2	1	1	2	1

25170 Radical resection of tumor, radius or ulna **T**

RVU		Global Days	Modifiers				
Mod	Non-Fac Total	Fac Total		51	50	62	80	MUE
	42.90	42.90	090	2	1	1	2	1

25210 Carpectomy; 1 bone **A2 T**

RVU		Global Days	Modifiers				
Mod	Non-Fac Total	Fac Total		51	50	62	80	MUE
	14.09	14.09	090	2	0	1	0	2

25215 Carpectomy; all bones of proximal row **A2 T**

RVU		Global Days	Modifiers				
Mod	Non-Fac Total	Fac Total		51	50	62	80	MUE
	17.84	17.84	090	2	1	1	2	1

25230 Radial styloidectomy (separate procedure) **A2 T**

RVU		Global Days	Modifiers				
Mod	Non-Fac Total	Fac Total		51	50	62	80	MUE
	12.50	12.50	090	2	1	1	1	1

25240 Excision distal ulna partial or complete (eg, Darrach type or matched resection) **A2 T**

RVU		Global Days	Modifiers				
Mod	Non-Fac Total	Fac Total		51	50	62	80	MUE
	12.35	12.35	090	2	1	1	0	1

Forearm/Wrist Introduction/Removal Procedures

25246 Injection procedure for wrist arthrography **N N**

RVU		Global Days	Modifiers				
Mod	Non-Fac Total	Fac Total		51	50	62	80	MUE
	4.60	2.17	000	2	1	0	1	1

AMA: Aug 15: 6

25248 Exploration with removal of deep foreign body, forearm or wrist **A2 T**

RVU		Global Days	Modifiers				
Mod	Non-Fac Total	Fac Total		51	50	62	80	MUE
	11.97	11.97	090	2	1	0	1	3

25250 Removal of wrist prosthesis; (separate procedure) **A2 Q2**

RVU		Global Days	Modifiers				
Mod	Non-Fac Total	Fac Total		51	50	62	80	MUE
	15.24	15.24	090	2	1	0	2	1

● New ▲ Revised Deleted ⊙ Moderate Sedation ✚ Add-on Codes ⊘ High Risk Denial ⒶAge Edit ♀ Female ♂ Male **AMA** *CPT® Assistant* **MUE** Medically Unlikely Edit
⊘ Modifier 51 Exempt ⊖ Modifier 63 Exempt ⊠ Unlisted **Modifiers:** *See Inside Back Cover* Ⓜ Maternity **A2–Z3** ASC Payment Indicators **A–Y** OPPS Status Indicators

Surgical Procedures

25251 – 25316

25251 Removal of wrist prosthesis; complicated, including total wrist `A 2 Q 2`

RVU			Global Days	Modifiers				
Mod	Non-Fac Total	Fac Total		51	50	62	80	MUE
	20.70	20.70	090	2	1	0	2	1

25259 Manipulation, wrist, under anesthesia `G 2 T`

RVU			Global Days	Modifiers				
Mod	Non-Fac Total	Fac Total		51	50	62	80	MUE
	11.98	11.98	090	2	1	0	1	1

AMA: Jan 04: 27, Jun 05: 12

Forearm/Wrist Repair/Revision/Reconstruction Procedures

25260 Repair, tendon or muscle, flexor, forearm and/or wrist; primary, single, each tendon or muscle `A 2 T`

RVU			Global Days	Modifiers				
Mod	Non-Fac Total	Fac Total		51	50	62	80	MUE
	18.22	18.22	090	2	0	0	1	9

25263 Repair, tendon or muscle, flexor, forearm and/or wrist; secondary, single, each tendon or muscle `A 2 T`

RVU			Global Days	Modifiers				
Mod	Non-Fac Total	Fac Total		51	50	62	80	MUE
	17.97	17.97	090	2	0	0	2	4

25265 Repair, tendon or muscle, flexor, forearm and/or wrist; secondary, with free graft (includes obtaining graft), each tendon or muscle `A 2 T`

RVU			Global Days	Modifiers				
Mod	Non-Fac Total	Fac Total		51	50	62	80	MUE
	21.59	21.59	090	2	0	0	2	4

25270 Repair, tendon or muscle, extensor, forearm and/or wrist; primary, single, each tendon or muscle `A 2 T`

RVU			Global Days	Modifiers				
Mod	Non-Fac Total	Fac Total		51	50	62	80	MUE
	14.13	14.13	090	2	0	0	0	8

25272 Repair, tendon or muscle, extensor, forearm and/or wrist; secondary, single, each tendon or muscle `A 2 T`

RVU			Global Days	Modifiers				
Mod	Non-Fac Total	Fac Total		51	50	62	80	MUE
	15.95	15.95	090	2	0	0	0	4

25274 Repair, tendon or muscle, extensor, forearm and/or wrist; secondary, with free graft (includes obtaining graft), each tendon or muscle `A 2 T`

RVU			Global Days	Modifiers				
Mod	Non-Fac Total	Fac Total		51	50	62	80	MUE
	19.20	19.20	090	2	0	1	0	4

25275 Repair, tendon sheath, extensor, forearm and/or wrist, with free graft (includes obtaining graft) (eg, for extensor carpi ulnaris subluxation) `A 2 T`

RVU			Global Days	Modifiers				
Mod	Non-Fac Total	Fac Total		51	50	62	80	MUE
	19.44	19.44	090	2	1	1	0	2

25280 Lengthening or shortening of flexor or extensor tendon, forearm and/or wrist, single, each tendon `A 2 T`

RVU			Global Days	Modifiers				
Mod	Non-Fac Total	Fac Total		51	50	62	80	MUE
	16.27	16.27	090	2	0	1	0	9

25290 Tenotomy, open, flexor or extensor tendon, forearm and/or wrist, single, each tendon `A 2 T`

RVU			Global Days	Modifiers				
Mod	Non-Fac Total	Fac Total		51	50	62	80	MUE
	12.63	12.63	090	2	0	0	1	12

25295 Tenolysis, flexor or extensor tendon, forearm and/or wrist, single, each tendon `A 2 T`

RVU			Global Days	Modifiers				
Mod	Non-Fac Total	Fac Total		51	50	62	80	MUE
	15.13	15.13	090	2	0	0	1	9

AMA: Apr 97: 11, Aug 98: 10

25300 Tenodesis at wrist; flexors of fingers `A 2 T`

RVU			Global Days	Modifiers				
Mod	Non-Fac Total	Fac Total		51	50	62	80	MUE
	19.70	19.70	090	2	1	0	2	1

25301 Tenodesis at wrist; extensors of fingers `A 2 T`

RVU			Global Days	Modifiers				
Mod	Non-Fac Total	Fac Total		51	50	62	80	MUE
	18.54	18.54	090	2	1	0	2	1

25310 Tendon transplantation or transfer, flexor or extensor, forearm and/or wrist, single; each tendon `A 2 T`

RVU			Global Days	Modifiers				
Mod	Non-Fac Total	Fac Total		51	50	62	80	MUE
	17.88	17.88	090	2	0	1	2	5

AMA: Jun 02: 11

25312 Tendon transplantation or transfer, flexor or extensor, forearm and/or wrist, single; with tendon graft(s) (includes obtaining graft), each tendon `A 2 T`

RVU			Global Days	Modifiers				
Mod	Non-Fac Total	Fac Total		51	50	62	80	MUE
	20.63	20.63	090	2	0	1	2	5

25315 Flexor origin slide (eg, for cerebral palsy, Volkmann contracture), forearm and/or wrist `A 2 T`

RVU			Global Days	Modifiers				
Mod	Non-Fac Total	Fac Total		51	50	62	80	MUE
	22.28	22.28	090	2	1	0	2	1

25316 Flexor origin slide (eg, for cerebral palsy, Volkmann contracture), forearm and/or wrist; with tendon(s) transfer `A 2 J 1`

RVU			Global Days	Modifiers				
Mod	Non-Fac Total	Fac Total		51	50	62	80	MUE
	26.43	26.43	090	2	1	0	2	1

● New   ▲ Revised   ✖ Deleted   ⊙ Moderate Sedation   ✚ Add-on Codes   ⊘ High Risk Denial   Ⓐ Age Edit   ♀ Female   ♂ Male   **AMA** *CPT® Assistant*   **MUE** Medically Unlikely Edit
⊘ Modifier 51 Exempt   ⊖ Modifier 63 Exempt   ✗ Unlisted   **Modifiers:** *See Inside Back Cover*   Ⓜ Maternity   A 2–Z 3 ASC Payment Indicators   A–Y OPPS Status Indicators

262   CPT © 2015 American Medical Association. All Rights Reserved.   © 2016 DecisionHealth

25320 Capsulorrhaphy or reconstruction, wrist, open (eg, capsulodesis, ligament repair, tendon transfer or graft) (includes synovectomy, capsulotomy and open reduction) for carpal instability   `A 2 T`

RVU			Global Days	Modifiers				
Mod	Non-Fac Total	Fac Total		51	50	62	80	MUE
	28.55	28.55	090	2	1	0	2	1

25332 Arthroplasty, wrist, with or without interposition, with or without external or internal fixation   `A 2 T`

RVU			Global Days	Modifiers				
Mod	Non-Fac Total	Fac Total		51	50	62	80	MUE
	24.35	24.35	090	2	1	0	2	1

AMA: Nov 96: 5, Jan 05: 8

25335 Centralization of wrist on ulna (eg, radial club hand)   `A 2 T`

RVU			Global Days	Modifiers				
Mod	Non-Fac Total	Fac Total		51	50	62	80	MUE
	23.20	23.20	090	2	1	0	2	1

25337 Reconstruction for stabilization of unstable distal ulna or distal radioulnar joint, secondary by soft tissue stabilization (eg, tendon transfer, tendon graft or weave, or tenodesis) with or without open reduction of distal radioulnar joint   `A 2 T`

RVU			Global Days	Modifiers				
Mod	Non-Fac Total	Fac Total		51	50	62	80	MUE
	25.78	25.78	090	2	1	0	1	1

25350 Osteotomy, radius; distal third   `A 2 J I`

RVU			Global Days	Modifiers				
Mod	Non-Fac Total	Fac Total		51	50	62	80	MUE
	19.49	19.49	090	2	1	0	2	1

25355 Osteotomy, radius; middle or proximal third   `A 2 T`

RVU			Global Days	Modifiers				
Mod	Non-Fac Total	Fac Total		51	50	62	80	MUE
	21.69	21.69	090	2	1	0	2	1

25360 Osteotomy; ulna   `A 2 J I`

RVU			Global Days	Modifiers				
Mod	Non-Fac Total	Fac Total		51	50	62	80	MUE
	18.85	18.85	090	2	1	1	2	1

25365 Osteotomy; radius AND ulna   `A 2 J I`

RVU			Global Days	Modifiers				
Mod	Non-Fac Total	Fac Total		51	50	62	80	MUE
	26.33	26.33	090	2	1	0	2	1

25370 Multiple osteotomies, with realignment on intramedullary rod (Sofield type procedure); radius OR ulna   `A 2 T`

RVU			Global Days	Modifiers				
Mod	Non-Fac Total	Fac Total		51	50	62	80	MUE
	29.17	29.17	090	2	1	0	2	1

25375 Multiple osteotomies, with realignment on intramedullary rod (Sofield type procedure); radius AND ulna   `⊗ A 2 T`

RVU			Global Days	Modifiers				
Mod	Non-Fac Total	Fac Total		51	50	62	80	MUE
	27.55	27.55	090	2	1	1	2	1

25390 Osteoplasty, radius OR ulna; shortening   `A 2 J I`

RVU			Global Days	Modifiers				
Mod	Non-Fac Total	Fac Total		51	50	62	80	MUE
	22.24	22.24	090	2	1	1	2	1

Osteoplasty, radius or ulna, shortening

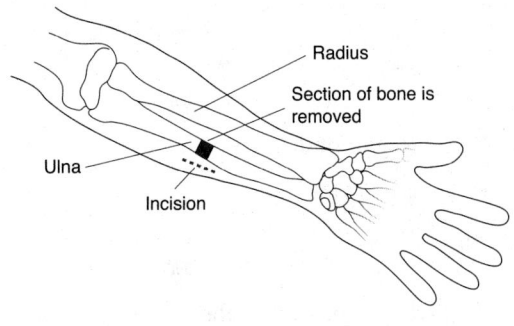

A section of bone is removed from the forearm and the two pieces of remaining bone are connected

25391 Osteoplasty, radius OR ulna; lengthening with autograft   `G 2 J I`

RVU			Global Days	Modifiers				
Mod	Non-Fac Total	Fac Total		51	50	62	80	MUE
	28.82	28.82	090	2	1	1	2	1

25392 Osteoplasty, radius AND ulna; shortening (excluding 64876)   `A 2 T`

RVU			Global Days	Modifiers				
Mod	Non-Fac Total	Fac Total		51	50	62	80	MUE
	25.02	25.02	090	2	1	0	2	1

25393 Osteoplasty, radius AND ulna; lengthening with autograft   `A 2 T`

RVU			Global Days	Modifiers				
Mod	Non-Fac Total	Fac Total		51	50	62	80	MUE
	33.09	33.09	090	2	1	0	2	1

25394 Osteoplasty, carpal bone, shortening   `G 2 T`

RVU			Global Days	Modifiers				
Mod	Non-Fac Total	Fac Total		51	50	62	80	MUE
	22.51	22.51	090	2	1	1	2	1

25400 Repair of nonunion or malunion, radius OR ulna; without graft (eg, compression technique)   `A 2 J I`

RVU			Global Days	Modifiers				
Mod	Non-Fac Total	Fac Total		51	50	62	80	MUE
	23.22	23.22	090	2	1	1	2	1

25405 Repair of nonunion or malunion, radius OR ulna; with autograft (includes obtaining graft)   `A 2 J I`

RVU			Global Days	Modifiers				
Mod	Non-Fac Total	Fac Total		51	50	62	80	MUE
	29.97	29.97	090	2	1	1	2	1

25415 Repair of nonunion or malunion, radius AND ulna; without graft (eg, compression technique)   `A 2 J I`

RVU			Global Days	Modifiers				
Mod	Non-Fac Total	Fac Total		51	50	62	80	MUE
	27.82	27.82	090	2	1	1	2	1

● New   ▲ Revised   Deleted   ⊙ Moderate Sedation   ✚ Add-on Codes   ⊗ High Risk Denial   Ⓐ Age Edit   ♀ Female   ♂ Male   **AMA** *CPT® Assistant*   **MUE** Medically Unlikely Edit
⊘ Modifier 51 Exempt   ⊖ Modifier 63 Exempt   ⊠ Unlisted   **Modifiers:** *See Inside Back Cover*   Ⓜ Maternity   `A 2`–`Z 3` ASC Payment Indicators   `A`–`Y` OPPS Status Indicators

25420 Repair of nonunion or malunion, radius AND ulna; with autograft (includes obtaining graft)　G 2 J 1

RVU			Global Days	Modifiers				
Mod	Non-Fac Total	Fac Total		51	50	62	80	MUE
	33.76	33.76	090	2	1	1	2	1

25425 Repair of defect with autograft; radius OR ulna　A 2 T

RVU			Global Days	Modifiers				
Mod	Non-Fac Total	Fac Total		51	50	62	80	MUE
	27.85	27.85	090	2	1	1	2	1

25426 Repair of defect with autograft; radius AND ulna　⊘ A 2 T

RVU			Global Days	Modifiers				
Mod	Non-Fac Total	Fac Total		51	50	62	80	MUE
	32.54	32.54	090	2	1	1	2	1

25430 Insertion of vascular pedicle into carpal bone (eg, Hori procedure)　G 2 T

RVU			Global Days	Modifiers				
Mod	Non-Fac Total	Fac Total		51	50	62	80	MUE
	21.12	21.12	090	2	1	0	1	1

25431 Repair of nonunion of carpal bone (excluding carpal scaphoid (navicular)) (includes obtaining graft and necessary fixation), each bone　G 2 J 1

RVU			Global Days	Modifiers				
Mod	Non-Fac Total	Fac Total		51	50	62	80	MUE
	22.70	22.70	090	2	1	1	2	1

25440 Repair of nonunion, scaphoid carpal (navicular) bone, with or without radial styloidectomy (includes obtaining graft and necessary fixation)　A 2 J 1

RVU			Global Days	Modifiers				
Mod	Non-Fac Total	Fac Total		51	50	62	80	MUE
	22.18	22.18	090	2	1	1	2	1

25441 Arthroplasty with prosthetic replacement; distal radius　J 8 J 1

RVU			Global Days	Modifiers				
Mod	Non-Fac Total	Fac Total		51	50	62	80	MUE
	27.28	27.28	090	2	1	1	2	1

AMA: Jan 05: 8, 9

25442 Arthroplasty with prosthetic replacement; distal ulna　J 8 J 1

RVU			Global Days	Modifiers				
Mod	Non-Fac Total	Fac Total		51	50	62	80	MUE
	23.34	23.34	090	2	1	1	2	1

AMA: Jan 05: 8, 9

25443 Arthroplasty with prosthetic replacement; scaphoid carpal (navicular)　A 2 J 1

RVU			Global Days	Modifiers				
Mod	Non-Fac Total	Fac Total		51	50	62	80	MUE
	22.57	22.57	090	2	1	1	2	1

AMA: Jan 05: 8, 9

25444 Arthroplasty with prosthetic replacement; lunate　J 8 J 1

RVU			Global Days	Modifiers				
Mod	Non-Fac Total	Fac Total		51	50	62	80	MUE
	23.88	23.88	090	2	1	0	2	1

AMA: Jan 05: 8, 10

25445 Arthroplasty with prosthetic replacement; trapezium　A 2 J 1

RVU			Global Days	Modifiers				
Mod	Non-Fac Total	Fac Total		51	50	62	80	MUE
	20.88	20.88	090	2	1	1	1	1

AMA: Jan 05: 8, 10

25446 Arthroplasty with prosthetic replacement; distal radius and partial or entire carpus (total wrist)　J 8 J 1

RVU			Global Days	Modifiers				
Mod	Non-Fac Total	Fac Total		51	50	62	80	MUE
	33.91	33.91	090	2	1	1	2	1

AMA: Jan 05: 8, 11

25447 Arthroplasty, interposition, intercarpal or carpometacarpal joints　A 2 T

RVU			Global Days	Modifiers				
Mod	Non-Fac Total	Fac Total		51	50	62	80	MUE
	23.94	23.94	090	2	1	1	2	4

AMA: Nov 98: 8, Jan 05: 8, 11, 12

25449 Revision of arthroplasty, including removal of implant, wrist joint　A 2 J 1

RVU			Global Days	Modifiers				
Mod	Non-Fac Total	Fac Total		51	50	62	80	MUE
	29.91	29.91	090	2	1	1	2	1

25450 Epiphyseal arrest by epiphysiodesis or stapling; distal radius OR ulna　A 2 T

RVU			Global Days	Modifiers				
Mod	Non-Fac Total	Fac Total		51	50	62	80	MUE
	14.88	14.88	090	2	1	0	1	1

25455 Epiphyseal arrest by epiphysiodesis or stapling; distal radius AND ulna　A 2 T

RVU			Global Days	Modifiers				
Mod	Non-Fac Total	Fac Total		51	50	62	80	MUE
	17.62	17.62	090	2	1	0	1	1

● New　▲ Revised　✖ Deleted　⊙ Moderate Sedation　✚ Add-on Codes　⊘ High Risk Denial　Ⓐ Age Edit　♀ Female　♂ Male　**AMA** *CPT® Assistant*　***MUE*** Medically Unlikely Edit
⊘ Modifier 51 Exempt　⊖ Modifier 63 Exempt　✗ Unlisted　**Modifiers:** *See Inside Back Cover*　Ⓜ Maternity　A2 – Z3 ASC Payment Indicators　A – Y OPPS Status Indicators

CPT © 2015 American Medical Association. All Rights Reserved.　© 2016 DecisionHealth

25490 Prophylactic treatment (nailing, pinning, plating or wiring) with or without methylmethacrylate; radius `A 2 T`

RVU			Global Days	Modifiers				
Mod	Non-Fac Total	Fac Total		51	50	62	80	MUE
	20.72	20.72	090	2	1	0	2	1

Prophylactic treatment with/without methylmethacrylate, radius and/or ulna

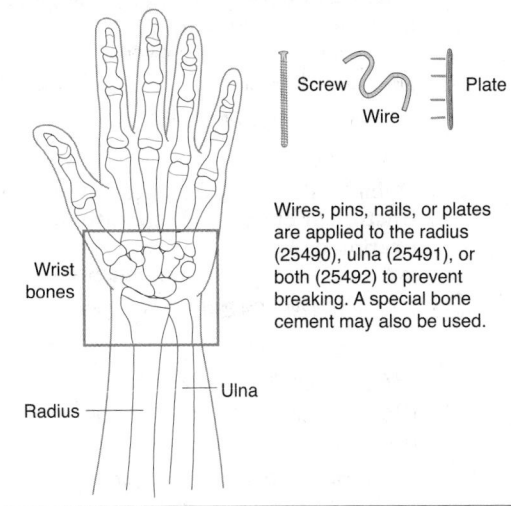

Screw   Wire   Plate

Wires, pins, nails, or plates are applied to the radius (25490), ulna (25491), or both (25492) to prevent breaking. A special bone cement may also be used.

Wrist bones

Radius   Ulna

25491 Prophylactic treatment (nailing, pinning, plating or wiring) with or without methylmethacrylate; ulna `A 2 J I`

RVU			Global Days	Modifiers				
Mod	Non-Fac Total	Fac Total		51	50	62	80	MUE
	21.37	21.37	090	2	1	0	2	1

25492 Prophylactic treatment (nailing, pinning, plating or wiring) with or without methylmethacrylate; radius AND ulna `A 2 T`

RVU			Global Days	Modifiers				
Mod	Non-Fac Total	Fac Total		51	50	62	80	MUE
	26.14	26.14	090	2	1	0	2	1

Forearm/Wrist Fracture/Dislocation Procedures

25500 Closed treatment of radial shaft fracture; without manipulation `P 2 T`

Coding tip: Closed treatment of ulnar shaft fracture - 25530

Coding tip: Closed treatment of radial shaft fracture with dislocation of radioulnar joint - 25520

RVU			Global Days	Modifiers				
Mod	Non-Fac Total	Fac Total		51	50	62	80	MUE
	7.81	7.18	090	2	1	0	1	1

25505 Closed treatment of radial shaft fracture; with manipulation `A 2 T`

Coding tip: Add modifier 77 for re-reduction of the fracture by another physician

Coding tip: Closed treatment of ulnar shaft fracture with manipulation - 25535

RVU			Global Days	Modifiers				
Mod	Non-Fac Total	Fac Total		51	50	62	80	MUE
	14.43	13.25	090	2	1	0	1	1

25515 Open treatment of radial shaft fracture, includes internal fixation, when performed `A 2 J I`

RVU			Global Days	Modifiers				
Mod	Non-Fac Total	Fac Total		51	50	62	80	MUE
	19.30	19.30	090	2	1	1	2	1

25520 Closed treatment of radial shaft fracture and closed treatment of dislocation of distal radioulnar joint (Galeazzi fracture/dislocation) `A 2 T`

RVU			Global Days	Modifiers				
Mod	Non-Fac Total	Fac Total		51	50	62	80	MUE
	16.03	15.23	090	2	1	0	1	1

25525 Open treatment of radial shaft fracture, includes internal fixation, when performed, and closed treatment of distal radioulnar joint dislocation (Galeazzi fracture/ dislocation), includes percutaneous skeletal fixation, when performed `A 2 J I`

RVU			Global Days	Modifiers				
Mod	Non-Fac Total	Fac Total		51	50	62	80	MUE
	22.66	22.66	090	2	1	2	2	1

25526 Open treatment of radial shaft fracture, includes internal fixation, when performed, and open treatment of distal radioulnar joint dislocation (Galeazzi fracture/ dislocation), includes internal fixation, when performed, includes repair of triangular fibrocartilage complex `A 2 J I`

RVU			Global Days	Modifiers				
Mod	Non-Fac Total	Fac Total		51	50	62	80	MUE
	27.49	27.49	090	2	1	2	2	1

25530 Closed treatment of ulnar shaft fracture; without manipulation `P 2 T`

Coding tip: Closed treatment of ulnar shaft fracture with radial shaft fracture - 25560

Coding tip: Closed treatment of radial shaft fracture - 25500

RVU			Global Days	Modifiers				
Mod	Non-Fac Total	Fac Total		51	50	62	80	MUE
	7.51	6.80	090	2	1	0	1	1

AMA: Apr 02: 14

25535 Closed treatment of ulnar shaft fracture; with manipulation `A 2 T`

Coding tip: Closed treatment of ulnar shaft fracture and radial shaft fracture with manipulation - 25565

Coding tip: Closed treatment of radial shaft fracture with manipulation - 25505

Coding tip: Add modifier 77 for re-reduction of the fracture by another physician

RVU			Global Days	Modifiers				
Mod	Non-Fac Total	Fac Total		51	50	62	80	MUE
	14.03	13.01	090	2	1	0	1	1

AMA: Sep 10: 7

25545 Open treatment of ulnar shaft fracture, includes internal fixation, when performed `A 2 J I`

RVU			Global Days	Modifiers				
Mod	Non-Fac Total	Fac Total		51	50	62	80	MUE
	17.97	17.97	090	2	1	1	2	1

AMA: Fall 93: 23, Oct 99: 5

● New   ▲ Revised   Deleted   ⊙ Moderate Sedation   ✚ Add-on Codes   ⊘ High Risk Denial   Ⓐ Age Edit   ♀ Female   ♂ Male   **AMA** *CPT® Assistant*   **MUE** Medically Unlikely Edit
⊘ Modifier 51 Exempt   ⊖ Modifier 63 Exempt   ⊠ Unlisted   **Modifiers:** *See Inside Back Cover*   Ⓜ Maternity   `A 2`–`Z 3` ASC Payment Indicators   `A`–`Y` OPPS Status Indicators

25560 **Closed treatment of radial and ulnar shaft fractures; without manipulation** `P 2 T`

Coding tip: *Closed treatment of ulnar shaft fracture alone - 25530*

Coding tip: *Closed treatment of radial shaft fracture alone - 25500*

RVU			Global Days	Modifiers				
Mod	Non-Fac Total	Fac Total		51	50	62	80	MUE
	7.94	7.19	090	2	1	0	1	1

25565 **Closed treatment of radial and ulnar shaft fractures; with manipulation** `A 2 T`

Coding tip: *Closed treatment of radial shaft fracture alone with manipulation - 25505*

Coding tip: *Add modifier 77 for re-reduction of the fractures by another physician*

Coding tip: *Closed treatment of ulnar shaft fracture alone with manipulation - 25535*

RVU			Global Days	Modifiers				
Mod	Non-Fac Total	Fac Total		51	50	62	80	MUE
	14.96	13.58	090	2	1	0	1	1

25574 **Open treatment of radial AND ulnar shaft fractures, with internal fixation, when performed; of radius OR ulna** `A 2 J I`

RVU			Global Days	Modifiers				
Mod	Non-Fac Total	Fac Total		51	50	62	80	MUE
	19.39	19.39	090	2	1	2	2	1

AMA: Fall 93: 23, Oct 99: 5

25575 **Open treatment of radial AND ulnar shaft fractures, with internal fixation, when performed; of radius AND ulna** `G 2 J I`

RVU			Global Days	Modifiers				
Mod	Non-Fac Total	Fac Total		51	50	62	80	MUE
	26.01	26.01	090	2	1	1	2	1

25600 **Closed treatment of distal radial fracture (eg, Colles or Smith type) or epiphyseal separation, includes closed treatment of fracture of ulnar styloid, when performed; without manipulation** `P 2 T`

RVU			Global Days	Modifiers				
Mod	Non-Fac Total	Fac Total		51	50	62	80	MUE
	9.41	8.92	090	2	1	0	1	1

AMA: Oct 07: 7, Apr 13: 10

25605 **Closed treatment of distal radial fracture (eg, Colles or Smith type) or epiphyseal separation, includes closed treatment of fracture of ulnar styloid, when performed; with manipulation** `A 2 T`

RVU			Global Days	Modifiers				
Mod	Non-Fac Total	Fac Total		51	50	62	80	MUE
	15.80	14.89	090	2	1	0	1	1

AMA: Oct 07: 7, Apr 13: 10

25606 **Percutaneous skeletal fixation of distal radial fracture or epiphyseal separation** `A 2 T`

RVU			Global Days	Modifiers				
Mod	Non-Fac Total	Fac Total		51	50	62	80	MUE
	19.13	19.13	090	2	1	0	1	1

25607 **Open treatment of distal radial extra-articular fracture or epiphyseal separation, with internal fixation** `A 2 J I`

RVU			Global Days	Modifiers				
Mod	Non-Fac Total	Fac Total		51	50	62	80	MUE
	21.21	21.21	090	2	1	0	2	1

AMA: Oct 07: 7, Nov 12: 13

25608 **Open treatment of distal radial intra-articular fracture or epiphyseal separation; with internal fixation of 2 fragments** `A 2 J I`

RVU			Global Days	Modifiers				
Mod	Non-Fac Total	Fac Total		51	50	62	80	MUE
	23.79	23.79	090	2	1	0	2	1

AMA: Oct 07: 7

25609 **Open treatment of distal radial intra-articular fracture or epiphyseal separation; with internal fixation of 3 or more fragments** `A 2 J I`

RVU			Global Days	Modifiers				
Mod	Non-Fac Total	Fac Total		51	50	62	80	MUE
	30.21	30.21	090	2	1	0	2	1

AMA: Oct 07: 7, Mar 13: 13, Dec 13: 14

25622 **Closed treatment of carpal scaphoid (navicular) fracture; without manipulation** `P 2 T`

Coding tip: *Closed treatment of other carpal bone fracture - 25630*

RVU			Global Days	Modifiers				
Mod	Non-Fac Total	Fac Total		51	50	62	80	MUE
	8.72	7.96	090	2	1	0	1	1

Closed treatment of carpal scaphoid (navicular) fracture; without manipulation

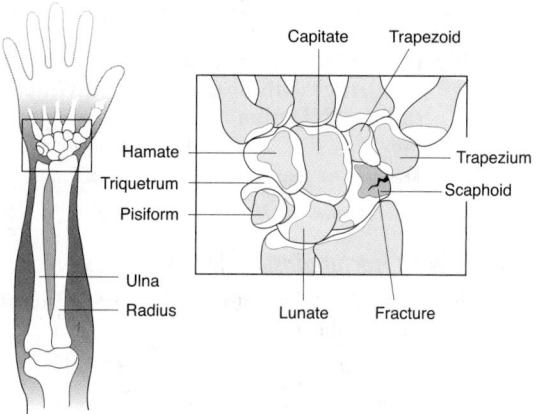

The physician treats a fracture of the wrist joint that lies directly over the outer bone of the forearm. The forearm and wrist are put in a cast.

25624 **Closed treatment of carpal scaphoid (navicular) fracture; with manipulation** `A 2 T`

Coding tip: *Closed treatment of other carpal bone fracture with manipulation - 25635*

Coding tip: *Add modifier 77 for re-reduction of the fracture by another physician*

RVU			Global Days	Modifiers				
Mod	Non-Fac Total	Fac Total		51	50	62	80	MUE
	13.62	12.43	090	2	1	0	0	1

● New   ▲ Revised   ✖ Deleted   ⊙ Moderate Sedation   ✚ Add-on Codes   ⊘ High Risk Denial   Ⓐ Age Edit   ♀ Female   ♂ Male   **AMA** CPT® Assistant   **MUE** Medically Unlikely Edit

⊘ Modifier 51 Exempt   ⊖ Modifier 63 Exempt   ✖ Unlisted   **Modifiers:** See Inside Back Cover   Ⓜ Maternity   `A 2`–`Z 3` ASC Payment Indicators   `A`–`Y` OPPS Status Indicators

CPT © 2015 American Medical Association. All Rights Reserved.   © 2016 DecisionHealth

25628 Open treatment of carpal scaphoid (navicular) fracture, includes internal fixation, when performed   `A 2 T`

RVU			Global Days	Modifiers				
Mod	Non-Fac Total	Fac Total		51	50	62	80	MUE
	20.83	20.83	090	2	1	0	2	1

25630 Closed treatment of carpal bone fracture (excluding carpal scaphoid [navicular]); without manipulation, each bone   `P 2 T`

Coding tip: Closed treatment of scaphoid (navicular) carpal bone - 25622

RVU			Global Days	Modifiers				
Mod	Non-Fac Total	Fac Total		51	50	62	80	MUE
	8.77	8.07	090	2	1	0	1	1

25635 Closed treatment of carpal bone fracture (excluding carpal scaphoid [navicular]); with manipulation, each bone   `A 2 T`

Coding tip: Closed treatment of scaphoid (navicular) carpal bone with manipulation - 25624

Coding tip: Add modifier 77 for re-reduction of the fracture by another physician

RVU			Global Days	Modifiers				
Mod	Non-Fac Total	Fac Total		51	50	62	80	MUE
	12.09	10.82	090	2	1	0	0	1

25645 Open treatment of carpal bone fracture (other than carpal scaphoid [navicular]), each bone   `A 2 T`

RVU			Global Days	Modifiers				
Mod	Non-Fac Total	Fac Total		51	50	62	80	MUE
	16.35	16.35	090	2	1	0	2	1

25650 Closed treatment of ulnar styloid fracture   `P 2 T`

RVU			Global Days	Modifiers				
Mod	Non-Fac Total	Fac Total		51	50	62	80	MUE
	9.18	8.63	090	2	1	0	1	1

AMA: Oct 07: 7, Apr 13: 10

25651 Percutaneous skeletal fixation of ulnar styloid fracture   `G 2 T`

RVU			Global Days	Modifiers				
Mod	Non-Fac Total	Fac Total		51	50	62	80	MUE
	13.89	13.89	090	2	1	0	0	1

25652 Open treatment of ulnar styloid fracture   `G 2 J 1`

RVU			Global Days	Modifiers				
Mod	Non-Fac Total	Fac Total		51	50	62	80	MUE
	18.02	18.02	090	2	1	1	1	1

AMA: Oct 07: 7

25660 Closed treatment of radiocarpal or intercarpal dislocation, 1 or more bones, with manipulation   `A 2 T`

RVU			Global Days	Modifiers				
Mod	Non-Fac Total	Fac Total		51	50	62	80	MUE
	11.72	11.72	090	2	1	0	0	1

25670 Open treatment of radiocarpal or intercarpal dislocation, 1 or more bones   `A 2 T`

RVU			Global Days	Modifiers				
Mod	Non-Fac Total	Fac Total		51	50	62	80	MUE
	17.38	17.38	090	2	1	1	2	1

25671 Percutaneous skeletal fixation of distal radioulnar dislocation   `A 2 T`

RVU			Global Days	Modifiers				
Mod	Non-Fac Total	Fac Total		51	50	62	80	MUE
	15.30	15.30	090	2	1	0	1	1

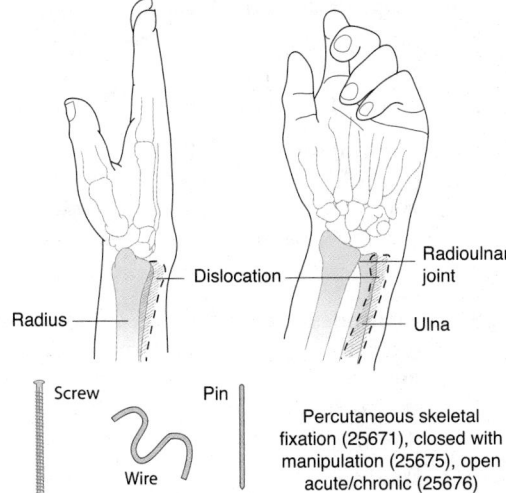

Treatment of distal radioulnar dislocation

Percutaneous skeletal fixation (25671), closed with manipulation (25675), open acute/chronic (25676)

25675 Closed treatment of distal radioulnar dislocation with manipulation   `A 2 T`

RVU			Global Days	Modifiers				
Mod	Non-Fac Total	Fac Total		51	50	62	80	MUE
	12.44	11.37	090	2	1	0	0	1

25676 Open treatment of distal radioulnar dislocation, acute or chronic   `A 2 J 1`

RVU			Global Days	Modifiers				
Mod	Non-Fac Total	Fac Total		51	50	62	80	MUE
	18.00	18.00	090	2	1	0	2	1

25680 Closed treatment of trans-scaphoperilunar type of fracture dislocation, with manipulation   `A 2 T`

RVU			Global Days	Modifiers				
Mod	Non-Fac Total	Fac Total		51	50	62	80	MUE
	13.57	13.57	090	2	1	0	0	1

25685 Open treatment of trans-scaphoperilunar type of fracture dislocation   `A 2 T`

RVU			Global Days	Modifiers				
Mod	Non-Fac Total	Fac Total		51	50	62	80	MUE
	21.19	21.19	090	2	1	0	2	1

25690 Closed treatment of lunate dislocation, with manipulation   `A 2 T`

RVU			Global Days	Modifiers				
Mod	Non-Fac Total	Fac Total		51	50	62	80	MUE
	13.67	13.67	090	2	1	0	0	1

25695 Open treatment of lunate dislocation   `A 2 T`

RVU			Global Days	Modifiers				
Mod	Non-Fac Total	Fac Total		51	50	62	80	MUE
	18.28	18.28	090	2	1	1	2	1

● New ▲ Revised Deleted ⊙ Moderate Sedation ✚ Add-on Codes ⊗ High Risk Denial Ⓐ Age Edit ♀ Female ♂ Male **AMA** *CPT® Assistant* *MUE* Medically Unlikely Edit
⊘ Modifier 51 Exempt ⊖ Modifier 63 Exempt ✗ Unlisted **Modifiers:** *See Inside Back Cover* Ⓜ Maternity `A 2`–`Z 3` ASC Payment Indicators `A`–`Y` OPPS Status Indicators

Surgical Procedures

25800 – 26011

Forearm/Wrist Arthrodesis

25800 Arthrodesis, wrist; complete, without bone graft (includes radiocarpal and/or intercarpal and/or carpometacarpal joints) `G 2 J I`

	RVU		Global Days	Modifiers				
Mod	Non-Fac Total	Fac Total		51	50	62	80	MUE
	21.15	21.15	090	2	1	1	2	1

AMA: Nov 98: 8

25805 Arthrodesis, wrist; with sliding graft `A 2 J I`

	RVU		Global Days	Modifiers				
Mod	Non-Fac Total	Fac Total		51	50	62	80	MUE
	24.42	24.42	090	2	1	1	2	1

25810 Arthrodesis, wrist; with iliac or other autograft (includes obtaining graft) `G 2 J I`

	RVU		Global Days	Modifiers				
Mod	Non-Fac Total	Fac Total		51	50	62	80	MUE
	25.09	25.09	090	2	1	1	2	1

25820 Arthrodesis, wrist; limited, without bone graft (eg, intercarpal or radiocarpal) `A 2 J I`

	RVU		Global Days	Modifiers				
Mod	Non-Fac Total	Fac Total		51	50	62	80	MUE
	17.76	17.76	090	2	1	1	2	1

AMA: Nov 98: 8

25825 Arthrodesis, wrist; with autograft (includes obtaining graft) `A 2 J I`

	RVU		Global Days	Modifiers				
Mod	Non-Fac Total	Fac Total		51	50	62	80	MUE
	21.91	21.91	090	2	1	1	2	1

AMA: Jul 12: 12

25830 Arthrodesis, distal radioulnar joint with segmental resection of ulna, with or without bone graft (eg, Sauve-Kapandji procedure) `A 2 J I`

	RVU		Global Days	Modifiers				
Mod	Non-Fac Total	Fac Total		51	50	62	80	MUE
	27.32	27.32	090	2	1	1	2	1

AMA: Nov 98: 8

Forearm/Wrist Amputation

25900 Amputation, forearm, through radius and ulna `C`

	RVU		Global Days	Modifiers				
Mod	Non-Fac Total	Fac Total		51	50	62	80	MUE
	20.48	20.48	090	2	1	0	0	1

25905 Amputation, forearm, through radius and ulna; open, circular (guillotine) `C`

	RVU		Global Days	Modifiers				
Mod	Non-Fac Total	Fac Total		51	50	62	80	MUE
	18.65	18.65	090	2	1	0	2	1

25907 Amputation, forearm, through radius and ulna; secondary closure or scar revision `⊗ A 2 T`

	RVU		Global Days	Modifiers				
Mod	Non-Fac Total	Fac Total		51	50	62	80	MUE
	16.76	16.76	090	2	1	0	2	1

25909 Amputation, forearm, through radius and ulna; re-amputation `T`

	RVU		Global Days	Modifiers				
Mod	Non-Fac Total	Fac Total		51	50	62	80	MUE
	19.78	19.78	090	2	1	0	2	1

25915 Krukenberg procedure `C`

	RVU		Global Days	Modifiers				
Mod	Non-Fac Total	Fac Total		51	50	62	80	MUE
	34.21	34.21	090	2	1	0	2	1

25920 Disarticulation through wrist `C`

	RVU		Global Days	Modifiers				
Mod	Non-Fac Total	Fac Total		51	50	62	80	MUE
	20.02	20.02	090	2	1	0	0	1

25922 Disarticulation through wrist; secondary closure or scar revision `A 2 T`

	RVU		Global Days	Modifiers				
Mod	Non-Fac Total	Fac Total		51	50	62	80	MUE
	16.26	16.26	090	2	1	0	2	1

25924 Disarticulation through wrist; re-amputation `C`

	RVU		Global Days	Modifiers				
Mod	Non-Fac Total	Fac Total		51	50	62	80	MUE
	17.48	17.48	090	2	1	0	2	1

25927 Transmetacarpal amputation `C`

	RVU		Global Days	Modifiers				
Mod	Non-Fac Total	Fac Total		51	50	62	80	MUE
	23.39	23.39	090	2	1	0	0	1

25929 Transmetacarpal amputation; secondary closure or scar revision `⊗ A 2 T`

	RVU		Global Days	Modifiers				
Mod	Non-Fac Total	Fac Total		51	50	62	80	MUE
	17.02	17.02	090	2	1	0	2	1

25931 Transmetacarpal amputation; re-amputation `G 2 T`

	RVU		Global Days	Modifiers				
Mod	Non-Fac Total	Fac Total		51	50	62	80	MUE
	19.03	19.03	090	2	1	0	1	1

Other Forearm/Wrist Procedures

25999 Unlisted procedure, forearm or wrist `x T`

	RVU		Global Days	Modifiers				
Mod	Non-Fac Total	Fac Total		51	50	62	80	MUE
	0.00	0.00	YYY	2	1	1	0	

Hand/Finger Procedures

Hand/Finger Incisional Procedures

26010 Drainage of finger abscess; simple `P 2 T`

Coding tip: Drainage of paronychia or onychia - 10060-10061

	RVU		Global Days	Modifiers				
Mod	Non-Fac Total	Fac Total		51	50	62	80	MUE
	7.51	3.93	010	2	0	0	1	2

26011 Drainage of finger abscess; complicated (eg, felon) `A 2 T`

	RVU		Global Days	Modifiers				
Mod	Non-Fac Total	Fac Total		51	50	62	80	MUE
	11.18	5.33	010	2	0	0	1	3

● New   ▲ Revised   ✖ Deleted   ⊙ Moderate Sedation   ✚ Add-on Codes   ⊖ High Risk Denial   Ⓐ Age Edit   ♀ Female   ♂ Male   **AMA** CPT® Assistant   **MUE** Medically Unlikely Edit
⊘ Modifier 51 Exempt   ⊖ Modifier 63 Exempt   ✖ Unlisted   **Modifiers:** See Inside Back Cover   Ⓜ Maternity   `A 2`–`Z 3` ASC Payment Indicators   `A`–`Y` OPPS Status Indicators

CPT © 2015 American Medical Association. All Rights Reserved.   © 2016 DecisionHealth

26020 Drainage of tendon sheath, digit and/or palm, each `A 2 T`

RVU			Global Days	Modifiers				
Mod	Non-Fac Total	Fac Total		51	50	62	80	MUE
	12.55	12.55	090	2	0	0	1	4

26025 Drainage of palmar bursa; single, bursa `A 2 T`

RVU			Global Days	Modifiers				
Mod	Non-Fac Total	Fac Total		51	50	62	80	MUE
	12.21	12.21	090	2	1	0	0	1

AMA: Nov 98: 8

26030 Drainage of palmar bursa; multiple bursa `A 2 T`

RVU			Global Days	Modifiers				
Mod	Non-Fac Total	Fac Total		51	50	62	80	MUE
	14.20	14.20	090	2	1	0	0	1

AMA: Nov 98: 8

26034 Incision, bone cortex, hand or finger (eg, osteomyelitis or bone abscess) `A 2 T`

RVU			Global Days	Modifiers				
Mod	Non-Fac Total	Fac Total		51	50	62	80	MUE
	15.53	15.53	090	2	0	0	1	2

AMA: Nov 98: 8

26035 Decompression fingers and/or hand, injection injury (eg, grease gun) `G 2 T`

RVU			Global Days	Modifiers				
Mod	Non-Fac Total	Fac Total		51	50	62	80	MUE
	24.79	24.79	090	2	0	0	0	1

26037 Decompressive fasciotomy, hand (excludes 26035) `G 2 T`

RVU			Global Days	Modifiers				
Mod	Non-Fac Total	Fac Total		51	50	62	80	MUE
	16.40	16.40	090	2	1	0	0	1

Decompressive fasciotomy

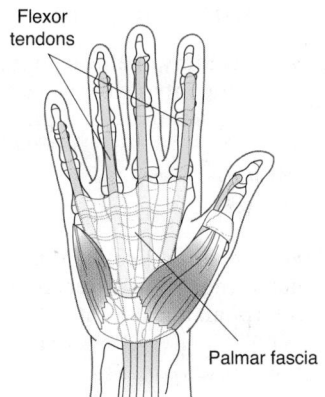

Flexor tendons

Palmar fascia

The membrane that surrounds the tissue in the palm of the hand is decompressed.

26040 Fasciotomy, palmar (eg, Dupuytren's contracture); percutaneous `A 2 T`

RVU			Global Days	Modifiers				
Mod	Non-Fac Total	Fac Total		51	50	62	80	MUE
	9.01	9.01	090	2	1	0	1	1

AMA: Nov 98: 8, Apr 10: 10, Oct 10: 10

26045 Fasciotomy, palmar (eg, Dupuytren's contracture); open, partial `A 2 T`

RVU			Global Days	Modifiers				
Mod	Non-Fac Total	Fac Total		51	50	62	80	MUE
	13.53	13.53	090	2	1	0	1	1

26055 Tendon sheath incision (eg, for trigger finger) `A 2 T`

RVU			Global Days	Modifiers				
Mod	Non-Fac Total	Fac Total		51	50	62	80	MUE
	16.04	8.94	090	2	0	0	1	5

26060 Tenotomy, percutaneous, single, each digit `A 2 T`

RVU			Global Days	Modifiers				
Mod	Non-Fac Total	Fac Total		51	50	62	80	MUE
	7.64	7.64	090	2	0	0	0	5

26070 Arthrotomy, with exploration, drainage, or removal of loose or foreign body; carpometacarpal joint `A 2 T`

RVU			Global Days	Modifiers				
Mod	Non-Fac Total	Fac Total		51	50	62	80	MUE
	8.93	8.93	090	2	1	0	1	2

AMA: Nov 98: 10

26075 Arthrotomy, with exploration, drainage, or removal of loose or foreign body; metacarpophalangeal joint, each `A 2 T`

RVU			Global Days	Modifiers				
Mod	Non-Fac Total	Fac Total		51	50	62	80	MUE
	9.55	9.55	090	2	1	0	1	4

AMA: Sep 12: 10

26080 Arthrotomy, with exploration, drainage, or removal of loose or foreign body; interphalangeal joint, each `A 2 T`

RVU			Global Days	Modifiers				
Mod	Non-Fac Total	Fac Total		51	50	62	80	MUE
	11.27	11.27	090	2	0	0	1	4

AMA: Sep 12: 10

Hand/Finger Excisional Procedures

26100 Arthrotomy with biopsy; carpometacarpal joint, each `A 2 T`

RVU			Global Days	Modifiers				
Mod	Non-Fac Total	Fac Total		51	50	62	80	MUE
	9.58	9.58	090	2	1	0	0	1

26105 Arthrotomy with biopsy; metacarpophalangeal joint, each `A 2 T`

RVU			Global Days	Modifiers				
Mod	Non-Fac Total	Fac Total		51	50	62	80	MUE
	9.60	9.60	090	2	1	0	0	2

26110 Arthrotomy with biopsy; interphalangeal joint, each `A 2 T`

RVU			Global Days	Modifiers				
Mod	Non-Fac Total	Fac Total		51	50	62	80	MUE
	9.26	9.26	090	2	0	0	1	3

● New   ▲ Revised   Deleted   ⊙ Moderate Sedation   ✚ Add-on Codes   ⊘ High Risk Denial   Ⓐ Age Edit   ♀ Female   ♂ Male   **AMA** *CPT® Assistant*   **MUE** Medically Unlikely Edit
⊘ Modifier 51 Exempt   ⊖ Modifier 63 Exempt   🗶 Unlisted   **Modifiers:** *See Inside Back Cover*   Ⓜ Maternity   A 2 – Z 3 ASC Payment Indicators   A – Y OPPS Status Indicators

26111 Excision, tumor or vascular malformation, soft tissue of hand or finger, subcutaneous; 1.5 cm or greater   G2 T

Coding tip: Code 26111 is listed out of numerical order in CPT. Related soft tissue tumor/vascular malformation excision procedures - 26115 (subcutaneous tissue); 26116, 26113 (subfascial).

RVU			Global Days	Modifiers				
Mod	Non-Fac Total	Fac Total		51	50	62	80	MUE
	12.09	12.09	090	2	0	0	2	4

26113 Excision, tumor, soft tissue, or vascular malformation, of hand or finger, subfascial (eg, intramuscular); 1.5 cm or greater   G2 T

Coding tip: Code 26113 is listed out of numerical order in CPT. Related soft tissue tumor/vascular malformation excision procedures - 26111, 26115 (subcutaneous tissue); 26116 (subfascial).

RVU			Global Days	Modifiers				
Mod	Non-Fac Total	Fac Total		51	50	62	80	MUE
	15.87	15.87	090	2	0	0	2	4

AMA: Apr 10: 3

26115 Excision, tumor or vascular malformation, soft tissue of hand or finger, subcutaneous; less than 1.5 cm   G2 T

Coding tip: Related soft tissue tumor/vascular malformation excision codes - 26111, 26113 and 26116

RVU			Global Days	Modifiers				
Mod	Non-Fac Total	Fac Total		51	50	62	80	MUE
	14.51	9.62	090	2	0	0	1	4

26116 Excision, tumor, soft tissue, or vascular malformation, of hand or finger, subfascial (eg, intramuscular); less than 1.5 cm   G2 T

Coding tip: Related soft tissue tumor/vascular malformation excision codes - 26111, 26113 and 26115

RVU			Global Days	Modifiers				
Mod	Non-Fac Total	Fac Total		51	50	62	80	MUE
	15.26	15.26	090	2	0	0	1	2

AMA: Apr 10: 3

26117 Radical resection of tumor (eg, sarcoma), soft tissue of hand or finger; less than 3 cm   G2 T

RVU			Global Days	Modifiers				
Mod	Non-Fac Total	Fac Total		51	50	62	80	MUE
	21.72	21.72	090	2	0	0	1	2

Radical resection of tumor

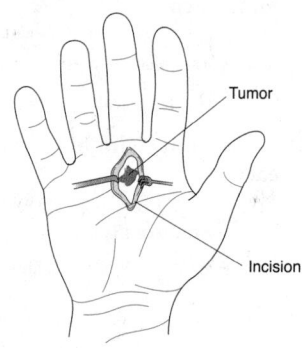

An incison is made into the soft tissue of the hand or finger to remove a tumor, less than 3 cm (26117), 3 cm or greater (26118)

26118 Radical resection of tumor (eg, sarcoma), soft tissue of hand or finger; 3 cm or greater   G2 T

RVU			Global Days	Modifiers				
Mod	Non-Fac Total	Fac Total		51	50	62	80	MUE
	30.45	30.45	090	2	0	0	2	1

26121 Fasciectomy, palm only, with or without Z-plasty, other local tissue rearrangement, or skin grafting (includes obtaining graft)   A2 T

RVU			Global Days	Modifiers				
Mod	Non-Fac Total	Fac Total		51	50	62	80	MUE
	17.27	17.27	090	2	1	0	1	1

AMA: Jun 11: 13, Oct 10: 10

26123 Fasciectomy, partial palmar with release of single digit including proximal interphalangeal joint, with or without Z-plasty, other local tissue rearrangement, or skin grafting (includes obtaining graft)   A2 T

RVU			Global Days	Modifiers				
Mod	Non-Fac Total	Fac Total		51	50	62	80	MUE
	24.16	24.16	090	2	1	0	1	1

AMA: Jan 05: 8, Jun 11: 13, Oct 10: 10

+ **26125** Fasciectomy, partial palmar with release of single digit including proximal interphalangeal joint, with or without Z-plasty, other local tissue rearrangement, or skin grafting (includes obtaining graft); each additional digit (List separately in addition to code for primary procedure)   N IN

RVU			Global Days	Modifiers				
Mod	Non-Fac Total	Fac Total		51	50	62	80	MUE
	7.98	7.98	ZZZ	0	0	0	1	4

AMA: Jan 05: 8, Jun 11: 13, Oct 10: 10

26130 Synovectomy, carpometacarpal joint   A2 T

RVU			Global Days	Modifiers				
Mod	Non-Fac Total	Fac Total		51	50	62	80	MUE
	13.32	13.32	090	2	1	0	1	1

26135 Synovectomy, metacarpophalangeal joint including intrinsic release and extensor hood reconstruction, each digit   A2 T

RVU			Global Days	Modifiers				
Mod	Non-Fac Total	Fac Total		51	50	62	80	MUE
	15.87	15.87	090	2	0	0	0	4

26140 Synovectomy, proximal interphalangeal joint, including extensor reconstruction, each interphalangeal joint   A2 T

RVU			Global Days	Modifiers				
Mod	Non-Fac Total	Fac Total		51	50	62	80	MUE
	14.59	14.59	090	2	0	0	1	3

26145 Synovectomy, tendon sheath, radical (tenosynovectomy), flexor tendon, palm and/or finger, each tendon   A2 T

RVU			Global Days	Modifiers				
Mod	Non-Fac Total	Fac Total		51	50	62	80	MUE
	14.79	14.79	090	2	0	0	1	6

AMA: Nov 98: 8

● New   ▲ Revised   ✖ Deleted   ☉ Moderate Sedation   ✚ Add-on Codes   ⊘ High Risk Denial   Ⓐ Age Edit   ♀ Female   ♂ Male   **AMA** CPT® Assistant   **MUE** Medically Unlikely Edit
⊘ Modifier 51 Exempt   ⊖ Modifier 63 Exempt   ☒ Unlisted   **Modifiers:** See Inside Back Cover   Ⓜ Maternity   A2–Z3 ASC Payment Indicators   A–Y OPPS Status Indicators

CPT © 2015 American Medical Association. All Rights Reserved.   © 2016 DecisionHealth

26160 Excision of lesion of tendon sheath or joint capsule (eg, cyst, mucous cyst, or ganglion), hand or finger　A 2 T

RVU			Global Days	Modifiers				
Mod	Non-Fac Total	Fac Total		51	50	62	80	MUE
	16.49	9.63	090	2	0	0	1	5

Excision of lesion of tendon sheath/joint capsule

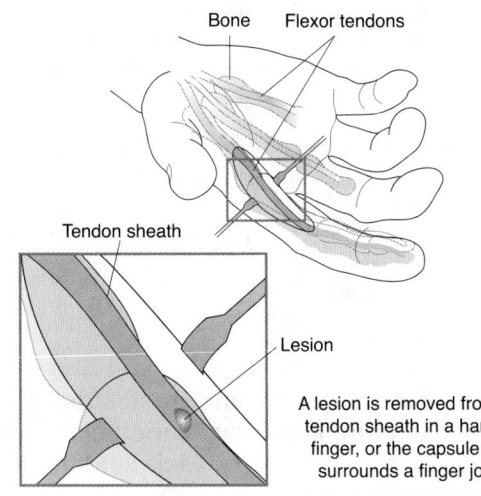

A lesion is removed from the tendon sheath in a hand or finger, or the capsule that surrounds a finger joint.

26170 Excision of tendon, palm, flexor or extensor, single, each tendon　A 2 T

RVU			Global Days	Modifiers				
Mod	Non-Fac Total	Fac Total		51	50	62	80	MUE
	11.70	11.70	090	2	0	0	0	5

AMA: Jun 13: 13

26180 Excision of tendon, finger, flexor or extensor, each tendon　A 2 T

RVU			Global Days	Modifiers				
Mod	Non-Fac Total	Fac Total		51	50	62	80	MUE
	12.81	12.81	090	2	0	0	0	4

AMA: Nov 98: 8

26185 Sesamoidectomy, thumb or finger (separate procedure)　A 2 T

RVU			Global Days	Modifiers				
Mod	Non-Fac Total	Fac Total		51	50	62	80	MUE
	15.83	15.83	090	2	1	0	2	1

26200 Excision or curettage of bone cyst or benign tumor of metacarpal　A 2 T

RVU			Global Days	Modifiers				
Mod	Non-Fac Total	Fac Total		51	50	62	80	MUE
	13.01	13.01	090	2	0	0	0	2

26205 Excision or curettage of bone cyst or benign tumor of metacarpal; with autograft (includes obtaining graft)　A 2 T

RVU			Global Days	Modifiers				
Mod	Non-Fac Total	Fac Total		51	50	62	80	MUE
	17.37	17.37	090	2	0	0	1	1

26210 Excision or curettage of bone cyst or benign tumor of proximal, middle, or distal phalanx of finger　A 2 T

RVU			Global Days	Modifiers				
Mod	Non-Fac Total	Fac Total		51	50	62	80	MUE
	12.79	12.79	090	2	0	0	1	2

26215 Excision or curettage of bone cyst or benign tumor of proximal, middle, or distal phalanx of finger; with autograft (includes obtaining graft)　A 2 T

RVU			Global Days	Modifiers				
Mod	Non-Fac Total	Fac Total		51	50	62	80	MUE
	16.24	16.24	090	2	0	0	1	2

26230 Partial excision (craterization, saucerization, or diaphysectomy) bone (eg, osteomyelitis); metacarpal　A 2 T

RVU			Global Days	Modifiers				
Mod	Non-Fac Total	Fac Total		51	50	62	80	MUE
	14.43	14.43	090	2	0	0	0	2

26235 Partial excision (craterization, saucerization, or diaphysectomy) bone (eg, osteomyelitis); proximal or middle phalanx of finger　A 2 T

RVU			Global Days	Modifiers				
Mod	Non-Fac Total	Fac Total		51	50	62	80	MUE
	14.29	14.29	090	2	0	0	0	2

26236 Partial excision (craterization, saucerization, or diaphysectomy) bone (eg, osteomyelitis); distal phalanx of finger　A 2 T

RVU			Global Days	Modifiers				
Mod	Non-Fac Total	Fac Total		51	50	62	80	MUE
	12.78	12.78	090	2	0	0	1	2

26250 Radical resection of tumor, metacarpal　A 2 T

RVU			Global Days	Modifiers				
Mod	Non-Fac Total	Fac Total		51	50	62	80	MUE
	31.31	31.31	090	2	0	0	0	2

AMA: Nov 98: 8

26260 Radical resection of tumor, proximal or middle phalanx of finger　A 2 T

RVU			Global Days	Modifiers				
Mod	Non-Fac Total	Fac Total		51	50	62	80	MUE
	23.24	23.24	090	2	0	0	2	1

AMA: Nov 98: 8

26262 Radical resection of tumor, distal phalanx of finger　A 2 T

RVU			Global Days	Modifiers				
Mod	Non-Fac Total	Fac Total		51	50	62	80	MUE
	18.23	18.23	090	2	0	0	2	1

AMA: Nov 98: 8

Hand/Finger Introduction/Removal Procedures

26320 Removal of implant from finger or hand　A 2 Q 2

RVU			Global Days	Modifiers				
Mod	Non-Fac Total	Fac Total		51	50	62	80	MUE
	10.03	10.03	090	2	0	0	1	4

● New　▲ Revised　Deleted　⊙ Moderate Sedation　✚ Add-on Codes　⊘ High Risk Denial　Ⓐ Age Edit　♀ Female　♂ Male　**AMA** *CPT® Assistant*　**MUE** Medically Unlikely Edit
⊘ Modifier 51 Exempt　⊖ Modifier 63 Exempt　✗ Unlisted　**Modifiers:** *See Inside Back Cover*　Ⓜ Maternity　A 2–Z 3 ASC Payment Indicators　A –Y OPPS Status Indicators

Hand/Finger Repair/Revision/Reconstruction Procedures

26340 Manipulation, finger joint, under anesthesia, each joint   `G2T`

RVU			Global Days	Modifiers				
Mod	Non-Fac Total	Fac Total		51	50	62	80	MUE
	9.64	9.64	090	2	1	0	1	4

AMA: Nov 02: 10

26341 Manipulation, palmar fascial cord (ie, Dupuytren's cord), post enzyme injection (eg, collagenase), single cord   `P3T`

RVU			Global Days	Modifiers				
Mod	Non-Fac Total	Fac Total		51	50	62	80	MUE
	2.85	2.17	010	2	1	0	1	2

AMA: Jul 12: 8, 14

26350 Repair or advancement, flexor tendon, not in zone 2 digital flexor tendon sheath (eg, no man's land); primary or secondary without free graft, each tendon   `A2T`

RVU			Global Days	Modifiers				
Mod	Non-Fac Total	Fac Total		51	50	62	80	MUE
	20.30	20.30	090	2	0	0	1	6

AMA: Nov 98: 8

Repair or advancement, flexor tendon, not in zone 2, digital flexor tendon sheath

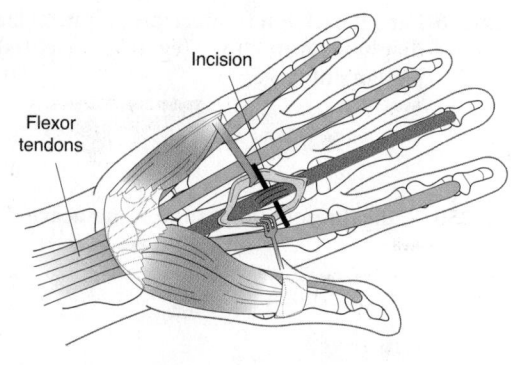

An incision is made and a tendon is pulled forward on the hand, primary (26350), secondary (26352)

26352 Repair or advancement, flexor tendon, not in zone 2 digital flexor tendon sheath (eg, no man's land); secondary with free graft (includes obtaining graft), each tendon   `A2T`

RVU			Global Days	Modifiers				
Mod	Non-Fac Total	Fac Total		51	50	62	80	MUE
	23.24	23.24	090	2	0	1	2	2

26356 Repair or advancement, flexor tendon, in zone 2 digital flexor tendon sheath (eg, no man's land); primary, without free graft, each tendon   `A2T`

RVU			Global Days	Modifiers				
Mod	Non-Fac Total	Fac Total		51	50	62	80	MUE
	24.99	24.99	090	2	0	0	1	4

AMA: Nov 98: 8, Dec 98: 9, Dec 08: 6, Sep 14: 13

26357 Repair or advancement, flexor tendon, in zone 2 digital flexor tendon sheath (eg, no man's land); secondary, without free graft, each tendon   `A2T`

RVU			Global Days	Modifiers				
Mod	Non-Fac Total	Fac Total		51	50	62	80	MUE
	24.75	24.75	090	2	0	0	2	2

26358 Repair or advancement, flexor tendon, in zone 2 digital flexor tendon sheath (eg, no man's land); secondary, with free graft (includes obtaining graft), each tendon   `A2T`

RVU			Global Days	Modifiers				
Mod	Non-Fac Total	Fac Total		51	50	62	80	MUE
	27.48	27.48	090	2	0	0	2	2

26370 Repair or advancement of profundus tendon, with intact superficialis tendon; primary, each tendon   `A2T`

RVU			Global Days	Modifiers				
Mod	Non-Fac Total	Fac Total		51	50	62	80	MUE
	21.59	21.59	090	2	0	0	0	3

AMA: Nov 98: 8, Dec 08: 6

Repair or advancement of profundus tendon, with intact superficialis tendon; primary, each tendon

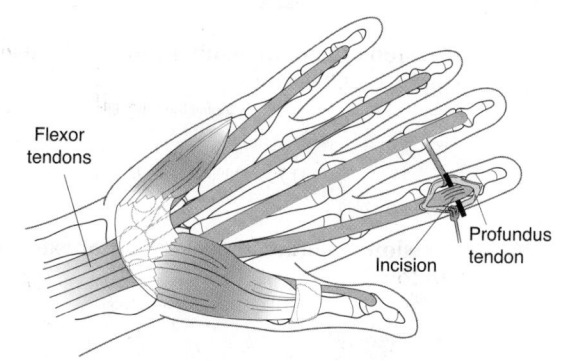

26372 Repair or advancement of profundus tendon, with intact superficialis tendon; secondary with free graft (includes obtaining graft), each tendon   `A2T`

RVU			Global Days	Modifiers				
Mod	Non-Fac Total	Fac Total		51	50	62	80	MUE
	24.96	24.96	090	2	0	0	2	1

AMA: Nov 98: 8

26373 Repair or advancement of profundus tendon, with intact superficialis tendon; secondary without free graft, each tendon   `A2T`

RVU			Global Days	Modifiers				
Mod	Non-Fac Total	Fac Total		51	50	62	80	MUE
	23.99	23.99	090	2	0	0	2	2

AMA: Nov 98: 8

● New   ▲ Revised   ✖ Deleted   ⊙ Moderate Sedation   ✚ Add-on Codes   ⊘ High Risk Denial   Ⓐ Age Edit   ♀ Female   ♂ Male   **AMA** *CPT® Assistant*   **MUE** Medically Unlikely Edit

⊘ Modifier 51 Exempt   ⊖ Modifier 63 Exempt   ✖ Unlisted   **Modifiers:** *See Inside Back Cover*   Ⓜ Maternity   A2–Z3 ASC Payment Indicators   A–Y OPPS Status Indicators

CPT © 2015 American Medical Association. All Rights Reserved.   © 2016 DecisionHealth

26390 Excision flexor tendon, with implantation of synthetic rod for delayed tendon graft, hand or finger, each rod A2 J I

RVU			Global Days	Modifiers				
Mod	Non-Fac Total	Fac Total		51	50	62	80	MUE
	23.82	23.82	090	2	0	1	2	2

AMA: Nov 98: 8

26392 Removal of synthetic rod and insertion of flexor tendon graft, hand or finger (includes obtaining graft), each rod A2 J I

RVU			Global Days	Modifiers				
Mod	Non-Fac Total	Fac Total		51	50	62	80	MUE
	27.51	27.51	090	2	0	1	2	2

AMA: Nov 98: 8

26410 Repair, extensor tendon, hand, primary or secondary; without free graft, each tendon A2 T

RVU			Global Days	Modifiers				
Mod	Non-Fac Total	Fac Total		51	50	62	80	MUE
	16.11	16.11	090	2	0	0	1	4

AMA: Nov 98: 8

26412 Repair, extensor tendon, hand, primary or secondary; with free graft (includes obtaining graft), each tendon A2 T

RVU			Global Days	Modifiers				
Mod	Non-Fac Total	Fac Total		51	50	62	80	MUE
	19.43	19.43	090	2	0	0	0	3

AMA: Nov 98: 8

26415 Excision of extensor tendon, with implantation of synthetic rod for delayed tendon graft, hand or finger, each rod ⊘A2 T

RVU			Global Days	Modifiers				
Mod	Non-Fac Total	Fac Total		51	50	62	80	MUE
	21.72	21.72	090	2	0	0	0	2

AMA: Nov 98: 8

26416 Removal of synthetic rod and insertion of extensor tendon graft (includes obtaining graft), hand or finger, each rod ⊘A2 T

RVU			Global Days	Modifiers				
Mod	Non-Fac Total	Fac Total		51	50	62	80	MUE
	20.44	20.44	090	2	0	0	1	2

AMA: Nov 99: 12

26418 Repair, extensor tendon, finger, primary or secondary; without free graft, each tendon A2 T

RVU			Global Days	Modifiers				
Mod	Non-Fac Total	Fac Total		51	50	62	80	MUE
	16.45	16.45	090	2	0	0	1	4

AMA: Nov 98: 8, Dec 99: 10, Dec 00: 14

26420 Repair, extensor tendon, finger, primary or secondary; with free graft (includes obtaining graft) each tendon A2 T

RVU			Global Days	Modifiers				
Mod	Non-Fac Total	Fac Total		51	50	62	80	MUE
	20.17	20.17	090	2	0	0	2	4

26426 Repair of extensor tendon, central slip, secondary (eg, boutonniere deformity); using local tissue(s), including lateral band(s), each finger A2 T

RVU			Global Days	Modifiers				
Mod	Non-Fac Total	Fac Total		51	50	62	80	MUE
	14.49	14.49	090	2	0	0	1	4

AMA: Nov 98: 8

26428 Repair of extensor tendon, central slip, secondary (eg, boutonniere deformity); with free graft (includes obtaining graft), each finger A2 T

RVU			Global Days	Modifiers				
Mod	Non-Fac Total	Fac Total		51	50	62	80	MUE
	21.44	21.44	090	2	0	0	0	2

26432 Closed treatment of distal extensor tendon insertion, with or without percutaneous pinning (eg, mallet finger) A2 T

RVU			Global Days	Modifiers				
Mod	Non-Fac Total	Fac Total		51	50	62	80	MUE
	14.20	14.20	090	2	0	0	1	2

AMA: Nov 98: 8

26433 Repair of extensor tendon, distal insertion, primary or secondary; without graft (eg, mallet finger) A2 T

RVU			Global Days	Modifiers				
Mod	Non-Fac Total	Fac Total		51	50	62	80	MUE
	15.14	15.14	090	2	0	0	1	2

AMA: Nov 98: 8

26434 Repair of extensor tendon, distal insertion, primary or secondary; with free graft (includes obtaining graft) A2 T

RVU			Global Days	Modifiers				
Mod	Non-Fac Total	Fac Total		51	50	62	80	MUE
	18.34	18.34	090	2	0	0	2	2

26437 Realignment of extensor tendon, hand, each tendon A2 T

RVU			Global Days	Modifiers				
Mod	Non-Fac Total	Fac Total		51	50	62	80	MUE
	17.77	17.77	090	2	0	0	1	4

AMA: Nov 98: 8

● New   ▲ Revised   Deleted   ⊙ Moderate Sedation   ✚ Add-on Codes   ⊘ High Risk Denial   Ⓐ Age Edit   ♀ Female   ♂ Male   **AMA** *CPT® Assistant*   **MUE** Medically Unlikely Edit
⊘ Modifier 51 Exempt   ⊖ Modifier 63 Exempt   ✗ Unlisted   **Modifiers:** *See Inside Back Cover*   Ⓜ Maternity   A2–Z3 ASC Payment Indicators   A–Y OPPS Status Indicators

26440 Tenolysis, flexor tendon; palm OR finger, each tendon
A 2 T

| RVU | | | Global Days | Modifiers | | | | |
Mod	Non-Fac Total	Fac Total		51	50	62	80	MUE
	17.67	17.67	090	2	0	0	1	6

AMA: Apr 02: 18, Jun 15: 10

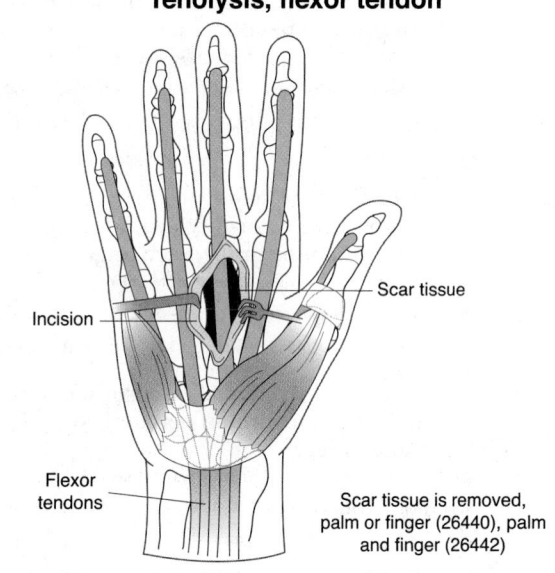

Tenolysis, flexor tendon

Incision

Scar tissue

Flexor tendons

Scar tissue is removed, palm or finger (26440), palm and finger (26442)

26442 Tenolysis, flexor tendon; palm AND finger, each tendon
A 2 T

| RVU | | | Global Days | Modifiers | | | | |
Mod	Non-Fac Total	Fac Total		51	50	62	80	MUE
	27.53	27.53	090	2	0	0	1	5

26445 Tenolysis, extensor tendon, hand OR finger, each tendon
A 2 T

| RVU | | | Global Days | Modifiers | | | | |
Mod	Non-Fac Total	Fac Total		51	50	62	80	MUE
	16.44	16.44	090	2	0	0	1	5

AMA: Nov 98: 8, Dec 02: 11, Mar 03: 20

26449 Tenolysis, complex, extensor tendon, finger, including forearm, each tendon
A 2 T

| RVU | | | Global Days | Modifiers | | | | |
Mod	Non-Fac Total	Fac Total		51	50	62	80	MUE
	20.09	20.09	090	2	0	0	0	5

AMA: Nov 98: 8

26450 Tenotomy, flexor, palm, open, each tendon
A 2 T

| RVU | | | Global Days | Modifiers | | | | |
Mod	Non-Fac Total	Fac Total		51	50	62	80	MUE
	11.60	11.60	090	2	0	0	0	6

AMA: Nov 98: 8

26455 Tenotomy, flexor, finger, open, each tendon
A 2 T

| RVU | | | Global Days | Modifiers | | | | |
Mod	Non-Fac Total	Fac Total		51	50	62	80	MUE
	11.41	11.41	090	2	0	0	0	6

AMA: Nov 98: 8

26460 Tenotomy, extensor, hand or finger, open, each tendon
A 2 T

| RVU | | | Global Days | Modifiers | | | | |
Mod	Non-Fac Total	Fac Total		51	50	62	80	MUE
	11.23	11.23	090	2	0	0	1	4

AMA: Nov 98: 8

26471 Tenodesis; of proximal interphalangeal joint, each joint
A 2 T

| RVU | | | Global Days | Modifiers | | | | |
Mod	Non-Fac Total	Fac Total		51	50	62	80	MUE
	17.49	17.49	090	2	0	0	0	4

AMA: Nov 98: 8

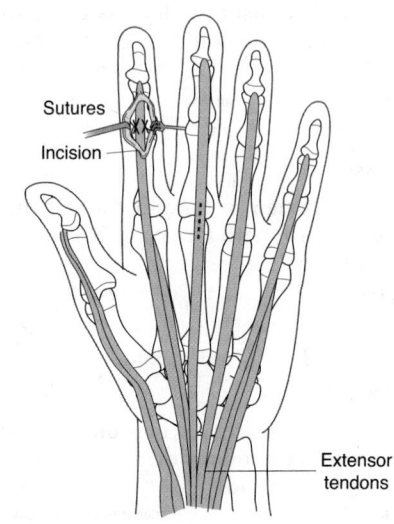

Tenodesis; each joint

Sutures

Incision

Extensor tendons

Proximal interphalangeal joint (26471), distal joint (26474)

26474 Tenodesis; of distal joint, each joint
A 2 T

| RVU | | | Global Days | Modifiers | | | | |
Mod	Non-Fac Total	Fac Total		51	50	62	80	MUE
	17.06	17.06	090	2	0	0	2	4

AMA: Nov 98: 8

26476 Lengthening of tendon, extensor, hand or finger, each tendon
A 2 T

| RVU | | | Global Days | Modifiers | | | | |
Mod	Non-Fac Total	Fac Total		51	50	62	80	MUE
	16.63	16.63	090	2	0	0	1	4

AMA: Nov 98: 8

26477 Shortening of tendon, extensor, hand or finger, each tendon
A 2 T

| RVU | | | Global Days | Modifiers | | | | |
Mod	Non-Fac Total	Fac Total		51	50	62	80	MUE
	16.59	16.59	090	2	0	1	1	4

AMA: Nov 98: 8

26478 Lengthening of tendon, flexor, hand or finger, each tendon
A 2 T

| RVU | | | Global Days | Modifiers | | | | |
Mod	Non-Fac Total	Fac Total		51	50	62	80	MUE
	17.67	17.67	090	2	0	0	0	6

AMA: Nov 98: 8, Dec 13: 16

● New   ▲ Revised   ✖ Deleted   ⊙ Moderate Sedation   ✚ Add-on Codes   ⊘ High Risk Denial   Ⓐ Age Edit   ♀ Female   ♂ Male   **AMA** CPT® Assistant   **MUE** Medically Unlikely Edit
⊘ Modifier 51 Exempt   ⊖ Modifier 63 Exempt   ☒ Unlisted   **Modifiers:** See Inside Back Cover   Ⓜ Maternity   A 2 – Z 3 ASC Payment Indicators   A – Y OPPS Status Indicators

CPT © 2015 American Medical Association. All Rights Reserved.   © 2016 DecisionHealth

26479 Shortening of tendon, flexor, hand or finger, each tendon A2T

Mod	Non-Fac Total	Fac Total	Global Days	51	50	62	80	MUE
	17.60	17.60	090	2	0	0	2	4

AMA: Nov 98: 8

26480 Transfer or transplant of tendon, carpometacarpal area or dorsum of hand; without free graft, each tendon A2T

Mod	Non-Fac Total	Fac Total	Global Days	51	50	62	80	MUE
	21.39	21.39	090	2	0	0	0	4

AMA: Nov 98: 8, Dec 13: 16

26483 Transfer or transplant of tendon, carpometacarpal area or dorsum of hand; with free tendon graft (includes obtaining graft), each tendon A2T

Mod	Non-Fac Total	Fac Total	Global Days	51	50	62	80	MUE
	24.03	24.03	090	2	0	1	2	4

26485 Transfer or transplant of tendon, palmar; without free tendon graft, each tendon A2T

Mod	Non-Fac Total	Fac Total	Global Days	51	50	62	80	MUE
	23.00	23.00	090	2	0	1	2	4

AMA: Nov 98: 8

26489 Transfer or transplant of tendon, palmar; with free tendon graft (includes obtaining graft), each tendon A2T

Mod	Non-Fac Total	Fac Total	Global Days	51	50	62	80	MUE
	26.18	26.18	090	2	0	0	0	3

26490 Opponensplasty; superficialis tendon transfer type, each tendon A2T

Mod	Non-Fac Total	Fac Total	Global Days	51	50	62	80	MUE
	22.46	22.46	090	2	0	0	0	3

26492 Opponensplasty; tendon transfer with graft (includes obtaining graft), each tendon A2T

Mod	Non-Fac Total	Fac Total	Global Days	51	50	62	80	MUE
	25.08	25.08	090	2	0	1	2	2

26494 Opponensplasty; hypothenar muscle transfer A2T

Mod	Non-Fac Total	Fac Total	Global Days	51	50	62	80	MUE
	22.45	22.45	090	2	0	1	2	1

26496 Opponensplasty; other methods A2T

Mod	Non-Fac Total	Fac Total	Global Days	51	50	62	80	MUE
	24.52	24.52	090	2	0	0	0	1

26497 Transfer of tendon to restore intrinsic function; ring and small finger A2T

Mod	Non-Fac Total	Fac Total	Global Days	51	50	62	80	MUE
	24.66	24.66	090	2	0	0	2	2

AMA: Nov 98: 8

26498 Transfer of tendon to restore intrinsic function; all 4 fingers A2T

Mod	Non-Fac Total	Fac Total	Global Days	51	50	62	80	MUE
	32.66	32.66	090	2	0	1	2	1

26499 Correction claw finger, other methods A2T

Mod	Non-Fac Total	Fac Total	Global Days	51	50	62	80	MUE
	23.63	23.63	090	2	0	1	2	2

26500 Reconstruction of tendon pulley, each tendon; with local tissues (separate procedure) A2T

Mod	Non-Fac Total	Fac Total	Global Days	51	50	62	80	MUE
	17.75	17.75	090	2	0	0	0	4

AMA: Nov 98: 8

26502 Reconstruction of tendon pulley, each tendon; with tendon or fascial graft (includes obtaining graft) (separate procedure) A2T

Mod	Non-Fac Total	Fac Total	Global Days	51	50	62	80	MUE
	20.01	20.01	090	2	0	0	2	3

26508 Release of thenar muscle(s) (eg, thumb contracture) A2T

Mod	Non-Fac Total	Fac Total	Global Days	51	50	62	80	MUE
	18.22	18.22	090	2	1	0	0	1

AMA: Nov 98: 8

26510 Cross intrinsic transfer, each tendon A2T

Mod	Non-Fac Total	Fac Total	Global Days	51	50	62	80	MUE
	16.88	16.88	090	2	0	0	0	4

26516 Capsulodesis, metacarpophalangeal joint; single digit A2T

Mod	Non-Fac Total	Fac Total	Global Days	51	50	62	80	MUE
	19.90	19.90	090	2	1	0	0	1

AMA: Nov 98: 8

26517 Capsulodesis, metacarpophalangeal joint; 2 digits A2T

Mod	Non-Fac Total	Fac Total	Global Days	51	50	62	80	MUE
	23.41	23.41	090	2	1	0	2	1

26518 Capsulodesis, metacarpophalangeal joint; 3 or 4 digits ⊘A2T

Mod	Non-Fac Total	Fac Total	Global Days	51	50	62	80	MUE
	23.72	23.72	090	2	1	1	2	1

26520 Capsulectomy or capsulotomy; metacarpophalangeal joint, each joint A2T

Mod	Non-Fac Total	Fac Total	Global Days	51	50	62	80	MUE
	18.55	18.55	090	2	0	0	1	4

AMA: Nov 98: 8

● New ▲ Revised Deleted ⊙ Moderate Sedation ✚ Add-on Codes ⊘ High Risk Denial Ⓐ Age Edit ♀ Female ♂ Male **AMA** *CPT® Assistant* **MUE** Medically Unlikely Edit
⃠ Modifier 51 Exempt ⊖ Modifier 63 Exempt ⊠ Unlisted **Modifiers:** *See Inside Back Cover* Ⓜ Maternity A2-Z3 ASC Payment Indicators A-Y OPPS Status Indicators

© 2016 DecisionHealth | CPT © 2015 American Medical Association. All Rights Reserved. | 275

26525 Capsulectomy or capsulotomy; interphalangeal joint, each joint A 2 T

RVU		Global Days	Modifiers				
Mod	Non-Fac Total Fac Total			51	50	62	80	MUE
	18.57 18.57	090		2	0	1	1	4

AMA: Nov 98: 8, Apr 02: 18, Mar 03: 20, Jun 15: 10

26530 Arthroplasty, metacarpophalangeal joint; each joint A 2 T

RVU		Global Days	Modifiers				
Mod	Non-Fac Total Fac Total			51	50	62	80	MUE
	15.47 15.47	090		2	0	0	2	4

AMA: Nov 98: 8

Arthroplasty, metacarpophalangeal joint

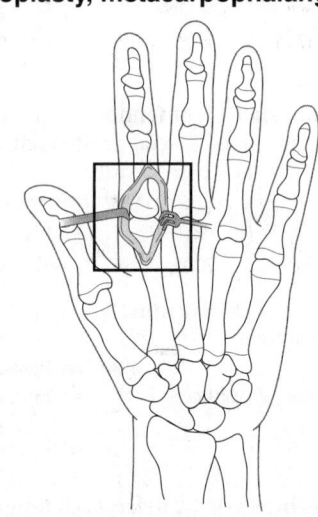

The metacarpophalangeal joint is reshaped, without prosthetic implant (26530), with prosthetic implant (26531)

26531 Arthroplasty, metacarpophalangeal joint; with prosthetic implant, each joint A 2 J I

RVU		Global Days	Modifiers				
Mod	Non-Fac Total Fac Total			51	50	62	80	MUE
	18.03 18.03	090		2	0	1	2	4

AMA: Nov 98: 8, Sep 11: 12

26535 Arthroplasty, interphalangeal joint; each joint A 2 T

RVU		Global Days	Modifiers				
Mod	Non-Fac Total Fac Total			51	50	62	80	MUE
	12.18 12.18	090		2	0	0	1	4

AMA: Nov 98: 8

26536 Arthroplasty, interphalangeal joint; with prosthetic implant, each joint A 2 J I

RVU		Global Days	Modifiers				
Mod	Non-Fac Total Fac Total			51	50	62	80	MUE
	20.32 20.32	090		2	0	0	0	4

AMA: Nov 98: 8

26540 Repair of collateral ligament, metacarpophalangeal or interphalangeal joint A 2 T

RVU		Global Days	Modifiers				
Mod	Non-Fac Total Fac Total			51	50	62	80	MUE
	18.73 18.73	090		2	0	1	0	4

AMA: Nov 96: 6

26541 Reconstruction, collateral ligament, metacarpophalangeal joint, single; with tendon or fascial graft (includes obtaining graft) A 2 T

RVU		Global Days	Modifiers				
Mod	Non-Fac Total Fac Total			51	50	62	80	MUE
	22.83 22.83	090		2	0	1	2	4

AMA: Jan 97: 3

26542 Reconstruction, collateral ligament, metacarpophalangeal joint, single; with local tissue (eg, adductor advancement) A 2 T

RVU		Global Days	Modifiers				
Mod	Non-Fac Total Fac Total			51	50	62	80	MUE
	19.31 19.31	090		2	0	0	0	4

AMA: Jan 97: 3

26545 Reconstruction, collateral ligament, interphalangeal joint, single, including graft, each joint A 2 T

RVU		Global Days	Modifiers				
Mod	Non-Fac Total Fac Total			51	50	62	80	MUE
	19.68 19.68	090		2	0	0	0	4

26546 Repair non-union, metacarpal or phalanx (includes obtaining bone graft with or without external or internal fixation) A 2 T

RVU		Global Days	Modifiers				
Mod	Non-Fac Total Fac Total			51	50	62	80	MUE
	28.32 28.32	090		2	1	0	2	2

AMA: Nov 96: 6

26548 Repair and reconstruction, finger, volar plate, interphalangeal joint A 2 T

RVU		Global Days	Modifiers				
Mod	Non-Fac Total Fac Total			51	50	62	80	MUE
	21.67 21.67	090		2	0	0	0	3

26550 Pollicization of a digit ⊙ A 2 T

RVU		Global Days	Modifiers				
Mod	Non-Fac Total Fac Total			51	50	62	80	MUE
	44.32 44.32	090		2	1	0	2	1

26551 Transfer, toe-to-hand with microvascular anastomosis; great toe wrap-around with bone graft C

RVU		Global Days	Modifiers				
Mod	Non-Fac Total Fac Total			51	50	62	80	MUE
	81.64 81.64	090		2	1	0	2	1

AMA: Nov 96: 6, Apr 97: 7, Jun 97: 9, Nov 98: 8, 10, 11

● New   ▲ Revised   ✖ Deleted   ⊙ Moderate Sedation   ✚ Add-on Codes   ⊗ High Risk Denial   Ⓐ Age Edit   ♀ Female   ♂ Male   **AMA** *CPT® Assistant*   **MUE** Medically Unlikely Edit
⊘ Modifier 51 Exempt   ⊖ Modifier 63 Exempt   ✗ Unlisted   **Modifiers:** *See Inside Back Cover*   Ⓜ Maternity   A 2 – Z 3 ASC Payment Indicators   A – Y OPPS Status Indicators

276   CPT © 2015 American Medical Association. All Rights Reserved.   © 2016 DecisionHealth

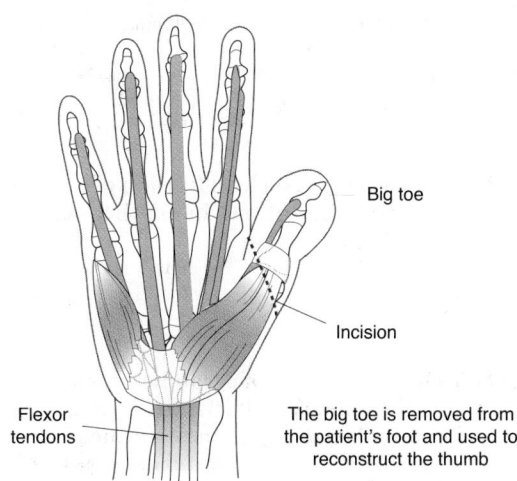

Transfer, toe-to-hand with microvascular anastomosis; great toe wrap around with bone graft

Big toe

Incision

Flexor tendons

The big toe is removed from the patient's foot and used to reconstruct the thumb

26553 Transfer, toe-to-hand with microvascular anastomosis; other than great toe, single   Ⓒ

RVU			Global Days	Modifiers				
Mod	Non-Fac Total	Fac Total		51	50	62	80	MUE
	94.48	94.48	090	2	1	1	2	1

AMA: Nov 96: 6, Apr 97: 7, Jun 97: 9, Nov 98: 8, 10, 11

26554 Transfer, toe-to-hand with microvascular anastomosis; other than great toe, double   Ⓒ

RVU			Global Days	Modifiers				
Mod	Non-Fac Total	Fac Total		51	50	62	80	MUE
	94.95	94.95	090	2	1	1	2	1

AMA: Nov 96: 6, Apr 97: 7, Jun 97: 9, Nov 98: 8, 10, 11

26555 Transfer, finger to another position without microvascular anastomosis   A 2 T

RVU			Global Days	Modifiers				
Mod	Non-Fac Total	Fac Total		51	50	62	80	MUE
	38.61	38.61	090	2	0	0	2	2

AMA: Nov 98: 8, 10, 11

26556 Transfer, free toe joint, with microvascular anastomosis   Ⓒ

RVU			Global Days	Modifiers				
Mod	Non-Fac Total	Fac Total		51	50	62	80	MUE
	80.59	80.59	090	2	0	1	2	2

AMA: Nov 96: 6, Apr 97: 7, Jun 97: 9, Nov 98: 8

26560 Repair of syndactyly (web finger) each web space; with skin flaps   A 2 T

RVU			Global Days	Modifiers				
Mod	Non-Fac Total	Fac Total		51	50	62	80	MUE
	15.98	15.98	090	2	0	0	2	2

26561 Repair of syndactyly (web finger) each web space; with skin flaps and grafts   A 2 T

RVU			Global Days	Modifiers				
Mod	Non-Fac Total	Fac Total		51	50	62	80	MUE
	26.64	26.64	090	2	0	1	2	2

26562 Repair of syndactyly (web finger) each web space; complex (eg, involving bone, nails)   ⊘ A 2 T

RVU			Global Days	Modifiers				
Mod	Non-Fac Total	Fac Total		51	50	62	80	MUE
	38.41	38.41	090	2	0	0	2	2

26565 Osteotomy; metacarpal, each   A 2 T

RVU			Global Days	Modifiers				
Mod	Non-Fac Total	Fac Total		51	50	62	80	MUE
	19.30	19.30	090	2	0	0	2	3

AMA: Nov 98: 9

26567 Osteotomy; phalanx of finger, each   A 2 T

RVU			Global Days	Modifiers				
Mod	Non-Fac Total	Fac Total		51	50	62	80	MUE
	19.42	19.42	090	2	0	0	0	3

AMA: Apr 12: 17

26568 Osteoplasty, lengthening, metacarpal or phalanx   A 2 T

RVU			Global Days	Modifiers				
Mod	Non-Fac Total	Fac Total		51	50	62	80	MUE
	25.59	25.59	090	2	0	0	2	2

26580 Repair cleft hand   A 2 T

RVU			Global Days	Modifiers				
Mod	Non-Fac Total	Fac Total		51	50	62	80	MUE
	42.12	42.12	090	2	1	0	2	1

26587 Reconstruction of polydactylous digit, soft tissue and bone   A 2 T

RVU			Global Days	Modifiers				
Mod	Non-Fac Total	Fac Total		51	50	62	80	MUE
	26.13	26.13	090	2	0	0	2	2

AMA: Oct 01: 10, Aug 03: 14, May 04: 16

26590 Repair macrodactylia, each digit   A 2 T

RVU			Global Days	Modifiers				
Mod	Non-Fac Total	Fac Total		51	50	62	80	MUE
	38.60	38.60	090	2	0	0	2	2

AMA: Oct 01: 10, Aug 03: 14, May 04: 16

26591 Repair, intrinsic muscles of hand, each muscle   A 2 T

RVU			Global Days	Modifiers				
Mod	Non-Fac Total	Fac Total		51	50	62	80	MUE
	12.40	12.40	090	2	0	0	0	4

AMA: May 98: 11, Jul 98: 11, Nov 98: 8, 11

26593 Release, intrinsic muscles of hand, each muscle   A 2 T

RVU			Global Days	Modifiers				
Mod	Non-Fac Total	Fac Total		51	50	62	80	MUE
	17.14	17.14	090	2	0	0	1	9

AMA: Nov 98: 8, 11

26596 Excision of constricting ring of finger, with multiple Z-plasties   A 2 T

RVU			Global Days	Modifiers				
Mod	Non-Fac Total	Fac Total		51	50	62	80	MUE
	21.69	21.69	090	2	0	0	2	1

● New   ▲ Revised   Deleted   ⊙ Moderate Sedation   ✚ Add-on Codes   ⊘ High Risk Denial   Ⓐ Age Edit   ♀ Female   ♂ Male   **AMA** *CPT® Assistant*   **MUE** Medically Unlikely Edit

⊘ Modifier 51 Exempt   ⊖ Modifier 63 Exempt   ⊠ Unlisted   **Modifiers:** *See Inside Back Cover*   Ⓜ Maternity   A 2 – Z 3 ASC Payment Indicators   A – Y OPPS Status Indicators

Surgical Procedures

26600 – 26686

Hand/Finger Fracture/Dislocation Procedures

26600 Closed treatment of metacarpal fracture, single; without manipulation, each bone `P 2 T`

RVU			Global Days	Modifiers				
Mod	Non-Fac Total	Fac Total		51	50	62	80	MUE
	8.44	7.96	090	2	0	1	2	

Closed treatment of metacarpal fracture

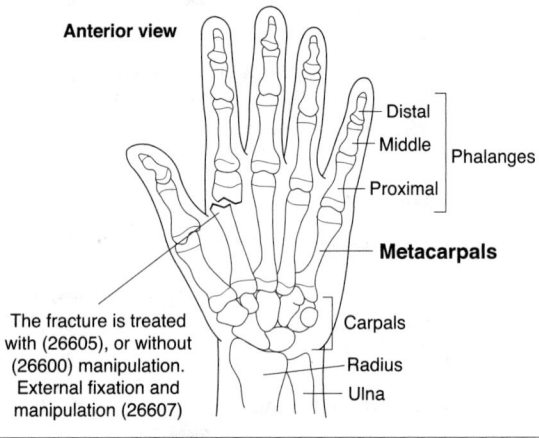

26605 Closed treatment of metacarpal fracture, single; with manipulation, each bone `A 2 T`

Coding tip: Add modifier 77 for re-reduction of the fracture by another physician

RVU			Global Days	Modifiers				
Mod	Non-Fac Total	Fac Total		51	50	62	80	MUE
	9.23	8.42	090	2	0	0	1	3

26607 Closed treatment of metacarpal fracture, with manipulation, with external fixation, each bone `A 2 T`

Coding tip: Adjustment or revision of external fixation system (new pins/wires/bars) requiring anesthesia - 20693

RVU			Global Days	Modifiers				
Mod	Non-Fac Total	Fac Total		51	50	62	80	MUE
	13.11	13.11	090	2	0	0	0	2

26608 Percutaneous skeletal fixation of metacarpal fracture, each bone `A 2 T`

RVU			Global Days	Modifiers				
Mod	Non-Fac Total	Fac Total		51	50	62	80	MUE
	13.74	13.74	090	2	0	0	0	5

26615 Open treatment of metacarpal fracture, single, includes internal fixation, when performed, each bone `A 2 T`

RVU			Global Days	Modifiers				
Mod	Non-Fac Total	Fac Total		51	50	62	80	MUE
	16.66	16.66	090	2	0	0	1	4

26641 Closed treatment of carpometacarpal dislocation, thumb, with manipulation `P 2 T`

Coding tip: Add modifier 77 for re-reduction of the dislocation by another physician

RVU			Global Days	Modifiers				
Mod	Non-Fac Total	Fac Total		51	50	62	80	MUE
	10.48	9.59	090	2	1	0	0	1

26645 Closed treatment of carpometacarpal fracture dislocation, thumb (Bennett fracture), with manipulation `A 2 T`

Coding tip: Closed treatment of thumb carpometacarpal dislocation only - 26641

Coding tip: Add modifier 77 for re-reduction of the fracture/dislocation by another physician

RVU			Global Days	Modifiers				
Mod	Non-Fac Total	Fac Total		51	50	62	80	MUE
	12.08	11.11	090	2	1	0	0	1

26650 Percutaneous skeletal fixation of carpometacarpal fracture dislocation, thumb (Bennett fracture), with manipulation `A 2 T`

RVU			Global Days	Modifiers				
Mod	Non-Fac Total	Fac Total		51	50	62	80	MUE
	13.78	13.78	090	2	1	0	1	1

26665 Open treatment of carpometacarpal fracture dislocation, thumb (Bennett fracture), includes internal fixation, when performed `A 2 T`

RVU			Global Days	Modifiers				
Mod	Non-Fac Total	Fac Total		51	50	62	80	MUE
	18.22	18.22	090	2	1	1	1	1

26670 Closed treatment of carpometacarpal dislocation, other than thumb, with manipulation, each joint; without anesthesia `P 2 T`

RVU			Global Days	Modifiers				
Mod	Non-Fac Total	Fac Total		51	50	62	80	MUE
	9.69	8.81	090	2	0	0	0	2

26675 Closed treatment of carpometacarpal dislocation, other than thumb, with manipulation, each joint; requiring anesthesia `A 2 T`

RVU			Global Days	Modifiers				
Mod	Non-Fac Total	Fac Total		51	50	62	80	MUE
	12.92	11.90	090	2	0	0	0	1

26676 Percutaneous skeletal fixation of carpometacarpal dislocation, other than thumb, with manipulation, each joint `A 2 T`

RVU			Global Days	Modifiers				
Mod	Non-Fac Total	Fac Total		51	50	62	80	MUE
	14.44	14.44	090	2	0	0	1	3

26685 Open treatment of carpometacarpal dislocation, other than thumb; includes internal fixation, when performed, each joint `A 2 T`

RVU			Global Days	Modifiers				
Mod	Non-Fac Total	Fac Total		51	50	62	80	MUE
	16.68	16.68	090	2	0	1	1	3

26686 Open treatment of carpometacarpal dislocation, other than thumb; complex, multiple, or delayed reduction `A 2 T`

RVU			Global Days	Modifiers				
Mod	Non-Fac Total	Fac Total		51	50	62	80	MUE
	17.99	17.99	090	2	0	0	2	3

● New   ▲ Revised   ✖ Deleted   ⊙ Moderate Sedation   ✚ Add-on Codes   ⊘ High Risk Denial   Ⓐ Age Edit   ♀ Female   ♂ Male   **AMA** *CPT® Assistant*   **MUE** Medically Unlikely Edit

⊘ Modifier 51 Exempt   ⊖ Modifier 63 Exempt   ✗ Unlisted   **Modifiers:** *See Inside Back Cover*   Ⓜ Maternity   `A 2`–`Z 3` ASC Payment Indicators   `A`–`Y` OPPS Status Indicators

26700 Closed treatment of metacarpophalangeal dislocation, single, with manipulation; without anesthesia   P 2 T

RVU			Global Days	Modifiers				
Mod	Non-Fac Total	Fac Total			51	50	62	80	MUE
	9.19	8.64	090		2	0	0	1	3

AMA: May 14: 10

26705 Closed treatment of metacarpophalangeal dislocation, single, with manipulation; requiring anesthesia   A 2 T

RVU			Global Days	Modifiers				
Mod	Non-Fac Total	Fac Total			51	50	62	80	MUE
	11.96	10.97	090		2	0	0	0	3

26706 Percutaneous skeletal fixation of metacarpophalangeal dislocation, single, with manipulation   A 2 T

RVU			Global Days	Modifiers				
Mod	Non-Fac Total	Fac Total			51	50	62	80	MUE
	12.71	12.71	090		2	0	0	1	4

26715 Open treatment of metacarpophalangeal dislocation, single, includes internal fixation, when performed   A 2 T

RVU			Global Days	Modifiers				
Mod	Non-Fac Total	Fac Total			51	50	62	80	MUE
	16.53	16.53	090		2	0	0	0	4

26720 Closed treatment of phalangeal shaft fracture, proximal or middle phalanx, finger or thumb; without manipulation, each   P 2 T

Coding tip: Closed treatment of distal phalangeal fracture - 26750

RVU			Global Days	Modifiers				
Mod	Non-Fac Total	Fac Total			51	50	62	80	MUE
	5.67	5.28	090		2	0	0	1	4

Closed treatment of phalangeal shaft fracture

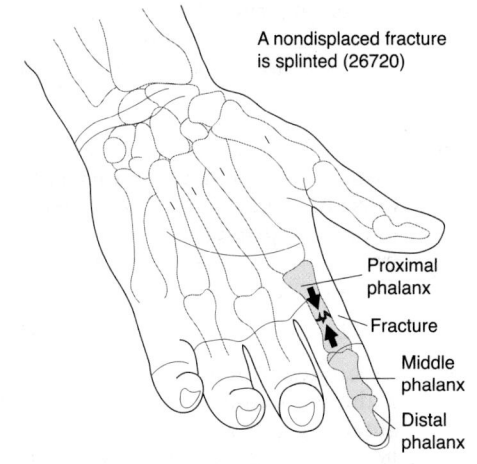

A nondisplaced fracture is splinted (26720)

Proximal phalanx

Fracture

Middle phalanx

Distal phalanx

The bone is pushed back into place, and the finger may be put in traction directly on the skin or into the bone (26725).

26725 Closed treatment of phalangeal shaft fracture, proximal or middle phalanx, finger or thumb; with manipulation, with or without skin or skeletal traction, each   P 2 T

Coding tip: Add modifier 77 for re-reduction of the fracture by another physician

Coding tip: Skeletal traction requires the use of a wire, pin, screw, or clamp attached through the bone, which is included in the initial placement - code separately only when a subsequent traction device is placed

Coding tip: Closed treatment of distal phalangeal fracture with manipulation - 26755

Coding tip: Removal of the initial traction device is included - code separately only when a subsequent traction device is removed

RVU			Global Days	Modifiers				
Mod	Non-Fac Total	Fac Total			51	50	62	80	MUE
	9.68	8.75	090		2	0	0	1	4

26727 Percutaneous skeletal fixation of unstable phalangeal shaft fracture, proximal or middle phalanx, finger or thumb, with manipulation, each   A 2 T

RVU			Global Days	Modifiers				
Mod	Non-Fac Total	Fac Total			51	50	62	80	MUE
	13.54	13.54	090		2	0	0	1	4

26735 Open treatment of phalangeal shaft fracture, proximal or middle phalanx, finger or thumb, includes internal fixation, when performed, each   A 2 T

RVU			Global Days	Modifiers				
Mod	Non-Fac Total	Fac Total			51	50	62	80	MUE
	17.25	17.25	090		2	0	0	1	4

26740 Closed treatment of articular fracture, involving metacarpophalangeal or interphalangeal joint; without manipulation, each   P 2 T

RVU			Global Days	Modifiers				
Mod	Non-Fac Total	Fac Total			51	50	62	80	MUE
	6.60	6.20	090		2	0	0	1	3

26742 Closed treatment of articular fracture, involving metacarpophalangeal or interphalangeal joint; with manipulation, each   A 2 T

RVU			Global Days	Modifiers				
Mod	Non-Fac Total	Fac Total			51	50	62	80	MUE
	10.58	9.62	090		2	0	0	1	3

26746 Open treatment of articular fracture, involving metacarpophalangeal or interphalangeal joint, includes internal fixation, when performed, each   A 2 T

RVU			Global Days	Modifiers				
Mod	Non-Fac Total	Fac Total			51	50	62	80	MUE
	21.48	21.48	090		2	0	0	1	3

26750 Closed treatment of distal phalangeal fracture, finger or thumb; without manipulation, each   P 2 T

Coding tip: Closed treatment of phalangeal shaft fracture - 26720

RVU			Global Days	Modifiers				
Mod	Non-Fac Total	Fac Total			51	50	62	80	MUE
	5.28	5.30	090		2	0	0	1	3

● New   ▲ Revised   Deleted   ⊙ Moderate Sedation   ✚ Add-on Codes   ⊘ High Risk Denial   Ⓐ Age Edit   ♀ Female   ♂ Male   **AMA** *CPT® Assistant*   **MUE** Medically Unlikely Edit
⊘ Modifier 51 Exempt   ⊖ Modifier 63 Exempt   ☒ Unlisted   **Modifiers:** *See Inside Back Cover*   Ⓜ Maternity   A 2 – Z 3 ASC Payment Indicators   A – Y OPPS Status Indicators

© 2016 DecisionHealth   CPT © 2015 American Medical Association. All Rights Reserved.   **279**

26755 Closed treatment of distal phalangeal fracture, finger or thumb; with manipulation, each `G 2 T`

Coding tip: Add modifier 77 for re-reduction of the fracture by another physician

Coding tip: Closed treatment of phalangeal shaft fracture with manipulation - 26725

RVU			Global Days	Modifiers				
Mod	Non-Fac Total	Fac Total		51	50	62	80	MUE
	9.02	7.86	090	2	0	0	1	3

26756 Percutaneous skeletal fixation of distal phalangeal fracture, finger or thumb, each `A 2 T`

RVU			Global Days	Modifiers				
Mod	Non-Fac Total	Fac Total		51	50	62	80	MUE
	12.05	12.05	090	2	0	0	0	3

26765 Open treatment of distal phalangeal fracture, finger or thumb, includes internal fixation, when performed, each `A 2 T`

RVU			Global Days	Modifiers				
Mod	Non-Fac Total	Fac Total		51	50	62	80	MUE
	14.47	14.47	090	2	0	0	1	5

26770 Closed treatment of interphalangeal joint dislocation, single, with manipulation; without anesthesia `G 2 T`

Coding tip: Add modifier 77 for re-reduction of the dislocation by another physician

RVU			Global Days	Modifiers				
Mod	Non-Fac Total	Fac Total		51	50	62	80	MUE
	7.79	7.23	090	2	0	0	1	3

26775 Closed treatment of interphalangeal joint dislocation, single, with manipulation; requiring anesthesia `P 2 S`

Coding tip: Add modifier 77 for re-reduction of the dislocation by another physician

RVU			Global Days	Modifiers				
Mod	Non-Fac Total	Fac Total		51	50	62	80	MUE
	10.96	9.93	090	2	0	0	1	4

26776 Percutaneous skeletal fixation of interphalangeal joint dislocation, single, with manipulation `A 2 T`

RVU			Global Days	Modifiers				
Mod	Non-Fac Total	Fac Total		51	50	62	80	MUE
	12.78	12.78	090	2	0	0	1	4

26785 Open treatment of interphalangeal joint dislocation, includes internal fixation, when performed, single `A 2 T`

RVU			Global Days	Modifiers				
Mod	Non-Fac Total	Fac Total		51	50	62	80	MUE
	15.83	15.83	090	2	0	0	1	3

Hand/Finger Arthrodesis

26820 Fusion in opposition, thumb, with autogenous graft (includes obtaining graft) `A 2 T`

RVU			Global Days	Modifiers				
Mod	Non-Fac Total	Fac Total		51	50	62	80	MUE
	22.35	22.35	090	2	1	1	2	1

26841 Arthrodesis, carpometacarpal joint, thumb, with or without internal fixation `A 2 T`

RVU			Global Days	Modifiers				
Mod	Non-Fac Total	Fac Total		51	50	62	80	MUE
	20.65	20.65	090	2	1	1	0	1

26842 Arthrodesis, carpometacarpal joint, thumb, with or without internal fixation; with autograft (includes obtaining graft) `A 2 J 1`

RVU			Global Days	Modifiers				
Mod	Non-Fac Total	Fac Total		51	50	62	80	MUE
	22.35	22.35	090	2	1	1	2	1

26843 Arthrodesis, carpometacarpal joint, digit, other than thumb, each `A 2 J 1`

RVU			Global Days	Modifiers				
Mod	Non-Fac Total	Fac Total		51	50	62	80	MUE
	21.01	21.01	090	2	0	1	2	2

26844 Arthrodesis, carpometacarpal joint, digit, other than thumb, each; with autograft (includes obtaining graft) `A 2 J 1`

RVU			Global Days	Modifiers				
Mod	Non-Fac Total	Fac Total		51	50	62	80	MUE
	23.32	23.32	090	2	0	1	2	2

26850 Arthrodesis, metacarpophalangeal joint, with or without internal fixation `A 2 T`

RVU			Global Days	Modifiers				
Mod	Non-Fac Total	Fac Total		51	50	62	80	MUE
	19.72	19.72	090	2	0	0	0	5

26852 Arthrodesis, metacarpophalangeal joint, with or without internal fixation; with autograft (includes obtaining graft) `A 2 T`

RVU			Global Days	Modifiers				
Mod	Non-Fac Total	Fac Total		51	50	62	80	MUE
	22.66	22.66	090	2	0	1	2	2

26860 Arthrodesis, interphalangeal joint, with or without internal fixation `A 2 T`

RVU			Global Days	Modifiers				
Mod	Non-Fac Total	Fac Total		51	50	62	80	MUE
	16.09	16.09	090	2	0	0	1	1

+ **26861 Arthrodesis, interphalangeal joint, with or without internal fixation; each additional interphalangeal joint (List separately in addition to code for primary procedure)** `N 1 N`

RVU			Global Days	Modifiers				
Mod	Non-Fac Total	Fac Total		51	50	62	80	MUE
	3.01	3.01	ZZZ	0	0	0	1	4

26862 Arthrodesis, interphalangeal joint, with or without internal fixation; with autograft (includes obtaining graft) `A 2 T`

RVU			Global Days	Modifiers				
Mod	Non-Fac Total	Fac Total		51	50	62	80	MUE
	20.71	20.71	090	2	0	1	2	1

● New   ▲ Revised   ✖ Deleted   ⊙ Moderate Sedation   ✚ Add-on Codes   ⊗ High Risk Denial   ⒶAge Edit   ♀ Female   ♂ Male   **AMA** *CPT® Assistant*   *MUE* Medically Unlikely Edit

⊘ Modifier 51 Exempt   ⊖ Modifier 63 Exempt   ✗ Unlisted   **Modifiers:** *See Inside Back Cover*   Ⓜ Maternity   `A 2`–`Z 3` ASC Payment Indicators   `A`–`Y` OPPS Status Indicators

CPT © 2015 American Medical Association. All Rights Reserved.   © 2016 DecisionHealth

+ 26863 Arthrodesis, interphalangeal joint, with or without internal fixation; with autograft (includes obtaining graft), each additional joint (List separately in addition to code for primary procedure) `NIN`

Mod	Non-Fac Total	Fac Total	Global Days	51	50	62	80	MUE
	6.68	6.68	ZZZ	0	0	0	2	3

Hand/Finger Amputation

26910 Amputation, metacarpal, with finger or thumb (ray amputation), single, with or without interosseous transfer `A2 T`

Mod	Non-Fac Total	Fac Total	Global Days	51	50	62	80	MUE
	20.54	20.54	090	2	0	0	1	4

26951 Amputation, finger or thumb, primary or secondary, any joint or phalanx, single, including neurectomies; with direct closure `A2 T`

Mod	Non-Fac Total	Fac Total	Global Days	51	50	62	80	MUE
	18.65	18.65	090	2	0	0	1	8

26952 Amputation, finger or thumb, primary or secondary, any joint or phalanx, single, including neurectomies; with local advancement flaps (V-Y, hood) `A2 T`

Mod	Non-Fac Total	Fac Total	Global Days	51	50	62	80	MUE
	18.42	18.42	090	2	0	0	1	5

Other Hand/Finger Procedures

26989 Unlisted procedure, hands or fingers `⊘ x T`

Mod	Non-Fac Total	Fac Total	Global Days	51	50	62	80	MUE
	0.00	0.00	YYY	2	0	1	1	

Pelvic/Hip Procedures

Pelvic/Hip Incisional Procedures

26990 Incision and drainage, pelvis or hip joint area; deep abscess or hematoma `A2 T`

Mod	Non-Fac Total	Fac Total	Global Days	51	50	62	80	MUE
	18.01	18.01	090	2	0	0	1	2

26991 Incision and drainage, pelvis or hip joint area; infected bursa `A2 T`

Mod	Non-Fac Total	Fac Total	Global Days	51	50	62	80	MUE
	20.17	15.03	090	2	0	0	0	1

26992 Incision, bone cortex, pelvis and/or hip joint (eg, osteomyelitis or bone abscess) `C`

Mod	Non-Fac Total	Fac Total	Global Days	51	50	62	80	MUE
	27.70	27.70	090	2	0	0	0	2

AMA: Jan 02: 10, Oct 12: 14

27000 Tenotomy, adductor of hip, percutaneous (separate procedure) `A2 T`

Mod	Non-Fac Total	Fac Total	Global Days	51	50	62	80	MUE
	11.60	11.60	090	2	1	1	1	1

27001 Tenotomy, adductor of hip, open `A2 T`

Mod	Non-Fac Total	Fac Total	Global Days	51	50	62	80	MUE
	15.41	15.41	090	2	1	1	2	1

27003 Tenotomy, adductor, subcutaneous, open, with obturator neurectomy `A2 T`

Mod	Non-Fac Total	Fac Total	Global Days	51	50	62	80	MUE
	17.17	17.17	090	2	1	1	1	1

27005 Tenotomy, hip flexor(s), open (separate procedure) `C`

Mod	Non-Fac Total	Fac Total	Global Days	51	50	62	80	MUE
	20.78	20.78	090	2	1	1	2	1

27006 Tenotomy, abductors and/or extensor(s) of hip, open (separate procedure) `T`

Mod	Non-Fac Total	Fac Total	Global Days	51	50	62	80	MUE
	21.18	21.18	090	2	1	1	2	1

27025 Fasciotomy, hip or thigh, any type `C`

Mod	Non-Fac Total	Fac Total	Global Days	51	50	62	80	MUE
	26.36	26.36	090	2	1	1	0	1

27027 Decompression fasciotomy(ies), pelvic (buttock) compartment(s) (eg, gluteus medius-minimus, gluteus maximus, iliopsoas, and/or tensor fascia lata muscle), unilateral `T`

Mod	Non-Fac Total	Fac Total	Global Days	51	50	62	80	MUE
	26.04	26.04	090	2	1	0	0	1

27030 Arthrotomy, hip, with drainage (eg, infection) `C`

Mod	Non-Fac Total	Fac Total	Global Days	51	50	62	80	MUE
	27.06	27.06	090	2	1	1	1	1

AMA: Nov 98: 8

27033 Arthrotomy, hip, including exploration or removal of loose or foreign body `A2 T`

Mod	Non-Fac Total	Fac Total	Global Days	51	50	62	80	MUE
	28.06	28.06	090	2	1	1	2	1

AMA: Spring 92: 11

27035 Denervation, hip joint, intrapelvic or extrapelvic intra-articular branches of sciatic, femoral, or obturator nerves `⊘ A2 T`

Mod	Non-Fac Total	Fac Total	Global Days	51	50	62	80	MUE
	33.20	33.20	090	2	1	1	2	1

AMA: Nov 98: 8, Mar 14: 13

● New ▲ Revised Deleted ⊙ Moderate Sedation ✛ Add-on Codes ⊘ High Risk Denial Ⓐ Age Edit ♀ Female ♂ Male **AMA** CPT® Assistant **MUE** Medically Unlikely Edit
⊘ Modifier 51 Exempt ⊖ Modifier 63 Exempt ✗ Unlisted **Modifiers:** See Inside Back Cover Ⓜ Maternity A2–Z3 ASC Payment Indicators A –Y OPPS Status Indicators

27036 Capsulectomy or capsulotomy, hip, with or without excision of heterotopic bone, with release of hip flexor muscles (ie, gluteus medius, gluteus minimus, tensor fascia latae, rectus femoris, sartorius, iliopsoas)   C

Mod	Non-Fac Total	Fac Total	Global Days	51	50	62	80	MUE
	29.06	29.06	090	2	1	1	2	1

AMA: Jan 05: 8

Pelvic/Hip Excisional Procedures

27040 Biopsy, soft tissue of pelvis and hip area; superficial   A2 T

Coding tip: Code 99000 for specimen transfer from office setting to an outside laboratory

Mod	Non-Fac Total	Fac Total	Global Days	51	50	62	80	MUE
	9.79	5.75	010	2	1	0	1	2

27041 Biopsy, soft tissue of pelvis and hip area; deep, subfascial or intramuscular   A2 T

Mod	Non-Fac Total	Fac Total	Global Days	51	50	62	80	MUE
	19.71	19.71	090	2	1	0	1	3

AMA: Nov 98: 8

27043 Excision, tumor, soft tissue of pelvis and hip area, subcutaneous; 3 cm or greater   G2 T

Coding tip: Code 27043 is listed out of numerical order in CPT. Related soft tissue tumor excision procedures - 27047 (subcutaneous tissue); 27048, 27043 (subfascial).

Mod	Non-Fac Total	Fac Total	Global Days	51	50	62	80	MUE
	13.59	13.59	090	2	1	0	1	3

27045 Excision, tumor, soft tissue of pelvis and hip area, subfascial (eg, intramuscular); 5 cm or greater   G2 T

Coding tip: Code 27045 is listed out of numerical order in CPT. Related soft tissue tumor excision procedures - 27043, 27047 (subcutaneous tissue); 27048 (subfascial).

Mod	Non-Fac Total	Fac Total	Global Days	51	50	62	80	MUE
	21.62	21.62	090	2	1	1	2	3

27047 Excision, tumor, soft tissue of pelvis and hip area, subcutaneous; less than 3 cm   G2 T

Coding tip: Related soft tissue excision codes - 27043, 27045, and 27048

Mod	Non-Fac Total	Fac Total	Global Days	51	50	62	80	MUE
	13.37	10.44	090	2	1	0	1	4

AMA: Nov 98: 8

27048 Excision, tumor, soft tissue of pelvis and hip area, subfascial (eg, intramuscular); less than 5 cm   G2 T

Coding tip: Related soft tissue excision codes - 27043, 27045, and 27047

Mod	Non-Fac Total	Fac Total	Global Days	51	50	62	80	MUE
	17.59	17.59	090	2	1	1	2	2

27049 Radical resection of tumor (eg, sarcoma), soft tissue of pelvis and hip area; less than 5 cm   G2 T

Coding tip: Related radical resection of soft tissue tumor code - 27059

Mod	Non-Fac Total	Fac Total	Global Days	51	50	62	80	MUE
	39.03	39.03	090	2	1	1	2	1

AMA: Nov 98: 8

27050 Arthrotomy, with biopsy; sacroiliac joint   A2 T

Mod	Non-Fac Total	Fac Total	Global Days	51	50	62	80	MUE
	10.93	10.93	090	2	1	1	0	1

27052 Arthrotomy, with biopsy; hip joint   A2 T

Mod	Non-Fac Total	Fac Total	Global Days	51	50	62	80	MUE
	16.60	16.60	090	2	1	1	2	1

27054 Arthrotomy with synovectomy, hip joint   C

Mod	Non-Fac Total	Fac Total	Global Days	51	50	62	80	MUE
	19.67	19.67	090	2	1	1	2	1

27057 Decompression fasciotomy(ies), pelvic (buttock) compartment(s) (eg, gluteus medius-minimus, gluteus maximus, iliopsoas, and/or tensor fascia lata muscle) with debridement of nonviable muscle, unilateral   T

Mod	Non-Fac Total	Fac Total	Global Days	51	50	62	80	MUE
	29.38	29.38	090	2	1	0	0	1

27059 Radical resection of tumor (eg, sarcoma), soft tissue of pelvis and hip area; 5 cm or greater   G2 T

Coding tip: Code 27059 is listed out of numerical order in CPT. Related radical resection of soft tissue tumor procedures - 27049

Mod	Non-Fac Total	Fac Total	Global Days	51	50	62	80	MUE
	52.71	52.71	090	2	1	1	2	1

27060 Excision; ischial bursa   A2 T

Mod	Non-Fac Total	Fac Total	Global Days	51	50	62	80	MUE
	13.34	13.34	090	2	1	0	1	1

27062 Excision; trochanteric bursa or calcification   A2 T

Mod	Non-Fac Total	Fac Total	Global Days	51	50	62	80	MUE
	13.18	13.18	090	2	1	1	1	1

27065 Excision of bone cyst or benign tumor, wing of ilium, symphysis pubis, or greater trochanter of femur; superficial, includes autograft, when performed   A2 T

Mod	Non-Fac Total	Fac Total	Global Days	51	50	62	80	MUE
	14.69	14.69	090	2	1	1	2	1

● New   ▲ Revised   ✖ Deleted   ⊙ Moderate Sedation   ✚ Add-on Codes   ⊘ High Risk Denial   Ⓐ Age Edit   ♀ Female   ♂ Male   **AMA** CPT® Assistant   **MUE** Medically Unlikely Edit

⊘ Modifier 51 Exempt   ⊖ Modifier 63 Exempt   ☒ Unlisted   **Modifiers:** See Inside Back Cover   Ⓜ Maternity   A2–Z3 ASC Payment Indicators   A–Y OPPS Status Indicators

27066 Excision of bone cyst or benign tumor, wing of ilium, symphysis pubis, or greater trochanter of femur; deep (subfascial), includes autograft, when performed A 2 T

RVU			Global Days	Modifiers				
Mod	Non-Fac Total	Fac Total		51	50	62	80	MUE
	23.29	23.29	090	2	1	1	2	1

27067 Excision of bone cyst or benign tumor, wing of ilium, symphysis pubis, or greater trochanter of femur; with autograft requiring separate incision A 2 T

RVU			Global Days	Modifiers				
Mod	Non-Fac Total	Fac Total		51	50	62	80	MUE
	29.32	29.32	090	2	1	0	2	1

27070 Partial excision, wing of ilium, symphysis pubis, or greater trochanter of femur, (craterization, saucerization) (eg, osteomyelitis or bone abscess); superficial C

RVU			Global Days	Modifiers				
Mod	Non-Fac Total	Fac Total		51	50	62	80	MUE
	24.45	24.45	090	2	1	1	2	1

27071 Partial excision, wing of ilium, symphysis pubis, or greater trochanter of femur, (craterization, saucerization) (eg, osteomyelitis or bone abscess); deep (subfascial or intramuscular) C

RVU			Global Days	Modifiers				
Mod	Non-Fac Total	Fac Total		51	50	62	80	MUE
	26.44	26.44	090	2	1	1	2	1

27075 Radical resection of tumor; wing of ilium, 1 pubic or ischial ramus or symphysis pubis C

RVU			Global Days	Modifiers				
Mod	Non-Fac Total	Fac Total		51	50	62	80	MUE
	60.76	60.76	090	2	0	1	2	1

27076 Radical resection of tumor; ilium, including acetabulum, both pubic rami, or ischium and acetabulum C

RVU			Global Days	Modifiers				
Mod	Non-Fac Total	Fac Total		51	50	62	80	MUE
	73.29	73.29	090	2	0	1	2	1

27077 Radical resection of tumor; innominate bone, total C

RVU			Global Days	Modifiers				
Mod	Non-Fac Total	Fac Total		51	50	62	80	MUE
	82.53	82.53	090	2	0	1	2	1

27078 Radical resection of tumor; ischial tuberosity and greater trochanter of femur C

RVU			Global Days	Modifiers				
Mod	Non-Fac Total	Fac Total		51	50	62	80	MUE
	59.88	59.88	090	2	1	1	2	1

27080 Coccygectomy, primary A 2 T

RVU			Global Days	Modifiers				
Mod	Non-Fac Total	Fac Total		51	50	62	80	MUE
	14.85	14.85	090	2	0	1	2	1

Pelvic/Hip Introduction/Removal Procedures

27086 Removal of foreign body, pelvis or hip; subcutaneous tissue A 2 T

RVU			Global Days	Modifiers				
Mod	Non-Fac Total	Fac Total		51	50	62	80	MUE
	8.31	4.78	010	2	1	0	0	1

AMA: Jul 98: 8

27087 Removal of foreign body, pelvis or hip; deep (subfascial or intramuscular) A 2 T

RVU			Global Days	Modifiers				
Mod	Non-Fac Total	Fac Total		51	50	62	80	MUE
	18.07	18.07	090	2	1	1	2	1

AMA: Nov 98: 8

27090 Removal of hip prosthesis; (separate procedure) C

RVU			Global Days	Modifiers				
Mod	Non-Fac Total	Fac Total		51	50	62	80	MUE
	23.95	23.95	090	2	1	1	2	1

27091 Removal of hip prosthesis; complicated, including total hip prosthesis, methylmethacrylate with or without insertion of spacer C

RVU			Global Days	Modifiers				
Mod	Non-Fac Total	Fac Total		51	50	62	80	MUE
	46.17	46.17	090	2	1	1	2	1

27093 Injection procedure for hip arthrography; without anesthesia N I N

RVU			Global Days	Modifiers				
Mod	Non-Fac Total	Fac Total		51	50	62	80	MUE
	5.34	2.03	000	2	1	0	1	1

AMA: Jun 12: 14, Aug 15: 6

27095 Injection procedure for hip arthrography; with anesthesia N I N

RVU			Global Days	Modifiers				
Mod	Non-Fac Total	Fac Total		51	50	62	80	MUE
	6.90	2.39	000	2	1	0	1	1

AMA: Jun 12: 14, Aug 15: 6

27096 Injection procedure for sacroiliac joint, anesthetic/steroid, with image guidance (fluoroscopy or CT) including arthrography when performed B

RVU			Global Days	Modifiers				
Mod	Non-Fac Total	Fac Total		51	50	62	80	MUE
	4.62	2.44	000	2	1	0	1	1

AMA: Nov 99: 12, Apr 03: 8, Apr 04: 15, Jul 08: 9, Jan 12: 3, Aug 15: 6

● New   ▲ Revised   Deleted   ⊙ Moderate Sedation   ✚ Add-on Codes   ⊘ High Risk Denial   Ⓐ Age Edit   ♀ Female   ♂ Male   **AMA** CPT® Assistant   **MUE** Medically Unlikely Edit
⊘ Modifier 51 Exempt   ⊖ Modifier 63 Exempt   ☒ Unlisted   **Modifiers:** See Inside Back Cover   Ⓜ Maternity   A2–Z3 ASC Payment Indicators   A–Y OPPS Status Indicators

Surgical Procedures

27097 – 27146

Pelvic/Hip Repair/Revision/Reconstruction Procedures

27097   Release or recession, hamstring, proximal   A2 T

RVU			Global Days	Modifiers				
Mod	Non-Fac Total	Fac Total		51	50	62	80	MUE
	19.35	19.35	090	2	1	0	2	1

AMA: Nov 98: 8

Hamstring release or recession

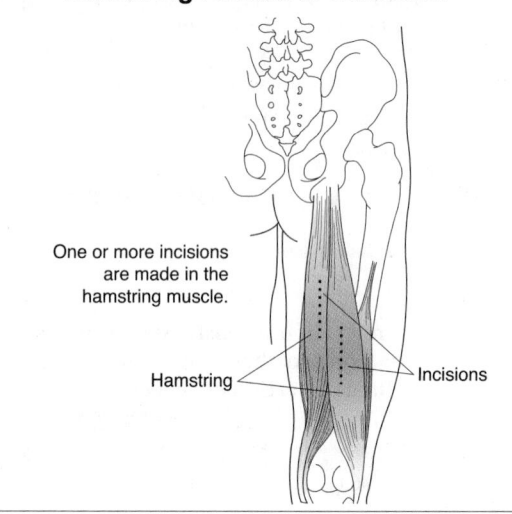

One or more incisions are made in the hamstring muscle.

Hamstring   Incisions

27098   Transfer, adductor to ischium   A2 T

RVU			Global Days	Modifiers				
Mod	Non-Fac Total	Fac Total		51	50	62	80	MUE
	19.29	19.29	090	2	1	0	2	1

AMA: Nov 98: 8

27100   Transfer external oblique muscle to greater trochanter including fascial or tendon extension (graft)   A2 J1

RVU			Global Days	Modifiers				
Mod	Non-Fac Total	Fac Total		51	50	62	80	MUE
	23.53	23.53	090	2	1	1	2	1

27105   Transfer paraspinal muscle to hip (includes fascial or tendon extension graft)   A2 T

RVU			Global Days	Modifiers				
Mod	Non-Fac Total	Fac Total		51	50	62	80	MUE
	25.06	25.06	090	2	1	0	2	1

27110   Transfer iliopsoas; to greater trochanter of femur   A2 T

RVU			Global Days	Modifiers				
Mod	Non-Fac Total	Fac Total		51	50	62	80	MUE
	27.98	27.98	090	2	1	1	2	1

27111   Transfer iliopsoas; to femoral neck   A2 T

RVU			Global Days	Modifiers				
Mod	Non-Fac Total	Fac Total		51	50	62	80	MUE
	26.03	26.03	090	2	1	1	2	1

27120   Acetabuloplasty; (eg, Whitman, Colonna, Haygroves, or cup type)   C

RVU			Global Days	Modifiers				
Mod	Non-Fac Total	Fac Total		51	50	62	80	MUE
	37.70	37.70	090	2	1	1	2	1

27122   Acetabuloplasty; resection, femoral head (eg, Girdlestone procedure)   C

RVU			Global Days	Modifiers				
Mod	Non-Fac Total	Fac Total		51	50	62	80	MUE
	31.79	31.79	090	2	1	1	2	1

27125   Hemiarthroplasty, hip, partial (eg, femoral stem prosthesis, bipolar arthroplasty)   C

RVU			Global Days	Modifiers				
Mod	Non-Fac Total	Fac Total		51	50	62	80	MUE
	32.81	32.81	090	2	1	1	2	1

AMA: Spring 92: 8, Feb 98: 11, Nov 98: 8

27130   Arthroplasty, acetabular and proximal femoral prosthetic replacement (total hip arthroplasty), with or without autograft or allograft   C

RVU			Global Days	Modifiers				
Mod	Non-Fac Total	Fac Total		51	50	62	80	MUE
	39.17	39.17	090	2	1	1	2	1

AMA: Spring 92: 8, Jan 07: 1, Dec 11: 14

27132   Conversion of previous hip surgery to total hip arthroplasty, with or without autograft or allograft   C

RVU			Global Days	Modifiers				
Mod	Non-Fac Total	Fac Total		51	50	62	80	MUE
	48.37	48.37	090	2	1	1	2	1

AMA: Spring 92: 11, Dec 08: 3

27134   Revision of total hip arthroplasty; both components, with or without autograft or allograft   C

RVU			Global Days	Modifiers				
Mod	Non-Fac Total	Fac Total		51	50	62	80	MUE
	55.26	55.26	090	2	1	1	2	1

AMA: Spring 92: 7, Dec 08: 3

27137   Revision of total hip arthroplasty; acetabular component only, with or without autograft or allograft   C

RVU			Global Days	Modifiers				
Mod	Non-Fac Total	Fac Total		51	50	62	80	MUE
	42.48	42.48	090	2	1	1	2	1

AMA: Spring 92: 7

27138   Revision of total hip arthroplasty; femoral component only, with or without allograft   C

RVU			Global Days	Modifiers				
Mod	Non-Fac Total	Fac Total		51	50	62	80	MUE
	44.16	44.16	090	2	1	1	2	1

AMA: Spring 92: 7

27140   Osteotomy and transfer of greater trochanter of femur (separate procedure)   C

RVU			Global Days	Modifiers				
Mod	Non-Fac Total	Fac Total		51	50	62	80	MUE
	25.75	25.75	090	2	1	1	2	1

27146   Osteotomy, iliac, acetabular or innominate bone   C

RVU			Global Days	Modifiers				
Mod	Non-Fac Total	Fac Total		51	50	62	80	MUE
	37.29	37.29	090	2	1	1	2	1

AMA: Feb 99: 10

● New   ▲ Revised   ✖ Deleted   ⊙ Moderate Sedation   ✚ Add-on Codes   ⊘ High Risk Denial   Ⓐ Age Edit   ♀ Female   ♂ Male   **AMA** CPT® Assistant   **MUE** Medically Unlikely Edit

⊘ Modifier 51 Exempt   ⊖ Modifier 63 Exempt   ✗ Unlisted   **Modifiers:** See Inside Back Cover   Ⓜ Maternity   A2–Z3 ASC Payment Indicators   A–Y OPPS Status Indicators

284   CPT © 2015 American Medical Association. All Rights Reserved.   © 2016 DecisionHealth

27147 Osteotomy, iliac, acetabular or innominate bone; with open reduction of hip ⓒ

RVU			Global Days	Modifiers				
Mod	Non-Fac Total	Fac Total		51	50	62	80	MUE
	42.67	42.67	090	2	1	1	2	1

27151 Osteotomy, iliac, acetabular or innominate bone; with femoral osteotomy ⓒ

RVU			Global Days	Modifiers				
Mod	Non-Fac Total	Fac Total		51	50	62	80	MUE
	46.07	46.07	090	2	1	1	2	1

27156 Osteotomy, iliac, acetabular or innominate bone; with femoral osteotomy and with open reduction of hip ⓒ

RVU			Global Days	Modifiers				
Mod	Non-Fac Total	Fac Total		51	50	62	80	MUE
	49.82	49.82	090	2	1	1	2	1

27158 Osteotomy, pelvis, bilateral (eg, congenital malformation) ⓒ

RVU			Global Days	Modifiers				
Mod	Non-Fac Total	Fac Total		51	50	62	80	MUE
	41.34	41.34	090	2	2	0	2	1

27161 Osteotomy, femoral neck (separate procedure) ⓒ

RVU			Global Days	Modifiers				
Mod	Non-Fac Total	Fac Total		51	50	62	80	MUE
	35.00	35.00	090	2	1	1	2	1

27165 Osteotomy, intertrochanteric or subtrochanteric including internal or external fixation and/or cast ⓒ

RVU			Global Days	Modifiers				
Mod	Non-Fac Total	Fac Total		51	50	62	80	MUE
	39.70	39.70	090	2	1	1	2	1

AMA: Spring 92: 11

27170 Bone graft, femoral head, neck, intertrochanteric or subtrochanteric area (includes obtaining bone graft) ⓒ

RVU			Global Days	Modifiers				
Mod	Non-Fac Total	Fac Total		51	50	62	80	MUE
	33.96	33.96	090	2	1	1	2	1

AMA: Spring 92: 11

27175 Treatment of slipped femoral epiphysis; by traction, without reduction ⓒ

RVU			Global Days	Modifiers				
Mod	Non-Fac Total	Fac Total		51	50	62	80	MUE
	19.29	19.29	090	2	1	0	0	1

27176 Treatment of slipped femoral epiphysis; by single or multiple pinning, in situ ⓒ

RVU			Global Days	Modifiers				
Mod	Non-Fac Total	Fac Total		51	50	62	80	MUE
	26.01	26.01	090	2	1	1	2	1

27177 Open treatment of slipped femoral epiphysis; single or multiple pinning or bone graft (includes obtaining graft) ⓒ

RVU			Global Days	Modifiers				
Mod	Non-Fac Total	Fac Total		51	50	62	80	MUE
	32.28	32.28	090	2	1	1	2	1

27178 Open treatment of slipped femoral epiphysis; closed manipulation with single or multiple pinning ⓒ

RVU			Global Days	Modifiers				
Mod	Non-Fac Total	Fac Total		51	50	62	80	MUE
	26.57	26.57	090	2	1	1	2	1

27179 Open treatment of slipped femoral epiphysis; osteoplasty of femoral neck (Heyman type procedure) J1

RVU			Global Days	Modifiers				
Mod	Non-Fac Total	Fac Total		51	50	62	80	MUE
	28.27	28.27	090	2	1	0	2	1

27181 Open treatment of slipped femoral epiphysis; osteotomy and internal fixation ⓒ

RVU			Global Days	Modifiers				
Mod	Non-Fac Total	Fac Total		51	50	62	80	MUE
	27.79	27.79	090	2	1	0	2	1

27185 Epiphyseal arrest by epiphysiodesis or stapling, greater trochanter of femur ⓒ

RVU			Global Days	Modifiers				
Mod	Non-Fac Total	Fac Total		51	50	62	80	MUE
	17.52	17.52	090	2	1	1	1	1

27187 Prophylactic treatment (nailing, pinning, plating or wiring) with or without methylmethacrylate, femoral neck and proximal femur ⓒ

RVU			Global Days	Modifiers				
Mod	Non-Fac Total	Fac Total		51	50	62	80	MUE
	28.61	28.61	090	2	1	1	2	1

Pelvic/Hip Fracture/Dislocation Procedures

27193 Closed treatment of pelvic ring fracture, dislocation, diastasis or subluxation; without manipulation A2T

RVU			Global Days	Modifiers				
Mod	Non-Fac Total	Fac Total		51	50	62	80	MUE
	13.57	13.76	090	2	0	0	1	1

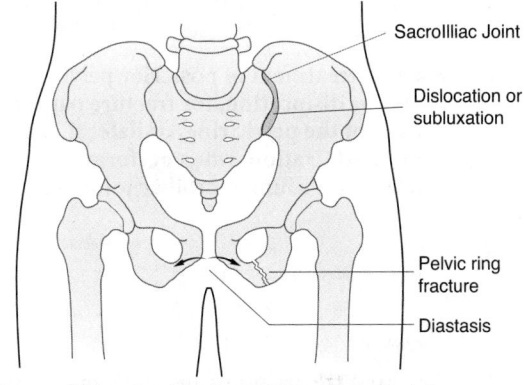

Closed treatment of pelvic ring fracture, disclocation, diastasis or subluxation

SacroIlliac Joint

Dislocation or subluxation

Pelvic ring fracture

Diastasis

Without manipulation (27193), with manipulation and more than local anesthesia (27194)

● New   ▲ Revised   Deleted   ⊙ Moderate Sedation   ✛ Add-on Codes   ⊘ High Risk Denial   Ⓐ Age Edit   ♀ Female   ♂ Male   **AMA** CPT® Assistant   **MUE** Medically Unlikely Edit
◌ Modifier 51 Exempt   ⊖ Modifier 63 Exempt   ✗ Unlisted   **Modifiers:** See Inside Back Cover   Ⓜ Maternity   A2–Z3 ASC Payment Indicators   A–Y OPPS Status Indicators

27194 Closed treatment of pelvic ring fracture, dislocation, diastasis or subluxation; with manipulation, requiring more than local anesthesia   A 2 T

RVU			Global Days	Modifiers				
Mod	Non-Fac Total	Fac Total		51	50	62	80	MUE
	20.25	20.25	090	2	0	2	0	1

27200 Closed treatment of coccygeal fracture   P 2 T

RVU			Global Days	Modifiers				
Mod	Non-Fac Total	Fac Total		51	50	62	80	MUE
	5.19	5.41	090	2	0	0	1	1

27202 Open treatment of coccygeal fracture   A 2 T

RVU			Global Days	Modifiers				
Mod	Non-Fac Total	Fac Total		51	50	62	80	MUE
	15.30	15.30	090	2	0	0	2	1

27215 Open treatment of iliac spine(s), tuberosity avulsion, or iliac wing fracture(s), unilateral, for pelvic bone fracture patterns that do not disrupt the pelvic ring, includes internal fixation, when performed   ⊘ E

RVU			Global Days	Modifiers				
Mod	Non-Fac Total	Fac Total		51	50	62	80	MUE
	17.97	17.97	090	9	9	9	9	

27216 Percutaneous skeletal fixation of posterior pelvic bone fracture and/or dislocation, for fracture patterns that disrupt the pelvic ring, unilateral (includes ipsilateral ilium, sacroiliac joint and/or sacrum)   ⊘ E

RVU			Global Days	Modifiers				
Mod	Non-Fac Total	Fac Total		51	50	62	80	MUE
	26.64	26.64	090	9	9	9	9	

AMA: Sep 13: 19, Mar 14: 4

27217 Open treatment of anterior pelvic bone fracture and/or dislocation for fracture patterns that disrupt the pelvic ring, unilateral, includes internal fixation, when performed (includes pubic symphysis and/or ipsilateral superior/inferior rami)   ⊘ E

RVU			Global Days	Modifiers				
Mod	Non-Fac Total	Fac Total		51	50	62	80	MUE
	24.99	24.99	090	9	9	9	9	

27218 Open treatment of posterior pelvic bone fracture and/or dislocation, for fracture patterns that disrupt the pelvic ring, unilateral, includes internal fixation, when performed (includes ipsilateral ilium, sacroiliac joint and/or sacrum)   ⊘ E

RVU			Global Days	Modifiers				
Mod	Non-Fac Total	Fac Total		51	50	62	80	MUE
	34.56	34.56	090	9	9	9	9	

AMA: Mar 14: 4

27220 Closed treatment of acetabulum (hip socket) fracture(s); without manipulation   G 2 T

RVU			Global Days	Modifiers				
Mod	Non-Fac Total	Fac Total		51	50	62	80	MUE
	15.30	15.18	090	2	1	0	1	1

27222 Closed treatment of acetabulum (hip socket) fracture(s); with manipulation, with or without skeletal traction   C

RVU			Global Days	Modifiers				
Mod	Non-Fac Total	Fac Total		51	50	62	80	MUE
	28.32	28.32	090	2	1	0	1	1

27226 Open treatment of posterior or anterior acetabular wall fracture, with internal fixation   C

RVU			Global Days	Modifiers				
Mod	Non-Fac Total	Fac Total		51	50	62	80	MUE
	30.53	30.53	090	2	1	2	2	1

27227 Open treatment of acetabular fracture(s) involving anterior or posterior (one) column, or a fracture running transversely across the acetabulum, with internal fixation   C

RVU			Global Days	Modifiers				
Mod	Non-Fac Total	Fac Total		51	50	62	80	MUE
	48.02	48.02	090	2	1	2	2	1

27228 Open treatment of acetabular fracture(s) involving anterior and posterior (two) columns, includes T-fracture and both column fracture with complete articular detachment, or single column or transverse fracture with associated acetabular wall fracture, with internal fixation   C

RVU			Global Days	Modifiers				
Mod	Non-Fac Total	Fac Total		51	50	62	80	MUE
	54.67	54.67	090	2	1	2	2	1

27230 Closed treatment of femoral fracture, proximal end, neck; without manipulation   A 2 T

RVU			Global Days	Modifiers				
Mod	Non-Fac Total	Fac Total		51	50	62	80	MUE
	13.70	13.61	090	2	1	0	1	1

27232 Closed treatment of femoral fracture, proximal end, neck; with manipulation, with or without skeletal traction   C

RVU			Global Days	Modifiers				
Mod	Non-Fac Total	Fac Total		51	50	62	80	MUE
	21.89	21.89	090	2	1	0	1	1

27235 Percutaneous skeletal fixation of femoral fracture, proximal end, neck   J 1

RVU			Global Days	Modifiers				
Mod	Non-Fac Total	Fac Total		51	50	62	80	MUE
	26.34	26.34	090	2	1	1	1	1

27236 Open treatment of femoral fracture, proximal end, neck, internal fixation or prosthetic replacement   C

RVU			Global Days	Modifiers				
Mod	Non-Fac Total	Fac Total		51	50	62	80	MUE
	34.63	34.63	090	2	1	1	2	1

AMA: Spring 92: 10, Feb 98: 11, Jan 07: 1

27238 Closed treatment of intertrochanteric, peritrochanteric, or subtrochanteric femoral fracture; without manipulation   A 2 T

RVU			Global Days	Modifiers				
Mod	Non-Fac Total	Fac Total		51	50	62	80	MUE
	13.27	13.27	090	2	1	0	1	1

● New   ▲ Revised   ✖ Deleted   ⊙ Moderate Sedation   ✚ Add-on Codes   ⊘ High Risk Denial   Ⓐ Age Edit   ♀ Female   ♂ Male   **AMA** *CPT® Assistant*   **MUE** Medically Unlikely Edit
⊘ Modifier 51 Exempt   ⊖ Modifier 63 Exempt   ⊠ Unlisted   **Modifiers:** *See Inside Back Cover*   Ⓜ Maternity   A 2 – Z 3 ASC Payment Indicators   A – Y OPPS Status Indicators

CPT © 2015 American Medical Association. All Rights Reserved.   © 2016 DecisionHealth

AMA: Summer 93: 12

27240 Closed treatment of intertrochanteric, peritrochanteric, or subtrochanteric femoral fracture; with manipulation, with or without skin or skeletal traction C

RVU			Global Days	Modifiers				
Mod	Non-Fac Total	Fac Total		51	50	62	80	MUE
	27.76	27.76	090	2	1	0	1	1

AMA: Summer 93: 12

27244 Treatment of intertrochanteric, peritrochanteric, or subtrochanteric femoral fracture; with plate/screw type implant, with or without cerclage C

RVU			Global Days	Modifiers				
Mod	Non-Fac Total	Fac Total		51	50	62	80	MUE
	35.68	35.68	090	2	1	1	2	1

AMA: Summer 93: 12

27245 Treatment of intertrochanteric, peritrochanteric, or subtrochanteric femoral fracture; with intramedullary implant, with or without interlocking screws and/or cerclage C

RVU			Global Days	Modifiers				
Mod	Non-Fac Total	Fac Total		51	50	62	80	MUE
	35.67	35.67	090	2	1	2	2	1

AMA: Summer 93: 12, Sep 13: 17

27246 Closed treatment of greater trochanteric fracture, without manipulation A2T

RVU			Global Days	Modifiers				
Mod	Non-Fac Total	Fac Total		51	50	62	80	MUE
	11.11	11.16	090	2	1	0	1	1

27248 Open treatment of greater trochanteric fracture, includes internal fixation, when performed C

RVU			Global Days	Modifiers				
Mod	Non-Fac Total	Fac Total		51	50	62	80	MUE
	21.47	21.47	090	2	1	1	2	1

27250 Closed treatment of hip dislocation, traumatic; without anesthesia A2T

RVU			Global Days	Modifiers				
Mod	Non-Fac Total	Fac Total		51	50	62	80	MUE
	5.21	5.21	000	2	1	0	1	1

27252 Closed treatment of hip dislocation, traumatic; requiring anesthesia A2T

RVU			Global Days	Modifiers				
Mod	Non-Fac Total	Fac Total		51	50	62	80	MUE
	22.00	22.00	090	2	1	0	1	1

27253 Open treatment of hip dislocation, traumatic, without internal fixation C

RVU			Global Days	Modifiers				
Mod	Non-Fac Total	Fac Total		51	50	62	80	MUE
	27.17	27.17	090	2	1	1	2	1

27254 Open treatment of hip dislocation, traumatic, with acetabular wall and femoral head fracture, with or without internal or external fixation C

RVU			Global Days	Modifiers				
Mod	Non-Fac Total	Fac Total		51	50	62	80	MUE
	36.64	36.64	090	2	1	1	2	1

27256 Treatment of spontaneous hip dislocation (developmental, including congenital or pathological), by abduction, splint or traction; without anesthesia, without manipulation G2T

RVU			Global Days	Modifiers				
Mod	Non-Fac Total	Fac Total		51	50	62	80	MUE
	8.57	6.74	010	2	1	0	0	1

27257 Treatment of spontaneous hip dislocation (developmental, including congenital or pathological), by abduction, splint or traction; with manipulation, requiring anesthesia A2T

RVU			Global Days	Modifiers				
Mod	Non-Fac Total	Fac Total		51	50	62	80	MUE
	10.52	10.52	010	2	1	0	0	1

27258 Open treatment of spontaneous hip dislocation (developmental, including congenital or pathological), replacement of femoral head in acetabulum (including tenotomy, etc) C

RVU			Global Days	Modifiers				
Mod	Non-Fac Total	Fac Total		51	50	62	80	MUE
	32.17	32.17	090	2	1	1	2	1

27259 Open treatment of spontaneous hip dislocation (developmental, including congenital or pathological), replacement of femoral head in acetabulum (including tenotomy, etc); with femoral shaft shortening C

RVU			Global Days	Modifiers				
Mod	Non-Fac Total	Fac Total		51	50	62	80	MUE
	45.07	45.07	090	2	1	0	2	1

27265 Closed treatment of post hip arthroplasty dislocation; without anesthesia A2T

RVU			Global Days	Modifiers				
Mod	Non-Fac Total	Fac Total		51	50	62	80	MUE
	11.49	11.49	090	2	1	0	1	1

27266 Closed treatment of post hip arthroplasty dislocation; requiring regional or general anesthesia A2T

RVU			Global Days	Modifiers				
Mod	Non-Fac Total	Fac Total		51	50	62	80	MUE
	16.79	16.79	090	2	1	0	1	1

27267 Closed treatment of femoral fracture, proximal end, head; without manipulation G2T

RVU			Global Days	Modifiers				
Mod	Non-Fac Total	Fac Total		51	50	62	80	MUE
	12.59	12.59	090	2	1	1	2	1

AMA: Jan 08: 4

27268 Closed treatment of femoral fracture, proximal end, head; with manipulation C

RVU			Global Days	Modifiers				
Mod	Non-Fac Total	Fac Total		51	50	62	80	MUE
	15.34	15.34	090	2	1	1	2	1

AMA: Jan 08: 4

● New ▲ Revised Deleted ⊙ Moderate Sedation ✚ Add-on Codes ⊘ High Risk Denial Ⓐ Age Edit ♀ Female ♂ Male AMA CPT® Assistant MUE Medically Unlikely Edit
⊘ Modifier 51 Exempt ⊖ Modifier 63 Exempt ☒ Unlisted Modifiers: See Inside Back Cover Ⓜ Maternity A2–Z3 ASC Payment Indicators A–Y OPPS Status Indicators

27269 Open treatment of femoral fracture, proximal end, head, includes internal fixation, when performed   C

RVU			Global Days	Modifiers				
Mod	Non-Fac Total	Fac Total		51	50	62	80	MUE
	35.87	35.87	090	2	1	1	2	1

AMA: Jan 08: 4, Dec 08: 3

Pelvic/Hip Manipulation

27275 Manipulation, hip joint, requiring general anesthesia   A2T

RVU			Global Days	Modifiers				
Mod	Non-Fac Total	Fac Total		51	50	62	80	MUE
	5.25	5.25	010	2	0	0	1	2

Hip joint manipulation

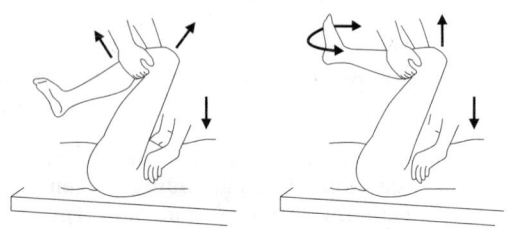

The hip joint is manipulated by moving the leg.

27279 Arthrodesis, sacroiliac joint, percutaneous or minimally invasive (indirect visualization), with image guidance, includes obtaining bone graft when performed, and placement of transfixing device   J8JI

RVU			Global Days	Modifiers				
Mod	Non-Fac Total	Fac Total		51	50	62	80	MUE
	20.15	20.15	090	2	1	1	2	1

Arthrodesis, sacroiliac joint, percutaneous or minimally invasive,
with image guidance, includes obtaining bone graft when performed, and placement of transfixing device

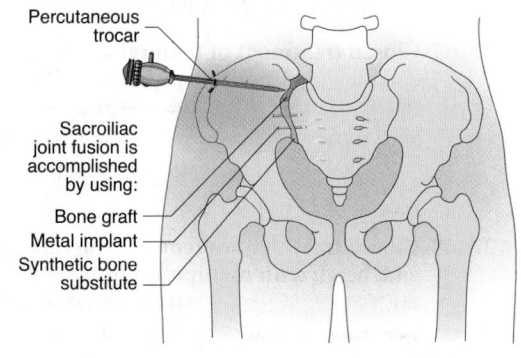

Percutaneous trocar

Sacroiliac joint fusion is accomplished by using:

Bone graft
Metal implant
Synthetic bone substitute

Pelvic/Hip Arthrodesis

27280 Arthrodesis, open, sacroiliac joint, including obtaining bone graft, including instrumentation, when performed   C

RVU			Global Days	Modifiers				
Mod	Non-Fac Total	Fac Total		51	50	62	80	MUE
	39.50	39.50	090	2	1	1	2	1

AMA: Sep 13: 19, Mar 14: 4

27282 Arthrodesis, symphysis pubis (including obtaining graft)   C

RVU			Global Days	Modifiers				
Mod	Non-Fac Total	Fac Total		51	50	62	80	MUE
	23.83	23.83	090	2	0	1	2	1

27284 Arthrodesis, hip joint (including obtaining graft)   C

RVU			Global Days	Modifiers				
Mod	Non-Fac Total	Fac Total		51	50	62	80	MUE
	45.02	45.02	090	2	1	1	2	1

27286 Arthrodesis, hip joint (including obtaining graft); with subtrochanteric osteotomy   C

RVU			Global Days	Modifiers				
Mod	Non-Fac Total	Fac Total		51	50	62	80	MUE
	47.39	47.39	090	2	1	1	2	1

Pelvic/Hip Amputation

27290 Interpelviabdominal amputation (hindquarter amputation)   C

RVU			Global Days	Modifiers				
Mod	Non-Fac Total	Fac Total		51	50	62	80	MUE
	46.68	46.68	090	2	0	1	2	1

27295 Disarticulation of hip   C

RVU			Global Days	Modifiers				
Mod	Non-Fac Total	Fac Total		51	50	62	80	MUE
	36.44	36.44	090	2	1	1	2	1

Other Pelvic/Hip Procedures

27299 Unlisted procedure, pelvis or hip joint   T

RVU			Global Days	Modifiers				
Mod	Non-Fac Total	Fac Total		51	50	62	80	MUE
	0.00	0.00	YYY	2	1	1	2	

AMA: Jan 02: 10, Dec 05: 9, Dec 08: 3, Oct 12: 14, Nov 12: 13, Mar 14: 13

Thigh Region/Knee Procedures

Thigh Region/Knee Incisional Procedures

27301 Incision and drainage, deep abscess, bursa, or hematoma, thigh or knee region   A2T

RVU			Global Days	Modifiers				
Mod	Non-Fac Total	Fac Total		51	50	62	80	MUE
	19.31	14.49	090	2	1	0	1	3

AMA: Nov 98: 9, Dec 08: 3

27303 Incision, deep, with opening of bone cortex, femur or knee (eg, osteomyelitis or bone abscess)   C

RVU			Global Days	Modifiers				
Mod	Non-Fac Total	Fac Total		51	50	62	80	MUE
	18.34	18.34	090	2	1	1	2	2

AMA: Nov 98: 8

● New   ▲ Revised   ✖ Deleted   ⊙ Moderate Sedation   ✚ Add-on Codes   ⊘ High Risk Denial   Ⓐ Age Edit   ♀ Female   ♂ Male   **AMA** CPT® Assistant   **MUE** Medically Unlikely Edit
⊘ Modifier 51 Exempt   ⊖ Modifier 63 Exempt   ⊠ Unlisted   **Modifiers:** See Inside Back Cover   Ⓜ Maternity   A2–Z3 ASC Payment Indicators   A–Y OPPS Status Indicators

CPT © 2015 American Medical Association. All Rights Reserved.   © 2016 DecisionHealth

27305 Fasciotomy, iliotibial (tenotomy), open `A 2 T`

RVU			Global Days	Modifiers				
Mod	Non-Fac Total	Fac Total		51	50	62	80	MUE
	13.83	13.83	090	2	1	1	2	1

27306 Tenotomy, percutaneous, adductor or hamstring; single tendon (separate procedure) `A 2 T`

RVU			Global Days	Modifiers				
Mod	Non-Fac Total	Fac Total		51	50	62	80	MUE
	10.13	10.13	090	2	1	0	2	1

AMA: Nov 98: 8

27307 Tenotomy, percutaneous, adductor or hamstring; multiple tendons `A 2 T`

RVU			Global Days	Modifiers				
Mod	Non-Fac Total	Fac Total		51	50	62	80	MUE
	13.26	13.26	090	2	1	1	0	1

AMA: Nov 98: 8

27310 Arthrotomy, knee, with exploration, drainage, or removal of foreign body (eg, infection) `A 2 T`

RVU			Global Days	Modifiers				
Mod	Non-Fac Total	Fac Total		51	50	62	80	MUE
	21.11	21.11	090	2	1	1	2	1

AMA: Nov 98: 8, Dec 08: 3

Thigh Region/Knee Excisional Procedures

27323 Biopsy, soft tissue of thigh or knee area; superficial `A 2 T`

Coding tip: Code 99000 for specimen transfer from office setting to an outside laboratory

RVU			Global Days	Modifiers				
Mod	Non-Fac Total	Fac Total		51	50	62	80	MUE
	7.75	5.13	010	2	1	0	1	2

AMA: Jun 97: 12

27324 Biopsy, soft tissue of thigh or knee area; deep (subfascial or intramuscular) `A 2 T`

RVU			Global Days	Modifiers				
Mod	Non-Fac Total	Fac Total		51	50	62	80	MUE
	11.45	11.45	090	2	1	0	1	3

AMA: Mar 97: 4, Nov 98: 8

27325 Neurectomy, hamstring muscle `A 2 T`

RVU			Global Days	Modifiers				
Mod	Non-Fac Total	Fac Total		51	50	62	80	MUE
	15.82	15.82	090	2	1	0	2	1

27326 Neurectomy, popliteal (gastrocnemius) `A 2 T`

RVU			Global Days	Modifiers				
Mod	Non-Fac Total	Fac Total		51	50	62	80	MUE
	14.98	14.98	090	2	1	1	2	1

27327 Excision, tumor, soft tissue of thigh or knee area, subcutaneous; less than 3 cm `G 2 T`

Coding tip: Related soft tissue excision codes - 27328, 27337, and 27339

RVU			Global Days	Modifiers				
Mod	Non-Fac Total	Fac Total		51	50	62	80	MUE
	13.18	9.06	090	2	1	0	1	5

27328 Excision, tumor, soft tissue of thigh or knee area, subfascial (eg, intramuscular); less than 5 cm `G 2 T`

Coding tip: Related soft tissue excision codes - 27327, 27337, and 27339

RVU			Global Days	Modifiers				
Mod	Non-Fac Total	Fac Total		51	50	62	80	MUE
	17.93	17.93	090	2	1	0	1	4

27329 Radical resection of tumor (eg, sarcoma), soft tissue of thigh or knee area; less than 5 cm `G 2 T`

Coding tip: Code 27329 is listed out of numerical order in CPT. Related radical resection of soft tissue tumor procedure - 27364

RVU			Global Days	Modifiers				
Mod	Non-Fac Total	Fac Total		51	50	62	80	MUE
	30.00	30.00	090	2	1	1	2	1

27330 Arthrotomy, knee; with synovial biopsy only `A 2 T`

RVU			Global Days	Modifiers				
Mod	Non-Fac Total	Fac Total		51	50	62	80	MUE
	12.06	12.06	090	2	1	1	1	1

AMA: Mar 12: 9

27331 Arthrotomy, knee; including joint exploration, biopsy, or removal of loose or foreign bodies `A 2 T`

RVU			Global Days	Modifiers				
Mod	Non-Fac Total	Fac Total		51	50	62	80	MUE
	13.68	13.68	090	2	1	1	2	1

AMA: May 96: 6, Nov 98: 8, Nov 12: 13

27332 Arthrotomy, with excision of semilunar cartilage (meniscectomy) knee; medial OR lateral `A 2 T`

RVU			Global Days	Modifiers				
Mod	Non-Fac Total	Fac Total		51	50	62	80	MUE
	18.43	18.43	090	2	1	1	2	1

AMA: Nov 98: 8

27333 Arthrotomy, with excision of semilunar cartilage (meniscectomy) knee; medial AND lateral `A 2 T`

RVU			Global Days	Modifiers				
Mod	Non-Fac Total	Fac Total		51	50	62	80	MUE
	16.91	16.91	090	2	1	1	2	1

AMA: Mar 12: 9

27334 Arthrotomy, with synovectomy, knee; anterior OR posterior `A 2 T`

RVU			Global Days	Modifiers				
Mod	Non-Fac Total	Fac Total		51	50	62	80	MUE
	19.65	19.65	090	2	1	1	2	1

AMA: Nov 98: 8

27335 Arthrotomy, with synovectomy, knee; anterior AND posterior including popliteal area `A 2 J 1`

RVU			Global Days	Modifiers				
Mod	Non-Fac Total	Fac Total		51	50	62	80	MUE
	21.95	21.95	090	2	1	1	2	1

27337 Excision, tumor, soft tissue of thigh or knee area, subcutaneous; 3 cm or greater `G 2 T`

Coding tip: Code 27337 is listed out of numerical order in CPT. Related soft tissue tumor excision procedures - 27327 (subcutaneous tissue); 27328, 27339 (subfascial).

RVU			Global Days	Modifiers				
Mod	Non-Fac Total	Fac Total		51	50	62	80	MUE
	12.09	12.09	090	2	1	0	2	4

● New ▲ Revised Deleted ⊙ Moderate Sedation ✚ Add-on Codes ⊘ High Risk Denial Ⓐ Age Edit ♀ Female ♂ Male **AMA** CPT® Assistant **MUE** Medically Unlikely Edit
⊗ Modifier 51 Exempt ⊖ Modifier 63 Exempt Ⓧ Unlisted **Modifiers:** See Inside Back Cover Ⓜ Maternity A 2–Z 3 ASC Payment Indicators A–Y OPPS Status Indicators

Surgical Procedures

27339 – 27386

27339 Excision, tumor, soft tissue of thigh or knee area, subfascial (eg, intramuscular); 5 cm or greater G2T

Coding tip: *Code 27339 is listed out of numerical order in CPT. Related soft tissue tumor excision procedures - 27327, 27337 (subcutaneous tissue); 27328 (subfascial)*

RVU			Global Days	Modifiers				
Mod	Non-Fac Total	Fac Total		51	50	62	80	MUE
	21.79	21.79	090	2	1	0	2	4

27340 Excision, prepatellar bursa A2T

RVU			Global Days	Modifiers				
Mod	Non-Fac Total	Fac Total		51	50	62	80	MUE
	10.72	10.72	090	2	1	0	1	1

27345 Excision of synovial cyst of popliteal space (eg, Baker's cyst) A2T

RVU			Global Days	Modifiers				
Mod	Non-Fac Total	Fac Total		51	50	62	80	MUE
	13.80	13.80	090	2	1	2	1	

27347 Excision of lesion of meniscus or capsule (eg, cyst, ganglion), knee A2T

RVU			Global Days	Modifiers				
Mod	Non-Fac Total	Fac Total		51	50	62	80	MUE
	15.25	15.25	090	2	1	1	2	1

AMA: Nov 98: 11

27350 Patellectomy or hemipatellectomy A2T

RVU			Global Days	Modifiers				
Mod	Non-Fac Total	Fac Total		51	50	62	80	MUE
	18.73	18.73	090	2	1	1	2	1

27355 Excision or curettage of bone cyst or benign tumor of femur A2T

RVU			Global Days	Modifiers				
Mod	Non-Fac Total	Fac Total		51	50	62	80	MUE
	17.29	17.29	090	2	1	1	2	1

27356 Excision or curettage of bone cyst or benign tumor of femur; with allograft J8JI

RVU			Global Days	Modifiers				
Mod	Non-Fac Total	Fac Total		51	50	62	80	MUE
	21.21	21.21	090	2	1	1	2	1

27357 Excision or curettage of bone cyst or benign tumor of femur; with autograft (includes obtaining graft) A2JI

RVU			Global Days	Modifiers				
Mod	Non-Fac Total	Fac Total		51	50	62	80	MUE
	23.48	23.48	090	2	1	1	2	1

AMA: Dec 02: 11

+ 27358 Excision or curettage of bone cyst or benign tumor of femur; with internal fixation (List in addition to code for primary procedure) NIN

RVU			Global Days	Modifiers				
Mod	Non-Fac Total	Fac Total		51	50	62	80	MUE
	8.09	8.09	ZZZ	0	0	0	2	1

27360 Partial excision (craterization, saucerization, or diaphysectomy) bone, femur, proximal tibia and/ or fibula (eg, osteomyelitis or bone abscess) A2T

RVU			Global Days	Modifiers				
Mod	Non-Fac Total	Fac Total		51	50	62	80	MUE
	24.54	24.54	090	2	1	1	2	2

AMA: Nov 98: 8

27364 Radical resection of tumor (eg, sarcoma), soft tissue of thigh or knee area; 5 cm or greater G2T

Coding tip: *Related radial resection of soft tissue tumor code - 27329*

RVU			Global Days	Modifiers				
Mod	Non-Fac Total	Fac Total		51	50	62	80	MUE
	45.29	45.29	090	2	1	1	2	1

27365 Radical resection of tumor, femur or knee C

RVU			Global Days	Modifiers				
Mod	Non-Fac Total	Fac Total		51	50	62	80	MUE
	59.91	59.91	090	2	1	1	2	1

Thigh Region/Knee Introduction/Removal Procedures

27370 Injection of contrast for knee arthrography NIN

RVU			Global Days	Modifiers				
Mod	Non-Fac Total	Fac Total		51	50	62	80	MUE
	4.40	1.46	000	2	1	0	1	1

AMA: Feb 15: 6, Aug 15: 6

27372 Removal of foreign body, deep, thigh region or knee area A2T

RVU			Global Days	Modifiers				
Mod	Non-Fac Total	Fac Total		51	50	62	80	MUE
	17.40	11.64	090	2	1	0	0	2

Thigh Region/Knee Repair/Revision/Reconstruction Procedures

27380 Suture of infrapatellar tendon; primary A2T

RVU			Global Days	Modifiers				
Mod	Non-Fac Total	Fac Total		51	50	62	80	MUE
	17.08	17.08	090	2	1	1	2	2

27381 Suture of infrapatellar tendon; secondary reconstruction, including fascial or tendon graft A2JI

RVU			Global Days	Modifiers				
Mod	Non-Fac Total	Fac Total		51	50	62	80	MUE
	22.92	22.92	090	2	1	1	2	2

27385 Suture of quadriceps or hamstring muscle rupture; primary A2T

RVU			Global Days	Modifiers				
Mod	Non-Fac Total	Fac Total		51	50	62	80	MUE
	16.54	16.54	090	2	1	1	2	2

27386 Suture of quadriceps or hamstring muscle rupture; secondary reconstruction, including fascial or tendon graft A2JI

RVU			Global Days	Modifiers				
Mod	Non-Fac Total	Fac Total		51	50	62	80	MUE
	23.88	23.88	090	2	1	1	2	2

● New   ▲ Revised   ✖ Deleted   ⊙ Moderate Sedation   ✚ Add-on Codes   ⊘ High Risk Denial   Ⓐ Age Edit   ♀ Female   ♂ Male   **AMA** *CPT® Assistant*   **MUE** Medically Unlikely Edit

⊘ Modifier 51 Exempt   ⊖ Modifier 63 Exempt   ✖ Unlisted   **Modifiers:** *See Inside Back Cover*   Ⓜ Maternity   A2–Z3 ASC Payment Indicators   A–Y OPPS Status Indicators

290   CPT © 2015 American Medical Association. All Rights Reserved.   © 2016 DecisionHealth

27390   Tenotomy, open, hamstring, knee to hip; single tendon   `A 2 T`

RVU			Global Days	Modifiers				
Mod	Non-Fac Total	Fac Total		51	50	62	80	MUE
	12.91	12.91	090	2	1	0	2	1

AMA: Nov 98: 8

27391   Tenotomy, open, hamstring, knee to hip; multiple tendons, 1 leg   `A 2 T`

RVU			Global Days	Modifiers				
Mod	Non-Fac Total	Fac Total		51	50	62	80	MUE
	16.64	16.64	090	2	0	1	0	1

AMA: Nov 98: 8

27392   Tenotomy, open, hamstring, knee to hip; multiple tendons, bilateral   `A 2 T`

RVU			Global Days	Modifiers				
Mod	Non-Fac Total	Fac Total		51	50	62	80	MUE
	20.49	20.49	090	2	2	1	2	1

AMA: Nov 98: 8

27393   Lengthening of hamstring tendon; single tendon   `A 2 T`

RVU			Global Days	Modifiers				
Mod	Non-Fac Total	Fac Total		51	50	62	80	MUE
	14.48	14.48	090	2	1	1	2	1

AMA: Nov 98: 8

27394   Lengthening of hamstring tendon; multiple tendons, 1 leg   `A 2 T`

RVU			Global Days	Modifiers				
Mod	Non-Fac Total	Fac Total		51	50	62	80	MUE
	18.23	18.23	090	2	0	0	2	1

AMA: Nov 98: 8

27395   Lengthening of hamstring tendon; multiple tendons, bilateral   `A 2 T`

RVU			Global Days	Modifiers				
Mod	Non-Fac Total	Fac Total		51	50	62	80	MUE
	25.41	25.41	090	2	2	1	2	1

AMA: Nov 98: 8

Pub 100-04, 12, 40.7

27396   Transplant or transfer (with muscle redirection or rerouting), thigh (eg, extensor to flexor); single tendon   `A 2 T`

RVU			Global Days	Modifiers				
Mod	Non-Fac Total	Fac Total		51	50	62	80	MUE
	17.78	17.78	090	2	1	1	2	1

AMA: Nov 98: 8

27397   Transplant or transfer (with muscle redirection or rerouting), thigh (eg, extensor to flexor); multiple tendons   `A 2 T`

RVU			Global Days	Modifiers				
Mod	Non-Fac Total	Fac Total		51	50	62	80	MUE
	26.12	26.12	090	2	1	0	2	1

AMA: Nov 98: 8

27400   Transfer, tendon or muscle, hamstrings to femur (eg, Egger's type procedure)   `A 2 T`

RVU			Global Days	Modifiers				
Mod	Non-Fac Total	Fac Total		51	50	62	80	MUE
	20.06	20.06	090	2	1	1	2	1

AMA: Nov 98: 8

27403   Arthrotomy with meniscus repair, knee   `A 2 T`

RVU			Global Days	Modifiers				
Mod	Non-Fac Total	Fac Total		51	50	62	80	MUE
	18.39	18.39	090	2	1	1	2	1

AMA: Nov 98: 8

27405   Repair, primary, torn ligament and/or capsule, knee; collateral   `A 2 T`

RVU			Global Days	Modifiers				
Mod	Non-Fac Total	Fac Total		51	50	62	80	MUE
	19.40	19.40	090	2	1	1	2	2

AMA: Dec 12: 12

27407   Repair, primary, torn ligament and/or capsule, knee; cruciate   `A 2 J 1`

RVU			Global Days	Modifiers				
Mod	Non-Fac Total	Fac Total		51	50	62	80	MUE
	22.59	22.59	090	2	1	1	2	2

27409   Repair, primary, torn ligament and/or capsule, knee; collateral and cruciate ligaments   `A 2 T`

RVU			Global Days	Modifiers				
Mod	Non-Fac Total	Fac Total		51	50	62	80	MUE
	27.54	27.54	090	2	1	1	2	1

27412   Autologous chondrocyte implantation, knee   `⊙ J 1`

RVU			Global Days	Modifiers				
Mod	Non-Fac Total	Fac Total		51	50	62	80	MUE
	47.96	47.96	090	2	1	1	2	1

27415   Osteochondral allograft, knee, open   `G2 J 1`

RVU			Global Days	Modifiers				
Mod	Non-Fac Total	Fac Total		51	50	62	80	MUE
	39.72	39.72	090	2	1	1	2	1

27416   Osteochondral autograft(s), knee, open (eg, mosaicplasty) (includes harvesting of autograft[s])   `G2 J 1`

RVU			Global Days	Modifiers				
Mod	Non-Fac Total	Fac Total		51	50	62	80	MUE
	28.32	28.32	090	2	1	0	2	1

AMA: Jan 08: 4

27418   Anterior tibial tubercleplasty (eg, Maquet type procedure)   `A 2 J 1`

RVU			Global Days	Modifiers				
Mod	Non-Fac Total	Fac Total		51	50	62	80	MUE
	23.89	23.89	090	2	1	1	2	1

AMA: Feb 10: 13

27420   Reconstruction of dislocating patella; (eg, Hauser type procedure)   `A 2 J 1`

RVU			Global Days	Modifiers				
Mod	Non-Fac Total	Fac Total		51	50	62	80	MUE
	21.44	21.44	090	2	1	1	2	1

AMA: Nov 12: 13

● New   ▲ Revised   Deleted   ⊙ Moderate Sedation   ✚ Add-on Codes   ⊘ High Risk Denial   ⓐ Age Edit   ♀ Female   ♂ Male   **AMA** *CPT® Assistant*   ***MUE*** Medically Unlikely Edit
⊘ Modifier 51 Exempt   ⊖ Modifier 63 Exempt   Ⓧ Unlisted   **Modifiers:** *See Inside Back Cover*   Ⓜ Maternity   `A 2`–`Z 3` ASC Payment Indicators   `A`–`Y` OPPS Status Indicators

27422 Reconstruction of dislocating patella; with extensor realignment and/or muscle advancement or release (eg, Campbell, Goldwaite type procedure) A2T

RVU		Global Days	Modifiers				
Mod	Non-Fac Total	Fac Total		51	50	62	80	MUE
	21.35	21.35	090	2	1	1	2	1

AMA: Mar 11: 9

27424 Reconstruction of dislocating patella; with patellectomy A2T

RVU		Global Days	Modifiers				
Mod	Non-Fac Total	Fac Total		51	50	62	80	MUE
	21.63	21.63	090	2	1	1	2	1

27425 Lateral retinacular release, open A2T

RVU		Global Days	Modifiers				
Mod	Non-Fac Total	Fac Total		51	50	62	80	MUE
	12.93	12.93	090	2	1	1	1	1

AMA: Nov 00: 11, Mar 11: 9

Lateral retinacular release

Iliotibial band
Patella
Lateral patellar retinaculum is incised
Patellar tendon

An incision is made in one of the two ligaments on either side of the knee to prevent the kneecap from being pulled too far to one side.

Normal alignment   Poor alignment

27427 Ligamentous reconstruction (augmentation), knee; extra-articular A2J1

RVU		Global Days	Modifiers				
Mod	Non-Fac Total	Fac Total		51	50	62	80	MUE
	20.49	20.49	090	2	1	1	2	1

AMA: Nov 99: 13, Dec 12: 12

27428 Ligamentous reconstruction (augmentation), knee; intra-articular (open) G2J1

RVU		Global Days	Modifiers				
Mod	Non-Fac Total	Fac Total		51	50	62	80	MUE
	32.13	32.13	090	2	1	1	2	1

AMA: Nov 99: 13, Apr 09: 8

27429 Ligamentous reconstruction (augmentation), knee; intra-articular (open) and extra-articular G2J1

RVU		Global Days	Modifiers				
Mod	Non-Fac Total	Fac Total		51	50	62	80	MUE
	35.76	35.76	090	2	1	1	2	1

AMA: Nov 99: 13, Apr 09: 8

27430 Quadricepsplasty (eg, Bennett or Thompson type) A2T

RVU		Global Days	Modifiers				
Mod	Non-Fac Total	Fac Total		51	50	62	80	MUE
	21.25	21.25	090	2	1	1	2	1

27435 Capsulotomy, posterior capsular release, knee A2T

RVU		Global Days	Modifiers				
Mod	Non-Fac Total	Fac Total		51	50	62	80	MUE
	23.10	23.10	090	2	1	1	2	1

AMA: Nov 98: 8

27437 Arthroplasty, patella; without prosthesis A2J1

RVU		Global Days	Modifiers				
Mod	Non-Fac Total	Fac Total		51	50	62	80	MUE
	19.03	19.03	090	2	1	1	1	1

27438 Arthroplasty, patella; with prosthesis J8J1

RVU		Global Days	Modifiers				
Mod	Non-Fac Total	Fac Total		51	50	62	80	MUE
	24.25	24.25	090	2	1	1	2	1

27440 Arthroplasty, knee, tibial plateau J8J1

RVU		Global Days	Modifiers				
Mod	Non-Fac Total	Fac Total		51	50	62	80	MUE
	23.09	23.09	090	2	1	1	2	1

27441 Arthroplasty, knee, tibial plateau; with debridement and partial synovectomy J8J1

RVU		Global Days	Modifiers				
Mod	Non-Fac Total	Fac Total		51	50	62	80	MUE
	23.80	23.80	090	2	1	1	2	1

27442 Arthroplasty, femoral condyles or tibial plateau(s), knee J8J1

RVU		Global Days	Modifiers				
Mod	Non-Fac Total	Fac Total		51	50	62	80	MUE
	25.04	25.04	090	2	1	1	2	1

AMA: Nov 99: 13

27443 Arthroplasty, femoral condyles or tibial plateau(s), knee; with debridement and partial synovectomy G2J1

RVU		Global Days	Modifiers				
Mod	Non-Fac Total	Fac Total		51	50	62	80	MUE
	23.31	23.31	090	2	1	1	2	1

27445 Arthroplasty, knee, hinge prosthesis (eg, Walldius type) C

RVU		Global Days	Modifiers				
Mod	Non-Fac Total	Fac Total		51	50	62	80	MUE
	36.07	36.07	090	2	1	1	2	1

AMA: Nov 98: 8

27446 Arthroplasty, knee, condyle and plateau; medial OR lateral compartment J8J1

RVU		Global Days	Modifiers				
Mod	Non-Fac Total	Fac Total		51	50	62	80	MUE
	33.44	33.44	090	2	1	1	2	1

● New   ▲ Revised   ✖ Deleted   ⊙ Moderate Sedation   ✚ Add-on Codes   ⊘ High Risk Denial   Ⓐ Age Edit   ♀ Female   ♂ Male   **AMA** *CPT® Assistant*   **MUE** Medically Unlikely Edit
⊘ Modifier 51 Exempt   ⊖ Modifier 63 Exempt   ✗ Unlisted   **Modifiers:** *See Inside Back Cover*   Ⓜ Maternity   A2–Z3 ASC Payment Indicators   A–Y OPPS Status Indicators

CPT © 2015 American Medical Association. All Rights Reserved.
© 2016 DecisionHealth

27447 Arthroplasty, knee, condyle and plateau; medial AND lateral compartments with or without patella resurfacing (total knee arthroplasty) ▣C

RVU			Global Days	Modifiers				
Mod	Non-Fac Total	Fac Total		51	50	62	80	MUE
	39.17	39.17	090	2	1	1	2	1

AMA: Jan 07: 1

27448 Osteotomy, femur, shaft or supracondylar; without fixation ▣C

RVU			Global Days	Modifiers				
Mod	Non-Fac Total	Fac Total		51	50	62	80	MUE
	22.09	22.09	090	2	1	1	2	1

27450 Osteotomy, femur, shaft or supracondylar; with fixation ▣C

RVU			Global Days	Modifiers				
Mod	Non-Fac Total	Fac Total		51	50	62	80	MUE
	29.12	29.12	090	2	1	1	2	1

27454 Osteotomy, multiple, with realignment on intramedullary rod, femoral shaft (eg, Sofield type procedure) ▣C

RVU			Global Days	Modifiers				
Mod	Non-Fac Total	Fac Total		51	50	62	80	MUE
	37.69	37.69	090	2	1	1	2	1

AMA: Nov 98: 8

27455 Osteotomy, proximal tibia, including fibular excision or osteotomy (includes correction of genu varus [bowleg] or genu valgus [knock-knee]); before epiphyseal closure ▣C

RVU			Global Days	Modifiers				
Mod	Non-Fac Total	Fac Total		51	50	62	80	MUE
	27.23	27.23	090	2	1	1	2	1

27457 Osteotomy, proximal tibia, including fibular excision or osteotomy (includes correction of genu varus [bowleg] or genu valgus [knock-knee]); after epiphyseal closure ▣C

RVU			Global Days	Modifiers				
Mod	Non-Fac Total	Fac Total		51	50	62	80	MUE
	27.22	27.22	090	2	1	1	2	1

27465 Osteoplasty, femur; shortening (excluding 64876) ▣C

RVU			Global Days	Modifiers				
Mod	Non-Fac Total	Fac Total		51	50	62	80	MUE
	35.57	35.57	090	2	1	1	2	1

27466 Osteoplasty, femur; lengthening ▣C

RVU			Global Days	Modifiers				
Mod	Non-Fac Total	Fac Total		51	50	62	80	MUE
	33.85	33.85	090	2	1	1	2	1

27468 Osteoplasty, femur; combined, lengthening and shortening with femoral segment transfer ▣C

RVU			Global Days	Modifiers				
Mod	Non-Fac Total	Fac Total		51	50	62	80	MUE
	35.62	35.62	090	2	1	1	2	1

27470 Repair, nonunion or malunion, femur, distal to head and neck; without graft (eg, compression technique) ▣C

RVU			Global Days	Modifiers				
Mod	Non-Fac Total	Fac Total		51	50	62	80	MUE
	33.95	33.95	090	2	1	1	2	1

27472 Repair, nonunion or malunion, femur, distal to head and neck; with iliac or other autogenous bone graft (includes obtaining graft) ▣C

RVU			Global Days	Modifiers				
Mod	Non-Fac Total	Fac Total		51	50	62	80	MUE
	36.48	36.48	090	2	1	1	2	1

27475 Arrest, epiphyseal, any method (eg, epiphysiodesis); distal femur ▣G2T

RVU			Global Days	Modifiers				
Mod	Non-Fac Total	Fac Total		51	50	62	80	MUE
	19.11	19.11	090	2	1	1	1	1

AMA: Nov 98: 8

27477 Arrest, epiphyseal, any method (eg, epiphysiodesis); tibia and fibula, proximal ⊘T

RVU			Global Days	Modifiers				
Mod	Non-Fac Total	Fac Total		51	50	62	80	MUE
	21.14	21.14	090	2	1	1	1	1

27479 Arrest, epiphyseal, any method (eg, epiphysiodesis); combined distal femur, proximal tibia and fibula ▣G2T

RVU			Global Days	Modifiers				
Mod	Non-Fac Total	Fac Total		51	50	62	80	MUE
	22.71	22.71	090	2	1	0	2	1

27485 Arrest, hemiepiphyseal, distal femur or proximal tibia or fibula (eg, genu varus or valgus) ⊘T

RVU			Global Days	Modifiers				
Mod	Non-Fac Total	Fac Total		51	50	62	80	MUE
	19.37	19.37	090	2	1	0	1	1

AMA: Nov 98: 8

27486 Revision of total knee arthroplasty, with or without allograft; 1 component ▣C

RVU			Global Days	Modifiers				
Mod	Non-Fac Total	Fac Total		51	50	62	80	MUE
	40.59	40.59	090	2	1	1	2	1

AMA: Dec 13: 16, Jul 15: 10

27487 Revision of total knee arthroplasty, with or without allograft; femoral and entire tibial component ▣C

RVU			Global Days	Modifiers				
Mod	Non-Fac Total	Fac Total		51	50	62	80	MUE
	50.68	50.68	090	2	1	1	2	1

AMA: Nov 98: 8, Jul 13: 6

27488 Removal of prosthesis, including total knee prosthesis, methylmethacrylate with or without insertion of spacer, knee ▣C

RVU			Global Days	Modifiers				
Mod	Non-Fac Total	Fac Total		51	50	62	80	MUE
	34.69	34.69	090	2	1	1	2	1

AMA: Nov 98: 8, Jul 13: 6

● New ▲ Revised Deleted ⊙ Moderate Sedation ✚ Add-on Codes ⊘ High Risk Denial Ⓐ Age Edit ♀ Female ♂ Male **AMA** *CPT® Assistant* **MUE** Medically Unlikely Edit ⊘ Modifier 51 Exempt ⊖ Modifier 63 Exempt ✗ Unlisted **Modifiers:** *See Inside Back Cover* Ⓜ Maternity A2–Z3 ASC Payment Indicators A–Y OPPS Status Indicators

27495 Prophylactic treatment (nailing, pinning, plating, or wiring) with or without methylmethacrylate, femur   C

RVU			Global Days	Modifiers				
Mod	Non-Fac Total	Fac Total		51	50	62	80	MUE
	32.58	32.58	090	2	1	1	2	1

27496 Decompression fasciotomy, thigh and/or knee, 1 compartment (flexor or extensor or adductor)   A2T

RVU			Global Days	Modifiers				
Mod	Non-Fac Total	Fac Total		51	50	62	80	MUE
	15.62	15.62	090	2	1	0	1	1

27497 Decompression fasciotomy, thigh and/or knee, 1 compartment (flexor or extensor or adductor); with debridement of nonviable muscle and/or nerve   A2T

RVU			Global Days	Modifiers				
Mod	Non-Fac Total	Fac Total		51	50	62	80	MUE
	16.71	16.71	090	2	1	2	0	1

27498 Decompression fasciotomy, thigh and/or knee, multiple compartments   A2T

RVU			Global Days	Modifiers				
Mod	Non-Fac Total	Fac Total		51	50	62	80	MUE
	18.62	18.62	090	2	1	2	2	1

27499 Decompression fasciotomy, thigh and/or knee, multiple compartments; with debridement of nonviable muscle and/or nerve   A2T

RVU			Global Days	Modifiers				
Mod	Non-Fac Total	Fac Total		51	50	62	80	MUE
	20.16	20.16	090	2	1	2	2	1

Thigh Region/Knee Fracture/Dislocation Procedures

27500 Closed treatment of femoral shaft fracture, without manipulation   A2T

Coding tip: Closed treatment of femoral shaft fracture with manipulation - 27502

RVU			Global Days	Modifiers				
Mod	Non-Fac Total	Fac Total		51	50	62	80	MUE
	14.97	13.89	090	2	1	0	1	1

27501 Closed treatment of supracondylar or transcondylar femoral fracture with or without intercondylar extension, without manipulation   A2T

Coding tip: Closed treatment of femoral supracondylar/transcondylar fracture with manipulation - 27503

RVU			Global Days	Modifiers				
Mod	Non-Fac Total	Fac Total		51	50	62	80	MUE
	14.53	14.42	090	2	1	0	0	1

27502 Closed treatment of femoral shaft fracture, with manipulation, with or without skin or skeletal traction   A2T

Coding tip: Skeletal traction requires the use of a wire, pin, screw, or clamp attached through the bone, which is included in the initial placement - code separately only when a subsequent traction device is placed

Coding tip: Add modifier 77 for re-reduction of the fracture by another physician

Coding tip: Removal of the initial traction device is included - code separately only when a subsequent traction device is removed

RVU			Global Days	Modifiers				
Mod	Non-Fac Total	Fac Total		51	50	62	80	MUE
	22.36	22.36	090	2	1	0	1	1

AMA: Fall 93: 22, Oct 99: 5

Closed treatment, femoral shaft fracture

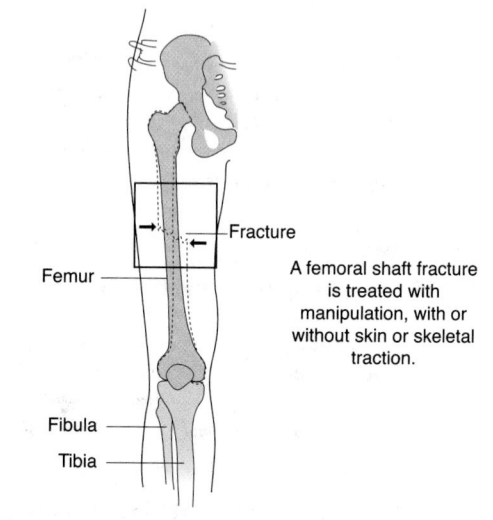

A femoral shaft fracture is treated with manipulation, with or without skin or skeletal traction.

27503 Closed treatment of supracondylar or transcondylar femoral fracture with or without intercondylar extension, with manipulation, with or without skin or skeletal traction   A2T

RVU			Global Days	Modifiers				
Mod	Non-Fac Total	Fac Total		51	50	62	80	MUE
	23.23	23.23	090	2	1	0	0	1

27506 Open treatment of femoral shaft fracture, with or without external fixation, with insertion of intramedullary implant, with or without cerclage and/or locking screws   C

RVU			Global Days	Modifiers				
Mod	Non-Fac Total	Fac Total		51	50	62	80	MUE
	38.71	38.71	090	2	1	1	2	1

AMA: Winter 92: 10, Jun 09: 7

27507 Open treatment of femoral shaft fracture with plate/screws, with or without cerclage   C

RVU			Global Days	Modifiers				
Mod	Non-Fac Total	Fac Total		51	50	62	80	MUE
	28.08	28.08	090	2	1	2	2	1

● New   ▲ Revised   ✖ Deleted   ⊙ Moderate Sedation   ✚ Add-on Codes   ⊘ High Risk Denial   Ⓐ Age Edit   ♀ Female   ♂ Male   **AMA** CPT® Assistant   **MUE** Medically Unlikely Edit
⊘ Modifier 51 Exempt   ⊖ Modifier 63 Exempt   ✗ Unlisted   **Modifiers:** See Inside Back Cover   Ⓜ Maternity   A2–Z3 ASC Payment Indicators   A–Y OPPS Status Indicators

CPT © 2015 American Medical Association. All Rights Reserved.   © 2016 DecisionHealth

27508   Closed treatment of femoral fracture, distal end, medial or lateral condyle, without manipulation   A 2 T

Coding tip: Closed treatment of distal femoral fracture with manipulation - 27510

RVU			Global Days	Modifiers				
Mod	Non-Fac Total	Fac Total		51	50	62	80	MUE
	15.16	14.29	090	2	1	0	1	1

27509   Percutaneous skeletal fixation of femoral fracture, distal end, medial or lateral condyle, or supracondylar or transcondylar, with or without intercondylar extension, or distal femoral epiphyseal separation   A 2 J 1

RVU			Global Days	Modifiers				
Mod	Non-Fac Total	Fac Total		51	50	62	80	MUE
	18.51	18.51	090	2	1	0	0	1

27510   Closed treatment of femoral fracture, distal end, medial or lateral condyle, with manipulation   A 2 T

Coding tip: Closed treatment of distal femoral fracture without manipulation - 27508

Coding tip: Add modifier 77 for re-reduction of the fracture by another physician

RVU			Global Days	Modifiers				
Mod	Non-Fac Total	Fac Total		51	50	62	80	MUE
	19.94	19.94	090	2	1	0	1	1

27511   Open treatment of femoral supracondylar or transcondylar fracture without intercondylar extension, includes internal fixation, when performed   C

RVU			Global Days	Modifiers				
Mod	Non-Fac Total	Fac Total		51	50	62	80	MUE
	28.84	28.84	090	2	1	2	2	1

AMA: May 96: 6

Open treatment of femoral supracondylar or transcondylar fracture

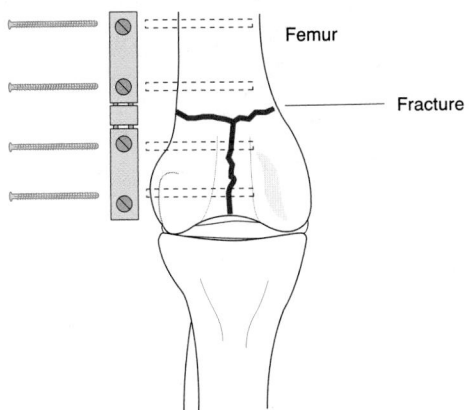

Use (27511) when the fracture does not extend into the intercondylar region. Use (27513) when a fracture of the intercondylar region is treated and an arthrotomy is done

27513   Open treatment of femoral supracondylar or transcondylar fracture with intercondylar extension, includes internal fixation, when performed   C

RVU			Global Days	Modifiers				
Mod	Non-Fac Total	Fac Total		51	50	62	80	MUE
	35.90	35.90	090	2	1	2	2	1

27514   Open treatment of femoral fracture, distal end, medial or lateral condyle, includes internal fixation, when performed   C

RVU			Global Days	Modifiers				
Mod	Non-Fac Total	Fac Total		51	50	62	80	MUE
	27.98	27.98	090	2	1	1	2	1

27516   Closed treatment of distal femoral epiphyseal separation; without manipulation   A 2 T

RVU			Global Days	Modifiers				
Mod	Non-Fac Total	Fac Total		51	50	62	80	MUE
	14.63	13.76	090	2	1	0	1	1

27517   Closed treatment of distal femoral epiphyseal separation; with manipulation, with or without skin or skeletal traction   A 2 T

Coding tip: Skeletal traction requires the use of a wire, pin, screw, or clamp attached through the bone, which is included in the initial placement - code separately only when a subsequent traction device is placed

Coding tip: Add modifier 77 for re-reduction by another physician

Coding tip: Removal of the initial traction device is included - code separately only when a subsequent traction device is removed

RVU			Global Days	Modifiers				
Mod	Non-Fac Total	Fac Total		51	50	62	80	MUE
	19.44	19.44	090	2	1	0	0	1

27519   Open treatment of distal femoral epiphyseal separation, includes internal fixation, when performed   C

RVU			Global Days	Modifiers				
Mod	Non-Fac Total	Fac Total		51	50	62	80	MUE
	25.84	25.84	090	2	1	1	2	1

27520   Closed treatment of patellar fracture, without manipulation   A 2 T

RVU			Global Days	Modifiers				
Mod	Non-Fac Total	Fac Total		51	50	62	80	MUE
	9.26	8.47	090	2	1	0	1	1

27524   Open treatment of patellar fracture, with internal fixation and/or partial or complete patellectomy and soft tissue repair   G 2 T

RVU			Global Days	Modifiers				
Mod	Non-Fac Total	Fac Total		51	50	62	80	MUE
	21.72	21.72	090	2	1	1	2	1

27530   Closed treatment of tibial fracture, proximal (plateau); without manipulation   A 2 T

RVU			Global Days	Modifiers				
Mod	Non-Fac Total	Fac Total		51	50	62	80	MUE
	8.66	8.05	090	2	1	0	1	1

● New   ▲ Revised   Deleted   ⊙ Moderate Sedation   ✚ Add-on Codes   ⊘ High Risk Denial   Ⓐ Age Edit   ♀ Female   ♂ Male   **AMA** CPT® Assistant   **MUE** Medically Unlikely Edit
⊘ Modifier 51 Exempt   ⊖ Modifier 63 Exempt   ✘ Unlisted   **Modifiers:** See Inside Back Cover   Ⓜ Maternity   A 2 - Z 3 ASC Payment Indicators   A - Y OPPS Status Indicators

27532 Closed treatment of tibial fracture, proximal (plateau); with or without manipulation, with skeletal traction A2T

RVU			Global Days	Modifiers				
Mod	Non-Fac Total	Fac Total		51	50	62	80	MUE
	17.70	16.63	090	2	1	0	1	1

27535 Open treatment of tibial fracture, proximal (plateau); unicondylar, includes internal fixation, when performed C

RVU			Global Days	Modifiers				
Mod	Non-Fac Total	Fac Total		51	50	62	80	MUE
	25.96	25.96	090	2	1	2	2	1

27536 Open treatment of tibial fracture, proximal (plateau); bicondylar, with or without internal fixation C

RVU			Global Days	Modifiers				
Mod	Non-Fac Total	Fac Total		51	50	62	80	MUE
	34.40	34.40	090	2	1	1	2	1

27538 Closed treatment of intercondylar spine(s) and/or tuberosity fracture(s) of knee, with or without manipulation A2T

RVU			Global Days	Modifiers				
Mod	Non-Fac Total	Fac Total		51	50	62	80	MUE
	13.57	12.73	090	2	1	0	0	1

27540 Open treatment of intercondylar spine(s) and/or tuberosity fracture(s) of the knee, includes internal fixation, when performed C

RVU			Global Days	Modifiers				
Mod	Non-Fac Total	Fac Total		51	50	62	80	MUE
	23.36	23.36	090	2	1	1	2	1

27550 Closed treatment of knee dislocation; without anesthesia A2T

RVU			Global Days	Modifiers				
Mod	Non-Fac Total	Fac Total		51	50	62	80	MUE
	14.62	13.60	090	2	1	0	0	1

27552 Closed treatment of knee dislocation; requiring anesthesia A2T

RVU			Global Days	Modifiers				
Mod	Non-Fac Total	Fac Total		51	50	62	80	MUE
	18.05	18.05	090	2	1	0	0	1

27556 Open treatment of knee dislocation, includes internal fixation, when performed; without primary ligamentous repair or augmentation/reconstruction C

RVU			Global Days	Modifiers				
Mod	Non-Fac Total	Fac Total		51	50	62	80	MUE
	25.28	25.28	090	2	1	1	2	1

27557 Open treatment of knee dislocation, includes internal fixation, when performed; with primary ligamentous repair C

RVU			Global Days	Modifiers				
Mod	Non-Fac Total	Fac Total		51	50	62	80	MUE
	30.39	30.39	090	2	1	1	2	1

27558 Open treatment of knee dislocation, includes internal fixation, when performed; with primary ligamentous repair, with augmentation/reconstruction C

RVU			Global Days	Modifiers				
Mod	Non-Fac Total	Fac Total		51	50	62	80	MUE
	34.50	34.50	090	2	1	2	2	1

27560 Closed treatment of patellar dislocation; without anesthesia A2T

RVU			Global Days	Modifiers				
Mod	Non-Fac Total	Fac Total		51	50	62	80	MUE
	10.42	9.64	090	2	1	0	1	1

AMA: Apr 02: 15

27562 Closed treatment of patellar dislocation; requiring anesthesia A2T

RVU			Global Days	Modifiers				
Mod	Non-Fac Total	Fac Total		51	50	62	80	MUE
	13.52	13.52	090	2	1	0	0	1

27566 Open treatment of patellar dislocation, with or without partial or total patellectomy A2T

RVU			Global Days	Modifiers				
Mod	Non-Fac Total	Fac Total		51	50	62	80	MUE
	25.76	25.76	090	2	1	1	2	1

Thigh Region/Knee Manipulation

27570 Manipulation of knee joint under general anesthesia (includes application of traction or other fixation devices) A2T

RVU			Global Days	Modifiers				
Mod	Non-Fac Total	Fac Total		51	50	62	80	MUE
	4.36	4.36	010	2	1	0	1	1

AMA: Mar 11: 9

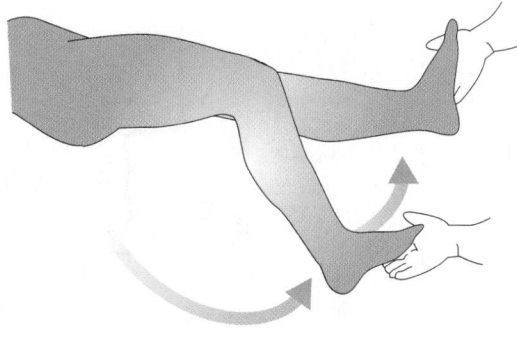

Manipulation of knee joint under general anesthesia

Under general anesthesia, the physician flexes the knee joint to increase its range of motion.

Thigh Region/Knee Arthrodesis

27580 Arthrodesis, knee, any technique C

RVU			Global Days	Modifiers				
Mod	Non-Fac Total	Fac Total		51	50	62	80	MUE
	41.50	41.50	090	2	1	1	2	1

● New ▲ Revised ✖ Deleted ⊙ Moderate Sedation ✚ Add-on Codes ⊘ High Risk Denial Ⓐ Age Edit ♀ Female ♂ Male **AMA** *CPT® Assistant* **MUE** Medically Unlikely Edit ⊘ Modifier 51 Exempt ⊖ Modifier 63 Exempt ✗ Unlisted **Modifiers:** *See Inside Back Cover* Ⓜ Maternity A2–Z3 ASC Payment Indicators A–Y OPPS Status Indicators

CPT © 2015 American Medical Association. All Rights Reserved. © 2016 DecisionHealth

Thigh Region/Knee Amputation

27590 Amputation, thigh, through femur, any level   C

RVU			Global Days	Modifiers				
Mod	Non-Fac Total	Fac Total		51	50	62	80	MUE
	23.45	23.45	090	2	1	1	2	1

27591 Amputation, thigh, through femur, any level; immediate fitting technique including first cast   C

RVU			Global Days	Modifiers				
Mod	Non-Fac Total	Fac Total		51	50	62	80	MUE
	27.92	27.92	090	2	1	1	2	1

27592 Amputation, thigh, through femur, any level; open, circular (guillotine)   C

RVU			Global Days	Modifiers				
Mod	Non-Fac Total	Fac Total		51	50	62	80	MUE
	19.91	19.91	090	2	1	1	2	1

27594 Amputation, thigh, through femur, any level; secondary closure or scar revision   A 2 T

RVU			Global Days	Modifiers				
Mod	Non-Fac Total	Fac Total		51	50	62	80	MUE
	14.76	14.76	090	2	1	0	1	1

27596 Amputation, thigh, through femur, any level; re-amputation   C

RVU			Global Days	Modifiers				
Mod	Non-Fac Total	Fac Total		51	50	62	80	MUE
	21.08	21.08	090	2	1	1	1	1

27598 Disarticulation at knee   C

RVU			Global Days	Modifiers				
Mod	Non-Fac Total	Fac Total		51	50	62	80	MUE
	21.05	21.05	090	2	1	1	2	1

Other Thigh Region/Knee Procedures

27599 Unlisted procedure, femur or knee   x T

RVU			Global Days	Modifiers				
Mod	Non-Fac Total	Fac Total		51	50	62	80	MUE
	0.00	0.00	YYY	2	1	1	2	

AMA: Mar 08: 14, Dec 12: 13, Jan 14: 9, Jan 15: 13

Lower Leg/Ankle Procedures

Lower Leg/Ankle Incisional Procedures

27600 Decompression fasciotomy, leg; anterior and/or lateral compartments only   A 2 T

RVU			Global Days	Modifiers				
Mod	Non-Fac Total	Fac Total		51	50	62	80	MUE
	12.05	12.05	090	2	1	1	1	1

27601 Decompression fasciotomy, leg; posterior compartment(s) only   A 2 T

RVU			Global Days	Modifiers				
Mod	Non-Fac Total	Fac Total		51	50	62	80	MUE
	12.71	12.71	090	2	1	0	1	1

27602 Decompression fasciotomy, leg; anterior and/or lateral, and posterior compartment(s)   A 2 T

RVU			Global Days	Modifiers				
Mod	Non-Fac Total	Fac Total		51	50	62	80	MUE
	14.47	14.47	090	2	1	1	2	1

27603 Incision and drainage, leg or ankle; deep abscess or hematoma   A 2 T

RVU			Global Days	Modifiers				
Mod	Non-Fac Total	Fac Total		51	50	62	80	MUE
	15.24	11.22	090	2	1	0	1	2

27604 Incision and drainage, leg or ankle; infected bursa   A 2 T

RVU			Global Days	Modifiers				
Mod	Non-Fac Total	Fac Total		51	50	62	80	MUE
	14.18	9.96	090	2	1	0	0	2

27605 Tenotomy, percutaneous, Achilles tendon (separate procedure); local anesthesia   A 2 T

RVU			Global Days	Modifiers				
Mod	Non-Fac Total	Fac Total		51	50	62	80	MUE
	9.80	5.31	010	2	1	0	0	1

27606 Tenotomy, percutaneous, Achilles tendon (separate procedure); general anesthesia   A 2 T

RVU			Global Days	Modifiers				
Mod	Non-Fac Total	Fac Total		51	50	62	80	MUE
	8.14	8.14	010	2	1	1	1	1

27607 Incision (eg, osteomyelitis or bone abscess), leg or ankle   A 2 T

RVU			Global Days	Modifiers				
Mod	Non-Fac Total	Fac Total		51	50	62	80	MUE
	17.53	17.53	090	2	1	0	1	2

27610 Arthrotomy, ankle, including exploration, drainage, or removal of foreign body   A 2 T

RVU			Global Days	Modifiers				
Mod	Non-Fac Total	Fac Total		51	50	62	80	MUE
	18.80	18.80	090	2	1	0	1	1

AMA: Nov 98: 9

27612 Arthrotomy, posterior capsular release, ankle, with or without Achilles tendon lengthening   A 2 T

RVU			Global Days	Modifiers				
Mod	Non-Fac Total	Fac Total		51	50	62	80	MUE
	16.02	16.02	090	2	1	1	2	1

AMA: Nov 98: 8

Lower Leg/Ankle Excisional Procedures

27613 Biopsy, soft tissue of leg or ankle area; superficial   P 3 T

Coding tip: Code 99000 for specimen transfer from office setting to an outside laboratory

RVU			Global Days	Modifiers				
Mod	Non-Fac Total	Fac Total		51	50	62	80	MUE
	7.20	4.68	010	2	1	0	1	4

27614 Biopsy, soft tissue of leg or ankle area; deep (subfascial or intramuscular)   A 2 T

RVU			Global Days	Modifiers				
Mod	Non-Fac Total	Fac Total		51	50	62	80	MUE
	16.53	11.62	090	2	1	0	1	3

AMA: Nov 98: 8

● New   ▲ Revised   Deleted   ⊙ Moderate Sedation   ✚ Add-on Codes   ⊗ High Risk Denial   Ⓐ Age Edit   ♀ Female   ♂ Male   **AMA** CPT® Assistant   **MUE** Medically Unlikely Edit
⊘ Modifier 51 Exempt   ⊖ Modifier 63 Exempt   ✗ Unlisted   **Modifiers:** See Inside Back Cover   Ⓜ Maternity   A2 – Z3 ASC Payment Indicators   A – Y OPPS Status Indicators

27615 Radical resection of tumor (eg, sarcoma), soft tissue of leg or ankle area; less than 5 cm `G2 T`

Mod	Non-Fac Total	Fac Total	Global Days	51	50	62	80	MUE
	29.67	29.67	090	2	1	1	0	1

27616 Radical resection of tumor (eg, sarcoma), soft tissue of leg or ankle area; 5 cm or greater `G2 T`

Mod	Non-Fac Total	Fac Total	Global Days	51	50	62	80	MUE
	36.91	36.91	090	2	1	1	0	1

27618 Excision, tumor, soft tissue of leg or ankle area, subcutaneous; less than 3 cm `G2 T`

Coding tip: Related soft tissue tumor excision - 27619, 27632, 27634

Mod	Non-Fac Total	Fac Total	Global Days	51	50	62	80	MUE
	12.87	8.86	090	2	1	0	1	4

27619 Excision, tumor, soft tissue of leg or ankle area, subfascial (eg, intramuscular); less than 5 cm `G2 T`

Coding tip: Related soft tissue tumor excision - 27618, 27632, 27634

Mod	Non-Fac Total	Fac Total	Global Days	51	50	62	80	MUE
	13.56	13.56	090	2	1	0	1	4

27620 Arthrotomy, ankle, with joint exploration, with or without biopsy, with or without removal of loose or foreign body `A2 T`

Mod	Non-Fac Total	Fac Total	Global Days	51	50	62	80	MUE
	13.13	13.13	090	2	1	1	2	1

27625 Arthrotomy, with synovectomy, ankle `A2 T`

Mod	Non-Fac Total	Fac Total	Global Days	51	50	62	80	MUE
	16.86	16.86	090	2	1	1	2	1

AMA: Nov 98: 8

27626 Arthrotomy, with synovectomy, ankle; including tenosynovectomy `A2 T`

Mod	Non-Fac Total	Fac Total	Global Days	51	50	62	80	MUE
	17.78	17.78	090	2	1	0	2	1

27630 Excision of lesion of tendon sheath or capsule (eg, cyst or ganglion), leg and/or ankle `A2 T`

Mod	Non-Fac Total	Fac Total	Global Days	51	50	62	80	MUE
	16.12	10.55	090	2	1	0	1	2

27632 Excision, tumor, soft tissue of leg or ankle area, subcutaneous; 3 cm or greater `G2 T`

Coding tip: Code 27632 is listed out of numerical order in CPT. Related soft tissue tumor excision procedures - 27618 (subcutaneous tissue); 27619, 27634 (subfascial)

Mod	Non-Fac Total	Fac Total	Global Days	51	50	62	80	MUE
	11.99	11.99	090	2	1	0	2	4

AMA: Apr 10: 3

27634 Excision, tumor, soft tissue of leg or ankle area, subfascial (eg, intramuscular); 5 cm or greater `G2 T`

Coding tip: Code 27634 is listed out of numerical order in CPT. Related soft tissue tumor excision procedures - 27618, 27632 (subcutaneous tissue); 27619 (subfascial)

Mod	Non-Fac Total	Fac Total	Global Days	51	50	62	80	MUE
	19.87	19.87	090	2	1	0	2	2

27635 Excision or curettage of bone cyst or benign tumor, tibia or fibula `A2 T`

Mod	Non-Fac Total	Fac Total	Global Days	51	50	62	80	MUE
	16.93	16.93	090	2	1	1	1	1

AMA: Apr 12: 17

27637 Excision or curettage of bone cyst or benign tumor, tibia or fibula; with autograft (includes obtaining graft) `A2 J1`

Mod	Non-Fac Total	Fac Total	Global Days	51	50	62	80	MUE
	21.52	21.52	090	2	1	1	2	1

27638 Excision or curettage of bone cyst or benign tumor, tibia or fibula; with allograft `A2 J1`

Mod	Non-Fac Total	Fac Total	Global Days	51	50	62	80	MUE
	21.98	21.98	090	2	1	1	2	1

27640 Partial excision (craterization, saucerization, or diaphysectomy), bone (eg, osteomyelitis); tibia `A2 T`

Mod	Non-Fac Total	Fac Total	Global Days	51	50	62	80	MUE
	24.10	24.10	090	2	1	1	1	1

AMA: Apr 12: 17

27641 Partial excision (craterization, saucerization, or diaphysectomy), bone (eg, osteomyelitis); fibula `A2 T`

Mod	Non-Fac Total	Fac Total	Global Days	51	50	62	80	MUE
	19.29	19.29	090	2	1	1	1	1

27645 Radical resection of tumor; tibia `C`

Mod	Non-Fac Total	Fac Total	Global Days	51	50	62	80	MUE
	51.47	51.47	090	2	1	1	2	1

27646 Radical resection of tumor; fibula `C`

Mod	Non-Fac Total	Fac Total	Global Days	51	50	62	80	MUE
	44.62	44.62	090	2	1	1	2	1

27647 Radical resection of tumor; talus or calcaneus `A2 T`

Mod	Non-Fac Total	Fac Total	Global Days	51	50	62	80	MUE
	29.51	29.51	090	2	1	0	2	1

● New   ▲ Revised   ✖ Deleted   ⊙ Moderate Sedation   ✚ Add-on Codes   ⊘ High Risk Denial   Ⓐ Age Edit   ♀ Female   ♂ Male   **AMA** CPT® Assistant   **MUE** Medically Unlikely Edit   ⊘ Modifier 51 Exempt   ⊖ Modifier 63 Exempt   Ⓧ Unlisted   **Modifiers:** See Inside Back Cover   Ⓜ Maternity   A2–Z3 ASC Payment Indicators   A–Y OPPS Status Indicators

CPT © 2015 American Medical Association. All Rights Reserved.   © 2016 DecisionHealth

Lower Leg/Ankle Introduction/Removal Procedures

27648 Injection procedure for ankle arthrography N I N

RVU			Global Days	Modifiers				
Mod	Non-Fac Total	Fac Total		51	50	62	80	MUE
	4.68	1.52	000	2	1	0	0	1

AMA: Aug 15: 6

Lower Leg/Ankle Repair/Revision/Reconstruction Procedures

27650 Repair, primary, open or percutaneous, ruptured Achilles tendon A 2 T

RVU			Global Days	Modifiers				
Mod	Non-Fac Total	Fac Total		51	50	62	80	MUE
	19.01	19.01	090	2	1	1	2	1

AMA: Jul 14: 5

27652 Repair, primary, open or percutaneous, ruptured Achilles tendon; with graft (includes obtaining graft) A 2 J I

RVU			Global Days	Modifiers				
Mod	Non-Fac Total	Fac Total		51	50	62	80	MUE
	19.72	19.72	090	2	1	1	1	1

AMA: Jul 14: 5

27654 Repair, secondary, Achilles tendon, with or without graft A 2 J I

RVU			Global Days	Modifiers				
Mod	Non-Fac Total	Fac Total		51	50	62	80	MUE
	20.34	20.34	090	2	1	1	2	1

AMA: Jul 14: 5

27656 Repair, fascial defect of leg A 2 T

RVU			Global Days	Modifiers				
Mod	Non-Fac Total	Fac Total		51	50	62	80	MUE
	18.29	11.45	090	2	1	0	2	1

27658 Repair, flexor tendon, leg; primary, without graft, each tendon A 2 T

RVU			Global Days	Modifiers				
Mod	Non-Fac Total	Fac Total		51	50	62	80	MUE
	10.72	10.72	090	2	0	1	2	2

AMA: Nov 98: 8

27659 Repair, flexor tendon, leg; secondary, with or without graft, each tendon A 2 T

RVU			Global Days	Modifiers				
Mod	Non-Fac Total	Fac Total		51	50	62	80	MUE
	13.82	13.82	090	2	0	1	2	2

AMA: Jan 15: 13

27664 Repair, extensor tendon, leg; primary, without graft, each tendon A 2 T

RVU			Global Days	Modifiers				
Mod	Non-Fac Total	Fac Total		51	50	62	80	MUE
	10.39	10.39	090	2	0	0	0	2

AMA: Nov 98: 8, Jan 15: 13

27665 Repair, extensor tendon, leg; secondary, with or without graft, each tendon A 2 J I

RVU			Global Days	Modifiers				
Mod	Non-Fac Total	Fac Total		51	50	62	80	MUE
	11.79	11.79	090	2	0	1	2	2

AMA: Nov 98: 8

27675 Repair, dislocating peroneal tendons; without fibular osteotomy A 2 T

RVU			Global Days	Modifiers				
Mod	Non-Fac Total	Fac Total		51	50	62	80	MUE
	13.99	13.99	090	2	1	1	2	1

27676 Repair, dislocating peroneal tendons; with fibular osteotomy A 2 T

RVU			Global Days	Modifiers				
Mod	Non-Fac Total	Fac Total		51	50	62	80	MUE
	17.36	17.36	090	2	1	0	2	1

27680 Tenolysis, flexor or extensor tendon, leg and/or ankle; single, each tendon A 2 T

RVU			Global Days	Modifiers				
Mod	Non-Fac Total	Fac Total		51	50	62	80	MUE
	12.28	12.28	090	2	0	1	1	3

AMA: Nov 98: 8

27681 Tenolysis, flexor or extensor tendon, leg and/or ankle; multiple tendons (through separate incision[s]) A 2 T

RVU			Global Days	Modifiers				
Mod	Non-Fac Total	Fac Total		51	50	62	80	MUE
	15.74	15.74	090	2	1	1	1	1

AMA: Nov 98: 8

27685 Lengthening or shortening of tendon, leg or ankle; single tendon (separate procedure) A 2 T

RVU			Global Days	Modifiers				
Mod	Non-Fac Total	Fac Total		51	50	62	80	MUE
	19.02	13.32	090	2	1	1	2	2

AMA: Nov 98: 8, Sep 09: 11

27686 Lengthening or shortening of tendon, leg or ankle; multiple tendons (through same incision), each A 2 T

RVU			Global Days	Modifiers				
Mod	Non-Fac Total	Fac Total		51	50	62	80	MUE
	16.07	16.07	090	2	1	1	1	3

AMA: Nov 98: 8, Sep 09: 11

27687 Gastrocnemius recession (eg, Strayer procedure) A 2 T

RVU			Global Days	Modifiers				
Mod	Non-Fac Total	Fac Total		51	50	62	80	MUE
	13.06	13.06	090	2	1	1	2	1

27690 Transfer or transplant of single tendon (with muscle redirection or rerouting); superficial (eg, anterior tibial extensors into midfoot) A 2 T

RVU			Global Days	Modifiers				
Mod	Non-Fac Total	Fac Total		51	50	62	80	MUE
	18.07	18.07	090	2	1	1	2	2

27691 Transfer or transplant of single tendon (with muscle redirection or rerouting); deep (eg, anterior tibial or posterior tibial through interosseous space, flexor digitorum longus, flexor hallucis longus, or peroneal tendon to midfoot or hindfoot) A 2 T

RVU			Global Days	Modifiers				
Mod	Non-Fac Total	Fac Total		51	50	62	80	MUE
	21.61	21.61	090	2	1	1	2	2

● New   ▲ Revised   Deleted   ⊙ Moderate Sedation   ✚ Add-on Codes   ⊗ High Risk Denial   Ⓐ Age Edit   ♀ Female   ♂ Male   **AMA** CPT® Assistant   **MUE** Medically Unlikely Edit
⊘ Modifier 51 Exempt   ⊖ Modifier 63 Exempt   ✗ Unlisted   **Modifiers:** See Inside Back Cover   Ⓜ Maternity   A 2 – Z 3 ASC Payment Indicators   A – Y OPPS Status Indicators

© 2016 DecisionHealth   CPT © 2015 American Medical Association. All Rights Reserved.

+ 27692 Transfer or transplant of single tendon (with muscle redirection or rerouting); each additional tendon (List separately in addition to code for primary procedure)   N I N

RVU			Global Days	Modifiers				
Mod	Non-Fac Total	Fac Total		51	50	62	80	MUE
	3.02	3.02	ZZZ	0	0	1	2	4

27695 Repair, primary, disrupted ligament, ankle; collateral   A 2 T

RVU			Global Days	Modifiers				
Mod	Non-Fac Total	Fac Total		51	50	62	80	MUE
	13.51	13.51	090	2	1	1	1	1

AMA: Mar 14: 14

27696 Repair, primary, disrupted ligament, ankle; both collateral ligaments   A 2 T

RVU			Global Days	Modifiers				
Mod	Non-Fac Total	Fac Total		51	50	62	80	MUE
	16.00	16.00	090	2	1	1	1	1

AMA: Mar 14: 14

27698 Repair, secondary, disrupted ligament, ankle, collateral (eg, Watson-Jones procedure)   A 2 T

RVU			Global Days	Modifiers				
Mod	Non-Fac Total	Fac Total		51	50	62	80	MUE
	18.40	18.40	090	2	1	1	2	2

AMA: Mar 14: 14

27700 Arthroplasty, ankle   A 2 J I

RVU			Global Days	Modifiers				
Mod	Non-Fac Total	Fac Total		51	50	62	80	MUE
	17.14	17.14	090	2	1	1	2	1

27702 Arthroplasty, ankle; with implant (total ankle) ⊙ C

RVU			Global Days	Modifiers				
Mod	Non-Fac Total	Fac Total		51	50	62	80	MUE
	27.89	27.89	090	2	1	1	2	1

27703 Arthroplasty, ankle; revision, total ankle   C

RVU			Global Days	Modifiers				
Mod	Non-Fac Total	Fac Total		51	50	62	80	MUE
	32.05	32.05	090	2	1	0	2	1

27704 Removal of ankle implant   A 2 Q 2

RVU			Global Days	Modifiers				
Mod	Non-Fac Total	Fac Total		51	50	62	80	MUE
	16.68	16.68	090	2	1	1	1	1

27705 Osteotomy; tibia   A 2 T

RVU			Global Days	Modifiers				
Mod	Non-Fac Total	Fac Total		51	50	62	80	MUE
	21.83	21.83	090	2	1	1	2	1

27707 Osteotomy; fibula   A 2 T

RVU			Global Days	Modifiers				
Mod	Non-Fac Total	Fac Total		51	50	62	80	MUE
	11.65	11.65	090	2	1	1	1	1

27709 Osteotomy; tibia and fibula   A 2 J I

RVU			Global Days	Modifiers				
Mod	Non-Fac Total	Fac Total		51	50	62	80	MUE
	33.74	33.74	090	2	1	1	2	1

27712 Osteotomy; multiple, with realignment on intramedullary rod (eg, Sofield type procedure) C

RVU			Global Days	Modifiers				
Mod	Non-Fac Total	Fac Total		51	50	62	80	MUE
	31.89	31.89	090	2	1	1	2	1

27715 Osteoplasty, tibia and fibula, lengthening or shortening   C

RVU			Global Days	Modifiers				
Mod	Non-Fac Total	Fac Total		51	50	62	80	MUE
	31.03	31.03	090	2	1	1	2	1

27720 Repair of nonunion or malunion, tibia; without graft, (eg, compression technique)   G 2 J I

RVU			Global Days	Modifiers				
Mod	Non-Fac Total	Fac Total		51	50	62	80	MUE
	25.25	25.25	090	2	1	1	2	1

27722 Repair of nonunion or malunion, tibia; with sliding graft   J I

RVU			Global Days	Modifiers				
Mod	Non-Fac Total	Fac Total		51	50	62	80	MUE
	25.44	25.44	090	2	1	1	2	1

27724 Repair of nonunion or malunion, tibia; with iliac or other autograft (includes obtaining graft)   C

RVU			Global Days	Modifiers				
Mod	Non-Fac Total	Fac Total		51	50	62	80	MUE
	36.54	36.54	090	2	1	1	2	1

AMA: May 12: 11

27725 Repair of nonunion or malunion, tibia; by synostosis, with fibula, any method   C

RVU			Global Days	Modifiers				
Mod	Non-Fac Total	Fac Total		51	50	62	80	MUE
	34.84	34.84	090	2	1	1	2	1

27726 Repair of fibula nonunion and/or malunion with internal fixation   G 2 J I

RVU			Global Days	Modifiers				
Mod	Non-Fac Total	Fac Total		51	50	62	80	MUE
	28.04	28.04	090	2	1	1	1	1

AMA: Jan 08: 4, Apr 09: 9

27727 Repair of congenital pseudarthrosis, tibia   C

RVU			Global Days	Modifiers				
Mod	Non-Fac Total	Fac Total		51	50	62	80	MUE
	30.03	30.03	090	2	1	1	2	1

27730 Arrest, epiphyseal (epiphysiodesis), open; distal tibia   A 2 T

RVU			Global Days	Modifiers				
Mod	Non-Fac Total	Fac Total		51	50	62	80	MUE
	16.46	16.46	090	2	1	1	1	1

AMA: Nov 98: 8

27732 Arrest, epiphyseal (epiphysiodesis), open; distal fibula   A 2 T

RVU			Global Days	Modifiers				
Mod	Non-Fac Total	Fac Total		51	50	62	80	MUE
	11.70	11.70	090	2	1	0	1	1

● New   ▲ Revised   ✖ Deleted   ⊙ Moderate Sedation   ✚ Add-on Codes   ⊘ High Risk Denial   Ⓐ Age Edit   ♀ Female   ♂ Male   **AMA** *CPT® Assistant*   **MUE** Medically Unlikely Edit
⊘ Modifier 51 Exempt   ⊖ Modifier 63 Exempt   ✗ Unlisted   **Modifiers:** *See Inside Back Cover*   Ⓜ Maternity   A 2 – Z 3 ASC Payment Indicators   A – Y OPPS Status Indicators

CPT © 2015 American Medical Association. All Rights Reserved.   © 2016 DecisionHealth

27734 Arrest, epiphyseal (epiphysiodesis), open; distal tibia and fibula   `A 2 T`

RVU			Global Days	Modifiers				
Mod	Non-Fac Total	Fac Total		51	50	62	80	MUE
	18.95	18.95	090	2	1	0	1	1

27740 Arrest, epiphyseal (epiphysiodesis), any method, combined, proximal and distal tibia and fibula   `A 2 T`

RVU			Global Days	Modifiers				
Mod	Non-Fac Total	Fac Total		51	50	62	80	MUE
	20.47	20.47	090	2	1	0	2	1

AMA: Nov 98: 8

27742 Arrest, epiphyseal (epiphysiodesis), any method, combined, proximal and distal tibia and fibula; and distal femur   `A 2 T`

RVU			Global Days	Modifiers				
Mod	Non-Fac Total	Fac Total		51	50	62	80	MUE
	22.63	22.63	090	2	1	1	2	1

27745 Prophylactic treatment (nailing, pinning, plating or wiring) with or without methylmethacrylate, tibia   `G 2 J I`

RVU			Global Days	Modifiers				
Mod	Non-Fac Total	Fac Total		51	50	62	80	MUE
	21.78	21.78	090	2	1	1	2	1

Lower Leg/Ankle Fracture/Dislocation Procedures

27750 Closed treatment of tibial shaft fracture (with or without fibular fracture); without manipulation   `A 2 T`

RVU			Global Days	Modifiers				
Mod	Non-Fac Total	Fac Total		51	50	62	80	MUE
	9.94	9.14	090	2	1	0	1	1

AMA: Winter 92: 10, Fall 93: 21, Mar 96: 10

Closed treatment of tibial shaft fracture

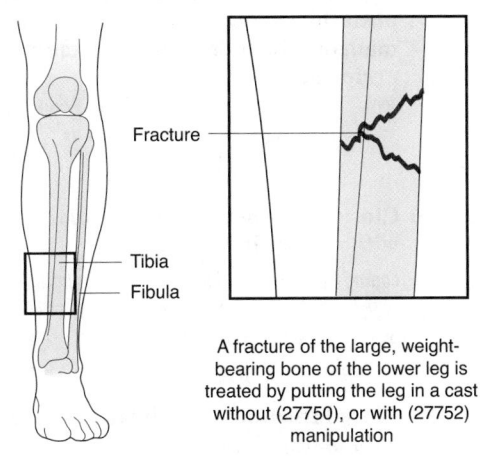

Fracture

Tibia

Fibula

A fracture of the large, weight-bearing bone of the lower leg is treated by putting the leg in a cast without (27750), or with (27752) manipulation

27752 Closed treatment of tibial shaft fracture (with or without fibular fracture); with manipulation, with or without skeletal traction   `A 2 T`

Coding tip: Add modifier 77 for re-reduction of the fracture by another physician

Coding tip: Skeletal traction requires the use of a wire, pin, screw, or clamp attached through the bone, which is included in the initial placement - code separately only when a subsequent traction device is placed

Coding tip: Removal of the initial traction device is included - code separately only when a subsequent traction device is removed

RVU			Global Days	Modifiers				
Mod	Non-Fac Total	Fac Total		51	50	62	80	MUE
	15.51	14.35	090	2	1	0	1	1

AMA: Winter 92: 10, Fall 93: 21, Feb 96: 3, Mar 96: 10

27756 Percutaneous skeletal fixation of tibial shaft fracture (with or without fibular fracture) (eg, pins or screws)   `A 2 J I`

RVU			Global Days	Modifiers				
Mod	Non-Fac Total	Fac Total		51	50	62	80	MUE
	16.49	16.49	090	2	1	1	2	1

AMA: Winter 92: 10

27758 Open treatment of tibial shaft fracture (with or without fibular fracture), with plate/screws, with or without cerclage   `G 2 J I`

RVU			Global Days	Modifiers				
Mod	Non-Fac Total	Fac Total		51	50	62	80	MUE
	25.71	25.71	090	2	1	1	2	1

AMA: Winter 92: 10, Mar 00: 11

27759 Treatment of tibial shaft fracture (with or without fibular fracture) by intramedullary implant, with or without interlocking screws and/or cerclage   `G 2 J I`

RVU			Global Days	Modifiers				
Mod	Non-Fac Total	Fac Total		51	50	62	80	MUE
	28.88	28.88	090	2	1	2	2	1

AMA: Winter 92: 10

27760 Closed treatment of medial malleolus fracture; without manipulation   `A 2 T`

Coding tip: Closed treatment of posterior malleolus fracture - 27767

RVU			Global Days	Modifiers				
Mod	Non-Fac Total	Fac Total		51	50	62	80	MUE
	9.57	8.74	090	2	1	0	1	1

27762 Closed treatment of medial malleolus fracture; with manipulation, with or without skin or skeletal traction   `A 2 T`

Coding tip: Add modifier 77 for re-reduction of the fracture by another physician

Coding tip: Skeletal traction requires the use of a wire, pin, screw, or clamp attached through the bone, which is included in the initial placement - code separately only when a subsequent traction device is placed

Coding tip: Closed treatment of posterior malleolus fracture with manipulation - 27768

Coding tip: Removal of the initial traction device is included - code separately only when a subsequent traction device is removed

RVU			Global Days	Modifiers				
Mod	Non-Fac Total	Fac Total		51	50	62	80	MUE
	13.66	12.49	090	2	1	0	1	1

● New   ▲ Revised   Deleted   ⊙ Moderate Sedation   ✚ Add-on Codes   ⊘ High Risk Denial   Ⓐ Age Edit   ♀ Female   ♂ Male   **AMA** *CPT® Assistant*   **MUE** Medically Unlikely Edit

⊘ Modifier 51 Exempt   ⊖ Modifier 63 Exempt   ☒ Unlisted   **Modifiers:** *See Inside Back Cover*   Ⓜ Maternity   `A 2`–`Z 3` ASC Payment Indicators   `A`–`Y` OPPS Status Indicators

Surgical Procedures

27766 – 27818

27766 Open treatment of medial malleolus fracture, includes internal fixation, when performed `A 2 T`

Mod	Non-Fac Total	Fac Total	Global Days	51	50	62	80	MUE
	17.62	17.62	090	2	1	1	1	1

27767 Closed treatment of posterior malleolus fracture; without manipulation `P 2 T`

Coding tip: Closed treatment of medial malleolus fracture - 27760

Mod	Non-Fac Total	Fac Total	Global Days	51	50	62	80	MUE
	8.04	8.08	090	2	1	0	1	1

27768 Closed treatment of posterior malleolus fracture; with manipulation `G 2 T`

Coding tip: Add modifier 77 for re-reduction of the fracture by another physician

Coding tip: Closed treatment of medial malleolus fracture with manipulation - 27762

Mod	Non-Fac Total	Fac Total	Global Days	51	50	62	80	MUE
	12.68	12.68	090	2	1	0	1	1

27769 Open treatment of posterior malleolus fracture, includes internal fixation, when performed `G 2 J I`

Mod	Non-Fac Total	Fac Total	Global Days	51	50	62	80	MUE
	21.20	21.20	090	2	1	0	1	1

27780 Closed treatment of proximal fibula or shaft fracture; without manipulation `A 2 T`

Coding tip: Closed treatment of distal fibular fracture - 27786

Mod	Non-Fac Total	Fac Total	Global Days	51	50	62	80	MUE
	8.78	7.99	090	2	1	0	1	1

AMA: Winter 92: 11

27781 Closed treatment of proximal fibula or shaft fracture; with manipulation `A 2 T`

Coding tip: Add modifier 77 for re-reduction of the fracture by another physician

Coding tip: Closed treatment of distal fibular fracture with manipulation - 27788

Mod	Non-Fac Total	Fac Total	Global Days	51	50	62	80	MUE
	12.05	11.19	090	2	1	0	1	1

27784 Open treatment of proximal fibula or shaft fracture, includes internal fixation, when performed `A 2 J I`

Mod	Non-Fac Total	Fac Total	Global Days	51	50	62	80	MUE
	20.68	20.68	090	2	1	1	1	1

AMA: Mar 00: 11

27786 Closed treatment of distal fibular fracture (lateral malleolus); without manipulation `A 2 T`

Coding tip: Closed treatment of proximal or shaft fibular fracture - 27780

Mod	Non-Fac Total	Fac Total	Global Days	51	50	62	80	MUE
	9.08	8.23	090	2	1	0	1	1

27788 Closed treatment of distal fibular fracture (lateral malleolus); with manipulation `A 2 T`

Coding tip: Add modifier 77 for re-reduction of the fracture by another physician

Coding tip: Closed treatment of proximal or shaft fibular fracture with manipulation - 27781

Mod	Non-Fac Total	Fac Total	Global Days	51	50	62	80	MUE
	12.11	11.09	090	2	1	0	1	1

27792 Open treatment of distal fibular fracture (lateral malleolus), includes internal fixation, when performed `A 2 J I`

Mod	Non-Fac Total	Fac Total	Global Days	51	50	62	80	MUE
	18.85	18.85	090	2	1	1	1	1

27808 Closed treatment of bimalleolar ankle fracture (eg, lateral and medial malleoli, or lateral and posterior malleoli or medial and posterior malleoli); without manipulation `A 2 T`

Coding tip: Closed treatment of trimalleolar fracture - 27816

Mod	Non-Fac Total	Fac Total	Global Days	51	50	62	80	MUE
	9.59	8.64	090	2	1	0	1	1

27810 Closed treatment of bimalleolar ankle fracture (eg, lateral and medial malleoli, or lateral and posterior malleoli or medial and posterior malleoli); with manipulation `A 2 T`

Coding tip: Closed treatment of trimalleolar fracture with manipulation - 27818

Coding tip: Add modifier 77 for re-reduction of the fracture by another physician

Mod	Non-Fac Total	Fac Total	Global Days	51	50	62	80	MUE
	13.46	12.26	090	2	1	0	1	1

27814 Open treatment of bimalleolar ankle fracture (eg, lateral and medial malleoli, or lateral and posterior malleoli, or medial and posterior malleoli), includes internal fixation, when performed `A 2 J I`

Mod	Non-Fac Total	Fac Total	Global Days	51	50	62	80	MUE
	22.31	22.31	090	2	1	1	2	1

27816 Closed treatment of trimalleolar ankle fracture; without manipulation `A 2 T`

Coding tip: Closed treatment of bimalleolar fracture - 27808

Mod	Non-Fac Total	Fac Total	Global Days	51	50	62	80	MUE
	9.19	8.25	090	2	1	0	1	1

27818 Closed treatment of trimalleolar ankle fracture; with manipulation `A 2 T`

Coding tip: Closed treatment of bimalleolar fracture with manipulation - 27810

Coding tip: Add modifier 77 for re-reduction of the fracture by another physician

Mod	Non-Fac Total	Fac Total	Global Days	51	50	62	80	MUE
	13.93	12.54	090	2	1	0	1	1

● New   ▲ Revised   ✖ Deleted   ⊙ Moderate Sedation   ✚ Add-on Codes   ⊖ High Risk Denial   Ⓐ Age Edit   ♀ Female   ♂ Male   **AMA** *CPT® Assistant*   **MUE** Medically Unlikely Edit

⊘ Modifier 51 Exempt   ⊖ Modifier 63 Exempt   ✗ Unlisted   **Modifiers:** *See Inside Back Cover*   Ⓜ Maternity   `A 2–Z 3` ASC Payment Indicators   `A–Y` OPPS Status Indicators

302   CPT © 2015 American Medical Association. All Rights Reserved.   © 2016 DecisionHealth

27822 Open treatment of trimalleolar ankle fracture, includes internal fixation, when performed, medial and/or lateral malleolus; without fixation of posterior lip   A 2 J I

RVU			Global Days	Modifiers				
Mod	Non-Fac Total	Fac Total		51	50	62	80	MUE
	24.28	24.28	090	2	1	1	2	1

27823 Open treatment of trimalleolar ankle fracture, includes internal fixation, when performed, medial and/or lateral malleolus; with fixation of posterior lip   G 2 J I

RVU			Global Days	Modifiers				
Mod	Non-Fac Total	Fac Total		51	50	62	80	MUE
	27.58	27.58	090	2	1	1	2	1

27824 Closed treatment of fracture of weight bearing articular portion of distal tibia (eg, pilon or tibial plafond), with or without anesthesia; without manipulation   A 2 T

RVU			Global Days	Modifiers				
Mod	Non-Fac Total	Fac Total		51	50	62	80	MUE
	9.01	8.76	090	2	1	0	1	1

27825 Closed treatment of fracture of weight bearing articular portion of distal tibia (eg, pilon or tibial plafond), with or without anesthesia; with skeletal traction and/or requiring manipulation   A 2 T

RVU			Global Days	Modifiers				
Mod	Non-Fac Total	Fac Total		51	50	62	80	MUE
	15.60	14.16	090	2	1	0	0	1

27826 Open treatment of fracture of weight bearing articular surface/portion of distal tibia (eg, pilon or tibial plafond), with internal fixation, when performed; of fibula only   A 2 J I

RVU			Global Days	Modifiers				
Mod	Non-Fac Total	Fac Total		51	50	62	80	MUE
	24.05	24.05	090	2	1	2	2	1

27827 Open treatment of fracture of weight bearing articular surface/portion of distal tibia (eg, pilon or tibial plafond), with internal fixation, when performed; of tibia only   G 2 J I

RVU			Global Days	Modifiers				
Mod	Non-Fac Total	Fac Total		51	50	62	80	MUE
	31.22	31.22	090	2	1	2	2	1

27828 Open treatment of fracture of weight bearing articular surface/portion of distal tibia (eg, pilon or tibial plafond), with internal fixation, when performed; of both tibia and fibula   G 2 J I

RVU			Global Days	Modifiers				
Mod	Non-Fac Total	Fac Total		51	50	62	80	MUE
	37.40	37.40	090	2	1	2	2	1

AMA: Apr 14: 10

27829 Open treatment of distal tibiofibular joint (syndesmosis) disruption, includes internal fixation, when performed   A 2 T

RVU			Global Days	Modifiers				
Mod	Non-Fac Total	Fac Total		51	50	62	80	MUE
	19.72	19.72	090	2	1	2	2	1

AMA: Winter 92: 11, Mar 09: 10

27830 Closed treatment of proximal tibiofibular joint dislocation; without anesthesia   A 2 T

Coding tip: Closed treatment of ankle dislocation - 27840

RVU			Global Days	Modifiers				
Mod	Non-Fac Total	Fac Total		51	50	62	80	MUE
	10.93	10.19	090	2	1	0	0	1

27831 Closed treatment of proximal tibiofibular joint dislocation; requiring anesthesia   A 2 T

Coding tip: Closed treatment of ankle dislocation requiring anesthesia - 27842

RVU			Global Days	Modifiers				
Mod	Non-Fac Total	Fac Total		51	50	62	80	MUE
	11.31	11.31	090	2	1	0	0	1

27832 Open treatment of proximal tibiofibular joint dislocation, includes internal fixation, when performed, or with excision of proximal fibula   A 2 J I

RVU			Global Days	Modifiers				
Mod	Non-Fac Total	Fac Total		51	50	62	80	MUE
	21.89	21.89	090	2	1	1	2	1

27840 Closed treatment of ankle dislocation; without anesthesia   A 2 T

RVU			Global Days	Modifiers				
Mod	Non-Fac Total	Fac Total		51	50	62	80	MUE
	10.53	10.53	090	2	1	0	1	1

Closed treatment of ankle dislocation

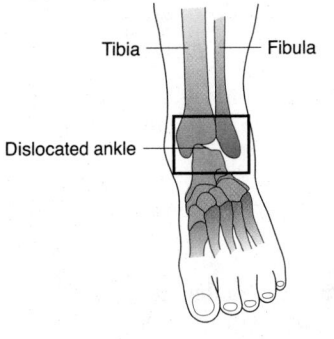

Without anesthesia (27840), with anesthesia and with or without percutaneous skeletal fixation (27842)

27842 Closed treatment of ankle dislocation; requiring anesthesia, with or without percutaneous skeletal fixation   A 2 T

RVU			Global Days	Modifiers				
Mod	Non-Fac Total	Fac Total		51	50	62	80	MUE
	14.31	14.31	090	2	1	0	1	1

27846 Open treatment of ankle dislocation, with or without percutaneous skeletal fixation; without repair or internal fixation   A 2 T

RVU			Global Days	Modifiers				
Mod	Non-Fac Total	Fac Total		51	50	62	80	MUE
	20.94	20.94	090	2	1	1	2	1

● New   ▲ Revised   Deleted   ⊙ Moderate Sedation   ✚ Add-on Codes   ⊘ High Risk Denial   Ⓐ Age Edit   ♀ Female   ♂ Male   **AMA** CPT® Assistant   **MUE** Medically Unlikely Edit

⊘ Modifier 51 Exempt   ⊖ Modifier 63 Exempt   ☒ Unlisted   **Modifiers:** See Inside Back Cover   Ⓜ Maternity   A 2 – Z 3 ASC Payment Indicators   A – Y OPPS Status Indicators

Surgical Procedures

27848 – 28002

27848 Open treatment of ankle dislocation, with or without percutaneous skeletal fixation; with repair or internal or external fixation `A2 T`

Mod	Non-Fac Total	Fac Total	Global Days	51	50	62	80	MUE
	23.40	23.40	090	2	1	1	2	1

Lower Leg/Ankle Manipulation

27860 Manipulation of ankle under general anesthesia (includes application of traction or other fixation apparatus) `A2 T`

Mod	Non-Fac Total	Fac Total	Global Days	51	50	62	80	MUE
	5.02	5.02	010	2	1	0	0	1

Lower Leg/Ankle Arthrodesis

27870 Arthrodesis, ankle, open `J8 J1`

Mod	Non-Fac Total	Fac Total	Global Days	51	50	62	80	MUE
	29.76	29.76	090	2	1	1	2	1

27871 Arthrodesis, tibiofibular joint, proximal or distal `G2 J1`

Mod	Non-Fac Total	Fac Total	Global Days	51	50	62	80	MUE
	19.67	19.67	090	2	1	1	2	1

Lower Leg/Ankle Amputation

27880 Amputation, leg, through tibia and fibula `C`

Mod	Non-Fac Total	Fac Total	Global Days	51	50	62	80	MUE
	26.81	26.81	090	2	1	1	2	1

27881 Amputation, leg, through tibia and fibula; with immediate fitting technique including application of first cast `C`

Mod	Non-Fac Total	Fac Total	Global Days	51	50	62	80	MUE
	25.39	25.39	090	2	1	1	2	1

27882 Amputation, leg, through tibia and fibula; open, circular (guillotine) `C`

Mod	Non-Fac Total	Fac Total	Global Days	51	50	62	80	MUE
	17.57	17.57	090	2	1	1	0	1

27884 Amputation, leg, through tibia and fibula; secondary closure or scar revision `A2 T`

Mod	Non-Fac Total	Fac Total	Global Days	51	50	62	80	MUE
	16.84	16.84	090	2	1	0	1	1

27886 Amputation, leg, through tibia and fibula; re-amputation `C`

Mod	Non-Fac Total	Fac Total	Global Days	51	50	62	80	MUE
	19.24	19.24	090	2	1	1	1	1

27888 Amputation, ankle, through malleoli of tibia and fibula (eg, Syme, Pirogoff type procedures), with plastic closure and resection of nerves `C`

Mod	Non-Fac Total	Fac Total	Global Days	51	50	62	80	MUE
	19.85	19.85	090	2	1	1	2	1

27889 Ankle disarticulation `A2 T`

Mod	Non-Fac Total	Fac Total	Global Days	51	50	62	80	MUE
	19.01	19.01	090	2	1	1	1	1

Other Lower Leg/Ankle Procedures

27892 Decompression fasciotomy, leg; anterior and/or lateral compartments only, with debridement of nonviable muscle and/or nerve `A2 T`

Mod	Non-Fac Total	Fac Total	Global Days	51	50	62	80	MUE
	15.98	15.98	090	2	1	0	0	1

27893 Decompression fasciotomy, leg; posterior compartment(s) only, with debridement of nonviable muscle and/or nerve `A2 T`

Mod	Non-Fac Total	Fac Total	Global Days	51	50	62	80	MUE
	17.48	17.48	090	2	1	0	0	1

27894 Decompression fasciotomy, leg; anterior and/or lateral, and posterior compartment(s), with debridement of nonviable muscle and/or nerve `A2 T`

Mod	Non-Fac Total	Fac Total	Global Days	51	50	62	80	MUE
	24.86	24.86	090	2	1	0	2	1

27899 Unlisted procedure, leg or ankle `x T`

Mod	Non-Fac Total	Fac Total	Global Days	51	50	62	80	MUE
	0.00	0.00	YYY	2	1	1	0	

AMA: Aug 00: 11

Foot/Toe Procedures

Foot/Toe Incisional Procedures

28001 Incision and drainage, bursa, foot `P3 T`

Mod	Non-Fac Total	Fac Total	Global Days	51	50	62	80	MUE
	7.98	4.88	010	2	0	0	1	2

AMA: Nov 98: 9

28002 Incision and drainage below fascia, with or without tendon sheath involvement, foot; single bursal space `A2 T`

Mod	Non-Fac Total	Fac Total	Global Days	51	50	62	80	MUE
	12.76	9.17	010	2	0	0	1	3

AMA: Nov 98: 8

● New   ▲ Revised   ✖ Deleted   ⊙ Moderate Sedation   ✚ Add-on Codes   ⊗ High Risk Denial   ⓐ Age Edit   ♀ Female   ♂ Male   **AMA** *CPT® Assistant*   **MUE** Medically Unlikely Edit
⊘ Modifier 51 Exempt   ⊖ Modifier 63 Exempt   ✗ Unlisted   **Modifiers:** *See Inside Back Cover*   Ⓜ Maternity   A2–Z3 ASC Payment Indicators   A–Y OPPS Status Indicators

304   CPT © 2015 American Medical Association. All Rights Reserved.   © 2016 DecisionHealth

28003 Incision and drainage below fascia, with or without tendon sheath involvement, foot; multiple areas   A 2 T

RVU			Global Days	Modifiers				
Mod	Non-Fac Total	Fac Total		51	50	62	80	MUE
	20.53	16.41	090	2	0	0	1	2

AMA: Nov 98: 9

28005 Incision, bone cortex (eg, osteomyelitis or bone abscess), foot   A 2 T

RVU			Global Days	Modifiers				
Mod	Non-Fac Total	Fac Total		51	50	62	80	MUE
	16.71	16.71	090	2	0	0	1	3

AMA: Nov 98: 9

28008 Fasciotomy, foot and/or toe   A 2 T

Coding tip: Do not report 28060, 28062, 28250 and 29893 with 28008; these codes should not be reported together if performed on the same foot at the same surgical session

RVU			Global Days	Modifiers				
Mod	Non-Fac Total	Fac Total		51	50	62	80	MUE
	12.42	8.41	090	2	1	0	1	2

28010 Tenotomy, percutaneous, toe; single tendon   P 3 T

RVU			Global Days	Modifiers				
Mod	Non-Fac Total	Fac Total		51	50	62	80	MUE
	6.63	5.97	090	2	0	0	1	

AMA: Nov 98: 8

28011 Tenotomy, percutaneous, toe; multiple tendons   A 2 T

RVU			Global Days	Modifiers				
Mod	Non-Fac Total	Fac Total		51	50	62	80	MUE
	9.23	8.24	090	2	0	0	1	

AMA: Nov 98: 8

28020 Arthrotomy, including exploration, drainage, or removal of loose or foreign body; intertarsal or tarsometatarsal joint   A 2 T

RVU			Global Days	Modifiers				
Mod	Non-Fac Total	Fac Total		51	50	62	80	MUE
	15.59	10.40	090	2	0	1	1	2

28022 Arthrotomy, including exploration, drainage, or removal of loose or foreign body; metatarsophalangeal joint   A 2 T

RVU			Global Days	Modifiers				
Mod	Non-Fac Total	Fac Total		51	50	62	80	MUE
	14.23	9.44	090	2	0	0	1	4

28024 Arthrotomy, including exploration, drainage, or removal of loose or foreign body; interphalangeal joint   A 2 T

RVU			Global Days	Modifiers				
Mod	Non-Fac Total	Fac Total		51	50	62	80	MUE
	13.37	8.80	090	2	0	0	1	4

28035 Release, tarsal tunnel (posterior tibial nerve decompression)   A 2 T

RVU			Global Days	Modifiers				
Mod	Non-Fac Total	Fac Total		51	50	62	80	MUE
	15.21	10.21	090	2	1	1	1	1

AMA: Nov 98: 8

Foot/Toe Excisional Procedures

28039 Excision, tumor, soft tissue of foot or toe, subcutaneous; 1.5 cm or greater   G 2 T

Coding tip: Code 28039 is listed out of numerical order in CPT. Related soft tissue tumor excision procedures - 28043 (subcutaneous); 28045, 28041 (subfascial)

RVU			Global Days	Modifiers				
Mod	Non-Fac Total	Fac Total		51	50	62	80	MUE
	14.78	10.14	090	2	1	0	2	3

28041 Excision, tumor, soft tissue of foot or toe, subfascial (eg, intramuscular); 1.5 cm or greater   G 2 T

Coding tip: Code 28041 is listed out of numerical order in CPT. Related soft tissue tumor excision procedures - 28043, 28039 (subcutaneous); 28045 (subfascial)

RVU			Global Days	Modifiers				
Mod	Non-Fac Total	Fac Total		51	50	62	80	MUE
	13.34	13.34	090	2	1	0	0	3

28043 Excision, tumor, soft tissue of foot or toe, subcutaneous; less than 1.5 cm   G 2 T

Coding tip: Related soft tissue tumor excision codes - 28039, 28041, 28045

RVU			Global Days	Modifiers				
Mod	Non-Fac Total	Fac Total		51	50	62	80	MUE
	11.54	7.55	090	2	1	0	1	4

28045 Excision, tumor, soft tissue of foot or toe, subfascial (eg, intramuscular); less than 1.5 cm   G 2 T

Coding tip: Related soft tissue tumor excision codes - 28039, 28041, 28043

RVU			Global Days	Modifiers				
Mod	Non-Fac Total	Fac Total		51	50	62	80	MUE
	14.33	10.01	090	2	1	0	0	4

28046 Radical resection of tumor (eg, sarcoma), soft tissue of foot or toe; less than 3 cm   G 2 T

RVU			Global Days	Modifiers				
Mod	Non-Fac Total	Fac Total		51	50	62	80	MUE
	21.04	21.04	090	2	1	1	1	1

28047 Radical resection of tumor (eg, sarcoma), soft tissue of foot or toe; 3 cm or greater   G 2 T

RVU			Global Days	Modifiers				
Mod	Non-Fac Total	Fac Total		51	50	62	80	MUE
	31.00	31.00	090	2	1	1	2	1

28050 Arthrotomy with biopsy; intertarsal or tarsometatarsal joint   A 2 T

RVU			Global Days	Modifiers				
Mod	Non-Fac Total	Fac Total		51	50	62	80	MUE
	12.28	8.06	090	2	1	1	1	2

28052 Arthrotomy with biopsy; metatarsophalangeal joint   A 2 T

RVU			Global Days	Modifiers				
Mod	Non-Fac Total	Fac Total		51	50	62	80	MUE
	13.16	8.34	090	2	1	1	1	2

● New   ▲ Revised   Deleted   ⊙ Moderate Sedation   ✚ Add-on Codes   ⊘ High Risk Denial   Ⓐ Age Edit   ♀ Female   ♂ Male   **AMA** *CPT® Assistant*   **MUE** Medically Unlikely Edit

⊘ Modifier 51 Exempt   ⊖ Modifier 63 Exempt   ✗ Unlisted   **Modifiers:** *See Inside Back Cover*   Ⓜ Maternity   A 2 – Z 3 ASC Payment Indicators   A – Y OPPS Status Indicators

© 2016 DecisionHealth   CPT © 2015 American Medical Association. All Rights Reserved.   **305**

28054 Arthrotomy with biopsy; interphalangeal joint
A2 T

RVU			Global Days	Modifiers				
Mod	Non-Fac Total	Fac Total		51	50	62	80	MUE
	11.41	7.09	090	2	1	0	0	2

28055 Neurectomy, intrinsic musculature of foot
A2 T

RVU			Global Days	Modifiers				
Mod	Non-Fac Total	Fac Total		51	50	62	80	MUE
	10.83	10.83	090	2	1	0	0	1

28060 Fasciectomy, plantar fascia; partial (separate procedure)
A2 T

Coding tip: Do not report 28008, 28062, 28250 and 29893 with 28060; these codes should not be reported together if performed on the same foot at the same surgical session

RVU			Global Days	Modifiers				
Mod	Non-Fac Total	Fac Total		51	50	62	80	MUE
	14.96	10.26	090	2	1	0	1	1

AMA: Mar 08: 14

28062 Fasciectomy, plantar fascia; radical (separate procedure)
A2 T

Coding tip: Do not report 28008, 28060, 28250 and 29893 with 28062; these codes should not be reported together if performed on the same foot at the same surgical session

RVU			Global Days	Modifiers				
Mod	Non-Fac Total	Fac Total		51	50	62	80	MUE
	16.97	11.74	090	2	1	1	1	1

28070 Synovectomy; intertarsal or tarsometatarsal joint, each

RVU			Global Days	Modifiers				
Mod	Non-Fac Total	Fac Total		51	50	62	80	MUE
	15.30	10.18	090	2	0	0	1	2

28072 Synovectomy; metatarsophalangeal joint, each
A2 T

RVU			Global Days	Modifiers				
Mod	Non-Fac Total	Fac Total		51	50	62	80	MUE
	14.68	9.58	090	2	0	0	1	4

28080 Excision, interdigital (Morton) neuroma, single, each
A2 T

RVU			Global Days	Modifiers				
Mod	Non-Fac Total	Fac Total		51	50	62	80	MUE
	15.19	10.58	090	2	0	0	0	4

28086 Synovectomy, tendon sheath, foot; flexor
A2 T

RVU			Global Days	Modifiers				
Mod	Non-Fac Total	Fac Total		51	50	62	80	MUE
	15.82	10.39	090	2	1	1	2	2

28088 Synovectomy, tendon sheath, foot; extensor
A2 T

RVU			Global Days	Modifiers				
Mod	Non-Fac Total	Fac Total		51	50	62	80	MUE
	12.91	8.11	090	2	1	0	0	2

28090 Excision of lesion, tendon, tendon sheath, or capsule (including synovectomy) (eg, cyst or ganglion); foot
A2 T

RVU			Global Days	Modifiers				
Mod	Non-Fac Total	Fac Total		51	50	62	80	MUE
	13.64	8.89	090	2	1	0	1	2

AMA: Nov 98: 8

28092 Excision of lesion, tendon, tendon sheath, or capsule (including synovectomy) (eg, cyst or ganglion); toe(s), each
A2 T

RVU			Global Days	Modifiers				
Mod	Non-Fac Total	Fac Total		51	50	62	80	MUE
	12.24	7.74	090	2	0	0	1	2

28100 Excision or curettage of bone cyst or benign tumor, talus or calcaneus
A2 T

RVU			Global Days	Modifiers				
Mod	Non-Fac Total	Fac Total		51	50	62	80	MUE
	17.49	11.86	090	2	1	1	2	1

28102 Excision or curettage of bone cyst or benign tumor, talus or calcaneus; with iliac or other autograft (includes obtaining graft)
A2 J 1

RVU			Global Days	Modifiers				
Mod	Non-Fac Total	Fac Total		51	50	62	80	MUE
	17.46	17.46	090	2	1	0	2	1

28103 Excision or curettage of bone cyst or benign tumor, talus or calcaneus; with allograft
A2 J 1

RVU			Global Days	Modifiers				
Mod	Non-Fac Total	Fac Total		51	50	62	80	MUE
	11.29	11.29	090	2	1	0	2	1

28104 Excision or curettage of bone cyst or benign tumor, tarsal or metatarsal, except talus or calcaneus
A2 T

RVU			Global Days	Modifiers				
Mod	Non-Fac Total	Fac Total		51	50	62	80	MUE
	15.31	10.20	090	2	0	1	2	2

28106 Excision or curettage of bone cyst or benign tumor, tarsal or metatarsal, except talus or calcaneus; with iliac or other autograft (includes obtaining graft)
A2 T

RVU			Global Days	Modifiers				
Mod	Non-Fac Total	Fac Total		51	50	62	80	MUE
	13.44	13.44	090	2	0	1	2	1

28107 Excision or curettage of bone cyst or benign tumor, tarsal or metatarsal, except talus or calcaneus; with allograft
A2 J 1

RVU			Global Days	Modifiers				
Mod	Non-Fac Total	Fac Total		51	50	62	80	MUE
	16.31	10.85	090	2	0	0	2	1

28108 Excision or curettage of bone cyst or benign tumor, phalanges of foot
A2 T

RVU			Global Days	Modifiers				
Mod	Non-Fac Total	Fac Total		51	50	62	80	MUE
	12.74	8.30	090	2	0	0	1	2

● New ▲ Revised ✖ Deleted ⊙ Moderate Sedation ✚ Add-on Codes ⊖ High Risk Denial Ⓐ Age Edit ♀ Female ♂ Male **AMA** *CPT® Assistant* ***MUE*** Medically Unlikely Edit
⊘ Modifier 51 Exempt ⊖ Modifier 63 Exempt ⊠ Unlisted **Modifiers:** *See Inside Back Cover* Ⓜ Maternity A2–Z3 ASC Payment Indicators A–Y OPPS Status Indicators

306 CPT © 2015 American Medical Association. All Rights Reserved. © 2016 DecisionHealth

28110 Ostectomy, partial excision, fifth metatarsal head (bunionette) (separate procedure) A 2 T

RVU			Global Days	Modifiers				MUE
Mod	Non-Fac Total	Fac Total		51	50	62	80	
	13.38	8.32	090	2	1	1	1	1

AMA: Oct 98: 10, Sep 00: 9, Dec 10: 17

28111 Ostectomy, complete excision; first metatarsal head A 2 T

RVU			Global Days	Modifiers				MUE
Mod	Non-Fac Total	Fac Total		51	50	62	80	
	14.26	9.41	090	2	1	1	1	1

28112 Ostectomy, complete excision; other metatarsal head (second, third or fourth) A 2 T

RVU			Global Days	Modifiers				MUE
Mod	Non-Fac Total	Fac Total		51	50	62	80	
	14.04	8.96	090	2	1	1	1	4

28113 Ostectomy, complete excision; fifth metatarsal head A 2 T

RVU			Global Days	Modifiers				MUE
Mod	Non-Fac Total	Fac Total		51	50	62	80	
	17.05	12.22	090	2	1	0	0	1

28114 Ostectomy, complete excision; all metatarsal heads, with partial proximal phalangectomy, excluding first metatarsal (eg, Clayton type procedure) A 2 T

RVU			Global Days	Modifiers				MUE
Mod	Non-Fac Total	Fac Total		51	50	62	80	
	31.12	24.21	090	2	1	1	2	1

28116 Ostectomy, excision of tarsal coalition A 2 T

RVU			Global Days	Modifiers				MUE
Mod	Non-Fac Total	Fac Total		51	50	62	80	
	21.75	16.40	090	2	1	0	1	1

28118 Ostectomy, calcaneus A 2 T

RVU			Global Days	Modifiers				MUE
Mod	Non-Fac Total	Fac Total		51	50	62	80	
	17.13	11.88	090	2	1	1	2	1

AMA: May 11: 9, Jan 15: 13

28119 Ostectomy, calcaneus; for spur, with or without plantar fascial release A 2 T

RVU			Global Days	Modifiers				MUE
Mod	Non-Fac Total	Fac Total		51	50	62	80	
	15.19	10.39	090	2	1	1	1	1

AMA: May 11: 9

28120 Partial excision (craterization, saucerization, sequestrectomy, or diaphysectomy) bone (eg, osteomyelitis or bossing); talus or calcaneus A 2 T

RVU			Global Days	Modifiers				MUE
Mod	Non-Fac Total	Fac Total		51	50	62	80	
	19.44	14.25	090	2	1	1	1	2

AMA: May 11: 9

28122 Partial excision (craterization, saucerization, sequestrectomy, or diaphysectomy) bone (eg, osteomyelitis or bossing); tarsal or metatarsal bone, except talus or calcaneus A 2 T

RVU			Global Days	Modifiers				MUE
Mod	Non-Fac Total	Fac Total		51	50	62	80	
	17.30	12.67	090	2	1	1	2	4

AMA: Nov 98: 11

28124 Partial excision (craterization, saucerization, sequestrectomy, or diaphysectomy) bone (eg, osteomyelitis or bossing); phalanx of toe P 3 T

RVU			Global Days	Modifiers				MUE
Mod	Non-Fac Total	Fac Total		51	50	62	80	
	13.78	9.49	090	2	1	0	1	4

28126 Resection, partial or complete, phalangeal base, each toe A 2 T

RVU			Global Days	Modifiers				MUE
Mod	Non-Fac Total	Fac Total		51	50	62	80	
	11.41	7.14	090	2	0	0	1	4

AMA: Nov 98: 8, Mar 15: 9

28130 Talectomy (astragalectomy) A 2 T

RVU			Global Days	Modifiers				MUE
Mod	Non-Fac Total	Fac Total		51	50	62	80	
	18.45	18.45	090	2	1	1	2	1

28140 Metatarsectomy A 2 T

RVU			Global Days	Modifiers				MUE
Mod	Non-Fac Total	Fac Total		51	50	62	80	
	17.31	12.74	090	2	0	1	1	4

28150 Phalangectomy, toe, each toe A 2 T

RVU			Global Days	Modifiers				MUE
Mod	Non-Fac Total	Fac Total		51	50	62	80	
	12.36	8.10	090	2	0	0	1	4

AMA: Nov 98: 8

28153 Resection, condyle(s), distal end of phalanx, each toe A 2 T

RVU			Global Days	Modifiers				MUE
Mod	Non-Fac Total	Fac Total		51	50	62	80	
	11.79	7.53	090	2	0	0	1	6

AMA: Nov 98: 8, Dec 11: 15

28160 Hemiphalangectomy or interphalangeal joint excision, toe, proximal end of phalanx, each A 2 T

RVU			Global Days	Modifiers				MUE
Mod	Non-Fac Total	Fac Total		51	50	62	80	
	12.14	7.75	090	2	0	0	1	5

AMA: Nov 98: 8

28171 Radical resection of tumor; tarsal (except talus or calcaneus) A 2 T

RVU			Global Days	Modifiers				MUE
Mod	Non-Fac Total	Fac Total		51	50	62	80	
	24.46	24.46	090	2	0	0	2	1

28173 Radical resection of tumor; metatarsal A 2 T

RVU			Global Days	Modifiers				MUE
Mod	Non-Fac Total	Fac Total		51	50	62	80	
	22.05	22.05	090	2	0	1	1	2

● New   ▲ Revised   Deleted   ⊙ Moderate Sedation   ✚ Add-on Codes   ⊘ High Risk Denial   Ⓐ Age Edit   ♀ Female   ♂ Male   **AMA** *CPT® Assistant*   **MUE** Medically Unlikely Edit
⊘ Modifier 51 Exempt   ⊖ Modifier 63 Exempt   ☒ Unlisted   **Modifiers:** *See Inside Back Cover*   Ⓜ Maternity   A 2 – Z 3 ASC Payment Indicators   A – Y OPPS Status Indicators

© 2016 DecisionHealth   CPT © 2015 American Medical Association. All Rights Reserved.   **307**

28175 Radical resection of tumor; phalanx of toe A 2 T

RVU			Global Days	Modifiers				
Mod	Non-Fac Total	Fac Total		51	50	62	80	MUE
	14.12	14.12	090	2	0	1	1	2

Foot/Toe Introduction/Removal Procedures

28190 Removal of foreign body, foot; subcutaneous P 3 T

RVU			Global Days	Modifiers				
Mod	Non-Fac Total	Fac Total		51	50	62	80	MUE
	7.42	3.86	010	2	1	0	1	3

AMA: Dec 13: 16

Removal of foreign body, foot

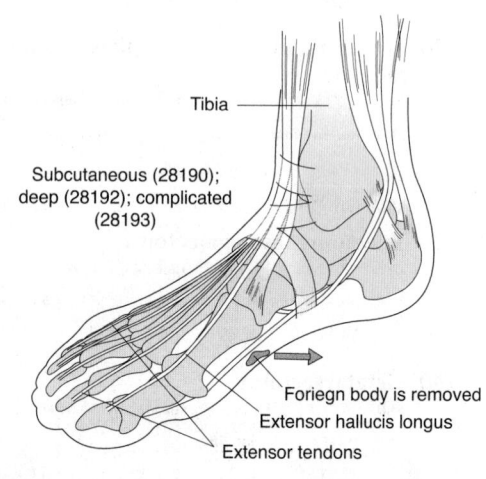

Tibia

Subcutaneous (28190); deep (28192); complicated (28193)

Foriegn body is removed

Extensor hallucis longus

Extensor tendons

28192 Removal of foreign body, foot; deep A 2 T

RVU			Global Days	Modifiers				
Mod	Non-Fac Total	Fac Total		51	50	62	80	MUE
	13.66	9.07	090	2	1	0	1	2

AMA: Dec 13: 16

28193 Removal of foreign body, foot; complicated A 2 T

RVU			Global Days	Modifiers				
Mod	Non-Fac Total	Fac Total		51	50	62	80	MUE
	15.34	10.62	090	2	1	0	1	2

Foot/Toe Repair/Revision/Reconstruction Procedures

28200 Repair, tendon, flexor, foot; primary or secondary, without free graft, each tendon A 2 T

RVU			Global Days	Modifiers				
Mod	Non-Fac Total	Fac Total		51	50	62	80	MUE
	14.18	9.26	090	2	0	1	1	4

AMA: Nov 98: 8, Jul 14: 5

28202 Repair, tendon, flexor, foot; secondary with free graft, each tendon (includes obtaining graft) A 2 J I

RVU			Global Days	Modifiers				
Mod	Non-Fac Total	Fac Total		51	50	62	80	MUE
	17.29	12.30	090	2	0	1	2	2

28208 Repair, tendon, extensor, foot; primary or secondary, each tendon A 2 T

RVU			Global Days	Modifiers				
Mod	Non-Fac Total	Fac Total		51	50	62	80	MUE
	13.80	9.03	090	2	0	1	1	4

AMA: Nov 98: 8

28210 Repair, tendon, extensor, foot; secondary with free graft, each tendon (includes obtaining graft) A 2 J I

RVU			Global Days	Modifiers				
Mod	Non-Fac Total	Fac Total		51	50	62	80	MUE
	16.54	11.75	090	2	0	0	2	2

28220 Tenolysis, flexor, foot; single tendon P 3 T

RVU			Global Days	Modifiers				
Mod	Non-Fac Total	Fac Total		51	50	62	80	MUE
	12.92	8.63	090	2	1	0	1	1

AMA: Nov 98: 8

28222 Tenolysis, flexor, foot; multiple tendons A 2 T

RVU			Global Days	Modifiers				
Mod	Non-Fac Total	Fac Total		51	50	62	80	MUE
	14.59	10.01	090	2	1	0	1	1

AMA: Nov 98: 8

28225 Tenolysis, extensor, foot; single tendon A 2 T

RVU			Global Days	Modifiers				
Mod	Non-Fac Total	Fac Total		51	50	62	80	MUE
	11.67	7.37	090	2	1	1	1	1

AMA: Nov 98: 8

28226 Tenolysis, extensor, foot; multiple tendons A 2 T

RVU			Global Days	Modifiers				
Mod	Non-Fac Total	Fac Total		51	50	62	80	MUE
	17.62	11.33	090	2	1	0	1	1

AMA: Nov 98: 8

28230 Tenotomy, open, tendon flexor; foot, single or multiple tendon(s) (separate procedure) P 3 T

RVU			Global Days	Modifiers				
Mod	Non-Fac Total	Fac Total		51	50	62	80	MUE
	12.42	8.06	090	2	1	0	1	1

AMA: Nov 98: 8

28232 Tenotomy, open, tendon flexor; toe, single tendon (separate procedure) P 3 T

RVU			Global Days	Modifiers				
Mod	Non-Fac Total	Fac Total		51	50	62	80	MUE
	11.07	6.92	090	2	0	0	1	6

AMA: Nov 98: 8, Mar 15: 9

28234 Tenotomy, open, extensor, foot or toe, each tendon A 2 T

RVU			Global Days	Modifiers				
Mod	Non-Fac Total	Fac Total		51	50	62	80	MUE
	11.58	7.46	090	2	0	0	1	6

AMA: Nov 98: 8, Sep 10: 9

CPT © 2015 American Medical Association. All Rights Reserved.   © 2016 DecisionHealth

28238 Reconstruction (advancement), posterior tibial tendon with excision of accessory tarsal navicular bone (eg, Kidner type procedure) `A 2 T`

	RVU		Global Days	Modifiers				
Mod	Non-Fac Total	Fac Total		51	50	62	80	MUE
	19.40	14.03	090	2	1	1	2	1

28240 Tenotomy, lengthening, or release, abductor hallucis muscle `A 2 T`

	RVU		Global Days	Modifiers				
Mod	Non-Fac Total	Fac Total		51	50	62	80	MUE
	12.65	8.28	090	2	1	0	1	1

28250 Division of plantar fascia and muscle (eg, Steindler stripping) (separate procedure) `A 2 T`

Coding tip: Do not report 28008, 28060, 28062 and 29893 with 28250; these codes should not be reported together if performed on the same foot at the same surgical session

	RVU		Global Days	Modifiers				
Mod	Non-Fac Total	Fac Total		51	50	62	80	MUE
	16.69	11.61	090	2	1	1	2	1

28260 Capsulotomy, midfoot; medial release only (separate procedure) `A 2 T`

	RVU		Global Days	Modifiers				
Mod	Non-Fac Total	Fac Total		51	50	62	80	MUE
	19.79	14.66	090	2	1	1	2	1

28261 Capsulotomy, midfoot; with tendon lengthening `A 2 T`

	RVU		Global Days	Modifiers				
Mod	Non-Fac Total	Fac Total		51	50	62	80	MUE
	28.25	22.30	090	2	1	0	0	1

28262 Capsulotomy, midfoot; extensive, including posterior talotibial capsulotomy and tendon(s) lengthening (eg, resistant clubfoot deformity) `A 2 J 1`

	RVU		Global Days	Modifiers				
Mod	Non-Fac Total	Fac Total		51	50	62	80	MUE
	42.64	34.30	090	2	1	1	2	1

28264 Capsulotomy, midtarsal (eg, Heyman type procedure) `A 2 T`

	RVU		Global Days	Modifiers				
Mod	Non-Fac Total	Fac Total		51	50	62	80	MUE
	29.00	22.08	090	2	1	0	2	1

28270 Capsulotomy; metatarsophalangeal joint, with or without tenorrhaphy, each joint (separate procedure) `A 2 T`

	RVU		Global Days	Modifiers				
Mod	Non-Fac Total	Fac Total		51	50	62	80	MUE
	14.08	9.52	090	2	1	0	1	6

AMA: Sep 11: 11, Sep 10: 9, Sep 14: 13

28272 Capsulotomy; interphalangeal joint, each joint (separate procedure) `P 3 T`

	RVU		Global Days	Modifiers				
Mod	Non-Fac Total	Fac Total		51	50	62	80	MUE
	11.38	7.30	090	2	1	0	1	6

AMA: Dec 02: 11

28280 Syndactylization, toes (eg, webbing or Kelikian type procedure) `A 2 T`

	RVU		Global Days	Modifiers				
Mod	Non-Fac Total	Fac Total		51	50	62	80	MUE
	14.98	10.08	090	2	1	0	0	1

AMA: Nov 98: 8

28285 Correction, hammertoe (eg, interphalangeal fusion, partial or total phalangectomy) `A 2 T`

	RVU		Global Days	Modifiers				
Mod	Non-Fac Total	Fac Total		51	50	62	80	MUE
	15.34	10.79	090	2	1	1	1	4

AMA: Nov 98: 8, May 06: 18, Sep 11: 11, Sep 10: 9, Mar 15: 9

28286 Correction, cock-up fifth toe, with plastic skin closure (eg, Ruiz-Mora type procedure) `A 2 T`

	RVU		Global Days	Modifiers				
Mod	Non-Fac Total	Fac Total		51	50	62	80	MUE
	13.09	8.63	090	2	1	0	1	1

AMA: Nov 98: 8

28288 Ostectomy, partial, exostectomy or condylectomy, metatarsal head, each metatarsal head `A 2 T`

	RVU		Global Days	Modifiers				
Mod	Non-Fac Total	Fac Total		51	50	62	80	MUE
	17.43	12.34	090	2	0	0	1	5

28289 Hallux rigidus correction with cheilectomy, debridement and capsular release of the first metatarsophalangeal joint `A 2 T`

	RVU		Global Days	Modifiers				
Mod	Non-Fac Total	Fac Total		51	50	62	80	MUE
	21.20	15.78	090	2	1	1	2	1

AMA: Nov 98: 11, May 11: 3

28290 Correction, hallux valgus (bunion), with or without sesamoidectomy; simple exostectomy (eg, Silver type procedure) `A 2 T`

	RVU		Global Days	Modifiers				
Mod	Non-Fac Total	Fac Total		51	50	62	80	MUE
	16.85	11.29	090	2	1	0	1	1

AMA: Dec 96: 5, Nov 98: 8, Jan 07: 31, May 10: 9

Hallux valgus correction

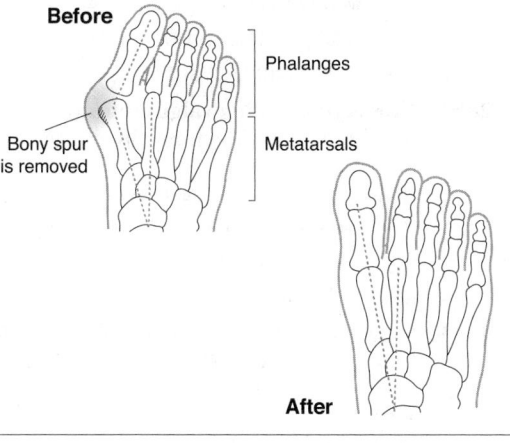

Before
Phalanges
Bony spur is removed
Metatarsals
After

● New   ▲ Revised   Deleted   ⊙ Moderate Sedation   ✚ Add-on Codes   ⊘ High Risk Denial   Ⓐ Age Edit   ♀ Female   ♂ Male   **AMA** CPT® Assistant   **MUE** Medically Unlikely Edit
⊘ Modifier 51 Exempt   ⊖ Modifier 63 Exempt   ✗ Unlisted   **Modifiers:** See Inside Back Cover   Ⓜ Maternity   `A 2`–`Z 3` ASC Payment Indicators   `A`–`Y` OPPS Status Indicators

28292 Correction, hallux valgus (bunion), with or without sesamoidectomy; Keller, McBride, or Mayo type procedure `A 2 T`

RVU		Global Days	Modifiers				
Mod	Non-Fac Total	Fac Total		51	50	62	80	MUE
	22.78	17.30	090	2	1	1	2	1

AMA: Dec 96: 5, Sep 00: 9, Jan 07: 31, Dec 10: 12, May 10: 9

28293 Correction, hallux valgus (bunion), with or without sesamoidectomy; resection of joint with implant `A 2 J I`

RVU		Global Days	Modifiers				
Mod	Non-Fac Total	Fac Total		51	50	62	80	MUE
	30.34	20.46	090	2	1	1	2	1

AMA: Dec 96: 6, Jan 07: 31, May 10: 9

28294 Correction, hallux valgus (bunion), with or without sesamoidectomy; with tendon transplants (eg, Joplin type procedure) `A 2 T`

RVU		Global Days	Modifiers				
Mod	Non-Fac Total	Fac Total		51	50	62	80	MUE
	22.20	15.76	090	2	1	1	2	1

AMA: Dec 96: 6, Jan 07: 31, May 10: 9

28296 Correction, hallux valgus (bunion), with or without sesamoidectomy; with metatarsal osteotomy (eg, Mitchell, Chevron, or concentric type procedures) `A 2 T`

RVU		Global Days	Modifiers				
Mod	Non-Fac Total	Fac Total		51	50	62	80	MUE
	20.63	15.02	090	2	1	1	2	1

AMA: Dec 96: 6, Jan 97: 10, Jan 07: 31, May 10: 9, Sep 13: 17

28297 Correction, hallux valgus (bunion), with or without sesamoidectomy; Lapidus-type procedure `A 2 J I`

RVU		Global Days	Modifiers				
Mod	Non-Fac Total	Fac Total		51	50	62	80	MUE
	23.48	16.78	090	2	1	1	2	1

AMA: Dec 96: 6, Jan 07: 31, May 10: 9

28298 Correction, hallux valgus (bunion), with or without sesamoidectomy; by phalanx osteotomy `A 2 T`

RVU		Global Days	Modifiers				
Mod	Non-Fac Total	Fac Total		51	50	62	80	MUE
	20.88	14.59	090	2	1	1	2	1

AMA: Dec 96: 7, Jan 07: 31, May 10: 9, Oct 13: 18

28299 Correction, hallux valgus (bunion), with or without sesamoidectomy; by double osteotomy `A 2 T`

RVU		Global Days	Modifiers				
Mod	Non-Fac Total	Fac Total		51	50	62	80	MUE
	25.95	19.54	090	2	1	1	2	1

AMA: Dec 96: 7, Jan 07: 31, May 10: 9, Sep 13: 17, Oct 13: 18

28300 Osteotomy; calcaneus (eg, Dwyer or Chambers type procedure), with or without internal fixation `A 2 J I`

RVU		Global Days	Modifiers				
Mod	Non-Fac Total	Fac Total		51	50	62	80	MUE
	18.67	18.67	090	2	1	1	2	1

28302 Osteotomy; talus `A 2 T`

RVU		Global Days	Modifiers				
Mod	Non-Fac Total	Fac Total		51	50	62	80	MUE
	20.69	20.69	090	2	1	1	2	1

28304 Osteotomy, tarsal bones, other than calcaneus or talus `A 2 J I`

RVU		Global Days	Modifiers				
Mod	Non-Fac Total	Fac Total		51	50	62	80	MUE
	23.41	17.17	090	2	1	1	2	1

AMA: Nov 98: 8

28305 Osteotomy, tarsal bones, other than calcaneus or talus; with autograft (includes obtaining graft) (eg, Fowler type) `A 2 J I`

RVU		Global Days	Modifiers				
Mod	Non-Fac Total	Fac Total		51	50	62	80	MUE
	19.00	19.00	090	2	1	1	2	1

28306 Osteotomy, with or without lengthening, shortening or angular correction, metatarsal; first metatarsal `A 2 T`

RVU		Global Days	Modifiers				
Mod	Non-Fac Total	Fac Total		51	50	62	80	MUE
	17.61	11.54	090	2	1	1	2	1

AMA: Nov 98: 8, Dec 99: 7, Dec 10: 12

28307 Osteotomy, with or without lengthening, shortening or angular correction, metatarsal; first metatarsal with autograft (other than first toe) `A 2 T`

RVU		Global Days	Modifiers				
Mod	Non-Fac Total	Fac Total		51	50	62	80	MUE
	19.72	13.00	090	2	1	0	0	1

AMA: Nov 98: 9

28308 Osteotomy, with or without lengthening, shortening or angular correction, metatarsal; other than first metatarsal, each `A 2 T`

RVU		Global Days	Modifiers				
Mod	Non-Fac Total	Fac Total		51	50	62	80	MUE
	16.27	10.80	090	2	1	1	2	4

28309 Osteotomy, with or without lengthening, shortening or angular correction, metatarsal; multiple (eg, Swanson type cavus foot procedure) `A 2 J I`

RVU		Global Days	Modifiers				
Mod	Non-Fac Total	Fac Total		51	50	62	80	MUE
	26.21	26.21	090	2	1	0	0	1

AMA: Nov 98: 8, Dec 99: 7

28310 Osteotomy, shortening, angular or rotational correction; proximal phalanx, first toe (separate procedure) `A 2 T`

RVU		Global Days	Modifiers				
Mod	Non-Fac Total	Fac Total		51	50	62	80	MUE
	15.85	10.32	090	2	1	1	1	1

AMA: Sep 13: 17

● New   ▲ Revised   ✖ Deleted   ⊙ Moderate Sedation   ✚ Add-on Codes   ⊘ High Risk Denial   Ⓐ Age Edit   ♀ Female   ♂ Male   **AMA** CPT® Assistant   **MUE** Medically Unlikely Edit
⊘ Modifier 51 Exempt   ⊖ Modifier 63 Exempt   ⵙ Unlisted   **Modifiers:** See Inside Back Cover   Ⓜ Maternity   `A 2`–`Z 3` ASC Payment Indicators   `A`–`Y` OPPS Status Indicators

CPT © 2015 American Medical Association. All Rights Reserved.   © 2016 DecisionHealth

28312 Osteotomy, shortening, angular or rotational correction; other phalanges, any toe `A 2 T`

RVU			Global Days	Modifiers				
Mod	Non-Fac Total	Fac Total		51	50	62	80	MUE
	14.68	9.16	090	2	0	1	1	4

28313 Reconstruction, angular deformity of toe, soft tissue procedures only (eg, overlapping second toe, fifth toe, curly toes) `A 2 T`

RVU			Global Days	Modifiers				
Mod	Non-Fac Total	Fac Total		51	50	62	80	MUE
	14.95	10.12	090	2	0	0	1	4

AMA: Nov 98: 8

28315 Sesamoidectomy, first toe (separate procedure) `A 2 T`

RVU			Global Days	Modifiers				
Mod	Non-Fac Total	Fac Total		51	50	62	80	MUE
	13.90	9.35	090	2	1	1	1	1

28320 Repair, nonunion or malunion; tarsal bones `G 2 J 1`

RVU			Global Days	Modifiers				
Mod	Non-Fac Total	Fac Total		51	50	62	80	MUE
	17.56	17.56	090	2	1	1	2	1

AMA: Nov 98: 9

28322 Repair, nonunion or malunion; metatarsal, with or without bone graft (includes obtaining graft) `A 2 J 1`

RVU			Global Days	Modifiers				
Mod	Non-Fac Total	Fac Total		51	50	62	80	MUE
	22.90	16.71	090	2	0	1	2	2

28340 Reconstruction, toe, macrodactyly; soft tissue resection `A 2 T`

RVU			Global Days	Modifiers				
Mod	Non-Fac Total	Fac Total		51	50	62	80	MUE
	16.75	11.91	090	2	0	0	1	2

28341 Reconstruction, toe, macrodactyly; requiring bone resection `A 2 T`

RVU			Global Days	Modifiers				
Mod	Non-Fac Total	Fac Total		51	50	62	80	MUE
	19.43	14.17	090	2	0	0	1	2

28344 Reconstruction, toe(s); polydactyly `A 2 T`

RVU			Global Days	Modifiers				
Mod	Non-Fac Total	Fac Total		51	50	62	80	MUE
	13.40	8.96	090	2	1	1	1	1

28345 Reconstruction, toe(s); syndactyly, with or without skin graft(s), each web `A 2 T`

RVU			Global Days	Modifiers				
Mod	Non-Fac Total	Fac Total		51	50	62	80	MUE
	15.13	10.51	090	2	0	0	0	2

28360 Reconstruction, cleft foot `J 1`

RVU			Global Days	Modifiers				
Mod	Non-Fac Total	Fac Total		51	50	62	80	MUE
	26.56	26.56	090	2	1	0	2	1

Foot/Toe Fracture/Dislocation Procedures

28400 Closed treatment of calcaneal fracture; without manipulation `A 2 T`

RVU			Global Days	Modifiers				
Mod	Non-Fac Total	Fac Total		51	50	62	80	MUE
	7.15	6.54	090	2	1	0	1	1

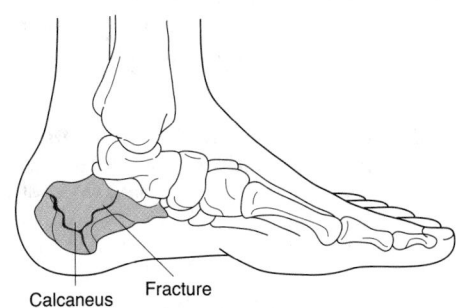

Closed treatment of calcaneal fracture

Calcaneus   Fracture

A fracture of the heel bone is repaired without (28400), or with (28405) manipulation

28405 Closed treatment of calcaneal fracture; with manipulation `A 2 T`

Coding tip: Add modifier 77 for re-reduction of the fracture by another physician

RVU			Global Days	Modifiers				
Mod	Non-Fac Total	Fac Total		51	50	62	80	MUE
	11.26	10.22	090	2	1	0	0	1

28406 Percutaneous skeletal fixation of calcaneal fracture, with manipulation `A 2 T`

RVU			Global Days	Modifiers				
Mod	Non-Fac Total	Fac Total		51	50	62	80	MUE
	15.10	15.10	090	2	1	0	0	1

28415 Open treatment of calcaneal fracture, includes internal fixation, when performed `A 2 J 1`

RVU			Global Days	Modifiers				
Mod	Non-Fac Total	Fac Total		51	50	62	80	MUE
	31.95	31.95	090	2	1	1	2	1

28420 Open treatment of calcaneal fracture, includes internal fixation, when performed; with primary iliac or other autogenous bone graft (includes obtaining graft) `J 8 J 1`

RVU			Global Days	Modifiers				
Mod	Non-Fac Total	Fac Total		51	50	62	80	MUE
	36.34	36.34	090	2	1	1	2	1

28430 Closed treatment of talus fracture; without manipulation `P 2 T`

RVU			Global Days	Modifiers				
Mod	Non-Fac Total	Fac Total		51	50	62	80	MUE
	6.81	6.06	090	2	1	0	1	1

● New   ▲ Revised   Deleted   ⊙ Moderate Sedation   ✛ Add-on Codes   ⊘ High Risk Denial   Ⓐ Age Edit   ♀ Female   ♂ Male   **AMA** *CPT® Assistant*   ***MUE*** Medically Unlikely Edit
⊘ Modifier 51 Exempt   ⊖ Modifier 63 Exempt   ☒ Unlisted   **Modifiers:** *See Inside Back Cover*   Ⓜ Maternity   `A 2`–`Z 3` ASC Payment Indicators   `A`–`Y` OPPS Status Indicators

Surgical Procedures

28435 – 28515

28435 Closed treatment of talus fracture; with manipulation   A2T

Coding tip: Add modifier 77 for re-reduction of the fracture by another physician

Mod	Non-Fac Total	Fac Total	Global Days	51	50	62	80	MUE
	9.12	8.15	090	2	1	0	0	1

28436 Percutaneous skeletal fixation of talus fracture, with manipulation   A2T

Mod	Non-Fac Total	Fac Total	Global Days	51	50	62	80	MUE
	12.97	12.97	090	2	1	0	1	1

28445 Open treatment of talus fracture, includes internal fixation, when performed   A2JI

Mod	Non-Fac Total	Fac Total	Global Days	51	50	62	80	MUE
	30.67	30.67	090	2	1	1	2	1

28446 Open osteochondral autograft, talus (includes obtaining graft[s])   G2JI

Mod	Non-Fac Total	Fac Total	Global Days	51	50	62	80	MUE
	35.08	35.08	090	2	1	1	2	1

AMA: Jan 08: 4, Dec 08: 6

28450 Treatment of tarsal bone fracture (except talus and calcaneus); without manipulation, each   P2T

Mod	Non-Fac Total	Fac Total	Global Days	51	50	62	80	MUE
	6.19	5.51	090	2	0	0	1	2

AMA: Dec 01: 7

28455 Treatment of tarsal bone fracture (except talus and calcaneus); with manipulation, each   P3T

Coding tip: Add modifier 77 for re-reduction of the fracture by another physician

Mod	Non-Fac Total	Fac Total	Global Days	51	50	62	80	MUE
	8.29	7.46	090	2	0	0	0	3

28456 Percutaneous skeletal fixation of tarsal bone fracture (except talus and calcaneus), with manipulation, each   A2JI

Mod	Non-Fac Total	Fac Total	Global Days	51	50	62	80	MUE
	9.21	9.21	090	2	0	0	1	2

28465 Open treatment of tarsal bone fracture (except talus and calcaneus), includes internal fixation, when performed, each   A2JI

Mod	Non-Fac Total	Fac Total	Global Days	51	50	62	80	MUE
	17.87	17.87	090	2	0	0	1	3

28470 Closed treatment of metatarsal fracture; without manipulation, each   P2T

Mod	Non-Fac Total	Fac Total	Global Days	51	50	62	80	MUE
	6.30	5.89	090	2	0	0	1	2

28475 Closed treatment of metatarsal fracture; with manipulation, each   P2T

Coding tip: Add modifier 77 for re-reduction of the fracture by another physician

Mod	Non-Fac Total	Fac Total	Global Days	51	50	62	80	MUE
	7.38	6.55	090	2	0	0	1	5

28476 Percutaneous skeletal fixation of metatarsal fracture, with manipulation, each   A2T

Mod	Non-Fac Total	Fac Total	Global Days	51	50	62	80	MUE
	10.14	10.14	090	2	0	0	0	4

28485 Open treatment of metatarsal fracture, includes internal fixation, when performed, each   A2T

Mod	Non-Fac Total	Fac Total	Global Days	51	50	62	80	MUE
	15.10	15.10	090	2	0	1	1	5

28490 Closed treatment of fracture great toe, phalanx or phalanges; without manipulation   P2T

Coding tip: Closed treatment of phalangeal fracture of other toes - 28510

Mod	Non-Fac Total	Fac Total	Global Days	51	50	62	80	MUE
	4.15	3.59	090	2	1	0	1	1

28495 Closed treatment of fracture great toe, phalanx or phalanges; with manipulation   P2T

Coding tip: Add modifier 77 for re-reduction of the fracture by another physician

Coding tip: Closed treatment of phalangeal fracture of other toes with manipulation - 28515

Mod	Non-Fac Total	Fac Total	Global Days	51	50	62	80	MUE
	5.09	4.28	090	2	1	0	1	1

28496 Percutaneous skeletal fixation of fracture great toe, phalanx or phalanges, with manipulation   A2T

Mod	Non-Fac Total	Fac Total	Global Days	51	50	62	80	MUE
	12.69	6.74	090	2	1	0	1	1

28505 Open treatment of fracture, great toe, phalanx or phalanges, includes internal fixation, when performed   A2T

Mod	Non-Fac Total	Fac Total	Global Days	51	50	62	80	MUE
	19.34	14.43	090	2	1	0	1	1

28510 Closed treatment of fracture, phalanx or phalanges, other than great toe; without manipulation, each   P3T

Coding tip: Closed treatment of phalangeal fracture of great toe - 28490

Mod	Non-Fac Total	Fac Total	Global Days	51	50	62	80	MUE
	3.54	3.44	090	2	0	0	1	4

28515 Closed treatment of fracture, phalanx or phalanges, other than great toe; with manipulation, each   P3T

Coding tip: Closed treatment of phalangeal fracture of great toe with manipulation - 28495

● New   ▲ Revised   ✖ Deleted   ⊙ Moderate Sedation   ✚ Add-on Codes   ⊘ High Risk Denial   Ⓐ Age Edit   ♀ Female   ♂ Male   **AMA** *CPT® Assistant*   **MUE** Medically Unlikely Edit

⊘ Modifier 51 Exempt   ⊖ Modifier 63 Exempt   ✗ Unlisted   **Modifiers:** *See Inside Back Cover*   Ⓜ Maternity   A2–Z3 ASC Payment Indicators   A–Y OPPS Status Indicators

312   CPT © 2015 American Medical Association. All Rights Reserved.   © 2016 DecisionHealth

Coding tip: Add modifier 77 for re-reduction of the fracture by another physician

RVU Mod	Non-Fac Total	Fac Total	Global Days	51	50	62	80	MUE
	4.61	4.08	090	2	0	0	1	4

28525 Open treatment of fracture, phalanx or phalanges, other than great toe, includes internal fixation, when performed, each   A2 T

RVU Mod	Non-Fac Total	Fac Total	Global Days	51	50	62	80	MUE
	16.22	11.38	090	2	0	0	0	4

28530 Closed treatment of sesamoid fracture   P3 T

RVU Mod	Non-Fac Total	Fac Total	Global Days	51	50	62	80	MUE
	3.33	2.95	090	2	1	0	0	1

28531 Open treatment of sesamoid fracture, with or without internal fixation   A2 T

RVU Mod	Non-Fac Total	Fac Total	Global Days	51	50	62	80	MUE
	10.00	5.30	090	2	1	2	1	1

28540 Closed treatment of tarsal bone dislocation, other than talotarsal; without anesthesia   P2 T

RVU Mod	Non-Fac Total	Fac Total	Global Days	51	50	62	80	MUE
	5.93	5.34	090	2	1	0	0	1

28545 Closed treatment of tarsal bone dislocation, other than talotarsal; requiring anesthesia   A2 T

RVU Mod	Non-Fac Total	Fac Total	Global Days	51	50	62	80	MUE
	8.38	7.43	090	2	1	0	0	1

28546 Percutaneous skeletal fixation of tarsal bone dislocation, other than talotarsal, with manipulation   A2 T

RVU Mod	Non-Fac Total	Fac Total	Global Days	51	50	62	80	MUE
	16.05	9.45	090	2	1	0	0	1

28555 Open treatment of tarsal bone dislocation, includes internal fixation, when performed   A2 J I

RVU Mod	Non-Fac Total	Fac Total	Global Days	51	50	62	80	MUE
	25.34	19.20	090	2	1	1	2	1

28570 Closed treatment of talotarsal joint dislocation; without anesthesia   P2 T

RVU Mod	Non-Fac Total	Fac Total	Global Days	51	50	62	80	MUE
	6.41	5.43	090	2	1	0	0	1

28575 Closed treatment of talotarsal joint dislocation; requiring anesthesia   A2 T

RVU Mod	Non-Fac Total	Fac Total	Global Days	51	50	62	80	MUE
	10.54	9.53	090	2	1	0	0	1

28576 Percutaneous skeletal fixation of talotarsal joint dislocation, with manipulation   A2 T

RVU Mod	Non-Fac Total	Fac Total	Global Days	51	50	62	80	MUE
	11.16	11.16	090	2	1	0	0	1

28585 Open treatment of talotarsal joint dislocation, includes internal fixation, when performed   A2 T

RVU Mod	Non-Fac Total	Fac Total	Global Days	51	50	62	80	MUE
	24.47	19.17	090	2	1	1	2	1

AMA: Sep 11: 12

28600 Closed treatment of tarsometatarsal joint dislocation; without anesthesia   P2 T

RVU Mod	Non-Fac Total	Fac Total	Global Days	51	50	62	80	MUE
	6.25	5.38	090	2	0	0	0	2

28605 Closed treatment of tarsometatarsal joint dislocation; requiring anesthesia   A2 T

RVU Mod	Non-Fac Total	Fac Total	Global Days	51	50	62	80	MUE
	9.40	8.46	090	2	0	0	0	2

28606 Percutaneous skeletal fixation of tarsometatarsal joint dislocation, with manipulation   A2 T

RVU Mod	Non-Fac Total	Fac Total	Global Days	51	50	62	80	MUE
	11.32	11.32	090	2	0	0	1	3

28615 Open treatment of tarsometatarsal joint dislocation, includes internal fixation, when performed   A2 J I

RVU Mod	Non-Fac Total	Fac Total	Global Days	51	50	62	80	MUE
	22.71	22.71	090	2	0	1	2	5

28630 Closed treatment of metatarsophalangeal joint dislocation; without anesthesia   P3 T

Coding tip: Closed treatment of interphalangeal joint dislocation - 28660

RVU Mod	Non-Fac Total	Fac Total	Global Days	51	50	62	80	MUE
	4.49	3.15	010	2	0	0	0	2

28635 Closed treatment of metatarsophalangeal joint dislocation; requiring anesthesia   A2 T

Coding tip: Closed treatment of interphalangeal joint dislocation with anesthesia - 28665

RVU Mod	Non-Fac Total	Fac Total	Global Days	51	50	62	80	MUE
	5.01	3.78	010	2	0	0	0	2

28636 Percutaneous skeletal fixation of metatarsophalangeal joint dislocation, with manipulation   A2 T

RVU Mod	Non-Fac Total	Fac Total	Global Days	51	50	62	80	MUE
	8.17	5.24	010	2	0	2	1	4

● New   ▲ Revised   Deleted   ⊙ Moderate Sedation   ✚ Add-on Codes   ⊘ High Risk Denial   Ⓐ Age Edit   ♀ Female   ♂ Male   **AMA** *CPT® Assistant*   ***MUE*** Medically Unlikely Edit
⊘ Modifier 51 Exempt   ⊖ Modifier 63 Exempt   ✗ Unlisted   **Modifiers:** *See Inside Back Cover*   Ⓜ Maternity   A2–Z3 ASC Payment Indicators   A–Y OPPS Status Indicators

© 2016 DecisionHealth   CPT © 2015 American Medical Association. All Rights Reserved.   **313**

28645 **Open treatment of metatarsophalangeal joint dislocation, includes internal fixation, when performed** `A 2 T`

RVU			Global Days	Modifiers				
Mod	Non-Fac Total	Fac Total		51	50	62	80	MUE
	18.98	13.97	090	2	0	1	1	4

AMA: Sep 14: 13

28660 **Closed treatment of interphalangeal joint dislocation; without anesthesia** `P 3 T`

Coding tip: Closed treatment of metatarsophalangeal joint dislocation - 28630

RVU			Global Days	Modifiers				
Mod	Non-Fac Total	Fac Total		51	50	62	80	MUE
	3.34	2.55	010	2	0	0	1	4

28665 **Closed treatment of interphalangeal joint dislocation; requiring anesthesia** `A 2 S`

Coding tip: Closed treatment of metatarsophalangeal joint dislocation with anesthesia - 28635

RVU			Global Days	Modifiers				
Mod	Non-Fac Total	Fac Total		51	50	62	80	MUE
	4.42	3.76	010	2	0	0	0	4

28666 **Percutaneous skeletal fixation of interphalangeal joint dislocation, with manipulation** `A 2 T`

RVU			Global Days	Modifiers				
Mod	Non-Fac Total	Fac Total		51	50	62	80	MUE
	5.41	5.41	010	2	0	2	1	4

28675 **Open treatment of interphalangeal joint dislocation, includes internal fixation, when performed** `A 2 T`

RVU			Global Days	Modifiers				
Mod	Non-Fac Total	Fac Total		51	50	62	80	MUE
	16.96	11.91	090	2	0	0	1	4

Foot/Toe Arthrodesis

28705 **Arthrodesis; pantalar** `J 8 J I`

RVU			Global Days	Modifiers				
Mod	Non-Fac Total	Fac Total		51	50	62	80	MUE
	36.18	36.18	090	2	1	1	2	1

28715 **Arthrodesis; triple** `J 8 J I`

RVU			Global Days	Modifiers				
Mod	Non-Fac Total	Fac Total		51	50	62	80	MUE
	27.07	27.07	090	2	1	1	2	1

28725 **Arthrodesis; subtalar** `G 2 J I`

RVU			Global Days	Modifiers				
Mod	Non-Fac Total	Fac Total		51	50	62	80	MUE
	22.43	22.43	090	2	1	1	2	1

AMA: Sep 11: 11

28730 **Arthrodesis, midtarsal or tarsometatarsal, multiple or transverse** `G 2 J I`

RVU			Global Days	Modifiers				
Mod	Non-Fac Total	Fac Total		51	50	62	80	MUE
	21.17	21.17	090	2	1	1	2	1

28735 **Arthrodesis, midtarsal or tarsometatarsal, multiple or transverse; with osteotomy (eg, flatfoot correction)** `J 8 J I`

RVU			Global Days	Modifiers				
Mod	Non-Fac Total	Fac Total		51	50	62	80	MUE
	22.55	22.55	090	2	1	1	2	1

28737 **Arthrodesis, with tendon lengthening and advancement, midtarsal, tarsal navicular-cuneiform (eg, Miller type procedure)** `G 2 J I`

RVU			Global Days	Modifiers				
Mod	Non-Fac Total	Fac Total		51	50	62	80	MUE
	19.77	19.77	090	2	1	1	2	1

28740 **Arthrodesis, midtarsal or tarsometatarsal, single joint** `G 2 J I`

RVU			Global Days	Modifiers				
Mod	Non-Fac Total	Fac Total		51	50	62	80	MUE
	24.37	17.89	090	2	0	1	2	5

28750 **Arthrodesis, great toe; metatarsophalangeal joint** `A 2 J I`

RVU			Global Days	Modifiers				
Mod	Non-Fac Total	Fac Total		51	50	62	80	MUE
	23.59	17.09	090	2	1	0	0	1

AMA: Dec 96: 7

28755 **Arthrodesis, great toe; interphalangeal joint** `A 2 T`

RVU			Global Days	Modifiers				
Mod	Non-Fac Total	Fac Total		51	50	62	80	MUE
	14.71	9.51	090	2	1	1	1	1

28760 **Arthrodesis, with extensor hallucis longus transfer to first metatarsal neck, great toe, interphalangeal joint (eg, Jones type procedure)** `A 2 J I`

RVU			Global Days	Modifiers				
Mod	Non-Fac Total	Fac Total		51	50	62	80	MUE
	22.85	16.66	090	2	1	1	2	1

AMA: Nov 98: 8

Foot/Toe Amputation

28800 **Amputation, foot; midtarsal (eg, Chopart type procedure)** `C`

RVU			Global Days	Modifiers				
Mod	Non-Fac Total	Fac Total		51	50	62	80	MUE
	15.72	15.72	090	2	1	1	2	1

28805 **Amputation, foot; transmetatarsal** `T`

RVU			Global Days	Modifiers				
Mod	Non-Fac Total	Fac Total		51	50	62	80	MUE
	21.26	21.26	090	2	1	0	0	1

AMA: May 97: 8

28810 **Amputation, metatarsal, with toe, single** `A 2 T`

RVU			Global Days	Modifiers				
Mod	Non-Fac Total	Fac Total		51	50	62	80	MUE
	12.56	12.56	090	2	0	0	0	6

28820 **Amputation, toe; metatarsophalangeal joint** `A 2 T`

RVU			Global Days	Modifiers				
Mod	Non-Fac Total	Fac Total		51	50	62	80	MUE
	16.45	11.49	090	2	0	0	1	6

AMA: May 97: 8

● New ▲ Revised ✖ Deleted ⊙ Moderate Sedation ✚ Add-on Codes ⊘ High Risk Denial Ⓐ Age Edit ♀ Female ♂ Male **AMA** *CPT® Assistant* **MUE** Medically Unlikely Edit
⊘ Modifier 51 Exempt ⊖ Modifier 63 Exempt ⓧ Unlisted **Modifiers:** *See Inside Back Cover* Ⓜ Maternity `A 2`–`Z 3` ASC Payment Indicators `A`–`Y` OPPS Status Indicators

28825 Amputation, toe; interphalangeal joint `A 2 T`

RVU			Global Days	Modifiers				
Mod	Non-Fac Total	Fac Total		51	50	62	80	MUE
	15.67	10.74	090	2	0	0	1	10

Other Foot/Toe Procedures

28890 Extracorporeal shock wave, high energy, performed by a physician or other qualified health care professional, requiring anesthesia other than local, including ultrasound guidance, involving the plantar fascia `P 3 T`

RVU			Global Days	Modifiers				
Mod	Non-Fac Total	Fac Total		51	50	62	80	MUE
	9.31	6.46	090	2	1	1	1	1

AMA: Dec 05: 10, Mar 06: 1

28899 Unlisted procedure, foot or toes `x T`

RVU			Global Days	Modifiers				
Mod	Non-Fac Total	Fac Total		51	50	62	80	MUE
	0.00	0.00	YYY	2	0	1	0	

AMA: Sep 11: 12

Casting/Strapping Procedures

Body/Upper Extremity Cast/Splints/Straps

Coding Guidance

Application of casting/splinting/strapping is not reported when any kind of treatment or restorative service aimed at correcting, protecting, or stabilizing the fracture or dislocation is concurrently done. Use application codes only as an initial service done without any restorative treatment or as a replacement service during or after follow-up care. Casting/strapping/splinting is not used for reporting a dressing application after a therapeutic procedure, such as an anesthetic injected into a peripheral nerve or an aspiration procedure.

29000 Application of halo type body cast (see 20661-20663 for insertion) `G 2 S`

RVU			Global Days	Modifiers				
Mod	Non-Fac Total	Fac Total		51	50	62	80	MUE
	8.47	5.15	000	2	0	0	0	1

AMA: Feb 96: 3, 5, Apr 02: 13

Application of halo type body cast

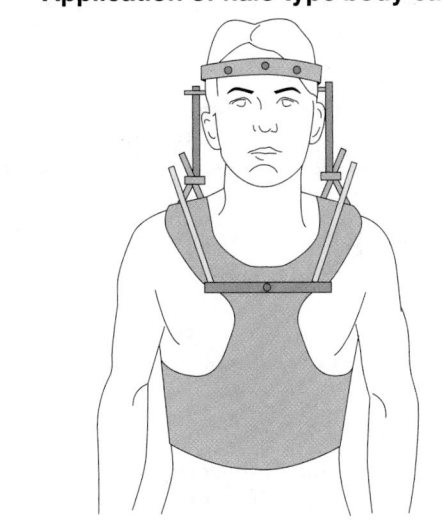

29010 Application of Risser jacket, localizer, body; only `⊘ P 2 S`

RVU			Global Days	Modifiers				
Mod	Non-Fac Total	Fac Total		51	50	62	80	MUE
	6.82	4.25	000	2	0	0	0	1

AMA: Feb 96: 3, Apr 02: 13

29015 Application of Risser jacket, localizer, body; including head `⊘ P 2 S`

RVU			Global Days	Modifiers				
Mod	Non-Fac Total	Fac Total		51	50	62	80	MUE
	8.19	5.16	000	2	0	0	0	1

AMA: Feb 96: 3, Apr 02: 13

29035 Application of body cast, shoulder to hips `P 2 S`

RVU			Global Days	Modifiers				
Mod	Non-Fac Total	Fac Total		51	50	62	80	MUE
	5.57	3.45	000	2	0	0	0	1

AMA: Feb 96: 3, Apr 02: 13

29040 Application of body cast, shoulder to hips; including head, Minerva type `G 2 S`

RVU			Global Days	Modifiers				
Mod	Non-Fac Total	Fac Total		51	50	62	80	MUE
	6.46	4.20	000	2	0	0	0	1

AMA: Feb 96: 3, Apr 02: 13

29044 Application of body cast, shoulder to hips; including 1 thigh `P 2 S`

RVU			Global Days	Modifiers				
Mod	Non-Fac Total	Fac Total		51	50	62	80	MUE
	8.09	4.40	000	2	0	0	0	1

AMA: Feb 96: 3, Apr 02: 13

29046 Application of body cast, shoulder to hips; including both thighs `G 2 S`

RVU			Global Days	Modifiers				
Mod	Non-Fac Total	Fac Total		51	50	62	80	MUE
	6.95	4.56	000	2	0	0	0	1

AMA: Feb 96: 3, Apr 02: 13

29049 Application, cast; figure-of-eight `P 3 S`

RVU			Global Days	Modifiers				
Mod	Non-Fac Total	Fac Total		51	50	62	80	MUE
	2.41	1.79	000	2	0	0	0	1

AMA: Feb 96: 3, Apr 02: 13

29055 Application, cast; shoulder spica `P 2 S`

RVU			Global Days	Modifiers				
Mod	Non-Fac Total	Fac Total		51	50	62	80	MUE
	6.41	4.02	000	2	0	0	0	1

AMA: Feb 96: 3, Apr 02: 13

29058 Application, cast; plaster Velpeau `P 3 S`

RVU			Global Days	Modifiers				
Mod	Non-Fac Total	Fac Total		51	50	62	80	MUE
	3.53	2.69	000	2	0	0	0	1

AMA: Feb 96: 3, Apr 02: 13

29065 Application, cast; shoulder to hand (long arm) `P 3 S`

RVU			Global Days	Modifiers				
Mod	Non-Fac Total	Fac Total		51	50	62	80	MUE
	2.78	1.98	000	2	1	0	1	1

AMA: Feb 96: 3, Apr 02: 13

● New ▲ Revised Deleted ⊙ Moderate Sedation ✚ Add-on Codes ⊘ High Risk Denial Ⓐ Age Edit ♀ Female ♂ Male **AMA** *CPT® Assistant* **MUE** Medically Unlikely Edit
⊘ Modifier 51 Exempt ⊖ Modifier 63 Exempt ✗ Unlisted **Modifiers:** *See Inside Back Cover* Ⓜ Maternity `A 2`–`Z 3` ASC Payment Indicators `A`–`Y` OPPS Status Indicators

Surgical Procedures

28825 – 29065

29075 Application, cast; elbow to finger (short arm) P 3 S

Mod	Non-Fac Total	Fac Total	Global Days	51	50	62	80	MUE
	2.51	1.81	000	2	1	0	1	1

AMA: Feb 96: 3, 4, Apr 02: 13

29085 Application, cast; hand and lower forearm (gauntlet) P 3 S

Mod	Non-Fac Total	Fac Total	Global Days	51	50	62	80	MUE
	2.76	1.96	000	2	1	0	1	1

AMA: Feb 96: 3, Apr 02: 13, Dec 02: 11

29086 Application, cast; finger (eg, contracture) P 3 S

Mod	Non-Fac Total	Fac Total	Global Days	51	50	62	80	MUE
	2.25	1.48	000	2	1	0	1	2

AMA: Apr 02: 13

29105 Application of long arm splint (shoulder to hand) P 3 S

Mod	Non-Fac Total	Fac Total	Global Days	51	50	62	80	MUE
	2.52	1.71	000	2	1	0	1	1

AMA: Feb 96: 3, Apr 02: 13, May 09: 8

29125 Application of short arm splint (forearm to hand); static N 1 Q 1

Mod	Non-Fac Total	Fac Total	Global Days	51	50	62	80	MUE
	1.85	1.13	000	2	1	0	1	1

AMA: Feb 96: 3, 4, Apr 02: 13

29126 Application of short arm splint (forearm to hand); dynamic N 1 Q 1

Mod	Non-Fac Total	Fac Total	Global Days	51	50	62	80	MUE
	2.20	1.40	000	2	1	0	1	1

AMA: Feb 96: 3, Apr 02: 13

29130 Application of finger splint; static N 1 Q 1

Mod	Non-Fac Total	Fac Total	Global Days	51	50	62	80	MUE
	1.18	0.82	000	2	1	0	1	3

AMA: Feb 96: 3, Apr 02: 13

29131 Application of finger splint; dynamic N 1 Q 1

Mod	Non-Fac Total	Fac Total	Global Days	51	50	62	80	MUE
	1.46	0.95	000	2	1	0	1	2

AMA: Feb 96: 3, Apr 02: 13

29200 Strapping; thorax P 3 S

Mod	Non-Fac Total	Fac Total	Global Days	51	50	62	80	MUE
	0.84	0.52	000	2	0	0	1	1

AMA: Feb 96: 3, Apr 02: 13

29240 Strapping; shoulder (eg, Velpeau) N 1 Q 1

Mod	Non-Fac Total	Fac Total	Global Days	51	50	62	80	MUE
	0.82	0.53	000	2	1	0	1	1

AMA: Feb 96: 3, Apr 02: 13, Jun 10: 8

29260 Strapping; elbow or wrist N 1 Q 1

Mod	Non-Fac Total	Fac Total	Global Days	51	50	62	80	MUE
	0.83	0.56	000	2	1	0	1	1

AMA: Feb 96: 3, Apr 02: 13

29280 Strapping; hand or finger N 1 Q 1

Mod	Non-Fac Total	Fac Total	Global Days	51	50	62	80	MUE
	0.84	0.58	000	2	1	0	1	2

AMA: Feb 96: 3, Apr 02: 13

Lower Extremity Cast/Splints/Straps

29305 Application of hip spica cast; 1 leg P 2 S

Mod	Non-Fac Total	Fac Total	Global Days	51	50	62	80	MUE
	7.11	4.62	000	2	0	0	0	1

AMA: Feb 96: 3, Apr 02: 13

29325 Application of hip spica cast; 1 and one-half spica or both legs P 2 S

Mod	Non-Fac Total	Fac Total	Global Days	51	50	62	80	MUE
	7.81	5.14	000	2	0	0	0	1

AMA: Feb 96: 3, Apr 02: 13

29345 Application of long leg cast (thigh to toes) P 3 S

Mod	Non-Fac Total	Fac Total	Global Days	51	50	62	80	MUE
	3.93	2.92	000	2	1	0	1	1

AMA: Feb 96: 3, Apr 02: 13, Sep 11: 11

29355 Application of long leg cast (thigh to toes); walker or ambulatory type P 3 S

Mod	Non-Fac Total	Fac Total	Global Days	51	50	62	80	MUE
	4.05	3.07	000	2	1	0	1	1

AMA: Feb 96: 3, Apr 02: 13, Sep 11: 11

29358 Application of long leg cast brace P 3 S

Mod	Non-Fac Total	Fac Total	Global Days	51	50	62	80	MUE
	4.62	3.01	000	2	1	0	1	1

AMA: Feb 96: 3, Apr 02: 13, Sep 11: 11

29365 Application of cylinder cast (thigh to ankle) P 3 S

Mod	Non-Fac Total	Fac Total	Global Days	51	50	62	80	MUE
	3.53	2.53	000	2	1	0	1	1

AMA: Feb 96: 3, Apr 02: 13, Sep 11: 11

29405 Application of short leg cast (below knee to toes) P 3 S

Mod	Non-Fac Total	Fac Total	Global Days	51	50	62	80	MUE
	2.35	1.73	000	2	1	0	1	1

AMA: Feb 96: 3, Apr 02: 13, Mar 03: 17, Sep 11: 11

29425 Application of short leg cast (below knee to toes); walking or ambulatory type P 3 S

Mod	Non-Fac Total	Fac Total	Global Days	51	50	62	80	MUE
	2.25	1.63	000	2	1	0	1	1

AMA: Feb 96: 3, Apr 02: 13, Sep 11: 11

● New   ▲ Revised   ✖ Deleted   ⊙ Moderate Sedation   ✚ Add-on Codes   ⊖ High Risk Denial   Ⓐ Age Edit   ♀ Female   ♂ Male   **AMA** *CPT® Assistant*   **MUE** Medically Unlikely Edit
⊘ Modifier 51 Exempt   ⊖ Modifier 63 Exempt   ✗ Unlisted   **Modifiers:** *See Inside Back Cover*   Ⓜ Maternity   A 2 – Z 3 ASC Payment Indicators   A – Y OPPS Status Indicators

CPT © 2015 American Medical Association. All Rights Reserved.   © 2016 DecisionHealth

29435 Application of patellar tendon bearing (PTB) cast [P 3 S]

Mod	Non-Fac Total	Fac Total	Global Days	51	50	62	80	MUE
	3.35	2.39	000	2	1	0	1	1

AMA: Feb 96: 3, Apr 02: 13, Sep 11: 11

29440 Adding walker to previously applied cast [P 3 S]

Mod	Non-Fac Total	Fac Total	Global Days	51	50	62	80	MUE
	1.25	0.83	000	2	1	0	1	1

AMA: Feb 96: 3, Apr 02: 13

29445 Application of rigid total contact leg cast [P 3 S]

Mod	Non-Fac Total	Fac Total	Global Days	51	50	62	80	MUE
	3.86	2.99	000	2	1	0	1	1

AMA: Feb 96: 3, Apr 02: 13, Sep 11: 11

29450 Application of clubfoot cast with molding or manipulation, long or short leg [P 3 S]

Mod	Non-Fac Total	Fac Total	Global Days	51	50	62	80	MUE
	4.11	3.23	000	2	1	0	1	1

AMA: Feb 96: 3, Apr 02: 13

29505 Application of long leg splint (thigh to ankle or toes) [P 3 S]

Mod	Non-Fac Total	Fac Total	Global Days	51	50	62	80	MUE
	2.38	1.43	000	2	1	0	1	1

AMA: Feb 96: 3, Apr 02: 13, May 09: 8

29515 Application of short leg splint (calf to foot) [P 3 S]

Mod	Non-Fac Total	Fac Total	Global Days	51	50	62	80	MUE
	2.05	1.43	000	2	1	0	1	1

AMA: Feb 96: 3, Apr 02: 13, Mar 03: 18

29520 Strapping; hip [N1 Q1]

Mod	Non-Fac Total	Fac Total	Global Days	51	50	62	80	MUE
	0.89	0.53	000	2	1	0	0	1

AMA: Feb 96: 3, Apr 02: 13

29530 Strapping; knee [N1 Q1]

Mod	Non-Fac Total	Fac Total	Global Days	51	50	62	80	MUE
	0.82	0.53	000	2	1	0	1	1

AMA: Feb 96: 3, Apr 02: 13, Aug 10: 15, Jun 10: 8

29540 Strapping; ankle and/or foot [P 3 S]

Mod	Non-Fac Total	Fac Total	Global Days	51	50	62	80	MUE
	0.74	0.52	000	2	1	0	1	1

AMA: Feb 96: 3, Apr 02: 13, Mar 03: 17, Jun 10: 8, Aug 10: 15, Mar 14: 4

29550 Strapping; toes [N1 Q1]

Mod	Non-Fac Total	Fac Total	Global Days	51	50	62	80	MUE
	0.54	0.33	000	2	1	0	1	1

AMA: Feb 96: 3, Apr 02: 13

29580 Strapping; Unna boot [P 3 S]

Mod	Non-Fac Total	Fac Total	Global Days	51	50	62	80	MUE
	1.50	1.02	000	2	1	0	1	1

AMA: Feb 96: 3, Jul 99: 10, Apr 02: 13, Mar 14: 4

29581 Application of multi-layer compression system; leg (below knee), including ankle and foot [P 3 S]

Mod	Non-Fac Total	Fac Total	Global Days	51	50	62	80	MUE
	1.75	0.36	000	2	1	0	0	1

AMA: May 11: 11, Sep 12: 16, Mar 15: 10, Sep 13: 17, Mar 14: 4, Oct 14: 6

29582 Application of multi-layer compression system; thigh and leg, including ankle and foot, when performed [P 3 S]

Mod	Non-Fac Total	Fac Total	Global Days	51	50	62	80	MUE
	1.99	0.45	000	2	1	0	0	1

AMA: Mar 14: 4, Mar 15: 10, Oct 14: 6

29583 Application of multi-layer compression system; upper arm and forearm [P 3 S]

Mod	Non-Fac Total	Fac Total	Global Days	51	50	62	80	MUE
	1.24	0.32	000	2	1	0	0	1

AMA: Mar 15: 10

29584 Application of multi-layer compression system; upper arm, forearm, hand, and fingers [P 3 S]

Mod	Non-Fac Total	Fac Total	Global Days	51	50	62	80	MUE
	1.99	0.45	000	2	1	0	0	1

AMA: Mar 15: 10

Cast Removal/Repair

Coding Guidance

Codes 29700-29750 for removal or repair of casts/splints/strapping are included in the application procedure when performed by the same provider. Removal or repair codes may only be reported by a different provider than the one who performed the initial application.

29700 Removal or bivalving; gauntlet, boot or body cast [P 3 S]

Mod	Non-Fac Total	Fac Total	Global Days	51	50	62	80	MUE
	1.79	0.96	000	2	0	0	1	2

AMA: Apr 02: 13

29705 Removal or bivalving; full arm or full leg cast [P 3 S]

Mod	Non-Fac Total	Fac Total	Global Days	51	50	62	80	MUE
	1.92	1.36	000	2	1	0	1	1

AMA: Apr 02: 13

29710 Removal or bivalving; shoulder or hip spica, Minerva, or Risser jacket, etc. [P 3 S]

Mod	Non-Fac Total	Fac Total	Global Days	51	50	62	80	MUE
	3.51	2.40	000	2	1	0	0	1

AMA: Apr 02: 13

● New ▲ Revised Deleted ⊙ Moderate Sedation ✚ Add-on Codes ⊘ High Risk Denial Ⓐ Age Edit ♀ Female ♂ Male AMA CPT® Assistant MUE Medically Unlikely Edit
⊘ Modifier 51 Exempt ⊖ Modifier 63 Exempt ✗ Unlisted Modifiers: See Inside Back Cover Ⓜ Maternity A2–Z3 ASC Payment Indicators A–Y OPPS Status Indicators

Surgical Procedures

29435 – 29710

Surgical Procedures

29720 – 29823

29720 Repair of spica, body cast or jacket P 3 S

RVU			Global Days	Modifiers				
Mod	Non-Fac Total	Fac Total		51	50	62	80	MUE
	2.45	1.28	000	2	0	0	1	1

AMA: Apr 02: 13

29730 Windowing of cast P 3 S

RVU			Global Days	Modifiers				
Mod	Non-Fac Total	Fac Total		51	50	62	80	MUE
	1.86	1.30	000	2	0	0	1	1

AMA: Apr 02: 13

29740 Wedging of cast (except clubfoot casts) P 3 S

RVU			Global Days	Modifiers				
Mod	Non-Fac Total	Fac Total		51	50	62	80	MUE
	2.86	2.04	000	2	0	0	1	1

AMA: Apr 02: 13

29750 Wedging of clubfoot cast P 3 S

RVU			Global Days	Modifiers				
Mod	Non-Fac Total	Fac Total		51	50	62	80	MUE
	2.56	1.93	000	2	1	0	0	1

AMA: Apr 02: 13

Other Casting/Strapping Procedures

29799 Unlisted procedure, casting or strapping ⊘ x S

RVU			Global Days	Modifiers				
Mod	Non-Fac Total	Fac Total		51	50	62	80	MUE
	0.00	0.00	YYY	2	0	1	0	

AMA: Sep 12: 16

Musculoskeletal Endoscopy/Arthroscopy Procedures

Coding Guidance

When an arthroscopic procedure is done and an open procedure follows directly during the same session, only the main service is reported, which generally is the open procedure. If the arthroscopic procedure is done at one site with an open procedure performed at another location, both services may be reported with the appropriate modifier indicating different anatomic sites.

29800 Arthroscopy, temporomandibular joint, diagnostic, with or without synovial biopsy (separate procedure) A 2 T

RVU			Global Days	Modifiers				
Mod	Non-Fac Total	Fac Total		51	50	62	80	MUE
	14.74	14.74	090	2	1	0	0	1

AMA: May 13: 12

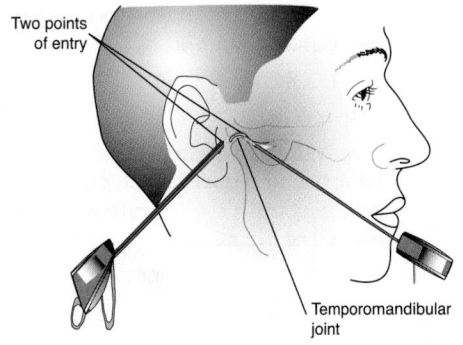

Arthroscopy, temporomandibular joint

Two points of entry

Temporomandibular joint

Diagnostic, with or without synovial biopsy (29800); surgical (29804)

29804 Arthroscopy, temporomandibular joint, surgical A 2 T

RVU			Global Days	Modifiers				
Mod	Non-Fac Total	Fac Total		51	50	62	80	MUE
	18.71	18.71	090	2	1	1	2	1

AMA: May 13: 12

29805 Arthroscopy, shoulder, diagnostic, with or without synovial biopsy (separate procedure) A 2 T

RVU			Global Days	Modifiers				
Mod	Non-Fac Total	Fac Total		51	50	62	80	MUE
	13.66	13.66	090	2	1	1	1	1

AMA: May 13: 12, Jun 15: 10

29806 Arthroscopy, shoulder, surgical; capsulorrhaphy A 2 J 1

RVU			Global Days	Modifiers				
Mod	Non-Fac Total	Fac Total		51	50	62	80	MUE
	30.75	30.75	090	3	1	1	1	1

AMA: Mar 15: 7, May 13: 12, Jul 15: 10

29807 Arthroscopy, shoulder, surgical; repair of SLAP lesion A 2 J 1

RVU			Global Days	Modifiers				
Mod	Non-Fac Total	Fac Total		51	50	62	80	MUE
	30.02	30.02	090	3	1	1	1	1

AMA: Mar 15: 7, May 13: 12

29819 Arthroscopy, shoulder, surgical; with removal of loose body or foreign body A 2 T

RVU			Global Days	Modifiers				
Mod	Non-Fac Total	Fac Total		51	50	62	80	MUE
	16.95	16.95	090	3	1	1	1	1

AMA: Mar 15: 7, May 13: 12

29820 Arthroscopy, shoulder, surgical; synovectomy, partial A 2 T

RVU			Global Days	Modifiers				
Mod	Non-Fac Total	Fac Total		51	50	62	80	MUE
	15.45	15.45	090	3	1	1	2	1

AMA: Mar 15: 7, May 13: 12, Jun 13: 13

29821 Arthroscopy, shoulder, surgical; synovectomy, complete A 2 T

RVU			Global Days	Modifiers				
Mod	Non-Fac Total	Fac Total		51	50	62	80	MUE
	16.86	16.86	090	3	1	1	2	1

AMA: Mar 15: 7, May 13: 12, Jun 13: 13

29822 Arthroscopy, shoulder, surgical; debridement, limited A 2 T

RVU			Global Days	Modifiers				
Mod	Non-Fac Total	Fac Total		51	50	62	80	MUE
	16.37	16.37	090	3	1	0	2	1

AMA: May 01: 9, Mar 15: 7, Apr 12: 17, Sep 12: 16, May 13: 12

29823 Arthroscopy, shoulder, surgical; debridement, extensive A 2 T

RVU			Global Days	Modifiers				
Mod	Non-Fac Total	Fac Total		51	50	62	80	MUE
	17.87	17.87	090	3	1	1	2	1

AMA: Mar 15: 7, Apr 12: 17, Sep 12: 16, May 13: 12

● New   ▲ Revised   ✖ Deleted   ⊙ Moderate Sedation   ✚ Add-on Codes   ⊘ High Risk Denial   Ⓐ Age Edit   ♀ Female   ♂ Male   **AMA** *CPT® Assistant*   **MUE** Medically Unlikely Edit
⊘ Modifier 51 Exempt   ⊖ Modifier 63 Exempt   ✗ Unlisted   **Modifiers:** *See Inside Back Cover*   Ⓜ Maternity   A2–Z3 ASC Payment Indicators   A–Y OPPS Status Indicators

318   CPT © 2015 American Medical Association. All Rights Reserved.   © 2016 DecisionHealth

29824 Arthroscopy, shoulder, surgical; distal claviculectomy including distal articular surface (Mumford procedure) `A2 T`

RVU			Global Days	Modifiers				
Mod	Non-Fac Total	Fac Total		51	50	62	80	MUE
	19.30	19.30	090	3	1	1	2	1

AMA: Mar 15: 7, May 13: 12

29825 Arthroscopy, shoulder, surgical; with lysis and resection of adhesions, with or without manipulation `A2 T`

RVU			Global Days	Modifiers				
Mod	Non-Fac Total	Fac Total		51	50	62	80	MUE
	16.70	16.70	090	3	1	1	2	1

AMA: Mar 15: 7, May 13: 12

+ **29826** Arthroscopy, shoulder, surgical; decompression of subacromial space with partial acromioplasty, with coracoacromial ligament (ie, arch) release, when performed (List separately in addition to code for primary procedure) `N I N`

RVU			Global Days	Modifiers				
Mod	Non-Fac Total	Fac Total		51	50	62	80	MUE
	5.03	5.03	ZZZ	0	1	1	2	1

AMA: May 01: 9, Aug 02: 10, Mar 15: 7, May 13: 12

29827 Arthroscopy, shoulder, surgical; with rotator cuff repair `A2 J I`

RVU			Global Days	Modifiers				
Mod	Non-Fac Total	Fac Total		51	50	62	80	MUE
	30.57	30.57	090	3	1	1	2	1

AMA: Mar 08: 14, Mar 15: 7, May 13: 12

29828 Arthroscopy, shoulder, surgical; biceps tenodesis `G2 J I`

RVU			Global Days	Modifiers				
Mod	Non-Fac Total	Fac Total		51	50	62	80	MUE
	26.44	26.44	090	3	1	1	2	1

AMA: Feb 08: 9, Mar 15: 7, May 13: 12

29830 Arthroscopy, elbow, diagnostic, with or without synovial biopsy (separate procedure) `A2 T`

RVU			Global Days	Modifiers				
Mod	Non-Fac Total	Fac Total		51	50	62	80	MUE
	13.18	13.18	090	2	1	0	1	1

AMA: May 13: 12

29834 Arthroscopy, elbow, surgical; with removal of loose body or foreign body `A2 T`

RVU			Global Days	Modifiers				
Mod	Non-Fac Total	Fac Total		51	50	62	80	MUE
	14.06	14.06	090	3	1	1	2	1

AMA: May 13: 12

29835 Arthroscopy, elbow, surgical; synovectomy, partial `A2 T`

RVU			Global Days	Modifiers				
Mod	Non-Fac Total	Fac Total		51	50	62	80	MUE
	14.62	14.62	090	3	1	1	2	1

AMA: May 13: 12

29836 Arthroscopy, elbow, surgical; synovectomy, complete `A2 T`

RVU			Global Days	Modifiers				
Mod	Non-Fac Total	Fac Total		51	50	62	80	MUE
	16.44	16.44	090	3	1	1	2	1

AMA: May 13: 12

29837 Arthroscopy, elbow, surgical; debridement, limited `A2 T`

RVU			Global Days	Modifiers				
Mod	Non-Fac Total	Fac Total		51	50	62	80	MUE
	15.13	15.13	090	3	1	1	2	1

AMA: May 13: 12

29838 Arthroscopy, elbow, surgical; debridement, extensive `A2 T`

RVU			Global Days	Modifiers				
Mod	Non-Fac Total	Fac Total		51	50	62	80	MUE
	16.96	16.96	090	3	1	0	0	1

AMA: May 13: 12

29840 Arthroscopy, wrist, diagnostic, with or without synovial biopsy (separate procedure) `A2 T`

RVU			Global Days	Modifiers				
Mod	Non-Fac Total	Fac Total		51	50	62	80	MUE
	13.08	13.08	090	2	1	0	0	1

AMA: May 13: 12

29843 Arthroscopy, wrist, surgical; for infection, lavage and drainage `A2 T`

RVU			Global Days	Modifiers				
Mod	Non-Fac Total	Fac Total		51	50	62	80	MUE
	14.01	14.01	090	3	1	1	2	1

AMA: May 13: 12

29844 Arthroscopy, wrist, surgical; synovectomy, partial `A2 T`

RVU			Global Days	Modifiers				
Mod	Non-Fac Total	Fac Total		51	50	62	80	MUE
	14.35	14.35	090	3	1	0	2	1

AMA: May 13: 12

29845 Arthroscopy, wrist, surgical; synovectomy, complete `A2 T`

RVU			Global Days	Modifiers				
Mod	Non-Fac Total	Fac Total		51	50	62	80	MUE
	16.67	16.67	090	3	1	1	2	1

AMA: Dec 03: 11, May 13: 12

29846 Arthroscopy, wrist, surgical; excision and/or repair of triangular fibrocartilage and/or joint debridement `A2 T`

RVU			Global Days	Modifiers				
Mod	Non-Fac Total	Fac Total		51	50	62	80	MUE
	15.09	15.09	090	3	1	0	0	1

AMA: Dec 03: 11, May 13: 12

29847 Arthroscopy, wrist, surgical; internal fixation for fracture or instability `A2 T`

RVU			Global Days	Modifiers				
Mod	Non-Fac Total	Fac Total		51	50	62	80	MUE
	15.44	15.44	090	3	1	0	2	1

AMA: May 13: 12

● New   ▲ Revised   Deleted   ⊙ Moderate Sedation   ✚ Add-on Codes   ⊗ High Risk Denial   Ⓐ Age Edit   ♀ Female   ♂ Male   **AMA** CPT® Assistant   **MUE** Medically Unlikely Edit
⊘ Modifier 51 Exempt   ⊖ Modifier 63 Exempt   ☒ Unlisted   **Modifiers:** See Inside Back Cover   Ⓜ Maternity   `A2`–`Z3` ASC Payment Indicators   `A`–`Y` OPPS Status Indicators

Coding Guidance

Code 29848 may not be reported in addition to code 64721 for the same wrist at the same encounter, since code 64721 includes open release of the transverse carpal ligament. When an endoscopic release of the transverse carpal ligament is converted to an open release, only the open procedure may be reported.

29848   **Endoscopy, wrist, surgical, with release of transverse carpal ligament**   `A 2 T`

RVU			Global Days	Modifiers				
Mod	Non-Fac Total	Fac Total		51	50	62	80	MUE
	14.82	14.82	090	2	1	0	1	1

AMA: Dec 99: 7, May 13: 12, Jul 15: 10

Surgical wrist arthroscopy

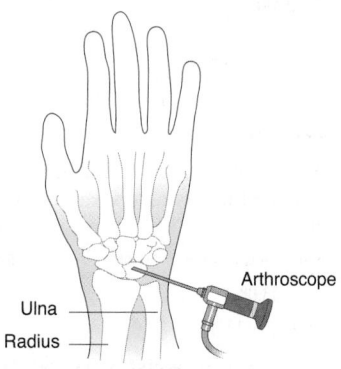

Arthroscope

Ulna

Radius

An arthroscope is inserted into the wrist and severs the ligament which runs across the small bones of the wrist.

29850   **Arthroscopically aided treatment of intercondylar spine(s) and/or tuberosity fracture(s) of the knee, with or without manipulation; without internal or external fixation (includes arthroscopy)**   `A 2 T`

RVU			Global Days	Modifiers				
Mod	Non-Fac Total	Fac Total		51	50	62	80	MUE
	17.83	17.83	090	2	1	2	0	1

AMA: May 13: 12

29851   **Arthroscopically aided treatment of intercondylar spine(s) and/or tuberosity fracture(s) of the knee, with or without manipulation; with internal or external fixation (includes arthroscopy)**   `A 2 T`

RVU			Global Days	Modifiers				
Mod	Non-Fac Total	Fac Total		51	50	62	80	MUE
	25.62	25.62	090	2	1	2	2	1

AMA: May 13: 12

29855   **Arthroscopically aided treatment of tibial fracture, proximal (plateau); unicondylar, includes internal fixation, when performed (includes arthroscopy)**   `A 2 J I`

RVU			Global Days	Modifiers				
Mod	Non-Fac Total	Fac Total		51	50	62	80	MUE
	22.55	22.55	090	2	1	2	2	1

AMA: May 13: 12

29856   **Arthroscopically aided treatment of tibial fracture, proximal (plateau); bicondylar, includes internal fixation, when performed (includes arthroscopy)**   `A 2 J I`

RVU			Global Days	Modifiers				
Mod	Non-Fac Total	Fac Total		51	50	62	80	MUE
	28.91	28.91	090	2	1	2	2	1

AMA: May 13: 12

Coding Guidance

Additional surgical arthroscopy procedures of the hip are listed out of numerical order in CPT. Report surgical arthroscopy of the hip with code 29914 for femoroplasty, code 29914 for acetabuloplasty, code 29916 for labral repair.

29860   **Arthroscopy, hip, diagnostic with or without synovial biopsy (separate procedure)**   `A 2 T`

RVU			Global Days	Modifiers				
Mod	Non-Fac Total	Fac Total		51	50	62	80	MUE
	19.08	19.08	090	2	1	1	2	1

AMA: Nov 97: 15, Jul 98: 8, Sep 11: 6, May 13: 12

29861   **Arthroscopy, hip, surgical; with removal of loose body or foreign body**   `A 2 T`

RVU			Global Days	Modifiers				
Mod	Non-Fac Total	Fac Total		51	50	62	80	MUE
	20.80	20.80	090	3	1	1	2	1

AMA: Nov 97: 15, Jul 98: 8, Sep 11: 5, May 13: 12

29862   **Arthroscopy, hip, surgical; with debridement/shaving of articular cartilage (chondroplasty), abrasion arthroplasty, and/or resection of labrum**   `A 2 J I`

RVU			Global Days	Modifiers				
Mod	Non-Fac Total	Fac Total		51	50	62	80	MUE
	23.33	23.33	090	3	1	1	2	1

AMA: Nov 97: 15, Jul 98: 8, Sep 11: 5, May 13: 12

29863   **Arthroscopy, hip, surgical; with synovectomy**   `A 2 T`

RVU			Global Days	Modifiers				
Mod	Non-Fac Total	Fac Total		51	50	62	80	MUE
	23.34	23.34	090	3	1	1	2	1

AMA: Nov 97: 15, Jul 98: 8, Sep 11: 5, May 13: 12

29866   **Arthroscopy, knee, surgical; osteochondral autograft(s) (eg, mosaicplasty) (includes harvesting of the autograft[s])**   `G 2 J I`

RVU			Global Days	Modifiers				
Mod	Non-Fac Total	Fac Total		51	50	62	80	MUE
	30.19	30.19	090	2	1	0	0	1

AMA: May 13: 12

29867   **Arthroscopy, knee, surgical; osteochondral allograft (eg, mosaicplasty)**   `J I`

RVU			Global Days	Modifiers				
Mod	Non-Fac Total	Fac Total		51	50	62	80	MUE
	36.61	36.61	090	2	1	0	0	1

AMA: May 13: 12

29868   **Arthroscopy, knee, surgical; meniscal transplantation (includes arthrotomy for meniscal insertion), medial or lateral**   `J I`

RVU			Global Days	Modifiers				
Mod	Non-Fac Total	Fac Total		51	50	62	80	MUE
	46.54	46.54	090	2	1	0	0	1

AMA: May 13: 12

● New   ▲ Revised   ✖ Deleted   ⊙ Moderate Sedation   ✚ Add-on Codes   ⊘ High Risk Denial   Ⓐ Age Edit   ♀ Female   ♂ Male   **AMA** *CPT® Assistant*   *MUE* Medically Unlikely Edit
⊘ Modifier 51 Exempt   ⊖ Modifier 63 Exempt   ✗ Unlisted   **Modifiers:** *See Inside Back Cover*   Ⓜ Maternity   `A 2` – `Z 3` ASC Payment Indicators   `A` – `Y` OPPS Status Indicators

29870 Arthroscopy, knee, diagnostic, with or without synovial biopsy (separate procedure) `A 2 T`

RVU		Global Days	Modifiers				
Mod	Non-Fac Total	Fac Total		51	50	62	80	MUE
	16.84	11.93	090	2	1	1	1	1

AMA: Dec 07: 10, Mar 11: 9, May 13: 12

29871 Arthroscopy, knee, surgical; for infection, lavage and drainage `A 2 T`

RVU		Global Days	Modifiers				
Mod	Non-Fac Total	Fac Total		51	50	62	80	MUE
	14.90	14.90	090	3	1	0	1	1

AMA: Aug 01: 6, May 13: 12

29873 Arthroscopy, knee, surgical; with lateral release `A 2 T`

RVU		Global Days	Modifiers				
Mod	Non-Fac Total	Fac Total		51	50	62	80	MUE
	15.19	15.19	090	3	1	1	1	1

AMA: Dec 07: 10, May 13: 12, Aug 09: 11

29874 Arthroscopy, knee, surgical; for removal of loose body or foreign body (eg, osteochondritis dissecans fragmentation, chondral fragmentation) `⊘ A 2 T`

RVU		Global Days	Modifiers				
Mod	Non-Fac Total	Fac Total		51	50	62	80	MUE
	15.54	15.54	090	3	1	0	0	1

AMA: Aug 01: 6, Apr 03: 12, May 13: 12

29875 Arthroscopy, knee, surgical; synovectomy, limited (eg, plica or shelf resection) (separate procedure) `A 2 T`

RVU		Global Days	Modifiers				
Mod	Non-Fac Total	Fac Total		51	50	62	80	MUE
	14.34	14.34	090	3	1	0	0	1

AMA: Aug 01: 6, May 13: 12, May 14: 10

29876 Arthroscopy, knee, surgical; synovectomy, major, 2 or more compartments (eg, medial or lateral) `A 2 T`

RVU		Global Days	Modifiers				
Mod	Non-Fac Total	Fac Total		51	50	62	80	MUE
	19.04	19.04	090	3	1	0	1	1

AMA: Aug 01: 6, May 13: 12

29877 Arthroscopy, knee, surgical; debridement/shaving of articular cartilage (chondroplasty) `⊘ A 2 T`

RVU		Global Days	Modifiers				
Mod	Non-Fac Total	Fac Total		51	50	62	80	MUE
	18.00	18.00	090	3	1	0	0	1

AMA: Feb 96: 9, Jun 99: 11, Aug 01: 7, Apr 03: 7, Apr 05: 14, Dec 07: 10, May 13: 12

29879 Arthroscopy, knee, surgical; abrasion arthroplasty (includes chondroplasty where necessary) or multiple drilling or microfracture `A 2 T`

RVU		Global Days	Modifiers				
Mod	Non-Fac Total	Fac Total		51	50	62	80	MUE
	19.17	19.17	090	3	1	0	0	1

AMA: Nov 99: 13, Aug 01: 7, May 13: 12

29880 Arthroscopy, knee, surgical; with meniscectomy (medial AND lateral, including any meniscal shaving) including debridement/shaving of articular cartilage (chondroplasty), same or separate compartment(s), when performed `A 2 T`

RVU		Global Days	Modifiers				
Mod	Non-Fac Total	Fac Total		51	50	62	80	MUE
	16.26	16.26	090	3	1	1	0	1

AMA: Jun 99: 11, Aug 01: 7, Jan 12: 3, May 13: 12

29881 Arthroscopy, knee, surgical; with meniscectomy (medial OR lateral, including any meniscal shaving) including debridement/shaving of articular cartilage (chondroplasty), same or separate compartment(s), when performed `A 2 T`

RVU		Global Days	Modifiers				
Mod	Non-Fac Total	Fac Total		51	50	62	80	MUE
	15.67	15.67	090	3	1	0	0	1

AMA: Feb 96: 9, Jun 99: 11, Aug 01: 7, Oct 03: 11, Apr 05: 14, Dec 07: 10, Jan 12: 3, May 13: 12, May 14: 10

29882 Arthroscopy, knee, surgical; with meniscus repair (medial OR lateral) `A 2 T`

RVU		Global Days	Modifiers				
Mod	Non-Fac Total	Fac Total		51	50	62	80	MUE
	20.29	20.29	090	3	1	0	1	1

AMA: Aug 01: 7, Sep 04: 12, Dec 07: 10, Dec 11: 15, May 13: 12

29883 Arthroscopy, knee, surgical; with meniscus repair (medial AND lateral) `A 2 T`

RVU		Global Days	Modifiers				
Mod	Non-Fac Total	Fac Total		51	50	62	80	MUE
	24.37	24.37	090	3	1	0	0	1

AMA: Aug 01: 7, Sep 04: 12, Dec 07: 10, Dec 11: 15, May 13: 12

29884 Arthroscopy, knee, surgical; with lysis of adhesions, with or without manipulation (separate procedure) `A 2 T`

RVU		Global Days	Modifiers				
Mod	Non-Fac Total	Fac Total		51	50	62	80	MUE
	17.78	17.78	090	3	1	1	2	1

AMA: Aug 01: 7, Mar 11: 9, May 13: 12

29885 Arthroscopy, knee, surgical; drilling for osteochondritis dissecans with bone grafting, with or without internal fixation (including debridement of base of lesion) `A 2 J 1`

RVU		Global Days	Modifiers				
Mod	Non-Fac Total	Fac Total		51	50	62	80	MUE
	21.77	21.77	090	3	1	1	2	1

AMA: Aug 01: 7, May 13: 12

29886 Arthroscopy, knee, surgical; drilling for intact osteochondritis dissecans lesion `A 2 T`

RVU		Global Days	Modifiers				
Mod	Non-Fac Total	Fac Total		51	50	62	80	MUE
	18.44	18.44	090	3	1	0	1	1

AMA: Aug 01: 12, May 13: 12

● New   ▲ Revised   Deleted   ⊙ Moderate Sedation   ✚ Add-on Codes   ⊘ High Risk Denial   Ⓐ Age Edit   ♀ Female   ♂ Male   **AMA** CPT® Assistant   **MUE** Medically Unlikely Edit
⊘ Modifier 51 Exempt   ⊖ Modifier 63 Exempt   ⊠ Unlisted   **Modifiers:** See Inside Back Cover   Ⓜ Maternity   A 2 – Z 3 ASC Payment Indicators   A – Y OPPS Status Indicators

29887 Arthroscopy, knee, surgical; drilling for intact osteochondritis dissecans lesion with internal fixation `A2T`

RVU			Global Days	Modifiers				
Mod	Non-Fac Total	Fac Total		51	50	62	80	MUE
	21.62	21.62	090	3	1	1	2	1

AMA: Aug 01: 12, May 13: 12

29888 Arthroscopically aided anterior cruciate ligament repair/augmentation or reconstruction `A2J I`

RVU			Global Days	Modifiers				
Mod	Non-Fac Total	Fac Total		51	50	62	80	MUE
	28.46	28.46	090	2	1	1	2	1

AMA: Oct 03: 11, Dec 07: 10, May 13: 12

29889 Arthroscopically aided posterior cruciate ligament repair/augmentation or reconstruction `J8J I`

RVU			Global Days	Modifiers				
Mod	Non-Fac Total	Fac Total		51	50	62	80	MUE
	35.38	35.38	090	2	1	1	2	1

AMA: Sep 96: 9, Oct 98: 11, Aug 01: 8, Dec 07: 10, May 13: 12

29891 Arthroscopy, ankle, surgical, excision of osteochondral defect of talus and/or tibia, including drilling of the defect `A2T`

RVU			Global Days	Modifiers				
Mod	Non-Fac Total	Fac Total		51	50	62	80	MUE
	19.53	19.53	090	2	1	0	2	1

AMA: Nov 97: 15, May 13: 12

29892 Arthroscopically aided repair of large osteochondritis dissecans lesion, talar dome fracture, or tibial plafond fracture, with or without internal fixation (includes arthroscopy) `A2T`

RVU			Global Days	Modifiers				
Mod	Non-Fac Total	Fac Total		51	50	62	80	MUE
	16.83	16.83	090	2	1	0	2	1

AMA: Nov 97: 15, Dec 08: 6, May 13: 12

29893 Endoscopic plantar fasciotomy `A2T`

Coding tip: Do not report 28008, 28060, 28062, and 28250 with 29893; codes from this group should not be reported together if performed on the same foot at the same surgical session

RVU			Global Days	Modifiers				
Mod	Non-Fac Total	Fac Total		51	50	62	80	MUE
	17.66	12.32	090	2	1	1	1	1

AMA: Nov 97: 15, May 13: 12

29894 Arthroscopy, ankle (tibiotalar and fibulotalar joints), surgical; with removal of loose body or foreign body `A2T`

RVU			Global Days	Modifiers				
Mod	Non-Fac Total	Fac Total		51	50	62	80	MUE
	14.39	14.39	090	2	1	1	2	1

AMA: May 13: 12

29895 Arthroscopy, ankle (tibiotalar and fibulotalar joints), surgical; synovectomy, partial `A2T`

RVU			Global Days	Modifiers				
Mod	Non-Fac Total	Fac Total		51	50	62	80	MUE
	13.75	13.75	090	2	1	1	2	1

AMA: May 13: 12

29897 Arthroscopy, ankle (tibiotalar and fibulotalar joints), surgical; debridement, limited `A2T`

RVU			Global Days	Modifiers				
Mod	Non-Fac Total	Fac Total		51	50	62	80	MUE
	14.66	14.66	090	2	1	0	2	1

AMA: May 13: 12

29898 Arthroscopy, ankle (tibiotalar and fibulotalar joints), surgical; debridement, extensive `A2T`

RVU			Global Days	Modifiers				
Mod	Non-Fac Total	Fac Total		51	50	62	80	MUE
	16.29	16.29	090	2	1	1	2	1

AMA: May 13: 12

29899 Arthroscopy, ankle (tibiotalar and fibulotalar joints), surgical; with ankle arthrodesis `G2J I`

RVU			Global Days	Modifiers				
Mod	Non-Fac Total	Fac Total		51	50	62	80	MUE
	29.93	29.93	090	2	1	1	2	1

AMA: May 13: 12

29900 Arthroscopy, metacarpophalangeal joint, diagnostic, includes synovial biopsy `A2T`

RVU			Global Days	Modifiers				
Mod	Non-Fac Total	Fac Total		51	50	62	80	MUE
	13.15	13.15	090	2	1	0	0	2

AMA: May 13: 12

29901 Arthroscopy, metacarpophalangeal joint, surgical; with debridement `A2T`

RVU			Global Days	Modifiers				
Mod	Non-Fac Total	Fac Total		51	50	62	80	MUE
	15.41	15.41	090	2	1	0	0	2

AMA: May 13: 12

29902 Arthroscopy, metacarpophalangeal joint, surgical; with reduction of displaced ulnar collateral ligament (eg, Stenar lesion) ⊘`A2T`

RVU			Global Days	Modifiers				
Mod	Non-Fac Total	Fac Total		51	50	62	80	MUE
	16.41	16.41	090	2	1	0	0	2

AMA: May 13: 12

29904 Arthroscopy, subtalar joint, surgical; with removal of loose body or foreign body `G2T`

RVU			Global Days	Modifiers				
Mod	Non-Fac Total	Fac Total		51	50	62	80	MUE
	18.47	18.47	090	2	1	0	2	1

AMA: May 13: 12

29905 Arthroscopy, subtalar joint, surgical; with synovectomy `G2T`

RVU			Global Days	Modifiers				
Mod	Non-Fac Total	Fac Total		51	50	62	80	MUE
	19.85	19.85	090	2	1	0	2	1

AMA: May 13: 12

29906 Arthroscopy, subtalar joint, surgical; with debridement `G2T`

RVU			Global Days	Modifiers				
Mod	Non-Fac Total	Fac Total		51	50	62	80	MUE
	20.84	20.84	090	2	1	0	2	1

AMA: May 13: 12

● New   ▲ Revised   ✖ Deleted   ⊙ Moderate Sedation   ✚ Add-on Codes   ⊘ High Risk Denial   Ⓐ Age Edit   ♀ Female   ♂ Male   **AMA** *CPT® Assistant*   **MUE** Medically Unlikely Edit
⊘ Modifier 51 Exempt   ⊖ Modifier 63 Exempt   ✗ Unlisted   **Modifiers:** *See Inside Back Cover*   Ⓜ Maternity   `A2`–`Z3` ASC Payment Indicators   `A`–`Y` OPPS Status Indicators

CPT © 2015 American Medical Association. All Rights Reserved.   © 2016 DecisionHealth

29907 Arthroscopy, subtalar joint, surgical; with subtalar arthrodesis G2 J I

RVU			Global Days	Modifiers				
Mod	Non-Fac Total	Fac Total		51	50	62	80	MUE
	25.40	25.40	090	2	1	0	2	1

AMA: May 13: 12

29914 Arthroscopy, hip, surgical; with femoroplasty (ie, treatment of cam lesion) G2 J I

Coding tip: *Code 29914 is listed out of numerical order in CPT. Related diagnostic/surgical hip arthroscopy procedures - 29860-29863, 29915, 29916*

RVU			Global Days	Modifiers				
Mod	Non-Fac Total	Fac Total		51	50	62	80	MUE
	28.82	28.82	090	3	1	1	2	1

AMA: Sep 11: 5

Arthroscopy, hip, surgical, with femoroplasty

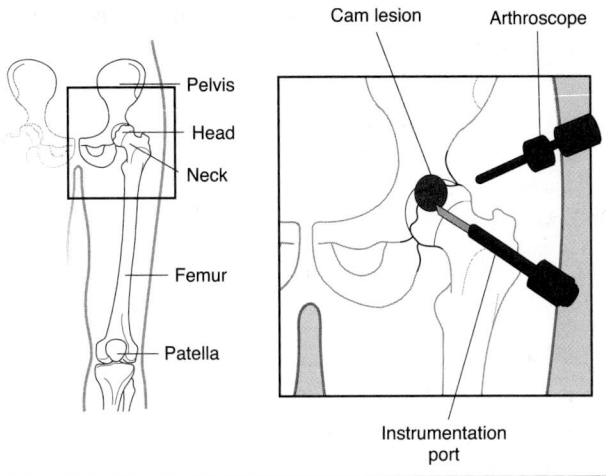

Pelvis
Head
Neck
Femur
Patella

Cam lesion
Arthroscope
Instrumentation port

29915 Arthroscopy, hip, surgical; with acetabuloplasty (ie, treatment of pincer lesion) G2 J I

Coding tip: *Code 29915 is listed out of numerical order in CPT. Related diagnostic/surgical hip arthroscopy procedures - 29860-29863, 29914, 29916*

RVU			Global Days	Modifiers				
Mod	Non-Fac Total	Fac Total		51	50	62	80	MUE
	29.31	29.31	090	3	1	1	2	1

AMA: Sep 11: 5

29916 Arthroscopy, hip, surgical; with labral repair G2 J I

Coding tip: *Code 29916 is listed out of numerical order in CPT. Related diagnostic/surgical hip arthroscopy procedures - 29860-29863, 29914, 29915*

RVU			Global Days	Modifiers				
Mod	Non-Fac Total	Fac Total		51	50	62	80	MUE
	29.34	29.34	090	3	1	1	2	1

AMA: Sep 11: 5

29999 Unlisted procedure, arthroscopy X T

RVU			Global Days	Modifiers				
Mod	Non-Fac Total	Fac Total		51	50	62	80	MUE
	0.00	0.00	YYY	2	1	1	0	

AMA: Aug 02: 10, Sep 04: 12, Nov 08: 10, Mar 09: 10, Dec 11: 15, Apr 12: 17, May 13: 12

● New   ▲ Revised   Deleted   ⊙ Moderate Sedation   ✚ Add-on Codes   ⊘ High Risk Denial   Ⓐ Age Edit   ♀ Female   ♂ Male   **AMA** *CPT® Assistant*   **MUE** Medically Unlikely Edit
⊘ Modifier 51 Exempt   ⊖ Modifier 63 Exempt   Ⓧ Unlisted   **Modifiers:** *See Inside Back Cover*   Ⓜ Maternity   A 2 – Z 3 ASC Payment Indicators   A – Y OPPS Status Indicators

Respiratory Procedures

Respiratory codes cover the nose, sinuses, larynx, trachea, bronchi, lungs and pleura by type of procedure and the method by which it is performed—openly or endoscopically.

Lung transplant codes, including codes for distinct work components, such as backbench preparation are reported with 32850-32856.

Therapeutic surgical collapse and thoracoplasty are coded 32900-32960.

Nasal Procedures

Nasal Incisional Procedures

30000 Drainage abscess or hematoma, nasal, internal approach   P 2 T

RVU			Global Days	Modifiers				
Mod	Non-Fac Total	Fac Total		51	50	62	80	MUE
	6.58	3.39	010	2	0	0	0	1

Drainage abscess or hematoma

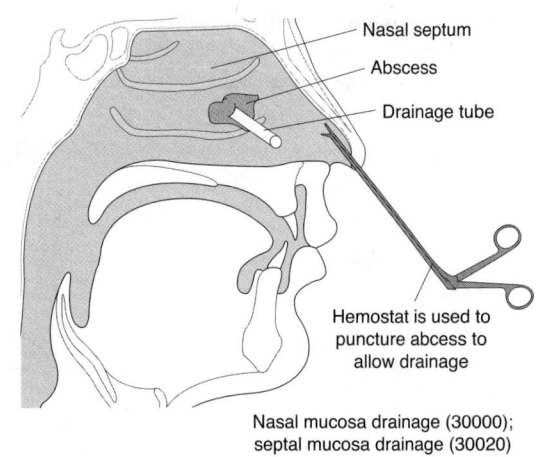

Nasal septum
Abscess
Drainage tube

Hemostat is used to puncture abcess to allow drainage

Nasal mucosa drainage (30000);
septal mucosa drainage (30020)

30020 Drainage abscess or hematoma, nasal septum P 2 T

RVU			Global Days	Modifiers				
Mod	Non-Fac Total	Fac Total		51	50	62	80	MUE
	6.68	3.43	010	2	0	0	1	1

Nasal Excisional Procedures

30100 Biopsy, intranasal   P 3 T

Coding tip: Code 99000 for specimen transfer from office setting to an outside laboratory

RVU			Global Days	Modifiers				
Mod	Non-Fac Total	Fac Total		51	50	62	80	MUE
	4.04	1.98	000	2	0	0	1	2

30110 Excision, nasal polyp(s), simple   P 3 T

RVU			Global Days	Modifiers				
Mod	Non-Fac Total	Fac Total		51	50	62	80	MUE
	6.60	3.74	010	2	1	0	1	1

30115 Excision, nasal polyp(s), extensive   A 2 T

RVU			Global Days	Modifiers				
Mod	Non-Fac Total	Fac Total		51	50	62	80	MUE
	12.40	12.40	090	2	1	0	1	1

30117 Excision or destruction (eg, laser), intranasal lesion; internal approach   A 2 T

RVU			Global Days	Modifiers				
Mod	Non-Fac Total	Fac Total		51	50	62	80	MUE
	25.14	9.78	090	2	0	0	1	2

30118 Excision or destruction (eg, laser), intranasal lesion; external approach (lateral rhinotomy)   A 2 T

RVU			Global Days	Modifiers				
Mod	Non-Fac Total	Fac Total		51	50	62	80	MUE
	22.10	22.10	090	2	0	1	1	1

30120 Excision or surgical planing of skin of nose for rhinophyma   A 2 T

RVU			Global Days	Modifiers				
Mod	Non-Fac Total	Fac Total		51	50	62	80	MUE
	14.96	12.64	090	2	0	0	1	1

AMA: May 07: 9

Excision/surgical planing; rhinophyma

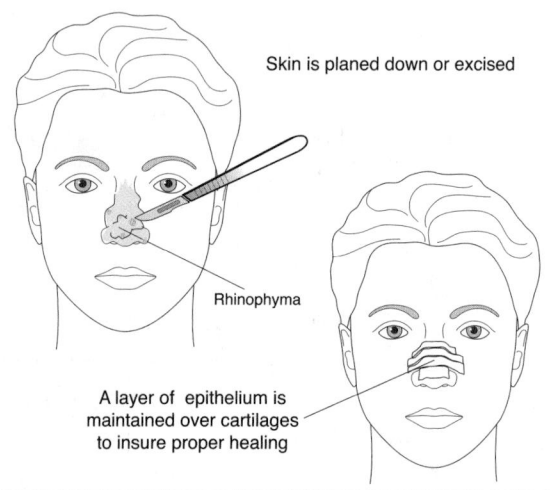

Skin is planed down or excised

Rhinophyma

A layer of epithelium is maintained over cartilages to insure proper healing

30124 Excision dermoid cyst, nose; simple, skin, subcutaneous   R 2 T

RVU			Global Days	Modifiers				
Mod	Non-Fac Total	Fac Total		51	50	62	80	MUE
	8.20	8.20	090	2	0	0	1	2

30125 Excision dermoid cyst, nose; complex, under bone or cartilage   A 2 J I

RVU			Global Days	Modifiers				
Mod	Non-Fac Total	Fac Total		51	50	62	80	MUE
	17.46	17.46	090	2	0	0	2	1

● New   ▲ Revised   ✖ Deleted   ⊙ Moderate Sedation   ✚ Add-on Codes   ⊘ High Risk Denial   Ⓐ Age Edit   ♀ Female   ♂ Male   **AMA** CPT® Assistant   **MUE** Medically Unlikely Edit
⊘ Modifier 51 Exempt   ⊖ Modifier 63 Exempt   ✗ Unlisted   **Modifiers:** See Inside Back Cover   Ⓜ Maternity   A 2 – Z 3 ASC Payment Indicators   A – Y OPPS Status Indicators

30130 Excision inferior turbinate, partial or complete, any method `A 2 T`

RVU			Global Days	Modifiers				
Mod	Non-Fac Total	Fac Total		51	50	62	80	MUE
	10.89	10.89	090	2	1	0	1	1

AMA: Feb 98: 11, Nov 98: 11, Sep 01: 10, May 03: 5

30140 Submucous resection inferior turbinate, partial or complete, any method `A 2 T`

RVU			Global Days	Modifiers				
Mod	Non-Fac Total	Fac Total		51	50	62	80	MUE
	12.64	12.64	090	2	1	0	1	1

AMA: Nov 98: 11, Dec 02: 10, Apr 03: 26, May 03: 5, Dec 04: 18, Mar 08: 14

30150 Rhinectomy; partial `A 2 J 1`

RVU			Global Days	Modifiers				
Mod	Non-Fac Total	Fac Total		51	50	62	80	MUE
	22.12	22.12	090	2	0	1	1	1

30160 Rhinectomy; total `A 2 J 1`

RVU			Global Days	Modifiers				
Mod	Non-Fac Total	Fac Total		51	50	62	80	MUE
	22.16	22.16	090	2	0	1	2	1

Nasal Introduction Procedures

30200 Injection into turbinate(s), therapeutic `P 3 T`

Coding tip: *This procedure is considered bilateral. Do not append modifier 50*

RVU			Global Days	Modifiers				
Mod	Non-Fac Total	Fac Total		51	50	62	80	MUE
	3.25	1.71	000	2	0	0	1	1

AMA: Dec 04: 19

Injection into turbinate(s), therapeutic

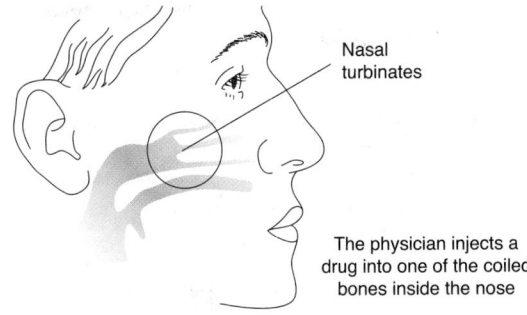

Nasal turbinates

The physician injects a drug into one of the coiled bones inside the nose

30210 Displacement therapy (Proetz type) `P 3 T`

RVU			Global Days	Modifiers				
Mod	Non-Fac Total	Fac Total		51	50	62	80	MUE
	4.29	2.86	010	2	0	0	1	1

30220 Insertion, nasal septal prosthesis (button) `A 2 T`

RVU			Global Days	Modifiers				
Mod	Non-Fac Total	Fac Total		51	50	62	80	MUE
	8.69	3.60	010	2	0	0	1	1

Nasal Foreign Body Removal

30300 Removal foreign body, intranasal; office type procedure `N I Q 1`

RVU			Global Days	Modifiers				
Mod	Non-Fac Total	Fac Total		51	50	62	80	MUE
	5.31	3.03	010	2	0	0	1	1

AMA: Jan 12: 13

Removal foreign body, intranasal

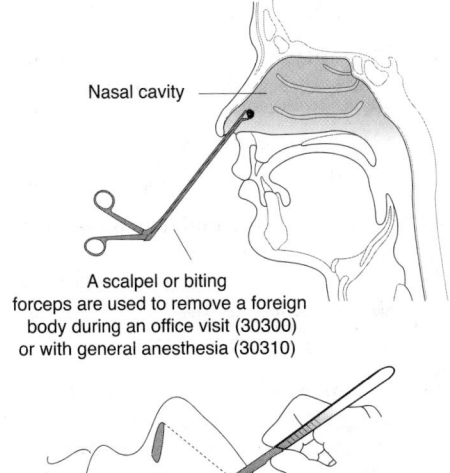

Nasal cavity

A scalpel or biting forceps are used to remove a foreign body during an office visit (30300) or with general anesthesia (30310)

Report code (30320) when the foreign body is accessed by lateral rhinotomy.

30310 Removal foreign body, intranasal; requiring general anesthesia `A 2 T`

RVU			Global Days	Modifiers				
Mod	Non-Fac Total	Fac Total		51	50	62	80	MUE
	5.91	5.91	010	2	0	0	0	1

30320 Removal foreign body, intranasal; by lateral rhinotomy `A 2 T`

Coding tip: *Lateral rhinotomy for intranasal lesion - 30118*

RVU			Global Days	Modifiers				
Mod	Non-Fac Total	Fac Total		51	50	62	80	MUE
	12.70	12.70	090	2	0	0	0	1

Nasal Repair Procedures

30400 Rhinoplasty, primary; lateral and alar cartilages and/or elevation of nasal tip `A 2 T`

RVU			Global Days	Modifiers				
Mod	Non-Fac Total	Fac Total		51	50	62	80	MUE
	29.01	29.01	090	2	0	0	0	1

30410 Rhinoplasty, primary; complete, external parts including bony pyramid, lateral and alar cartilages, and/or elevation of nasal tip `A 2 J 1`

RVU			Global Days	Modifiers				
Mod	Non-Fac Total	Fac Total		51	50	62	80	MUE
	33.92	33.92	090	2	0	0	2	1

● New   ▲ Revised   Deleted   ⊙ Moderate Sedation   ✚ Add-on Codes   ⊘ High Risk Denial   Ⓐ Age Edit   ♀ Female   ♂ Male   **AMA** *CPT® Assistant*   ***MUE*** Medically Unlikely Edit
⊘ Modifier 51 Exempt   ⊖ Modifier 63 Exempt   ✗ Unlisted   **Modifiers:** *See Inside Back Cover*   Ⓜ Maternity   `A 2`–`Z 3` ASC Payment Indicators   `A`–`Y` OPPS Status Indicators

30420 Rhinoplasty, primary; including major septal repair `A2 J I`

Mod	Non-Fac Total	Fac Total	Global Days	Modifiers 51	50	62	80	MUE
	39.40	39.40	090	2	0	0	1	1

30430 Rhinoplasty, secondary; minor revision (small amount of nasal tip work) `A2 T`

Mod	Non-Fac Total	Fac Total	Global Days	Modifiers 51	50	62	80	MUE
	27.88	27.88	090	2	0	0	2	1

30435 Rhinoplasty, secondary; intermediate revision (bony work with osteotomies) `A2 J I`

Mod	Non-Fac Total	Fac Total	Global Days	Modifiers 51	50	62	80	MUE
	31.83	31.83	090	2	0	0	2	1

30450 Rhinoplasty, secondary; major revision (nasal tip work and osteotomies) `A2 J I`

Mod	Non-Fac Total	Fac Total	Global Days	Modifiers 51	50	62	80	MUE
	42.89	42.89	090	2	0	0	2	1

30460 Rhinoplasty for nasal deformity secondary to congenital cleft lip and/or palate, including columellar lengthening; tip only ⊘`A2 J I`

Mod	Non-Fac Total	Fac Total	Global Days	Modifiers 51	50	62	80	MUE
	20.47	20.47	090	2	0	2	2	1

AMA: Dec 14: 18

Rhinoplasty, nasal deformity, secondary to cleft lip/palate, with columellar lengthening

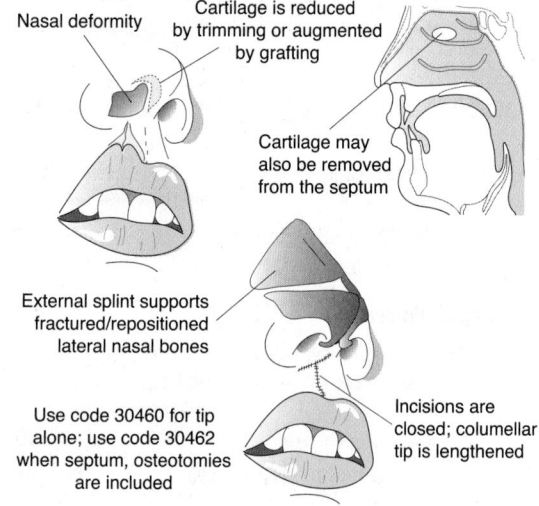

Nasal deformity

Cartilage is reduced by trimming or augmented by grafting

Cartilage may also be removed from the septum

External splint supports fractured/repositioned lateral nasal bones

Use code 30460 for tip alone; use code 30462 when septum, osteotomies are included

Incisions are closed; columellar tip is lengthened

30462 Rhinoplasty for nasal deformity secondary to congenital cleft lip and/or palate, including columellar lengthening; tip, septum, osteotomies `A2 J I`

Mod	Non-Fac Total	Fac Total	Global Days	Modifiers 51	50	62	80	MUE
	45.20	45.20	090	2	0	2	2	1

AMA: Dec 14: 18

30465 Repair of nasal vestibular stenosis (eg, spreader grafting, lateral nasal wall reconstruction) `A2 J I`

Mod	Non-Fac Total	Fac Total	Global Days	Modifiers 51	50	62	80	MUE
	28.18	28.18	090	2	0	0	0	1

30520 Septoplasty or submucous resection, with or without cartilage scoring, contouring or replacement with graft `A2 T`

Mod	Non-Fac Total	Fac Total	Global Days	Modifiers 51	50	62	80	MUE
	17.89	17.89	090	2	0	0	1	1

AMA: Oct 97: 11, Dec 02: 10, Mar 12: 9, Jul 15: 10

30540 Repair choanal atresia; intranasal ⊖`A2 J I`

Mod	Non-Fac Total	Fac Total	Global Days	Modifiers 51	50	62	80	MUE
	19.91	19.91	090	2	0	0	2	1

30545 Repair choanal atresia; transpalatine ⊗⊖`A2 J I`

Mod	Non-Fac Total	Fac Total	Global Days	Modifiers 51	50	62	80	MUE
	25.22	25.22	090	2	0	0	2	1

30560 Lysis intranasal synechia `A2 T`

Mod	Non-Fac Total	Fac Total	Global Days	Modifiers 51	50	62	80	MUE
	7.69	3.93	010	2	0	0	1	1

30580 Repair fistula; oromaxillary (combine with 31030 if antrotomy is included) `A2 J I`

Mod	Non-Fac Total	Fac Total	Global Days	Modifiers 51	50	62	80	MUE
	18.88	14.83	090	2	0	0	1	2

30600 Repair fistula; oronasal `A2 J I`

Mod	Non-Fac Total	Fac Total	Global Days	Modifiers 51	50	62	80	MUE
	16.99	12.89	090	2	0	0	0	1

30620 Septal or other intranasal dermatoplasty (does not include obtaining graft) `A2 J I`

Mod	Non-Fac Total	Fac Total	Global Days	Modifiers 51	50	62	80	MUE
	17.93	17.93	090	2	0	0	1	1

30630 Repair nasal septal perforations `A2 T`

Mod	Non-Fac Total	Fac Total	Global Days	Modifiers 51	50	62	80	MUE
	17.87	17.87	090	2	0	0	0	1

AMA: Aug 12: 13

Nasal Cautery/Ablation Procedures

30801 Ablation, soft tissue of inferior turbinates, unilateral or bilateral, any method (eg, electrocautery, radiofrequency ablation, or tissue volume reduction); superficial `A2 T`

Mod	Non-Fac Total	Fac Total	Global Days	Modifiers 51	50	62	80	MUE
	6.56	3.91	010	2	2	0	1	1

● New   ▲ Revised   ✖ Deleted   ⊙ Moderate Sedation   ✚ Add-on Codes   ⊘ High Risk Denial   Ⓐ Age Edit   ♀ Female   ♂ Male   **AMA** CPT® Assistant   **MUE** Medically Unlikely Edit
⊘ Modifier 51 Exempt   ⊖ Modifier 63 Exempt   ✗ Unlisted   **Modifiers:** See Inside Back Cover   Ⓜ Maternity   `A2`–`Z3` ASC Payment Indicators   `A`–`Y` OPPS Status Indicators

CPT © 2015 American Medical Association. All Rights Reserved.   © 2016 DecisionHealth

30802 Ablation, soft tissue of inferior turbinates, unilateral or bilateral, any method (eg, electrocautery, radiofrequency ablation, or tissue volume reduction); intramural (ie, submucosal) `A 2 T`

RVU			Global Days	Modifiers				
Mod	Non-Fac Total	Fac Total		51	50	62	80	MUE
	8.33	5.45	010	2	2	0	1	1

AMA: Mar 08: 14, Sep 10: 10

Other Nasal Procedures

Coding Guidance

Bleeding control is an integral part of endoscopic procedures and is not reported separately. Control of nasal hemorrhage codes should not be reported with nasal/sinus endoscopy procedures (e.g. 31235). Bleeding that occurs as a later complication and requires significant, separate treatment after a procedure's completion would be reported. Modifier 78 may be used to show that control of nasal hemorrhage requiring a return to the operating room is a related procedure to treat a complication during a postoperative period.

30901 Control nasal hemorrhage, anterior, simple (limited cautery and/or packing) any method `N I Q 1`

RVU			Global Days	Modifiers				
Mod	Non-Fac Total	Fac Total		51	50	62	80	MUE
	2.72	1.63	000	2	1	0	1	1

Control, nasal hemorrhage

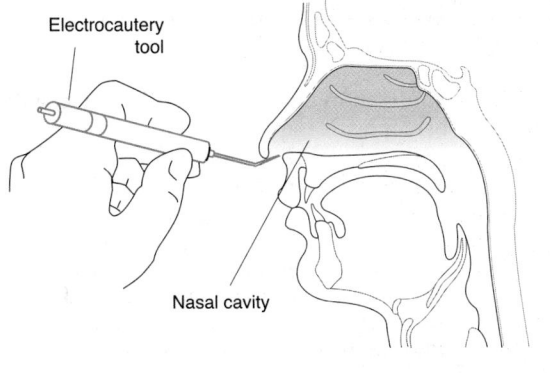

Electrocautery tool

Nasal cavity

Packing and/or cautery is used to seal nasal hemorrhaging; anterior, simple (30901) or complex (30903); posterior, initial (30905) or subsequent (30906).

30903 Control nasal hemorrhage, anterior, complex (extensive cautery and/or packing) any method `A 2 T`

RVU			Global Days	Modifiers				
Mod	Non-Fac Total	Fac Total		51	50	62	80	MUE
	6.31	2.32	000	2	1	0	1	1

30905 Control nasal hemorrhage, posterior, with posterior nasal packs and/or cautery, any method; initial `A 2 T`

RVU			Global Days	Modifiers				
Mod	Non-Fac Total	Fac Total		51	50	62	80	MUE
	7.74	3.08	000	2	2	0	1	1

AMA: Sep 10: 7

30906 Control nasal hemorrhage, posterior, with posterior nasal packs and/or cautery, any method; subsequent `A 2 T`

RVU			Global Days	Modifiers				
Mod	Non-Fac Total	Fac Total		51	50	62	80	MUE
	9.96	3.96	000	2	2	0	1	1

30915 Ligation arteries; ethmoidal `A 2 T`

RVU			Global Days	Modifiers				
Mod	Non-Fac Total	Fac Total		51	50	62	80	MUE
	16.53	16.53	090	2	0	0	1	1

30920 Ligation arteries; internal maxillary artery, transantral `A 2 T`

RVU			Global Days	Modifiers				
Mod	Non-Fac Total	Fac Total		51	50	62	80	MUE
	23.98	23.98	090	2	0	0	1	1

30930 Fracture nasal inferior turbinate(s), therapeutic `A 2 T`

RVU			Global Days	Modifiers				
Mod	Non-Fac Total	Fac Total		51	50	62	80	MUE
	3.54	3.54	010	2	1	0	1	1

AMA: Jul 01: 11, Dec 02: 10, Jul 03: 15, Aug 03: 14, Dec 04: 18, Sep 10: 10

30999 Unlisted procedure, nose `⊘ x T`

RVU			Global Days	Modifiers				
Mod	Non-Fac Total	Fac Total		51	50	62	80	MUE
	0.00	0.00	YYY	2	0	1	0	

AMA: Feb 13: 13

Sinus Procedures

Sinus Incisional Procedures

31000 Lavage by cannulation; maxillary sinus (antrum puncture or natural ostium) `P 3 T`

RVU			Global Days	Modifiers				
Mod	Non-Fac Total	Fac Total		51	50	62	80	MUE
	5.26	3.04	010	2	1	0	1	1

AMA: Apr 14: 10

31002 Lavage by cannulation; sphenoid sinus `R 2 T`

RVU			Global Days	Modifiers				
Mod	Non-Fac Total	Fac Total		51	50	62	80	MUE
	5.54	5.54	010	2	1	0	0	1

31020 Sinusotomy, maxillary (antrotomy); intranasal `A 2 T`

RVU			Global Days	Modifiers				
Mod	Non-Fac Total	Fac Total		51	50	62	80	MUE
	13.89	10.31	090	2	1	0	1	1

31030 Sinusotomy, maxillary (antrotomy); radical (Caldwell-Luc) without removal of antrochoanal polyps `A 2 J 1`

RVU			Global Days	Modifiers				
Mod	Non-Fac Total	Fac Total		51	50	62	80	MUE
	19.89	15.24	090	2	1	0	1	1

● New   ▲ Revised   Deleted   ⊙ Moderate Sedation   ✚ Add-on Codes   ⊘ High Risk Denial   Ⓐ Age Edit   ♀ Female   ♂ Male   **AMA** CPT® Assistant   **MUE** Medically Unlikely Edit
⊘ Modifier 51 Exempt   ⊖ Modifier 63 Exempt   ✗ Unlisted   **Modifiers:** See Inside Back Cover   Ⓜ Maternity   A2–Z3 ASC Payment Indicators   A–Y OPPS Status Indicators

Surgical Procedures

30802 – 31030

31032 Sinusotomy, maxillary (antrotomy); radical (Caldwell-Luc) with removal of antrochoanal polyps   `A 2 J I`

RVU			Global Days	Modifiers				
Mod	Non-Fac Total	Fac Total		51	50	62	80	MUE
	16.51	16.51	090	2	1	0	1	1

31040 Pterygomaxillary fossa surgery, any approach   `R 2 T`

RVU			Global Days	Modifiers				
Mod	Non-Fac Total	Fac Total		51	50	62	80	MUE
	21.87	21.87	090	2	1	1	1	1

31050 Sinusotomy, sphenoid, with or without biopsy   `A 2 J I`

RVU			Global Days	Modifiers				
Mod	Non-Fac Total	Fac Total		51	50	62	80	MUE
	13.98	13.98	090	2	1	0	1	1

31051 Sinusotomy, sphenoid, with or without biopsy; with mucosal stripping or removal of polyp(s)   `A 2 J I`

RVU			Global Days	Modifiers				
Mod	Non-Fac Total	Fac Total		51	50	62	80	MUE
	18.52	18.52	090	2	1	0	1	1

31070 Sinusotomy frontal; external, simple (trephine operation)   `A 2 J I`

RVU			Global Days	Modifiers				
Mod	Non-Fac Total	Fac Total		51	50	62	80	MUE
	12.59	12.59	090	2	1	0	1	1

Sinusotomy, frontal; simple

Bur is used to drill opening into frontal sinus

Frontal sinus

Catheters are used to irrigate sinus

The wound is closed. Catheters are sutured to the skin and removed after healing

31075 Sinusotomy frontal; transorbital, unilateral (for mucocele or osteoma, Lynch type)   `A 2 J I`

RVU			Global Days	Modifiers				
Mod	Non-Fac Total	Fac Total		51	50	62	80	MUE
	22.55	22.55	090	2	1	1	2	1

31080 Sinusotomy frontal; obliterative without osteoplastic flap, brow incision (includes ablation)   `A 2 J I`

RVU			Global Days	Modifiers				
Mod	Non-Fac Total	Fac Total		51	50	62	80	MUE
	29.74	29.74	090	2	1	0	2	1

31081 Sinusotomy frontal; obliterative, without osteoplastic flap, coronal incision (includes ablation)   `A 2 J I`

RVU			Global Days	Modifiers				
Mod	Non-Fac Total	Fac Total		51	50	62	80	MUE
	42.54	42.54	090	2	1	1	2	1

31084 Sinusotomy frontal; obliterative, with osteoplastic flap, brow incision   `A 2 J I`

RVU			Global Days	Modifiers				
Mod	Non-Fac Total	Fac Total		51	50	62	80	MUE
	33.25	33.25	090	2	1	1	2	1

31085 Sinusotomy frontal; obliterative, with osteoplastic flap, coronal incision   `A 2 J I`

RVU			Global Days	Modifiers				
Mod	Non-Fac Total	Fac Total		51	50	62	80	MUE
	45.41	45.41	090	2	1	1	2	1

31086 Sinusotomy frontal; nonobliterative, with osteoplastic flap, brow incision   `A 2 J I`

RVU			Global Days	Modifiers				
Mod	Non-Fac Total	Fac Total		51	50	62	80	MUE
	32.38	32.38	090	2	1	0	2	1

31087 Sinusotomy frontal; nonobliterative, with osteoplastic flap, coronal incision   `A 2 J I`

RVU			Global Days	Modifiers				
Mod	Non-Fac Total	Fac Total		51	50	62	80	MUE
	31.12	31.12	090	2	1	1	2	1

31090 Sinusotomy, unilateral, 3 or more paranasal sinuses (frontal, maxillary, ethmoid, sphenoid)   `A 2 J I`

RVU			Global Days	Modifiers				
Mod	Non-Fac Total	Fac Total		51	50	62	80	MUE
	29.34	29.34	090	2	1	0	1	1

AMA: Nov 97: 15, Nov 98: 11

Sinus Excisional Procedures

31200 Ethmoidectomy; intranasal, anterior   `A 2 J I`

RVU			Global Days	Modifiers				
Mod	Non-Fac Total	Fac Total		51	50	62	80	MUE
	16.22	16.22	090	2	1	0	1	1

31201 Ethmoidectomy; intranasal, total   `A 2 T`

RVU			Global Days	Modifiers				
Mod	Non-Fac Total	Fac Total		51	50	62	80	MUE
	21.20	21.20	090	2	1	0	1	1

31205 Ethmoidectomy; extranasal, total   `A 2 T`

RVU			Global Days	Modifiers				
Mod	Non-Fac Total	Fac Total		51	50	62	80	MUE
	25.64	25.64	090	2	1	1	2	1

● New   ▲ Revised   ✖ Deleted   ⊙ Moderate Sedation   ✚ Add-on Codes   ⊗ High Risk Denial   Ⓐ Age Edit   ♀ Female   ♂ Male   **AMA** *CPT® Assistant*   **MUE** Medically Unlikely Edit
⊘ Modifier 51 Exempt   ⊖ Modifier 63 Exempt   ✗ Unlisted   **Modifiers:** *See Inside Back Cover*   Ⓜ Maternity   `A 2`–`Z 3` ASC Payment Indicators   `A`–`Y` OPPS Status Indicators

CPT © 2015 American Medical Association. All Rights Reserved.   © 2016 DecisionHealth

31225 Maxillectomy; without orbital exenteration   C

RVU			Global Days	Modifiers				
Mod	Non-Fac Total	Fac Total		51	50	62	80	MUE
	53.94	53.94	090	2	1	1	2	1

31230 Maxillectomy; with orbital exenteration (en bloc)   C

RVU			Global Days	Modifiers				
Mod	Non-Fac Total	Fac Total		51	50	62	80	MUE
	59.87	59.87	090	2	1	1	2	1

Endoscopic Sinus Procedures

Coding Guidance

When a diagnostic endoscopy is done to determine that a non-endoscopic, surgical procedure is necessary, the diagnostic procedure may be reported separately as a distinct, diagnostic service. Modifier 58 may be used to note that the surgical procedure deemed necessary as a result of the diagnostic endoscopy, and the diagnostic endoscopy itself are planned or staged procedures. When an open surgical procedure is accompanied by a diagnostic endoscopy to evaluate the patient's respiratory system anatomy or determine surgical efficacy, the endoscopy is not reported.

31231 Nasal endoscopy, diagnostic, unilateral or bilateral (separate procedure)   P 2 T

Coding tip: Report only for diagnostic nasal inspection performed alone as an endoscopic procedure

Coding tip: Do not report with 31237-31297

RVU			Global Days	Modifiers				
Mod	Non-Fac Total	Fac Total		51	50	62	80	MUE
	6.00	1.88	000	2	2	0	1	1

AMA: Winter 93: 22, Jan 97: 4

Nasal endoscopy, diagnostic, unilateral or bilateral

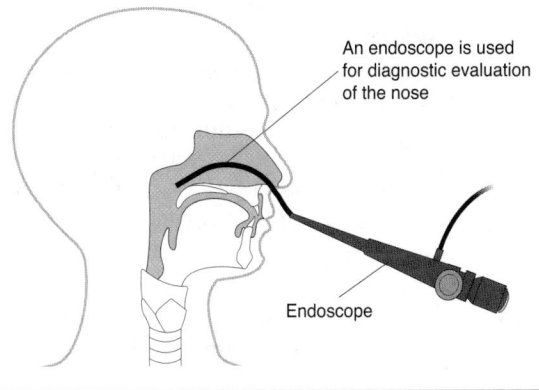

An endoscope is used for diagnostic evaluation of the nose

Endoscope

31233 Nasal/sinus endoscopy, diagnostic with maxillary sinusoscopy (via inferior meatus or canine fossa puncture)   A 2 T

RVU			Global Days	Modifiers				
Mod	Non-Fac Total	Fac Total		51	50	62	80	MUE
	7.53	3.94	000	2	1	0	0	1

AMA: Winter 93: 22, Jan 97: 4, Jun 11: 11

31235 Nasal/sinus endoscopy, diagnostic with sphenoid sinusoscopy (via puncture of sphenoidal face or cannulation of ostium)   A 2 T

RVU			Global Days	Modifiers				
Mod	Non-Fac Total	Fac Total		51	50	62	80	MUE
	8.58	4.67	000	2	1	0	0	1

AMA: Winter 93: 22, Jan 97: 4

31237 Nasal/sinus endoscopy, surgical; with biopsy, polypectomy or debridement (separate procedure)   A 2 T

Coding tip: Code 99001 for specimen transfer from a facility to an outside laboratory

RVU			Global Days	Modifiers				
Mod	Non-Fac Total	Fac Total		51	50	62	80	MUE
	7.41	4.66	000	2	1	0	1	1

AMA: Winter 93: 23, Jan 97: 4, Dec 01: 6, May 03: 5, Dec 11: 13, Jan 15: 13

31238 Nasal/sinus endoscopy, surgical; with control of nasal hemorrhage   A 2 T

Coding tip: Do not code with 31231

Coding tip: This includes diagnostic nasal inspection done before surgical control of hemorrhage

RVU			Global Days	Modifiers				
Mod	Non-Fac Total	Fac Total		51	50	62	80	MUE
	7.40	4.88	000	2	1	0	0	1

AMA: Winter 93: 23, Jan 97: 4

31239 Nasal/sinus endoscopy, surgical; with dacryocystorhinostomy   A 2 T

RVU			Global Days	Modifiers				
Mod	Non-Fac Total	Fac Total		51	50	62	80	MUE
	17.66	17.66	010	2	1	0	0	1

AMA: Winter 93: 23, Jan 97: 4

31240 Nasal/sinus endoscopy, surgical; with concha bullosa resection   A 2 T

RVU			Global Days	Modifiers				
Mod	Non-Fac Total	Fac Total		51	50	62	80	MUE
	4.65	4.65	000	2	1	0	0	1

AMA: Winter 93: 23, Jan 97: 4, May 03: 5

Coding Guidance

A separate code for nasal/sinus endoscopy with biopsy (31237) performed in conjunction with a polypectomy/ethmoidectomy is not to be reported with the main surgical code because biopsy tissue is procured as part of the procedure.

31254 Nasal/sinus endoscopy, surgical; with ethmoidectomy, partial (anterior)   A 2 T

RVU			Global Days	Modifiers				
Mod	Non-Fac Total	Fac Total		51	50	62	80	MUE
	7.88	7.88	000	2	1	0	1	1

AMA: Winter 93: 23, Jan 97: 4, Sep 97: 10, Oct 97: 5, Dec 01: 6, May 03: 5, Jul 11: 13

31255 Nasal/sinus endoscopy, surgical; with ethmoidectomy, total (anterior and posterior)   A 2 T

RVU			Global Days	Modifiers				
Mod	Non-Fac Total	Fac Total		51	50	62	80	MUE
	11.58	11.58	000	2	1	0	1	1

AMA: Winter 93: 23, Jan 97: 4, Dec 02: 10, May 03: 5, Jul 11: 13

Coding Guidance

A separate code for nasal/sinus endoscopy with biopsy (31237) performed in conjunction with a maxillary antrostomy is not to be reported with the main surgical code when biopsy tissue is procured as part of the procedure.

● New   ▲ Revised   Deleted   ⊙ Moderate Sedation   ✚ Add-on Codes   ⊘ High Risk Denial   Ⓐ Age Edit   ♀ Female   ♂ Male   **AMA** *CPT® Assistant*   **MUE** Medically Unlikely Edit
⊘ Modifier 51 Exempt   ⊖ Modifier 63 Exempt   ✗ Unlisted   **Modifiers:** *See Inside Back Cover*   Ⓜ Maternity   A2-Z3 ASC Payment Indicators   A-Y OPPS Status Indicators

Surgical Procedures

31225 – 31255

31256 Nasal/sinus endoscopy, surgical, with maxillary antrostomy A 2 T

RVU			Global Days	Modifiers				
Mod	Non-Fac Total	Fac Total		51	50	62	80	MUE
	5.72	5.72	000	2	1	0	1	1

AMA: Winter 93: 23, Jan 97: 4, Jun 11: 11, Jul 11: 13, Jun 13: 13

31267 Nasal/sinus endoscopy, surgical, with maxillary antrostomy; with removal of tissue from maxillary sinus A 2 T

RVU			Global Days	Modifiers				
Mod	Non-Fac Total	Fac Total		51	50	62	80	MUE
	9.18	9.18	000	2	1	0	1	1

AMA: Jan 97: 4, Dec 01: 6, Jun 11: 11, Jul 11: 13

Coding Guidance

A separate code for nasal/sinus endoscopy with biopsy (31237) performed in conjunction with frontal sinus exploration is not to be reported with the main surgical code when biopsy tissue is procured as part of the procedure.

31276 Nasal/sinus endoscopy, surgical with frontal sinus exploration, with or without removal of tissue from frontal sinus A 2 T

RVU			Global Days	Modifiers				
Mod	Non-Fac Total	Fac Total		51	50	62	80	MUE
	14.60	14.60	000	2	1	0	1	1

AMA: Winter 93: 24, Jan 97: 4, Jan 10: 11, Jun 11: 13

Nasal/sinus endoscopy, with frontal sinus exploration/tissue removal

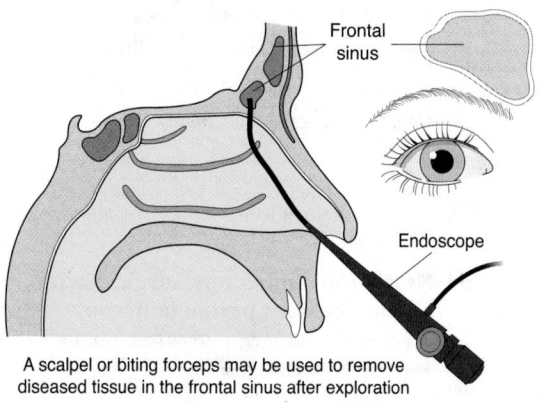

Frontal sinus

Endoscope

A scalpel or biting forceps may be used to remove diseased tissue in the frontal sinus after exploration

Coding Guidance

A separate code for nasal/sinus endoscopy with biopsy (31237) performed in conjunction with a sphenoidotomy is not to be reported with the main surgical code when biopsy tissue is procured as part of the procedure.

31287 Nasal/sinus endoscopy, surgical, with sphenoidotomy A 2 T

RVU			Global Days	Modifiers				
Mod	Non-Fac Total	Fac Total		51	50	62	80	MUE
	6.71	6.71	000	2	1	0	0	1

AMA: Winter 93: 24, Jan 97: 4, Jun 11: 11

31288 Nasal/sinus endoscopy, surgical, with sphenoidotomy; with removal of tissue from the sphenoid sinus A 2 T

RVU			Global Days	Modifiers				
Mod	Non-Fac Total	Fac Total		51	50	62	80	MUE
	7.76	7.76	000	2	1	0	0	1

AMA: Winter 93: 24, Jan 97: 4, Jun 11: 11

31290 Nasal/sinus endoscopy, surgical, with repair of cerebrospinal fluid leak; ethmoid region C

RVU			Global Days	Modifiers				
Mod	Non-Fac Total	Fac Total		51	50	62	80	MUE
	33.37	33.37	010	2	1	0	0	1

AMA: Winter 93: 24, Jan 97: 4, Jul 11: 13

31291 Nasal/sinus endoscopy, surgical, with repair of cerebrospinal fluid leak; sphenoid region C

RVU			Global Days	Modifiers				
Mod	Non-Fac Total	Fac Total		51	50	62	80	MUE
	35.64	35.64	010	2	1	0	0	1

AMA: Winter 93: 24, Jan 97: 4, Jul 11: 13

31292 Nasal/sinus endoscopy, surgical; with medial or inferior orbital wall decompression T

RVU			Global Days	Modifiers				
Mod	Non-Fac Total	Fac Total		51	50	62	80	MUE
	28.88	28.88	010	2	1	0	0	1

AMA: Winter 93: 24, Jan 97: 4, Jul 11: 13

31293 Nasal/sinus endoscopy, surgical; with medial orbital wall and inferior orbital wall decompression T

RVU			Global Days	Modifiers				
Mod	Non-Fac Total	Fac Total		51	50	62	80	MUE
	31.34	31.34	010	2	1	0	0	1

AMA: Winter 93: 24, Jan 97: 4, Jul 11: 13

31294 Nasal/sinus endoscopy, surgical; with optic nerve decompression T

RVU			Global Days	Modifiers				
Mod	Non-Fac Total	Fac Total		51	50	62	80	MUE
	35.80	35.80	010	2	1	0	0	1

AMA: Winter 93: 24, Jan 97: 4, Jul 11: 13

31295 Nasal/sinus endoscopy, surgical; with dilation of maxillary sinus ostium (eg, balloon dilation), transnasal or via canine fossa P 2 T

RVU			Global Days	Modifiers				
Mod	Non-Fac Total	Fac Total		51	50	62	80	MUE
	58.44	4.74	000	2	1	0	2	1

AMA: Jun 11: 11

Nasal/sinus endoscopy, with ostium dilation

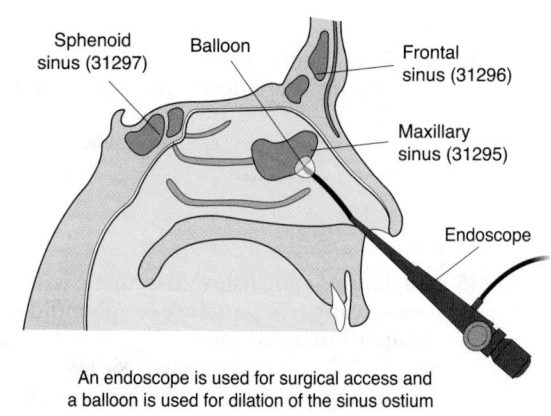

Sphenoid sinus (31297)   Balloon   Frontal sinus (31296)

Maxillary sinus (31295)

Endoscope

An endoscope is used for surgical access and a balloon is used for dilation of the sinus ostium

● New   ▲ Revised   ✖ Deleted   ⊙ Moderate Sedation   ✚ Add-on Codes   ⊘ High Risk Denial   Ⓐ Age Edit   ♀ Female   ♂ Male   **AMA** CPT® Assistant   **MUE** Medically Unlikely Edit
⊘ Modifier 51 Exempt   ⊖ Modifier 63 Exempt   ✗ Unlisted   **Modifiers:** See Inside Back Cover   Ⓜ Maternity   A2–Z3 ASC Payment Indicators   A–Y OPPS Status Indicators

CPT © 2015 American Medical Association. All Rights Reserved.   © 2016 DecisionHealth

31296 Nasal/sinus endoscopy, surgical; with dilation of frontal sinus ostium (eg, balloon dilation) P 2 T

| RVU | | | Global Days | Modifiers | | | | |
Mod	Non-Fac Total	Fac Total		51	50	62	80	MUE
	59.57	5.68	000	2	1	0	2	1

AMA: Jun 11: 11

31297 Nasal/sinus endoscopy, surgical; with dilation of sphenoid sinus ostium (eg, balloon dilation) P 2 T

| RVU | | | Global Days | Modifiers | | | | |
Mod	Non-Fac Total	Fac Total		51	50	62	80	MUE
	58.53	4.64	000	2	1	0	0	1

AMA: Jun 11: 11

Other Sinus Procedures

31299 Unlisted procedure, accessory sinuses ✗T

| RVU | | | Global Days | Modifiers | | | | |
Mod	Non-Fac Total	Fac Total		51	50	62	80	MUE
	0.00	0.00	YYY	2	0	1	0	

AMA: Jun 11: 11, Jan 10: 11, Jun 13: 13, Jul 15: 10

Laryngeal Procedures

Excisional Laryngeal Procedures

31300 Laryngotomy (thyrotomy, laryngofissure); with removal of tumor or laryngocele, cordectomy A 2 T

| RVU | | | Global Days | Modifiers | | | | |
Mod	Non-Fac Total	Fac Total		51	50	62	80	MUE
	37.69	37.69	090	2	0	1	2	1

31320 Laryngotomy (thyrotomy, laryngofissure); diagnostic A 2 J I

| RVU | | | Global Days | Modifiers | | | | |
Mod	Non-Fac Total	Fac Total		51	50	62	80	MUE
	20.13	20.13	090	2	0	0	0	1

31360 Laryngectomy; total, without radical neck dissection C

| RVU | | | Global Days | Modifiers | | | | |
Mod	Non-Fac Total	Fac Total		51	50	62	80	MUE
	61.12	61.12	090	2	0	1	2	1

AMA: Aug 10: 4

31365 Laryngectomy; total, with radical neck dissection C

| RVU | | | Global Days | Modifiers | | | | |
Mod	Non-Fac Total	Fac Total		51	50	62	80	MUE
	75.41	75.41	090	2	0	1	2	1

AMA: Oct 01: 10, Aug 10: 4

31367 Laryngectomy; subtotal supraglottic, without radical neck dissection C

| RVU | | | Global Days | Modifiers | | | | |
Mod	Non-Fac Total	Fac Total		51	50	62	80	MUE
	64.75	64.75	090	2	0	1	2	1

AMA: Aug 10: 4

31368 Laryngectomy; subtotal supraglottic, with radical neck dissection C

| RVU | | | Global Days | Modifiers | | | | |
Mod	Non-Fac Total	Fac Total		51	50	62	80	MUE
	72.28	72.28	090	2	0	1	2	1

31370 Partial laryngectomy (hemilaryngectomy); horizontal C

| RVU | | | Global Days | Modifiers | | | | |
Mod	Non-Fac Total	Fac Total		51	50	62	80	MUE
	61.00	61.00	090	2	0	1	2	1

31375 Partial laryngectomy (hemilaryngectomy); laterovertical C

| RVU | | | Global Days | Modifiers | | | | |
Mod	Non-Fac Total	Fac Total		51	50	62	80	MUE
	57.61	57.61	090	2	0	1	2	1

31380 Partial laryngectomy (hemilaryngectomy); anterovertical C

| RVU | | | Global Days | Modifiers | | | | |
Mod	Non-Fac Total	Fac Total		51	50	62	80	MUE
	57.01	57.01	090	2	0	1	2	1

31382 Partial laryngectomy (hemilaryngectomy); antero-latero-vertical C

| RVU | | | Global Days | Modifiers | | | | |
Mod	Non-Fac Total	Fac Total		51	50	62	80	MUE
	62.81	62.81	090	2	0	1	2	1

31390 Pharyngolaryngectomy, with radical neck dissection; without reconstruction C

| RVU | | | Global Days | Modifiers | | | | |
Mod	Non-Fac Total	Fac Total		51	50	62	80	MUE
	84.13	84.13	090	2	0	1	2	1

31395 Pharyngolaryngectomy, with radical neck dissection; with reconstruction C

| RVU | | | Global Days | Modifiers | | | | |
Mod	Non-Fac Total	Fac Total		51	50	62	80	MUE
	88.89	88.89	090	2	0	1	2	1

31400 Arytenoidectomy or arytenoidopexy, external approach A 2 J I

| RVU | | | Global Days | Modifiers | | | | |
Mod	Non-Fac Total	Fac Total		51	50	62	80	MUE
	28.16	28.16	090	2	0	0	2	1

31420 Epiglottidectomy A 2 J I

| RVU | | | Global Days | Modifiers | | | | |
Mod	Non-Fac Total	Fac Total		51	50	62	80	MUE
	24.03	24.03	090	2	0	1	2	1

Epiglottidectomy

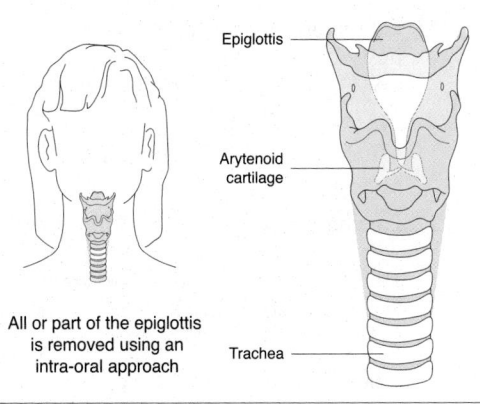

All or part of the epiglottis is removed using an intra-oral approach

Epiglottis

Arytenoid cartilage

Trachea

● New   ▲ Revised   Deleted   ⊙ Moderate Sedation   ✚ Add-on Codes   ⊘ High Risk Denial   Ⓐ Age Edit   ♀ Female   ♂ Male   **AMA** *CPT® Assistant*   **MUE** Medically Unlikely Edit
⊘ Modifier 51 Exempt   ⊖ Modifier 63 Exempt   ✗ Unlisted   **Modifiers:** *See Inside Back Cover*   Ⓜ Maternity   A 2 - Z 3 ASC Payment Indicators   A - Y OPPS Status Indicators

Surgical Procedures

Laryngeal Introduction Procedures

Coding Guidance

Do not report 31500 for elective intubation for non-emergency reasons, such as bronchoscopy or general anesthesia.

⊘ 31500 Intubation, endotracheal, emergency procedure

G 2 T

> **Coding tip:** *See also emergency tracheostomy procedure - 31603-31605*

RVU		Global Days	Modifiers				
Mod	Non-Fac Total	Fac Total		51	50	62	80	MUE
	3.17	3.17	000	0	0	0	1	2

AMA: Nov 99: 32, 33, Oct 03: 2, Aug 04: 8, Jul 06: 4, Jul 07: 1, Dec 09: 10
Pub 100-04, 12, 30.6.12

31502 Tracheotomy tube change prior to establishment of fistula tract

G 2 T

RVU		Global Days	Modifiers				
Mod	Non-Fac Total	Fac Total		51	50	62	80	MUE
	1.01	1.01	000	2	0	0	1	1

AMA: Winter 90: 6

Endoscopic Laryngeal Procedures

Coding Guidance

When a diagnostic laryngoscopy is done to determine that a non-endoscopic, surgical procedure is necessary, the diagnostic procedure may be reported separately as a distinct, diagnostic service. Modifier 58 may be used to note that the surgical procedure deemed necessary as a result of the diagnostic endoscopy, and the diagnostic endoscopy itself are planned or staged procedures. When an open surgical procedure is accompanied by a diagnostic endoscopy to evaluate the patient's respiratory system anatomy or determine surgical efficacy, the endoscopy is not reported. If the larynx is viewed during esophagoscopy through the esophagoscope, it cannot be reported. However, if it is viewed through a separate laryngoscope, both the laryngoscopy and the esophagoscopy may be reported.

31505 Laryngoscopy, indirect; diagnostic (separate procedure)

P 3 T

> **Coding tip:** *Report only when diagnostic laryngoscopy alone is performed*
> **Coding tip:** *Direct diagnostic laryngoscopy - 31525; with operating microscope - 31526*

RVU		Global Days	Modifiers				
Mod	Non-Fac Total	Fac Total		51	50	62	80	MUE
	2.38	1.42	000	2	0	0	1	1

AMA: Nov 99: 13

31510 Laryngoscopy, indirect; with biopsy

A 2 T

RVU		Global Days	Modifiers				
Mod	Non-Fac Total	Fac Total		51	50	62	80	MUE
	6.05	3.51	000	3	0	0	0	1

AMA: Nov 99: 13

31511 Laryngoscopy, indirect; with removal of foreign body

A 2 T

RVU		Global Days	Modifiers				
Mod	Non-Fac Total	Fac Total		51	50	62	80	MUE
	6.07	3.77	000	3	0	0	1	1

AMA: Nov 99: 13

31512 Laryngoscopy, indirect; with removal of lesion

A 2 T

RVU		Global Days	Modifiers				
Mod	Non-Fac Total	Fac Total		51	50	62	80	MUE
	5.86	3.74	000	3	0	0	0	1

AMA: Nov 99: 13

31513 Laryngoscopy, indirect; with vocal cord injection

A 2 T

RVU		Global Days	Modifiers				
Mod	Non-Fac Total	Fac Total		51	50	62	80	MUE
	3.82	3.82	000	3	0	0	0	1

AMA: Nov 99: 13

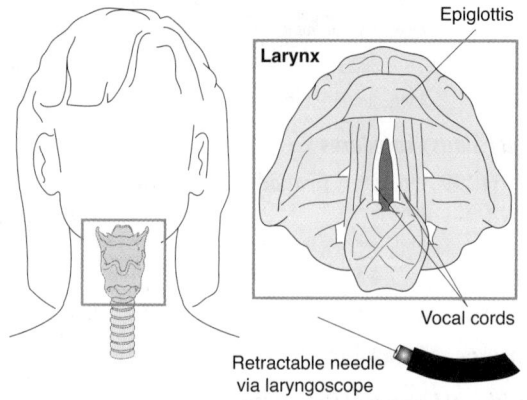

Laryngoscopy, indirect; with injection

The physician examines the vocal cords, the tongue, and the top of the throat and injects the vocal cords to treat paralysis/atrophy

31515 Laryngoscopy direct, with or without tracheoscopy; for aspiration

A 2 T

RVU		Global Days	Modifiers				
Mod	Non-Fac Total	Fac Total		51	50	62	80	MUE
	5.28	3.03	000	2	0	0	1	1

Coding Guidance

When a diagnostic laryngoscopy is done to determine that a non-endoscopic, surgical procedure is necessary, the diagnostic procedure may be reported separately as a distinct, diagnostic service. Modifier 58 may be used to note that the surgical procedure deemed necessary as a result of the diagnostic endoscopy, and the diagnostic endoscopy itself are planned or staged procedures. When an open surgical procedure is accompanied by a diagnostic endoscopy to evaluate the patient's respiratory system anatomy or determine surgical efficacy, the endoscopy is not reported.

31520 Laryngoscopy direct, with or without tracheoscopy; diagnostic, newborn

⊘ Ⓐ ⊖ G 2 T

RVU		Global Days	Modifiers				
Mod	Non-Fac Total	Fac Total		51	50	62	80	MUE
	4.53	4.53	000	2	0	0	0	1

31525 Laryngoscopy direct, with or without tracheoscopy; diagnostic, except newborn

A 2 T

RVU		Global Days	Modifiers				
Mod	Non-Fac Total	Fac Total		51	50	62	80	MUE
	7.27	4.65	000	2	0	0	1	1

AMA: Aug 10: 3

31526 Laryngoscopy direct, with or without tracheoscopy; diagnostic, with operating microscope or telescope

A 2 T

RVU		Global Days	Modifiers				
Mod	Non-Fac Total	Fac Total		51	50	62	80	MUE
	4.57	4.57	000	2	0	0	1	1

AMA: Nov 98: 11, 12

● New   ▲ Revised   ✖ Deleted   ⊙ Moderate Sedation   ✚ Add-on Codes   ⊘ High Risk Denial   Ⓐ Age Edit   ♀ Female   ♂ Male   **AMA** *CPT® Assistant*   **MUE** Medically Unlikely Edit
⊘ Modifier 51 Exempt   ⊖ Modifier 63 Exempt   Ⓧ Unlisted   **Modifiers:** *See Inside Back Cover*   Ⓜ Maternity   A 2 – Z 3 ASC Payment Indicators   A – Y OPPS Status Indicators

332   CPT © 2015 American Medical Association. All Rights Reserved.   © 2016 DecisionHealth

31527 Laryngoscopy direct, with or without tracheoscopy; with insertion of obturator A2 T

Mod	Non-Fac Total	Fac Total	Global Days	51	50	62	80	MUE
	5.65	5.65	000	3	0	0	0	1

31528 Laryngoscopy direct, with or without tracheoscopy; with dilation, initial A2 T

Mod	Non-Fac Total	Fac Total	Global Days	51	50	62	80	MUE
	4.20	4.20	000	3	0	0	0	1

31529 Laryngoscopy direct, with or without tracheoscopy; with dilation, subsequent A2 T

Mod	Non-Fac Total	Fac Total	Global Days	51	50	62	80	MUE
	4.71	4.71	000	3	0	0	0	1

31530 Laryngoscopy, direct, operative, with foreign body removal A2 T

Mod	Non-Fac Total	Fac Total	Global Days	51	50	62	80	MUE
	5.75	5.75	000	3	0	0	1	1

31531 Laryngoscopy, direct, operative, with foreign body removal; with operating microscope or telescope A2 T

Mod	Non-Fac Total	Fac Total	Global Days	51	50	62	80	MUE
	6.19	6.19	000	3	0	0	0	1

AMA: Nov 98: 11, 12

31535 Laryngoscopy, direct, operative, with biopsy A2 T

Coding tip: Code 99001 for specimen transfer from a facility to an outside laboratory

Mod	Non-Fac Total	Fac Total	Global Days	51	50	62	80	MUE
	5.52	5.52	000	3	0	0	1	1

31536 Laryngoscopy, direct, operative, with biopsy; with operating microscope or telescope A2 T

Mod	Non-Fac Total	Fac Total	Global Days	51	50	62	80	MUE
	6.14	6.14	000	3	0	0	1	1

AMA: Nov 98: 11, 12

31540 Laryngoscopy, direct, operative, with excision of tumor and/or stripping of vocal cords or epiglottis A2 T

Mod	Non-Fac Total	Fac Total	Global Days	51	50	62	80	MUE
	7.04	7.04	000	3	0	0	1	1

31541 Laryngoscopy, direct, operative, with excision of tumor and/or stripping of vocal cords or epiglottis; with operating microscope or telescope A2 T

Mod	Non-Fac Total	Fac Total	Global Days	51	50	62	80	MUE
	7.67	7.67	000	3	0	0	1	1

AMA: Nov 98: 11, 12

31545 Laryngoscopy, direct, operative, with operating microscope or telescope, with submucosal removal of non-neoplastic lesion(s) of vocal cord; reconstruction with local tissue flap(s) A2 T

Mod	Non-Fac Total	Fac Total	Global Days	51	50	62	80	MUE
	10.56	10.56	000	3	1	0	1	1

31546 Laryngoscopy, direct, operative, with operating microscope or telescope, with submucosal removal of non-neoplastic lesion(s) of vocal cord; reconstruction with graft(s) (includes obtaining autograft) A2 T

Mod	Non-Fac Total	Fac Total	Global Days	51	50	62	80	MUE
	16.07	16.07	000	3	1	0	1	1

31560 Laryngoscopy, direct, operative, with arytenoidectomy A2 T

Mod	Non-Fac Total	Fac Total	Global Days	51	50	62	80	MUE
	9.12	9.12	000	3	0	0	0	1

31561 Laryngoscopy, direct, operative, with arytenoidectomy; with operating microscope or telescope A2 T

Mod	Non-Fac Total	Fac Total	Global Days	51	50	62	80	MUE
	9.99	9.99	000	3	0	0	0	1

AMA: Nov 98: 11, 12

31570 Laryngoscopy, direct, with injection into vocal cord(s), therapeutic A2 T

Mod	Non-Fac Total	Fac Total	Global Days	51	50	62	80	MUE
	9.76	6.68	000	3	0	0	1	1

AMA: Jan 14: 6

31571 Laryngoscopy, direct, with injection into vocal cord(s), therapeutic; with operating microscope or telescope A2 T

Mod	Non-Fac Total	Fac Total	Global Days	51	50	62	80	MUE
	7.27	7.27	000	3	0	0	1	1

AMA: Nov 98: 11, 12, Nov 12: 14, Jan 14: 6

31575 Laryngoscopy, flexible fiberoptic; diagnostic P3 T

Mod	Non-Fac Total	Fac Total	Global Days	51	50	62	80	MUE
	3.27	2.21	000	2	0	0	1	1

31576 Laryngoscopy, flexible fiberoptic; with biopsy A2 T

Mod	Non-Fac Total	Fac Total	Global Days	51	50	62	80	MUE
	6.43	3.58	000	3	0	0	1	1

31577 Laryngoscopy, flexible fiberoptic; with removal of foreign body A2 T

Mod	Non-Fac Total	Fac Total	Global Days	51	50	62	80	MUE
	6.94	4.34	000	3	0	0	0	1

● New ▲ Revised Deleted ⊙ Moderate Sedation ✚ Add-on Codes ⊘ High Risk Denial Ⓐ Age Edit ♀ Female ♂ Male **AMA** CPT® Assistant **MUE** Medically Unlikely Edit
⃠ Modifier 51 Exempt ⊖ Modifier 63 Exempt ✗ Unlisted **Modifiers:** See Inside Back Cover Ⓜ Maternity A2–Z3 ASC Payment Indicators A–Y OPPS Status Indicators
© 2016 DecisionHealth CPT © 2015 American Medical Association. All Rights Reserved. **333**

31578 Laryngoscopy, flexible fiberoptic; with removal of lesion A 2 T

| RVU | | | Global Days | Modifiers | | | | |
Mod	Non-Fac Total	Fac Total		51	50	62	80	MUE
	8.01	4.99	000	3	0	0	0	1

31579 Laryngoscopy, flexible or rigid fiberoptic, with stroboscopy P 3 T

| RVU | | | Global Days | Modifiers | | | | |
Mod	Non-Fac Total	Fac Total		51	50	62	80	MUE
	6.03	4.08	000	3	0	0	1	1

Laryngeal Repair Procedures

31580 Laryngoplasty; for laryngeal web, 2-stage, with keel insertion and removal A 2 J I

| RVU | | | Global Days | Modifiers | | | | |
Mod	Non-Fac Total	Fac Total		51	50	62	80	MUE
	35.19	35.19	090	2	0	1	2	1

31582 Laryngoplasty; for laryngeal stenosis, with graft or core mold, including tracheotomy A 2 J I

| RVU | | | Global Days | Modifiers | | | | |
Mod	Non-Fac Total	Fac Total		51	50	62	80	MUE
	54.62	54.62	090	2	0	1	1	1

31584 Laryngoplasty; with open reduction of fracture C

| RVU | | | Global Days | Modifiers | | | | |
Mod	Non-Fac Total	Fac Total		51	50	62	80	MUE
	43.61	43.61	090	2	0	1	2	1

31587 Laryngoplasty, cricoid split C

| RVU | | | Global Days | Modifiers | | | | |
Mod	Non-Fac Total	Fac Total		51	50	62	80	MUE
	28.88	28.88	090	2	0	1	2	1

31588 Laryngoplasty, not otherwise specified (eg, for burns, reconstruction after partial laryngectomy) A 2 J I

| RVU | | | Global Days | Modifiers | | | | |
Mod	Non-Fac Total	Fac Total		51	50	62	80	MUE
	32.84	32.84	090	2	0	0	2	1

AMA: Aug 04: 11

31590 Laryngeal reinnervation by neuromuscular pedicle A 2 J I

| RVU | | | Global Days | Modifiers | | | | |
Mod	Non-Fac Total	Fac Total		51	50	62	80	MUE
	25.79	25.79	090	2	0	1	2	1

Laryngeal Destruction Procedures

31595 Section recurrent laryngeal nerve, therapeutic (separate procedure), unilateral A 2 J I

| RVU | | | Global Days | Modifiers | | | | |
Mod	Non-Fac Total	Fac Total		51	50	62	80	MUE
	22.02	22.02	090	2	1	1	2	1

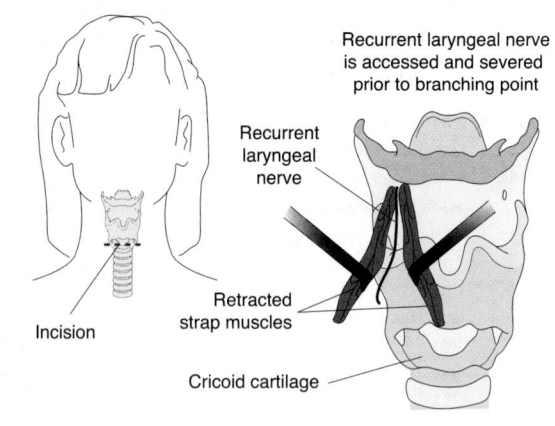

Section recurrent laryngeal nerve

Recurrent laryngeal nerve is accessed and severed prior to branching point

Recurrent laryngeal nerve

Incision

Retracted strap muscles

Cricoid cartilage

Other Laryngeal Procedures

31599 Unlisted procedure, larynx x T

| RVU | | | Global Days | Modifiers | | | | |
Mod	Non-Fac Total	Fac Total		51	50	62	80	MUE
	0.00	0.00	YYY	2	0	1	0	

AMA: Nov 12: 14

Tracheal/Bronchial Procedures

Incisional Tracheal/Bronchial Procedures

Coding Guidance

Tracheostomies that are routinely placed or performed as an essential part of another procedure, such as a laryngectomy or laryngoplasty, are not coded separately. If a laryngoscopy is required for tracheostomy placement, the tracheostomy code is reported without the laryngoscopy. Do not report a separate tracheostomy code together with 61576 (transoral approach to the skull base), as a tracheostomy is included in the code descriptor.

31600 Tracheostomy, planned (separate procedure) T

| RVU | | | Global Days | Modifiers | | | | |
Mod	Non-Fac Total	Fac Total		51	50	62	80	MUE
	11.53	11.53	000	2	0	0	1	1

AMA: Aug 10: 5

31601 Tracheostomy, planned (separate procedure); younger than 2 years A T

| RVU | | | Global Days | Modifiers | | | | |
Mod	Non-Fac Total	Fac Total		51	50	62	80	MUE
	7.30	7.30	000	2	0	1	2	1

31603 Tracheostomy, emergency procedure; transtracheal A 2 T

| RVU | | | Global Days | Modifiers | | | | |
Mod	Non-Fac Total	Fac Total		51	50	62	80	MUE
	6.50	6.50	000	2	0	0	1	1

31605 Tracheostomy, emergency procedure; cricothyroid membrane G 2 T

| RVU | | | Global Days | Modifiers | | | | |
Mod	Non-Fac Total	Fac Total		51	50	62	80	MUE
	5.30	5.30	000	2	0	0	1	1

● New   ▲ Revised   ✖ Deleted   ⊙ Moderate Sedation   ✚ Add-on Codes   ⊘ High Risk Denial   Ⓐ Age Edit   ♀ Female   ♂ Male   **AMA** *CPT® Assistant*   **MUE** Medically Unlikely Edit   ⊘ Modifier 51 Exempt   ⊖ Modifier 63 Exempt   ✖ Unlisted   **Modifiers:** *See Inside Back Cover*   Ⓜ Maternity   A 2 – Z 3 ASC Payment Indicators   A – Y OPPS Status Indicators

CPT © 2015 American Medical Association. All Rights Reserved.   © 2016 DecisionHealth

31610 Tracheostomy, fenestration procedure with skin flaps `J1`

RVU			Global Days	Modifiers				
Mod	Non-Fac Total	Fac Total		51	50	62	80	MUE
	20.63	20.63	090	2	0	0	1	1

31611 Construction of tracheoesophageal fistula and subsequent insertion of an alaryngeal speech prosthesis (eg, voice button, Blom-Singer prosthesis) `A2T`

RVU			Global Days	Modifiers				
Mod	Non-Fac Total	Fac Total		51	50	62	80	MUE
	15.56	15.56	090	2	0	1	2	1

31612 Tracheal puncture, percutaneous with transtracheal aspiration and/or injection `A2J1`

RVU			Global Days	Modifiers				
Mod	Non-Fac Total	Fac Total		51	50	62	80	MUE
	2.39	1.40	000	2	0	0	0	1

31613 Tracheostoma revision; simple, without flap rotation `A2T`

RVU			Global Days	Modifiers				
Mod	Non-Fac Total	Fac Total		51	50	62	80	MUE
	13.10	13.10	090	2	0	0	1	1

31614 Tracheostoma revision; complex, with flap rotation `A2J1`

RVU			Global Days	Modifiers				
Mod	Non-Fac Total	Fac Total		51	50	62	80	MUE
	21.75	21.75	090	2	0	0	1	1

Endoscopic Tracheal/Bronchial Procedures

⊙ 31615 Tracheobronchoscopy through established tracheostomy incision `A2T`

RVU			Global Days	Modifiers				
Mod	Non-Fac Total	Fac Total		51	50	62	80	MUE
	5.21	3.72	000	2	0	0	1	1

AMA: Feb 10: 6, Nov 12: 14

✕ ~~31620 Endobronchial ultrasound (EBUS) during bronchoscopic diagnostic or therapeutic intervention(s) (List separately in addition to code for primary procedure[s])~~

Coding Guidance

Fiberoptic bronchoscopies include a routine, limited inspection of the nasal cavity, pharynx, and larynx. Other codes for nasal/pharyngeal/laryngeal endoscopies are incidental and are not reported. When a diagnostic bronchoscopy is done to determine that a non-endoscopic, surgical procedure is necessary, the diagnostic procedure may be reported separately as a distinct, diagnostic service. Modifier 58 may be used to note that the surgical procedure deemed necessary as a result of the diagnostic endoscopy, and the diagnostic endoscopy itself are planned or staged procedures. When an open surgical procedure is accompanied by a diagnostic endoscopy to evaluate the patient's respiratory system anatomy or determine surgical efficacy, the endoscopy is not reported.

⊙ 31622 Bronchoscopy, rigid or flexible, including fluoroscopic guidance, when performed; diagnostic, with cell washing, when performed (separate procedure) `A2T`

RVU			Global Days	Modifiers				
Mod	Non-Fac Total	Fac Total		51	50	62	80	MUE
	8.65	4.15	000	2	0	0	1	1

AMA: Jul 96: 11, Nov 98: 12, Dec 98: 8, Mar 99: 3, Apr 00: 10, Jun 01: 10, Jan 02: 10, Sep 04: 8, 12, Aug 05: 4, Apr 10: 5, Feb 10: 6, Dec 09: 10, Feb 11: 8

⊙ 31623 Bronchoscopy, rigid or flexible, including fluoroscopic guidance, when performed; with brushing or protected brushings `A2T`

RVU			Global Days	Modifiers				
Mod	Non-Fac Total	Fac Total		51	50	62	80	MUE
	9.42	4.22	000	3	0	0	1	1

AMA: Nov 98: 12, Mar 99: 3, Nov 99: 13, Jan 02: 10, Sep 04: 8, Aug 05: 4, May 08: 15, Mar 13: 8, Apr 10: 5

⊙ 31624 Bronchoscopy, rigid or flexible, including fluoroscopic guidance, when performed; with bronchial alveolar lavage `A2T`

RVU			Global Days	Modifiers				
Mod	Non-Fac Total	Fac Total		51	50	62	80	MUE
	8.92	4.26	000	3	0	0	1	1

AMA: Nov 98: 12, Feb 99: 9, Mar 99: 3, 11, Jan 02: 10, Sep 04: 8, Aug 05: 4, May 08: 15, Mar 13: 8, Feb 10: 6, Apr 10: 5

⊙ 31625 Bronchoscopy, rigid or flexible, including fluoroscopic guidance, when performed; with bronchial or endobronchial biopsy(s), single or multiple sites `A2T`

RVU			Global Days	Modifiers				
Mod	Non-Fac Total	Fac Total		51	50	62	80	MUE
	11.26	4.88	000	3	0	0	1	1

AMA: Spring 91: 2, Jan 02: 10, Jun 02: 10, Sep 03: 15, Sep 04: 9, Aug 05: 4, Mar 13: 8, Apr 10: 5, Feb 10: 6

⊙ 31626 Bronchoscopy, rigid or flexible, including fluoroscopic guidance, when performed; with placement of fiducial markers, single or multiple `G2T`

RVU			Global Days	Modifiers				
Mod	Non-Fac Total	Fac Total		51	50	62	80	MUE
	25.90	6.10	000	2	0	0	0	1

AMA: Mar 13: 8, Jan 11: 6, Feb 10: 6, Apr 10: 5, Jun 15: 6

⊙+31627 Bronchoscopy, rigid or flexible, including fluoroscopic guidance, when performed; with computer-assisted, image-guided navigation (List separately in addition to code for primary procedure[s]) `N1N`

RVU			Global Days	Modifiers				
Mod	Non-Fac Total	Fac Total		51	50	62	80	MUE
	40.19	2.81	ZZZ	0	0	0	0	1

AMA: Mar 13: 8, Jan 11: 6, Feb 10: 6, Apr 10: 5

⊙ 31628 Bronchoscopy, rigid or flexible, including fluoroscopic guidance, when performed; with transbronchial lung biopsy(s), single lobe `A2T`

Coding tip: Code 99001 for specimen transfer from a facility to an outside laboratory

RVU			Global Days	Modifiers				
Mod	Non-Fac Total	Fac Total		51	50	62	80	MUE
	11.86	5.43	000	3	0	0	1	1

AMA: Jun 01: 10, Jan 02: 10, Sep 04: 9, Aug 05: 4, May 08: 15, Apr 10: 5, Feb 10: 6, Mar 13: 8

● New ▲ Revised Deleted ⊙ Moderate Sedation ✚ Add-on Codes ⊘ High Risk Denial Ⓐ Age Edit ♀ Female ♂ Male **AMA** CPT® Assistant **MUE** Medically Unlikely Edit
⊘ Modifier 51 Exempt ⊖ Modifier 63 Exempt Ⓧ Unlisted **Modifiers:** See Inside Back Cover Ⓜ Maternity A2-Z3 ASC Payment Indicators A-Y OPPS Status Indicators

Surgical Procedures

31610 – 31628

Surgical Procedures

31629 – 31641

⊙ **31629** Bronchoscopy, rigid or flexible, including fluoroscopic guidance, when performed; with transbronchial needle aspiration biopsy(s), trachea, main stem and/or lobar bronchus(i) `A2 T`

RVU		Global Days	Modifiers				
Mod	Non-Fac Total	Fac Total		51	50	62	80	MUE
	14.16	5.75	000	3	0	0	1	1

AMA: Apr 00: 10, Jan 02: 10, Sep 03: 15, May 04: 15, Jul 04: 13, Aug 05: 4, Apr 10: 5, Feb 10: 6, Nov 09: 8, Apr 11: 12, Mar 13: 8

31630 Bronchoscopy, rigid or flexible, including fluoroscopic guidance, when performed; with tracheal/bronchial dilation or closed reduction of fracture `A2 T`

RVU		Global Days	Modifiers				
Mod	Non-Fac Total	Fac Total		51	50	62	80	MUE
	5.78	5.78	000	3	0	0	1	1

AMA: Jan 02: 10, Aug 05: 4, Apr 10: 5, Feb 10: 6, Mar 13: 8

31631 Bronchoscopy, rigid or flexible, including fluoroscopic guidance, when performed; with placement of tracheal stent(s) (includes tracheal/bronchial dilation as required) `A2 T`

RVU		Global Days	Modifiers				
Mod	Non-Fac Total	Fac Total		51	50	62	80	MUE
	6.65	6.65	000	3	0	0	1	1

AMA: Jan 02: 10, Aug 05: 4, Apr 10: 5, Feb 10: 6, Mar 13: 8

⊙✚▲**31632** Bronchoscopy, rigid or flexible, including fluoroscopic guidance, when performed; with transbronchial lung biopsy(s), each additional lobe (List separately in addition to code for primary procedure) `N1 N`

RVU		Global Days	Modifiers				
Mod	Non-Fac Total	Fac Total		51	50	62	80	MUE
	2.13	1.42	ZZZ	0	0	0	1	2

AMA: Jan 02: 10, Sep 04: 9, Aug 05: 4, Mar 13: 8

⊙✚▲ **31633** Bronchoscopy, rigid or flexible, including fluoroscopic guidance, when performed; with transbronchial needle aspiration biopsy(s), each additional lobe (List separately in addition to code for primary procedure) `N1 N`

RVU		Global Days	Modifiers				
Mod	Non-Fac Total	Fac Total		51	50	62	80	MUE
	2.63	1.83	ZZZ	0	0	0	1	2

AMA: Jan 02: 10, May 04: 15, Jul 04: 13, Sep 04: 10, Aug 05: 4, Nov 09: 8, Apr 11: 12, Mar 13: 8

⊙ **31634** Bronchoscopy, rigid or flexible, including fluoroscopic guidance, when performed; with balloon occlusion, with assessment of air leak, with administration of occlusive substance (eg, fibrin glue), if performed `G2 T`

RVU		Global Days	Modifiers				
Mod	Non-Fac Total	Fac Total		51	50	62	80	MUE
	52.94	5.96	000	3	0	0	2	1

AMA: Jan 11: 6, Mar 13: 8

⊙ **31635** Bronchoscopy, rigid or flexible, including fluoroscopic guidance, when performed; with removal of foreign body `A2 T`

RVU		Global Days	Modifiers				
Mod	Non-Fac Total	Fac Total		51	50	62	80	MUE
	9.95	5.45	000	3	0	0	1	1

AMA: Jan 02: 10, Jun 02: 10, Apr 10: 5, Feb 10: 6, Jan 11: 6, Mar 13: 8

31636 Bronchoscopy, rigid or flexible, including fluoroscopic guidance, when performed; with placement of bronchial stent(s) (includes tracheal/bronchial dilation as required), initial bronchus `A2 T`

RVU		Global Days	Modifiers				
Mod	Non-Fac Total	Fac Total		51	50	62	80	MUE
	6.41	6.41	000	3	0	0	1	1

AMA: Aug 05: 4, Apr 10: 5, Mar 13: 8

✚ **31637** Bronchoscopy, rigid or flexible, including fluoroscopic guidance, when performed; each additional major bronchus stented (List separately in addition to code for primary procedure) `N1 N`

RVU		Global Days	Modifiers				
Mod	Non-Fac Total	Fac Total		51	50	62	80	MUE
	2.14	2.14	ZZZ	0	0	0	1	2

AMA: Aug 05: 4, Mar 13: 8

31638 Bronchoscopy, rigid or flexible, including fluoroscopic guidance, when performed; with revision of tracheal or bronchial stent inserted at previous session (includes tracheal/bronchial dilation as required) `A2 T`

RVU		Global Days	Modifiers				
Mod	Non-Fac Total	Fac Total		51	50	62	80	MUE
	7.31	7.31	000	3	0	0	1	1

AMA: Aug 05: 4, Apr 10: 5, Mar 13: 8

31640 Bronchoscopy, rigid or flexible, including fluoroscopic guidance, when performed; with excision of tumor `A2 T`

RVU		Global Days	Modifiers				
Mod	Non-Fac Total	Fac Total		51	50	62	80	MUE
	7.35	7.35	000	3	0	0	1	1

AMA: Jan 02: 10, Aug 05: 4, Apr 10: 5, Mar 13: 8

31641 Bronchoscopy, rigid or flexible, including fluoroscopic guidance, when performed; with destruction of tumor or relief of stenosis by any method other than excision (eg, laser therapy, cryotherapy) `A2 T`

RVU		Global Days	Modifiers				
Mod	Non-Fac Total	Fac Total		51	50	62	80	MUE
	7.45	7.45	000	3	0	0	1	1

AMA: Nov 99: 13, Sep 00: 5, Jan 02: 10, Aug 05: 4, Apr 10: 5, Oct 11: 11, Mar 13: 8, Apr 13: 8

● New   ▲ Revised   ✖ Deleted   ⊙ Moderate Sedation   ✚ Add-on Codes   ⊘ High Risk Denial   Ⓐ Age Edit   ♀ Female   ♂ Male   **AMA** *CPT® Assistant*   **MUE** Medically Unlikely Edit
⊘ Modifier 51 Exempt   ⊖ Modifier 63 Exempt   ✗ Unlisted   **Modifiers:** *See Inside Back Cover*   Ⓜ Maternity   `A2`–`Z3` ASC Payment Indicators   `A`–`Y` OPPS Status Indicators

31643 **Bronchoscopy, rigid or flexible, including fluoroscopic guidance, when performed; with placement of catheter(s) for intracavitary radioelement application** `A2T`

RVU			Global Days	Modifiers				
Mod	Non-Fac Total	Fac Total		51	50	62	80	MUE
	5.10	5.10	000	2	0	0	1	1

AMA: Nov 98: 12, Mar 99: 3, Jan 02: 10, Aug 05: 4, Apr 09: 3, Mar 13: 8

⊙ 31645 **Bronchoscopy, rigid or flexible, including fluoroscopic guidance, when performed; with therapeutic aspiration of tracheobronchial tree, initial (eg, drainage of lung abscess)** `A2T`

RVU			Global Days	Modifiers				
Mod	Non-Fac Total	Fac Total		51	50	62	80	MUE
	9.21	4.65	000	3	0	0	1	1

AMA: Jan 02: 10, Aug 05: 4, Mar 13: 8

⊙ 31646 **Bronchoscopy, rigid or flexible, including fluoroscopic guidance, when performed; with therapeutic aspiration of tracheobronchial tree, subsequent** `A2T`

RVU			Global Days	Modifiers				
Mod	Non-Fac Total	Fac Total		51	50	62	80	MUE
	8.27	4.02	000	2	0	0	1	2

AMA: Jan 02: 10, Aug 05: 4, Mar 13: 8

⊙ 31647 **Bronchoscopy, rigid or flexible, including fluoroscopic guidance, when performed; with balloon occlusion, when performed, assessment of air leak, airway sizing, and insertion of bronchial valve(s), initial lobe** `G2T`

RVU			Global Days	Modifiers				
Mod	Non-Fac Total	Fac Total		51	50	62	80	MUE
	6.39	6.39	000	3	0	0	1	1

AMA: Mar 13: 8

⊙ 31648 **Bronchoscopy, rigid or flexible, including fluoroscopic guidance, when performed; with removal of bronchial valve(s), initial lobe** `G2T`

RVU			Global Days	Modifiers				
Mod	Non-Fac Total	Fac Total		51	50	62	80	MUE
	5.91	5.91	000	3	0	0	1	1

AMA: Mar 13: 8

⊙✚31649 **Bronchoscopy, rigid or flexible, including fluoroscopic guidance, when performed; with removal of bronchial valve(s), each additional lobe (List separately in addition to code for primary procedure)** `G2Q2`

RVU			Global Days	Modifiers				
Mod	Non-Fac Total	Fac Total		51	50	62	80	MUE
	2.01	2.01	ZZZ	0	0	0	1	2

AMA: Mar 13: 8

⊙✚31651 **Bronchoscopy, rigid or flexible, including fluoroscopic guidance, when performed; with balloon occlusion, when performed, assessment of air leak, airway sizing, and insertion of bronchial valve(s), each additional lobe (List separately in addition to code for primary procedure[s])** `NIN`

RVU			Global Days	Modifiers				
Mod	Non-Fac Total	Fac Total		51	50	62	80	MUE
	2.29	2.29	ZZZ	0	0	0	1	3

AMA: Mar 13: 8

⊙● 31652 **Bronchoscopy, rigid or flexible, including fluoroscopic guidance, when performed; with endobronchial ultrasound (EBUS) guided transtracheal and/or transbronchial sampling (eg, aspiration[s]/biopsy[ies]), one or two mediastinal and/or hilar lymph node stations or structures** `G2T`

RVU			Global Days	Modifiers				
Mod	Non-Fac Total	Fac Total		51	50	62	80	MUE
	25.70	6.75	000	2	0	0	1	1

⊙● 31653 **Bronchoscopy, rigid or flexible, including fluoroscopic guidance, when performed; with endobronchial ultrasound (EBUS) guided transtracheal and/or transbronchial sampling (eg, aspiration[s]/biopsy[ies]), 3 or more mediastinal and/or hilar lymph node stations or structures** `G2T`

RVU			Global Days	Modifiers				
Mod	Non-Fac Total	Fac Total		51	50	62	80	MUE
	27.31	7.45	000	2	0	0	1	1

⊙✚● 31654 **Bronchoscopy, rigid or flexible, including fluoroscopic guidance, when performed; with transendoscopic endobronchial ultrasound (EBUS) during bronchoscopic diagnostic or therapeutic intervention(s) for peripheral lesion(s) (List separately in addition to code for primary procedure[s])** `NIN`

RVU			Global Days	Modifiers				
Mod	Non-Fac Total	Fac Total		51	50	62	80	MUE
	3.09	1.95	ZZZ	0	0	0	1	1

Thermoplasty

⊙ 31660 **Bronchoscopy, rigid or flexible, including fluoroscopic guidance, when performed; with bronchial thermoplasty, 1 lobe** `T`

RVU			Global Days	Modifiers				
Mod	Non-Fac Total	Fac Total		51	50	62	80	MUE
	6.05	6.05	000	3	0	0	1	1

AMA: Mar 13: 8

● New   ▲ Revised   Deleted   ⊙ Moderate Sedation   ✚ Add-on Codes   ⊘ High Risk Denial   Ⓐ Age Edit   ♀ Female   ♂ Male   **AMA** CPT® Assistant   **MUE** Medically Unlikely Edit
⊘ Modifier 51 Exempt   ⊖ Modifier 63 Exempt   ✗ Unlisted   **Modifiers:** See Inside Back Cover   Ⓜ Maternity   A2–Z3 ASC Payment Indicators   A–Y OPPS Status Indicators

⊙ **31661 Bronchoscopy, rigid or flexible, including fluoroscopic guidance, when performed; with bronchial thermoplasty, 2 or more lobes** T

RVU Mod	Non-Fac Total	Fac Total	Global Days	Modifiers 51	50	62	80	MUE
	6.34	6.34	000	3	0	0	1	1

AMA: Mar 13: 8

31717 Catheterization with bronchial brush biopsy A2 T

RVU Mod	Non-Fac Total	Fac Total	Global Days	Modifiers 51	50	62	80	MUE
	7.41	3.12	000	2	0	0	1	1

AMA: Feb 01: 11

Catheterization with bronchial brush biopsy

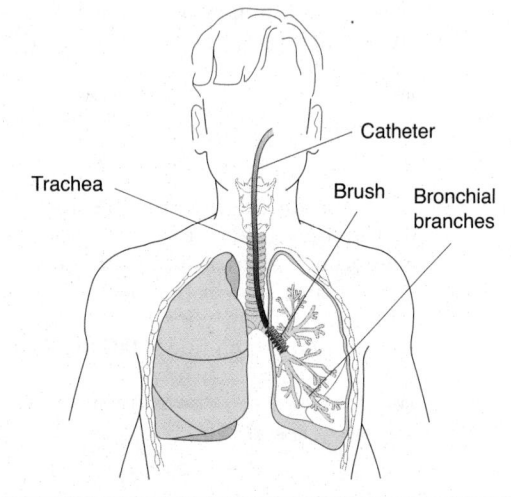

31720 Catheter aspiration (separate procedure); nasotracheal ⊘ N I Q1

Coding tip: Tracheobronchial therapeutic aspiration - 31645-31646

RVU Mod	Non-Fac Total	Fac Total	Global Days	Modifiers 51	50	62	80	MUE
	1.48	1.48	000	2	0	0	1	1

⊙ **31725 Catheter aspiration (separate procedure); tracheobronchial with fiberscope, bedside** C

Coding tip: Tracheobronchial therapeutic aspiration - 31645-31646

RVU Mod	Non-Fac Total	Fac Total	Global Days	Modifiers 51	50	62	80	MUE
	2.60	2.60	000	2	0	0	1	1

31730 Transtracheal (percutaneous) introduction of needle wire dilator/stent or indwelling tube for oxygen therapy A2 T

Coding tip: Tracheostomy procedures - 31600-31610

RVU Mod	Non-Fac Total	Fac Total	Global Days	Modifiers 51	50	62	80	MUE
	35.33	4.30	000	2	0	0	1	1

Tracheal/Bronchial Excisional/Repair Procedures

31750 Tracheoplasty; cervical A2 J1

RVU Mod	Non-Fac Total	Fac Total	Global Days	Modifiers 51	50	62	80	MUE
	40.78	40.78	090	2	0	1	2	1

AMA: Jul 11: 12

31755 Tracheoplasty; tracheopharyngeal fistulization, each stage A2 J1

RVU Mod	Non-Fac Total	Fac Total	Global Days	Modifiers 51	50	62	80	MUE
	51.00	51.00	090	2	0	1	2	1

Tracheopharyngeal fistulization

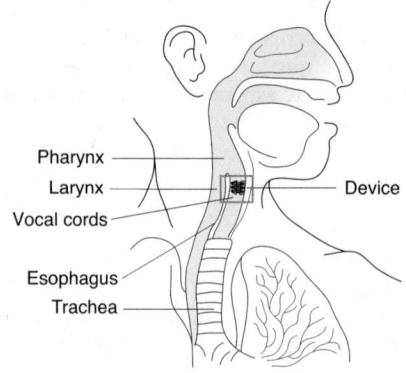

A passage is created between the trachea and pharynx to allow speech in a laryngectomy patient. A prosthetic speech device may be inserted.

31760 Tracheoplasty; intrathoracic C

RVU Mod	Non-Fac Total	Fac Total	Global Days	Modifiers 51	50	62	80	MUE
	40.62	40.62	090	2	0	1	2	1

31766 Carinal reconstruction C

RVU Mod	Non-Fac Total	Fac Total	Global Days	Modifiers 51	50	62	80	MUE
	52.12	52.12	090	2	0	1	2	1

31770 Bronchoplasty; graft repair C

RVU Mod	Non-Fac Total	Fac Total	Global Days	Modifiers 51	50	62	80	MUE
	39.12	39.12	090	2	0	1	2	2

31775 Bronchoplasty; excision stenosis and anastomosis C

RVU Mod	Non-Fac Total	Fac Total	Global Days	Modifiers 51	50	62	80	MUE
	37.40	37.40	090	2	0	0	2	1

31780 Excision tracheal stenosis and anastomosis; cervical C

RVU Mod	Non-Fac Total	Fac Total	Global Days	Modifiers 51	50	62	80	MUE
	34.26	34.26	090	2	0	1	2	1

31781 Excision tracheal stenosis and anastomosis; cervicothoracic C

RVU Mod	Non-Fac Total	Fac Total	Global Days	Modifiers 51	50	62	80	MUE
	41.95	41.95	090	2	0	1	2	1

31785 Excision of tracheal tumor or carcinoma; cervical T

RVU Mod	Non-Fac Total	Fac Total	Global Days	Modifiers 51	50	62	80	MUE
	31.50	31.50	090	2	0	1	2	1

● New   ▲ Revised   ✖ Deleted   ⊙ Moderate Sedation   ✚ Add-on Codes   ⊘ High Risk Denial   Ⓐ Age Edit   ♀ Female   ♂ Male   **AMA** CPT® Assistant   **MUE** Medically Unlikely Edit   ⊘ Modifier 51 Exempt   ⊖ Modifier 63 Exempt   ✖ Unlisted   **Modifiers:** See Inside Back Cover   Ⓜ Maternity   A2-Z3 ASC Payment Indicators   A-Y OPPS Status Indicators

31786 Excision of tracheal tumor or carcinoma; thoracic C

Mod	RVU Non-Fac Total	Fac Total	Global Days	Modifiers 51	50	62	80	MUE
	42.01	42.01	090	2	0	1	2	1

31800 Suture of tracheal wound or injury; cervical C

Mod	RVU Non-Fac Total	Fac Total	Global Days	Modifiers 51	50	62	80	MUE
	21.24	21.24	090	2	0	0	0	1

31805 Suture of tracheal wound or injury; intrathoracic C

Mod	RVU Non-Fac Total	Fac Total	Global Days	Modifiers 51	50	62	80	MUE
	24.07	24.07	090	2	0	1	2	1

31820 Surgical closure tracheostomy or fistula; without plastic repair A2 T

Mod	RVU Non-Fac Total	Fac Total	Global Days	Modifiers 51	50	62	80	MUE
	12.49	9.48	090	2	0	0	0	1

31825 Surgical closure tracheostomy or fistula; with plastic repair A2 T

Mod	RVU Non-Fac Total	Fac Total	Global Days	Modifiers 51	50	62	80	MUE
	17.28	13.85	090	2	0	0	0	1

31830 Revision of tracheostomy scar A2 T

Mod	RVU Non-Fac Total	Fac Total	Global Days	Modifiers 51	50	62	80	MUE
	12.77	9.93	090	2	0	0	0	1

Other Tracheal/Bronchial Procedures

31899 Unlisted procedure, trachea, bronchi X T

Mod	RVU Non-Fac Total	Fac Total	Global Days	Modifiers 51	50	62	80	MUE
	0.00	0.00	YYY	2	0	1	0	

AMA: Jan 10: 11, May 14: 10

Lung/Pleural Procedures

Incisional Lung/Pleural Procedures

32035 Thoracostomy; with rib resection for empyema C

Mod	RVU Non-Fac Total	Fac Total	Global Days	Modifiers 51	50	62	80	MUE
	20.91	20.91	090	2	1	1	2	1

32036 Thoracostomy; with open flap drainage for empyema C

Mod	RVU Non-Fac Total	Fac Total	Global Days	Modifiers 51	50	62	80	MUE
	22.56	22.56	090	2	1	1	2	1

32096 Thoracotomy, with diagnostic biopsy(ies) of lung infiltrate(s) (eg, wedge, incisional), unilateral C

Coding tip: For thoracoscopic lung biopsy(ies) - 32607-32608
Coding tip: For a diagnostic open wedge resection followed by an anatomic lung resection - 32507
Coding tip: This procedure is only reported for a wedge biopsy. For a thoracotomy with a therapeutic wedge resection - 32505-32506

Mod	RVU Non-Fac Total	Fac Total	Global Days	Modifiers 51	50	62	80	MUE
	23.48	23.48	090	2	0	1	2	1

AMA: Sep 12: 3

32097 Thoracotomy, with diagnostic biopsy(ies) of lung nodule(s) or mass(es) (eg, wedge, incisional), unilateral C

Coding tip: For thoracoscopic lung biopsy(ies) - 32607-32608
Coding tip: For a diagnostic open wedge resection followed by an anatomic lung resection - 32507
Coding tip: This procedure is only reported for a wedge biopsy. For a thoracotomy with a therapeutic wedge resection - 32505-32506

Mod	RVU Non-Fac Total	Fac Total	Global Days	Modifiers 51	50	62	80	MUE
	23.44	23.44	090	2	0	1	2	1

AMA: Sep 12: 3

32098 Thoracotomy, with biopsy(ies) of pleura C

Coding tip: For thoracoscopic biopsy(ies) of the pleura - 32609

Mod	RVU Non-Fac Total	Fac Total	Global Days	Modifiers 51	50	62	80	MUE
	22.25	22.25	090	2	0	1	2	1

AMA: Sep 12: 3

32100 Thoracotomy; with exploration C

Mod	RVU Non-Fac Total	Fac Total	Global Days	Modifiers 51	50	62	80	MUE
	23.55	23.55	090	2	0	1	2	1

AMA: Mar 07: 1, Sep 12: 3, Jan 13: 6

32110 Thoracotomy; with control of traumatic hemorrhage and/or repair of lung tear C

Mod	RVU Non-Fac Total	Fac Total	Global Days	Modifiers 51	50	62	80	MUE
	42.53	42.53	090	2	0	1	2	1

AMA: Sep 12: 3

32120 Thoracotomy; for postoperative complications C

Mod	RVU Non-Fac Total	Fac Total	Global Days	Modifiers 51	50	62	80	MUE
	25.35	25.35	090	2	0	1	2	1

32124 Thoracotomy; with open intrapleural pneumonolysis C

Mod	RVU Non-Fac Total	Fac Total	Global Days	Modifiers 51	50	62	80	MUE
	26.91	26.91	090	2	0	1	2	1

AMA: Sep 12: 3

32140 Thoracotomy; with cyst(s) removal, includes pleural procedure when performed C

Mod	RVU Non-Fac Total	Fac Total	Global Days	Modifiers 51	50	62	80	MUE
	29.10	29.10	090	2	0	1	2	1

AMA: Sep 12: 3

Surgical Procedures

31786 – 32140

32141 Thoracotomy; with resection-plication of bullae, includes any pleural procedure when performed ⓒ

RVU			Global Days	Modifiers				
Mod	Non-Fac Total	Fac Total		51	50	62	80	MUE
	44.48	44.48	090	2	0	1	2	1

AMA: Sep 12: 3

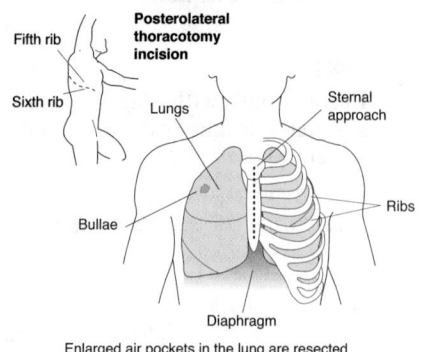

Thoracotomy; with resection-plication of bullae

Fifth rib

Posterolateral thoracotomy incision

Sixth rib

Lungs

Sternal approach

Bullae

Ribs

Diaphragm

Enlarged air pockets in the lung are resected and stapled, and the lung is reinflated

32150 Thoracotomy; with removal of intrapleural foreign body or fibrin deposit ⓒ

RVU			Global Days	Modifiers				
Mod	Non-Fac Total	Fac Total		51	50	62	80	MUE
	29.28	29.28	090	2	0	1	2	1

AMA: Sep 12: 3

32151 Thoracotomy; with removal of intrapulmonary foreign body ⓒ

RVU			Global Days	Modifiers				
Mod	Non-Fac Total	Fac Total		51	50	62	80	MUE
	29.28	29.28	090	2	0	1	2	1

32160 Thoracotomy; with cardiac massage ⓒ

RVU			Global Days	Modifiers				
Mod	Non-Fac Total	Fac Total		51	50	62	80	MUE
	22.99	22.99	090	2	0	1	2	1

32200 Pneumonostomy, with open drainage of abscess or cyst ⓒ

RVU			Global Days	Modifiers				
Mod	Non-Fac Total	Fac Total		51	50	62	80	MUE
	33.05	33.05	090	2	0	1	2	2

AMA: Nov 97: 15

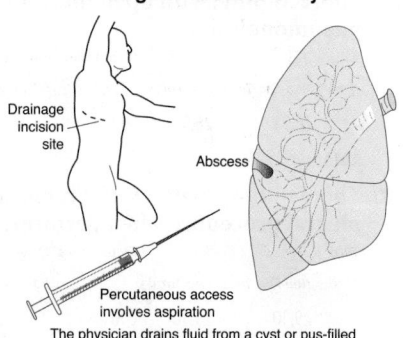

Pneumonostomy; with open drainage of abscess or cyst

Drainage incision site

Abscess

Percutaneous access involves aspiration

The physician drains fluid from a cyst or pus-filled sac (abscess) within the lung tissue through an open incision made in the chest wall over the site.

32215 Pleural scarification for repeat pneumothorax ⓒ

RVU			Global Days	Modifiers				
Mod	Non-Fac Total	Fac Total		51	50	62	80	MUE
	23.13	23.13	090	2	1	1	2	1

32220 Decortication, pulmonary (separate procedure); total ⓒ

RVU			Global Days	Modifiers				
Mod	Non-Fac Total	Fac Total		51	50	62	80	MUE
	46.06	46.06	090	2	1	1	2	1

32225 Decortication, pulmonary (separate procedure); partial ⓒ

RVU			Global Days	Modifiers				
Mod	Non-Fac Total	Fac Total		51	50	62	80	MUE
	28.92	28.92	090	2	1	1	2	1

Excisional Lung/Pleural Procedures

32310 Pleurectomy, parietal (separate procedure) ⓒ

RVU			Global Days	Modifiers				
Mod	Non-Fac Total	Fac Total		51	50	62	80	MUE
	26.40	26.40	090	2	0	1	2	1

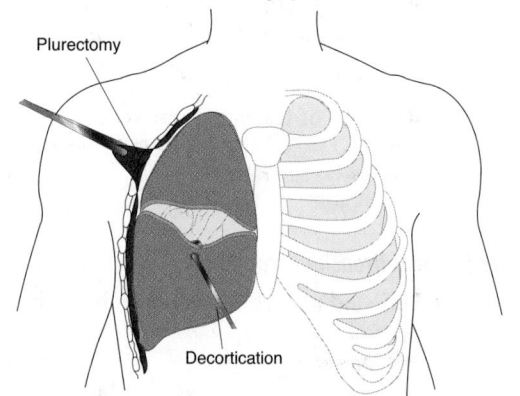

Pleurectomy, parietal

Plurectomy

Decortication

The parietal pleura only is removed (32310), or along with the fibrin layer around the lungs (decortication) (32320)

32320 Decortication and parietal pleurectomy ⓒ

RVU			Global Days	Modifiers				
Mod	Non-Fac Total	Fac Total		51	50	62	80	MUE
	46.52	46.52	090	2	0	1	2	1

32400 Biopsy, pleura, percutaneous needle   A2T

Coding tip: Report an additional code for radiological needle guidance - ultrasound 76942, fluoroscopy 77002, CT 77012, MRI 77021

RVU			Global Days	Modifiers				
Mod	Non-Fac Total	Fac Total		51	50	62	80	MUE
	4.30	2.52	000	2	0	0	1	2

AMA: Fall 94: 1, 2

⊙ 32405 Biopsy, lung or mediastinum, percutaneous needle   A2T

Coding tip: Report an additional code for radiological needle guidance - ultrasound 76942, fluoroscopy 77002, CT 77012, MRI 77021

RVU			Global Days	Modifiers				
Mod	Non-Fac Total	Fac Total		51	50	62	80	MUE
	12.77	3.00	000	2	0	0	1	2

AMA: Fall 94: 1, 2, Mar 97: 4, Aug 02: 10

● New   ▲ Revised   ✖ Deleted   ⊙ Moderate Sedation   ✚ Add-on Codes   ⊘ High Risk Denial   Ⓐ Age Edit   ♀ Female   ♂ Male   **AMA** *CPT® Assistant*   **MUE** Medically Unlikely Edit

⊘ Modifier 51 Exempt   ⊖ Modifier 63 Exempt   ✖ Unlisted   **Modifiers:** *See Inside Back Cover*   Ⓜ Maternity   A2–Z3 ASC Payment Indicators   A–Y OPPS Status Indicators

CPT © 2015 American Medical Association. All Rights Reserved.   © 2016 DecisionHealth

32440 Removal of lung, pneumonectomy [C]

RVU			Global Days	Modifiers				
Mod	Non-Fac Total	Fac Total		51	50	62	80	MUE
	45.61	45.61	090	2	0	1	2	1

AMA: Fall 94: 1, Sep 12: 3

32442 Removal of lung, pneumonectomy; with resection of segment of trachea followed by broncho-tracheal anastomosis (sleeve pneumonectomy) [C]

RVU			Global Days	Modifiers				
Mod	Non-Fac Total	Fac Total		51	50	62	80	MUE
	93.31	93.31	090	2	0	1	2	1

AMA: Fall 94: 1, 3

32445 Removal of lung, pneumonectomy; extrapleural [C]

RVU			Global Days	Modifiers				
Mod	Non-Fac Total	Fac Total		51	50	62	80	MUE
	103.54	103.54	090	2	0	1	2	1

AMA: Fall 94: 1, 3, Sep 12: 3

32480 Removal of lung, other than pneumonectomy; single lobe (lobectomy) [C]

RVU			Global Days	Modifiers				
Mod	Non-Fac Total	Fac Total		51	50	62	80	MUE
	43.01	43.01	090	2	0	1	2	1

AMA: Spring 91: 5, Fall 94: 1, 4, Sep 12: 3

32482 Removal of lung, other than pneumonectomy; 2 lobes (bilobectomy) [C]

RVU			Global Days	Modifiers				
Mod	Non-Fac Total	Fac Total		51	50	62	80	MUE
	46.02	46.02	090	2	0	1	2	1

AMA: Fall 94: 1, 4, Jan 07: 31, Sep 12: 3

32484 Removal of lung, other than pneumonectomy; single segment (segmentectomy) [C]

RVU			Global Days	Modifiers				
Mod	Non-Fac Total	Fac Total		51	50	62	80	MUE
	41.88	41.88	090	2	0	1	2	2

AMA: Fall 94: 1, 4, Sep 12: 3

Removal of lung, other than pneumonectomy

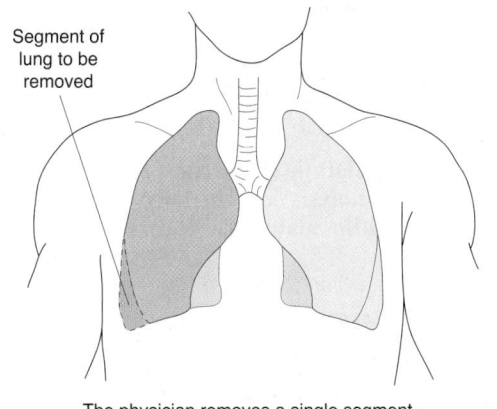

Segment of lung to be removed

The physician removes a single segment from a diseased or damaged lung

32486 Removal of lung, other than pneumonectomy; with circumferential resection of segment of bronchus followed by broncho-bronchial anastomosis (sleeve lobectomy) [C]

RVU			Global Days	Modifiers				
Mod	Non-Fac Total	Fac Total		51	50	62	80	MUE
	68.58	68.58	090	2	0	1	2	1

AMA: Fall 94: 1, 4

32488 Removal of lung, other than pneumonectomy; with all remaining lung following previous removal of a portion of lung (completion pneumonectomy) [C]

RVU			Global Days	Modifiers				
Mod	Non-Fac Total	Fac Total		51	50	62	80	MUE
	69.75	69.75	090	2	0	1	2	1

AMA: Fall 94: 1, 4, Sep 12: 3

32491 Removal of lung, other than pneumonectomy; with resection-plication of emphysematous lung(s) (bullous or non-bullous) for lung volume reduction, sternal split or transthoracic approach, includes any pleural procedure, when performed [C]

RVU			Global Days	Modifiers				
Mod	Non-Fac Total	Fac Total		51	50	62	80	MUE
	43.04	43.04	090	2	1	1	2	1

AMA: Nov 96: 7, Sep 12: 3

+ 32501 Resection and repair of portion of bronchus (bronchoplasty) when performed at time of lobectomy or segmentectomy (List separately in addition to code for primary procedure) [C]

RVU			Global Days	Modifiers				
Mod	Non-Fac Total	Fac Total		51	50	62	80	MUE
	7.11	7.11	ZZZ	0	0	1	2	1

32503 Resection of apical lung tumor (eg, Pancoast tumor), including chest wall resection, rib(s) resection(s), neurovascular dissection, when performed; without chest wall reconstruction(s) [C]

RVU			Global Days	Modifiers				
Mod	Non-Fac Total	Fac Total		51	50	62	80	MUE
	52.57	52.57	090	2	0	1	2	1

32504 Resection of apical lung tumor (eg, Pancoast tumor), including chest wall resection, rib(s) resection(s), neurovascular dissection, when performed; with chest wall reconstruction [C]

RVU			Global Days	Modifiers				
Mod	Non-Fac Total	Fac Total		51	50	62	80	MUE
	60.14	60.14	090	2	0	1	2	1

32505 Thoracotomy; with therapeutic wedge resection (eg, mass, nodule), initial [C]

Coding tip: If only an open wedge biopsy is performed without therapeutic treatment - 32096-32097

Coding tip: For thoracoscopic therapeutic wedge resection - 32607-32608

RVU			Global Days	Modifiers				
Mod	Non-Fac Total	Fac Total		51	50	62	80	MUE
	27.15	27.15	090	2	0	1	2	1

AMA: Sep 12: 3

● New   ▲ Revised   Deleted   ⊙ Moderate Sedation   ✚ Add-on Codes   ⊘ High Risk Denial   Ⓐ Age Edit   ♀ Female   ♂ Male   **AMA** *CPT® Assistant*   **MUE** Medically Unlikely Edit
⊘ Modifier 51 Exempt   ⊖ Modifier 63 Exempt   ✗ Unlisted   **Modifiers:** *See Inside Back Cover*   Ⓜ Maternity   A2–Z3 ASC Payment Indicators   A–Y OPPS Status Indicators

Surgical Procedures

32506 – 32562

+ **32506 Thoracotomy; with therapeutic wedge resection (eg, mass or nodule), each additional resection, ipsilateral (List separately in addition to code for primary procedure)**   C

Coding tip: For thoracoscopic therapeutic wedge resection - 32607-32608

Coding tip: If only an open wedge biopsy is performed without therapeutic treatment - 32096-32097

RVU			Global Days	Modifiers				
Mod	Non-Fac Total	Fac Total		51	50	62	80	MUE
	4.53	4.53	ZZZ	0	0	1	2	3

AMA: Sep 12: 3·

+ **32507 Thoracotomy; with diagnostic wedge resection followed by anatomic lung resection (List separately in addition to code for primary procedure)**   C

Coding tip: For thoracoscopic diagnostic wedge resection with anatomic lung resection - 32668

RVU			Global Days	Modifiers				
Mod	Non-Fac Total	Fac Total		51	50	62	80	MUE
	4.49	4.49	ZZZ	0	0	1	2	2

AMA: Sep 12: 3

32540 Extrapleural enucleation of empyema (empyemectomy)   C

RVU			Global Days	Modifiers				
Mod	Non-Fac Total	Fac Total		51	50	62	80	MUE
	50.66	50.66	090	2	0	1	2	1

Lung/Pleural Introduction Procedures

⊙ **32550 Insertion of indwelling tunneled pleural catheter with cuff**   G2T

Coding tip: If radiological guidance is performed - 75989

RVU			Global Days	Modifiers				
Mod	Non-Fac Total	Fac Total		51	50	62	80	MUE
	22.27	6.44	000	0	0	0	1	2

AMA: Jul 10: 10, Mar 14: 14, May 14: 3

⊙ **32551 Tube thoracostomy, includes connection to drainage system (eg, water seal), when performed, open (separate procedure)**   T

Coding tip: If radiological guidance is performed - 75989

RVU			Global Days	Modifiers				
Mod	Non-Fac Total	Fac Total		51	50	62	80	MUE
	4.91	4.91	000	2	1	0	1	2

AMA: Aug 11: 4, Sep 10: 6, Feb 09: 7, Nov 12: 3, May 14: 3

32552 Removal of indwelling tunneled pleural catheter with cuff   G2Q2

RVU			Global Days	Modifiers				
Mod	Non-Fac Total	Fac Total		51	50	62	80	MUE
	5.31	4.61	010	2	0	0	0	2

AMA: Feb 10: 6

⊙ **32553 Placement of interstitial device(s) for radiation therapy guidance (eg, fiducial markers, dosimeter), percutaneous, intra-thoracic, single or multiple**   G2S

Coding tip: Report an additional code for radiological guidance in placing the interstitial devices - ultrasound 76942; fluoroscopy 77002; CT 77012; MRI 77021

RVU			Global Days	Modifiers				
Mod	Non-Fac Total	Fac Total		51	50	62	80	MUE
	16.80	5.61	000	2	0	0	2	1

AMA: Feb 10: 6, 7, Jun 15: 6

32554 Thoracentesis, needle or catheter, aspiration of the pleural space; without imaging guidance   G2T

RVU			Global Days	Modifiers				
Mod	Non-Fac Total	Fac Total		51	50	62	80	MUE
	5.69	2.59	000	2	1	0	1	2

AMA: Nov 12: 3, May 14: 3

32555 Thoracentesis, needle or catheter, aspiration of the pleural space; with imaging guidance   G2T

RVU			Global Days	Modifiers				
Mod	Non-Fac Total	Fac Total		51	50	62	80	MUE
	8.23	3.25	000	2	1	0	1	2

AMA: Nov 12: 3

32556 Pleural drainage, percutaneous, with insertion of indwelling catheter; without imaging guidance   G2T

RVU			Global Days	Modifiers				
Mod	Non-Fac Total	Fac Total		51	50	62	80	MUE
	15.34	3.57	000	2	1	0	1	2

32557 Pleural drainage, percutaneous, with insertion of indwelling catheter; with imaging guidance   G2T

RVU			Global Days	Modifiers				
Mod	Non-Fac Total	Fac Total		51	50	62	80	MUE
	14.65	4.44	000	2	1	0	1	2

AMA: Nov 12: 3, May 14: 3

Lung/Pleural Destruction Procedures

32560 Instillation, via chest tube/catheter, agent for pleurodesis (eg, talc for recurrent or persistent pneumothorax)   T

RVU			Global Days	Modifiers				
Mod	Non-Fac Total	Fac Total		51	50	62	80	MUE
	6.95	2.25	000	2	0	0	1	1

AMA: Feb 10: 6

32561 Instillation(s), via chest tube/catheter, agent for fibrinolysis (eg, fibrinolytic agent for break up of multiloculated effusion); initial day   T

RVU			Global Days	Modifiers				
Mod	Non-Fac Total	Fac Total		51	50	62	80	MUE
	2.65	1.98	000	2	0	0	2	1

AMA: Feb 10: 6

32562 Instillation(s), via chest tube/catheter, agent for fibrinolysis (eg, fibrinolytic agent for break up of multiloculated effusion); subsequent day   T

RVU			Global Days	Modifiers				
Mod	Non-Fac Total	Fac Total		51	50	62	80	MUE
	2.39	1.79	000	2	0	0	2	1

AMA: Feb 10: 6

● New   ▲ Revised   ✖ Deleted   ⊙ Moderate Sedation   ✚ Add-on Codes   ⊘ High Risk Denial   Ⓐ Age Edit   ♀ Female   ♂ Male   **AMA** *CPT® Assistant*   **MUE** Medically Unlikely Edit
⊘ Modifier 51 Exempt   ⊖ Modifier 63 Exempt   🗷 Unlisted   **Modifiers:** *See Inside Back Cover*   Ⓜ Maternity   A2–Z3 ASC Payment Indicators   A–Y OPPS Status Indicators

CPT © 2015 American Medical Association. All Rights Reserved.   © 2016 DecisionHealth

Endoscopic Lung/Pleural Procedures

Coding Guidance

When a diagnostic thoracoscopy is done to determine that a non-endoscopic, surgical procedure is necessary, the diagnostic procedure may be reported separately as a distinct, diagnostic service. Modifier 58 may be used to note that the surgical procedure deemed necessary as a result of the diagnostic endoscopy, and the diagnostic endoscopy itself are planned or staged procedures. When an open surgical procedure is accompanied by a diagnostic endoscopy to evaluate the patient's respiratory system anatomy or determine surgical efficacy, the endoscopy is not reported.

32601   **Thoracoscopy, diagnostic (separate procedure); lungs, pericardial sac, mediastinal or pleural space, without biopsy**   🅣

RVU		Global Days	Modifiers				
Mod	Non-Fac Total	Fac Total		51	50	62	80	MUE
	9.01	9.01	000	2	0	0	0	1

AMA: Fall 94: 1, 4, Sep 12: 3, Aug 13: 14

Thoracoscopy, diagnostic

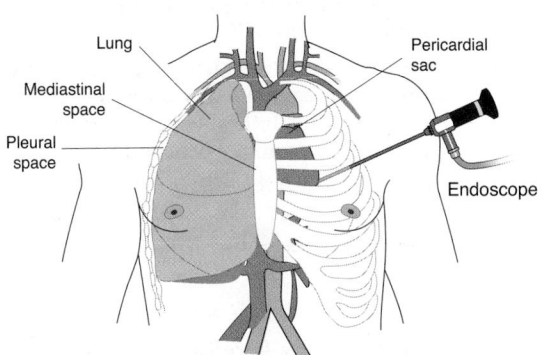

A thoracoscopy is performed to visualize the lungs, pericardial sac, mediastinal or pleural space, without biopsy

32604   **Thoracoscopy, diagnostic (separate procedure); pericardial sac, with biopsy**   🅣

RVU		Global Days	Modifiers				
Mod	Non-Fac Total	Fac Total		51	50	62	80	MUE
	14.09	14.09	000	2	0	0	0	1

AMA: Fall 94: 1, 4, Aug 13: 14

32606   **Thoracoscopy, diagnostic (separate procedure); mediastinal space, with biopsy**   🅣

RVU		Global Days	Modifiers				
Mod	Non-Fac Total	Fac Total		51	50	62	80	MUE
	13.50	13.50	000	2	0	0	0	1

AMA: Fall 94: 1, 5, Aug 13: 14

32607   **Thoracoscopy; with diagnostic biopsy(ies) of lung infiltrate(s) (eg, wedge, incisional), unilateral**   🅣

Coding tip: For open biopsy(ies) of lung - 32096-32097

RVU		Global Days	Modifiers				
Mod	Non-Fac Total	Fac Total		51	50	62	80	MUE
	9.03	9.03	000	2	0	0	0	1

AMA: Sep 12: 3, Aug 13: 14

32608   **Thoracoscopy; with diagnostic biopsy(ies) of lung nodule(s) or mass(es) (eg, wedge, incisional), unilateral**   🅣

Coding tip: For open biopsy(ies) of lung - 32096-32097

RVU		Global Days	Modifiers				
Mod	Non-Fac Total	Fac Total		51	50	62	80	MUE
	11.06	11.06	000	2	0	0	0	1

AMA: Sep 12: 3, Aug 13: 14

32609   **Thoracoscopy; with biopsy(ies) of pleura**   🅣

Coding tip: For open biopsy(ies) of the pleura - 32098

RVU		Global Days	Modifiers				
Mod	Non-Fac Total	Fac Total		51	50	62	80	MUE
	7.57	7.57	000	2	0	0	0	1

AMA: Sep 12: 3, Aug 13: 14

Coding Guidance

An open thoracotomy includes a surgical thoracoscopy when done at the same session. If the decision to perform an open thoracostomy depends on the initial diagnosis from a diagnostic thoracoscopy, then both procedures may be reported with the appropriate modifier showing them to be staged or planned procedures.

32650   **Thoracoscopy, surgical; with pleurodesis (eg, mechanical or chemical)**   🅒

RVU		Global Days	Modifiers				
Mod	Non-Fac Total	Fac Total		51	50	62	80	MUE
	19.36	19.36	090	2	1	1	2	1

AMA: Fall 94: 1, 6, Aug 13: 14

Surgical thoracoscopy; with pleurodesis

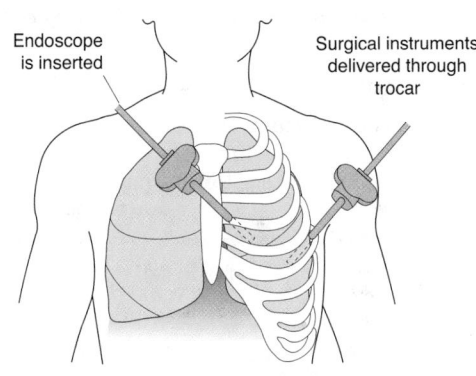

Video assisted thoracoscopic surgery is done to induce mechanical or chemical scarring and adherence of the pleurae

32651   **Thoracoscopy, surgical; with partial pulmonary decortication**   🅒

RVU		Global Days	Modifiers				
Mod	Non-Fac Total	Fac Total		51	50	62	80	MUE
	31.98	31.98	090	2	1	1	2	1

AMA: Fall 94: 1, 6, Aug 13: 14

32652   **Thoracoscopy, surgical; with total pulmonary decortication, including intrapleural pneumonolysis**   🅒

RVU		Global Days	Modifiers				
Mod	Non-Fac Total	Fac Total		51	50	62	80	MUE
	48.44	48.44	090	2	1	1	2	1

AMA: Fall 94: 1, 6, Aug 13: 14

● New   ▲ Revised   Deleted   ⊙ Moderate Sedation   ✚ Add-on Codes   ⊘ High Risk Denial   Ⓐ Age Edit   ♀ Female   ♂ Male   **AMA** *CPT® Assistant*   **MUE** Medically Unlikely Edit
⊘ Modifier 51 Exempt   ⊖ Modifier 63 Exempt   ☒ Unlisted   **Modifiers:** *See Inside Back Cover*   Ⓜ Maternity   🄰🄰2–🅉3 ASC Payment Indicators   🄰–🅈 OPPS Status Indicators

© 2016 DecisionHealth   CPT © 2015 American Medical Association. All Rights Reserved.

Surgical Procedures

32653 – 32671

32653 Thoracoscopy, surgical; with removal of intrapleural foreign body or fibrin deposit   [C]

RVU			Global Days	Modifiers				
Mod	Non-Fac Total	Fac Total		51	50	62	80	MUE
	30.87	30.87	090	2	0	1	2	1

AMA: Fall 94: 1, 6, Aug 13: 14

32654 Thoracoscopy, surgical; with control of traumatic hemorrhage   [C]

RVU			Global Days	Modifiers				
Mod	Non-Fac Total	Fac Total		51	50	62	80	MUE
	34.34	34.34	090	2	1	1	2	1

AMA: Fall 94: 1, 6, Aug 13: 14

32655 Thoracoscopy, surgical; with resection-plication of bullae, includes any pleural procedure when performed   [C]

RVU			Global Days	Modifiers				
Mod	Non-Fac Total	Fac Total		51	50	62	80	MUE
	27.87	27.87	090	2	1	1	2	1

AMA: Fall 94: 1, 6, Aug 05: 15, Aug 13: 14

32656 Thoracoscopy, surgical; with parietal pleurectomy   [C]

RVU			Global Days	Modifiers				
Mod	Non-Fac Total	Fac Total		51	50	62	80	MUE
	23.36	23.36	090	2	1	1	2	1

AMA: Fall 94: 1, 6, Aug 13: 14

32658 Thoracoscopy, surgical; with removal of clot or foreign body from pericardial sac   [C]

RVU			Global Days	Modifiers				
Mod	Non-Fac Total	Fac Total		51	50	62	80	MUE
	20.85	20.85	090	2	0	1	2	1

AMA: Fall 94: 1, 6, Aug 13: 14

32659 Thoracoscopy, surgical; with creation of pericardial window or partial resection of pericardial sac for drainage   [C]

RVU			Global Days	Modifiers				
Mod	Non-Fac Total	Fac Total		51	50	62	80	MUE
	21.28	21.28	090	2	0	1	2	1

AMA: Fall 94: 1, 6, Aug 13: 14

32661 Thoracoscopy, surgical; with excision of pericardial cyst, tumor, or mass   [C]

RVU			Global Days	Modifiers				
Mod	Non-Fac Total	Fac Total		51	50	62	80	MUE
	23.39	23.39	090	2	0	1	2	1

AMA: Fall 94: 1, 6, Aug 13: 14

32662 Thoracoscopy, surgical; with excision of mediastinal cyst, tumor, or mass   [C]

RVU			Global Days	Modifiers				
Mod	Non-Fac Total	Fac Total		51	50	62	80	MUE
	25.98	25.98	090	2	0	1	2	1

AMA: Fall 94: 1, 6, Aug 13: 14

32663 Thoracoscopy, surgical; with lobectomy (single lobe)   [C]

RVU			Global Days	Modifiers				
Mod	Non-Fac Total	Fac Total		51	50	62	80	MUE
	40.78	40.78	090	2	0	1	2	1

AMA: Fall 94: 1, 6, Sep 12: 3, Aug 13: 14

32664 Thoracoscopy, surgical; with thoracic sympathectomy   [C]

RVU			Global Days	Modifiers				
Mod	Non-Fac Total	Fac Total		51	50	62	80	MUE
	24.81	24.81	090	2	1	1	2	1

AMA: Fall 94: 1, Oct 99: 10, Aug 13: 14

32665 Thoracoscopy, surgical; with esophagomyotomy (Heller type)   [C]

RVU			Global Days	Modifiers				
Mod	Non-Fac Total	Fac Total		51	50	62	80	MUE
	35.76	35.76	090	2	0	1	2	1

AMA: Fall 94: 1, 6, Aug 13: 14

32666 Thoracoscopy, surgical; with therapeutic wedge resection (eg, mass, nodule), initial unilateral   [C]

Coding tip: For open therapeutic wedge resection - 32505-32506

RVU			Global Days	Modifiers				
Mod	Non-Fac Total	Fac Total		51	50	62	80	MUE
	25.37	25.37	090	2	0	1	2	1

AMA: Sep 12: 3, Aug 13: 14

+ 32667 Thoracoscopy, surgical; with therapeutic wedge resection (eg, mass or nodule), each additional resection, ipsilateral (List separately in addition to code for primary procedure)   [C]

Coding tip: For open therapeutic wedge resection - 32505-32506

RVU			Global Days	Modifiers				
Mod	Non-Fac Total	Fac Total		51	50	62	80	MUE
	4.53	4.53	ZZZ	0	0	1	2	3

AMA: Sep 12: 3, Aug 13: 14

+ 32668 Thoracoscopy, surgical; with diagnostic wedge resection followed by anatomic lung resection (List separately in addition to code for primary procedure)   [C]

Coding tip: For open diagnostic wedge resection followed by anatomic lung resection - 32507

RVU			Global Days	Modifiers				
Mod	Non-Fac Total	Fac Total		51	50	62	80	MUE
	4.53	4.53	ZZZ	0	0	1	2	2

AMA: Sep 12: 3, Aug 13: 14

32669 Thoracoscopy, surgical; with removal of a single lung segment (segmentectomy)   [C]

RVU			Global Days	Modifiers				
Mod	Non-Fac Total	Fac Total		51	50	62	80	MUE
	39.26	39.26	090	2	0	1	2	2

AMA: Sep 12: 3, Aug 13: 14

32670 Thoracoscopy, surgical; with removal of two lobes (bilobectomy)   [C]

RVU			Global Days	Modifiers				
Mod	Non-Fac Total	Fac Total		51	50	62	80	MUE
	46.58	46.58	090	2	0	1	2	1

AMA: Sep 12: 3, Aug 13: 14

32671 Thoracoscopy, surgical; with removal of lung (pneumonectomy)   [C]

RVU			Global Days	Modifiers				
Mod	Non-Fac Total	Fac Total		51	50	62	80	MUE
	51.74	51.74	090	2	0	1	2	1

AMA: Sep 12: 3, Aug 13: 14

● New   ▲ Revised   ✖ Deleted   ⊙ Moderate Sedation   ✛ Add-on Codes   ⊘ High Risk Denial   Ⓐ Age Edit   ♀ Female   ♂ Male   **AMA** *CPT® Assistant*   **MUE** Medically Unlikely Edit
⊘ Modifier 51 Exempt   ⊖ Modifier 63 Exempt   ✗ Unlisted   **Modifiers:** *See Inside Back Cover*   Ⓜ Maternity   A2–Z3 ASC Payment Indicators   A–Y OPPS Status Indicators

CPT © 2015 American Medical Association. All Rights Reserved.   © 2016 DecisionHealth

32672 Thoracoscopy, surgical; with resection-plication for emphysematous lung (bullous or non-bullous) for lung volume reduction (LVRS), unilateral includes any pleural procedure, when performed C

| RVU | | | Global Days | Modifiers | | | | |
Mod	Non-Fac Total	Fac Total		51	50	62	80	MUE
	44.41	44.41	090	2	0	1	2	1

AMA: Sep 12: 3, Aug 13: 14

32673 Thoracoscopy, surgical; with resection of thymus, unilateral or bilateral C

| RVU | | | Global Days | Modifiers | | | | |
Mod	Non-Fac Total	Fac Total		51	50	62	80	MUE
	35.52	35.52	090	2	0	1	2	1

AMA: Sep 12: 3, Aug 13: 14

+ 32674 Thoracoscopy, surgical; with mediastinal and regional lymphadenectomy (List separately in addition to code for primary procedure) C

| RVU | | | Global Days | Modifiers | | | | |
Mod	Non-Fac Total	Fac Total		51	50	62	80	MUE
	6.23	6.23	ZZZ	0	0	1	2	1

AMA: Sep 12: 3, Aug 13: 14, May 14: 3

Thoracic Stereotactic Body Radiation

32701 Thoracic target(s) delineation for stereotactic body radiation therapy (SRS/SBRT), (photon or particle beam), entire course of treatment B

| RVU | | | Global Days | Modifiers | | | | |
Mod	Non-Fac Total	Fac Total		51	50	62	80	MUE
	6.36	6.36	XXX	0	0	1	0	1

AMA: Jun 15: 6

Thoracic target(s) delineation for stereotactic body radiation therapy SRS/SBRT

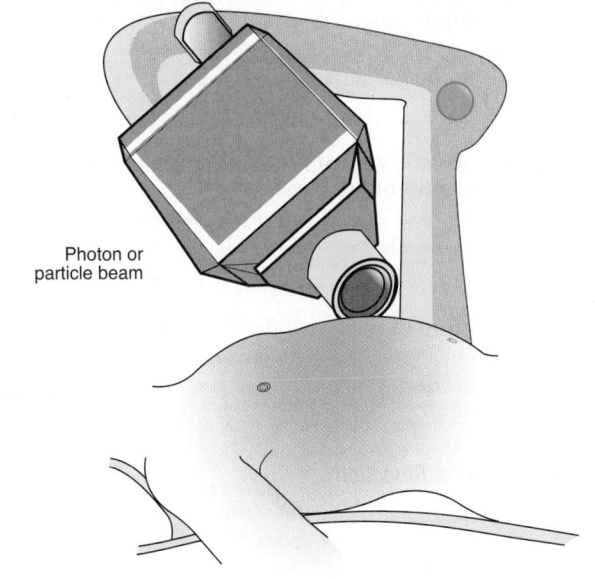

Photon or particle beam

Lung/Pleural Repair Procedures

32800 Repair lung hernia through chest wall C

| RVU | | | Global Days | Modifiers | | | | |
Mod	Non-Fac Total	Fac Total		51	50	62	80	MUE
	27.60	27.60	090	2	0	1	2	1

32810 Closure of chest wall following open flap drainage for empyema (Clagett type procedure) C

| RVU | | | Global Days | Modifiers | | | | |
Mod	Non-Fac Total	Fac Total		51	50	62	80	MUE
	26.32	26.32	090	2	0	0	2	1

32815 Open closure of major bronchial fistula C

| RVU | | | Global Days | Modifiers | | | | |
Mod	Non-Fac Total	Fac Total		51	50	62	80	MUE
	81.73	81.73	090	2	0	1	2	1

32820 Major reconstruction, chest wall (posttraumatic) C

| RVU | | | Global Days | Modifiers | | | | |
Mod	Non-Fac Total	Fac Total		51	50	62	80	MUE
	39.00	39.00	090	2	0	1	2	1

Lung Transplant Procedures

32850 Donor pneumonectomy(s) (including cold preservation), from cadaver donor ⊘C

| RVU | | | Global Days | Modifiers | | | | |
Mod	Non-Fac Total	Fac Total		51	50	62	80	MUE
	0.00	0.00	XXX	9	9	9	9	1

32851 Lung transplant, single; without cardiopulmonary bypass C

| RVU | | | Global Days | Modifiers | | | | |
Mod	Non-Fac Total	Fac Total		51	50	62	80	MUE
	96.28	96.28	090	2	0	1	2	1

32852 Lung transplant, single; with cardiopulmonary bypass C

| RVU | | | Global Days | Modifiers | | | | |
Mod	Non-Fac Total	Fac Total		51	50	62	80	MUE
	105.42	105.42	090	2	0	1	2	1

32853 Lung transplant, double (bilateral sequential or en bloc); without cardiopulmonary bypass C

| RVU | | | Global Days | Modifiers | | | | |
Mod	Non-Fac Total	Fac Total		51	50	62	80	MUE
	134.14	134.14	090	2	2	1	2	1

32854 Lung transplant, double (bilateral sequential or en bloc); with cardiopulmonary bypass C

| RVU | | | Global Days | Modifiers | | | | |
Mod	Non-Fac Total	Fac Total		51	50	62	80	MUE
	142.62	142.62	090	2	2	1	2	1

32855 Backbench standard preparation of cadaver donor lung allograft prior to transplantation, including dissection of allograft from surrounding soft tissues to prepare pulmonary venous/atrial cuff, pulmonary artery, and bronchus; unilateral C

| RVU | | | Global Days | Modifiers | | | | |
Mod	Non-Fac Total	Fac Total		51	50	62	80	MUE
	0.00	0.00	XXX	2	0	1	2	1

● New ▲ Revised Deleted ⊙ Moderate Sedation ✚ Add-on Codes ⊘ High Risk Denial Ⓐ Age Edit ♀ Female ♂ Male **AMA** CPT® Assistant **MUE** Medically Unlikely Edit
⊘ Modifier 51 Exempt ⊖ Modifier 63 Exempt ✗ Unlisted **Modifiers:** See Inside Back Cover Ⓜ Maternity A2–Z3 ASC Payment Indicators A–Y OPPS Status Indicators

Surgical Procedures

32856 – 33120

32856 Backbench standard preparation of cadaver donor lung allograft prior to transplantation, including dissection of allograft from surrounding soft tissues to prepare pulmonary venous/atrial cuff, pulmonary artery, and bronchus; bilateral   C

RVU			Global Days	Modifiers				
Mod	Non-Fac Total	Fac Total		51	50	62	80	MUE
	0.00	0.00	XXX	2	0	1	2	1

Therapeutic Collapse/Thoracoplasty

32900 Resection of ribs, extrapleural, all stages   C

RVU			Global Days	Modifiers				
Mod	Non-Fac Total	Fac Total		51	50	62	80	MUE
	40.68	40.68	090	2	0	1	2	1

32905 Thoracoplasty, Schede type or extrapleural (all stages)   C

RVU			Global Days	Modifiers				
Mod	Non-Fac Total	Fac Total		51	50	62	80	MUE
	39.19	39.19	090	2	0	1	2	1

32906 Thoracoplasty, Schede type or extrapleural (all stages); with closure of bronchopleural fistula   C

RVU			Global Days	Modifiers				
Mod	Non-Fac Total	Fac Total		51	50	62	80	MUE
	48.41	48.41	090	2	0	1	2	1

32940 Pneumonolysis, extraperiosteal, including filling or packing procedures   C

RVU			Global Days	Modifiers				
Mod	Non-Fac Total	Fac Total		51	50	62	80	MUE
	36.04	36.04	090	2	0	1	2	1

32960 Pneumothorax, therapeutic, intrapleural injection of air   G2T

RVU			Global Days	Modifiers				
Mod	Non-Fac Total	Fac Total		51	50	62	80	MUE
	4.06	2.89	000	2	0	0	1	1

Other Lung/Pleural Procedures

32997 Total lung lavage (unilateral)   C

RVU			Global Days	Modifiers				
Mod	Non-Fac Total	Fac Total		51	50	62	80	MUE
	9.91	9.91	000	2	1	0	1	1

AMA: Nov 98: 13, Nov 99: 14

32998 Ablation therapy for reduction or eradication of 1 or more pulmonary tumor(s) including pleura or chest wall when involved by tumor extension, percutaneous, radiofrequency, unilateral   G2T

Coding tip: Ablation therapy with ultrasound guidance and monitoring - 32998, 76940; with CT guidance and monitoring - 32998, 77013; with magnetic resonance guidance and monitoring - 32998, 77022

RVU			Global Days	Modifiers				
Mod	Non-Fac Total	Fac Total		51	50	62	80	MUE
	67.93	8.23	000	2	1	0	2	1

32999 Unlisted procedure, lungs and pleura   T

RVU			Global Days	Modifiers				
Mod	Non-Fac Total	Fac Total		51	50	62	80	MUE
	0.00	0.00	YYY	2	0	1	1	

AMA: Jan 02: 11, Feb 02: 11, Jul 08: 10, Apr 10: 10, Aug 11: 9, Jun 15: 6

Cardiovascular Procedures

Heart/Pericardial Procedures

Pericardial Procedures

⊙ **33010** Pericardiocentesis; initial   A2T

Coding tip: Pericardiocentesis with ultrasonic guidance - 33010, 76930

RVU			Global Days	Modifiers				
Mod	Non-Fac Total	Fac Total		51	50	62	80	MUE
	3.49	3.49	000	2	0	1	1	1

AMA: Feb 15: 11

⊙ **33011** Pericardiocentesis; subsequent   A2T

Coding tip: Pericardiocentesis with ultrasonic guidance - 33011, 76930

RVU			Global Days	Modifiers				
Mod	Non-Fac Total	Fac Total		51	50	62	80	MUE
	3.50	3.50	000	2	0	0	0	1

AMA: Sep 10: 7, Feb 15: 11

33015 Tube pericardiostomy   C

RVU			Global Days	Modifiers				
Mod	Non-Fac Total	Fac Total		51	50	62	80	MUE
	14.75	14.75	090	2	0	0	1	1

AMA: Aug 14: 14

33020 Pericardiotomy for removal of clot or foreign body (primary procedure)   C

RVU			Global Days	Modifiers				
Mod	Non-Fac Total	Fac Total		51	50	62	80	MUE
	25.64	25.64	090	2	0	1	2	1

33025 Creation of pericardial window or partial resection for drainage   C

RVU			Global Days	Modifiers				
Mod	Non-Fac Total	Fac Total		51	50	62	80	MUE
	23.30	23.30	090	2	0	1	2	1

33030 Pericardiectomy, subtotal or complete; without cardiopulmonary bypass   C

RVU			Global Days	Modifiers				
Mod	Non-Fac Total	Fac Total		51	50	62	80	MUE
	58.41	58.41	090	2	0	1	2	1

33031 Pericardiectomy, subtotal or complete; with cardiopulmonary bypass   C

RVU			Global Days	Modifiers				
Mod	Non-Fac Total	Fac Total		51	50	62	80	MUE
	72.04	72.04	090	2	0	1	2	1

33050 Resection of pericardial cyst or tumor   C

RVU			Global Days	Modifiers				
Mod	Non-Fac Total	Fac Total		51	50	62	80	MUE
	29.06	29.06	090	2	0	1	2	1

Heart Tumor Excision/Resection

33120 Excision of intracardiac tumor, resection with cardiopulmonary bypass   C

RVU			Global Days	Modifiers				
Mod	Non-Fac Total	Fac Total		51	50	62	80	MUE
	61.04	61.04	090	2	0	1	2	1

AMA: Mar 07: 1

● New   ▲ Revised   ✖ Deleted   ⊙ Moderate Sedation   ✚ Add-on Codes   ⊘ High Risk Denial   Ⓐ Age Edit   ♀ Female   ♂ Male   **AMA** *CPT® Assistant*   **MUE** Medically Unlikely Edit
⊘ Modifier 51 Exempt   ⊖ Modifier 63 Exempt   ✗ Unlisted   **Modifiers:** *See Inside Back Cover*   Ⓜ Maternity   A2–Z3 ASC Payment Indicators   A–Y OPPS Status Indicators

CPT © 2015 American Medical Association. All Rights Reserved.   © 2016 DecisionHealth

33130 Resection of external cardiac tumor   C

RVU			Global Days	Modifiers				
Mod	Non-Fac Total	Fac Total		51	50	62	80	MUE
	40.32	40.32	090	2	0	1	2	1

AMA: Mar 07: 1

Transmyocardial Laser Revascularization

33140 Transmyocardial laser revascularization, by thoracotomy; (separate procedure)   C

RVU			Global Days	Modifiers				
Mod	Non-Fac Total	Fac Total		51	50	62	80	MUE
	46.01	46.01	090	2	0	0	2	1

AMA: Nov 99: 14, Nov 00: 5, Apr 01: 7

+ 33141 Transmyocardial laser revascularization, by thoracotomy; performed at the time of other open cardiac procedure(s) (List separately in addition to code for primary procedure)   C

RVU			Global Days	Modifiers				
Mod	Non-Fac Total	Fac Total		51	50	62	80	MUE
	3.79	3.79	ZZZ	0	0	1	2	1

AMA: Apr 01: 7

Pacemaker/Cardioverter-Defibrillator Insertion/Revision/Removal

Coding Guidance

Placing catheters intravascularly into coronary vessels or chambers of the heart is often necessary for pacemaker/pacing cardioverter defibrillator procedures. Cardiac or selective catheterization codes should not be reported with these procedures. A separately reported cardiac catheterization code may be used when it is medically needed and performed as a distinct service on the same day or different patient encounter. Fluoroscopy and ultrasound are not reportable with the procedures described in 33202-33249, 33262-33264.

33202 Insertion of epicardial electrode(s); open incision (eg, thoracotomy, median sternotomy, subxiphoid approach)   C

RVU			Global Days	Modifiers				
Mod	Non-Fac Total	Fac Total		51	50	62	80	MUE
	22.65	22.65	090	2	0	0	1	1

AMA: Jun 12: 5, Nov 14: 5, May 15: 3

33203 Insertion of epicardial electrode(s); endoscopic approach (eg, thoracoscopy, pericardioscopy)   C

RVU			Global Days	Modifiers				
Mod	Non-Fac Total	Fac Total		51	50	62	80	MUE
	23.50	23.50	090	2	0	0	1	1

AMA: Jun 12: 4, Nov 14: 5, May 15: 3

⊙ 33206 Insertion of new or replacement of permanent pacemaker with transvenous electrode(s); atrial   J8J1

RVU			Global Days	Modifiers				
Mod	Non-Fac Total	Fac Total		51	50	62	80	MUE
	13.38	13.38	090	2	0	2	1	1

AMA: Summer 94: 10, 17, Oct 96: 9, Nov 99: 15, Jun 08: 14, Jun 12: 3, Apr 13: 10, Nov 14: 5, May 15: 3

Pub 100-04, 32, 320.4.2, 320.4.3, 320.4.5, 320.4.6, 320.4.7

⊙ 33207 Insertion of new or replacement of permanent pacemaker with transvenous electrode(s); ventricular   J8J1

RVU			Global Days	Modifiers				
Mod	Non-Fac Total	Fac Total		51	50	62	80	MUE
	14.27	14.27	090	2	0	2	1	1

AMA: Summer 94: 10, 17, Oct 96: 9, Nov 99: 15, Jun 08: 14, Jun 12: 3, Apr 13: 10, May 15: 3

Pub 100-04, 32, 320.4.2, 320.4.3, 320.4.5, 320.4.6, 320.4.7

⊙ 33208 Insertion of new or replacement of permanent pacemaker with transvenous electrode(s); atrial and ventricular   J8J1

RVU			Global Days	Modifiers				
Mod	Non-Fac Total	Fac Total		51	50	62	80	MUE
	15.46	15.46	090	2	0	2	1	1

AMA: Summer 94: 10, 17, Jul 96: 10, Nov 99: 15, Jun 08: 14, Jun 12: 3, Apr 13: 10, Nov 14: 5, May 15: 3

Pub 100-04, 32, 320.4.2, 320.4.3, 320.4.5, 320.4.6, 320.4.7

⊙ 33210 Insertion or replacement of temporary transvenous single chamber cardiac electrode or pacemaker catheter (separate procedure)   J8J1

RVU			Global Days	Modifiers				
Mod	Non-Fac Total	Fac Total		51	50	62	80	MUE
	5.21	5.21	000	2	0	0	1	1

AMA: Summer 94: 10, 17, Mar 07: 1, Aug 11: 4, Jun 12: 3, Jan 13: 6, May 15: 3

⊙ 33211 Insertion or replacement of temporary transvenous dual chamber pacing electrodes (separate procedure)   J8J1

RVU			Global Days	Modifiers				
Mod	Non-Fac Total	Fac Total		51	50	62	80	MUE
	5.32	5.32	000	2	0	0	1	1

AMA: Summer 94: 10, 17, Mar 07: 1, Aug 11: 4, Jun 12: 3, May 15: 3

⊙ 33212 Insertion of pacemaker pulse generator only; with existing single lead   J8J1

Coding tip: Insertion pacemaker pulse generator only with existing multiple leads - 33221

RVU			Global Days	Modifiers				
Mod	Non-Fac Total	Fac Total		51	50	62	80	MUE
	9.67	9.67	090	2	0	0	1	1

AMA: Summer 94: 10, 18, Fall 94: 24, May 04: 15, Jun 08: 14, Jun 12: 3, Nov 14: 5, May 15: 3

⊙ 33213 Insertion of pacemaker pulse generator only; with existing dual leads   J8J1

Coding tip: Insertion pacemaker pulse generator only with existing multiple leads - 33221

RVU			Global Days	Modifiers				
Mod	Non-Fac Total	Fac Total		51	50	62	80	MUE
	10.09	10.09	090	2	0	0	1	1

AMA: Summer 94: 10, 18, Oct 96: 10, Feb 98: 11, Jun 12: 3, Nov 14: 5, May 15: 3

⊙ 33214 Upgrade of implanted pacemaker system, conversion of single chamber system to dual chamber system (includes removal of previously placed pulse generator, testing of existing lead, insertion of new lead, insertion of new pulse generator)   J8J1

RVU			Global Days	Modifiers				
Mod	Non-Fac Total	Fac Total		51	50	62	80	MUE
	14.19	14.19	090	2	0	2	0	1

AMA: Summer 94: 10, 18, Fall 94: 24, Jun 08: 14, Jun 12: 3, Nov 14: 5

33215 Repositioning of previously implanted transvenous pacemaker or implantable defibrillator (right atrial or right ventricular) electrode `G2T`

RVU			Global Days	Modifiers				
Mod	Non-Fac Total	Fac Total		51	50	62	80	MUE
	8.98	8.98	090	2	0	0	1	2

AMA: Jun 12: 3, Nov 14: 5

Repositioning of implanted transvenous pacemaker/defibrillator electrode

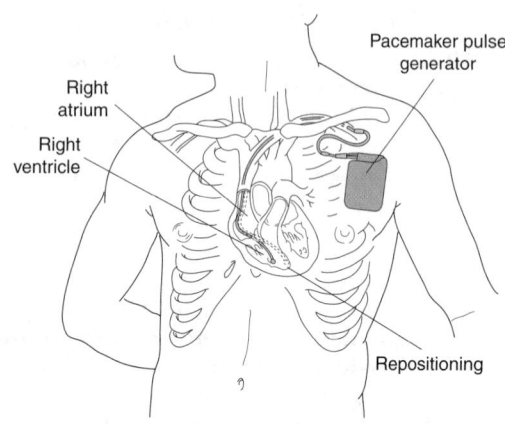

An already existing wire of a permanent pacemaker or implantable defibrillator is repositioned in the right atrium or the right ventricle

⊙ 33216 Insertion of a single transvenous electrode, permanent pacemaker or implantable defibrillator `J8J1`

RVU			Global Days	Modifiers				
Mod	Non-Fac Total	Fac Total		51	50	62	80	MUE
	11.09	11.09	090	2	0	0	1	1

AMA: Summer 94: 10, 18, Jul 96: 10, Nov 99: 15, 16

⊙ 33217 Insertion of 2 transvenous electrodes, permanent pacemaker or implantable defibrillator `J8J1`

RVU			Global Days	Modifiers				
Mod	Non-Fac Total	Fac Total		51	50	62	80	MUE
	10.88	10.88	090	2	0	0	1	1

AMA: Summer 94: 10, 18, Jul 96: 10, Nov 99: 15, 16, Jul 00: 5, Apr 09: 8, Jun 12: 3

⊙ 33218 Repair of single transvenous electrode, permanent pacemaker or implantable defibrillator `G2T`

RVU			Global Days	Modifiers				
Mod	Non-Fac Total	Fac Total		51	50	62	80	MUE
	11.61	11.61	090	2	0	0	1	1

AMA: Summer 94: 10, 19, Oct 96: 9, Nov 99: 15, 16, Jun 12: 3

⊙ 33220 Repair of 2 transvenous electrodes for permanent pacemaker or implantable defibrillator `G2T`

RVU			Global Days	Modifiers				
Mod	Non-Fac Total	Fac Total		51	50	62	80	MUE
	11.63	11.63	090	2	0	0	1	1

AMA: Summer 94: 10, 19, Oct 96: 9, Nov 99: 15, 16, Jun 08: 14, Jun 12: 3

⊙ 33221 Insertion of pacemaker pulse generator only; with existing multiple leads `J8J1`

Coding tip: Code 33221 is listed out of numerical order in CPT. Related pulse generation insertion only codes - 33212 existing single lead; 33213 existing dual leads

RVU			Global Days	Modifiers				
Mod	Non-Fac Total	Fac Total		51	50	62	80	MUE
	10.81	10.81	090	2	0	0	1	1

AMA: Jun 12: 3, Nov 14: 5, May 15: 3

⊙ 33222 Relocation of skin pocket for pacemaker `⊙A2T`

RVU			Global Days	Modifiers				
Mod	Non-Fac Total	Fac Total		51	50	62	80	MUE
	10.11	10.11	090	2	0	0	1	1

AMA: Spring 94: 30, Summer 94: 10, Nov 99: 15, 16, Jun 08: 14, Jun 12: 3, Nov 14: 5, May 15: 3

Revision or relocation of skin pocket for pacemaker or implantable defibrillator

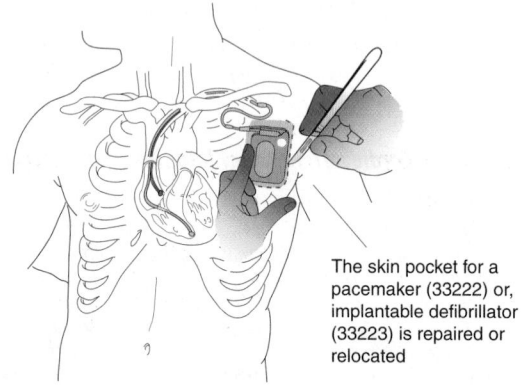

The skin pocket for a pacemaker (33222) or, implantable defibrillator (33223) is repaired or relocated

⊙ 33223 Relocation of skin pocket for implantable defibrillator `⊙A2T`

RVU			Global Days	Modifiers				
Mod	Non-Fac Total	Fac Total		51	50	62	80	MUE
	12.18	12.18	090	2	0	0	0	1

AMA: Summer 94: 10, 19, Nov 99: 15, 16, Jun 08: 14, Jun 12: 3, Nov 14: 5

33224 Insertion of pacing electrode, cardiac venous system, for left ventricular pacing, with attachment to previously placed pacemaker or implantable defibrillator pulse generator (including revision of pocket, removal, insertion, and/or replacement of existing generator) `J8J1`

RVU			Global Days	Modifiers				
Mod	Non-Fac Total	Fac Total		51	50	62	80	MUE
	14.96	14.96	000	2	0	0	1	1

AMA: Dec 07: 16, Jun 12: 3, Nov 14: 5, May 15: 3

+ 33225 Insertion of pacing electrode, cardiac venous system, for left ventricular pacing, at time of insertion of implantable defibrillator or pacemaker pulse generator (eg, for upgrade to dual chamber system) (List separately in addition to code for primary procedure) `N1N`

RVU			Global Days	Modifiers				
Mod	Non-Fac Total	Fac Total		51	50	62	80	MUE
	13.59	13.59	ZZZ	0	0	0	1	1

AMA: Dec 07: 16, Jun 12: 3, Nov 14: 5, May 15: 3

● New   ▲ Revised   ✖ Deleted   ⊙ Moderate Sedation   ✚ Add-on Codes   ⊘ High Risk Denial   Ⓐ Age Edit   ♀ Female   ♂ Male   **AMA** CPT® Assistant   **MUE** Medically Unlikely Edit
⊘ Modifier 51 Exempt   ⊖ Modifier 63 Exempt   ✗ Unlisted   **Modifiers:** See Inside Back Cover   Ⓜ Maternity   `A2`–`Z3` ASC Payment Indicators   `A`–`Y` OPPS Status Indicators

CPT © 2015 American Medical Association. All Rights Reserved.   © 2016 DecisionHealth

33226 Repositioning of previously implanted cardiac venous system (left ventricular) electrode (including removal, insertion and/or replacement of existing generator) `G2T`

RVU			Global Days	Modifiers				
Mod	Non-Fac Total	Fac Total		51	50	62	80	MUE
	14.34	14.34	000	2	0	0	1	1

AMA: Jun 12: 3, Nov 14: 5, May 15: 3

⊙ **33227 Removal of permanent pacemaker pulse generator with replacement of pacemaker pulse generator; single lead system** `J8J1`

Coding tip: Code 33227 is listed out of numerical order in CPT. Related removal permanent pacemaker pulse generator codes - 33233 removal only; 33228, 33229 removal with replacement

RVU			Global Days	Modifiers				
Mod	Non-Fac Total	Fac Total		51	50	62	80	MUE
	10.17	10.17	090	2	0	0	1	1

AMA: Jun 12: 3, Apr 13: 10, Nov 14: 5

Pub 100-04, 32, 320.4.2

⊙ **33228 Removal of permanent pacemaker pulse generator with replacement of pacemaker pulse generator; dual lead system** `J8J1`

Coding tip: Code 33228 is listed out of numerical order in CPT. Related removal permanent pacemaker pulse generator codes - 33233 removal only; 33227, 33229 removal with replacement

RVU			Global Days	Modifiers				
Mod	Non-Fac Total	Fac Total		51	50	62	80	MUE
	10.60	10.60	090	2	0	0	1	1

AMA: Jun 12: 3, Apr 13: 10

Pub 100-04, 32, 320.4.2

⊙ **33229 Removal of permanent pacemaker pulse generator with replacement of pacemaker pulse generator; multiple lead system** `J8J1`

Coding tip: Code 33229 is listed out of numerical order in CPT. Related removal permanent pacemaker pulse generator codes - 33233 removal only; 33227, 33228 removal with replacement

RVU			Global Days	Modifiers				
Mod	Non-Fac Total	Fac Total		51	50	62	80	MUE
	11.17	11.17	090	2	0	0	1	1

AMA: Jun 12: 3, Apr 13: 10, Nov 14: 5

⊙ **33230 Insertion of implantable defibrillator pulse generator only; with existing dual leads** `J8J1`

Coding tip: Code 33230 is listed out of numerical order in CPT. Related codes for pacing cardioverter-defibrillator insertion with existing leads - 33240 existing single lead; 33231 existing multiple leads

RVU			Global Days	Modifiers				
Mod	Non-Fac Total	Fac Total		51	50	62	80	MUE
	11.51	11.51	090	2	0	0	1	1

AMA: Jun 12: 3, Nov 14: 5

⊙ **33231 Insertion of implantable defibrillator pulse generator only; with existing multiple leads** `J8J1`

Coding tip: Code 33231 is listed out of numerical order in CPT. Related codes for pacing cardioverter-defibrillator insertion with existing leads - 33240 existing single lead; 33230 existing dual leads

RVU			Global Days	Modifiers				
Mod	Non-Fac Total	Fac Total		51	50	62	80	MUE
	11.98	11.98	090	2	0	0	1	1

AMA: Jun 12: 3, Nov 14: 5

⊙ **33233 Removal of permanent pacemaker pulse generator only** `J8Q2`

Coding tip: Removal permanent pacemaker pulse generator with replacement - 33227, 33228, 33229

RVU			Global Days	Modifiers				
Mod	Non-Fac Total	Fac Total		51	50	62	80	MUE
	7.02	7.02	090	2	0	0	1	1

AMA: Summer 94: 10, 19, Fall 94: 24, Oct 96: 10, Jun 12: 3, Nov 14: 5

⊙ **33234 Removal of transvenous pacemaker electrode(s); single lead system, atrial or ventricular** `G2Q2`

RVU			Global Days	Modifiers				
Mod	Non-Fac Total	Fac Total		51	50	62	80	MUE
	14.40	14.40	090	2	0	0	1	1

AMA: Summer 94: 10, 19, Nov 99: 16, Jun 12: 3, Oct 12: 15, Nov 14: 5

⊙ **33235 Removal of transvenous pacemaker electrode(s); dual lead system** `G2Q2`

RVU			Global Days	Modifiers				
Mod	Non-Fac Total	Fac Total		51	50	62	80	MUE
	18.78	18.78	090	2	0	0	1	1

AMA: Summer 94: 10, 19, Nov 99: 16, Jun 12: 3, Oct 12: 15, Dec 13: 14, Nov 14: 5

33236 Removal of permanent epicardial pacemaker and electrodes by thoracotomy; single lead system, atrial or ventricular `C`

RVU			Global Days	Modifiers				
Mod	Non-Fac Total	Fac Total		51	50	62	80	MUE
	22.89	22.89	090	2	0	2	0	1

AMA: Summer 94: 10, 19, Nov 99: 16, Jun 12: 3

33237 Removal of permanent epicardial pacemaker and electrodes by thoracotomy; dual lead system `C`

RVU			Global Days	Modifiers				
Mod	Non-Fac Total	Fac Total		51	50	62	80	MUE
	24.57	24.57	090	2	0	2	0	1

AMA: Summer 94: 10, 19, Nov 99: 16, Jun 12: 3

33238 Removal of permanent transvenous electrode(s) by thoracotomy `C`

RVU			Global Days	Modifiers				
Mod	Non-Fac Total	Fac Total		51	50	62	80	MUE
	27.19	27.19	090	2	0	2	0	1

AMA: Summer 94: 10, 19, Nov 99: 16, Jun 12: 3, Nov 14: 5

⊙ **33240 Insertion of implantable defibrillator pulse generator only; with existing single lead** `J8J1`

RVU			Global Days	Modifiers				
Mod	Non-Fac Total	Fac Total		51	50	62	80	MUE
	10.96	10.96	090	2	0	0	1	1

AMA: Summer 94: 40, Jun 96: 10, Nov 99: 16, 17, Jul 00: 5, Apr 04: 6, Jun 08: 14, Jun 12: 3, Nov 14: 5

Pub 100-04, 32, 270.1

● New ▲ Revised Deleted ⊙ Moderate Sedation ➕ Add-on Codes ⊘ High Risk Denial ⒶAge Edit ♀ Female ♂ Male **AMA** *CPT® Assistant* **MUE** Medically Unlikely Edit
⊘ Modifier 51 Exempt ⊖ Modifier 63 Exempt ⊠ Unlisted **Modifiers:** *See Inside Back Cover* Ⓜ Maternity A2–Z3 ASC Payment Indicators A–Y OPPS Status Indicators

© 2016 DecisionHealth | CPT © 2015 American Medical Association. All Rights Reserved. | **349**

Surgical Procedures

33226 – 33240

Surgical Procedures

33241 – 33258

⊙ **33241 Removal of implantable defibrillator pulse generator only**   G2 Q2

Coding tip: Removal of pacing cardioverter-defibrillator pulse generator with replacement - 33262 single lead system; 33263 dual lead system; 33264 multiple lead system

RVU		Global Days	Modifiers				
Mod	Non-Fac Total	Fac Total		51	50	62	80	MUE
	6.60	6.60	090	2	0	0	1	1

AMA: Summer 94: 40, Nov 99: 16, 17, Jun 12: 3, Nov 14: 5

Pub 100-04, 32, 270.1

33243 Removal of single or dual chamber implantable defibrillator electrode(s); by thoracotomy   C

RVU		Global Days	Modifiers				
Mod	Non-Fac Total	Fac Total		51	50	62	80	MUE
	39.81	39.81	090	2	0	1	2	1

AMA: Summer 94: 40, Nov 99: 16, 17, Jun 12: 3, Nov 14: 5

Pub 100-04, 32, 270.1

⊙ **33244 Removal of single or dual chamber implantable defibrillator electrode(s); by transvenous extraction**   Q2

RVU		Global Days	Modifiers				
Mod	Non-Fac Total	Fac Total		51	50	62	80	MUE
	25.23	25.23	090	2	0	1	1	1

AMA: Summer 94: 40, Nov 99: 16, 17, Jul 00: 5, Jun 12: 3, Nov 14: 5

Pub 100-04, 32, 270.1

⊙ **33249 Insertion or replacement of permanent implantable defibrillator system, with transvenous lead(s), single or dual chamber**   J8 J1

RVU		Global Days	Modifiers				
Mod	Non-Fac Total	Fac Total		51	50	62	80	MUE
	26.89	26.89	090	2	0	1	1	1

AMA: Summer 94: 21, Nov 99: 16, 17, Apr 04: 6, May 08: 14, Jun 08: 14, Jun 12: 3, Nov 14: 5

Pub 100-04, 32, 270.1

Electrophysiological Operative Ablation

33250 Operative ablation of supraventricular arrhythmogenic focus or pathway (eg, Wolff-Parkinson-White, atrioventricular node re-entry), tract(s) and/or focus (foci); without cardiopulmonary bypass   C

RVU		Global Days	Modifiers				
Mod	Non-Fac Total	Fac Total		51	50	62	80	MUE
	42.88	42.88	090	2	0	1	2	1

AMA: Summer 94: 16, Nov 99: 17, 18

33251 Operative ablation of supraventricular arrhythmogenic focus or pathway (eg, Wolff-Parkinson-White, atrioventricular node re-entry), tract(s) and/or focus (foci); with cardiopulmonary bypass   C

RVU		Global Days	Modifiers				
Mod	Non-Fac Total	Fac Total		51	50	62	80	MUE
	47.25	47.25	090	2	0	1	2	1

AMA: Summer 94: 16, Nov 99: 17, 18

33254 Operative tissue ablation and reconstruction of atria, limited (eg, modified maze procedure)   C

RVU		Global Days	Modifiers				
Mod	Non-Fac Total	Fac Total		51	50	62	80	MUE
	40.10	40.10	090	2	0	1	2	1

AMA: Mar 07: 1

Operative tissue ablation and reconstruction of atria, limited

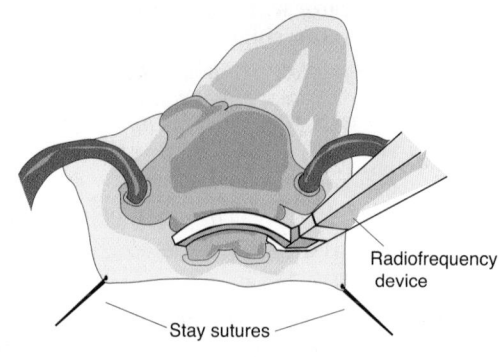

Limited ablation is done to disrupt electrical conduction pathways

33255 Operative tissue ablation and reconstruction of atria, extensive (eg, maze procedure); without cardiopulmonary bypass   C

RVU		Global Days	Modifiers				
Mod	Non-Fac Total	Fac Total		51	50	62	80	MUE
	47.12	47.12	090	2	0	1	2	1

AMA: Mar 07: 1

33256 Operative tissue ablation and reconstruction of atria, extensive (eg, maze procedure); with cardiopulmonary bypass   ⊘C

RVU		Global Days	Modifiers				
Mod	Non-Fac Total	Fac Total		51	50	62	80	MUE
	57.12	57.12	090	2	0	1	2	1

AMA: Mar 07: 1

✚ **33257 Operative tissue ablation and reconstruction of atria, performed at the time of other cardiac procedure(s), limited (eg, modified maze procedure) (List separately in addition to code for primary procedure)**   C

RVU		Global Days	Modifiers				
Mod	Non-Fac Total	Fac Total		51	50	62	80	MUE
	17.00	17.00	ZZZ	0	0	0	2	1

✚ **33258 Operative tissue ablation and reconstruction of atria, performed at the time of other cardiac procedure(s), extensive (eg, maze procedure), without cardiopulmonary bypass (List separately in addition to code for primary procedure)**   C

RVU		Global Days	Modifiers				
Mod	Non-Fac Total	Fac Total		51	50	62	80	MUE
	19.03	19.03	ZZZ	0	0	0	2	1

● New   ▲ Revised   ✖ Deleted   ⊙ Moderate Sedation   ✚ Add-on Codes   ⊘ High Risk Denial   Ⓐ Age Edit   ♀ Female   ♂ Male   **AMA** *CPT® Assistant*   **MUE** Medically Unlikely Edit

⊘ Modifier 51 Exempt   ⊖ Modifier 63 Exempt   ⓧ Unlisted   **Modifiers:** *See Inside Back Cover*   Ⓜ Maternity   A2–Z3 ASC Payment Indicators   A–Y OPPS Status Indicators

CPT © 2015 American Medical Association. All Rights Reserved.   © 2016 DecisionHealth

+ 33259 Operative tissue ablation and reconstruction of atria, performed at the time of other cardiac procedure(s), extensive (eg, maze procedure), with cardiopulmonary bypass (List separately in addition to code for primary procedure) **C**

RVU			Global Days	Modifiers				
Mod	Non-Fac Total	Fac Total		51	50	62	80	MUE
	24.60	24.60	ZZZ	0	0	0	2	1

33261 Operative ablation of ventricular arrhythmogenic focus with cardiopulmonary bypass **C**

RVU			Global Days	Modifiers				
Mod	Non-Fac Total	Fac Total		51	50	62	80	MUE
	47.66	47.66	090	2	0	1	2	1

AMA: Summer 94: 16

Operative ablation of ventricular arrhythmogenic focus with cardiopulmonary bypass

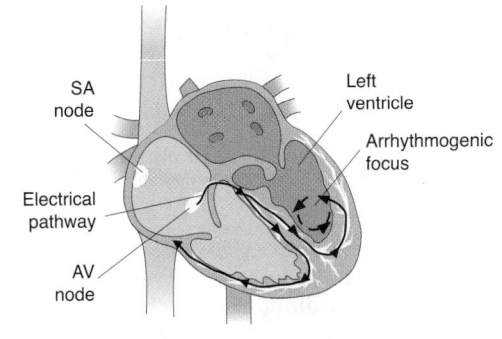

SA node
Left ventricle
Arrhythmogenic focus
Electrical pathway
AV node

The abnormal electrical pathway is interrupted by incision or ablation

⊙ **33262** Removal of implantable defibrillator pulse generator with replacement of implantable defibrillator pulse generator; single lead system **J 8 J I**

Coding tip: Code 33262 is listed out of numerical order in CPT. Related removal of pacing cardioverter-defibrillator pulse generator codes - 33241 removal only; 33263 removal with replacement dual lead system; 33264 removal with replacement multiple lead system

RVU			Global Days	Modifiers				
Mod	Non-Fac Total	Fac Total		51	50	62	80	MUE
	11.16	11.16	090	2	0	0	1	1

AMA: Jun 12: 3, Nov 14: 5

⊙ **33263** Removal of implantable defibrillator pulse generator with replacement of implantable defibrillator pulse generator; dual lead system **J 8 J I**

Coding tip: Code 33263 is listed out of numerical order in CPT. Related removal of pacing cardioverter-defibrillator pulse generator codes - 33241 removal only; 33262 removal with replacement single lead system; 33264 removal with replacement multiple lead system

RVU			Global Days	Modifiers				
Mod	Non-Fac Total	Fac Total		51	50	62	80	MUE
	11.60	11.60	090	2	0	0	1	1

AMA: Jun 12: 3, Dec 13: 17, Nov 14: 5

⊙ **33264** Removal of implantable defibrillator pulse generator with replacement of implantable defibrillator pulse generator; multiple lead system **J 8 J I**

Coding tip: Code 33262 is listed out of numerical order in CPT. Related removal of pacing cardioverter-defibrillator pulse generator codes - 33241 removal only; 33262 removal with replacement single lead system; 33263 removal with replacement dual lead system

RVU			Global Days	Modifiers				
Mod	Non-Fac Total	Fac Total		51	50	62	80	MUE
	12.09	12.09	090	2	0	0	1	1

AMA: Jun 12: 3, Dec 13: 17, Nov 14: 5

Endoscopic Electrophysiological Operative Ablation

33265 Endoscopy, surgical; operative tissue ablation and reconstruction of atria, limited (eg, modified maze procedure), without cardiopulmonary bypass **C**

RVU			Global Days	Modifiers				
Mod	Non-Fac Total	Fac Total		51	50	62	80	MUE
	39.53	39.53	090	2	0	1	2	1

AMA: Mar 07: 1

33266 Endoscopy, surgical; operative tissue ablation and reconstruction of atria, extensive (eg, maze procedure), without cardiopulmonary bypass **C**

RVU			Global Days	Modifiers				
Mod	Non-Fac Total	Fac Total		51	50	62	80	MUE
	53.78	53.78	090	2	0	1	2	1

AMA: Mar 07: 1

33270 Insertion or replacement of permanent subcutaneous implantable defibrillator system, with subcutaneous electrode, including defibrillation threshold evaluation, induction of arrhythmia, evaluation of sensing for arrhythmia termination, and programming or reprogramming of sensing or therapeutic parameters, when performed **J 8 J I**

RVU			Global Days	Modifiers				
Mod	Non-Fac Total	Fac Total		51	50	62	80	MUE
	17.15	17.15	090	2	0	0	1	1

AMA: Nov 14: 5

Insertion or replacement, permanent implantable defibrillator system with electrode, subcutaneous

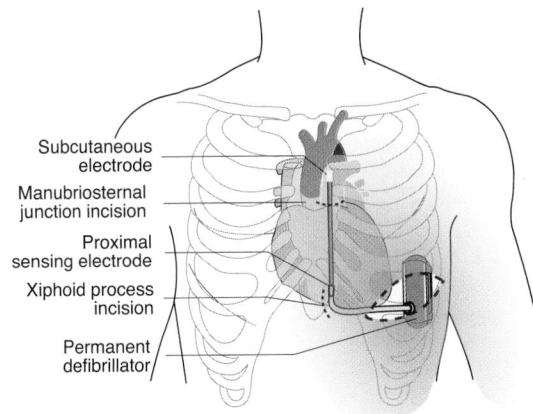

Subcutaneous electrode
Manubriosternal junction incision
Proximal sensing electrode
Xiphoid process incision
Permanent defibrillator

● New   ▲ Revised   Deleted   ⊙ Moderate Sedation   ✚ Add-on Codes   ⊘ High Risk Denial   Ⓐ Age Edit   ♀ Female   ♂ Male   **AMA** *CPT® Assistant*   **MUE** Medically Unlikely Edit
⊘ Modifier 51 Exempt   ⊖ Modifier 63 Exempt   Ⓧ Unlisted   **Modifiers:** *See Inside Back Cover*   Ⓜ Maternity   A2–Z3 ASC Payment Indicators   A–Y OPPS Status Indicators

33271 Insertion of subcutaneous implantable defibrillator electrode J 8 J I

RVU			Global Days	Modifiers				
Mod	Non-Fac Total	Fac Total		51	50	62	80	MUE
	14.44	14.44	090	2	0	0	1	1

AMA: Nov 14: 5

33272 Removal of subcutaneous implantable defibrillator electrode Q2

RVU			Global Days	Modifiers				
Mod	Non-Fac Total	Fac Total		51	50	62	80	MUE
	10.19	10.19	090	2	0	0	1	1

AMA: Nov 14: 5

33273 Repositioning of previously implanted subcutaneous implantable defibrillator electrode G2T

RVU			Global Days	Modifiers				
Mod	Non-Fac Total	Fac Total		51	50	62	80	MUE
	11.68	11.68	090	2	0	0	1	1

AMA: Nov 14: 5

Insertion/Removal Event Recorder (Patient-Activated)

⊙ **33282 Implantation of patient-activated cardiac event recorder** J 8 J I

RVU			Global Days	Modifiers				
Mod	Non-Fac Total	Fac Total		51	50	62	80	MUE
	6.90	6.90	090	2	0	0	1	1

AMA: Nov 99: 17, 18, Jul 00: 5, Jun 08: 14

⊙ **33284 Removal of an implantable, patient-activated cardiac event recorder** G2Q2

RVU			Global Days	Modifiers				
Mod	Non-Fac Total	Fac Total		51	50	62	80	MUE
	6.11	6.11	090	2	0	0	1	1

AMA: Nov 99: 17, 18, Jul 00: 5

Heart/Great Vessel Wound Repair

33300 Repair of cardiac wound; without bypass C

RVU			Global Days	Modifiers				
Mod	Non-Fac Total	Fac Total		51	50	62	80	MUE
	71.59	71.59	090	2	0	1	2	1

33305 Repair of cardiac wound; with cardiopulmonary bypass C

RVU			Global Days	Modifiers				
Mod	Non-Fac Total	Fac Total		51	50	62	80	MUE
	119.78	119.78	090	2	0	1	2	1

33310 Cardiotomy, exploratory (includes removal of foreign body, atrial or ventricular thrombus); without bypass C

RVU			Global Days	Modifiers				
Mod	Non-Fac Total	Fac Total		51	50	62	80	MUE
	34.42	34.42	090	2	0	1	2	1

Cardiotomy, exploratory

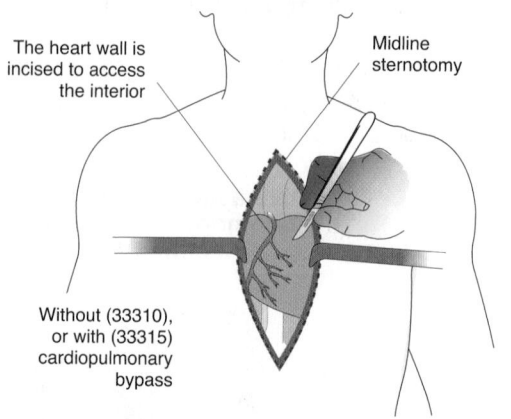

The heart wall is incised to access the interior

Midline sternotomy

Without (33310), or with (33315) cardiopulmonary bypass

The heart is accessed and explored. A ventricle or atrial foreign body or thrombus is removed

33315 Cardiotomy, exploratory (includes removal of foreign body, atrial or ventricular thrombus); with cardiopulmonary bypass C

RVU			Global Days	Modifiers				
Mod	Non-Fac Total	Fac Total		51	50	62	80	MUE
	55.59	55.59	090	2	0	1	2	1

AMA: Oct 10: 12, Dec 10: 12

33320 Suture repair of aorta or great vessels; without shunt or cardiopulmonary bypass C

RVU			Global Days	Modifiers				
Mod	Non-Fac Total	Fac Total		51	50	62	80	MUE
	30.94	30.94	090	2	0	1	2	1

AMA: Fall 91: 7

33321 Suture repair of aorta or great vessels; with shunt bypass C

RVU			Global Days	Modifiers				
Mod	Non-Fac Total	Fac Total		51	50	62	80	MUE
	35.94	35.94	090	2	0	1	2	1

AMA: Fall 91: 7

33322 Suture repair of aorta or great vessels; with cardiopulmonary bypass C

RVU			Global Days	Modifiers				
Mod	Non-Fac Total	Fac Total		51	50	62	80	MUE
	40.47	40.47	090	2	0	1	2	1

AMA: Fall 91: 7

33330 Insertion of graft, aorta or great vessels; without shunt, or cardiopulmonary bypass C

RVU			Global Days	Modifiers				
Mod	Non-Fac Total	Fac Total		51	50	62	80	MUE
	41.63	41.63	090	2	0	1	2	1

● New　▲ Revised　✖ Deleted　⊙ Moderate Sedation　✚ Add-on Codes　⊘ High Risk Denial　Ⓐ Age Edit　♀ Female　♂ Male　**AMA** CPT® Assistant　**MUE** Medically Unlikely Edit
⊘ Modifier 51 Exempt　⊖ Modifier 63 Exempt　✗ Unlisted　**Modifiers:** See Inside Back Cover　Ⓜ Maternity　A2–Z3 ASC Payment Indicators　A–Y OPPS Status Indicators

CPT © 2015 American Medical Association. All Rights Reserved.　© 2016 DecisionHealth

33335 Insertion of graft, aorta or great vessels; with cardiopulmonary bypass   C

RVU			Global Days	Modifiers				
Mod	Non-Fac Total	Fac Total		51	50	62	80	MUE
	54.35	54.35	090	2	0	1	2	1

33361 Transcatheter aortic valve replacement (TAVR/TAVI) with prosthetic valve; percutaneous femoral artery approach   C

RVU			Global Days	Modifiers				
Mod	Non-Fac Total	Fac Total		51	50	62	80	MUE
	39.65	39.65	000	2	0	2	0	1

AMA: Jan 13: 6, Jan 14: 5, Jul 14: 8, Mar 15: 9

Pub 100-04, 32, 290.1.1, 290.2

Transcatheter aortic valve replacement (TAVR/TAVI) with prosthetic valve; percutaneous femoral artery approach

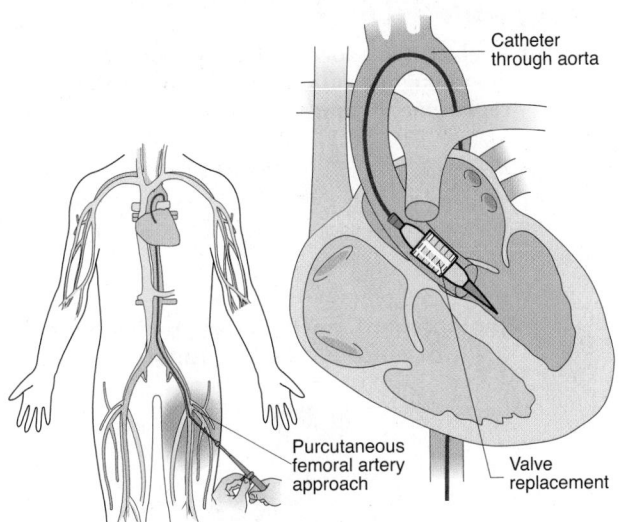

Catheter through aorta

Purcutaneous femoral artery approach

Valve replacement

33362 Transcatheter aortic valve replacement (TAVR/TAVI) with prosthetic valve; open femoral artery approach   C

RVU			Global Days	Modifiers				
Mod	Non-Fac Total	Fac Total		51	50	62	80	MUE
	43.36	43.36	000	2	0	2	0	1

AMA: Jan 13: 6, Jan 14: 5, Mar 15: 9

Pub 100-04, 32, 290.1.1, 290.2

33363 Transcatheter aortic valve replacement (TAVR/TAVI) with prosthetic valve; open axillary artery approach   C

RVU			Global Days	Modifiers				
Mod	Non-Fac Total	Fac Total		51	50	62	80	MUE
	45.04	45.04	000	2	0	2	0	1

AMA: Jan 13: 6, Jan 14: 5, Mar 15: 9

Pub 100-04, 32, 290.1.1, 290.2

33364 Transcatheter aortic valve replacement (TAVR/TAVI) with prosthetic valve; open iliac artery approach   C

RVU			Global Days	Modifiers				
Mod	Non-Fac Total	Fac Total		51	50	62	80	MUE
	47.22	47.22	000	2	0	2	0	1

AMA: Jan 13: 6, Jan 14: 5, Mar 15: 9

Pub 100-04, 32, 290.1.1, 290.2

33365 Transcatheter aortic valve replacement (TAVR/TAVI) with prosthetic valve; transaortic approach (eg, median sternotomy, mediastinotomy)   C

RVU			Global Days	Modifiers				
Mod	Non-Fac Total	Fac Total		51	50	62	80	MUE
	51.98	51.98	000	2	0	2	0	1

AMA: Jan 13: 6, Jan 14: 5, Mar 15: 9

Pub 100-04, 32, 290.1.1, 290.2

33366 Transcatheter aortic valve replacement (TAVR/TAVI) with prosthetic valve; transapical exposure (eg, left thoracotomy)   C

RVU			Global Days	Modifiers				
Mod	Non-Fac Total	Fac Total		51	50	62	80	MUE
	56.24	56.24	000	2	0	2	0	1

AMA: Jan 14: 5, Jul 14: 8, Mar 15: 9

Pub 100-04, 32, 290.2

TAVR/TAVI with prosthetic valve;
Transapical exposure (eg, left thoracotomy)

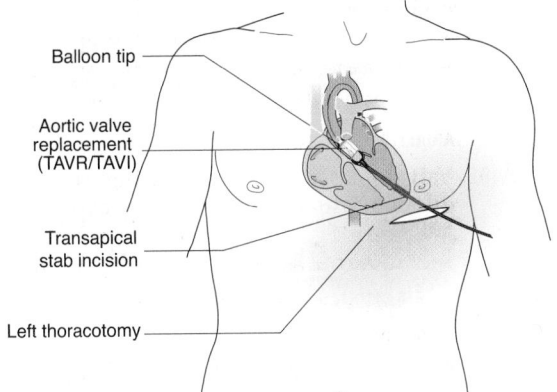

Balloon tip

Aortic valve replacement (TAVR/TAVI)

Transapical stab incision

Left thoracotomy

+ 33367 Transcatheter aortic valve replacement (TAVR/TAVI) with prosthetic valve; cardiopulmonary bypass support with percutaneous peripheral arterial and venous cannulation (eg, femoral vessels) (List separately in addition to code for primary procedure)   ⊘C

RVU			Global Days	Modifiers				
Mod	Non-Fac Total	Fac Total		51	50	62	80	MUE
	18.27	18.27	ZZZ	0	0	0	0	1

AMA: Jan 13: 6

● New   ▲ Revised   Deleted   ⊙ Moderate Sedation   ✚ Add-on Codes   ⊘ High Risk Denial   Ⓐ Age Edit   ♀ Female   ♂ Male   **AMA** *CPT® Assistant*   **MUE** Medically Unlikely Edit
⊘ Modifier 51 Exempt   ⊖ Modifier 63 Exempt   ✗ Unlisted   **Modifiers:** *See Inside Back Cover*   Ⓜ Maternity   A2–Z3 ASC Payment Indicators   A–Y OPPS Status Indicators

Surgical Procedures

33368 – 33415

+ 33368 Transcatheter aortic valve replacement (TAVR/TAVI) with prosthetic valve; cardiopulmonary bypass support with open peripheral arterial and venous cannulation (eg, femoral, iliac, axillary vessels) (List separately in addition to code for primary procedure) 🄲

RVU			Global Days	Modifiers				
Mod	Non-Fac Total	Fac Total		51	50	62	80	MUE
	21.91	21.91	ZZZ	0	0	0	0	1

AMA: Jan 13: 6

+ 33369 Transcatheter aortic valve replacement (TAVR/TAVI) with prosthetic valve; cardiopulmonary bypass support with central arterial and venous cannulation (eg, aorta, right atrium, pulmonary artery) (List separately in addition to code for primary procedure) ⊘🄲

RVU			Global Days	Modifiers				
Mod	Non-Fac Total	Fac Total		51	50	62	80	MUE
	28.95	28.95	ZZZ	0	0	0	0	1

AMA: Jan 13: 6

Cardiac Valve Procedures

33400 Valvuloplasty, aortic valve; open, with cardiopulmonary bypass 🄲

RVU			Global Days	Modifiers				
Mod	Non-Fac Total	Fac Total		51	50	62	80	MUE
	66.25	66.25	090	2	0	1	2	1

AMA: Feb 05: 14, Mar 07: 1

33401 Valvuloplasty, aortic valve; open, with inflow occlusion ⊖🄲

RVU			Global Days	Modifiers				
Mod	Non-Fac Total	Fac Total		51	50	62	80	MUE
	42.79	42.79	090	2	0	1	2	1

AMA: Feb 05: 14

33403 Valvuloplasty, aortic valve; using transventricular dilation, with cardiopulmonary bypass ⊖🄲

RVU			Global Days	Modifiers				
Mod	Non-Fac Total	Fac Total		51	50	62	80	MUE
	43.41	43.41	090	2	0	1	2	1

AMA: Feb 05: 14

33404 Construction of apical-aortic conduit 🄲

RVU			Global Days	Modifiers				
Mod	Non-Fac Total	Fac Total		51	50	62	80	MUE
	51.54	51.54	090	2	0	1	2	1

AMA: Jan 04: 28, Feb 05: 14

33405 Replacement, aortic valve, with cardiopulmonary bypass; with prosthetic valve other than homograft or stentless valve 🄲

RVU			Global Days	Modifiers				
Mod	Non-Fac Total	Fac Total		51	50	62	80	MUE
	66.10	66.10	090	2	0	1	2	1

AMA: Nov 99: 18, Feb 05: 14, Aug 11: 3, Jan 13: 6

33406 Replacement, aortic valve, with cardiopulmonary bypass; with allograft valve (freehand) 🄲

RVU			Global Days	Modifiers				
Mod	Non-Fac Total	Fac Total		51	50	62	80	MUE
	83.68	83.68	090	2	0	1	2	1

AMA: Nov 99: 18, Feb 05: 14, Aug 11: 3

33410 Replacement, aortic valve, with cardiopulmonary bypass; with stentless tissue valve 🄲

RVU			Global Days	Modifiers				
Mod	Non-Fac Total	Fac Total		51	50	62	80	MUE
	73.72	73.72	090	2	0	1	2	1

AMA: Nov 99: 18, Feb 05: 14, Aug 11: 3

33411 Replacement, aortic valve; with aortic annulus enlargement, noncoronary sinus 🄲

RVU			Global Days	Modifiers				
Mod	Non-Fac Total	Fac Total		51	50	62	80	MUE
	97.77	97.77	090	2	0	0	2	1

AMA: Feb 05: 14, Aug 11: 3

33412 Replacement, aortic valve; with transventricular aortic annulus enlargement (Konno procedure) 🄲

RVU			Global Days	Modifiers				
Mod	Non-Fac Total	Fac Total		51	50	62	80	MUE
	92.80	92.80	090	2	0	1	2	1

AMA: Feb 05: 14, Aug 11: 3

33413 Replacement, aortic valve; by translocation of autologous pulmonary valve with allograft replacement of pulmonary valve (Ross procedure) 🄲

RVU			Global Days	Modifiers				
Mod	Non-Fac Total	Fac Total		51	50	62	80	MUE
	95.20	95.20	090	2	0	1	2	1

AMA: Feb 05: 14, Aug 11: 3

Replacement, aortic valve; by translocation of autologous pulmonary valve

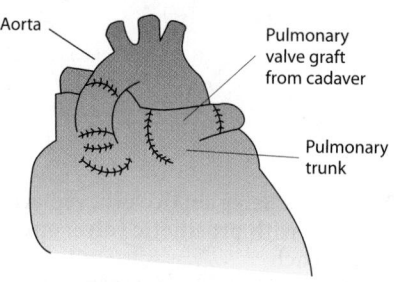

Aorta

Pulmonary valve graft from cadaver

Pulmonary trunk

A stenosed aortic valve is replaced by relocating the patient's pulmonary valve

33414 Repair of left ventricular outflow tract obstruction by patch enlargement of the outflow tract 🄲

RVU			Global Days	Modifiers				
Mod	Non-Fac Total	Fac Total		51	50	62	80	MUE
	62.91	62.91	090	2	0	1	2	1

AMA: Feb 05: 14

33415 Resection or incision of subvalvular tissue for discrete subvalvular aortic stenosis 🄲

RVU			Global Days	Modifiers				
Mod	Non-Fac Total	Fac Total		51	50	62	80	MUE
	58.87	58.87	090	2	0	1	2	1

AMA: Feb 05: 14

● New   ▲ Revised   ✖ Deleted   ⊙ Moderate Sedation   ✚ Add-on Codes   ⊘ High Risk Denial   Ⓐ Age Edit   ♀ Female   ♂ Male   **AMA** CPT® Assistant   **MUE** Medically Unlikely Edit
⊘ Modifier 51 Exempt   ⊖ Modifier 63 Exempt   ✖ Unlisted   **Modifiers:** See Inside Back Cover   Ⓜ Maternity   A2–Z3 ASC Payment Indicators   A–Y OPPS Status Indicators

CPT © 2015 American Medical Association. All Rights Reserved.   © 2016 DecisionHealth

33416 Ventriculomyotomy (-myectomy) for idiopathic hypertrophic subaortic stenosis (eg, asymmetric septal hypertrophy) [C]

RVU Mod	Non-Fac Total	Fac Total	Global Days	Modifiers 51	50	62	80	MUE
	59.05	59.05	090	2	0	1	2	1

AMA: Feb 05: 14

33417 Aortoplasty (gusset) for supravalvular stenosis [C]

RVU Mod	Non-Fac Total	Fac Total	Global Days	Modifiers 51	50	62	80	MUE
	48.84	48.84	090	2	0	1	2	1

AMA: Feb 05: 14

33418 Transcatheter mitral valve repair, percutaneous approach, including transseptal puncture when performed; initial prosthesis [C]

RVU Mod	Non-Fac Total	Fac Total	Global Days	Modifiers 51	50	62	80	MUE
	52.30	52.30	090	2	0	1	2	1

Pub 100-04, 32, 340, 340.2

Transcatheter mitral valve repair, percutaneous approach, including transseptal puncture

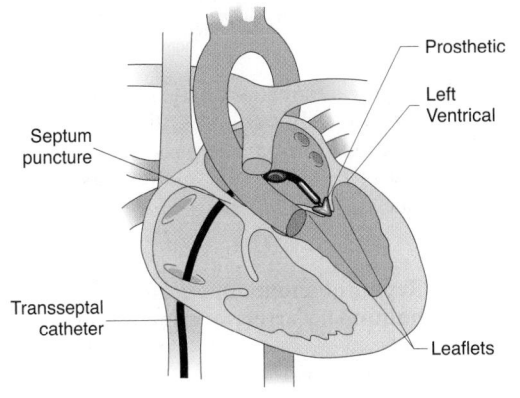

- Prosthetic
- Left Ventrical
- Septum puncture
- Transseptal catheter
- Leaflets

+ 33419 Transcatheter mitral valve repair, percutaneous approach, including transseptal puncture when performed; additional prosthesis(es) during same session (List separately in addition to code for primary procedure) [N] [I] [N]

RVU Mod	Non-Fac Total	Fac Total	Global Days	Modifiers 51	50	62	80	MUE
	12.31	12.31	ZZZ	0	0	1	2	1

Pub 100-04, 32, 340, 340.2

33420 Valvotomy, mitral valve; closed heart [C]

RVU Mod	Non-Fac Total	Fac Total	Global Days	Modifiers 51	50	62	80	MUE
	45.42	45.42	090	2	0	1	1	1

AMA: Feb 05: 14

33422 Valvotomy, mitral valve; open heart, with cardiopulmonary bypass [C]

RVU Mod	Non-Fac Total	Fac Total	Global Days	Modifiers 51	50	62	80	MUE
	48.81	48.81	090	2	0	1	2	1

AMA: Feb 05: 14

33425 Valvuloplasty, mitral valve, with cardiopulmonary bypass [C]

RVU Mod	Non-Fac Total	Fac Total	Global Days	Modifiers 51	50	62	80	MUE
	79.67	79.67	090	2	0	1	2	1

AMA: May 03: 19, Feb 05: 14

33426 Valvuloplasty, mitral valve, with cardiopulmonary bypass; with prosthetic ring [C]

RVU Mod	Non-Fac Total	Fac Total	Global Days	Modifiers 51	50	62	80	MUE
	69.34	69.34	090	2	0	1	2	1

AMA: Feb 05: 14

33427 Valvuloplasty, mitral valve, with cardiopulmonary bypass; radical reconstruction, with or without ring [C]

RVU Mod	Non-Fac Total	Fac Total	Global Days	Modifiers 51	50	62	80	MUE
	71.13	71.13	090	2	0	1	2	1

AMA: Feb 05: 14

33430 Replacement, mitral valve, with cardiopulmonary bypass [C]

RVU Mod	Non-Fac Total	Fac Total	Global Days	Modifiers 51	50	62	80	MUE
	81.56	81.56	090	2	0	1	2	1

AMA: Feb 05: 14

33460 Valvectomy, tricuspid valve, with cardiopulmonary bypass [C]

RVU Mod	Non-Fac Total	Fac Total	Global Days	Modifiers 51	50	62	80	MUE
	71.44	71.44	090	2	0	1	2	1

AMA: Feb 05: 14

33463 Valvuloplasty, tricuspid valve; without ring insertion [C]

RVU Mod	Non-Fac Total	Fac Total	Global Days	Modifiers 51	50	62	80	MUE
	90.21	90.21	090	2	0	1	2	1

AMA: Feb 05: 14

33464 Valvuloplasty, tricuspid valve; with ring insertion [C]

RVU Mod	Non-Fac Total	Fac Total	Global Days	Modifiers 51	50	62	80	MUE
	71.13	71.13	090	2	0	1	2	1

AMA: Feb 05: 14

33465 Replacement, tricuspid valve, with cardiopulmonary bypass [C]

RVU Mod	Non-Fac Total	Fac Total	Global Days	Modifiers 51	50	62	80	MUE
	80.47	80.47	090	2	0	1	2	1

AMA: Feb 05: 14

● New ▲ Revised Deleted ⊙ Moderate Sedation ✚ Add-on Codes ⊘ High Risk Denial Ⓐ Age Edit ♀ Female ♂ Male **AMA** *CPT Assistant* **MUE** Medically Unlikely Edit
⊘ Modifier 51 Exempt ⊖ Modifier 63 Exempt ✗ Unlisted **Modifiers:** *See Inside Back Cover* Ⓜ Maternity A2-Z3 ASC Payment Indicators A-Y OPPS Status Indicators
© 2016 DecisionHealth | CPT © 2015 American Medical Association. All Rights Reserved. | **355**

33468 Tricuspid valve repositioning and plication for Ebstein anomaly [C]

	RVU		Global Days	Modifiers				
Mod	Non-Fac Total	Fac Total		51	50	62	80	MUE
	71.74	71.74	090	2	0	1	2	1

AMA: Feb 05: 14

33470 Valvotomy, pulmonary valve, closed heart; transventricular ⊙⊖[C]

	RVU		Global Days	Modifiers				
Mod	Non-Fac Total	Fac Total		51	50	62	80	MUE
	37.82	37.82	090	2	0	0	2	1

AMA: Feb 05: 14

33471 Valvotomy, pulmonary valve, closed heart; via pulmonary artery [C]

	RVU		Global Days	Modifiers				
Mod	Non-Fac Total	Fac Total		51	50	62	80	MUE
	40.42	40.42	090	2	0	1	2	1

AMA: Feb 05: 14

33474 Valvotomy, pulmonary valve, open heart, with cardiopulmonary bypass [C]

	RVU		Global Days	Modifiers				
Mod	Non-Fac Total	Fac Total		51	50	62	80	MUE
	63.97	63.97	090	2	0	1	2	1

AMA: Feb 05: 14

33475 Replacement, pulmonary valve [C]

	RVU		Global Days	Modifiers				
Mod	Non-Fac Total	Fac Total		51	50	62	80	MUE
	67.96	67.96	090	2	0	1	2	1

AMA: Feb 05: 14

33476 Right ventricular resection for infundibular stenosis, with or without commissurotomy [C]

	RVU		Global Days	Modifiers				
Mod	Non-Fac Total	Fac Total		51	50	62	80	MUE
	44.79	44.79	090	2	0	1	2	1

AMA: Feb 05: 14

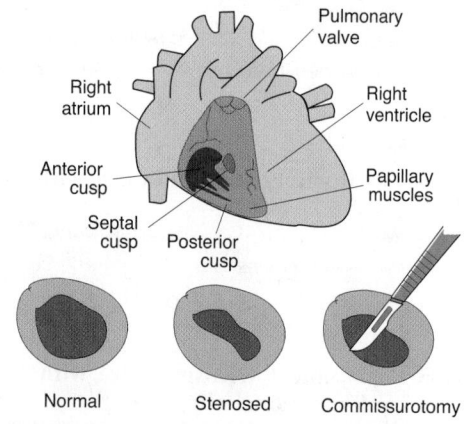

Right ventricular resection for infundibular stenosis

Pulmonary valve
Right atrium
Right ventricle
Anterior cusp
Papillary muscles
Septal cusp
Posterior cusp

Normal   Stenosed   Commissurotomy

Obstructed blood flow from the right ventricle is corrected

● 33477 Transcatheter pulmonary valve implantation, percutaneous approach, including pre-stenting of the valve delivery site, when performed [C]

	RVU		Global Days	Modifiers				
Mod	Non-Fac Total	Fac Total		51	50	62	80	MUE
	37.59	37.59	000	2	0	1	0	1

33478 Outflow tract augmentation (gusset), with or without commissurotomy or infundibular resection [C]

	RVU		Global Days	Modifiers				
Mod	Non-Fac Total	Fac Total		51	50	62	80	MUE
	45.86	45.86	090	2	0	1	2	1

AMA: Feb 05: 14

Other Valve Procedures

33496 Repair of non-structural prosthetic valve dysfunction with cardiopulmonary bypass (separate procedure) [C]

	RVU		Global Days	Modifiers				
Mod	Non-Fac Total	Fac Total		51	50	62	80	MUE
	48.92	48.92	090	2	0	1	2	1

AMA: Nov 97: 16, Feb 05: 14

Coronary Artery Aberration Procedures

33500 Repair of coronary arteriovenous or arteriocardiac chamber fistula; with cardiopulmonary bypass [C]

	RVU		Global Days	Modifiers				
Mod	Non-Fac Total	Fac Total		51	50	62	80	MUE
	45.75	45.75	090	2	0	1	2	1

33501 Repair of coronary arteriovenous or arteriocardiac chamber fistula; without cardiopulmonary bypass [C]

	RVU		Global Days	Modifiers				
Mod	Non-Fac Total	Fac Total		51	50	62	80	MUE
	33.16	33.16	090	2	0	2	2	1

33502 Repair of anomalous coronary artery from pulmonary artery origin; by ligation ⊖[C]

	RVU		Global Days	Modifiers				
Mod	Non-Fac Total	Fac Total		51	50	62	80	MUE
	37.25	37.25	090	2	0	1	2	1

33503 Repair of anomalous coronary artery from pulmonary artery origin; by graft, without cardiopulmonary bypass ⊖[C]

	RVU		Global Days	Modifiers				
Mod	Non-Fac Total	Fac Total		51	50	62	80	MUE
	39.02	39.02	090	2	0	1	0	1

33504 Repair of anomalous coronary artery from pulmonary artery origin; by graft, with cardiopulmonary bypass [C]

	RVU		Global Days	Modifiers				
Mod	Non-Fac Total	Fac Total		51	50	62	80	MUE
	43.42	43.42	090	2	0	1	2	1

33505 Repair of anomalous coronary artery from pulmonary artery origin; with construction of intrapulmonary artery tunnel (Takeuchi procedure) ⊖[C]

	RVU		Global Days	Modifiers				
Mod	Non-Fac Total	Fac Total		51	50	62	80	MUE
	60.73	60.73	090	2	0	1	2	1

● New　▲ Revised　✖ Deleted　⊙ Moderate Sedation　✚ Add-on Codes　⊖ High Risk Denial　Ⓐ Age Edit　♀ Female　♂ Male　**AMA** CPT® Assistant　**MUE** Medically Unlikely Edit
⊘ Modifier 51 Exempt　⊖ Modifier 63 Exempt　✗ Unlisted　**Modifiers:** See Inside Back Cover　Ⓜ Maternity　A2-Z3 ASC Payment Indicators　A-Y OPPS Status Indicators

CPT © 2015 American Medical Association. All Rights Reserved.

© 2016 DecisionHealth

33506 Repair of anomalous coronary artery from pulmonary artery origin; by translocation from pulmonary artery to aorta ⊖Ⓒ

RVU			Global Days	Modifiers				
Mod	Non-Fac Total	Fac Total		51	50	62	80	MUE
	61.39	61.39	090	2	0	1	2	1

33507 Repair of anomalous (eg, intramural) aortic origin of coronary artery by unroofing or translocation Ⓒ

RVU			Global Days	Modifiers				
Mod	Non-Fac Total	Fac Total		51	50	62	80	MUE
	50.31	50.31	090	2	0	1	2	1

AMA: Mar 07: 1

Endoscopic Vein Harvest

✚ **33508 Endoscopy, surgical, including video-assisted harvest of vein(s) for coronary artery bypass procedure (List separately in addition to code for primary procedure)** Ⓝ Ⓘ Ⓝ

RVU			Global Days	Modifiers				
Mod	Non-Fac Total	Fac Total		51	50	62	80	MUE
	0.46	0.46	ZZZ	0	0	1	2	1

Coronary Artery Bypass Venous Grafting

Coding Guidance

Ligation, division, and stripping of saphenous veins are not reported in addition to coronary artery bypass procedures 33510-33523, since the placement of a venous graft is integral to the bypass. If venous grafting alone is done, report only one code from 33510-33516.

33510 Coronary artery bypass, vein only; single coronary venous graft Ⓒ

RVU			Global Days	Modifiers				
Mod	Non-Fac Total	Fac Total		51	50	62	80	MUE
	56.08	56.08	090	2	0	0	2	1

AMA: Fall 91: 5, Winter 92: 12, Jul 99: 11, Apr 01: 7, Feb 05: 14, Jan 07: 7, Mar 07: 1, Aug 14: 14

Coronary artery bypass, vein only; single coronary venous graft

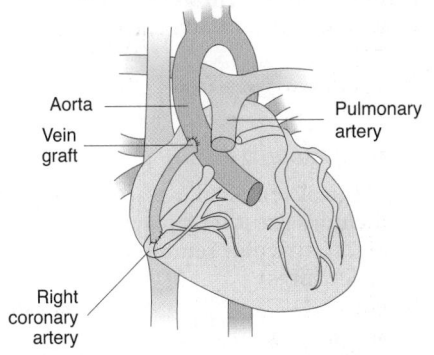

Aorta — Pulmonary artery
Vein graft
Right coronary artery

The heart is accessed by opening the sternum.

33511 Coronary artery bypass, vein only; 2 coronary venous grafts Ⓒ

RVU			Global Days	Modifiers				
Mod	Non-Fac Total	Fac Total		51	50	62	80	MUE
	61.76	61.76	090	2	0	0	2	1

AMA: Fall 91: 5, Winter 92: 12, Jul 99: 11, Apr 01: 7, Feb 05: 14, Jan 07: 7, Mar 07: 1

33512 Coronary artery bypass, vein only; 3 coronary venous grafts Ⓒ

RVU			Global Days	Modifiers				
Mod	Non-Fac Total	Fac Total		51	50	62	80	MUE
	70.30	70.30	090	2	0	0	2	1

AMA: Fall 91: 5, Winter 92: 12, Apr 01: 7, Feb 05: 14, Jan 07: 7, Mar 07: 1

33513 Coronary artery bypass, vein only; 4 coronary venous grafts Ⓒ

RVU			Global Days	Modifiers				
Mod	Non-Fac Total	Fac Total		51	50	62	80	MUE
	72.35	72.35	090	2	0	0	2	1

AMA: Fall 91: 5, Winter 92: 12, Apr 01: 7, Feb 05: 14, Jan 07: 7, Mar 07: 1

33514 Coronary artery bypass, vein only; 5 coronary venous grafts Ⓒ

RVU			Global Days	Modifiers				
Mod	Non-Fac Total	Fac Total		51	50	62	80	MUE
	76.19	76.19	090	2	0	0	2	1

AMA: Fall 91: 5, Winter 92: 12, Apr 01: 7, Feb 05: 14, Jan 07: 7, Mar 07: 1

33516 Coronary artery bypass, vein only; 6 or more coronary venous grafts Ⓒ

RVU			Global Days	Modifiers				
Mod	Non-Fac Total	Fac Total		51	50	62	80	MUE
	79.88	79.88	090	2	0	0	2	1

AMA: Fall 91: 5, Winter 92: 12, Jul 99: 11, Apr 01: 7, Feb 05: 14, Jan 07: 7, Mar 07: 1, Aug 14: 14

Coronary Artery Bypass Arterial-Venous Grafting

Coding Guidance

Combined arterial-venous grafting codes for coronary artery bypass cannot be reported alone. The most comprehensive code from the combined grafting group of bypass codes (33517-33523) must be reported together with one code from the group 33533-33536 for arterial grafting bypass.

✚ **33517 Coronary artery bypass, using venous graft(s) and arterial graft(s); single vein graft (List separately in addition to code for primary procedure)** Ⓒ

RVU			Global Days	Modifiers				
Mod	Non-Fac Total	Fac Total		51	50	62	80	MUE
	5.44	5.44	ZZZ	0	0	0	2	1

AMA: Fall 91: 5, Winter 92: 13, Nov 99: 18, Apr 01: 7, Feb 05: 14

Coronary artery bypass, using venous graft(s) and arterial graft(s)

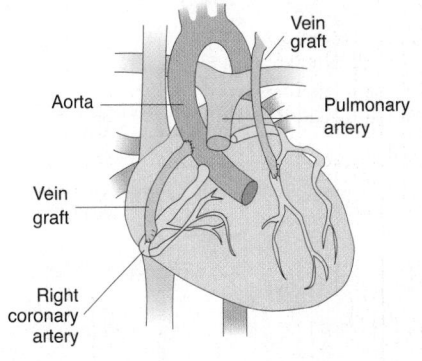

Vein graft
Aorta — Pulmonary artery
Vein graft
Right coronary artery

Coronary artery bypass graft (CABG) is performed using a combination of venous and arterial grafts

---

● New   ▲ Revised   Deleted   ⊙ Moderate Sedation   ✚ Add-on Codes   ⊘ High Risk Denial   Ⓐ Age Edit   ♀ Female   ♂ Male   **AMA** *CPT® Assistant*   **MUE** Medically Unlikely Edit
⊘ Modifier 51 Exempt   ⊖ Modifier 63 Exempt   ✗ Unlisted   **Modifiers:** *See Inside Back Cover*   Ⓜ Maternity   Ⓐ2–Ⓩ3 ASC Payment Indicators   Ⓐ–Ⓨ OPPS Status Indicators

✛ **33518** Coronary artery bypass, using venous graft(s) and arterial graft(s); 2 venous grafts (List separately in addition to code for primary procedure) **C**

RVU			Global Days	Modifiers				
Mod	Non-Fac Total	Fac Total		51	50	62	80	MUE
	11.94	11.94	ZZZ	0	0	0	2	1

AMA: Fall 91: 5, Winter 92: 13, Apr 01: 7, Feb 05: 14, Jan 07: 7, Mar 07: 1

✛ **33519** Coronary artery bypass, using venous graft(s) and arterial graft(s); 3 venous grafts (List separately in addition to code for primary procedure) **C**

RVU			Global Days	Modifiers				
Mod	Non-Fac Total	Fac Total		51	50	62	80	MUE
	15.75	15.75	ZZZ	0	0	0	2	1

AMA: Fall 91: 5, Winter 92: 13, Apr 01: 7, Feb 05: 14, Jan 07: 7, Mar 07: 1

✛ **33521** Coronary artery bypass, using venous graft(s) and arterial graft(s); 4 venous grafts (List separately in addition to code for primary procedure) **C**

RVU			Global Days	Modifiers				
Mod	Non-Fac Total	Fac Total		51	50	62	80	MUE
	18.85	18.85	ZZZ	0	0	0	2	1

AMA: Fall 91: 5, Winter 92: 13, Apr 01: 7, Feb 05: 14, Jan 07: 7, Mar 07: 1

✛ **33522** Coronary artery bypass, using venous graft(s) and arterial graft(s); 5 venous grafts (List separately in addition to code for primary procedure) **C**

RVU			Global Days	Modifiers				
Mod	Non-Fac Total	Fac Total		51	50	62	80	MUE
	21.18	21.18	ZZZ	0	0	0	2	1

AMA: Fall 91: 5, Winter 92: 13, Apr 01: 7, Feb 05: 14, Jan 07: 7, Mar 07: 1

✛ **33523** Coronary artery bypass, using venous graft(s) and arterial graft(s); 6 or more venous grafts (List separately in addition to code for primary procedure) **C**

RVU			Global Days	Modifiers				
Mod	Non-Fac Total	Fac Total		51	50	62	80	MUE
	24.20	24.20	ZZZ	0	0	0	2	1

AMA: Fall 91: 5, Winter 92: 13, Apr 01: 7, Feb 05: 14, Jan 07: 7, Mar 07: 1

✛ **33530** Reoperation, coronary artery bypass procedure or valve procedure, more than 1 month after original operation (List separately in addition to code for primary procedure) **C**

RVU			Global Days	Modifiers				
Mod	Non-Fac Total	Fac Total		51	50	62	80	MUE
	15.22	15.22	ZZZ	0	0	0	2	1

AMA: Winter 90: 6, Fall 91: 5, Winter 92: 13, Apr 01: 7, Jul 01: 11, Feb 05: 13, 14, Jan 07: 7, Feb 11: 8

Reoperation, coronary artery bypass procedure or valve procedure

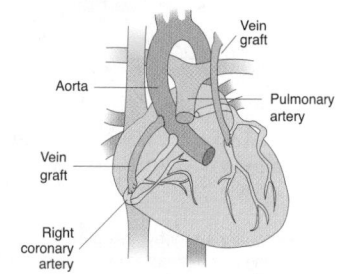

A previous coronary bypass procedure or valve operation is redone after a month has passed

Coronary Artery Bypass Arterial Grafting

Coding Guidance

When coronary artery bypass is done using arterial grafts alone, only the most comprehensive code from the arterial grafting group of bypass codes may be reported.

33533 Coronary artery bypass, using arterial graft(s); single arterial graft **C**

RVU			Global Days	Modifiers				
Mod	Non-Fac Total	Fac Total		51	50	62	80	MUE
	54.47	54.47	090	2	0	0	2	1

AMA: Winter 92: 12, Nov 99: 18, Apr 01: 7, Feb 05: 14, Jan 07: 7, Mar 07: 1, Nov 14: 14

33534 Coronary artery bypass, using arterial graft(s); 2 coronary arterial grafts **C**

RVU			Global Days	Modifiers				
Mod	Non-Fac Total	Fac Total		51	50	62	80	MUE
	63.99	63.99	090	2	0	0	2	1

AMA: Winter 92: 12, Apr 01: 7, Feb 05: 14, Jan 07: 7, Mar 07: 1

33535 Coronary artery bypass, using arterial graft(s); 3 coronary arterial grafts **C**

RVU			Global Days	Modifiers				
Mod	Non-Fac Total	Fac Total		51	50	62	80	MUE
	71.25	71.25	090	2	0	0	2	1

AMA: Winter 92: 12, Apr 01: 7, Feb 05: 14, Jan 07: 7, Mar 07: 1

33536 Coronary artery bypass, using arterial graft(s); 4 or more coronary arterial grafts **C**

RVU			Global Days	Modifiers				
Mod	Non-Fac Total	Fac Total		51	50	62	80	MUE
	76.72	76.72	090	2	0	0	2	1

AMA: Winter 92: 12, Apr 01: 7, Feb 05: 14, Jan 07: 7, Mar 07: 1, Nov 14: 14

33542 Myocardial resection (eg, ventricular aneurysmectomy) **C**

RVU			Global Days	Modifiers				
Mod	Non-Fac Total	Fac Total		51	50	62	80	MUE
	76.61	76.61	090	2	0	1	2	1

AMA: Winter 92: 12, Mar 07: 1

33545 Repair of postinfarction ventricular septal defect, with or without myocardial resection **C**

RVU			Global Days	Modifiers				
Mod	Non-Fac Total	Fac Total		51	50	62	80	MUE
	90.51	90.51	090	2	0	1	2	1

AMA: Winter 92: 12, Mar 07: 1

33548 Surgical ventricular restoration procedure, includes prosthetic patch, when performed (eg, ventricular remodeling, SVR, SAVER, Dor procedures) **C**

RVU			Global Days	Modifiers				
Mod	Non-Fac Total	Fac Total		51	50	62	80	MUE
	86.44	86.44	090	2	0	1	2	1

AMA: Nov 06: 21, Dec 06: 10, Mar 07: 1

● New   ▲ Revised   ✖ Deleted   ☉ Moderate Sedation   ✛ Add-on Codes   ⊘ High Risk Denial   Ⓐ Age Edit   ♀ Female   ♂ Male   **AMA** *CPT® Assistant*   **MUE** Medically Unlikely Edit

⊘ Modifier 51 Exempt   ⊖ Modifier 63 Exempt   ✗ Unlisted   **Modifiers:** *See Inside Back Cover*   Ⓜ Maternity   A2–Z3 ASC Payment Indicators   A–Y OPPS Status Indicators

CPT © 2015 American Medical Association. All Rights Reserved.   © 2016 DecisionHealth

Coronary Endarterectomy Procedures

✛ **33572** Coronary endarterectomy, open, any method, of left anterior descending, circumflex, or right coronary artery performed in conjunction with coronary artery bypass graft procedure, each vessel (List separately in addition to primary procedure) ⓒ

RVU			Global Days	Modifiers				
Mod	Non-Fac Total	Fac Total		51	50	62	80	MUE
	6.61	6.61	ZZZ	0	0	0	2	3

Ventricle/Complex Cardiac Anomaly Procedures

33600 Closure of atrioventricular valve (mitral or tricuspid) by suture or patch ⓒ

RVU			Global Days	Modifiers				
Mod	Non-Fac Total	Fac Total		51	50	62	80	MUE
	50.14	50.14	090	2	0	1	2	1

AMA: Mar 07: 1

33602 Closure of semilunar valve (aortic or pulmonary) by suture or patch ⓒ

RVU			Global Days	Modifiers				
Mod	Non-Fac Total	Fac Total		51	50	62	80	MUE
	49.48	49.48	090	2	0	1	2	1

33606 Anastomosis of pulmonary artery to aorta (Damus-Kaye-Stansel procedure) ⓒ

RVU			Global Days	Modifiers				
Mod	Non-Fac Total	Fac Total		51	50	62	80	MUE
	54.54	54.54	090	2	0	1	2	1

Anastomosis of pulmonary artery to aorta

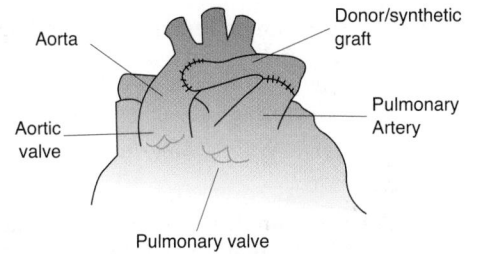

The aorta and pulmonary artery are connected in an end to side anastomosis

33608 Repair of complex cardiac anomaly other than pulmonary atresia with ventricular septal defect by construction or replacement of conduit from right or left ventricle to pulmonary artery ⒶⒸ

RVU			Global Days	Modifiers				
Mod	Non-Fac Total	Fac Total		51	50	62	80	MUE
	52.62	52.62	090	2	0	1	2	1

33610 Repair of complex cardiac anomalies (eg, single ventricle with subaortic obstruction) by surgical enlargement of ventricular septal defect Ⓐ⊖Ⓒ

RVU			Global Days	Modifiers				
Mod	Non-Fac Total	Fac Total		51	50	62	80	MUE
	55.67	55.67	090	2	0	1	2	1

33611 Repair of double outlet right ventricle with intraventricular tunnel repair Ⓐ⊖Ⓒ

RVU			Global Days	Modifiers				
Mod	Non-Fac Total	Fac Total		51	50	62	80	MUE
	60.23	60.23	090	2	0	1	2	1

33612 Repair of double outlet right ventricle with intraventricular tunnel repair; with repair of right ventricular outflow tract obstruction ⒶⒸ

RVU			Global Days	Modifiers				
Mod	Non-Fac Total	Fac Total		51	50	62	80	MUE
	58.98	58.98	090	2	0	1	2	1

33615 Repair of complex cardiac anomalies (eg, tricuspid atresia) by closure of atrial septal defect and anastomosis of atria or vena cava to pulmonary artery (simple Fontan procedure) ⒶⒸ

RVU			Global Days	Modifiers				
Mod	Non-Fac Total	Fac Total		51	50	62	80	MUE
	59.71	59.71	090	2	0	1	2	1

33617 Repair of complex cardiac anomalies (eg, single ventricle) by modified Fontan procedure ⓒ

RVU			Global Days	Modifiers				
Mod	Non-Fac Total	Fac Total		51	50	62	80	MUE
	63.27	63.27	090	2	0	1	2	1

33619 Repair of single ventricle with aortic outflow obstruction and aortic arch hypoplasia (hypoplastic left heart syndrome) (eg, Norwood procedure) Ⓐ⊖Ⓒ

RVU			Global Days	Modifiers				
Mod	Non-Fac Total	Fac Total		51	50	62	80	MUE
	80.23	80.23	090	2	0	1	2	1

AMA: Mar 07: 1, Apr 11: 6, May 12: 14

33620 Application of right and left pulmonary artery bands (eg, hybrid approach stage 1) ⓒ

RVU			Global Days	Modifiers				
Mod	Non-Fac Total	Fac Total		51	50	62	80	MUE
	45.13	45.13	090	2	0	1	2	1

AMA: Apr 11: 3, May 12: 14

33621 Transthoracic insertion of catheter for stent placement with catheter removal and closure (eg, hybrid approach stage 1) ⊘Ⓒ

RVU			Global Days	Modifiers				
Mod	Non-Fac Total	Fac Total		51	50	62	80	MUE
	27.39	27.39	090	2	0	1	2	1

AMA: Apr 11: 3

● New ▲ Revised Deleted ⊙ Moderate Sedation ✛ Add-on Codes ⊘ High Risk Denial Ⓐ Age Edit ♀ Female ♂ Male **AMA** *CPT® Assistant* **MUE** Medically Unlikely Edit
⊘ Modifier 51 Exempt ⊖ Modifier 63 Exempt ✗ Unlisted **Modifiers:** *See Inside Back Cover* Ⓜ Maternity A2-Z3 ASC Payment Indicators A-Y OPPS Status Indicators

33622 Reconstruction of complex cardiac anomaly (eg, single ventricle or hypoplastic left heart) with palliation of single ventricle with aortic outflow obstruction and aortic arch hypoplasia, creation of cavopulmonary anastomosis, and removal of right and left pulmonary bands (eg, hybrid approach stage 2, Norwood, bidirectional Glenn, pulmonary artery debanding)   C

RVU			Global Days	Modifiers				
Mod	Non-Fac Total	Fac Total		51	50	62	80	MUE
	106.42	106.42	090	2	0	1	2	1

AMA: Apr 11: 3, May 12: 14

Reconstruction of complex cardiac anomaly (hybrid approach stage 2)

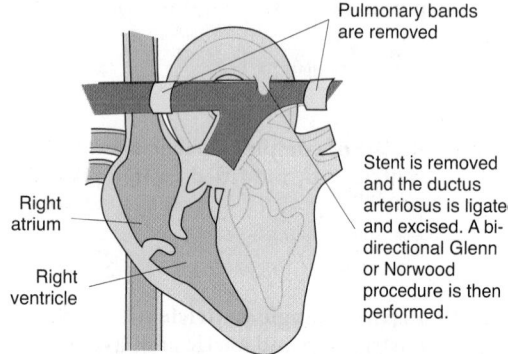

Pulmonary bands are removed

Right atrium

Right ventricle

Stent is removed and the ductus arteriosus is ligated and excised. A bi-directional Glenn or Norwood procedure is then performed.

Stage 2 of a cardiac anomaly reconstruction is completed through a median sternotomy

Septal Defect Procedures

33641 Repair atrial septal defect, secundum, with cardiopulmonary bypass, with or without patch C

RVU			Global Days	Modifiers				
Mod	Non-Fac Total	Fac Total		51	50	62	80	MUE
	48.16	48.16	090	2	0	1	2	1

AMA: Mar 07: 1, Dec 10: 12

33645 Direct or patch closure, sinus venosus, with or without anomalous pulmonary venous drainage C

RVU			Global Days	Modifiers				
Mod	Non-Fac Total	Fac Total		51	50	62	80	MUE
	50.68	50.68	090	2	0	1	2	1

33647 Repair of atrial septal defect and ventricular septal defect, with direct or patch closure ⊖C

RVU			Global Days	Modifiers				
Mod	Non-Fac Total	Fac Total		51	50	62	80	MUE
	53.72	53.72	090	2	0	1	2	1

33660 Repair of incomplete or partial atrioventricular canal (ostium primum atrial septal defect), with or without atrioventricular valve repair C

RVU			Global Days	Modifiers				
Mod	Non-Fac Total	Fac Total		51	50	62	80	MUE
	50.83	50.83	090	2	0	1	2	1

33665 Repair of intermediate or transitional atrioventricular canal, with or without atrioventricular valve repair ⊖C

RVU			Global Days	Modifiers				
Mod	Non-Fac Total	Fac Total		51	50	62	80	MUE
	56.01	56.01	090	2	0	1	2	1

33670 Repair of complete atrioventricular canal, with or without prosthetic valve ⊖C

RVU			Global Days	Modifiers				
Mod	Non-Fac Total	Fac Total		51	50	62	80	MUE
	58.05	58.05	090	2	0	1	2	1

33675 Closure of multiple ventricular septal defects C

RVU			Global Days	Modifiers				
Mod	Non-Fac Total	Fac Total		51	50	62	80	MUE
	57.78	57.78	090	2	0	1	2	1

AMA: Mar 07: 1

33676 Closure of multiple ventricular septal defects; with pulmonary valvotomy or infundibular resection (acyanotic) C

RVU			Global Days	Modifiers				
Mod	Non-Fac Total	Fac Total		51	50	62	80	MUE
	62.49	62.49	090	2	0	1	2	1

AMA: Mar 07: 1

33677 Closure of multiple ventricular septal defects; with removal of pulmonary artery band, with or without gusset C

RVU			Global Days	Modifiers				
Mod	Non-Fac Total	Fac Total		51	50	62	80	MUE
	64.93	64.93	090	2	0	1	2	1

AMA: Mar 07: 1

33681 Closure of single ventricular septal defect, with or without patch C

RVU			Global Days	Modifiers				
Mod	Non-Fac Total	Fac Total		51	50	62	80	MUE
	53.91	53.91	090	2	0	1	2	1

AMA: Mar 07: 1

33684 Closure of single ventricular septal defect, with or without patch; with pulmonary valvotomy or infundibular resection (acyanotic) ⊗C

RVU			Global Days	Modifiers				
Mod	Non-Fac Total	Fac Total		51	50	62	80	MUE
	58.27	58.27	090	2	0	1	2	1

33688 Closure of single ventricular septal defect, with or without patch; with removal of pulmonary artery band, with or without gusset C

RVU			Global Days	Modifiers				
Mod	Non-Fac Total	Fac Total		51	50	62	80	MUE
	55.24	55.24	090	2	0	1	2	1

● New   ▲ Revised   ✖ Deleted   ⊙ Moderate Sedation   ✚ Add-on Codes   ⊗ High Risk Denial   Ⓐ Age Edit   ♀ Female   ♂ Male   **AMA** CPT® Assistant   **MUE** Medically Unlikely Edit
⊘ Modifier 51 Exempt   ⊖ Modifier 63 Exempt   ✗ Unlisted   **Modifiers:** See Inside Back Cover   Ⓜ Maternity   A2–Z3 ASC Payment Indicators   A–Y OPPS Status Indicators

CPT © 2015 American Medical Association. All Rights Reserved.   © 2016 DecisionHealth

33690 Banding of pulmonary artery ⊖C

Mod	Non-Fac Total	Fac Total	Global Days	51	50	62	80	MUE
	32.48	32.48	090	2	0	1	2	1

AMA: Apr 11: 4, May 12: 14

Banding of pulmonary artery

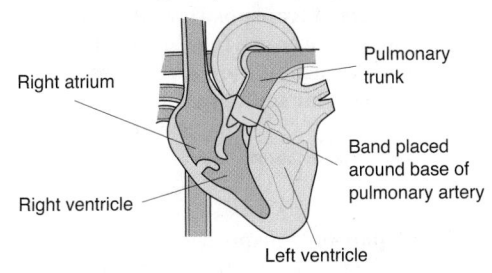

Right atrium
Pulmonary trunk
Band placed around base of pulmonary artery
Right ventricle
Left ventricle

Pulmonary artery banding (PAB) is performed as an initial staged intervention for cardiac defects with left-to-right shunting to control pulmonary overcirculation

33692 Complete repair tetralogy of Fallot without pulmonary atresia ⒶC

Mod	Non-Fac Total	Fac Total	Global Days	51	50	62	80	MUE
	60.56	60.56	090	2	0	1	2	1

33694 Complete repair tetralogy of Fallot without pulmonary atresia; with transannular patch Ⓐ⊖C

Mod	Non-Fac Total	Fac Total	Global Days	51	50	62	80	MUE
	60.23	60.23	090	2	0	1	2	1

33697 Complete repair tetralogy of Fallot with pulmonary atresia including construction of conduit from right ventricle to pulmonary artery and closure of ventricular septal defect ⒶC

Mod	Non-Fac Total	Fac Total	Global Days	51	50	62	80	MUE
	61.18	61.18	090	2	0	1	2	1

AMA: Mar 07: 1

Sinus of Valsalva Procedures

33702 Repair sinus of Valsalva fistula, with cardiopulmonary bypass C

Mod	Non-Fac Total	Fac Total	Global Days	51	50	62	80	MUE
	45.21	45.21	090	2	0	1	2	1

AMA: Mar 07: 1

33710 Repair sinus of Valsalva fistula, with cardiopulmonary bypass; with repair of ventricular septal defect C

Mod	Non-Fac Total	Fac Total	Global Days	51	50	62	80	MUE
	63.36	63.36	090	2	0	0	2	1

33720 Repair sinus of Valsalva aneurysm, with cardiopulmonary bypass C

Mod	Non-Fac Total	Fac Total	Global Days	51	50	62	80	MUE
	45.52	45.52	090	2	0	1	2	1

33722 Closure of aortico-left ventricular tunnel C

Mod	Non-Fac Total	Fac Total	Global Days	51	50	62	80	MUE
	49.67	49.67	090	2	0	1	2	1

AMA: Mar 07: 1

Venous Anomaly Procedures

33724 Repair of isolated partial anomalous pulmonary venous return (eg, Scimitar Syndrome) C

Mod	Non-Fac Total	Fac Total	Global Days	51	50	62	80	MUE
	45.21	45.21	090	2	0	1	2	1

AMA: Mar 07: 1

33726 Repair of pulmonary venous stenosis C

Mod	Non-Fac Total	Fac Total	Global Days	51	50	62	80	MUE
	58.61	58.61	090	2	0	1	2	1

AMA: Mar 07: 1

33730 Complete repair of anomalous pulmonary venous return (supracardiac, intracardiac, or infracardiac types) ⊖C

Mod	Non-Fac Total	Fac Total	Global Days	51	50	62	80	MUE
	60.12	60.12	090	2	0	1	2	1

AMA: Mar 07: 1

33732 Repair of cor triatriatum or supravalvular mitral ring by resection of left atrial membrane ⊖C

Mod	Non-Fac Total	Fac Total	Global Days	51	50	62	80	MUE
	48.49	48.49	090	2	0	1	2	1

AMA: Mar 07: 1

Shunt Procedures

33735 Atrial septectomy or septostomy; closed heart (Blalock-Hanlon type operation) ⊖C

Mod	Non-Fac Total	Fac Total	Global Days	51	50	62	80	MUE
	37.66	37.66	090	2	0	0	2	1

AMA: Mar 07: 1

33736 Atrial septectomy or septostomy; open heart with cardiopulmonary bypass ⊖C

Mod	Non-Fac Total	Fac Total	Global Days	51	50	62	80	MUE
	41.09	41.09	090	2	0	1	2	1

33737 Atrial septectomy or septostomy; open heart, with inflow occlusion C

Mod	Non-Fac Total	Fac Total	Global Days	51	50	62	80	MUE
	39.63	39.63	090	2	0	1	2	1

33750 Shunt; subclavian to pulmonary artery (Blalock-Taussig type operation) ⊖C

Mod	Non-Fac Total	Fac Total	Global Days	51	50	62	80	MUE
	36.93	36.93	090	2	0	1	2	1

● New ▲ Revised Deleted ⊙ Moderate Sedation ✚ Add-on Codes ⊘ High Risk Denial Ⓐ Age Edit ♀ Female ♂ Male **AMA** CPT® Assistant **MUE** Medically Unlikely Edit
⊘ Modifier 51 Exempt ⊖ Modifier 63 Exempt ✗ Unlisted **Modifiers:** See Inside Back Cover Ⓜ Maternity A2–Z3 ASC Payment Indicators A–Y OPPS Status Indicators

Surgical Procedures

33690 – 33750

Surgical Procedures

33755 – 33782

33755 Shunt; ascending aorta to pulmonary artery (Waterston type operation) ⊖ C

Mod	RVU		Global Days	Modifiers				
	Non-Fac Total	Fac Total		51	50	62	80	MUE
	38.47	38.47	090	2	0	1	2	1

33762 Shunt; descending aorta to pulmonary artery (Potts-Smith type operation) ⊘ ⊖ C

Mod	RVU		Global Days	Modifiers				
	Non-Fac Total	Fac Total		51	50	62	80	MUE
	39.28	39.28	090	2	0	1	2	1

33764 Shunt; central, with prosthetic graft C

Mod	RVU		Global Days	Modifiers				
	Non-Fac Total	Fac Total		51	50	62	80	MUE
	38.73	38.73	090	2	0	1	2	1

33766 Shunt; superior vena cava to pulmonary artery for flow to 1 lung (classical Glenn procedure) C

Mod	RVU		Global Days	Modifiers				
	Non-Fac Total	Fac Total		51	50	62	80	MUE
	38.83	38.83	090	2	0	1	2	1

33767 Shunt; superior vena cava to pulmonary artery for flow to both lungs (bidirectional Glenn procedure) C

Mod	RVU		Global Days	Modifiers				
	Non-Fac Total	Fac Total		51	50	62	80	MUE
	41.87	41.87	090	2	0	1	2	1

AMA: Apr 11: 6

+ 33768 Anastomosis, cavopulmonary, second superior vena cava (List separately in addition to primary procedure) C

Mod	RVU		Global Days	Modifiers				
	Non-Fac Total	Fac Total		51	50	62	80	MUE
	12.21	12.21	ZZZ	0	0	2	2	1

AMA: Mar 07: 1, Apr 11: 6

Great Vessel Transposition Procedures

33770 Repair of transposition of the great arteries with ventricular septal defect and subpulmonary stenosis; without surgical enlargement of ventricular septal defect Ⓐ C

Mod	RVU		Global Days	Modifiers				
	Non-Fac Total	Fac Total		51	50	62	80	MUE
	65.49	65.49	090	2	0	1	2	1

AMA: Mar 07: 1

33771 Repair of transposition of the great arteries with ventricular septal defect and subpulmonary stenosis; with surgical enlargement of ventricular septal defect Ⓐ C

Mod	RVU		Global Days	Modifiers				
	Non-Fac Total	Fac Total		51	50	62	80	MUE
	67.53	67.53	090	2	0	1	2	1

33774 Repair of transposition of the great arteries, atrial baffle procedure (eg, Mustard or Senning type) with cardiopulmonary bypass Ⓐ C

Mod	RVU		Global Days	Modifiers				
	Non-Fac Total	Fac Total		51	50	62	80	MUE
	52.95	52.95	090	2	0	1	2	1

33775 Repair of transposition of the great arteries, atrial baffle procedure (eg, Mustard or Senning type) with cardiopulmonary bypass; with removal of pulmonary band ⊘ Ⓐ C

Mod	RVU		Global Days	Modifiers				
	Non-Fac Total	Fac Total		51	50	62	80	MUE
	56.90	56.90	090	2	0	0	2	1

33776 Repair of transposition of the great arteries, atrial baffle procedure (eg, Mustard or Senning type) with cardiopulmonary bypass; with closure of ventricular septal defect Ⓐ C

Mod	RVU		Global Days	Modifiers				
	Non-Fac Total	Fac Total		51	50	62	80	MUE
	60.10	60.10	090	2	0	1	2	1

33777 Repair of transposition of the great arteries, atrial baffle procedure (eg, Mustard or Senning type) with cardiopulmonary bypass; with repair of subpulmonic obstruction Ⓐ C

Mod	RVU		Global Days	Modifiers				
	Non-Fac Total	Fac Total		51	50	62	80	MUE
	58.24	58.24	090	2	0	0	2	1

33778 Repair of transposition of the great arteries, aortic pulmonary artery reconstruction (eg, Jatene type) Ⓐ ⊖ C

Mod	RVU		Global Days	Modifiers				
	Non-Fac Total	Fac Total		51	50	62	80	MUE
	72.45	72.45	090	2	0	1	2	1

33779 Repair of transposition of the great arteries, aortic pulmonary artery reconstruction (eg, Jatene type); with removal of pulmonary band Ⓐ C

Mod	RVU		Global Days	Modifiers				
	Non-Fac Total	Fac Total		51	50	62	80	MUE
	72.06	72.06	090	2	0	1	2	1

33780 Repair of transposition of the great arteries, aortic pulmonary artery reconstruction (eg, Jatene type); with closure of ventricular septal defect Ⓐ C

Mod	RVU		Global Days	Modifiers				
	Non-Fac Total	Fac Total		51	50	62	80	MUE
	69.78	69.78	090	2	0	1	2	1

33781 Repair of transposition of the great arteries, aortic pulmonary artery reconstruction (eg, Jatene type); with repair of subpulmonic obstruction Ⓐ C

Mod	RVU		Global Days	Modifiers				
	Non-Fac Total	Fac Total		51	50	62	80	MUE
	71.74	71.74	090	2	0	0	2	1

AMA: Mar 07: 1

33782 Aortic root translocation with ventricular septal defect and pulmonary stenosis repair (ie, Nikaidoh procedure); without coronary ostium reimplantation Ⓐ C

Mod	RVU		Global Days	Modifiers				
	Non-Fac Total	Fac Total		51	50	62	80	MUE
	95.12	95.12	090	2	0	1	2	1

● New   ▲ Revised   ✖ Deleted   ⊙ Moderate Sedation   ✚ Add-on Codes   ⊘ High Risk Denial   Ⓐ Age Edit   ♀ Female   ♂ Male   **AMA** *CPT® Assistant*   **MUE** Medically Unlikely Edit
⊘ Modifier 51 Exempt   ⊖ Modifier 63 Exempt   ✗ Unlisted   **Modifiers:** *See Inside Back Cover*   Ⓜ Maternity   A2-Z3 ASC Payment Indicators   A-Y OPPS Status Indicators

362   CPT © 2015 American Medical Association. All Rights Reserved.   © 2016 DecisionHealth

33783 Aortic root translocation with ventricular septal defect and pulmonary stenosis repair (ie, Nikaidoh procedure); with reimplantation of 1 or both coronary ostia Ⓐ©

Mod	Non-Fac Total	Fac Total	Global Days	Modifiers 51	50	62	80	MUE
	108.17	108.17	090	2	0	1	2	1

Truncus Arteriosus Procedures

33786 Total repair, truncus arteriosus (Rastelli type operation) ⊖©

Mod	Non-Fac Total	Fac Total	Global Days	Modifiers 51	50	62	80	MUE
	67.01	67.01	090	2	0	1	2	1

AMA: Mar 07: 1

33788 Reimplantation of an anomalous pulmonary artery ©

Mod	Non-Fac Total	Fac Total	Global Days	Modifiers 51	50	62	80	MUE
	47.10	47.10	090	2	0	1	2	1

AMA: Mar 07: 1

Aorta Anomaly Procedures

33800 Aortic suspension (aortopexy) for tracheal decompression (eg, for tracheomalacia) (separate procedure) ©

Mod	Non-Fac Total	Fac Total	Global Days	Modifiers 51	50	62	80	MUE
	27.78	27.78	090	2	0	2	2	1

AMA: Mar 07: 1

33802 Division of aberrant vessel (vascular ring) ©

Mod	Non-Fac Total	Fac Total	Global Days	Modifiers 51	50	62	80	MUE
	31.55	31.55	090	2	0	1	2	1

33803 Division of aberrant vessel (vascular ring); with reanastomosis ©

Mod	Non-Fac Total	Fac Total	Global Days	Modifiers 51	50	62	80	MUE
	33.65	33.65	090	2	0	1	2	1

33813 Obliteration of aortopulmonary septal defect; without cardiopulmonary bypass ©

Mod	Non-Fac Total	Fac Total	Global Days	Modifiers 51	50	62	80	MUE
	37.83	37.83	090	2	0	1	2	1

33814 Obliteration of aortopulmonary septal defect; with cardiopulmonary bypass ©

Mod	Non-Fac Total	Fac Total	Global Days	Modifiers 51	50	62	80	MUE
	46.89	46.89	090	2	0	1	2	1

33820 Repair of patent ductus arteriosus; by ligation ©

Mod	Non-Fac Total	Fac Total	Global Days	Modifiers 51	50	62	80	MUE
	28.48	28.48	090	2	0	0	2	1

AMA: Mar 07: 1

33822 Repair of patent ductus arteriosus; by division, younger than 18 years Ⓐ©

Mod	Non-Fac Total	Fac Total	Global Days	Modifiers 51	50	62	80	MUE
	31.21	31.21	090	2	0	1	2	1

AMA: Mar 07: 1, Apr 11: 6

33824 Repair of patent ductus arteriosus; by division, 18 years and older Ⓐ©

Mod	Non-Fac Total	Fac Total	Global Days	Modifiers 51	50	62	80	MUE
	35.60	35.60	090	2	0	1	2	1

33840 Excision of coarctation of aorta, with or without associated patent ductus arteriosus; with direct anastomosis ©

Mod	Non-Fac Total	Fac Total	Global Days	Modifiers 51	50	62	80	MUE
	37.70	37.70	090	2	0	1	2	1

AMA: Apr 11: 6

33845 Excision of coarctation of aorta, with or without associated patent ductus arteriosus; with graft ©

Mod	Non-Fac Total	Fac Total	Global Days	Modifiers 51	50	62	80	MUE
	38.97	38.97	090	2	0	1	2	1

AMA: Apr 11: 6

33851 Excision of coarctation of aorta, with or without associated patent ductus arteriosus; repair using either left subclavian artery or prosthetic material as gusset for enlargement ©

Mod	Non-Fac Total	Fac Total	Global Days	Modifiers 51	50	62	80	MUE
	33.85	33.85	090	2	0	1	2	1

AMA: Apr 11: 6

33852 Repair of hypoplastic or interrupted aortic arch using autogenous or prosthetic material; without cardiopulmonary bypass ©

Mod	Non-Fac Total	Fac Total	Global Days	Modifiers 51	50	62	80	MUE
	41.15	41.15	090	2	0	0	2	1

33853 Repair of hypoplastic or interrupted aortic arch using autogenous or prosthetic material; with cardiopulmonary bypass ©

Mod	Non-Fac Total	Fac Total	Global Days	Modifiers 51	50	62	80	MUE
	53.94	53.94	090	2	0	1	2	1

AMA: Mar 07: 1, Apr 11: 6

Thoracic Aorta Aneurysm Procedures

33860 Ascending aorta graft, with cardiopulmonary bypass, includes valve suspension, when performed ©

Mod	Non-Fac Total	Fac Total	Global Days	Modifiers 51	50	62	80	MUE
	93.53	93.53	090	2	0	1	2	1

AMA: Mar 07: 1, Aug 11: 3

● New   ▲ Revised   Deleted   ⊙ Moderate Sedation   ✚ Add-on Codes   ⊘ High Risk Denial   Ⓐ Age Edit   ♀ Female   ♂ Male   **AMA** CPT® Assistant   **MUE** Medically Unlikely Edit
⊘ Modifier 51 Exempt   ⊖ Modifier 63 Exempt   ✗ Unlisted   **Modifiers:** See Inside Back Cover   Ⓜ Maternity   Ⓐ2–Z3 ASC Payment Indicators   Ⓐ–Ⓨ OPPS Status Indicators

33863 Ascending aorta graft, with cardiopulmonary bypass, with aortic root replacement using valved conduit and coronary reconstruction (eg, Bentall) Ⓒ

Mod	Non-Fac Total	Fac Total	Global Days	Modifiers 51	50	62	80	MUE
	91.75	91.75	090	2	0	1	2	1

AMA: Feb 05: 14, Mar 07: 1, Aug 11: 3

33864 Ascending aorta graft, with cardiopulmonary bypass with valve suspension, with coronary reconstruction and valve-sparing aortic root remodeling (eg, David Procedure, Yacoub Procedure) Ⓒ

Mod	Non-Fac Total	Fac Total	Global Days	Modifiers 51	50	62	80	MUE
	93.82	93.82	090	2	0	1	2	1

AMA: Aug 11: 3

33870 Transverse arch graft, with cardiopulmonary bypass Ⓒ

Mod	Non-Fac Total	Fac Total	Global Days	Modifiers 51	50	62	80	MUE
	73.32	73.32	090	2	0	1	2	1

Transverse arch graft

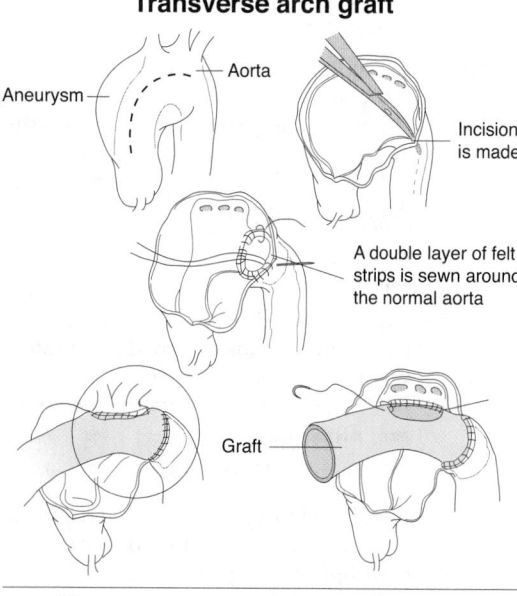

Aneurysm — Aorta — Incision is made — A double layer of felt strips is sewn around the normal aorta — Graft

33875 Descending thoracic aorta graft, with or without bypass Ⓒ

Mod	Non-Fac Total	Fac Total	Global Days	Modifiers 51	50	62	80	MUE
	80.36	80.36	090	2	0	2	2	1

33877 Repair of thoracoabdominal aortic aneurysm with graft, with or without cardiopulmonary bypass Ⓒ

Mod	Non-Fac Total	Fac Total	Global Days	Modifiers 51	50	62	80	MUE
	106.56	106.56	090	2	0	2	2	1

Descending Thoracic Aorta Endovascular Repair

33880 Endovascular repair of descending thoracic aorta (eg, aneurysm, pseudoaneurysm, dissection, penetrating ulcer, intramural hematoma, or traumatic disruption); involving coverage of left subclavian artery origin, initial endoprosthesis plus descending thoracic aortic extension(s), if required, to level of celiac artery origin Ⓒ

Mod	Non-Fac Total	Fac Total	Global Days	Modifiers 51	50	62	80	MUE
	52.97	52.97	090	2	2	2	2	1

33881 Endovascular repair of descending thoracic aorta (eg, aneurysm, pseudoaneurysm, dissection, penetrating ulcer, intramural hematoma, or traumatic disruption); not involving coverage of left subclavian artery origin, initial endoprosthesis plus descending thoracic aortic extension(s), if required, to level of celiac artery origin Ⓒ

Mod	Non-Fac Total	Fac Total	Global Days	Modifiers 51	50	62	80	MUE
	45.48	45.48	090	2	2	2	2	1

33883 Placement of proximal extension prosthesis for endovascular repair of descending thoracic aorta (eg, aneurysm, pseudoaneurysm, dissection, penetrating ulcer, intramural hematoma, or traumatic disruption); initial extension Ⓒ

Mod	Non-Fac Total	Fac Total	Global Days	Modifiers 51	50	62	80	MUE
	32.90	32.90	090	2	0	2	2	1

+ 33884 Placement of proximal extension prosthesis for endovascular repair of descending thoracic aorta (eg, aneurysm, pseudoaneurysm, dissection, penetrating ulcer, intramural hematoma, or traumatic disruption); each additional proximal extension (List separately in addition to code for primary procedure) Ⓒ

Mod	Non-Fac Total	Fac Total	Global Days	Modifiers 51	50	62	80	MUE
	12.02	12.02	ZZZ	0	0	2	2	2

33886 Placement of distal extension prosthesis(s) delayed after endovascular repair of descending thoracic aorta Ⓒ

Mod	Non-Fac Total	Fac Total	Global Days	Modifiers 51	50	62	80	MUE
	28.43	28.43	090	2	0	2	2	1

33889 Open subclavian to carotid artery transposition performed in conjunction with endovascular repair of descending thoracic aorta, by neck incision, unilateral Ⓒ

Mod	Non-Fac Total	Fac Total	Global Days	Modifiers 51	50	62	80	MUE
	23.24	23.24	000	2	1	2	2	1

● New   ▲ Revised   ✖ Deleted   ⊙ Moderate Sedation   ✚ Add-on Codes   ⊘ High Risk Denial   ⓐ Age Edit   ♀ Female   ♂ Male   **AMA** *CPT® Assistant*   **MUE** Medically Unlikely Edit
⊘ Modifier 51 Exempt   ⊖ Modifier 63 Exempt   ☒ Unlisted   **Modifiers:** *See Inside Back Cover*   Ⓜ Maternity   A2–Z3 ASC Payment Indicators   A–Y OPPS Status Indicators

364   CPT © 2015 American Medical Association. All Rights Reserved.   © 2016 DecisionHealth

33891 Bypass graft, with other than vein, transcervical retropharyngeal carotid-carotid, performed in conjunction with endovascular repair of descending thoracic aorta, by neck incision   C

	RVU			Global Days	Modifiers				
Mod	Non-Fac Total	Fac Total			51	50	62	80	MUE
	28.57	28.57	000		2	1	2	2	1

Pulmonary Artery Procedures

33910 Pulmonary artery embolectomy; with cardiopulmonary bypass   C

	RVU			Global Days	Modifiers				
Mod	Non-Fac Total	Fac Total			51	50	62	80	MUE
	76.85	76.85	090		2	0	1	2	1

AMA: Mar 07: 1

33915 Pulmonary artery embolectomy; without cardiopulmonary bypass   C

	RVU			Global Days	Modifiers				
Mod	Non-Fac Total	Fac Total			51	50	62	80	MUE
	36.96	36.96	090		2	0	1	2	1

AMA: Mar 07: 1

33916 Pulmonary endarterectomy, with or without embolectomy, with cardiopulmonary bypass   C

	RVU			Global Days	Modifiers				
Mod	Non-Fac Total	Fac Total			51	50	62	80	MUE
	123.36	123.36	090		2	0	1	2	1

AMA: Mar 07: 1

33917 Repair of pulmonary artery stenosis by reconstruction with patch or graft   C

	RVU			Global Days	Modifiers				
Mod	Non-Fac Total	Fac Total			51	50	62	80	MUE
	42.40	42.40	090		2	0	1	2	1

AMA: Mar 07: 1, Apr 11: 6

Repair of pulmonary artery stenosis

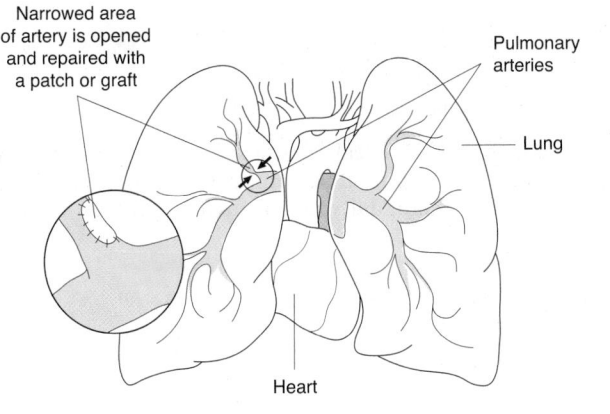

Narrowed area of artery is opened and repaired with a patch or graft

Pulmonary arteries

Lung

Heart

33920 Repair of pulmonary atresia with ventricular septal defect, by construction or replacement of conduit from right or left ventricle to pulmonary artery   C

	RVU			Global Days	Modifiers				
Mod	Non-Fac Total	Fac Total			51	50	62	80	MUE
	55.74	55.74	090		2	0	1	2	1

AMA: Mar 07: 1

33922 Transection of pulmonary artery with cardiopulmonary bypass   ⊖C

	RVU			Global Days	Modifiers				
Mod	Non-Fac Total	Fac Total			51	50	62	80	MUE
	40.81	40.81	090		2	0	1	2	1

+ 33924 Ligation and takedown of a systemic-to-pulmonary artery shunt, performed in conjunction with a congenital heart procedure (List separately in addition to code for primary procedure)   C

	RVU			Global Days	Modifiers				
Mod	Non-Fac Total	Fac Total			51	50	62	80	MUE
	8.39	8.39	ZZZ		0	0	1	2	1

33925 Repair of pulmonary artery arborization anomalies by unifocalization; without cardiopulmonary bypass   ⊗C

	RVU			Global Days	Modifiers				
Mod	Non-Fac Total	Fac Total			51	50	62	80	MUE
	50.60	50.60	090		2	0	1	2	1

33926 Repair of pulmonary artery arborization anomalies by unifocalization; with cardiopulmonary bypass   C

	RVU			Global Days	Modifiers				
Mod	Non-Fac Total	Fac Total			51	50	62	80	MUE
	74.82	74.82	090		2	0	1	2	1

Heart/Lung Transplant Procedures

33930 Donor cardiectomy-pneumonectomy (including cold preservation)   ⊗C

	RVU			Global Days	Modifiers				
Mod	Non-Fac Total	Fac Total			51	50	62	80	MUE
	0.00	0.00	XXX		9	9	9	9	1

33933 Backbench standard preparation of cadaver donor heart/lung allograft prior to transplantation, including dissection of allograft from surrounding soft tissues to prepare aorta, superior vena cava, inferior vena cava, and trachea for implantation   C

	RVU			Global Days	Modifiers				
Mod	Non-Fac Total	Fac Total			51	50	62	80	MUE
	0.00	0.00	XXX		2	0	1	2	1

● New   ▲ Revised   Deleted   ⊙ Moderate Sedation   ✚ Add-on Codes   ⊘ High Risk Denial   Ⓐ Age Edit   ♀ Female   ♂ Male   **AMA** *CPT® Assistant*   **MUE** Medically Unlikely Edit
⊘ Modifier 51 Exempt   ⊖ Modifier 63 Exempt   ✗ Unlisted   **Modifiers:** *See Inside Back Cover*   Ⓜ Maternity   A2–Z3 ASC Payment Indicators   A – Y OPPS Status Indicators

Surgical Procedures

33935 – 33949

33935 Heart-lung transplant with recipient cardiectomy-pneumonectomy ⊗🅒

RVU			Global Days	Modifiers				
Mod	Non-Fac Total	Fac Total		51	50	62	80	MUE
	146.34	146.34	090	2	0	1	2	1

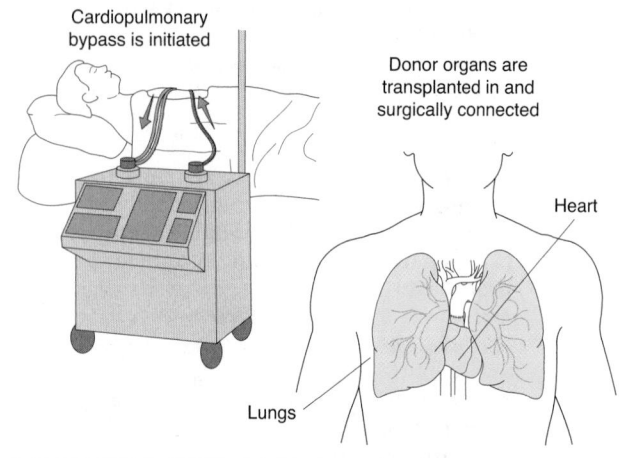

Heart-lung transplant
with recipient cardiectomy-pneumonectomy

Cardiopulmonary bypass is initiated

Donor organs are transplanted in and surgically connected

Heart

Lungs

33940 Donor cardiectomy (including cold preservation) ⊗🅒

RVU			Global Days	Modifiers				
Mod	Non-Fac Total	Fac Total		51	50	62	80	MUE
	0.00	0.00	XXX	9	9	9	9	1

AMA: Apr 05: 10, 11

33944 Backbench standard preparation of cadaver donor heart allograft prior to transplantation, including dissection of allograft from surrounding soft tissues to prepare aorta, superior vena cava, inferior vena cava, pulmonary artery, and left atrium for implantation 🅒

RVU			Global Days	Modifiers				
Mod	Non-Fac Total	Fac Total		51	50	62	80	MUE
	0.00	0.00	XXX	2	0	1	2	1

33945 Heart transplant, with or without recipient cardiectomy 🅒

RVU			Global Days	Modifiers				
Mod	Non-Fac Total	Fac Total		51	50	62	80	MUE
	142.19	142.19	090	2	0	1	2	1

AMA: Fall 92: 20

33946 Extracorporeal membrane oxygenation (ECMO)/ extracorporeal life support (ECLS) provided by physician; initiation, veno-venous ⊖🅒

RVU			Global Days	Modifiers				
Mod	Non-Fac Total	Fac Total		51	50	62	80	MUE
	8.96	8.96	XXX	0	0	0	1	1

AMA: Jul 15: 3

Extracorporeal membrane oxygenation (ECMO)/extracorporeal life support (ECLS) initiation
veno-venous (33946), veno-arterial (33947)

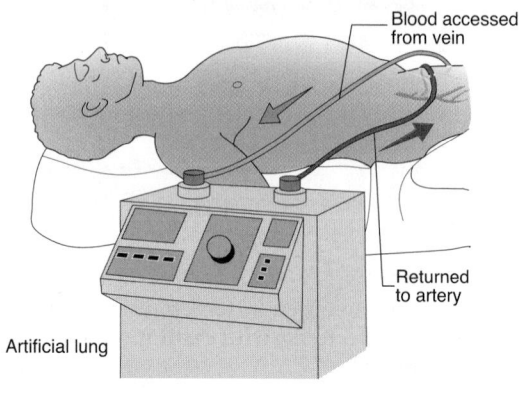

Blood accessed from vein

Returned to artery

Artificial lung

33947 Extracorporeal membrane oxygenation (ECMO)/ extracorporeal life support (ECLS) provided by physician; initiation, veno-arterial ⊖🅒

RVU			Global Days	Modifiers				
Mod	Non-Fac Total	Fac Total		51	50	62	80	MUE
	9.91	9.91	XXX	0	0	0	1	1

AMA: Jul 15: 4

33948 Extracorporeal membrane oxygenation (ECMO)/ extracorporeal life support (ECLS) provided by physician; daily management, each day, veno-venous 🅒

RVU			Global Days	Modifiers				
Mod	Non-Fac Total	Fac Total		51	50	62	80	MUE
	7.06	7.06	XXX	0	0	0	1	1

AMA: Jul 15: 4

33949 Extracorporeal membrane oxygenation (ECMO)/ extracorporeal life support (ECLS) provided by physician; daily management, each day, veno-arterial ⊖🅒

RVU			Global Days	Modifiers				
Mod	Non-Fac Total	Fac Total		51	50	62	80	MUE
	6.87	6.87	XXX	0	0	0	1	1

AMA: Jul 15: 4

● New   ▲ Revised   ✖ Deleted   ⊙ Moderate Sedation   ➕ Add-on Codes   ⊘ High Risk Denial   Ⓐ Age Edit   ♀ Female   ♂ Male   **AMA** *CPT® Assistant*   **MUE** Medically Unlikely Edit
⊘ Modifier 51 Exempt   ⊖ Modifier 63 Exempt   ✗ Unlisted   **Modifiers:** *See Inside Back Cover*   Ⓜ Maternity   A 2 – Z 3 ASC Payment Indicators   A – Y OPPS Status Indicators

366   CPT © 2015 American Medical Association. All Rights Reserved.   © 2016 DecisionHealth

33951 Extracorporeal membrane oxygenation (ECMO)/ extracorporeal life support (ECLS) provided by physician; insertion of peripheral (arterial and/or venous) cannula(e), percutaneous, birth through 5 years of age (includes fluoroscopic guidance, when performed)   **C**

RVU			Global Days	Modifiers				
Mod	Non-Fac Total	Fac Total		51	50	62	80	MUE
	12.16	12.16	000	2	0	0	0	1

AMA: Jul 15: 4

Extracorporeal membrane oxygenation (ECMO)/extracorporeal life support (ECLS) peripheral cannula(e) insertion, percutaneous

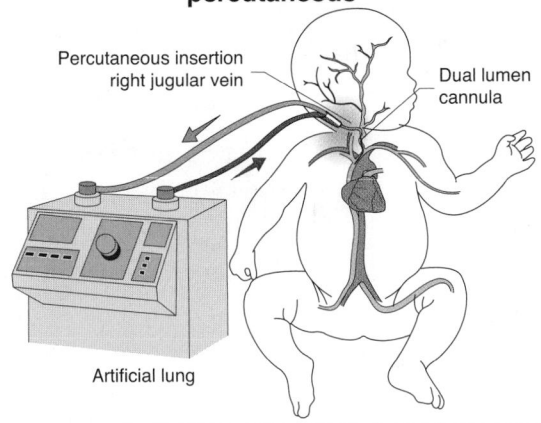

Percutaneous insertion right jugular vein

Dual lumen cannula

Artificial lung

33952 Extracorporeal membrane oxygenation (ECMO)/ extracorporeal life support (ECLS) provided by physician; insertion of peripheral (arterial and/or venous) cannula(e), percutaneous, 6 years and older (includes fluoroscopic guidance, when performed)   **C**

RVU			Global Days	Modifiers				
Mod	Non-Fac Total	Fac Total		51	50	62	80	MUE
	12.58	12.58	000	2	0	0	0	1

AMA: Jul 15: 4

33953 Extracorporeal membrane oxygenation (ECMO)/ extracorporeal life support (ECLS) provided by physician; insertion of peripheral (arterial and/or venous) cannula(e), open, birth through 5 years of age   **C**

RVU			Global Days	Modifiers				
Mod	Non-Fac Total	Fac Total		51	50	62	80	MUE
	13.58	13.58	000	2	0	0	0	1

AMA: Jul 15: 4

33954 Extracorporeal membrane oxygenation (ECMO)/ extracorporeal life support (ECLS) provided by physician; insertion of peripheral (arterial and/or venous) cannula(e), open, 6 years and older   **C**

RVU			Global Days	Modifiers				
Mod	Non-Fac Total	Fac Total		51	50	62	80	MUE
	14.06	14.06	000	2	0	0	0	1

AMA: Jul 15: 4

33955 Extracorporeal membrane oxygenation (ECMO)/ extracorporeal life support (ECLS) provided by physician; insertion of central cannula(e) by sternotomy or thoracotomy, birth through 5 years of age   **C**

RVU			Global Days	Modifiers				
Mod	Non-Fac Total	Fac Total		51	50	62	80	MUE
	24.43	24.43	000	2	0	1	0	1

AMA: Jul 15: 4

33956 Extracorporeal membrane oxygenation (ECMO)/ extracorporeal life support (ECLS) provided by physician; insertion of central cannula(e) by sternotomy or thoracotomy, 6 years and older   **C**

RVU			Global Days	Modifiers				
Mod	Non-Fac Total	Fac Total		51	50	62	80	MUE
	24.56	24.56	000	2	0	1	0	1

AMA: Jul 15: 5

33957 Extracorporeal membrane oxygenation (ECMO)/ extracorporeal life support (ECLS) provided by physician; reposition peripheral (arterial and/or venous) cannula(e), percutaneous, birth through 5 years of age (includes fluoroscopic guidance, when performed)   **C**

RVU			Global Days	Modifiers				
Mod	Non-Fac Total	Fac Total		51	50	62	80	MUE
	5.42	5.42	000	2	0	0	0	1

AMA: Jul 15: 5

33958 Extracorporeal membrane oxygenation (ECMO)/ extracorporeal life support (ECLS) provided by physician; reposition peripheral (arterial and/or venous) cannula(e), percutaneous, 6 years and older (includes fluoroscopic guidance, when performed)   **C**

RVU			Global Days	Modifiers				
Mod	Non-Fac Total	Fac Total		51	50	62	80	MUE
	5.35	5.35	000	2	0	0	0	1

AMA: Jul 15: 5

33959 Extracorporeal membrane oxygenation (ECMO)/ extracorporeal life support (ECLS) provided by physician; reposition peripheral (arterial and/or venous) cannula(e), open, birth through 5 years of age (includes fluoroscopic guidance, when performed)   **C**

RVU			Global Days	Modifiers				
Mod	Non-Fac Total	Fac Total		51	50	62	80	MUE
	6.88	6.88	000	2	0	0	0	1

AMA: Jul 15: 5

33962 Extracorporeal membrane oxygenation (ECMO)/ extracorporeal life support (ECLS) provided by physician; reposition peripheral (arterial and/or venous) cannula(e), open, 6 years and older (includes fluoroscopic guidance, when performed)   **C**

RVU			Global Days	Modifiers				
Mod	Non-Fac Total	Fac Total		51	50	62	80	MUE
	7.00	7.00	000	2	0	0	0	1

AMA: Jul 15: 5

● New   ▲ Revised   Deleted   ⊙ Moderate Sedation   ✚ Add-on Codes   ⊘ High Risk Denial   ⒶAge Edit   ♀ Female   ♂ Male   **AMA** CPT® Assistant   **MUE** Medically Unlikely Edit
⊘ Modifier 51 Exempt   ⊖ Modifier 63 Exempt   ✗ Unlisted   **Modifiers:** See Inside Back Cover   Ⓜ Maternity   Ⓐ2–Z3 ASC Payment Indicators   Ⓐ–Y OPPS Status Indicators

33963 Extracorporeal membrane oxygenation (ECMO)/ extracorporeal life support (ECLS) provided by physician; reposition of central cannula(e) by sternotomy or thoracotomy, birth through 5 years of age (includes fluoroscopic guidance, when performed) C

RVU			Global Days	Modifiers				
Mod	Non-Fac Total	Fac Total		51	50	62	80	MUE
	13.78	13.78	000	2	0	1	0	1

AMA: Jul 15: 5

33964 Extracorporeal membrane oxygenation (ECMO)/ extracorporeal life support (ECLS) provided by physician; reposition central cannula(e) by sternotomy or thoracotomy, 6 years and older (includes fluoroscopic guidance, when performed) C

RVU			Global Days	Modifiers				
Mod	Non-Fac Total	Fac Total		51	50	62	80	MUE
	14.34	14.34	000	2	0	1	0	1

AMA: Jul 15: 5

33965 Extracorporeal membrane oxygenation (ECMO)/ extracorporeal life support (ECLS) provided by physician; removal of peripheral (arterial and/or venous) cannula(e), percutaneous, birth through 5 years of age C

RVU			Global Days	Modifiers				
Mod	Non-Fac Total	Fac Total		51	50	62	80	MUE
	5.42	5.42	000	2	0	0	0	1

AMA: Jul 15: 5

33966 Extracorporeal membrane oxygenation (ECMO)/ extracorporeal life support (ECLS) provided by physician; removal of peripheral (arterial and/ or venous) cannula(e), percutaneous, 6 years and older C

RVU			Global Days	Modifiers				
Mod	Non-Fac Total	Fac Total		51	50	62	80	MUE
	6.91	6.91	000	2	0	0	0	1

AMA: Jul 15: 5

33967 Insertion of intra-aortic balloon assist device, percutaneous C

RVU			Global Days	Modifiers				
Mod	Non-Fac Total	Fac Total		51	50	62	80	MUE
	7.57	7.57	000	2	0	0	0	1

AMA: Feb 02: 2, Nov 11: 8, Mar 13: 10

33968 Removal of intra-aortic balloon assist device, percutaneous C

RVU			Global Days	Modifiers				
Mod	Non-Fac Total	Fac Total		51	50	62	80	MUE
	0.98	0.98	000	0	0	0	1	1

AMA: Nov 99: 19, Jan 00: 10, Nov 11: 8

33969 Extracorporeal membrane oxygenation (ECMO)/ extracorporeal life support (ECLS) provided by physician; removal of peripheral (arterial and/or venous) cannula(e), open, birth through 5 years of age C

RVU			Global Days	Modifiers				
Mod	Non-Fac Total	Fac Total		51	50	62	80	MUE
	8.03	8.03	000	2	0	0	0	1

AMA: Jul 15: 5

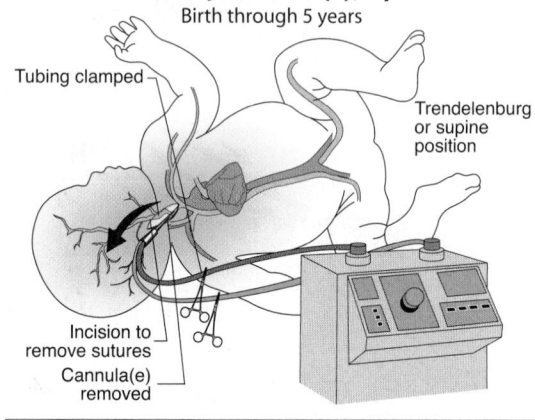

Extracorporeal membrane oxygenation (ECMO)/extracorporeal life support (ECLS) Removal of peripheral (arterial and/or venous) cannula(e), open

Birth through 5 years

Tubing clamped

Trendelenburg or supine position

Incision to remove sutures

Cannula(e) removed

33970 Insertion of intra-aortic balloon assist device through the femoral artery, open approach C

RVU			Global Days	Modifiers				
Mod	Non-Fac Total	Fac Total		51	50	62	80	MUE
	10.38	10.38	000	2	0	1	2	1

AMA: Nov 99: 19, Nov 11: 8, Mar 13: 10

33971 Removal of intra-aortic balloon assist device including repair of femoral artery, with or without graft C

RVU			Global Days	Modifiers				
Mod	Non-Fac Total	Fac Total		51	50	62	80	MUE
	20.74	20.74	090	2	0	0	1	1

AMA: Nov 11: 8

33973 Insertion of intra-aortic balloon assist device through the ascending aorta C

RVU			Global Days	Modifiers				
Mod	Non-Fac Total	Fac Total		51	50	62	80	MUE
	15.02	15.02	000	2	0	1	2	1

AMA: Nov 11: 8, Mar 13: 10

33974 Removal of intra-aortic balloon assist device from the ascending aorta, including repair of the ascending aorta, with or without graft C

RVU			Global Days	Modifiers				
Mod	Non-Fac Total	Fac Total		51	50	62	80	MUE
	25.87	25.87	090	2	0	0	1	1

AMA: Nov 11: 8

● New   ▲ Revised   ✖ Deleted   ⊙ Moderate Sedation   ✚ Add-on Codes   ⊘ High Risk Denial   Ⓐ Age Edit   ♀ Female   ♂ Male   **AMA** CPT® Assistant   **MUE** Medically Unlikely Edit
⊘ Modifier 51 Exempt   ⊖ Modifier 63 Exempt   ✖ Unlisted   **Modifiers:** See Inside Back Cover   Ⓜ Maternity   A2–Z3 ASC Payment Indicators   A–Y OPPS Status Indicators

CPT © 2015 American Medical Association. All Rights Reserved.   © 2016 DecisionHealth

33975 Insertion of ventricular assist device; extracorporeal, single ventricle ☒

RVU			Global Days	Modifiers				
Mod	Non-Fac Total	Fac Total		51	50	62	80	MUE
	38.44	38.44	XXX	2	0	0	2	1

AMA: Feb 92: 2, Jan 04: 28, Nov 09: 10, Jan 10: 11, Apr 10: 6, Mar 13: 10

33976 Insertion of ventricular assist device; extracorporeal, biventricular ☒

RVU			Global Days	Modifiers				
Mod	Non-Fac Total	Fac Total		51	50	62	80	MUE
	46.80	46.80	XXX	2	2	0	2	1

AMA: Feb 02: 2, Apr 10: 6, Nov 09: 10, Jan 10: 11, Mar 13: 10

33977 Removal of ventricular assist device; extracorporeal, single ventricle ☒

RVU			Global Days	Modifiers				
Mod	Non-Fac Total	Fac Total		51	50	62	80	MUE
	32.97	32.97	XXX	2	0	0	2	1

AMA: Feb 02: 2, Nov 09: 10, Jan 10: 11, Apr 10: 6, Mar 13: 10

33978 Removal of ventricular assist device; extracorporeal, biventricular ☒

RVU			Global Days	Modifiers				
Mod	Non-Fac Total	Fac Total		51	50	62	80	MUE
	39.22	39.22	XXX	2	2	0	2	1

AMA: Feb 02: 2, Nov 09: 10, Jan 10: 11, Apr 10: 6, Mar 13: 10

33979 Insertion of ventricular assist device, implantable intracorporeal, single ventricle ☒

RVU			Global Days	Modifiers				
Mod	Non-Fac Total	Fac Total		51	50	62	80	MUE
	56.99	56.99	XXX	2	0	0	2	1

AMA: Feb 02: 3, Jan 04: 28, Nov 09: 10, Jan 10: 11, Apr 10: 6, Mar 13: 10

33980 Removal of ventricular assist device, implantable intracorporeal, single ventricle ☒

RVU			Global Days	Modifiers				
Mod	Non-Fac Total	Fac Total		51	50	62	80	MUE
	52.19	52.19	XXX	2	0	0	2	1

AMA: Feb 02: 3, Nov 09: 10, Apr 10: 6, Mar 13: 10

33981 Replacement of extracorporeal ventricular assist device, single or biventricular, pump(s), single or each pump ☒

RVU			Global Days	Modifiers				
Mod	Non-Fac Total	Fac Total		51	50	62	80	MUE
	24.55	24.55	XXX	2	0	0	2	1

AMA: Apr 10: 6

33982 Replacement of ventricular assist device pump(s); implantable intracorporeal, single ventricle, without cardiopulmonary bypass ☒

RVU			Global Days	Modifiers				
Mod	Non-Fac Total	Fac Total		51	50	62	80	MUE
	58.05	58.05	XXX	2	0	0	2	1

AMA: Apr 10: 6

33983 Replacement of ventricular assist device pump(s); implantable intracorporeal, single ventricle, with cardiopulmonary bypass ☒

RVU			Global Days	Modifiers				
Mod	Non-Fac Total	Fac Total		51	50	62	80	MUE
	67.70	67.70	XXX	2	0	0	2	1

AMA: Apr 10: 6

33984 Extracorporeal membrane oxygenation (ECMO)/extracorporeal life support (ECLS) provided by physician; removal of peripheral (arterial and/or venous) cannula(e), open, 6 years and older ☒

RVU			Global Days	Modifiers				
Mod	Non-Fac Total	Fac Total		51	50	62	80	MUE
	8.37	8.37	000	2	0	0	0	1

AMA: Jul 15: 6

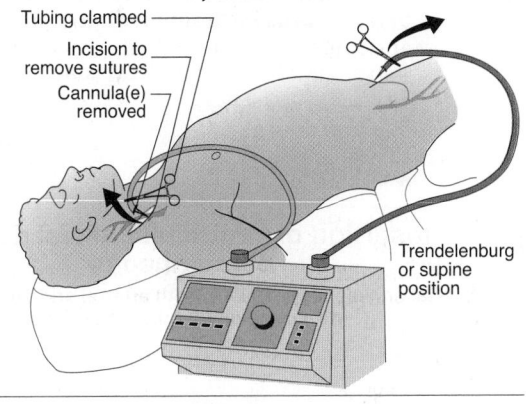

Extracorporeal membrane oxygenation (ECMO)/extracorporeal life support (ECLS) Removal of peripheral (arterial and/or venous) cannula(e), open
6 years and older

Tubing clamped
Incision to remove sutures
Cannula(e) removed
Trendelenburg or supine position

33985 Extracorporeal membrane oxygenation (ECMO)/extracorporeal life support (ECLS) provided by physician; removal of central cannula(e) by sternotomy or thoracotomy, birth through 5 years of age ☒

RVU			Global Days	Modifiers				
Mod	Non-Fac Total	Fac Total		51	50	62	80	MUE
	15.13	15.13	000	2	0	1	0	1

AMA: Jul 15: 6

33986 Extracorporeal membrane oxygenation (ECMO)/extracorporeal life support (ECLS) provided by physician; removal of central cannula(e) by sternotomy or thoracotomy, 6 years and older ☒

RVU			Global Days	Modifiers				
Mod	Non-Fac Total	Fac Total		51	50	62	80	MUE
	15.53	15.53	000	2	0	1	0	1

AMA: Jul 15: 6

+ **33987** Arterial exposure with creation of graft conduit (eg, chimney graft) to facilitate arterial perfusion for ECMO/ECLS (List separately in addition to code for primary procedure) ☒

RVU			Global Days	Modifiers				
Mod	Non-Fac Total	Fac Total		51	50	62	80	MUE
	6.11	6.11	ZZZ	0	0	1	0	1

AMA: Jul 15: 6

● New   ▲ Revised   Deleted   ⊙ Moderate Sedation   ✚ Add-on Codes   ⊘ High Risk Denial   Ⓐ Age Edit   ♀ Female   ♂ Male   **AMA** CPT® Assistant   **MUE** Medically Unlikely Edit
⊘ Modifier 51 Exempt   ⊖ Modifier 63 Exempt   Ⓧ Unlisted   **Modifiers:** See Inside Back Cover   Ⓜ Maternity   A2–Z3 ASC Payment Indicators   A–Y OPPS Status Indicators

33988 Insertion of left heart vent by thoracic incision (eg, sternotomy, thoracotomy) for ECMO/ECLS ◪

RVU			Global Days	Modifiers				
Mod	Non-Fac Total	Fac Total		51	50	62	80	MUE
	22.79	22.79	000	2	0	1	0	1

AMA: Jul 15: 6

33989 Removal of left heart vent by thoracic incision (eg, sternotomy, thoracotomy) for ECMO/ECLS ◪

RVU			Global Days	Modifiers				
Mod	Non-Fac Total	Fac Total		51	50	62	80	MUE
	14.73	14.73	000	2	0	1	0	1

AMA: Jul 15: 6

⊙ **33990** Insertion of ventricular assist device, percutaneous including radiological supervision and interpretation; arterial access only ◪

RVU			Global Days	Modifiers				
Mod	Non-Fac Total	Fac Total		51	50	62	80	MUE
	12.81	12.81	XXX	2	0	0	2	1

AMA: Mar 13: 10, Oct 14: 15

Insertion of ventricular assist device, percutaneous

Arterial access only (33990), both arterial and venous access, with transseptal puncture (33991)

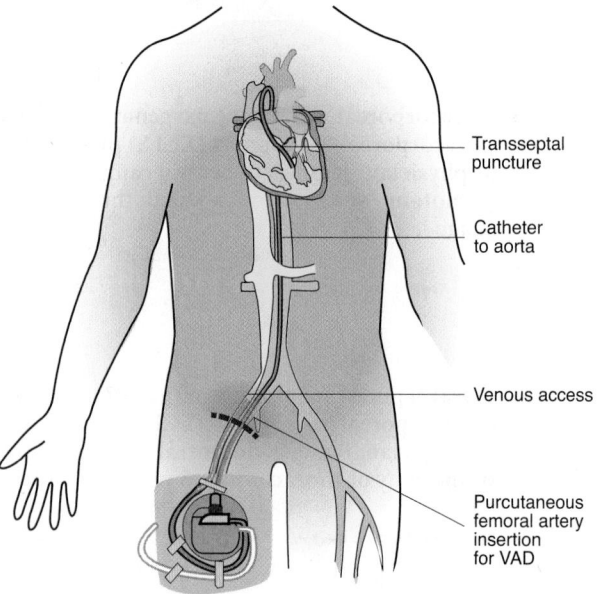

- Transseptal puncture
- Catheter to aorta
- Venous access
- Purcutaneous femoral artery insertion for VAD

⊙ **33991** Insertion of ventricular assist device, percutaneous including radiological supervision and interpretation; both arterial and venous access, with transseptal puncture ◪

RVU			Global Days	Modifiers				
Mod	Non-Fac Total	Fac Total		51	50	62	80	MUE
	18.66	18.66	XXX	2	0	0	2	1

AMA: Mar 13: 10

⊙ **33992** Removal of percutaneous ventricular assist device at separate and distinct session from insertion ◪

RVU			Global Days	Modifiers				
Mod	Non-Fac Total	Fac Total		51	50	62	80	MUE
	6.08	6.08	XXX	2	0	0	2	1

AMA: Mar 13: 10

Removal of percutaneous ventricular assist device at separate and distinct session from insertion

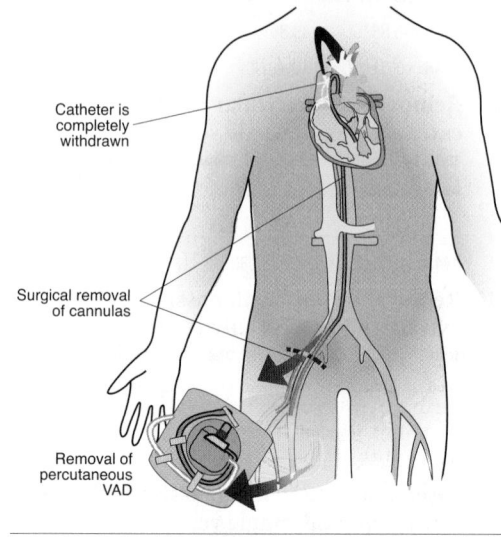

- Catheter is completely withdrawn
- Surgical removal of cannulas
- Removal of percutaneous VAD

⊙ **33993** Repositioning of percutaneous ventricular assist device with imaging guidance at separate and distinct session from insertion ◪

RVU			Global Days	Modifiers				
Mod	Non-Fac Total	Fac Total		51	50	62	80	MUE
	5.33	5.33	XXX	2	0	0	2	1

AMA: Mar 13: 10

Repositioning of percutaneous ventricular assist device at separate and distinct session

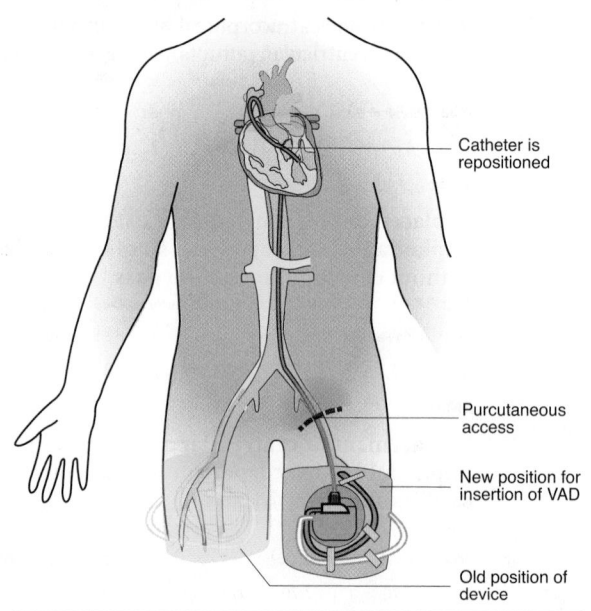

- Catheter is repositioned
- Purcutaneous access
- New position for insertion of VAD
- Old position of device

● New   ▲ Revised   ✖ Deleted   ⊙ Moderate Sedation   ✚ Add-on Codes   ⊘ High Risk Denial   Ⓐ Age Edit   ♀ Female   ♂ Male   **AMA** *CPT® Assistant*   **MUE** Medically Unlikely Edit
⊘ Modifier 51 Exempt   ⊖ Modifier 63 Exempt   ✖ Unlisted   **Modifiers:** *See Inside Back Cover*   Ⓜ Maternity   A2–Z3 ASC Payment Indicators   A–Y OPPS Status Indicators

Other Cardiac Surgery

33999 Unlisted procedure, cardiac surgery ✗🅣

RVU			Global Days	Modifiers				
Mod	Non-Fac Total	Fac Total		51	50	62	80	MUE
	0.00	0.00	YYY	2	0	1	2	

AMA: Oct 99: 11, Jan 04: 7, Mar 07: 1, Nov 09: 10, Jan 10: 11, Apr 10: 6, Feb 13: 13, Mar 13: 10, Dec 13: 14, Dec 14: 17

Arterial/Venous Procedures

Embolus/Thrombus Procedures

Coding Guidance

Embolectomy, thrombectomy, endarterectomy may be performed alone as a separate procedure or in combination with thromboendarterectomy (35301-35372) to treat vascular obstruction. Report only the more comprehensive code describing the service at a given site; do not report a code from both groups for the same operative session.

34001 Embolectomy or thrombectomy, with or without catheter; carotid, subclavian or innominate artery, by neck incision 🅒

RVU			Global Days	Modifiers				
Mod	Non-Fac Total	Fac Total		51	50	62	80	MUE
	28.85	28.85	090	2	1	1	2	1

34051 Embolectomy or thrombectomy, with or without catheter; innominate, subclavian artery, by thoracic incision 🅒

RVU			Global Days	Modifiers				
Mod	Non-Fac Total	Fac Total		51	50	62	80	MUE
	29.05	29.05	090	2	1	1	2	1

34101 Embolectomy or thrombectomy, with or without catheter; axillary, brachial, innominate, subclavian artery, by arm incision 🅣

RVU			Global Days	Modifiers				
Mod	Non-Fac Total	Fac Total		51	50	62	80	MUE
	17.78	17.78	090	2	1	1	2	1

34111 Embolectomy or thrombectomy, with or without catheter; radial or ulnar artery, by arm incision 🅣

RVU			Global Days	Modifiers				
Mod	Non-Fac Total	Fac Total		51	50	62	80	MUE
	17.74	17.74	090	2	1	1	2	2

34151 Embolectomy or thrombectomy, with or without catheter; renal, celiac, mesentery, aortoiliac artery, by abdominal incision 🅒

RVU			Global Days	Modifiers				
Mod	Non-Fac Total	Fac Total		51	50	62	80	MUE
	41.35	41.35	090	2	1	1	2	2

34201 Embolectomy or thrombectomy, with or without catheter; femoropopliteal, aortoiliac artery, by leg incision 🅣

RVU			Global Days	Modifiers				
Mod	Non-Fac Total	Fac Total		51	50	62	80	MUE
	30.47	30.47	090	2	1	1	2	1

AMA: Aug 11: 9

34203 Embolectomy or thrombectomy, with or without catheter; popliteal-tibio-peroneal artery, by leg incision 🅣

RVU			Global Days	Modifiers				
Mod	Non-Fac Total	Fac Total		51	50	62	80	MUE
	28.23	28.23	090	2	1	1	2	1

34401 Thrombectomy, direct or with catheter; vena cava, iliac vein, by abdominal incision 🅒

RVU			Global Days	Modifiers				
Mod	Non-Fac Total	Fac Total		51	50	62	80	MUE
	42.62	42.62	090	2	1	1	2	1

34421 Thrombectomy, direct or with catheter; vena cava, iliac, femoropopliteal vein, by leg incision 🅣

RVU			Global Days	Modifiers				
Mod	Non-Fac Total	Fac Total		51	50	62	80	MUE
	21.58	21.58	090	2	1	1	2	1

AMA: Spring 94: 30

34451 Thrombectomy, direct or with catheter; vena cava, iliac, femoropopliteal vein, by abdominal and leg incision 🅒

RVU			Global Days	Modifiers				
Mod	Non-Fac Total	Fac Total		51	50	62	80	MUE
	42.65	42.65	090	2	1	1	2	1

34471 Thrombectomy, direct or with catheter; subclavian vein, by neck incision 🅣

RVU			Global Days	Modifiers				
Mod	Non-Fac Total	Fac Total		51	50	62	80	MUE
	31.91	31.91	090	2	1	1	1	1

34490 Thrombectomy, direct or with catheter; axillary and subclavian vein, by arm incision G2🅣

RVU			Global Days	Modifiers				
Mod	Non-Fac Total	Fac Total		51	50	62	80	MUE
	18.15	18.15	090	2	1	0	1	1

Venous Reconstruction Procedures

34501 Valvuloplasty, femoral vein 🅣

RVU			Global Days	Modifiers				
Mod	Non-Fac Total	Fac Total		51	50	62	80	MUE
	28.88	28.88	090	2	1	1	2	1

34502 Reconstruction of vena cava, any method 🅒

RVU			Global Days	Modifiers				
Mod	Non-Fac Total	Fac Total		51	50	62	80	MUE
	45.08	45.08	090	2	0	0	2	1

34510 Venous valve transposition, any vein donor 🅣

RVU			Global Days	Modifiers				
Mod	Non-Fac Total	Fac Total		51	50	62	80	MUE
	35.00	35.00	090	2	1	1	2	2

34520 Cross-over vein graft to venous system 🅣

RVU			Global Days	Modifiers				
Mod	Non-Fac Total	Fac Total		51	50	62	80	MUE
	29.64	29.64	090	2	1	1	2	1

34530 Saphenopopliteal vein anastomosis 🅣

RVU			Global Days	Modifiers				
Mod	Non-Fac Total	Fac Total		51	50	62	80	MUE
	32.14	32.14	090	2	1	1	2	1

● New ▲ Revised Deleted ⊙ Moderate Sedation ✚ Add-on Codes ⊘ High Risk Denial Ⓐ Age Edit ♀ Female ♂ Male **AMA** *CPT® Assistant* **MUE** Medically Unlikely Edit
⊘ Modifier 51 Exempt ⊖ Modifier 63 Exempt ✗ Unlisted **Modifiers:** *See Inside Back Cover* Ⓜ Maternity A2–Z3 ASC Payment Indicators A–Y OPPS Status Indicators

Surgical Procedures

34800 – 34831

Abdominal Aortic Aneurysm Endovascular Repair

34800 Endovascular repair of infrarenal abdominal aortic aneurysm or dissection; using aorto-aortic tube prosthesis   Ⓒ

RVU			Global Days	Modifiers				
Mod	Non-Fac Total	Fac Total		51	50	62	80	MUE
	33.38	33.38	090	2	0	2	2	1

AMA: Dec 00: 1, 4, Sep 02: 3, Feb 03: 2, Nov 03: 5, Dec 04: 18, Apr 12: 3, Dec 13: 8

34802 Endovascular repair of infrarenal abdominal aortic aneurysm or dissection; using modular bifurcated prosthesis (1 docking limb)   Ⓒ

RVU			Global Days	Modifiers				
Mod	Non-Fac Total	Fac Total		51	50	62	80	MUE
	36.79	36.79	090	2	0	2	2	1

AMA: Dec 00: 1, 4, Sep 02: 3, Feb 03: 2, Dec 04: 18, Apr 12: 3, Dec 13: 8

34803 Endovascular repair of infrarenal abdominal aortic aneurysm or dissection; using modular bifurcated prosthesis (2 docking limbs)   Ⓒ

RVU			Global Days	Modifiers				
Mod	Non-Fac Total	Fac Total		51	50	62	80	MUE
	37.99	37.99	090	2	2	2	2	1

AMA: Apr 12: 3

34804 Endovascular repair of infrarenal abdominal aortic aneurysm or dissection; using unibody bifurcated prosthesis   Ⓒ

RVU			Global Days	Modifiers				
Mod	Non-Fac Total	Fac Total		51	50	62	80	MUE
	36.76	36.76	090	2	0	2	2	1

AMA: Dec 00: 5, Sep 02: 3, Feb 03: 2, Apr 12: 3

34805 Endovascular repair of infrarenal abdominal aortic aneurysm or dissection; using aorto-uniiliac or aorto-unifemoral prosthesis   Ⓒ

RVU			Global Days	Modifiers				
Mod	Non-Fac Total	Fac Total		51	50	62	80	MUE
	35.21	35.21	090	2	0	2	2	1

AMA: Jun 04: 9, Dec 04: 18, Apr 12: 3, Dec 13: 8

+ 34806 Transcatheter placement of wireless physiologic sensor in aneurysmal sac during endovascular repair, including radiological supervision and interpretation, instrument calibration, and collection of pressure data (List separately in addition to code for primary procedure)   Ⓒ

RVU			Global Days	Modifiers				
Mod	Non-Fac Total	Fac Total		51	50	62	80	MUE
	2.95	2.95	ZZZ	0	0	2	1	1

AMA: Apr 12: 3

+ 34808 Endovascular placement of iliac artery occlusion device (List separately in addition to code for primary procedure)   Ⓒ

RVU			Global Days	Modifiers				
Mod	Non-Fac Total	Fac Total		51	50	62	80	MUE
	6.11	6.11	ZZZ	0	0	2	1	1

AMA: Dec 00: 6, Sep 02: 3, Apr 12: 3

34812 Open femoral artery exposure for delivery of endovascular prosthesis, by groin incision, unilateral   Ⓒ

RVU			Global Days	Modifiers				
Mod	Non-Fac Total	Fac Total		51	50	62	80	MUE
	9.97	9.97	000	2	1	2	2	1

AMA: Dec 00: 6, Sep 02: 3, Feb 03: 2, Mar 04: 10, Jul 06: 7, Mar 13: 10, Dec 13: 8

+ 34813 Placement of femoral-femoral prosthetic graft during endovascular aortic aneurysm repair (List separately in addition to code for primary procedure)   Ⓒ

RVU			Global Days	Modifiers				
Mod	Non-Fac Total	Fac Total		51	50	62	80	MUE
	6.98	6.98	ZZZ	0	0	2	2	1

AMA: Dec 00: 6, Sep 02: 3, Apr 12: 3

34820 Open iliac artery exposure for delivery of endovascular prosthesis or iliac occlusion during endovascular therapy, by abdominal or retroperitoneal incision, unilateral   Ⓒ

RVU			Global Days	Modifiers				
Mod	Non-Fac Total	Fac Total		51	50	62	80	MUE
	14.54	14.54	000	2	1	2	2	1

AMA: Dec 00: 7, 8, Sep 02: 3, Feb 03: 4, Aug 04: 10, Jul 06: 7

34825 Placement of proximal or distal extension prosthesis for endovascular repair of infrarenal abdominal aortic or iliac aneurysm, false aneurysm, or dissection; initial vessel   Ⓒ

RVU			Global Days	Modifiers				
Mod	Non-Fac Total	Fac Total		51	50	62	80	MUE
	20.48	20.48	090	2	0	2	2	2

AMA: Dec 00: 5, Sep 02: 3, Feb 03: 3, Apr 12: 3, Dec 13: 8

+ 34826 Placement of proximal or distal extension prosthesis for endovascular repair of infrarenal abdominal aortic or iliac aneurysm, false aneurysm, or dissection; each additional vessel (List separately in addition to code for primary procedure)   Ⓒ

RVU			Global Days	Modifiers				
Mod	Non-Fac Total	Fac Total		51	50	62	80	MUE
	6.03	6.03	ZZZ	0	0	2	2	4

AMA: Dec 00: 6, Sep 02: 3, Feb 03: 3, Apr 12: 3, Dec 13: 8

34830 Open repair of infrarenal aortic aneurysm or dissection, plus repair of associated arterial trauma, following unsuccessful endovascular repair; tube prosthesis   Ⓒ

RVU			Global Days	Modifiers				
Mod	Non-Fac Total	Fac Total		51	50	62	80	MUE
	52.17	52.17	090	2	0	2	2	1

AMA: Dec 00: 6, Sep 02: 3, Oct 08: 10

34831 Open repair of infrarenal aortic aneurysm or dissection, plus repair of associated arterial trauma, following unsuccessful endovascular repair; aorto-bi-iliac prosthesis   Ⓒ

RVU			Global Days	Modifiers				
Mod	Non-Fac Total	Fac Total		51	50	62	80	MUE
	56.22	56.22	090	2	0	2	2	1

AMA: Dec 00: 6, Sep 02: 3, Oct 08: 10

● New ▲ Revised ✖ Deleted ⊙ Moderate Sedation ✚ Add-on Codes ⊘ High Risk Denial Ⓐ Age Edit ♀ Female ♂ Male **AMA** *CPT® Assistant* **MUE** Medically Unlikely Edit
⊘ Modifier 51 Exempt ⊖ Modifier 63 Exempt Ⓧ Unlisted **Modifiers:** *See Inside Back Cover* Ⓜ Maternity Ⓐ2–Ⓩ3 ASC Payment Indicators Ⓐ–Ⓨ OPPS Status Indicators

372   CPT © 2015 American Medical Association. All Rights Reserved.   © 2016 DecisionHealth

34832 Open repair of infrarenal aortic aneurysm or dissection, plus repair of associated arterial trauma, following unsuccessful endovascular repair; aorto-bifemoral prosthesis ☐C

RVU			Global Days	Modifiers				
Mod	Non-Fac Total	Fac Total		51	50	62	80	MUE
	55.78	55.78	090	2	0	2	2	1

AMA: Dec 00: 6, Sep 02: 3, Oct 08: 10

34833 Open iliac artery exposure with creation of conduit for delivery of aortic or iliac endovascular prosthesis, by abdominal or retroperitoneal incision, unilateral ☐C

RVU			Global Days	Modifiers				
Mod	Non-Fac Total	Fac Total		51	50	62	80	MUE
	17.99	17.99	000	2	1	2	2	1

AMA: Aug 04: 10, Feb 03: 4, Jul 06: 7

34834 Open brachial artery exposure to assist in the deployment of aortic or iliac endovascular prosthesis by arm incision, unilateral ☐C

RVU			Global Days	Modifiers				
Mod	Non-Fac Total	Fac Total		51	50	62	80	MUE
	8.07	8.07	000	2	1	2	2	1

AMA: Feb 03: 4, Jul 06: 7

34839 Physician planning of a patient-specific fenestrated visceral aortic endograft requiring a minimum of 90 minutes of physician time ☐B

RVU			Global Days	Modifiers				
Mod	Non-Fac Total	Fac Total		51	50	62	80	MUE
	0.00	0.00	YYY	0	0	0	0	1

Physician planning of a patient-specific fenestrated visceral aortic endograft
requiring a minimum of 90 minutes of physician time

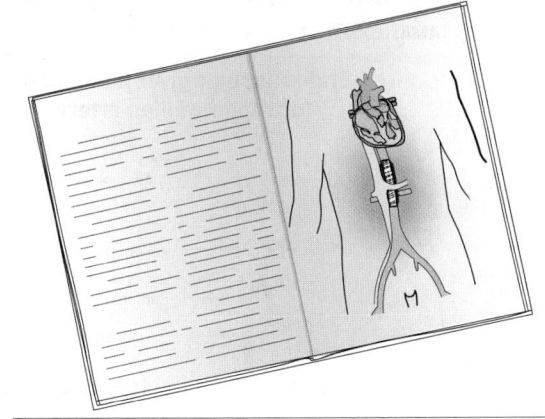

34841 Endovascular repair of visceral aorta (eg, aneurysm, pseudoaneurysm, dissection, penetrating ulcer, intramural hematoma, or traumatic disruption) by deployment of a fenestrated visceral aortic endograft and all associated radiological supervision and interpretation, including target zone angioplasty, when performed; including one visceral artery endoprosthesis (superior mesenteric, celiac or renal artery) ☐C

RVU			Global Days	Modifiers				
Mod	Non-Fac Total	Fac Total		51	50	62	80	MUE
	0.00	0.00	YYY	2	0	2	2	1

AMA: Dec 13: 8

34842 Endovascular repair of visceral aorta (eg, aneurysm, pseudoaneurysm, dissection, penetrating ulcer, intramural hematoma, or traumatic disruption) by deployment of a fenestrated visceral aortic endograft and all associated radiological supervision and interpretation, including target zone angioplasty, when performed; including two visceral artery endoprostheses (superior mesenteric, celiac and/or renal artery[s]) ☐C

RVU			Global Days	Modifiers				
Mod	Non-Fac Total	Fac Total		51	50	62	80	MUE
	0.00	0.00	YYY	2	0	2	2	1

AMA: Dec 13: 8

34843 Endovascular repair of visceral aorta (eg, aneurysm, pseudoaneurysm, dissection, penetrating ulcer, intramural hematoma, or traumatic disruption) by deployment of a fenestrated visceral aortic endograft and all associated radiological supervision and interpretation, including target zone angioplasty, when performed; including three visceral artery endoprostheses (superior mesenteric, celiac and/or renal artery[s]) ☐C

RVU			Global Days	Modifiers				
Mod	Non-Fac Total	Fac Total		51	50	62	80	MUE
	0.00	0.00	YYY	2	0	2	2	1

AMA: Dec 13: 8

34844 Endovascular repair of visceral aorta (eg, aneurysm, pseudoaneurysm, dissection, penetrating ulcer, intramural hematoma, or traumatic disruption) by deployment of a fenestrated visceral aortic endograft and all associated radiological supervision and interpretation, including target zone angioplasty, when performed; including four or more visceral artery endoprostheses (superior mesenteric, celiac and/or renal artery[s]) ☐C

RVU			Global Days	Modifiers				
Mod	Non-Fac Total	Fac Total		51	50	62	80	MUE
	0.00	0.00	YYY	2	0	2	2	1

AMA: Dec 13: 8

34845 Endovascular repair of visceral aorta and infrarenal abdominal aorta (eg, aneurysm, pseudoaneurysm, dissection, penetrating ulcer, intramural hematoma, or traumatic disruption) with a fenestrated visceral aortic endograft and concomitant unibody or modular infrarenal aortic endograft and all associated radiological supervision and interpretation, including target zone angioplasty, when performed; including one visceral artery endoprosthesis (superior mesenteric, celiac or renal artery) **C**

RVU			Global Days	Modifiers				
Mod	Non-Fac Total	Fac Total		51	50	62	80	MUE
	0.00	0.00	YYY	2	0	2	2	1

AMA: Dec 13: 8

Endovascular repair of visceral aorta and infrarenal abdominal aorta
One endoprosthesis (34845), two (34846), three (34847), four or more (34848)

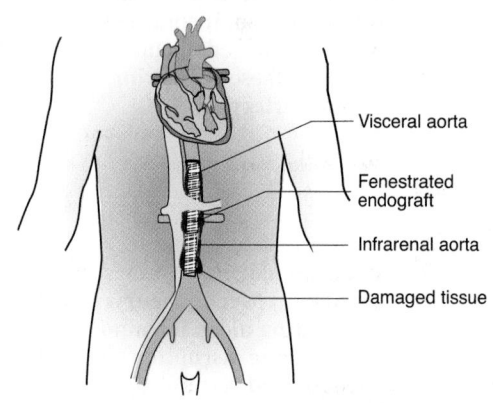

- Visceral aorta
- Fenestrated endograft
- Infrarenal aorta
- Damaged tissue

34846 Endovascular repair of visceral aorta and infrarenal abdominal aorta (eg, aneurysm, pseudoaneurysm, dissection, penetrating ulcer, intramural hematoma, or traumatic disruption) with a fenestrated visceral aortic endograft and concomitant unibody or modular infrarenal aortic endograft and all associated radiological supervision and interpretation, including target zone angioplasty, when performed; including two visceral artery endoprostheses (superior mesenteric, celiac and/or renal artery[s]) **C**

RVU			Global Days	Modifiers				
Mod	Non-Fac Total	Fac Total		51	50	62	80	MUE
	0.00	0.00	YYY	2	0	2	2	1

AMA: Dec 13: 8

34847 Endovascular repair of visceral aorta and infrarenal abdominal aorta (eg, aneurysm, pseudoaneurysm, dissection, penetrating ulcer, intramural hematoma, or traumatic disruption) with a fenestrated visceral aortic endograft and concomitant unibody or modular infrarenal aortic endograft and all associated radiological supervision and interpretation, including target zone angioplasty, when performed; including three visceral artery endoprostheses (superior mesenteric, celiac and/or renal artery[s]) **C**

RVU			Global Days	Modifiers				
Mod	Non-Fac Total	Fac Total		51	50	62	80	MUE
	0.00	0.00	YYY	2	0	2	2	1

AMA: Dec 13: 8

34848 Endovascular repair of visceral aorta and infrarenal abdominal aorta (eg, aneurysm, pseudoaneurysm, dissection, penetrating ulcer, intramural hematoma, or traumatic disruption) with a fenestrated visceral aortic endograft and concomitant unibody or modular infrarenal aortic endograft and all associated radiological supervision and interpretation, including target zone angioplasty, when performed; including four or more visceral artery endoprostheses (superior mesenteric, celiac and/or renal artery[s]) **C**

RVU			Global Days	Modifiers				
Mod	Non-Fac Total	Fac Total		51	50	62	80	MUE
	0.00	0.00	YYY	2	0	2	2	1

AMA: Dec 13: 8

Iliac Aneurysm Endovascular Repair

34900 Endovascular repair of iliac artery (eg, aneurysm, pseudoaneurysm, arteriovenous malformation, trauma) using ilio-iliac tube endoprosthesis **C**

RVU			Global Days	Modifiers				
Mod	Non-Fac Total	Fac Total		51	50	62	80	MUE
	26.45	26.45	090	2	1	2	2	1

AMA: Feb 93: 2, Apr 12: 3

Endovascular graft placement for repair of iliac artery

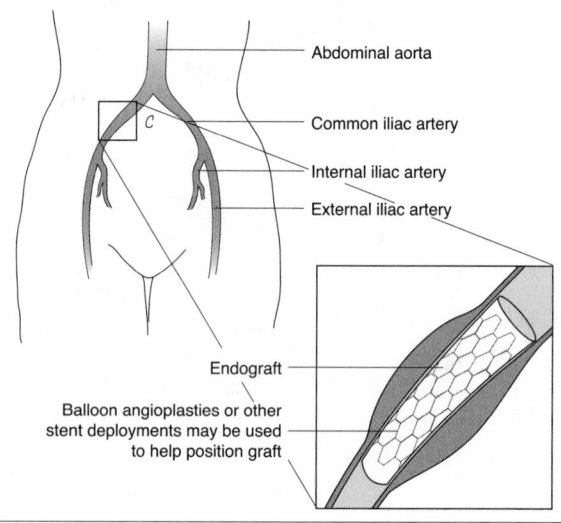

- Abdominal aorta
- Common iliac artery
- Internal iliac artery
- External iliac artery
- Endograft
- Balloon angioplasties or other stent deployments may be used to help position graft

---

● New   ▲ Revised   ✖ Deleted   ⊙ Moderate Sedation   ✚ Add-on Codes   ⊘ High Risk Denial   Ⓐ Age Edit   ♀ Female   ♂ Male   **AMA** *CPT® Assistant*   **MUE** Medically Unlikely Edit
⊘ Modifier 51 Exempt   ⊖ Modifier 63 Exempt   ✗ Unlisted   **Modifiers:** *See Inside Back Cover*   Ⓜ Maternity   A2–Z3 ASC Payment Indicators   A–Y OPPS Status Indicators

374   CPT © 2015 American Medical Association. All Rights Reserved.   © 2016 DecisionHealth

Aneursym/Pseudoaneurysm/Occlusive Disease Repair/Excision and Grafting

35001 Direct repair of aneurysm, pseudoaneurysm, or excision (partial or total) and graft insertion, with or without patch graft; for aneurysm and associated occlusive disease, carotid, subclavian artery, by neck incision ◾C

RVU			Global Days	Modifiers				
Mod	Non-Fac Total	Fac Total		51	50	62	80	MUE
	33.05	33.05	090	2	1	1	2	1

35002 Direct repair of aneurysm, pseudoaneurysm, or excision (partial or total) and graft insertion, with or without patch graft; for ruptured aneurysm, carotid, subclavian artery, by neck incision ◾C

RVU			Global Days	Modifiers				
Mod	Non-Fac Total	Fac Total		51	50	62	80	MUE
	33.58	33.58	090	2	1	1	2	1

35005 Direct repair of aneurysm, pseudoaneurysm, or excision (partial or total) and graft insertion, with or without patch graft; for aneurysm, pseudoaneurysm, and associated occlusive disease, vertebral artery ◾C

RVU			Global Days	Modifiers				
Mod	Non-Fac Total	Fac Total		51	50	62	80	MUE
	31.96	31.96	090	2	1	1	2	1

35011 Direct repair of aneurysm, pseudoaneurysm, or excision (partial or total) and graft insertion, with or without patch graft; for aneurysm and associated occlusive disease, axillary-brachial artery, by arm incision ◾T

RVU			Global Days	Modifiers				
Mod	Non-Fac Total	Fac Total		51	50	62	80	MUE
	29.62	29.62	090	2	1	1	2	1

35013 Direct repair of aneurysm, pseudoaneurysm, or excision (partial or total) and graft insertion, with or without patch graft; for ruptured aneurysm, axillary-brachial artery, by arm incision ◾C

RVU			Global Days	Modifiers				
Mod	Non-Fac Total	Fac Total		51	50	62	80	MUE
	37.10	37.10	090	2	1	1	2	1

35021 Direct repair of aneurysm, pseudoaneurysm, or excision (partial or total) and graft insertion, with or without patch graft; for aneurysm, pseudoaneurysm, and associated occlusive disease, innominate, subclavian artery, by thoracic incision ◾C

RVU			Global Days	Modifiers				
Mod	Non-Fac Total	Fac Total		51	50	62	80	MUE
	37.00	37.00	090	2	1	1	2	1

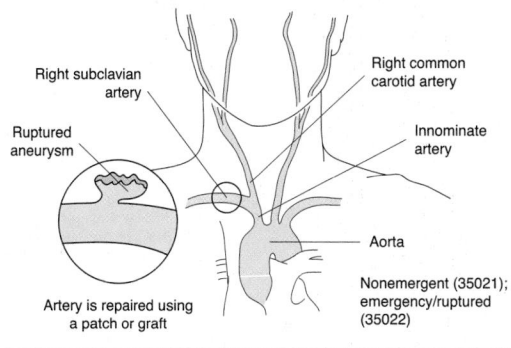

Repair of aneurysm, subclavian/innominate artery, thoracic approach

Right subclavian artery
Right common carotid artery
Ruptured aneurysm
Innominate artery
Aorta
Nonemergent (35021); emergency/ruptured (35022)
Artery is repaired using a patch or graft

35022 Direct repair of aneurysm, pseudoaneurysm, or excision (partial or total) and graft insertion, with or without patch graft; for ruptured aneurysm, innominate, subclavian artery, by thoracic incision ◾C

RVU			Global Days	Modifiers				
Mod	Non-Fac Total	Fac Total		51	50	62	80	MUE
	40.98	40.98	090	2	1	1	2	1

35045 Direct repair of aneurysm, pseudoaneurysm, or excision (partial or total) and graft insertion, with or without patch graft; for aneurysm, pseudoaneurysm, and associated occlusive disease, radial or ulnar artery ◾T

RVU			Global Days	Modifiers				
Mod	Non-Fac Total	Fac Total		51	50	62	80	MUE
	29.33	29.33	090	2	1	1	2	2

35081 Direct repair of aneurysm, pseudoaneurysm, or excision (partial or total) and graft insertion, with or without patch graft; for aneurysm, pseudoaneurysm, and associated occlusive disease, abdominal aorta ◾C

RVU			Global Days	Modifiers				
Mod	Non-Fac Total	Fac Total		51	50	62	80	MUE
	51.68	51.68	090	2	0	1	2	1

AMA: Dec 00: 2, Dec 01: 7, Dec 13: 8

35082 Direct repair of aneurysm, pseudoaneurysm, or excision (partial or total) and graft insertion, with or without patch graft; for ruptured aneurysm, abdominal aorta ◾C

RVU			Global Days	Modifiers				
Mod	Non-Fac Total	Fac Total		51	50	62	80	MUE
	65.00	65.00	090	2	0	1	2	1

● New   ▲ Revised   Deleted   ⊙ Moderate Sedation   ✚ Add-on Codes   ⊘ High Risk Denial   Ⓐ Age Edit   ♀ Female   ♂ Male   **AMA** *CPT® Assistant*   **MUE** Medically Unlikely Edit
⊘ Modifier 51 Exempt   ⊖ Modifier 63 Exempt   ☒ Unlisted   **Modifiers:** *See Inside Back Cover*   Ⓜ Maternity   A2–Z3 ASC Payment Indicators   A–Y OPPS Status Indicators

35091 Direct repair of aneurysm, pseudoaneurysm, or excision (partial or total) and graft insertion, with or without patch graft; for aneurysm, pseudoaneurysm, and associated occlusive disease, abdominal aorta involving visceral vessels (mesenteric, celiac, renal) Ⓒ

RVU			Global Days	Modifiers				
Mod	Non-Fac Total	Fac Total		51	50	62	80	MUE
	53.08	53.08	090	2	1	1	2	1

AMA: Dec 00: 2

Direct repair of aortic aneurysm

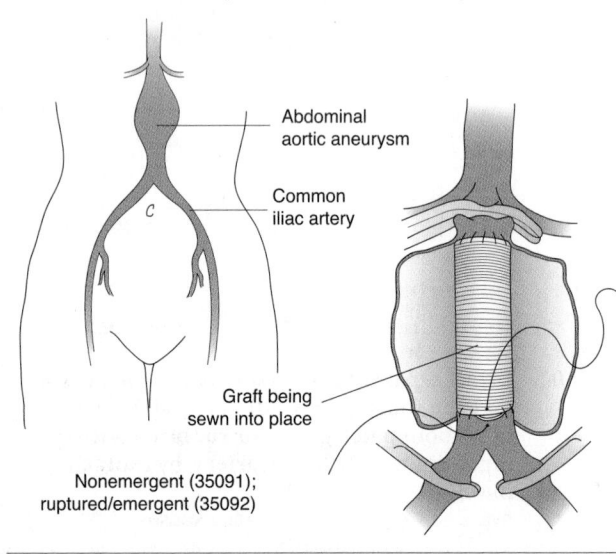

Abdominal aortic aneurysm

Common iliac artery

Graft being sewn into place

Nonemergent (35091);
ruptured/emergent (35092)

35092 Direct repair of aneurysm, pseudoaneurysm, or excision (partial or total) and graft insertion, with or without patch graft; for ruptured aneurysm, abdominal aorta involving visceral vessels (mesenteric, celiac, renal) Ⓒ

RVU			Global Days	Modifiers				
Mod	Non-Fac Total	Fac Total		51	50	62	80	MUE
	76.96	76.96	090	2	1	1	2	1

35102 Direct repair of aneurysm, pseudoaneurysm, or excision (partial or total) and graft insertion, with or without patch graft; for aneurysm, pseudoaneurysm, and associated occlusive disease, abdominal aorta involving iliac vessels (common, hypogastric, external) Ⓒ

RVU			Global Days	Modifiers				
Mod	Non-Fac Total	Fac Total		51	50	62	80	MUE
	55.91	55.91	090	2	1	1	2	1

AMA: Dec 13: 8

35103 Direct repair of aneurysm, pseudoaneurysm, or excision (partial or total) and graft insertion, with or without patch graft; for ruptured aneurysm, abdominal aorta involving iliac vessels (common, hypogastric, external) Ⓒ

RVU			Global Days	Modifiers				
Mod	Non-Fac Total	Fac Total		51	50	62	80	MUE
	66.52	66.52	090	2	1	1	2	1

35111 Direct repair of aneurysm, pseudoaneurysm, or excision (partial or total) and graft insertion, with or without patch graft; for aneurysm, pseudoaneurysm, and associated occlusive disease, splenic artery Ⓒ

RVU			Global Days	Modifiers				
Mod	Non-Fac Total	Fac Total		51	50	62	80	MUE
	44.98	44.98	090	2	1	1	2	1

35112 Direct repair of aneurysm, pseudoaneurysm, or excision (partial or total) and graft insertion, with or without patch graft; for ruptured aneurysm, splenic artery Ⓒ

RVU			Global Days	Modifiers				
Mod	Non-Fac Total	Fac Total		51	50	62	80	MUE
	54.37	54.37	090	2	1	1	2	1

35121 Direct repair of aneurysm, pseudoaneurysm, or excision (partial or total) and graft insertion, with or without patch graft; for aneurysm, pseudoaneurysm, and associated occlusive disease, hepatic, celiac, renal, or mesenteric artery Ⓒ

RVU			Global Days	Modifiers				
Mod	Non-Fac Total	Fac Total		51	50	62	80	MUE
	48.64	48.64	090	2	1	0	2	1

35122 Direct repair of aneurysm, pseudoaneurysm, or excision (partial or total) and graft insertion, with or without patch graft; for ruptured aneurysm, hepatic, celiac, renal, or mesenteric artery Ⓒ

RVU			Global Days	Modifiers				
Mod	Non-Fac Total	Fac Total		51	50	62	80	MUE
	63.41	63.41	090	2	1	1	2	1

35131 Direct repair of aneurysm, pseudoaneurysm, or excision (partial or total) and graft insertion, with or without patch graft; for aneurysm, pseudoaneurysm, and associated occlusive disease, iliac artery (common, hypogastric, external) Ⓒ

RVU			Global Days	Modifiers				
Mod	Non-Fac Total	Fac Total		51	50	62	80	MUE
	41.06	41.06	090	2	1	1	2	1

AMA: Feb 03: 2

35132 Direct repair of aneurysm, pseudoaneurysm, or excision (partial or total) and graft insertion, with or without patch graft; for ruptured aneurysm, iliac artery (common, hypogastric, external) Ⓒ

RVU			Global Days	Modifiers				
Mod	Non-Fac Total	Fac Total		51	50	62	80	MUE
	48.23	48.23	090	2	1	1	2	1

35141 Direct repair of aneurysm, pseudoaneurysm, or excision (partial or total) and graft insertion, with or without patch graft; for aneurysm, pseudoaneurysm, and associated occlusive disease, common femoral artery (profunda femoris, superficial femoral) Ⓒ

RVU			Global Days	Modifiers				
Mod	Non-Fac Total	Fac Total		51	50	62	80	MUE
	32.74	32.74	090	2	1	1	2	1

● New   ▲ Revised   ✖ Deleted   ⊙ Moderate Sedation   ✚ Add-on Codes   ⊘ High Risk Denial   Ⓐ Age Edit   ♀ Female   ♂ Male   **AMA** *CPT® Assistant*   ***MUE*** Medically Unlikely Edit
⊗ Modifier 51 Exempt   ⊖ Modifier 63 Exempt   Ⓧ Unlisted   **Modifiers:** *See Inside Back Cover*   Ⓜ Maternity   Ⓐ2–Ⓩ3 ASC Payment Indicators   Ⓐ–Ⓨ OPPS Status Indicators

CPT © 2015 American Medical Association. All Rights Reserved.   © 2016 DecisionHealth

35142 Direct repair of aneurysm, pseudoaneurysm, or excision (partial or total) and graft insertion, with or without patch graft; for ruptured aneurysm, common femoral artery (profunda femoris, superficial femoral)   C

RVU			Global Days	Modifiers				
Mod	Non-Fac Total	Fac Total		51	50	62	80	MUE
	39.14	39.14	090	2	1	1	2	1

35151 Direct repair of aneurysm, pseudoaneurysm, or excision (partial or total) and graft insertion, with or without patch graft; for aneurysm, pseudoaneurysm, and associated occlusive disease, popliteal artery   C

RVU			Global Days	Modifiers				
Mod	Non-Fac Total	Fac Total		51	50	62	80	MUE
	36.75	36.75	090	2	1	1	2	1

35152 Direct repair of aneurysm, pseudoaneurysm, or excision (partial or total) and graft insertion, with or without patch graft; for ruptured aneurysm, popliteal artery   C

RVU			Global Days	Modifiers				
Mod	Non-Fac Total	Fac Total		51	50	62	80	MUE
	41.44	41.44	090	2	1	1	2	1

Arteriovenous Fistula Repair

35180 Repair, congenital arteriovenous fistula; head and neck   T

RVU			Global Days	Modifiers				
Mod	Non-Fac Total	Fac Total		51	50	62	80	MUE
	27.50	27.50	090	2	0	1	2	2

AMA: Aug 11: 9

35182 Repair, congenital arteriovenous fistula; thorax and abdomen   C

RVU			Global Days	Modifiers				
Mod	Non-Fac Total	Fac Total		51	50	62	80	MUE
	51.31	51.31	090	2	0	1	2	2

AMA: Apr 11: 9

35184 Repair, congenital arteriovenous fistula; extremities   T

RVU			Global Days	Modifiers				
Mod	Non-Fac Total	Fac Total		51	50	62	80	MUE
	30.80	30.80	090	2	0	1	2	2

AMA: Apr 11: 9

35188 Repair, acquired or traumatic arteriovenous fistula; head and neck   A2 T

RVU			Global Days	Modifiers				
Mod	Non-Fac Total	Fac Total		51	50	62	80	MUE
	34.14	34.14	090	2	0	1	2	2

AMA: Apr 11: 9

35189 Repair, acquired or traumatic arteriovenous fistula; thorax and abdomen   C

RVU			Global Days	Modifiers				
Mod	Non-Fac Total	Fac Total		51	50	62	80	MUE
	45.24	45.24	090	2	0	1	2	1

AMA: Apr 11: 9

35190 Repair, acquired or traumatic arteriovenous fistula; extremities   T

RVU			Global Days	Modifiers				
Mod	Non-Fac Total	Fac Total		51	50	62	80	MUE
	22.46	22.46	090	2	0	1	2	2

AMA: Aug 11: 9

Other Blood Vessel Repair

Coding Guidance
Repair of blood vessels is not reported in addition to a primary vascular procedure; it is included in the closure and repair.

35201 Repair blood vessel, direct; neck   T

RVU			Global Days	Modifiers				
Mod	Non-Fac Total	Fac Total		51	50	62	80	MUE
	28.00	28.00	090	2	1	1	2	2

AMA: Apr 14: 10, Mar 14: 8

35206 Repair blood vessel, direct; upper extremity   T

RVU			Global Days	Modifiers				
Mod	Non-Fac Total	Fac Total		51	50	62	80	MUE
	22.83	22.83	090	2	1	1	2	2

AMA: Oct 00: 3, Nov 03: 5, Apr 12: 4, Apr 14: 10

35207 Repair blood vessel, direct; hand, finger   A2 T

RVU			Global Days	Modifiers				
Mod	Non-Fac Total	Fac Total		51	50	62	80	MUE
	22.12	22.12	090	2	1	1	1	3

35211 Repair blood vessel, direct; intrathoracic, with bypass   C

RVU			Global Days	Modifiers				
Mod	Non-Fac Total	Fac Total		51	50	62	80	MUE
	40.19	40.19	090	2	1	1	2	3

35216 Repair blood vessel, direct; intrathoracic, without bypass   C

RVU			Global Days	Modifiers				
Mod	Non-Fac Total	Fac Total		51	50	62	80	MUE
	60.09	60.09	090	2	1	1	2	2

AMA: Apr 05: 10, 11

35221 Repair blood vessel, direct; intra-abdominal   C

RVU			Global Days	Modifiers				
Mod	Non-Fac Total	Fac Total		51	50	62	80	MUE
	42.64	42.64	090	2	1	1	2	3

35226 Repair blood vessel, direct; lower extremity   T

RVU			Global Days	Modifiers				
Mod	Non-Fac Total	Fac Total		51	50	62	80	MUE
	24.58	24.58	090	2	1	1	2	3

AMA: Apr 12: 8, 9, Mar 13: 10, Dec 13: 8

35231 Repair blood vessel with vein graft; neck   T

RVU			Global Days	Modifiers				
Mod	Non-Fac Total	Fac Total		51	50	62	80	MUE
	35.43	35.43	090	2	1	1	2	2

35236 Repair blood vessel with vein graft; upper extremity   T

RVU			Global Days	Modifiers				
Mod	Non-Fac Total	Fac Total		51	50	62	80	MUE
	28.86	28.86	090	2	1	1	2	2

AMA: Oct 04: 8

● New   ▲ Revised   Deleted   ⊙ Moderate Sedation   ✚ Add-on Codes   ⊘ High Risk Denial   Ⓐ Age Edit   ♀ Female   ♂ Male   **AMA** *CPT® Assistant*   **MUE** Medically Unlikely Edit
⦸ Modifier 51 Exempt   ⊖ Modifier 63 Exempt   ✗ Unlisted   **Modifiers:** *See Inside Back Cover*   Ⓜ Maternity   A2 –Z3 ASC Payment Indicators   A –Y OPPS Status Indicators

35241 Repair blood vessel with vein graft; intrathoracic, with bypass   C

RVU			Global Days	Modifiers				
Mod	Non-Fac Total	Fac Total		51	50	62	80	MUE
	40.03	40.03	090	2	1	1	2	2

35246 Repair blood vessel with vein graft; intrathoracic, without bypass   C

RVU			Global Days	Modifiers				
Mod	Non-Fac Total	Fac Total		51	50	62	80	MUE
	46.32	46.32	090	2	1	1	2	2

35251 Repair blood vessel with vein graft; intra-abdominal   C

RVU			Global Days	Modifiers				
Mod	Non-Fac Total	Fac Total		51	50	62	80	MUE
	50.04	50.04	090	2	1	1	2	2

35256 Repair blood vessel with vein graft; lower extremity   T

RVU			Global Days	Modifiers				
Mod	Non-Fac Total	Fac Total		51	50	62	80	MUE
	30.12	30.12	090	2	1	1	2	2

35261 Repair blood vessel with graft other than vein; neck   T

RVU			Global Days	Modifiers				
Mod	Non-Fac Total	Fac Total		51	50	62	80	MUE
	31.01	31.01	090	2	1	1	2	1

35266 Repair blood vessel with graft other than vein; upper extremity   T

RVU			Global Days	Modifiers				
Mod	Non-Fac Total	Fac Total		51	50	62	80	MUE
	25.76	25.76	090	2	1	1	2	2

35271 Repair blood vessel with graft other than vein; intrathoracic, with bypass   C

RVU			Global Days	Modifiers				
Mod	Non-Fac Total	Fac Total		51	50	62	80	MUE
	40.04	40.04	090	2	1	1	2	2

35276 Repair blood vessel with graft other than vein; intrathoracic, without bypass   C

RVU			Global Days	Modifiers				
Mod	Non-Fac Total	Fac Total		51	50	62	80	MUE
	42.84	42.84	090	2	1	1	2	2

35281 Repair blood vessel with graft other than vein; intra-abdominal   C

RVU			Global Days	Modifiers				
Mod	Non-Fac Total	Fac Total		51	50	62	80	MUE
	47.63	47.63	090	2	1	1	2	2

35286 Repair blood vessel with graft other than vein; lower extremity   T

RVU			Global Days	Modifiers				
Mod	Non-Fac Total	Fac Total		51	50	62	80	MUE
	27.68	27.68	090	2	1	1	2	2

AMA: Apr 12: 8, 9, Mar 13: 10, Dec 13: 8, Apr 14: 10

Thromboendarterectomy

Coding Guidance

When a thromboendarterectomy is done at the site of an aneurysm for which direct repair or graft insertion is necessary, the thromboendarterectomy is included and is not reported as a separate service. If a vascular occlusion necessitates thromboendarterectomy at the same session on a different vessel, the appropriate code is reported with a modifier to denote another noncontiguous vessel site of the thromboendarterectomy. Closure and repair of the blood vessel is included when an open thromboendartectomy is performed. If a balloon thrombectomy fails and is followed by an open thromboendarterectomy, report only the more comprehensive, open service.

35301 Thromboendarterectomy, including patch graft, if performed; carotid, vertebral, subclavian, by neck incision   C

RVU			Global Days	Modifiers				
Mod	Non-Fac Total	Fac Total		51	50	62	80	MUE
	33.44	33.44	090	2	1	1	2	2

AMA: Jan 07: 7, Sep 10: 7

Thromboendarterectomy, including patch graft, if performed; carotid/vertebral/subclavian

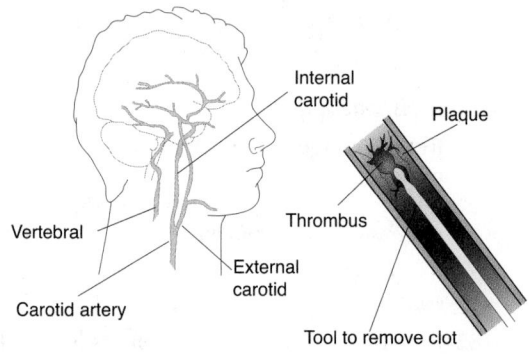

Internal carotid

Plaque

Vertebral

Thrombus

External carotid

Carotid artery

Tool to remove clot

The neck vessel is opened and the blood clot or plaque and inner lining are removed. The vessel is closed. A graft may be used to enlarge its diameter.

35302 Thromboendarterectomy, including patch graft, if performed; superficial femoral artery   C

RVU			Global Days	Modifiers				
Mod	Non-Fac Total	Fac Total		51	50	62	80	MUE
	33.27	33.27	090	2	1	1	2	1

AMA: Jan 07: 7, May 07: 9

● New   ▲ Revised   ✖ Deleted   ⊙ Moderate Sedation   ✚ Add-on Codes   ⊘ High Risk Denial   Ⓐ Age Edit   ♀ Female   ♂ Male   **AMA** *CPT® Assistant*   **MUE** Medically Unlikely Edit
⊘ Modifier 51 Exempt   ⊖ Modifier 63 Exempt   ✗ Unlisted   **Modifiers:** *See Inside Back Cover*   Ⓜ Maternity   A2–Z3 ASC Payment Indicators   A–Y OPPS Status Indicators

378   CPT © 2015 American Medical Association. All Rights Reserved.   © 2016 DecisionHealth

35303 Thromboendarterectomy, including patch graft, if performed; popliteal artery   C

RVU			Global Days	Modifiers				
Mod	Non-Fac Total	Fac Total		51	50	62	80	MUE
	36.83	36.83	090	2	1	1	2	1

AMA: Jan 07: 7, May 07: 9

Thromboendarterectomy, including patch graft, if performed; popliteal artery

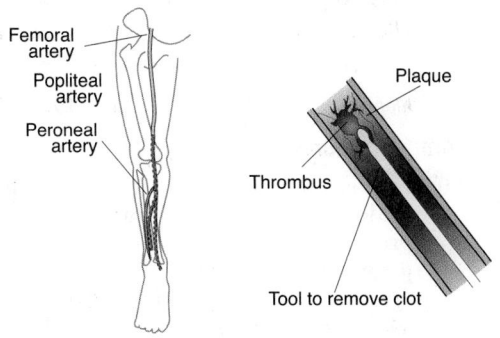

The popliteal artery is opened and the clot/plaque
and inner lining of the vessel are removed

35304 Thromboendarterectomy, including patch graft, if performed; tibioperoneal trunk artery   C

RVU			Global Days	Modifiers				
Mod	Non-Fac Total	Fac Total		51	50	62	80	MUE
	37.90	37.90	090	2	1	1	2	1

AMA: Jan 07: 7, May 07: 9

35305 Thromboendarterectomy, including patch graft, if performed; tibial or peroneal artery, initial vessel   C

RVU			Global Days	Modifiers				
Mod	Non-Fac Total	Fac Total		51	50	62	80	MUE
	36.32	36.32	090	2	1	1	2	1

AMA: May 07: 9

+ 35306 Thromboendarterectomy, including patch graft, if performed; each additional tibial or peroneal artery (List separately in addition to code for primary procedure)   C

RVU			Global Days	Modifiers				
Mod	Non-Fac Total	Fac Total		51	50	62	80	MUE
	13.42	13.42	ZZZ	0	0	1	2	2

AMA: Jan 07: 7, May 07: 9

35311 Thromboendarterectomy, including patch graft, if performed; subclavian, innominate, by thoracic incision   C

RVU			Global Days	Modifiers				
Mod	Non-Fac Total	Fac Total		51	50	62	80	MUE
	43.11	43.11	090	2	1	1	2	1

35321 Thromboendarterectomy, including patch graft, if performed; axillary-brachial   T

RVU			Global Days	Modifiers				
Mod	Non-Fac Total	Fac Total		51	50	62	80	MUE
	26.34	26.34	090	2	1	1	2	1

35331 Thromboendarterectomy, including patch graft, if performed; abdominal aorta   C

RVU			Global Days	Modifiers				
Mod	Non-Fac Total	Fac Total		51	50	62	80	MUE
	42.83	42.83	090	2	1	1	2	1

35341 Thromboendarterectomy, including patch graft, if performed; mesenteric, celiac, or renal   C

RVU			Global Days	Modifiers				
Mod	Non-Fac Total	Fac Total		51	50	62	80	MUE
	40.41	40.41	090	2	1	1	2	3

35351 Thromboendarterectomy, including patch graft, if performed; iliac   C

RVU			Global Days	Modifiers				
Mod	Non-Fac Total	Fac Total		51	50	62	80	MUE
	37.86	37.86	090	2	1	1	2	1

35355 Thromboendarterectomy, including patch graft, if performed; iliofemoral   C

RVU			Global Days	Modifiers				
Mod	Non-Fac Total	Fac Total		51	50	62	80	MUE
	30.65	30.65	090	2	1	1	2	1

35361 Thromboendarterectomy, including patch graft, if performed; combined aortoiliac   C

RVU			Global Days	Modifiers				
Mod	Non-Fac Total	Fac Total		51	50	62	80	MUE
	45.50	45.50	090	2	1	1	2	1

35363 Thromboendarterectomy, including patch graft, if performed; combined aortoiliofemoral   C

RVU			Global Days	Modifiers				
Mod	Non-Fac Total	Fac Total		51	50	62	80	MUE
	51.89	51.89	090	2	1	1	2	1

35371 Thromboendarterectomy, including patch graft, if performed; common femoral   C

RVU			Global Days	Modifiers				
Mod	Non-Fac Total	Fac Total		51	50	62	80	MUE
	24.22	24.22	090	2	1	1	2	1

AMA: Jan 07: 7

35372 Thromboendarterectomy, including patch graft, if performed; deep (profunda) femoral   C

RVU			Global Days	Modifiers				
Mod	Non-Fac Total	Fac Total		51	50	62	80	MUE
	29.02	29.02	090	2	1	1	2	1

AMA: Jan 07: 7

+ 35390 Reoperation, carotid, thromboendarterectomy, more than 1 month after original operation (List separately in addition to code for primary procedure)   C

RVU			Global Days	Modifiers				
Mod	Non-Fac Total	Fac Total		51	50	62	80	MUE
	4.66	4.66	ZZZ	0	0	1	2	1

AMA: Nov 97: 16

● New   ▲ Revised   Deleted   ⊙ Moderate Sedation   ✚ Add-on Codes   ⊘ High Risk Denial   Ⓐ Age Edit   ♀ Female   ♂ Male   **AMA** *CPT® Assistant*   **MUE** Medically Unlikely Edit
⊘ Modifier 51 Exempt   ⊖ Modifier 63 Exempt   🗷 Unlisted   **Modifiers:** *See Inside Back Cover*   Ⓜ Maternity   A2–Z3 ASC Payment Indicators   A–Y OPPS Status Indicators

Non-coronary Angioscopy

+ 35400 Angioscopy (noncoronary vessels or grafts) during therapeutic intervention (List separately in addition to code for primary procedure) C

RVU			Global Days	Modifiers				
Mod	Non-Fac Total	Fac Total		51	50	62	80	MUE
	4.41	4.41	ZZZ	0	0	1	0	1

AMA: Nov 97: 16

Transluminal Angioplasty Procedures

Coding Guidance

When a percutaneous vascular procedure (percutaneous transluminal angioplasty/thrombectomy/embolectomy) is unsuccessful and requires a similar open procedure at the same session (open transluminal angioplasty or thromboendarterectomy), only the more extensive, successful procedure is reported. A percutaneous procedure performed at one site with an open procedure performed at a separate site during the same session may both be reported with the appropriate modifier when the locations are in distinct, anatomically different vessels.

35450 Transluminal balloon angioplasty, open; renal or other visceral artery C

RVU			Global Days	Modifiers				
Mod	Non-Fac Total	Fac Total		51	50	62	80	MUE
	14.95	14.95	000	2	1	1	2	2

AMA: Feb 97: 2, 3

35452 Transluminal balloon angioplasty, open; aortic C

RVU			Global Days	Modifiers				
Mod	Non-Fac Total	Fac Total		51	50	62	80	MUE
	10.08	10.08	000	2	1	1	2	1

AMA: Feb 97: 2, 3, Dec 13: 8

35458 Transluminal balloon angioplasty, open; brachiocephalic trunk or branches, each vessel J 1

RVU			Global Days	Modifiers				
Mod	Non-Fac Total	Fac Total		51	50	62	80	MUE
	14.58	14.58	000	2	1	1	2	2

AMA: Feb 97: 2, 3, May 01: 11, Mar 14: 8

35460 Transluminal balloon angioplasty, open; venous G 2 J 1

RVU			Global Days	Modifiers				
Mod	Non-Fac Total	Fac Total		51	50	62	80	MUE
	9.29	9.29	000	2	1	1	1	2

AMA: Feb 97: 2, 3

⊙ **35471 Transluminal balloon angioplasty, percutaneous; renal or visceral artery** J 1

RVU			Global Days	Modifiers				
Mod	Non-Fac Total	Fac Total		51	50	62	80	MUE
	72.67	15.33	000	2	1	0	1	3

AMA: Aug 96: 3, Feb 97: 2, 3

⊙ **35472 Transluminal balloon angioplasty, percutaneous; aortic** J 1

RVU			Global Days	Modifiers				
Mod	Non-Fac Total	Fac Total		51	50	62	80	MUE
	52.38	10.45	000	2	1	1	0	1

AMA: Aug 96: 3, Feb 97: 2, 3, Dec 13: 8

⊙ **35475 Transluminal balloon angioplasty, percutaneous; brachiocephalic trunk or branches, each vessel** P 3 J 1

RVU			Global Days	Modifiers				
Mod	Non-Fac Total	Fac Total		51	50	62	80	MUE
	44.26	9.74	000	2	1	0	1	4

AMA: Aug 96: 3, Feb 97: 2, 3, May 01: 4, Sep 08: 10

⊙ **35476 Transluminal balloon angioplasty, percutaneous; venous** P 3 J 1

RVU			Global Days	Modifiers				
Mod	Non-Fac Total	Fac Total		51	50	62	80	MUE
	40.57	7.87	000	2	1	0	1	5

AMA: Aug 96: 3, Feb 97: 2, 3, May 01: 4, Dec 03: 2, Dec 11: 16, Apr 12: 5

Bypass Graft Procedures

+ 35500 Harvest of upper extremity vein, 1 segment, for lower extremity or coronary artery bypass procedure (List separately in addition to code for primary procedure) N

RVU			Global Days	Modifiers				
Mod	Non-Fac Total	Fac Total		51	50	62	80	MUE
	9.37	9.37	ZZZ	0	0	1	2	2

AMA: Nov 98: 13, Mar 99: 6, Nov 99: 19, Jan 07: 7, Apr 12: 4

Coding Guidance

Only one type of bypass (venous/nonvenous) can be reported for a given site of obstruction. The different types of peripheral vascular bypass grafting codes are mutually exclusive. When different vessels have different bypass methodologies employed, then separate codes may be reported. When the same vessel requires different bypass techniques for multiple obstructions in more than one area, then different procedure codes may be reported with modifiers to indicate the separate procedures. When placing a bypass graft requires an endarterectomy, only the bypass code may be reported.

35501 Bypass graft, with vein; common carotid-ipsilateral internal carotid C

RVU			Global Days	Modifiers				
Mod	Non-Fac Total	Fac Total		51	50	62	80	MUE
	44.26	44.26	090	2	1	1	2	1

AMA: Apr 99: 11

35506 Bypass graft, with vein; carotid-subclavian or subclavian-carotid C

RVU			Global Days	Modifiers				
Mod	Non-Fac Total	Fac Total		51	50	62	80	MUE
	37.73	37.73	090	2	1	1	2	1

AMA: Oct 04: 6, Jan 07: 7

35508 Bypass graft, with vein; carotid-vertebral C

RVU			Global Days	Modifiers				
Mod	Non-Fac Total	Fac Total		51	50	62	80	MUE
	40.08	40.08	090	2	1	1	2	1

● New ▲ Revised ✖ Deleted ⊙ Moderate Sedation + Add-on Codes ⊘ High Risk Denial Ⓐ Age Edit ♀ Female ♂ Male **AMA** CPT® Assistant **MUE** Medically Unlikely Edit

⊘ Modifier 51 Exempt ⊖ Modifier 63 Exempt Ⓧ Unlisted **Modifiers:** See Inside Back Cover Ⓜ Maternity A 2 – Z 3 ASC Payment Indicators A – Y OPPS Status Indicators

380 | CPT © 2015 American Medical Association. All Rights Reserved. | © 2016 DecisionHealth

35509 Bypass graft, with vein; carotid-contralateral carotid   C

RVU			Global Days	Modifiers				
Mod	Non-Fac Total	Fac Total		51	50	62	80	MUE
	41.76	41.76	090	2	1	1	2	1

AMA: Jan 07: 7, May 07: 9

**Bypass graft, with vein;
carotid-contralateral carotid**

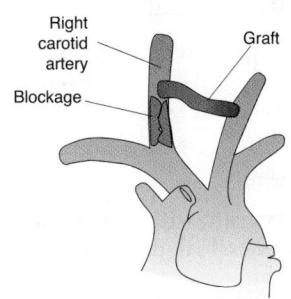

Right carotid artery — Graft
Blockage

The damaged or blocked portion of the carotid is bypassed
with a harvested vein, restoring adequate blood flow from
the carotid artery on the other side.

35510 Bypass graft, with vein; carotid-brachial   C

RVU			Global Days	Modifiers				
Mod	Non-Fac Total	Fac Total		51	50	62	80	MUE
	36.44	36.44	090	2	1	1	2	1

AMA: Oct 04: 6, Nov 07: 8

35511 Bypass graft, with vein; subclavian-subclavian   C

RVU			Global Days	Modifiers				
Mod	Non-Fac Total	Fac Total		51	50	62	80	MUE
	33.19	33.19	090	2	1	1	2	1

35512 Bypass graft, with vein; subclavian-brachial   C

RVU			Global Days	Modifiers				
Mod	Non-Fac Total	Fac Total		51	50	62	80	MUE
	36.11	36.11	090	2	1	1	2	1

AMA: Oct 04: 7

35515 Bypass graft, with vein; subclavian-vertebral   C

RVU			Global Days	Modifiers				
Mod	Non-Fac Total	Fac Total		51	50	62	80	MUE
	42.47	42.47	090	2	1	1	2	1

**Bypass graft, with vein;
subclavian-vertebral**

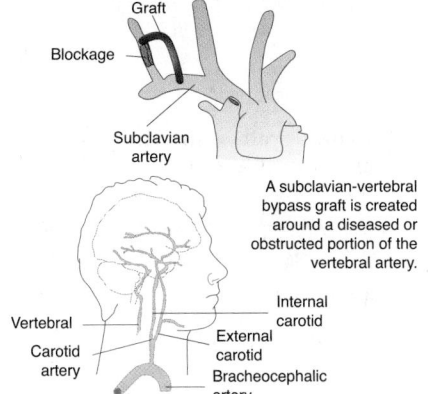

Graft
Blockage
Subclavian artery

A subclavian-vertebral
bypass graft is created
around a diseased or
obstructed portion of the
vertebral artery.

Vertebral
Carotid artery
Internal carotid
External carotid
Bracheocephalic artery

35516 Bypass graft, with vein; subclavian-axillary   C

RVU			Global Days	Modifiers				
Mod	Non-Fac Total	Fac Total		51	50	62	80	MUE
	36.13	36.13	090	2	1	1	2	1

35518 Bypass graft, with vein; axillary-axillary   C

RVU			Global Days	Modifiers				
Mod	Non-Fac Total	Fac Total		51	50	62	80	MUE
	34.36	34.36	090	2	1	1	2	1

AMA: Oct 04: 9

35521 Bypass graft, with vein; axillary-femoral   C

RVU			Global Days	Modifiers				
Mod	Non-Fac Total	Fac Total		51	50	62	80	MUE
	36.57	36.57	090	2	1	1	2	1

35522 Bypass graft, with vein; axillary-brachial   C

RVU			Global Days	Modifiers				
Mod	Non-Fac Total	Fac Total		51	50	62	80	MUE
	35.74	35.74	090	2	1	1	2	1

AMA: Oct 04: 9

35523 Bypass graft, with vein; brachial-ulnar or -radial   C

RVU			Global Days	Modifiers				
Mod	Non-Fac Total	Fac Total		51	50	62	80	MUE
	37.95	37.95	090	2	1	1	2	1

35525 Bypass graft, with vein; brachial-brachial   C

RVU			Global Days	Modifiers				
Mod	Non-Fac Total	Fac Total		51	50	62	80	MUE
	33.87	33.87	090	2	1	1	2	1

AMA: Oct 04: 10

35526 Bypass graft, with vein; aortosubclavian, aortoinnominate, or aortocarotid   C

RVU			Global Days	Modifiers				
Mod	Non-Fac Total	Fac Total		51	50	62	80	MUE
	50.32	50.32	090	2	1	1	2	1

**Bypass graft, with vein; aortosubclavian/
aortoinnominate or aortocarotid**

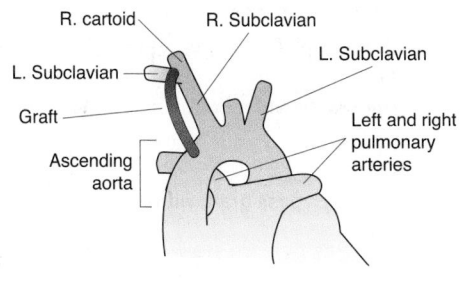

R. cartoid
R. Subclavian
L. Subclavian
L. Subclavian
Graft
Left and right pulmonary arteries
Ascending aorta

A damaged or blocked portion of artery
is bypassed using a harvested vein

35531 Bypass graft, with vein; aortoceliac or aortomesenteric   C

RVU			Global Days	Modifiers				
Mod	Non-Fac Total	Fac Total		51	50	62	80	MUE
	59.94	59.94	090	2	1	1	2	2

● New   ▲ Revised   Deleted   ⊙ Moderate Sedation   ✚ Add-on Codes   ⊗ High Risk Denial   Ⓐ Age Edit   ♀ Female   ♂ Male   **AMA** CPT® Assistant   **MUE** Medically Unlikely Edit
⊘ Modifier 51 Exempt   ⊖ Modifier 63 Exempt   ✗ Unlisted   **Modifiers:** See Inside Back Cover   Ⓜ Maternity   A2–Z3 ASC Payment Indicators   A–Y OPPS Status Indicators

Surgical Procedures

35533 – 35571

35533   Bypass graft, with vein; axillary-femoral-femoral   C

RVU			Global Days	Modifiers				
Mod	Non-Fac Total	Fac Total		51	50	62	80	MUE
	44.33	44.33	090	2	1	1	2	1

35535   Bypass graft, with vein; hepatorenal   C

RVU			Global Days	Modifiers				
Mod	Non-Fac Total	Fac Total		51	50	62	80	MUE
	56.72	56.72	090	2	1	1	2	1

35536   Bypass graft, with vein; splenorenal   C

RVU			Global Days	Modifiers				
Mod	Non-Fac Total	Fac Total		51	50	62	80	MUE
	50.03	50.03	090	2	1	1	2	1

AMA: Jun 99: 10

35537   Bypass graft, with vein; aortoiliac   C

RVU			Global Days	Modifiers				
Mod	Non-Fac Total	Fac Total		51	50	62	80	MUE
	64.71	64.71	090	2	0	1	2	1

AMA: Jan 07: 7

35538   Bypass graft, with vein; aortobi-iliac   C

RVU			Global Days	Modifiers				
Mod	Non-Fac Total	Fac Total		51	50	62	80	MUE
	69.45	69.45	090	2	0	1	2	1

AMA: Jan 07: 7

35539   Bypass graft, with vein; aortofemoral   C

RVU			Global Days	Modifiers				
Mod	Non-Fac Total	Fac Total		51	50	62	80	MUE
	65.00	65.00	090	2	1	1	2	1

AMA: Jan 07: 7

35540   Bypass graft, with vein; aortobifemoral   C

RVU			Global Days	Modifiers				
Mod	Non-Fac Total	Fac Total		51	50	62	80	MUE
	72.64	72.64	090	2	1	1	1	1

AMA: Jan 07: 7

35556   Bypass graft, with vein; femoral-popliteal   C

RVU			Global Days	Modifiers				
Mod	Non-Fac Total	Fac Total		51	50	62	80	MUE
	41.42	41.42	090	2	1	1	2	1

AMA: Fall 92: 20, May 97: 10, Jan 07: 7, Nov 07: 8

35558   Bypass graft, with vein; femoral-femoral   C

RVU			Global Days	Modifiers				
Mod	Non-Fac Total	Fac Total		51	50	62	80	MUE
	36.54	36.54	090	2	1	1	2	1

Bypass graft, with vein; femoral-femoral

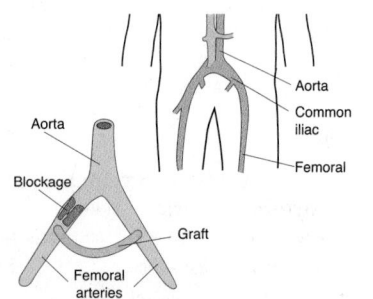

The damaged or blocked portion of the femoral artery is bypassed with a harvested vein, creating adequate blood flow from the femoral artery to the opposite femoral artery.

35560   Bypass graft, with vein; aortorenal   C

RVU			Global Days	Modifiers				
Mod	Non-Fac Total	Fac Total		51	50	62	80	MUE
	50.80	50.80	090	2	1	1	2	1

AMA: Jun 99: 10

35563   Bypass graft, with vein; ilioiliac   C

RVU			Global Days	Modifiers				
Mod	Non-Fac Total	Fac Total		51	50	62	80	MUE
	39.21	39.21	090	2	1	1	2	1

35565   Bypass graft, with vein; iliofemoral   C

RVU			Global Days	Modifiers				
Mod	Non-Fac Total	Fac Total		51	50	62	80	MUE
	39.23	39.23	090	2	1	1	2	1

AMA: Oct 04: 8

35566   Bypass graft, with vein; femoral-anterior tibial, posterior tibial, peroneal artery or other distal vessels   C

RVU			Global Days	Modifiers				
Mod	Non-Fac Total	Fac Total		51	50	62	80	MUE
	49.45	49.45	090	2	1	1	2	1

AMA: Jan 07: 7, Nov 07: 8

35570   Bypass graft, with vein; tibial-tibial, peroneal-tibial, or tibial/peroneal trunk-tibial   C

RVU			Global Days	Modifiers				
Mod	Non-Fac Total	Fac Total		51	50	62	80	MUE
	45.02	45.02	090	2	1	1	2	1

AMA: Apr 12: 4

Bypass graft, with vein; tibial-tibial, peroneal-tibial, or tibial/peroneal trunk-tibial

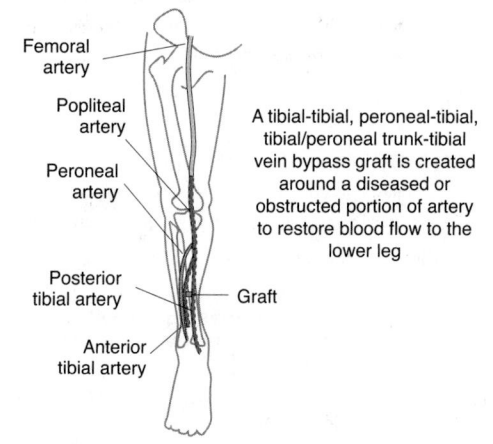

A tibial-tibial, peroneal-tibial, tibial/peroneal trunk-tibial vein bypass graft is created around a diseased or obstructed portion of artery to restore blood flow to the lower leg

35571   Bypass graft, with vein; popliteal-tibial, -peroneal artery or other distal vessels   C

RVU			Global Days	Modifiers				
Mod	Non-Fac Total	Fac Total		51	50	62	80	MUE
	39.36	39.36	090	2	1	1	2	2

AMA: Jan 07: 7, Nov 07: 8

● New   ▲ Revised   ✖ Deleted   ⊙ Moderate Sedation   ✚ Add-on Codes   ⊘ High Risk Denial   ⒶAge Edit   ♀ Female   ♂ Male   **AMA** *CPT® Assistant*   **MUE** Medically Unlikely Edit
⊘ Modifier 51 Exempt   ⊖ Modifier 63 Exempt   ✄ Unlisted   **Modifiers:** *See Inside Back Cover*   Ⓜ Maternity   A2–Z3 ASC Payment Indicators   A–Y OPPS Status Indicators

CPT © 2015 American Medical Association. All Rights Reserved.   © 2016 DecisionHealth

+ **35572** Harvest of femoropopliteal vein, 1 segment, for vascular reconstruction procedure (eg, aortic, vena caval, coronary, peripheral artery) (List separately in addition to code for primary procedure) N I N

RVU			Global Days	Modifiers				
Mod	Non-Fac Total	Fac Total		51	50	62	80	MUE
	10.19	10.19	ZZZ	0	0	0	2	2

AMA: Jan 07: 28

35583 In-situ vein bypass; femoral-popliteal   C

RVU			Global Days	Modifiers				
Mod	Non-Fac Total	Fac Total		51	50	62	80	MUE
	42.83	42.83	090	2	1	1	2	1

AMA: Jan 07: 7, Nov 07: 8

35585 In-situ vein bypass; femoral-anterior tibial, posterior tibial, or peroneal artery   C

RVU			Global Days	Modifiers				
Mod	Non-Fac Total	Fac Total		51	50	62	80	MUE
	49.68	49.68	090	2	1	1	2	2

AMA: Jan 07: 7, Nov 07: 8

35587 In-situ vein bypass; popliteal-tibial, peroneal   C

RVU			Global Days	Modifiers				
Mod	Non-Fac Total	Fac Total		51	50	62	80	MUE
	40.43	40.43	090	2	1	1	2	2

AMA: Apr 99: 11, Jan 07: 7, Nov 07: 8

+ **35600** Harvest of upper extremity artery, 1 segment, for coronary artery bypass procedure (List separately in addition to code for primary procedure)   C

RVU			Global Days	Modifiers				
Mod	Non-Fac Total	Fac Total		51	50	62	80	MUE
	7.36	7.36	ZZZ	0	0	1	2	2

AMA: Apr 07: 12

35601 Bypass graft, with other than vein; common carotid-ipsilateral internal carotid   C

RVU			Global Days	Modifiers				
Mod	Non-Fac Total	Fac Total		51	50	62	80	MUE
	41.53	41.53	090	2	1	1	2	1

AMA: Jul 06: 7, Jan 07: 7

35606 Bypass graft, with other than vein; carotid-subclavian   C

RVU			Global Days	Modifiers				
Mod	Non-Fac Total	Fac Total		51	50	62	80	MUE
	34.74	34.74	090	2	1	1	2	1

35612 Bypass graft, with other than vein; subclavian-subclavian   C

RVU			Global Days	Modifiers				
Mod	Non-Fac Total	Fac Total		51	50	62	80	MUE
	31.83	31.83	090	2	1	1	2	1

35616 Bypass graft, with other than vein; subclavian-axillary   C

RVU			Global Days	Modifiers				
Mod	Non-Fac Total	Fac Total		51	50	62	80	MUE
	32.67	32.67	090	2	1	1	2	1

35621 Bypass graft, with other than vein; axillary-femoral   C

RVU			Global Days	Modifiers				
Mod	Non-Fac Total	Fac Total		51	50	62	80	MUE
	32.57	32.57	090	2	1	1	2	1

AMA: Jan 07: 7

35623 Bypass graft, with other than vein; axillary-popliteal or -tibial   C

RVU			Global Days	Modifiers				
Mod	Non-Fac Total	Fac Total		51	50	62	80	MUE
	38.92	38.92	090	2	1	1	2	1

35626 Bypass graft, with other than vein; aortosubclavian, aortoinnominate, or aortocarotid   C

RVU			Global Days	Modifiers				
Mod	Non-Fac Total	Fac Total		51	50	62	80	MUE
	46.49	46.49	090	2	1	1	2	3

35631 Bypass graft, with other than vein; aortoceliac, aortomesenteric, aortorenal   C

RVU			Global Days	Modifiers				
Mod	Non-Fac Total	Fac Total		51	50	62	80	MUE
	54.80	54.80	090	2	1	1	2	4

35632 Bypass graft, with other than vein; ilio-celiac   C

RVU			Global Days	Modifiers				
Mod	Non-Fac Total	Fac Total		51	50	62	80	MUE
	53.33	53.33	090	2	1	1	2	1

35633 Bypass graft, with other than vein; ilio-mesenteric   C

RVU			Global Days	Modifiers				
Mod	Non-Fac Total	Fac Total		51	50	62	80	MUE
	59.38	59.38	090	2	1	1	2	1

35634 Bypass graft, with other than vein; iliorenal   C

RVU			Global Days	Modifiers				
Mod	Non-Fac Total	Fac Total		51	50	62	80	MUE
	52.26	52.26	090	2	1	1	2	1

35636 Bypass graft, with other than vein; splenorenal (splenic to renal arterial anastomosis)   C

RVU			Global Days	Modifiers				
Mod	Non-Fac Total	Fac Total		51	50	62	80	MUE
	47.67	47.67	090	2	1	1	2	1

35637 Bypass graft, with other than vein; aortoiliac   C

RVU			Global Days	Modifiers				
Mod	Non-Fac Total	Fac Total		51	50	62	80	MUE
	51.15	51.15	090	2	0	1	2	1

AMA: Jan 07: 7

35638 Bypass graft, with other than vein; aortobi-iliac   C

RVU			Global Days	Modifiers				
Mod	Non-Fac Total	Fac Total		51	50	62	80	MUE
	52.26	52.26	090	2	0	1	2	1

AMA: Jan 07: 7

● New   ▲ Revised   Deleted   ⊙ Moderate Sedation   ✚ Add-on Codes   ⊘ High Risk Denial   Ⓐ Age Edit   ♀ Female   ♂ Male   **AMA** CPT® Assistant   **MUE** Medically Unlikely Edit
⊘ Modifier 51 Exempt   ⊖ Modifier 63 Exempt   ✗ Unlisted   **Modifiers:** See Inside Back Cover   Ⓜ Maternity   A2–Z3 ASC Payment Indicators   A–Y OPPS Status Indicators

© 2016 DecisionHealth   CPT © 2015 American Medical Association. All Rights Reserved.   **383**

35642 Bypass graft, with other than vein; carotid-vertebral ⊗C

RVU			Global Days	Modifiers				
Mod	Non-Fac Total	Fac Total		51	50	62	80	MUE
	29.18	29.18	090	2	1	1	2	1

35645 Bypass graft, with other than vein; subclavian-vertebral C

RVU			Global Days	Modifiers				
Mod	Non-Fac Total	Fac Total		51	50	62	80	MUE
	30.29	30.29	090	2	1	1	2	1

35646 Bypass graft, with other than vein; aortobifemoral C

RVU			Global Days	Modifiers				
Mod	Non-Fac Total	Fac Total		51	50	62	80	MUE
	50.87	50.87	090	2	0	1	2	1

AMA: Jan 07: 7

35647 Bypass graft, with other than vein; aortofemoral C

RVU			Global Days	Modifiers				
Mod	Non-Fac Total	Fac Total		51	50	62	80	MUE
	46.21	46.21	090	2	1	1	2	1

AMA: Jan 07: 7

35650 Bypass graft, with other than vein; axillary-axillary C

RVU			Global Days	Modifiers				
Mod	Non-Fac Total	Fac Total		51	50	62	80	MUE
	31.89	31.89	090	2	1	1	2	1

35654 Bypass graft, with other than vein; axillary-femoral-femoral C

RVU			Global Days	Modifiers				
Mod	Non-Fac Total	Fac Total		51	50	62	80	MUE
	40.59	40.59	090	2	0	1	2	1

AMA: Jan 07: 7

35656 Bypass graft, with other than vein; femoral-popliteal C

RVU			Global Days	Modifiers				
Mod	Non-Fac Total	Fac Total		51	50	62	80	MUE
	32.12	32.12	090	2	1	1	2	1

AMA: Nov 07: 8

35661 Bypass graft, with other than vein; femoral-femoral C

RVU			Global Days	Modifiers				
Mod	Non-Fac Total	Fac Total		51	50	62	80	MUE
	32.16	32.16	090	2	1	1	2	1

AMA: Dec 04: 6, Jan 07: 7

35663 Bypass graft, with other than vein; ilioiliac C

RVU			Global Days	Modifiers				
Mod	Non-Fac Total	Fac Total		51	50	62	80	MUE
	37.27	37.27	090	2	1	1	2	1

35665 Bypass graft, with other than vein; iliofemoral C

RVU			Global Days	Modifiers				
Mod	Non-Fac Total	Fac Total		51	50	62	80	MUE
	34.76	34.76	090	2	1	1	2	1

AMA: Jan 07: 7

35666 Bypass graft, with other than vein; femoral-anterior tibial, posterior tibial, or peroneal artery C

RVU			Global Days	Modifiers				
Mod	Non-Fac Total	Fac Total		51	50	62	80	MUE
	37.57	37.57	090	2	1	1	2	2

AMA: Nov 07: 8

35671 Bypass graft, with other than vein; popliteal-tibial or -peroneal artery C

RVU			Global Days	Modifiers				
Mod	Non-Fac Total	Fac Total		51	50	62	80	MUE
	33.11	33.11	090	2	1	1	2	2

Harvest/Anastomosis Composite Grafts

+ 35681 Bypass graft; composite, prosthetic and vein (List separately in addition to code for primary procedure) C

RVU			Global Days	Modifiers				
Mod	Non-Fac Total	Fac Total		51	50	62	80	MUE
	2.33	2.33	ZZZ	0	0	1	2	1

AMA: Nov 98: 13, 14, Mar 99: 6, Apr 99: 11

+ 35682 Bypass graft; autogenous composite, 2 segments of veins from 2 locations (List separately in addition to code for primary procedure) C

RVU			Global Days	Modifiers				
Mod	Non-Fac Total	Fac Total		51	50	62	80	MUE
	10.47	10.47	ZZZ	0	0	1	0	1

AMA: Nov 98: 13, 14, Mar 99: 6, Apr 99: 11, Sep 02: 4

+ 35683 Bypass graft; autogenous composite, 3 or more segments of vein from 2 or more locations (List separately in addition to code for primary procedure) C

RVU			Global Days	Modifiers				
Mod	Non-Fac Total	Fac Total		51	50	62	80	MUE
	12.20	12.20	ZZZ	0	0	1	0	1

AMA: Nov 98: 13, 14, Mar 99: 6, Apr 99: 11, Sep 02: 4

Other Bypass Procedures

+ 35685 Placement of vein patch or cuff at distal anastomosis of bypass graft, synthetic conduit (List separately in addition to code for primary procedure) N

RVU			Global Days	Modifiers				
Mod	Non-Fac Total	Fac Total		51	50	62	80	MUE
	5.86	5.86	ZZZ	0	0	1	2	2

AMA: Sep 02: 3

+ 35686 Creation of distal arteriovenous fistula during lower extremity bypass surgery (non-hemodialysis) (List separately in addition to code for primary procedure) N

RVU			Global Days	Modifiers				
Mod	Non-Fac Total	Fac Total		51	50	62	80	MUE
	4.78	4.78	ZZZ	0	0	1	2	1

AMA: Sep 02: 3, Apr 12: 4

● New   ▲ Revised   ✖ Deleted   ⊙ Moderate Sedation   ✛ Add-on Codes   ⊗ High Risk Denial   ⓐ Age Edit   ♀ Female   ♂ Male   **AMA** CPT® Assistant   **MUE** Medically Unlikely Edit
⊘ Modifier 51 Exempt   ⊖ Modifier 63 Exempt   ✖ Unlisted   **Modifiers:** See Inside Back Cover   Ⓜ Maternity   A2–Z3 ASC Payment Indicators   A–Y OPPS Status Indicators

384   CPT © 2015 American Medical Association. All Rights Reserved.   © 2016 DecisionHealth

Arterial Transposition Procedures

35691   Transposition and/or reimplantation; vertebral to carotid artery   **C**

RVU			Global Days	Modifiers				
Mod	Non-Fac Total	Fac Total		51	50	62	80	MUE
	28.47	28.47	090	2	1	1	2	1

Transposition/reimplantation; vertebral to carotid/subclavian artery

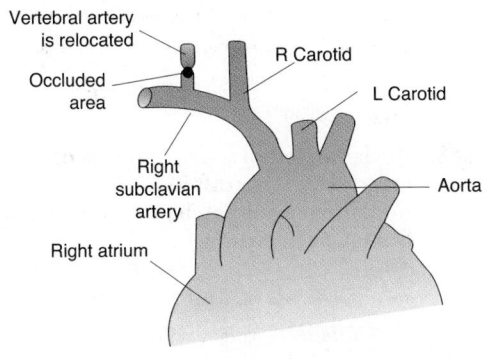

The vertebral artery is divided above the stenotic area and repositioned/reimplanted onto the carotid (35691), or subclavian (35693) artery

35693   Transposition and/or reimplantation; vertebral to subclavian artery   **C**

RVU			Global Days	Modifiers				
Mod	Non-Fac Total	Fac Total		51	50	62	80	MUE
	24.09	24.09	090	2	1	1	2	1

35694   Transposition and/or reimplantation; subclavian to carotid artery   **C**

RVU			Global Days	Modifiers				
Mod	Non-Fac Total	Fac Total		51	50	62	80	MUE
	29.32	29.32	090	2	1	1	2	1

35695   Transposition and/or reimplantation; carotid to subclavian artery   **C**

RVU			Global Days	Modifiers				
Mod	Non-Fac Total	Fac Total		51	50	62	80	MUE
	31.11	31.11	090	2	1	1	2	1

+ 35697   Reimplantation, visceral artery to infrarenal aortic prosthesis, each artery (List separately in addition to code for primary procedure)   **C**

RVU			Global Days	Modifiers				
Mod	Non-Fac Total	Fac Total		51	50	62	80	MUE
	4.34	4.34	ZZZ	0	0	2	2	2

Excisional/Exploration/Repair/Revision Procedures

+ 35700   Reoperation, femoral-popliteal or femoral (popliteal)-anterior tibial, posterior tibial, peroneal artery, or other distal vessels, more than 1 month after original operation (List separately in addition to code for primary procedure)   **C**

RVU			Global Days	Modifiers				
Mod	Non-Fac Total	Fac Total		51	50	62	80	MUE
	4.49	4.49	ZZZ	0	0	1	2	2

AMA: Apr 12: 4

Vessel reoperation

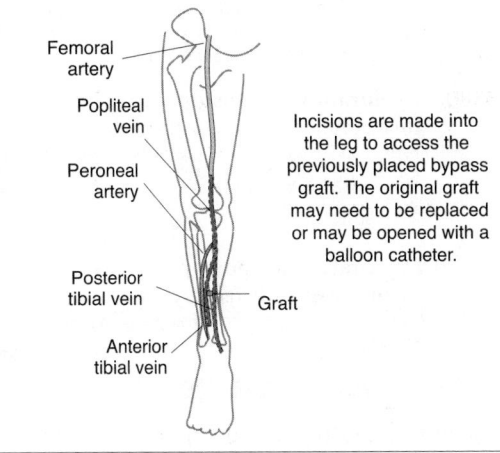

Incisions are made into the leg to access the previously placed bypass graft. The original graft may need to be replaced or may be opened with a balloon catheter.

35701   Exploration (not followed by surgical repair), with or without lysis of artery; carotid artery   **C**

RVU			Global Days	Modifiers				
Mod	Non-Fac Total	Fac Total		51	50	62	80	MUE
	16.54	16.54	090	2	1	1	2	1

Exploration, with or without lysis of artery

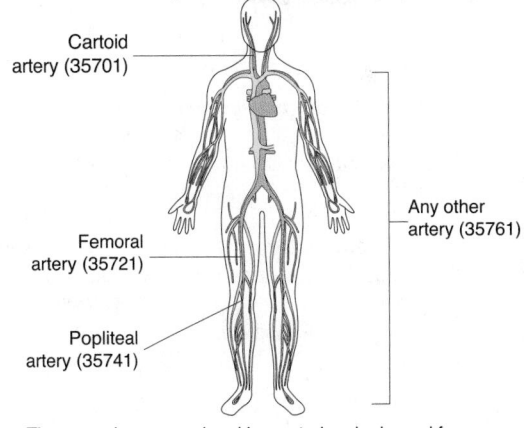

The artery is accessed and inspected and released from surrounding tissue (lysis) if needed

35721   Exploration (not followed by surgical repair), with or without lysis of artery; femoral artery   **C**

RVU			Global Days	Modifiers				
Mod	Non-Fac Total	Fac Total		51	50	62	80	MUE
	13.38	13.38	090	2	1	1	2	1

AMA: Jun 96: 8

● New   ▲ Revised   Deleted   ⊙ Moderate Sedation   ✚ Add-on Codes   ⊘ High Risk Denial   Ⓐ Age Edit   ♀ Female   ♂ Male   **AMA** CPT® Assistant   **MUE** Medically Unlikely Edit

⊗ Modifier 51 Exempt   ⊖ Modifier 63 Exempt   ☒ Unlisted   **Modifiers:** See Inside Back Cover   Ⓜ Maternity   A2–Z3 ASC Payment Indicators   A–Y OPPS Status Indicators

Surgical Procedures

35741 – 35907

35741 Exploration (not followed by surgical repair), with or without lysis of artery; popliteal artery   **C**

RVU			Global Days	Modifiers				
Mod	Non-Fac Total	Fac Total		51	50	62	80	MUE
	15.11	15.11	090	2	1	1	2	1

35761 Exploration (not followed by surgical repair), with or without lysis of artery; other vessels   **G2 T**

RVU			Global Days	Modifiers				
Mod	Non-Fac Total	Fac Total		51	50	62	80	MUE
	11.40	11.40	090	2	1	1	2	2

Coding Guidance

Codes 35800-35860 are for a return to the operating room due to postoperative hemorrhaging, not for bleeding that occurs in the initial operative session. A modifier is usually reported to denote a return to the operating room for a related procedure within the postoperative period.

35800 Exploration for postoperative hemorrhage, thrombosis or infection; neck   **C**

RVU			Global Days	Modifiers				
Mod	Non-Fac Total	Fac Total		51	50	62	80	MUE
	20.99	20.99	090	2	0	1	2	2

35820 Exploration for postoperative hemorrhage, thrombosis or infection; chest   **C**

RVU			Global Days	Modifiers				
Mod	Non-Fac Total	Fac Total		51	50	62	80	MUE
	58.84	58.84	090	2	0	1	2	2

35840 Exploration for postoperative hemorrhage, thrombosis or infection; abdomen   **C**

RVU			Global Days	Modifiers				
Mod	Non-Fac Total	Fac Total		51	50	62	80	MUE
	34.84	34.84	090	2	0	1	2	2

AMA: May 97: 8

35860 Exploration for postoperative hemorrhage, thrombosis or infection; extremity   **T**

RVU			Global Days	Modifiers				
Mod	Non-Fac Total	Fac Total		51	50	62	80	MUE
	24.86	24.86	090	2	0	1	2	2

AMA: Fall 92: 21, Apr 14: 10

35870 Repair of graft-enteric fistula   **C**

RVU			Global Days	Modifiers				
Mod	Non-Fac Total	Fac Total		51	50	62	80	MUE
	36.82	36.82	090	2	0	1	2	1

35875 Thrombectomy of arterial or venous graft (other than hemodialysis graft or fistula)   **A2 T**

RVU			Global Days	Modifiers				
Mod	Non-Fac Total	Fac Total		51	50	62	80	MUE
	17.64	17.64	090	2	0	1	1	2

AMA: Nov 98: 14, Feb 99: 6, Mar 99: 6, Apr 00: 10

35876 Thrombectomy of arterial or venous graft (other than hemodialysis graft or fistula); with revision of arterial or venous graft   **A2 T**

RVU			Global Days	Modifiers				
Mod	Non-Fac Total	Fac Total		51	50	62	80	MUE
	27.95	27.95	090	2	0	1	2	2

AMA: Nov 98: 14

35879 Revision, lower extremity arterial bypass, without thrombectomy, open; with vein patch angioplasty   **T**

RVU			Global Days	Modifiers				
Mod	Non-Fac Total	Fac Total		51	50	62	80	MUE
	27.31	27.31	090	2	1	1	2	2

AMA: Nov 99: 19

35881 Revision, lower extremity arterial bypass, without thrombectomy, open; with segmental vein interposition   **T**

RVU			Global Days	Modifiers				
Mod	Non-Fac Total	Fac Total		51	50	62	80	MUE
	30.18	30.18	090	2	1	1	2	2

AMA: Nov 99: 19

35883 Revision, femoral anastomosis of synthetic arterial bypass graft in groin, open; with nonautogenous patch graft (eg, Dacron, ePTFE, bovine pericardium)   **T**

RVU			Global Days	Modifiers				
Mod	Non-Fac Total	Fac Total		51	50	62	80	MUE
	35.76	35.76	090	2	1	1	2	1

AMA: Jan 07: 7

35884 Revision, femoral anastomosis of synthetic arterial bypass graft in groin, open; with autogenous vein patch graft   **T**

RVU			Global Days	Modifiers				
Mod	Non-Fac Total	Fac Total		51	50	62	80	MUE
	36.66	36.66	090	2	1	1	2	1

AMA: Jan 07: 7

35901 Excision of infected graft; neck   **C**

RVU			Global Days	Modifiers				
Mod	Non-Fac Total	Fac Total		51	50	62	80	MUE
	13.97	13.97	090	2	0	1	2	1

35903 Excision of infected graft; extremity   **T**

RVU			Global Days	Modifiers				
Mod	Non-Fac Total	Fac Total		51	50	62	80	MUE
	16.70	16.70	090	2	0	1	2	2

35905 Excision of infected graft; thorax   **C**

RVU			Global Days	Modifiers				
Mod	Non-Fac Total	Fac Total		51	50	62	80	MUE
	49.85	49.85	090	2	0	1	2	1

35907 Excision of infected graft; abdomen   **C**

RVU			Global Days	Modifiers				
Mod	Non-Fac Total	Fac Total		51	50	62	80	MUE
	56.66	56.66	090	2	0	1	2	1

Vascular Injections

Intravenous Procedures

Coding Guidance

The service described in 36000 should not be reported if it is related to the delivery of anesthesia. Intravenous access that is routinely obtained or necessary for completing a procedure is not reported separately. The work value of gaining intravenous access is inherent in the work value for the primary procedure. If an intravenous line is placed to prepare an access in case of a problem with a procedure or to administer contrast, it is considered part of the procedure.

● New   ▲ Revised   ✖ Deleted   ⊙ Moderate Sedation   ✚ Add-on Codes   ⊘ High Risk Denial   Ⓐ Age Edit   ♀ Female   ♂ Male   **AMA** *CPT® Assistant*   **MUE** Medically Unlikely Edit
⊘ Modifier 51 Exempt   ⊖ Modifier 63 Exempt   ✖ Unlisted   **Modifiers:** *See Inside Back Cover*   Ⓜ Maternity   **A2–Z3** ASC Payment Indicators   **A–Y** OPPS Status Indicators

CPT © 2015 American Medical Association. All Rights Reserved.   © 2016 DecisionHealth

36000 Introduction of needle or intracatheter, vein ⊘N I N

Coding tip: Report this procedure separately only when performed alone, or distinct from other procedures on the same day

Coding tip: Routine venipuncture for collection of venous blood - 36415

Coding tip: Venipuncture requiring the skill of a physician or other qualified health care professional - 36400-36410

Coding tip: Introduction of needles or catheters is usually included as a component of a more complex procedure(s)

Coding tip: Do not code with injection procedures, which include introduction of needle/catheter

RVU			Global Days	Modifiers				
Mod	Non-Fac Total	Fac Total		51	50	62	80	MUE
	0.73	0.27	XXX	9	9	9	9	4

AMA: Summer 95: 2, Apr 98: 1, 3, 7, Jul 98: 1, Apr 03: 26, Oct 03: 2, Jul 06: 4, Feb 07: 10, Jul 07: 1, Dec 08: 7, Sep 14: 13, May 14: 4, Oct 14: 6

Pub 100-04, 12, 30.6.12

Introduction of needle or intracatheter, vein

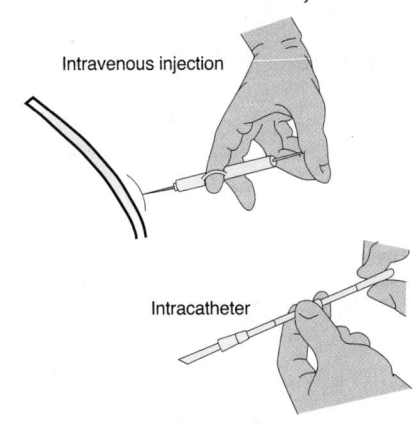

Intravenous injection

Intracatheter

Introduction of needle or intracatheter, vein

36002 Injection procedures (eg, thrombin) for percutaneous treatment of extremity pseudoaneurysm G 2 S

Coding tip: Report an additional code with injection procedures that require radiological needle guidance - ultrasound 76942; fluoroscopy 77002; CT 77012; MRI 77021

RVU			Global Days	Modifiers				
Mod	Non-Fac Total	Fac Total		51	50	62	80	MUE
	4.63	3.09	000	2	1	0	1	2

AMA: Nov 13: 6, Oct 14: 6

36005 Injection procedure for extremity venography (including introduction of needle or intracatheter) N I N

Coding tip: Bilateral injection of contrast with bilateral radiologic supervision - add modifier 50 and code 75822

Coding tip: Injection procedure with unilateral radiologic supervision - 36005, 75820

RVU			Global Days	Modifiers				
Mod	Non-Fac Total	Fac Total		51	50	62	80	MUE
	9.28	1.40	000	2	1	0	0	2

AMA: Oct 14: 6

⊙ 36010 Introduction of catheter, superior or inferior vena cava N I N

RVU			Global Days	Modifiers				
Mod	Non-Fac Total	Fac Total		51	50	62	80	MUE
	14.14	3.56	XXX	2	1	0	1	2

AMA: Aug 96: 2, Apr 98: 7, Sep 00: 11, May 01: 10, Jul 03: 12, Oct 08: 11, Jan 09: 7, Apr 12: 4

Coding Guidance

Only one selective catheter placement code may be reported per site when a noncoronary percutaneous intravascular interventional procedure is done in conjunction with a diagnostic angiogram (venous or arterial). Diagnostic angiograms performed on the same service date before the percutaneous intravascular interventional procedure to define the anatomy and pathology should be reported separately with the appropriate modifier.

36011 Selective catheter placement, venous system; first order branch (eg, renal vein, jugular vein) N I N

RVU			Global Days	Modifiers				
Mod	Non-Fac Total	Fac Total		51	50	62	80	MUE
	23.55	4.57	XXX	2	1	0	1	4

AMA: Aug 96: 11, Apr 98: 7, Jul 03: 12, Dec 03: 2, Apr 12: 5

Selective catheter placement, venous system

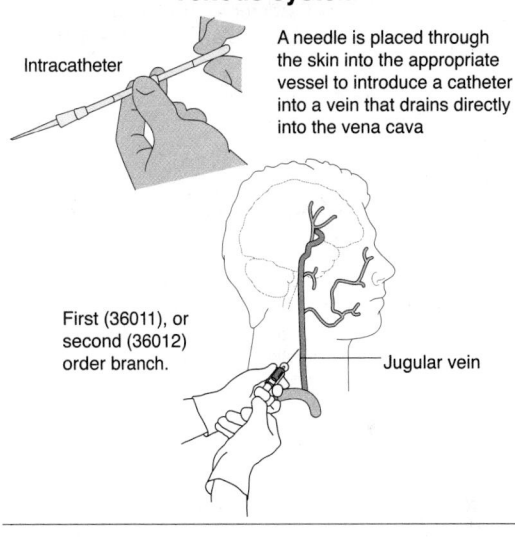

Intracatheter

A needle is placed through the skin into the appropriate vessel to introduce a catheter into a vein that drains directly into the vena cava

First (36011), or second (36012) order branch.

Jugular vein

36012 Selective catheter placement, venous system; second order, or more selective, branch (eg, left adrenal vein, petrosal sinus) N I N

RVU			Global Days	Modifiers				
Mod	Non-Fac Total	Fac Total		51	50	62	80	MUE
	24.47	5.09	XXX	2	1	0	1	4

AMA: Aug 96: 11, Sep 98: 7, Jul 03: 12, Apr 12: 5

36013 Introduction of catheter, right heart or main pulmonary artery N I N

RVU			Global Days	Modifiers				
Mod	Non-Fac Total	Fac Total		51	50	62	80	MUE
	22.54	3.70	XXX	2	0	0	1	2

AMA: Aug 96: 11, Oct 08: 11, Jan 09: 7

© 2016 DecisionHealth   CPT © 2015 American Medical Association. All Rights Reserved.

Surgical Procedures

36000 – 36013

36014 Selective catheter placement, left or right pulmonary artery   N|N

RVU			Global Days	Modifiers				
Mod	Non-Fac Total	Fac Total		51	50	62	80	MUE
	23.08	4.36	XXX	2	1	0	1	2

AMA: Aug 96: 11, Apr 98: 7

36015 Selective catheter placement, segmental or subsegmental pulmonary artery   N|N

RVU			Global Days	Modifiers				
Mod	Non-Fac Total	Fac Total		51	50	62	80	MUE
	24.69	4.99	XXX	2	1	0	1	4

AMA: Aug 96: 11, Sep 00: 11, Mar 12: 10

Intra-Arterial/Aortic Procedures

36100 Introduction of needle or intracatheter, carotid or vertebral artery   N|N

RVU			Global Days	Modifiers				
Mod	Non-Fac Total	Fac Total		51	50	62	80	MUE
	13.87	4.51	XXX	2	1	0	1	2

AMA: Aug 96: 11

Introduction of needle or intracatheter

Catheter is inserted into artery after needle and guidewire insertion

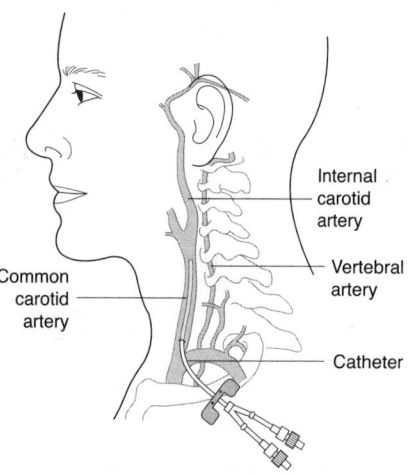

- Internal carotid artery
- Vertebral artery
- Common carotid artery
- Catheter

36120 Introduction of needle or intracatheter; retrograde brachial artery   N|N

RVU			Global Days	Modifiers				
Mod	Non-Fac Total	Fac Total		51	50	62	80	MUE
	11.97	2.93	XXX	2	0	0	1	2

AMA: Fall 93: 16, Aug 96: 3, Jun 09: 10

⊙ 36140 Introduction of needle or intracatheter; extremity artery   N|N

RVU			Global Days	Modifiers				
Mod	Non-Fac Total	Fac Total		51	50	62	80	MUE
	12.33	3.00	XXX	2	0	0	1	3

AMA: Fall 93: 16, Aug 96: 3, Nov 99: 32, 33, Oct 03: 2, Jul 06: 4, 7, Jul 07: 1, Dec 07: 10, 11, Jun 09: 10, Jul 11: 5

⊙ 36147 Introduction of needle and/or catheter, arteriovenous shunt created for dialysis (graft/fistula); initial access with complete radiological evaluation of dialysis access, including fluoroscopy, image documentation and report (includes access of shunt, injection[s] of contrast, and all necessary imaging from the arterial anastomosis and adjacent artery through entire venous outflow including the inferior or superior vena cava)   P 2 T

RVU			Global Days	Modifiers				
Mod	Non-Fac Total	Fac Total		51	50	62	80	MUE
	23.80	5.42	XXX	2	0	0	2	2

AMA: Dec 11: 15, Apr 12: 5, Mar 10: 3

⊙+36148 Introduction of needle and/or catheter, arteriovenous shunt created for dialysis (graft/fistula); additional access for therapeutic intervention (List separately in addition to code for primary procedure)   N|N

RVU			Global Days	Modifiers				
Mod	Non-Fac Total	Fac Total		51	50	62	80	MUE
	7.44	1.43	ZZZ	0	0	0	2	1

AMA: Apr 12: 5, Mar 10: 3

36160 Introduction of needle or intracatheter, aortic, translumbar   N|N

RVU			Global Days	Modifiers				
Mod	Non-Fac Total	Fac Total		51	50	62	80	MUE
	14.01	3.59	XXX	2	0	0	1	2

AMA: Aug 96: 3

⊙ 36200 Introduction of catheter, aorta   N|N

RVU			Global Days	Modifiers				
Mod	Non-Fac Total	Fac Total		51	50	62	80	MUE
	17.73	4.48	000	2	1	0	1	2

AMA: Fall 93: 16, Aug 96: 3, Jul 06: 7, Dec 07: 10, 14, Apr 08: 11, Dec 09: 13, Jul 11: 5, Oct 11: 9, Apr 12: 4, Feb 13: 16

36215 Selective catheter placement, arterial system; each first order thoracic or brachiocephalic branch, within a vascular family   N|N

RVU			Global Days	Modifiers				
Mod	Non-Fac Total	Fac Total		51	50	62	80	MUE
	31.98	6.85	XXX	2	0	0	1	6

AMA: Fall 93: 15, Aug 96: 3, Nov 97: 16, Apr 98: 9, Sep 00: 11, Oct 00: 4, Feb 03: 3, Apr 12: 4

Selective catheter placement, arterial system; thoracic/brachiocephalic

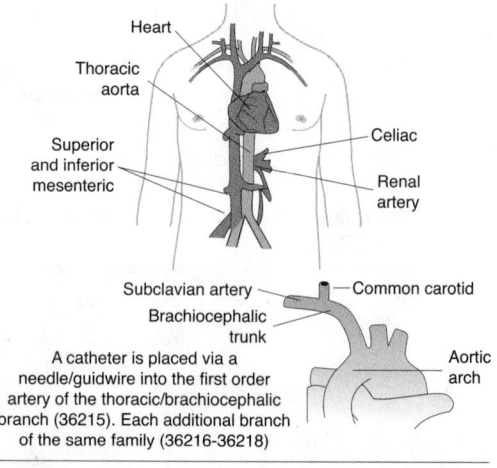

- Heart
- Thoracic aorta
- Celiac
- Superior and inferior mesenteric
- Renal artery
- Subclavian artery
- Common carotid
- Brachiocephalic trunk
- Aortic arch

A catheter is placed via a needle/guidwire into the first order artery of the thoracic/brachiocephalic branch (36215). Each additional branch of the same family (36216-36218)

● New   ▲ Revised   ✖ Deleted   ⊙ Moderate Sedation   ✚ Add-on Codes   ⊘ High Risk Denial   Ⓐ Age Edit   ♀ Female   ♂ Male   **AMA** *CPT® Assistant*   **MUE** Medically Unlikely Edit
⊘ Modifier 51 Exempt   ⊖ Modifier 63 Exempt   ✗ Unlisted   **Modifiers:** *See Inside Back Cover*   Ⓜ Maternity   A 2 – Z 3 ASC Payment Indicators   A – Y OPPS Status Indicators

CPT © 2015 American Medical Association. All Rights Reserved.   © 2016 DecisionHealth

Surgical Procedures

36216 Selective catheter placement, arterial system; initial second order thoracic or brachiocephalic branch, within a vascular family   N1N

Mod	Non-Fac Total	Fac Total	Global Days	51	50	62	80	MUE
	34.21	8.10	XXX	2	0	0	1	4

AMA: Fall 93: 15, Aug 96: 3, Oct 00: 4, Dec 07: 10, Dec 11: 12, Apr 12: 4, Nov 13: 14

36217 Selective catheter placement, arterial system; initial third order or more selective thoracic or brachiocephalic branch, within a vascular family   N1N

Mod	Non-Fac Total	Fac Total	Global Days	51	50	62	80	MUE
	57.14	9.65	XXX	2	0	0	1	2

AMA: Fall 93: 15, Aug 96: 3, Oct 00: 4, Dec 07: 10, Dec 11: 12, Apr 12: 5

+ 36218 Selective catheter placement, arterial system; additional second order, third order, and beyond, thoracic or brachiocephalic branch, within a vascular family (List in addition to code for initial second or third order vessel as appropriate)   N1N

Mod	Non-Fac Total	Fac Total	Global Days	51	50	62	80	MUE
	5.48	1.55	ZZZ	0	0	0	1	6

AMA: Fall 93: 15, Aug 96: 3, Oct 00: 4, Jul 06: 7, Dec 07: 10, May 13: 3, Apr 12: 5

⊙ **36221** Non-selective catheter placement, thoracic aorta, with angiography of the extracranial carotid, vertebral, and/or intracranial vessels, unilateral or bilateral, and all associated radiological supervision and interpretation, includes angiography of the cervicocerebral arch, when performed   N1Q2

Mod	Non-Fac Total	Fac Total	Global Days	51	50	62	80	MUE
	31.19	6.29	000	2	2	0	1	1

AMA: May 13: 3, Feb 13: 16, Jun 13: 12, Oct 13: 18, Mar 14: 8, May 15: 7

⊙ **36222** Selective catheter placement, common carotid or innominate artery, unilateral, any approach, with angiography of the ipsilateral extracranial carotid circulation and all associated radiological supervision and interpretation, includes angiography of the cervicocerebral arch, when performed   N1Q2

Mod	Non-Fac Total	Fac Total	Global Days	51	50	62	80	MUE
	37.43	8.63	000	2	1	0	1	1

AMA: May 13: 3, Feb 13: 17, Jun 13: 12, Oct 13: 18, Nov 13: 14, Mar 14: 8, May 15: 7

⊙ **36223** Selective catheter placement, common carotid or innominate artery, unilateral, any approach, with angiography of the ipsilateral intracranial carotid circulation and all associated radiological supervision and interpretation, includes angiography of the extracranial carotid and cervicocerebral arch, when performed   N1Q2

Mod	Non-Fac Total	Fac Total	Global Days	51	50	62	80	MUE
	43.79	9.43	000	2	1	0	1	1

AMA: May 13: 3, Feb 13: 17, Jun 13: 12, Oct 13: 18, Mar 14: 8

⊙ **36224** Selective catheter placement, internal carotid artery, unilateral, with angiography of the ipsilateral intracranial carotid circulation and all associated radiological supervision and interpretation, includes angiography of the extracranial carotid and cervicocerebral arch, when performed   N1Q2

Mod	Non-Fac Total	Fac Total	Global Days	51	50	62	80	MUE
	51.65	10.49	000	2	1	0	1	1

AMA: May 13: 3, Feb 13: 17, Jun 13: 12, Oct 13: 18, Mar 14: 8

⊙ **36225** Selective catheter placement, subclavian or innominate artery, unilateral, with angiography of the ipsilateral vertebral circulation and all associated radiological supervision and interpretation, includes angiography of the cervicocerebral arch, when performed   N1Q2

Mod	Non-Fac Total	Fac Total	Global Days	51	50	62	80	MUE
	42.77	9.29	000	2	1	0	1	1

AMA: May 13: 3, Jun 13: 12, Oct 13: 18, Nov 13: 14, Mar 14: 8

⊙ **36226** Selective catheter placement, vertebral artery, unilateral, with angiography of the ipsilateral vertebral circulation and all associated radiological supervision and interpretation, includes angiography of the cervicocerebral arch, when performed   N1Q2

Mod	Non-Fac Total	Fac Total	Global Days	51	50	62	80	MUE
	52.43	10.53	000	2	1	0	1	1

AMA: May 13: 3, Jun 13: 12, Oct 13: 18, Mar 14: 8

⊙+ **36227** Selective catheter placement, external carotid artery, unilateral, with angiography of the ipsilateral external carotid circulation and all associated radiological supervision and interpretation (List separately in addition to code for primary procedure)   N1N

Mod	Non-Fac Total	Fac Total	Global Days	51	50	62	80	MUE
	7.18	3.32	ZZZ	0	1	0	1	1

AMA: May 13: 3, Feb 13: 17, Jun 13: 12, Oct 13: 18, Mar 14: 8

● New   ▲ Revised   Deleted   ⊙ Moderate Sedation   ✚ Add-on Codes   ⊘ High Risk Denial   Ⓐ Age Edit   ♀ Female   ♂ Male   **AMA** *CPT® Assistant*   **MUE** Medically Unlikely Edit
⊘ Modifier 51 Exempt   ⊖ Modifier 63 Exempt   Ⓧ Unlisted   **Modifiers:** *See Inside Back Cover*   Ⓜ Maternity   A2–Z3 ASC Payment Indicators   A–Y OPPS Status Indicators

© 2016 DecisionHealth   CPT © 2015 American Medical Association. All Rights Reserved.   **389**

⊙✛**36228** Selective catheter placement, each intracranial branch of the internal carotid or vertebral arteries, unilateral, with angiography of the selected vessel circulation and all associated radiological supervision and interpretation (eg, middle cerebral artery, posterior inferior cerebellar artery) (List separately in addition to code for primary procedure)   N I N

RVU			Global Days	Modifiers				
Mod	Non-Fac Total	Fac Total		51	50	62	80	MUE
	34.66	6.81	ZZZ	0	1	0	1	4

AMA: May 13: 3, Feb 13: 17, Jun 13: 12, Oct 13: 18

⊙ **36245** Selective catheter placement, arterial system; each first order abdominal, pelvic, or lower extremity artery branch, within a vascular family   N I N

RVU			Global Days	Modifiers				
Mod	Non-Fac Total	Fac Total		51	50	62	80	MUE
	38.98	7.36	XXX	2	1	0	1	6

AMA: Fall 93: 15, Aug 96: 3, Jan 01: 14, Jan 07: 7, Dec 07: 10, Apr 12: 4, Jul 11: 5, Oct 11: 9, Nov 13: 14

⊙ **36246** Selective catheter placement, arterial system; initial second order abdominal, pelvic, or lower extremity artery branch, within a vascular family   N I N

RVU			Global Days	Modifiers				
Mod	Non-Fac Total	Fac Total		51	50	62	80	MUE
	25.35	7.86	000	2	1	0	1	4

AMA: Fall 93: 15, Aug 96: 3, Jan 01: 14, Jan 07: 7, Dec 07: 10, 11, Apr 12: 4, Jul 11: 5, Oct 11: 9, Nov 13: 14

⊙ **36247** Selective catheter placement, arterial system; initial third order or more selective abdominal, pelvic, or lower extremity artery branch, within a vascular family   N I N

RVU			Global Days	Modifiers				
Mod	Non-Fac Total	Fac Total		51	50	62	80	MUE
	44.84	9.31	000	2	1	0	1	3

AMA: Fall 93: 15, Aug 96: 3, Jan 01: 14, Jan 07: 7, Dec 07: 10, Jul 11: 5, Apr 12: 4, Nov 13: 14

⊙✛**36248** Selective catheter placement, arterial system; additional second order, third order, and beyond, abdominal, pelvic, or lower extremity artery branch, within a vascular family (List in addition to code for initial second or third order vessel as appropriate)   N I N

RVU			Global Days	Modifiers				
Mod	Non-Fac Total	Fac Total		51	50	62	80	MUE
	4.35	1.44	ZZZ	0	0	0	1	6

AMA: Fall 93: 15, Aug 96: 3, Apr 98: 1, 7, Oct 00: 4, Jan 01: 14, Jan 07: 7, Jul 11: 5, Apr 12: 4

Coding Guidance

Sometimes during cardiac catheterization, a small amount of dye may be injected upon catheter withdrawal to examine the renal arteries. Renal angiography, codes 36251-36254, should not be reported unless a complete study is performed and interpreted, just as it would without the concomitant cardiac catheterization.

⊙ **36251** Selective catheter placement (first-order), main renal artery and any accessory renal artery(s) for renal angiography, including arterial puncture and catheter placement(s), fluoroscopy, contrast injection(s), image postprocessing, permanent recording of images, and radiological supervision and interpretation, including pressure gradient measurements when performed, and flush aortogram when performed; unilateral   N I Q2

RVU			Global Days	Modifiers				
Mod	Non-Fac Total	Fac Total		51	50	62	80	MUE
	40.55	8.21	000	2	0	0	1	1

AMA: Apr 12: 6, Aug 12: 13, Nov 13: 14

⊙ **36252** Selective catheter placement (first-order), main renal artery and any accessory renal artery(s) for renal angiography, including arterial puncture and catheter placement(s), fluoroscopy, contrast injection(s), image postprocessing, permanent recording of images, and radiological supervision and interpretation, including pressure gradient measurements when performed, and flush aortogram when performed; bilateral   N I Q2

RVU			Global Days	Modifiers				
Mod	Non-Fac Total	Fac Total		51	50	62	80	MUE
	43.98	10.95	000	2	2	0	1	1

AMA: Apr 12: 6

⊙ **36253** Superselective catheter placement (one or more second order or higher renal artery branches) renal artery and any accessory renal artery(s) for renal angiography, including arterial puncture, catheterization, fluoroscopy, contrast injection(s), image postprocessing, permanent recording of images, and radiological supervision and interpretation, including pressure gradient measurements when performed, and flush aortogram when performed; unilateral   N I Q2

RVU			Global Days	Modifiers				
Mod	Non-Fac Total	Fac Total		51	50	62	80	MUE
	64.34	11.02	000	2	0	0	1	1

AMA: Apr 12: 6, Aug 12: 13, Nov 13: 14

● New   ▲ Revised   ✖ Deleted   ⊙ Moderate Sedation   ✛ Add-on Codes   ⊖ High Risk Denial   Ⓐ Age Edit   ♀ Female   ♂ Male   **AMA** *CPT® Assistant*   **MUE** Medically Unlikely Edit

⊘ Modifier 51 Exempt   ⊖ Modifier 63 Exempt   ☒ Unlisted   **Modifiers:** *See Inside Back Cover*   Ⓜ Maternity   A2–Z3 ASC Payment Indicators   A–Y OPPS Status Indicators

390   CPT © 2015 American Medical Association. All Rights Reserved.   © 2016 DecisionHealth

⊙ **36254** **Superselective catheter placement (one or more second order or higher renal artery branches) renal artery and any accessory renal artery(s) for renal angiography, including arterial puncture, catheterization, fluoroscopy, contrast injection(s), image postprocessing, permanent recording of images, and radiological supervision and interpretation, including pressure gradient measurements when performed, and flush aortogram when performed; bilateral** N 1 Q 2

RVU			Global Days	Modifiers				
Mod	Non-Fac Total	Fac Total		51	50	62	80	MUE
	62.65	12.72	000	2	2	0	1	1

AMA: Apr 12: 6, Aug 12: 13

36260 **Insertion of implantable intra-arterial infusion pump (eg, for chemotherapy of liver)** A 2 T

RVU			Global Days	Modifiers				
Mod	Non-Fac Total	Fac Total		51	50	62	80	MUE
	18.35	18.35	090	2	0	0	1	1

AMA: Fall 95: 5

Insertion of implantable intra-arterial infusion pump

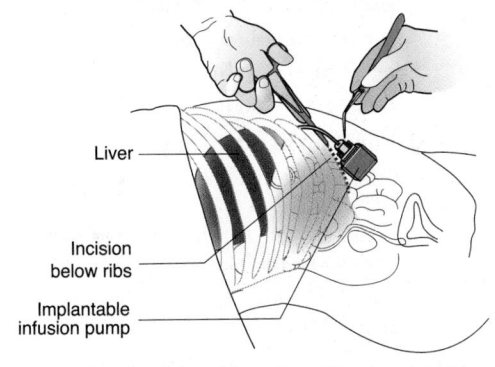

Liver

Incision below ribs

Implantable infusion pump

Insertion (36260); revision (36261); removal (36262)

36261 **Revision of implanted intra-arterial infusion pump** G 2 T

RVU			Global Days	Modifiers				
Mod	Non-Fac Total	Fac Total		51	50	62	80	MUE
	10.66	10.66	090	2	0	0	2	1

36262 **Removal of implanted intra-arterial infusion pump** ⊗ G 2 Q 2

RVU			Global Days	Modifiers				
Mod	Non-Fac Total	Fac Total		51	50	62	80	MUE
	8.88	8.88	090	2	0	0	1	1

36299 **Unlisted procedure, vascular injection** ✗ N

RVU			Global Days	Modifiers				
Mod	Non-Fac Total	Fac Total		51	50	62	80	MUE
	0.00	0.00	YYY	2	0	1	0	

Diagnostic/Therapeutic Venipuncture

Venous

Coding Guidance

Services reported with 36406 and 36410 should not be reported if related to the delivery of anesthesia. Intravenous access that is routinely obtained or necessary for completing a procedure is not reported separately. The work value of gaining intravenous access is inherent in the work value for the primary procedure.

36400 **Venipuncture, younger than age 3 years, necessitating the skill of a physician or other qualified health care professional, not to be used for routine venipuncture; femoral or jugular vein** ⊗ Ⓐ N I N

Coding tip: *Do not code 79101*

RVU			Global Days	Modifiers				
Mod	Non-Fac Total	Fac Total		51	50	62	80	MUE
	0.85	0.58	XXX	2	0	0	1	1

AMA: Jul 06: 4, Jul 07: 1, Dec 08: 7, May 14: 4

Venipuncture younger than age three

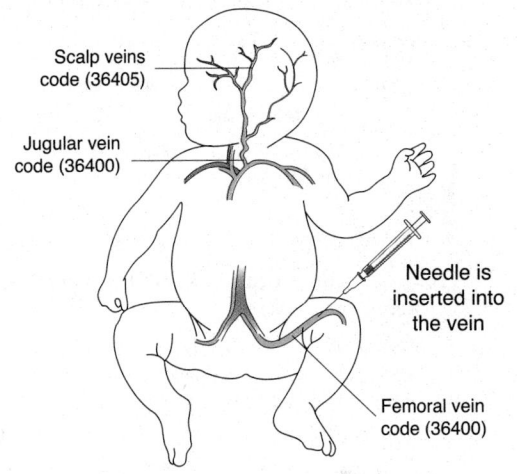

Scalp veins code (36405)

Jugular vein code (36400)

Needle is inserted into the vein

Femoral vein code (36400)

For other vein, use code (36406)

36405 **Venipuncture, younger than age 3 years, necessitating the skill of a physician or other qualified health care professional, not to be used for routine venipuncture; scalp vein** ⊗ Ⓐ N I N

RVU			Global Days	Modifiers				
Mod	Non-Fac Total	Fac Total		51	50	62	80	MUE
	0.74	0.47	XXX	2	0	0	1	1

AMA: Jul 06: 4, Jul 07: 1, Dec 08: 7, May 14: 4

36406 **Venipuncture, younger than age 3 years, necessitating the skill of a physician or other qualified health care professional, not to be used for routine venipuncture; other vein** ⊗ Ⓐ N I N

RVU			Global Days	Modifiers				
Mod	Non-Fac Total	Fac Total		51	50	62	80	MUE
	0.48	0.24	XXX	2	0	0	1	1

AMA: Jul 06: 4, Jul 07: 1, May 14: 4

● New　▲ Revised　Deleted　⊙ Moderate Sedation　✚ Add-on Codes　⊗ High Risk Denial　Ⓐ Age Edit　♀ Female　♂ Male　**AMA** CPT® Assistant　**MUE** Medically Unlikely Edit
⃠ Modifier 51 Exempt　⊖ Modifier 63 Exempt　✗ Unlisted　**Modifiers:** *See Inside Back Cover*　Ⓜ Maternity　A 2 – Z 3 ASC Payment Indicators　A – Y OPPS Status Indicators

© 2016 DecisionHealth　　　　CPT © 2015 American Medical Association. All Rights Reserved.　　　　**391**

Coding Guidance

Code 36410 describes a service that may be utilized for pain management purposes. Medicare global surgery rules block payment for postoperative pain management services provided by the same physician who performed the surgery. The service described by 36410 may be reported by the physician performing the surgery only if it is for purposes unrelated to the procedure, postoperative pain management, or anesthesia for the procedure.

36410 Venipuncture, age 3 years or older, necessitating the skill of a physician or other qualified health care professional (separate procedure), for diagnostic or therapeutic purposes (not to be used for routine venipuncture) N1N

Coding tip: Do not code 79101

RVU			Global Days	Modifiers				
Mod	Non-Fac Total	Fac Total		51	50	62	80	MUE
	0.48	0.27	XXX	2	0	0	1	3

AMA: Jun 96: 10, May 01: 11, Aug 02: 2, Oct 03: 10, Feb 07: 10, Jul 07: 1, Dec 08: 7, Sep 13: 18, Oct 14: 6

Pub 100-04, 12, 30.6.12

36415 Collection of venous blood by venipuncture ⊖N1Q4

Coding tip: Blood collection from completely implantable venous access device - 36591; from established arterial catheter - 37799

Coding tip: Use this code for routine venipuncture

RVU			Global Days	Modifiers				
Mod	Non-Fac Total	Fac Total		51	50	62	80	MUE
	0.00	0.00	XXX	9	9	9	9	4

AMA: Jun 96: 10, Mar 98: 10, Oct 99: 11, Aug 00: 2, Feb 07: 10, Jul 07: 1, Dec 08: 7, May 14: 4

Pub 100-04, 12, 30.6.12; 100-04, 16, 60.1.4

36416 Collection of capillary blood specimen (eg, finger, heel, ear stick) ⊘N1N

Coding tip: Routine venipuncture - 36415

Coding tip: Capillary blood specimen is most often taken from finger stick

RVU			Global Days	Modifiers				
Mod	Non-Fac Total	Fac Total		51	50	62	80	MUE
	0.00	0.00	XXX	9	9	9	9	

36420 Venipuncture, cutdown; younger than age 1 year ⊘Ⓐ⊖N1Q1

RVU			Global Days	Modifiers				
Mod	Non-Fac Total	Fac Total		51	50	62	80	MUE
	1.51	1.51	XXX	2	0	0	0	2

AMA: Nov 99: 32, 33, Aug 00: 2, Oct 03: 2, Jul 06: 4

36425 Venipuncture, cutdown; age 1 or over N1Q1

RVU			Global Days	Modifiers				
Mod	Non-Fac Total	Fac Total		51	50	62	80	MUE
	1.15	1.15	XXX	2	0	0	1	2

AMA: Oct 14: 6

Pub 100-04, 13, 70.2

36430 Transfusion, blood or blood components P3S

Coding tip: Exchange transfusion of blood - 36450, 36455

RVU			Global Days	Modifiers				
Mod	Non-Fac Total	Fac Total		51	50	62	80	MUE
	0.98	0.98	XXX	0	0	0	1	1

AMA: Aug 97: 18, Nov 99: 32, 33, Aug 00: 2, Mar 01: 10, Oct 03: 2, Jul 06: 4, Jul 07: 1

36440 Push transfusion, blood, 2 years or younger ⒶR2S

RVU			Global Days	Modifiers				
Mod	Non-Fac Total	Fac Total		51	50	62	80	MUE
	1.65	1.65	XXX	2	0	0	0	1

AMA: Aug 00: 2, Oct 03: 2, Jul 06: 4, Jul 07: 1

36450 Exchange transfusion, blood; newborn ⊘Ⓐ⊖R2S

RVU			Global Days	Modifiers				
Mod	Non-Fac Total	Fac Total		51	50	62	80	MUE
	3.37	3.37	XXX	2	0	0	0	1

36455 Exchange transfusion, blood; other than newborn G2S

RVU			Global Days	Modifiers				
Mod	Non-Fac Total	Fac Total		51	50	62	80	MUE
	3.66	3.66	XXX	2	0	0	1	1

36460 Transfusion, intrauterine, fetal ♀⊖MS

RVU			Global Days	Modifiers				
Mod	Non-Fac Total	Fac Total		51	50	62	80	MUE
	9.99	9.99	XXX	2	0	0	2	2

36468 Single or multiple injections of sclerosing solutions, spider veins (telangiectasia), limb or trunk ⊘N1Q1

Coding tip: Sclerosing injection into a single vein - 36470; multiple veins - 36471

RVU			Global Days	Modifiers				
Mod	Non-Fac Total	Fac Total		51	50	62	80	MUE
	0.00	0.00	000	2	0	0	0	1

AMA: Aug 14: 14, Oct 14: 6, Apr 15: 10

36470 Injection of sclerosing solution; single vein P3T

Coding tip: See also intralesional injection (non-chemotherapeutic) - 11900-11901

RVU			Global Days	Modifiers				
Mod	Non-Fac Total	Fac Total		51	50	62	80	MUE
	4.25	2.42	010	2	1	0	1	1

AMA: Oct 14: 6, Apr 15: 10

36471 Injection of sclerosing solution; multiple veins, same leg P3T

RVU			Global Days	Modifiers				
Mod	Non-Fac Total	Fac Total		51	50	62	80	MUE
	4.98	2.91	010	2	1	0	1	1

AMA: Oct 14: 6, Apr 15: 10, Aug 15: 8

36475 Endovenous ablation therapy of incompetent vein, extremity, inclusive of all imaging guidance and monitoring, percutaneous, radiofrequency; first vein treated A2T

RVU			Global Days	Modifiers				
Mod	Non-Fac Total	Fac Total		51	50	62	80	MUE
	43.74	8.22	000	2	1	0	1	1

AMA: Jul 10: 11, Mar 14: 4, Oct 14: 6, Apr 15: 10

+ 36476 Endovenous ablation therapy of incompetent vein, extremity, inclusive of all imaging guidance and monitoring, percutaneous, radiofrequency; second and subsequent veins treated in a single extremity, each through separate access sites (List separately in addition to code for primary procedure) N1N

RVU			Global Days	Modifiers				
Mod	Non-Fac Total	Fac Total		51	50	62	80	MUE
	8.49	3.97	ZZZ	0	1	0	1	2

AMA: Jul 10: 11, Mar 14: 4, Oct 14: 6, Apr 15: 10

● New ▲ Revised ✖ Deleted ⊙ Moderate Sedation ✚ Add-on Codes ⊘ High Risk Denial Ⓐ Age Edit ♀ Female ♂ Male **AMA** CPT® Assistant **MUE** Medically Unlikely Edit
⊘ Modifier 51 Exempt ⊖ Modifier 63 Exempt ✖ Unlisted **Modifiers:** See Inside Back Cover M Maternity A2–Z3 ASC Payment Indicators A–Y OPPS Status Indicators

392 | CPT © 2015 American Medical Association. All Rights Reserved. | © 2016 DecisionHealth

36478 Endovenous ablation therapy of incompetent vein, extremity, inclusive of all imaging guidance and monitoring, percutaneous, laser; first vein treated `A2T`

RVU			Global Days	Modifiers				
Mod	Non-Fac Total	Fac Total		51	50	62	80	MUE
	34.36	8.18	000	2	1	0	1	1

AMA: Jul 12: 12, Mar 14: 4, Oct 14: 6, Apr 15: 10

✚ 36479 Endovenous ablation therapy of incompetent vein, extremity, inclusive of all imaging guidance and monitoring, percutaneous, laser; second and subsequent veins treated in a single extremity, each through separate access sites (List separately in addition to code for primary procedure) `NIN`

RVU			Global Days	Modifiers				
Mod	Non-Fac Total	Fac Total		51	50	62	80	MUE
	8.83	3.99	ZZZ	0	1	0	1	2

AMA: Jul 10: 11, Jul 12: 12, Mar 14: 4, Aug 14: 14, Oct 14: 6, Apr 15: 10

⊙ 36481 Percutaneous portal vein catheterization by any method `NIN`

RVU			Global Days	Modifiers				
Mod	Non-Fac Total	Fac Total		51	50	62	80	MUE
	57.90	10.12	000	2	0	0	1	1

AMA: Oct 96: 1, Mar 02: 10, Dec 03: 2

Coding Guidance

Code 36500 may be reported for venous blood sampling through a catheter specifically placed for the sole purpose of obtaining the venous blood sample. When the catheter is placed for a purpose other than venous blood sampling, reporting 75893 or 36500 for venous blood sampling, in addition to the code for the other venous procedure is a misuse of this code. Code 36500 is not for blood sampling during an arterial procedure.

36500 Venous catheterization for selective organ blood sampling `NIN`

RVU			Global Days	Modifiers				
Mod	Non-Fac Total	Fac Total		51	50	62	80	MUE
	5.31	5.31	000	2	0	0	1	4

Venous catheterization for selective organ blood sampling

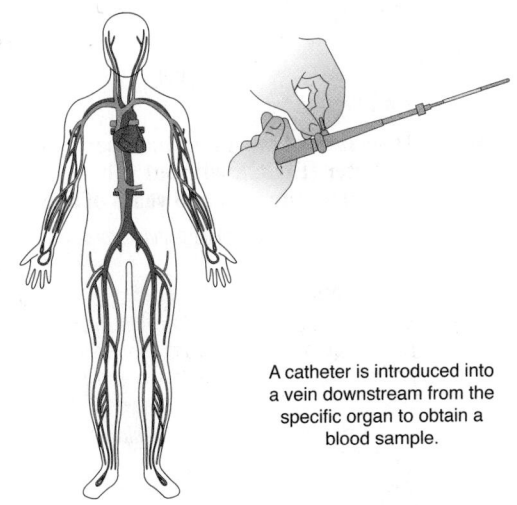

A catheter is introduced into a vein downstream from the specific organ to obtain a blood sample.

36510 Catheterization of umbilical vein for diagnosis or therapy, newborn ⊙Ⓐ⊖`NIN`

RVU			Global Days	Modifiers				
Mod	Non-Fac Total	Fac Total		51	50	62	80	MUE
	2.58	1.60	000	2	0	0	0	1

AMA: Nov 99: 5, 6, Aug 00: 2, Oct 03: 2, Jul 06: 4, Jul 07: 1

36511 Therapeutic apheresis; for white blood cells `G2S`

RVU			Global Days	Modifiers				
Mod	Non-Fac Total	Fac Total		51	50	62	80	MUE
	2.69	2.69	000	2	0	0	1	1

AMA: Oct 13: 3

36512 Therapeutic apheresis; for red blood cells `G2S`

RVU			Global Days	Modifiers				
Mod	Non-Fac Total	Fac Total		51	50	62	80	MUE
	2.71	2.71	000	2	0	0	1	1

AMA: Oct 13: 3

36513 Therapeutic apheresis; for platelets `G2S`

RVU			Global Days	Modifiers				
Mod	Non-Fac Total	Fac Total		51	50	62	80	MUE
	2.79	2.79	000	2	0	0	1	1

AMA: Oct 13: 3

36514 Therapeutic apheresis; for plasma pheresis `G2S`

RVU			Global Days	Modifiers				
Mod	Non-Fac Total	Fac Total		51	50	62	80	MUE
	15.26	2.67	000	2	0	0	1	1

AMA: Oct 13: 3

36515 Therapeutic apheresis; with extracorporeal immunoadsorption and plasma reinfusion `P2S`

RVU			Global Days	Modifiers				
Mod	Non-Fac Total	Fac Total		51	50	62	80	MUE
	58.36	2.52	000	2	0	0	1	1

AMA: Oct 13: 3

36516 Therapeutic apheresis; with extracorporeal selective adsorption or selective filtration and plasma reinfusion `P2S`

RVU			Global Days	Modifiers				
Mod	Non-Fac Total	Fac Total		51	50	62	80	MUE
	58.99	2.01	000	2	0	0	1	1

AMA: Oct 13: 3

36522 Photopheresis, extracorporeal `G2S`

RVU			Global Days	Modifiers				
Mod	Non-Fac Total	Fac Total		51	50	62	80	MUE
	39.73	2.93	000	2	0	0	1	1

AMA: Fall 93: 25, Jun 09: 3, Sep 09: 3, Aug 10: 12, Oct 13: 3

Pub 100-04, 32, 190.2, 190.3

● New   ▲ Revised   Deleted   ⊙ Moderate Sedation   ✚ Add-on Codes   ⊗ High Risk Denial   Ⓐ Age Edit   ♀ Female   ♂ Male   **AMA** *CPT® Assistant*   **MUE** Medically Unlikely Edit
⊘ Modifier 51 Exempt   ⊖ Modifier 63 Exempt   🄴 Unlisted   **Modifiers:** *See Inside Back Cover*   Ⓜ Maternity   `A2`–`Z3` ASC Payment Indicators   `A`–`Y` OPPS Status Indicators

© 2016 DecisionHealth   CPT © 2015 American Medical Association. All Rights Reserved.   **393**

Central Venous Access Device Procedures

Central Venous Procedures

⊙ **36555 Insertion of non-tunneled centrally inserted central venous catheter; younger than 5 years of age** ⊘Ⓐ A2 T

Coding tip: Ultrasound image guidance for accessing/evaluating the venous entry site - 76937

Coding tip: Fluoroscopic image guidance for central venous catheter insertion - 77001

RVU		Global Days	Modifiers				
Mod	Non-Fac Total	Fac Total		51	50	62	80	MUE
	7.62	3.47	000	0	0	0	1	2

AMA: Dec 04: 7, Jul 06: 4, Jul 07: 1, Jun 08: 8

36556 Insertion of non-tunneled centrally inserted central venous catheter; age 5 years or older A2 T

Coding tip: Ultrasound image guidance for accessing/evaluating the venous entry site - 76937

Coding tip: Fluoroscopic image guidance for central venous catheter insertion - 77001

RVU		Global Days	Modifiers				
Mod	Non-Fac Total	Fac Total		51	50	62	80	MUE
	6.72	3.51	000	0	0	0	1	2

AMA: Dec 04: 7, Jun 08: 8

⊙ **36557 Insertion of tunneled centrally inserted central venous catheter, without subcutaneous port or pump; younger than 5 years of age** ⊘Ⓐ A2 T

Coding tip: Fluoroscopic image guidance for central venous catheter insertion - 77001

Coding tip: Ultrasound image guidance for accessing/evaluating the venous entry site - 76937

RVU		Global Days	Modifiers				
Mod	Non-Fac Total	Fac Total		51	50	62	80	MUE
	28.75	9.56	010	2	1	0	0	2

AMA: Dec 04: 7, Jun 08: 8

⊙ **36558 Insertion of tunneled centrally inserted central venous catheter, without subcutaneous port or pump; age 5 years or older** A2 T

Coding tip: Ultrasound image guidance for accessing/evaluating the venous entry site - 76937

Coding tip: Fluoroscopic image guidance for central venous catheter insertion - 77001

RVU		Global Days	Modifiers				
Mod	Non-Fac Total	Fac Total		51	50	62	80	MUE
	22.25	8.01	010	2	1	0	0	2

AMA: Dec 04: 7, Jun 08: 8, Jan 15: 13

⊙ **36560 Insertion of tunneled centrally inserted central venous access device, with subcutaneous port; younger than 5 years of age** ⊘Ⓐ A2 T

Coding tip: Ultrasound image guidance for accessing/evaluating the venous entry site - 76937

Coding tip: Fluoroscopic image guidance for CVAD insertion - 77001

RVU		Global Days	Modifiers				
Mod	Non-Fac Total	Fac Total		51	50	62	80	MUE
	38.36	11.33	010	2	1	0	0	2

AMA: Dec 04: 7, Jun 08: 8, Dec 09: 11

⊙ **36561 Insertion of tunneled centrally inserted central venous access device, with subcutaneous port; age 5 years or older** A2 T

Coding tip: Ultrasound image guidance for accessing/evaluating the venous entry site - 76937

Coding tip: Fluoroscopic image guidance for CVAD insertion - 77001

RVU		Global Days	Modifiers				
Mod	Non-Fac Total	Fac Total		51	50	62	80	MUE
	33.51	10.30	010	2	1	0	0	2

AMA: Dec 04: 7, Jun 08: 8, Dec 09: 11

⊙ **36563 Insertion of tunneled centrally inserted central venous access device with subcutaneous pump** A2 T

Coding tip: Fluoroscopic image guidance for CVAD insertion - 77001

Coding tip: Ultrasound image guidance for accessing/evaluating the venous entry site - 76937

RVU		Global Days	Modifiers				
Mod	Non-Fac Total	Fac Total		51	50	62	80	MUE
	37.99	11.13	010	2	0	0	0	1

AMA: Dec 04: 8, Jun 08: 8

⊙ **36565 Insertion of tunneled centrally inserted central venous access device, requiring 2 catheters via 2 separate venous access sites; without subcutaneous port or pump (eg, Tesio type catheter)** A2 T

Coding tip: Ultrasound image guidance for accessing/evaluating the venous entry site - 76937

Coding tip: Fluoroscopic image guidance for CVAD insertion - 77001

RVU		Global Days	Modifiers				
Mod	Non-Fac Total	Fac Total		51	50	62	80	MUE
	27.80	10.18	010	2	1	0	0	1

AMA: Dec 04: 8, Jun 08: 8

⊙ **36566 Insertion of tunneled centrally inserted central venous access device, requiring 2 catheters via 2 separate venous access sites; with subcutaneous port(s)** A2 T

Coding tip: Fluoroscopic image guidance for CVAD insertion - 77001

Coding tip: Ultrasound image guidance for accessing/evaluating the venous entry site - 76937

RVU		Global Days	Modifiers				
Mod	Non-Fac Total	Fac Total		51	50	62	80	MUE
	155.37	11.22	010	2	1	0	0	1

AMA: Dec 04: 8, Jun 08: 8

⊙ **36568 Insertion of peripherally inserted central venous catheter (PICC), without subcutaneous port or pump; younger than 5 years of age** ⊘Ⓐ A2 T

Coding tip: Ultrasound image guidance for accessing/evaluating the venous entry site - 76937

Coding tip: Do not code 99143-99145

Coding tip: Codes 99148-99150 may be reported when a second physician or other qualified health care professional (other than the one performing the procedure) provides moderate sedation in a facility setting only

Coding tip: Fluoroscopic image guidance for central venous catheter insertion - 77001

RVU		Global Days	Modifiers				
Mod	Non-Fac Total	Fac Total		51	50	62	80	MUE
	8.59	2.81	000	0	0	0	1	2

AMA: Oct 04: 14, Dec 04: 8, May 05: 13, Jun 08: 8, Nov 12: 14

● New   ▲ Revised   ✖ Deleted   ⊙ Moderate Sedation   ✚ Add-on Codes   ⊘ High Risk Denial   Ⓐ Age Edit   ♀ Female   ♂ Male   **AMA** *CPT® Assistant*   **MUE** Medically Unlikely Edit
⊘ Modifier 51 Exempt   ⊖ Modifier 63 Exempt   ✖ Unlisted   **Modifiers:** *See Inside Back Cover*   Ⓜ Maternity   A2–Z3 ASC Payment Indicators   A–Y OPPS Status Indicators

394   CPT © 2015 American Medical Association. All Rights Reserved.   © 2016 DecisionHealth

36569 Insertion of peripherally inserted central venous catheter (PICC), without subcutaneous port or pump; age 5 years or older   A 2 T

Coding tip: Ultrasound image guidance for accessing/evaluating the venous entry site - 76937

Coding tip: Fluoroscopic image guidance for central venous catheter insertion - 77001

RVU			Global Days	Modifiers				
Mod	Non-Fac Total	Fac Total		51	50	62	80	MUE
	7.11	2.65	000	0	0	0	1	2

AMA: Oct 04: 14, Dec 04: 8, May 05: 13, Jun 08: 8, Nov 12: 14, Sep 13: 18, Sep 14: 13

⊙ **36570** Insertion of peripherally inserted central venous access device, with subcutaneous port; younger than 5 years of age   ⊘ⒶA 2 T

Coding tip: Fluoroscopic image guidance for CVAD insertion - 77001

Coding tip: Codes 99148-99150 may be reported when a second physician or other qualified health care professional (other than the one performing the procedure) provides moderate sedation in a facility setting only

Coding tip: Ultrasound image guidance for accessing/evaluating the venous entry site - 76937

Coding tip: Do not code 99143-99145

RVU			Global Days	Modifiers				
Mod	Non-Fac Total	Fac Total		51	50	62	80	MUE
	32.98	9.01	010	2	1	0	0	2

AMA: Dec 04: 8, Jun 08: 8, Dec 09: 11

⊙ **36571** Insertion of peripherally inserted central venous access device, with subcutaneous port; age 5 years or older   A 2 T

Coding tip: Fluoroscopic image guidance for CVAD insertion - 77001

Coding tip: Ultrasound image guidance for accessing/evaluating the venous entry site - 76937

RVU			Global Days	Modifiers				
Mod	Non-Fac Total	Fac Total		51	50	62	80	MUE
	37.24	9.41	010	2	1	0	0	2

AMA: Dec 04: 9, Jun 08: 8, Dec 09: 11

36575 Repair of tunneled or non-tunneled central venous access catheter, without subcutaneous port or pump, central or peripheral insertion site   A 2 T

RVU			Global Days	Modifiers				
Mod	Non-Fac Total	Fac Total		51	50	62	80	MUE
	4.73	1.02	000	2	0	0	0	2

⊙ **36576** Repair of central venous access device, with subcutaneous port or pump, central or peripheral insertion site   A 2 T

RVU			Global Days	Modifiers				
Mod	Non-Fac Total	Fac Total		51	50	62	80	MUE
	11.11	5.75	010	2	0	0	0	2

AMA: Dec 04: 9, Jun 08: 8

⊙ **36578** Replacement, catheter only, of central venous access device, with subcutaneous port or pump, central or peripheral insertion site   A 2 T

Coding tip: Fluoroscopic image guidance for CVAD catheter only replacement - 77001

RVU			Global Days	Modifiers				
Mod	Non-Fac Total	Fac Total		51	50	62	80	MUE
	14.84	6.29	010	2	0	0	0	2

AMA: Dec 04: 10, Jun 08: 8

36580 Replacement, complete, of a non-tunneled centrally inserted central venous catheter, without subcutaneous port or pump, through same venous access   A 2 T

Coding tip: Fluoroscopic image guidance for CVAD complete replacement - 77001

RVU			Global Days	Modifiers				
Mod	Non-Fac Total	Fac Total		51	50	62	80	MUE
	6.11	1.94	000	0	0	0	1	2

AMA: Dec 04: 10, Jun 08: 8

⊙ **36581** Replacement, complete, of a tunneled centrally inserted central venous catheter, without subcutaneous port or pump, through same venous access   A 2 T

Coding tip: Fluoroscopic image guidance for CVAD complete replacement - 77001

RVU			Global Days	Modifiers				
Mod	Non-Fac Total	Fac Total		51	50	62	80	MUE
	21.82	5.69	010	2	0	0	0	2

AMA: Dec 04: 10, Jun 08: 8

⊙ **36582** Replacement, complete, of a tunneled centrally inserted central venous access device, with subcutaneous port, through same venous access   A 2 T

Coding tip: Fluoroscopic image guidance for CVAD complete replacement - 77001

RVU			Global Days	Modifiers				
Mod	Non-Fac Total	Fac Total		51	50	62	80	MUE
	31.40	8.90	010	2	0	0	0	2

AMA: Dec 04: 10, Jun 08: 8

⊙ **36583** Replacement, complete, of a tunneled centrally inserted central venous access device, with subcutaneous pump, through same venous access   A 2 T

Coding tip: Fluoroscopic image guidance for CVAD complete replacement - 77001

RVU			Global Days	Modifiers				
Mod	Non-Fac Total	Fac Total		51	50	62	80	MUE
	39.00	9.87	010	2	0	0	0	2

AMA: Dec 04: 10, 11, Jun 08: 8

● New   ▲ Revised   Deleted   ⊙ Moderate Sedation   ✚ Add-on Codes   ⊘ High Risk Denial   Ⓐ Age Edit   ♀ Female   ♂ Male   **AMA** *CPT® Assistant*   **MUE** Medically Unlikely Edit   ⊘ Modifier 51 Exempt   ⊖ Modifier 63 Exempt   ✗ Unlisted   **Modifiers:** *See Inside Back Cover*   Ⓜ Maternity   A 2 - Z 3 ASC Payment Indicators   A - Y OPPS Status Indicators

36584 **Replacement, complete, of a peripherally inserted central venous catheter (PICC), without subcutaneous port or pump, through same venous access** `A 2 T`

Coding tip: Local anesthesia is included.

Coding tip: Fluoroscopic image guidance for CVAD complete replacement - 77001

RVU			Global Days	Modifiers				
Mod	Non-Fac Total	Fac Total		51	50	62	80	MUE
	5.82	1.92	000	0	0	0	1	2

AMA: Dec 04: 11, Jun 08: 8

Replacement, complete, of a peripherally inserted central venous catheter (PICC)

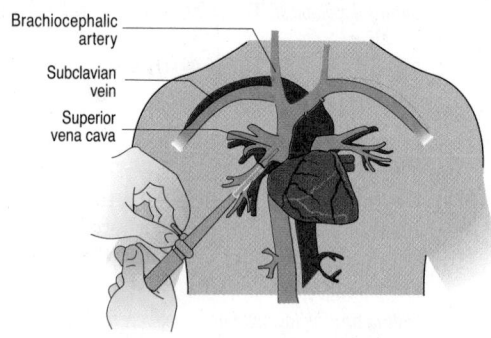

Brachiocephalic artery
Subclavian vein
Superior vena cava

Without subcutaneous port or pump, through same venous access (36584); with subcutaneous port, through same venous access (36585)

⊙ **36585** **Replacement, complete, of a peripherally inserted central venous access device, with subcutaneous port, through same venous access** `A 2 T`

Coding tip: Fluoroscopic image guidance for CVAD complete replacement - 77001

Coding tip: The newly replaced catheter and port connection includes verification with injection

Coding tip: Do not code 99143-99145

Coding tip: Codes 99148-99150 may be reported when a second physician or qualified health care professional (other than the one performing the procedure) provides moderate sedation in a facility setting only

RVU			Global Days	Modifiers				
Mod	Non-Fac Total	Fac Total		51	50	62	80	MUE
	32.79	8.25	010	2	0	0	0	2

AMA: Dec 04: 11, Jun 08: 8

36589 **Removal of tunneled central venous catheter, without subcutaneous port or pump** `A 2 Q 2`

Coding tip: Fluoroscopic image guidance for central venous catheter removal - 77001

RVU			Global Days	Modifiers				
Mod	Non-Fac Total	Fac Total		51	50	62	80	MUE
	4.73	3.99	010	2	0	0	0	2

AMA: Dec 04: 11, Jun 08: 8

⊙ **36590** **Removal of tunneled central venous access device, with subcutaneous port or pump, central or peripheral insertion** `A 2 Q 2`

Coding tip: Fluoroscopic image guidance for CVAD removal - 77001

RVU			Global Days	Modifiers				
Mod	Non-Fac Total	Fac Total		51	50	62	80	MUE
	8.40	5.95	010	2	0	0	0	2

AMA: Dec 04: 11, Jun 08: 8, Jul 10: 10

36591 **Collection of blood specimen from a completely implantable venous access device** `N I Q 1`

RVU			Global Days	Modifiers				
Mod	Non-Fac Total	Fac Total		51	50	62	80	MUE
	0.66	0.66	XXX	0	0	0	0	2

AMA: Apr 08: 9, Jul 11: 16, May 14: 4

Pub 100-04, 12, 30.6.12

36592 **Collection of blood specimen using established central or peripheral catheter, venous, not otherwise specified** `N I Q 1`

RVU			Global Days	Modifiers				
Mod	Non-Fac Total	Fac Total		51	50	62	80	MUE
	0.74	0.74	XXX	0	0	0	0	1

AMA: Apr 08: 9, Jul 11: 16

36593 **Declotting by thrombolytic agent of implanted vascular access device or catheter** `P 3 T`

RVU			Global Days	Modifiers				
Mod	Non-Fac Total	Fac Total		51	50	62	80	MUE
	0.88	0.88	XXX	0	0	0	0	2

AMA: Apr 08: 9, Dec 09: 11, Aug 11: 9, Feb 13: 3

36595 **Mechanical removal of pericatheter obstructive material (eg, fibrin sheath) from central venous device via separate venous access** `P 3 T`

Coding tip: Mechanical removal of pericatheter obstructive material with radiological supervision - 36595, 75901

RVU			Global Days	Modifiers				
Mod	Non-Fac Total	Fac Total		51	50	62	80	MUE
	16.64	5.34	000	2	0	0	1	2

AMA: Dec 04: 9, 12

36596 **Mechanical removal of intraluminal (intracatheter) obstructive material from central venous device through device lumen** `G 2 T`

Coding tip: Mechanical removal of intraluminal obstructive material with radiological supervision - 36596, 75902

RVU			Global Days	Modifiers				
Mod	Non-Fac Total	Fac Total		51	50	62	80	MUE
	3.80	1.30	000	2	0	0	1	2

AMA: Dec 04: 9, 12

36597 **Repositioning of previously placed central venous catheter under fluoroscopic guidance** `G 2 T`

RVU			Global Days	Modifiers				
Mod	Non-Fac Total	Fac Total		51	50	62	80	MUE
	3.63	1.78	000	2	0	0	1	2

AMA: Dec 04: 12, Sep 14: 5

36598 **Contrast injection(s) for radiologic evaluation of existing central venous access device, including fluoroscopy, image documentation and report** `P 3 T`

RVU			Global Days	Modifiers				
Mod	Non-Fac Total	Fac Total		51	50	62	80	MUE
	3.14	1.07	000	2	1	0	0	2

● New   ▲ Revised   ✖ Deleted   ⊙ Moderate Sedation   ✚ Add-on Codes   ⊘ High Risk Denial   Ⓐ Age Edit   ♀ Female   ♂ Male   **AMA** CPT® Assistant   **MUE** Medically Unlikely Edit

⊘ Modifier 51 Exempt   ⊖ Modifier 63 Exempt   ✗ Unlisted   **Modifiers:** See Inside Back Cover   Ⓜ Maternity   `A 2`–`Z 3` ASC Payment Indicators   `A`–`Y` OPPS Status Indicators

CPT © 2015 American Medical Association. All Rights Reserved.   © 2016 DecisionHealth

Arterial Procedures

36600 Arterial puncture, withdrawal of blood for diagnosis   N I Q I

Coding tip: Report separately only when performed alone, or distinct from other procedures on the same day

Coding tip: Venipuncture for collection of blood - 36415

RVU			Global Days	Modifiers				
Mod	Non-Fac Total	Fac Total		51	50	62	80	MUE
	0.90	0.45	XXX	2	0	0	1	4

AMA: Fall 95: 7, Aug 00: 2, Oct 03: 2, Jul 05: 11, Jul 06: 4, Feb 07: 10, Jul 07: 1, May 14: 4

Pub 100-04, 12, 30.6.12

Arterial puncture, for blood sampling

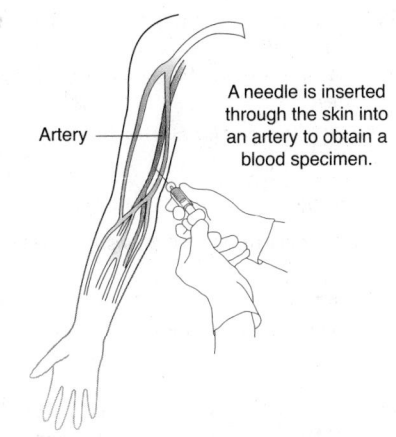

Artery

A needle is inserted through the skin into an artery to obtain a blood specimen.

⊘ 36620 Arterial catheterization or cannulation for sampling, monitoring or transfusion (separate procedure); percutaneous   N I N

Coding tip: Report separately only when performed alone, or distinct from other procedures on the same day

Coding tip: Introduction of catheter into a vein - 36000

Coding tip: Arterial catheterization or cannulization is usually included as a component of more complex procedures

RVU			Global Days	Modifiers				
Mod	Non-Fac Total	Fac Total		51	50	62	80	MUE
	1.49	1.49	000	0	0	0	1	3

AMA: Fall 95: 7, Apr 98: 3, Nov 99: 32, 33, Aug 00: 2, Oct 03: 2, Jul 06: 4, Jul 07: 1

36625 Arterial catheterization or cannulation for sampling, monitoring or transfusion (separate procedure); cutdown   N I N

RVU			Global Days	Modifiers				
Mod	Non-Fac Total	Fac Total		51	50	62	80	MUE
	3.03	3.03	000	0	0	0	1	2

AMA: Fall 95: 7

36640 Arterial catheterization for prolonged infusion therapy (chemotherapy), cutdown   A 2 T

RVU			Global Days	Modifiers				
Mod	Non-Fac Total	Fac Total		51	50	62	80	MUE
	3.42	3.42	000	2	0	0	1	1

AMA: Fall 95: 7

36660 Catheterization, umbilical artery, newborn, for diagnosis or therapy   ⊙Ⓐ⊖Ⓒ

Coding tip: This procedure has significant pre- and post-service time associated with it and has been removed from the Modifier 51 exempt codes. Use modifier 51 when reporting 36660 in addition to other procedures

RVU			Global Days	Modifiers				
Mod	Non-Fac Total	Fac Total		51	50	62	80	MUE
	1.86	1.86	000	2	0	0	0	1

AMA: Fall 95: 8, Oct 03: 2, Jul 06: 4, Jul 07: 1

Intraosseous Infusion

36680 Placement of needle for intraosseous infusion   N I Q I

Coding tip: Report drugs or medicinal substances separately

RVU			Global Days	Modifiers				
Mod	Non-Fac Total	Fac Total		51	50	62	80	MUE
	1.69	1.69	000	2	0	0	0	1

Hemodialysis Access/Intervascular Cannulation/Shunt Insertion

Coding Guidance

Intravascular cannulation or shunt insertion procedures, recognized as separate procedures, are not reported when done as part of another procedure at the same site requiring vascular revision.

36800 Insertion of cannula for hemodialysis, other purpose (separate procedure); vein to vein   A 2 T

RVU			Global Days	Modifiers				
Mod	Non-Fac Total	Fac Total		51	50	62	80	MUE
	3.58	3.58	000	2	0	0	1	1

AMA: Fall 93: 3

36810 Insertion of cannula for hemodialysis, other purpose (separate procedure); arteriovenous, external (Scribner type)   A 2 T

RVU			Global Days	Modifiers				
Mod	Non-Fac Total	Fac Total		51	50	62	80	MUE
	6.34	6.34	000	2	0	0	1	1

AMA: Fall 93: 3, May 97: 10

36815 Insertion of cannula for hemodialysis, other purpose (separate procedure); arteriovenous, external revision, or closure   A 2 T

RVU			Global Days	Modifiers				
Mod	Non-Fac Total	Fac Total		51	50	62	80	MUE
	4.27	4.27	000	2	0	0	1	1

AMA: Fall 93: 3

36818 Arteriovenous anastomosis, open; by upper arm cephalic vein transposition   A 2 T

RVU			Global Days	Modifiers				
Mod	Non-Fac Total	Fac Total		51	50	62	80	MUE
	20.47	20.47	090	2	0	1	2	1

AMA: Jul 05: 9

36819 Arteriovenous anastomosis, open; by upper arm basilic vein transposition   A 2 T

RVU			Global Days	Modifiers				
Mod	Non-Fac Total	Fac Total		51	50	62	80	MUE
	21.63	21.63	090	2	0	1	2	1

AMA: Nov 99: 20, Jul 05: 9

● New   ▲ Revised   Deleted   ⊙ Moderate Sedation   ✚ Add-on Codes   ⊘ High Risk Denial   Ⓐ Age Edit   ♀ Female   ♂ Male   **AMA** CPT® Assistant   **MUE** Medically Unlikely Edit
⊘ Modifier 51 Exempt   ⊖ Modifier 63 Exempt   🅇 Unlisted   **Modifiers:** See Inside Back Cover   Ⓜ Maternity   A2–Z3 ASC Payment Indicators   A–Y OPPS Status Indicators

Surgical Procedures

36820 – 36870

36820 Arteriovenous anastomosis, open; by forearm vein transposition A2 T

RVU			Global Days	Modifiers				
Mod	Non-Fac Total	Fac Total		51	50	62	80	MUE
	21.59	21.59	090	2	1	1	2	1

AMA: Fall 93: 4, Jul 05: 9

36821 Arteriovenous anastomosis, open; direct, any site (eg, Cimino type) (separate procedure) A2 T

RVU			Global Days	Modifiers				
Mod	Non-Fac Total	Fac Total		51	50	62	80	MUE
	19.61	19.61	090	2	0	1	2	2

AMA: Fall 93: 3, Feb 97: 2, Nov 99: 20, Jul 05: 9, Aug 15: 8

36823 Insertion of arterial and venous cannula(s) for isolated extracorporeal circulation including regional chemotherapy perfusion to an extremity, with or without hyperthermia, with removal of cannula(s) and repair of arteriotomy and venotomy sites C

RVU			Global Days	Modifiers				
Mod	Non-Fac Total	Fac Total		51	50	62	80	MUE
	39.37	39.37	090	2	0	0	1	1

AMA: Nov 98: 14, 15

Insertion of arterial and venous cannula(s) for isolated extracorporeal circulation

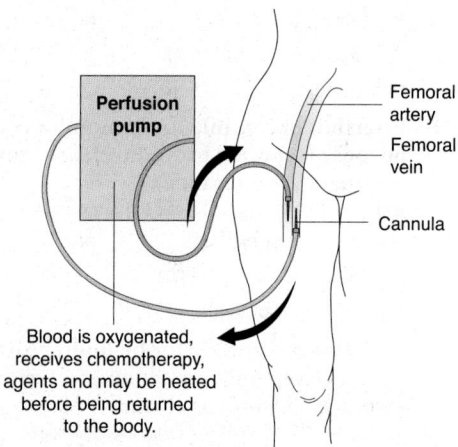

Perfusion pump

Femoral artery

Femoral vein

Cannula

Blood is oxygenated, receives chemotherapy, agents and may be heated before being returned to the body.

36825 Creation of arteriovenous fistula by other than direct arteriovenous anastomosis (separate procedure); autogenous graft A2 T

RVU			Global Days	Modifiers				
Mod	Non-Fac Total	Fac Total		51	50	62	80	MUE
	23.67	23.67	090	2	0	1	2	1

AMA: Fall 93: 3, Feb 97: 2, Jul 05: 9

36830 Creation of arteriovenous fistula by other than direct arteriovenous anastomosis (separate procedure); nonautogenous graft (eg, biological collagen, thermoplastic graft) A2 T

RVU			Global Days	Modifiers				
Mod	Non-Fac Total	Fac Total		51	50	62	80	MUE
	19.68	19.68	090	2	0	1	2	2

AMA: Fall 93: 3, Feb 97: 2, Jul 05: 9, Jan 15: 13

36831 Thrombectomy, open, arteriovenous fistula without revision, autogenous or nonautogenous dialysis graft (separate procedure) A2 T

RVU			Global Days	Modifiers				
Mod	Non-Fac Total	Fac Total		51	50	62	80	MUE
	18.24	18.24	090	2	0	1	2	1

AMA: Nov 98: 14, 15, Feb 99: 6, Mar 99: 6, Apr 99: 11

36832 Revision, open, arteriovenous fistula; without thrombectomy, autogenous or nonautogenous dialysis graft (separate procedure) A2 T

RVU			Global Days	Modifiers				
Mod	Non-Fac Total	Fac Total		51	50	62	80	MUE
	22.36	22.36	090	2	0	1	2	2

AMA: Fall 93: 3, Feb 97: 2, Nov 98: 15, Feb 99: 6, Mar 99: 6, Apr 99: 11, Nov 99: 20, 21

36833 Revision, open, arteriovenous fistula; with thrombectomy, autogenous or nonautogenous dialysis graft (separate procedure) A2 T

RVU			Global Days	Modifiers				
Mod	Non-Fac Total	Fac Total		51	50	62	80	MUE
	23.96	23.96	090	2	0	1	2	1

AMA: Nov 98: 15, Feb 99: 6, Apr 99: 11

36835 Insertion of Thomas shunt (separate procedure) A2 T

RVU			Global Days	Modifiers				
Mod	Non-Fac Total	Fac Total		51	50	62	80	MUE
	14.52	14.52	090	2	0	0	1	1

36838 Distal revascularization and interval ligation (DRIL), upper extremity hemodialysis access (steal syndrome) T

RVU			Global Days	Modifiers				
Mod	Non-Fac Total	Fac Total		51	50	62	80	MUE
	33.78	33.78	090	2	1	1	2	1

36860 External cannula declotting (separate procedure); without balloon catheter A2 T

RVU			Global Days	Modifiers				
Mod	Non-Fac Total	Fac Total		51	50	62	80	MUE
	5.92	3.19	000	2	0	0	1	2

AMA: Fall 93: 3, Feb 97: 2, Nov 98: 15, Feb 99: 6, May 01: 3

36861 External cannula declotting (separate procedure); with balloon catheter A2 T

RVU			Global Days	Modifiers				
Mod	Non-Fac Total	Fac Total		51	50	62	80	MUE
	3.85	3.85	000	2	0	0	1	2

AMA: Fall 93: 3, Feb 97: 2, May 01: 3

⊙ 36870 Thrombectomy, percutaneous, arteriovenous fistula, autogenous or nonautogenous graft (includes mechanical thrombus extraction and intra-graft thrombolysis) A2 J1 T

RVU			Global Days	Modifiers				
Mod	Non-Fac Total	Fac Total		51	50	62	80	MUE
	52.11	8.71	090	2	1	2	1	2

AMA: May 01: 3, Dec 11: 16, Feb 13: 3

● New   ▲ Revised   ✖ Deleted   ⊙ Moderate Sedation   ✚ Add-on Codes   ⊖ High Risk Denial   Ⓐ Age Edit   ♀ Female   ♂ Male   **AMA** *CPT® Assistant*   **MUE** Medically Unlikely Edit
⊘ Modifier 51 Exempt   ⊖ Modifier 63 Exempt   ⊠ Unlisted   **Modifiers:** *See Inside Back Cover*   Ⓜ Maternity   A2-Z3 ASC Payment Indicators   A-Y OPPS Status Indicators

398   CPT © 2015 American Medical Association. All Rights Reserved.   © 2016 DecisionHealth

Portal Decompression

37140 Venous anastomosis, open; portocaval ⊗C

Mod	Non-Fac Total	Fac Total	Global Days	Modifiers 51	50	62	80	MUE
	66.74	66.74	090	2	0	1	1	1

37145 Venous anastomosis, open; renoportal C

Mod	Non-Fac Total	Fac Total	Global Days	Modifiers 51	50	62	80	MUE
	62.64	62.64	090	2	0	0	2	1

37160 Venous anastomosis, open; caval-mesenteric C

Mod	Non-Fac Total	Fac Total	Global Days	Modifiers 51	50	62	80	MUE
	64.33	64.33	090	2	0	1	2	1

37180 Venous anastomosis, open; splenorenal, proximal C

Mod	Non-Fac Total	Fac Total	Global Days	Modifiers 51	50	62	80	MUE
	59.26	59.26	090	2	0	1	2	1

37181 Venous anastomosis, open; splenorenal, distal (selective decompression of esophagogastric varices, any technique) C

Mod	Non-Fac Total	Fac Total	Global Days	Modifiers 51	50	62	80	MUE
	67.68	67.68	090	2	0	1	2	1

37182 Insertion of transvenous intrahepatic portosystemic shunt(s) (TIPS) (includes venous access, hepatic and portal vein catheterization, portography with hemodynamic evaluation, intrahepatic tract formation/dilatation, stent placement and all associated imaging guidance and documentation) C

Mod	Non-Fac Total	Fac Total	Global Days	Modifiers 51	50	62	80	MUE
	24.23	24.23	000	2	0	0	0	1

AMA: Dec 03: 2, Sep 13: 17

⊙ **37183 Revision of transvenous intrahepatic portosystemic shunt(s) (TIPS) (includes venous access, hepatic and portal vein catheterization, portography with hemodynamic evaluation, intrahepatic tract recanulization/dilatation, stent placement and all associated imaging guidance and documentation)** J1

Mod	Non-Fac Total	Fac Total	Global Days	Modifiers 51	50	62	80	MUE
	167.98	11.43	000	2	0	0	0	1

AMA: Dec 03: 2

Transcatheter Procedures

Arterial Mechanical Thrombus Procedure

⊙▲ **37184 Primary percutaneous transluminal mechanical thrombectomy, noncoronary, non-intracranial, arterial or arterial bypass graft, including fluoroscopic guidance and intraprocedural pharmacological thrombolytic injection(s); initial vessel** G2T

Mod	Non-Fac Total	Fac Total	Global Days	Modifiers 51	50	62	80	MUE
	64.62	13.46	000	2	1	2	1	1

AMA: Nov 11: 11, Feb 13: 3, Apr 15: 10

⊙+▲ **37185 Primary percutaneous transluminal mechanical thrombectomy, noncoronary, non-intracranial, arterial or arterial bypass graft, including fluoroscopic guidance and intraprocedural pharmacological thrombolytic injection(s); second and all subsequent vessel(s) within the same vascular family (List separately in addition to code for primary mechanical thrombectomy procedure)** NIN

Mod	Non-Fac Total	Fac Total	Global Days	Modifiers 51	50	62	80	MUE
	20.56	4.92	ZZZ	0	2	2	1	2

AMA: Nov 11: 11, Feb 13: 3, Apr 15: 10

⊙+▲ **37186 Secondary percutaneous transluminal thrombectomy (eg, nonprimary mechanical, snare basket, suction technique), noncoronary, non-intracranial, arterial or arterial bypass graft, including fluoroscopic guidance and intraprocedural pharmacological thrombolytic injections, provided in conjunction with another percutaneous intervention other than primary mechanical thrombectomy (List separately in addition to code for primary procedure)** NIN

Mod	Non-Fac Total	Fac Total	Global Days	Modifiers 51	50	62	80	MUE
	39.23	7.32	ZZZ	0	2	2	1	2

AMA: Jul 11: 11, Nov 11: 9, Feb 13: 3

Venous Mechanical Thrombus Procedure

⊙ **37187 Percutaneous transluminal mechanical thrombectomy, vein(s), including intraprocedural pharmacological thrombolytic injections and fluoroscopic guidance** G2T

Mod	Non-Fac Total	Fac Total	Global Days	Modifiers 51	50	62	80	MUE
	58.55	11.91	000	2	1	2	1	1

AMA: Nov 11: 11, Feb 13: 3

⊙ **37188 Percutaneous transluminal mechanical thrombectomy, vein(s), including intraprocedural pharmacological thrombolytic injections and fluoroscopic guidance, repeat treatment on subsequent day during course of thrombolytic therapy** G2T

Mod	Non-Fac Total	Fac Total	Global Days	Modifiers 51	50	62	80	MUE
	50.56	8.56	000	2	1	2	1	1

AMA: Nov 11: 11, Feb 13: 3

● New   ▲ Revised   Deleted   ⊙ Moderate Sedation   ✚ Add-on Codes   ⊗ High Risk Denial   ⊛ Age Edit   ♀ Female   ♂ Male   **AMA** CPT® Assistant   **MUE** Medically Unlikely Edit   ⊘ Modifier 51 Exempt   ⊖ Modifier 63 Exempt   ✗ Unlisted   **Modifiers:** See Inside Back Cover   Ⓜ Maternity   A2–Z3 ASC Payment Indicators   A–Y OPPS Status Indicators

© 2016 DecisionHealth   CPT © 2015 American Medical Association. All Rights Reserved.   **399**

⊙ **37191** **Insertion of intravascular vena cava filter, endovascular approach including vascular access, vessel selection, and radiological supervision and interpretation, intraprocedural roadmapping, and imaging guidance (ultrasound and fluoroscopy), when performed** T

Coding tip: For supply of vena cava filter, refer to HCPCS Level II code C1880, but only for hospital outpatient departments under the Medicare outpatient prospective payment system (OPPS)

RVU			Global Days	Modifiers				
Mod	Non-Fac Total	Fac Total		51	50	62	80	MUE
	74.83	6.97	000	2	0	0	1	1

AMA: Apr 12: 8, Feb 13: 3

⊙ **37192** **Repositioning of intravascular vena cava filter, endovascular approach including vascular access, vessel selection, and radiological supervision and interpretation, intraprocedural roadmapping, and imaging guidance (ultrasound and fluoroscopy), when performed** T

RVU			Global Days	Modifiers				
Mod	Non-Fac Total	Fac Total		51	50	62	80	MUE
	44.08	10.74	000	2	0	0	1	1

AMA: Apr 12: 8, Feb 13: 3

⊙ **37193** **Retrieval (removal) of intravascular vena cava filter, endovascular approach including vascular access, vessel selection, and radiological supervision and interpretation, intraprocedural roadmapping, and imaging guidance (ultrasound and fluoroscopy), when performed** T

RVU			Global Days	Modifiers				
Mod	Non-Fac Total	Fac Total		51	50	62	80	MUE
	45.53	10.69	000	2	0	0	1	1

AMA: Apr 12: 8, Feb 13: 3

Other Transcatheter Procedures

37195 **Thrombolysis, cerebral, by intravenous infusion** ⊙ T

RVU			Global Days	Modifiers				
Mod	Non-Fac Total	Fac Total		51	50	62	80	MUE
	0.00	0.00	XXX	0	0	0	0	1

AMA: Nov 97: 16

⊙ **37197** **Transcatheter retrieval, percutaneous, of intravascular foreign body (eg, fractured venous or arterial catheter), includes radiological supervision and interpretation, and imaging guidance (ultrasound or fluoroscopy), when performed** G2 T

RVU			Global Days	Modifiers				
Mod	Non-Fac Total	Fac Total		51	50	62	80	MUE
	43.27	9.24	000	2	0	0	1	2

AMA: Feb 13: 3

37200 **Transcatheter biopsy** G2 T

RVU			Global Days	Modifiers				
Mod	Non-Fac Total	Fac Total		51	50	62	80	MUE
	6.39	6.39	000	2	0	0	1	2

✖ ~~37202~~ ~~Transcatheter therapy, infusion other than for thrombolysis, any type (eg, spasmolytic, vasoconstrictive)~~

⊙▲**37211** **Transcatheter therapy, arterial infusion for thrombolysis other than coronary or intracranial, any method, including radiological supervision and interpretation, initial treatment day** G2 T

Coding tip: Code 37211 is listed out of numerical order in CPT. Related transcatheter arterial/venous infusion procedures - 37202 infusion other than for thrombolysis; 37212 venous infusion for thrombolysis initial day; 37213 arterial/venous infusion for thrombolysis other than coronary subsequent day

RVU			Global Days	Modifiers				
Mod	Non-Fac Total	Fac Total		51	50	62	80	MUE
	11.69	11.69	000	2	1	0	1	1

AMA: Feb 13: 3

⊙ **37212** **Transcatheter therapy, venous infusion for thrombolysis, any method, including radiological supervision and interpretation, initial treatment day** G2 T

Coding tip: Code 37212 is listed out of numerical order in CPT. Related transcatheter arterial/venous infusion procedures - 37202 infusion other than for thrombolysis; 37211 arterial infusion for thrombolysis other than coronary initial day; 37213 arterial/venous infusion for thrombolysis other than coronary subsequent day

RVU			Global Days	Modifiers				
Mod	Non-Fac Total	Fac Total		51	50	62	80	MUE
	10.28	10.28	000	2	1	0	1	1

AMA: Feb 13: 3

⊙ **37213** **Transcatheter therapy, arterial or venous infusion for thrombolysis other than coronary, any method, including radiological supervision and interpretation, continued treatment on subsequent day during course of thrombolytic therapy, including follow-up catheter contrast injection, position change, or exchange, when performed** T

Coding tip: Code 37213 is listed out of numerical order in CPT. Related transcatheter arterial/venous infusion procedures - 37202 infusion other than for thrombolysis; 37211 arterial infusion for thrombolysis other than coronary initial day; 37212 venous infusion for thrombolysis initial day

RVU			Global Days	Modifiers				
Mod	Non-Fac Total	Fac Total		51	50	62	80	MUE
	7.22	7.22	000	2	0	0	1	1

AMA: Feb 13: 3

⊙ **37214** **Transcatheter therapy, arterial or venous infusion for thrombolysis other than coronary, any method, including radiological supervision and interpretation, continued treatment on subsequent day during course of thrombolytic therapy, including follow-up catheter contrast injection, position change, or exchange, when performed; cessation of thrombolysis including removal of catheter and vessel closure by any method** T

RVU			Global Days	Modifiers				
Mod	Non-Fac Total	Fac Total		51	50	62	80	MUE
	3.95	3.95	000	2	0	0	1	1

AMA: Feb 13: 3

Coding Guidance

Codes 37215 and 37216 include all necessary selective carotid artery catheterization(s), diagnostic cervical and cerebral carotid arteriography(ies), and all radiological supervision and interpretation on the same side. Code 75962 is not appropriate to use with these codes since radiological supervision

---

● New   ▲ Revised   ✖ Deleted   ⊙ Moderate Sedation   ⊘ High Risk Denial   ⊛ Age Edit   ♀ Female   ♂ Male   **AMA** *CPT® Assistant*   *MUE* Medically Unlikely Edit

⊘ Modifier 51 Exempt   ⊖ Modifier 63 Exempt   ✗ Unlisted   **Modifiers:** *See Inside Back Cover*   Ⓜ Maternity   A2 – Z3 ASC Payment Indicators   A – Y OPPS Status Indicators

400   CPT © 2015 American Medical Association. All Rights Reserved.   © 2016 DecisionHealth

and interpretation for angioplasty is included and the cervical carotid artery is not a peripheral artery.

⊙ **37215** Transcatheter placement of intravascular stent(s), cervical carotid artery, open or percutaneous, including angioplasty, when performed, and radiological supervision and interpretation; with distal embolic protection **C**

RVU			Global Days	Modifiers				
Mod	Non-Fac Total	Fac Total		51	50	62	80	MUE
	29.41	29.41	090	2	1	0	0	1

AMA: May 05: 7, Feb 13: 3, Mar 14: 8

Transcatheter placement of intravascular stent(s), cervical carotid artery

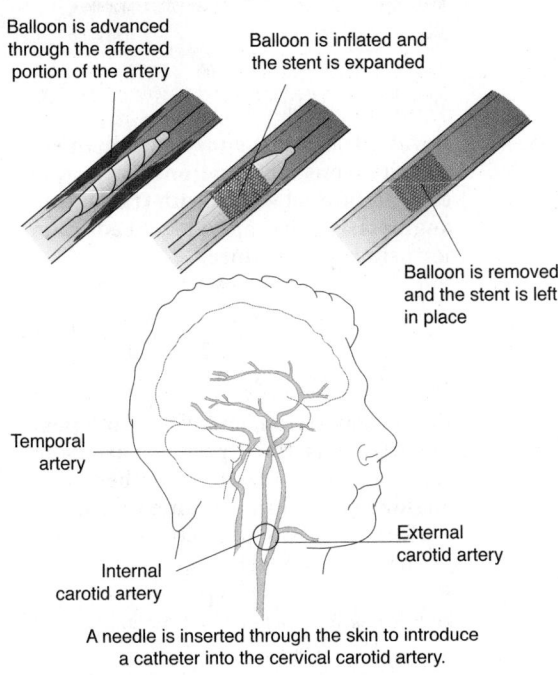

Balloon is advanced through the affected portion of the artery

Balloon is inflated and the stent is expanded

Balloon is removed and the stent is left in place

Temporal artery

Internal carotid artery

External carotid artery

A needle is inserted through the skin to introduce a catheter into the cervical carotid artery.

⊙ **37216** Transcatheter placement of intravascular stent(s), cervical carotid artery, open or percutaneous, including angioplasty, when performed, and radiological supervision and interpretation; without distal embolic protection ⊘**E**

RVU			Global Days	Modifiers				
Mod	Non-Fac Total	Fac Total		51	50	62	80	MUE
	0.00	0.00	090	9	9	9	9	

AMA: May 05: 7, Feb 13: 3, Mar 14: 8

37217 Transcatheter placement of intravascular stent(s), intrathoracic common carotid artery or innominate artery by retrograde treatment, open ipsilateral cervical carotid artery exposure, including angioplasty, when performed, and radiological supervision and interpretation **C**

RVU			Global Days	Modifiers				
Mod	Non-Fac Total	Fac Total		51	50	62	80	MUE
	32.09	32.09	090	2	1	0	0	1

AMA: Mar 14: 8, May 15: 7

Transcatheter placement intravascular stent(s), retrograde approach
intrathoracic common carotid or innominate artery

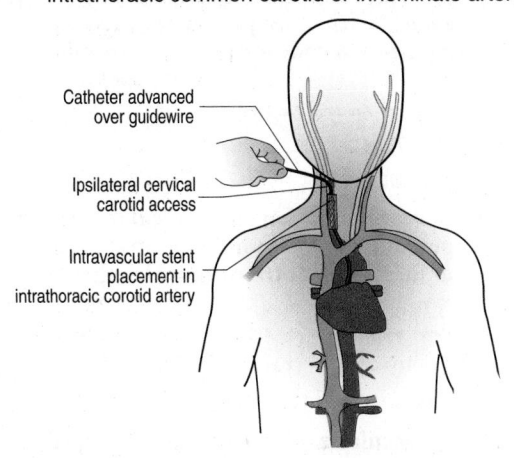

Catheter advanced over guidewire

Ipsilateral cervical carotid access

Intravascular stent placement in intrathoracic corotid artery

⊙ **37218** Transcatheter placement of intravascular stent(s), intrathoracic common carotid artery or innominate artery, open or percutaneous antegrade approach, including angioplasty, when performed, and radiological supervision and interpretation **C**

RVU			Global Days	Modifiers				
Mod	Non-Fac Total	Fac Total		51	50	62	80	MUE
	24.07	24.07	090	2	1	0	0	1

AMA: May 15: 7

Lower Extremity Endovascular Revascularization

⊙ **37220** Revascularization, endovascular, open or percutaneous, iliac artery, unilateral, initial vessel; with transluminal angioplasty **G2J1**

RVU			Global Days	Modifiers				
Mod	Non-Fac Total	Fac Total		51	50	62	80	MUE
	89.86	12.22	000	2	1	0	1	2

AMA: Jul 11: 3, Oct 11: 9, Dec 13: 8

⊙ **37221** Revascularization, endovascular, open or percutaneous, iliac artery, unilateral, initial vessel; with transluminal stent placement(s), includes angioplasty within the same vessel, when performed **J8J1**

RVU			Global Days	Modifiers				
Mod	Non-Fac Total	Fac Total		51	50	62	80	MUE
	132.42	15.01	000	2	1	0	0	2

AMA: Jul 11: 3, Oct 11: 9, Jan 15: 13

⊙➕ **37222** Revascularization, endovascular, open or percutaneous, iliac artery, each additional ipsilateral iliac vessel; with transluminal angioplasty (List separately in addition to code for primary procedure) **NIN**

RVU			Global Days	Modifiers				
Mod	Non-Fac Total	Fac Total		51	50	62	80	MUE
	25.24	5.51	ZZZ	0	1	0	0	2

AMA: Jul 11: 3, Oct 11: 9

● New　▲ Revised　Deleted　⊙ Moderate Sedation　➕ Add-on Codes　⊘ High Risk Denial　Ⓐ Age Edit　♀ Female　♂ Male　**AMA** *CPT Assistant*　**MUE** Medically Unlikely Edit
⊘ Modifier 51 Exempt　⊖ Modifier 63 Exempt　Ⓧ Unlisted　**Modifiers:** *See Inside Back Cover*　Ⓜ Maternity　**A2–Z3** ASC Payment Indicators　**A–Y** OPPS Status Indicators

⊙+**37223** Revascularization, endovascular, open or percutaneous, iliac artery, each additional ipsilateral iliac vessel; with transluminal stent placement(s), includes angioplasty within the same vessel, when performed (List separately in addition to code for primary procedure) N I N

	RVU		Global Days	Modifiers				
Mod	Non-Fac Total	Fac Total		51	50	62	80	MUE
	73.64	6.32	ZZZ	0	1	0	0	2

AMA: Jul 11: 3, Oct 11: 9, Apr 12: 8, Dec 13: 8

⊙ **37224** Revascularization, endovascular, open or percutaneous, femoral, popliteal artery(s), unilateral; with transluminal angioplasty G 2 J I

	RVU		Global Days	Modifiers				
Mod	Non-Fac Total	Fac Total		51	50	62	80	MUE
	109.00	13.44	000	2	1	0	0	2

AMA: Jul 11: 3, Oct 11: 9, Dec 11: 15

⊙ **37225** Revascularization, endovascular, open or percutaneous, femoral, popliteal artery(s), unilateral; with atherectomy, includes angioplasty within the same vessel, when performed J 8 J I

	RVU		Global Days	Modifiers				
Mod	Non-Fac Total	Fac Total		51	50	62	80	MUE
	313.15	18.23	000	2	1	0	0	2

AMA: Jul 11: 3, Oct 11: 9, Nov 11: 9

⊙ **37226** Revascularization, endovascular, open or percutaneous, femoral, popliteal artery(s), unilateral; with transluminal stent placement(s), includes angioplasty within the same vessel, when performed J 8 J I

	RVU		Global Days	Modifiers				
Mod	Non-Fac Total	Fac Total		51	50	62	80	MUE
	257.45	15.80	000	2	1	0	0	2

AMA: Jul 11: 3, Oct 11: 9, Dec 11: 15

⊙ **37227** Revascularization, endovascular, open or percutaneous, femoral, popliteal artery(s), unilateral; with transluminal stent placement(s) and atherectomy, includes angioplasty within the same vessel, when performed J 8 J I

	RVU		Global Days	Modifiers				
Mod	Non-Fac Total	Fac Total		51	50	62	80	MUE
	422.88	21.94	000	2	1	0	0	2

AMA: Jul 11: 3, Oct 11: 9, Nov 11: 9

⊙ **37228** Revascularization, endovascular, open or percutaneous, tibial, peroneal artery, unilateral, initial vessel; with transluminal angioplasty J 8 J I

	RVU		Global Days	Modifiers				
Mod	Non-Fac Total	Fac Total		51	50	62	80	MUE
	154.86	16.43	000	2	1	0	0	2

AMA: Jul 11: 3, Oct 11: 9

⊙ **37229** Revascularization, endovascular, open or percutaneous, tibial, peroneal artery, unilateral, initial vessel; with atherectomy, includes angioplasty within the same vessel, when performed J 8 J I

	RVU		Global Days	Modifiers				
Mod	Non-Fac Total	Fac Total		51	50	62	80	MUE
	308.55	21.26	000	2	1	0	0	2

AMA: Jul 11: 3, Oct 11: 9, Nov 11: 9

⊙ **37230** Revascularization, endovascular, open or percutaneous, tibial, peroneal artery, unilateral, initial vessel; with transluminal stent placement(s), includes angioplasty within the same vessel, when performed J 8 J I

	RVU		Global Days	Modifiers				
Mod	Non-Fac Total	Fac Total		51	50	62	80	MUE
	236.02	20.95	000	2	1	0	0	2

AMA: Jul 11: 3, Oct 11: 9

⊙ **37231** Revascularization, endovascular, open or percutaneous, tibial, peroneal artery, unilateral, initial vessel; with transluminal stent placement(s) and atherectomy, includes angioplasty within the same vessel, when performed J 8 J I

	RVU		Global Days	Modifiers				
Mod	Non-Fac Total	Fac Total		51	50	62	80	MUE
	379.70	22.77	000	2	1	0	0	2

AMA: Jul 11: 3, Oct 11: 9, Nov 11: 9

⊙+**37232** Revascularization, endovascular, open or percutaneous, tibial/peroneal artery, unilateral, each additional vessel; with transluminal angioplasty (List separately in addition to code for primary procedure) N I N

	RVU		Global Days	Modifiers				
Mod	Non-Fac Total	Fac Total		51	50	62	80	MUE
	34.51	5.97	ZZZ	0	1	0	0	2

AMA: Jul 11: 3, Oct 11: 9, Apr 12: 8

⊙+**37233** Revascularization, endovascular, open or percutaneous, tibial/peroneal artery, unilateral, each additional vessel; with atherectomy, includes angioplasty within the same vessel, when performed (List separately in addition to code for primary procedure) N I N

	RVU		Global Days	Modifiers				
Mod	Non-Fac Total	Fac Total		51	50	62	80	MUE
	41.69	9.72	ZZZ	0	1	0	0	2

AMA: Jul 11: 3, Oct 11: 9, Nov 11: 9, Apr 12: 8

⊙+**37234** Revascularization, endovascular, open or percutaneous, tibial/peroneal artery, unilateral, each additional vessel; with transluminal stent placement(s), includes angioplasty within the same vessel, when performed (List separately in addition to code for primary procedure) N I N

	RVU		Global Days	Modifiers				
Mod	Non-Fac Total	Fac Total		51	50	62	80	MUE
	110.26	8.38	ZZZ	0	1	0	0	2

AMA: Jul 11: 3, Oct 11: 9, Apr 12: 9

⊙+**37235** Revascularization, endovascular, open or percutaneous, tibial/peroneal artery, unilateral, each additional vessel; with transluminal stent placement(s) and atherectomy, includes angioplasty within the same vessel, when performed (List separately in addition to code for primary procedure) N I N

	RVU		Global Days	Modifiers				
Mod	Non-Fac Total	Fac Total		51	50	62	80	MUE
	116.09	11.90	ZZZ	0	1	0	0	2

AMA: Jul 11: 3, Oct 11: 9, Nov 11: 9

● New   ▲ Revised   ✖ Deleted   ⊙ Moderate Sedation   ✚ Add-on Codes   ⊘ High Risk Denial   ⓐ Age Edit   ♀ Female   ♂ Male   **AMA** *CPT® Assistant*   **MUE** Medically Unlikely Edit

⊘ Modifier 51 Exempt   ⊖ Modifier 63 Exempt   ⊠ Unlisted   **Modifiers:** *See Inside Back Cover*   Ⓜ Maternity   A 2 – Z 3 ASC Payment Indicators   A – Y OPPS Status Indicators

37236 Transcatheter placement of an intravascular stent(s) (except lower extremity artery(s) for occlusive disease, cervical carotid, extracranial vertebral or intrathoracic carotid, intracranial, or coronary), open or percutaneous, including radiological supervision and interpretation and including all angioplasty within the same vessel, when performed; initial artery `J 8 J 1`

RVU			Global Days	Modifiers				
Mod	Non-Fac Total	Fac Total		51	50	62	80	MUE
	116.96	13.30	000	2	1	0	0	1

AMA: Dec 13: 8, May 15: 7

+37237 Transcatheter placement of an intravascular stent(s) (except lower extremity artery(s) for occlusive disease, cervical carotid, extracranial vertebral or intrathoracic carotid, intracranial, or coronary), open or percutaneous, including radiological supervision and interpretation and including all angioplasty within the same vessel, when performed; each additional artery (List separately in addition to code for primary procedure) `N I N`

RVU			Global Days	Modifiers				
Mod	Non-Fac Total	Fac Total		51	50	62	80	MUE
	69.92	6.27	ZZZ	0	1	0	0	2

AMA: Dec 13: 8

37238 Transcatheter placement of an intravascular stent(s), open or percutaneous, including radiological supervision and interpretation and including angioplasty within the same vessel, when performed; initial vein `J 8 J 1`

RVU			Global Days	Modifiers				
Mod	Non-Fac Total	Fac Total		51	50	62	80	MUE
	119.20	9.21	000	2	1	0	0	1

Transcatheter placement of intravascular venous stent(s), open or percutaneous

Initial vein (37238), Each additional vein (37239)

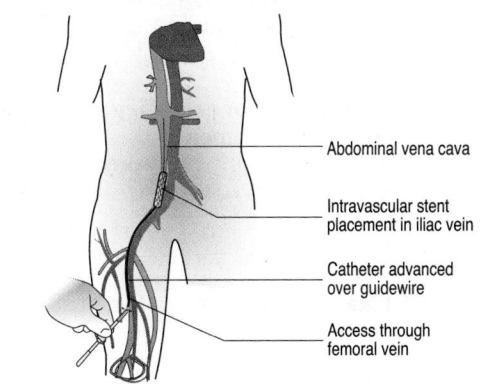

- Abdominal vena cava
- Intravascular stent placement in iliac vein
- Catheter advanced over guidewire
- Access through femoral vein

+37239 Transcatheter placement of an intravascular stent(s), open or percutaneous, including radiological supervision and interpretation and including angioplasty within the same vessel, when performed; each additional vein (List separately in addition to code for primary procedure) `N I N`

RVU			Global Days	Modifiers				
Mod	Non-Fac Total	Fac Total		51	50	62	80	MUE
	57.70	4.39	ZZZ	0	1	0	0	2

37241 Vascular embolization or occlusion, inclusive of all radiological supervision and interpretation, intraprocedural roadmapping, and imaging guidance necessary to complete the intervention; venous, other than hemorrhage (eg, congenital or acquired venous malformations, venous and capillary hemangiomas, varices, varicoceles) `J 8 J 1`

RVU			Global Days	Modifiers				
Mod	Non-Fac Total	Fac Total		51	50	62	80	MUE
	135.96	13.20	000	2	0	0	1	2

AMA: Nov 13: 6, Aug 14: 14, Oct 14: 6, Apr 15: 10, Aug 15: 8

37242 Vascular embolization or occlusion, inclusive of all radiological supervision and interpretation, intraprocedural roadmapping, and imaging guidance necessary to complete the intervention; arterial, other than hemorrhage or tumor (eg, congenital or acquired arterial malformations, arteriovenous malformations, arteriovenous fistulas, aneurysms, pseudoaneurysms) `J 8 J 1`

RVU			Global Days	Modifiers				
Mod	Non-Fac Total	Fac Total		51	50	62	80	MUE
	217.87	14.42	000	2	0	0	1	2

AMA: Nov 13: 6, Oct 14: 6

37243 Vascular embolization or occlusion, inclusive of all radiological supervision and interpretation, intraprocedural roadmapping, and imaging guidance necessary to complete the intervention; for tumors, organ ischemia, or infarction `J 8 J 1`

RVU			Global Days	Modifiers				
Mod	Non-Fac Total	Fac Total		51	50	62	80	MUE
	276.66	17.01	000	2	0	0	1	1

AMA: Nov 13: 7, Oct 14: 6

37244 Vascular embolization or occlusion, inclusive of all radiological supervision and interpretation, intraprocedural roadmapping, and imaging guidance necessary to complete the intervention; for arterial or venous hemorrhage or lymphatic extravasation `J 1`

RVU			Global Days	Modifiers				
Mod	Non-Fac Total	Fac Total		51	50	62	80	MUE
	192.79	19.93	000	2	0	0	1	2

AMA: Nov 13: 7, Aug 14: 14, Oct 14: 6

● New ▲ Revised Deleted ⊙ Moderate Sedation ✚ Add-on Codes ⊘ High Risk Denial ⒶAge Edit ♀ Female ♂ Male **AMA** CPT® Assistant **MUE** Medically Unlikely Edit ⊘ Modifier 51 Exempt ⊖ Modifier 63 Exempt ✗ Unlisted **Modifiers:** See Inside Back Cover Ⓜ Maternity A 2 – Z 3 ASC Payment Indicators A – Y OPPS Status Indicators

© 2016 DecisionHealth | CPT © 2015 American Medical Association. All Rights Reserved. | **403**

✖ 37250 Intravascular ultrasound (non coronary vessel) during diagnostic evaluation and/or therapeutic intervention, initial vessel

✖ 37251 Intravascular ultrasound (non coronary vessel) during diagnostic evaluation and/or therapeutic intervention, each additional vessel

⊙✚● **37252** Intravascular ultrasound (noncoronary vessel) during diagnostic evaluation and/or therapeutic intervention, including radiological supervision and interpretation; initial noncoronary vessel (List separately in addition to code for primary procedure) **N I N**

RVU				Global Days	Modifiers			
Mod	Non-Fac Total	Fac Total			51	50	62	80	MUE
	39.70	2.70	ZZZ		0	0	1	0	1

⊙✚● **37253** Intravascular ultrasound (noncoronary vessel) during diagnostic evaluation and/or therapeutic intervention, including radiological supervision and interpretation; each additional noncoronary vessel (List separately in addition to code for primary procedure) **N I N**

RVU				Global Days	Modifiers			
Mod	Non-Fac Total	Fac Total			51	50	62	80	MUE
	6.17	2.16	ZZZ		0	0	1	0	

Vascular Endoscopic Procedures

37500 Vascular endoscopy, surgical, with ligation of perforator veins, subfascial (SEPS) **A 2 T**

RVU				Global Days	Modifiers			
Mod	Non-Fac Total	Fac Total			51	50	62	80	MUE
	22.28	22.28	090		2	1	1	1	1

AMA: Jul 10: 6

37501 Unlisted vascular endoscopy procedure **✖ T**

RVU				Global Days	Modifiers			
Mod	Non-Fac Total	Fac Total			51	50	62	80	MUE
	0.00	0.00	YYY		2	1	1	1	

Vascular Ligation Procedures

37565 Ligation, internal jugular vein **T**

RVU				Global Days	Modifiers			
Mod	Non-Fac Total	Fac Total			51	50	62	80	MUE
	21.14	21.14	090		2	1	1	0	1

37600 Ligation; external carotid artery **T**

RVU				Global Days	Modifiers			
Mod	Non-Fac Total	Fac Total			51	50	62	80	MUE
	20.76	20.76	090		2	0	1	2	1

37605 Ligation; internal or common carotid artery **T**

RVU				Global Days	Modifiers			
Mod	Non-Fac Total	Fac Total			51	50	62	80	MUE
	23.61	23.61	090		2	0	1	2	1

37606 Ligation; internal or common carotid artery, with gradual occlusion, as with Selverstone or Crutchfield clamp **T**

RVU				Global Days	Modifiers			
Mod	Non-Fac Total	Fac Total			51	50	62	80	MUE
	17.00	17.00	090		2	0	0	2	1

37607 Ligation or banding of angioaccess arteriovenous fistula **A 2 T**

RVU				Global Days	Modifiers			
Mod	Non-Fac Total	Fac Total			51	50	62	80	MUE
	11.07	11.07	090		2	0	1	1	1

37609 Ligation or biopsy, temporal artery **A 2 T**

RVU				Global Days	Modifiers			
Mod	Non-Fac Total	Fac Total			51	50	62	80	MUE
	8.91	6.03	010		2	1	0	1	1

Ligation or biopsy, temporal artery

An incision is made into the skin in front of the ear to access the temporal artery.

Temporal artery

Artery is tied off with suture or wire or tissue is removed for diagnosis

37615 Ligation, major artery (eg, post-traumatic, rupture); neck **T**

RVU				Global Days	Modifiers			
Mod	Non-Fac Total	Fac Total			51	50	62	80	MUE
	14.89	14.89	090		2	0	1	2	2

37616 Ligation, major artery (eg, post-traumatic, rupture); chest **C**

RVU				Global Days	Modifiers			
Mod	Non-Fac Total	Fac Total			51	50	62	80	MUE
	32.20	32.20	090		2	0	1	2	1

37617 Ligation, major artery (eg, post-traumatic, rupture); abdomen **C**

RVU				Global Days	Modifiers			
Mod	Non-Fac Total	Fac Total			51	50	62	80	MUE
	39.12	39.12	090		2	0	1	2	3

AMA: Aug 13: 14

37618 Ligation, major artery (eg, post-traumatic, rupture); extremity **C**

RVU				Global Days	Modifiers			
Mod	Non-Fac Total	Fac Total			51	50	62	80	MUE
	11.26	11.26	090		2	0	1	2	2

37619 Ligation of inferior vena cava **T**

RVU				Global Days	Modifiers			
Mod	Non-Fac Total	Fac Total			51	50	62	80	MUE
	47.95	47.95	090		2	0	0	2	1

AMA: Apr 12: 8

● New   ▲ Revised   ✖ Deleted   ⊙ Moderate Sedation   ✚ Add-on Codes   ⊘ High Risk Denial   Ⓐ Age Edit   ♀ Female   ♂ Male   **AMA** CPT® Assistant   **MUE** Medically Unlikely Edit

⊘ Modifier 51 Exempt   ⊖ Modifier 63 Exempt   ✖ Unlisted   **Modifiers:** See Inside Back Cover   Ⓜ Maternity   **A 2**–**Z 3** ASC Payment Indicators   **A**–**Y** OPPS Status Indicators

37650 Ligation of femoral vein   A 2 T

Mod	Non-Fac Total	Fac Total	Global Days	51	50	62	80	MUE
	14.97	14.97	090	2	1	1	1	1

37660 Ligation of common iliac vein   C

Mod	Non-Fac Total	Fac Total	Global Days	51	50	62	80	MUE
	34.11	34.11	090	2	1	1	2	1

Coding Guidance

Ligation, division, and stripping of saphenous veins are not reported in addition to coronary artery bypass procedures 33510-33523, since the placement of a venous graft is integral to the bypass.

37700 Ligation and division of long saphenous vein at saphenofemoral junction, or distal interruptions   A 2 T

Mod	Non-Fac Total	Fac Total	Global Days	51	50	62	80	MUE
	7.33	7.33	090	2	1	0	1	1

AMA: Aug 96: 10

37718 Ligation, division, and stripping, short saphenous vein   A 2 T

Mod	Non-Fac Total	Fac Total	Global Days	51	50	62	80	MUE
	12.89	12.89	090	2	1	1	1	1

37722 Ligation, division, and stripping, long (greater) saphenous veins from saphenofemoral junction to knee or below   A 2 T

Mod	Non-Fac Total	Fac Total	Global Days	51	50	62	80	MUE
	14.12	14.12	090	2	1	1	1	1

37735 Ligation and division and complete stripping of long or short saphenous veins with radical excision of ulcer and skin graft and/or interruption of communicating veins of lower leg, with excision of deep fascia   A 2 T

Mod	Non-Fac Total	Fac Total	Global Days	51	50	62	80	MUE
	20.19	20.19	090	2	1	1	1	1

37760 Ligation of perforator veins, subfascial, radical (Linton type), including skin graft, when performed, open, 1 leg   A 2 T

Mod	Non-Fac Total	Fac Total	Global Days	51	50	62	80	MUE
	18.19	18.19	090	2	1	1	1	1

AMA: Jul 10: 6

37761 Ligation of perforator vein(s), subfascial, open, including ultrasound guidance, when performed, 1 leg   R 2 T

Mod	Non-Fac Total	Fac Total	Global Days	51	50	62	80	MUE
	16.22	16.22	090	2	1	1	2	1

AMA: Jul 10: 6

37765 Stab phlebectomy of varicose veins, 1 extremity; 10-20 stab incisions   P 3 T

Mod	Non-Fac Total	Fac Total	Global Days	51	50	62	80	MUE
	18.89	13.21	090	2	1	1	1	1

AMA: Aug 04: 6, Nov 10: 9, Oct 14: 6

37766 Stab phlebectomy of varicose veins, 1 extremity; more than 20 incisions   P 3 T

Mod	Non-Fac Total	Fac Total	Global Days	51	50	62	80	MUE
	22.45	16.12	090	2	1	1	1	1

AMA: Aug 04: 6, Sep 13: 17, Oct 14: 6

37780 Ligation and division of short saphenous vein at saphenopopliteal junction (separate procedure)   A 2 T

Mod	Non-Fac Total	Fac Total	Global Days	51	50	62	80	MUE
	7.47	7.47	090	2	1	1	1	1

AMA: Aug 96: 10

37785 Ligation, division, and/or excision of varicose vein cluster(s), 1 leg   A 2 T

Mod	Non-Fac Total	Fac Total	Global Days	51	50	62	80	MUE
	10.32	7.70	090	2	1	0	1	1

AMA: Aug 04: 5, Nov 10: 9

Other Vascular Procedures

37788 Penile revascularization, artery, with or without vein graft   ⊗ ♂ C

Mod	Non-Fac Total	Fac Total	Global Days	51	50	62	80	MUE
	37.26	37.26	090	2	0	1	2	1

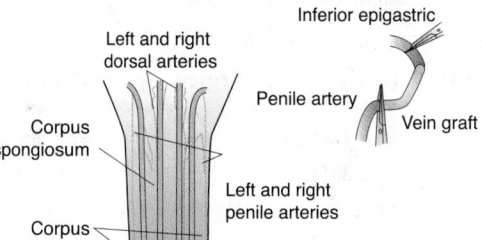

Penile revascularization, artery, with or without vein graft

A small incision is made at the base of the penis to access the penile artery and surrounding vessels.

37790 Penile venous occlusive procedure   A 2 T

Mod	Non-Fac Total	Fac Total	Global Days	51	50	62	80	MUE
	14.55	14.55	090	2	0	0	0	1

37799 Unlisted procedure, vascular surgery   ✗ T

Mod	Non-Fac Total	Fac Total	Global Days	51	50	62	80	MUE
	0.00	0.00	YYY	2	0	1	0	

AMA: Spring 93: 12, Fall 93: 3, Feb 97: 10, Sep 97: 10, May 01: 11, Oct 04: 16, Aug 11: 9, Nov 10: 9, Nov 13: 14, Mar 14: 8, Aug 14: 14, Oct 14: 6, Apr 15: 10

● New   ▲ Revised   Deleted   ⊙ Moderate Sedation   ✚ Add-on Codes   ⊘ High Risk Denial   Ⓐ Age Edit   ♀ Female   ♂ Male   **AMA** *CPT® Assistant*   ***MUE*** Medically Unlikely Edit
⊘ Modifier 51 Exempt   ⊖ Modifier 63 Exempt   ✗ Unlisted   **Modifiers:** *See Inside Back Cover*   Ⓜ Maternity   A 2 – Z 3 ASC Payment Indicators   A – Y OPPS Status Indicators

Surgical Procedures

38100 – 38212

Hemic/Lymphatic Procedures

Spleen Procedures

Excisional Spleen Procedures

38100 Splenectomy; total (separate procedure)   C

Mod	RVU Non-Fac Total	Fac Total	Global Days	51	50	62	80	MUE
	33.55	33.55	090	2	0	1	2	1

AMA: July 93: 9, Summer 93: 10, Sep 12: 11

38101 Splenectomy; partial (separate procedure)   C

Mod	RVU Non-Fac Total	Fac Total	Global Days	51	50	62	80	MUE
	33.63	33.63	090	2	0	1	2	1

AMA: Summer 93: 10, Sep 12: 11

+ 38102 Splenectomy; total, en bloc for extensive disease, in conjunction with other procedure (List in addition to code for primary procedure)   C

Mod	RVU Non-Fac Total	Fac Total	Global Days	51	50	62	80	MUE
	7.62	7.62	ZZZ	0	0	1	2	1

AMA: Summer 93: 10, Sep 12: 11

Spleen Repair Procedures

38115 Repair of ruptured spleen (splenorrhaphy) with or without partial splenectomy   C

Mod	RVU Non-Fac Total	Fac Total	Global Days	51	50	62	80	MUE
	36.80	36.80	090	2	0	1	2	1

AMA: Summer 93: 10, Sep 12: 11

Laparoscopic Spleen Procedures

38120 Laparoscopy, surgical, splenectomy   J1

Mod	RVU Non-Fac Total	Fac Total	Global Days	51	50	62	80	MUE
	30.57	30.57	090	2	0	1	2	1

AMA: Nov 99: 20, 21, Mar 00: 8, Sep 12: 11

38129 Unlisted laparoscopy procedure, spleen   ⊘x J1

Mod	RVU Non-Fac Total	Fac Total	Global Days	51	50	62	80	MUE
	0.00	0.00	YYY	2	0	1	2	

AMA: Nov 99: 20, 21, Mar 00: 8, Sep 12: 11

Spleen Introduction Procedures

38200 Injection procedure for splenoportography   N1N

Mod	RVU Non-Fac Total	Fac Total	Global Days	51	50	62	80	MUE
	3.36	3.36	000	2	0	0	0	1

Bone Marrow/Stem Cell Services/Procedures

38204 Management of recipient hematopoietic progenitor cell donor search and cell acquisition   ⊘N1N

Mod	RVU Non-Fac Total	Fac Total	Global Days	51	50	62	80	MUE
	3.04	3.04	XXX	9	9	9	9	

AMA: Oct 13: 3

38205 Blood-derived hematopoietic progenitor cell harvesting for transplantation, per collection; allogeneic   B

Mod	RVU Non-Fac Total	Fac Total	Global Days	51	50	62	80	MUE
	2.37	2.37	000	2	0	0	0	1

AMA: Oct 13: 3

38206 Blood-derived hematopoietic progenitor cell harvesting for transplantation, per collection; autologous   G2 S

Mod	RVU Non-Fac Total	Fac Total	Global Days	51	50	62	80	MUE
	2.39	2.39	000	2	0	0	0	1

AMA: Oct 13: 3

38207 Transplant preparation of hematopoietic progenitor cells; cryopreservation and storage   ⊘S

Mod	RVU Non-Fac Total	Fac Total	Global Days	51	50	62	80	MUE
	1.35	1.35	XXX	9	9	9	9	

AMA: Jul 03: 9, Jun 09: 3, Oct 13: 3

38208 Transplant preparation of hematopoietic progenitor cells; thawing of previously frozen harvest, without washing, per donor   ⊘S

Mod	RVU Non-Fac Total	Fac Total	Global Days	51	50	62	80	MUE
	0.85	0.85	XXX	9	9	9	9	0

AMA: Jul 03: 9, Jun 09: 3, Oct 13: 3

38209 Transplant preparation of hematopoietic progenitor cells; thawing of previously frozen harvest, with washing, per donor   ⊘S

Mod	RVU Non-Fac Total	Fac Total	Global Days	51	50	62	80	MUE
	0.36	0.36	XXX	9	9	9	9	0

AMA: Oct 13: 3

38210 Transplant preparation of hematopoietic progenitor cells; specific cell depletion within harvest, T-cell depletion   S

Mod	RVU Non-Fac Total	Fac Total	Global Days	51	50	62	80	MUE
	2.38	2.38	XXX	9	9	9	9	0

AMA: Oct 13: 3

38211 Transplant preparation of hematopoietic progenitor cells; tumor cell depletion   S

Mod	RVU Non-Fac Total	Fac Total	Global Days	51	50	62	80	MUE
	2.15	2.15	XXX	9	9	9	9	0

AMA: Oct 13: 3

38212 Transplant preparation of hematopoietic progenitor cells; red blood cell removal   S

Mod	RVU Non-Fac Total	Fac Total	Global Days	51	50	62	80	MUE
	1.43	1.43	XXX	9	9	9	9	0

AMA: Oct 13: 3

● New   ▲ Revised   ✖ Deleted   ⊙ Moderate Sedation   ✚ Add-on Codes   ⊘ High Risk Denial   Ⓐ Age Edit   ♀ Female   ♂ Male   **AMA** *CPT® Assistant*   **MUE** Medically Unlikely Edit
⊗ Modifier 51 Exempt   ⊖ Modifier 63 Exempt   ⋈ Unlisted   **Modifiers:** *See Inside Back Cover*   Ⓜ Maternity   A2–Z3 ASC Payment Indicators   A–Y OPPS Status Indicators

406   CPT © 2015 American Medical Association. All Rights Reserved.   © 2016 DecisionHealth

38213 Transplant preparation of hematopoietic progenitor cells; platelet depletion S

RVU			Global Days	Modifiers				
Mod	Non-Fac Total	Fac Total		51	50	62	80	MUE
	0.36	0.36	XXX	9	9	9	9	0

AMA: Oct 13: 3

38214 Transplant preparation of hematopoietic progenitor cells; plasma (volume) depletion ⊘S

RVU			Global Days	Modifiers				
Mod	Non-Fac Total	Fac Total		51	50	62	80	MUE
	1.23	1.23	XXX	9	9	9	9	0

AMA: Oct 13: 3

38215 Transplant preparation of hematopoietic progenitor cells; cell concentration in plasma, mononuclear, or buffy coat layer ⊘S

RVU			Global Days	Modifiers				
Mod	Non-Fac Total	Fac Total		51	50	62	80	MUE
	1.43	1.43	XXX	9	9	9	9	0

AMA: Oct 13: 3

Coding Guidance

Codes 38220 and 38221 can only be reported together when these two procedures are done at separate sites or encounters. Separate site reporting requires that aspiration and biopsy are done in different bones, or through two different skin incisions at different sites on the same bone. When both an aspiration and a biopsy are done on the same bone through the same access incision, report only the biopsy code.

38220 Bone marrow; aspiration only P 3 T

RVU			Global Days	Modifiers				
Mod	Non-Fac Total	Fac Total		51	50	62	80	MUE
	4.68	1.77	XXX	2	1	0	0	1

AMA: Jan 04: 26, Jun 07: 10, Apr 12: 15, May 12: 11, Oct 13: 3, Mar 15: 9
Pub 100-04, 12, 60

Bone marrow aspiration

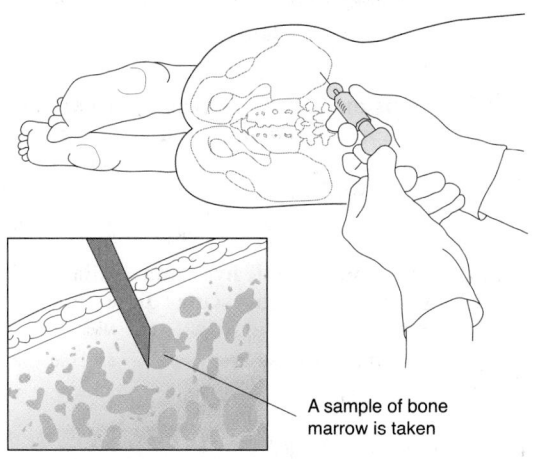

A sample of bone marrow is taken

Coding Guidance

Do not report code 38221 for bone marrow biopsy together with code 20220 for bone biopsy. When it is necessary to evaluate both bone matrix structure and bone marrow, only one code can be reported: either 38221 or 20220. If two separate biopsies are required at separate sites, both codes may be reported using modifier 59 on one code. If only one specimen is submitted for pathological evaluation, only one interpretation code may be reported, whether or not the report includes a morphological evaluation of both bone structure and bone marrow.

38221 Bone marrow; biopsy, needle or trocar P 3 T

Coding tip: Code 99001 for specimen transfer from a facility to an outside laboratory

Coding tip: If a powered biopsy needle is used, report HCPCS Level II code C1830 (OPPS only).

RVU			Global Days	Modifiers				
Mod	Non-Fac Total	Fac Total		51	50	62	80	MUE
	4.75	2.15	XXX	2	1	0	0	1

AMA: Mar 15: 9
Pub 100-04, 12, 60

38230 Bone marrow harvesting for transplantation; allogeneic ⊘G2S

RVU			Global Days	Modifiers				
Mod	Non-Fac Total	Fac Total		51	50	62	80	MUE
	5.73	5.73	000	2	0	0	0	1

AMA: Apr 96: 1, Jun 09: 3, May 12: 11, Oct 13: 3

38232 Bone marrow harvesting for transplantation; autologous ⊘G2S

RVU			Global Days	Modifiers				
Mod	Non-Fac Total	Fac Total		51	50	62	80	MUE
	5.71	5.71	000	2	0	0	0	1

AMA: Oct 13: 3

Hematopoietic Progenitor Cell Transplant/Lymphocyte Infusion

38240 Hematopoietic progenitor cell (HPC); allogeneic transplantation per donor S

Coding tip: HPC boost - 38243

RVU			Global Days	Modifiers				
Mod	Non-Fac Total	Fac Total		51	50	62	80	MUE
	6.42	6.42	XXX	2	0	0	0	1

AMA: Apr 96: 2, Nov 98: 15, Nov 99: 21, Jun 09: 3, Oct 13: 3
Pub 100-04, 32, 90.2, 90.6

38241 Hematopoietic progenitor cell (HPC); autologous transplantation G2S

Coding tip: HPC boost - 38243

RVU			Global Days	Modifiers				
Mod	Non-Fac Total	Fac Total		51	50	62	80	MUE
	4.81	4.81	XXX	2	0	0	0	1

AMA: Apr 96: 2, Nov 98: 15, Nov 99: 21, Jun 09: 3, Oct 13: 3, Feb 15: 10
Pub 100-04, 32, 90.2, 90.4

38242 Allogeneic lymphocyte infusions R 2 S

RVU			Global Days	Modifiers				
Mod	Non-Fac Total	Fac Total		51	50	62	80	MUE
	3.38	3.38	000	2	0	0	0	1

AMA: Jun 13: 13, Oct 13: 3

38243 Hematopoietic progenitor cell (HPC); HPC boost R 2 S

RVU			Global Days	Modifiers				
Mod	Non-Fac Total	Fac Total		51	50	62	80	MUE
	3.37	3.37	000	2	0	0	0	1

AMA: Jun 13: 13, Oct 13: 3, Feb 15: 10

● New   ▲ Revised   Deleted   ⊙ Moderate Sedation   ✚ Add-on Codes   ⊘ High Risk Denial   Ⓐ Age Edit   ♀ Female   ♂ Male   **AMA** *CPT® Assistant*   **MUE** Medically Unlikely Edit
⦸ Modifier 51 Exempt   ⊖ Modifier 63 Exempt   ✗ Unlisted   **Modifiers:** *See Inside Back Cover*   Ⓜ Maternity   A 2 – Z 3 ASC Payment Indicators   A – Y OPPS Status Indicators

Lymph Node/Lymphatic Channel Procedures

Incisional Lymph Node/Lymphatic Channel Procedures

38300 Drainage of lymph node abscess or lymphadenitis; simple `A 2 T`

Coding tip: Drainage of skin or subcutaneous abscess, simple - 10060; complicated - 10061

Coding tip: Drainage of hematoma or seroma - 10140

	RVU		Global Days	Modifiers				
Mod	Non-Fac Total	Fac Total		51	50	62	80	MUE
	7.87	5.30	010	2	0	0	1	1

38305 Drainage of lymph node abscess or lymphadenitis; extensive `A 2 T`

	RVU		Global Days	Modifiers				
Mod	Non-Fac Total	Fac Total		51	50	62	80	MUE
	13.78	13.78	090	2	0	0	1	1

38308 Lymphangiotomy or other operations on lymphatic channels `A 2 T`

	RVU		Global Days	Modifiers				
Mod	Non-Fac Total	Fac Total		51	50	62	80	MUE
	12.78	12.78	090	2	0	1	2	1

38380 Suture and/or ligation of thoracic duct; cervical approach `C`

	RVU		Global Days	Modifiers				
Mod	Non-Fac Total	Fac Total		51	50	62	80	MUE
	16.47	16.47	090	2	0	1	2	1

38381 Suture and/or ligation of thoracic duct; thoracic approach `C`

	RVU		Global Days	Modifiers				
Mod	Non-Fac Total	Fac Total		51	50	62	80	MUE
	23.33	23.33	090	2	0	1	2	1

38382 Suture and/or ligation of thoracic duct; abdominal approach `C`

	RVU		Global Days	Modifiers				
Mod	Non-Fac Total	Fac Total		51	50	62	80	MUE
	17.88	17.88	090	2	0	1	2	1

Excisional Lymph Node/Lymphatic Channel Procedures

Coding Guidance

Open biopsy or excision of sentinel lymph node(s) are specific to site. Sentinel node biopsy or excision involves removal of one or more discretely identified lymph nodes. For axillary node(s) use 38500 or 38525; deep cervical node(s) use 38510; internal mammary use 38530. Code 38740 should not be reported for a sentinel lymph node excision of superficial axillary node(s) because it requires removal of all superficial axillary adipose tissue with all lymph nodes in the adipose tissue. Code 38500 is the appropriate code for open biopsy or excision of one or more discrete superficial lymph nodes in the axillary region.

38500 Biopsy or excision of lymph node(s); open, superficial `A 2 T`

	RVU		Global Days	Modifiers				
Mod	Non-Fac Total	Fac Total		51	50	62	80	MUE
	9.55	7.37	010	2	1	0	1	2

AMA: Jun 97: 5, Jul 99: 7, Oct 05: 23, Dec 07: 8, Sep 08: 5, Jan 09: 7, Jun 12: 15

38505 Biopsy or excision of lymph node(s); by needle, superficial (eg, cervical, inguinal, axillary) `A 2 T`

	RVU		Global Days	Modifiers				
Mod	Non-Fac Total	Fac Total		51	50	62	80	MUE
	3.61	2.06	000	2	1	0	1	3

AMA: Jul 99: 6, Jan 09: 7

38510 Biopsy or excision of lymph node(s); open, deep cervical node(s) `A 2 T`

	RVU		Global Days	Modifiers				
Mod	Non-Fac Total	Fac Total		51	50	62	80	MUE
	14.99	12.20	010	2	1	0	1	1

AMA: May 98: 10, Jul 99: 6, Jun 12: 15

38520 Biopsy or excision of lymph node(s); open, deep cervical node(s) with excision scalene fat pad `A 2 T`

	RVU		Global Days	Modifiers				
Mod	Non-Fac Total	Fac Total		51	50	62	80	MUE
	13.45	13.45	090	2	1	0	1	1

AMA: May 98: 10, Jul 99: 6

38525 Biopsy or excision of lymph node(s); open, deep axillary node(s) `A 2 T`

	RVU		Global Days	Modifiers				
Mod	Non-Fac Total	Fac Total		51	50	62	80	MUE
	12.67	12.67	090	2	1	0	1	1

AMA: May 98: 10, Jul 99: 7, Oct 05: 23, Dec 07: 8, Sep 08: 5, Mar 15: 5, Apr 14: 11

38530 Biopsy or excision of lymph node(s); open, internal mammary node(s) `A 2 T`

	RVU		Global Days	Modifiers				
Mod	Non-Fac Total	Fac Total		51	50	62	80	MUE
	15.95	15.95	090	2	1	1	2	1

AMA: May 98: 10, Jul 99: 6, Aug 10: 6, Apr 14: 11

38542 Dissection, deep jugular node(s) `A 2 J 1`

	RVU		Global Days	Modifiers				
Mod	Non-Fac Total	Fac Total		51	50	62	80	MUE
	15.03	15.03	090	2	1	1	2	1

AMA: Jul 99: 7, Aug 10: 6

38550 Excision of cystic hygroma, axillary or cervical; without deep neurovascular dissection `A 2 T`

	RVU		Global Days	Modifiers				
Mod	Non-Fac Total	Fac Total		51	50	62	80	MUE
	14.65	14.65	090	2	0	0	0	1

38555 Excision of cystic hygroma, axillary or cervical; with deep neurovascular dissection `A 2 T`

	RVU		Global Days	Modifiers				
Mod	Non-Fac Total	Fac Total		51	50	62	80	MUE
	29.13	29.13	090	2	0	1	2	1

Staging Lymphadenectomy

38562 Limited lymphadenectomy for staging (separate procedure); pelvic and para-aortic `C`

	RVU		Global Days	Modifiers				
Mod	Non-Fac Total	Fac Total		51	50	62	80	MUE
	20.31	20.31	090	2	2	1	2	1

AMA: Mar 01: 10

● New ▲ Revised ✖ Deleted ⊙ Moderate Sedation ✚ Add-on Codes ⊘ High Risk Denial Ⓐ Age Edit ♀ Female ♂ Male **AMA** *CPT® Assistant* **MUE** Medically Unlikely Edit
⊘ Modifier 51 Exempt ⊖ Modifier 63 Exempt ☒ Unlisted **Modifiers:** *See Inside Back Cover* Ⓜ Maternity `A 2`–`Z 3` ASC Payment Indicators `A`–`Y` OPPS Status Indicators

CPT © 2015 American Medical Association. All Rights Reserved.

© 2016 DecisionHealth

38564 Limited lymphadenectomy for staging (separate procedure); retroperitoneal (aortic and/or splenic) `C`

RVU			Global Days	Modifiers				
Mod	Non-Fac Total	Fac Total		51	50	62	80	MUE
	20.44	20.44	090	2	0	1	2	1

Laparoscopic Lymph Node/Lymphatic Channel Procedures

38570 Laparoscopy, surgical; with retroperitoneal lymph node sampling (biopsy), single or multiple `A2 J1`

RVU			Global Days	Modifiers				
Mod	Non-Fac Total	Fac Total		51	50	62	80	MUE
	14.56	14.56	010	3	0	2	2	1

AMA: Nov 99: 21, Mar 00: 8

38571 Laparoscopy, surgical; with bilateral total pelvic lymphadenectomy `A2 J1`

RVU			Global Days	Modifiers				
Mod	Non-Fac Total	Fac Total		51	50	62	80	MUE
	19.20	19.20	010	3	2	2	2	1

AMA: Nov 99: 21, Mar 00: 8

38572 Laparoscopy, surgical; with bilateral total pelvic lymphadenectomy and peri-aortic lymph node sampling (biopsy), single or multiple `A2 J1`

RVU			Global Days	Modifiers				
Mod	Non-Fac Total	Fac Total		51	50	62	80	MUE
	26.80	26.80	010	3	2	2	2	1

AMA: Nov 99: 21, Jan 15: 14

38589 Unlisted laparoscopy procedure, lymphatic system `x J1`

RVU			Global Days	Modifiers				
Mod	Non-Fac Total	Fac Total		51	50	62	80	MUE
	0.00	0.00	YYY	2	1	1	2	

AMA: Nov 99: 21, Mar 00: 8

Radical Lymphadenectomy Procedures

38700 Suprahyoid lymphadenectomy `G2 T`

RVU			Global Days	Modifiers				
Mod	Non-Fac Total	Fac Total		51	50	62	80	MUE
	23.38	23.38	090	2	1	1	2	1

AMA: Aug 02: 8, Aug 10: 3

38720 Cervical lymphadenectomy (complete) `T`

RVU			Global Days	Modifiers				
Mod	Non-Fac Total	Fac Total		51	50	62	80	MUE
	39.07	39.07	090	2	1	1	2	1

AMA: Oct 01: 10, Aug 02: 8, Aug 10: 4

38724 Cervical lymphadenectomy (modified radical neck dissection) `C`

RVU			Global Days	Modifiers				
Mod	Non-Fac Total	Fac Total		51	50	62	80	MUE
	42.22	42.22	090	2	1	1	2	1

AMA: Jan 01: 13, Aug 02: 8, Aug 10: 4, Dec 12: 3

Coding Guidance
Superficial axillary lymphadenectomy is not to be coded for a sentinel lymph node biopsy. Biopsy or excision of a sentinel lymph node of the superficial axillary node(s) is reported as 38500. Coding 38740 requires complete removal of all adipose tissue and lymph nodes within the superficial axillary region.

38740 Axillary lymphadenectomy; superficial `A2 J1`

RVU			Global Days	Modifiers				
Mod	Non-Fac Total	Fac Total		51	50	62	80	MUE
	20.13	20.13	090	2	1	1	2	1

AMA: Apr 14: 11

38745 Axillary lymphadenectomy; complete `A2 J1`

RVU			Global Days	Modifiers				
Mod	Non-Fac Total	Fac Total		51	50	62	80	MUE
	25.40	25.40	090	2	1	1	2	1

+ 38746 Thoracic lymphadenectomy by thoracotomy, mediastinal and regional lymphadenectomy (List separately in addition to code for primary procedure) `C`

RVU			Global Days	Modifiers				
Mod	Non-Fac Total	Fac Total		51	50	62	80	MUE
	6.20	6.20	ZZZ	0	0	1	2	1

AMA: Sep 12: 3, May 14: 3

Thoracic lymphadenectomy, by thoracotomy, mediastinal and regional,

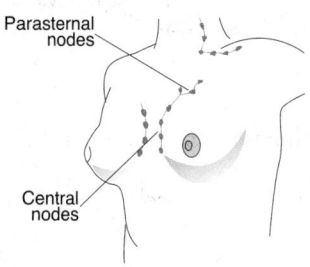

The involved lymph nodes are dissected from the surrounding tissue during a seperately reported thoracic procedure

+ 38747 Abdominal lymphadenectomy, regional, including celiac, gastric, portal, peripancreatic, with or without para-aortic and vena caval nodes (List separately in addition to code for primary procedure) `C`

RVU			Global Days	Modifiers				
Mod	Non-Fac Total	Fac Total		51	50	62	80	MUE
	7.74	7.74	ZZZ	0	0	1	2	1

AMA: Nov 98: 15

38760 Inguinofemoral lymphadenectomy, superficial, including Cloquets node (separate procedure) `A2 T`

RVU			Global Days	Modifiers				
Mod	Non-Fac Total	Fac Total		51	50	62	80	MUE
	24.39	24.39	090	2	1	1	2	1

38765 Inguinofemoral lymphadenectomy, superficial, in continuity with pelvic lymphadenectomy, including external iliac, hypogastric, and obturator nodes (separate procedure) `C`

RVU			Global Days	Modifiers				
Mod	Non-Fac Total	Fac Total		51	50	62	80	MUE
	37.49	37.49	090	2	1	1	2	1

● New   ▲ Revised   Deleted   ⊙ Moderate Sedation   ✚ Add-on Codes   ⊘ High Risk Denial   ⒶAge Edit   ♀ Female   ♂ Male   **AMA** *CPT® Assistant*   **MUE** Medically Unlikely Edit
⊘ Modifier 51 Exempt   ⊖ Modifier 63 Exempt   x Unlisted   **Modifiers:** *See Inside Back Cover*   Ⓜ Maternity   A2–Z3 ASC Payment Indicators   A–Y OPPS Status Indicators

© 2016 DecisionHealth   CPT © 2015 American Medical Association. All Rights Reserved.   **409**

38770 Pelvic lymphadenectomy, including external iliac, hypogastric, and obturator nodes (separate procedure) C

RVU			Global Days	Modifiers				
Mod	Non-Fac Total	Fac Total		51	50	62	80	MUE
	23.32	23.32	090	2	1	1	2	1

38780 Retroperitoneal transabdominal lymphadenectomy, extensive, including pelvic, aortic, and renal nodes (separate procedure) C

RVU			Global Days	Modifiers				
Mod	Non-Fac Total	Fac Total		51	50	62	80	MUE
	29.60	29.60	090	2	0	1	2	1

Introduction Lymph Node/Lymphatic Channel Procedures

38790 Injection procedure; lymphangiography NIN

RVU			Global Days	Modifiers				
Mod	Non-Fac Total	Fac Total		51	50	62	80	MUE
	2.41	2.41	000	2	1	0	1	1

AMA: Jul 99: 6

38792 Injection procedure; radioactive tracer for identification of sentinel node NIQI

RVU			Global Days	Modifiers				
Mod	Non-Fac Total	Fac Total		51	50	62	80	MUE
	1.13	1.13	000	2	1	0	1	1

AMA: Nov 98: 15, Jul 99: 6, Dec 99: 8, Sep 08: 5, Mar 15: 5

38794 Cannulation, thoracic duct NIN

RVU			Global Days	Modifiers				
Mod	Non-Fac Total	Fac Total		51	50	62	80	MUE
	8.59	8.59	090	2	0	0	0	1

Other Lymph Node/Lymphatic Channel Procedures

+ 38900 Intraoperative identification (eg, mapping) of sentinel lymph node(s) includes injection of non-radioactive dye, when performed (List separately in addition to code for primary procedure) NIN

RVU			Global Days	Modifiers				
Mod	Non-Fac Total	Fac Total		51	50	62	80	MUE
	4.01	4.01	ZZZ	0	1	1	2	1

AMA: Mar 15: 5

38999 Unlisted procedure, hemic or lymphatic system ⊗S

RVU			Global Days	Modifiers				
Mod	Non-Fac Total	Fac Total		51	50	62	80	MUE
	0.00	0.00	YYY	2	0	1	0	

AMA: May 98: 10

Mediastinum/Diaphragm Procedures

Mediastinum

Incisional Mediastinum Procedures

39000 Mediastinotomy with exploration, drainage, removal of foreign body, or biopsy; cervical approach C

RVU			Global Days	Modifiers				
Mod	Non-Fac Total	Fac Total		51	50	62	80	MUE
	14.46	14.46	090	2	0	1	2	1

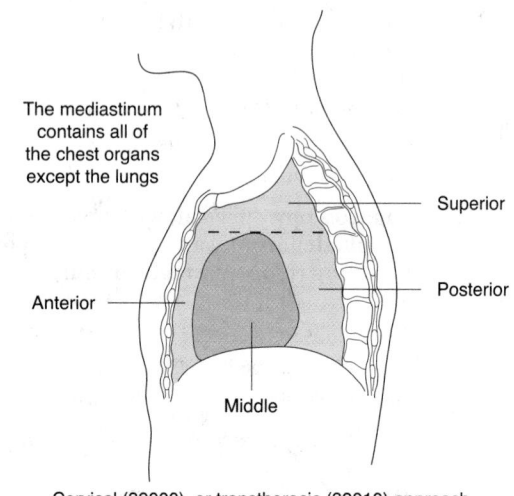

Mediastinotomy

Mediastinum exploration includes the drainage of fluids, removal of a foreign body, or removal of tissue for biopsy

The mediastinum contains all of the chest organs except the lungs

Superior

Posterior

Anterior

Middle

Cervical (39000), or transthoracic (39010) approach

39010 Mediastinotomy with exploration, drainage, removal of foreign body, or biopsy; transthoracic approach, including either transthoracic or median sternotomy C

RVU			Global Days	Modifiers				
Mod	Non-Fac Total	Fac Total		51	50	62	80	MUE
	22.93	22.93	090	2	0	1	2	1

AMA: Jan 13: 6, Jan 14: 5

Excisional Mediastinum Procedures

39200 Resection of mediastinal cyst C

RVU			Global Days	Modifiers				
Mod	Non-Fac Total	Fac Total		51	50	62	80	MUE
	25.75	25.75	090	2	0	1	2	1

39220 Resection of mediastinal tumor C

RVU			Global Days	Modifiers				
Mod	Non-Fac Total	Fac Total		51	50	62	80	MUE
	33.13	33.13	090	2	0	1	2	1

✖ ~~39400 Mediastinoscopy, includes biopsy(ies), when performed~~

● New　▲ Revised　✖ Deleted　⊙ Moderate Sedation　✚ Add-on Codes　⊘ High Risk Denial　Ⓐ Age Edit　♀ Female　♂ Male　**AMA** *CPT® Assistant*　**MUE** Medically Unlikely Edit
⊘ Modifier 51 Exempt　⊖ Modifier 63 Exempt　⊠ Unlisted　**Modifiers:** *See Inside Back Cover*　Ⓜ Maternity　A2–Z3 ASC Payment Indicators　A–Y OPPS Status Indicators

CPT © 2015 American Medical Association. All Rights Reserved.　　© 2016 DecisionHealth

● 39401 **Mediastinoscopy; includes biopsy(ies) of mediastinal mass (eg, lymphoma), when performed** Ⓣ

RVU			Global Days	Modifiers				
Mod	Non-Fac Total	Fac Total		51	50	62	80	MUE
	9.10	9.10	000	2	0	0	1	1

● 39402 **Mediastinoscopy; with lymph node biopsy(ies) (eg, lung cancer staging)** Ⓣ

RVU			Global Days	Modifiers				
Mod	Non-Fac Total	Fac Total		51	50	62	80	MUE
	11.87	11.87	000	2	0	0	1	1

Other Mediastinum Procedures

39499 **Unlisted procedure, mediastinum** ⓍⒸ

RVU			Global Days	Modifiers				
Mod	Non-Fac Total	Fac Total		51	50	62	80	MUE
	0.00	0.00	YYY	2	0	1	2	

Diaphragm

Diaphragm Repair Procedures

39501 **Repair, laceration of diaphragm, any approach** Ⓒ

RVU			Global Days	Modifiers				
Mod	Non-Fac Total	Fac Total		51	50	62	80	MUE
	24.58	24.58	090	2	0	1	2	1

AMA: Nov 00: 3, Dec 14: 16

39503 **Repair, neonatal diaphragmatic hernia, with or without chest tube insertion and with or without creation of ventral hernia** Ⓐ⊖Ⓒ

RVU			Global Days	Modifiers				
Mod	Non-Fac Total	Fac Total		51	50	62	80	MUE
	178.97	178.97	090	2	0	1	2	1

AMA: Feb 12: 3

Neonatal diaphragmatic hernia repair

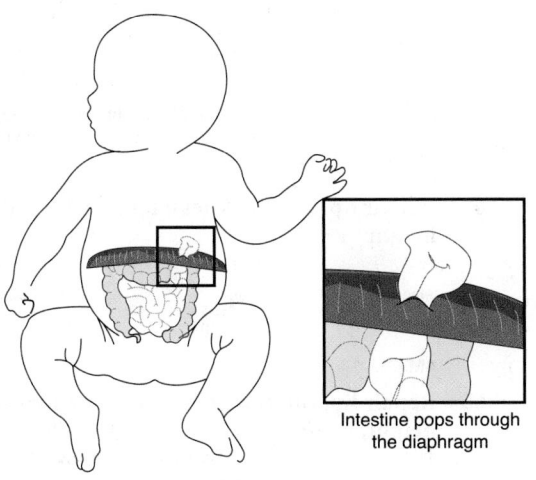

Intestine pops through the diaphragm

Abdominal contents are returned to their normal position and the defect is repaired.

39540 **Repair, diaphragmatic hernia (other than neonatal), traumatic; acute** Ⓒ

RVU			Global Days	Modifiers				
Mod	Non-Fac Total	Fac Total		51	50	62	80	MUE
	25.12	25.12	090	2	0	1	2	1

AMA: Nov 00: 9, Jun 08: 3

39541 **Repair, diaphragmatic hernia (other than neonatal), traumatic; chronic** Ⓒ

RVU			Global Days	Modifiers				
Mod	Non-Fac Total	Fac Total		51	50	62	80	MUE
	27.40	27.40	090	2	0	1	2	1

39545 **Imbrication of diaphragm for eventration, transthoracic or transabdominal, paralytic or nonparalytic** Ⓒ

RVU			Global Days	Modifiers				
Mod	Non-Fac Total	Fac Total		51	50	62	80	MUE
	26.04	26.04	090	2	0	1	2	1

AMA: Nov 00: 3

39560 **Resection, diaphragm; with simple repair (eg, primary suture)** Ⓒ

RVU			Global Days	Modifiers				
Mod	Non-Fac Total	Fac Total		51	50	62	80	MUE
	23.09	23.09	090	2	0	1	2	1

AMA: Nov 99: 21, Nov 00: 3

39561 **Resection, diaphragm; with complex repair (eg, prosthetic material, local muscle flap)** Ⓒ

RVU			Global Days	Modifiers				
Mod	Non-Fac Total	Fac Total		51	50	62	80	MUE
	36.07	36.07	090	2	0	1	2	1

AMA: Nov 99: 21, Nov 00: 3

Other Diaphragm Procedures

39599 **Unlisted procedure, diaphragm** ⓍⒸ

RVU			Global Days	Modifiers				
Mod	Non-Fac Total	Fac Total		51	50	62	80	MUE
	0.00	0.00	YYY	2	0	1	2	

● New   ▲ Revised   Deleted   ⊙ Moderate Sedation   ✚ Add-on Codes   ⊘ High Risk Denial   Ⓐ Age Edit   ♀ Female   ♂ Male   **AMA** *CPT® Assistant*   **MUE** Medically Unlikely Edit
⊘ Modifier 51 Exempt   ⊖ Modifier 63 Exempt   Ⓧ Unlisted   **Modifiers:** *See Inside Back Cover*   Ⓜ Maternity   Ⓐ2–Ⓩ3 ASC Payment Indicators   Ⓐ–Ⓨ OPPS Status Indicators

© 2016 DecisionHealth   CPT © 2015 American Medical Association. All Rights Reserved.   **411**

Digestive System Procedures

Digestive system services follow the alimentary tract and begin with procedures on the lips, mouth, tongue, and teeth and also include the salivary glands and ducts, tonsils, adenoids, pharynx, esophagus as well as the stomach and intestines. The different types of services are broadly determined by approach, whether open, endoscopic, or laparoscopic.

Procedures on other organs necessary to the digestive process, such as the liver, gallbladder, bile ducts, and pancreas, are also included along with related transplantation services. Codes for the abdomen, peritoneum, and omentum are generally organized by open or laparoscopic method and include hernia repairs, categorized by the type of hernia, age of the patient, and initial or recurrent status.

Lip Procedures

Excisional Lip Procedures

40490 Biopsy of lip   P 3 T

Coding tip: Biopsy of vestibule of mouth - 40808

Coding tip: Code 99000 for specimen transfer from office setting to an outside laboratory

RVU			Global Days	Modifiers				
Mod	Non-Fac Total	Fac Total		51	50	62	80	MUE
	3.69	2.12	000	2	0	0	1	3

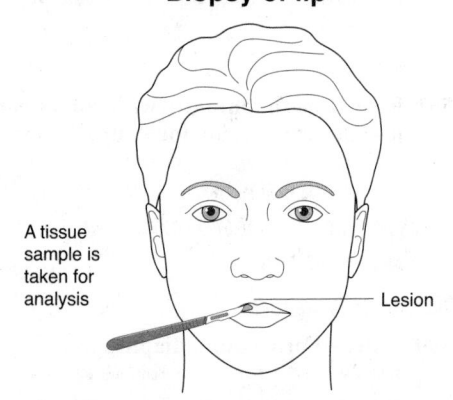

Biopsy of lip

A tissue sample is taken for analysis — Lesion

40500 Vermilionectomy (lip shave), with mucosal advancement   A 2 T

Coding tip: Other procedures on lesions of the lips - 11310-11313, 11440-11446, 11640-11646, 17280-17286

RVU			Global Days	Modifiers				
Mod	Non-Fac Total	Fac Total		51	50	62	80	MUE
	14.66	10.62	090	2	0	0	1	2

40510 Excision of lip; transverse wedge excision with primary closure   A 2 T

RVU			Global Days	Modifiers				
Mod	Non-Fac Total	Fac Total		51	50	62	80	MUE
	14.06	10.41	090	2	0	0	1	2

40520 Excision of lip; V-excision with primary direct linear closure   A 2 T

RVU			Global Days	Modifiers				
Mod	Non-Fac Total	Fac Total		51	50	62	80	MUE
	14.22	10.48	090	2	0	0	1	2

40525 Excision of lip; full thickness, reconstruction with local flap (eg, Estlander or fan)   A 2 T

RVU			Global Days	Modifiers				
Mod	Non-Fac Total	Fac Total		51	50	62	80	MUE
	16.12	16.12	090	2	0	0	1	2

40527 Excision of lip; full thickness, reconstruction with cross lip flap (Abbe-Estlander)   A 2 J 1

RVU			Global Days	Modifiers				
Mod	Non-Fac Total	Fac Total		51	50	62	80	MUE
	17.97	17.97	090	2	0	0	0	2

40530 Resection of lip, more than one-fourth, without reconstruction   A 2 T

RVU			Global Days	Modifiers				
Mod	Non-Fac Total	Fac Total		51	50	62	80	MUE
	15.68	11.78	090	2	0	0	1	2

Lip Repair

40650 Repair lip, full thickness; vermilion only   A 2 T

RVU			Global Days	Modifiers				
Mod	Non-Fac Total	Fac Total		51	50	62	80	MUE
	12.78	8.70	090	2	0	0	0	2

AMA: Jul 00: 10

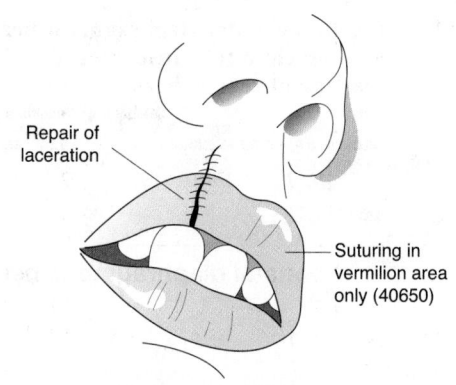

Lip repair, full thickness

Repair of laceration

Suturing in vermilion area only (40650)

Up to half vertical height of lip (40652)
Over one half vertical height of lip (complex) (40654)

40652 Repair lip, full thickness; up to half vertical height   A 2 T

RVU			Global Days	Modifiers				
Mod	Non-Fac Total	Fac Total		51	50	62	80	MUE
	14.15	10.27	090	2	0	0	0	2

AMA: Jul 00: 10

40654 Repair lip, full thickness; over one-half vertical height, or complex   A 2 T

RVU			Global Days	Modifiers				
Mod	Non-Fac Total	Fac Total		51	50	62	80	MUE
	16.59	12.45	090	2	0	0	1	2

● New   ▲ Revised   ✖ Deleted   ⊙ Moderate Sedation   ✚ Add-on Codes   ⊘ High Risk Denial   Ⓐ Age Edit   ♀ Female   ♂ Male   **AMA** *CPT® Assistant*   **MUE** Medically Unlikely Edit

⊘ Modifier 51 Exempt   ⊖ Modifier 63 Exempt   ✖ Unlisted   **Modifiers:** *See Inside Back Cover*   Ⓜ Maternity   A 2 – Z 3 ASC Payment Indicators   A – Y OPPS Status Indicators

412   CPT © 2015 American Medical Association. All Rights Reserved.   © 2016 DecisionHealth

40700 Plastic repair of cleft lip/nasal deformity; primary, partial or complete, unilateral `A 2 J 1`

RVU			Global Days	Modifiers				
Mod	Non-Fac Total	Fac Total		51	50	62	80	MUE
	26.28	26.28	090	2	0	0	0	1

AMA: Dec 14: 18

Plastic repair of cleft lip/nasal deformity; primary, partial or complete, unilateral

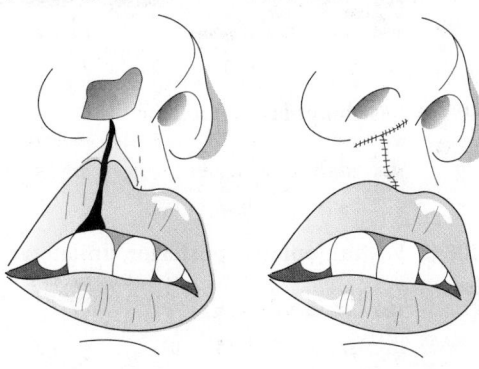

Unilateral cleft margins are incised

Incisions are closed in layers, correcting deformity

40701 Plastic repair of cleft lip/nasal deformity; primary bilateral, 1-stage procedure `⊙ A 2 J 1`

RVU			Global Days	Modifiers				
Mod	Non-Fac Total	Fac Total		51	50	62	80	MUE
	29.46	29.46	090	2	2	0	2	1

40702 Plastic repair of cleft lip/nasal deformity; primary bilateral, 1 of 2 stages `⊙ R 2 J 1`

RVU			Global Days	Modifiers				
Mod	Non-Fac Total	Fac Total		51	50	62	80	MUE
	24.70	24.70	090	2	2	0	2	1

40720 Plastic repair of cleft lip/nasal deformity; secondary, by recreation of defect and reclosure `A 2 J 1`

RVU			Global Days	Modifiers				
Mod	Non-Fac Total	Fac Total		51	50	62	80	MUE
	29.90	29.90	090	2	1	0	0	1

AMA: Dec 14: 18

40761 Plastic repair of cleft lip/nasal deformity; with cross lip pedicle flap (Abbe-Estlander type), including sectioning and inserting of pedicle `A 2 J 1`

RVU			Global Days	Modifiers				
Mod	Non-Fac Total	Fac Total		51	50	62	80	MUE
	31.64	31.64	090	2	0	0	1	1

Other Lip Procedures

40799 Unlisted procedure, lips `⊘ x T`

RVU			Global Days	Modifiers				
Mod	Non-Fac Total	Fac Total		51	50	62	80	MUE
	0.00	0.00	YYY	2	0	1	2	

Mouth - Vestibule Procedures

Incisional Vestibule of Mouth Procedures

40800 Drainage of abscess, cyst, hematoma, vestibule of mouth; simple `P 2 T`

Coding tip: Drainage of skin or subcutaneous abscess/cyst - 10060; hematoma or seroma - 10140

RVU			Global Days	Modifiers				
Mod	Non-Fac Total	Fac Total		51	50	62	80	MUE
	6.23	3.88	010	2	0	0	1	2

40801 Drainage of abscess, cyst, hematoma, vestibule of mouth; complicated `A 2 T`

RVU			Global Days	Modifiers				
Mod	Non-Fac Total	Fac Total		51	50	62	80	MUE
	9.27	6.57	010	2	0	0	1	2

40804 Removal of embedded foreign body, vestibule of mouth; simple `N 1 Q 1`

RVU			Global Days	Modifiers				
Mod	Non-Fac Total	Fac Total		51	50	62	80	MUE
	5.57	3.44	010	2	0	0	0	2

Removal of embedded foreign body, vestibule of mouth

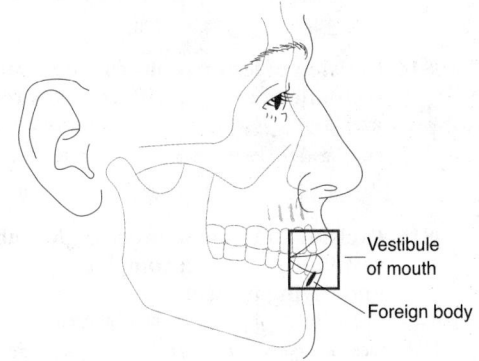

Vestibule of mouth

Foreign body

A foreign body is removed from the area between the opening of the mouth and the teeth. Simple (40804), Complex (40805)

40805 Removal of embedded foreign body, vestibule of mouth; complicated `P 3 T`

Coding tip: Any necessary closure is included

RVU			Global Days	Modifiers				
Mod	Non-Fac Total	Fac Total		51	50	62	80	MUE
	10.66	6.50	010	2	0	0	0	2

40806 Incision of labial frenum (frenotomy) `P 3 T`

Coding tip: Frenoplasty - 41520

RVU			Global Days	Modifiers				
Mod	Non-Fac Total	Fac Total		51	50	62	80	MUE
	3.27	0.94	000	2	0	0	0	2

Surgical Procedures

40808 – 40899

Excisional/Destruction Vestibule of Mouth Procedures

40808 Biopsy, vestibule of mouth   `P 3 T`

Coding tip: Code 99000 for specimen transfer from office setting to an outside laboratory

Coding tip: Biopsy of lip - 40490

Coding tip: Do not report separately if done as part of another more complex procedure, such as lesion excision

RVU			Global Days	Modifiers				
Mod	Non-Fac Total	Fac Total		51	50	62	80	MUE
	5.47	3.20	010	2	0	0	1	4

40810 Excision of lesion of mucosa and submucosa, vestibule of mouth; without repair   `P 3 T`

Coding tip: Local anesthesia is included

RVU			Global Days	Modifiers				
Mod	Non-Fac Total	Fac Total		51	50	62	80	MUE
	6.04	3.77	010	2	0	0	1	4

40812 Excision of lesion of mucosa and submucosa, vestibule of mouth; with simple repair   `P 3 T`

Coding tip: Local anesthesia is included

Coding tip: Chemical or electrical cauterization may be done as simple repair

RVU			Global Days	Modifiers				
Mod	Non-Fac Total	Fac Total		51	50	62	80	MUE
	8.48	5.84	010	2	0	0	1	4

40814 Excision of lesion of mucosa and submucosa, vestibule of mouth; with complex repair   `A 2 T`

RVU			Global Days	Modifiers				
Mod	Non-Fac Total	Fac Total		51	50	62	80	MUE
	11.32	9.03	090	2	0	0	1	4

40816 Excision of lesion of mucosa and submucosa, vestibule of mouth; complex, with excision of underlying muscle   `A 2 T`

RVU			Global Days	Modifiers				
Mod	Non-Fac Total	Fac Total		51	50	62	80	MUE
	11.82	9.36	090	2	0	0	1	2

40818 Excision of mucosa of vestibule of mouth as donor graft   `A 2 T`

RVU			Global Days	Modifiers				
Mod	Non-Fac Total	Fac Total		51	50	62	80	MUE
	10.48	8.02	090	2	0	0	0	2

40819 Excision of frenum, labial or buccal (frenumectomy, frenulectomy, frenectomy)   `A 2 T`

RVU			Global Days	Modifiers				
Mod	Non-Fac Total	Fac Total		51	50	62	80	MUE
	9.32	7.11	090	2	0	0	0	2

40820 Destruction of lesion or scar of vestibule of mouth by physical methods (eg, laser, thermal, cryo, chemical)   `P 3 T`

RVU			Global Days	Modifiers				
Mod	Non-Fac Total	Fac Total		51	50	62	80	MUE
	7.78	5.07	010	2	0	0	1	5

Vestibule of Mouth Repair

40830 Closure of laceration, vestibule of mouth; 2.5 cm or less   `G 2 T`

RVU			Global Days	Modifiers				
Mod	Non-Fac Total	Fac Total		51	50	62	80	MUE
	7.76	4.85	010	2	0	0	0	2

40831 Closure of laceration, vestibule of mouth; over 2.5 cm or complex   `A 2 T`

RVU			Global Days	Modifiers				
Mod	Non-Fac Total	Fac Total		51	50	62	80	MUE
	9.90	6.60	010	2	0	0	0	2

40840 Vestibuloplasty; anterior   `A 2 T`

RVU			Global Days	Modifiers				
Mod	Non-Fac Total	Fac Total		51	50	62	80	MUE
	23.75	18.46	090	2	0	0	2	1

40842 Vestibuloplasty; posterior, unilateral   `A 2 J I`

RVU			Global Days	Modifiers				
Mod	Non-Fac Total	Fac Total		51	50	62	80	MUE
	22.74	17.63	090	2	0	0	0	1

40843 Vestibuloplasty; posterior, bilateral   `A 2 T`

RVU			Global Days	Modifiers				
Mod	Non-Fac Total	Fac Total		51	50	62	80	MUE
	31.64	24.94	090	2	2	0	2	1

40844 Vestibuloplasty; entire arch   `⊘ A 2 J I`

RVU			Global Days	Modifiers				
Mod	Non-Fac Total	Fac Total		51	50	62	80	MUE
	37.89	30.68	090	2	0	0	2	1

40845 Vestibuloplasty; complex (including ridge extension, muscle repositioning)   `A 2 J I`

RVU			Global Days	Modifiers				
Mod	Non-Fac Total	Fac Total		51	50	62	80	MUE
	42.67	35.90	090	2	0	0	0	1

Vestibuloplasty; complex

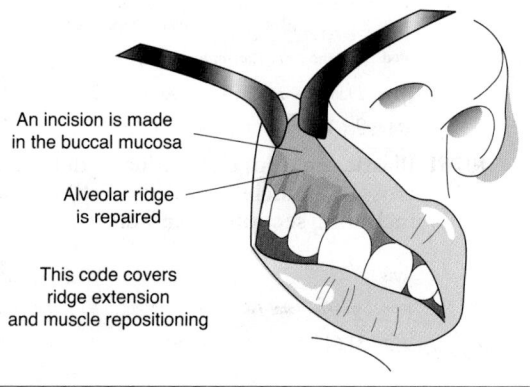

An incision is made in the buccal mucosa

Alveolar ridge is repaired

This code covers ridge extension and muscle repositioning

Other Vestibule of Mouth Procedures

40899 Unlisted procedure, vestibule of mouth   `⊘ x T`

RVU			Global Days	Modifiers				
Mod	Non-Fac Total	Fac Total		51	50	62	80	MUE
	0.00	0.00	YYY	2	0	1	0	

● New   ▲ Revised   ✖ Deleted   ⊙ Moderate Sedation   ✚ Add-on Codes   ⊘ High Risk Denial   ⒶAge Edit   ♀ Female   ♂ Male   **AMA** *CPT® Assistant*   **MUE** Medically Unlikely Edit

⦸ Modifier 51 Exempt   ⊖ Modifier 63 Exempt   ✗ Unlisted   **Modifiers:** *See Inside Back Cover*   Ⓜ Maternity   `A 2`–`Z 3` ASC Payment Indicators   `A`–`Y` OPPS Status Indicators

CPT © 2015 American Medical Association. All Rights Reserved.   © 2016 DecisionHealth

Tongue/Floor of Mouth Procedures

Incisional Tongue/Floor of Mouth Procedures

41000 Intraoral incision and drainage of abscess, cyst, or hematoma of tongue or floor of mouth; lingual   P 3 T

Coding tip: Drainage of abscess/cyst/hematoma of vestibule of mouth - 40800, 40801

Mod	Non-Fac Total	Fac Total	Global Days	51	50	62	80	MUE
	4.75	3.31	010	2	0	0	1	2

41005 Intraoral incision and drainage of abscess, cyst, or hematoma of tongue or floor of mouth; sublingual, superficial   A 2 T

Mod	Non-Fac Total	Fac Total	Global Days	51	50	62	80	MUE
	6.64	3.68	010	2	0	0	0	2

41006 Intraoral incision and drainage of abscess, cyst, or hematoma of tongue or floor of mouth; sublingual, deep, supramylohyoid   A 2 T

Mod	Non-Fac Total	Fac Total	Global Days	51	50	62	80	MUE
	10.46	7.39	090	2	0	0	0	2

41007 Intraoral incision and drainage of abscess, cyst, or hematoma of tongue or floor of mouth; submental space   A 2 T

Mod	Non-Fac Total	Fac Total	Global Days	51	50	62	80	MUE
	10.22	7.12	090	2	0	0	0	2

41008 Intraoral incision and drainage of abscess, cyst, or hematoma of tongue or floor of mouth; submandibular space   A 2 T

Mod	Non-Fac Total	Fac Total	Global Days	51	50	62	80	MUE
	11.13	7.97	090	2	0	0	0	2

41009 Intraoral incision and drainage of abscess, cyst, or hematoma of tongue or floor of mouth; masticator space   A 2 T

Mod	Non-Fac Total	Fac Total	Global Days	51	50	62	80	MUE
	11.82	8.64	090	2	0	0	0	2

41010 Incision of lingual frenum (frenotomy)   A 2 T

Mod	Non-Fac Total	Fac Total	Global Days	51	50	62	80	MUE
	5.91	3.18	010	2	0	0	0	1

41015 Extraoral incision and drainage of abscess, cyst, or hematoma of floor of mouth; sublingual   A 2 T

Mod	Non-Fac Total	Fac Total	Global Days	51	50	62	80	MUE
	13.34	10.39	090	2	0	0	0	2

41016 Extraoral incision and drainage of abscess, cyst, or hematoma of floor of mouth; submental   A 2 T

Mod	Non-Fac Total	Fac Total	Global Days	51	50	62	80	MUE
	12.96	10.40	090	2	0	0	0	2

41017 Extraoral incision and drainage of abscess, cyst, or hematoma of floor of mouth; submandibular   A 2 T

Mod	Non-Fac Total	Fac Total	Global Days	51	50	62	80	MUE
	13.09	10.47	090	2	0	0	0	2

41018 Extraoral incision and drainage of abscess, cyst, or hematoma of floor of mouth; masticator space   A 2 T

Mod	Non-Fac Total	Fac Total	Global Days	51	50	62	80	MUE
	14.91	12.24	090	2	0	0	0	2

41019 Placement of needles, catheters, or other device(s) into the head and/or neck region (percutaneous, transoral, or transnasal) for subsequent interstitial radioelement application   G 2 T

Coding tip: Report an additional code when correct placement of the needles or catheters requires radiological guidance - ultrasound 76942; fluoroscopy 77002; CT 77012; MRI 77021

Mod	Non-Fac Total	Fac Total	Global Days	51	50	62	80	MUE
	13.52	13.52	000	2	0	1	0	1

Excisional Tongue/Floor of Mouth Procedures

41100 Biopsy of tongue; anterior two-thirds   P 3 T

Mod	Non-Fac Total	Fac Total	Global Days	51	50	62	80	MUE
	4.91	3.17	010	2	0	0	1	3

41105 Biopsy of tongue; posterior one-third   P 3 T

Mod	Non-Fac Total	Fac Total	Global Days	51	50	62	80	MUE
	5.00	3.29	010	2	0	0	1	3

41108 Biopsy of floor of mouth   P 3 T

Mod	Non-Fac Total	Fac Total	Global Days	51	50	62	80	MUE
	4.32	2.66	010	2	0	0	1	2

41110 Excision of lesion of tongue without closure   P 3 T

Mod	Non-Fac Total	Fac Total	Global Days	51	50	62	80	MUE
	6.20	3.87	010	2	0	0	1	2

41112 Excision of lesion of tongue with closure; anterior two-thirds   A 2 T

Mod	Non-Fac Total	Fac Total	Global Days	51	50	62	80	MUE
	9.83	7.47	090	2	0	0	1	2

41113 Excision of lesion of tongue with closure; posterior one-third   A 2 T

Mod	Non-Fac Total	Fac Total	Global Days	51	50	62	80	MUE
	10.76	8.28	090	2	0	0	1	2

41114 Excision of lesion of tongue with closure; with local tongue flap   A 2 T

Mod	Non-Fac Total	Fac Total	Global Days	51	50	62	80	MUE
	18.67	18.67	090	2	0	0	0	2

● New   ▲ Revised   Deleted   ⊙ Moderate Sedation   ✚ Add-on Codes   ⊘ High Risk Denial   Ⓐ Age Edit   ♀ Female   ♂ Male   **AMA** *CPT® Assistant*   **MUE** Medically Unlikely Edit

⊘ Modifier 51 Exempt   ⊖ Modifier 63 Exempt   ✗ Unlisted   **Modifiers:** *See Inside Back Cover*   Ⓜ Maternity   A 2 – Z 3 ASC Payment Indicators   A – Y OPPS Status Indicators

© 2016 DecisionHealth   CPT © 2015 American Medical Association. All Rights Reserved.

41115 Excision of lingual frenum (frenectomy) `P 3 T`

RVU			Global Days	Modifiers				
Mod	Non-Fac Total	Fac Total		51	50	62	80	MUE
	7.26	4.50	010	2	0	0	0	1

41116 Excision, lesion of floor of mouth `A 2 T`

RVU			Global Days	Modifiers				
Mod	Non-Fac Total	Fac Total		51	50	62	80	MUE
	9.73	6.50	090	2	0	0	1	2

41120 Glossectomy; less than one-half tongue `A 2 J I`

RVU			Global Days	Modifiers				
Mod	Non-Fac Total	Fac Total		51	50	62	80	MUE
	31.82	31.82	090	2	0	1	2	1

AMA: Aug 10: 10

41130 Glossectomy; hemiglossectomy `C`

RVU			Global Days	Modifiers				
Mod	Non-Fac Total	Fac Total		51	50	62	80	MUE
	39.15	39.15	090	2	0	1	2	1

AMA: Aug 10: 5

41135 Glossectomy; partial, with unilateral radical neck dissection `C`

RVU			Global Days	Modifiers				
Mod	Non-Fac Total	Fac Total		51	50	62	80	MUE
	64.15	64.15	090	2	0	1	2	1

AMA: Aug 10: 5

41140 Glossectomy; complete or total, with or without tracheostomy, without radical neck dissection `C`

RVU			Global Days	Modifiers				
Mod	Non-Fac Total	Fac Total		51	50	62	80	MUE
	64.70	64.70	090	2	0	1	2	1

AMA: Aug 10: 5

41145 Glossectomy; complete or total, with or without tracheostomy, with unilateral radical neck dissection `C`

RVU			Global Days	Modifiers				
Mod	Non-Fac Total	Fac Total		51	50	62	80	MUE
	82.22	82.22	090	2	0	1	2	1

AMA: Aug 10: 5

41150 Glossectomy; composite procedure with resection floor of mouth and mandibular resection, without radical neck dissection `C`

RVU			Global Days	Modifiers				
Mod	Non-Fac Total	Fac Total		51	50	62	80	MUE
	65.11	65.11	090	2	0	1	2	1

AMA: Aug 10: 5

41153 Glossectomy; composite procedure with resection floor of mouth, with suprahyoid neck dissection `C`

RVU			Global Days	Modifiers				
Mod	Non-Fac Total	Fac Total		51	50	62	80	MUE
	70.95	70.95	090	2	0	1	2	1

AMA: Aug 10: 3

41155 Glossectomy; composite procedure with resection floor of mouth, mandibular resection, and radical neck dissection (Commando type) `C`

RVU			Global Days	Modifiers				
Mod	Non-Fac Total	Fac Total		51	50	62	80	MUE
	88.93	88.93	090	2	0	1	2	1

AMA: Jan 01: 13, Aug 10: 3

Tongue/Floor of Mouth Repair

41250 Repair of laceration 2.5 cm or less; floor of mouth and/or anterior two-thirds of tongue `N I Q I`

Coding tip: Repair of laceration of vestibule of mouth - 40830-40831

RVU			Global Days	Modifiers				
Mod	Non-Fac Total	Fac Total		51	50	62	80	MUE
	7.78	4.49	010	2	0	0	0	2

41251 Repair of laceration 2.5 cm or less; posterior one-third of tongue `A 2 T`

RVU			Global Days	Modifiers				
Mod	Non-Fac Total	Fac Total		51	50	62	80	MUE
	8.48	5.33	010	2	0	0	0	2

41252 Repair of laceration of tongue, floor of mouth, over 2.6 cm or complex `A 2 T`

Coding tip: Repair of laceration of palate - 42180-42182

RVU			Global Days	Modifiers				
Mod	Non-Fac Total	Fac Total		51	50	62	80	MUE
	9.20	6.15	010	2	0	0	0	2

Other Tongue/Floor of Mouth Procedures

41500 Fixation of tongue, mechanical, other than suture (eg, K-wire) `A 2 T`

RVU			Global Days	Modifiers				
Mod	Non-Fac Total	Fac Total		51	50	62	80	MUE
	12.09	12.09	090	2	0	0	0	1

AMA: Aug 10: 11

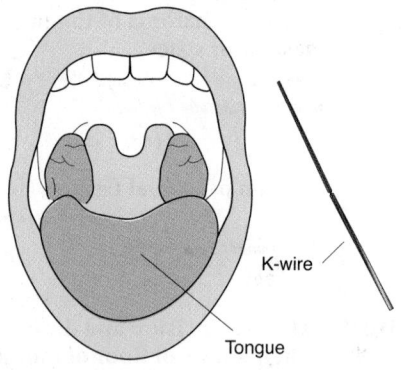

Mechanical fixation of tongue

K-wire

Tongue

A device is placed inside the mouth to immobilize the tongue

41510 Suture of tongue to lip for micrognathia (Douglas type procedure) `A 2 T`

RVU			Global Days	Modifiers				
Mod	Non-Fac Total	Fac Total		51	50	62	80	MUE
	12.38	12.38	090	2	0	0	0	1

AMA: Aug 10: 11

41512 Tongue base suspension, permanent suture technique `G 2 J I`

RVU			Global Days	Modifiers				
Mod	Non-Fac Total	Fac Total		51	50	62	80	MUE
	19.50	19.50	090	2	0	0	0	1

AMA: Aug 10: 11, Aug 12: 13

41520 Frenoplasty (surgical revision of frenum, eg, with Z-plasty) `A 2 J I`

RVU			Global Days	Modifiers				
Mod	Non-Fac Total	Fac Total		51	50	62	80	MUE
	10.39	7.63	090	2	0	0	0	1

41530 Submucosal ablation of the tongue base, radiofrequency, 1 or more sites, per session `R 2 T`

RVU			Global Days	Modifiers				
Mod	Non-Fac Total	Fac Total		51	50	62	80	MUE
	28.65	11.05	000	2	0	0	0	1

AMA: Aug 10: 10

41599 Unlisted procedure, tongue, floor of mouth `X T`

RVU			Global Days	Modifiers				
Mod	Non-Fac Total	Fac Total		51	50	62	80	MUE
	0.00	0.00	YYY	2	0	1	0	

AMA: Dec 00: 14

Dentoalveolar Procedures

Incisional Dentoalveolar Procedures

41800 Drainage of abscess, cyst, hematoma from dentoalveolar structures `C N I Q I`

RVU			Global Days	Modifiers				
Mod	Non-Fac Total	Fac Total		51	50	62	80	MUE
	7.93	4.31	010	2	0	0	1	2

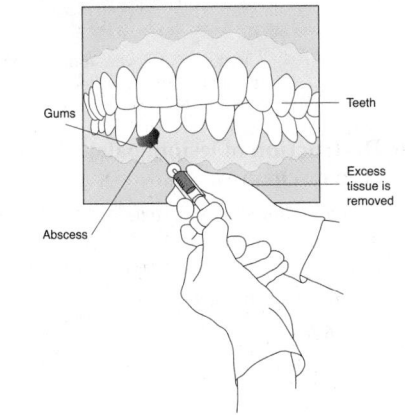

Drainage of abscess, cyst, hematoma from dentoalveolar structures

Gums

Teeth

Excess tissue is removed

Abscess

Fluid is drained from a lesion or abscess located on the gums

41805 Removal of embedded foreign body from dentoalveolar structures; soft tissues `P 3 T`

RVU			Global Days	Modifiers				
Mod	Non-Fac Total	Fac Total		51	50	62	80	MUE
	7.58	5.16	010	2	0	0	0	3

41806 Removal of embedded foreign body from dentoalveolar structures; bone `C P 3 T`

RVU			Global Days	Modifiers				
Mod	Non-Fac Total	Fac Total		51	50	62	80	MUE
	10.42	7.71	010	2	0	0	0	3

Excisional/Destruction Dentoalveolar Procedures

41820 Gingivectomy, excision gingiva, each quadrant `C R 2 T`

RVU			Global Days	Modifiers				
Mod	Non-Fac Total	Fac Total		51	50	62	80	MUE
	0.00	0.00	000	2	0	0	0	4

41821 Operculectomy, excision pericoronal tissues `C G 2 T`

RVU			Global Days	Modifiers				
Mod	Non-Fac Total	Fac Total		51	50	62	80	MUE
	0.00	0.00	000	2	0	0	0	2

41822 Excision of fibrous tuberosities, dentoalveolar structures `C P 3 T`

RVU			Global Days	Modifiers				
Mod	Non-Fac Total	Fac Total		51	50	62	80	MUE
	8.62	5.40	010	2	0	0	0	1

41823 Excision of osseous tuberosities, dentoalveolar structures `C P 3 J I`

RVU			Global Days	Modifiers				
Mod	Non-Fac Total	Fac Total		51	50	62	80	MUE
	12.59	9.58	090	2	0	0	0	1

41825 Excision of lesion or tumor (except listed above), dentoalveolar structures; without repair `P 3 T`

RVU			Global Days	Modifiers				
Mod	Non-Fac Total	Fac Total		51	50	62	80	MUE
	6.23	3.63	010	2	0	0	1	2

41826 Excision of lesion or tumor (except listed above), dentoalveolar structures; with simple repair `P 3 T`

Coding tip: Chemical or electrical cauterization may be done as a simple repair

RVU			Global Days	Modifiers				
Mod	Non-Fac Total	Fac Total		51	50	62	80	MUE
	9.29	6.31	010	2	0	0	1	2

41827 Excision of lesion or tumor (except listed above), dentoalveolar structures; with complex repair `A 2 J I`

RVU			Global Days	Modifiers				
Mod	Non-Fac Total	Fac Total		51	50	62	80	MUE
	12.98	9.11	090	2	0	0	1	2

41828 Excision of hyperplastic alveolar mucosa, each quadrant (specify) `C P 3 T`

RVU			Global Days	Modifiers				
Mod	Non-Fac Total	Fac Total		51	50	62	80	MUE
	9.09	6.29	010	2	0	0	0	4

41830 Alveolectomy, including curettage of osteitis or sequestrectomy `C P 3 T`

RVU			Global Days	Modifiers				
Mod	Non-Fac Total	Fac Total		51	50	62	80	MUE
	11.60	8.45	010	2	0	0	0	2

● New ▲ Revised Deleted ⊙ Moderate Sedation ✚ Add-on Codes ⊘ High Risk Denial Ⓐ Age Edit ♀ Female ♂ Male **AMA** CPT® Assistant **MUE** Medically Unlikely Edit
⊘ Modifier 51 Exempt ⊖ Modifier 63 Exempt ✗ Unlisted **Modifiers:** See Inside Back Cover Ⓜ Maternity A2–Z3 ASC Payment Indicators A–Y OPPS Status Indicators

41850 Destruction of lesion (except excision), dentoalveolar structures `CR 2 T`

RVU			Global Days	Modifiers				
Mod	Non-Fac Total	Fac Total		51	50	62	80	MUE
	0.00	0.00	000	2	0	0	0	2

Other Dentoalveolar Procedures

41870 Periodontal mucosal grafting `CG 2 J I`

RVU			Global Days	Modifiers				
Mod	Non-Fac Total	Fac Total		51	50	62	80	MUE
	0.00	0.00	000	2	0	0	0	2

41872 Gingivoplasty, each quadrant (specify) `CP 3 J I`

RVU			Global Days	Modifiers				
Mod	Non-Fac Total	Fac Total		51	50	62	80	MUE
	10.77	7.60	090	2	0	0	0	4

41874 Alveoloplasty, each quadrant (specify) `CP 3 T`

RVU			Global Days	Modifiers				
Mod	Non-Fac Total	Fac Total		51	50	62	80	MUE
	11.10	7.60	090	2	0	0	0	4

41899 Unlisted procedure, dentoalveolar structures `x T`

RVU			Global Days	Modifiers				
Mod	Non-Fac Total	Fac Total		51	50	62	80	MUE
	0.00	0.00	YYY	2	0	1	0	

Palate/Uvula Procedures

Incisional Palate/Uvula Procedures

42000 Drainage of abscess of palate, uvula `A 2 T`

Coding tip: Drainage of abscess of tongue or lingual floor of mouth - 41000

RVU			Global Days	Modifiers				
Mod	Non-Fac Total	Fac Total		51	50	62	80	MUE
	4.64	3.05	010	2	0	0	0	1

Excisional Palate/Uvula Procedures

42100 Biopsy of palate, uvula `P 3 T`

Coding tip: Do not report separately if done as part of another more complex procedure, such as lesion excision

Coding tip: Code 99000 for specimen transfer from office setting to an outside laboratory

RVU			Global Days	Modifiers				
Mod	Non-Fac Total	Fac Total		51	50	62	80	MUE
	4.39	3.23	010	2	0	0	1	3

42104 Excision, lesion of palate, uvula; without closure `P 3 T`

RVU			Global Days	Modifiers				
Mod	Non-Fac Total	Fac Total		51	50	62	80	MUE
	6.31	4.10	010	2	0	0	1	3

42106 Excision, lesion of palate, uvula; with simple primary closure `P 3 T`

Coding tip: Chemical or electrical cauterization may be done as a simple repair

RVU			Global Days	Modifiers				
Mod	Non-Fac Total	Fac Total		51	50	62	80	MUE
	8.05	5.28	010	2	0	0	1	2

42107 Excision, lesion of palate, uvula; with local flap closure `A 2 J I`

RVU			Global Days	Modifiers				
Mod	Non-Fac Total	Fac Total		51	50	62	80	MUE
	13.55	10.23	090	2	0	0	1	2

42120 Resection of palate or extensive resection of lesion `A 2 T`

RVU			Global Days	Modifiers				
Mod	Non-Fac Total	Fac Total		51	50	62	80	MUE
	29.99	29.99	090	2	0	1	2	1

42140 Uvulectomy, excision of uvula `A 2 T`

RVU			Global Days	Modifiers				
Mod	Non-Fac Total	Fac Total		51	50	62	80	MUE
	7.38	4.53	090	2	0	0	1	1

42145 Palatopharyngoplasty (eg, uvulopalatopharyngoplasty, uvulopharyngoplasty) `A 2 J I`

RVU			Global Days	Modifiers				
Mod	Non-Fac Total	Fac Total		51	50	62	80	MUE
	20.55	20.55	090	2	0	0	1	1

AMA: Dec 04: 19

Palatopharyngoplasty

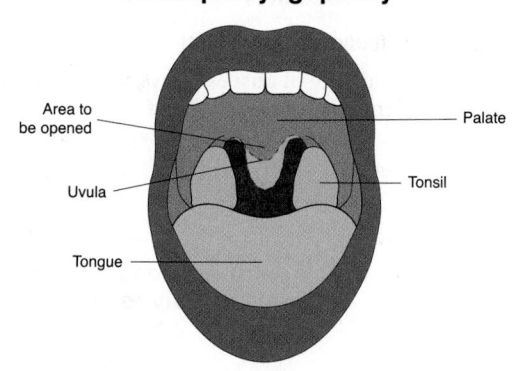

Tissue is removed from the top of the throat to create a wider airway opening

42160 Destruction of lesion, palate or uvula (thermal, cryo or chemical) `P 3 T`

Coding tip: Use an office visit code for initiation/follow-up of topical chemotherapy agents

RVU			Global Days	Modifiers				
Mod	Non-Fac Total	Fac Total		51	50	62	80	MUE
	6.78	4.32	010	2	0	0	0	2

AMA: Apr 10: 10

● New   ▲ Revised   ✖ Deleted   ⊙ Moderate Sedation   ✚ Add-on Codes   ⊘ High Risk Denial   Ⓐ Age Edit   ♀ Female   ♂ Male   **AMA** *CPT® Assistant*   **MUE** Medically Unlikely Edit

⊘ Modifier 51 Exempt   ⊖ Modifier 63 Exempt   ✗ Unlisted   **Modifiers:** *See Inside Back Cover*   Ⓜ Maternity   `A 2`–`Z 3` ASC Payment Indicators   `A`–`Y` OPPS Status Indicators

CPT © 2015 American Medical Association. All Rights Reserved.   © 2016 DecisionHealth

Surgical Procedures

42180 – 42300

Palate/Uvula Repair

42180 Repair, laceration of palate; up to 2 cm   `A 2 T`

Coding tip: Repair of laceration of tongue/floor of mouth - 41250-41251

Coding tip: Repair of laceration of vestibule of mouth - 40830-40831

RVU			Global Days	Modifiers				
Mod	Non-Fac Total	Fac Total		51	50	62	80	MUE
	7.11	5.38	010	2	0	0	0	1

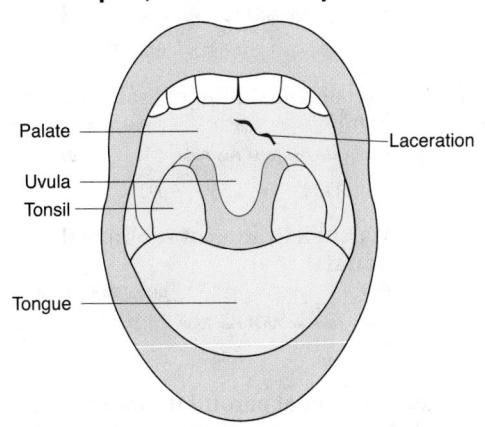

Repair, laceration of palate

A laceration located on the roof of the mouth is repaired, up to 2 cm use code (42180), over 2 cm use code (42182)

42182 Repair, laceration of palate; over 2 cm or complex   `A 2 T`

RVU			Global Days	Modifiers				
Mod	Non-Fac Total	Fac Total		51	50	62	80	MUE
	9.33	7.47	010	2	0	0	0	1

42200 Palatoplasty for cleft palate, soft and/or hard palate only   `A 2 J I`

RVU			Global Days	Modifiers				
Mod	Non-Fac Total	Fac Total		51	50	62	80	MUE
	24.86	24.86	090	2	0	0	2	1

AMA: Jul 14: 8, Mar 15: 9

42205 Palatoplasty for cleft palate, with closure of alveolar ridge; soft tissue only   `A 2 J I`

RVU			Global Days	Modifiers				
Mod	Non-Fac Total	Fac Total		51	50	62	80	MUE
	25.84	25.84	090	2	0	0	2	1

42210 Palatoplasty for cleft palate, with closure of alveolar ridge; with bone graft to alveolar ridge (includes obtaining graft)   `A 2 J I`

RVU			Global Days	Modifiers				
Mod	Non-Fac Total	Fac Total		51	50	62	80	MUE
	28.94	28.94	090	2	0	0	2	1

42215 Palatoplasty for cleft palate; major revision   `A 2 J I`

RVU			Global Days	Modifiers				
Mod	Non-Fac Total	Fac Total		51	50	62	80	MUE
	19.23	19.23	090	2	0	0	2	1

42220 Palatoplasty for cleft palate; secondary lengthening procedure   `A 2 J I`

RVU			Global Days	Modifiers				
Mod	Non-Fac Total	Fac Total		51	50	62	80	MUE
	14.51	14.51	090	2	0	0	2	1

42225 Palatoplasty for cleft palate; attachment pharyngeal flap   `G 2 J I`

RVU			Global Days	Modifiers				
Mod	Non-Fac Total	Fac Total		51	50	62	80	MUE
	25.64	25.64	090	2	0	0	2	1

42226 Lengthening of palate, and pharyngeal flap   `A 2 J I`

RVU			Global Days	Modifiers				
Mod	Non-Fac Total	Fac Total		51	50	62	80	MUE
	26.24	26.24	090	2	0	0	2	1

42227 Lengthening of palate, with island flap   `G 2 J I`

RVU			Global Days	Modifiers				
Mod	Non-Fac Total	Fac Total		51	50	62	80	MUE
	24.85	24.85	090	2	0	0	2	1

42235 Repair of anterior palate, including vomer flap   `A 2 J I`

RVU			Global Days	Modifiers				
Mod	Non-Fac Total	Fac Total		51	50	62	80	MUE
	21.44	21.44	090	2	0	0	2	1

AMA: Jul 14: 8, Mar 15: 9

42260 Repair of nasolabial fistula   `A 2 T`

RVU			Global Days	Modifiers				
Mod	Non-Fac Total	Fac Total		51	50	62	80	MUE
	23.76	19.42	090	2	0	0	2	1

42280 Maxillary impression for palatal prosthesis   `P 3 T`

RVU			Global Days	Modifiers				
Mod	Non-Fac Total	Fac Total		51	50	62	80	MUE
	4.85	3.25	010	2	0	0	0	1

42281 Insertion of pin-retained palatal prosthesis   `G 2 T`

RVU			Global Days	Modifiers				
Mod	Non-Fac Total	Fac Total		51	50	62	80	MUE
	5.97	4.42	010	2	0	0	0	1

Other Palate/Uvula Procedures

42299 Unlisted procedure, palate, uvula   `⊗ x T`

RVU			Global Days	Modifiers				
Mod	Non-Fac Total	Fac Total		51	50	62	80	MUE
	0.00	0.00	YYY	2	0	1	2	

AMA: Dec 04: 19, Apr 10: 10, Nov 10: 9, Jul 14: 8

Salivary Gland/Duct Procedures

Incisional Salivary Gland/Duct Procedures

42300 Drainage of abscess; parotid, simple   `A 2 T`

Coding tip: Drainage of abscess/cyst/hematoma of vestibule of mouth - 40800-40801

Coding tip: Intraoral drainage of abscess of tongue or lingual floor of mouth - 41000

Coding tip: Drainage of abscess of palate/uvula - 42000

RVU			Global Days	Modifiers				
Mod	Non-Fac Total	Fac Total		51	50	62	80	MUE
	6.10	4.47	010	2	0	0	1	2

● New   ▲ Revised   Deleted   ⊙ Moderate Sedation   ✚ Add-on Codes   ⊘ High Risk Denial   Ⓐ Age Edit   ♀ Female   ♂ Male   **AMA** CPT® Assistant   **MUE** Medically Unlikely Edit

⊘ Modifier 51 Exempt   ⊖ Modifier 63 Exempt   🗵 Unlisted   **Modifiers:** See Inside Back Cover   Ⓜ Maternity   `A 2`–`Z 3` ASC Payment Indicators   `A`–`Y` OPPS Status Indicators

Surgical Procedures

42305 Drainage of abscess; parotid, complicated `A 2 T`

RVU			Global Days	Modifiers				
Mod	Non-Fac Total	Fac Total		51	50	62	80	MUE
	12.60	12.60	090	2	0	0	0	2

42310 Drainage of abscess; submaxillary or sublingual, intraoral `A 2 T`

Coding tip: Drainage of abscess of palate/uvula - 42000

Coding tip: Intraoral drainage of abscess of tongue or lingual floor of mouth - 41000; sublingual - 41005-41006

Coding tip: Drainage of abscess/cyst/hematoma of vestibule of mouth - 40800-40801

RVU			Global Days	Modifiers				
Mod	Non-Fac Total	Fac Total		51	50	62	80	MUE
	4.68	3.62	010	2	0	0	0	2

Drainage of abscess; submaxillary or sublingual, intraoral/external

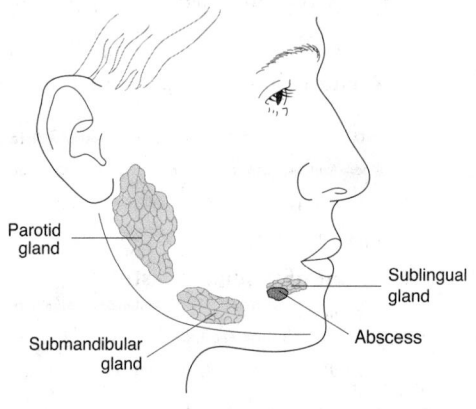

Parotid gland

Submandibular gland

Sublingual gland

Abscess

Fluid is drained from an abscess on the salivary gland intraorally (42310), or externally (42320)

42320 Drainage of abscess; submaxillary, external `A 2 T`

RVU			Global Days	Modifiers				
Mod	Non-Fac Total	Fac Total		51	50	62	80	MUE
	7.27	5.12	010	2	0	0	0	2

42330 Sialolithotomy; submandibular (submaxillary), sublingual or parotid, uncomplicated, intraoral `P 3 T`

RVU			Global Days	Modifiers				
Mod	Non-Fac Total	Fac Total		51	50	62	80	MUE
	6.77	4.82	010	2	0	0	1	2

42335 Sialolithotomy; submandibular (submaxillary), complicated, intraoral `P 3 T`

RVU			Global Days	Modifiers				
Mod	Non-Fac Total	Fac Total		51	50	62	80	MUE
	10.94	7.55	090	2	0	0	1	2

42340 Sialolithotomy; parotid, extraoral or complicated intraoral `A 2 T`

RVU			Global Days	Modifiers				
Mod	Non-Fac Total	Fac Total		51	50	62	80	MUE
	13.51	9.81	090	2	1	0	0	1

Excisional Salivary Gland/Duct Procedures

42400 Biopsy of salivary gland; needle `P 3 T`

Coding tip: Report an additional code for radiological needle guidance - ultrasound 76942, fluoroscopy 77002, CT 77012, MRI 77021

RVU			Global Days	Modifiers				
Mod	Non-Fac Total	Fac Total		51	50	62	80	MUE
	3.07	1.60	000	2	0	0	1	2

42405 Biopsy of salivary gland; incisional `A 2 T`

RVU			Global Days	Modifiers				
Mod	Non-Fac Total	Fac Total		51	50	62	80	MUE
	8.68	6.59	010	2	0	0	1	2

42408 Excision of sublingual salivary cyst (ranula) `A 2 T`

RVU			Global Days	Modifiers				
Mod	Non-Fac Total	Fac Total		51	50	62	80	MUE
	13.14	9.50	090	2	0	0	0	1

42409 Marsupialization of sublingual salivary cyst (ranula) `A 2 T`

RVU			Global Days	Modifiers				
Mod	Non-Fac Total	Fac Total		51	50	62	80	MUE
	9.68	6.46	090	2	0	0	2	1

42410 Excision of parotid tumor or parotid gland; lateral lobe, without nerve dissection `A 2 J 1`

RVU			Global Days	Modifiers				
Mod	Non-Fac Total	Fac Total		51	50	62	80	MUE
	18.12	18.12	090	2	1	1	2	1

42415 Excision of parotid tumor or parotid gland; lateral lobe, with dissection and preservation of facial nerve `A 2 J 1`

RVU			Global Days	Modifiers				
Mod	Non-Fac Total	Fac Total		51	50	62	80	MUE
	30.74	30.74	090	2	1	1	2	1

42420 Excision of parotid tumor or parotid gland; total, with dissection and preservation of facial nerve `A 2 J 1`

RVU			Global Days	Modifiers				
Mod	Non-Fac Total	Fac Total		51	50	62	80	MUE
	34.53	34.53	090	2	1	1	2	1

AMA: Aug 10: 4

42425 Excision of parotid tumor or parotid gland; total, en bloc removal with sacrifice of facial nerve `A 2 J 1`

RVU			Global Days	Modifiers				
Mod	Non-Fac Total	Fac Total		51	50	62	80	MUE
	24.33	24.33	090	2	1	1	2	1

42426 Excision of parotid tumor or parotid gland; total, with unilateral radical neck dissection `C`

RVU			Global Days	Modifiers				
Mod	Non-Fac Total	Fac Total		51	50	62	80	MUE
	39.26	39.26	090	2	1	1	2	1

● New   ▲ Revised   ✖ Deleted   ⊙ Moderate Sedation   ✚ Add-on Codes   ⊘ High Risk Denial   Ⓐ Age Edit   ♀ Female   ♂ Male   **AMA** CPT® Assistant   **MUE** Medically Unlikely Edit
⊘ Modifier 51 Exempt   ⊖ Modifier 63 Exempt   ✗ Unlisted   **Modifiers:** See Inside Back Cover   Ⓜ Maternity   `A 2`-`Z 3` ASC Payment Indicators   `A`-`Y` OPPS Status Indicators

420   CPT © 2015 American Medical Association. All Rights Reserved.   © 2016 DecisionHealth

42440 Excision of submandibular (submaxillary) gland

A2 J I

RVU			Global Days	Modifiers				
Mod	Non-Fac Total	Fac Total		51	50	62	80	MUE
	12.01	12.01	090	2	1	1	2	1

Excision of submandibular gland

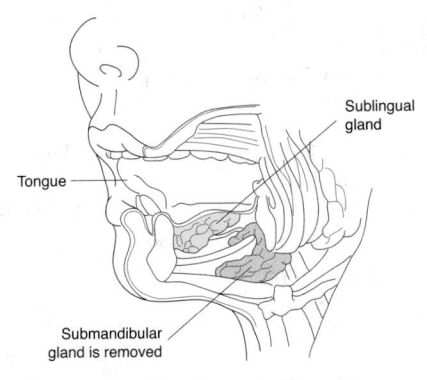

42450 Excision of sublingual gland

A2 J I

RVU			Global Days	Modifiers				
Mod	Non-Fac Total	Fac Total		51	50	62	80	MUE
	13.16	10.47	090	2	0	0	0	2

Salivary Gland/Duct repair

42500 Plastic repair of salivary duct, sialodochoplasty; primary or simple

A2 T

RVU			Global Days	Modifiers				
Mod	Non-Fac Total	Fac Total		51	50	62	80	MUE
	12.64	10.01	090	2	0	0	0	2

42505 Plastic repair of salivary duct, sialodochoplasty; secondary or complicated

A2 J I

RVU			Global Days	Modifiers				
Mod	Non-Fac Total	Fac Total		51	50	62	80	MUE
	16.21	13.27	090	2	0	0	1	2

42507 Parotid duct diversion, bilateral (Wilke type procedure)

A2 J I

RVU			Global Days	Modifiers				
Mod	Non-Fac Total	Fac Total		51	50	62	80	MUE
	15.05	15.05	090	2	2	0	2	1

Bilateral parotid duct diversion

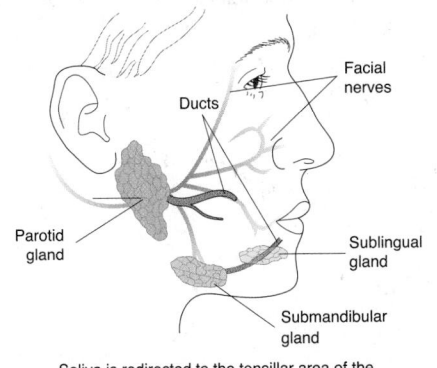

Saliva is redirected to the tonsillar area of the throat (42507) with removal of one (42508), or both (42509) submandibular glands, or duct ligation (42510)

42509 Parotid duct diversion, bilateral (Wilke type procedure); with excision of both submandibular glands

A2 J I

RVU			Global Days	Modifiers				
Mod	Non-Fac Total	Fac Total		51	50	62	80	MUE
	24.64	24.64	090	2	2	0	0	1

42510 Parotid duct diversion, bilateral (Wilke type procedure); with ligation of both submandibular (Wharton's) ducts

A2 J I

RVU			Global Days	Modifiers				
Mod	Non-Fac Total	Fac Total		51	50	62	80	MUE
	18.79	18.79	090	2	2	1	2	1

Other Salivary Gland/Duct Procedures

42550 Injection procedure for sialography

N I N

Coding tip: Procedure with radiologic supervision - 42550, 70390

RVU			Global Days	Modifiers				
Mod	Non-Fac Total	Fac Total		51	50	62	80	MUE
	3.85	1.83	000	2	0	0	1	2

42600 Closure salivary fistula

A2 T

RVU			Global Days	Modifiers				
Mod	Non-Fac Total	Fac Total		51	50	62	80	MUE
	13.93	10.15	090	2	0	0	0	2

Salivary fistula closure

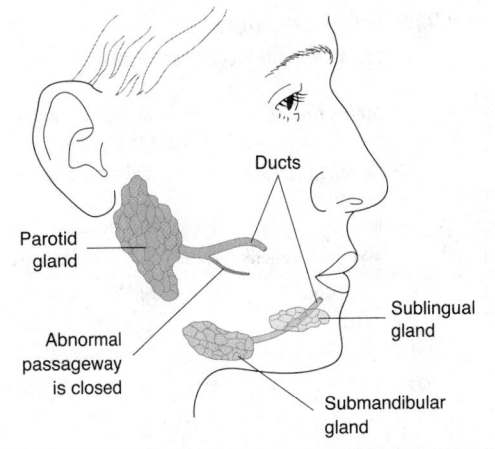

42650 Dilation salivary duct

P 3 T

RVU			Global Days	Modifiers				
Mod	Non-Fac Total	Fac Total		51	50	62	80	MUE
	2.44	1.72	000	2	0	0	1	2

42660 Dilation and catheterization of salivary duct, with or without injection

P 3 T

RVU			Global Days	Modifiers				
Mod	Non-Fac Total	Fac Total		51	50	62	80	MUE
	3.72	2.61	000	2	0	0	0	2

42665 Ligation salivary duct, intraoral

A2 J I

RVU			Global Days	Modifiers				
Mod	Non-Fac Total	Fac Total		51	50	62	80	MUE
	8.96	5.95	090	2	0	0	0	2

● New   ▲ Revised   Deleted   ⊙ Moderate Sedation   ✚ Add-on Codes   ⊘ High Risk Denial   ⒶAge Edit   ♀ Female   ♂ Male   **AMA** *CPT® Assistant*   **MUE** Medically Unlikely Edit
⊘ Modifier 51 Exempt   ⊖ Modifier 63 Exempt   ☒ Unlisted   **Modifiers:** *See Inside Back Cover*   Ⓜ Maternity   A2–Z3 ASC Payment Indicators   A–Y OPPS Status Indicators

42699 Unlisted procedure, salivary glands or ducts ✗T

RVU			Global Days	Modifiers				
Mod	Non-Fac Total	Fac Total		51	50	62	80	MUE
	0.00	0.00	YYY	2	0	1	2	

Pharyngeal/Adenoid/Tonsil Procedures

Incisional Pharyngeal/Adenoid/Tonsil Procedures

42700 Incision and drainage abscess; peritonsillar A2T

Coding tip: Drainage of abscess of tongue or lingual floor of mouth - 41000; sublingual - 41005-41006; palate/uvula - 42000; parotid gland - 42300-42305; submaxillary gland - 42310-42320

RVU			Global Days	Modifiers				
Mod	Non-Fac Total	Fac Total		51	50	62	80	MUE
	5.51	3.96	010	2	0	0	1	2

42720 Incision and drainage abscess; retropharyngeal or parapharyngeal, intraoral approach A2T

RVU			Global Days	Modifiers				
Mod	Non-Fac Total	Fac Total		51	50	62	80	MUE
	13.23	11.45	010	2	0	0	0	1

42725 Incision and drainage abscess; retropharyngeal or parapharyngeal, external approach A2JI

RVU			Global Days	Modifiers				
Mod	Non-Fac Total	Fac Total		51	50	62	80	MUE
	23.84	23.84	090	2	0	1	2	1

Excisional Pharyngeal/Adenoid/Tonsil Procedures

42800 Biopsy; oropharynx P3T

Coding tip: Code 99000 for specimen transfer from office setting to an outside laboratory

Coding tip: Report this procedure separately only when performed alone, or distinct from other procedures on the same day

Coding tip: Biopsy is usually included as a component of a more complex procedure

RVU			Global Days	Modifiers				
Mod	Non-Fac Total	Fac Total		51	50	62	80	MUE
	4.60	3.27	010	2	0	0	1	3

Biopsy

Oropharynx(42800);
nasopharynx, visible lesion, simple (42804);
nasopharynx, survey for unknown primary lesion (42806)

42804 Biopsy; nasopharynx, visible lesion, simple A2T

RVU			Global Days	Modifiers				
Mod	Non-Fac Total	Fac Total		51	50	62	80	MUE
	5.68	3.31	010	2	0	0	1	3

42806 Biopsy; nasopharynx, survey for unknown primary lesion A2T

Coding tip: Do not report separately if done as part of another more complex procedure, such as lesion excision

RVU			Global Days	Modifiers				
Mod	Non-Fac Total	Fac Total		51	50	62	80	MUE
	6.38	3.86	010	2	0	0	1	1

42808 Excision or destruction of lesion of pharynx, any method A2T

RVU			Global Days	Modifiers				
Mod	Non-Fac Total	Fac Total		51	50	62	80	MUE
	6.60	4.73	010	2	0	0	1	2

42809 Removal of foreign body from pharynx NIQI

RVU			Global Days	Modifiers				
Mod	Non-Fac Total	Fac Total		51	50	62	80	MUE
	5.87	3.56	010	2	0	0	1	1

42810 Excision branchial cleft cyst or vestige, confined to skin and subcutaneous tissues A2T

RVU			Global Days	Modifiers				
Mod	Non-Fac Total	Fac Total		51	50	62	80	MUE
	11.26	8.43	090	2	1	0	2	1

42815 Excision branchial cleft cyst, vestige, or fistula, extending beneath subcutaneous tissues and/or into pharynx A2JI

RVU			Global Days	Modifiers				
Mod	Non-Fac Total	Fac Total		51	50	62	80	MUE
	16.30	16.30	090	2	1	1	2	1

42820 Tonsillectomy and adenoidectomy; younger than age 12 Ⓐ A2T

Coding tip: Removal of tonsils alone - 42825; adenoids alone - 42830, 42835

RVU			Global Days	Modifiers				
Mod	Non-Fac Total	Fac Total		51	50	62	80	MUE
	8.45	8.45	090	2	0	0	0	1

AMA: Feb 98: 11, Mar 08: 15, May 08: 14

42821 Tonsillectomy and adenoidectomy; age 12 or over A2T

RVU			Global Days	Modifiers				
Mod	Non-Fac Total	Fac Total		51	50	62	80	MUE
	8.77	8.77	090	2	0	0	0	1

AMA: Aug 97: 18, Feb 98: 11, Mar 08: 15, May 08: 14

● New   ▲ Revised   ✖ Deleted   ⊙ Moderate Sedation   ✚ Add-on Codes   ⊘ High Risk Denial   Ⓐ Age Edit   ♀ Female   ♂ Male   **AMA** CPT® Assistant   **MUE** Medically Unlikely Edit
⊘ Modifier 51 Exempt   ⊖ Modifier 63 Exempt   ✗ Unlisted   **Modifiers:** See Inside Back Cover   Ⓜ Maternity   A2–Z3 ASC Payment Indicators   A–Y OPPS Status Indicators

422   CPT © 2015 American Medical Association. All Rights Reserved.   © 2016 DecisionHealth

42825 Tonsillectomy, primary or secondary; younger than age 12 ⊘ⒶA 2 J 1

Coding tip: Excision of tonsil tags - 42860

RVU			Global Days	Modifiers				
Mod	Non-Fac Total	Fac Total		51	50	62	80	MUE
	7.63	7.63	090	2	0	0	0	1

AMA: Aug 97: 18, Feb 98: 11, Mar 08: 15

Tonsillectomy

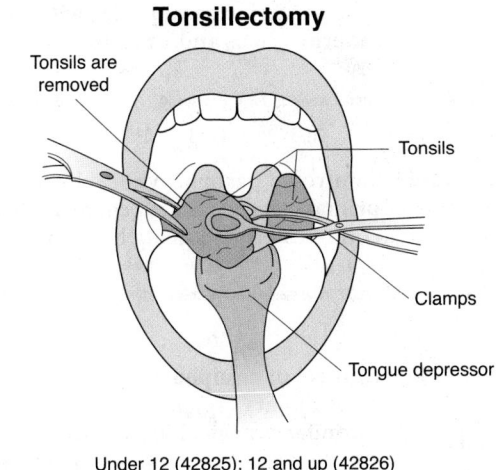

Tonsils are removed

Tonsils

Clamps

Tongue depressor

Under 12 (42825); 12 and up (42826)

42826 Tonsillectomy, primary or secondary; age 12 or over A 2 T

Coding tip: Tonsillectomy with adenoidectomy - 42821

RVU			Global Days	Modifiers				
Mod	Non-Fac Total	Fac Total		51	50	62	80	MUE
	7.32	7.32	090	2	0	0	1	1

AMA: Aug 97: 18, Feb 98: 11, Mar 08: 15, Apr 10: 10

42830 Adenoidectomy, primary; younger than age 12 ⊘ⒶA 2 J 1

RVU			Global Days	Modifiers				
Mod	Non-Fac Total	Fac Total		51	50	62	80	MUE
	6.03	6.03	090	2	0	0	0	1

42831 Adenoidectomy, primary; age 12 or over A 2 T

RVU			Global Days	Modifiers				
Mod	Non-Fac Total	Fac Total		51	50	62	80	MUE
	6.52	6.52	090	2	0	0	0	1

42835 Adenoidectomy, secondary; younger than age 12 ⒶA 2 T

RVU			Global Days	Modifiers				
Mod	Non-Fac Total	Fac Total		51	50	62	80	MUE
	5.60	5.60	090	2	0	0	0	1

42836 Adenoidectomy, secondary; age 12 or over A 2 T

Coding tip: Adenoidectomy with tonsillectomy - 42821

RVU			Global Days	Modifiers				
Mod	Non-Fac Total	Fac Total		51	50	62	80	MUE
	7.01	7.01	090	2	0	0	0	1

AMA: Feb 98: 11, Nov 10: 9

42842 Radical resection of tonsil, tonsillar pillars, and/or retromolar trigone; without closure J 1

RVU			Global Days	Modifiers				
Mod	Non-Fac Total	Fac Total		51	50	62	80	MUE
	29.92	29.92	090	2	0	0	0	1

AMA: Aug 10: 6

42844 Radical resection of tonsil, tonsillar pillars, and/or retromolar trigone; closure with local flap (eg, tongue, buccal) J 1

RVU			Global Days	Modifiers				
Mod	Non-Fac Total	Fac Total		51	50	62	80	MUE
	40.98	40.98	090	2	0	1	2	1

AMA: Aug 10: 6

42845 Radical resection of tonsil, tonsillar pillars, and/or retromolar trigone; closure with other flap C

RVU			Global Days	Modifiers				
Mod	Non-Fac Total	Fac Total		51	50	62	80	MUE
	66.00	66.00	090	2	0	1	2	1

AMA: Aug 10: 6

42860 Excision of tonsil tags A 2 J 1

Coding tip: Excision of tonsils alone - 42825-42826; excision of lingual tonsil - 42870

RVU			Global Days	Modifiers				
Mod	Non-Fac Total	Fac Total		51	50	62	80	MUE
	5.48	5.48	090	2	0	0	0	1

42870 Excision or destruction lingual tonsil, any method (separate procedure) A 2 T

Coding tip: Do not report separately if done as part of another more complex procedure, such as lesion excision

RVU			Global Days	Modifiers				
Mod	Non-Fac Total	Fac Total		51	50	62	80	MUE
	17.64	17.64	090	2	0	0	0	1

Excision or destruction of lingual tonsil

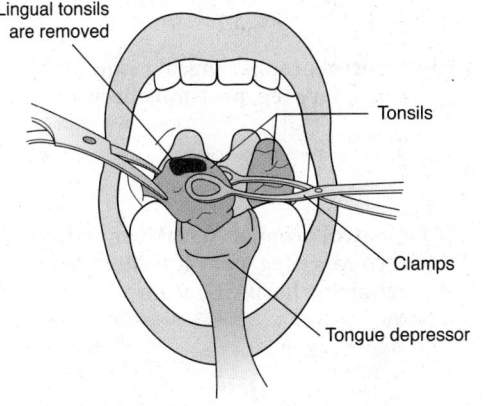

Lingual tonsils are removed

Tonsils

Clamps

Tongue depressor

The lingual tonsil is cut out or destroyed by any method. The lingual tonsil is a collection of lymphoid tissue located at the back or base of the tongue.

42890 Limited pharyngectomy A 2 J 1

RVU			Global Days	Modifiers				
Mod	Non-Fac Total	Fac Total		51	50	62	80	MUE
	42.28	42.28	090	2	0	1	2	1

● New   ▲ Revised   Deleted   ⊙ Moderate Sedation   ✚ Add-on Codes   ⊘ High Risk Denial   Ⓐ Age Edit   ♀ Female   ♂ Male   **AMA** *CPT® Assistant*   **MUE** Medically Unlikely Edit   ⊘ Modifier 51 Exempt   ⊖ Modifier 63 Exempt   ⊠ Unlisted   **Modifiers:** *See Inside Back Cover*   Ⓜ Maternity   A 2 – Z 3 ASC Payment Indicators   A – Y OPPS Status Indicators

© 2016 DecisionHealth   CPT © 2015 American Medical Association. All Rights Reserved.   **423**

42892 Resection of lateral pharyngeal wall or pyriform sinus, direct closure by advancement of lateral and posterior pharyngeal walls A 2 J I

	RVU		Global Days	Modifiers				
Mod	Non-Fac Total	Fac Total		51	50	62	80	MUE
	55.80	55.80	090	2	0	1	2	1

AMA: Aug 10: 6

42894 Resection of pharyngeal wall requiring closure with myocutaneous or fasciocutaneous flap or free muscle, skin, or fascial flap with microvascular anastomosis C

	RVU		Global Days	Modifiers				
Mod	Non-Fac Total	Fac Total		51	50	62	80	MUE
	70.16	70.16	090	2	0	1	2	1

AMA: Nov 07: 8, Aug 10: 6

Pharyngeal/Adenoid/Tonsil Repair

42900 Suture pharynx for wound or injury A 2 T

	RVU		Global Days	Modifiers				
Mod	Non-Fac Total	Fac Total		51	50	62	80	MUE
	9.83	9.83	010	2	0	0	0	1

42950 Pharyngoplasty (plastic or reconstructive operation on pharynx) A 2 J I

	RVU		Global Days	Modifiers				
Mod	Non-Fac Total	Fac Total		51	50	62	80	MUE
	24.15	24.15	090	2	0	1	2	1

42953 Pharyngoesophageal repair C

	RVU		Global Days	Modifiers				
Mod	Non-Fac Total	Fac Total		51	50	62	80	MUE
	29.09	29.09	090	2	0	0	2	1

Other Pharyngeal/Adenoid/Tonsil Procedures

42955 Pharyngostomy (fistulization of pharynx, external for feeding) A 2 T

	RVU		Global Days	Modifiers				
Mod	Non-Fac Total	Fac Total		51	50	62	80	MUE
	22.77	22.77	090	2	0	0	2	1

42960 Control oropharyngeal hemorrhage, primary or secondary (eg, post-tonsillectomy); simple A 2 T

	RVU		Global Days	Modifiers				
Mod	Non-Fac Total	Fac Total		51	50	62	80	MUE
	4.96	4.96	010	2	0	0	0	1

42961 Control oropharyngeal hemorrhage, primary or secondary (eg, post-tonsillectomy); complicated, requiring hospitalization C

	RVU		Global Days	Modifiers				
Mod	Non-Fac Total	Fac Total		51	50	62	80	MUE
	12.36	12.36	090	2	0	0	2	1

42962 Control oropharyngeal hemorrhage, primary or secondary (eg, post-tonsillectomy); with secondary surgical intervention A 2 T

	RVU		Global Days	Modifiers				
Mod	Non-Fac Total	Fac Total		51	50	62	80	MUE
	15.14	15.14	090	2	0	0	1	1

42970 Control of nasopharyngeal hemorrhage, primary or secondary (eg, postadenoidectomy); simple, with posterior nasal packs, with or without anterior packs and/or cautery R 2 T

	RVU		Global Days	Modifiers				
Mod	Non-Fac Total	Fac Total		51	50	62	80	MUE
	11.73	11.73	090	2	0	0	1	1

42971 Control of nasopharyngeal hemorrhage, primary or secondary (eg, postadenoidectomy); complicated, requiring hospitalization C

	RVU		Global Days	Modifiers				
Mod	Non-Fac Total	Fac Total		51	50	62	80	MUE
	13.32	13.32	090	2	0	0	2	1

42972 Control of nasopharyngeal hemorrhage, primary or secondary (eg, postadenoidectomy); with secondary surgical intervention A 2 T

	RVU		Global Days	Modifiers				
Mod	Non-Fac Total	Fac Total		51	50	62	80	MUE
	14.91	14.91	090	2	0	0	2	1

42999 Unlisted procedure, pharynx, adenoids, or tonsils x T

	RVU		Global Days	Modifiers				
Mod	Non-Fac Total	Fac Total		51	50	62	80	MUE
	0.00	0.00	YYY	2	0	1	0	

AMA: Feb 14: 11

Esophageal Procedures

Incisional Esophageal Procedures

43020 Esophagotomy, cervical approach, with removal of foreign body T

	RVU		Global Days	Modifiers				
Mod	Non-Fac Total	Fac Total		51	50	62	80	MUE
	15.42	15.42	090	2	0	1	2	1

43030 Cricopharyngeal myotomy G 2 J I

	RVU		Global Days	Modifiers				
Mod	Non-Fac Total	Fac Total		51	50	62	80	MUE
	15.11	15.11	090	2	0	1	2	1

43045 Esophagotomy, thoracic approach, with removal of foreign body C

	RVU		Global Days	Modifiers				
Mod	Non-Fac Total	Fac Total		51	50	62	80	MUE
	38.17	38.17	090	2	0	1	2	1

● New   ▲ Revised   ✖ Deleted   ⊙ Moderate Sedation   ✚ Add-on Codes   ⊘ High Risk Denial   Ⓐ Age Edit   ♀ Female   ♂ Male   **AMA** CPT® Assistant   **MUE** Medically Unlikely Edit
⊘ Modifier 51 Exempt   ⊖ Modifier 63 Exempt   ✖ Unlisted   **Modifiers:** See Inside Back Cover   Ⓜ Maternity   A 2 – Z 3 ASC Payment Indicators   A – Y OPPS Status Indicators

CPT © 2015 American Medical Association. All Rights Reserved.   © 2016 DecisionHealth

Excisional Esophageal Procedures

43100 Excision of lesion, esophagus, with primary repair; cervical approach   C

RVU			Global Days	Modifiers				
Mod	Non-Fac Total	Fac Total		51	50	62	80	MUE
	18.16	18.16	090	2	0	1	2	1

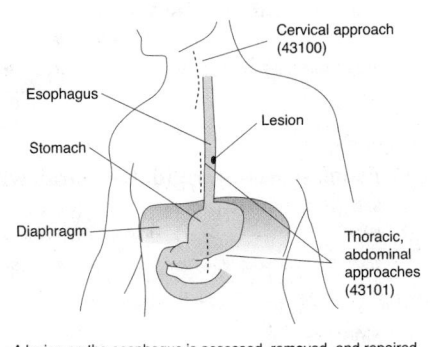

Excision of esophageal lesion, with primary repair

A lesion on the esophagus is accessed, removed, and repaired

43101 Excision of lesion, esophagus, with primary repair; thoracic or abdominal approach   C

RVU			Global Days	Modifiers				
Mod	Non-Fac Total	Fac Total		51	50	62	80	MUE
	29.77	29.77	090	2	0	1	2	1

AMA: Aug 10: 4

43107 Total or near total esophagectomy, without thoracotomy; with pharyngogastrostomy or cervical esophagogastrostomy, with or without pyloroplasty (transhiatal)   C

RVU			Global Days	Modifiers				
Mod	Non-Fac Total	Fac Total		51	50	62	80	MUE
	74.59	74.59	090	2	0	1	2	1

AMA: Aug 10: 4

43108 Total or near total esophagectomy, without thoracotomy; with colon interposition or small intestine reconstruction, including intestine mobilization, preparation and anastomosis(es)   C

RVU			Global Days	Modifiers				
Mod	Non-Fac Total	Fac Total		51	50	62	80	MUE
	133.73	133.73	090	2	0	1	2	1

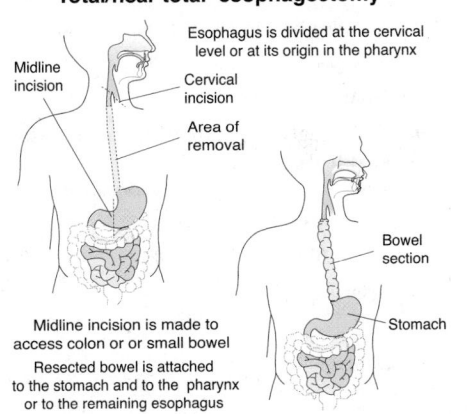

Total/near total esophagectomy

Esophagus is divided at the cervical level or at its origin in the pharynx

Midline incision

Cervical incision

Area of removal

Bowel section

Stomach

Midline incision is made to access colon or or small bowel

Resected bowel is attached to the stomach and to the pharynx or to the remaining esophagus

43112 Total or near total esophagectomy, with thoracotomy; with pharyngogastrostomy or cervical esophagogastrostomy, with or without pyloroplasty   C

RVU			Global Days	Modifiers				
Mod	Non-Fac Total	Fac Total		51	50	62	80	MUE
	78.76	78.76	090	2	0	2	2	1

AMA: Aug 13: 14

43113 Total or near total esophagectomy, with thoracotomy; with colon interposition or small intestine reconstruction, including intestine mobilization, preparation, and anastomosis(es)   C

RVU			Global Days	Modifiers				
Mod	Non-Fac Total	Fac Total		51	50	62	80	MUE
	132.27	132.27	090	2	0	2	2	1

43116 Partial esophagectomy, cervical, with free intestinal graft, including microvascular anastomosis, obtaining the graft and intestinal reconstruction   C

RVU			Global Days	Modifiers				
Mod	Non-Fac Total	Fac Total		51	50	62	80	MUE
	147.70	147.70	090	2	0	1	2	1

AMA: Nov 97: 17, Nov 98: 16, Aug 10: 4

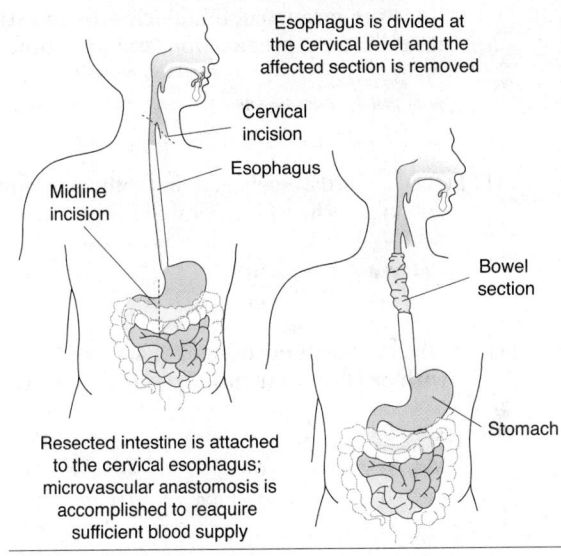

Partial esophagectomy

Esophagus is divided at the cervical level and the affected section is removed

Cervical incision

Esophagus

Midline incision

Bowel section

Stomach

Resected intestine is attached to the cervical esophagus; microvascular anastomosis is accomplished to reacquire sufficient blood supply

43117 Partial esophagectomy, distal two-thirds, with thoracotomy and separate abdominal incision, with or without proximal gastrectomy; with thoracic esophagogastrostomy, with or without pyloroplasty (Ivor Lewis)   C

RVU			Global Days	Modifiers				
Mod	Non-Fac Total	Fac Total		51	50	62	80	MUE
	72.07	72.07	090	2	0	2	2	1

● New   ▲ Revised   Deleted   ⊙ Moderate Sedation   ✚ Add-on Codes   ⊗ High Risk Denial   Ⓐ Age Edit   ♀ Female   ♂ Male   **AMA** *CPT® Assistant*   **MUE** Medically Unlikely Edit

⊘ Modifier 51 Exempt   ⊖ Modifier 63 Exempt   ☒ Unlisted   **Modifiers:** *See Inside Back Cover*   Ⓜ Maternity   A 2 – Z 3 ASC Payment Indicators   A – Y OPPS Status Indicators

Surgical Procedures

43100 – 43117

43118 Partial esophagectomy, distal two-thirds, with thoracotomy and separate abdominal incision, with or without proximal gastrectomy; with colon interposition or small intestine reconstruction, including intestine mobilization, preparation, and anastomosis(es)   **C**

RVU			Global Days	Modifiers				
Mod	Non-Fac Total	Fac Total		51	50	62	80	MUE
	107.90	107.90	090	2	0	2	2	1

43121 Partial esophagectomy, distal two-thirds, with thoracotomy only, with or without proximal gastrectomy, with thoracic esophagogastrostomy, with or without pyloroplasty   **C**

RVU			Global Days	Modifiers				
Mod	Non-Fac Total	Fac Total		51	50	62	80	MUE
	84.09	84.09	090	2	0	2	2	1

43122 Partial esophagectomy, thoracoabdominal or abdominal approach, with or without proximal gastrectomy; with esophagogastrostomy, with or without pyloroplasty   **C**

RVU			Global Days	Modifiers				
Mod	Non-Fac Total	Fac Total		51	50	62	80	MUE
	74.91	74.91	090	2	0	1	2	1

43123 Partial esophagectomy, thoracoabdominal or abdominal approach, with or without proximal gastrectomy; with colon interposition or small intestine reconstruction, including intestine mobilization, preparation, and anastomosis(es)   **C**

RVU			Global Days	Modifiers				
Mod	Non-Fac Total	Fac Total		51	50	62	80	MUE
	138.02	138.02	090	2	0	1	2	1

43124 Total or partial esophagectomy, without reconstruction (any approach), with cervical esophagostomy   **C**

RVU			Global Days	Modifiers				
Mod	Non-Fac Total	Fac Total		51	50	62	80	MUE
	112.07	112.07	090	2	0	1	2	1

43130 Diverticulectomy of hypopharynx or esophagus, with or without myotomy; cervical approach   **G2 J1**

RVU			Global Days	Modifiers				
Mod	Non-Fac Total	Fac Total		51	50	62	80	MUE
	22.92	22.92	090	2	0	1	2	1

AMA: Oct 10: 12, Dec 10: 12

43135 Diverticulectomy of hypopharynx or esophagus, with or without myotomy; thoracic approach   **C**

RVU			Global Days	Modifiers				
Mod	Non-Fac Total	Fac Total		51	50	62	80	MUE
	43.36	43.36	090	2	0	1	2	1

AMA: Oct 10: 12, Dec 10: 12

43180 Esophagoscopy, rigid, transoral with diverticulectomy of hypopharynx or cervical esophagus (eg, Zenker's diverticulum), with cricopharyngeal myotomy, includes use of telescope or operating microscope and repair, when performed   **G2 T**

RVU			Global Days	Modifiers				
Mod	Non-Fac Total	Fac Total		51	50	62	80	MUE
	16.01	16.01	090	2	0	0	1	1

43191 Esophagoscopy, rigid, transoral; diagnostic, including collection of specimen(s) by brushing or washing when performed (separate procedure)   **G2 T**

RVU			Global Days	Modifiers				
Mod	Non-Fac Total	Fac Total		51	50	62	80	MUE
	4.49	4.49	000	2	0	0	1	1

AMA: Dec 13: 3, Feb 14: 9, 11

43192 Esophagoscopy, rigid, transoral; with directed submucosal injection(s), any substance   **G2 T**

RVU			Global Days	Modifiers				
Mod	Non-Fac Total	Fac Total		51	50	62	80	MUE
	4.95	4.95	000	3	0	0	1	1

AMA: Dec 13: 3

43193 Esophagoscopy, rigid, transoral; with biopsy, single or multiple   **G2 T**

RVU			Global Days	Modifiers				
Mod	Non-Fac Total	Fac Total		51	50	62	80	MUE
	4.94	4.94	000	3	0	0	1	1

AMA: Dec 13: 3

43194 Esophagoscopy, rigid, transoral; with removal of foreign body(s)   **G2 T**

RVU			Global Days	Modifiers				
Mod	Non-Fac Total	Fac Total		51	50	62	80	MUE
	5.62	5.62	000	3	0	0	1	1

AMA: Dec 13: 3

43195 Esophagoscopy, rigid, transoral; with balloon dilation (less than 30 mm diameter)   **G2 T**

RVU			Global Days	Modifiers				
Mod	Non-Fac Total	Fac Total		51	50	62	80	MUE
	5.37	5.37	000	3	0	0	1	1

AMA: Dec 13: 3

43196 Esophagoscopy, rigid, transoral; with insertion of guide wire followed by dilation over guide wire   **G2 T**

RVU			Global Days	Modifiers				
Mod	Non-Fac Total	Fac Total		51	50	62	80	MUE
	5.75	5.75	000	3	0	0	1	1

AMA: Dec 13: 3, Feb 14: 9

43197 Esophagoscopy, flexible, transnasal; diagnostic, including collection of specimen(s) by brushing or washing, when performed (separate procedure)   **P3 T**

RVU			Global Days	Modifiers				
Mod	Non-Fac Total	Fac Total		51	50	62	80	MUE
	5.41	2.41	000	2	0	0	1	1

AMA: Dec 13: 3, Feb 14: 9

43198 Esophagoscopy, flexible, transnasal; with biopsy, single or multiple   **P3 T**

RVU			Global Days	Modifiers				
Mod	Non-Fac Total	Fac Total		51	50	62	80	MUE
	6.01	2.89	000	3	0	0	1	1

AMA: Dec 13: 3, Feb 14: 9

● New   ▲ Revised   ✖ Deleted   ⊙ Moderate Sedation   ✚ Add-on Codes   ⊘ High Risk Denial   Ⓐ Age Edit   ♀ Female   ♂ Male   **AMA** *CPT® Assistant*   **MUE** Medically Unlikely Edit
⊘ Modifier 51 Exempt   ⊖ Modifier 63 Exempt   ✗ Unlisted   **Modifiers:** *See Inside Back Cover*   Ⓜ Maternity   **A2–Z3** ASC Payment Indicators   **A–Y** OPPS Status Indicators

CPT © 2015 American Medical Association. All Rights Reserved.   © 2016 DecisionHealth

Endoscopic Esophageal Procedures

Coding Guidance

When a surgical endoscopy directly follows a diagnostic endoscopy, the diagnostic portion is included. When a diagnostic endoscopic service is provided in conjunction with therapeutic endoscopic services, report only the more comprehensive endoscopy code that desribes the service. If different therapeutic endoscopic services performed are not adequately described by a comprehensive service code, the appropriate multiple GI endoscopy codes can be used. When an endoscopy is performed to confirm or establish anatomical landmarks as a scout endoscopy, the procedure is not reported separately. When an endoscopy is done as a diagnostic procedure for basing the decision to do a more extensive open surgical procedure, the endoscopy may be separately reported. Control of bleeding resulting from an endoscopy and performed at the time of the service is included. If it becomes necessary to repeat an endoscopy in order to control bleeding, then a procedure code for endoscopic control of bleeding may be reported with a modifier identifying a return to the operative room in the postoperative period. If the larynx is viewed during esophagoscopy through the esophagoscope, it cannot be reported. However, if it is viewed through a separate laryngoscope, both the laryngoscopy and the esophagoscopy may be reported.

⊙ **43200 Esophagoscopy, flexible, transoral; diagnostic, including collection of specimen(s) by brushing or washing, when performed (separate procedure)** `A2T`

Coding tip: Report this procedure separately only when performed alone, or distinct from other procedures on the same day

Coding tip: Do not report with any surgical esophagoscopy

Coding tip: Esophagoscopy, flexible, transoral, diagnostic, with collection of specimen(s) by brushing or washing, with endoscopic mucosal resection - 43211

Coding tip: Esophagoscopy, flexible, transoral, diagnostic, with dilation of esophagus with balloon (30mm or larger) (includes fluoroscopic guidance when performed) - 43214

Coding tip: Codes 99148-99150 may be reported when a second physician or qualified health care professional (other than the one performing the procedure) provides moderate sedation in a facility setting only

Coding tip: Esophagoscopy, flexible, transoral, diagnostic, with dilation of esophagus with balloon or dilator, retrograde (includes fluoroscopic guidance, when performed) - 43213

Coding tip: Do not code 99143-99145

Coding tip: Esophagoscopy, flexible, transoral, diagnostic, with placement of endoscopic stent, including pre- and post- dilation, and guide wire - 43212

RVU		Global Days	Modifiers				
Mod	Non-Fac Total Fac Total		51	50	62	80	MUE
	7.75 2.73	000	2	0	0	1	1

AMA: Spring 91: 7, Spring 94: 1, Jun 98: 10, Nov 99: 21, Sep 03: 3, Oct 08: 6, Jan 13: 11, Feb 13: 16, Dec 13: 3, Feb 14: 9

Esophagoscopy, diagnostic

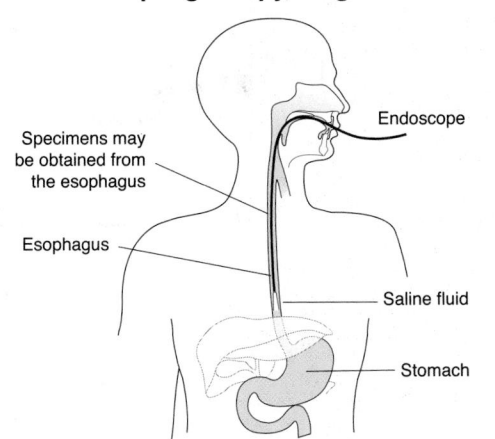

Specimens may be obtained from the esophagus

Endoscope

Esophagus

Saline fluid

Stomach

A flexible or rigid endoscope is inserted through the mouth or nose

⊙ **43201 Esophagoscopy, flexible, transoral; with directed submucosal injection(s), any substance** `A2T`

RVU		Global Days	Modifiers				
Mod	Non-Fac Total Fac Total		51	50	62	80	MUE
	7.88 3.19	000	3	0	0	1	1

AMA: Jun 10: 4, Jan 13: 11, Dec 13: 3

⊙ **43202 Esophagoscopy, flexible, transoral; with biopsy, single or multiple** `A2T`

Coding tip: Code 99000 for specimen transfer from office setting to an outside laboratory

RVU		Global Days	Modifiers				
Mod	Non-Fac Total Fac Total		51	50	62	80	MUE
	10.32 3.19	000	3	0	0	1	1

AMA: Spring 94: 1, Oct 08: 6, Jan 13: 11, Dec 13: 3

Pub 100-04, 12, 40.6

⊙ **43204 Esophagoscopy, flexible, transoral; with injection sclerosis of esophageal varices** `A2T`

RVU		Global Days	Modifiers				
Mod	Non-Fac Total Fac Total		51	50	62	80	MUE
	4.12 4.12	000	3	0	0	1	1

AMA: Spring 94: 1, Oct 08: 6, Jun 10: 5, Jan 13: 11, Dec 13: 3

⊙ **43205 Esophagoscopy, flexible, transoral; with band ligation of esophageal varices** `A2T`

RVU		Global Days	Modifiers				
Mod	Non-Fac Total Fac Total		51	50	62	80	MUE
	4.30 4.30	000	3	0	0	1	1

AMA: Spring 94: 1, Oct 08: 6, Jan 13: 11, Dec 13: 3

⊙ **43206 Esophagoscopy, flexible, transoral; with optical endomicroscopy** `G2T`

RVU		Global Days	Modifiers				
Mod	Non-Fac Total Fac Total		51	50	62	80	MUE
	9.40 4.12	000	3	0	0	1	1

AMA: Jan 13: 11, Aug 13: 5, Dec 13: 3

Esophagoscopy, flexible, transoral with optical endomicroscopy

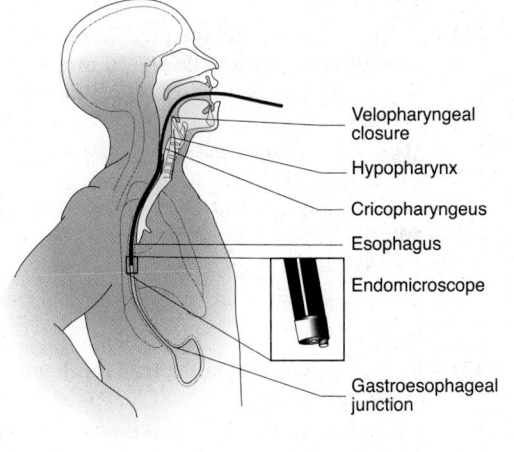

Velopharyngeal closure

Hypopharynx

Cricopharyngeus

Esophagus

Endomicroscope

Gastroesophageal junction

● New   ▲ Revised   Deleted   ⊙ Moderate Sedation   ⊘ High Risk Denial   Ⓐ Age Edit   ♀ Female   ♂ Male   **AMA** *CPT® Assistant*   *MUE* Medically Unlikely Edit
⊗ Modifier 51 Exempt   ⊖ Modifier 63 Exempt   ✗ Unlisted   **Modifiers:** *See Inside Back Cover*   Ⓜ Maternity   `A2`–`Z3` ASC Payment Indicators   `A`–`Y` OPPS Status Indicators

© 2016 DecisionHealth   CPT © 2015 American Medical Association. All Rights Reserved.   **427**

● **43210** **Esophagogastroduodenoscopy, flexible, transoral; with esophagogastric fundoplasty, partial or complete, includes duodenoscopy when performed** G2 J I

RVU			Global Days	Modifiers				
Mod	Non-Fac Total	Fac Total		51	50	62	80	MUE
	12.43	12.43	YYY	3	0	0	1	1

⊙ **43211** **Esophagoscopy, flexible, transoral; with endoscopic mucosal resection** G2 T

Coding tip: Code 43211 is listed out of numerical order in CPT. Related codes for esophagoscopy, flexible, transoral - 43200-43206, 43212-43214, 43215-43217, 43220, 43226-43232

RVU			Global Days	Modifiers				
Mod	Non-Fac Total	Fac Total		51	50	62	80	MUE
	7.08	7.08	000	3	0	0	1	1

AMA: Dec 13: 3

⊙ **43212** **Esophagoscopy, flexible, transoral; with placement of endoscopic stent (includes pre- and post-dilation and guide wire passage, when performed)** G2 J I

Coding tip: Code 43212 is listed out of numerical order in CPT. Related codes for esophagoscopy, flexible, transoral - 43200-43206, 43211, 43213-43214, 43215-43217, 43220, 43226-43232

RVU			Global Days	Modifiers				
Mod	Non-Fac Total	Fac Total		51	50	62	80	MUE
	5.74	5.74	000	3	0	0	1	1

AMA: Dec 13: 3

⊙ **43213** **Esophagoscopy, flexible, transoral; with dilation of esophagus, by balloon or dilator, retrograde (includes fluoroscopic guidance, when performed)** G2 T

Coding tip: Code 43213 is listed out of numerical order in CPT. Related codes for esophagoscopy, flexible, transoral - 43200-43206, 43211-43212, 43214, 43215-43217, 43220, 43226-43232

RVU			Global Days	Modifiers				
Mod	Non-Fac Total	Fac Total		51	50	62	80	MUE
	34.81	7.73	000	3	0	0	1	1

AMA: Dec 13: 3

⊙ **43214** **Esophagoscopy, flexible, transoral; with dilation of esophagus with balloon (30 mm diameter or larger) (includes fluoroscopic guidance, when performed)** G2 T

Coding tip: Code 43214 is listed out of numerical order in CPT. Related codes for esophagoscopy, flexible, transoral - 43200-43206, 43211-43213, 43215-43217, 43220, 43226-43232

RVU			Global Days	Modifiers				
Mod	Non-Fac Total	Fac Total		51	50	62	80	MUE
	5.79	5.79	000	3	0	0	1	1

AMA: Dec 13: 3

⊙ **43215** **Esophagoscopy, flexible, transoral; with removal of foreign body(s)** A2 T

Coding tip: Foreign body removal with radiological supervision - add 74235

RVU			Global Days	Modifiers				
Mod	Non-Fac Total	Fac Total		51	50	62	80	MUE
	11.93	4.32	000	3	0	0	1	1

AMA: Spring 94: 1, Oct 08: 6, Dec 13: 3

Esophagoscopy, with foreign body removal

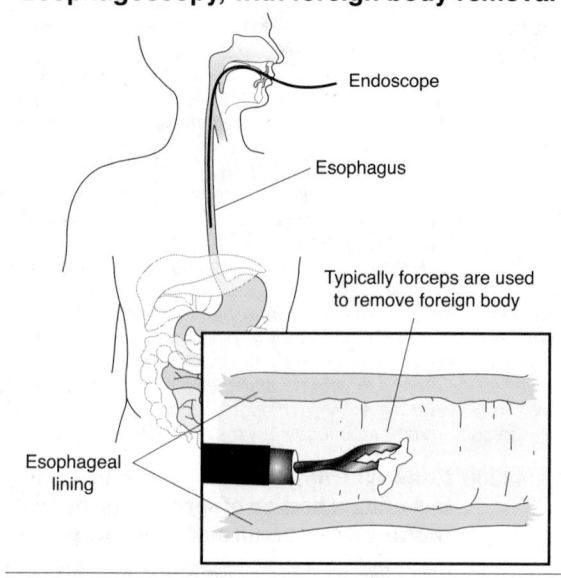

Endoscope

Esophagus

Typically forceps are used to remove foreign body

Esophageal lining

⊙ **43216** **Esophagoscopy, flexible, transoral; with removal of tumor(s), polyp(s), or other lesion(s) by hot biopsy forceps** A2 T

Coding tip: Code 99001 for specimen transfer from a facility to an outside laboratory

RVU			Global Days	Modifiers				
Mod	Non-Fac Total	Fac Total		51	50	62	80	MUE
	11.78	4.09	000	3	0	0	1	1

AMA: Spring 94: 1, Oct 08: 6, Jan 13: 11, Dec 13: 3

Esophagoscopy, with tumor/polyp/lesion removal

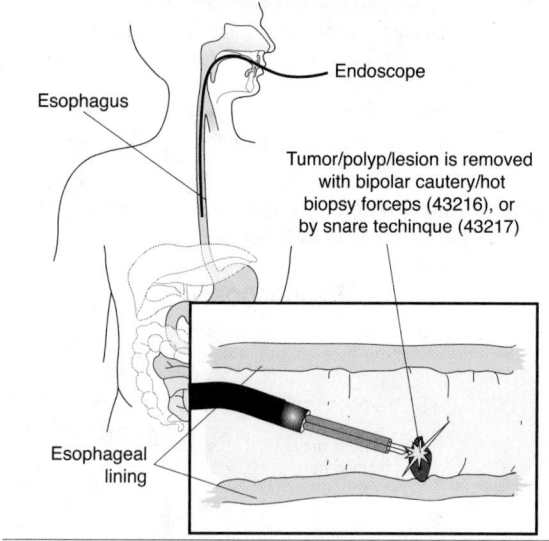

Endoscope

Esophagus

Tumor/polyp/lesion is removed with bipolar cautery/hot biopsy forceps (43216), or by snare techinque (43217)

Esophageal lining

● New   ▲ Revised   ✖ Deleted   ⊙ Moderate Sedation   ✚ Add-on Codes   ⊘ High Risk Denial   Ⓐ Age Edit   ♀ Female   ♂ Male   **AMA** CPT® Assistant   **MUE** Medically Unlikely Edit

⊘ Modifier 51 Exempt   ⊖ Modifier 63 Exempt   ✖ Unlisted   **Modifiers:** See Inside Back Cover   Ⓜ Maternity   A2–Z3 ASC Payment Indicators   A–Y OPPS Status Indicators

CPT © 2015 American Medical Association. All Rights Reserved.   © 2016 DecisionHealth

⊙ **43217** **Esophagoscopy, flexible, transoral; with removal of tumor(s), polyp(s), or other lesion(s) by snare technique** `A 2 T`

RVU			Global Days	Modifiers				
Mod	Non-Fac Total	Fac Total		51	50	62	80	MUE
	12.72	4.88	000	3	0	0	1	1

AMA: Spring 94: 1, Oct 08: 6, Jan 13: 11, Dec 13: 3

Pub 100-04, 12, 40.6

⊙ **43220** **Esophagoscopy, flexible, transoral; with transendoscopic balloon dilation (less than 30 mm diameter)** `A 2 T`

Coding tip: Balloon dilation with imaging guidance - add 74360

RVU			Global Days	Modifiers				
Mod	Non-Fac Total	Fac Total		51	50	62	80	MUE
	32.23	3.62	000	3	0	0	1	1

AMA: Spring 94: 2, Jan 97: 10, May 05: 3, Oct 08: 6, Jan 13: 11, Dec 13: 3

⊙ **43226** **Esophagoscopy, flexible, transoral; with insertion of guide wire followed by passage of dilator(s) over guide wire** `A 2 T`

Coding tip: Dilation over guide wire with imaging guidance - add 74360

RVU			Global Days	Modifiers				
Mod	Non-Fac Total	Fac Total		51	50	62	80	MUE
	10.84	4.00	000	3	0	0	1	1

AMA: Spring 94: 2, Jan 13: 11, Dec 13: 3

⊙ **43227** **Esophagoscopy, flexible, transoral; with control of bleeding, any method** `A 2 T`

RVU			Global Days	Modifiers				
Mod	Non-Fac Total	Fac Total		51	50	62	80	MUE
	19.77	5.01	000	3	0	0	1	1

AMA: Spring 94: 2, Oct 08: 6, Jun 10: 4, Jan 13: 11, Dec 13: 3, Feb 14: 11

⊙ **43229** **Esophagoscopy, flexible, transoral; with ablation of tumor(s), polyp(s), or other lesion(s) (includes pre- and post-dilation and guide wire passage, when performed)** `G 2 T`

RVU			Global Days	Modifiers				
Mod	Non-Fac Total	Fac Total		51	50	62	80	MUE
	20.54	5.96	000	3	0	0	1	1

AMA: Dec 13: 3

⊙ **43231** **Esophagoscopy, flexible, transoral; with endoscopic ultrasound examination** `A 2 T`

RVU			Global Days	Modifiers				
Mod	Non-Fac Total	Fac Total		51	50	62	80	MUE
	11.40	4.86	000	3	0	2	1	1

AMA: Oct 01: 4, May 04: 6, Oct 08: 6, Mar 09: 8, Jan 13: 11, Dec 13: 3

⊙ **43232** **Esophagoscopy, flexible, transoral; with transendoscopic ultrasound-guided intramural or transmural fine needle aspiration/biopsy(s)** `A 2 T`

RVU			Global Days	Modifiers				
Mod	Non-Fac Total	Fac Total		51	50	62	80	MUE
	13.61	5.98	000	3	0	2	1	1

AMA: Oct 01: 4, Mar 04: 11, May 04: 6, Oct 08: 6, Mar 09: 8, Jan 13: 11, Dec 13: 3, Feb 14: 9

⊙ **43233** **Esophagogastroduodenoscopy, flexible, transoral; with dilation of esophagus with balloon (30 mm diameter or larger) (includes fluoroscopic guidance, when performed)** `G 2 T`

Coding tip: Code 43233 is listed out of numerical order in CPT. Related codes for flexible esophagogastroduodenoscopy - 43235-43273

RVU			Global Days	Modifiers				
Mod	Non-Fac Total	Fac Total		51	50	62	80	MUE
	6.85	6.85	000	3	0	0	1	1

AMA: Dec 13: 3

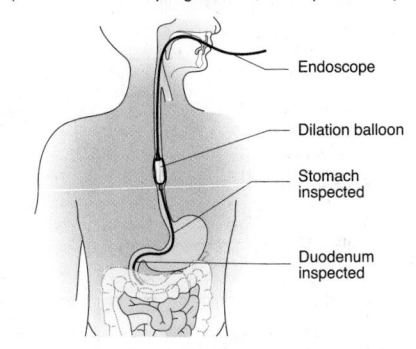

Esophagogastroduodenoscopy, flexible, transoral
With dilation of esophagus with balloon (30 mm diameter or larger) (includes fluoroscopic guidance, when performed)

Endoscope
Dilation balloon
Stomach inspected
Duodenum inspected

⊙ **43235** **Esophagogastroduodenoscopy, flexible, transoral; diagnostic, including collection of specimen(s) by brushing or washing, when performed (separate procedure)** `A 2 T`

Coding tip: Do not code 99143-99145

Coding tip: Report this procedure separately only when performed alone, or distinct from other procedures on the same day

Coding tip: Esophagogastroduodenoscopy, flexible, transoral; with endoscopic stent placement, with pre- and post-dilation and guide wire passage, when performed - 43266

Coding tip: Do not report with any surgical esophagoscopy

Coding tip: Esophagogastroduodenoscopy, flexible, transoral; including ablation of tumor(s), polyp(s), or other lesion(s) with pre- and post-dilation and guide wire passage, when performed - 43270

Coding tip: Codes 99148-99150 may be reported when a second physician or qualified health care professional (other than the one performing the procedure) provides moderate sedation in a facility setting only

Coding tip: Esophagogastroduodenoscopy, flexible, transoral; with dilation of esophagus with balloon (30 mm diameter or larger) (includes fluoroscopic guidance, when performed) - 43233

RVU			Global Days	Modifiers				
Mod	Non-Fac Total	Fac Total		51	50	62	80	MUE
	8.85	3.76	000	2	0	0	1	1

AMA: Spring 94: 4, Dec 97: 11, Jun 03: 11, Sep 03: 3, Oct 08: 6, May 09: 8, Jan 13: 11, Dec 13: 3

⊙ **43236** **Esophagogastroduodenoscopy, flexible, transoral; with directed submucosal injection(s), any substance** `A 2 T`

RVU			Global Days	Modifiers				
Mod	Non-Fac Total	Fac Total		51	50	62	80	MUE
	11.01	4.23	000	3	0	0	1	1

AMA: Jun 10: 4, Jan 13: 11, Dec 13: 3

● New ▲ Revised Deleted ⊙ Moderate Sedation ✚ Add-on Codes ⊘ High Risk Denial Ⓐ Age Edit ♀ Female ♂ Male **AMA** *CPT® Assistant* **MUE** Medically Unlikely Edit
⊘ Modifier 51 Exempt ⊖ Modifier 63 Exempt Ⓧ Unlisted **Modifiers:** *See Inside Back Cover* Ⓜ Maternity A2-Z3 ASC Payment Indicators A-Y OPPS Status Indicators

© 2016 DecisionHealth | CPT © 2015 American Medical Association. All Rights Reserved. | **429**

Surgical Procedures

43237 – 43246

⊙ **43237** **Esophagogastroduodenoscopy, flexible, transoral; with endoscopic ultrasound examination limited to the esophagus, stomach or duodenum, and adjacent structures** A2 T

RVU			Global Days	Modifiers				
Mod	Non-Fac Total	Fac Total		51	50	62	80	MUE
	5.91	5.91	000	3	0	0	1	1

AMA: Jan 13: 11, Dec 13: 3

Endoscopy, upper gastrointestinal

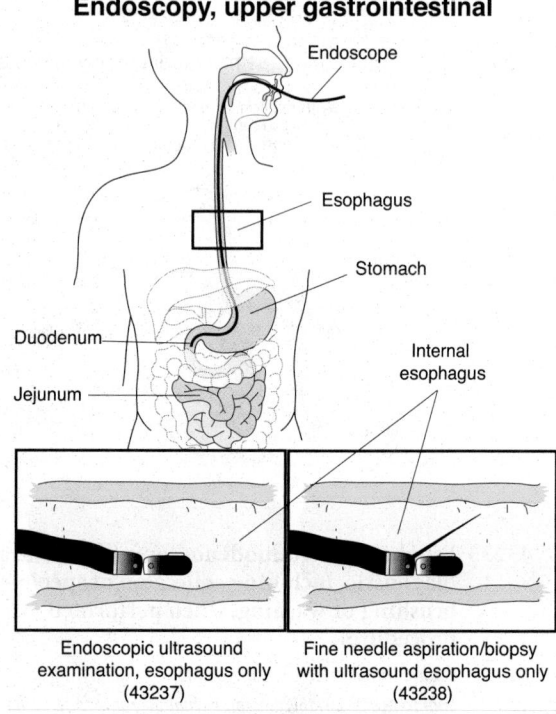

Endoscopic ultrasound examination, esophagus only (43237)

Fine needle aspiration/biopsy with ultrasound esophagus only (43238)

⊙ **43238** **Esophagogastroduodenoscopy, flexible, transoral; with transendoscopic ultrasound-guided intramural or transmural fine needle aspiration/ biopsy(s), (includes endoscopic ultrasound examination limited to the esophagus, stomach or duodenum, and adjacent structures)** A2 T

RVU			Global Days	Modifiers				
Mod	Non-Fac Total	Fac Total		51	50	62	80	MUE
	7.00	7.00	000	3	0	0	1	1

AMA: Jan 13: 11, Dec 13: 3

⊙ **43239** **Esophagogastroduodenoscopy, flexible, transoral; with biopsy, single or multiple** A2 T

Coding tip: Code 99001 for specimen transfer from a facility to an outside laboratory

RVU			Global Days	Modifiers				
Mod	Non-Fac Total	Fac Total		51	50	62	80	MUE
	11.29	4.22	000	3	0	0	1	1

AMA: Spring 94: 4, Apr 98: 14, Feb 99: 11, Oct 01: 4, Nov 07: 9, Jan 13: 11, Dec 13: 3

⊙ **43240** **Esophagogastroduodenoscopy, flexible, transoral; with transmural drainage of pseudocyst (includes placement of transmural drainage catheter[s]/ stent[s], when performed, and endoscopic ultrasound, when performed)** A2 T

RVU			Global Days	Modifiers				
Mod	Non-Fac Total	Fac Total		51	50	62	80	MUE
	11.71	11.71	000	3	0	0	1	1

AMA: Oct 01: 4, Jan 13: 11, Dec 13: 3

⊙ **43241** **Esophagogastroduodenoscopy, flexible, transoral; with insertion of intraluminal tube or catheter** A2 T

RVU			Global Days	Modifiers				
Mod	Non-Fac Total	Fac Total		51	50	62	80	MUE
	4.34	4.34	000	3	0	0	1	1

AMA: Spring 94: 4, Nov 01: 7, Apr 09: 3, Jan 13: 11, Dec 13: 3

⊙ **43242** **Esophagogastroduodenoscopy, flexible, transoral; with transendoscopic ultrasound-guided intramural or transmural fine needle aspiration/ biopsy(s) (includes endoscopic ultrasound examination of the esophagus, stomach, and either the duodenum or a surgically altered stomach where the jejunum is examined distal to the anastomosis)** A2 T

RVU			Global Days	Modifiers				
Mod	Non-Fac Total	Fac Total		51	50	62	80	MUE
	7.89	7.89	000	3	0	0	1	1

AMA: Oct 01: 4, Mar 09: 8, Jan 13: 11, Dec 13: 3

⊙ **43243** **Esophagogastroduodenoscopy, flexible, transoral; with injection sclerosis of esophageal/gastric varices** A2 T

RVU			Global Days	Modifiers				
Mod	Non-Fac Total	Fac Total		51	50	62	80	MUE
	7.13	7.13	000	3	0	0	1	1

AMA: Spring 94: 4, Jun 10: 5, Jan 13: 11, Dec 13: 3

⊙ **43244** **Esophagogastroduodenoscopy, flexible, transoral; with band ligation of esophageal/gastric varices** A2 T

RVU			Global Days	Modifiers				
Mod	Non-Fac Total	Fac Total		51	50	62	80	MUE
	7.38	7.38	000	3	0	0	1	1

AMA: Spring 94: 4, Jun 11: 13, Jan 13: 11, Dec 13: 3

⊙ **43245** **Esophagogastroduodenoscopy, flexible, transoral; with dilation of gastric/duodenal stricture(s) (eg, balloon, bougie)** A2 T

Coding tip: Dilation with imaging guidance - add 74360

RVU			Global Days	Modifiers				
Mod	Non-Fac Total	Fac Total		51	50	62	80	MUE
	17.45	5.32	000	3	0	0	1	1

AMA: Spring 94: 4, Oct 01: 4, Jan 04: 26, Jan 13: 11, Dec 13: 3

⊙ **43246** **Esophagogastroduodenoscopy, flexible, transoral; with directed placement of percutaneous gastrostomy tube** A2 T

RVU			Global Days	Modifiers				
Mod	Non-Fac Total	Fac Total		51	50	62	80	MUE
	6.04	6.04	000	3	0	2	0	1

AMA: Spring 94: 4, Feb 97: 10, Mar 10: 10, Jan 13: 11, May 13: 12, Dec 13: 3

● New   ▲ Revised   ✖ Deleted   ⊙ Moderate Sedation   ✚ Add-on Codes   ⊖ High Risk Denial   Ⓐ Age Edit   ♀ Female   ♂ Male   **AMA** *CPT® Assistant*   **MUE** Medically Unlikely Edit

⊘ Modifier 51 Exempt   ⊖ Modifier 63 Exempt   ✗ Unlisted   **Modifiers:** *See Inside Back Cover*   Ⓜ Maternity   A2–Z3 ASC Payment Indicators   A–Y OPPS Status Indicators

CPT © 2015 American Medical Association. All Rights Reserved.   © 2016 DecisionHealth

Coding Guidance
Upper gastrointestinal endoscopy with removal of foreign body is not appropriate to bill separately for routine removal of previously placed therapeutic devices, such as a G-tube.

⊙ **43247 Esophagogastroduodenoscopy, flexible, transoral; with removal of foreign body(s)** A2T

Coding tip: Removal of esophageal foreign body with radiological supervision - add 74235

RVU			Global Days	Modifiers				
Mod	Non-Fac Total	Fac Total			51	50	62	80	MUE
	11.83	5.37	000		3	0	0	1	1

AMA: Spring 94: 4, Jan 13: 11, Dec 13: 3

Endoscopy, upper gastrointestinal

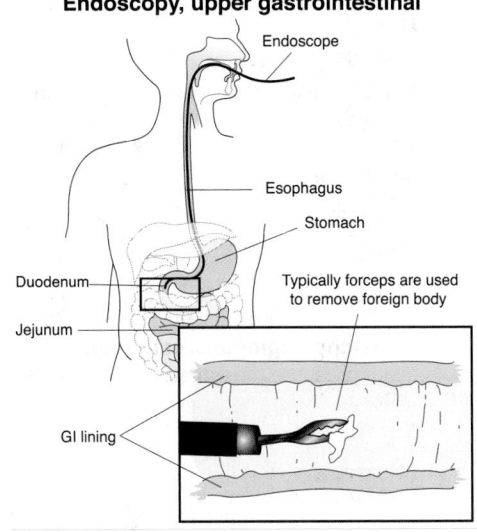

Endoscope
Esophagus
Stomach
Duodenum
Jejunum
Typically forceps are used to remove foreign body
GI lining

⊙ **43248 Esophagogastroduodenoscopy, flexible, transoral; with insertion of guide wire followed by passage of dilator(s) through esophagus over guide wire** A2T

Coding tip: Dilation of esophagus over guidewire with imaging guidance - add 74360

RVU			Global Days	Modifiers				
Mod	Non-Fac Total	Fac Total			51	50	62	80	MUE
	11.61	5.04	000		3	0	0	1	1

AMA: Spring 94: 4, Dec 97: 11, Oct 08: 6, Jan 13: 11, Dec 13: 3

⊙ **43249 Esophagogastroduodenoscopy, flexible, transoral; with transendoscopic balloon dilation of esophagus (less than 30 mm diameter)** A2T

Coding tip: Balloon dilation of esophagus with imaging guidance - add 74360

RVU			Global Days	Modifiers				
Mod	Non-Fac Total	Fac Total			51	50	62	80	MUE
	30.52	4.67	000		3	0	0	1	1

AMA: May 05: 3, Jan 13: 11, Dec 13: 3

⊙ **43250 Esophagogastroduodenoscopy, flexible, transoral; with removal of tumor(s), polyp(s), or other lesion(s) by hot biopsy forceps** A2T

Coding tip: Code 99001 for specimen transfer from a facility to an outside laboratory

RVU			Global Days	Modifiers				
Mod	Non-Fac Total	Fac Total			51	50	62	80	MUE
	12.96	5.15	000		3	0	0	1	1

AMA: Spring 94: 4, Feb 99: 11, Nov 07: 9, Jan 13: 11, Dec 13: 3

⊙ **43251 Esophagogastroduodenoscopy, flexible, transoral; with removal of tumor(s), polyp(s), or other lesion(s) by snare technique** A2T

RVU			Global Days	Modifiers				
Mod	Non-Fac Total	Fac Total			51	50	62	80	MUE
	14.19	5.93	000		3	0	0	1	1

AMA: Spring 94: 4, Oct 04: 12, Nov 07: 9, Jun 11: 13, Jan 13: 11, Dec 13: 3

⊙ **43252 Esophagogastroduodenoscopy, flexible, transoral; with optical endomicroscopy** G2T

RVU			Global Days	Modifiers				
Mod	Non-Fac Total	Fac Total			51	50	62	80	MUE
	10.45	5.10	000		3	0	0	1	1

AMA: Jan 13: 11, Aug 13: 5, Dec 13: 3

Esophagogastroduodenoscopy, flexible, transoral; with optical endomicroscopy

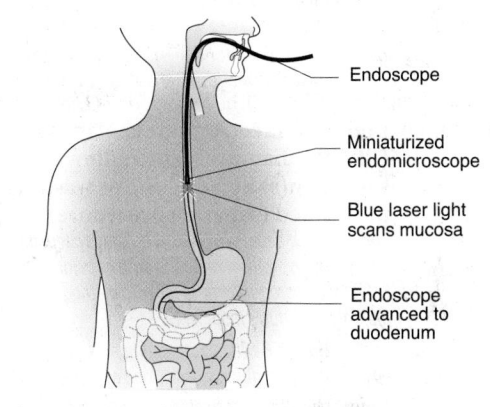

Endoscope
Miniaturized endomicroscope
Blue laser light scans mucosa
Endoscope advanced to duodenum

⊙ **43253 Esophagogastroduodenoscopy, flexible, transoral; with transendoscopic ultrasound-guided transmural injection of diagnostic or therapeutic substance(s) (eg, anesthetic, neurolytic agent) or fiducial marker(s) (includes endoscopic ultrasound examination of the esophagus, stomach, and either the duodenum or a surgically altered stomach where the jejunum is examined distal to the anastomosis)** G2T

RVU			Global Days	Modifiers				
Mod	Non-Fac Total	Fac Total			51	50	62	80	MUE
	7.87	7.87	000		3	0	0	1	1

AMA: Dec 13: 3

⊙ **43254 Esophagogastroduodenoscopy, flexible, transoral; with endoscopic mucosal resection** G2T

RVU			Global Days	Modifiers				
Mod	Non-Fac Total	Fac Total			51	50	62	80	MUE
	8.11	8.11	000		3	0	0	1	1

AMA: Dec 13: 3

⊙ **43255 Esophagogastroduodenoscopy, flexible, transoral; with control of bleeding, any method** A2T

RVU			Global Days	Modifiers				
Mod	Non-Fac Total	Fac Total			51	50	62	80	MUE
	20.74	6.06	000		3	0	0	1	2

AMA: Spring 94: 4, Jun 10: 4, Dec 13: 3

● New   ▲ Revised   Deleted   ⊙ Moderate Sedation   ✚ Add-on Codes   ⊘ High Risk Denial   Ⓐ Age Edit   ♀ Female   ♂ Male   **AMA** CPT® Assistant   **MUE** Medically Unlikely Edit
⊘ Modifier 51 Exempt   ⊖ Modifier 63 Exempt   ✗ Unlisted   **Modifiers:** See Inside Back Cover   Ⓜ Maternity   A2–Z3 ASC Payment Indicators   A–Y OPPS Status Indicators

43247 – 43255

⊙ **43257** **Esophagogastroduodenoscopy, flexible, transoral; with delivery of thermal energy to the muscle of lower esophageal sphincter and/or gastric cardia, for treatment of gastroesophageal reflux disease** A2 T

RVU			Global Days	Modifiers				
Mod	Non-Fac Total	Fac Total		51	50	62	80	MUE
	7.01	7.01	000	3	0	0	1	1

AMA: May 05: 3, Jan 13: 11, Dec 13: 3

⊙ **43259** **Esophagogastroduodenoscopy, flexible, transoral; with endoscopic ultrasound examination, including the esophagus, stomach, and either the duodenum or a surgically altered stomach where the jejunum is examined distal to the anastomosis** A2 T

RVU			Global Days	Modifiers				
Mod	Non-Fac Total	Fac Total		51	50	62	80	MUE
	6.81	6.81	000	3	0	0	1	1

AMA: Spring 94: 4, May 04: 7, Mar 09: 8, Jan 13: 11, Dec 13: 3

Pub 100-04, 12, 30.1

Coding Guidance

When imaging guidance is used for ERCP procedures reported with 43260-43272, add 74328 for biliary duct catheterization guidance, 74329 for pancreatic duct catheterization guidance, and 74330 for both combined.

⊙ **43260** **Endoscopic retrograde cholangiopancreatography (ERCP); diagnostic, including collection of specimen(s) by brushing or washing, when performed (separate procedure)** A2 T

Coding tip: If hepatic/biliary/pancreatic system diagnostic endoscopy requires using multiple methods, such as biliary T-tube endoscopy and ERCP, then appropriate codes for each method may be reported with a multiple procedures modifier

Coding tip: ERCP with ablation of tumors, polyps, lesions, with pre- and post-dilation and guidewire passage when performed - 43278

Coding tip: ERCP with foreign body or stents removal from biliary or pancreatic duct(s) - 43275

Coding tip: ERCP with trans-endoscopic balloon dilation of biliary or pancreatic duct(s), or sphincteroplasty (ampulla) including sphincterotomy when performed (each duct) - 43277

Coding tip: ERCP with stent placement into biliary or pancreatic duct with pre- and post-dilation, guide wire passage, and sphincterotomy when performed - 43274

Coding tip: ERCP with stent removal and exchange (each stent) from biliary or pancreatic duct with pre- and post-dilation, guide wire passage, and sphincterotomy when performed - 43276

RVU			Global Days	Modifiers				
Mod	Non-Fac Total	Fac Total		51	50	62	80	MUE
	9.64	9.64	000	2	0	0	1	1

AMA: Spring 94: 5, Oct 04: 13, May 08: 14, Aug 08: 12, Jan 12: 12, Jan 13: 11, Dec 13: 3

Endoscopic retrograde cholangiopancreatography (ERCP)

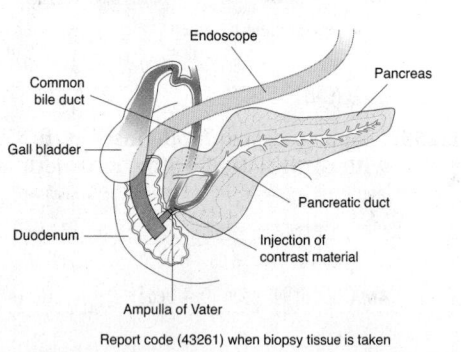

Report code (43261) when biopsy tissue is taken

⊙ **43261** **Endoscopic retrograde cholangiopancreatography (ERCP); with biopsy, single or multiple** A2 T

Coding tip: Code 99001 for specimen transfer from a facility to an outside laboratory

RVU			Global Days	Modifiers				
Mod	Non-Fac Total	Fac Total		51	50	62	80	MUE
	10.13	10.13	000	3	0	0	1	1

AMA: Spring 94: 5, Aug 08: 12, Jun 11: 13, Jan 13: 11

⊙ **43262** **Endoscopic retrograde cholangiopancreatography (ERCP); with sphincterotomy/papillotomy** A2 T

RVU			Global Days	Modifiers				
Mod	Non-Fac Total	Fac Total		51	50	62	80	MUE
	10.67	10.67	000	3	0	0	1	2

AMA: Spring 94: 5, Oct 04: 13, Jul 09: 10, Jan 13: 11

⊙ **43263** **Endoscopic retrograde cholangiopancreatography (ERCP); with pressure measurement of sphincter of Oddi** A2 T

RVU			Global Days	Modifiers				
Mod	Non-Fac Total	Fac Total		51	50	62	80	MUE
	10.69	10.69	000	3	0	0	1	1

AMA: Spring 94: 5, Oct 04: 13, Jan 13: 11, Dec 13: 3

Endoscopic retrograde cholangiopancreatography (ERCP)
(with pressure measurement of sphincter of Oddi)

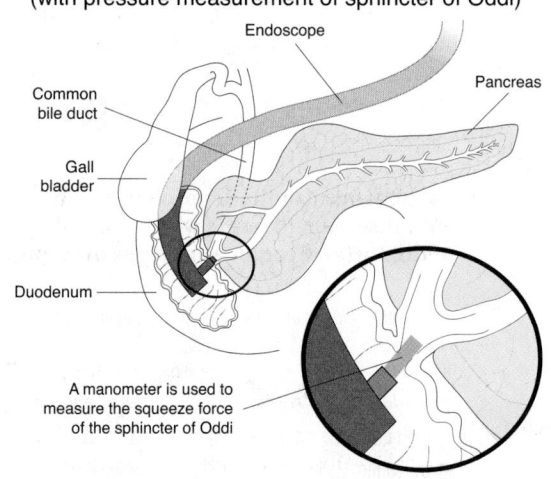

A manometer is used to measure the squeeze force of the sphincter of Oddi

⊙ **43264** **Endoscopic retrograde cholangiopancreatography (ERCP); with removal of calculi/debris from biliary/pancreatic duct(s)** A2 T

RVU			Global Days	Modifiers				
Mod	Non-Fac Total	Fac Total		51	50	62	80	MUE
	10.87	10.87	000	3	0	0	1	1

AMA: Spring 94: 5, Jan 13: 11, Dec 13: 3

⊙ **43265** **Endoscopic retrograde cholangiopancreatography (ERCP); with destruction of calculi, any method (eg, mechanical, electrohydraulic, lithotripsy)** A2 T

RVU			Global Days	Modifiers				
Mod	Non-Fac Total	Fac Total		51	50	62	80	MUE
	12.92	12.92	000	3	0	0	1	1

AMA: Spring 94: 5, Jan 13: 11, Dec 13: 3

● New   ▲ Revised   ✖ Deleted   ⊙ Moderate Sedation   ✚ Add-on Codes   ⊘ High Risk Denial   Ⓐ Age Edit   ♀ Female   ♂ Male   **AMA** *CPT® Assistant*   *MUE* Medically Unlikely Edit
⊗ Modifier 51 Exempt   ⊖ Modifier 63 Exempt   ✗ Unlisted   **Modifiers:** *See Inside Back Cover*   Ⓜ Maternity   A2–Z3 ASC Payment Indicators   A–Y OPPS Status Indicators

432   CPT © 2015 American Medical Association. All Rights Reserved.   © 2016 DecisionHealth

⊙ **43266** **Esophagogastroduodenoscopy, flexible, transoral; with placement of endoscopic stent (includes pre- and post-dilation and guide wire passage, when performed)**   G2 J 1

Coding tip: Code 43266 is listed out of numerical order in CPT. Related codes for flexible esophagogastroduodenoscopy - 43235-43259, 43270

RVU			Global Days	Modifiers				
Mod	Non-Fac Total	Fac Total		51	50	62	80	MUE
	6.81	6.81	000	3	0	0	1	1

AMA: Dec 13: 3

Esophagogastroduodenoscopy, flexible, transoral; with placement of endoscopic stent

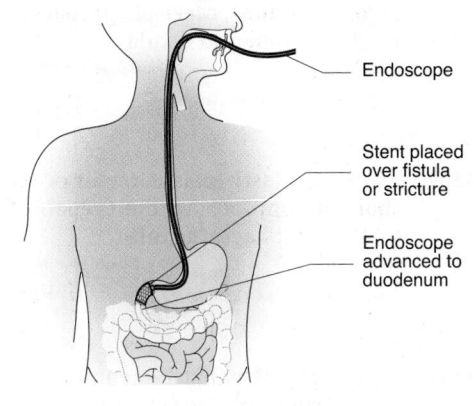

Endoscope

Stent placed over fistula or stricture

Endoscope advanced to duodenum

⊙ **43270** **Esophagogastroduodenoscopy, flexible, transoral; with ablation of tumor(s), polyp(s), or other lesion(s) (includes pre- and post-dilation and guide wire passage, when performed)**   G2 T

Coding tip: Code 43270 is listed out of numerical order in CPT. Related codes for flexible esophagogastroduodenoscopy - 43235-43259, 43266

RVU			Global Days	Modifiers				
Mod	Non-Fac Total	Fac Total		51	50	62	80	MUE
	21.36	7.00	000	3	0	0	1	1

AMA: Dec 13: 3

⊙+**43273** **Endoscopic cannulation of papilla with direct visualization of pancreatic/common bile duct(s) (List separately in addition to code(s) for primary procedure)**   N 1 N

RVU			Global Days	Modifiers				
Mod	Non-Fac Total	Fac Total		51	50	62	80	MUE
	3.52	3.52	ZZZ	0	0	0	0	1

AMA: Jan 13: 11, Dec 13: 3

⊙ **43274** **Endoscopic retrograde cholangiopancreatography (ERCP); with placement of endoscopic stent into biliary or pancreatic duct, including pre- and post-dilation and guide wire passage, when performed, including sphincterotomy, when performed, each stent**   G2 J 1

Coding tip: Code 43274 is listed out of numerical order in CPT. Related codes for ERCP - 43260-43265, 43273, 43275-43278

RVU			Global Days	Modifiers				
Mod	Non-Fac Total	Fac Total		51	50	62	80	MUE
	13.79	13.79	000	3	0	0	1	2

AMA: Dec 13: 3

Endoscopic retrograde cholangiopancreatography (ERCP); with placement of endoscopic stent into biliary or pancreatic duct, including sphincterotomy, when performed

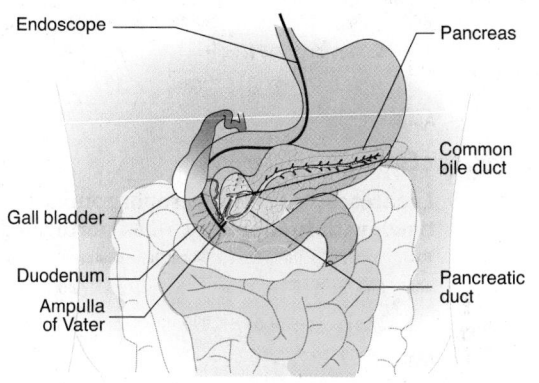

Endoscope

Pancreas

Common bile duct

Gall bladder

Duodenum

Ampulla of Vater

Pancreatic duct

⊙ **43275** **Endoscopic retrograde cholangiopancreatography (ERCP); with removal of foreign body(s) or stent(s) from biliary/pancreatic duct(s)**   G2 T

Coding tip: Code 43275 is listed out of numerical order in CPT. Related codes for ERCP - 43260-43265, 43273-43274, 43276-43278

RVU			Global Days	Modifiers				
Mod	Non-Fac Total	Fac Total		51	50	62	80	MUE
	11.24	11.24	000	3	0	0	1	1

AMA: Dec 13: 3

⊙ **43276** **Endoscopic retrograde cholangiopancreatography (ERCP); with removal and exchange of stent(s), biliary or pancreatic duct, including pre- and post-dilation and guide wire passage, when performed, including sphincterotomy, when performed, each stent exchanged**   G2 J 1

Coding tip: Code 43276 is listed out of numerical order in CPT. Related codes for ERCP - 43260-43265, 43273-43275, 43277-43278

RVU			Global Days	Modifiers				
Mod	Non-Fac Total	Fac Total		51	50	62	80	MUE
	14.35	14.35	000	3	0	0	1	2

AMA: Dec 13: 3

43266 – 43276

● New   ▲ Revised   Deleted   ⊙ Moderate Sedation   ✚ Add-on Codes   ⊘ High Risk Denial   ⒶAge Edit   ♀ Female   ♂ Male   **AMA** *CPT® Assistant*   **MUE** Medically Unlikely Edit
⊘ Modifier 51 Exempt   ⊖ Modifier 63 Exempt   ✗ Unlisted   **Modifiers:** *See Inside Back Cover*   Ⓜ Maternity   A2–Z3 ASC Payment Indicators   A–Y OPPS Status Indicators

Surgical Procedures

43277 – 43325

⊙ **43277 Endoscopic retrograde cholangiopancreatography (ERCP); with trans-endoscopic balloon dilation of biliary/pancreatic duct(s) or of ampulla (sphincteroplasty), including sphincterotomy, when performed, each duct** G2T

Coding tip: Code 43277 is listed out of numerical order in CPT. Related codes for ERCP - 43260-43265, 43273-43276, 43278

RVU		Global Days	Modifiers				
Mod	*Non-Fac Total*	*Fac Total*		51	50	62	80	MUE
	11.30	11.30	000	3	0	0	1	3

AMA: Dec 13: 3

⊙ **43278 Endoscopic retrograde cholangiopancreatography (ERCP); with ablation of tumor(s), polyp(s), or other lesion(s), including pre- and post-dilation and guide wire passage, when performed** G2T

Coding tip: Code 43278 is listed out of numerical order in CPT. Related codes for ERCP - 43260-43265, 43273-43277

RVU		Global Days	Modifiers				
Mod	*Non-Fac Total*	*Fac Total*		51	50	62	80	MUE
	12.91	12.91	000	3	0	0	1	1

AMA: Dec 13: 3

Laparoscopic Esophageal Procedures

43279 Laparoscopy, surgical, esophagomyotomy (Heller type), with fundoplasty, when performed C

RVU		Global Days	Modifiers				
Mod	*Non-Fac Total*	*Fac Total*		51	50	62	80	MUE
	37.61	37.61	090	2	0	1	2	1

AMA: Feb 12: 3

43280 Laparoscopy, surgical, esophagogastric fundoplasty (eg, Nissen, Toupet procedures) J1

RVU		Global Days	Modifiers				
Mod	*Non-Fac Total*	*Fac Total*		51	50	62	80	MUE
	31.39	31.39	090	2	0	1	2	1

AMA: Nov 99: 22, Mar 00: 8, Dec 02: 2, Jun 11: 8, Feb 12: 3, Dec 14: 16

43281 Laparoscopy, surgical, repair of paraesophageal hernia, includes fundoplasty, when performed; without implantation of mesh J1

RVU		Global Days	Modifiers				
Mod	*Non-Fac Total*	*Fac Total*		51	50	62	80	MUE
	44.82	44.82	090	2	0	1	2	1

AMA: Jun 11: 9, Feb 12: 3, Dec 14: 16

43282 Laparoscopy, surgical, repair of paraesophageal hernia, includes fundoplasty, when performed; with implantation of mesh C

RVU		Global Days	Modifiers				
Mod	*Non-Fac Total*	*Fac Total*		51	50	62	80	MUE
	50.37	50.37	090	2	0	1	2	1

AMA: Jun 11: 9, Feb 12: 3, Dec 14: 16

✚ **43283 Laparoscopy, surgical, esophageal lengthening procedure (eg, Collis gastroplasty or wedge gastroplasty) (List separately in addition to code for primary procedure)** C

RVU		Global Days	Modifiers				
Mod	*Non-Fac Total*	*Fac Total*		51	50	62	80	MUE
	4.60	4.60	ZZZ	0	0	1	2	1

AMA: Jun 11: 9, Feb 12: 3

43289 Unlisted laparoscopy procedure, esophagus ✗ J1

RVU		Global Days	Modifiers				
Mod	*Non-Fac Total*	*Fac Total*		51	50	62	80	MUE
	0.00	0.00	YYY	2	1	1	2	

AMA: Nov 99: 22, Mar 00: 8, Dec 14: 16

Esophageal Repair

43300 Esophagoplasty (plastic repair or reconstruction), cervical approach; without repair of tracheoesophageal fistula C

RVU		Global Days	Modifiers				
Mod	*Non-Fac Total*	*Fac Total*		51	50	62	80	MUE
	17.94	17.94	090	2	0	1	2	1

43305 Esophagoplasty (plastic repair or reconstruction), cervical approach; with repair of tracheoesophageal fistula C

RVU		Global Days	Modifiers				
Mod	*Non-Fac Total*	*Fac Total*		51	50	62	80	MUE
	31.97	31.97	090	2	0	1	2	1

43310 Esophagoplasty (plastic repair or reconstruction), thoracic approach; without repair of tracheoesophageal fistula C

RVU		Global Days	Modifiers				
Mod	*Non-Fac Total*	*Fac Total*		51	50	62	80	MUE
	43.54	43.54	090	2	0	1	2	1

43312 Esophagoplasty (plastic repair or reconstruction), thoracic approach; with repair of tracheoesophageal fistula C

RVU		Global Days	Modifiers				
Mod	*Non-Fac Total*	*Fac Total*		51	50	62	80	MUE
	47.22	47.22	090	2	0	1	2	1

43313 Esophagoplasty for congenital defect (plastic repair or reconstruction), thoracic approach; without repair of congenital tracheoesophageal fistula ⊖C

RVU		Global Days	Modifiers				
Mod	*Non-Fac Total*	*Fac Total*		51	50	62	80	MUE
	78.71	78.71	090	2	0	1	2	1

43314 Esophagoplasty for congenital defect (plastic repair or reconstruction), thoracic approach; with repair of congenital tracheoesophageal fistula ⊖C

RVU		Global Days	Modifiers				
Mod	*Non-Fac Total*	*Fac Total*		51	50	62	80	MUE
	89.98	89.98	090	2	0	1	2	1

43320 Esophagogastrostomy (cardioplasty), with or without vagotomy and pyloroplasty, transabdominal or transthoracic approach C

RVU		Global Days	Modifiers				
Mod	*Non-Fac Total*	*Fac Total*		51	50	62	80	MUE
	40.51	40.51	090	2	0	1	2	1

43325 Esophagogastric fundoplasty, with fundic patch (Thal-Nissen procedure) C

RVU		Global Days	Modifiers				
Mod	*Non-Fac Total*	*Fac Total*		51	50	62	80	MUE
	38.95	38.95	090	2	0	1	2	1

AMA: Winter 90: 6

● New   ▲ Revised   ✖ Deleted   ⊙ Moderate Sedation   ✚ Add-on Codes   ⊘ High Risk Denial   Ⓐ Age Edit   ♀ Female   ♂ Male   **AMA** *CPT® Assistant*   **MUE** Medically Unlikely Edit

⊘ Modifier 51 Exempt   ⊖ Modifier 63 Exempt   ✗ Unlisted   **Modifiers:** *See Inside Back Cover*   Ⓜ Maternity   A2–Z3 ASC Payment Indicators   A–Y OPPS Status Indicators

CPT © 2015 American Medical Association. All Rights Reserved.   © 2016 DecisionHealth

43327 Esophagogastric fundoplasty partial or complete; laparotomy C

RVU			Global Days	Modifiers				
Mod	Non-Fac Total	Fac Total		51	50	62	80	MUE
	23.84	23.84	090	2	0	1	2	1

AMA: Jun 11: 8, Feb 12: 3

43328 Esophagogastric fundoplasty partial or complete; thoracotomy C

RVU			Global Days	Modifiers				
Mod	Non-Fac Total	Fac Total		51	50	62	80	MUE
	33.09	33.09	090	2	0	1	2	1

AMA: Jun 11: 8, Feb 12: 3

43330 Esophagomyotomy (Heller type); abdominal approach C

RVU			Global Days	Modifiers				
Mod	Non-Fac Total	Fac Total		51	50	62	80	MUE
	38.67	38.67	090	2	0	1	2	1

AMA: Nov 99: 22

Esophagomyotomy (Heller type)

Esophagus
Stomach
Diaphragm
Thoracic (43331), abdominal (43330), approaches
Esophagus
Incision
Diaphragm

Small incisions are made in the muscles surrounding the bottom of the esophagus

43331 Esophagomyotomy (Heller type); thoracic approach C

RVU			Global Days	Modifiers				
Mod	Non-Fac Total	Fac Total		51	50	62	80	MUE
	39.34	39.34	090	2	0	1	2	1

AMA: Nov 99: 22

43332 Repair, paraesophageal hiatal hernia (including fundoplication), via laparotomy, except neonatal; without implantation of mesh or other prosthesis C

RVU			Global Days	Modifiers				
Mod	Non-Fac Total	Fac Total		51	50	62	80	MUE
	33.75	33.75	090	2	0	1	2	1

AMA: Feb 12: 3

43333 Repair, paraesophageal hiatal hernia (including fundoplication), via laparotomy, except neonatal; with implantation of mesh or other prosthesis C

RVU			Global Days	Modifiers				
Mod	Non-Fac Total	Fac Total		51	50	62	80	MUE
	36.81	36.81	090	2	0	1	2	1

AMA: Feb 12: 3

43334 Repair, paraesophageal hiatal hernia (including fundoplication), via thoracotomy, except neonatal; without implantation of mesh or other prosthesis C

RVU			Global Days	Modifiers				
Mod	Non-Fac Total	Fac Total		51	50	62	80	MUE
	36.61	36.61	090	2	0	1	2	1

AMA: Feb 12: 3

43335 Repair, paraesophageal hiatal hernia (including fundoplication), via thoracotomy, except neonatal; with implantation of mesh or other prosthesis C

RVU			Global Days	Modifiers				
Mod	Non-Fac Total	Fac Total		51	50	62	80	MUE
	39.30	39.30	090	2	0	1	2	1

AMA: Feb 12: 3

43336 Repair, paraesophageal hiatal hernia, (including fundoplication), via thoracoabdominal incision, except neonatal; without implantation of mesh or other prosthesis C

RVU			Global Days	Modifiers				
Mod	Non-Fac Total	Fac Total		51	50	62	80	MUE
	44.05	44.05	090	2	0	1	2	1

AMA: Feb 12: 3

43337 Repair, paraesophageal hiatal hernia, (including fundoplication), via thoracoabdominal incision, except neonatal; with implantation of mesh or other prosthesis C

RVU			Global Days	Modifiers				
Mod	Non-Fac Total	Fac Total		51	50	62	80	MUE
	47.51	47.51	090	2	0	1	2	1

AMA: Feb 12: 3

+ 43338 Esophageal lengthening procedure (eg, Collis gastroplasty or wedge gastroplasty) (List separately in addition to code for primary procedure) C

RVU			Global Days	Modifiers				
Mod	Non-Fac Total	Fac Total		51	50	62	80	MUE
	3.39	3.39	ZZZ	0	0	1	2	1

AMA: Jun 11: 10, Feb 12: 3

43340 Esophagojejunostomy (without total gastrectomy); abdominal approach C

RVU			Global Days	Modifiers				
Mod	Non-Fac Total	Fac Total		51	50	62	80	MUE
	39.64	39.64	090	2	0	1	2	1

43341 Esophagojejunostomy (without total gastrectomy); thoracic approach ⊘C

RVU			Global Days	Modifiers				
Mod	Non-Fac Total	Fac Total		51	50	62	80	MUE
	43.06	43.06	090	2	0	1	2	1

43351 Esophagostomy, fistulization of esophagus, external; thoracic approach C

RVU			Global Days	Modifiers				
Mod	Non-Fac Total	Fac Total		51	50	62	80	MUE
	37.58	37.58	090	2	0	1	2	1

● New ▲ Revised Deleted ⊙ Moderate Sedation ✚ Add-on Codes ⊘ High Risk Denial Ⓐ Age Edit ♀ Female ♂ Male **AMA** CPT® Assistant **MUE** Medically Unlikely Edit ⊘ Modifier 51 Exempt ⊖ Modifier 63 Exempt Ⓧ Unlisted **Modifiers:** See Inside Back Cover Ⓜ Maternity A2–Z3 ASC Payment Indicators A–Y OPPS Status Indicators

© 2016 DecisionHealth CPT © 2015 American Medical Association. All Rights Reserved. **435**

43352 Esophagostomy, fistulization of esophagus, external; cervical approach   C

RVU			Global Days	Modifiers				
Mod	Non-Fac Total	Fac Total		51	50	62	80	MUE
	31.29	31.29	090	2	0	1	2	1

43360 Gastrointestinal reconstruction for previous esophagectomy, for obstructing esophageal lesion or fistula, or for previous esophageal exclusion; with stomach, with or without pyloroplasty   C

RVU			Global Days	Modifiers				
Mod	Non-Fac Total	Fac Total		51	50	62	80	MUE
	68.94	68.94	090	2	0	1	2	1

43361 Gastrointestinal reconstruction for previous esophagectomy, for obstructing esophageal lesion or fistula, or for previous esophageal exclusion; with colon interposition or small intestine reconstruction, including intestine mobilization, preparation, and anastomosis(es)   C

RVU			Global Days	Modifiers				
Mod	Non-Fac Total	Fac Total		51	50	62	80	MUE
	74.77	74.77	090	2	0	1	2	1

43400 Ligation, direct, esophageal varices   C

RVU			Global Days	Modifiers				
Mod	Non-Fac Total	Fac Total		51	50	62	80	MUE
	43.19	43.19	090	2	0	1	2	1

Ligation of esophageal varices

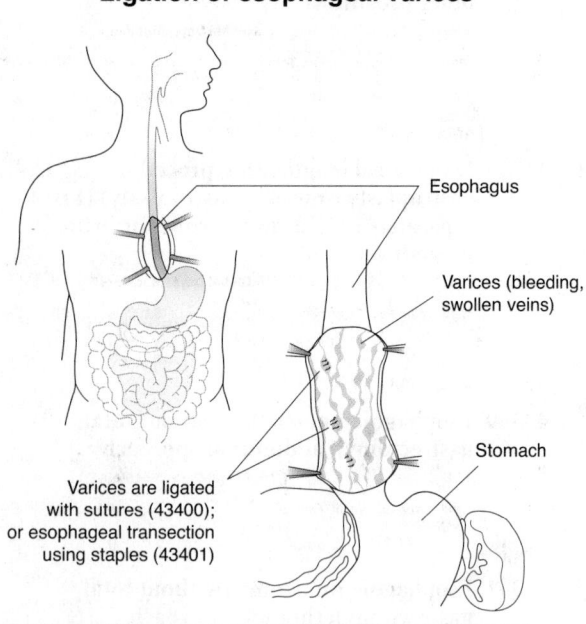

Esophagus

Varices (bleeding, swollen veins)

Stomach

Varices are ligated with sutures (43400); or esophageal transection using staples (43401)

43401 Transection of esophagus with repair, for esophageal varices   C

RVU			Global Days	Modifiers				
Mod	Non-Fac Total	Fac Total		51	50	62	80	MUE
	45.61	45.61	090	2	0	1	2	1

43405 Ligation or stapling at gastroesophageal junction for pre-existing esophageal perforation   C

RVU			Global Days	Modifiers				
Mod	Non-Fac Total	Fac Total		51	50	62	80	MUE
	42.72	42.72	090	2	0	1	2	1

43410 Suture of esophageal wound or injury; cervical approach   C

RVU			Global Days	Modifiers				
Mod	Non-Fac Total	Fac Total		51	50	62	80	MUE
	30.59	30.59	090	2	0	1	2	1

AMA: Jun 96: 7

43415 Suture of esophageal wound or injury; transthoracic or transabdominal approach   C

RVU			Global Days	Modifiers				
Mod	Non-Fac Total	Fac Total		51	50	62	80	MUE
	75.16	75.16	090	2	0	1	2	1

43420 Closure of esophagostomy or fistula; cervical approach   T

RVU			Global Days	Modifiers				
Mod	Non-Fac Total	Fac Total		51	50	62	80	MUE
	29.57	29.57	090	2	0	1	0	1

43425 Closure of esophagostomy or fistula; transthoracic or transabdominal approach   C

RVU			Global Days	Modifiers				
Mod	Non-Fac Total	Fac Total		51	50	62	80	MUE
	42.07	42.07	090	2	0	1	2	1

Esophageal Manipulation

Coding Guidance

If dilation of the esophagus in codes 43450-43458 is unsuccessful and an endoscopic esophageal dilation procedure then succeeds, only the endoscopic procedure should be reported.

43450 Dilation of esophagus, by unguided sound or bougie, single or multiple passes   A2 T

Coding tip: *Dilation with imaging guidance - add 74360*

RVU			Global Days	Modifiers				
Mod	Non-Fac Total	Fac Total		51	50	62	80	MUE
	6.02	2.48	000	2	0	0	1	1

AMA: Spring 94: 1, Jan 97: 10, Apr 98: 14, Jun 98: 10, Dec 13: 3

Dilation of esophagus

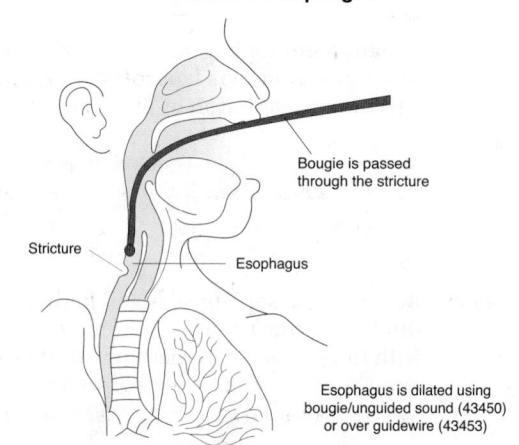

Bougie is passed through the stricture

Stricture

Esophagus

Esophagus is dilated using bougie/unguided sound (43450) or over guidewire (43453)

● New   ▲ Revised   ✖ Deleted   ⊙ Moderate Sedation   ✚ Add-on Codes   ⊘ High Risk Denial   Ⓐ Age Edit   ♀ Female   ♂ Male   **AMA** *CPT® Assistant*   **MUE** Medically Unlikely Edit

⊘ Modifier 51 Exempt   ⊖ Modifier 63 Exempt   Ⓧ Unlisted   **Modifiers:** *See Inside Back Cover*   Ⓜ Maternity   A2–Z3 ASC Payment Indicators   A–Y OPPS Status Indicators

436

CPT © 2015 American Medical Association. All Rights Reserved.   © 2016 DecisionHealth

⊙ **43453** **Dilation of esophagus, over guide wire** `A 2 T`

Coding tip: *Dilation with imaging guidance - add 74360*

RVU			Global Days	Modifiers				
Mod	Non-Fac Total	Fac Total		51	50	62	80	MUE
	27.45	2.67	000	2	0	0	1	1

AMA: Spring 94: 1, Jan 97: 10, Dec 97: 11

43460 **Esophagogastric tamponade, with balloon (Sengstaken type)** `C`

RVU			Global Days	Modifiers				
Mod	Non-Fac Total	Fac Total		51	50	62	80	MUE
	6.26	6.26	000	2	0	0	1	1

Other Esophageal Procedures

43496 **Free jejunum transfer with microvascular anastomosis** `C`

RVU			Global Days	Modifiers				
Mod	Non-Fac Total	Fac Total		51	50	62	80	MUE
	0.00	0.00	090	2	0	1	2	1

AMA: Nov 96: 8, Apr 97: 4, Jun 97: 10, Nov 97: 17, Nov 98: 16

43499 **Unlisted procedure, esophagus** `x T`

RVU			Global Days	Modifiers				
Mod	Non-Fac Total	Fac Total		51	50	62	80	MUE
	0.00	0.00	YYY	2	0	1	1	

AMA: May 07: 10, May 11: 9, Dec 11: 19, Oct 10: 12, Dec 10: 12, Mar 13: 13

Stomach Procedures

Incisional Stomach Procedures

43500 **Gastrotomy; with exploration or foreign body removal** `C`

RVU			Global Days	Modifiers				
Mod	Non-Fac Total	Fac Total		51	50	62	80	MUE
	22.75	22.75	090	2	0	1	2	1

43501 **Gastrotomy; with suture repair of bleeding ulcer** `C`

RVU			Global Days	Modifiers				
Mod	Non-Fac Total	Fac Total		51	50	62	80	MUE
	39.07	39.07	090	2	0	1	2	1

43502 **Gastrotomy; with suture repair of pre-existing esophagogastric laceration (eg, Mallory-Weiss)** `C`

RVU			Global Days	Modifiers				
Mod	Non-Fac Total	Fac Total		51	50	62	80	MUE
	44.26	44.26	090	2	0	1	2	1

43510 **Gastrotomy; with esophageal dilation and insertion of permanent intraluminal tube (eg, Celestin or Mousseaux-Barbin)** `T`

RVU			Global Days	Modifiers				
Mod	Non-Fac Total	Fac Total		51	50	62	80	MUE
	27.45	27.45	090	2	0	1	2	1

43520 **Pyloromyotomy, cutting of pyloric muscle (Fredet-Ramstedt type operation)** `⊖ C`

RVU			Global Days	Modifiers				
Mod	Non-Fac Total	Fac Total		51	50	62	80	MUE
	20.01	20.01	090	2	0	1	2	1

Excisional Stomach Procedures

43605 **Biopsy of stomach, by laparotomy** `C`

RVU			Global Days	Modifiers				
Mod	Non-Fac Total	Fac Total		51	50	62	80	MUE
	24.32	24.32	090	2	0	1	2	1

43610 **Excision, local; ulcer or benign tumor of stomach** `C`

RVU			Global Days	Modifiers				
Mod	Non-Fac Total	Fac Total		51	50	62	80	MUE
	28.46	28.46	090	2	0	1	2	2

43611 **Excision, local; malignant tumor of stomach** `C`

RVU			Global Days	Modifiers				
Mod	Non-Fac Total	Fac Total		51	50	62	80	MUE
	35.59	35.59	090	2	0	1	2	2

43620 **Gastrectomy, total; with esophagoenterostomy** `C`

RVU			Global Days	Modifiers				
Mod	Non-Fac Total	Fac Total		51	50	62	80	MUE
	56.94	56.94	090	2	0	1	2	1

43621 **Gastrectomy, total; with Roux-en-Y reconstruction** `C`

RVU			Global Days	Modifiers				
Mod	Non-Fac Total	Fac Total		51	50	62	80	MUE
	66.12	66.12	090	2	0	1	2	1

43622 **Gastrectomy, total; with formation of intestinal pouch, any type** `C`

RVU			Global Days	Modifiers				
Mod	Non-Fac Total	Fac Total		51	50	62	80	MUE
	67.40	67.40	090	2	0	1	2	1

43631 **Gastrectomy, partial, distal; with gastroduodenostomy** `C`

RVU			Global Days	Modifiers				
Mod	Non-Fac Total	Fac Total		51	50	62	80	MUE
	42.12	42.12	090	2	0	1	2	1

Gastrectomy, partial, distal with gastoduodenostomy/gastrojejunostomy

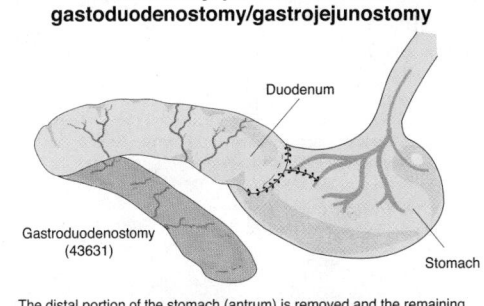

Gastroduodenostomy (43631)

Duodenum

Stomach

The distal portion of the stomach (antrum) is removed and the remaining stomach is anastomosed to the duodenum (43631) or to the jejunum (43632)

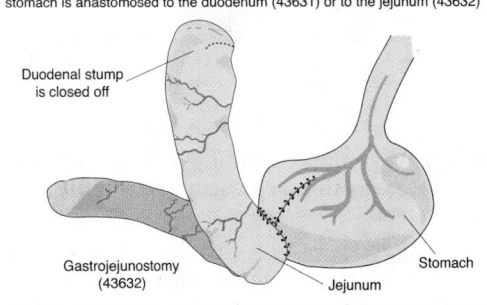

Duodenal stump is closed off

Gastrojejunostomy (43632)

Jejunum

Stomach

● New ▲ Revised Deleted ⊙ Moderate Sedation ➕ Add-on Codes ⊗ High Risk Denial Ⓐ Age Edit ♀ Female ♂ Male **AMA** *CPT® Assistant* **MUE** Medically Unlikely Edit
⊘ Modifier 51 Exempt ⊖ Modifier 63 Exempt ✗ Unlisted **Modifiers:** *See Inside Back Cover* Ⓜ Maternity `A2`–`Z3` ASC Payment Indicators `A`–`Y` OPPS Status Indicators
© 2016 DecisionHealth CPT © 2015 American Medical Association. All Rights Reserved.

43632 Gastrectomy, partial, distal; with gastrojejunostomy ⒞

RVU			Global Days	Modifiers				
Mod	Non-Fac Total	Fac Total		51	50	62	80	MUE
	59.08	59.08	090	2	0	1	2	1

43633 Gastrectomy, partial, distal; with Roux-en-Y reconstruction ⒞

RVU			Global Days	Modifiers				
Mod	Non-Fac Total	Fac Total		51	50	62	80	MUE
	55.82	55.82	090	2	0	1	2	1

43634 Gastrectomy, partial, distal; with formation of intestinal pouch ⒞

RVU			Global Days	Modifiers				
Mod	Non-Fac Total	Fac Total		51	50	62	80	MUE
	61.57	61.57	090	2	0	1	2	1

Coding Guidance

When vagotomy is performed at the time of gastric or esophageal surgery, only the most appropriate comprehensive code is reported. CPT codes 43635-43641 report procedures done with vagotomy as part of the service. They should not be reported with codes from 64752-64760, which report services as separate vagotomy procedures.

✚ 43635 Vagotomy when performed with partial distal gastrectomy (List separately in addition to code[s] for primary procedure) ⒞

RVU			Global Days	Modifiers				
Mod	Non-Fac Total	Fac Total		51	50	62	80	MUE
	3.26	3.26	ZZZ	0	0	1	2	1

AMA: Nov 97: 17

43640 Vagotomy including pyloroplasty, with or without gastrostomy; truncal or selective ⒞

RVU			Global Days	Modifiers				
Mod	Non-Fac Total	Fac Total		51	50	62	80	MUE
	34.23	34.23	090	2	0	1	2	1

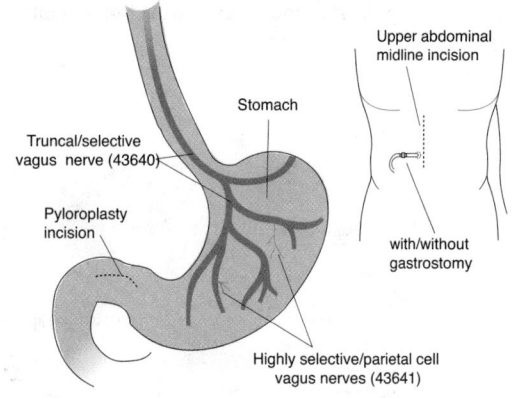

Vagotomy including pyloroplasty, with/without gastrostomy; truncal/selective/parietal cell

Upper abdominal midline incision

Stomach

Truncal/selective vagus nerve (43640)

Pyloroplasty incision

with/without gastrostomy

Highly selective/parietal cell vagus nerves (43641)

43641 Vagotomy including pyloroplasty, with or without gastrostomy; parietal cell (highly selective) ⒞

RVU			Global Days	Modifiers				
Mod	Non-Fac Total	Fac Total		51	50	62	80	MUE
	34.48	34.48	090	2	0	1	2	1

Laparoscopic Stomach Procedures

43644 Laparoscopy, surgical, gastric restrictive procedure; with gastric bypass and Roux-en-Y gastroenterostomy (roux limb 150 cm or less) ⒞

Coding tip: Open procedure with gastric bypass and Roux-en-Y gastroenterostomy- 43846

RVU			Global Days	Modifiers				
Mod	Non-Fac Total	Fac Total		51	50	62	80	MUE
	50.21	50.21	090	2	0	1	2	1

AMA: May 05: 3

Pub 100-04, 32, 150.2

43645 Laparoscopy, surgical, gastric restrictive procedure; with gastric bypass and small intestine reconstruction to limit absorption ⒞

Coding tip: Open procedure with gastric bypass and small intestine reconstruction - 43847

RVU			Global Days	Modifiers				
Mod	Non-Fac Total	Fac Total		51	50	62	80	MUE
	53.63	53.63	090	2	0	1	2	1

AMA: May 05: 3

Pub 100-04, 32, 150.2

43647 Laparoscopy, surgical; implantation or replacement of gastric neurostimulator electrodes, antrum J1

Coding tip: Open implantation or replacement of gastric neurostimulator electrodes, antrum - 43881

RVU			Global Days	Modifiers				
Mod	Non-Fac Total	Fac Total		51	50	62	80	MUE
	0.00	0.00	YYY	2	0	1	2	1

AMA: Mar 07: 4

43648 Laparoscopy, surgical; revision or removal of gastric neurostimulator electrodes, antrum J1

Coding tip: Open revision or removal of gastric neurostimulator electrodes, antrum - 43882

RVU			Global Days	Modifiers				
Mod	Non-Fac Total	Fac Total		51	50	62	80	MUE
	0.00	0.00	YYY	2	0	1	2	1

AMA: Mar 07: 4

43651 Laparoscopy, surgical; transection of vagus nerves, truncal J1

RVU			Global Days	Modifiers				
Mod	Non-Fac Total	Fac Total		51	50	62	80	MUE
	18.95	18.95	090	2	0	1	2	1

AMA: Nov 99: 22, Mar 00: 8

43652 Laparoscopy, surgical; transection of vagus nerves, selective or highly selective J1

RVU			Global Days	Modifiers				
Mod	Non-Fac Total	Fac Total		51	50	62	80	MUE
	22.23	22.23	090	2	0	1	2	1

AMA: Nov 99: 22, Mar 00: 8

43653 Laparoscopy, surgical; gastrostomy, without construction of gastric tube (eg, Stamm procedure) (separate procedure) A2 J1

RVU			Global Days	Modifiers				
Mod	Non-Fac Total	Fac Total		51	50	62	80	MUE
	16.60	16.60	090	2	0	1	2	1

AMA: Nov 99: 22, Mar 00: 8

● New   ▲ Revised   ✖ Deleted   ⊙ Moderate Sedation   ✚ Add-on Codes   ⊘ High Risk Denial   Ⓐ Age Edit   ♀ Female   ♂ Male   **AMA** *CPT® Assistant*   *MUE* Medically Unlikely Edit
Ⓢ Modifier 51 Exempt   ⊖ Modifier 63 Exempt   ✗ Unlisted   **Modifiers:** *See Inside Back Cover*   Ⓜ Maternity   A2–Z3 ASC Payment Indicators   A–Y OPPS Status Indicators

438   CPT © 2015 American Medical Association. All Rights Reserved.   © 2016 DecisionHealth

43659 Unlisted laparoscopy procedure, stomach ⊠▉J▉1

RVU			Global Days	Modifiers				
Mod	Non-Fac Total	Fac Total		51	50	62	80	MUE
	0.00	0.00	YYY	2	1	1		2

AMA: Nov 99: 22, Mar 00: 8, Apr 06: 19, Jun 06: 16, Dec 07: 12, Dec 11: 19, Jun 11: 8, Feb 13: 13, Jun 13: 13

Introduction Stomach Procedures

43752 Naso- or oro-gastric tube placement, requiring physician's skill and fluoroscopic guidance (includes fluoroscopy, image documentation and report) ▉G▉2▉Q▉3

RVU			Global Days	Modifiers				
Mod	Non-Fac Total	Fac Total		51	50	62	80	MUE
	1.18	1.18	000	0	0	0	1	2

AMA: Jan 02: 11, Apr 03: 7, Oct 03: 2, Jul 06: 4, Feb 07: 10, Jul 07: 1, Aug 08: 7, Sep 11: 4, May 14: 4

Pub 100-04, 12, 30.6.12

Nasogastric/orogastric tube placement

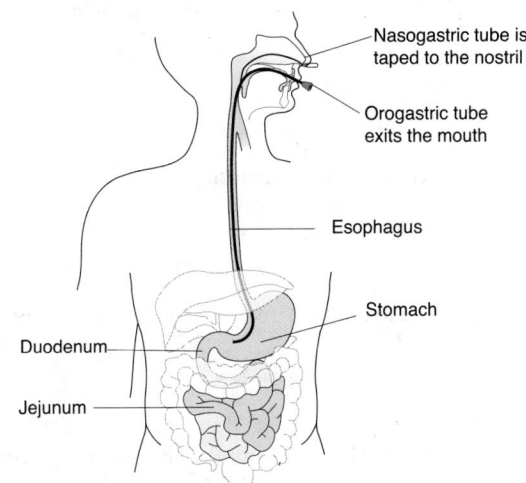

Nasogastric tube is taped to the nostril

Orogastric tube exits the mouth

Esophagus

Stomach

Duodenum

Jejunum

The feeding tube is placed into the stomach through the mouth or nose

43753 Gastric intubation and aspiration(s) therapeutic, necessitating physician's skill (eg, for gastrointestinal hemorrhage), including lavage if performed ▉N▉I▉Q▉1

RVU			Global Days	Modifiers				
Mod	Non-Fac Total	Fac Total		51	50	62	80	MUE
	0.63	0.63	000	0	0	0	2	1

AMA: Sep 11: 3, May 14: 4

43754 Gastric intubation and aspiration, diagnostic; single specimen (eg, acid analysis) ▉C▉N▉I▉Q▉1

RVU			Global Days	Modifiers				
Mod	Non-Fac Total	Fac Total		51	50	62	80	MUE
	3.02	0.95	000	0	0	0	2	1

AMA: Sep 11: 3, Dec 10: 10

43755 Gastric intubation and aspiration, diagnostic; collection of multiple fractional specimens with gastric stimulation, single or double lumen tube (gastric secretory study) (eg, histamine, insulin, pentagastrin, calcium, secretin), includes drug administration ▉G▉2▉S

RVU			Global Days	Modifiers				
Mod	Non-Fac Total	Fac Total		51	50	62	80	MUE
	4.02	1.78	000	0	0	0	2	1

AMA: Sep 11: 3, Dec 10: 10

43756 Duodenal intubation and aspiration, diagnostic, includes image guidance; single specimen (eg, bile study for crystals or afferent loop culture) ▉G▉2▉Q▉1

RVU			Global Days	Modifiers				
Mod	Non-Fac Total	Fac Total		51	50	62	80	MUE
	5.85	1.49	000	0	0	0	2	1

AMA: Sep 11: 3, Dec 10: 10

43757 Duodenal intubation and aspiration, diagnostic, includes image guidance; collection of multiple fractional specimens with pancreatic or gallbladder stimulation, single or double lumen tube, includes drug administration ▉G▉2▉T

RVU			Global Days	Modifiers				
Mod	Non-Fac Total	Fac Total		51	50	62	80	MUE
	8.26	2.25	000	0	0	0	2	1

AMA: Sep 11: 3, Dec 10: 10

43760 Change of gastrostomy tube, percutaneous, without imaging or endoscopic guidance ▉A▉2▉T

RVU			Global Days	Modifiers				
Mod	Non-Fac Total	Fac Total		51	50	62	80	MUE
	13.87	1.36	000	2	0	0	1	2

AMA: Apr 08: 11, Aug 08: 7, Sep 10: 9

Change of gastrostomy tube

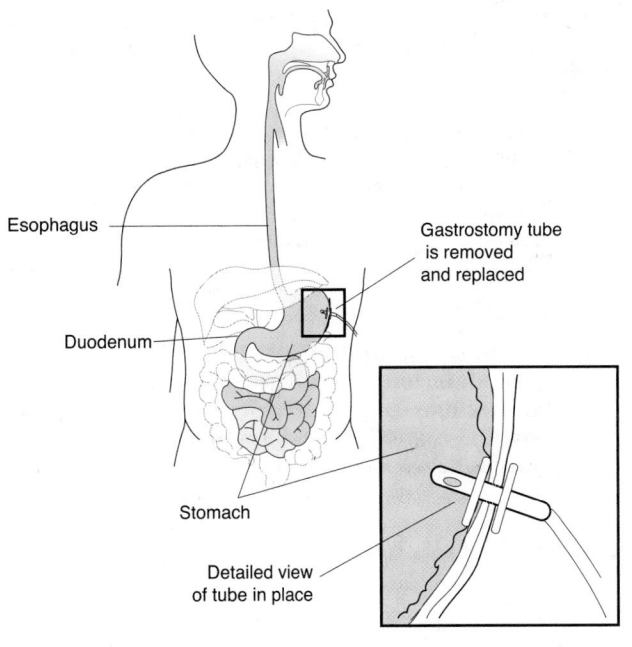

Esophagus

Duodenum

Gastrostomy tube is removed and replaced

Stomach

Detailed view of tube in place

● New ▲ Revised Deleted ⊙ Moderate Sedation ✚ Add-on Codes ⊘ High Risk Denial ⊛ Age Edit ♀ Female ♂ Male **AMA** *CPT® Assistant* **MUE** Medically Unlikely Edit
⊘ Modifier 51 Exempt ⊖ Modifier 63 Exempt ⊠ Unlisted **Modifiers:** *See Inside Back Cover* Ⓜ Maternity ▉A▉2–▉Z▉3 ASC Payment Indicators ▉A–▉Y OPPS Status Indicators
© 2016 DecisionHealth   CPT © 2015 American Medical Association. All Rights Reserved.

43761 Repositioning of a naso- or oro-gastric feeding tube, through the duodenum for enteric nutrition [A2][T]

Coding tip: Separate fluoroscopic guidance - 76000

Mod	RVU Non-Fac Total	Fac Total	Global Days	Modifiers 51	50	62	80	MUE
	3.34	2.97	000	2	0	0	1	2

AMA: Oct 96: 9, Nov 99: 22, Jun 08: 8, Aug 08: 7

Bariatric Procedures

Laparoscopic Bariatric Procedures

43770 Laparoscopy, surgical, gastric restrictive procedure; placement of adjustable gastric restrictive device (eg, gastric band and subcutaneous port components) [J][I]

Mod	RVU Non-Fac Total	Fac Total	Global Days	Modifiers 51	50	62	80	MUE
	32.47	32.47	090	2	0	1	2	1

AMA: Dec 10: 13

Pub 100-04, 32, 150.2

43771 Laparoscopy, surgical, gastric restrictive procedure; revision of adjustable gastric restrictive device component only [C]

Mod	RVU Non-Fac Total	Fac Total	Global Days	Modifiers 51	50	62	80	MUE
	36.96	36.96	090	2	0	1	2	1

43772 Laparoscopy, surgical, gastric restrictive procedure; removal of adjustable gastric restrictive device component only [C]

Mod	RVU Non-Fac Total	Fac Total	Global Days	Modifiers 51	50	62	80	MUE
	27.51	27.51	090	2	0	1	2	1

43773 Laparoscopy, surgical, gastric restrictive procedure; removal and replacement of adjustable gastric restrictive device component only [C]

Mod	RVU Non-Fac Total	Fac Total	Global Days	Modifiers 51	50	62	80	MUE
	36.83	36.83	090	2	0	1	2	1

43774 Laparoscopy, surgical, gastric restrictive procedure; removal of adjustable gastric restrictive device and subcutaneous port components [C]

Mod	RVU Non-Fac Total	Fac Total	Global Days	Modifiers 51	50	62	80	MUE
	27.81	27.81	090	2	0	1	2	1

43775 Laparoscopy, surgical, gastric restrictive procedure; longitudinal gastrectomy (ie, sleeve gastrectomy) [C]

Mod	RVU Non-Fac Total	Fac Total	Global Days	Modifiers 51	50	62	80	MUE
	35.56	35.56	090	2	0	1	2	1

Pub 100-04, 32, 150.2

Other Bariatric Procedures

43800 Pyloroplasty [C]

Mod	RVU Non-Fac Total	Fac Total	Global Days	Modifiers 51	50	62	80	MUE
	26.98	26.98	090	2	0	1	2	1

Pyloroplasty

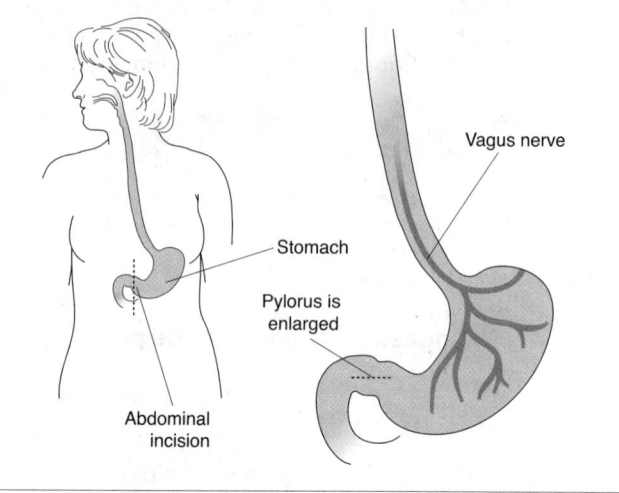

Vagus nerve

Stomach

Pylorus is enlarged

Abdominal incision

43810 Gastroduodenostomy [C]

Mod	RVU Non-Fac Total	Fac Total	Global Days	Modifiers 51	50	62	80	MUE
	29.54	29.54	090	2	0	1	2	1

43820 Gastrojejunostomy; without vagotomy [C]

Mod	RVU Non-Fac Total	Fac Total	Global Days	Modifiers 51	50	62	80	MUE
	38.99	38.99	090	2	0	1	2	1

43825 Gastrojejunostomy; with vagotomy, any type [C]

Mod	RVU Non-Fac Total	Fac Total	Global Days	Modifiers 51	50	62	80	MUE
	37.95	37.95	090	2	0	1	2	1

43830 Gastrostomy, open; without construction of gastric tube (eg, Stamm procedure) (separate procedure) [T]

Mod	RVU Non-Fac Total	Fac Total	Global Days	Modifiers 51	50	62	80	MUE
	20.30	20.30	090	2	0	1	2	1

AMA: Nov 99: 22

43831 Gastrostomy, open; neonatal, for feeding [A][⊖][T]

Mod	RVU Non-Fac Total	Fac Total	Global Days	Modifiers 51	50	62	80	MUE
	16.91	16.91	090	2	0	1	2	1

AMA: Nov 99: 22

43832 Gastrostomy, open; with construction of gastric tube (eg, Janeway procedure) [C]

Mod	RVU Non-Fac Total	Fac Total	Global Days	Modifiers 51	50	62	80	MUE
	30.18	30.18	090	2	0	1	2	1

AMA: Nov 99: 22

● New ▲ Revised ✖ Deleted ⊙ Moderate Sedation ✚ Add-on Codes ⊘ High Risk Denial Ⓐ Age Edit ♀ Female ♂ Male **AMA** *CPT® Assistant* **MUE** Medically Unlikely Edit ⊘ Modifier 51 Exempt ⊖ Modifier 63 Exempt ⌧ Unlisted **Modifiers:** *See Inside Back Cover* Ⓜ Maternity [A2]-[Z3] ASC Payment Indicators [A]-[Y] OPPS Status Indicators

440

CPT © 2015 American Medical Association. All Rights Reserved. © 2016 DecisionHealth

Surgical Procedures

43761 – 43832

43840 Gastrorrhaphy, suture of perforated duodenal or gastric ulcer, wound, or injury C

RVU			Global Days	Modifiers				
Mod	Non-Fac Total	Fac Total		51	50	62	80	MUE
	39.50	39.50	090	2	0	1	2	2

43842 Gastric restrictive procedure, without gastric bypass, for morbid obesity; vertical-banded gastroplasty C E

RVU			Global Days	Modifiers				
Mod	Non-Fac Total	Fac Total		51	50	62	80	MUE
	34.52	34.52	090	9	9	9	9	

AMA: May 98: 5

Pub 100-04, 32, 150.2

43843 Gastric restrictive procedure, without gastric bypass, for morbid obesity; other than vertical-banded gastroplasty C

RVU			Global Days	Modifiers				
Mod	Non-Fac Total	Fac Total		51	50	62	80	MUE
	37.15	37.15	090	2	0	2	2	1

AMA: May 98: 5

43845 Gastric restrictive procedure with partial gastrectomy, pylorus-preserving duodenoileostomy and ileoileostomy (50 to 100 cm common channel) to limit absorption (biliopancreatic diversion with duodenal switch) C

RVU			Global Days	Modifiers				
Mod	Non-Fac Total	Fac Total		51	50	62	80	MUE
	56.99	56.99	090	2	0	1	2	1

AMA: May 05: 3

Pub 100-04, 32, 150.2

43846 Gastric restrictive procedure, with gastric bypass for morbid obesity; with short limb (150 cm or less) Roux-en-Y gastroenterostomy C

Coding tip: Laparoscopic approach - 43644

RVU			Global Days	Modifiers				
Mod	Non-Fac Total	Fac Total		51	50	62	80	MUE
	46.81	46.81	090	2	0	1	2	1

AMA: May 98: 5, May 05: 3

Pub 100-04, 32, 150.2

43847 Gastric restrictive procedure, with gastric bypass for morbid obesity; with small intestine reconstruction to limit absorption C

Coding tip: Laparoscopic procedure - 43645

RVU			Global Days	Modifiers				
Mod	Non-Fac Total	Fac Total		51	50	62	80	MUE
	51.59	51.59	090	2	0	1	2	1

AMA: May 98: 5, May 02: 7

Pub 100-04, 32, 150.2

43848 Revision, open, of gastric restrictive procedure for morbid obesity, other than adjustable gastric restrictive device (separate procedure) C

Coding tip: Open revision of gastric restrictive port component alone - 43886

Coding tip: Laparoscopic revision of adjustable gastric restrictive device - 43771

RVU			Global Days	Modifiers				
Mod	Non-Fac Total	Fac Total		51	50	62	80	MUE
	55.92	55.92	090	2	0	1	2	1

AMA: May 98: 5, Apr 06: 1

43850 Revision of gastroduodenal anastomosis (gastroduodenostomy) with reconstruction; without vagotomy C

RVU			Global Days	Modifiers				
Mod	Non-Fac Total	Fac Total		51	50	62	80	MUE
	47.15	47.15	090	2	0	1	2	1

43855 Revision of gastroduodenal anastomosis (gastroduodenostomy) with reconstruction; with vagotomy C

RVU			Global Days	Modifiers				
Mod	Non-Fac Total	Fac Total		51	50	62	80	MUE
	47.71	47.71	090	2	0	1	2	1

43860 Revision of gastrojejunal anastomosis (gastrojejunostomy) with reconstruction, with or without partial gastrectomy or intestine resection; without vagotomy C

RVU			Global Days	Modifiers				
Mod	Non-Fac Total	Fac Total		51	50	62	80	MUE
	47.51	47.51	090	2	0	1	2	1

43865 Revision of gastrojejunal anastomosis (gastrojejunostomy) with reconstruction, with or without partial gastrectomy or intestine resection; with vagotomy C

RVU			Global Days	Modifiers				
Mod	Non-Fac Total	Fac Total		51	50	62	80	MUE
	49.51	49.51	090	2	0	1	2	1

43870 Closure of gastrostomy, surgical A2 T

RVU			Global Days	Modifiers				
Mod	Non-Fac Total	Fac Total		51	50	62	80	MUE
	20.65	20.65	090	2	0	1	2	1

43880 Closure of gastrocolic fistula C

RVU			Global Days	Modifiers				
Mod	Non-Fac Total	Fac Total		51	50	62	80	MUE
	46.45	46.45	090	2	0	1	2	1

43881 Implantation or replacement of gastric neurostimulator electrodes, antrum, open C

Coding tip: Laparoscopic procedure - 43647

RVU			Global Days	Modifiers				
Mod	Non-Fac Total	Fac Total		51	50	62	80	MUE
	0.00	0.00	YYY	2	0	1	2	1

AMA: Mar 07: 4

● New   ▲ Revised   Deleted   ⊙ Moderate Sedation   ✚ Add-on Codes   ⊘ High Risk Denial   Ⓐ Age Edit   ♀ Female   ♂ Male   **AMA** *CPT® Assistant*   **MUE** Medically Unlikely Edit
⊘ Modifier 51 Exempt   ⊖ Modifier 63 Exempt   ⊠ Unlisted   **Modifiers:** *See Inside Back Cover*   Ⓜ Maternity   A2 – Z3 ASC Payment Indicators   A – Y OPPS Status Indicators

Surgical Procedures

43882 – 44050

43882 Revision or removal of gastric neurostimulator electrodes, antrum, open C

Coding tip: Laparoscopic revision or removal - 43648

	RVU		Global Days	Modifiers				
Mod	Non-Fac Total	Fac Total		51	50	62	80	MUE
	0.00	0.00	YYY	2	0	1	2	1

AMA: Mar 07: 4

43886 Gastric restrictive procedure, open; revision of subcutaneous port component only G2 T

Coding tip: Revision, open, of gastric restrictive procedure, other than adjustable device - 43848

	RVU		Global Days	Modifiers				
Mod	Non-Fac Total	Fac Total		51	50	62	80	MUE
	10.47	10.47	090	2	0	1	2	1

43887 Gastric restrictive procedure, open; removal of subcutaneous port component only G2 Q2

Coding tip: When port component and restrictive device are both removed laparoscopically, report 43774

	RVU		Global Days	Modifiers				
Mod	Non-Fac Total	Fac Total		51	50	62	80	MUE
	9.37	9.37	090	2	0	1	2	1

43888 Gastric restrictive procedure, open; removal and replacement of subcutaneous port component only G2 T

	RVU		Global Days	Modifiers				
Mod	Non-Fac Total	Fac Total		51	50	62	80	MUE
	13.27	13.27	090	2	0	1	2	1

43999 Unlisted procedure, stomach x T

	RVU		Global Days	Modifiers				
Mod	Non-Fac Total	Fac Total		51	50	62	80	MUE
	0.00	0.00	YYY	2	0	1	0	

AMA: Jun 11: 13, Mar 10: 10, Feb 13: 13
Pub 100-04, 32, 150.2

Intestinal Procedures (Excluding Rectum)

Incisional Intestinal Procedures

Coding Guidance

As a separate procedure, open enterolysis is not reportable with other intra-abdominal or pelvic procedures. If an extensive, time-consuming enterolysis is performed in conjunction with another procedure, modifier 22 may be appended to the CPT code for the intra-abdominal or pelvic procedure.

44005 Enterolysis (freeing of intestinal adhesion) (separate procedure) C

Coding tip: Laparoscopic enterolysis - 44180

	RVU		Global Days	Modifiers				
Mod	Non-Fac Total	Fac Total		51	50	62	80	MUE
	31.78	31.78	090	2	0	1	2	1

AMA: Winter 90: 6, Nov 97: 17, Nov 99: 23, Jan 00: 11, Apr 00: 10

Enterolysis (freeing of intestinal adhesion)

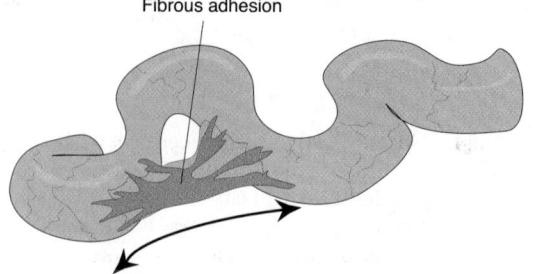

Fibrous adhesion

The bowel is accessed by abdominal incision and freed from the adhesion to itself, or to another structure

44010 Duodenotomy, for exploration, biopsy(s), or foreign body removal C

	RVU		Global Days	Modifiers				
Mod	Non-Fac Total	Fac Total		51	50	62	80	MUE
	25.04	25.04	090	2	0	1	2	1

+ 44015 Tube or needle catheter jejunostomy for enteral alimentation, intraoperative, any method (List separately in addition to primary procedure) C

	RVU		Global Days	Modifiers				
Mod	Non-Fac Total	Fac Total		51	50	62	80	MUE
	4.14	4.14	ZZZ	0	0	1	2	1

AMA: Mar 02: 10, Jul 10: 10

44020 Enterotomy, small intestine, other than duodenum; for exploration, biopsy(s), or foreign body removal C

	RVU		Global Days	Modifiers				
Mod	Non-Fac Total	Fac Total		51	50	62	80	MUE
	28.31	28.31	090	2	0	1	2	2

44021 Enterotomy, small intestine, other than duodenum; for decompression (eg, Baker tube) C

	RVU		Global Days	Modifiers				
Mod	Non-Fac Total	Fac Total		51	50	62	80	MUE
	28.30	28.30	090	2	0	1	2	1

44025 Colotomy, for exploration, biopsy(s), or foreign body removal C

	RVU		Global Days	Modifiers				
Mod	Non-Fac Total	Fac Total		51	50	62	80	MUE
	28.65	28.65	090	2	0	1	2	1

44050 Reduction of volvulus, intussusception, internal hernia, by laparotomy C

	RVU		Global Days	Modifiers				
Mod	Non-Fac Total	Fac Total		51	50	62	80	MUE
	27.19	27.19	090	2	0	1	2	1

● New ▲ Revised ✖ Deleted ⊙ Moderate Sedation ✚ Add-on Codes ⊘ High Risk Denial ⓐ Age Edit ♀ Female ♂ Male **AMA** *CPT® Assistant* **MUE** Medically Unlikely Edit
⊘ Modifier 51 Exempt ⊖ Modifier 63 Exempt ✖ Unlisted **Modifiers:** *See Inside Back Cover* Ⓜ Maternity A2-Z3 ASC Payment Indicators A-Y OPPS Status Indicators

442
CPT © 2015 American Medical Association. All Rights Reserved.
© 2016 DecisionHealth

44055 Correction of malrotation by lysis of duodenal bands and/or reduction of midgut volvulus (eg, Ladd procedure) ⊖C

RVU			Global Days	Modifiers				
Mod	Non-Fac Total	Fac Total		51	50	62	80	MUE
	43.36	43.36	090	2	0	1	2	1

Excisional Intestinal Procedures

44100 Biopsy of intestine by capsule, tube, peroral (1 or more specimens) A 2 T

RVU			Global Days	Modifiers				
Mod	Non-Fac Total	Fac Total		51	50	62	80	MUE
	3.16	3.16	000	2	0	0	1	1

44110 Excision of 1 or more lesions of small or large intestine not requiring anastomosis, exteriorization, or fistulization; single enterotomy C

RVU			Global Days	Modifiers				
Mod	Non-Fac Total	Fac Total		51	50	62	80	MUE
	24.74	24.74	090	2	0	1	2	1

44111 Excision of 1 or more lesions of small or large intestine not requiring anastomosis, exteriorization, or fistulization; multiple enterotomies C

RVU			Global Days	Modifiers				
Mod	Non-Fac Total	Fac Total		51	50	62	80	MUE
	28.61	28.61	090	2	0	1	2	1

44120 Enterectomy, resection of small intestine; single resection and anastomosis C

RVU			Global Days	Modifiers				
Mod	Non-Fac Total	Fac Total		51	50	62	80	MUE
	35.57	35.57	090	2	0	1	2	1

AMA: Mar 04: 3, Aug 08: 7

Enterectomy, resection of small intestine with anastomosis

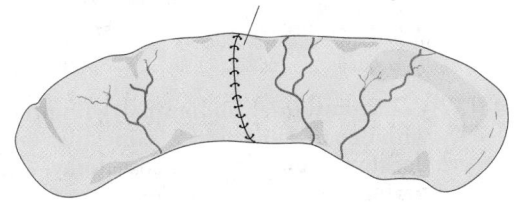

A section of bowel is removed and anastomosed to restore continuity

Single resection/anastomosis (44120); each additional resection/anastomosis (44121)

+ 44121 Enterectomy, resection of small intestine; each additional resection and anastomosis (List separately in addition to code for primary procedure) C

RVU			Global Days	Modifiers				
Mod	Non-Fac Total	Fac Total		51	50	62	80	MUE
	7.04	7.04	ZZZ	0	0	1	2	4

44125 Enterectomy, resection of small intestine; with enterostomy C

RVU			Global Days	Modifiers				
Mod	Non-Fac Total	Fac Total		51	50	62	80	MUE
	34.32	34.32	090	2	0	1	2	1

44126 Enterectomy, resection of small intestine for congenital atresia, single resection and anastomosis of proximal segment of intestine; without tapering Ⓐ⊖C

RVU			Global Days	Modifiers				
Mod	Non-Fac Total	Fac Total		51	50	62	80	MUE
	71.74	71.74	090	2	0	1	2	1

44127 Enterectomy, resection of small intestine for congenital atresia, single resection and anastomosis of proximal segment of intestine; with tapering Ⓐ⊖C

RVU			Global Days	Modifiers				
Mod	Non-Fac Total	Fac Total		51	50	62	80	MUE
	82.35	82.35	090	2	0	1	2	1

+ 44128 Enterectomy, resection of small intestine for congenital atresia, single resection and anastomosis of proximal segment of intestine; each additional resection and anastomosis (List separately in addition to code for primary procedure) ⊗⊖C

RVU			Global Days	Modifiers				
Mod	Non-Fac Total	Fac Total		51	50	62	80	MUE
	7.15	7.15	ZZZ	0	0	1	2	2

44130 Enteroenterostomy, anastomosis of intestine, with or without cutaneous enterostomy (separate procedure) C

RVU			Global Days	Modifiers				
Mod	Non-Fac Total	Fac Total		51	50	62	80	MUE
	38.16	38.16	090	2	0	1	2	3

44132 Donor enterectomy (including cold preservation), open; from cadaver donor ⊗C

RVU			Global Days	Modifiers				
Mod	Non-Fac Total	Fac Total		51	50	62	80	MUE
	0.00	0.00	XXX	0	0	0	0	1

44133 Donor enterectomy (including cold preservation), open; partial, from living donor C

RVU			Global Days	Modifiers				
Mod	Non-Fac Total	Fac Total		51	50	62	80	MUE
	0.00	0.00	XXX	0	0	0	0	1

44135 Intestinal allotransplantation; from cadaver donor ⊗C

RVU			Global Days	Modifiers				
Mod	Non-Fac Total	Fac Total		51	50	62	80	MUE
	0.00	0.00	XXX	0	0	0	0	1

44136 Intestinal allotransplantation; from living donor C

RVU			Global Days	Modifiers				
Mod	Non-Fac Total	Fac Total		51	50	62	80	MUE
	0.00	0.00	XXX	0	0	0	0	1

● New ▲ Revised Deleted ⊙ Moderate Sedation ✚ Add-on Codes ⊘ High Risk Denial Ⓐ Age Edit ♀ Female ♂ Male **AMA** CPT® Assistant **MUE** Medically Unlikely Edit
⊘ Modifier 51 Exempt ⊖ Modifier 63 Exempt ☒ Unlisted **Modifiers:** See Inside Back Cover Ⓜ Maternity A 2 – Z 3 ASC Payment Indicators A – Y OPPS Status Indicators

Surgical Procedures

44137 – 44158

44137 Removal of transplanted intestinal allograft, complete   C

RVU			Global Days	Modifiers				
Mod	Non-Fac Total	Fac Total		51	50	62	80	MUE
	0.00	0.00	XXX	2	0	1	2	1

Removal of transplanted intestinal allograft, complete

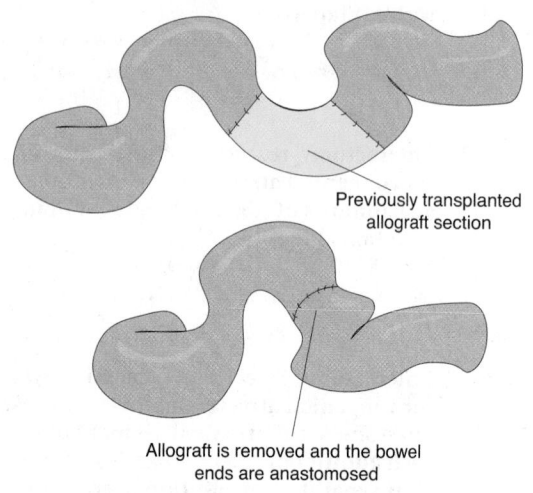

Previously transplanted allograft section

Allograft is removed and the bowel ends are anastomosed

+ 44139 Mobilization (take-down) of splenic flexure performed in conjunction with partial colectomy (List separately in addition to primary procedure)   C

RVU			Global Days	Modifiers				
Mod	Non-Fac Total	Fac Total		51	50	62	80	MUE
	3.51	3.51	ZZZ	0	0	1	2	1

44140 Colectomy, partial; with anastomosis   C

Coding tip: Laparoscopic partial colectomy with anastomosis - 44204

RVU			Global Days	Modifiers				
Mod	Non-Fac Total	Fac Total		51	50	62	80	MUE
	38.97	38.97	090	2	0	1	2	2

AMA: Fall 92: 23, Aug 08: 7, Nov 08: 7, Sep 10: 7

44141 Colectomy, partial; with skin level cecostomy or colostomy   C

RVU			Global Days	Modifiers				
Mod	Non-Fac Total	Fac Total		51	50	62	80	MUE
	53.06	53.06	090	2	0	1	2	1

AMA: Fall 92: 24, Nov 08: 7

44143 Colectomy, partial; with end colostomy and closure of distal segment (Hartmann type procedure)   C

RVU			Global Days	Modifiers				
Mod	Non-Fac Total	Fac Total		51	50	62	80	MUE
	48.38	48.38	090	2	0	1	2	1

AMA: Fall 92: 24, Nov 08: 7

44144 Colectomy, partial; with resection, with colostomy or ileostomy and creation of mucofistula   C

RVU			Global Days	Modifiers				
Mod	Non-Fac Total	Fac Total		51	50	62	80	MUE
	51.48	51.48	090	2	0	1	2	1

AMA: Fall 92: 24, Nov 08: 7

44145 Colectomy, partial; with coloproctostomy (low pelvic anastomosis)   C

RVU			Global Days	Modifiers				
Mod	Non-Fac Total	Fac Total		51	50	62	80	MUE
	48.17	48.17	090	2	0	1	2	1

AMA: Fall 92: 24

44146 Colectomy, partial; with coloproctostomy (low pelvic anastomosis), with colostomy   C

RVU			Global Days	Modifiers				
Mod	Non-Fac Total	Fac Total		51	50	62	80	MUE
	61.52	61.52	090	2	0	1	2	1

AMA: Fall 92: 24, Nov 08: 7

44147 Colectomy, partial; abdominal and transanal approach   C

RVU			Global Days	Modifiers				
Mod	Non-Fac Total	Fac Total		51	50	62	80	MUE
	56.49	56.49	090	2	0	1	2	1

AMA: Fall 92: 24, Nov 08: 7

44150 Colectomy, total, abdominal, without proctectomy; with ileostomy or ileoproctostomy   C

RVU			Global Days	Modifiers				
Mod	Non-Fac Total	Fac Total		51	50	62	80	MUE
	54.33	54.33	090	2	0	1	2	1

44151 Colectomy, total, abdominal, without proctectomy; with continent ileostomy   C

RVU			Global Days	Modifiers				
Mod	Non-Fac Total	Fac Total		51	50	62	80	MUE
	62.18	62.18	090	2	0	1	2	1

44155 Colectomy, total, abdominal, with proctectomy; with ileostomy   C

RVU			Global Days	Modifiers				
Mod	Non-Fac Total	Fac Total		51	50	62	80	MUE
	60.50	60.50	090	2	0	1	2	1

44156 Colectomy, total, abdominal, with proctectomy; with continent ileostomy   C

RVU			Global Days	Modifiers				
Mod	Non-Fac Total	Fac Total		51	50	62	80	MUE
	66.80	66.80	090	2	0	1	2	1

44157 Colectomy, total, abdominal, with proctectomy; with ileoanal anastomosis, includes loop ileostomy, and rectal mucosectomy, when performed   C

RVU			Global Days	Modifiers				
Mod	Non-Fac Total	Fac Total		51	50	62	80	MUE
	62.62	62.62	090	2	0	1	2	1

44158 Colectomy, total, abdominal, with proctectomy; with ileoanal anastomosis, creation of ileal reservoir (S or J), includes loop ileostomy, and rectal mucosectomy, when performed   C

RVU			Global Days	Modifiers				
Mod	Non-Fac Total	Fac Total		51	50	62	80	MUE
	61.90	61.90	090	2	0	1	2	1

● New   ▲ Revised   ✖ Deleted   ⊙ Moderate Sedation   ✚ Add-on Codes   ⊘ High Risk Denial   Ⓐ Age Edit   ♀ Female   ♂ Male   **AMA** CPT® Assistant   **MUE** Medically Unlikely Edit   ⊘ Modifier 51 Exempt   ⊖ Modifier 63 Exempt   🗵 Unlisted   **Modifiers:** See Inside Back Cover   Ⓜ Maternity   A2–Z3 ASC Payment Indicators   A–Y OPPS Status Indicators

CPT © 2015 American Medical Association. All Rights Reserved.   © 2016 DecisionHealth

44160 Colectomy, partial, with removal of terminal ileum with ileocolostomy ☐C

RVU			Global Days	Modifiers				
Mod	Non-Fac Total	Fac Total		51	50	62	80	MUE
	36.09	36.09	090	2	0	1	2	1

Laparoscopic Intestinal Procedures

Coding Guidance

As a separate procedure, laparoscopic enterolysis is not reportable with other intra-abdominal or pelvic procedures. If an extensive, time-consuming enterolysis is performed in conjunction with another procedure, modifier 22 may be appended to the CPT code for the intra-abdominal or pelvic procedure.

44180 Laparoscopy, surgical, enterolysis (freeing of intestinal adhesion) (separate procedure) JI

RVU			Global Days	Modifiers				
Mod	Non-Fac Total	Fac Total		51	50	62	80	MUE
	26.65	26.65	090	2	0	1	2	1

Laparoscopic enterolysis

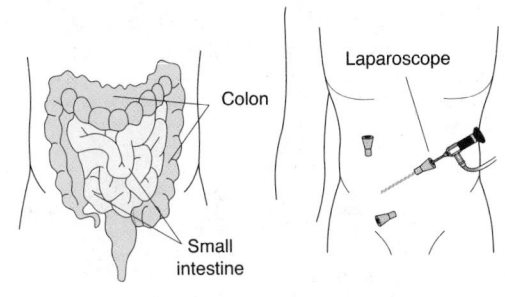

Colon — Laparoscope — Small intestine

Intestines which have become stuck together or to another structure are surgically separated

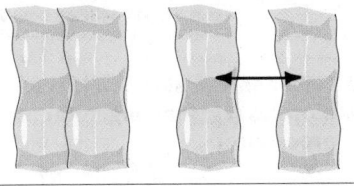

44186 Laparoscopy, surgical; jejunostomy (eg, for decompression or feeding) JI

RVU			Global Days	Modifiers				
Mod	Non-Fac Total	Fac Total		51	50	62	80	MUE
	18.96	18.96	090	2	0	1	2	1

44187 Laparoscopy, surgical; ileostomy or jejunostomy, non-tube ☐C

RVU			Global Days	Modifiers				
Mod	Non-Fac Total	Fac Total		51	50	62	80	MUE
	32.16	32.16	090	2	0	1	2	1

44188 Laparoscopy, surgical, colostomy or skin level cecostomy ☐C

RVU			Global Days	Modifiers				
Mod	Non-Fac Total	Fac Total		51	50	62	80	MUE
	35.59	35.59	090	2	0	1	2	1

44202 Laparoscopy, surgical; enterectomy, resection of small intestine, single resection and anastomosis ⊗C

RVU			Global Days	Modifiers				
Mod	Non-Fac Total	Fac Total		51	50	62	80	MUE
	40.26	40.26	090	2	0	1	2	1

AMA: Nov 99: 23, Mar 00: 9, May 03: 2, Apr 06: 1

+ 44203 Laparoscopy, surgical; each additional small intestine resection and anastomosis (List separately in addition to code for primary procedure) ☐C

RVU			Global Days	Modifiers				
Mod	Non-Fac Total	Fac Total		51	50	62	80	MUE
	7.03	7.03	ZZZ	0	0	1	2	2

AMA: May 03: 2

44204 Laparoscopy, surgical; colectomy, partial, with anastomosis ☐C

RVU			Global Days	Modifiers				
Mod	Non-Fac Total	Fac Total		51	50	62	80	MUE
	44.65	44.65	090	2	0	1	2	2

AMA: May 03: 3, Apr 06: 1, 19

44205 Laparoscopy, surgical; colectomy, partial, with removal of terminal ileum with ileocolostomy ☐C

RVU			Global Days	Modifiers				
Mod	Non-Fac Total	Fac Total		51	50	62	80	MUE
	38.85	38.85	090	2	0	1	2	1

AMA: May 03: 3, Apr 06: 1

44206 Laparoscopy, surgical; colectomy, partial, with end colostomy and closure of distal segment (Hartmann type procedure) ☐C

RVU			Global Days	Modifiers				
Mod	Non-Fac Total	Fac Total		51	50	62	80	MUE
	50.95	50.95	090	2	0	1	2	1

AMA: May 03: 3, Apr 06: 1

44207 Laparoscopy, surgical; colectomy, partial, with anastomosis, with coloproctostomy (low pelvic anastomosis) ☐C

RVU			Global Days	Modifiers				
Mod	Non-Fac Total	Fac Total		51	50	62	80	MUE
	52.88	52.88	090	2	0	1	2	1

AMA: May 03: 3, Apr 06: 1

44208 Laparoscopy, surgical; colectomy, partial, with anastomosis, with coloproctostomy (low pelvic anastomosis) with colostomy ☐C

RVU			Global Days	Modifiers				
Mod	Non-Fac Total	Fac Total		51	50	62	80	MUE
	57.73	57.73	090	2	0	1	2	1

AMA: May 03: 3, Apr 06: 1

44210 Laparoscopy, surgical; colectomy, total, abdominal, without proctectomy, with ileostomy or ileoproctostomy ☐C

RVU			Global Days	Modifiers				
Mod	Non-Fac Total	Fac Total		51	50	62	80	MUE
	51.74	51.74	090	2	0	1	2	1

AMA: May 03: 3

● New ▲ Revised Deleted ⊙ Moderate Sedation ✚ Add-on Codes ⊗ High Risk Denial ⒶAge Edit ♀ Female ♂ Male **AMA** *CPT® Assistant* **MUE** Medically Unlikely Edit
⊘ Modifier 51 Exempt ⊖ Modifier 63 Exempt ✗ Unlisted **Modifiers:** *See Inside Back Cover* Ⓜ Maternity A2–Z3 ASC Payment Indicators A–Y OPPS Status Indicators

44211 Laparoscopy, surgical; colectomy, total, abdominal, with proctectomy, with ileoanal anastomosis, creation of ileal reservoir (S or J), with loop ileostomy, includes rectal mucosectomy, when performed   C

RVU			Global Days	Modifiers				
Mod	Non-Fac Total	Fac Total		51	50	62	80	MUE
	63.41	63.41	090	2	0	1	2	1

AMA: May 03: 3

44212 Laparoscopy, surgical; colectomy, total, abdominal, with proctectomy, with ileostomy   C

RVU			Global Days	Modifiers				
Mod	Non-Fac Total	Fac Total		51	50	62	80	MUE
	59.49	59.49	090	2	0	1	2	1

AMA: May 03: 3

+ 44213 Laparoscopy, surgical, mobilization (take-down) of splenic flexure performed in conjunction with partial colectomy (List separately in addition to primary procedure)   C

RVU			Global Days	Modifiers				
Mod	Non-Fac Total	Fac Total		51	50	62	80	MUE
	5.46	5.46	ZZZ	0	0	1	2	1

44227 Laparoscopy, surgical, closure of enterostomy, large or small intestine, with resection and anastomosis   C

RVU			Global Days	Modifiers				
Mod	Non-Fac Total	Fac Total		51	50	62	80	MUE
	48.47	48.47	090	2	0	1	2	1

44238 Unlisted laparoscopy procedure, intestine (except rectum)   x J 1

RVU			Global Days	Modifiers				
Mod	Non-Fac Total	Fac Total		51	50	62	80	MUE
	0.00	0.00	YYY	2	1	1	2	

AMA: May 03: 4

Enterostomy Creation/Revision Procedures

44300 Placement, enterostomy or cecostomy, tube open (eg, for feeding or decompression) (separate procedure)   C

RVU			Global Days	Modifiers				
Mod	Non-Fac Total	Fac Total		51	50	62	80	MUE
	24.45	24.45	090	2	0	1	2	1

AMA: Mar 02: 10, Aug 08: 7

44310 Ileostomy or jejunostomy, non-tube   C

RVU			Global Days	Modifiers				
Mod	Non-Fac Total	Fac Total		51	50	62	80	MUE
	30.35	30.35	090	2	0	1	2	2

AMA: Mar 02: 10, Apr 06: 1

44312 Revision of ileostomy; simple (release of superficial scar) (separate procedure)   A 2 T

RVU			Global Days	Modifiers				
Mod	Non-Fac Total	Fac Total		51	50	62	80	MUE
	17.06	17.06	090	2	0	0	0	1

AMA: Spring 93: 35

44314 Revision of ileostomy; complicated (reconstruction in-depth) (separate procedure)   C

RVU			Global Days	Modifiers				
Mod	Non-Fac Total	Fac Total		51	50	62	80	MUE
	29.10	29.10	090	2	0	1	2	1

44316 Continent ileostomy (Kock procedure) (separate procedure)   C

RVU			Global Days	Modifiers				
Mod	Non-Fac Total	Fac Total		51	50	62	80	MUE
	41.18	41.18	090	2	0	1	2	1

44320 Colostomy or skin level cecostomy   C

RVU			Global Days	Modifiers				
Mod	Non-Fac Total	Fac Total		51	50	62	80	MUE
	34.90	34.90	090	2	0	1	2	1

Colostomy or skin level cecostomy

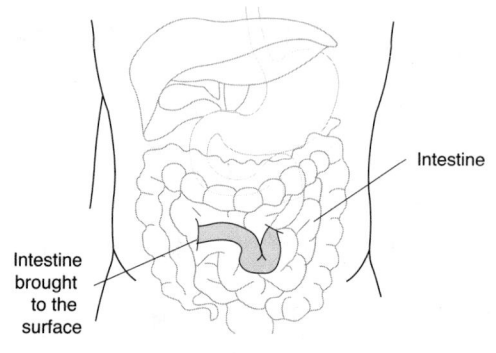

For 44320, a loop of the large intestine or the end of the large intestine is brought to the skin surface for the elimination of waste. Report 44322 for multiple biopsies.

44322 Colostomy or skin level cecostomy; with multiple biopsies (eg, for congenital megacolon) (separate procedure)   C

RVU			Global Days	Modifiers				
Mod	Non-Fac Total	Fac Total		51	50	62	80	MUE
	28.97	28.97	090	2	0	1	2	1

44340 Revision of colostomy; simple (release of superficial scar) (separate procedure)   A 2 T

RVU			Global Days	Modifiers				
Mod	Non-Fac Total	Fac Total		51	50	62	80	MUE
	18.15	18.15	090	2	0	1	1	1

Pub 100-04, 20, 130.1

44345 Revision of colostomy; complicated (reconstruction in-depth) (separate procedure)   C

RVU			Global Days	Modifiers				
Mod	Non-Fac Total	Fac Total		51	50	62	80	MUE
	30.55	30.55	090	2	0	1	2	1

44346 Revision of colostomy; with repair of paracolostomy hernia (separate procedure)   C

RVU			Global Days	Modifiers				
Mod	Non-Fac Total	Fac Total		51	50	62	80	MUE
	34.35	34.35	090	2	0	1	2	1

Pub 100-04, 20, 130.1

● New   ▲ Revised   ✖ Deleted   ⊙ Moderate Sedation   ✚ Add-on Codes   ⊘ High Risk Denial   Ⓐ Age Edit   ♀ Female   ♂ Male   **AMA** CPT® Assistant   **MUE** Medically Unlikely Edit
⊘ Modifier 51 Exempt   ⊖ Modifier 63 Exempt   ✗ Unlisted   **Modifiers:** See Inside Back Cover   Ⓜ Maternity   A 2–Z 3 ASC Payment Indicators   A –Y OPPS Status Indicators

CPT © 2015 American Medical Association. All Rights Reserved.   © 2016 DecisionHealth

Endoscopic Small Intestine/Stomal Procedures

Coding Guidance

When a surgical endoscopy directly follows a diagnostic endoscopy, the diagnostic portion is included. When a diagnostic endoscopic service is provided in conjunction with therapeutic endoscopic services, report only the more comprehensive endoscopy code that describes the service. If different therapeutic endoscopic services performed are not adequately described by a comprehensive service code, the appropriate multiple GI endoscopy codes can be used. When an endoscopy is performed to confirm or establish anatomical landmarks as a scout endoscopy, the procedure is not reported separately. When an endoscopy is done as a diagnostic procedure for basing the decision to do a more extensive open surgical procedure, the endoscopy may be separately reported. Control of bleeding resulting from an endoscopy and performed at the time of the service is included. If it becomes necessary to repeat an endoscopy in order to control bleeding, then a procedure code for endoscopic control of bleeding may be reported with a modifier identifying a return to the operative room in the postoperative period.

⊙ **44360** Small intestinal endoscopy, enteroscopy beyond second portion of duodenum, not including ileum; diagnostic, including collection of specimen(s) by brushing or washing, when performed (separate procedure) `A2 T`

RVU Mod	Non-Fac Total	Fac Total	Global Days	Modifiers 51	50	62	80	MUE
	4.38	4.38	000	2	0	0	1	1

AMA: Spring 94: 7, Mar 11: 10, Dec 13: 3, Nov 14: 3

Small intestinal endoscopy

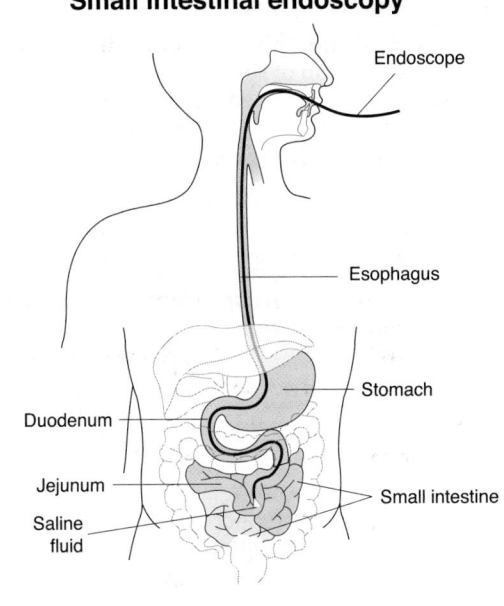

Report code (44361) when biopsy(s) are taken by endoscopic instrument

⊙ **44361** Small intestinal endoscopy, enteroscopy beyond second portion of duodenum, not including ileum; with biopsy, single or multiple `A2 T`

Coding tip: *Code 99001 for specimen transfer from a facility to an outside laboratory*

RVU Mod	Non-Fac Total	Fac Total	Global Days	Modifiers 51	50	62	80	MUE
	4.83	4.83	000	3	0	0	1	1

⊙ **44363** Small intestinal endoscopy, enteroscopy beyond second portion of duodenum, not including ileum; with removal of foreign body(s) `A2 T`

RVU Mod	Non-Fac Total	Fac Total	Global Days	Modifiers 51	50	62	80	MUE
	5.79	5.79	000	3	0	0	0	1

Small intestine endoscopy

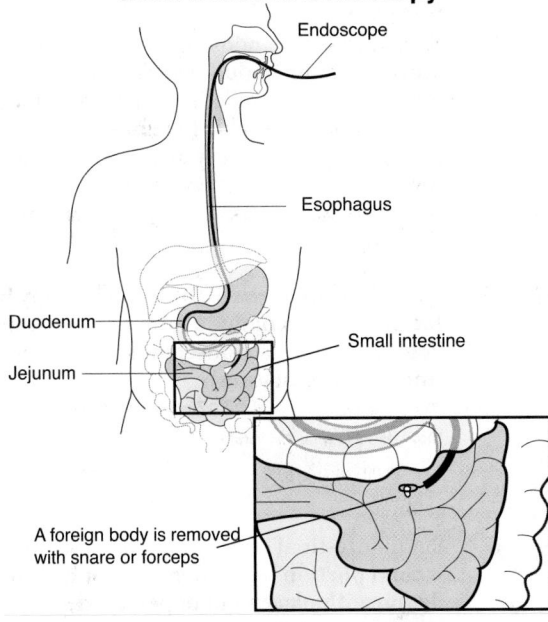

A foreign body is removed with snare or forceps

⊙ **44364** Small intestinal endoscopy, enteroscopy beyond second portion of duodenum, not including ileum; with removal of tumor(s), polyp(s), or other lesion(s) by snare technique `A2 T`

RVU Mod	Non-Fac Total	Fac Total	Global Days	Modifiers 51	50	62	80	MUE
	6.16	6.16	000	3	0	0	0	1

⊙ **44365** Small intestinal endoscopy, enteroscopy beyond second portion of duodenum, not including ileum; with removal of tumor(s), polyp(s), or other lesion(s) by hot biopsy forceps or bipolar cautery   `A 2 T`

RVU			Global Days	Modifiers				
Mod	Non-Fac Total	Fac Total		51	50	62	80	MUE
	5.42	5.42	000	3	0	0	0	1

⊙ **44366** Small intestinal endoscopy, enteroscopy beyond second portion of duodenum, not including ileum; with control of bleeding (eg, injection, bipolar cautery, unipolar cautery, laser, heater probe, stapler, plasma coagulator)   `A 2 T`

RVU			Global Days	Modifiers				
Mod	Non-Fac Total	Fac Total		51	50	62	80	MUE
	7.22	7.22	000	3	0	0	1	1

AMA: Jun 10: 4

⊙ **44369** Small intestinal endoscopy, enteroscopy beyond second portion of duodenum, not including ileum; with ablation of tumor(s), polyp(s), or other lesion(s) not amenable to removal by hot biopsy forceps, bipolar cautery or snare technique   `A 2 T`

RVU			Global Days	Modifiers				
Mod	Non-Fac Total	Fac Total		51	50	62	80	MUE
	7.39	7.39	000	3	0	0	0	1

⊙ **44370** Small intestinal endoscopy, enteroscopy beyond second portion of duodenum, not including ileum; with transendoscopic stent placement (includes predilation)   `A 2 J I`

RVU			Global Days	Modifiers				
Mod	Non-Fac Total	Fac Total		51	50	62	80	MUE
	8.00	8.00	000	3	0	0	0	1

AMA: Nov 01: 7

⊙ **44372** Small intestinal endoscopy, enteroscopy beyond second portion of duodenum, not including ileum; with placement of percutaneous jejunostomy tube   `A 2 T`

RVU			Global Days	Modifiers				
Mod	Non-Fac Total	Fac Total		51	50	62	80	MUE
	7.22	7.22	000	3	0	0	1	1

AMA: Spring 94: 7

⊙ **44373** Small intestinal endoscopy, enteroscopy beyond second portion of duodenum, not including ileum; with conversion of percutaneous gastrostomy tube to percutaneous jejunostomy tube   `A 2 T`

RVU			Global Days	Modifiers				
Mod	Non-Fac Total	Fac Total		51	50	62	80	MUE
	5.80	5.80	000	3	0	0	1	1

AMA: Spring 94: 7, Dec 13: 3

⊙ **44376** Small intestinal endoscopy, enteroscopy beyond second portion of duodenum, including ileum; diagnostic, with or without collection of specimen(s) by brushing or washing (separate procedure)   `A 2 T`

RVU			Global Days	Modifiers				
Mod	Non-Fac Total	Fac Total		51	50	62	80	MUE
	8.51	8.51	000	2	0	0	0	1

AMA: Spring 94: 7, Mar 11: 10, Dec 13: 3

⊙ **44377** Small intestinal endoscopy, enteroscopy beyond second portion of duodenum, including ileum; with biopsy, single or multiple   `A 2 T`

Coding tip: *Code 99001 for specimen transfer from a facility to an outside laboratory*

RVU			Global Days	Modifiers				
Mod	Non-Fac Total	Fac Total		51	50	62	80	MUE
	8.98	8.98	000	3	0	0	0	1

AMA: Spring 94: 7

⊙ **44378** Small intestinal endoscopy, enteroscopy beyond second portion of duodenum, including ileum; with control of bleeding (eg, injection, bipolar cautery, unipolar cautery, laser, heater probe, stapler, plasma coagulator)   `A 2 T`

RVU			Global Days	Modifiers				
Mod	Non-Fac Total	Fac Total		51	50	62	80	MUE
	11.48	11.48	000	3	0	0	0	1

AMA: Spring 94: 7, Apr 12: 17, Jun 10: 4, Dec 13: 3

⊙ **44379** Small intestinal endoscopy, enteroscopy beyond second portion of duodenum, including ileum; with transendoscopic stent placement (includes predilation)   `A 2 J I`

RVU			Global Days	Modifiers				
Mod	Non-Fac Total	Fac Total		51	50	62	80	MUE
	12.23	12.23	000	3	0	0	0	1

AMA: Nov 01: 7, Nov 14: 3

⊙ **44380** Ileoscopy, through stoma; diagnostic, including collection of specimen(s) by brushing or washing, when performed (separate procedure)   `A 2 T`

RVU			Global Days	Modifiers				
Mod	Non-Fac Total	Fac Total		51	50	62	80	MUE
	6.26	1.81	000	2	0	0	1	1

AMA: Dec 13: 3, Nov 14: 3, Dec 14: 3

Pub 100-04, 20, 130.1

⊙ **44381** Ileoscopy, through stoma; with transendoscopic balloon dilation   `G 2 T`

RVU			Global Days	Modifiers				
Mod	Non-Fac Total	Fac Total		51	50	62	80	MUE
	28.41	2.65	000	3	0	0	1	1

AMA: Nov 14: 3

**Ileoscopy, through stoma;
with transendoscopic balloon dilation**

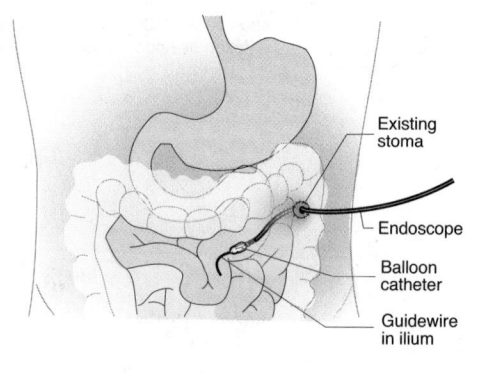

Existing stoma
Endoscope
Balloon catheter
Guidewire in ilium

● New   ▲ Revised   ✖ Deleted   ⊙ Moderate Sedation   ✚ Add-on Codes   ⊘ High Risk Denial   Ⓐ Age Edit   ♀ Female   ♂ Male   **AMA** *CPT® Assistant*   **MUE** Medically Unlikely Edit

⊘ Modifier 51 Exempt   ⊖ Modifier 63 Exempt   ✘ Unlisted   **Modifiers:** *See Inside Back Cover*   Ⓜ Maternity   `A 2`–`Z 3` ASC Payment Indicators   `A`–`Y` OPPS Status Indicators

CPT © 2015 American Medical Association. All Rights Reserved.   © 2016 DecisionHealth

⊙ **44382 Ileoscopy, through stoma; with biopsy, single or multiple** `A2T`

Coding tip: Code 99001 for specimen transfer from a facility to an outside laboratory

Mod	RVU Non-Fac Total	Fac Total	Global Days	51	50	62	80	MUE
	9.09	2.30	000	3	0	0	1	1

AMA: Dec 13: 3

Pub 100-04, 20, 130.1

⊙ **44384 Ileoscopy, through stoma; with placement of endoscopic stent (includes pre- and post-dilation and guide wire passage, when performed)** `G2J1`

Mod	RVU Non-Fac Total	Fac Total	Global Days	51	50	62	80	MUE
	4.59	4.59	000	3	0	0	1	1

AMA: Nov 14: 3

⊙ **44385 Endoscopic evaluation of small intestinal pouch (eg, Kock pouch, ileal reservoir [S or J]); diagnostic, including collection of specimen(s) by brushing or washing, when performed (separate procedure)** `A2T`

Mod	RVU Non-Fac Total	Fac Total	Global Days	51	50	62	80	MUE
	6.91	2.24	000	2	0	0	1	1

⊙ **44386 Endoscopic evaluation of small intestinal pouch (eg, Kock pouch, ileal reservoir [S or J]); with biopsy, single or multiple** `A2T`

Coding tip: Code 99001 for specimen transfer from a facility to an outside laboratory

Mod	RVU Non-Fac Total	Fac Total	Global Days	51	50	62	80	MUE
	9.73	2.77	000	2	0	0	1	1

AMA: Dec 13: 3

⊙ **44388 Colonoscopy through stoma; diagnostic, including collection of specimen(s) by brushing or washing, when performed (separate procedure)** `A2T`

Mod	RVU Non-Fac Total	Fac Total	Global Days	51	50	62	80	MUE
	10.04	4.75	000	2	0	0	1	1
53	4.98	2.34	000	2	0	0	1	1

AMA: Nov 07: 8, Dec 13: 3, Nov 14: 3

Pub 100-04, 20, 130.1

⊙ **44389 Colonoscopy through stoma; with biopsy, single or multiple** `A2T`

Coding tip: Code 99001 for specimen transfer from a facility to an outside laboratory

Mod	RVU Non-Fac Total	Fac Total	Global Days	51	50	62	80	MUE
	12.66	5.21	000	3	0	0	1	1

AMA: Dec 14: 3

⊙ **44390 Colonoscopy through stoma; with removal of foreign body(s)** `A2T`

Mod	RVU Non-Fac Total	Fac Total	Global Days	51	50	62	80	MUE
	12.64	6.35	000	3	0	0	1	1

⊙ **44391 Colonoscopy through stoma; with control of bleeding, any method** `A2T`

Mod	RVU Non-Fac Total	Fac Total	Global Days	51	50	62	80	MUE
	21.80	6.94	000	3	0	0	1	1

AMA: Jun 10: 4

⊙ **44392 Colonoscopy through stoma; with removal of tumor(s), polyp(s), or other lesion(s) by hot biopsy forceps** `A2T`

Mod	RVU Non-Fac Total	Fac Total	Global Days	51	50	62	80	MUE
	11.89	5.98	000	3	0	0	1	1

Pub 100-04, 20, 130.1

⊙ **44394 Colonoscopy through stoma; with removal of tumor(s), polyp(s), or other lesion(s) by snare technique** `A2T`

Mod	RVU Non-Fac Total	Fac Total	Global Days	51	50	62	80	MUE
	13.40	6.79	000	3	0	0	1	1

⊙ **44401 Colonoscopy through stoma; with ablation of tumor(s), polyp(s), or other lesion(s) (includes pre-and post-dilation and guide wire passage, when performed)** `G2T`

Mod	RVU Non-Fac Total	Fac Total	Global Days	51	50	62	80	MUE
	92.54	7.28	000	3	0	0	1	1

AMA: Nov 14: 3

Colonoscopy through stoma; with ablation of tumor(s), polyp(s), or other lesion(s)

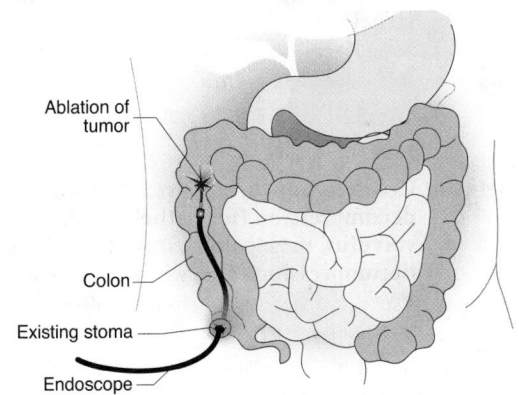

Ablation of tumor

Colon

Existing stoma

Endoscope

⊙ **44402 Colonoscopy through stoma; with endoscopic stent placement (including pre- and post-dilation and guide wire passage, when performed)** `G2J1`

Mod	RVU Non-Fac Total	Fac Total	Global Days	51	50	62	80	MUE
	7.89	7.89	000	3	0	0	1	1

AMA: Nov 14: 3

● New   ▲ Revised   Deleted   ⊙ Moderate Sedation   ✚ Add-on Codes   ⊘ High Risk Denial   Ⓐ Age Edit   ♀ Female   ♂ Male   **AMA** *CPT® Assistant*   *MUE* Medically Unlikely Edit
⊘ Modifier 51 Exempt   ⊖ Modifier 63 Exempt   ✗ Unlisted   **Modifiers:** *See Inside Back Cover*   Ⓜ Maternity   `A2`–`Z3` ASC Payment Indicators   `A`–`Y` OPPS Status Indicators

© 2016 DecisionHealth   CPT © 2015 American Medical Association. All Rights Reserved.   **449**

Surgical Procedures

44382 – 44402

Surgical Procedures

44403 – 44604

⊙ **44403 Colonoscopy through stoma; with endoscopic mucosal resection** `G2T`

RVU			Global Days	Modifiers				
Mod	Non-Fac Total	Fac Total		51	50	62	80	MUE
	9.05	9.05	000	3	0	0	1	1

AMA: Nov 14: 3

⊙ **44404 Colonoscopy through stoma; with directed submucosal injection(s), any substance** `G2T`

RVU			Global Days	Modifiers				
Mod	Non-Fac Total	Fac Total		51	50	62	80	MUE
	12.13	5.22	000	3	0	0	1	1

AMA: Nov 14: 3

⊙ **44405 Colonoscopy through stoma; with transendoscopic balloon dilation** `G2T`

RVU			Global Days	Modifiers				
Mod	Non-Fac Total	Fac Total		51	50	62	80	MUE
	17.39	5.55	000	3	0	0	1	1

AMA: Nov 14: 3

⊙ **44406 Colonoscopy through stoma; with endoscopic ultrasound examination, limited to the sigmoid, descending, transverse, or ascending colon and cecum and adjacent structures** `G2T`

RVU			Global Days	Modifiers				
Mod	Non-Fac Total	Fac Total		51	50	62	80	MUE
	6.91	6.91	000	3	0	0	1	1

AMA: Nov 14: 3

⊙ **44407 Colonoscopy through stoma; with transendoscopic ultrasound guided intramural or transmural fine needle aspiration/biopsy(s), includes endoscopic ultrasound examination limited to the sigmoid, descending, transverse, or ascending colon and cecum and adjacent structures** `G2T`

RVU			Global Days	Modifiers				
Mod	Non-Fac Total	Fac Total		51	50	62	80	MUE
	8.27	8.27	000	3	0	0	1	1

AMA: Nov 14: 3, Dec 14: 3

⊙ **44408 Colonoscopy through stoma; with decompression (for pathologic distention) (eg, volvulus, megacolon), including placement of decompression tube, when performed** `G2T`

RVU			Global Days	Modifiers				
Mod	Non-Fac Total	Fac Total		51	50	62	80	MUE
	6.98	6.98	000	3	0	0	1	1

AMA: Nov 14: 3, Dec 14: 3

Introduction Intestinal Procedures

⊙⃠ **44500 Introduction of long gastrointestinal tube (eg, Miller-Abbott) (separate procedure)** `G2T`

Coding tip: For radiological portion of procedure - 74340

Coding tip: Codes 99148-99150 may be reported when a second physician or other qualified health care professional (other than the one performing the procedure) provides moderate sedation in a facility setting only

RVU			Global Days	Modifiers				
Mod	Non-Fac Total	Fac Total		51	50	62	80	MUE
	0.71	0.71	000	0	0	0	0	1

Introduction of long gastrointestinal tube

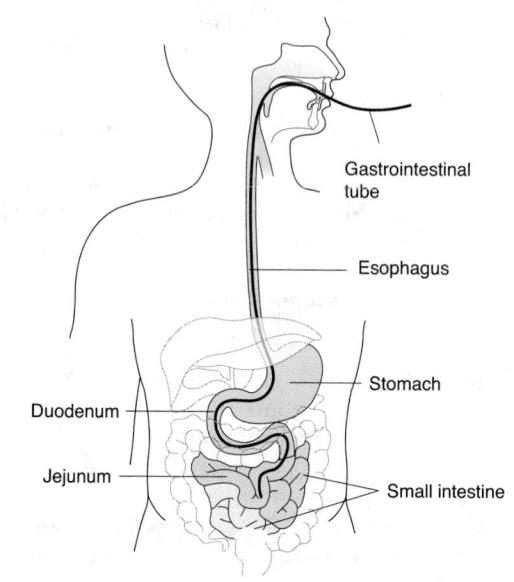

A long tube is inserted through the mouth or nose and into the gastrointestinal tract. The tube may travel as far as the intestines.

Intestinal Repair

44602 Suture of small intestine (enterorrhaphy) for perforated ulcer, diverticulum, wound, injury or rupture; single perforation `C`

RVU			Global Days	Modifiers				
Mod	Non-Fac Total	Fac Total		51	50	62	80	MUE
	41.09	41.09	090	2	0	1	2	1

44603 Suture of small intestine (enterorrhaphy) for perforated ulcer, diverticulum, wound, injury or rupture; multiple perforations `C`

RVU			Global Days	Modifiers				
Mod	Non-Fac Total	Fac Total		51	50	62	80	MUE
	47.09	47.09	090	2	0	1	2	1

44604 Suture of large intestine (colorrhaphy) for perforated ulcer, diverticulum, wound, injury or rupture (single or multiple perforations); without colostomy `C`

RVU			Global Days	Modifiers				
Mod	Non-Fac Total	Fac Total		51	50	62	80	MUE
	30.72	30.72	090	2	0	1	2	1

● New   ▲ Revised   ✖ Deleted   ⊙ Moderate Sedation   ✚ Add-on Codes   ⊘ High Risk Denial   Ⓐ Age Edit   ♀ Female   ♂ Male   **AMA** *CPT® Assistant*   **MUE** Medically Unlikely Edit

⃠ Modifier 51 Exempt   ⊖ Modifier 63 Exempt   ✘ Unlisted   **Modifiers:** *See Inside Back Cover*   Ⓜ Maternity   `A2`–`Z3` ASC Payment Indicators   `A`–`Y` OPPS Status Indicators

450   CPT © 2015 American Medical Association. All Rights Reserved.   © 2016 DecisionHealth

44605 Suture of large intestine (colorrhaphy) for perforated ulcer, diverticulum, wound, injury or rupture (single or multiple perforations); with colostomy ☒

RVU		Global Days	Modifiers				
Mod	Non-Fac Total	Fac Total		51	50	62	80	MUE
	37.96	37.96	090	2	0	1	2	1

44615 Intestinal stricturoplasty (enterotomy and enterorrhaphy) with or without dilation, for intestinal obstruction ☒

RVU		Global Days	Modifiers				
Mod	Non-Fac Total	Fac Total		51	50	62	80	MUE
	31.27	31.27	090	2	0	1	2	4

44620 Closure of enterostomy, large or small intestine ☒

RVU		Global Days	Modifiers				
Mod	Non-Fac Total	Fac Total		51	50	62	80	MUE
	25.20	25.20	090	2	0	1	2	2

AMA: Nov 97: 17, May 02: 7

44625 Closure of enterostomy, large or small intestine; with resection and anastomosis other than colorectal ☒

RVU		Global Days	Modifiers				
Mod	Non-Fac Total	Fac Total		51	50	62	80	MUE
	29.55	29.55	090	2	0	1	2	1

AMA: Nov 97: 17

44626 Closure of enterostomy, large or small intestine; with resection and colorectal anastomosis (eg, closure of Hartmann type procedure) ☒

RVU		Global Days	Modifiers				
Mod	Non-Fac Total	Fac Total		51	50	62	80	MUE
	46.61	46.61	090	2	0	1	2	1

AMA: Nov 97: 17

44640 Closure of intestinal cutaneous fistula ☒

RVU		Global Days	Modifiers				
Mod	Non-Fac Total	Fac Total		51	50	62	80	MUE
	40.78	40.78	090	2	0	1	2	2

44650 Closure of enteroenteric or enterocolic fistula ☒

RVU		Global Days	Modifiers				
Mod	Non-Fac Total	Fac Total		51	50	62	80	MUE
	42.18	42.18	090	2	0	1	2	2

44660 Closure of enterovesical fistula; without intestinal or bladder resection ☒

RVU		Global Days	Modifiers				
Mod	Non-Fac Total	Fac Total		51	50	62	80	MUE
	38.42	38.42	090	2	0	1	2	1

44661 Closure of enterovesical fistula; with intestine and/or bladder resection ☒

Coding tip: This code includes resection and anastomosis of a bowel segment when enteric resection is necessary for enterovesical fistula closure.

RVU		Global Days	Modifiers				
Mod	Non-Fac Total	Fac Total		51	50	62	80	MUE
	45.06	45.06	090	2	0	1	2	1

44680 Intestinal plication (separate procedure) ☒

RVU		Global Days	Modifiers				
Mod	Non-Fac Total	Fac Total		51	50	62	80	MUE
	30.95	30.95	090	2	0	1	2	1

Other Intestinal Procedures

44700 Exclusion of small intestine from pelvis by mesh or other prosthesis, or native tissue (eg, bladder or omentum) ☒

RVU		Global Days	Modifiers				
Mod	Non-Fac Total	Fac Total		51	50	62	80	MUE
	29.62	29.62	090	2	0	1	2	1

AMA: Nov 97: 18

✚ 44701 Intraoperative colonic lavage (List separately in addition to code for primary procedure) ☒ N I N

RVU		Global Days	Modifiers				
Mod	Non-Fac Total	Fac Total		51	50	62	80	MUE
	4.88	4.88	ZZZ	0	0	1	2	1

44705 Preparation of fecal microbiota for instillation, including assessment of donor specimen ☒ B

RVU		Global Days	Modifiers				
Mod	Non-Fac Total	Fac Total		51	50	62	80	MUE
	0.00	0.00	XXX	9	9	9	9	1

AMA: Jan 13: 11, May 13: 12

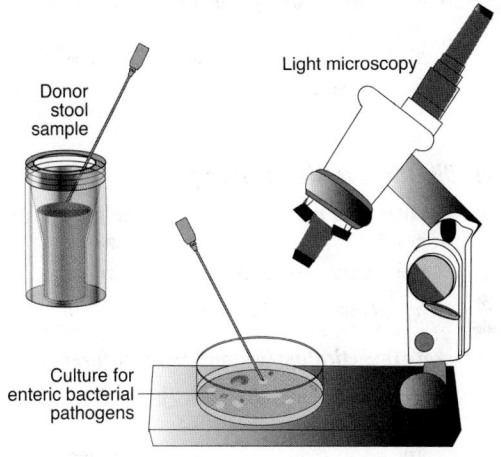

Preparation of fecal microbiota for instillation, including assessment of donor specimen

Donor stool sample

Light microscopy

Culture for enteric bacterial pathogens

44715 Backbench standard preparation of cadaver or living donor intestine allograft prior to transplantation, including mobilization and fashioning of the superior mesenteric artery and vein ☒

RVU		Global Days	Modifiers				
Mod	Non-Fac Total	Fac Total		51	50	62	80	MUE
	0.00	0.00	XXX	2	0	1	2	1

● New   ▲ Revised   Deleted   ⊙ Moderate Sedation   ✚ Add-on Codes   ⊘ High Risk Denial   Ⓐ Age Edit   ♀ Female   ♂ Male   **AMA** CPT® Assistant   **MUE** Medically Unlikely Edit
⊘ Modifier 51 Exempt   ⊖ Modifier 63 Exempt   Ⓧ Unlisted   **Modifiers:** See Inside Back Cover   Ⓜ Maternity   A 2 – Z 3 ASC Payment Indicators   A – Y OPPS Status Indicators

© 2016 DecisionHealth   CPT © 2015 American Medical Association. All Rights Reserved.   **451**

44605 – 44715

Surgical Procedures

44720 – 45000

44720 Backbench reconstruction of cadaver or living donor intestine allograft prior to transplantation; venous anastomosis, each   C

RVU			Global Days	Modifiers				
Mod	Non-Fac Total	Fac Total		51	50	62	80	MUE
	8.03	8.03	XXX	2	0	1	2	2

44721 Backbench reconstruction of cadaver or living donor intestine allograft prior to transplantation; arterial anastomosis, each   C

RVU			Global Days	Modifiers				
Mod	Non-Fac Total	Fac Total		51	50	62	80	MUE
	11.22	11.22	XXX	2	0	1	2	2

AMA: Apr 05: 10, 11

44799 Unlisted procedure, small intestine   ✗T

RVU			Global Days	Modifiers				
Mod	Non-Fac Total	Fac Total		51	50	62	80	MUE
	0.00	0.00	XXX	2	0	1		1

AMA: Dec 00: 14, May 08: 15, Nov 08: 11, Mar 10: 10, Mar 11: 10, May 11: 9, Jul 10: 10, May 13: 12, Nov 14: 3

Meckel's Diverticulum/Mesentery Procedures

Excisional Meckel's Diverticulum/Mesentery Procedures

44800 Excision of Meckel's diverticulum (diverticulectomy) or omphalomesenteric duct   C

RVU			Global Days	Modifiers				
Mod	Non-Fac Total	Fac Total		51	50	62	80	MUE
	22.12	22.12	090	2	0	1	2	1

44820 Excision of lesion of mesentery (separate procedure)   ⊘C

RVU			Global Days	Modifiers				
Mod	Non-Fac Total	Fac Total		51	50	62	80	MUE
	24.37	24.37	090	2	0	1	2	1

Meckel's Diverticulum/Mesentery Repair

44850 Suture of mesentery (separate procedure)   ⊘C

RVU			Global Days	Modifiers				
Mod	Non-Fac Total	Fac Total		51	50	62	80	MUE
	21.80	21.80	090	2	0	1	2	1

Other Meckel's Diverticulum/Mesentery Procedures

44899 Unlisted procedure, Meckel's diverticulum and the mesentery   ✗C

RVU			Global Days	Modifiers				
Mod	Non-Fac Total	Fac Total		51	50	62	80	MUE
	0.00	0.00	YYY	2	0	1	2	

Appendix Procedures

Incisional Appendix Procedures

44900 Incision and drainage of appendiceal abscess, open   C

RVU			Global Days	Modifiers				
Mod	Non-Fac Total	Fac Total		51	50	62	80	MUE
	22.39	22.39	090	2	0	1	2	1

AMA: Nov 97: 18

Excisional Appendix Procedures

Coding Guidance

Appendectomies are commonly done as an incidental procedure during intra-abdominal surgery and are not reported separately, but are included in the major surgery. The appendectomy is reported separately if medically necessary as a distinct service and may require the appropriate modifier if not reported alone.

44950 Appendectomy   T

RVU			Global Days	Modifiers				
Mod	Non-Fac Total	Fac Total		51	50	62	80	MUE
	18.65	18.65	090	2	0	1	2	1

AMA: Aug 02: 2, Nov 08: 7, Feb 92: 22, Sep 96: 4

✚ 44955 Appendectomy; when done for indicated purpose at time of other major procedure (not as separate procedure) (List separately in addition to code for primary procedure)   N

RVU			Global Days	Modifiers				
Mod	Non-Fac Total	Fac Total		51	50	62	80	MUE
	2.43	2.43	ZZZ	0	0	1	2	1

AMA: Fall 92: 22, Sep 96: 4, Apr 97: 3, Nov 08: 7, Jan 12: 13

44960 Appendectomy; for ruptured appendix with abscess or generalized peritonitis   C

RVU			Global Days	Modifiers				
Mod	Non-Fac Total	Fac Total		51	50	62	80	MUE
	25.41	25.41	090	2	0	1	2	1

AMA: Fall 92: 22, Nov 08: 7

Laparoscopic Appendix Procedures

44970 Laparoscopy, surgical, appendectomy   J1

Coding tip: *Removal of a normal appendix with another laparoscopic procedure is not separately reportable and should not be reported for an incidental laparoscopic appendectomy. Code 44970 may be reported separately with another laparoscopic procedure code when a diseased appendix is removed.*

RVU			Global Days	Modifiers				
Mod	Non-Fac Total	Fac Total		51	50	62	80	MUE
	17.44	17.44	090	2	0	2	2	1

AMA: Nov 99: 23, Mar 00: 9, Apr 06: 1, 20, Mar 15: 3

44979 Unlisted laparoscopy procedure, appendix   ✗J1

RVU			Global Days	Modifiers				
Mod	Non-Fac Total	Fac Total		51	50	62	80	MUE
	0.00	0.00	YYY	2	1	1	2	

AMA: Nov 99: 23, Mar 00: 9, Jan 12: 13

Rectal Procedures

Incisional Rectal Procedures

45000 Transrectal drainage of pelvic abscess   A2 T

RVU			Global Days	Modifiers				
Mod	Non-Fac Total	Fac Total		51	50	62	80	MUE
	12.23	12.23	090	2	0	0	1	1

● New   ▲ Revised   ✖ Deleted   ⊙ Moderate Sedation   ✚ Add-on Codes   ⊖ High Risk Denial   Ⓐ Age Edit   ♀ Female   ♂ Male   **AMA** *CPT® Assistant*   **MUE** Medically Unlikely Edit
⊘ Modifier 51 Exempt   ⊖ Modifier 63 Exempt   ✖ Unlisted   **Modifiers:** *See Inside Back Cover*   Ⓜ Maternity   A2–Z3 ASC Payment Indicators   A–Y OPPS Status Indicators

452   CPT © 2015 American Medical Association. All Rights Reserved.   © 2016 DecisionHealth

45005 Incision and drainage of submucosal abscess, rectum

A 2 T

Mod	Non-Fac Total	Fac Total	Global Days	Modifiers				MUE
				51	50	62	80	
	7.85	4.66	010	2	0	0	1	1

Incision and drainage of abscess, rectum/pelvirectal/retrorectal

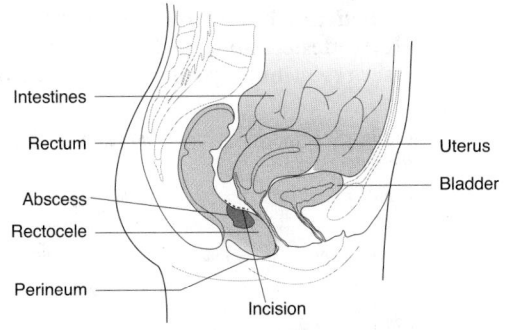

For submucosal abscess of the rectum use code (45005)
For deep pelvirectal/retrorectal abscess use code (45020)

45020 Incision and drainage of deep supralevator, pelvirectal, or retrorectal abscess

A 2 T

Coding tip: Incision and drainage of ischiorectal/perirectal abscess - 46040

Mod	Non-Fac Total	Fac Total	Global Days	Modifiers				MUE
				51	50	62	80	
	16.54	16.54	090	2	0	0	1	1

Excisional Rectal Procedures

45100 Biopsy of anorectal wall, anal approach (eg, congenital megacolon)

A 2 T

Coding tip: Do not report separately if done as part of another more complex procedure, such as lesion excision

Coding tip: Code 99000 for specimen transfer from office setting to an outside laboratory

Mod	Non-Fac Total	Fac Total	Global Days	Modifiers				MUE
				51	50	62	80	
	8.66	8.66	090	2	0	0	1	2

Biopsy of anorectal wall, anal approach

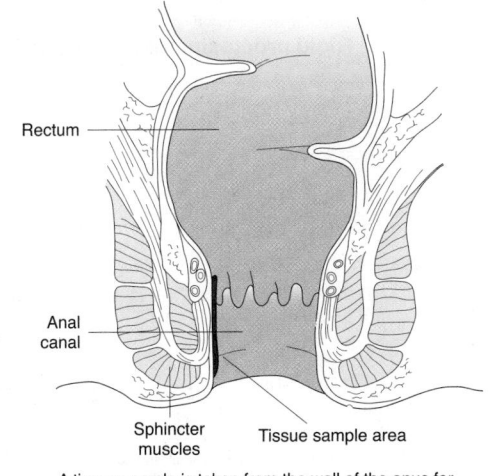

A tissue sample is taken from the wall of the anus for examination and diagnosis.

45108 Anorectal myomectomy

A 2 T

Mod	Non-Fac Total	Fac Total	Global Days	Modifiers				MUE
				51	50	62	80	
	10.60	10.60	090	2	0	1	1	1

45110 Proctectomy; complete, combined abdominoperineal, with colostomy

C

Mod	Non-Fac Total	Fac Total	Global Days	Modifiers				MUE
				51	50	62	80	
	53.65	53.65	090	2	0	1	2	1

45111 Proctectomy; partial resection of rectum, transabdominal approach

C

Mod	Non-Fac Total	Fac Total	Global Days	Modifiers				MUE
				51	50	62	80	
	31.55	31.55	090	2	0	1	2	1

45112 Proctectomy, combined abdominoperineal, pull-through procedure (eg, colo-anal anastomosis)

C

Mod	Non-Fac Total	Fac Total	Global Days	Modifiers				MUE
				51	50	62	80	
	54.56	54.56	090	2	0	1	2	1

AMA: Nov 97: 18

45113 Proctectomy, partial, with rectal mucosectomy, ileoanal anastomosis, creation of ileal reservoir (S or J), with or without loop ileostomy

C

Mod	Non-Fac Total	Fac Total	Global Days	Modifiers				MUE
				51	50	62	80	
	54.99	54.99	090	2	0	1	2	1

45114 Proctectomy, partial, with anastomosis; abdominal and transsacral approach

C

Mod	Non-Fac Total	Fac Total	Global Days	Modifiers				MUE
				51	50	62	80	
	52.85	52.85	090	2	0	1	2	1

45116 Proctectomy, partial, with anastomosis; transsacral approach only (Kraske type)

C

Mod	Non-Fac Total	Fac Total	Global Days	Modifiers				MUE
				51	50	62	80	
	47.82	47.82	090	2	0	1	2	1

45119 Proctectomy, combined abdominoperineal pull-through procedure (eg, colo-anal anastomosis), with creation of colonic reservoir (eg, J-pouch), with diverting enterostomy when performed

C

Mod	Non-Fac Total	Fac Total	Global Days	Modifiers				MUE
				51	50	62	80	
	56.54	56.54	090	2	0	1	2	1

AMA: Nov 97: 18, Apr 06: 1

45120 Proctectomy, complete (for congenital megacolon), abdominal and perineal approach; with pull-through procedure and anastomosis (eg, Swenson, Duhamel, or Soave type operation)

C

Mod	Non-Fac Total	Fac Total	Global Days	Modifiers				MUE
				51	50	62	80	
	43.64	43.64	090	2	0	1	2	1

● New   ▲ Revised   Deleted   ⊙ Moderate Sedation   ✚ Add-on Codes   ⊘ High Risk Denial   Ⓐ Age Edit   ♀ Female   ♂ Male   **AMA** *CPT® Assistant*   **MUE** Medically Unlikely Edit
⊘ Modifier 51 Exempt   ⊖ Modifier 63 Exempt   ✗ Unlisted   **Modifiers:** *See Inside Back Cover*   Ⓜ Maternity   A 2–Z 3 ASC Payment Indicators   A–Y OPPS Status Indicators

45121 Proctectomy, complete (for congenital megacolon), abdominal and perineal approach; with subtotal or total colectomy, with multiple biopsies   C

Mod	RVU Non-Fac Total	Fac Total	Global Days	Modifiers 51	50	62	80	MUE
	50.49	50.49	090	2	0	1	2	1

45123 Proctectomy, partial, without anastomosis, perineal approach   C

Mod	RVU Non-Fac Total	Fac Total	Global Days	Modifiers 51	50	62	80	MUE
	32.51	32.51	090	2	0	1	2	1

45126 Pelvic exenteration for colorectal malignancy, with proctectomy (with or without colostomy), with removal of bladder and ureteral transplantations, and/or hysterectomy, or cervicectomy, with or without removal of tube(s), with or without removal of ovary(s), or any combination thereof   C

Mod	RVU Non-Fac Total	Fac Total	Global Days	Modifiers 51	50	62	80	MUE
	81.25	81.25	090	2	0	1	2	1

AMA: Nov 98: 16

45130 Excision of rectal procidentia, with anastomosis; perineal approach   C

Mod	RVU Non-Fac Total	Fac Total	Global Days	Modifiers 51	50	62	80	MUE
	31.56	31.56	090	2	0	1	2	1

45135 Excision of rectal procidentia, with anastomosis; abdominal and perineal approach   C

Mod	RVU Non-Fac Total	Fac Total	Global Days	Modifiers 51	50	62	80	MUE
	39.77	39.77	090	2	0	1	2	1

45136 Excision of ileoanal reservoir with ileostomy   C

Mod	RVU Non-Fac Total	Fac Total	Global Days	Modifiers 51	50	62	80	MUE
	52.52	52.52	090	2	0	1	2	1

45150 Division of stricture of rectum   A 2 T

Mod	RVU Non-Fac Total	Fac Total	Global Days	Modifiers 51	50	62	80	MUE
	11.30	11.30	090	2	0	0	0	1

45160 Excision of rectal tumor by proctotomy, transsacral or transcoccygeal approach   A 2 T

Mod	RVU Non-Fac Total	Fac Total	Global Days	Modifiers 51	50	62	80	MUE
	29.67	29.67	090	2	0	1	2	1

45171 Excision of rectal tumor, transanal approach; not including muscularis propria (ie, partial thickness)   G 2 T

Mod	RVU Non-Fac Total	Fac Total	Global Days	Modifiers 51	50	62	80	MUE
	17.39	17.39	090	2	0	1	2	2

AMA: Jun 10: 3

45172 Excision of rectal tumor, transanal approach; including muscularis propria (ie, full thickness)   G 2 T

Mod	RVU Non-Fac Total	Fac Total	Global Days	Modifiers 51	50	62	80	MUE
	23.44	23.44	090	2	0	1	2	2

AMA: Jun 10: 3

Rectal Destruction Procedures

45190 Destruction of rectal tumor (eg, electrodesiccation, electrosurgery, laser ablation, laser resection, cryosurgery) transanal approach   A 2 T

Coding tip: Report for any method used to accomplish destruction of the tumor

Coding tip: Do not code local anesthesia

Mod	RVU Non-Fac Total	Fac Total	Global Days	Modifiers 51	50	62	80	MUE
	20.07	20.07	090	2	0	1	1	1

AMA: Jun 10: 3

Endoscopic Rectal Procedures

45300 Proctosigmoidoscopy, rigid; diagnostic, with or without collection of specimen(s) by brushing or washing (separate procedure)   P 3 T

Coding tip: Do not report with any surgical proctosigmoidoscopy

Coding tip: Report this procedure separately only when performed alone, or distinct from other procedures on the same day

Mod	RVU Non-Fac Total	Fac Total	Global Days	Modifiers 51	50	62	80	MUE
	3.50	1.56	000	2	0	0	1	1

AMA: Spring 94: 8, Oct 97: 6, Apr 06: 1

⊙ **45303** Proctosigmoidoscopy, rigid; with dilation (eg, balloon, guide wire, bougie)   P 2 T

Coding tip: Dilation with imaging guidance - add 74360

Coding tip: Codes 99148-99150 may be reported when a second physician or qualified health care professional (other than the one performing the procedure) provides moderate sedation in a facility setting only

Mod	RVU Non-Fac Total	Fac Total	Global Days	Modifiers 51	50	62	80	MUE
	27.33	2.68	000	3	0	0	1	1

AMA: Spring 94: 8, Oct 97: 6, Apr 06: 1

Rigid proctosigmoidoscopy with dilation

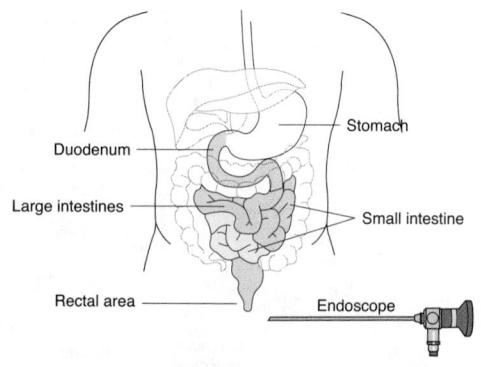

The physician inserts an endoscope into the rectal cavity to visualize the rectum and the last section of the large intestine, and dilate strictures.

● New   ▲ Revised   ✖ Deleted   ⊙ Moderate Sedation   ✚ Add-on Codes   ⊘ High Risk Denial   Ⓐ Age Edit   ♀ Female   ♂ Male   **AMA** *CPT® Assistant*   **MUE** Medically Unlikely Edit
⊘ Modifier 51 Exempt   ⊖ Modifier 63 Exempt   ✗ Unlisted   **Modifiers:** *See Inside Back Cover*   Ⓜ Maternity   A 2 – Z 3 ASC Payment Indicators   A – Y OPPS Status Indicators

CPT © 2015 American Medical Association. All Rights Reserved.   © 2016 DecisionHealth

⊙ **45305 Proctosigmoidoscopy, rigid; with biopsy, single or multiple** A 2 T

Coding tip: Do not report when the entire lesion/tumor/polyp is removed

Coding tip: Code 99000 for specimen transfer from office setting to an outside laboratory

Coding tip: Do not report more than once for all biopsy specimens taken

RVU			Global Days	Modifiers				
Mod	*Non-Fac Total*	*Fac Total*		51	50	62	80	MUE
	5.55	2.27	000	3	0	0	1	1

AMA: Spring 94: 8, Oct 97: 6, Apr 06: 1

⊙ **45307 Proctosigmoidoscopy, rigid; with removal of foreign body** A 2 T

RVU			Global Days	Modifiers				
Mod	*Non-Fac Total*	*Fac Total*		51	50	62	80	MUE
	6.66	3.08	000	3	0	0	0	1

AMA: Spring 94: 8, Oct 97: 6, Apr 06: 1

⊙ **45308 Proctosigmoidoscopy, rigid; with removal of single tumor, polyp, or other lesion by hot biopsy forceps or bipolar cautery** A 2 T

Coding tip: Ablation of tumors, polyps, or other lesions - 45320

RVU			Global Days	Modifiers				
Mod	*Non-Fac Total*	*Fac Total*		51	50	62	80	MUE
	6.14	2.58	000	3	0	0	1	1

AMA: Spring 94: 8, Oct 97: 6, Apr 06: 1

⊙ **45309 Proctosigmoidoscopy, rigid; with removal of single tumor, polyp, or other lesion by snare technique** A 2 T

RVU			Global Days	Modifiers				
Mod	*Non-Fac Total*	*Fac Total*		51	50	62	80	MUE
	6.44	2.75	000	3	0	0	1	1

AMA: Spring 94: 8, Oct 97: 6, Apr 06: 1

⊙ **45315 Proctosigmoidoscopy, rigid; with removal of multiple tumors, polyps, or other lesions by hot biopsy forceps, bipolar cautery or snare technique** A 2 T

RVU			Global Days	Modifiers				
Mod	*Non-Fac Total*	*Fac Total*		51	50	62	80	MUE
	6.43	3.03	000	3	0	0	1	1

AMA: Spring 94: 8, Oct 97: 6, Apr 06: 1

⊙ **45317 Proctosigmoidoscopy, rigid; with control of bleeding (eg, injection, bipolar cautery, unipolar cautery, laser, heater probe, stapler, plasma coagulator)** A 2 T

RVU			Global Days	Modifiers				
Mod	*Non-Fac Total*	*Fac Total*		51	50	62	80	MUE
	6.94	3.41	000	3	0	0	1	1

AMA: Spring 94: 8, Oct 97: 6, Apr 06: 1

⊙ **45320 Proctosigmoidoscopy, rigid; with ablation of tumor(s), polyp(s), or other lesion(s) not amenable to removal by hot biopsy forceps, bipolar cautery or snare technique (eg, laser)** A 2 T

Coding tip: For removal of tumors, polyps, or lesions - 45308-45315

RVU			Global Days	Modifiers				
Mod	*Non-Fac Total*	*Fac Total*		51	50	62	80	MUE
	6.94	3.20	000	3	0	0	1	1

AMA: Spring 94: 8, Oct 97: 6, Apr 06: 1

⊙ **45321 Proctosigmoidoscopy, rigid; with decompression of volvulus** A 2 T

RVU			Global Days	Modifiers				
Mod	*Non-Fac Total*	*Fac Total*		51	50	62	80	MUE
	3.11	3.11	000	3	0	0	1	1

AMA: Spring 94: 8, Oct 97: 6, Apr 06: 1

⊙ **45327 Proctosigmoidoscopy, rigid; with transendoscopic stent placement (includes predilation)** A 2 J 1

RVU			Global Days	Modifiers				
Mod	*Non-Fac Total*	*Fac Total*		51	50	62	80	MUE
	3.54	3.54	000	3	0	0	1	1

AMA: Nov 01: 7, Apr 06: 1

45330 Sigmoidoscopy, flexible; diagnostic, including collection of specimen(s) by brushing or washing, when performed (separate procedure) P 3 T

Coding tip: Do not report with any surgical sigmoidoscopy

Coding tip: Report this procedure separately only when performed alone, or distinct from other procedures on the same day

RVU			Global Days	Modifiers				
Mod	*Non-Fac Total*	*Fac Total*		51	50	62	80	MUE
	4.74	1.63	000	2	0	0	1	1

AMA: Spring 94: 9, May 05: 3, May 07: 10, Nov 07: 8, Dec 13: 3, Dec 14: 3, 19

Pub 100-04, 12, 30.1

45331 Sigmoidoscopy, flexible; with biopsy, single or multiple A 2 T

Coding tip: Code 99000 for specimen transfer from office setting to an outside laboratory

Coding tip: Do not report more than once for all biopsy specimens taken

Coding tip: Do not report when the entire lesion/tumor/polyp is removed

RVU			Global Days	Modifiers				
Mod	*Non-Fac Total*	*Fac Total*		51	50	62	80	MUE
	7.28	2.11	000	3	0	0	1	1

AMA: Spring 94: 9, Sep 96: 6, Jan 07: 28

Flexible sigmoidoscopy with biopsy

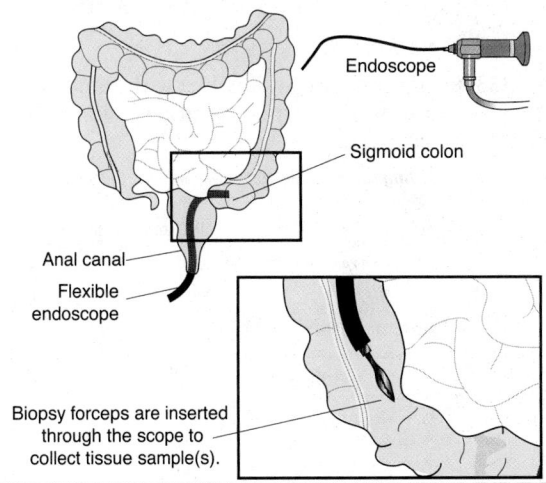

Endoscope

Sigmoid colon

Anal canal

Flexible endoscope

Biopsy forceps are inserted through the scope to collect tissue sample(s).

● New   ▲ Revised   Deleted   ⊙ Moderate Sedation   ✚ Add-on Codes   ⊘ High Risk Denial   Ⓐ Age Edit   ♀ Female   ♂ Male   **AMA** *CPT® Assistant*   **MUE** Medically Unlikely Edit

⊘ Modifier 51 Exempt   ⊖ Modifier 63 Exempt   ✗ Unlisted   **Modifiers:** *See Inside Back Cover*   Ⓜ Maternity   A 2 - Z 3 ASC Payment Indicators   A - Y OPPS Status Indicators

⊙ **45332 Sigmoidoscopy, flexible; with removal of foreign body(s)** `A 2 T`

Coding tip: Do not code 99143-99145

Coding tip: Codes 99148-99150 may be reported when a second physician or qualified health care professional (other than the one performing the procedure) provides moderate sedation in a facility setting only

RVU			Global Days	Modifiers				
Mod	Non-Fac Total	Fac Total		51	50	62	80	MUE
	8.83	3.25	000	3	0	0	1	1

AMA: Winter 90: 3, Spring 94: 9, Dec 14: 3

⊙ **45333 Sigmoidoscopy, flexible; with removal of tumor(s), polyp(s), or other lesion(s) by hot biopsy forceps** `A 2 T`

RVU			Global Days	Modifiers				
Mod	Non-Fac Total	Fac Total		51	50	62	80	MUE
	9.91	2.91	000	3	0	0	1	1

AMA: Winter 90: 3, Spring 94: 9, Dec 14: 3

⊙ **45334 Sigmoidoscopy, flexible; with control of bleeding, any method** `A 2 T`

Coding tip: Proctosigmoidoscopy with control of bleeding - 45317

RVU			Global Days	Modifiers				
Mod	Non-Fac Total	Fac Total		51	50	62	80	MUE
	17.32	3.61	000	3	0	0	1	1

AMA: Spring 94: 9, Sep 96: 6, Jan 07: 28, Jun 10: 5, Dec 14: 3

⊙ **45335 Sigmoidoscopy, flexible; with directed submucosal injection(s), any substance** `A 2 T`

RVU			Global Days	Modifiers				
Mod	Non-Fac Total	Fac Total		51	50	62	80	MUE
	8.21	2.10	000	3	0	0	1	1

AMA: Mar 03: 22, Jun 10: 5

⊙ **45337 Sigmoidoscopy, flexible; with decompression (for pathologic distention) (eg, volvulus, megacolon), including placement of decompression tube, when performed** `A 2 T`

RVU			Global Days	Modifiers				
Mod	Non-Fac Total	Fac Total		51	50	62	80	MUE
	3.54	3.54	000	3	0	0	1	1

AMA: Spring 94: 9, Dec 14: 3

⊙ **45338 Sigmoidoscopy, flexible; with removal of tumor(s), polyp(s), or other lesion(s) by snare technique** `A 2 T`

Coding tip: Proctosigmoidoscopy with removal of tumors, polyps, lesions - 45308-45315

RVU			Global Days	Modifiers				
Mod	Non-Fac Total	Fac Total		51	50	62	80	MUE
	9.22	3.69	000	3	0	0	1	1

AMA: Spring 94: 9

⊙ **45340 Sigmoidoscopy, flexible; with transendoscopic balloon dilation** `A 2 T`

Coding tip: Dilation with imaging guidance - add 74360

RVU			Global Days	Modifiers				
Mod	Non-Fac Total	Fac Total		51	50	62	80	MUE
	13.92	2.44	000	3	0	0	1	1

AMA: Dec 14: 3

⊙ **45341 Sigmoidoscopy, flexible; with endoscopic ultrasound examination** `A 2 T`

RVU			Global Days	Modifiers				
Mod	Non-Fac Total	Fac Total		51	50	62	80	MUE
	3.80	3.80	000	3	0	0	1	1

AMA: Oct 01: 4, May 05: 3, Dec 13: 3

⊙ **45342 Sigmoidoscopy, flexible; with transendoscopic ultrasound guided intramural or transmural fine needle aspiration/biopsy(s)** `A 2 T`

RVU			Global Days	Modifiers				
Mod	Non-Fac Total	Fac Total		51	50	62	80	MUE
	5.15	5.15	000	3	0	0	1	1

AMA: Oct 01: 4, May 05: 3, Dec 13: 3

⊙ **45346 Sigmoidoscopy, flexible; with ablation of tumor(s), polyp(s), or other lesion(s) (includes pre- and post-dilation and guide wire passage, when performed)** `G 2 T`

RVU			Global Days	Modifiers				
Mod	Non-Fac Total	Fac Total		51	50	62	80	MUE
	88.64	4.86	000	3	0	0	1	1

AMA: Dec 14: 3

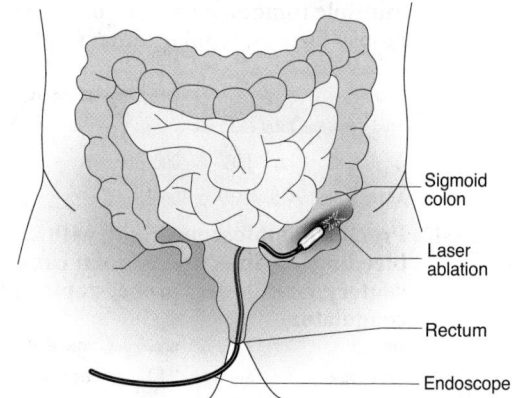

Sigmoidoscopy, flexible; with ablation of tumor(s), polyp(s), or other lesion(s)

Sigmoid colon

Laser ablation

Rectum

Endoscope

⊙ **45347 Sigmoidoscopy, flexible; with placement of endoscopic stent (includes pre- and post-dilation and guide wire passage, when performed)** `G 2 J I`

RVU			Global Days	Modifiers				
Mod	Non-Fac Total	Fac Total		51	50	62	80	MUE
	4.69	4.69	000	3	0	0	1	1

AMA: Dec 14: 3

● New   ▲ Revised   ✖ Deleted   ⊙ Moderate Sedation   ✚ Add-on Codes   ⊘ High Risk Denial   Ⓐ Age Edit   ♀ Female   ♂ Male   **AMA** *CPT® Assistant*   **MUE** Medically Unlikely Edit

⊘ Modifier 51 Exempt   ⊖ Modifier 63 Exempt   ✖ Unlisted   **Modifiers:** *See Inside Back Cover*   Ⓜ Maternity   `A 2`–`Z 3` ASC Payment Indicators   `A`–`Y` OPPS Status Indicators

CPT © 2015 American Medical Association. All Rights Reserved.   © 2016 DecisionHealth

⊙ **45349 Sigmoidoscopy, flexible; with endoscopic mucosal resection** `G2T`

RVU			Global Days	Modifiers				
Mod	Non-Fac Total	Fac Total		51	50	62	80	MUE
	5.98	5.98	000	3	0	0	1	1

AMA: Dec 14: 3

⊙ **45350 Sigmoidoscopy, flexible; with band ligation(s) (eg, hemorrhoids)** `G2T`

RVU			Global Days	Modifiers				
Mod	Non-Fac Total	Fac Total		51	50	62	80	MUE
	16.58	3.10	000	3	0	0	1	1

AMA: Dec 14: 3

⊙ **45378 Colonoscopy, flexible; diagnostic, including collection of specimen(s) by brushing or washing, when performed (separate procedure)** `A2T`

Coding tip: Report this procedure separately only when performed alone, or distinct from other procedures on the same day

Coding tip: Do not report with any surgical colonoscopy

Coding tip: Do not code 99143-99145

Coding tip: Codes 99148-99150 may be reported when a second physician or qualified health care professional (other than the one performing the procedure) provides moderate sedation in a facility setting only

RVU			Global Days	Modifiers				
Mod	Non-Fac Total	Fac Total		51	50	62	80	MUE
	10.78	5.59	000	2	0	0	1	1
53	5.38	2.79	000	2	0	0	1	1

AMA: Spring 94: 9, Aug 99: 3, Jan 02: 12, Jan 04: 4, May 05: 3, Dec 10: 3, Apr 11: 12, Jan 13: 11, Nov 14: 3, Dec 14: 3

Pub 100-04, 12, 30.1; 100-04, 18, 60.2.2

Colonoscopy

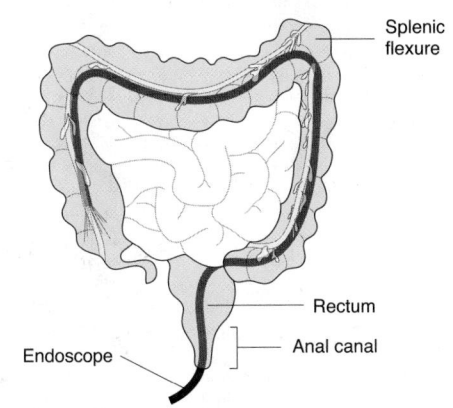

Splenic flexure

Rectum

Anal canal

Endoscope

⊙ **45379 Colonoscopy, flexible; with removal of foreign body(s)** `A2T`

RVU			Global Days	Modifiers				
Mod	Non-Fac Total	Fac Total		51	50	62	80	MUE
	13.60	7.19	000	3	0	0	1	1

AMA: Spring 94: 9, Aug 99: 3, Dec 14: 3

⊙ **45380 Colonoscopy, flexible; with biopsy, single or multiple** `A2T`

Coding tip: Code 99001 for specimen transfer from a facility setting to an outside laboratory

RVU			Global Days	Modifiers				
Mod	Non-Fac Total	Fac Total		51	50	62	80	MUE
	13.33	6.06	000	3	0	0	1	1

AMA: Spring 94: 9, Jan 96: 7, Feb 99: 11, Aug 99: 3, Jan 04: 7, Jul 04: 15, Dec 14: 3

⊙ **45381 Colonoscopy, flexible; with directed submucosal injection(s), any substance** `A2T`

RVU			Global Days	Modifiers				
Mod	Non-Fac Total	Fac Total		51	50	62	80	MUE
	12.82	6.05	000	3	0	0	1	1

AMA: Mar 03: 22, Jan 04: 7, Jun 10: 5

⊙ **45382 Colonoscopy, flexible; with control of bleeding, any method** `A2T`

RVU			Global Days	Modifiers				
Mod	Non-Fac Total	Fac Total		51	50	62	80	MUE
	22.55	7.78	000	3	0	0	1	1

AMA: Spring 94: 9, Aug 99: 3, Jun 10: 5, Dec 14: 3

⊙ **45384 Colonoscopy, flexible; with removal of tumor(s), polyp(s), or other lesion(s) by hot biopsy forceps** `A2T`

RVU			Global Days	Modifiers				
Mod	Non-Fac Total	Fac Total		51	50	62	80	MUE
	14.63	6.87	000	3	0	0	1	1

AMA: Spring 94: 9, Jul 98: 10, Feb 99: 11, Aug 99: 3, Jan 04: 6, Jul 04: 15, Apr 11: 12, Dec 14: 3, Jun 15: 10

⊙ **45385 Colonoscopy, flexible; with removal of tumor(s), polyp(s), or other lesion(s) by snare technique** `A2T`

Documentation Finder: Documentation should support a snare cautery technique where a wire loop is placed around the desired piece of tissue or polyp and is heated to shave off the lesion. Larger lesions may be removed with a single application of the snare or can be removed with several applications of the snare in pieces frequently described as "piecemeal." You should not report this code if the documentation states that the provider removed polyps using forceps.

RVU			Global Days	Modifiers				
Mod	Non-Fac Total	Fac Total		51	50	62	80	MUE
	13.98	7.65	000	3	0	0	1	1

AMA: Spring 94: 9, Jan 96: 7, Jul 98: 10, Aug 99: 3, Jan 04: 5, Jul 04: 15, Jun 10: 5

⊙ **45386 Colonoscopy, flexible; with transendoscopic balloon dilation** `A2T`

Coding tip: Dilation with imaging guidance - add 74360

RVU			Global Days	Modifiers				
Mod	Non-Fac Total	Fac Total		51	50	62	80	MUE
	18.63	6.39	000	3	0	0	1	1

AMA: Dec 14: 3

● New   ▲ Revised   Deleted   ⊙ Moderate Sedation   ✚ Add-on Codes   ⊘ High Risk Denial   Ⓐ Age Edit   ♀ Female   ♂ Male   **AMA** CPT® Assistant   **MUE** Medically Unlikely Edit
⊗ Modifier 51 Exempt   ⊖ Modifier 63 Exempt   ✗ Unlisted   **Modifiers:** See Inside Back Cover   Ⓜ Maternity   `A2`-`Z3` ASC Payment Indicators   `A`-`Y` OPPS Status Indicators

© 2016 DecisionHealth   CPT © 2015 American Medical Association. All Rights Reserved.   **457**

⊙ **45388** Colonoscopy, flexible; with ablation of tumor(s), polyp(s), or other lesion(s) (includes pre- and post-dilation and guide wire passage, when performed)   G2 T

RVU			Global Days	Modifiers				
Mod	Non-Fac Total	Fac Total		51	50	62	80	MUE
	93.10	8.12	000	3	0	0	1	1

AMA: Dec 14: 3

Colonoscopy, flexible; with ablation of tumor(s), polyp(s), or other lesion(s)

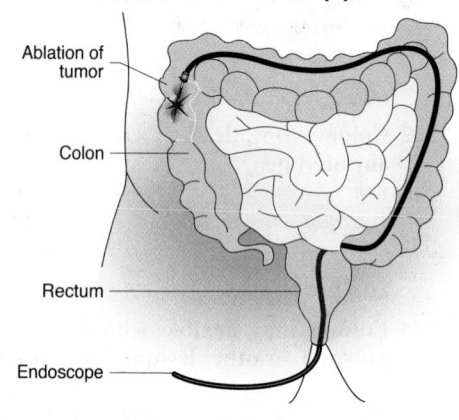

Ablation of tumor
Colon
Rectum
Endoscope

⊙ **45389** Colonoscopy, flexible; with endoscopic stent placement (includes pre- and post-dilation and guide wire passage, when performed)   G2 J T

RVU			Global Days	Modifiers				
Mod	Non-Fac Total	Fac Total		51	50	62	80	MUE
	8.69	8.69	000	3	0	0	1	1

AMA: Dec 14: 3

⊙ **45390** Colonoscopy, flexible; with endoscopic mucosal resection   G2 T

RVU			Global Days	Modifiers				
Mod	Non-Fac Total	Fac Total		51	50	62	80	MUE
	9.92	9.92	000	3	0	0	1	1

AMA: Dec 14: 3

⊙ **45391** Colonoscopy, flexible; with endoscopic ultrasound examination limited to the rectum, sigmoid, descending, transverse, or ascending colon and cecum, and adjacent structures   A2 T

RVU			Global Days	Modifiers				
Mod	Non-Fac Total	Fac Total		51	50	62	80	MUE
	7.73	7.73	000	3	0	0	1	1

AMA: May 05: 3, Dec 13: 3, Dec 14: 3

⊙ **45392** Colonoscopy, flexible; with transendoscopic ultrasound guided intramural or transmural fine needle aspiration/biopsy(s), includes endoscopic ultrasound examination limited to the rectum, sigmoid, descending, transverse, or ascending colon and cecum, and adjacent structures   A2 T

RVU			Global Days	Modifiers				
Mod	Non-Fac Total	Fac Total		51	50	62	80	MUE
	9.11	9.11	000	3	0	0	1	1

AMA: May 05: 3, Dec 13: 3, Dec 14: 3

⊙ **45393** Colonoscopy, flexible; with decompression (for pathologic distention) (eg, volvulus, megacolon), including placement of decompression tube, when performed   G2 T

RVU			Global Days	Modifiers				
Mod	Non-Fac Total	Fac Total		51	50	62	80	MUE
	7.59	7.59	000	3	0	0	1	1

AMA: Dec 14: 4

Laparoscopic Rectal Procedures

45395 Laparoscopy, surgical; proctectomy, complete, combined abdominoperineal, with colostomy   C

RVU			Global Days	Modifiers				
Mod	Non-Fac Total	Fac Total		51	50	62	80	MUE
	57.43	57.43	090	2	0	1	2	1

45397 Laparoscopy, surgical; proctectomy, combined abdominoperineal pull-through procedure (eg, colo-anal anastomosis), with creation of colonic reservoir (eg, J-pouch), with diverting enterostomy, when performed   C

RVU			Global Days	Modifiers				
Mod	Non-Fac Total	Fac Total		51	50	62	80	MUE
	62.54	62.54	090	2	0	1	2	1

⊙ **45398** Colonoscopy, flexible; with band ligation(s) (eg, hemorrhoids)   G2 T

RVU			Global Days	Modifiers				
Mod	Non-Fac Total	Fac Total		51	50	62	80	MUE
	20.82	7.07	000	3	0	0	1	1

AMA: Dec 14: 3

Colonoscopy, flexible; with band ligation(s) (eg, hemorrhoids)

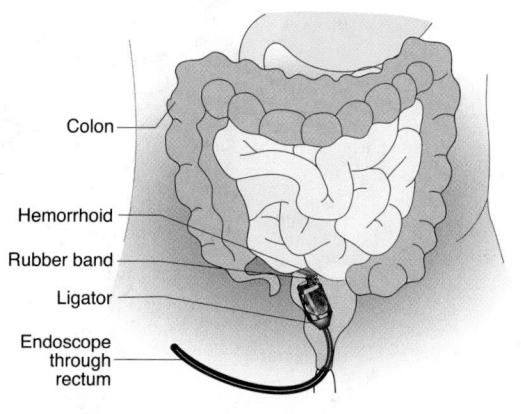

Colon
Hemorrhoid
Rubber band
Ligator
Endoscope through rectum

45399 Unlisted procedure, colon   T

RVU			Global Days	Modifiers				
Mod	Non-Fac Total	Fac Total		51	50	62	80	MUE
	0.00	0.00	XXX	2	0	1	1	

AMA: Nov 14: 3, Dec 14: 4

45400 Laparoscopy, surgical; proctopexy (for prolapse)   C

RVU			Global Days	Modifiers				
Mod	Non-Fac Total	Fac Total		51	50	62	80	MUE
	33.08	33.08	090	2	0	1	2	1

● New   ▲ Revised   ✖ Deleted   ⊙ Moderate Sedation   ➕ Add-on Codes   ⊘ High Risk Denial   Ⓐ Age Edit   ♀ Female   ♂ Male   **AMA** CPT® Assistant   **MUE** Medically Unlikely Edit
⊘ Modifier 51 Exempt   ⊖ Modifier 63 Exempt   ✗ Unlisted   **Modifiers:** *See Inside Back Cover*   Ⓜ Maternity   A2–Z3 ASC Payment Indicators   A–Y OPPS Status Indicators

458   CPT © 2015 American Medical Association. All Rights Reserved.   © 2016 DecisionHealth

45402 Laparoscopy, surgical; proctopexy (for prolapse), with sigmoid resection `C`

RVU			Global Days	Modifiers				
Mod	Non-Fac Total	Fac Total		51	50	62	80	MUE
	44.10	44.10	090	2	0	1	2	1

45499 Unlisted laparoscopy procedure, rectum `xJ1T`

RVU			Global Days	Modifiers				
Mod	Non-Fac Total	Fac Total		51	50	62	80	MUE
	0.00	0.00	YYY	2	0	1	2	

Rectal Repair

45500 Proctoplasty; for stenosis `A2T`

RVU			Global Days	Modifiers				
Mod	Non-Fac Total	Fac Total		51	50	62	80	MUE
	15.08	15.08	090	2	0	0	0	1

45505 Proctoplasty; for prolapse of mucous membrane `A2T`

RVU			Global Days	Modifiers				
Mod	Non-Fac Total	Fac Total		51	50	62	80	MUE
	17.15	17.15	090	2	0	0	1	1

AMA: Mar 15: 10, Oct 13: 19

45520 Perirectal injection of sclerosing solution for prolapse `NIQIT`

Coding tip: Do not report more than one time per session, regardless of the number of injections

RVU			Global Days	Modifiers				
Mod	Non-Fac Total	Fac Total		51	50	62	80	MUE
	4.47	1.17	000	2	0	0	1	1

AMA: Jul 01: 11, Aug 01: 10

Perirectal injection of sclerosing solution for prolapse

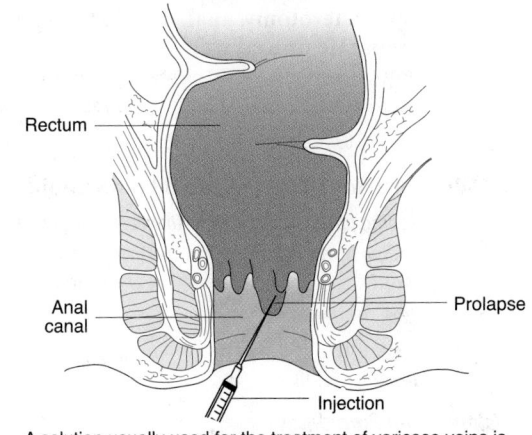

A solution usually used for the treatment of varicose veins is used to treat a condition in which the rectum protrudes through the anus.

45540 Proctopexy (eg, for prolapse); abdominal approach `C`

RVU			Global Days	Modifiers				
Mod	Non-Fac Total	Fac Total		51	50	62	80	MUE
	30.71	30.71	090	2	0	1	2	1

45541 Proctopexy (eg, for prolapse); perineal approach `G2T`

RVU			Global Days	Modifiers				
Mod	Non-Fac Total	Fac Total		51	50	62	80	MUE
	27.36	27.36	090	2	0	1	2	1

45550 Proctopexy (eg, for prolapse); with sigmoid resection, abdominal approach `C`

RVU			Global Days	Modifiers				
Mod	Non-Fac Total	Fac Total		51	50	62	80	MUE
	42.32	42.32	090	2	0	1	2	1

45560 Repair of rectocele (separate procedure) `A2T`

RVU			Global Days	Modifiers				
Mod	Non-Fac Total	Fac Total		51	50	62	80	MUE
	19.86	19.86	090	2	0	1	2	1

45562 Exploration, repair, and presacral drainage for rectal injury `C`

RVU			Global Days	Modifiers				
Mod	Non-Fac Total	Fac Total		51	50	62	80	MUE
	32.56	32.56	090	2	0	1	2	1

45563 Exploration, repair, and presacral drainage for rectal injury; with colostomy `C`

RVU			Global Days	Modifiers				
Mod	Non-Fac Total	Fac Total		51	50	62	80	MUE
	47.90	47.90	090	2	0	1	2	1

45800 Closure of rectovesical fistula `C`

RVU			Global Days	Modifiers				
Mod	Non-Fac Total	Fac Total		51	50	62	80	MUE
	34.59	34.59	090	2	0	1	2	1

45805 Closure of rectovesical fistula; with colostomy `C`

RVU			Global Days	Modifiers				
Mod	Non-Fac Total	Fac Total		51	50	62	80	MUE
	42.52	42.52	090	2	0	1	2	1

45820 Closure of rectourethral fistula `C`

RVU			Global Days	Modifiers				
Mod	Non-Fac Total	Fac Total		51	50	62	80	MUE
	34.54	34.54	090	2	0	1	2	1

45825 Closure of rectourethral fistula; with colostomy `C`

RVU			Global Days	Modifiers				
Mod	Non-Fac Total	Fac Total		51	50	62	80	MUE
	40.08	40.08	090	2	0	1	2	1

Rectal Manipulation Procedures

45900 Reduction of procidentia (separate procedure) under anesthesia `A2T`

RVU			Global Days	Modifiers				
Mod	Non-Fac Total	Fac Total		51	50	62	80	MUE
	5.88	5.88	010	2	0	0	0	1

45905 Dilation of anal sphincter (separate procedure) under anesthesia other than local `A2T`

RVU			Global Days	Modifiers				
Mod	Non-Fac Total	Fac Total		51	50	62	80	MUE
	4.91	4.91	010	2	0	0	1	1

● New ▲ Revised Deleted ⊙ Moderate Sedation ✚ Add-on Codes ⊘ High Risk Denial Ⓐ Age Edit ♀ Female ♂ Male **AMA** *CPT® Assistant* ***MUE*** Medically Unlikely Edit

⊘ Modifier 51 Exempt ⊖ Modifier 63 Exempt ✗ Unlisted **Modifiers:** *See Inside Back Cover* Ⓜ Maternity `A2`–`Z3` ASC Payment Indicators `A`–`Y` OPPS Status Indicators

Surgical Procedures

45402 – 45905

Surgical Procedures

45910 – 46200

45910 Dilation of rectal stricture (separate procedure) under anesthesia other than local   A 2 T

RVU			Global Days	Modifiers				
Mod	Non-Fac Total	Fac Total		51	50	62	80	MUE
	5.62	5.62	010	2	0	0	1	1

45915 Removal of fecal impaction or foreign body (separate procedure) under anesthesia   A 2 T

Coding tip: Report this procedure separately only when performed alone, or distinct from other procedures on the same day

RVU			Global Days	Modifiers				
Mod	Non-Fac Total	Fac Total		51	50	62	80	MUE
	9.47	6.52	010	2	0	0	1	1

Other Rectal Procedures

45990 Anorectal exam, surgical, requiring anesthesia (general, spinal, or epidural), diagnostic   A 2 T

Coding tip: Do not code any individual components included in the exam separately

RVU			Global Days	Modifiers				
Mod	Non-Fac Total	Fac Total		51	50	62	80	MUE
	3.13	3.13	000	2	0	1	0	1

45999 Unlisted procedure, rectum   ⊗ x T

RVU			Global Days	Modifiers				
Mod	Non-Fac Total	Fac Total		51	50	62	80	MUE
	0.00	0.00	YYY	2	0	1	0	

Anal Procedures

Incisional Anal Procedures

46020 Placement of seton   A 2 T

RVU			Global Days	Modifiers				
Mod	Non-Fac Total	Fac Total		51	50	62	80	MUE
	7.93	6.76	010	2	0	0	1	2

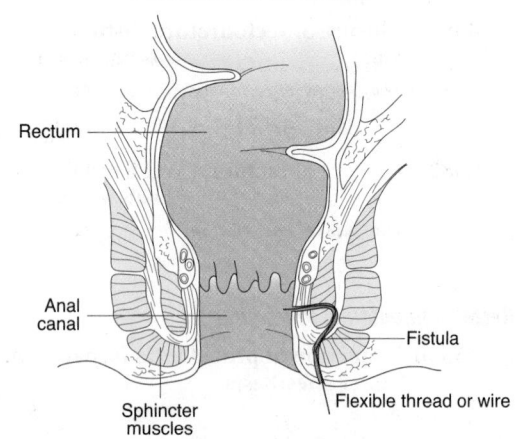

Placement of seton

A flexible thread or wire is placed in the tract of an abscess or fistula that has developed in the walls of the anus.

Labels: Rectum, Anal canal, Sphincter muscles, Fistula, Flexible thread or wire

46030 Removal of anal seton, other marker   A 2 T

RVU			Global Days	Modifiers				
Mod	Non-Fac Total	Fac Total		51	50	62	80	MUE
	3.98	2.60	010	2	0	0	0	1

46040 Incision and drainage of ischiorectal and/or perirectal abscess (separate procedure)   A 2 T

Coding tip: Inicison and drainage of submucosal rectal abscess - 45005
Coding tip: Subcutaneous treatment of anal fistula - 46270

RVU			Global Days	Modifiers				
Mod	Non-Fac Total	Fac Total		51	50	62	80	MUE
	15.36	11.97	090	2	0	0	1	2

46045 Incision and drainage of intramural, intramuscular, or submucosal abscess, transanal, under anesthesia   A 2 T

Coding tip: Inicison and drainage of pelvirectal or retrorectal abscess - 45020

RVU			Global Days	Modifiers				
Mod	Non-Fac Total	Fac Total		51	50	62	80	MUE
	12.53	12.53	090	2	0	0	1	2

46050 Incision and drainage, perianal abscess, superficial   A 2 T

RVU			Global Days	Modifiers				
Mod	Non-Fac Total	Fac Total		51	50	62	80	MUE
	5.74	2.80	010	2	0	0	1	2

46060 Incision and drainage of ischiorectal or intramural abscess, with fistulectomy or fistulotomy, submuscular, with or without placement of seton   A 2 T

RVU			Global Days	Modifiers				
Mod	Non-Fac Total	Fac Total		51	50	62	80	MUE
	13.77	13.77	090	2	0	0	1	2

46070 Incision, anal septum (infant)   Ⓐ ⊖ G 2 T

RVU			Global Days	Modifiers				
Mod	Non-Fac Total	Fac Total		51	50	62	80	MUE
	6.53	6.53	090	2	0	0	0	1

46080 Sphincterotomy, anal, division of sphincter (separate procedure)   A 2 T

RVU			Global Days	Modifiers				
Mod	Non-Fac Total	Fac Total		51	50	62	80	MUE
	7.09	4.60	010	2	0	0	1	1

46083 Incision of thrombosed hemorrhoid, external   P 2 T

Coding tip: Excision of external thrombosed hemorrhoid - 46320
Coding tip: Excision of external anal tags or papillae - 46230

RVU			Global Days	Modifiers				
Mod	Non-Fac Total	Fac Total		51	50	62	80	MUE
	5.01	3.06	010	2	0	0	1	2

AMA: Jun 97: 10

Excisional Anal Procedures

Coding Guidance

Hemorrhoidectomy, internal, by ligation other than rubber band is reported with code 46495 (single hemorrhoid column/group) or 46946 (2 or more hemorrhoid columns/groups). Hemorrhoidopexy is reported with code 46947.

46200 Fissurectomy, including sphincterotomy, when performed   A 2 T

RVU			Global Days	Modifiers				
Mod	Non-Fac Total	Fac Total		51	50	62	80	MUE
	12.71	9.35	090	2	0	0	1	1

● New   ▲ Revised   ✖ Deleted   ⊙ Moderate Sedation   ✚ Add-on Codes   ⊗ High Risk Denial   Ⓐ Age Edit   ♀ Female   ♂ Male   **AMA** *CPT® Assistant*   **MUE** Medically Unlikely Edit
⊘ Modifier 51 Exempt   ⊖ Modifier 63 Exempt   ⊠ Unlisted   **Modifiers:** *See Inside Back Cover*   Ⓜ Maternity   A 2 – Z 3 ASC Payment Indicators   A – Y OPPS Status Indicators

460   CPT © 2015 American Medical Association. All Rights Reserved.   © 2016 DecisionHealth

46220 Excision of single external papilla or tag, anus `A 2 T`

> **Coding tip:** *Code 46220 is listed out of numeric order in CPT. Related codes - 46200-46262, 46320, 46945-46946*
>
> **Coding tip:** *Excision of multiple papillae or tags - 46230*

RVU		Global Days	Modifiers				
Mod	*Non-Fac Total*	*Fac Total*		51	50	62	80	MUE
	5.89	3.43	010	2	0	0	1	1

Coding Guidance

Only the more extensive procedure necessary to accomplish the hemorrhoidectomy is reported. If an abscess is identified and drained during the hemorrhoidectomy, a separate code is not reported for the incision and drainage. If the abscess occurred at a different location than the hemorrhoidectomy, then an incision and drainage may be reported with the appropriate modifier.

46221 Hemorrhoidectomy, internal, by rubber band ligation(s) `P 3 T`

> **Coding tip:** *Ligation other than rubber band - 46945-46946*

RVU		Global Days	Modifiers				
Mod	*Non-Fac Total*	*Fac Total*		51	50	62	80	MUE
	7.66	5.47	010	2	0	0	1	1

AMA: Oct 97: 8, Dec 14: 3, Apr 15: 10

46230 Excision of multiple external papillae or tags, anus `A 2 T`

> **Coding tip:** *Excision single external papilla or tag - 46220*

RVU		Global Days	Modifiers				
Mod	*Non-Fac Total*	*Fac Total*		51	50	62	80	MUE
	7.80	4.98	010	2	0	0	1	1

46250 Hemorrhoidectomy, external, 2 or more columns/groups `A 2 T`

> **Coding tip:** *Incision of thrombosed hemorrhoid - 46083*
>
> **Coding tip:** *Excision external thrombosed hemorrhoid - 46320*
>
> **Coding tip:** *For single external column/group - 46999*

RVU		Global Days	Modifiers				
Mod	*Non-Fac Total*	*Fac Total*		51	50	62	80	MUE
	13.29	9.11	090	2	0	0	1	1

Hemorrhoidectomy

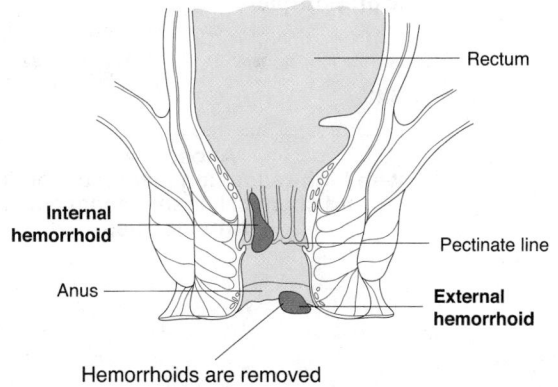

Rectum

Internal hemorrhoid

Pectinate line

Anus

External hemorrhoid

Hemorrhoids are removed

46255 Hemorrhoidectomy, internal and external, single column/group `A 2 T`

RVU		Global Days	Modifiers				
Mod	*Non-Fac Total*	*Fac Total*		51	50	62	80	MUE
	14.53	10.23	090	2	0	0	1	1

AMA: Oct 14: 15

46257 Hemorrhoidectomy, internal and external, single column/group; with fissurectomy `A 2 T`

RVU		Global Days	Modifiers				
Mod	*Non-Fac Total*	*Fac Total*		51	50	62	80	MUE
	12.18	12.18	090	2	0	0	1	1

46258 Hemorrhoidectomy, internal and external, single column/group; with fistulectomy, including fissurectomy, when performed `A 2 T`

RVU		Global Days	Modifiers				
Mod	*Non-Fac Total*	*Fac Total*		51	50	62	80	MUE
	13.49	13.49	090	2	0	0	0	1

46260 Hemorrhoidectomy, internal and external, 2 or more columns/groups `A 2 T`

RVU		Global Days	Modifiers				
Mod	*Non-Fac Total*	*Fac Total*		51	50	62	80	MUE
	13.75	13.75	090	2	0	0	1	1

46261 Hemorrhoidectomy, internal and external, 2 or more columns/groups; with fissurectomy `A 2 T`

RVU		Global Days	Modifiers				
Mod	*Non-Fac Total*	*Fac Total*		51	50	62	80	MUE
	15.09	15.09	090	2	0	0	1	1

46262 Hemorrhoidectomy, internal and external, 2 or more columns/groups; with fistulectomy, including fissurectomy, when performed `A 2 T`

RVU		Global Days	Modifiers				
Mod	*Non-Fac Total*	*Fac Total*		51	50	62	80	MUE
	15.93	15.93	090	2	0	0	1	1

AMA: May 05: 3

46270 Surgical treatment of anal fistula (fistulectomy/fistulotomy); subcutaneous `A 2 T`

RVU		Global Days	Modifiers				
Mod	*Non-Fac Total*	*Fac Total*		51	50	62	80	MUE
	14.59	11.33	090	2	0	0	1	1

46275 Surgical treatment of anal fistula (fistulectomy/fistulotomy); intersphincteric `A 2 T`

RVU		Global Days	Modifiers				
Mod	*Non-Fac Total*	*Fac Total*		51	50	62	80	MUE
	15.43	11.94	090	2	0	0	1	1

46280 Surgical treatment of anal fistula (fistulectomy/fistulotomy); transsphincteric, suprasphincteric, extrasphincteric or multiple, including placement of seton, when performed `A 2 T`

RVU		Global Days	Modifiers				
Mod	*Non-Fac Total*	*Fac Total*		51	50	62	80	MUE
	13.55	13.55	090	2	0	0	1	1

46285 Surgical treatment of anal fistula (fistulectomy/fistulotomy); second stage `A 2 T`

RVU		Global Days	Modifiers				
Mod	*Non-Fac Total*	*Fac Total*		51	50	62	80	MUE
	15.29	11.91	090	2	0	0	1	1

● New   ▲ Revised   Deleted   ⊙ Moderate Sedation   ✚ Add-on Codes   ⊖ High Risk Denial   Ⓐ Age Edit   ♀ Female   ♂ Male   **AMA** *CPT® Assistant*   **MUE** Medically Unlikely Edit
⊘ Modifier 51 Exempt   ⊖ Modifier 63 Exempt   ✗ Unlisted   **Modifiers:** *See Inside Back Cover*   Ⓜ Maternity   `A 2`–`Z 3` ASC Payment Indicators   `A`–`Y` OPPS Status Indicators

© 2016 DecisionHealth   CPT © 2015 American Medical Association. All Rights Reserved.   **461**

Surgical Procedures

46220 — 46285

46288 Closure of anal fistula with rectal advancement flap

`A 2 T`

RVU			Global Days	Modifiers				
Mod	Non-Fac Total	Fac Total		51	50	62	80	MUE
	15.89	15.89	090	2	0	0	1	1

46320 Excision of thrombosed hemorrhoid, external

`P 3 T`

Coding tip: Code 46320 is listed out of numeric order in CPT. Related codes - 46200-46262, 46945-46946

RVU			Global Days	Modifiers				
Mod	Non-Fac Total	Fac Total		51	50	62	80	MUE
	5.23	3.20	010	2	0	0	1	2

Introduction/Injection Anal Procedures

46500 Injection of sclerosing solution, hemorrhoids `P 3 T`

Coding tip: Other hemorrhoid procedures: excision - 46250-46262; destruction - 46930; ligation - 46945-46946; hemorrhoidopexy - 46947

RVU			Global Days	Modifiers				
Mod	Non-Fac Total	Fac Total		51	50	62	80	MUE
	5.54	3.55	010	2	0	0	1	1

AMA: May 05: 3

46505 Chemodenervation of internal anal sphincter `G 2 T`

RVU			Global Days	Modifiers				
Mod	Non-Fac Total	Fac Total		51	50	62	80	MUE
	8.17	6.88	010	2	1	0	1	1

Endoscopic Anal Procedures

46600 Anoscopy; diagnostic, including collection of specimen(s) by brushing or washing, when performed (separate procedure)

`N 1 Q 1`

RVU			Global Days	Modifiers				
Mod	Non-Fac Total	Fac Total		51	50	62	80	MUE
	2.52	1.18	000	2	0	0	1	1

AMA: Spring 94: 9, Oct 97: 6, Apr 06: 1, Aug 11: 9, Jun 10: 3

46601 Anoscopy; diagnostic, with high-resolution magnification (HRA) (eg, colposcope, operating microscope) and chemical agent enhancement, including collection of specimen(s) by brushing or washing, when performed

`N 1 Q 1`

RVU			Global Days	Modifiers				
Mod	Non-Fac Total	Fac Total		51	50	62	80	MUE
	3.90	2.70	000	3	0	0	1	1

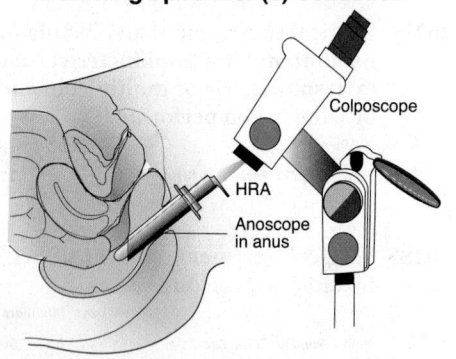

Anoscopy; diagnostic, with high-resolution magnification (HRA) and chemical agent enhancement including specimen(s) collection

46604 Anoscopy; with dilation (eg, balloon, guide wire, bougie)

`P 3 T`

Coding tip: Dilation with proctosigmoidoscopy - 45303; with sigmoidoscopy - 45340

RVU			Global Days	Modifiers				
Mod	Non-Fac Total	Fac Total		51	50	62	80	MUE
	17.62	1.92	000	3	0	0	1	1

AMA: Spring 94: 9, Oct 97: 6

46606 Anoscopy; with biopsy, single or multiple `P 3 T`

Coding tip: Do not report more than once for all biopsy specimens taken

Coding tip: Biopsy with proctosigmoidoscopy - 45305; with sigmoidoscopy - 45331

Coding tip: Code 99000 for specimen transfer from office setting to an outside laboratory

Coding tip: Do not report when the entire lesion/tumor/polyp is removed

RVU			Global Days	Modifiers				
Mod	Non-Fac Total	Fac Total		51	50	62	80	MUE
	6.43	2.20	000	3	0	0	1	1

AMA: Spring 94: 9, Oct 97: 6

Pub 100-04, 12, 40.6

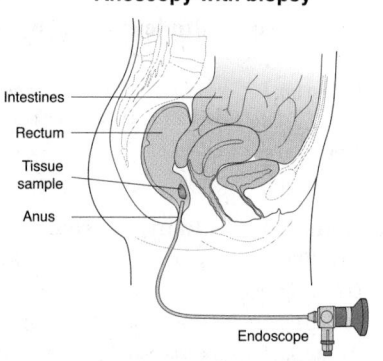

Anoscopy with biopsy

Intestines
Rectum
Tissue sample
Anus
Endoscope

The physician inserts an endoscope into the anus to check for disease or injury. One or more tissue samples are taken for examination/diagnosis.

46607 Anoscopy; with high-resolution magnification (HRA) (eg, colposcope, operating microscope) and chemical agent enhancement, with biopsy, single or multiple

`G 2 T`

RVU			Global Days	Modifiers				
Mod	Non-Fac Total	Fac Total		51	50	62	80	MUE
	5.44	3.64	000	3	0	0	1	1

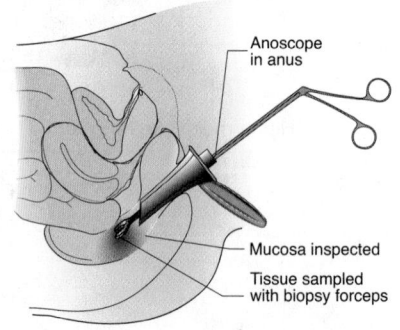

Anoscopy; with high-resolution magnification (HRA) and chemical agent enhancement, with biopsies

Anoscope in anus
Mucosa inspected
Tissue sampled with biopsy forceps

● New   ▲ Revised   ✖ Deleted   ☉ Moderate Sedation   ✚ Add-on Codes   ⊘ High Risk Denial   Ⓐ Age Edit   ♀ Female   ♂ Male   **AMA** CPT® Assistant   **MUE** Medically Unlikely Edit

⊘ Modifier 51 Exempt   ⊖ Modifier 63 Exempt   ✗ Unlisted   **Modifiers:** See Inside Back Cover   Ⓜ Maternity   `A 2`–`Z 3` ASC Payment Indicators   `A`–`Y` OPPS Status Indicators

CPT © 2015 American Medical Association. All Rights Reserved.   © 2016 DecisionHealth

46608 Anoscopy; with removal of foreign body `A2 T`

Coding tip: Removal of foreign body with proctosigmoidoscopy - 45307; with sigmoidoscopy - 45332

RVU		Global Days	Modifiers				
Mod	Non-Fac Total	Fac Total		51	50	62	80	MUE
	6.61	2.34	000	3	0	0	1	1

AMA: Spring 94: 9, Oct 97: 6

Pub 100-04, 12, 40.6

46610 Anoscopy; with removal of single tumor, polyp, or other lesion by hot biopsy forceps or bipolar cautery `A2 T`

Coding tip: Removal of single tumor/polyp/lesion with proctosigmoidoscopy - 45308-45309; with sigmoidoscopy - 45333, 45338

RVU		Global Days	Modifiers				
Mod	Non-Fac Total	Fac Total		51	50	62	80	MUE
	6.43	2.34	000	3	0	0	1	1

AMA: Spring 94: 10, Oct 97: 6

46611 Anoscopy; with removal of single tumor, polyp, or other lesion by snare technique `A2 T`

RVU		Global Days	Modifiers				
Mod	Non-Fac Total	Fac Total		51	50	62	80	MUE
	5.00	2.35	000	3	0	0	1	1

AMA: Spring 94: 10, Oct 97: 6

46612 Anoscopy; with removal of multiple tumors, polyps, or other lesions by hot biopsy forceps, bipolar cautery or snare technique `A2 T`

Coding tip: Removal of multiple tumors/polyps/lesions with proctosigmoidoscopy - 45315; sigmoidoscopy - 45333, 45338

RVU		Global Days	Modifiers				
Mod	Non-Fac Total	Fac Total		51	50	62	80	MUE
	7.33	2.70	000	3	0	0	1	1

AMA: Spring 94: 10, Oct 97: 6

46614 Anoscopy; with control of bleeding (eg, injection, bipolar cautery, unipolar cautery, laser, heater probe, stapler, plasma coagulator) `P3 T`

Coding tip: Control of bleeding with proctosigmoidoscopy - 45317; with sigmoidoscopy - 45334

RVU		Global Days	Modifiers				
Mod	Non-Fac Total	Fac Total		51	50	62	80	MUE
	3.65	1.87	000	3	0	0	1	1

AMA: Spring 94: 10, Oct 97: 6

46615 Anoscopy; with ablation of tumor(s), polyp(s), or other lesion(s) not amenable to removal by hot biopsy forceps, bipolar cautery or snare technique `A2 T`

Coding tip: Ablation of tumors/polyps/lesions with proctosigmoidoscopy - 45320; with sigmoidoscopy - 45339

RVU		Global Days	Modifiers				
Mod	Non-Fac Total	Fac Total		51	50	62	80	MUE
	4.11	2.68	000	3	0	0	1	1

AMA: Spring 94: 10, Oct 97: 6

Anal Repair

46700 Anoplasty, plastic operation for stricture; adult `Ⓐ A2 T`

RVU		Global Days	Modifiers				
Mod	Non-Fac Total	Fac Total		51	50	62	80	MUE
	18.88	18.88	090	2	0	0	1	1

46705 Anoplasty, plastic operation for stricture; infant `Ⓐ ⊖ C`

RVU		Global Days	Modifiers				
Mod	Non-Fac Total	Fac Total		51	50	62	80	MUE
	14.47	14.47	090	2	0	1	2	1

46706 Repair of anal fistula with fibrin glue `A2 T`

RVU		Global Days	Modifiers				
Mod	Non-Fac Total	Fac Total		51	50	62	80	MUE
	4.79	4.79	010	2	0	0	1	1

46707 Repair of anorectal fistula with plug (eg, porcine small intestine submucosa [SIS]) `G2 T`

RVU		Global Days	Modifiers				
Mod	Non-Fac Total	Fac Total		51	50	62	80	MUE
	13.77	13.77	090	2	0	0	0	1

AMA: Jan 12: 10, Oct 13: 15

46710 Repair of ileoanal pouch fistula/sinus (eg, perineal or vaginal), pouch advancement; transperineal approach `C`

RVU		Global Days	Modifiers				
Mod	Non-Fac Total	Fac Total		51	50	62	80	MUE
	30.47	30.47	090	2	0	1	2	1

46712 Repair of ileoanal pouch fistula/sinus (eg, perineal or vaginal), pouch advancement; combined transperineal and transabdominal approach `C`

RVU		Global Days	Modifiers				
Mod	Non-Fac Total	Fac Total		51	50	62	80	MUE
	61.96	61.96	090	2	0	1	2	1

46715 Repair of low imperforate anus; with anoperineal fistula (cut-back procedure) `Ⓐ ⊖ C`

RVU		Global Days	Modifiers				
Mod	Non-Fac Total	Fac Total		51	50	62	80	MUE
	15.68	15.68	090	2	0	0	2	1

46716 Repair of low imperforate anus; with transposition of anoperineal or anovestibular fistula `Ⓐ ⊖ C`

RVU		Global Days	Modifiers				
Mod	Non-Fac Total	Fac Total		51	50	62	80	MUE
	32.03	32.03	090	2	0	1	2	1

46730 Repair of high imperforate anus without fistula; perineal or sacroperineal approach `⊗ Ⓐ ⊖ C`

RVU		Global Days	Modifiers				
Mod	Non-Fac Total	Fac Total		51	50	62	80	MUE
	52.69	52.69	090	2	0	1	2	1

46735 Repair of high imperforate anus without fistula; combined transabdominal and sacroperineal approaches `Ⓐ ⊖ C`

RVU		Global Days	Modifiers				
Mod	Non-Fac Total	Fac Total		51	50	62	80	MUE
	61.07	61.07	090	2	0	1	2	1

● New   ▲ Revised   Deleted   ⊙ Moderate Sedation   ✚ Add-on Codes   ⊘ High Risk Denial   Ⓐ Age Edit   ♀ Female   ♂ Male   **AMA** CPT® Assistant   **MUE** Medically Unlikely Edit
⊘ Modifier 51 Exempt   ⊖ Modifier 63 Exempt   ⌧ Unlisted   **Modifiers:** See Inside Back Cover   Ⓜ Maternity   A2–Z3 ASC Payment Indicators   A–Y OPPS Status Indicators

46740 Repair of high imperforate anus with rectourethral or rectovaginal fistula; perineal or sacroperineal approach   Ⓐ⊖Ⓒ

RVU			Global Days	Modifiers				
Mod	Non-Fac Total	Fac Total		51	50	62	80	MUE
	62.31	62.31	090	2	0	1	2	1

46742 Repair of high imperforate anus with rectourethral or rectovaginal fistula; combined transabdominal and sacroperineal approaches   Ⓐ⊖Ⓒ

RVU			Global Days	Modifiers				
Mod	Non-Fac Total	Fac Total		51	50	62	80	MUE
	70.47	70.47	090	2	0	1	2	1

46744 Repair of cloacal anomaly by anorectovaginoplasty and urethroplasty, sacroperineal approach   Ⓐ♀⊖Ⓒ

RVU			Global Days	Modifiers				
Mod	Non-Fac Total	Fac Total		51	50	62	80	MUE
	102.47	102.47	090	2	0	1	2	1

46746 Repair of cloacal anomaly by anorectovaginoplasty and urethroplasty, combined abdominal and sacroperineal approach   Ⓐ♀Ⓒ

RVU			Global Days	Modifiers				
Mod	Non-Fac Total	Fac Total		51	50	62	80	MUE
	105.75	105.75	090	2	0	1	2	1

46748 Repair of cloacal anomaly by anorectovaginoplasty and urethroplasty, combined abdominal and sacroperineal approach; with vaginal lengthening by intestinal graft or pedicle flaps   Ⓐ♀Ⓒ

RVU			Global Days	Modifiers				
Mod	Non-Fac Total	Fac Total		51	50	62	80	MUE
	114.85	114.85	090	2	0	1	2	1

46750 Sphincteroplasty, anal, for incontinence or prolapse; adult   ⒶA2T

RVU			Global Days	Modifiers				
Mod	Non-Fac Total	Fac Total		51	50	62	80	MUE
	21.80	21.80	090	2	0	1	2	1

46751 Sphincteroplasty, anal, for incontinence or prolapse; child   ⒶⒸ

RVU			Global Days	Modifiers				
Mod	Non-Fac Total	Fac Total		51	50	62	80	MUE
	17.23	17.23	090	2	0	1	2	1

46753 Graft (Thiersch operation) for rectal incontinence and/or prolapse   A2T

RVU			Global Days	Modifiers				
Mod	Non-Fac Total	Fac Total		51	50	62	80	MUE
	17.69	17.69	090	2	0	0	1	1

46754 Removal of Thiersch wire or suture, anal canal   A2T

RVU			Global Days	Modifiers				
Mod	Non-Fac Total	Fac Total		51	50	62	80	MUE
	8.35	6.53	010	2	0	0	0	1

46760 Sphincteroplasty, anal, for incontinence, adult; muscle transplant   A2T

RVU			Global Days	Modifiers				
Mod	Non-Fac Total	Fac Total		51	50	62	80	MUE
	31.57	31.57	090	2	0	1	2	1

46761 Sphincteroplasty, anal, for incontinence, adult; levator muscle imbrication (Park posterior anal repair)   A2T

RVU			Global Days	Modifiers				
Mod	Non-Fac Total	Fac Total		51	50	62	80	MUE
	26.54	26.54	090	2	0	1	2	1

46762 Sphincteroplasty, anal, for incontinence, adult; implantation artificial sphincter   A2J1

RVU			Global Days	Modifiers				
Mod	Non-Fac Total	Fac Total		51	50	62	80	MUE
	26.79	26.79	090	2	0	1	2	1

Anal Destruction Procedures

46900 Destruction of lesion(s), anus (eg, condyloma, papilloma, molluscum contagiosum, herpetic vesicle), simple; chemical   P2T

Coding tip: Destruction of lesion(s), anus, extensive - 46924

Coding tip: Destruction of rectal tumor - 45190

RVU			Global Days	Modifiers				
Mod	Non-Fac Total	Fac Total		51	50	62	80	MUE
	6.92	3.96	010	2	0	0	1	1

Destruction of anal lesion(s)

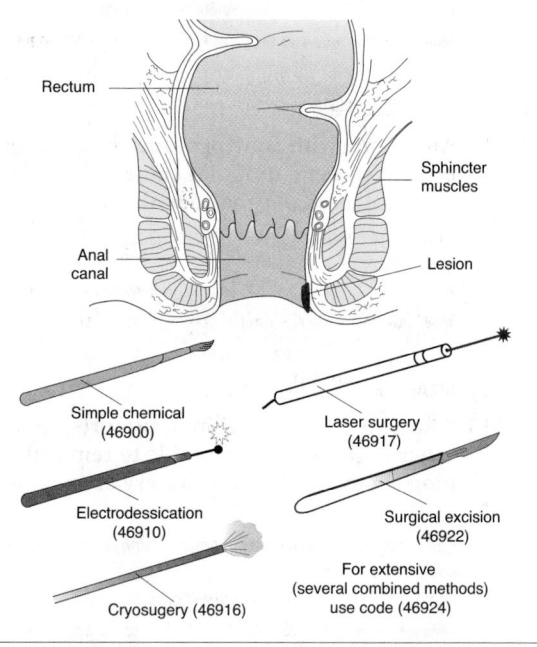

Rectum

Anal canal

Sphincter muscles

Lesion

Simple chemical (46900)

Laser surgery (46917)

Electrodessication (46910)

Surgical excision (46922)

Cryosugery (46916)

For extensive (several combined methods) use code (46924)

46910 Destruction of lesion(s), anus (eg, condyloma, papilloma, molluscum contagiosum, herpetic vesicle), simple; electrodesiccation   P3T

RVU			Global Days	Modifiers				
Mod	Non-Fac Total	Fac Total		51	50	62	80	MUE
	7.32	3.87	010	2	0	0	1	1

● New   ▲ Revised   ✖ Deleted   ⊙ Moderate Sedation   ✚ Add-on Codes   ⊘ High Risk Denial   Ⓐ Age Edit   ♀ Female   ♂ Male   **AMA** CPT® Assistant   **MUE** Medically Unlikely Edit
⊘ Modifier 51 Exempt   ⊖ Modifier 63 Exempt   ✗ Unlisted   **Modifiers:** See Inside Back Cover   Ⓜ Maternity   A2–Z3 ASC Payment Indicators   Ⓐ–Ⓨ OPPS Status Indicators

CPT © 2015 American Medical Association. All Rights Reserved.   © 2016 DecisionHealth

46916 Destruction of lesion(s), anus (eg, condyloma, papilloma, molluscum contagiosum, herpetic vesicle), simple; cryosurgery   P2T

RVU			Global Days	Modifiers				
Mod	Non-Fac Total	Fac Total		51	50	62	80	MUE
	6.56	4.13	010	2	0	0	1	1

46917 Destruction of lesion(s), anus (eg, condyloma, papilloma, molluscum contagiosum, herpetic vesicle), simple; laser surgery   A2T

RVU			Global Days	Modifiers				
Mod	Non-Fac Total	Fac Total		51	50	62	80	MUE
	12.85	3.80	010	2	0	0	1	1

46922 Destruction of lesion(s), anus (eg, condyloma, papilloma, molluscum contagiosum, herpetic vesicle), simple; surgical excision   A2T

RVU			Global Days	Modifiers				
Mod	Non-Fac Total	Fac Total		51	50	62	80	MUE
	7.62	3.91	010	2	0	0	1	1

46924 Destruction of lesion(s), anus (eg, condyloma, papilloma, molluscum contagiosum, herpetic vesicle), extensive (eg, laser surgery, electrosurgery, cryosurgery, chemosurgery)   A2T

Coding tip: Destruction of lesion(s), anus, simple - 46900-46922

Coding tip: Do not code local anesthesia

RVU			Global Days	Modifiers				
Mod	Non-Fac Total	Fac Total		51	50	62	80	MUE
	15.20	5.30	010	2	0	0	1	1

46930 Destruction of internal hemorrhoid(s) by thermal energy (eg, infrared coagulation, cautery, radiofrequency)   P3T

Coding tip: See also other hemorrhoid procedures: incision, external thrombosed hemorrhoids - 46083; injection - 46500; excision - 46250-46262, 46320; ligation - 46221, 46945-46946; hemorrhoidopexy - 46947

RVU			Global Days	Modifiers				
Mod	Non-Fac Total	Fac Total		51	50	62	80	MUE
	5.86	4.21	090	2	0	0	0	1

AMA: Apr 15: 10

46940 Curettage or cautery of anal fissure, including dilation of anal sphincter (separate procedure); initial   P3T

Coding tip: Do not report separately if done as part of another more complex procedure

Coding tip: Report this procedure separately only when performed alone, or distinct from other procedures on the same day

RVU			Global Days	Modifiers				
Mod	Non-Fac Total	Fac Total		51	50	62	80	MUE
	6.53	4.22	010	2	0	0	1	1

46942 Curettage or cautery of anal fissure, including dilation of anal sphincter (separate procedure); subsequent   P3T

RVU			Global Days	Modifiers				
Mod	Non-Fac Total	Fac Total		51	50	62	80	MUE
	6.17	3.79	010	2	0	0	0	1

Other Anal Procedures

46945 Hemorrhoidectomy, internal, by ligation other than rubber band; single hemorrhoid column/group   P3T

Coding tip: Code 46945 is listed out of numeric order in CPT. Related codes - 46200-46262, 46320, 46946

RVU			Global Days	Modifiers				
Mod	Non-Fac Total	Fac Total		51	50	62	80	MUE
	8.83	6.49	090	2	0	0	1	1

AMA: Apr 15: 10

46946 Hemorrhoidectomy, internal, by ligation other than rubber band; 2 or more hemorrhoid columns/groups   A2T

Coding tip: Code 46946 is listed out of numeric order in CPT. Related codes - 46200-46262, 46320, 46945

RVU			Global Days	Modifiers				
Mod	Non-Fac Total	Fac Total		51	50	62	80	MUE
	8.96	6.48	090	2	0	0	1	1

AMA: Apr 15: 10

46947 Hemorrhoidopexy (eg, for prolapsing internal hemorrhoids) by stapling   A2T

Coding tip: Code 46947 is listed out of numerical order in CPT. Additional anal/sphincter repair codes - 46700-46762

RVU			Global Days	Modifiers				
Mod	Non-Fac Total	Fac Total		51	50	62	80	MUE
	11.06	11.06	090	2	0	0	1	1

AMA: May 05: 3, 14

46999 Unlisted procedure, anus   ⨉T

RVU			Global Days	Modifiers				
Mod	Non-Fac Total	Fac Total		51	50	62	80	MUE
	0.00	0.00	YYY	2	0	1	0	

AMA: Oct 97: 8, Apr 15: 10

Liver Procedures

Incisional Liver Procedures

⊙ **47000** Biopsy of liver, needle; percutaneous   A2T

Coding tip: Report an additional code for radiological needle guidance - ultrasound 76942, fluoroscopy 77002, CT 77012, MRI 77021

RVU			Global Days	Modifiers				
Mod	Non-Fac Total	Fac Total		51	50	62	80	MUE
	10.30	2.98	000	2	0	0	1	3

AMA: Fall 93: 12

+ **47001** Biopsy of liver, needle; when done for indicated purpose at time of other major procedure (List separately in addition to code for primary procedure)   NIN

Coding tip: Radiological needle guidance - ultrasound 76942, fluoroscopy 77002

RVU			Global Days	Modifiers				
Mod	Non-Fac Total	Fac Total		51	50	62	80	MUE
	3.02	3.02	ZZZ	0	0	1	1	3

AMA: Jun 07: 10

47010 Hepatotomy, for open drainage of abscess or cyst, 1 or 2 stages   C

RVU			Global Days	Modifiers				
Mod	Non-Fac Total	Fac Total		51	50	62	80	MUE
	34.94	34.94	090	2	0	1	2	3

AMA: Nov 97: 18

● New   ▲ Revised   Deleted   ⊙ Moderate Sedation   ✚ Add-on Codes   ⊘ High Risk Denial   Ⓐ Age Edit   ♀ Female   ♂ Male   **AMA** CPT® Assistant   **MUE** Medically Unlikely Edit
⊘ Modifier 51 Exempt   ⊖ Modifier 63 Exempt   ⨉ Unlisted   **Modifiers:** See Inside Back Cover   Ⓜ Maternity   A2-Z3 ASC Payment Indicators   A-Y OPPS Status Indicators

© 2016 DecisionHealth   CPT © 2015 American Medical Association. All Rights Reserved.   **465**

47015 Laparotomy, with aspiration and/or injection of hepatic parasitic (eg, amoebic or echinococcal) cyst(s) or abscess(es) ⓒ

RVU			Global Days	Modifiers				
Mod	Non-Fac Total	Fac Total		51	50	62	80	MUE
	33.18	33.18	090	2	0	1	2	1

Excisional Liver Procedures

47100 Biopsy of liver, wedge ⓒ

RVU			Global Days	Modifiers				
Mod	Non-Fac Total	Fac Total		51	50	62	80	MUE
	24.49	24.49	090	2	0	1	2	3

Coding Guidance

Hepatectomy includes gallbladder removal; a cholecystectomy code is not reportable with hepatectomy codes.

47120 Hepatectomy, resection of liver; partial lobectomy ⓒ

RVU			Global Days	Modifiers				
Mod	Non-Fac Total	Fac Total		51	50	62	80	MUE
	67.76	67.76	090	2	0	1	2	2

AMA: May 98: 10, Sep 14: 14

47122 Hepatectomy, resection of liver; trisegmentectomy ⓒ

RVU			Global Days	Modifiers				
Mod	Non-Fac Total	Fac Total		51	50	62	80	MUE
	100.02	100.02	090	2	0	1	2	1

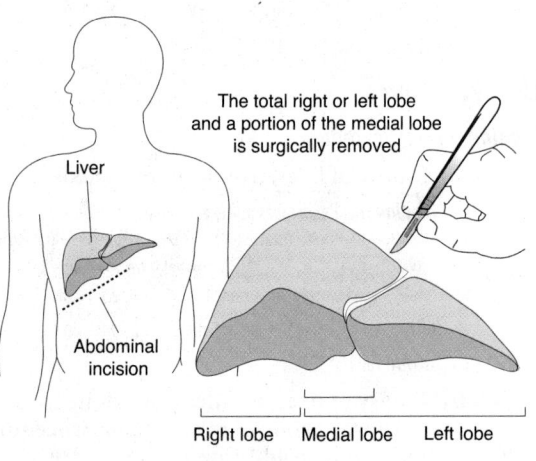

Hepatectomy, resection of liver; trisegmentectomy

The total right or left lobe and a portion of the medial lobe is surgically removed

Liver

Abdominal incision

Right lobe   Medial lobe   Left lobe

47125 Hepatectomy, resection of liver; total left lobectomy ⓒ

RVU			Global Days	Modifiers				
Mod	Non-Fac Total	Fac Total		51	50	62	80	MUE
	89.39	89.39	090	2	0	1	2	1

47130 Hepatectomy, resection of liver; total right lobectomy ⓒ

RVU			Global Days	Modifiers				
Mod	Non-Fac Total	Fac Total		51	50	62	80	MUE
	96.06	96.06	090	2	0	1	2	1

47133 Donor hepatectomy (including cold preservation), from cadaver donor ⓒⓒ

RVU			Global Days	Modifiers				
Mod	Non-Fac Total	Fac Total		51	50	62	80	MUE
	0.00	0.00	XXX	9	9	9	9	1

Liver Transplant Procedures

47135 Liver allotransplantation, orthotopic, partial or whole, from cadaver or living donor, any age ⓒ

RVU			Global Days	Modifiers				
Mod	Non-Fac Total	Fac Total		51	50	62	80	MUE
	156.05	156.05	090	2	0	1	2	1

AMA: Dec 11: 16

✖ ~~47136 Liver allotransplantation; heterotopic, partial or whole, from cadaver or living donor, any age~~

47140 Donor hepatectomy (including cold preservation), from living donor; left lateral segment only (segments II and III) ⓒⓒ

RVU			Global Days	Modifiers				
Mod	Non-Fac Total	Fac Total		51	50	62	80	MUE
	103.88	103.88	090	2	0	1	2	1

AMA: Aug 11: 9

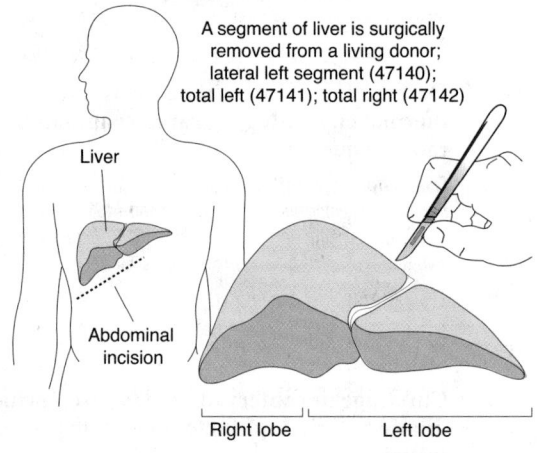

Donor hepatectomy, living donor; left lateral/total left/total right

A segment of liver is surgically removed from a living donor; lateral left segment (47140); total left (47141); total right (47142)

Liver

Abdominal incision

Right lobe   Left lobe

47141 Donor hepatectomy (including cold preservation), from living donor; total left lobectomy (segments II, III and IV) ⓒ

RVU			Global Days	Modifiers				
Mod	Non-Fac Total	Fac Total		51	50	62	80	MUE
	124.16	124.16	090	2	0	1	2	1

47142 Donor hepatectomy (including cold preservation), from living donor; total right lobectomy (segments V, VI, VII and VIII) ⓒ

RVU			Global Days	Modifiers				
Mod	Non-Fac Total	Fac Total		51	50	62	80	MUE
	136.89	136.89	090	2	0	1	2	1

● New   ▲ Revised   ✖ Deleted   ⊙ Moderate Sedation   ✚ Add-on Codes   ⊘ High Risk Denial   Ⓐ Age Edit   ♀ Female   ♂ Male   **AMA** *CPT® Assistant*   **MUE** Medically Unlikely Edit
⊘ Modifier 51 Exempt   ⊖ Modifier 63 Exempt   ☒ Unlisted   **Modifiers:** *See Inside Back Cover*   Ⓜ Maternity   Ⓐ2–Ⓩ3 ASC Payment Indicators   Ⓐ–Ⓨ OPPS Status Indicators

CPT © 2015 American Medical Association. All Rights Reserved.   © 2016 DecisionHealth

47143 Backbench standard preparation of cadaver donor whole liver graft prior to allotransplantation, including cholecystectomy, if necessary, and dissection and removal of surrounding soft tissues to prepare the vena cava, portal vein, hepatic artery, and common bile duct for implantation; without trisegment or lobe split ▣

	RVU		Global Days	Modifiers				
Mod	Non-Fac Total	Fac Total		51	50	62	80	MUE
	0.00	0.00	XXX	2	0	1	2	1

AMA: Apr 05: 10, 12

47144 Backbench standard preparation of cadaver donor whole liver graft prior to allotransplantation, including cholecystectomy, if necessary, and dissection and removal of surrounding soft tissues to prepare the vena cava, portal vein, hepatic artery, and common bile duct for implantation; with trisegment split of whole liver graft into 2 partial liver grafts (ie, left lateral segment [segments II and III] and right trisegment [segments I and IV through VIII]) ▣

	RVU		Global Days	Modifiers				
Mod	Non-Fac Total	Fac Total		51	50	62	80	MUE
	0.00	0.00	090	2	0	1	2	1

47145 Backbench standard preparation of cadaver donor whole liver graft prior to allotransplantation, including cholecystectomy, if necessary, and dissection and removal of surrounding soft tissues to prepare the vena cava, portal vein, hepatic artery, and common bile duct for implantation; with lobe split of whole liver graft into 2 partial liver grafts (ie, left lobe [segments II, III, and IV] and right lobe [segments I and V through VIII]) ▣

	RVU		Global Days	Modifiers				
Mod	Non-Fac Total	Fac Total		51	50	62	80	MUE
	0.00	0.00	XXX	2	0	1	2	1

47146 Backbench reconstruction of cadaver or living donor liver graft prior to allotransplantation; venous anastomosis, each ▣

	RVU		Global Days	Modifiers				
Mod	Non-Fac Total	Fac Total		51	50	62	80	MUE
	9.61	9.61	XXX	2	0	1	2	3

47147 Backbench reconstruction of cadaver or living donor liver graft prior to allotransplantation; arterial anastomosis, each ▣

	RVU		Global Days	Modifiers				
Mod	Non-Fac Total	Fac Total		51	50	62	80	MUE
	11.17	11.17	XXX	2	0	1	2	2

Liver Repair

47300 Marsupialization of cyst or abscess of liver ▣

	RVU		Global Days	Modifiers				
Mod	Non-Fac Total	Fac Total		51	50	62	80	MUE
	32.89	32.89	090	2	0	1	2	2

47350 Management of liver hemorrhage; simple suture of liver wound or injury ▣

	RVU		Global Days	Modifiers				
Mod	Non-Fac Total	Fac Total		51	50	62	80	MUE
	39.80	39.80	090	2	0	1	2	1

47360 Management of liver hemorrhage; complex suture of liver wound or injury, with or without hepatic artery ligation ▣

	RVU		Global Days	Modifiers				
Mod	Non-Fac Total	Fac Total		51	50	62	80	MUE
	54.03	54.03	090	2	0	1	2	1

47361 Management of liver hemorrhage; exploration of hepatic wound, extensive debridement, coagulation and/or suture, with or without packing of liver ▣

	RVU		Global Days	Modifiers				
Mod	Non-Fac Total	Fac Total		51	50	62	80	MUE
	87.83	87.83	090	2	0	1	2	1

47362 Management of liver hemorrhage; re-exploration of hepatic wound for removal of packing ▣

	RVU		Global Days	Modifiers				
Mod	Non-Fac Total	Fac Total		51	50	62	80	MUE
	42.11	42.11	090	2	0	1	2	1

Laparoscopic Liver Procedures

Coding Guidance
Report 76940 for ultrasound imaging guidance for liver tumor ablation procedures.

47370 Laparoscopy, surgical, ablation of 1 or more liver tumor(s); radiofrequency ▣J1

	RVU		Global Days	Modifiers				
Mod	Non-Fac Total	Fac Total		51	50	62	80	MUE
	36.24	36.24	090	2	0	1	2	1

AMA: Oct 02: 2

47371 Laparoscopy, surgical, ablation of 1 or more liver tumor(s); cryosurgical ▣J1

	RVU		Global Days	Modifiers				
Mod	Non-Fac Total	Fac Total		51	50	62	80	MUE
	32.67	32.67	090	2	0	1	2	1

47379 Unlisted laparoscopic procedure, liver xJ1

	RVU		Global Days	Modifiers				
Mod	Non-Fac Total	Fac Total		51	50	62	80	MUE
	0.00	0.00	YYY	2	0	1	2	

AMA: Aug 06: 10, Dec 07: 12, Dec 14: 18

Other Liver Procedures

47380 Ablation, open, of 1 or more liver tumor(s); radiofrequency ▣

	RVU		Global Days	Modifiers				
Mod	Non-Fac Total	Fac Total		51	50	62	80	MUE
	41.93	41.93	090	2	0	1	2	1

AMA: Oct 02: 1

47381 Ablation, open, of 1 or more liver tumor(s); cryosurgical ▣

	RVU		Global Days	Modifiers				
Mod	Non-Fac Total	Fac Total		51	50	62	80	MUE
	38.64	38.64	090	2	0	1	2	1

● New ▲ Revised — Deleted ⊙ Moderate Sedation ✛ Add-on Codes ⊖ High Risk Denial Ⓐ Age Edit ♀ Female ♂ Male **AMA** *CPT® Assistant* **MUE** Medically Unlikely Edit
⊘ Modifier 51 Exempt ⊖ Modifier 63 Exempt ✗ Unlisted **Modifiers:** *See Inside Back Cover* Ⓜ Maternity Ⓐ2–Ⓩ3 ASC Payment Indicators Ⓐ–Ⓨ OPPS Status Indicators

© 2016 DecisionHealth | CPT © 2015 American Medical Association. All Rights Reserved. | **467**

⊙ **47382** **Ablation, 1 or more liver tumor(s), percutaneous, radiofrequency** G2 T

Coding tip: *Report 76940 for ultrasound imaging guidance, 77013 for CT guidance, and 77022 for MRI guidance*

RVU			Global Days	Modifiers				
Mod	Non-Fac Total	Fac Total		51	50	62	80	MUE
	142.20	22.33	010	2	0	0	1	1

AMA: Oct 02: 1

Ablation, liver tumor(s) percutaneous, radiofrequency

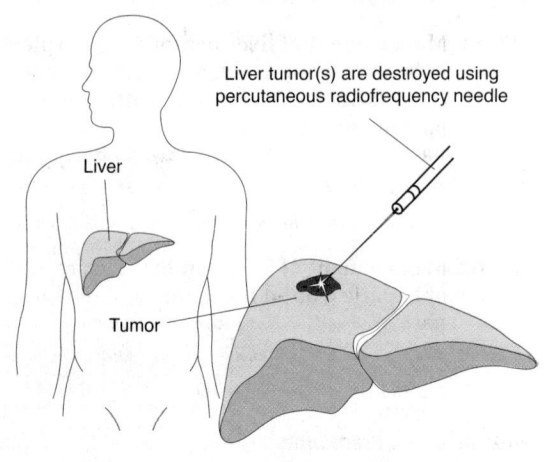

Liver tumor(s) are destroyed using percutaneous radiofrequency needle

Liver

Tumor

⊙ **47383** **Ablation, 1 or more liver tumor(s), percutaneous, cryoablation** G2 T

RVU			Global Days	Modifiers				
Mod	Non-Fac Total	Fac Total		51	50	62	80	MUE
	214.05	14.21	010	2	0	0	1	1

AMA: Dec 14: 18

Ablation, 1 or more liver tumor(s), percutaneous, cryoablation

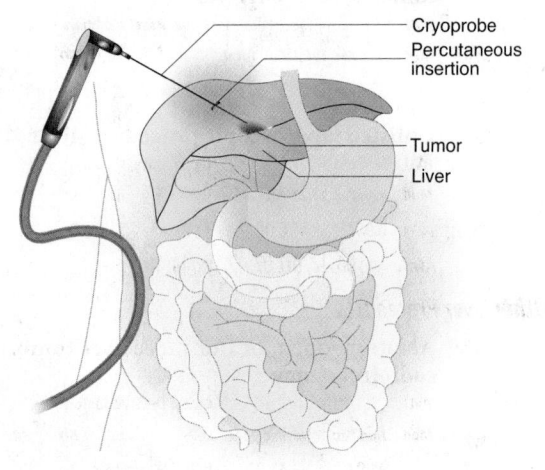

Cryoprobe
Percutaneous insertion
Tumor
Liver

47399 **Unlisted procedure, liver** ✗ T

RVU			Global Days	Modifiers				
Mod	Non-Fac Total	Fac Total		51	50	62	80	MUE
	0.00	0.00	YYY	2	0	1	1	

AMA: Dec 14: 18

Biliary Tract Procedures

Incisional Biliary Tract Procedures

47400 **Hepaticotomy or hepaticostomy with exploration, drainage, or removal of calculus** C

RVU			Global Days	Modifiers				
Mod	Non-Fac Total	Fac Total		51	50	62	80	MUE
	62.50	62.50	090	2	0	1	2	1

Hepaticotomy/hepaticostomy

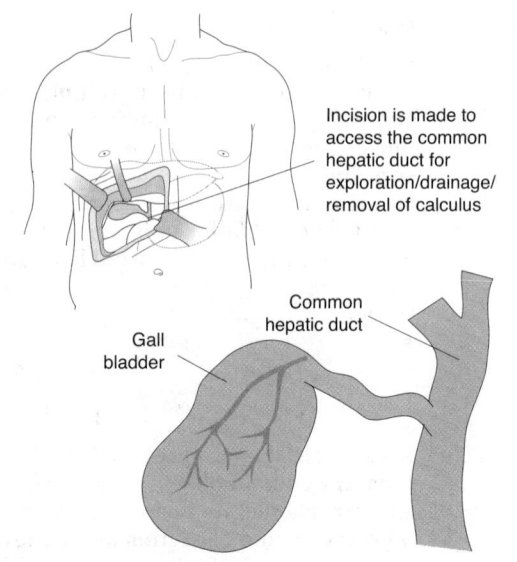

Incision is made to access the common hepatic duct for exploration/drainage/removal of calculus

Common hepatic duct

Gall bladder

Drainage tube may be brought to skin surface and left in place

47420 **Choledochotomy or choledochostomy with exploration, drainage, or removal of calculus, with or without cholecystotomy; without transduodenal sphincterotomy or sphincteroplasty** C

RVU			Global Days	Modifiers				
Mod	Non-Fac Total	Fac Total		51	50	62	80	MUE
	38.98	38.98	090	2	0	1	2	1

47425 **Choledochotomy or choledochostomy with exploration, drainage, or removal of calculus, with or without cholecystotomy; with transduodenal sphincterotomy or sphincteroplasty** C

RVU			Global Days	Modifiers				
Mod	Non-Fac Total	Fac Total		51	50	62	80	MUE
	39.33	39.33	090	2	0	1	2	1

47460 **Transduodenal sphincterotomy or sphincteroplasty, with or without transduodenal extraction of calculus (separate procedure)** C

RVU			Global Days	Modifiers				
Mod	Non-Fac Total	Fac Total		51	50	62	80	MUE
	36.39	36.39	090	2	0	1	2	1

● New ▲ Revised ✖ Deleted ⊙ Moderate Sedation ➕ Add-on Codes ⊘ High Risk Denial Ⓐ Age Edit ♀ Female ♂ Male **AMA** *CPT® Assistant* **MUE** Medically Unlikely Edit
⊘ Modifier 51 Exempt ⊖ Modifier 63 Exempt ✗ Unlisted **Modifiers:** *See Inside Back Cover* Ⓜ Maternity A2–Z3 ASC Payment Indicators A–Y OPPS Status Indicators

CPT © 2015 American Medical Association. All Rights Reserved. © 2016 DecisionHealth

47480 Cholecystotomy or cholecystostomy, open, with exploration, drainage, or removal of calculus (separate procedure) **C**

Mod	Non-Fac Total	Fac Total	Global Days	Modifiers 51	50	62	80	MUE
	25.37	25.37	090	2	0	1	2	1

AMA: Apr 11: 12

47490 Cholecystostomy, percutaneous, complete procedure, including imaging guidance, catheter placement, cholecystogram when performed, and radiological supervision and interpretation **T**

Mod	Non-Fac Total	Fac Total	Global Days	Modifiers 51	50	62	80	MUE
	9.58	9.58	010	2	0	0	1	1

AMA: Apr 11: 12

✗ 47500 ~~Injection procedure for percutaneous transhepatic cholangiography~~

✗ 47505 ~~Injection procedure for cholangiography through an existing catheter (eg, percutaneous transhepatic or T-tube)~~

✗ 47510 ~~Introduction of percutaneous transhepatic catheter for biliary drainage~~

✗ 47511 ~~Introduction of percutaneous transhepatic stent for internal and external biliary drainage~~

✗ 47525 ~~Change of percutaneous biliary drainage catheter~~

✗ 47530 ~~Revision and/or reinsertion of transhepatic tube~~

● 47531 Injection procedure for cholangiography, percutaneous, complete diagnostic procedure including imaging guidance (eg, ultrasound and/or fluoroscopy) and all associated radiological supervision and interpretation; existing access **N1 Q2**

Mod	Non-Fac Total	Fac Total	Global Days	Modifiers 51	50	62	80	MUE
	10.56	2.78	000	2	0	0	1	2

⊙● 47532 Injection procedure for cholangiography, percutaneous, complete diagnostic procedure including imaging guidance (eg, ultrasound and/or fluoroscopy) and all associated radiological supervision and interpretation; new access (eg, percutaneous transhepatic cholangiogram) **N1 Q2**

Mod	Non-Fac Total	Fac Total	Global Days	Modifiers 51	50	62	80	MUE
	23.23	6.26	000	2	0	0	1	1

⊙● 47533 Placement of biliary drainage catheter, percutaneous, including diagnostic cholangiography when performed, imaging guidance (eg, ultrasound and/or fluoroscopy), and all associated radiological supervision and interpretation; external **G2 T**

Mod	Non-Fac Total	Fac Total	Global Days	Modifiers 51	50	62	80	MUE
	37.92	8.88	000	2	0	0	1	1

⊙● 47534 Placement of biliary drainage catheter, percutaneous, including diagnostic cholangiography when performed, imaging guidance (eg, ultrasound and/or fluoroscopy), and all associated radiological supervision and interpretation; internal-external **G2 T**

Mod	Non-Fac Total	Fac Total	Global Days	Modifiers 51	50	62	80	MUE
	46.73	11.77	000	2	0	0	1	1

⊙● 47535 Conversion of external biliary drainage catheter to internal-external biliary drainage catheter, percutaneous, including diagnostic cholangiography when performed, imaging guidance (eg, fluoroscopy), and all associated radiological supervision and interpretation **G2 T**

Mod	Non-Fac Total	Fac Total	Global Days	Modifiers 51	50	62	80	MUE
	31.34	6.76	000	2	0	0	1	1

⊙● 47536 Exchange of biliary drainage catheter (eg, external, internal-external, or conversion of internal-external to external only), percutaneous, including diagnostic cholangiography when performed, imaging guidance (eg, fluoroscopy), and all associated radiological supervision and interpretation **G2 T**

Mod	Non-Fac Total	Fac Total	Global Days	Modifiers 51	50	62	80	MUE
	23.12	4.28	000	2	0	0	1	1

● 47537 Removal of biliary drainage catheter, percutaneous, requiring fluoroscopic guidance (eg, with concurrent indwelling biliary stents), including diagnostic cholangiography when performed, imaging guidance (eg, fluoroscopy), and all associated radiological supervision and interpretation **G2 Q2**

Mod	Non-Fac Total	Fac Total	Global Days	Modifiers 51	50	62	80	MUE
	11.44	2.89	000	2	0	0	1	1

⊙● 47538 Placement of stent(s) into a bile duct, percutaneous, including diagnostic cholangiography, imaging guidance (eg, fluoroscopy and/or ultrasound), balloon dilation, catheter exchange(s) and catheter removal(s) when performed, and all associated radiological supervision and interpretation, each stent; existing access **G2 T**

Mod	Non-Fac Total	Fac Total	Global Days	Modifiers 51	50	62	80	MUE
	127.56	9.53	000	2	0	0	1	

● New ▲ Revised Deleted ⊙ Moderate Sedation ✚ Add-on Codes ⊘ High Risk Denial ⒶＡge Edit ♀ Female ♂ Male **AMA** *CPT® Assistant* **MUE** Medically Unlikely Edit
⊘ Modifier 51 Exempt ⊖ Modifier 63 Exempt ✗ Unlisted **Modifiers:** *See Inside Back Cover* Ⓜ Maternity **A2–Z3** ASC Payment Indicators **A–Y** OPPS Status Indicators

⊙● **47539** Placement of stent(s) into a bile duct, percutaneous, including diagnostic cholangiography, imaging guidance (eg, fluoroscopy and/or ultrasound), balloon dilation, catheter exchange(s) and catheter removal(s) when performed, and all associated radiological supervision and interpretation, each stent; new access, without placement of separate biliary drainage catheter　　　G2T

RVU			Global Days	Modifiers				
Mod	Non-Fac Total	Fac Total		51	50	62	80	MUE
	139.43	12.89	000	2	0	0	1	

⊙● **47540** Placement of stent(s) into a bile duct, percutaneous, including diagnostic cholangiography, imaging guidance (eg, fluoroscopy and/or ultrasound), balloon dilation, catheter exchange(s) and catheter removal(s) when performed, and all associated radiological supervision and interpretation, each stent; new access, with placement of separate biliary drainage catheter (eg, external or internal-external)　　　G2T

RVU			Global Days	Modifiers				
Mod	Non-Fac Total	Fac Total		51	50	62	80	MUE
	144.99	15.40	000	2	0	0	1	

⊙● **47541** Placement of access through the biliary tree and into small bowel to assist with an endoscopic biliary procedure (eg, rendezvous procedure), percutaneous, including diagnostic cholangiography when performed, imaging guidance (eg, ultrasound and/or fluoroscopy), and all associated radiological supervision and interpretation, new access　　　G2T

RVU			Global Days	Modifiers				
Mod	Non-Fac Total	Fac Total		51	50	62	80	MUE
	33.48	8.20	000	2	0	0	1	1

⊙+● **47542** Balloon dilation of biliary duct(s) or of ampulla (sphincteroplasty), percutaneous, including imaging guidance (eg, fluoroscopy), and all associated radiological supervision and interpretation, each duct (List separately in addition to code for primary procedure)　　　NIN

RVU			Global Days	Modifiers				
Mod	Non-Fac Total	Fac Total		51	50	62	80	MUE
	14.65	3.87	ZZZ	0	0	0	1	2

⊙+● **47543** Endoluminal biopsy(ies) of biliary tree, percutaneous, any method(s) (eg, brush, forceps, and/or needle), including imaging guidance (eg, fluoroscopy), and all associated radiological supervision and interpretation, single or multiple (List separately in addition to code for primary procedure)　　　NIN

RVU			Global Days	Modifiers				
Mod	Non-Fac Total	Fac Total		51	50	62	80	MUE
	37.69	4.89	ZZZ	0	0	0	1	1

⊙+● **47544** Removal of calculi/debris from biliary duct(s) and/or gallbladder, percutaneous, including destruction of calculi by any method (eg, mechanical, electrohydraulic, lithotripsy) when performed, imaging guidance (eg, fluoroscopy), and all associated radiological supervision and interpretation (List separately in addition to code for primary procedure)　　　NIN

RVU			Global Days	Modifiers				
Mod	Non-Fac Total	Fac Total		51	50	62	80	MUE
	23.02	6.12	ZZZ	0	0	0	1	1

Endoscopic Biliary Tract Procedures

Coding Guidance

When a surgical endoscopy directly follows a diagnostic endoscopy, the diagnostic portion is included. When a diagnostic endscopic service is provided in conjunction with therapeutic endoscopic services, report only the more comprehensive endoscopy code that desribes the service. If different therapeutic endoscopic services performed are not adequately described by a comprehensive service code, the appropriate multiple GI endoscopy codes can be used. When an endoscopy is performed to confirm or establish anatomical landmarks as a scout endoscopy, the procedure is not reported separately. When an endoscopy is done as a diagnostic procedure for basing the decision to do a more extensive open surgical procedure, the endoscopy may be separately reported. Control of bleeding resulting from an endoscopy and performed at the time of the service is included. It if becomes necessary to repeat an endoscopy in order to control bleeding, then a procedure code for endoscopic control of bleeding may be reported with a modifier identifying a return to the operative room in the postoperative period.

+　**47550** Biliary endoscopy, intraoperative (choledochoscopy) (List separately in addition to code for primary procedure)　　　C

RVU			Global Days	Modifiers				
Mod	Non-Fac Total	Fac Total		51	50	62	80	MUE
	4.82	4.82	ZZZ	0	0	1	2	1

Biliary endoscopy, intraoperative

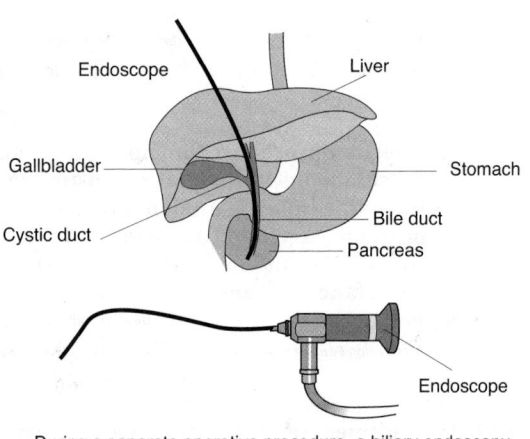

During a separate operative procedure, a biliary endoscopy (choledochoscopy) is performed.

Coding Guidance

If hepatic/biliary/pancreatic system diagnostic endoscopy requires using multiple methods, such as biliary T-tube endoscopy and ERCP, then appropriate codes for each method may be reported with a multiple procedures modifier.

47552 Biliary endoscopy, percutaneous via T-tube or other tract; diagnostic, with collection of specimen(s) by brushing and/or washing, when performed (separate procedure) `A2 T`

	RVU		Global Days	Modifiers				
Mod	Non-Fac Total	Fac Total		51	50	62	80	MUE
	9.01	9.01	000	2	0	1	1	1

47553 Biliary endoscopy, percutaneous via T-tube or other tract; with biopsy, single or multiple `A2 T`

	RVU		Global Days	Modifiers				
Mod	Non-Fac Total	Fac Total		51	50	62	80	MUE
	8.90	8.90	000	3	0	0	1	1

47554 Biliary endoscopy, percutaneous via T-tube or other tract; with removal of calculus/calculi `A2 T`

	RVU		Global Days	Modifiers				
Mod	Non-Fac Total	Fac Total		51	50	62	80	MUE
	13.88	13.88	000	3	0	1	1	1

47555 Biliary endoscopy, percutaneous via T-tube or other tract; with dilation of biliary duct stricture(s) without stent `A2 T`

Coding tip: Imaging guidance for percutaneous dilation of biliary duct strictures - 74363

	RVU		Global Days	Modifiers				
Mod	Non-Fac Total	Fac Total		51	50	62	80	MUE
	10.65	10.65	000	3	0	0	1	1

47556 Biliary endoscopy, percutaneous via T-tube or other tract; with dilation of biliary duct stricture(s) with stent `A2 T`

Coding tip: Imaging guidance for percutaneous dilation of biliary duct strictures - 74363

Coding tip: Imaging guidance for percutaneous placement of biliary stent - 75982

	RVU		Global Days	Modifiers				
Mod	Non-Fac Total	Fac Total		51	50	62	80	MUE
	12.13	12.13	000	3	0	0	1	1

✖ ~~47560 Laparoscopy, surgical; with guided transhepatic cholangiography, without biopsy~~

✖ ~~47561 Laparoscopy, surgical; with guided transhepatic cholangiography with biopsy~~

47562 Laparoscopy, surgical; cholecystectomy `G2 J 1`

Coding tip: Open cholecystectomy - 47600

	RVU		Global Days	Modifiers				
Mod	Non-Fac Total	Fac Total		51	50	62	80	MUE
	19.06	19.06	090	2	0	1	2	1

AMA: Nov 99: 23, Mar 00: 9, Sep 03: 3, Dec 07: 12

47563 Laparoscopy, surgical; cholecystectomy with cholangiography `G2 J 1`

Coding tip: Intraoperative cholangiography - 74300-74301

Coding tip: Open cholecystectomy with cholangiography - 47605

	RVU		Global Days	Modifiers				
Mod	Non-Fac Total	Fac Total		51	50	62	80	MUE
	20.70	20.70	090	2	0	1	2	1

AMA: Nov 99: 23, Mar 00: 9, Dec 00: 14, Dec 07: 12

47564 Laparoscopy, surgical; cholecystectomy with exploration of common duct `G2 J 1`

Coding tip: Open cholecystectomy with exploration of common duct - 47610

	RVU		Global Days	Modifiers				
Mod	Non-Fac Total	Fac Total		51	50	62	80	MUE
	32.30	32.30	090	2	0	1	2	1

AMA: Nov 99: 23, Mar 00: 9

47570 Laparoscopy, surgical; cholecystoenterostomy `C`

Coding tip: Direct cholecystoenterostomy - 47720

	RVU		Global Days	Modifiers				
Mod	Non-Fac Total	Fac Total		51	50	62	80	MUE
	22.24	22.24	090	2	0	1	2	1

AMA: Nov 99: 23, Mar 00: 9

47579 Unlisted laparoscopy procedure, biliary tract `✖ J 1`

	RVU		Global Days	Modifiers				
Mod	Non-Fac Total	Fac Total		51	50	62	80	MUE
	0.00	0.00	YYY	2	1	1	2	

AMA: Nov 99: 23, Mar 00: 9

Excisional Biliary Tract Procedures

47600 Cholecystectomy `C`

Coding tip: Laparoscopic cholecystectomy - 47562

	RVU		Global Days	Modifiers				
Mod	Non-Fac Total	Fac Total		51	50	62	80	MUE
	30.98	30.98	090	2	0	1	2	1

AMA: Fall 92: 19, Nov 99: 24

47605 Cholecystectomy; with cholangiography `C`

Coding tip: Intraoperative cholangiography - 74300-74301

Coding tip: Laparoscopic cholecystectomy with cholangiography - 47563

	RVU		Global Days	Modifiers				
Mod	Non-Fac Total	Fac Total		51	50	62	80	MUE
	32.63	32.63	090	2	0	1	2	1

AMA: Nov 99: 24, Apr 02: 19

47610 Cholecystectomy with exploration of common duct `C`

Coding tip: Laparoscopic cholecystectomy with exploration of common duct - 47564

	RVU		Global Days	Modifiers				
Mod	Non-Fac Total	Fac Total		51	50	62	80	MUE
	36.45	36.45	090	2	0	1	2	1

AMA: Apr 02: 19

47612 Cholecystectomy with exploration of common duct; with choledochoenterostomy `C`

	RVU		Global Days	Modifiers				
Mod	Non-Fac Total	Fac Total		51	50	62	80	MUE
	36.90	36.90	090	2	0	1	2	1

47620 Cholecystectomy with exploration of common duct; with transduodenal sphincterotomy or sphincteroplasty, with or without cholangiography `C`

	RVU		Global Days	Modifiers				
Mod	Non-Fac Total	Fac Total		51	50	62	80	MUE
	40.00	40.00	090	2	0	1	2	1

✖ ~~47630 Biliary duct stone extraction, percutaneous via T-tube tract, basket, or snare (eg, Burhenne technique)~~

● New   ▲ Revised   Deleted   ⊙ Moderate Sedation   ✚ Add-on Codes   ⊘ High Risk Denial   Ⓐ Age Edit   ♀ Female   ♂ Male   **AMA** CPT® Assistant   **MUE** Medically Unlikely Edit
⊘ Modifier 51 Exempt   ⊖ Modifier 63 Exempt   ✖ Unlisted   **Modifiers:** See Inside Back Cover   Ⓜ Maternity   A2–Z3 ASC Payment Indicators   A–Y OPPS Status Indicators

© 2016 DecisionHealth   CPT © 2015 American Medical Association. All Rights Reserved.   **471**

47700 Exploration for congenital atresia of bile ducts, without repair, with or without liver biopsy, with or without cholangiography ⊖🅲

RVU		Global Days	Modifiers				
Mod	Non-Fac Total	Fac Total		51	50	62	80	MUE
	30.06	30.06	090	2	0	1	2	1

47701 Portoenterostomy (eg, Kasai procedure) Ⓐ⊖🅲

RVU		Global Days	Modifiers				
Mod	Non-Fac Total	Fac Total		51	50	62	80	MUE
	49.24	49.24	090	2	0	0	0	1

Portoenterostomy

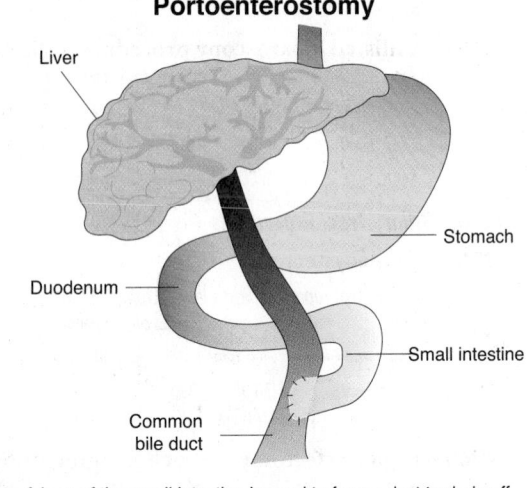

A loop of the small intestine is used to form a duct to drain off excess bile from the bile duct.

47711 Excision of bile duct tumor, with or without primary repair of bile duct; extrahepatic 🅲

RVU		Global Days	Modifiers				
Mod	Non-Fac Total	Fac Total		51	50	62	80	MUE
	45.20	45.20	090	2	0	1	2	1

47712 Excision of bile duct tumor, with or without primary repair of bile duct; intrahepatic 🅲

RVU		Global Days	Modifiers				
Mod	Non-Fac Total	Fac Total		51	50	62	80	MUE
	57.73	57.73	090	2	0	1	2	1

47715 Excision of choledochal cyst 🅲

RVU		Global Days	Modifiers				
Mod	Non-Fac Total	Fac Total		51	50	62	80	MUE
	38.70	38.70	090	2	0	1	2	1

Biliary Tract Repair

47720 Cholecystoenterostomy; direct 🅲

RVU		Global Days	Modifiers				
Mod	Non-Fac Total	Fac Total		51	50	62	80	MUE
	33.38	33.38	090	2	0	1	2	1

AMA: Nov 99: 24

47721 Cholecystoenterostomy; with gastroenterostomy 🅲

RVU		Global Days	Modifiers				
Mod	Non-Fac Total	Fac Total		51	50	62	80	MUE
	39.41	39.41	090	2	0	1	2	1

47740 Cholecystoenterostomy; Roux-en-Y 🅲

RVU		Global Days	Modifiers				
Mod	Non-Fac Total	Fac Total		51	50	62	80	MUE
	37.78	37.78	090	2	0	1	2	1

47741 Cholecystoenterostomy; Roux-en-Y with gastroenterostomy 🅲

RVU		Global Days	Modifiers				
Mod	Non-Fac Total	Fac Total		51	50	62	80	MUE
	42.63	42.63	090	2	0	1	2	1

47760 Anastomosis, of extrahepatic biliary ducts and gastrointestinal tract 🅲

RVU		Global Days	Modifiers				
Mod	Non-Fac Total	Fac Total		51	50	62	80	MUE
	65.66	65.66	090	2	0	1	2	1

47765 Anastomosis, of intrahepatic ducts and gastrointestinal tract 🅲

RVU		Global Days	Modifiers				
Mod	Non-Fac Total	Fac Total		51	50	62	80	MUE
	88.19	88.19	090	2	0	1	2	1

47780 Anastomosis, Roux-en-Y, of extrahepatic biliary ducts and gastrointestinal tract 🅲

RVU		Global Days	Modifiers				
Mod	Non-Fac Total	Fac Total		51	50	62	80	MUE
	71.87	71.87	090	2	0	1	2	1

47785 Anastomosis, Roux-en-Y, of intrahepatic biliary ducts and gastrointestinal tract 🅲

RVU		Global Days	Modifiers				
Mod	Non-Fac Total	Fac Total		51	50	62	80	MUE
	94.40	94.40	090	2	0	1	2	1

47800 Reconstruction, plastic, of extrahepatic biliary ducts with end-to-end anastomosis 🅲

RVU		Global Days	Modifiers				
Mod	Non-Fac Total	Fac Total		51	50	62	80	MUE
	45.73	45.73	090	2	0	1	2	1

47801 Placement of choledochal stent 🅲

RVU		Global Days	Modifiers				
Mod	Non-Fac Total	Fac Total		51	50	62	80	MUE
	28.62	28.62	090	2	0	1	2	1

AMA: Dec 10: 13

47802 U-tube hepaticoenterostomy 🅲

RVU		Global Days	Modifiers				
Mod	Non-Fac Total	Fac Total		51	50	62	80	MUE
	43.58	43.58	090	2	0	1	2	1

47900 Suture of extrahepatic biliary duct for pre-existing injury (separate procedure) 🅲

RVU		Global Days	Modifiers				
Mod	Non-Fac Total	Fac Total		51	50	62	80	MUE
	39.79	39.79	090	2	0	1	2	1

Other Biliary Tract Procedures

47999 Unlisted procedure, biliary tract ⊗x🆃

RVU		Global Days	Modifiers				
Mod	Non-Fac Total	Fac Total		51	50	62	80	MUE
	0.00	0.00	YYY	2	0	1	1	

AMA: May 11: 9

● New   ▲ Revised   ✖ Deleted   ⊙ Moderate Sedation   ✚ Add-on Codes   ⊘ High Risk Denial   Ⓐ Age Edit   ♀ Female   ♂ Male   **AMA** CPT® Assistant   **MUE** Medically Unlikely Edit
⊘ Modifier 51 Exempt   ⊖ Modifier 63 Exempt   🗵 Unlisted   **Modifiers:** See Inside Back Cover   Ⓜ Maternity   🅰2–🆉3 ASC Payment Indicators   🅰–🆈 OPPS Status Indicators

CPT © 2015 American Medical Association. All Rights Reserved.   © 2016 DecisionHealth

Pancreas Procedures

Incisional Pancreas Procedures

48000 Placement of drains, peripancreatic, for acute pancreatitis   **C**

Mod	RVU Non-Fac Total	Fac Total	Global Days	Modifiers 51	50	62	80	MUE
	54.42	54.42	090	2	0	1	2	1

48001 Placement of drains, peripancreatic, for acute pancreatitis; with cholecystostomy, gastrostomy, and jejunostomy   **C**

Mod	RVU Non-Fac Total	Fac Total	Global Days	Modifiers 51	50	62	80	MUE
	66.52	66.52	090	2	0	1	2	1

48020 Removal of pancreatic calculus   **C**

Mod	RVU Non-Fac Total	Fac Total	Global Days	Modifiers 51	50	62	80	MUE
	33.98	33.98	090	2	0	1	2	1

AMA: Spring 91: 7

Removal of pancreatic calculus

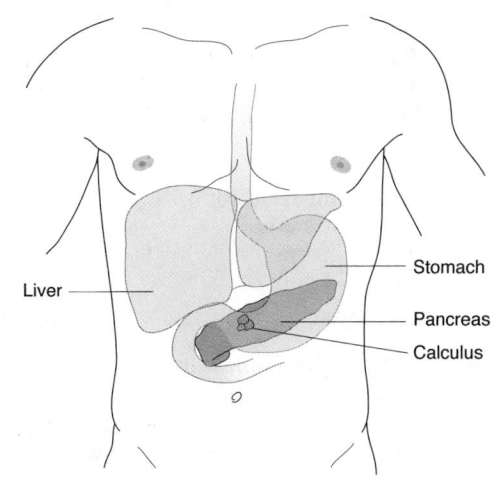

A calculus (stone) is removed from the pancreas. A subcostal or midline incision is made in the abdomen. The pancreas is inspected and the stone is identified.

Excisional Pancreas Procedures

48100 Biopsy of pancreas, open (eg, fine needle aspiration, needle core biopsy, wedge biopsy)   **C**

Mod	RVU Non-Fac Total	Fac Total	Global Days	Modifiers 51	50	62	80	MUE
	25.65	25.65	090	2	0	1	2	1

48102 Biopsy of pancreas, percutaneous needle   **A 2 T**

Coding tip: Radiological guidance for correct needle placement - ultrasound 76942; fluoroscopy 77002; CT 77012; MRI 77021

Mod	RVU Non-Fac Total	Fac Total	Global Days	Modifiers 51	50	62	80	MUE
	15.18	7.02	010	2	0	0	1	1

48105 Resection or debridement of pancreas and peripancreatic tissue for acute necrotizing pancreatitis   **C**

Mod	RVU Non-Fac Total	Fac Total	Global Days	Modifiers 51	50	62	80	MUE
	82.90	82.90	090	2	0	1	2	1

48120 Excision of lesion of pancreas (eg, cyst, adenoma)   **C**

Mod	RVU Non-Fac Total	Fac Total	Global Days	Modifiers 51	50	62	80	MUE
	32.20	32.20	090	2	0	1	2	1

48140 Pancreatectomy, distal subtotal, with or without splenectomy; without pancreaticojejunostomy   **C**

Mod	RVU Non-Fac Total	Fac Total	Global Days	Modifiers 51	50	62	80	MUE
	45.47	45.47	090	2	0	1	2	1

48145 Pancreatectomy, distal subtotal, with or without splenectomy; with pancreaticojejunostomy   **C**

Mod	RVU Non-Fac Total	Fac Total	Global Days	Modifiers 51	50	62	80	MUE
	47.29	47.29	090	2	0	1	2	1

48146 Pancreatectomy, distal, near-total with preservation of duodenum (Child-type procedure)   **C**

Mod	RVU Non-Fac Total	Fac Total	Global Days	Modifiers 51	50	62	80	MUE
	54.54	54.54	090	2	0	1	2	1

48148 Excision of ampulla of Vater   **C**

Mod	RVU Non-Fac Total	Fac Total	Global Days	Modifiers 51	50	62	80	MUE
	36.18	36.18	090	2	0	1	2	1

Coding Guidance

Codes 48150-48154, Whipple-type pancreatectomy procedures, include removal of the gallbladder; codes 47562-47564, 47600-47620 (cholecystectomy procedures) should not be reported separately.

48150 Pancreatectomy, proximal subtotal with total duodenectomy, partial gastrectomy, choledochoenterostomy and gastrojejunostomy (Whipple-type procedure); with pancreatojejunostomy   **C**

Mod	RVU Non-Fac Total	Fac Total	Global Days	Modifiers 51	50	62	80	MUE
	90.58	90.58	090	2	0	1	2	1

48152 Pancreatectomy, proximal subtotal with total duodenectomy, partial gastrectomy, choledochoenterostomy and gastrojejunostomy (Whipple-type procedure); without pancreatojejunostomy   **C**

Mod	RVU Non-Fac Total	Fac Total	Global Days	Modifiers 51	50	62	80	MUE
	83.44	83.44	090	2	0	1	2	1

● New   ▲ Revised   Deleted   ⊙ Moderate Sedation   ✚ Add-on Codes   ⊘ High Risk Denial   Ⓐ Age Edit   ♀ Female   ♂ Male   **AMA** *CPT® Assistant*   **MUE** Medically Unlikely Edit
⊘ Modifier 51 Exempt   ⊖ Modifier 63 Exempt   ✖ Unlisted   **Modifiers:** *See Inside Back Cover*   Ⓜ Maternity   **A 2–Z 3** ASC Payment Indicators   **A –Y** OPPS Status Indicators

48153 Pancreatectomy, proximal subtotal with near-total duodenectomy, choledochoenterostomy and duodenojejunostomy (pylorus-sparing, Whipple-type procedure); with pancreatojejunostomy C

RVU			Global Days	Modifiers				
Mod	Non-Fac Total	Fac Total		51	50	62	80	MUE
	90.01	90.01	090	2	0	1	2	1

48154 Pancreatectomy, proximal subtotal with near-total duodenectomy, choledochoenterostomy and duodenojejunostomy (pylorus-sparing, Whipple-type procedure); without pancreatojejunostomy C

RVU			Global Days	Modifiers				
Mod	Non-Fac Total	Fac Total		51	50	62	80	MUE
	84.45	84.45	090	2	0	1	2	1

48155 Pancreatectomy, total C

RVU			Global Days	Modifiers				
Mod	Non-Fac Total	Fac Total		51	50	62	80	MUE
	52.90	52.90	090	2	0	1	2	1

48160 Pancreatectomy, total or subtotal, with autologous transplantation of pancreas or pancreatic islet cells C E

RVU			Global Days	Modifiers				
Mod	Non-Fac Total	Fac Total		51	50	62	80	MUE
	0.00	0.00	XXX	9	9	9	9	

Introduction Pancreas Procedures

✚ **48400** Injection procedure for intraoperative pancreatography (List separately in addition to code for primary procedure) C

Coding tip: Pancreatography through existing catheter - 74305

Coding tip: Intraoperative pancreatography - 74300-74301

RVU			Global Days	Modifiers				
Mod	Non-Fac Total	Fac Total		51	50	62	80	MUE
	3.07	3.07	ZZZ	0	0	0	0	1

AMA: Dec 07: 12

Injection procedure for intraoperative pancreatography

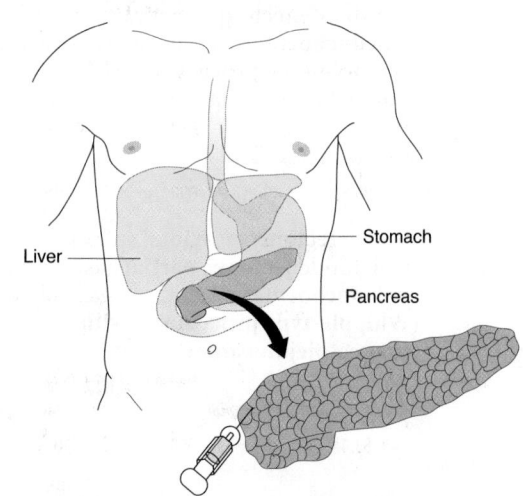

Liver   Stomach   Pancreas

The pancreatic ducts are visualized following injection of contrast (dye) during a separately reportable operative procedure. The distal pancreatic duct is identified.

Pancreas Repair

48500 Marsupialization of pancreatic cyst C

RVU			Global Days	Modifiers				
Mod	Non-Fac Total	Fac Total		51	50	62	80	MUE
	32.60	32.60	090	2	0	1	2	1

48510 External drainage, pseudocyst of pancreas, open C

RVU			Global Days	Modifiers				
Mod	Non-Fac Total	Fac Total		51	50	62	80	MUE
	31.61	31.61	090	2	0	1	2	1

AMA: Nov 97: 18

48520 Internal anastomosis of pancreatic cyst to gastrointestinal tract; direct C

RVU			Global Days	Modifiers				
Mod	Non-Fac Total	Fac Total		51	50	62	80	MUE
	31.77	31.77	090	2	0	1	2	1

48540 Internal anastomosis of pancreatic cyst to gastrointestinal tract; Roux-en-Y C

RVU			Global Days	Modifiers				
Mod	Non-Fac Total	Fac Total		51	50	62	80	MUE
	37.74	37.74	090	2	0	1	2	1

48545 Pancreatorrhaphy for injury C

RVU			Global Days	Modifiers				
Mod	Non-Fac Total	Fac Total		51	50	62	80	MUE
	38.73	38.73	090	2	0	1	2	1

48547 Duodenal exclusion with gastrojejunostomy for pancreatic injury C

RVU			Global Days	Modifiers				
Mod	Non-Fac Total	Fac Total		51	50	62	80	MUE
	52.00	52.00	090	2	0	1	2	1

48548 Pancreaticojejunostomy, side-to-side anastomosis (Puestow-type operation) C

RVU			Global Days	Modifiers				
Mod	Non-Fac Total	Fac Total		51	50	62	80	MUE
	48.38	48.38	090	2	0	1	2	1

Pancreas Transplant Procedures

48550 Donor pancreatectomy (including cold preservation), with or without duodenal segment for transplantation C E

RVU			Global Days	Modifiers				
Mod	Non-Fac Total	Fac Total		51	50	62	80	MUE
	0.00	0.00	XXX	9	9	9	9	1

AMA: Apr 05: 10, 12

48551 Backbench standard preparation of cadaver donor pancreas allograft prior to transplantation, including dissection of allograft from surrounding soft tissues, splenectomy, duodenotomy, ligation of bile duct, ligation of mesenteric vessels, and Y-graft arterial anastomoses from iliac artery to superior mesenteric artery and to splenic artery C

RVU			Global Days	Modifiers				
Mod	Non-Fac Total	Fac Total		51	50	62	80	MUE
	0.00	0.00	XXX	2	0	1	2	1

● New   ▲ Revised   ✖ Deleted   ⊙ Moderate Sedation   ✚ Add-on Codes   ⊘ High Risk Denial   Ⓐ Age Edit   ♀ Female   ♂ Male   **AMA** CPT® Assistant   **MUE** Medically Unlikely Edit
⊘ Modifier 51 Exempt   ⊖ Modifier 63 Exempt   ✗ Unlisted   **Modifiers:** See Inside Back Cover   Ⓜ Maternity   A2–Z3 ASC Payment Indicators   A–Y OPPS Status Indicators

474   CPT © 2015 American Medical Association. All Rights Reserved.   © 2016 DecisionHealth

48552 Backbench reconstruction of cadaver donor pancreas allograft prior to transplantation, venous anastomosis, each Ⓒ

RVU			Global Days	Modifiers				
Mod	Non-Fac Total	Fac Total		51	50	62	80	MUE
	6.86	6.86	XXX	2	0	1	2	2

Backbench reconstruction of cadaver donor pancreas allograft prior to transplantation

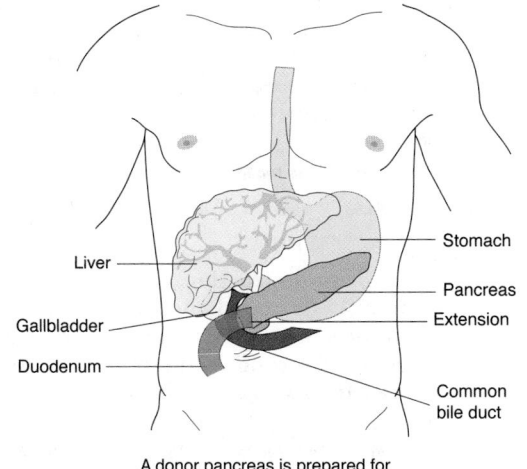

Liver · Gallbladder · Duodenum · Stomach · Pancreas · Extension · Common bile duct

A donor pancreas is prepared for transplant from a cadaver or living donor

48554 Transplantation of pancreatic allograft Ⓒ

RVU			Global Days	Modifiers				
Mod	Non-Fac Total	Fac Total		51	50	62	80	MUE
	74.18	74.18	090	2	0	2	2	1

48556 Removal of transplanted pancreatic allograft Ⓒ

RVU			Global Days	Modifiers				
Mod	Non-Fac Total	Fac Total		51	50	62	80	MUE
	36.82	36.82	090	2	0	2	2	1

Other Pancreas Procedures

48999 Unlisted procedure, pancreas ⓍⓉ

RVU			Global Days	Modifiers				
Mod	Non-Fac Total	Fac Total		51	50	62	80	MUE
	0.00	0.00	YYY	2	0	1	2	

AMA: Dec 07: 12, May 11: 9, Feb 13: 13

Abdominal/Peritoneum/Omentum Procedures

Incisional Abdominal/Peritoneum/Omentum Procedures

Coding Guidance

Exploratory laparotomy is not reported with an open abdominal procedure. Surgical field exploration to identify anatomical structures and anomalies is routine with open surgery. If abnormalities identified during open surgery through routine exploration require an enlarged surgical field and make the procedure unusual, then the appropriate modifier for an unusual service provided may be appended.

49000 Exploratory laparotomy, exploratory celiotomy with or without biopsy(s) (separate procedure) Ⓒ

RVU			Global Days	Modifiers				
Mod	Non-Fac Total	Fac Total		51	50	62	80	MUE
	22.36	22.36	090	2	0	1	2	1

AMA: Fall 92: 23, Mar 01: 10, Nov 08: 7, Sep 12: 11

Exploratory laparotomy, exploratory celiotomy with or without biopsy(s)

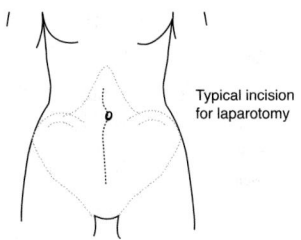

Typical incision for laparotomy

An access incision is made into the abdominal cavity for exploratory purposes. Biopsy samples may be collected during the surgical session.

49002 Reopening of recent laparotomy Ⓒ

RVU			Global Days	Modifiers				
Mod	Non-Fac Total	Fac Total		51	50	62	80	MUE
	30.39	30.39	090	2	0	1	2	1

AMA: Fall 92: 23, Nov 08: 7

49010 Exploration, retroperitoneal area with or without biopsy(s) (separate procedure) Ⓒ

RVU			Global Days	Modifiers				
Mod	Non-Fac Total	Fac Total		51	50	62	80	MUE
	27.11	27.11	090	2	0	1	2	1

49020 Drainage of peritoneal abscess or localized peritonitis, exclusive of appendiceal abscess, open Ⓒ

RVU			Global Days	Modifiers				
Mod	Non-Fac Total	Fac Total		51	50	62	80	MUE
	46.22	46.22	090	2	0	0	2	2

49040 Drainage of subdiaphragmatic or subphrenic abscess, open Ⓒ

RVU			Global Days	Modifiers				
Mod	Non-Fac Total	Fac Total		51	50	62	80	MUE
	29.01	29.01	090	2	0	1	2	2

AMA: Nov 97: 18

Drainage of subdiaphragmatic or subphrenic abscess; open

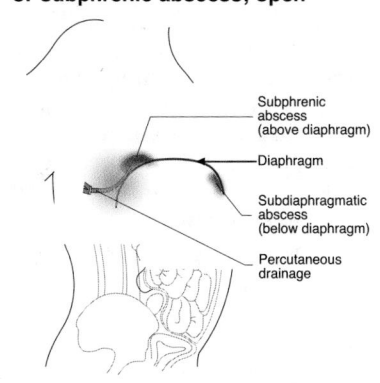

Subphrenic abscess (above diaphragm) · Diaphragm · Subdiaphragmatic abscess (below diaphragm) · Percutaneous drainage

● New ▲ Revised Deleted ⊙ Moderate Sedation ✚ Add-on Codes ⊘ High Risk Denial Ⓐ Age Edit ♀ Female ♂ Male **AMA** *CPT® Assistant* **MUE** Medically Unlikely Edit
⊘ Modifier 51 Exempt ⊖ Modifier 63 Exempt Ⓧ Unlisted **Modifiers:** *See Inside Back Cover* Ⓜ Maternity Ⓐ2–Ⓩ3 ASC Payment Indicators Ⓐ–Ⓨ OPPS Status Indicators

Surgical Procedures

49060 – 49255

49060 Drainage of retroperitoneal abscess, open   C

Mod	Non-Fac Total	Fac Total	Global Days	51	50	62	80	MUE
	31.89	31.89	090	2	0	1	1	2

AMA: Nov 97: 18, Nov 99: 24, Jul 01: 11, Aug 01: 10

49062 Drainage of extraperitoneal lymphocele to peritoneal cavity, open   C

Mod	Non-Fac Total	Fac Total	Global Days	51	50	62	80	MUE
	21.27	21.27	090	2	0	1	2	1

AMA: Nov 97: 19, Jul 01: 11, Aug 01: 10

49082 Abdominal paracentesis (diagnostic or therapeutic); without imaging guidance   G 2 T

Mod	Non-Fac Total	Fac Total	Global Days	51	50	62	80	MUE
	5.46	2.15	000	2	0	0	1	1

AMA: Dec 12: 9

49083 Abdominal paracentesis (diagnostic or therapeutic); with imaging guidance   G 2 T

Coding tip: All the radiologic services necessary for the procedure are included in this code; do not report an additional radiologic code for this procedure.

Mod	Non-Fac Total	Fac Total	Global Days	51	50	62	80	MUE
	8.33	3.15	000	2	0	0	1	2

AMA: Dec 12: 9, Mar 14: 14

49084 Peritoneal lavage, including imaging guidance, when performed   G 2 T

Coding tip: All the radiologic services necessary for the procedure are included in this code; do not report an additional radiologic code for this procedure.

Mod	Non-Fac Total	Fac Total	Global Days	51	50	62	80	MUE
	3.14	3.14	000	2	0	0	1	1

AMA: Dec 12: 9

Excisional/Destruction Abdominal/Peritoneum/Omentum Procedures

49180 Biopsy, abdominal or retroperitoneal mass, percutaneous needle   A 2 T

Coding tip: Radiological guidance for correct needle placement - ultrasound 76942; fluoroscopy 77002; CT 77012; MRI 77021

Mod	Non-Fac Total	Fac Total	Global Days	51	50	62	80	MUE
	4.65	2.48	000	2	0	0	1	2

AMA: Fall 93: 11

● 49185 Sclerotherapy of a fluid collection (eg, lymphocele, cyst, or seroma), percutaneous, including contrast injection(s), sclerosant injection(s), diagnostic study, imaging guidance (eg, ultrasound, fluoroscopy) and radiological supervision and interpretation when performed   T

Mod	Non-Fac Total	Fac Total	Global Days	51	50	62	80	MUE
	28.23	3.57	000	0	0	0	1	2

49203 Excision or destruction, open, intra-abdominal tumors, cysts or endometriomas, 1 or more peritoneal, mesenteric, or retroperitoneal primary or secondary tumors; largest tumor 5 cm diameter or less   C

Mod	Non-Fac Total	Fac Total	Global Days	51	50	62	80	MUE
	34.73	34.73	090	2	0	1	2	1

AMA: Dec 10: 16, Aug 08: 7

49204 Excision or destruction, open, intra-abdominal tumors, cysts or endometriomas, 1 or more peritoneal, mesenteric, or retroperitoneal primary or secondary tumors; largest tumor 5.1-10.0 cm diameter   C

Mod	Non-Fac Total	Fac Total	Global Days	51	50	62	80	MUE
	44.45	44.45	090	2	0	1	2	1

AMA: Dec 10: 16, Aug 08: 7

49205 Excision or destruction, open, intra-abdominal tumors, cysts or endometriomas, 1 or more peritoneal, mesenteric, or retroperitoneal primary or secondary tumors; largest tumor greater than 10.0 cm diameter   C

Mod	Non-Fac Total	Fac Total	Global Days	51	50	62	80	MUE
	51.06	51.06	090	2	0	1	2	1

AMA: Dec 10: 16, Aug 08: 7

49215 Excision of presacral or sacrococcygeal tumor ⊖ C

Mod	Non-Fac Total	Fac Total	Global Days	51	50	62	80	MUE
	64.42	64.42	090	2	0	1	2	1

49220 Staging laparotomy for Hodgkins disease or lymphoma (includes splenectomy, needle or open biopsies of both liver lobes, possibly also removal of abdominal nodes, abdominal node and/or bone marrow biopsies, ovarian repositioning)   C

Mod	Non-Fac Total	Fac Total	Global Days	51	50	62	80	MUE
	25.76	25.76	090	2	0	1	2	1

49250 Umbilectomy, omphalectomy, excision of umbilicus (separate procedure)   A A 2 T

Mod	Non-Fac Total	Fac Total	Global Days	51	50	62	80	MUE
	17.07	17.07	090	2	0	1	1	1

49255 Omentectomy, epiploectomy, resection of omentum (separate procedure)   C

Documentation Finder: Documentation will make reference to removal of the fat layer (omentum - an large apron of fatty tissue containing veins, arteries, lymphatics) where the bottom edge attaches to the stomach and then hangs down in front of the intestines.

Mod	Non-Fac Total	Fac Total	Global Days	51	50	62	80	MUE
	22.93	22.93	090	2	0	1	2	1

AMA: Nov 99: 24

● New   ▲ Revised   ✖ Deleted   ⊙ Moderate Sedation   ✚ Add-on Codes   ⊗ High Risk Denial   Ⓐ Age Edit   ♀ Female   ♂ Male   **AMA** CPT® Assistant   **MUE** Medically Unlikely Edit

⊘ Modifier 51 Exempt   ⊖ Modifier 63 Exempt   ✖ Unlisted   **Modifiers:** See Inside Back Cover   Ⓜ Maternity   A 2 – Z 3 ASC Payment Indicators   A – Y OPPS Status Indicators

476   CPT © 2015 American Medical Association. All Rights Reserved.   © 2016 DecisionHealth

Laparoscopic Abdominal/Peritoneum/Omentum Procedures

Coding Guidance

Code 49320 is included in all surgical laparoscopic, hysteroscopic, or peritoneoscopic procedures.

49320 Laparoscopy, abdomen, peritoneum, and omentum, diagnostic, with or without collection of specimen(s) by brushing or washing (separate procedure) `A2 J 1`

RVU				Global Days	Modifiers				
Mod	Non-Fac Total	Fac Total				51	50	62	80	MUE
	9.42	9.42		010		2	0	0	2	1

AMA: Nov 99: 24, Mar 00: 9, Apr 06: 19, Mar 07: 4, Nov 07: 1, Dec 08: 7, Jun 10: 7

Pub 100-04, 32, 150.2

49321 Laparoscopy, surgical; with biopsy (single or multiple) `A2 J 1`

RVU				Global Days	Modifiers				
Mod	Non-Fac Total	Fac Total				51	50	62	80	MUE
	10.00	10.00		010		3	0	2	2	1

AMA: Nov 99: 24, Mar 00: 9

49322 Laparoscopy, surgical; with aspiration of cavity or cyst (eg, ovarian cyst) (single or multiple) `A2 J 1`

RVU				Global Days	Modifiers				
Mod	Non-Fac Total	Fac Total				51	50	62	80	MUE
	10.65	10.65		010		3	0	2	2	1

AMA: Nov 99: 24, Mar 00: 9

49323 Laparoscopy, surgical; with drainage of lymphocele to peritoneal cavity `J 1`

RVU				Global Days	Modifiers				
Mod	Non-Fac Total	Fac Total				51	50	62	80	MUE
	18.41	18.41		090		3	0	2	2	1

AMA: Nov 99: 24, Mar 00: 9, May 00: 4, Jul 01: 11, Aug 01: 10

49324 Laparoscopy, surgical; with insertion of tunneled intraperitoneal catheter `G2 J 1`

RVU				Global Days	Modifiers				
Mod	Non-Fac Total	Fac Total				51	50	62	80	MUE
	11.31	11.31		010		3	0	2	2	1

49325 Laparoscopy, surgical; with revision of previously placed intraperitoneal cannula or catheter, with removal of intraluminal obstructive material if performed `G2 J 1`

RVU				Global Days	Modifiers				
Mod	Non-Fac Total	Fac Total				51	50	62	80	MUE
	12.07	12.07		010		3	0	2	2	1

+ 49326 Laparoscopy, surgical; with omentopexy (omental tacking procedure) (List separately in addition to code for primary procedure) `N N N`

RVU				Global Days	Modifiers				
Mod	Non-Fac Total	Fac Total				51	50	62	80	MUE
	5.49	5.49		ZZZ		0	0	1	2	1

+ 49327 Laparoscopy, surgical; with placement of interstitial device(s) for radiation therapy guidance (eg, fiducial markers, dosimeter), intra-abdominal, intrapelvic, and/or retroperitoneum, including imaging guidance, if performed, single or multiple (List separately in addition to code for primary procedure) `N N N`

RVU				Global Days	Modifiers				
Mod	Non-Fac Total	Fac Total				51	50	62	80	MUE
	3.81	3.81		ZZZ		0	0	1	2	1

49329 Unlisted laparoscopy procedure, abdomen, peritoneum and omentum `X J 1`

RVU				Global Days	Modifiers				
Mod	Non-Fac Total	Fac Total				51	50	62	80	MUE
	0.00	0.00		YYY		2	1	1	2	

AMA: Nov 99: 24, Mar 00: 9, Feb 06: 16, Dec 11: 16, Oct 13: 18

Introduction/Revision/Removal Abdominal/Peritoneum/Omentum Procedures

49400 Injection of air or contrast into peritoneal cavity (separate procedure) `N N N`

Coding tip: Peritoneogram - 74190

RVU				Global Days	Modifiers				
Mod	Non-Fac Total	Fac Total				51	50	62	80	MUE
	3.88	2.72		000		2	0	0	1	1

AMA: Dec 10: 13

49402 Removal of peritoneal foreign body from peritoneal cavity `A2 T`

RVU				Global Days	Modifiers				
Mod	Non-Fac Total	Fac Total				51	50	62	80	MUE
	24.85	24.85		090		2	0	1	1	1

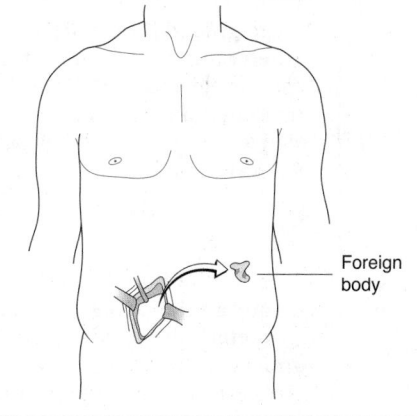

Removal of foreign body from peritoneal cavity

Foreign body

● New   ▲ Revised   Deleted   ⊙ Moderate Sedation   ✚ Add-on Codes   ⊘ High Risk Denial   Ⓐ Age Edit   ♀ Female   ♂ Male   **AMA** *CPT® Assistant*   **MUE** Medically Unlikely Edit
⊘ Modifier 51 Exempt   ⊖ Modifier 63 Exempt   ✗ Unlisted   **Modifiers:** *See Inside Back Cover*   Ⓜ Maternity   `A2`–`Z3` ASC Payment Indicators   `A`–`Y` OPPS Status Indicators

⊙ **49405** Image-guided fluid collection drainage by catheter (eg, abscess, hematoma, seroma, lymphocele, cyst); visceral (eg, kidney, liver, spleen, lung/mediastinum), percutaneous   🅣

RVU		Global Days	Modifiers				
Mod	Non-Fac Total	Fac Total		51	50	62	80	MUE
	24.83	6.13	000	2	0	0	1	2

AMA: May 14: 9

Image guided fluid collection drainage by catheter

Visceral-percutaneous (49405),
Peritoneal or retroperitoneal-percutaneous (49406),
Peritoneal or retroperitoneal-transvaginal or transrectal (49407)

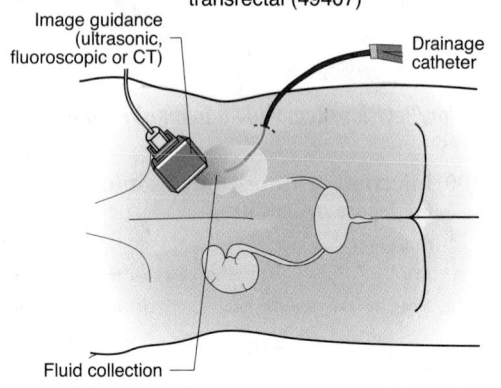

⊙ **49406** Image-guided fluid collection drainage by catheter (eg, abscess, hematoma, seroma, lymphocele, cyst); peritoneal or retroperitoneal, percutaneous   🅖2🅣

RVU		Global Days	Modifiers				
Mod	Non-Fac Total	Fac Total		51	50	62	80	MUE
	24.85	6.14	000	2	0	0	1	2

AMA: May 14: 9

⊙ **49407** Image-guided fluid collection drainage by catheter (eg, abscess, hematoma, seroma, lymphocele, cyst); peritoneal or retroperitoneal, transvaginal or transrectal   🅖2🅣

RVU		Global Days	Modifiers				
Mod	Non-Fac Total	Fac Total		51	50	62	80	MUE
	20.76	6.59	000	2	0	0	1	1

AMA: May 14: 9

⊙ **49411** Placement of interstitial device(s) for radiation therapy guidance (eg, fiducial markers, dosimeter), percutaneous, intra-abdominal, intra-pelvic (except prostate), and/or retroperitoneum, single or multiple   🅟3🅢

Coding tip: *Radiological guidance for correct placement - ultrasound 76942; fluoroscopy 77002; CT 77012; MRI 77021*

RVU		Global Days	Modifiers				
Mod	Non-Fac Total	Fac Total		51	50	62	80	MUE
	15.57	5.72	000	2	0	0	0	1

AMA: Feb 10: 7

✚ **49412** Placement of interstitial device(s) for radiation therapy guidance (eg, fiducial markers, dosimeter), open, intra-abdominal, intrapelvic, and/or retroperitoneum, including image guidance, if performed, single or multiple (List separately in addition to code for primary procedure)   🅒

RVU		Global Days	Modifiers				
Mod	Non-Fac Total	Fac Total		51	50	62	80	MUE
	2.41	2.41	ZZZ	0	0	1	0	1

⊙ **49418** Insertion of tunneled intraperitoneal catheter (eg, dialysis, intraperitoneal chemotherapy instillation, management of ascites), complete procedure, including imaging guidance, catheter placement, contrast injection when performed, and radiological supervision and interpretation, percutaneous   🅖2🅣

RVU		Global Days	Modifiers				
Mod	Non-Fac Total	Fac Total		51	50	62	80	MUE
	40.72	6.32	000	2	0	0	0	1

49419 Insertion of tunneled intraperitoneal catheter, with subcutaneous port (ie, totally implantable)   🅐2🅣

RVU		Global Days	Modifiers				
Mod	Non-Fac Total	Fac Total		51	50	62	80	MUE
	12.80	12.80	090	2	0	0	1	1

49421 Insertion of tunneled intraperitoneal catheter for dialysis, open   🅖2🅣

RVU		Global Days	Modifiers				
Mod	Non-Fac Total	Fac Total		51	50	62	80	MUE
	6.71	6.71	000	2	0	0	1	1

AMA: Fall 93: 2, Jul 06: 19

49422 Removal of tunneled intraperitoneal catheter   🅐2🅞2

RVU		Global Days	Modifiers				
Mod	Non-Fac Total	Fac Total		51	50	62	80	MUE
	11.05	11.05	010	2	0	0	1	1

49423 Exchange of previously placed abscess or cyst drainage catheter under radiological guidance (separate procedure)   🅖2🅣

Coding tip: *Guidance for change of drainage catheter - 75984*

RVU		Global Days	Modifiers				
Mod	Non-Fac Total	Fac Total		51	50	62	80	MUE
	15.59	2.09	000	2	0	0	0	2

AMA: Nov 97: 19, Mar 98: 8

49424 Contrast injection for assessment of abscess or cyst via previously placed drainage catheter or tube (separate procedure)   🅝🅝

Coding tip: *Radiology exam of abscess - 76080*

RVU		Global Days	Modifiers				
Mod	Non-Fac Total	Fac Total		51	50	62	80	MUE
	4.16	1.11	000	2	0	0	0	3

AMA: Nov 97: 19, Mar 98: 8, Nov 03: 14

49425 Insertion of peritoneal-venous shunt   🅒

RVU		Global Days	Modifiers				
Mod	Non-Fac Total	Fac Total		51	50	62	80	MUE
	21.18	21.18	090	2	0	1	2	1

● New   ▲ Revised   ✖ Deleted   ⊙ Moderate Sedation   ✚ Add-on Codes   ⊘ High Risk Denial   Ⓐ Age Edit   ♀ Female   ♂ Male   **AMA** *CPT® Assistant*   **MUE** Medically Unlikely Edit
⊘ Modifier 51 Exempt   ⊖ Modifier 63 Exempt   🅧 Unlisted   **Modifiers:** *See Inside Back Cover*   🅜 Maternity   🅐2–🅩3 ASC Payment Indicators   🅐–🅨 OPPS Status Indicators

49426 Revision of peritoneal-venous shunt   A2T

RVU			Global Days	Modifiers				
Mod	Non-Fac Total	Fac Total		51	50	62	80	MUE
	17.73	17.73	090	2	0	0	1	1

49427 Injection procedure (eg, contrast media) for evaluation of previously placed peritoneal-venous shunt   NIN

Coding tip: Shuntogram for investigation of nonvascular shunt - 75809
Coding tip: Peritoneal-venous shunt patency test - 78291

RVU			Global Days	Modifiers				
Mod	Non-Fac Total	Fac Total		51	50	62	80	MUE
	1.34	1.34	000	2	0	0	0	1

49428 Ligation of peritoneal-venous shunt   C

RVU			Global Days	Modifiers				
Mod	Non-Fac Total	Fac Total		51	50	62	80	MUE
	12.51	12.51	010	2	0	0	1	1

49429 Removal of peritoneal-venous shunt   G2Q2

RVU			Global Days	Modifiers				
Mod	Non-Fac Total	Fac Total		51	50	62	80	MUE
	13.30	13.30	010	2	0	0	1	1

+ 49435 Insertion of subcutaneous extension to intraperitoneal cannula or catheter with remote chest exit site (List separately in addition to code for primary procedure)   NIN

RVU			Global Days	Modifiers				
Mod	Non-Fac Total	Fac Total		51	50	62	80	MUE
	3.48	3.48	ZZZ	0	0	1	2	1

49436 Delayed creation of exit site from embedded subcutaneous segment of intraperitoneal cannula or catheter   G2T

RVU			Global Days	Modifiers				
Mod	Non-Fac Total	Fac Total		51	50	62	80	MUE
	5.41	5.41	010	2	0	1	2	1

⊙ **49440 Insertion of gastrostomy tube, percutaneous, under fluoroscopic guidance including contrast injection(s), image documentation and report**   G2T

RVU			Global Days	Modifiers				
Mod	Non-Fac Total	Fac Total		51	50	62	80	MUE
	29.51	6.42	010	2	0	0	0	1

AMA: Jan 08: 8, Jun 08: 8, Aug 08: 7, Sep 10: 9, Sep 14: 5, Dec 14: 18

⊙ **49441 Insertion of duodenostomy or jejunostomy tube, percutaneous, under fluoroscopic guidance including contrast injection(s), image documentation and report**   G2T

RVU			Global Days	Modifiers				
Mod	Non-Fac Total	Fac Total		51	50	62	80	MUE
	33.23	7.43	010	2	0	0	0	1

AMA: Jan 08: 8, Jun 08: 8, Aug 08: 7, Dec 14: 18

⊙ **49442 Insertion of cecostomy or other colonic tube, percutaneous, under fluoroscopic guidance including contrast injection(s), image documentation and report**   G2T

RVU			Global Days	Modifiers				
Mod	Non-Fac Total	Fac Total		51	50	62	80	MUE
	27.48	6.43	010	2	0	0	0	1

AMA: Jan 08: 8, Jun 08: 8, Aug 08: 7, Dec 14: 18

⊙ **49446 Conversion of gastrostomy tube to gastro-jejunostomy tube, percutaneous, under fluoroscopic guidance including contrast injection(s), image documentation and report**   G2T

RVU			Global Days	Modifiers				
Mod	Non-Fac Total	Fac Total		51	50	62	80	MUE
	28.41	4.71	000	2	0	0	0	1

Conversion of gastrostomy tube to gastro-jejunostomy tube

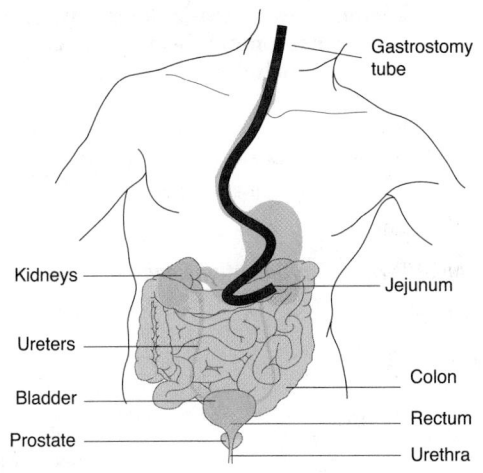

A gastrostomy tube is converted to a gastrojejunostomy tube using percutaneous technique under fluoroscopic guidance

49450 Replacement of gastrostomy or cecostomy (or other colonic) tube, percutaneous, under fluoroscopic guidance including contrast injection(s), image documentation and report   G2T

RVU			Global Days	Modifiers				
Mod	Non-Fac Total	Fac Total		51	50	62	80	MUE
	18.95	1.94	000	2	0	0	0	1

AMA: Sep 10: 9, Dec 13: 17

49451 Replacement of duodenostomy or jejunostomy tube, percutaneous, under fluoroscopic guidance including contrast injection(s), image documentation and report   G2T

RVU			Global Days	Modifiers				
Mod	Non-Fac Total	Fac Total		51	50	62	80	MUE
	20.67	2.64	000	2	0	0	0	1

AMA: Jan 08: 8, Jun 08: 8, Aug 08: 7, Jul 10: 10, Dec 14: 18

● New   ▲ Revised   Deleted   ⊙ Moderate Sedation   ✚ Add-on Codes   ⊘ High Risk Denial   Ⓐ Age Edit   ♀ Female   ♂ Male   **AMA** *CPT® Assistant*   ***MUE*** Medically Unlikely Edit
⊘ Modifier 51 Exempt   ⊖ Modifier 63 Exempt   ✖ Unlisted   **Modifiers:** *See Inside Back Cover*   Ⓜ Maternity   A2–Z3 ASC Payment Indicators   A–Y OPPS Status Indicators

© 2016 DecisionHealth   CPT © 2015 American Medical Association. All Rights Reserved.   **479**

49452 Replacement of gastro-jejunostomy tube, percutaneous, under fluoroscopic guidance including contrast injection(s), image documentation and report G2 T

RVU			Global Days	Modifiers				
Mod	Non-Fac Total	Fac Total		51	50	62	80	MUE
	25.56	4.06	000	2	0	0	0	1

AMA: Mar 10: 10

49460 Mechanical removal of obstructive material from gastrostomy, duodenostomy, jejunostomy, gastro-jejunostomy, or cecostomy (or other colonic) tube, any method, under fluoroscopic guidance including contrast injection(s), if performed, image documentation and report G2 T

RVU			Global Days	Modifiers				
Mod	Non-Fac Total	Fac Total		51	50	62	80	MUE
	20.84	1.40	000	2	0	0	0	1

49465 Contrast injection(s) for radiological evaluation of existing gastrostomy, duodenostomy, jejunostomy, gastro-jejunostomy, or cecostomy (or other colonic) tube, from a percutaneous approach including image documentation and report G2 Q I

RVU			Global Days	Modifiers				
Mod	Non-Fac Total	Fac Total		51	50	62	80	MUE
	4.63	0.90	000	2	0	0	0	1

AMA: Sep 14: 5

Abdominal/Peritoneum/Omentum Repair

Hernia Repair

Coding Guidance

An incidental hernia repair done during another open intra-abdominal surgery, or at the same incision site as another surgery, is not reported. The hernia repair is reportable if it is done at a site other than the incision for another open surgery. A recurrent hernia repair and an initial incisional hernia repair are not reported together unless both are performed at separately identified sites.

49491 Repair, initial inguinal hernia, preterm infant (younger than 37 weeks gestation at birth), performed from birth up to 50 weeks postconception age, with or without hydrocelectomy; reducible ⊗ A ⊖ T

RVU			Global Days	Modifiers				
Mod	Non-Fac Total	Fac Total		51	50	62	80	MUE
	21.25	21.25	090	2	1	1	2	1

AMA: Mar 04: 2, Jun 08: 3

49492 Repair, initial inguinal hernia, preterm infant (younger than 37 weeks gestation at birth), performed from birth up to 50 weeks postconception age, with or without hydrocelectomy; incarcerated or strangulated ⊗ A ⊖ T

RVU			Global Days	Modifiers				
Mod	Non-Fac Total	Fac Total		51	50	62	80	MUE
	27.80	27.80	090	2	1	1	2	1

AMA: Mar 04: 2, Jun 08: 3

49495 Repair, initial inguinal hernia, full term infant younger than age 6 months, or preterm infant older than 50 weeks postconception age and younger than age 6 months at the time of surgery, with or without hydrocelectomy; reducible ⊛ A ⊖ A2 T

RVU			Global Days	Modifiers				
Mod	Non-Fac Total	Fac Total		51	50	62	80	MUE
	11.04	11.04	090	2	1	1	2	1

AMA: Winter 93: 6, Winter 94: 13, Jan 04: 27, Mar 04: 10, May 04: 14, Nov 07: 9, Jun 08: 3

49496 Repair, initial inguinal hernia, full term infant younger than age 6 months, or preterm infant older than 50 weeks postconception age and younger than age 6 months at the time of surgery, with or without hydrocelectomy; incarcerated or strangulated ⊛ A ⊖ A2 T

RVU			Global Days	Modifiers				
Mod	Non-Fac Total	Fac Total		51	50	62	80	MUE
	17.83	17.83	090	2	1	1	2	1

AMA: Winter 93: 6, Winter 94: 13, Jan 04: 27, Mar 04: 10, May 04: 14, Jun 08: 3

49500 Repair initial inguinal hernia, age 6 months to younger than 5 years, with or without hydrocelectomy; reducible ⊗ A A2 T

RVU			Global Days	Modifiers				
Mod	Non-Fac Total	Fac Total		51	50	62	80	MUE
	10.40	10.40	090	2	1	1	2	1

AMA: Winter 94: 13, Jan 04: 27, Mar 04: 10, Nov 07: 9, Jun 08: 3, Nov 14: 14

49501 Repair initial inguinal hernia, age 6 months to younger than 5 years, with or without hydrocelectomy; incarcerated or strangulated ⊛ A A2 T

RVU			Global Days	Modifiers				
Mod	Non-Fac Total	Fac Total		51	50	62	80	MUE
	16.88	16.88	090	2	1	1	2	1

AMA: Winter 94: 13, Jan 04: 27, Mar 04: 12, Jun 08: 3

49505 Repair initial inguinal hernia, age 5 years or older; reducible A2 T

RVU			Global Days	Modifiers				
Mod	Non-Fac Total	Fac Total		51	50	62	80	MUE
	15.06	15.06	090	2	1	1	2	1

AMA: Winter 94: 13, Sep 00: 10, Jan 04: 27, Mar 04: 12, Jun 08: 3

49507 Repair initial inguinal hernia, age 5 years or older; incarcerated or strangulated A2 T

RVU			Global Days	Modifiers				
Mod	Non-Fac Total	Fac Total		51	50	62	80	MUE
	16.96	16.96	090	2	1	1	2	1

AMA: Winter 94: 13, Jan 04: 27, Mar 04: 10, Jun 08: 3

49520 Repair recurrent inguinal hernia, any age; reducible A2 T

RVU			Global Days	Modifiers				
Mod	Non-Fac Total	Fac Total		51	50	62	80	MUE
	18.31	18.31	090	2	1	1	2	1

AMA: Winter 94: 13, Sep 03: 3, Jan 04: 27, Mar 04: 3, Jun 08: 3

CPT © 2015 American Medical Association. All Rights Reserved.

© 2016 DecisionHealth

49521 Repair recurrent inguinal hernia, any age; incarcerated or strangulated　A 2 T

Mod	Non-Fac Total	Fac Total	Global Days	51	50	62	80	MUE
	20.74	20.74	090	2	1	1	2	1

AMA: Winter 94: 13, Jan 04: 27, Mar 04: 10, Jun 08: 3

49525 Repair inguinal hernia, sliding, any age　A 2 T

Mod	Non-Fac Total	Fac Total	Global Days	51	50	62	80	MUE
	16.60	16.60	090	2	1	1	2	1

AMA: Winter 94: 14, Jan 04: 27, Mar 04: 10, Nov 07: 9, Jun 08: 3

49540 Repair lumbar hernia　A 2 T

Mod	Non-Fac Total	Fac Total	Global Days	51	50	62	80	MUE
	19.45	19.45	090	2	1	1	2	1

AMA: Winter 94: 14, Jun 08: 3

49550 Repair initial femoral hernia, any age; reducible　A 2 T

Mod	Non-Fac Total	Fac Total	Global Days	51	50	62	80	MUE
	16.67	16.67	090	2	1	1	2	1

AMA: Winter 94: 14, Jun 08: 3

49553 Repair initial femoral hernia, any age; incarcerated or strangulated　A 2 T

Mod	Non-Fac Total	Fac Total	Global Days	51	50	62	80	MUE
	18.29	18.29	090	2	1	1	2	1

AMA: Winter 94: 14, Jun 08: 3

49555 Repair recurrent femoral hernia; reducible　A 2 T

Mod	Non-Fac Total	Fac Total	Global Days	51	50	62	80	MUE
	17.32	17.32	090	2	1	1	2	1

AMA: Winter 94: 14, Jun 08: 3

49557 Repair recurrent femoral hernia; incarcerated or strangulated　A 2 T

Mod	Non-Fac Total	Fac Total	Global Days	51	50	62	80	MUE
	20.98	20.98	090	2	1	1	2	1

AMA: Winter 94: 14, Jun 08: 3

49560 Repair initial incisional or ventral hernia; reducible　A 2 T

Mod	Non-Fac Total	Fac Total	Global Days	51	50	62	80	MUE
	21.35	21.35	090	2	1	1	2	2

AMA: Winter 93: 6, Winter 94: 14, Nov 97: 19, Jun 08: 3, Jan 12: 10, Oct 13: 15

49561 Repair initial incisional or ventral hernia; incarcerated or strangulated　A 2 T

Mod	Non-Fac Total	Fac Total	Global Days	51	50	62	80	MUE
	26.96	26.96	090	2	1	1	2	2

AMA: Winter 94: 14, Jun 08: 3, Jan 12: 10, Oct 13: 15

49565 Repair recurrent incisional or ventral hernia; reducible　A 2 T

Mod	Non-Fac Total	Fac Total	Global Days	51	50	62	80	MUE
	22.25	22.25	090	2	1	1	2	2

AMA: Winter 94: 14, Nov 97: 19, Jun 08: 3, Jan 12: 10, Oct 13: 15

49566 Repair recurrent incisional or ventral hernia; incarcerated or strangulated　A 2 T

Mod	Non-Fac Total	Fac Total	Global Days	51	50	62	80	MUE
	27.20	27.20	090	2	1	1	2	2

AMA: Winter 94: 14, Jun 08: 3, Jan 12: 10, Oct 13: 15

Coding Guidance

Add-on code 49568 is for use with other incisional or ventral hernia repair codes 49560-49566. The use of mesh or other prosthesis placed during other types of hernia repairs is a bundled service and is not separately reportable. Do not use 49568 with other types of hernia repairs. When an incisional or ventral hernia repair with mesh is performed at the same time as another type of hernia repair, use the appropriate modifier with code 49568 to report it outside bundling edits.

+ 49568 Implantation of mesh or other prosthesis for open incisional or ventral hernia repair or mesh for closure of debridement for necrotizing soft tissue infection (List separately in addition to code for the incisional or ventral hernia repair)　N1 N

Mod	Non-Fac Total	Fac Total	Global Days	51	50	62	80	MUE
	7.76	7.76	ZZZ	0	0	1	2	2

AMA: Winter 94: 14, Nov 97: 19, Sep 01: 11, Nov 05: 15, Nov 07: 9, Jun 08: 3, Jan 12: 10, Oct 13: 15

49570 Repair epigastric hernia (eg, preperitoneal fat); reducible (separate procedure)　A 2 T

Mod	Non-Fac Total	Fac Total	Global Days	51	50	62	80	MUE
	12.05	12.05	090	2	1	1	2	1

AMA: Winter 94: 15, Jun 08: 3

49572 Repair epigastric hernia (eg, preperitoneal fat); incarcerated or strangulated　A 2 T

Mod	Non-Fac Total	Fac Total	Global Days	51	50	62	80	MUE
	14.95	14.95	090	2	1	1	2	1

AMA: Winter 94: 15, Jun 08: 3

49580 Repair umbilical hernia, younger than age 5 years; reducible　⊗Ⓐ A 2 T

Mod	Non-Fac Total	Fac Total	Global Days	51	50	62	80	MUE
	9.62	9.62	090	2	0	1	2	1

AMA: Winter 94: 15, Jun 08: 3

49582 Repair umbilical hernia, younger than age 5 years; incarcerated or strangulated　⊗Ⓐ A 2 T

Mod	Non-Fac Total	Fac Total	Global Days	51	50	62	80	MUE
	14.00	14.00	090	2	0	1	2	1

AMA: Winter 94: 15, Jun 08: 3

● New　▲ Revised　Deleted　⊙ Moderate Sedation　✚ Add-on Codes　⊗ High Risk Denial　Ⓐ Age Edit　♀ Female　♂ Male　**AMA** *CPT® Assistant*　***MUE*** Medically Unlikely Edit　⊘ Modifier 51 Exempt　⊖ Modifier 63 Exempt　Ⓧ Unlisted　**Modifiers:** *See Inside Back Cover*　Ⓜ Maternity　A2–Z3 ASC Payment Indicators　A–Y OPPS Status Indicators

49585 Repair umbilical hernia, age 5 years or older; reducible `A 2 T`

| RVU | | | Global Days | Modifiers | | | | |
Mod	Non-Fac Total	Fac Total		51	50	62	80	MUE
	12.88	12.88	090	2	0	1	2	1

AMA: Winter 94: 15

49587 Repair umbilical hernia, age 5 years or older; incarcerated or strangulated `A 2 T`

| RVU | | | Global Days | Modifiers | | | | |
Mod	Non-Fac Total	Fac Total		51	50	62	80	MUE
	13.76	13.76	090	2	0	1	2	1

AMA: Winter 94: 15

49590 Repair spigelian hernia `A 2 T`

| RVU | | | Global Days | Modifiers | | | | |
Mod	Non-Fac Total	Fac Total		51	50	62	80	MUE
	16.57	16.57	090	2	1	1	2	1

AMA: Winter 94: 15

49600 Repair of small omphalocele, with primary closure `⊖ A 2 T`

| RVU | | | Global Days | Modifiers | | | | |
Mod	Non-Fac Total	Fac Total		51	50	62	80	MUE
	20.34	20.34	090	2	0	1	2	1

AMA: Winter 94: 15

Repair of small omphalocele

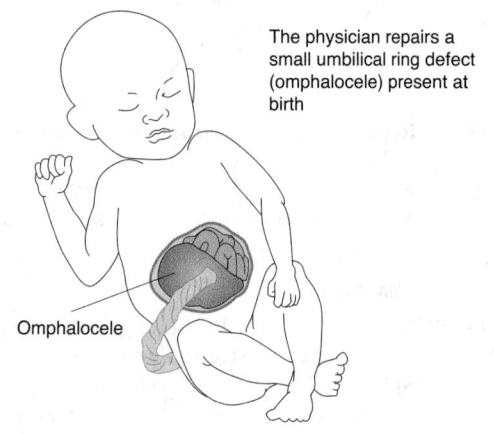

The physician repairs a small umbilical ring defect (omphalocele) present at birth

Omphalocele

49605 Repair of large omphalocele or gastroschisis; with or without prosthesis `Ⓐ ⊖ C`

| RVU | | | Global Days | Modifiers | | | | |
Mod	Non-Fac Total	Fac Total		51	50	62	80	MUE
	143.90	143.90	090	2	0	1	2	1

AMA: Winter 94: 15

49606 Repair of large omphalocele or gastroschisis; with removal of prosthesis, final reduction and closure, in operating room `Ⓐ ⊖ C`

| RVU | | | Global Days | Modifiers | | | | |
Mod	Non-Fac Total	Fac Total		51	50	62	80	MUE
	32.43	32.43	090	2	0	1	2	1

AMA: Winter 94: 15

49610 Repair of omphalocele (Gross type operation); first stage `Ⓐ ⊖ C`

| RVU | | | Global Days | Modifiers | | | | |
Mod	Non-Fac Total	Fac Total		51	50	62	80	MUE
	19.97	19.97	090	2	0	1	2	1

AMA: Winter 94: 15

49611 Repair of omphalocele (Gross type operation); second stage `Ⓐ ⊖ C`

| RVU | | | Global Days | Modifiers | | | | |
Mod	Non-Fac Total	Fac Total		51	50	62	80	MUE
	17.58	17.58	090	2	0	1	2	1

AMA: Winter 94: 15

Laparoscopic Hernia Repair

49650 Laparoscopy, surgical; repair initial inguinal hernia `A 2 J I`

| RVU | | | Global Days | Modifiers | | | | |
Mod	Non-Fac Total	Fac Total		51	50	62	80	MUE
	12.38	12.38	090	2	1	1	2	1

AMA: Nov 99: 24, Mar 00: 9, Jul 14: 5

49651 Laparoscopy, surgical; repair recurrent inguinal hernia `A 2 J I`

| RVU | | | Global Days | Modifiers | | | | |
Mod	Non-Fac Total	Fac Total		51	50	62	80	MUE
	16.08	16.08	090	2	1	1	2	1

AMA: Nov 99: 24, Mar 00: 9

49652 Laparoscopy, surgical, repair, ventral, umbilical, spigelian or epigastric hernia (includes mesh insertion, when performed); reducible `G 2 J I`

| RVU | | | Global Days | Modifiers | | | | |
Mod	Non-Fac Total	Fac Total		51	50	62	80	MUE
	21.55	21.55	090	2	1	1	2	2

49653 Laparoscopy, surgical, repair, ventral, umbilical, spigelian or epigastric hernia (includes mesh insertion, when performed); incarcerated or strangulated `G 2 J I`

| RVU | | | Global Days | Modifiers | | | | |
Mod	Non-Fac Total	Fac Total		51	50	62	80	MUE
	26.88	26.88	090	2	1	1	2	2

49654 Laparoscopy, surgical, repair, incisional hernia (includes mesh insertion, when performed); reducible `G 2 J I`

| RVU | | | Global Days | Modifiers | | | | |
Mod	Non-Fac Total	Fac Total		51	50	62	80	MUE
	24.47	24.47	090	2	1	1	2	2

49655 Laparoscopy, surgical, repair, incisional hernia (includes mesh insertion, when performed); incarcerated or strangulated `G 2 J I`

| RVU | | | Global Days | Modifiers | | | | |
Mod	Non-Fac Total	Fac Total		51	50	62	80	MUE
	29.88	29.88	090	2	1	1	2	2

49656 Laparoscopy, surgical, repair, recurrent incisional hernia (includes mesh insertion, when performed); reducible `G 2 J I`

| RVU | | | Global Days | Modifiers | | | | |
Mod	Non-Fac Total	Fac Total		51	50	62	80	MUE
	26.63	26.63	090	2	1	1	2	2

● New   ▲ Revised   ✖ Deleted   ⊙ Moderate Sedation   ✚ Add-on Codes   ⊘ High Risk Denial   Ⓐ Age Edit   ♀ Female   ♂ Male   **AMA** *CPT® Assistant*   **MUE** Medically Unlikely Edit
⊘ Modifier 51 Exempt   ⊖ Modifier 63 Exempt   ✗ Unlisted   **Modifiers:** *See Inside Back Cover*   Ⓜ Maternity   A 2 – Z 3 ASC Payment Indicators   A – Y OPPS Status Indicators

CPT © 2015 American Medical Association. All Rights Reserved.   © 2016 DecisionHealth

49657 Laparoscopy, surgical, repair, recurrent incisional hernia (includes mesh insertion, when performed); incarcerated or strangulated   `G2J1`

RVU			Global Days	Modifiers				
Mod	Non-Fac Total	Fac Total		51	50	62	80	MUE
	38.27	38.27	090	2	1	1	2	2

49659 Unlisted laparoscopy procedure, hernioplasty, herniorrhaphy, herniotomy   `xJ1`

RVU			Global Days	Modifiers				
Mod	Non-Fac Total	Fac Total		51	50	62	80	MUE
	0.00	0.00	YYY	2	1	1	2	

AMA: Nov 99: 25, Mar 00: 9, Sep 01: 11, Nov 05: 15, Feb 06: 16, Jan 09: 7, Jul 14: 5, Dec 14: 16

Abdominal/Peritoneum/Omentum Suture

49900 Suture, secondary, of abdominal wall for evisceration or dehiscence   `C`

RVU			Global Days	Modifiers				
Mod	Non-Fac Total	Fac Total		51	50	62	80	MUE
	23.61	23.61	090	2	0	1	2	1

AMA: Sep 10: 7

Other Abdominal/Peritoneum/Omentum Procedures

49904 Omental flap, extra-abdominal (eg, for reconstruction of sternal and chest wall defects)   `C`

RVU			Global Days	Modifiers				
Mod	Non-Fac Total	Fac Total		51	50	62	80	MUE
	41.75	41.75	090	2	0	1	1	1

Omental flap, intra/extra-abdominal

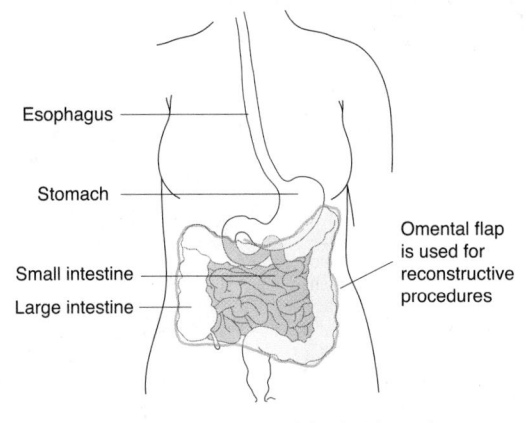

Esophagus

Stomach

Small intestine

Large intestine

Omental flap is used for reconstructive procedures

Use code 49904 for extra-abdominal (sternal or chest wall); use code 49905 for intra-abdominal; use code 49906 for free vascularized repair flap

+ 49905 Omental flap, intra-abdominal (List separately in addition to code for primary procedure)   `C`

RVU			Global Days	Modifiers				
Mod	Non-Fac Total	Fac Total		51	50	62	80	MUE
	10.25	10.25	ZZZ	0	0	2	2	1

AMA: Nov 00: 11

49906 Free omental flap with microvascular anastomosis   `CC`

RVU			Global Days	Modifiers				
Mod	Non-Fac Total	Fac Total		51	50	62	80	MUE
	0.00	0.00	090	2	0	1	1	1

AMA: Nov 96: 8, Apr 97: 8, Nov 98: 16

49999 Unlisted procedure, abdomen, peritoneum and omentum   `xT`

RVU			Global Days	Modifiers				
Mod	Non-Fac Total	Fac Total		51	50	62	80	MUE
	0.00	0.00	YYY	2	0	1	1	

AMA: Jul 06: 19, Sep 07: 10, Nov 07: 9, Aug 08: 7, Apr 10: 10, Jun 11: 13, Dec 10: 13, Jan 14: 9

● New   ▲ Revised   Deleted   ⊙ Moderate Sedation   ✚ Add-on Codes   ⊘ High Risk Denial   Ⓐ Age Edit   ♀ Female   ♂ Male   **AMA** *CPT® Assistant*   **MUE** Medically Unlikely Edit
⊘ Modifier 51 Exempt   ⊖ Modifier 63 Exempt   x⃞ Unlisted   **Modifiers:** *See Inside Back Cover*   Ⓜ Maternity   A2–Z3 ASC Payment Indicators   A–Y OPPS Status Indicators

Urinary Procedures

The urinary system encompasses the kidneys, ureters, bladder, urethra, and prostate. The main procedures organized under these sites are incision, excision, introduction, and repair. Procedures on the urinary system are very often accomplished laparoscopically or endoscopically. Many of these procedures are listed with different combinations of specific components as an endoscopic choice.

Kidney (Renal) Procedures

Incisional Kidney (Renal) Procedures

Coding Guidance

Genitourinary tract lesions requiring biopsy, excision, or destruction of the mucocutaneous border may have several CPT codes that describe the general nature of the biopsy. Only one biopsy code with one unit of service that most accurately describes the service should be reported. When excision or destruction is done immediately following a biopsy during the same session, only the most accurate, comprehensive code is reported. Separate CPT codes for lesion biopsy, excision, or destruction for both integumentary and genitourinary system procedures should not be reported unless the lesions are distinctly different and are located in both the genitourinary tract and in the skin.

50010 Renal exploration, not necessitating other specific procedures   C

RVU			Global Days	Modifiers				
Mod	Non-Fac Total	Fac Total		51	50	62	80	MUE
	21.30	21.30	090	2	1	1	2	1

50020 Drainage of perirenal or renal abscess, open   T

RVU			Global Days	Modifiers				
Mod	Non-Fac Total	Fac Total		51	50	62	80	MUE
	29.30	29.30	090	2	0	1	1	1

AMA: Nov 97: 19, Oct 01: 8, May 14: 9

50040 Nephrostomy, nephrotomy with drainage   C

RVU			Global Days	Modifiers				
Mod	Non-Fac Total	Fac Total		51	50	62	80	MUE
	26.60	26.60	090	2	1	1	1	1

AMA: Spring 93: 35, Oct 01: 8

50045 Nephrotomy, with exploration   C

RVU			Global Days	Modifiers				
Mod	Non-Fac Total	Fac Total		51	50	62	80	MUE
	27.78	27.78	090	2	1	1	2	1

AMA: Oct 01: 8

50060 Nephrolithotomy; removal of calculus   C

RVU			Global Days	Modifiers				
Mod	Non-Fac Total	Fac Total		51	50	62	80	MUE
	32.87	32.87	090	2	1	1	2	1

AMA: Oct 01: 8

50065 Nephrolithotomy; secondary surgical operation for calculus   C

RVU			Global Days	Modifiers				
Mod	Non-Fac Total	Fac Total		51	50	62	80	MUE
	34.76	34.76	090	2	1	0	2	1

AMA: Oct 01: 8

50070 Nephrolithotomy; complicated by congenital kidney abnormality   C

RVU			Global Days	Modifiers				
Mod	Non-Fac Total	Fac Total		51	50	62	80	MUE
	34.08	34.08	090	2	1	1	2	1

AMA: Oct 01: 8

50075 Nephrolithotomy; removal of large staghorn calculus filling renal pelvis and calyces (including anatrophic pyelolithotomy)   C

RVU			Global Days	Modifiers				
Mod	Non-Fac Total	Fac Total		51	50	62	80	MUE
	41.92	41.92	090	2	1	1	2	1

AMA: Oct 01: 8

50080 Percutaneous nephrostolithotomy or pyelostolithotomy, with or without dilation, endoscopy, lithotripsy, stenting, or basket extraction; up to 2 cm   J8J1

Coding Tip: *Additional fluoroscopic guidance - 76000, 76001*

RVU			Global Days	Modifiers				
Mod	Non-Fac Total	Fac Total		51	50	62	80	MUE
	24.99	24.99	090	2	1	0	1	1

AMA: Oct 01: 8, Dec 08: 7, Jun 09: 10

Percutaneous nephrostolithotomy or pyelostolithotomy

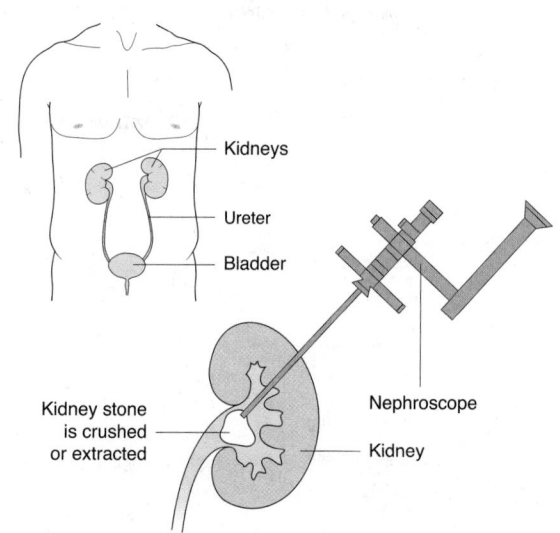

Kidneys
Ureter
Bladder
Nephroscope
Kidney stone is crushed or extracted
Kidney

50081 Percutaneous nephrostolithotomy or pyelostolithotomy, with or without dilation, endoscopy, lithotripsy, stenting, or basket extraction; over 2 cm   J8J1

Coding Tip: *Additional fluoroscopic guidance - 76000, 76001*

RVU			Global Days	Modifiers				
Mod	Non-Fac Total	Fac Total		51	50	62	80	MUE
	36.70	36.70	090	2	1	1	2	1

AMA: Oct 01: 8, Dec 08: 7, Jun 09: 10

● New   ▲ Revised   ✖ Deleted   ⊙ Moderate Sedation   ✚ Add-on Codes   ⊘ High Risk Denial   Ⓐ Age Edit   ♀ Female   ♂ Male   **AMA** *CPT® Assistant*   **MUE** Medically Unlikely Edit

⊘ Modifier 51 Exempt   ⊖ Modifier 63 Exempt   ✗ Unlisted   **Modifiers:** *See Inside Back Cover*   Ⓜ Maternity   A2—Z3 ASC Payment Indicators   A—Y OPPS Status Indicators

50100 Transection or repositioning of aberrant renal vessels (separate procedure) ⊘C

Mod	Non-Fac Total	Fac Total	Global Days	51	50	62	80	MUE
	30.45	30.45	090	2	1	1	2	1

AMA: Oct 01: 8

Transection or repositioning of aberrant renal vessels

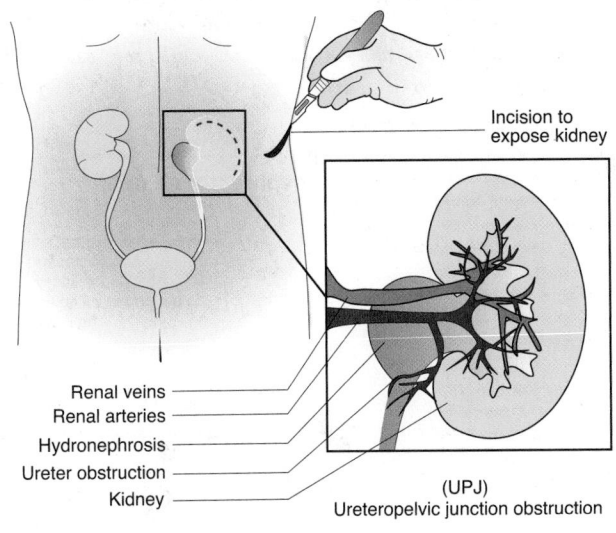

Incision to expose kidney

Renal veins
Renal arteries
Hydronephrosis
Ureter obstruction
Kidney

(UPJ)
Ureteropelvic junction obstruction

50120 Pyelotomy; with exploration C

Mod	Non-Fac Total	Fac Total	Global Days	51	50	62	80	MUE
	27.28	27.28	090	2	1	1	2	1

AMA: Oct 01: 8

50125 Pyelotomy; with drainage, pyelostomy C

Mod	Non-Fac Total	Fac Total	Global Days	51	50	62	80	MUE
	29.72	29.72	090	2	1	1	2	1

AMA: Oct 01: 8

50130 Pyelotomy; with removal of calculus (pyelolithotomy, pelviolithotomy, including coagulum pyelolithotomy) C

Mod	Non-Fac Total	Fac Total	Global Days	51	50	62	80	MUE
	29.69	29.69	090	2	1	1	2	1

AMA: Oct 01: 8

50135 Pyelotomy; complicated (eg, secondary operation, congenital kidney abnormality) C

Mod	Non-Fac Total	Fac Total	Global Days	51	50	62	80	MUE
	32.76	32.76	090	2	1	1	2	1

AMA: Oct 01: 8

Excisional Kidney (Renal) Procedures

⊙ 50200 Renal biopsy; percutaneous, by trocar or needle A2T

Coding Tip: Radiological guidance for correct needle placement - ultrasound 76942; fluoroscopy 77002; CT 77012; MRI 77021

Mod	Non-Fac Total	Fac Total	Global Days	51	50	62	80	MUE
	17.43	4.11	000	2	1	0	1	1

AMA: Fall 93: 13, Oct 01: 8, Feb 10: 7

Renal biopsy

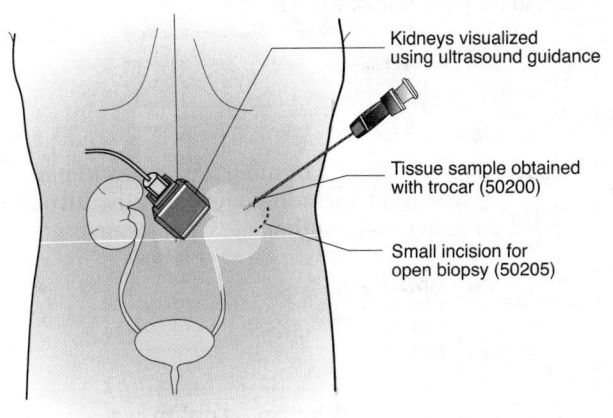

Kidneys visualized using ultrasound guidance

Tissue sample obtained with trocar (50200)

Small incision for open biopsy (50205)

Percutaneous by trocar or needle (50200);
by surgical exposure of kidney (50205)

50205 Renal biopsy; by surgical exposure of kidney C

Mod	Non-Fac Total	Fac Total	Global Days	51	50	62	80	MUE
	21.71	21.71	090	2	1	1	2	1

AMA: Oct 01: 8

50220 Nephrectomy, including partial ureterectomy, any open approach including rib resection C

Mod	Non-Fac Total	Fac Total	Global Days	51	50	62	80	MUE
	30.11	30.11	090	2	1	1	2	1

AMA: Oct 01: 8, Nov 02: 3, Aug 08: 7

50225 Nephrectomy, including partial ureterectomy, any open approach including rib resection; complicated because of previous surgery on same kidney C

Mod	Non-Fac Total	Fac Total	Global Days	51	50	62	80	MUE
	34.65	34.65	090	2	1	1	2	1

AMA: Oct 01: 8, Nov 02: 3

50230 Nephrectomy, including partial ureterectomy, any open approach including rib resection; radical, with regional lymphadenectomy and/or vena caval thrombectomy C

Mod	Non-Fac Total	Fac Total	Global Days	51	50	62	80	MUE
	36.90	36.90	090	2	1	2	2	1

AMA: Oct 01: 8, Nov 02: 3

● New   ▲ Revised   Deleted   ⊙ Moderate Sedation   ✚ Add-on Codes   ⊘ High Risk Denial   Ⓐ Age Edit   ♀ Female   ♂ Male   **AMA** CPT® Assistant   **MUE** Medically Unlikely Edit
⊘ Modifier 51 Exempt   ⊖ Modifier 63 Exempt   Ⓧ Unlisted   **Modifiers:** See Inside Back Cover   Ⓜ Maternity   A2–Z3 ASC Payment Indicators   A–Y OPPS Status Indicators

© 2016 DecisionHealth   CPT © 2015 American Medical Association. All Rights Reserved.

50234 Nephrectomy with total ureterectomy and bladder cuff; through same incision   C

RVU			Global Days	Modifiers				
Mod	Non-Fac Total	Fac Total		51	50	62	80	MUE
	37.40	37.40	090	2	1	1	2	1

AMA: Oct 01: 8, Nov 02: 3

50236 Nephrectomy with total ureterectomy and bladder cuff; through separate incision   C

RVU			Global Days	Modifiers				
Mod	Non-Fac Total	Fac Total		51	50	62	80	MUE
	42.24	42.24	090	2	1	1	2	1

AMA: Oct 01: 8, Nov 02: 3

50240 Nephrectomy, partial   C

RVU			Global Days	Modifiers				
Mod	Non-Fac Total	Fac Total		51	50	62	80	MUE
	38.07	38.07	090	2	1	1	2	1

AMA: Oct 01: 8, Nov 02: 3, Jan 03: 20, Apr 05: 10, 12, Aug 08: 7

50250 Ablation, open, 1 or more renal mass lesion(s), cryosurgical, including intraoperative ultrasound guidance and monitoring, if performed   C

RVU			Global Days	Modifiers				
Mod	Non-Fac Total	Fac Total		51	50	62	80	MUE
	34.98	34.98	090	2	0	1	2	1

AMA: May 06: 17

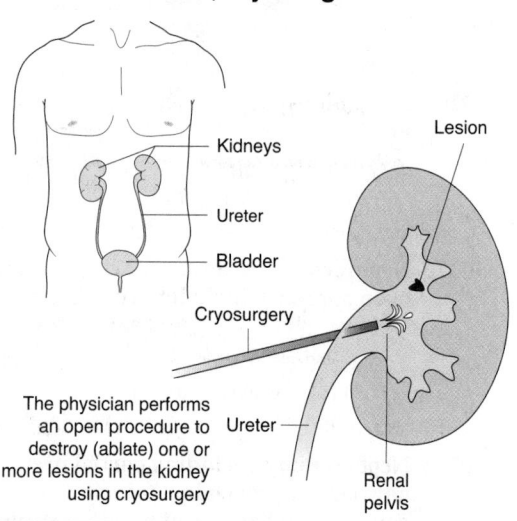

Ablation, renal mass lesion, cryosurgical

Kidneys
Ureter
Bladder
Lesion
Cryosurgery
Ureter
Renal pelvis

The physician performs an open procedure to destroy (ablate) one or more lesions in the kidney using cryosurgery

50280 Excision or unroofing of cyst(s) of kidney   C

RVU			Global Days	Modifiers				
Mod	Non-Fac Total	Fac Total		51	50	62	80	MUE
	27.45	27.45	090	2	1	1	2	1

AMA: Nov 99: 25, Oct 01: 8

50290 Excision of perinephric cyst   C

RVU			Global Days	Modifiers				
Mod	Non-Fac Total	Fac Total		51	50	62	80	MUE
	25.81	25.81	090	2	0	1	2	1

AMA: Oct 01: 8

Kidney (Renal) Transplant Procedures

50300 Donor nephrectomy (including cold preservation); from cadaver donor, unilateral or bilateral   C C

RVU			Global Days	Modifiers				
Mod	Non-Fac Total	Fac Total		51	50	62	80	MUE
	0.00	0.00	XXX	9	9	9	9	1

AMA: Nov 99: 25, Apr 05: 10, 12

50320 Donor nephrectomy (including cold preservation); open, from living donor   C

RVU			Global Days	Modifiers				
Mod	Non-Fac Total	Fac Total		51	50	62	80	MUE
	41.99	41.99	090	2	1	1	2	1

AMA: Nov 99: 25, May 00: 4

Donor nephrectomy; open

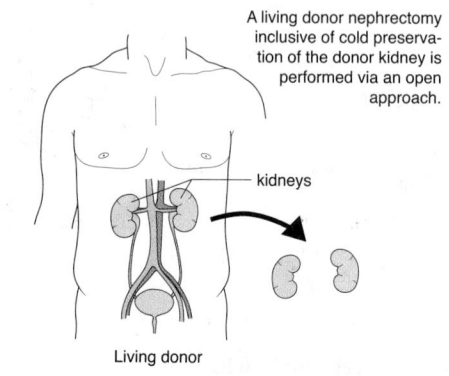

A living donor nephrectomy inclusive of cold preservation of the donor kidney is performed via an open approach.

kidneys

Living donor

50323 Backbench standard preparation of cadaver donor renal allograft prior to transplantation, including dissection and removal of perinephric fat, diaphragmatic and retroperitoneal attachments, excision of adrenal gland, and preparation of ureter(s), renal vein(s), and renal artery(s), ligating branches, as necessary   C

RVU			Global Days	Modifiers				
Mod	Non-Fac Total	Fac Total		51	50	62	80	MUE
	0.00	0.00	XXX	2	0	1	2	1

AMA: Apr 05: 10, 11

Backbench standard preparation of cadaver donor renal allograft prior to transplantation

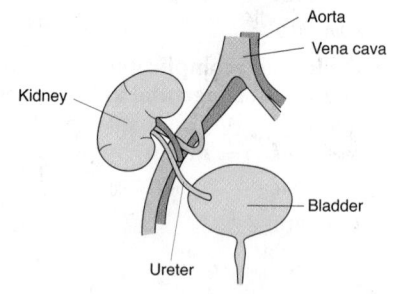

Aorta
Vena cava
Kidney
Bladder
Ureter

For 50323, a donor kidney is prepared for transplant from a cadaver or living donor. Report 50325, for removal of excess tissue and fat from the kidney(s) to be transplanted

---

● New   ▲ Revised   ✖ Deleted   ⊙ Moderate Sedation   ➕ Add-on Codes   ⊘ High Risk Denial   Ⓐ Age Edit   ♀ Female   ♂ Male   **AMA** CPT® Assistant   **MUE** Medically Unlikely Edit
⊘ Modifier 51 Exempt   ⊖ Modifier 63 Exempt   ☒ Unlisted   **Modifiers:** See Inside Back Cover   Ⓜ Maternity   A2–Z3 ASC Payment Indicators   A–Y OPPS Status Indicators

CPT © 2015 American Medical Association. All Rights Reserved.   © 2016 DecisionHealth

50325 Backbench standard preparation of living donor renal allograft (open or laparoscopic) prior to transplantation, including dissection and removal of perinephric fat and preparation of ureter(s), renal vein(s), and renal artery(s), ligating branches, as necessary ⒸC

RVU			Global Days	Modifiers				
Mod	Non-Fac Total	Fac Total		51	50	62	80	MUE
	0.00	0.00	XXX	2	0	1	2	1

50327 Backbench reconstruction of cadaver or living donor renal allograft prior to transplantation; venous anastomosis, each ⒸC

RVU			Global Days	Modifiers				
Mod	Non-Fac Total	Fac Total		51	50	62	80	MUE
	6.32	6.32	XXX	2	0	1	2	1

50328 Backbench reconstruction of cadaver or living donor renal allograft prior to transplantation; arterial anastomosis, each ⒸC

RVU			Global Days	Modifiers				
Mod	Non-Fac Total	Fac Total		51	50	62	80	MUE
	5.54	5.54	XXX	2	0	1	2	1

50329 Backbench reconstruction of cadaver or living donor renal allograft prior to transplantation; ureteral anastomosis, each ⒸC

RVU			Global Days	Modifiers				
Mod	Non-Fac Total	Fac Total		51	50	62	80	MUE
	5.18	5.18	XXX	2	0	1	2	1

50340 Recipient nephrectomy (separate procedure) ⒸC

RVU			Global Days	Modifiers				
Mod	Non-Fac Total	Fac Total		51	50	62	80	MUE
	27.13	27.13	090	2	1	1	2	1

50360 Renal allotransplantation, implantation of graft; without recipient nephrectomy ⒸC

RVU			Global Days	Modifiers				
Mod	Non-Fac Total	Fac Total		51	50	62	80	MUE
	70.21	70.21	090	2	0	2	2	1

50365 Renal allotransplantation, implantation of graft; with recipient nephrectomy ⒸC

RVU			Global Days	Modifiers				
Mod	Non-Fac Total	Fac Total		51	50	62	80	MUE
	82.05	82.05	090	2	1	2	2	1

AMA: Apr 05: 10, 11

50370 Removal of transplanted renal allograft ⒸC

RVU			Global Days	Modifiers				
Mod	Non-Fac Total	Fac Total		51	50	62	80	MUE
	34.77	34.77	090	2	0	1	2	1

50380 Renal autotransplantation, reimplantation of kidney ⒸC

RVU			Global Days	Modifiers				
Mod	Non-Fac Total	Fac Total		51	50	62	80	MUE
	57.64	57.64	090	2	0	1	2	1

AMA: Apr 05: 10, 12

Introduction Kidney (Renal) Procedures

Kidney (Renal) Catheter Procedures

⊙ **50382** Removal (via snare/capture) and replacement of internally dwelling ureteral stent via percutaneous approach, including radiological supervision and interpretation G2T

RVU			Global Days	Modifiers				
Mod	Non-Fac Total	Fac Total		51	50	62	80	MUE
	33.71	7.83	000	2	1	0	1	1

AMA: Sep 06: 1, 16, Oct 08: 8, Dec 09: 4

⊙ **50384** Removal (via snare/capture) of internally dwelling ureteral stent via percutaneous approach, including radiological supervision and interpretation G2Q2

RVU			Global Days	Modifiers				
Mod	Non-Fac Total	Fac Total		51	50	62	80	MUE
	26.88	7.11	000	2	1	0	1	1

AMA: Sep 06: 2, 16, Oct 08: 8

⊙ **50385** Removal (via snare/capture) and replacement of internally dwelling ureteral stent via transurethral approach, without use of cystoscopy, including radiological supervision and interpretation G2T

RVU			Global Days	Modifiers				
Mod	Non-Fac Total	Fac Total		51	50	62	80	MUE
	32.44	6.70	000	2	1	0	0	1

AMA: Oct 08: 8, Dec 09: 4

⊙ **50386** Removal (via snare/capture) of internally dwelling ureteral stent via transurethral approach, without use of cystoscopy, including radiological supervision and interpretation P3Q2

RVU			Global Days	Modifiers				
Mod	Non-Fac Total	Fac Total		51	50	62	80	MUE
	21.15	5.09	000	2	1	0	0	1

AMA: Oct 08: 8

⊙▲**50387** Removal and replacement of externally accessible nephroureteral catheter (eg, external/internal stent) requiring fluoroscopic guidance, including radiological supervision and interpretation G2T

RVU			Global Days	Modifiers				
Mod	Non-Fac Total	Fac Total		51	50	62	80	MUE
	15.46	2.81	000	2	1	0	0	1

AMA: Mar 12: 3, Sep 06: 2, 4, 16, Dec 09: 4

50389 Removal of nephrostomy tube, requiring fluoroscopic guidance (eg, with concurrent indwelling ureteral stent) G2Q2

RVU			Global Days	Modifiers				
Mod	Non-Fac Total	Fac Total		51	50	62	80	MUE
	8.42	1.57	000	2	1	0	1	1

AMA: Sep 06: 1, 2, 4

● New ▲ Revised Deleted ⊙ Moderate Sedation ➕ Add-on Codes ⊘ High Risk Denial Ⓐ Age Edit ♀ Female ♂ Male **AMA** *CPT® Assistant* **MUE** Medically Unlikely Edit
⊘ Modifier 51 Exempt ⊖ Modifier 63 Exempt ⊠ Unlisted **Modifiers:** *See Inside Back Cover* Ⓜ Maternity A2–Z3 ASC Payment Indicators A–Y OPPS Status Indicators

© 2016 DecisionHealth CPT © 2015 American Medical Association. All Rights Reserved. **487**

50390 Aspiration and/or injection of renal cyst or pelvis by needle, percutaneous `A 2 T`

Coding Tip: Antegrade pyelostogram/nephrostogram - 74425

Coding Tip: Radiological guidance for correct needle placement - ultrasound 76942; fluoroscopy 77002; CT 77012; MRI 77021

Coding Tip: Radiologic translumbar renal cyst examination - 74470

RVU			Global Days	Modifiers				
Mod	Non-Fac Total	Fac Total		51	50	62	80	MUE
	2.79	2.79	000	2	1	0	1	2

AMA: Fall 93: 14, Dec 97: 7, Oct 01: 8, Oct 05: 18, Oct 08: 8

50391 Instillation(s) of therapeutic agent into renal pelvis and/or ureter through established nephrostomy, pyelostomy or ureterostomy tube (eg, anticarcinogenic or antifungal agent) `P 3 T`

RVU			Global Days	Modifiers				
Mod	Non-Fac Total	Fac Total		51	50	62	80	MUE
	3.48	2.82	000	2	1	0	1	1

AMA: Oct 05: 18

✖ 50392 Introduction of intracatheter or catheter into renal pelvis for drainage and/or injection, percutaneous

✖ 50393 Introduction of ureteral catheter or stent into ureter through renal pelvis for drainage and/or injection, percutaneous

✖ 50394 Injection procedure for pyelography (as nephrostogram, pyelostogram, antegrade pyeloureterograms) through nephrostomy or pyelostomy tube, or indwelling ureteral catheter

50395 Introduction of guide into renal pelvis and/or ureter with dilation to establish nephrostomy tract, percutaneous `A 2 T`

Coding Tip: Radiological guidance for introduction into ureter through renal pelvis - 74480

Coding Tip: Dilation guidance - 74485

Coding Tip: Radiological guidance for introduction into renal pelvis - 74475

RVU			Global Days	Modifiers				
Mod	Non-Fac Total	Fac Total		51	50	62	80	MUE
	5.16	5.16	000	2	1	0	1	1

AMA: Oct 01: 8, Oct 05: 18, Sep 06: 1, Dec 08: 7, Jan 09: 7

50396 Manometric studies through nephrostomy or pyelostomy tube, or indwelling ureteral catheter `A 2 T`

Coding Tip: Antegrade pyelostogram/nephrostogram- 74425

Coding Tip: For manometric studies performed through ureterostomy or indwelling ureteral catheter, use 50686

Coding Tip: Radiological guidance for introduction into ureter through renal pelvis - 74480

Coding Tip: Radiological guidance for introduction into renal pelvis - 74475

RVU			Global Days	Modifiers				
Mod	Non-Fac Total	Fac Total		51	50	62	80	MUE
	3.40	3.40	000	2	1	0	0	1

AMA: Fall 93: 16, Dec 97: 7, Oct 01: 8

✖ 50398 Change of nephrostomy or pyelostomy tube

Kidney (Renal) Repair

Other Introduction Kidney (Renal) Procedures

50400 Pyeloplasty (Foley Y-pyeloplasty), plastic operation on renal pelvis, with or without plastic operation on ureter, nephropexy, nephrostomy, pyelostomy, or ureteral splinting; simple `C`

RVU			Global Days	Modifiers				
Mod	Non-Fac Total	Fac Total		51	50	62	80	MUE
	33.31	33.31	090	2	1	1	2	1

AMA: Nov 99: 25, May 00: 4, Oct 01: 8

50405 Pyeloplasty (Foley Y-pyeloplasty), plastic operation on renal pelvis, with or without plastic operation on ureter, nephropexy, nephrostomy, pyelostomy, or ureteral splinting; complicated (congenital kidney abnormality, secondary pyeloplasty, solitary kidney, calycoplasty) `C`

RVU			Global Days	Modifiers				
Mod	Non-Fac Total	Fac Total		51	50	62	80	MUE
	40.19	40.19	090	2	1	1	2	1

AMA: Nov 99: 25, May 00: 4, Oct 01: 8

⊙● **50430 Injection procedure for antegrade nephrostogram and/or ureterogram, complete diagnostic procedure including imaging guidance (eg, ultrasound and fluoroscopy) and all associated radiological supervision and interpretation; new access** `N I Q2`

RVU			Global Days	Modifiers				
Mod	Non-Fac Total	Fac Total		51	50	62	80	MUE
	14.78	4.83	000	2	1	0	1	2

● **50431 Injection procedure for antegrade nephrostogram and/or ureterogram, complete diagnostic procedure including imaging guidance (eg, ultrasound and fluoroscopy) and all associated radiological supervision and interpretation; existing access** `N I Q2`

RVU			Global Days	Modifiers				
Mod	Non-Fac Total	Fac Total		51	50	62	80	MUE
	4.59	1.92	000	2	1	0	1	2

⊙● **50432 Placement of nephrostomy catheter, percutaneous, including diagnostic nephrostogram and/or ureterogram when performed, imaging guidance (eg, ultrasound and/or fluoroscopy) and all associated radiological supervision and interpretation** `G 2 T`

RVU			Global Days	Modifiers				
Mod	Non-Fac Total	Fac Total		51	50	62	80	MUE
	23.95	6.38	000	2	1	0	1	2

⊙● **50433 Placement of nephroureteral catheter, percutaneous, including diagnostic nephrostogram and/or ureterogram when performed, imaging guidance (eg, ultrasound and/or fluoroscopy) and all associated radiological supervision and interpretation, new access** `G 2 T`

RVU			Global Days	Modifiers				
Mod	Non-Fac Total	Fac Total		51	50	62	80	MUE
	32.24	7.88	000	2	1	0	1	2

● New   ▲ Revised   ✖ Deleted   ⊙ Moderate Sedation   ✚ Add-on Codes   ⊘ High Risk Denial   Ⓐ Age Edit   ♀ Female   ♂ Male   **AMA** CPT® Assistant   **MUE** Medically Unlikely Edit
⃠ Modifier 51 Exempt   ⊖ Modifier 63 Exempt   🗵 Unlisted   **Modifiers:** See Inside Back Cover   Ⓜ Maternity   A 2 – Z 3 ASC Payment Indicators   A – Y OPPS Status Indicators

CPT © 2015 American Medical Association. All Rights Reserved.   © 2016 DecisionHealth

⊙● **50434** Convert nephrostomy catheter to nephroureteral catheter, percutaneous, including diagnostic nephrostogram and/or ureterogram when performed, imaging guidance (eg, ultrasound and/or fluoroscopy) and all associated radiological supervision and interpretation, via pre-existing nephrostomy tract   G2 T

RVU		Global Days	Modifiers				
Mod	Non-Fac Total	Fac Total		51	50	62	80	MUE
	25.52	6.04	000	2	1	0	1	2

● **50435** Exchange nephrostomy catheter, percutaneous, including diagnostic nephrostogram and/or ureterogram when performed, imaging guidance (eg, ultrasound and/or fluoroscopy) and all associated radiological supervision and interpretation   G2 T

RVU		Global Days	Modifiers				
Mod	Non-Fac Total	Fac Total		51	50	62	80	MUE
	13.39	2.93	000	2	1	0	1	2

50500 Nephrorrhaphy, suture of kidney wound or injury   ⊗ C

RVU		Global Days	Modifiers				
Mod	Non-Fac Total	Fac Total		51	50	62	80	MUE
	36.94	36.94	090	2	0	1	2	1

50520 Closure of nephrocutaneous or pyelocutaneous fistula   C

RVU		Global Days	Modifiers				
Mod	Non-Fac Total	Fac Total		51	50	62	80	MUE
	32.60	32.60	090	2	0	1	2	1

50525 Closure of nephrovisceral fistula (eg, renocolic), including visceral repair; abdominal approach   C

RVU		Global Days	Modifiers				
Mod	Non-Fac Total	Fac Total		51	50	62	80	MUE
	41.28	41.28	090	2	0	1	2	1

50526 Closure of nephrovisceral fistula (eg, renocolic), including visceral repair; thoracic approach   C

RVU		Global Days	Modifiers				
Mod	Non-Fac Total	Fac Total		51	50	62	80	MUE
	42.81	42.81	090	2	0	0	2	1

50540 Symphysiotomy for horseshoe kidney with or without pyeloplasty and/or other plastic procedure, unilateral or bilateral (1 operation)   C

RVU		Global Days	Modifiers				
Mod	Non-Fac Total	Fac Total		51	50	62	80	MUE
	33.09	33.09	090	2	2	1	2	1

Laparoscopic Kidney (Renal) Procedures

50541 Laparoscopy, surgical; ablation of renal cysts   J1

RVU		Global Days	Modifiers				
Mod	Non-Fac Total	Fac Total		51	50	62	80	MUE
	26.44	26.44	090	2	1	1	2	1

AMA: Nov 99: 25, May 00: 4, Oct 01: 8, Nov 02: 3, Jan 03: 20

50542 Laparoscopy, surgical; ablation of renal mass lesion(s), including intraoperative ultrasound guidance and monitoring, when performed   J1

RVU		Global Days	Modifiers				
Mod	Non-Fac Total	Fac Total		51	50	62	80	MUE
	33.55	33.55	090	2	1	1	2	1

AMA: Nov 02: 3, Jan 03: 21, Aug 04: 12

50543 Laparoscopy, surgical; partial nephrectomy   J1

RVU		Global Days	Modifiers				
Mod	Non-Fac Total	Fac Total		51	50	62	80	MUE
	42.76	42.76	090	2	1	1	2	1

AMA: Nov 02: 3, Jan 03: 21

50544 Laparoscopy, surgical; pyeloplasty   J1

RVU		Global Days	Modifiers				
Mod	Non-Fac Total	Fac Total		51	50	62	80	MUE
	35.79	35.79	090	2	1	1	2	1

AMA: Nov 99: 25, May 00: 4, Oct 01: 8

50545 Laparoscopy, surgical; radical nephrectomy (includes removal of Gerota's fascia and surrounding fatty tissue, removal of regional lymph nodes, and adrenalectomy)   C

RVU		Global Days	Modifiers				
Mod	Non-Fac Total	Fac Total		51	50	62	80	MUE
	38.55	38.55	090	2	1	1	2	1

AMA: Oct 01: 8

Surgical laparoscopy; radical nephrectomy

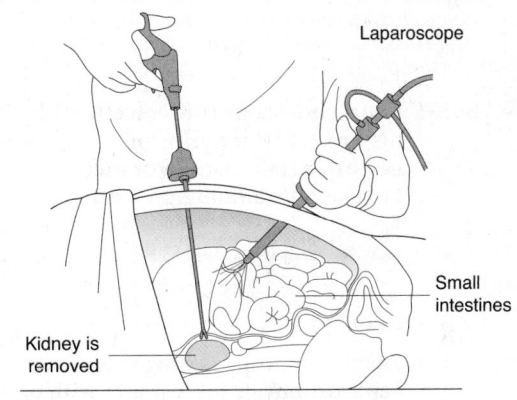

Laparoscope

Small intestines

Kidney is removed

50546 Laparoscopy, surgical; nephrectomy, including partial ureterectomy   C

RVU		Global Days	Modifiers				
Mod	Non-Fac Total	Fac Total		51	50	62	80	MUE
	34.61	34.61	090	2	1	1	2	1

AMA: Nov 99: 25, May 00: 4, Oct 01: 8

50547 Laparoscopy, surgical; donor nephrectomy (including cold preservation), from living donor   C

RVU		Global Days	Modifiers				
Mod	Non-Fac Total	Fac Total		51	50	62	80	MUE
	46.62	46.62	090	2	1	1	2	1

AMA: Nov 99: 25, May 00: 4, Oct 01: 8

● New   ▲ Revised   Deleted   ⊙ Moderate Sedation   ✚ Add-on Codes   ⊘ High Risk Denial   Ⓐ Age Edit   ♀ Female   ♂ Male   **AMA** *CPT® Assistant*   **MUE** Medically Unlikely Edit
⊘ Modifier 51 Exempt   ⊖ Modifier 63 Exempt   ✗ Unlisted   **Modifiers:** *See Inside Back Cover*   Ⓜ Maternity   A2-Z3 ASC Payment Indicators   A-Y OPPS Status Indicators

50548 Laparoscopy, surgical; nephrectomy with total ureterectomy C

Mod	Non-Fac Total	Fac Total	Global Days	51	50	62	80	MUE
	38.77	38.77	090	2	1	1	2	1

AMA: Nov 99: 25, May 00: 4, Oct 01: 8

50549 Unlisted laparoscopy procedure, renal xJ1

Mod	Non-Fac Total	Fac Total	Global Days	51	50	62	80	MUE
	0.00	0.00	YYY	2	1	1	2	

AMA: Nov 99: 25, Mar 00: 9, May 00: 4, Feb 06: 16

Endoscopic Kidney (Renal) Procedures

Coding Guidance

When a surgical endoscopy directly follows a diagnostic endoscopy, the diagnostic portion is included. If an endoscopy is done as part of an open surgical procedure, only the open procedure is reported. When a diagnostic endoscopic service is provided with a subsequent therapeutic endoscopic service in the same session, report the code with the highest level of specificity. If the code narrative does not include diagnostic endoscopy, and a separate diagnostic procedure was necessary, modifier 58 may be used to note that the diagnostic endoscopy and the subsequent therapeutic endoscopy were staged procedures. If multiple endoscopic services performed at the same session are not adequately described by a single comprehensive service code, the appropriate genitourinary endoscopy codes can be used with modifier 51. When an endoscopy is performed as confirmatory or to establish anatomical landmarks as a scout endoscopy, the procedure is considered as surgical field assessment and is not reported separately. When an endoscopy is done as a diagnostic procedure for basing the decision to do a more extensive open surgical procedure, the endoscopy may be separately reported. Control of bleeding resulting from the endoscopy and performed at the time of the service is included. It if becomes necessary to repeat an endoscopy in order to control bleeding, then a procedure code for endoscopic control of bleeding may be reported with a modifier identifying a return to the operative room in the postoperative period.

50551 Renal endoscopy through established nephrostomy or pyelostomy, with or without irrigation, instillation, or ureteropyelography, exclusive of radiologic service A2T

Mod	Non-Fac Total	Fac Total	Global Days	51	50	62	80	MUE
	10.29	8.49	000	2	1	0	0	1

AMA: Oct 01: 8, Jan 03: 21

50553 Renal endoscopy through established nephrostomy or pyelostomy, with or without irrigation, instillation, or ureteropyelography, exclusive of radiologic service; with ureteral catheterization, with or without dilation of ureter A2J1

Mod	Non-Fac Total	Fac Total	Global Days	51	50	62	80	MUE
	10.93	8.96	000	2	1	0	1	1

AMA: Oct 01: 8

50555 Renal endoscopy through established nephrostomy or pyelostomy, with or without irrigation, instillation, or ureteropyelography, exclusive of radiologic service; with biopsy A2T

Mod	Non-Fac Total	Fac Total	Global Days	51	50	62	80	MUE
	11.75	9.79	000	3	1	0	0	1

AMA: Oct 01: 8

50557 Renal endoscopy through established nephrostomy or pyelostomy, with or without irrigation, instillation, or ureteropyelography, exclusive of radiologic service; with fulguration and/or incision, with or without biopsy J8J1

Mod	Non-Fac Total	Fac Total	Global Days	51	50	62	80	MUE
	12.01	9.98	000	3	1	0	0	1

AMA: Oct 01: 8

50561 Renal endoscopy through established nephrostomy or pyelostomy, with or without irrigation, instillation, or ureteropyelography, exclusive of radiologic service; with removal of foreign body or calculus A2J1

Mod	Non-Fac Total	Fac Total	Global Days	51	50	62	80	MUE
	13.62	11.38	000	3	1	0	0	1

AMA: Oct 01: 8, Jan 03: 21

50562 Renal endoscopy through established nephrostomy or pyelostomy, with or without irrigation, instillation, or ureteropyelography, exclusive of radiologic service; with resection of tumor G2T

Mod	Non-Fac Total	Fac Total	Global Days	51	50	62	80	MUE
	16.73	16.73	090	2	0	1	2	1

AMA: Jan 03: 21

Coding Guidance

Endoscopic visualization of the urinary system is reported by the particular approach as defined in the CPT code descriptor (e.g., established ureterostomy, nephrotomy, pyelotomy). If multiple endoscopic approaches are necessary simultaneously to complete a given service, they may be coded separately with a multiple procedure modifier on the less extensive portions. If multiple approaches are necessary in attempting to successfully complete a given procedure, only the successful endoscopic approach should be reported.

50570 Renal endoscopy through nephrotomy or pyelotomy, with or without irrigation, instillation, or ureteropyelography, exclusive of radiologic service G2T

Mod	Non-Fac Total	Fac Total	Global Days	51	50	62	80	MUE
	14.17	14.17	000	2	1	0	0	1

AMA: Oct 01: 8

50572 Renal endoscopy through nephrotomy or pyelotomy, with or without irrigation, instillation, or ureteropyelography, exclusive of radiologic service; with ureteral catheterization, with or without dilation of ureter G2T

Mod	Non-Fac Total	Fac Total	Global Days	51	50	62	80	MUE
	15.33	15.33	000	3	1	0	0	1

AMA: Oct 01: 8

50574 Renal endoscopy through nephrotomy or pyelotomy, with or without irrigation, instillation, or ureteropyelography, exclusive of radiologic service; with biopsy G2T

Mod	Non-Fac Total	Fac Total	Global Days	51	50	62	80	MUE
	16.30	16.30	000	3	1	0	0	1

AMA: Oct 01: 8

● New ▲ Revised ✖ Deleted ⊙ Moderate Sedation ✚ Add-on Codes ⊘ High Risk Denial Ⓐ Age Edit ♀ Female ♂ Male **AMA** CPT® Assistant **MUE** Medically Unlikely Edit ⊘ Modifier 51 Exempt ⊖ Modifier 63 Exempt ✖ Unlisted **Modifiers:** See Inside Back Cover Ⓜ Maternity A2–Z3 ASC Payment Indicators A–Y OPPS Status Indicators

490 CPT © 2015 American Medical Association. All Rights Reserved. © 2016 DecisionHealth

50575 Renal endoscopy through nephrotomy or pyelotomy, with or without irrigation, instillation, or ureteropyelography, exclusive of radiologic service; with endopyelotomy (includes cystoscopy, ureteroscopy, dilation of ureter and ureteral pelvic junction, incision of ureteral pelvic junction and insertion of endopyelotomy stent)   G 2 J I

RVU			Global Days	Modifiers				
Mod	Non-Fac Total	Fac Total		51	50	62	80	MUE
	20.59	20.59	000	3	1	0	1	1

AMA: Oct 01: 8, Aug 02: 11

50576 Renal endoscopy through nephrotomy or pyelotomy, with or without irrigation, instillation, or ureteropyelography, exclusive of radiologic service; with fulguration and/or incision, with or without biopsy   G 2 T

RVU			Global Days	Modifiers				
Mod	Non-Fac Total	Fac Total		51	50	62	80	MUE
	16.29	16.29	000	3	1	0	0	1

AMA: Oct 01: 8

50580 Renal endoscopy through nephrotomy or pyelotomy, with or without irrigation, instillation, or ureteropyelography, exclusive of radiologic service; with removal of foreign body or calculus   G 2 T

RVU			Global Days	Modifiers				
Mod	Non-Fac Total	Fac Total		51	50	62	80	MUE
	17.55	17.55	000	3	1	0	0	1

AMA: Oct 01: 8

Other Kidney (Renal) Procedures

50590 Lithotripsy, extracorporeal shock wave   G 2 J I

RVU			Global Days	Modifiers				
Mod	Non-Fac Total	Fac Total		51	50	62	80	MUE
	20.53	16.32	090	2	1	0	1	1

AMA: Jul 01: 11, Aug 01: 10, Oct 01: 8, Jul 03: 16, Aug 03: 14

Coding Guidance
Radiological guidance for percutaneous renal tumor ablation, whether by cryotherapy or radiofrequency, is reported with 76940 for ultrasound, 77013 for CT, or 77022 for MRI.

⊙ **50592** Ablation, 1 or more renal tumor(s), percutaneous, unilateral, radiofrequency   G 2 T

RVU			Global Days	Modifiers				
Mod	Non-Fac Total	Fac Total		51	50	62	80	MUE
	72.24	10.43	010	2	1	0	1	1

⊙ **50593** Ablation, renal tumor(s), unilateral, percutaneous, cryotherapy   G 2 T

RVU			Global Days	Modifiers				
Mod	Non-Fac Total	Fac Total		51	50	62	80	MUE
	131.45	13.86	010	2	1	0	2	1

Ureteral Procedures

Incisional Ureteral Procedures

50600 Ureterotomy with exploration or drainage (separate procedure)   C

RVU			Global Days	Modifiers				
Mod	Non-Fac Total	Fac Total		51	50	62	80	MUE
	27.15	27.15	090	2	1	1	2	1

50605 Ureterotomy for insertion of indwelling stent, all types   C

RVU			Global Days	Modifiers				
Mod	Non-Fac Total	Fac Total		51	50	62	80	MUE
	28.14	28.14	090	2	1	1	2	1

AMA: Oct 01: 8, Dec 09: 4, Apr 12: 18

⊙+● **50606** Endoluminal biopsy of ureter and/or renal pelvis, non-endoscopic, including imaging guidance (eg, ultrasound and/or fluoroscopy) and all associated radiological supervision and interpretation (List separately in addition to code for primary procedure)   N I N

RVU			Global Days	Modifiers				
Mod	Non-Fac Total	Fac Total		51	50	62	80	MUE
	14.99	4.56	ZZZ	0	1	0	1	2

50610 Ureterolithotomy; upper one-third of ureter   C

RVU			Global Days	Modifiers				
Mod	Non-Fac Total	Fac Total		51	50	62	80	MUE
	28.26	28.26	090	2	1	1	2	1

AMA: Nov 99: 26, Oct 01: 8

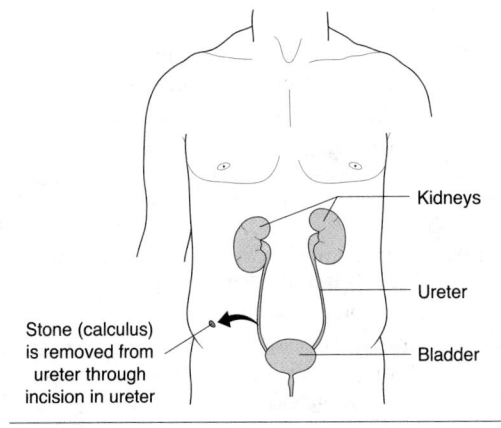

Ureterolithotomy

Stone (calculus) is removed from ureter through incision in ureter

Kidneys
Ureter
Bladder

50620 Ureterolithotomy; middle one-third of ureter   C

RVU			Global Days	Modifiers				
Mod	Non-Fac Total	Fac Total		51	50	62	80	MUE
	26.07	26.07	090	2	1	1	2	1

AMA: Nov 99: 26, Oct 01: 8

50630 Ureterolithotomy; lower one-third of ureter   C

RVU			Global Days	Modifiers				
Mod	Non-Fac Total	Fac Total		51	50	62	80	MUE
	25.61	25.61	090	2	1	1	2	1

AMA: Nov 99: 26, Oct 01: 8, May 14: 3

Surgical Procedures

50575 — 50630

● New   ▲ Revised   Deleted   ⊙ Moderate Sedation   ✚ Add-on Codes   ⊘ High Risk Denial   Ⓐ Age Edit   ♀ Female   ♂ Male   **AMA** *CPT® Assistant*   **MUE** Medically Unlikely Edit

⊘ Modifier 51 Exempt   ⊖ Modifier 63 Exempt   ✗ Unlisted   **Modifiers:** *See Inside Back Cover*   Ⓜ Maternity   A 2 – Z 3 ASC Payment Indicators   A – Y OPPS Status Indicators

Excisional Ureteral Procedures

Coding Guidance

Ureterectomy with bladder cuff is a separate procedure that is not reportable with other procedures in a related area on the ipsilateral (same side) ureter.

50650 Ureterectomy, with bladder cuff (separate procedure)   C

RVU			Global Days	Modifiers				
Mod	Non-Fac Total	Fac Total		51	50	62	80	MUE
	29.80	29.80	090	2	1	1	2	1

50660 Ureterectomy, total, ectopic ureter, combination abdominal, vaginal and/or perineal approach   C

RVU			Global Days	Modifiers				
Mod	Non-Fac Total	Fac Total		51	50	62	80	MUE
	33.06	33.06	090	2	0	1	2	1

Introduction Ureteral Procedures

50684 Injection procedure for ureterography or ureteropyelography through ureterostomy or indwelling ureteral catheter   N1N

Coding Tip: Urographic imaging portion of procedure - 74425

RVU			Global Days	Modifiers				
Mod	Non-Fac Total	Fac Total		51	50	62	80	MUE
	3.02	1.45	000	2	1	0	1	1

50686 Manometric studies through ureterostomy or indwelling ureteral catheter   P2S

Coding Tip: For manometric studies performed through nephrostomy or pyelostomy, use 50396

Coding Tip: Antegrade urographic imaging - 74425

RVU			Global Days	Modifiers				
Mod	Non-Fac Total	Fac Total		51	50	62	80	MUE
	4.11	2.58	000	2	0	0	0	2

50688 Change of ureterostomy tube or externally accessible ureteral stent via ileal conduit   A2T

Coding Tip: Imaging guidance for change of tube - 75984

RVU			Global Days	Modifiers				
Mod	Non-Fac Total	Fac Total		51	50	62	80	MUE
	2.29	2.29	010	2	0	0	1	2

50690 Injection procedure for visualization of ileal conduit and/or ureteropyelography, exclusive of radiologic service   N1N

Coding Tip: Urographic imaging portion of procedure - 74425

RVU			Global Days	Modifiers				
Mod	Non-Fac Total	Fac Total		51	50	62	80	MUE
	2.81	2.03	000	2	0	0	1	2

⊙● **50693 Placement of ureteral stent, percutaneous, including diagnostic nephrostogram and/or ureterogram when performed, imaging guidance (eg, ultrasound and/or fluoroscopy), and all associated radiological supervision and interpretation; pre-existing nephrostomy tract**   G2T

RVU			Global Days	Modifiers				
Mod	Non-Fac Total	Fac Total		51	50	62	80	MUE
	30.01	6.32	000	2	1	0	1	2

⊙● **50694 Placement of ureteral stent, percutaneous, including diagnostic nephrostogram and/or ureterogram when performed, imaging guidance (eg, ultrasound and/or fluoroscopy), and all associated radiological supervision and interpretation; new access, without separate nephrostomy catheter**   G2T

RVU			Global Days	Modifiers				
Mod	Non-Fac Total	Fac Total		51	50	62	80	MUE
	33.05	8.17	000	2	1	0	1	2

⊙● **50695 Placement of ureteral stent, percutaneous, including diagnostic nephrostogram and/or ureterogram when performed, imaging guidance (eg, ultrasound and/or fluoroscopy), and all associated radiological supervision and interpretation; new access, with separate nephrostomy catheter**   G2T

RVU			Global Days	Modifiers				
Mod	Non-Fac Total	Fac Total		51	50	62	80	MUE
	40.30	10.35	000	2	1	0	1	2

Ureteral Repair

50700 Ureteroplasty, plastic operation on ureter (eg, stricture)   C

RVU			Global Days	Modifiers				
Mod	Non-Fac Total	Fac Total		51	50	62	80	MUE
	26.76	26.76	090	2	1	1	2	1

⊙+● **50705 Ureteral embolization or occlusion, including imaging guidance (eg, ultrasound and/or fluoroscopy) and all associated radiological supervision and interpretation (List separately in addition to code for primary procedure)**   N1N

RVU			Global Days	Modifiers				
Mod	Non-Fac Total	Fac Total		51	50	62	80	MUE
	48.36	5.84	ZZZ	0	1	0	1	2

⊙+● **50706 Balloon dilation, ureteral stricture, including imaging guidance (eg, ultrasound and/or fluoroscopy) and all associated radiological supervision and interpretation (List separately in addition to code for primary procedure)**   N1N

RVU			Global Days	Modifiers				
Mod	Non-Fac Total	Fac Total		51	50	62	80	MUE
	21.69	5.42	ZZZ	0	1	0	1	2

50715 Ureterolysis, with or without repositioning of ureter for retroperitoneal fibrosis   C

RVU			Global Days	Modifiers				
Mod	Non-Fac Total	Fac Total		51	50	62	80	MUE
	35.21	35.21	090	2	1	1	2	1

● New   ▲ Revised   ✖ Deleted   ⊙ Moderate Sedation   ➕ Add-on Codes   ⊘ High Risk Denial   Ⓐ Age Edit   ♀ Female   ♂ Male   **AMA** *CPT® Assistant*   **MUE** Medically Unlikely Edit

⊘ Modifier 51 Exempt   ⊖ Modifier 63 Exempt   ✗ Unlisted   **Modifiers:** *See Inside Back Cover*   Ⓜ Maternity   A2–Z3 ASC Payment Indicators   A–Y OPPS Status Indicators

492   CPT © 2015 American Medical Association. All Rights Reserved.   © 2016 DecisionHealth

50722 Ureterolysis for ovarian vein syndrome ♀ⓒ

Mod	Non-Fac Total	Fac Total	Global Days	51	50	62	80	MUE
	29.43	29.43	090	2	0	1	2	1

Ureterolysis

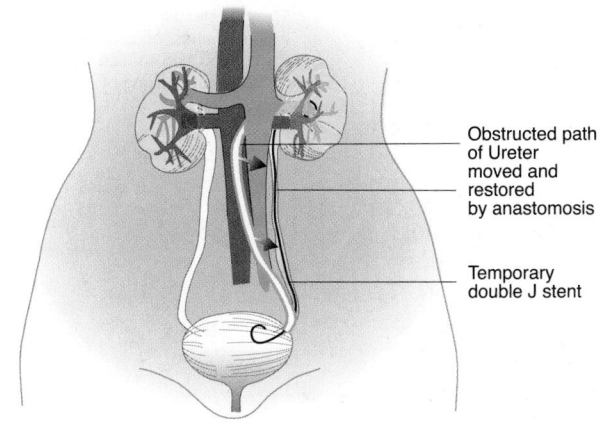

Obstructed path of Ureter moved and restored by anastomosis

Temporary double J stent

For ovarian vein syndrome (50722); for retrocaval ureter, with reanastomosis of upper urinary tract or vena cava (50725)

50725 Ureterolysis for retrocaval ureter, with reanastomosis of upper urinary tract or vena cava ⓒ

Mod	Non-Fac Total	Fac Total	Global Days	51	50	62	80	MUE
	32.52	32.52	090	2	0	1	2	1

50727 Revision of urinary-cutaneous anastomosis (any type urostomy) G2T

Mod	Non-Fac Total	Fac Total	Global Days	51	50	62	80	MUE
	14.58	14.58	090	2	0	2	2	1

50728 Revision of urinary-cutaneous anastomosis (any type urostomy); with repair of fascial defect and hernia ⓒ

Mod	Non-Fac Total	Fac Total	Global Days	51	50	62	80	MUE
	20.15	20.15	090	2	0	2	2	1

Coding Guidance
The ureteral anastomosis codes described in 50740-50780 and 50860 generally represent mutually exclusive procedures that cannot be reported together. Use the appropriate modifier if an anastomosis is performed on one ureter and a different anastomosis is done on the contralateral ureter.

50740 Ureteropyelostomy, anastomosis of ureter and renal pelvis ⓒ

Mod	Non-Fac Total	Fac Total	Global Days	51	50	62	80	MUE
	35.52	35.52	090	2	1	1	2	1

AMA: Oct 01: 8

50750 Ureterocalycostomy, anastomosis of ureter to renal calyx ⓒ

Mod	Non-Fac Total	Fac Total	Global Days	51	50	62	80	MUE
	33.16	33.16	090	2	1	0	2	1

AMA: Oct 01: 8

50760 Ureteroureterostomy ⓒ

Mod	Non-Fac Total	Fac Total	Global Days	51	50	62	80	MUE
	32.51	32.51	090	2	1	1	2	1

AMA: Oct 01: 8

Ureteroureterostomy/ Transureteroureterostomy

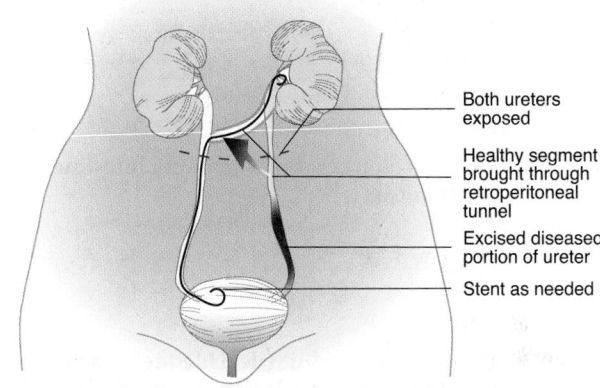

Both ureters exposed

Healthy segment brought through retroperitoneal tunnel

Excised diseased portion of ureter

Stent as needed

For ureteroureterostomy (50760); for transureteroureterostomy, anasomosis of ureter to contralateral ureter (50725)

50770 Transureteroureterostomy, anastomosis of ureter to contralateral ureter ⓒ

Mod	Non-Fac Total	Fac Total	Global Days	51	50	62	80	MUE
	33.11	33.11	090	2	0	1	2	1

50780 Ureteroneocystostomy; anastomosis of single ureter to bladder ⓒ

Mod	Non-Fac Total	Fac Total	Global Days	51	50	62	80	MUE
	31.89	31.89	090	2	1	1	2	1

AMA: Oct 01: 8

50782 Ureteroneocystostomy; anastomosis of duplicated ureter to bladder ⓒ

Mod	Non-Fac Total	Fac Total	Global Days	51	50	62	80	MUE
	30.35	30.35	090	2	1	2	2	1

AMA: Oct 01: 8

50783 Ureteroneocystostomy; with extensive ureteral tailoring ⓒ

Mod	Non-Fac Total	Fac Total	Global Days	51	50	62	80	MUE
	32.57	32.57	090	2	1	2	2	1

AMA: Oct 01: 8

● New   ▲ Revised   Deleted   ⊙ Moderate Sedation   ✚ Add-on Codes   ⊘ High Risk Denial   Ⓐ Age Edit   ♀ Female   ♂ Male   **AMA** *CPT® Assistant*   ***MUE*** Medically Unlikely Edit
⊘ Modifier 51 Exempt   ⊖ Modifier 63 Exempt   ⊠ Unlisted   **Modifiers:** *See Inside Back Cover*   Ⓜ Maternity   A2–Z3 ASC Payment Indicators   A–Y OPPS Status Indicators
© 2016 DecisionHealth   CPT © 2015 American Medical Association. All Rights Reserved.   **493**

50785 Ureteroneocystostomy; with vesico-psoas hitch or bladder flap   C

RVU			Global Days	Modifiers				
Mod	Non-Fac Total	Fac Total		51	50	62	80	MUE
	34.90	34.90	090	2	1	1	2	1

AMA: Oct 01: 8

50800 Ureteroenterostomy, direct anastomosis of ureter to intestine   C

RVU			Global Days	Modifiers				
Mod	Non-Fac Total	Fac Total		51	50	62	80	MUE
	26.57	26.57	090	2	1	1	2	1

AMA: Oct 01: 8

50810 Ureterosigmoidostomy, with creation of sigmoid bladder and establishment of abdominal or perineal colostomy, including intestine anastomosis   C

RVU			Global Days	Modifiers				
Mod	Non-Fac Total	Fac Total		51	50	62	80	MUE
	36.34	36.34	090	2	0	1	2	1

AMA: Oct 01: 8

50815 Ureterocolon conduit, including intestine anastomosis   C

RVU			Global Days	Modifiers				
Mod	Non-Fac Total	Fac Total		51	50	62	80	MUE
	35.21	35.21	090	2	1	1	2	1

AMA: Oct 01: 8

50820 Ureteroileal conduit (ileal bladder), including intestine anastomosis (Bricker operation)   C

RVU			Global Days	Modifiers				
Mod	Non-Fac Total	Fac Total		51	50	62	80	MUE
	37.83	37.83	090	2	1	1	2	1

AMA: Oct 01: 8

50825 Continent diversion, including intestine anastomosis using any segment of small and/or large intestine (Kock pouch or Camey enterocystoplasty)   C

RVU			Global Days	Modifiers				
Mod	Non-Fac Total	Fac Total		51	50	62	80	MUE
	47.67	47.67	090	2	0	1	2	1

AMA: Oct 01: 8

50830 Urinary undiversion (eg, taking down of ureteroileal conduit, ureterosigmoidostomy or ureteroenterostomy with ureteroureterostomy or ureteroneocystostomy)   C

RVU			Global Days	Modifiers				
Mod	Non-Fac Total	Fac Total		51	50	62	80	MUE
	52.11	52.11	090	2	0	1	2	1

AMA: Oct 01: 8

50840 Replacement of all or part of ureter by intestine segment, including intestine anastomosis   C

RVU			Global Days	Modifiers				
Mod	Non-Fac Total	Fac Total		51	50	62	80	MUE
	35.42	35.42	090	2	1	1	2	1

AMA: Oct 01: 8

50845 Cutaneous appendico-vesicostomy   C

	RVU		Global Days	Modifiers				
Mod	Non-Fac Total	Fac Total		51	50	62	80	MUE
	35.94	35.94	090	2	0	1	2	1

Cutaneous appendico-vesicostomy

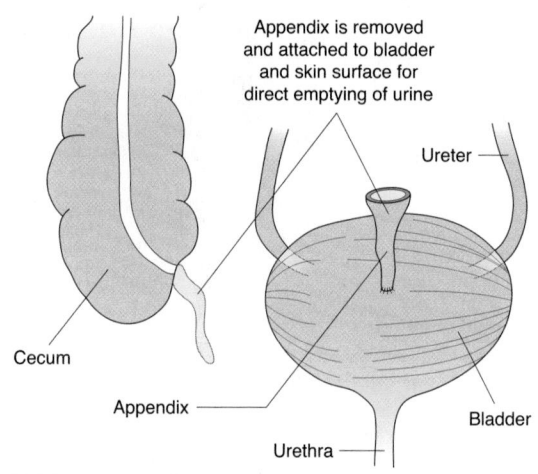

Appendix is removed and attached to bladder and skin surface for direct emptying of urine

Ureter

Cecum

Appendix

Bladder

Urethra

Coding Guidance

A ureterostomy to transplant the ureter to the skin is mutually exclusive of the procedures described in CPT codes 50800-50830, unless the ureterostomy is performed at a different location, in which case an anatomical modifier should be used.

50860 Ureterostomy, transplantation of ureter to skin   C

	RVU		Global Days	Modifiers				
Mod	Non-Fac Total	Fac Total		51	50	62	80	MUE
	27.15	27.15	090	2	1	1	2	1

50900 Ureterorrhaphy, suture of ureter (separate procedure)   C

	RVU		Global Days	Modifiers				
Mod	Non-Fac Total	Fac Total		51	50	62	80	MUE
	24.67	24.67	090	2	1	1	2	1

50920 Closure of ureterocutaneous fistula   C

	RVU		Global Days	Modifiers				
Mod	Non-Fac Total	Fac Total		51	50	62	80	MUE
	25.36	25.36	090	2	0	1	2	2

50930 Closure of ureterovisceral fistula (including visceral repair)   C

	RVU		Global Days	Modifiers				
Mod	Non-Fac Total	Fac Total		51	50	62	80	MUE
	34.02	34.02	090	2	0	1	2	2

50940 Deligation of ureter   C

	RVU		Global Days	Modifiers				
Mod	Non-Fac Total	Fac Total		51	50	62	80	MUE
	25.45	25.45	090	2	1	1	2	1

Laparoscopic Ureteral Procedures

50945 Laparoscopy, surgical; ureterolithotomy

	RVU		Global Days	Modifiers				
Mod	Non-Fac Total	Fac Total		51	50	62	80	MUE
	27.96	27.96	090	2	1	1	2	1

AMA: Nov 99: 26, May 00: 4, Oct 01: 8, Sep 06: 13

● New   ▲ Revised   ✖ Deleted   ⊙ Moderate Sedation   ✚ Add-on Codes   ⊖ High Risk Denial   Ⓐ Age Edit   ♀ Female   ♂ Male   **AMA** *CPT® Assistant*   **MUE** Medically Unlikely Edit
⊘ Modifier 51 Exempt   ⊖ Modifier 63 Exempt   ✗ Unlisted   **Modifiers:** *See Inside Back Cover*   Ⓜ Maternity   A-2 – Z-3 ASC Payment Indicators   A – Y OPPS Status Indicators

CPT © 2015 American Medical Association. All Rights Reserved.   © 2016 DecisionHealth

50947 **Laparoscopy, surgical; ureteroneocystostomy with cystoscopy and ureteral stent placement**

A 2 J I

RVU			Global Days	Modifiers				
Mod	Non-Fac Total	Fac Total		51	50	62	80	MUE
	39.96	39.96	090	2	1	1	2	1

AMA: Oct 01: 8

50948 **Laparoscopy, surgical; ureteroneocystostomy without cystoscopy and ureteral stent placement**

A 2 J I

RVU			Global Days	Modifiers				
Mod	Non-Fac Total	Fac Total		51	50	62	80	MUE
	36.73	36.73	090	2	1	1	2	1

AMA: Oct 01: 8

50949 **Unlisted laparoscopy procedure, ureter**

x J I

RVU			Global Days	Modifiers				
Mod	Non-Fac Total	Fac Total		51	50	62	80	MUE
	0.00	0.00	YYY	2	1	1	2	

AMA: Oct 01: 8

Endoscopic Ureteral Procedures

Coding Guidance

When a surgical endoscopy directly follows a diagnostic endoscopy, the diagnostic portion is included. If an endoscopy is done as part of an open surgical procedure, only the open procedure is reported. When a diagnostic endoscopic service is provided with a subsequent therapeutic endoscopic service in the same session, report the code with the highest level of specificity. If the code narrative does not include diagnostic endoscopy, and a separate diagnostic procedure was necessary, modifier 58 may be used to note that the diagnostic endoscopy and the subsequent therapeutic endoscopy were staged procedures. If multiple endoscopic services performed at the same session are not adequately described by a single comprehensive service code, the appropriate genitourinary endoscopy codes can be used with modifier 51. When an endoscopy is performed as confirmatory or to establish anatomical landmarks as a scout endoscopy, the procedure is considered as surgical field assessment and is not reported separately. When an endoscopy is done as a diagnostic procedure for basing the decision to do a more extensive open surgical procedure, the endoscopy may be separately reported. Control of bleeding resulting from the endoscopy and performed at the time of the service is included. If it becomes necessary to repeat an endoscopy in order to control bleeding, then a procedure code for endoscopic control of bleeding may be reported with a modifier identifying a return to the operative room in the postoperative period.

50951 **Ureteral endoscopy through established ureterostomy, with or without irrigation, instillation, or ureteropyelography, exclusive of radiologic service**

A 2 T

RVU			Global Days	Modifiers				
Mod	Non-Fac Total	Fac Total		51	50	62	80	MUE
	10.74	8.84	000	2	1	0	0	1

AMA: Oct 01: 8

50953 **Ureteral endoscopy through established ureterostomy, with or without irrigation, instillation, or ureteropyelography, exclusive of radiologic service; with ureteral catheterization, with or without dilation of ureter**

A 2 T

RVU			Global Days	Modifiers				
Mod	Non-Fac Total	Fac Total		51	50	62	80	MUE
	11.34	9.36	000	3	1	0	0	1

AMA: Oct 01: 8
Pub 100-04, 20, 130.1

50955 **Ureteral endoscopy through established ureterostomy, with or without irrigation, instillation, or ureteropyelography, exclusive of radiologic service; with biopsy**

A 2 T

RVU			Global Days	Modifiers				
Mod	Non-Fac Total	Fac Total		51	50	62	80	MUE
	12.16	10.16	000	3	1	0	0	1

AMA: Oct 01: 8
Pub 100-04, 20, 130.1

50957 **Ureteral endoscopy through established ureterostomy, with or without irrigation, instillation, or ureteropyelography, exclusive of radiologic service; with fulguration and/or incision, with or without biopsy**

A 2 J I

RVU			Global Days	Modifiers				
Mod	Non-Fac Total	Fac Total		51	50	62	80	MUE
	12.28	10.21	000	3	1	0	0	1

AMA: Oct 01: 8
Pub 100-04, 20, 130.1

50961 **Ureteral endoscopy through established ureterostomy, with or without irrigation, instillation, or ureteropyelography, exclusive of radiologic service; with removal of foreign body or calculus**

A 2 T

RVU			Global Days	Modifiers				
Mod	Non-Fac Total	Fac Total		51	50	62	80	MUE
	11.06	9.13	000	3	1	0	0	1

AMA: Oct 01: 8, Mar 07: 10, Apr 07: 12
Pub 100-04, 20, 130.1

Coding Guidance

Endoscopic visualization of the urinary system is reported by the particular approach as defined in the CPT code descriptor (e.g. established ureterostomy, nephrotomy, pyelotomy). If multiple endoscopic approaches are necessary simultaneously to complete a given service, they may be coded separately with a multiple procedure modifier on the less extensive portions. If multiple approaches are necessary in attempting to successfully complete a given procedure, only the successful endoscopic approach should be reported.

50970 **Ureteral endoscopy through ureterotomy, with or without irrigation, instillation, or ureteropyelography, exclusive of radiologic service**

A 2 T

RVU			Global Days	Modifiers				
Mod	Non-Fac Total	Fac Total		51	50	62	80	MUE
	10.72	10.72	000	2	1	0	0	1

AMA: Oct 01: 8

50972 **Ureteral endoscopy through ureterotomy, with or without irrigation, instillation, or ureteropyelography, exclusive of radiologic service; with ureteral catheterization, with or without dilation of ureter**

A 2 T

RVU			Global Days	Modifiers				
Mod	Non-Fac Total	Fac Total		51	50	62	80	MUE
	10.43	10.43	000	2	1	0	0	1

AMA: Oct 01: 8

● New   ▲ Revised   Deleted   ⊙ Moderate Sedation   ✚ Add-on Codes   ⊘ High Risk Denial   Ⓐ Age Edit   ♀ Female   ♂ Male   **AMA** *CPT® Assistant*   **MUE** Medically Unlikely Edit
⃠ Modifier 51 Exempt   ⊖ Modifier 63 Exempt   ☒ Unlisted   **Modifiers:** *See Inside Back Cover*   Ⓜ Maternity   A2–Z3 ASC Payment Indicators   A–Y OPPS Status Indicators

© 2016 DecisionHealth   CPT © 2015 American Medical Association. All Rights Reserved.

50974 Ureteral endoscopy through ureterotomy, with or without irrigation, instillation, or ureteropyelography, exclusive of radiologic service; with biopsy   A 2 J I

RVU			Global Days	Modifiers				
Mod	Non-Fac Total	Fac Total		51	50	62	80	MUE
	13.64	13.64	000	3	1	0	0	1

AMA: Oct 01: 8

50976 Ureteral endoscopy through ureterotomy, with or without irrigation, instillation, or ureteropyelography, exclusive of radiologic service; with fulguration and/or incision, with or without biopsy   A 2 J I

RVU			Global Days	Modifiers				
Mod	Non-Fac Total	Fac Total		51	50	62	80	MUE
	13.42	13.42	000	3	1	0	0	1

AMA: Oct 01: 8

50980 Ureteral endoscopy through ureterotomy, with or without irrigation, instillation, or ureteropyelography, exclusive of radiologic service; with removal of foreign body or calculus   A 2 T

RVU			Global Days	Modifiers				
Mod	Non-Fac Total	Fac Total		51	50	62	80	MUE
	10.20	10.20	000	2	1	0	0	1

AMA: Oct 01: 8

Bladder Procedures

Incisional Bladder Procedures

51020 Cystotomy or cystostomy; with fulguration and/or insertion of radioactive material   A 2 T

RVU			Global Days	Modifiers				
Mod	Non-Fac Total	Fac Total		51	50	62	80	MUE
	13.47	13.47	090	2	0	1	2	1

51030 Cystotomy or cystostomy; with cryosurgical destruction of intravesical lesion   A 2 T

RVU			Global Days	Modifiers				
Mod	Non-Fac Total	Fac Total		51	50	62	80	MUE
	13.69	13.69	090	2	0	0	0	1

51040 Cystostomy, cystotomy with drainage   A 2 T

RVU			Global Days	Modifiers				
Mod	Non-Fac Total	Fac Total		51	50	62	80	MUE
	8.29	8.29	090	2	0	1	2	1

51045 Cystotomy, with insertion of ureteral catheter or stent (separate procedure)   A 2 T

RVU			Global Days	Modifiers				
Mod	Non-Fac Total	Fac Total		51	50	62	80	MUE
	13.93	13.93	090	2	0	0	2	2

51050 Cystolithotomy, cystotomy with removal of calculus, without vesical neck resection   A 2 J I

RVU			Global Days	Modifiers				
Mod	Non-Fac Total	Fac Total		51	50	62	80	MUE
	13.55	13.55	090	2	0	1	2	1

51060 Transvesical ureterolithotomy   T

RVU			Global Days	Modifiers				
Mod	Non-Fac Total	Fac Total		51	50	62	80	MUE
	16.78	16.78	090	2	0	1	2	1

51065 Cystotomy, with calculus basket extraction and/or ultrasonic or electrohydraulic fragmentation of ureteral calculus   A 2 J I

RVU			Global Days	Modifiers				
Mod	Non-Fac Total	Fac Total		51	50	62	80	MUE
	16.61	16.61	090	2	0	0	0	1

51080 Drainage of perivesical or prevesical space abscess   A 2 T

RVU			Global Days	Modifiers				
Mod	Non-Fac Total	Fac Total		51	50	62	80	MUE
	11.78	11.78	090	2	0	1	2	1

Bladder Removal Procedures

51100 Aspiration of bladder; by needle   P 3 T

RVU			Global Days	Modifiers				
Mod	Non-Fac Total	Fac Total		51	50	62	80	MUE
	1.74	1.13	000	2	0	0	1	1

AMA: Jun 08: 11

51101 Aspiration of bladder; by trocar or intracatheter   P 3 S

RVU			Global Days	Modifiers				
Mod	Non-Fac Total	Fac Total		51	50	62	80	MUE
	3.53	1.50	000	2	0	0	1	1

AMA: Jun 08: 11

51102 Aspiration of bladder; with insertion of suprapubic catheter   A 2 T

RVU			Global Days	Modifiers				
Mod	Non-Fac Total	Fac Total		51	50	62	80	MUE
	6.45	4.16	000	2	0	0	1	1

AMA: Jun 08: 11

Excisional Bladder Procedures

51500 Excision of urachal cyst or sinus, with or without umbilical hernia repair   A 2 T

RVU			Global Days	Modifiers				
Mod	Non-Fac Total	Fac Total		51	50	62	80	MUE
	18.35	18.35	090	2	0	1	2	1

51520 Cystotomy; for simple excision of vesical neck (separate procedure)   A 2 T

RVU			Global Days	Modifiers				
Mod	Non-Fac Total	Fac Total		51	50	62	80	MUE
	17.20	17.20	090	2	0	1	2	1

51525 Cystotomy; for excision of bladder diverticulum, single or multiple (separate procedure)   C

RVU			Global Days	Modifiers				
Mod	Non-Fac Total	Fac Total		51	50	62	80	MUE
	24.67	24.67	090	2	0	1	2	1

51530 Cystotomy; for excision of bladder tumor   C

RVU			Global Days	Modifiers				
Mod	Non-Fac Total	Fac Total		51	50	62	80	MUE
	22.71	22.71	090	2	0	1	2	1

● New   ▲ Revised   ✖ Deleted   ⊙ Moderate Sedation   ✚ Add-on Codes   ⊘ High Risk Denial   Ⓐ Age Edit   ♀ Female   ♂ Male   **AMA** CPT® Assistant   **MUE** Medically Unlikely Edit
⊘ Modifier 51 Exempt   ⊖ Modifier 63 Exempt   ✄ Unlisted   **Modifiers:** See Inside Back Cover   Ⓜ Maternity   A 2 – Z 3 ASC Payment Indicators   A – Y OPPS Status Indicators

496   CPT © 2015 American Medical Association. All Rights Reserved.   © 2016 DecisionHealth

51535 Cystotomy for excision, incision, or repair of ureterocele   G2 T

Mod	Non-Fac Total	Fac Total	Global Days	51	50	62	80	MUE
	22.40	22.40	090	2	1	1	2	1

51550 Cystectomy, partial; simple   C

Mod	Non-Fac Total	Fac Total	Global Days	51	50	62	80	MUE
	27.61	27.61	090	2	0	1	2	1

51555 Cystectomy, partial; complicated (eg, postradiation, previous surgery, difficult location)   C

Mod	Non-Fac Total	Fac Total	Global Days	51	50	62	80	MUE
	36.46	36.46	090	2	0	1	2	1

51565 Cystectomy, partial, with reimplantation of ureter(s) into bladder (ureteroneocystostomy)   C

Mod	Non-Fac Total	Fac Total	Global Days	51	50	62	80	MUE
	37.41	37.41	090	2	0	1	2	1

51570 Cystectomy, complete; (separate procedure)   C

Mod	Non-Fac Total	Fac Total	Global Days	51	50	62	80	MUE
	42.52	42.52	090	2	0	1	2	1

AMA: Spring 93: 35

51575 Cystectomy, complete; with bilateral pelvic lymphadenectomy, including external iliac, hypogastric, and obturator nodes   C

Mod	Non-Fac Total	Fac Total	Global Days	51	50	62	80	MUE
	52.45	52.45	090	2	2	1	2	1

AMA: Spring 93: 35

51580 Cystectomy, complete, with ureterosigmoidostomy or ureterocutaneous transplantations   C

Mod	Non-Fac Total	Fac Total	Global Days	51	50	62	80	MUE
	54.51	54.51	090	2	0	1	2	1

51585 Cystectomy, complete, with ureterosigmoidostomy or ureterocutaneous transplantations; with bilateral pelvic lymphadenectomy, including external iliac, hypogastric, and obturator nodes   C

Mod	Non-Fac Total	Fac Total	Global Days	51	50	62	80	MUE
	60.68	60.68	090	2	2	1	2	1

51590 Cystectomy, complete, with ureteroileal conduit or sigmoid bladder, including intestine anastomosis   C

Mod	Non-Fac Total	Fac Total	Global Days	51	50	62	80	MUE
	55.66	55.66	090	2	0	1	2	1

51595 Cystectomy, complete, with ureteroileal conduit or sigmoid bladder, including intestine anastomosis; with bilateral pelvic lymphadenectomy, including external iliac, hypogastric, and obturator nodes   C

Mod	Non-Fac Total	Fac Total	Global Days	51	50	62	80	MUE
	62.95	62.95	090	2	2	1	2	1

51596 Cystectomy, complete, with continent diversion, any open technique, using any segment of small and/or large intestine to construct neobladder   C

Mod	Non-Fac Total	Fac Total	Global Days	51	50	62	80	MUE
	67.65	67.65	090	2	0	1	2	1

51597 Pelvic exenteration, complete, for vesical, prostatic or urethral malignancy, with removal of bladder and ureteral transplantations, with or without hysterectomy and/or abdominoperineal resection of rectum and colon and colostomy, or any combination thereof   C

Mod	Non-Fac Total	Fac Total	Global Days	51	50	62	80	MUE
	66.09	66.09	090	2	0	1	2	1

Complete pelvic exenteration

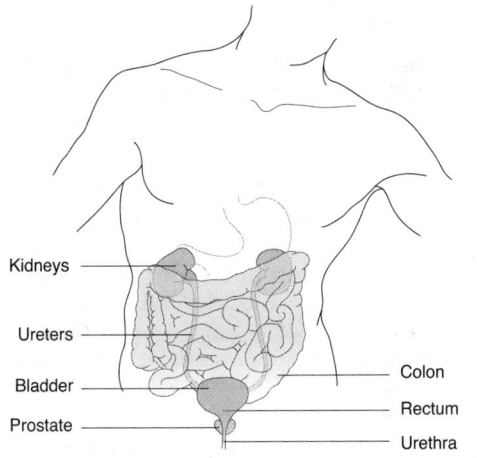

Lower urinary system is removed, including bladder, lower ureters, urethra, prostate, and lymph nodes. All or part of the uterus, rectum or colon may also be removed.

Introduction Bladder Procedures

51600 Injection procedure for cystography or voiding urethrocystography   N I N

Coding Tip: Cystography with at least 3 views - 74430
Coding Tip: Voiding urethrocystography - 74455

Mod	Non-Fac Total	Fac Total	Global Days	51	50	62	80	MUE
	5.19	1.27	000	2	0	0	1	1

51605 Injection procedure and placement of chain for contrast and/or chain urethrocystography   N I N

Mod	Non-Fac Total	Fac Total	Global Days	51	50	62	80	MUE
	1.10	1.10	000	2	0	0	1	1

● New   ▲ Revised   Deleted   ⊙ Moderate Sedation   ✚ Add-on Codes   ⊘ High Risk Denial   Ⓐ Age Edit   ♀ Female   ♂ Male   **AMA** CPT® Assistant   **MUE** Medically Unlikely Edit
⊘ Modifier 51 Exempt   ⊖ Modifier 63 Exempt   ✗ Unlisted   **Modifiers:** See Inside Back Cover   Ⓜ Maternity   A2–Z3 ASC Payment Indicators   A–Y OPPS Status Indicators

51610 Injection procedure for retrograde urethrocystography   `N I N`

RVU			Global Days	Modifiers				
Mod	Non-Fac Total	Fac Total		51	50	62	80	MUE
	3.03	1.85	000	2	0	0	1	1

Coding Guidance

Code 51700, bladder irrigation, is to be reported for independent therapeutic irrigation or instillation. Do not use 51700 when irrigation is performed as part of a more comprehensive procedure or for urinary system access or visualization purposes.

51700 Bladder irrigation, simple, lavage and/or instillation   `P 3 T`

Coding Tip: *Do not use for instillation of anticarcinogenic substance into bladder (51720)*

RVU			Global Days	Modifiers				
Mod	Non-Fac Total	Fac Total		51	50	62	80	MUE
	2.36	1.29	000	2	0	0	1	1

Coding Guidance

Catheters are often placed as an integral part of a surgical procedure. A urinary catheter is not reported when placed prior to or following surgery.

51701 Insertion of non-indwelling bladder catheter (eg, straight catheterization for residual urine)   `N I Q 1`

RVU			Global Days	Modifiers				
Mod	Non-Fac Total	Fac Total		51	50	62	80	MUE
	1.55	0.80	000	2	0	0	1	2

AMA: Jul 06: 4, Jan 07: 31, Jul 07: 1

51702 Insertion of temporary indwelling bladder catheter; simple (eg, Foley)   `N I Q 1`

RVU			Global Days	Modifiers				
Mod	Non-Fac Total	Fac Total		51	50	62	80	MUE
	2.00	0.87	000	2	0	0	1	2

AMA: Oct 03: 10, Jul 06: 4, Jan 07: 31, Jul 07: 1, May 14: 3

Insertion of temporary indwelling bladder catheter

A tube is inserted through the urethra into the bladder to drain urine. The tube is connected to a drainage bag and remains in place for a short while.

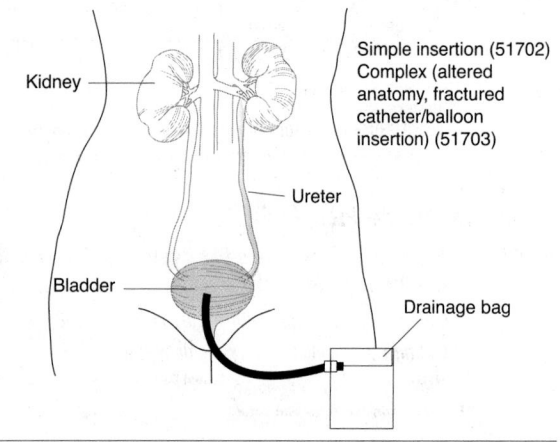

Kidney

Simple insertion (51702)
Complex (altered anatomy, fractured catheter/balloon insertion) (51703)

Ureter

Bladder

Drainage bag

51703 Insertion of temporary indwelling bladder catheter; complicated (eg, altered anatomy, fractured catheter/balloon)   `P 2 S`

RVU			Global Days	Modifiers				
Mod	Non-Fac Total	Fac Total		51	50	62	80	MUE
	3.68	2.34	000	2	0	0	1	2

AMA: Jan 07: 31

51705 Change of cystostomy tube; simple   `P 3 T`

RVU			Global Days	Modifiers				
Mod	Non-Fac Total	Fac Total		51	50	62	80	MUE
	2.58	1.49	000	2	0	0	1	1

AMA: Dec 07: 13

51710 Change of cystostomy tube; complicated   `A 2 T`

Coding Tip: *Imaging guidance for change of tube - 75984*

RVU			Global Days	Modifiers				
Mod	Non-Fac Total	Fac Total		51	50	62	80	MUE
	3.65	2.30	000	2	0	0	1	1

AMA: Dec 07: 13

51715 Endoscopic injection of implant material into the submucosal tissues of the urethra and/or bladder neck   `A 2 T`

RVU			Global Days	Modifiers				
Mod	Non-Fac Total	Fac Total		51	50	62	80	MUE
	8.26	5.75	000	2	0	0	0	1

51720 Bladder instillation of anticarcinogenic agent (including retention time)   `P 3 T`

RVU			Global Days	Modifiers				
Mod	Non-Fac Total	Fac Total		51	50	62	80	MUE
	3.09	2.30	000	2	0	0	1	1

AMA: Nov 02: 11

Bladder Urodynamic Procedures

51725 Simple cystometrogram (CMG) (eg, spinal manometer)   `P 3 T`

RVU			Global Days	Modifiers				
Mod	Non-Fac Total	Fac Total		51	50	62	80	MUE
	5.29	5.29	000	2	0	0	0	1
26	2.19	2.19	000	2	0	0	0	1
TC	3.10	3.10	000	2	0	0	0	1

AMA: Sep 02: 6, Feb 10: 7

51726 Complex cystometrogram (ie, calibrated electronic equipment)   `A 2 T`

RVU			Global Days	Modifiers				
Mod	Non-Fac Total	Fac Total		51	50	62	80	MUE
	7.43	7.43	000	2	0	0	1	1
26	2.45	2.45	000	2	0	0	1	1
TC	4.98	4.98	000	2	0	0	1	1

AMA: Sep 02: 6, Feb 10: 7

51727 Complex cystometrogram (ie, calibrated electronic equipment); with urethral pressure profile studies (ie, urethral closure pressure profile), any technique   `P 3 T`

RVU			Global Days	Modifiers				
Mod	Non-Fac Total	Fac Total		51	50	62	80	MUE
	8.82	8.82	000	2	0	0	0	1
26	3.07	3.07	000	2	0	0	0	1
TC	5.75	5.75	000	2	0	0	0	1

AMA: Feb 10: 7

● New   ▲ Revised   ✖ Deleted   ⊙ Moderate Sedation   ✚ Add-on Codes   ⊖ High Risk Denial   Ⓐ Age Edit   ♀ Female   ♂ Male   **AMA** *CPT® Assistant*   **MUE** Medically Unlikely Edit

⊘ Modifier 51 Exempt   ⊖ Modifier 63 Exempt   ✗ Unlisted   **Modifiers:** *See Inside Back Cover*   Ⓜ Maternity   `A 2`–`Z 3` ASC Payment Indicators   `A`–`Y` OPPS Status Indicators

CPT © 2015 American Medical Association. All Rights Reserved.   © 2016 DecisionHealth

51728 Complex cystometrogram (ie, calibrated electronic equipment); with voiding pressure studies (ie, bladder voiding pressure), any technique `P 3 T`

Coding Tip: Add intra-abdominal voiding pressure studies - 51797

RVU Mod	Non-Fac Total	Fac Total	Global Days	Modifiers 51	50	62	80	MUE
	8.88	8.88	000	2	0	0	0	1
26	3.00	3.00	000	2	0	0	0	1
TC	5.88	5.88	000	2	0	0	0	1

AMA: Feb 10: 7

51729 Complex cystometrogram (ie, calibrated electronic equipment); with voiding pressure studies (ie, bladder voiding pressure) and urethral pressure profile studies (ie, urethral closure pressure profile), any technique `P 3 T`

Coding Tip: Add intra-abdominal voiding pressure studies - 51797

RVU Mod	Non-Fac Total	Fac Total	Global Days	Modifiers 51	50	62	80	MUE
TC	5.98	5.98	000	2	0	0	0	1
	9.61	9.61	000	2	0	0	0	1
26	3.63	3.63	000	2	0	0	0	1

AMA: Feb 10: 7

51736 Simple uroflowmetry (UFR) (eg, stop-watch flow rate, mechanical uroflowmeter) `N I Q I`

RVU Mod	Non-Fac Total	Fac Total	Global Days	Modifiers 51	50	62	80	MUE
	0.44	0.44	XXX	2	0	0	0	1
26	0.24	0.24	XXX	2	0	0	0	1
TC	0.20	0.20	XXX	2	0	0	0	1

AMA: Sep 02: 6, Feb 10: 7

51741 Complex uroflowmetry (eg, calibrated electronic equipment) `N I Q I`

RVU Mod	Non-Fac Total	Fac Total	Global Days	Modifiers 51	50	62	80	MUE
	0.45	0.45	XXX	2	0	0	1	1
26	0.24	0.24	XXX	2	0	0	1	1
TC	0.21	0.21	XXX	2	0	0	1	1

AMA: Sep 02: 6, Feb 10: 7, Sep 14: 14

Coding Guidance

Use EMG codes 51784-51785 when the record supports that a significant, separately identifiable diagnostic EMG service was performed. Do not use these EMG codes when performed as part of a biofeedback session.

51784 Electromyography studies (EMG) of anal or urethral sphincter, other than needle, any technique `P 2 S`

RVU Mod	Non-Fac Total	Fac Total	Global Days	Modifiers 51	50	62	80	MUE
	5.43	5.43	000	2	0	0	1	1
26	2.20	2.20	000	2	0	0	1	1
TC	3.23	3.23	000	2	0	0	1	1

AMA: Sep 02: 6, Feb 10: 7, Feb 14: 11, Sep 14: 14

51785 Needle electromyography studies (EMG) of anal or urethral sphincter, any technique `A 2 T`

RVU Mod	Non-Fac Total	Fac Total	Global Days	Modifiers 51	50	62	80	MUE
	7.25	7.25	000	2	0	0	0	1
26	2.50	2.50	000	2	0	0	0	1
TC	4.75	4.75	000	2	0	0	0	1

AMA: Apr 02: 6, Sep 02: 6, Jul 04: 13, Feb 10: 7

51792 Stimulus evoked response (eg, measurement of bulbocavernosus reflex latency time) `N I Q I`

RVU Mod	Non-Fac Total	Fac Total	Global Days	Modifiers 51	50	62	80	MUE
	5.97	5.97	000	2	0	0	0	1
26	1.59	1.59	000	2	0	0	0	1
TC	4.38	4.38	000	2	0	0	0	1

AMA: Apr 02: 6, Sep 02: 6, Feb 10: 7, Feb 14: 11

+ 51797 Voiding pressure studies, intra-abdominal (ie, rectal, gastric, intraperitoneal) (List separately in addition to code for primary procedure) `N I N`

Coding Tip: Code 51797 is listed out of numerical order in CPT. Related primary procedure codes for complex cystometrogram with voiding pressure studies - 51728, 51729

RVU Mod	Non-Fac Total	Fac Total	Global Days	Modifiers 51	50	62	80	MUE
	3.16	3.16	ZZZ	0	0	0	0	1
26	1.15	1.15	ZZZ	0	0	0	0	1
TC	2.01	2.01	ZZZ	0	0	0	0	1

AMA: Dec 01: 7, Sep 02: 6, Feb 10: 7, Oct 09: 7

51798 Measurement of post-voiding residual urine and/or bladder capacity by ultrasound, non-imaging `N I Q I`

Coding Tip: This procedure represents technical component only, no physician work element, and replaces HCPCS code G0050

RVU Mod	Non-Fac Total	Fac Total	Global Days	Modifiers 51	50	62	80	MUE
	0.54	0.54	XXX	0	0	0	0	1

AMA: Dec 05: 3, Feb 10: 7

Bladder Repair

Coding Guidance

Cystoplasty or cystourethroplasty is included in the standard of practice for prostatectomy procedures. Code 51800 should not be reported separately with CPT codes 55801-55845.

51800 Cystoplasty or cystourethroplasty, plastic operation on bladder and/or vesical neck (anterior Y-plasty, vesical fundus resection), any procedure, with or without wedge resection of posterior vesical neck `C C`

RVU Mod	Non-Fac Total	Fac Total	Global Days	Modifiers 51	50	62	80	MUE
	29.96	29.96	090	2	0	1	2	1

51820 Cystourethroplasty with unilateral or bilateral ureteroneocystostomy `C`

RVU Mod	Non-Fac Total	Fac Total	Global Days	Modifiers 51	50	62	80	MUE
	32.05	32.05	090	2	2	1	2	1

Surgical Procedures

51840 – 51990

51840   Anterior vesicourethropexy, or urethropexy (eg, Marshall-Marchetti-Krantz, Burch); simple   **C**

RVU			Global Days	Modifiers				
Mod	Non-Fac Total	Fac Total		51	50	62	80	MUE
	18.88	18.88	090	2	0	1	2	1

AMA: Jan 97: 1, Nov 97: 19, Apr 98: 15, Jun 02: 7, May 06: 17, Jun 10: 6, Aug 12: 13

Anterior vesicourethropexy, or urethropexy

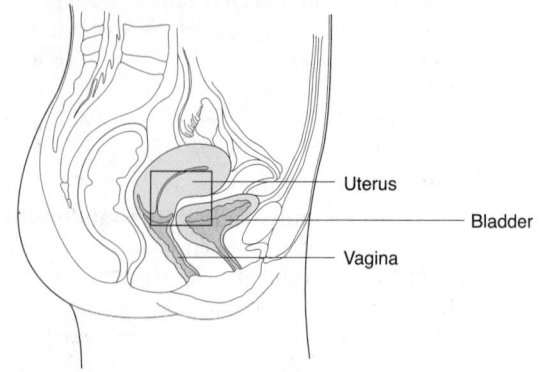

Uterus
Bladder
Vagina

The bladder is sutured to the pubic bone or the wall of the vagina.

51841   Anterior vesicourethropexy, or urethropexy (eg, Marshall-Marchetti-Krantz, Burch); complicated (eg, secondary repair)   **C**

RVU			Global Days	Modifiers				
Mod	Non-Fac Total	Fac Total		51	50	62	80	MUE
	22.37	22.37	090	2	0	1	2	1

AMA: Jan 97: 1, Jun 02: 7, Jun 10: 6, Aug 12: 13

51845   Abdomino-vaginal vesical neck suspension, with or without endoscopic control (eg, Stamey, Raz, modified Pereyra)   ♀ **J1**

RVU			Global Days	Modifiers				
Mod	Non-Fac Total	Fac Total		51	50	62	80	MUE
	16.82	16.82	090	2	0	1	2	1

AMA: Jan 97: 3

Abdomino-vaginal vesical neck suspension, with or without endoscopic control (eg, Stamey, Raz, modified Pereyra)

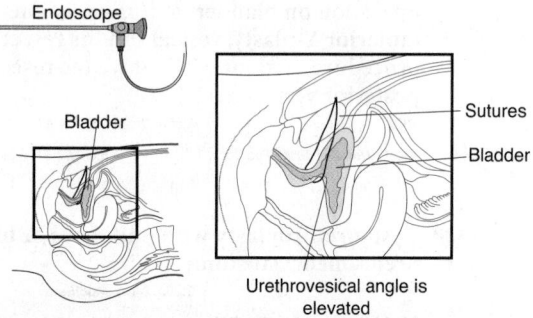

Endoscope
Bladder
Sutures
Bladder
Urethrovesical angle is elevated

The top portion of the bladder is sutured to the membrane which lines the abdomen. The physician may use an endoscope to assist with the procedure.

51860   Cystorrhaphy, suture of bladder wound, injury or rupture; simple   **J1**

RVU			Global Days	Modifiers				
Mod	Non-Fac Total	Fac Total		51	50	62	80	MUE
	21.29	21.29	090	2	0	1	2	1

51865   Cystorrhaphy, suture of bladder wound, injury or rupture; complicated   **C**

RVU			Global Days	Modifiers				
Mod	Non-Fac Total	Fac Total		51	50	62	80	MUE
	25.69	25.69	090	2	0	1	2	1

51880   Closure of cystostomy (separate procedure)   **A2 T**

RVU			Global Days	Modifiers				
Mod	Non-Fac Total	Fac Total		51	50	62	80	MUE
	13.42	13.42	090	2	0	1	2	1

51900   Closure of vesicovaginal fistula, abdominal approach   ⚭♀ **C**

RVU			Global Days	Modifiers				
Mod	Non-Fac Total	Fac Total		51	50	62	80	MUE
	23.97	23.97	090	2	0	1	2	1

51920   Closure of vesicouterine fistula   ♀ **C**

RVU			Global Days	Modifiers				
Mod	Non-Fac Total	Fac Total		51	50	62	80	MUE
	24.98	24.98	090	2	0	1	2	1

51925   Closure of vesicouterine fistula; with hysterectomy   ♀ **C**

RVU			Global Days	Modifiers				
Mod	Non-Fac Total	Fac Total		51	50	62	80	MUE
	31.66	31.66	090	2	0	1	2	1

51940   Closure, exstrophy of bladder   **C**

RVU			Global Days	Modifiers				
Mod	Non-Fac Total	Fac Total		51	50	62	80	MUE
	47.54	47.54	090	2	0	1	2	1

51960   Enterocystoplasty, including intestinal anastomosis   **C**

RVU			Global Days	Modifiers				
Mod	Non-Fac Total	Fac Total		51	50	62	80	MUE
	40.05	40.05	090	2	0	1	2	1

51980   Cutaneous vesicostomy   **C**

RVU			Global Days	Modifiers				
Mod	Non-Fac Total	Fac Total		51	50	62	80	MUE
	20.48	20.48	090	2	0	1	2	1

Laparoscopic Bladder Procedures

51990   Laparoscopy, surgical; urethral suspension for stress incontinence   **J1**

RVU			Global Days	Modifiers				
Mod	Non-Fac Total	Fac Total		51	50	62	80	MUE
	21.55	21.55	090	2	0	1	2	1

AMA: Nov 99: 26, May 00: 4, Jun 10: 6, Mar 12: 10, Aug 12: 13

● New   ▲ Revised   ✖ Deleted   ⊙ Moderate Sedation   ✚ Add-on Codes   ⊘ High Risk Denial   Ⓐ Age Edit   ♀ Female   ♂ Male   **AMA** *CPT® Assistant*   **MUE** Medically Unlikely Edit
⊘ Modifier 51 Exempt   ⊖ Modifier 63 Exempt   ⓧ Unlisted   **Modifiers:** *See Inside Back Cover*   Ⓜ Maternity   **A2–Z3** ASC Payment Indicators   **A–Y** OPPS Status Indicators

CPT © 2015 American Medical Association. All Rights Reserved.   © 2016 DecisionHealth

51992 Laparoscopy, surgical; sling operation for stress incontinence (eg, fascia or synthetic) `A 2 J 1`

Mod	RVU Non-Fac Total	Fac Total	Global Days	Modifiers 51	50	62	80	MUE
	24.16	24.16	090	2	0	1	2	1

AMA: Nov 99: 26, May 00: 4, Mar 12: 10, Aug 12: 13

Laparoscopy, surgical; urethral suspension for stress incontinence

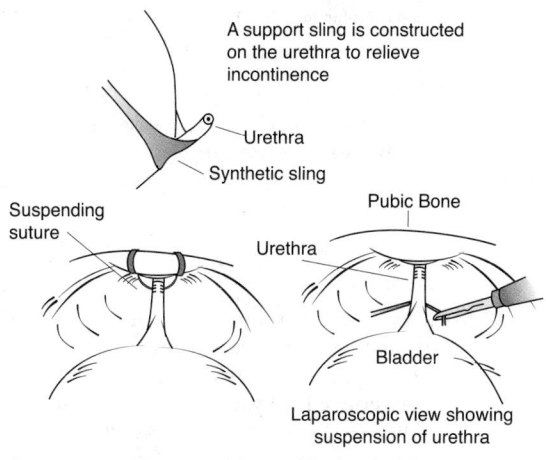

A support sling is constructed on the urethra to relieve incontinence

Urethra

Synthetic sling

Suspending suture

Pubic Bone

Urethra

Bladder

Laparoscopic view showing suspension of urethra

A laparoscope is inserted into the lower abdomen. The physician then suspends the lower part of the bladder and urethra to correct a condition in which a patient cannot control the release of urine.

51999 Unlisted laparoscopy procedure, bladder `x J 1`

Mod	RVU Non-Fac Total	Fac Total	Global Days	Modifiers 51	50	62	80	MUE
	0.00	0.00	YYY	0	0	1	0	

Endoscopic Bladder Procedures

52000 Cystourethroscopy (separate procedure) `A 2 T`

Mod	RVU Non-Fac Total	Fac Total	Global Days	Modifiers 51	50	62	80	MUE
	5.79	3.62	000	2	0	0	1	1

AMA: Oct 00: 7, May 01: 5, Sep 04: 11, Oct 05: 23, Nov 07: 9, Mar 13: 14, May 14: 3

Cystourethroscopy

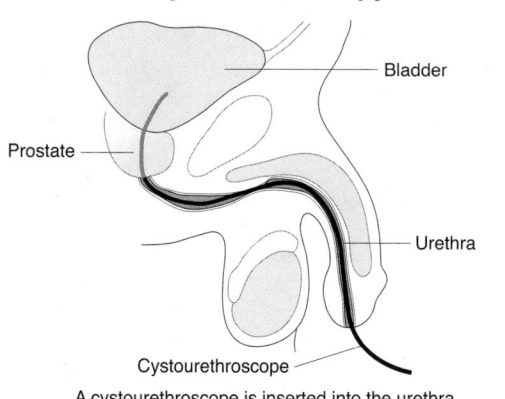

Bladder

Prostate

Urethra

Cystourethroscope

A cystourethroscope is inserted into the urethra and up into the bladder for diagnostic visualization.

52001 Cystourethroscopy with irrigation and evacuation of multiple obstructing clots `A 2 T`

Mod	RVU Non-Fac Total	Fac Total	Global Days	Modifiers 51	50	62	80	MUE
	10.58	8.28	000	3	0	0	1	1

Coding Guidance

Insertion and removal of a temporary ureteral catheter during the cystourethroscopy procedures described in codes 52320-52355 is already inclusive in the primary procedure.

52005 Cystourethroscopy, with ureteral catheterization, with or without irrigation, instillation, or ureteropyelography, exclusive of radiologic service `A 2 T`

Mod	RVU Non-Fac Total	Fac Total	Global Days	Modifiers 51	50	62	80	MUE
	7.52	3.83	000	3	0	0	1	2

AMA: Sep 00: 11, Jan 01: 13, May 01: 5, Oct 01: 8, Dec 10: 15
Pub 100-04, 12, 30.2

52007 Cystourethroscopy, with ureteral catheterization, with or without irrigation, instillation, or ureteropyelography, exclusive of radiologic service; with brush biopsy of ureter and/or renal pelvis `A 2 T`

Mod	RVU Non-Fac Total	Fac Total	Global Days	Modifiers 51	50	62	80	MUE
	12.53	4.77	000	3	1	0	1	1

AMA: May 01: 5, Oct 01: 8

52010 Cystourethroscopy, with ejaculatory duct catheterization, with or without irrigation, instillation, or duct radiography, exclusive of radiologic service `♂ A 2 T`

Coding Tip: *Radiographic service - 74440*

Mod	RVU Non-Fac Total	Fac Total	Global Days	Modifiers 51	50	62	80	MUE
	10.53	4.81	000	3	0	0	1	1

AMA: May 01: 5

Transurethral Procedures

Urethra/Bladder Procedures

52204 Cystourethroscopy, with biopsy(s) `A 2 T`

Coding Tip: *Code 99000 for specimen transfer from office setting to an outside laboratory*

Coding Tip: *Code 52204 includes all biopsies done at the time of the procedure and should only be reported with one unit of service.*

Coding Tip: *Code 99001 for specimen transfer from a facility to an outside laboratory*

Mod	RVU Non-Fac Total	Fac Total	Global Days	Modifiers 51	50	62	80	MUE
	10.41	4.08	000	3	0	0	1	1

AMA: May 01: 5, Sep 01: 1, Sep 03: 16, Aug 09: 6

52214 Cystourethroscopy, with fulguration (including cryosurgery or laser surgery) of trigone, bladder neck, prostatic fossa, urethra, or periurethral glands `A 2 T`

Mod	RVU Non-Fac Total	Fac Total	Global Days	Modifiers 51	50	62	80	MUE
	18.62	5.07	000	3	0	0	1	1

AMA: May 01: 5, Sep 01: 1, Aug 09: 6

● New　▲ Revised　Deleted　⊙ Moderate Sedation　✚ Add-on Codes　⊘ High Risk Denial　Ⓐ Age Edit　♀ Female　♂ Male　**AMA** *CPT® Assistant*　**MUE** Medically Unlikely Edit
⊘ Modifier 51 Exempt　⊖ Modifier 63 Exempt　Ⓧ Unlisted　**Modifiers:** *See Inside Back Cover*　Ⓜ Maternity　`A 2`–`Z 3` ASC Payment Indicators　`A`–`Y` OPPS Status Indicators

52224 Cystourethroscopy, with fulguration (including cryosurgery or laser surgery) or treatment of MINOR (less than 0.5 cm) lesion(s) with or without biopsy   A 2 T

Mod	RVU Non-Fac Total	Fac Total	Global Days	Modifiers 51	50	62	80	MUE
	19.49	5.87	000	3	0	0	1	1

AMA: May 01: 5, Sep 01: 1, Dec 07: 7, Aug 09: 6, Jun 09: 10

52234 Cystourethroscopy, with fulguration (including cryosurgery or laser surgery) and/or resection of; SMALL bladder tumor(s) (0.5 up to 2.0 cm)   A 2 T

Mod	RVU Non-Fac Total	Fac Total	Global Days	Modifiers 51	50	62	80	MUE
	7.09	7.09	000	3	0	0	1	1

AMA: May 01: 5, Sep 01: 1, Oct 02: 12, Jan 03: 21, Aug 09: 6, Jun 09: 10
Pub 100-04, 12, 30.2

52235 Cystourethroscopy, with fulguration (including cryosurgery or laser surgery) and/or resection of; MEDIUM bladder tumor(s) (2.0 to 5.0 cm)   A 2 T

Mod	RVU Non-Fac Total	Fac Total	Global Days	Modifiers 51	50	62	80	MUE
	8.31	8.31	000	3	0	0	1	1

AMA: May 01: 5, Sep 01: 1, Oct 02: 12, Jan 03: 21, Aug 09: 6, Jun 09: 10
Pub 100-04, 12, 30.2

52240 Cystourethroscopy, with fulguration (including cryosurgery or laser surgery) and/or resection of; LARGE bladder tumor(s)   A 2 T

Mod	RVU Non-Fac Total	Fac Total	Global Days	Modifiers 51	50	62	80	MUE
	11.30	11.30	000	3	0	0	1	1

AMA: May 01: 5, Sep 01: 1, Aug 09: 6, Jun 09: 10
Pub 100-04, 12, 30.2

52250 Cystourethroscopy with insertion of radioactive substance, with or without biopsy or fulguration   A 2 T

Mod	RVU Non-Fac Total	Fac Total	Global Days	Modifiers 51	50	62	80	MUE
	6.91	6.91	000	3	0	0	1	1

AMA: May 01: 5, Sep 01: 1

52260 Cystourethroscopy, with dilation of bladder for interstitial cystitis; general or conduction (spinal) anesthesia   A 2 T

Mod	RVU Non-Fac Total	Fac Total	Global Days	Modifiers 51	50	62	80	MUE
	6.06	6.06	000	3	0	0	1	1

AMA: May 01: 5, Sep 01: 1, Oct 05: 23

52265 Cystourethroscopy, with dilation of bladder for interstitial cystitis; local anesthesia   P 3 T

Mod	RVU Non-Fac Total	Fac Total	Global Days	Modifiers 51	50	62	80	MUE
	10.35	4.69	000	3	0	0	1	1

AMA: May 01: 5, Sep 01: 1

52270 Cystourethroscopy, with internal urethrotomy; female   ♀ A 2 T

Mod	RVU Non-Fac Total	Fac Total	Global Days	Modifiers 51	50	62	80	MUE
	10.06	5.23	000	3	0	0	1	1

AMA: May 01: 5, Sep 01: 1

52275 Cystourethroscopy, with internal urethrotomy; male   ♂ A 2 T

Mod	RVU Non-Fac Total	Fac Total	Global Days	Modifiers 51	50	62	80	MUE
	13.57	7.16	000	3	0	0	1	1

AMA: May 01: 5, Sep 01: 1

52276 Cystourethroscopy with direct vision internal urethrotomy   A 2 T

Mod	RVU Non-Fac Total	Fac Total	Global Days	Modifiers 51	50	62	80	MUE
	7.62	7.62	000	3	0	0	1	1

AMA: May 01: 5, Sep 01: 1, May 09: 8, Feb 10: 7

52277 Cystourethroscopy, with resection of external sphincter (sphincterotomy)   A 2 T

Mod	RVU Non-Fac Total	Fac Total	Global Days	Modifiers 51	50	62	80	MUE
	9.32	9.32	000	3	0	0	0	1

AMA: May 01: 5, Sep 01: 1

52281 Cystourethroscopy, with calibration and/or dilation of urethral stricture or stenosis, with or without meatotomy, with or without injection procedure for cystography, male or female   A 2 T

Mod	RVU Non-Fac Total	Fac Total	Global Days	Modifiers 51	50	62	80	MUE
	7.71	4.38	000	3	0	0	1	1

AMA: Nov 97: 20, May 01: 5, Sep 01: 1, Jun 07: 10

52282 Cystourethroscopy, with insertion of permanent urethral stent   A 2 T

Mod	RVU Non-Fac Total	Fac Total	Global Days	Modifiers 51	50	62	80	MUE
	9.69	9.69	000	3	0	0	1	1

AMA: Nov 97: 20, May 01: 5, Sep 01: 1, Feb 10: 7, Jun 15: 5

52283 Cystourethroscopy, with steroid injection into stricture   A 2 T

Mod	RVU Non-Fac Total	Fac Total	Global Days	Modifiers 51	50	62	80	MUE
	7.86	5.80	000	3	0	0	1	1

AMA: May 01: 5, Sep 01: 1, Mar 15: 9

Cystourethroscopy
With steroid injection into stricture

Bladder
Stricture injected with steroids
Prostate
Stricture
Urethra
Cystourethroscope

● New   ▲ Revised   ✖ Deleted   ⊙ Moderate Sedation   ✚ Add-on Codes   ⊘ High Risk Denial   Ⓐ Age Edit   ♀ Female   ♂ Male   **AMA** CPT® Assistant   **MUE** Medically Unlikely Edit
⊘ Modifier 51 Exempt   ⊖ Modifier 63 Exempt   ✗ Unlisted   **Modifiers:** See Inside Back Cover   Ⓜ Maternity   A 2 – Z 3 ASC Payment Indicators   A – Y OPPS Status Indicators

CPT © 2015 American Medical Association. All Rights Reserved.   © 2016 DecisionHealth

52285 Cystourethroscopy for treatment of the female urethral syndrome with any or all of the following: urethral meatotomy, urethral dilation, internal urethrotomy, lysis of urethrovaginal septal fibrosis, lateral incisions of the bladder neck, and fulguration of polyp(s) of urethra, bladder neck, and/or trigone ♀ A2 T

RVU			Global Days	Modifiers				
Mod	Non-Fac Total	Fac Total		51	50	62	80	MUE
	7.93	5.64	000	3	0	0	1	1

AMA: May 01: 5, Sep 01: 1

52287 Cystourethroscopy, with injection(s) for chemodenervation of the bladder G2 T

RVU			Global Days	Modifiers				
Mod	Non-Fac Total	Fac Total		51	50	62	80	MUE
	8.82	4.87	000	3	0	0	1	1

52290 Cystourethroscopy; with ureteral meatotomy, unilateral or bilateral A2 T

RVU			Global Days	Modifiers				
Mod	Non-Fac Total	Fac Total		51	50	62	80	MUE
	7.03	7.03	000	3	2	0	1	1

AMA: May 01: 5, Sep 01: 1
Pub 100-04, 12, 40.7

52300 Cystourethroscopy; with resection or fulguration of orthotopic ureterocele(s), unilateral or bilateral A2 T

RVU			Global Days	Modifiers				
Mod	Non-Fac Total	Fac Total		51	50	62	80	MUE
	8.08	8.08	000	3	2	0	0	1

AMA: May 01: 5, Sep 01: 1

52301 Cystourethroscopy; with resection or fulguration of ectopic ureterocele(s), unilateral or bilateral A2 T

RVU			Global Days	Modifiers				
Mod	Non-Fac Total	Fac Total		51	50	62	80	MUE
	8.36	8.36	000	3	2	0	0	1

AMA: May 01: 5, Sep 01: 1

52305 Cystourethroscopy; with incision or resection of orifice of bladder diverticulum, single or multiple A2 J1

RVU			Global Days	Modifiers				
Mod	Non-Fac Total	Fac Total		51	50	62	80	MUE
	8.04	8.04	000	3	0	0	1	1

AMA: May 01: 5, Sep 01: 1

52310 Cystourethroscopy, with removal of foreign body, calculus, or ureteral stent from urethra or bladder (separate procedure); simple A2 T

RVU			Global Days	Modifiers				
Mod	Non-Fac Total	Fac Total		51	50	62	80	MUE
	6.90	4.36	000	3	0	0	1	1

AMA: May 01: 5, Sep 01: 1

52315 Cystourethroscopy, with removal of foreign body, calculus, or ureteral stent from urethra or bladder (separate procedure); complicated A2 T

RVU			Global Days	Modifiers				
Mod	Non-Fac Total	Fac Total		51	50	62	80	MUE
	11.72	7.90	000	3	0	0	1	2

AMA: May 01: 5, Sep 01: 1

52317 Litholapaxy: crushing or fragmentation of calculus by any means in bladder and removal of fragments; simple or small (less than 2.5 cm) A2 T

RVU			Global Days	Modifiers				
Mod	Non-Fac Total	Fac Total		51	50	62	80	MUE
	22.73	10.01	000	3	0	0	1	1

AMA: May 01: 5, Sep 01: 1, Feb 12: 11

52318 Litholapaxy: crushing or fragmentation of calculus by any means in bladder and removal of fragments; complicated or large (over 2.5 cm) A2 J1

RVU			Global Days	Modifiers				
Mod	Non-Fac Total	Fac Total		51	50	62	80	MUE
	13.66	13.66	000	3	0	0	1	1

AMA: May 01: 5, Sep 01: 1, Feb 12: 11

Ureter/Kidney Pelvis Procedures

Coding Guidance
Inserting and removing a temporary stent or ureteral catheter placed during the procedures described in CPT codes 52320-52355 is included.

52320 Cystourethroscopy (including ureteral catheterization); with removal of ureteral calculus A2 T

RVU			Global Days	Modifiers				
Mod	Non-Fac Total	Fac Total		51	50	62	80	MUE
	7.10	7.10	000	3	1	0	1	1

AMA: Mar 96: 1, May 96: 11, Jan 01: 13, May 01: 5, Sep 01: 1, Oct 01: 8, May 14: 3

52325 Cystourethroscopy (including ureteral catheterization); with fragmentation of ureteral calculus (eg, ultrasonic or electro-hydraulic technique) A2 T

RVU			Global Days	Modifiers				
Mod	Non-Fac Total	Fac Total		51	50	62	80	MUE
	9.26	9.26	000	3	1	0	1	1

AMA: Mar 96: 1, May 96: 11, May 01: 5, Sep 01: 1, Oct 01: 8, Dec 07: 13

52327 Cystourethroscopy (including ureteral catheterization); with subureteric injection of implant material A2 T

RVU			Global Days	Modifiers				
Mod	Non-Fac Total	Fac Total		51	50	62	80	MUE
	7.55	7.55	000	3	1	0	1	1

AMA: Mar 96: 1, May 96: 11, May 01: 5, Sep 01: 1, Oct 01: 8

52330 Cystourethroscopy (including ureteral catheterization); with manipulation, without removal of ureteral calculus A2 T

RVU			Global Days	Modifiers				
Mod	Non-Fac Total	Fac Total		51	50	62	80	MUE
	13.97	7.60	000	3	1	0	1	1

AMA: Mar 96: 1, May 96: 11, Sep 00: 11, May 01: 5, Sep 01: 1, Oct 01: 8, May 14: 3

Coding Guidance
Code 52332 should not be used to report insertion and removal of a temporary stent during diagnostic or therapeutic procedures. Code 52332 may be used to report placement of a self-retaining, indwelling stent in addition to another primary procedure, using the appropriate modifier.

● New   ▲ Revised   Deleted   ⊙ Moderate Sedation   ✚ Add-on Codes   ⊘ High Risk Denial   Ⓐ Age Edit   ♀ Female   ♂ Male   **AMA** CPT® Assistant   **MUE** Medically Unlikely Edit
⊘ Modifier 51 Exempt   ⊖ Modifier 63 Exempt   ☒ Unlisted   **Modifiers:** See Inside Back Cover   Ⓜ Maternity   A2–Z3 ASC Payment Indicators   A–Y OPPS Status Indicators

© 2016 DecisionHealth   CPT © 2015 American Medical Association. All Rights Reserved.   **503**

52332 Cystourethroscopy, with insertion of indwelling ureteral stent (eg, Gibbons or double-J type) A 2 T

Mod	Non-Fac Total	Fac Total	Global Days	51	50	62	80	MUE
	13.80	4.48	000	3	1	0	1	1

AMA: Mar 96: 1, May 96: 11, Nov 96: 8, Jan 01: 13, May 01: 5, Sep 01: 1, Oct 01: 8, Oct 05: 18, Dec 09: 4, 12, May 14: 3

52334 Cystourethroscopy with insertion of ureteral guide wire through kidney to establish a percutaneous nephrostomy, retrograde A 2 T

Mod	Non-Fac Total	Fac Total	Global Days	51	50	62	80	MUE
	7.38	7.38	000	3	1	0	1	1

AMA: Mar 96: 11, May 96: 11, May 01: 5, Sep 01: 1, Oct 01: 8, May 14: 3

52341 Cystourethroscopy; with treatment of ureteral stricture (eg, balloon dilation, laser, electrocautery, and incision) A 2 T

Mod	Non-Fac Total	Fac Total	Global Days	51	50	62	80	MUE
	8.18	8.18	000	3	1	0	1	1

AMA: Nov 96: 9, Apr 01: 4, May 01: 5, Sep 01: 1, Oct 01: 8

52342 Cystourethroscopy; with treatment of ureteropelvic junction stricture (eg, balloon dilation, laser, electrocautery, and incision) A 2 T

Mod	Non-Fac Total	Fac Total	Global Days	51	50	62	80	MUE
	8.89	8.89	000	3	1	0	1	1

AMA: Apr 01: 4, May 01: 5, Sep 01: 1, Oct 01: 8, Aug 02: 11

52343 Cystourethroscopy; with treatment of intra-renal stricture (eg, balloon dilation, laser, electrocautery, and incision) A 2 T

Mod	Non-Fac Total	Fac Total	Global Days	51	50	62	80	MUE
	9.92	9.92	000	3	1	0	1	1

AMA: Apr 01: 4, May 01: 5, Sep 01: 1, Oct 01: 8, May 14: 3

52344 Cystourethroscopy with ureteroscopy; with treatment of ureteral stricture (eg, balloon dilation, laser, electrocautery, and incision) A 2 T

Mod	Non-Fac Total	Fac Total	Global Days	51	50	62	80	MUE
	10.65	10.65	000	3	1	0	1	1

AMA: Apr 01: 4, May 01: 5, Sep 01: 1, Oct 01: 8

52345 Cystourethroscopy with ureteroscopy; with treatment of ureteropelvic junction stricture (eg, balloon dilation, laser, electrocautery, and incision) A 2 T

Mod	Non-Fac Total	Fac Total	Global Days	51	50	62	80	MUE
	11.38	11.38	000	3	1	0	0	1

AMA: Apr 01: 4, May 01: 5, Sep 01: 1, Oct 01: 8

52346 Cystourethroscopy with ureteroscopy; with treatment of intra-renal stricture (eg, balloon dilation, laser, electrocautery, and incision) A 2 J 1

Mod	Non-Fac Total	Fac Total	Global Days	51	50	62	80	MUE
	12.87	12.87	000	3	1	0	0	1

AMA: Apr 01: 4, May 01: 5, Sep 01: 1, Oct 01: 8, May 14: 3

52351 Cystourethroscopy, with ureteroscopy and/or pyeloscopy; diagnostic A 2 T

Mod	Non-Fac Total	Fac Total	Global Days	51	50	62	80	MUE
	8.72	8.72	000	2	0	0	1	1

AMA: Apr 01: 4, May 01: 5, Sep 01: 1, Oct 01: 8, May 14: 3

52352 Cystourethroscopy, with ureteroscopy and/or pyeloscopy; with removal or manipulation of calculus (ureteral catheterization is included) A 2 T

Mod	Non-Fac Total	Fac Total	Global Days	51	50	62	80	MUE
	10.20	10.20	000	3	1	0	1	1

AMA: Apr 01: 4, May 01: 5, Sep 01: 1, Oct 01: 8, Jun 07: 10, Feb 10: 13, May 14: 3

52353 Cystourethroscopy, with ureteroscopy and/or pyeloscopy; with lithotripsy (ureteral catheterization is included) A 2 J 1

Mod	Non-Fac Total	Fac Total	Global Days	51	50	62	80	MUE
	11.30	11.30	000	3	1	0	1	1

AMA: Apr 01: 4, May 01: 5, Sep 01: 1, Oct 01: 8, Dec 07: 13, Apr 09: 8, May 14: 3

52354 Cystourethroscopy, with ureteroscopy and/or pyeloscopy; with biopsy and/or fulguration of ureteral or renal pelvic lesion A 2 T

Mod	Non-Fac Total	Fac Total	Global Days	51	50	62	80	MUE
	12.02	12.02	000	3	1	0	1	1

AMA: Apr 01: 4, May 01: 5, Sep 01: 1, Oct 01: 8, May 14: 3

52355 Cystourethroscopy, with ureteroscopy and/or pyeloscopy; with resection of ureteral or renal pelvic tumor A 2 J 1

Coding Tip: Cystourethroscopy with ureteroscopy and lithotripsy including insertion of indwelling ureteral stent - 52356

Mod	Non-Fac Total	Fac Total	Global Days	51	50	62	80	MUE
	13.48	13.48	000	3	1	0	1	1

AMA: Apr 01: 4, May 01: 5, Sep 01: 1, Oct 01: 8, Jan 03: 21, May 14: 3

52356 Cystourethroscopy, with ureteroscopy and/or pyeloscopy; with lithotripsy including insertion of indwelling ureteral stent (eg, Gibbons or double-J type) G 2 J 1

Coding Tip: Code 52356 is listed out of numerical order in CPT. Related code for cystourethroscopy with ureteroscopy and/or pyeloscopy, with lithotripsy û 52353

Mod	Non-Fac Total	Fac Total	Global Days	51	50	62	80	MUE
	11.98	11.98	000	3	1	0	1	1

AMA: May 14: 3

Vesical Neck/Prostate Procedures

52400 Cystourethroscopy with incision, fulguration, or resection of congenital posterior urethral valves, or congenital obstructive hypertrophic mucosal folds A 2 T

Mod	Non-Fac Total	Fac Total	Global Days	51	50	62	80	MUE
	13.76	13.76	090	3	0	0	1	1

AMA: Apr 01: 4

● New   ▲ Revised   ✖ Deleted   ⊙ Moderate Sedation   ✚ Add-on Codes   ⊘ High Risk Denial   Ⓐ Age Edit   ♀ Female   ♂ Male   **AMA** *CPT® Assistant*   **MUE** Medically Unlikely Edit
⊘ Modifier 51 Exempt   ⊖ Modifier 63 Exempt   ✗ Unlisted   **Modifiers:** *See Inside Back Cover*   Ⓜ Maternity   A2–Z3 ASC Payment Indicators   A–Y OPPS Status Indicators

CPT © 2015 American Medical Association. All Rights Reserved.

© 2016 DecisionHealth

52402 Cystourethroscopy with transurethral resection or incision of ejaculatory ducts ♂ A2 T

RVU			Global Days	Modifiers				
Mod	Non-Fac Total	Fac Total		51	50	62	80	MUE
	7.69	7.69	000	3	0	0	1	1

52441 Cystourethroscopy, with insertion of permanent adjustable transprostatic implant; single implant B

RVU			Global Days	Modifiers				
Mod	Non-Fac Total	Fac Total		51	50	62	80	MUE
	35.11	6.58	000	3	0	0	1	1

AMA: Jun 15: 5

+ 52442 Cystourethroscopy, with insertion of permanent adjustable transprostatic implant; each additional permanent adjustable transprostatic implant (List separately in addition to code for primary procedure) B

RVU			Global Days	Modifiers				
Mod	Non-Fac Total	Fac Total		51	50	62	80	MUE
	26.84	1.75	ZZZ	0	0	0	1	5

AMA: Jun 15: 5

52450 Transurethral incision of prostate ♂ A2 T

RVU			Global Days	Modifiers				
Mod	Non-Fac Total	Fac Total		51	50	62	80	MUE
	13.49	13.49	090	2	0	0	1	1

AMA: Apr 01: 4, Jul 05: 15, Jun 15: 5

52500 Transurethral resection of bladder neck (separate procedure) A2 T

RVU			Global Days	Modifiers				
Mod	Non-Fac Total	Fac Total		51	50	62	80	MUE
	14.01	14.01	090	2	0	0	1	1

AMA: Apr 01: 4, Jan 04: 27, Jul 05: 15, May 09: 8

Coding Guidance

Multiple methods of accomplishing a prostate service involving different approaches or procedures that are progressively more comprehensive cannot be reported at the same patient encounter. These prostate procedure codes are mutually exclusive of one another and only one method per given procedure should be reported.

52601 Transurethral electrosurgical resection of prostate, including control of postoperative bleeding, complete (vasectomy, meatotomy, cystourethroscopy, urethral calibration and/or dilation, and internal urethrotomy are included) ♂ A2 J I

RVU			Global Days	Modifiers				
Mod	Non-Fac Total	Fac Total		51	50	62	80	MUE
	24.30	24.30	090	2	0	0	1	1

AMA: Nov 97: 20, Apr 01: 4, Jun 03: 6, Oct 11: 10, Jun 15: 5

52630 Transurethral resection; residual or regrowth of obstructive prostate tissue including control of postoperative bleeding, complete (vasectomy, meatotomy, cystourethroscopy, urethral calibration and/or dilation, and internal urethrotomy are included) A2 J I

RVU			Global Days	Modifiers				
Mod	Non-Fac Total	Fac Total		51	50	62	80	MUE
	11.48	11.48	090	2	0	0	1	1

AMA: Apr 01: 4

52640 Transurethral resection; of postoperative bladder neck contracture A2 T

RVU			Global Days	Modifiers				
Mod	Non-Fac Total	Fac Total		51	50	62	80	MUE
	9.03	9.03	090	2	0	0	1	1

AMA: Apr 01: 4

52647 Laser coagulation of prostate, including control of postoperative bleeding, complete (vasectomy, meatotomy, cystourethroscopy, urethral calibration and/or dilation, and internal urethrotomy are included if performed) ♂ A2 J I

RVU			Global Days	Modifiers				
Mod	Non-Fac Total	Fac Total		51	50	62	80	MUE
	50.29	18.60	090	2	0	0	1	1

AMA: Nov 97: 20, Mar 98: 11, Apr 01: 4, Nov 06: 21

52648 Laser vaporization of prostate, including control of postoperative bleeding, complete (vasectomy, meatotomy, cystourethroscopy, urethral calibration and/or dilation, internal urethrotomy and transurethral resection of prostate are included if performed) ♂ A2 J I

RVU			Global Days	Modifiers				
Mod	Non-Fac Total	Fac Total		51	50	62	80	MUE
	51.77	19.84	090	2	0	0	1	1

AMA: Mar 98: 11, Apr 01: 5, Jul 05: 15, Nov 06: 21, Jun 15: 5

52649 Laser enucleation of the prostate with morcellation, including control of postoperative bleeding, complete (vasectomy, meatotomy, cystourethroscopy, urethral calibration and/or dilation, internal urethrotomy and transurethral resection of prostate are included if performed) ♂ G2 J I

RVU			Global Days	Modifiers				
Mod	Non-Fac Total	Fac Total		51	50	62	80	MUE
	23.63	23.63	090	2	0	0	0	1

AMA: Jun 15: 5

Coding Guidance

Transurethral drainage of a prostatic abscess is included in other transurethral prostatic procedures, such as removal (52601-52640) or destruction of the prostate (53850-53852), and is not reported separately.

52700 Transurethral drainage of prostatic abscess ♂ A2 T

RVU			Global Days	Modifiers				
Mod	Non-Fac Total	Fac Total		51	50	62	80	MUE
	12.66	12.66	090	2	0	0	0	1

AMA: Apr 01: 4

Urethral Procedures

Incisional Urethral Procedures

53000 Urethrotomy or urethrostomy, external (separate procedure); pendulous urethra A2 T

RVU			Global Days	Modifiers				
Mod	Non-Fac Total	Fac Total		51	50	62	80	MUE
	4.24	4.24	010	2	0	0	1	1

53010 Urethrotomy or urethrostomy, external (separate procedure); perineal urethra, external A2 J I

RVU			Global Days	Modifiers				
Mod	Non-Fac Total	Fac Total		51	50	62	80	MUE
	8.47	8.47	090	2	0	0	1	1

● New   ▲ Revised   Deleted   ⊙ Moderate Sedation   ✚ Add-on Codes   ⊘ High Risk Denial   Ⓐ Age Edit   ♀ Female   ♂ Male   **AMA** CPT® Assistant   **MUE** Medically Unlikely Edit

⊘ Modifier 51 Exempt   ⊖ Modifier 63 Exempt   ✗ Unlisted   **Modifiers:** See Inside Back Cover   Ⓜ Maternity   A2–Z3 ASC Payment Indicators   A–Y OPPS Status Indicators

53020 Meatotomy, cutting of meatus (separate procedure); except infant   `A 2 T`

Mod	Non-Fac Total	Fac Total	Global Days	51	50	62	80	MUE
	2.79	2.79	000	2	0	0	1	1

53025 Meatotomy, cutting of meatus (separate procedure); infant   `⊘ A ⊖ R 2 T`

Mod	Non-Fac Total	Fac Total	Global Days	51	50	62	80	MUE
	2.07	2.07	000	2	0	0	0	1

53040 Drainage of deep periurethral abscess   `A 2 T`

Mod	Non-Fac Total	Fac Total	Global Days	51	50	62	80	MUE
	11.26	11.26	090	2	0	0	0	1

53060 Drainage of Skene's gland abscess or cyst   `P 3 T`

Mod	Non-Fac Total	Fac Total	Global Days	51	50	62	80	MUE
	5.24	4.72	010	2	0	0	1	1

Drainage of Skene's gland abscess or cyst

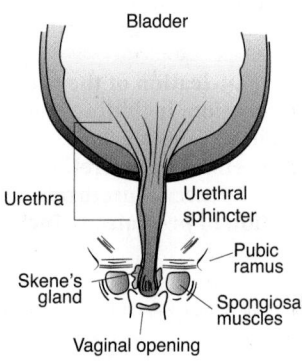

Fluid is drained from an abscess or cyst located just inside of and on the back side of the urethra in the female.

53080 Drainage of perineal urinary extravasation; uncomplicated (separate procedure)   `A 2 T`

Mod	Non-Fac Total	Fac Total	Global Days	51	50	62	80	MUE
	12.06	12.06	090	2	0	0	1	1

53085 Drainage of perineal urinary extravasation; complicated   `G 2 T`

Mod	Non-Fac Total	Fac Total	Global Days	51	50	62	80	MUE
	19.11	19.11	090	2	0	1	2	1

Excisional Urethral Procedures

53200 Biopsy of urethra   `A 2 T`

Mod	Non-Fac Total	Fac Total	Global Days	51	50	62	80	MUE
	4.47	4.09	000	2	0	0	1	1

53210 Urethrectomy, total, including cystostomy; female   `♀ A 2 J 1`

Mod	Non-Fac Total	Fac Total	Global Days	51	50	62	80	MUE
	22.12	22.12	090	2	0	1	2	1

53215 Urethrectomy, total, including cystostomy; male   `♂ A 2 J 1`

Mod	Non-Fac Total	Fac Total	Global Days	51	50	62	80	MUE
	26.71	26.71	090	2	0	1	2	1

53220 Excision or fulguration of carcinoma of urethra   `A 2 T`

Mod	Non-Fac Total	Fac Total	Global Days	51	50	62	80	MUE
	13.03	13.03	090	2	0	0	0	1

53230 Excision of urethral diverticulum (separate procedure); female   `♀ A 2 T`

Mod	Non-Fac Total	Fac Total	Global Days	51	50	62	80	MUE
	17.40	17.40	090	2	0	1	2	1

53235 Excision of urethral diverticulum (separate procedure); male   `♂ A 2 J 1`

Mod	Non-Fac Total	Fac Total	Global Days	51	50	62	80	MUE
	18.17	18.17	090	2	0	1	2	1

53240 Marsupialization of urethral diverticulum, male or female   `A 2 J 1`

Mod	Non-Fac Total	Fac Total	Global Days	51	50	62	80	MUE
	12.27	12.27	090	2	0	0	1	1

53250 Excision of bulbourethral gland (Cowper's gland)   `A 2 T`

Mod	Non-Fac Total	Fac Total	Global Days	51	50	62	80	MUE
	11.87	11.87	090	2	0	0	1	1

53260 Excision or fulguration; urethral polyp(s), distal urethra   `A 2 T`

Mod	Non-Fac Total	Fac Total	Global Days	51	50	62	80	MUE
	5.75	5.18	010	2	0	0	1	1

53265 Excision or fulguration; urethral caruncle   `A 2 T`

Mod	Non-Fac Total	Fac Total	Global Days	51	50	62	80	MUE
	6.21	5.34	010	2	0	0	1	1

53270 Excision or fulguration; Skene's glands   `A 2 T`

Mod	Non-Fac Total	Fac Total	Global Days	51	50	62	80	MUE
	5.94	5.34	010	2	0	0	1	1

53275 Excision or fulguration; urethral prolapse   `A 2 T`

Mod	Non-Fac Total	Fac Total	Global Days	51	50	62	80	MUE
	7.53	7.53	010	2	0	0	1	1

● New   ▲ Revised   ✖ Deleted   ⊙ Moderate Sedation   ✚ Add-on Codes   ⊘ High Risk Denial   Ⓐ Age Edit   ♀ Female   ♂ Male   **AMA** *CPT® Assistant*   **MUE** Medically Unlikely Edit
⊘ Modifier 51 Exempt   ⊖ Modifier 63 Exempt   ✗ Unlisted   **Modifiers:** *See Inside Back Cover*   Ⓜ Maternity   `A 2`–`Z 3` ASC Payment Indicators   `A`–`Y` OPPS Status Indicators

CPT © 2015 American Medical Association. All Rights Reserved.   © 2016 DecisionHealth

Urethral Repair

53400 Urethroplasty; first stage, for fistula, diverticulum, or stricture (eg, Johannsen type) A 2 J 1

RVU			Global Days	Modifiers				
Mod	Non-Fac Total	Fac Total		51	50	62	80	MUE
	23.02	23.02	090	2	0	1	2	1

53405 Urethroplasty; second stage (formation of urethra), including urinary diversion A 2 J 1

RVU			Global Days	Modifiers				
Mod	Non-Fac Total	Fac Total		51	50	62	80	MUE
	25.08	25.08	090	2	0	1	2	1

53410 Urethroplasty, 1-stage reconstruction of male anterior urethra ♂ A 2 J 1

RVU			Global Days	Modifiers				
Mod	Non-Fac Total	Fac Total		51	50	62	80	MUE
	28.10	28.10	090	2	0	1	2	1

53415 Urethroplasty, transpubic or perineal, 1-stage, for reconstruction or repair of prostatic or membranous urethra ♂ C

RVU			Global Days	Modifiers				
Mod	Non-Fac Total	Fac Total		51	50	62	80	MUE
	32.50	32.50	090	2	0	1	2	1

53420 Urethroplasty, 2-stage reconstruction or repair of prostatic or membranous urethra; first stage ♂ A 2 J 1

RVU			Global Days	Modifiers				
Mod	Non-Fac Total	Fac Total		51	50	62	80	MUE
	24.53	24.53	090	2	0	1	1	1

53425 Urethroplasty, 2-stage reconstruction or repair of prostatic or membranous urethra; second stage ♂ A 2 J 1

RVU			Global Days	Modifiers				
Mod	Non-Fac Total	Fac Total		51	50	62	80	MUE
	26.91	26.91	090	2	0	1	2	1

53430 Urethroplasty, reconstruction of female urethra ♀ A 2 T

RVU			Global Days	Modifiers				
Mod	Non-Fac Total	Fac Total		51	50	62	80	MUE
	27.70	27.70	090	2	0	1	2	1

53431 Urethroplasty with tubularization of posterior urethra and/or lower bladder for incontinence (eg, Tenago, Leadbetter procedure) A 2 J 1

RVU			Global Days	Modifiers				
Mod	Non-Fac Total	Fac Total		51	50	62	80	MUE
	33.30	33.30	090	2	0	1	2	1

53440 Sling operation for correction of male urinary incontinence (eg, fascia or synthetic) ♂ J 8 J 1

RVU			Global Days	Modifiers				
Mod	Non-Fac Total	Fac Total		51	50	62	80	MUE
	21.62	21.62	090	2	0	1	2	1

53442 Removal or revision of sling for male urinary incontinence (eg, fascia or synthetic) ♂ A 2 J 1

RVU			Global Days	Modifiers				
Mod	Non-Fac Total	Fac Total		51	50	62	80	MUE
	22.47	22.47	090	2	0	0	2	1

53444 Insertion of tandem cuff (dual cuff) J 8 J 1

RVU			Global Days	Modifiers				
Mod	Non-Fac Total	Fac Total		51	50	62	80	MUE
	22.77	22.77	090	2	0	1	2	1

53445 Insertion of inflatable urethral/bladder neck sphincter, including placement of pump, reservoir, and cuff J 8 J 1

RVU			Global Days	Modifiers				
Mod	Non-Fac Total	Fac Total		51	50	62	80	MUE
	21.61	21.61	090	2	0	1	2	1

53446 Removal of inflatable urethral/bladder neck sphincter, including pump, reservoir, and cuff A 2 Q 2

RVU			Global Days	Modifiers				
Mod	Non-Fac Total	Fac Total		51	50	62	80	MUE
	18.44	18.44	090	2	0	1	2	1

53447 Removal and replacement of inflatable urethral/bladder neck sphincter including pump, reservoir, and cuff at the same operative session J 8 J 1

RVU			Global Days	Modifiers				
Mod	Non-Fac Total	Fac Total		51	50	62	80	MUE
	23.21	23.21	090	2	0	1	2	1

53448 Removal and replacement of inflatable urethral/bladder neck sphincter including pump, reservoir, and cuff through an infected field at the same operative session including irrigation and debridement of infected tissue C

RVU			Global Days	Modifiers				
Mod	Non-Fac Total	Fac Total		51	50	62	80	MUE
	36.98	36.98	090	2	0	1	2	1

53449 Repair of inflatable urethral/bladder neck sphincter, including pump, reservoir, and cuff A 2 J 1

RVU			Global Days	Modifiers				
Mod	Non-Fac Total	Fac Total		51	50	62	80	MUE
	17.55	17.55	090	2	0	1	2	1

Repair of inflatable urethral/bladder neck sphincter

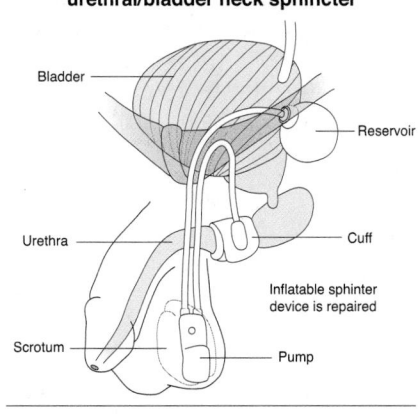

Bladder
Reservoir
Urethra
Cuff
Inflatable sphinter device is repaired
Scrotum
Pump

● New ▲ Revised Deleted ⊙ Moderate Sedation ✚ Add-on Codes ⊘ High Risk Denial Ⓐ Age Edit ♀ Female ♂ Male **AMA** CPT® Assistant **MUE** Medically Unlikely Edit
⊘ Modifier 51 Exempt ⊖ Modifier 63 Exempt ✗ Unlisted **Modifiers:** See Inside Back Cover Ⓜ Maternity A 2 – Z 3 ASC Payment Indicators A – Y OPPS Status Indicators

© 2016 DecisionHealth   CPT © 2015 American Medical Association. All Rights Reserved.   **507**

53450 Urethromeatoplasty, with mucosal advancement A2 T

RVU			Global Days	Modifiers				
Mod	Non-Fac Total	Fac Total		51	50	62	80	MUE
	11.73	11.73	090	2	0	0	1	1

AMA: Sep 12: 16

53460 Urethromeatoplasty, with partial excision of distal urethral segment (Richardson type procedure) A2 T

RVU			Global Days	Modifiers				
Mod	Non-Fac Total	Fac Total		51	50	62	80	MUE
	13.14	13.14	090	2	0	0	0	1

53500 Urethrolysis, transvaginal, secondary, open, including cystourethroscopy (eg, postsurgical obstruction, scarring) T

RVU			Global Days	Modifiers				
Mod	Non-Fac Total	Fac Total		51	50	62	80	MUE
	21.50	21.50	090	2	0	1	2	1

AMA: Sep 04: 11

Coding Guidance

Urethrorrhaphy codes 53502-53515 are for repair of urethral wounds or injury only. When a urethroplasty or reconstruction is done, the suture to repair a wound or injury is included.

53502 Urethrorrhaphy, suture of urethral wound or injury, female ♀A2 T

RVU			Global Days	Modifiers				
Mod	Non-Fac Total	Fac Total		51	50	62	80	MUE
	13.97	13.97	090	2	0	0	1	1

53505 Urethrorrhaphy, suture of urethral wound or injury; penile ♂A2 J I

RVU			Global Days	Modifiers				
Mod	Non-Fac Total	Fac Total		51	50	62	80	MUE
	14.02	14.02	090	2	0	0	2	1

53510 Urethrorrhaphy, suture of urethral wound or injury; perineal ♂A2 J I

RVU			Global Days	Modifiers				
Mod	Non-Fac Total	Fac Total		51	50	62	80	MUE
	18.14	18.14	090	2	0	1	2	1

53515 Urethrorrhaphy, suture of urethral wound or injury; prostatomembranous ♂A2 J I

RVU			Global Days	Modifiers				
Mod	Non-Fac Total	Fac Total		51	50	62	80	MUE
	22.85	22.85	090	2	0	1	2	1

53520 Closure of urethrostomy or urethrocutaneous fistula, male (separate procedure) ♂A2 J I

RVU			Global Days	Modifiers				
Mod	Non-Fac Total	Fac Total		51	50	62	80	MUE
	15.99	15.99	090	2	0	0	1	1

Urethral Manipulation

Coding Guidance

Radiologic guidance for all urethral dilations is reported with 74485.

53600 Dilation of urethral stricture by passage of sound or urethral dilator, male; initial ♂P3 T

RVU			Global Days	Modifiers				
Mod	Non-Fac Total	Fac Total		51	50	62	80	MUE
	2.36	1.83	000	2	0	0	1	1

53601 Dilation of urethral stricture by passage of sound or urethral dilator, male; subsequent ♂N I Q I

RVU			Global Days	Modifiers				
Mod	Non-Fac Total	Fac Total		51	50	62	80	MUE
	2.30	1.54	000	2	0	0	1	1

53605 Dilation of urethral stricture or vesical neck by passage of sound or urethral dilator, male, general or conduction (spinal) anesthesia ♂A2 T

RVU			Global Days	Modifiers				
Mod	Non-Fac Total	Fac Total		51	50	62	80	MUE
	1.86	1.86	000	2	0	0	1	1

53620 Dilation of urethral stricture by passage of filiform and follower, male; initial ♂P3 T

RVU			Global Days	Modifiers				
Mod	Non-Fac Total	Fac Total		51	50	62	80	MUE
	3.30	2.51	000	2	0	0	1	1

53621 Dilation of urethral stricture by passage of filiform and follower, male; subsequent ♂P3 T

RVU			Global Days	Modifiers				
Mod	Non-Fac Total	Fac Total		51	50	62	80	MUE
	3.11	2.07	000	2	0	0	1	1

53660 Dilation of female urethra including suppository and/or instillation; initial ♀P3 S

RVU			Global Days	Modifiers				
Mod	Non-Fac Total	Fac Total		51	50	62	80	MUE
	2.00	1.20	000	2	0	0	1	1

Dilation of female urethra, general or conduction (spinal) anesthesia

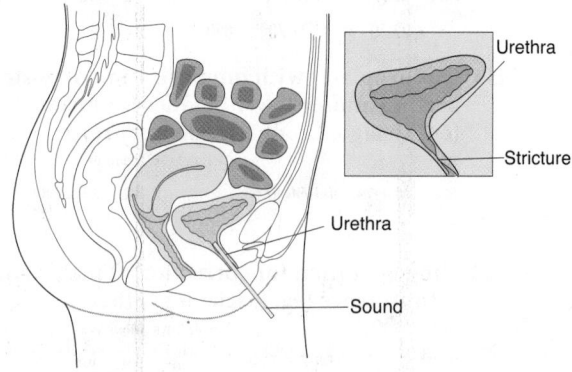

A device is inserted into the urethra of a female patient to widen a section of the urethra that has become constricted.

● New   ▲ Revised   ✖ Deleted   ⊙ Moderate Sedation   ✚ Add-on Codes   ⊘ High Risk Denial   Ⓐ Age Edit   ♀ Female   ♂ Male   **AMA** *CPT® Assistant*   **MUE** Medically Unlikely Edit
⊘ Modifier 51 Exempt   ⊖ Modifier 63 Exempt   ✗ Unlisted   **Modifiers:** *See Inside Back Cover*   Ⓜ Maternity   A2–Z3 ASC Payment Indicators   A–Y OPPS Status Indicators

CPT © 2015 American Medical Association. All Rights Reserved.   © 2016 DecisionHealth

53661 Dilation of female urethra including suppository and/or instillation; subsequent ♀N I Q I

RVU			Global Days	Modifiers				
Mod	Non-Fac Total	Fac Total		51	50	62	80	MUE
	1.96	1.16	000	2	0	0	1	1

53665 Dilation of female urethra, general or conduction (spinal) anesthesia ♀A 2 T

RVU			Global Days	Modifiers				
Mod	Non-Fac Total	Fac Total		51	50	62	80	MUE
	1.11	1.11	000	2	0	0	1	1

Other Urethral Procedures

53850 Transurethral destruction of prostate tissue; by microwave thermotherapy ♂P 2 T

RVU			Global Days	Modifiers				
Mod	Non-Fac Total	Fac Total		51	50	62	80	MUE
	58.50	17.43	090	2	0	0	1	1

AMA: Nov 97: 20, Apr 01: 6, Feb 10: 7, Jun 15: 5

53852 Transurethral destruction of prostate tissue; by radiofrequency thermotherapy ♂P 3 J I

RVU			Global Days	Modifiers				
Mod	Non-Fac Total	Fac Total		51	50	62	80	MUE
	53.93	17.88	090	2	0	0	1	1

AMA: Nov 97: 20, Apr 01: 6, Jun 15: 5

53855 Insertion of a temporary prostatic urethral stent, including urethral measurement ♂P 2 T

RVU			Global Days	Modifiers				
Mod	Non-Fac Total	Fac Total		51	50	62	80	MUE
	21.87	2.37	000	2	0	0	0	1

AMA: Feb 10: 7

53860 Transurethral radiofrequency micro-remodeling of the female bladder neck and proximal urethra for stress urinary incontinence ♀P 2 T

RVU			Global Days	Modifiers				
Mod	Non-Fac Total	Fac Total		51	50	62	80	MUE
	43.64	6.51	090	2	0	0	0	1

53899 Unlisted procedure, urinary system ⊘x T

RVU			Global Days	Modifiers				
Mod	Non-Fac Total	Fac Total		51	50	62	80	MUE
	0.00	0.00	YYY	2	0	1	0	

AMA: Aug 04: 12, Sep 04: 11, Oct 05: 18, 23, 24, Feb 06: 14, May 10: 10, Mar 15: 9, Jun 15: 5

Male Genital Procedures

Penis Procedures

Incisional Penis Procedures

54000 Slitting of prepuce, dorsal or lateral (separate procedure); newborn Ⓐ♂⊖A 2 T

RVU			Global Days	Modifiers				
Mod	Non-Fac Total	Fac Total		51	50	62	80	MUE
	4.20	3.10	010	2	0	0	0	1

Slitting of prepuce, dorsal or lateral (separate procedure)

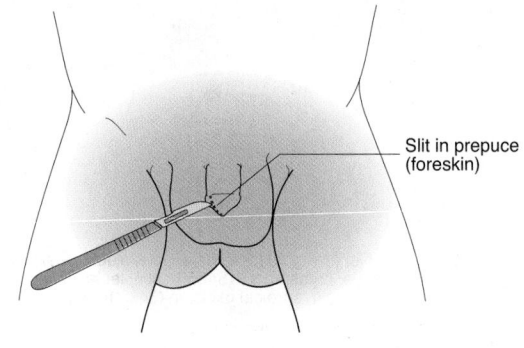

Slit in prepuce (foreskin)

Newborn (54000); other than newborn (54001)

54001 Slitting of prepuce, dorsal or lateral (separate procedure); except newborn ♂A 2 T

RVU			Global Days	Modifiers				
Mod	Non-Fac Total	Fac Total		51	50	62	80	MUE
	5.23	3.97	010	2	0	0	1	1

54015 Incision and drainage of penis, deep ♂A 2 T

RVU			Global Days	Modifiers				
Mod	Non-Fac Total	Fac Total		51	50	62	80	MUE
	8.90	8.90	010	2	0	0	0	1

Penile Destruction Procedures

Coding Guidance

Genitourinary tract lesions requiring biopsy, excision, or destruction of the mucocutaneous border may have several CPT codes that describe the general nature of the biopsy. Only one biopsy code as one unit of service should be reported that most accurately describes the service. When excision or destruction is done immediately following a biopsy during the same session, only the most accurate, comprehensive code is reported. Separate CPT codes for lesion biopsy, excision, or destruction for both integumentary and genitourinary system procedures should not be reported unless the lesions are distinctly different and are located in both the genitourinary tract and in the skin.

● New   ▲ Revised   Deleted   ⊙ Moderate Sedation   ✛ Add-on Codes   ⊖ High Risk Denial   Ⓐ Age Edit   ♀ Female   ♂ Male   **AMA** *CPT® Assistant*   **MUE** Medically Unlikely Edit
⊘ Modifier 51 Exempt   ⊖ Modifier 63 Exempt   ✗ Unlisted   **Modifiers:** *See Inside Back Cover*   Ⓜ Maternity   A 2–Z 3 ASC Payment Indicators   A–Y OPPS Status Indicators

© 2016 DecisionHealth   CPT © 2015 American Medical Association. All Rights Reserved.   **509**

54050 Destruction of lesion(s), penis (eg, condyloma, papilloma, molluscum contagiosum, herpetic vesicle), simple; chemical ♂ N I Q I

Coding Tip: Extensive destruction of lesion(s) of penis - 54065

RVU			Global Days	Modifiers				
Mod	Non-Fac Total	Fac Total		51	50	62	80	MUE
	3.75	3.01	010	2	0	0	1	1

Destruction of lesion(s), penis

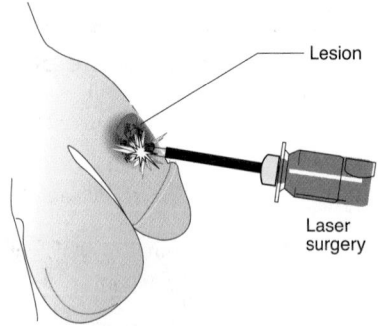

Lesion

Laser surgery

Simple, chemical (54050); simple, electrodesiccation (54055); simple, cryosurgery (54056); simple, laser surgery (54057); simple, surgical excision (54060); extensive (54065)

54055 Destruction of lesion(s), penis (eg, condyloma, papilloma, molluscum contagiosum, herpetic vesicle), simple; electrodesiccation ♂ P 3 T

RVU			Global Days	Modifiers				
Mod	Non-Fac Total	Fac Total		51	50	62	80	MUE
	3.38	2.66	010	2	0	0	1	1

54056 Destruction of lesion(s), penis (eg, condyloma, papilloma, molluscum contagiosum, herpetic vesicle), simple; cryosurgery ♂ N I Q I

RVU			Global Days	Modifiers				
Mod	Non-Fac Total	Fac Total		51	50	62	80	MUE
	4.04	3.19	010	2	0	0	1	1

54057 Destruction of lesion(s), penis (eg, condyloma, papilloma, molluscum contagiosum, herpetic vesicle), simple; laser surgery ♂ A 2 T

RVU			Global Days	Modifiers				
Mod	Non-Fac Total	Fac Total		51	50	62	80	MUE
	3.85	2.72	010	2	0	0	1	1

54060 Destruction of lesion(s), penis (eg, condyloma, papilloma, molluscum contagiosum, herpetic vesicle), simple; surgical excision ♂ A 2 T

Coding Tip: Do not code local anesthesia

Coding Tip: Report 99000 for transport of specimen to outside laboratory

RVU			Global Days	Modifiers				
Mod	Non-Fac Total	Fac Total		51	50	62	80	MUE
	5.09	3.74	010	2	0	0	1	1

54065 Destruction of lesion(s), penis (eg, condyloma, papilloma, molluscum contagiosum, herpetic vesicle), extensive (eg, laser surgery, electrosurgery, cryosurgery, chemosurgery) ♂ A 2 T

Coding Tip: Do not code local anesthesia

Coding Tip: Simple destuction of lesion of penis - 54050-54060

RVU			Global Days	Modifiers				
Mod	Non-Fac Total	Fac Total		51	50	62	80	MUE
	6.24	4.98	010	2	0	0	1	1

Excisional Penis Procedures

54100 Biopsy of penis; (separate procedure) ♂ A 2 T

Coding Tip: For surgical excision of the lesion - 54060

Coding Tip: Biopsy is usually included as a component of a more complex procedure

Coding Tip: Report this procedure separately only when performed alone, or distinct from other procedures on the same day

RVU			Global Days	Modifiers				
Mod	Non-Fac Total	Fac Total		51	50	62	80	MUE
	5.67	3.64	000	2	0	0	1	2

AMA: Nov 99: 26

54105 Biopsy of penis; deep structures ♂ A 2 T

Coding Tip: Code 99000 for specimen transfer from office setting to outside laboratory

Coding Tip: Do not code local anesthesia

RVU			Global Days	Modifiers				
Mod	Non-Fac Total	Fac Total		51	50	62	80	MUE
	7.52	6.12	010	2	0	0	1	2

54110 Excision of penile plaque (Peyronie disease) ♂ A 2 T

RVU			Global Days	Modifiers				
Mod	Non-Fac Total	Fac Total		51	50	62	80	MUE
	18.18	18.18	090	2	0	0	2	1

54111 Excision of penile plaque (Peyronie disease); with graft to 5 cm in length ♂ A 2 J 1

RVU			Global Days	Modifiers				
Mod	Non-Fac Total	Fac Total		51	50	62	80	MUE
	23.01	23.01	090	2	0	1	2	1

AMA: Aug 99: 5

54112 Excision of penile plaque (Peyronie disease); with graft greater than 5 cm in length ♂ J 8 T

RVU			Global Days	Modifiers				
Mod	Non-Fac Total	Fac Total		51	50	62	80	MUE
	26.99	26.99	090	2	0	1	2	1

54115 Removal foreign body from deep penile tissue (eg, plastic implant) ♂ A 2 T

RVU			Global Days	Modifiers				
Mod	Non-Fac Total	Fac Total		51	50	62	80	MUE
	12.95	12.20	090	2	0	0	2	1

54120 Amputation of penis; partial ♂ A 2 T

RVU			Global Days	Modifiers				
Mod	Non-Fac Total	Fac Total		51	50	62	80	MUE
	18.15	18.15	090	2	0	1	2	1

54125 Amputation of penis; complete ♂ C

RVU			Global Days	Modifiers				
Mod	Non-Fac Total	Fac Total		51	50	62	80	MUE
	23.34	23.34	090	2	0	1	2	1

● New   ▲ Revised   ✖ Deleted   ⊙ Moderate Sedation   ✚ Add-on Codes   ⊘ High Risk Denial   Ⓐ Age Edit   ♀ Female   ♂ Male   **AMA** CPT® Assistant   **MUE** Medically Unlikely Edit
⊘ Modifier 51 Exempt   ⊖ Modifier 63 Exempt   ✗ Unlisted   **Modifiers:** See Inside Back Cover   Ⓜ Maternity   A 2–Z 3 ASC Payment Indicators   A –Y OPPS Status Indicators

CPT © 2015 American Medical Association. All Rights Reserved.   © 2016 DecisionHealth

54130 Amputation of penis, radical; with bilateral inguinofemoral lymphadenectomy ♂🄲

RVU			Global Days	Modifiers				
Mod	Non-Fac Total	Fac Total		51	50	62	80	MUE
	34.23	34.23	090	2	2	1	2	1

54135 Amputation of penis, radical; in continuity with bilateral pelvic lymphadenectomy, including external iliac, hypogastric and obturator nodes ♂🄲

RVU			Global Days	Modifiers				
Mod	Non-Fac Total	Fac Total		51	50	62	80	MUE
	43.12	43.12	090	2	2	0	2	1

54150 Circumcision, using clamp or other device with regional dorsal penile or ring block ♂⊖A2T

RVU			Global Days	Modifiers				
Mod	Non-Fac Total	Fac Total		51	50	62	80	MUE
	4.38	2.81	000	2	0	0	0	1

AMA: Sep 96: 11, May 98: 11, Apr 03: 27, Aug 03: 6, May 07: 10, Jul 07: 5

Circumcision
Using clamp or other device with regional dorsal penile or ring block

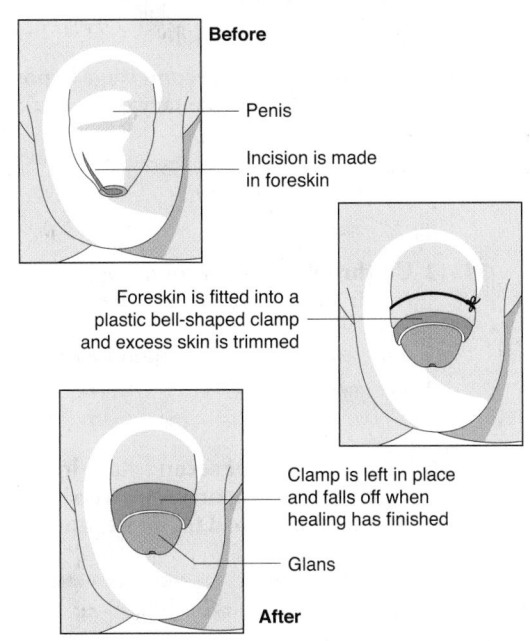

Before

Penis

Incision is made in foreskin

Foreskin is fitted into a plastic bell-shaped clamp and excess skin is trimmed

Clamp is left in place and falls off when healing has finished

Glans

After

54160 Circumcision, surgical excision other than clamp, device, or dorsal slit; neonate (28 days of age or less) ⊗🄰♂⊖A2T

RVU			Global Days	Modifiers				
Mod	Non-Fac Total	Fac Total		51	50	62	80	MUE
	6.33	4.19	010	2	0	0	1	1

AMA: Sep 96: 11, May 98: 11, May 07: 10, Jul 07: 5

54161 Circumcision, surgical excision other than clamp, device, or dorsal slit; older than 28 days of age ♂A2T

RVU			Global Days	Modifiers				
Mod	Non-Fac Total	Fac Total		51	50	62	80	MUE
	5.65	5.65	010	2	0	0	1	1

AMA: Sep 96: 11, Dec 96: 10, May 98: 11, Jul 07: 5

54162 Lysis or excision of penile post-circumcision adhesions ♂A2T

Coding Tip: *Lysis of preputial adhesions and stretching - 54450*

RVU			Global Days	Modifiers				
Mod	Non-Fac Total	Fac Total		51	50	62	80	MUE
	7.31	5.72	010	2	0	0	1	1

54163 Repair incomplete circumcision ♂A2T

RVU			Global Days	Modifiers				
Mod	Non-Fac Total	Fac Total		51	50	62	80	MUE
	6.26	6.26	010	2	0	0	1	1

Repair incomplete circumcision

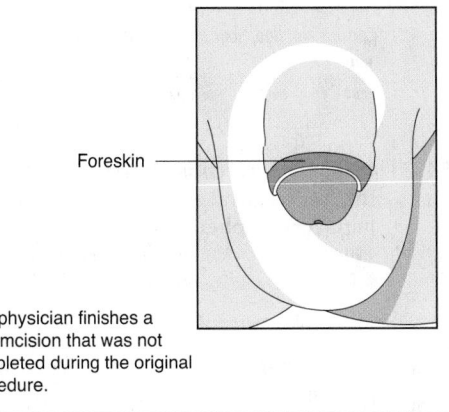

Foreskin

The physician finishes a circumcision that was not completed during the original procedure.

54164 Frenulotomy of penis ♂A2T

RVU			Global Days	Modifiers				
Mod	Non-Fac Total	Fac Total		51	50	62	80	MUE
	5.53	5.53	010	2	0	0	1	1

Introduction Penile Procedures

54200 Injection procedure for Peyronie disease ♂P3T

RVU			Global Days	Modifiers				
Mod	Non-Fac Total	Fac Total		51	50	62	80	MUE
	3.04	2.40	010	2	0	0	1	1

Injection procedure for Peyronie disease

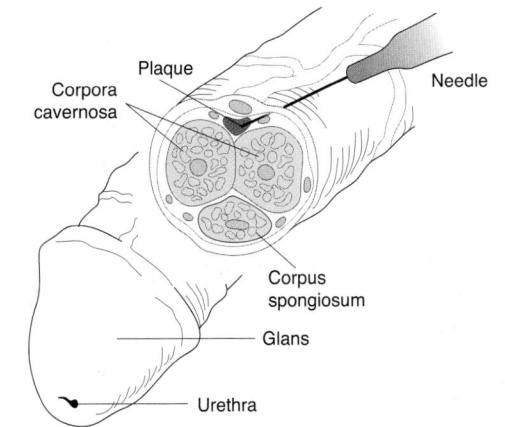

Plaque

Needle

Corpora cavernosa

Corpus spongiosum

Glans

Urethra

Medicine is injected into the penis to break down plaque build up in the spongy tissue. With surgical access (45205).

● New   ▲ Revised   Deleted   ⊙ Moderate Sedation   ✚ Add-on Codes   ⊗ High Risk Denial   🄰 Age Edit   ♀ Female   ♂ Male   **AMA** *CPT® Assistant*   **MUE** Medically Unlikely Edit
⊘ Modifier 51 Exempt   ⊖ Modifier 63 Exempt   🅇 Unlisted   **Modifiers:** *See Inside Back Cover*   🅜 Maternity   A2–Z3 ASC Payment Indicators   A–Y OPPS Status Indicators

54205 Injection procedure for Peyronie disease; with surgical exposure of plaque ♂ A 2 J 1

Coding Tip: *Surgical excision of plaque - 54110; with graft - 54111-54112*

RVU			Global Days	Modifiers				
Mod	Non-Fac Total	Fac Total		51	50	62	80	MUE
	15.29	15.29	090	2	0	0	2	1

54220 Irrigation of corpora cavernosa for priapism ♂ A 2 T

RVU			Global Days	Modifiers				
Mod	Non-Fac Total	Fac Total		51	50	62	80	MUE
	5.80	3.86	000	2	0	0	1	1

54230 Injection procedure for corpora cavernosography ♂ N I N

Coding Tip: *Radiological portion of corpora cavernosography - 74445*

RVU			Global Days	Modifiers				
Mod	Non-Fac Total	Fac Total		51	50	62	80	MUE
	2.75	2.29	000	2	0	0	1	1

54231 Dynamic cavernosometry, including intracavernosal injection of vasoactive drugs (eg, papaverine, phentolamine) ♂ P 3 T

RVU			Global Days	Modifiers				
Mod	Non-Fac Total	Fac Total		51	50	62	80	MUE
	4.00	3.34	000	2	0	0	1	1

54235 Injection of corpora cavernosa with pharmacologic agent(s) (eg, papaverine, phentolamine) ♂ P 3 T

RVU			Global Days	Modifiers				
Mod	Non-Fac Total	Fac Total		51	50	62	80	MUE
	2.57	2.11	000	2	0	0	1	1

AMA: Sep 96: 10

54240 Penile plethysmography ♂ P 3 S

RVU			Global Days	Modifiers				
Mod	Non-Fac Total	Fac Total		51	50	62	80	MUE
	2.91	2.91	000	0	0	0	0	1
26	1.92	1.92	000	0	0	0	0	1
TC	0.99	0.99	000	0	0	0	0	1

Penile plethysmography

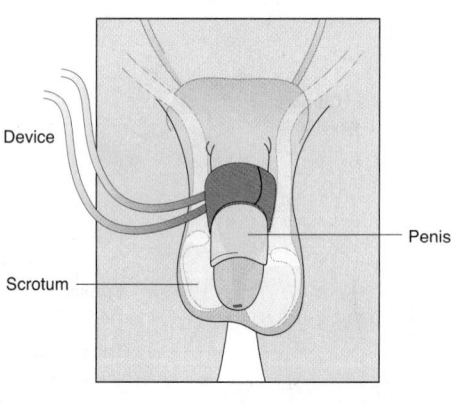

Device

Penis

Scrotum

A device is placed around the penis to measure
changes in diameter in response to stimulation.

54250 Nocturnal penile tumescence and/or rigidity test ♂ P 3 T

Coding Tip: *Application of monitoring device and recording is included*

RVU			Global Days	Modifiers				
Mod	Non-Fac Total	Fac Total		51	50	62	80	MUE
26	3.15	3.15	000	0	0	0	0	1
TC	0.31	0.31	000	0	0	0	0	1
	3.46	3.46	000	0	0	0	0	1

Pub 100-02, 15, 70

Penile Repair

54300 Plastic operation of penis for straightening of chordee (eg, hypospadias), with or without mobilization of urethra ♂ A 2 T

RVU			Global Days	Modifiers				
Mod	Non-Fac Total	Fac Total		51	50	62	80	MUE
	18.41	18.41	090	2	0	1	2	1

AMA: Dec 14: 16

54304 Plastic operation on penis for correction of chordee or for first stage hypospadias repair with or without transplantation of prepuce and/or skin flaps ♂ A 2 T

RVU			Global Days	Modifiers				
Mod	Non-Fac Total	Fac Total		51	50	62	80	MUE
	21.55	21.55	090	2	0	0	2	1

54308 Urethroplasty for second stage hypospadias repair (including urinary diversion); less than 3 cm ♂ A 2 J 1

RVU			Global Days	Modifiers				
Mod	Non-Fac Total	Fac Total		51	50	62	80	MUE
	20.55	20.55	090	2	0	1	2	1

54312 Urethroplasty for second stage hypospadias repair (including urinary diversion); greater than 3 cm ♂ A 2 T

RVU			Global Days	Modifiers				
Mod	Non-Fac Total	Fac Total		51	50	62	80	MUE
	24.76	24.76	090	2	0	1	2	1

54316 Urethroplasty for second stage hypospadias repair (including urinary diversion) with free skin graft obtained from site other than genitalia ♂ A 2 J 1

RVU			Global Days	Modifiers				
Mod	Non-Fac Total	Fac Total		51	50	62	80	MUE
	30.19	30.19	090	2	0	1	2	1

54318 Urethroplasty for third stage hypospadias repair to release penis from scrotum (eg, third stage Cecil repair) ⊗♂ A 2 T

RVU			Global Days	Modifiers				
Mod	Non-Fac Total	Fac Total		51	50	62	80	MUE
	21.51	21.51	090	2	0	1	2	1

54322 1-stage distal hypospadias repair (with or without chordee or circumcision); with simple meatal advancement (eg, Magpi, V-flap) ♂ A 2 T

RVU			Global Days	Modifiers				
Mod	Non-Fac Total	Fac Total		51	50	62	80	MUE
	22.16	22.16	090	2	0	0	2	1

CPT © 2015 American Medical Association. All Rights Reserved.   © 2016 DecisionHealth

54324 1-stage distal hypospadias repair (with or without chordee or circumcision); with urethroplasty by local skin flaps (eg, flip-flap, prepucial flap) ♂ A 2 T

RVU			Global Days	Modifiers				
Mod	Non-Fac Total	Fac Total			51	50	62	80	MUE
	28.67	28.67	090		2	0	1	2	1

54326 1-stage distal hypospadias repair (with or without chordee or circumcision); with urethroplasty by local skin flaps and mobilization of urethra

♂ A 2 J I

RVU			Global Days	Modifiers				
Mod	Non-Fac Total	Fac Total			51	50	62	80	MUE
	27.17	27.17	090		2	0	1	2	1

54328 1-stage distal hypospadias repair (with or without chordee or circumcision); with extensive dissection to correct chordee and urethroplasty with local skin flaps, skin graft patch, and/or island flap ♂ A 2 T

RVU			Global Days	Modifiers				
Mod	Non-Fac Total	Fac Total			51	50	62	80	MUE
	26.99	26.99	090		2	0	1	2	1

AMA: Oct 04: 15

54332 1-stage proximal penile or penoscrotal hypospadias repair requiring extensive dissection to correct chordee and urethroplasty by use of skin graft tube and/or island flap ♂ T

RVU			Global Days	Modifiers				
Mod	Non-Fac Total	Fac Total			51	50	62	80	MUE
	30.83	30.83	090		2	0	1	2	1

AMA: Mar 04: 11, Sep 04: 12

54336 1-stage perineal hypospadias repair requiring extensive dissection to correct chordee and urethroplasty by use of skin graft tube and/or island flap ♂ T

RVU			Global Days	Modifiers				
Mod	Non-Fac Total	Fac Total			51	50	62	80	MUE
	35.99	35.99	090		2	0	1	2	1

AMA: Oct 04: 15

54340 Repair of hypospadias complications (ie, fistula, stricture, diverticula); by closure, incision, or excision, simple ♂ A 2 T

RVU			Global Days	Modifiers				
Mod	Non-Fac Total	Fac Total			51	50	62	80	MUE
	16.37	16.37	090		2	0	1	2	1

54344 Repair of hypospadias complications (ie, fistula, stricture, diverticula); requiring mobilization of skin flaps and urethroplasty with flap or patch graft ♂ A 2 J I

RVU			Global Days	Modifiers				
Mod	Non-Fac Total	Fac Total			51	50	62	80	MUE
	29.95	29.95	090		2	0	1	2	1

54348 Repair of hypospadias complications (ie, fistula, stricture, diverticula); requiring extensive dissection and urethroplasty with flap, patch or tubed graft (includes urinary diversion) ♂ A 2 T

RVU			Global Days	Modifiers				
Mod	Non-Fac Total	Fac Total			51	50	62	80	MUE
	29.15	29.15	090		2	0	1	2	1

54352 Repair of hypospadias cripple requiring extensive dissection and excision of previously constructed structures including re-release of chordee and reconstruction of urethra and penis by use of local skin as grafts and island flaps and skin brought in as flaps or grafts ♂ A 2 J I

RVU			Global Days	Modifiers				
Mod	Non-Fac Total	Fac Total			51	50	62	80	MUE
	40.74	40.74	090		2	0	1	2	1

54360 Plastic operation on penis to correct angulation ♂ A 2 T

RVU			Global Days	Modifiers				
Mod	Non-Fac Total	Fac Total			51	50	62	80	MUE
	20.70	20.70	090		2	0	1	2	1

54380 Plastic operation on penis for epispadias distal to external sphincter ♂ A 2 T

RVU			Global Days	Modifiers				
Mod	Non-Fac Total	Fac Total			51	50	62	80	MUE
	22.95	22.95	090		2	0	1	2	1

54385 Plastic operation on penis for epispadias distal to external sphincter; with incontinence ⊙ ♂ A 2 T

RVU			Global Days	Modifiers				
Mod	Non-Fac Total	Fac Total			51	50	62	80	MUE
	28.08	28.08	090		2	0	1	2	1

54390 Plastic operation on penis for epispadias distal to external sphincter; with exstrophy of bladder ♂ C

RVU			Global Days	Modifiers				
Mod	Non-Fac Total	Fac Total			51	50	62	80	MUE
	37.53	37.53	090		2	0	1	2	1

54400 Insertion of penile prosthesis; non-inflatable (semi-rigid) ♂ J 8 J I

RVU			Global Days	Modifiers				
Mod	Non-Fac Total	Fac Total			51	50	62	80	MUE
	15.22	15.22	090		2	0	1	1	1

54401 Insertion of penile prosthesis; inflatable (self-contained) ♂ J 8 J I

RVU			Global Days	Modifiers				
Mod	Non-Fac Total	Fac Total			51	50	62	80	MUE
	18.84	18.84	090		2	0	1	1	1

54405 Insertion of multi-component, inflatable penile prosthesis, including placement of pump, cylinders, and reservoir ♂ J 8 J I

RVU			Global Days	Modifiers				
Mod	Non-Fac Total	Fac Total			51	50	62	80	MUE
	23.23	23.23	090		2	0	1	2	1

● New   ▲ Revised   Deleted   ⊙ Moderate Sedation   ✚ Add-on Codes   ⊘ High Risk Denial   Ⓐ Age Edit   ♀ Female   ♂ Male   **AMA** CPT® Assistant   **MUE** Medically Unlikely Edit

⊘ Modifier 51 Exempt   ⊖ Modifier 63 Exempt   Ⓧ Unlisted   **Modifiers:** See Inside Back Cover   Ⓜ Maternity   A 2 – Z 3 ASC Payment Indicators   A – Y OPPS Status Indicators

54406 Removal of all components of a multi-component, inflatable penile prosthesis without replacement of prosthesis ♂ A2 Q2

RVU		Global Days	Modifiers				
Mod	*Non-Fac Total*	*Fac Total*		**51**	**50**	**62**	**80**	**MUE**
	20.99	20.99	090	2	0	1	2	1

54408 Repair of component(s) of a multi-component, inflatable penile prosthesis ♂ A2 J1

RVU		Global Days	Modifiers				
Mod	*Non-Fac Total*	*Fac Total*		**51**	**50**	**62**	**80**	**MUE**
	22.68	22.68	090	2	0	1	2	1

54410 Removal and replacement of all component(s) of a multi-component, inflatable penile prosthesis at the same operative session ♂ J8 J1

RVU		Global Days	Modifiers				
Mod	*Non-Fac Total*	*Fac Total*		**51**	**50**	**62**	**80**	**MUE**
	24.67	24.67	090	2	0	1	2	1

54411 Removal and replacement of all components of a multi-component inflatable penile prosthesis through an infected field at the same operative session, including irrigation and debridement of infected tissue ♂ J1

RVU		Global Days	Modifiers				
Mod	*Non-Fac Total*	*Fac Total*		**51**	**50**	**62**	**80**	**MUE**
	29.47	29.47	090	2	0	1	2	1

54415 Removal of non-inflatable (semi-rigid) or inflatable (self-contained) penile prosthesis, without replacement of prosthesis ♂ A2 Q2

RVU		Global Days	Modifiers				
Mod	*Non-Fac Total*	*Fac Total*		**51**	**50**	**62**	**80**	**MUE**
	15.17	15.17	090	2	0	1	2	1

54416 Removal and replacement of non-inflatable (semi-rigid) or inflatable (self-contained) penile prosthesis at the same operative session ♂ J8 J1

RVU		Global Days	Modifiers				
Mod	*Non-Fac Total*	*Fac Total*		**51**	**50**	**62**	**80**	**MUE**
	20.38	20.38	090	2	0	1	2	1

54417 Removal and replacement of non-inflatable (semi-rigid) or inflatable (self-contained) penile prosthesis through an infected field at the same operative session, including irrigation and debridement of infected tissue ♂ J1

RVU		Global Days	Modifiers				
Mod	*Non-Fac Total*	*Fac Total*		**51**	**50**	**62**	**80**	**MUE**
	25.80	25.80	090	2	0	1	2	1

54420 Corpora cavernosa-saphenous vein shunt (priapism operation), unilateral or bilateral ♂ A2 T

RVU		Global Days	Modifiers				
Mod	*Non-Fac Total*	*Fac Total*		**51**	**50**	**62**	**80**	**MUE**
	20.25	20.25	090	2	0	0	2	1

54430 Corpora cavernosa-corpus spongiosum shunt (priapism operation), unilateral or bilateral ♂ C

RVU		Global Days	Modifiers				
Mod	*Non-Fac Total*	*Fac Total*		**51**	**50**	**62**	**80**	**MUE**
	18.39	18.39	090	2	2	0	2	1

54435 Corpora cavernosa-glans penis fistulization (eg, biopsy needle, Winter procedure, rongeur, or punch) for priapism ♂ A2 T

RVU		Global Days	Modifiers				
Mod	*Non-Fac Total*	*Fac Total*		**51**	**50**	**62**	**80**	**MUE**
	11.93	11.93	090	2	0	0	1	1

● **54437** Repair of traumatic corporeal tear(s) ♂ G2 T

RVU		Global Days	Modifiers				
Mod	*Non-Fac Total*	*Fac Total*		**51**	**50**	**62**	**80**	**MUE**
	19.59	19.59	090	2	0	1	2	1

● **54438** Replantation, penis, complete amputation including urethral repair ♂ C

RVU		Global Days	Modifiers				
Mod	*Non-Fac Total*	*Fac Total*		**51**	**50**	**62**	**80**	**MUE**
	39.52	39.52	090	2	0	1	2	1

54440 Plastic operation of penis for injury ♂ A2 T

RVU		Global Days	Modifiers				
Mod	*Non-Fac Total*	*Fac Total*		**51**	**50**	**62**	**80**	**MUE**
	0.00	0.00	090	2	0	1	2	1

Penile Foreskin Manipulation

54450 Foreskin manipulation including lysis of preputial adhesions and stretching ♂ A2 T

Coding Tip: Slitting of prepuce - 54000-54001

Coding Tip: Lysis of post-circumcision adhesions - 54162

RVU		Global Days	Modifiers				
Mod	*Non-Fac Total*	*Fac Total*		**51**	**50**	**62**	**80**	**MUE**
	2.00	1.66	000	2	0	0	1	1

Foreskin manipulation

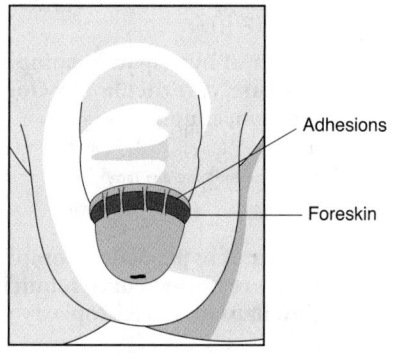

Adhesions

Foreskin

The foreskin is manually manipulated to break up adhesions

● New ▲ Revised ✖ Deleted ⊙ Moderate Sedation ✚ Add-on Codes ⊘ High Risk Denial Ⓐ Age Edit ♀ Female ♂ Male **AMA** *CPT® Assistant* **MUE** Medically Unlikely Edit
⊘ Modifier 51 Exempt ⊖ Modifier 63 Exempt ✗ Unlisted **Modifiers:** *See Inside Back Cover* Ⓜ Maternity A2–Z3 ASC Payment Indicators A–Y OPPS Status Indicators

514 CPT © 2015 American Medical Association. All Rights Reserved. © 2016 DecisionHealth

Testis Procedures

Excisional Testis Procedures

54500 Biopsy of testis, needle (separate procedure) ♂ A2 T

RVU			Global Days	Modifiers				
Mod	Non-Fac Total	Fac Total		51	50	62	80	MUE
	2.14	2.14	000	2	1	0	0	1

Biopsy of testis

Tissue mass

Incisional (54505)   Needle (54500)

54505 Biopsy of testis, incisional (separate procedure) ♂ A2 T

RVU			Global Days	Modifiers				
Mod	Non-Fac Total	Fac Total		51	50	62	80	MUE
	6.04	6.04	010	2	1	0	0	1

AMA: Oct 01: 8

54512 Excision of extraparenchymal lesion of testis ♂ A2 T

RVU			Global Days	Modifiers				
Mod	Non-Fac Total	Fac Total		51	50	62	80	MUE
	15.52	15.52	090	2	1	1	1	1

AMA: Oct 01: 8, Aug 05: 13

54520 Orchiectomy, simple (including subcapsular), with or without testicular prosthesis, scrotal or inguinal approach ♂ A2 T

RVU			Global Days	Modifiers				
Mod	Non-Fac Total	Fac Total		51	50	62	80	MUE
	9.32	9.32	090	2	1	0	1	1

AMA: Winter 94: 13, Oct 01: 8, Mar 04: 3

54522 Orchiectomy, partial ♂ A2 T

RVU			Global Days	Modifiers				
Mod	Non-Fac Total	Fac Total		51	50	62	80	MUE
	17.81	17.81	090	2	1	1	2	1

AMA: Oct 01: 8

54530 Orchiectomy, radical, for tumor; inguinal approach ♂ A2 T

RVU			Global Days	Modifiers				
Mod	Non-Fac Total	Fac Total		51	50	62	80	MUE
	14.51	14.51	090	2	1	1	2	1

AMA: Oct 01: 8

54535 Orchiectomy, radical, for tumor; with abdominal exploration ♂ T

RVU			Global Days	Modifiers				
Mod	Non-Fac Total	Fac Total		51	50	62	80	MUE
	21.36	21.36	090	2	1	0	2	1

AMA: Oct 01: 8

Testis Exploration

54550 Exploration for undescended testis (inguinal or scrotal area) ♂ A2 T

RVU			Global Days	Modifiers				
Mod	Non-Fac Total	Fac Total		51	50	62	80	MUE
	14.19	14.19	090	2	1	0	2	1

AMA: Oct 01: 8

54560 Exploration for undescended testis with abdominal exploration ♂ G2 T

RVU			Global Days	Modifiers				
Mod	Non-Fac Total	Fac Total		51	50	62	80	MUE
	19.74	19.74	090	2	1	1	2	1

AMA: Oct 01: 8

Testis Repair

54600 Reduction of torsion of testis, surgical, with or without fixation of contralateral testis ♂ A2 T

RVU			Global Days	Modifiers				
Mod	Non-Fac Total	Fac Total		51	50	62	80	MUE
	13.08	13.08	090	2	1	0	1	1

AMA: Aug 05: 13

54620 Fixation of contralateral testis (separate procedure) ♂ A2 T

RVU			Global Days	Modifiers				
Mod	Non-Fac Total	Fac Total		51	50	62	80	MUE
	8.65	8.65	010	2	1	0	1	1

Coding Guidance

A separate code for hernia repair may be reported with the appropriate modifier if the hernia repair is done at a different site through a separate incision.

54640 Orchiopexy, inguinal approach, with or without hernia repair ♂ A2 T

RVU			Global Days	Modifiers				
Mod	Non-Fac Total	Fac Total		51	50	62	80	MUE
	13.77	13.77	090	2	1	0	0	1

AMA: Oct 01: 8, Jan 04: 27, Mar 04: 10, Jun 08: 4

54650 Orchiopexy, abdominal approach, for intra-abdominal testis (eg, Fowler-Stephens) ♂ T

RVU			Global Days	Modifiers				
Mod	Non-Fac Total	Fac Total		51	50	62	80	MUE
	20.39	20.39	090	2	1	0	2	1

AMA: Nov 99: 26, May 00: 4, Oct 01: 8

54660 Insertion of testicular prosthesis (separate procedure) ♂ A2 J1

RVU			Global Days	Modifiers				
Mod	Non-Fac Total	Fac Total		51	50	62	80	MUE
	10.25	10.25	090	2	1	0	0	1

AMA: Oct 01: 8

54670 Suture or repair of testicular injury ♂ A2 T

© 2016 DecisionHealth CPT © 2015 American Medical Association. All Rights Reserved.

Coding Tip: *Bilateral procedure - add modifier 50*

Mod	Non-Fac Total	Fac Total	Global Days	51	50	62	80	MUE
	11.61	11.61	090	2	1	0	0	1

AMA: Oct 01: 8

54680 Transplantation of testis(es) to thigh (because of scrotal destruction) ♂ A2 T

Mod	Non-Fac Total	Fac Total	Global Days	51	50	62	80	MUE
	22.75	22.75	090	2	1	1	2	1

AMA: Oct 01: 8

Laparoscopic Testis Procedures

54690 Laparoscopy, surgical; orchiectomy ♂ A2 J1

Mod	Non-Fac Total	Fac Total	Global Days	51	50	62	80	MUE
	21.35	21.35	090	2	1	1	2	1

AMA: Nov 99: 26, Mar 00: 5, Oct 01: 8

54692 Laparoscopy, surgical; orchiopexy for intra-abdominal testis ♂ G2 J1

Mod	Non-Fac Total	Fac Total	Global Days	51	50	62	80	MUE
	24.69	24.69	090	2	1	0	1	1

AMA: Nov 99: 27, May 00: 4, Oct 01: 8

54699 Unlisted laparoscopy procedure, testis ♂ X J1

Mod	Non-Fac Total	Fac Total	Global Days	51	50	62	80	MUE
	0.00	0.00	YYY	2	1	1	2	

AMA: Nov 99: 27, Mar 00: 9

Epididymis Procedures

Epididymal Incision and Drainage

54700 Incision and drainage of epididymis, testis and/or scrotal space (eg, abscess or hematoma) ♂ A2 T

Mod	Non-Fac Total	Fac Total	Global Days	51	50	62	80	MUE
	6.15	6.15	010	2	1	0	1	1

AMA: Oct 01: 8

Excisional Epididymis Procedures

54800 Biopsy of epididymis, needle ♂ A2 T

Mod	Non-Fac Total	Fac Total	Global Days	51	50	62	80	MUE
	3.67	3.67	000	2	1	0	0	1

AMA: Oct 01: 8

54830 Excision of local lesion of epididymis ♂ A2 T

Mod	Non-Fac Total	Fac Total	Global Days	51	50	62	80	MUE
	10.70	10.70	090	2	1	0	0	1

AMA: Oct 01: 8

54840 Excision of spermatocele, with or without epididymectomy ♂ A2 T

Mod	Non-Fac Total	Fac Total	Global Days	51	50	62	80	MUE
	9.20	9.20	090	2	1	0	1	1

AMA: Oct 01: 8

54860 Epididymectomy; unilateral ♂ A2 T

Mod	Non-Fac Total	Fac Total	Global Days	51	50	62	80	MUE
	12.03	12.03	090	2	0	0	1	1

54861 Epididymectomy; bilateral ♂ A2 T

Mod	Non-Fac Total	Fac Total	Global Days	51	50	62	80	MUE
	16.28	16.28	090	2	0	0	0	1

Epididymal Exploration

54865 Exploration of epididymis, with or without biopsy ♂ A2 T

Mod	Non-Fac Total	Fac Total	Global Days	51	50	62	80	MUE
	10.29	10.29	090	2	0	0	0	1

Epididymal Repair

54900 Epididymovasostomy, anastomosis of epididymis to vas deferens; unilateral ♂⚥ A2 T

Mod	Non-Fac Total	Fac Total	Global Days	51	50	62	80	MUE
	24.21	24.21	090	2	0	0	0	1

AMA: Nov 98: 16, Jun 04: 11

54901 Epididymovasostomy, anastomosis of epididymis to vas deferens; bilateral ♂ A2 T

Mod	Non-Fac Total	Fac Total	Global Days	51	50	62	80	MUE
	31.95	31.95	090	2	2	0	0	1

AMA: Nov 98: 16, Jun 04: 11

Tunica Vaginalis Procedures

Incisional Tunica Vaginalis Procedures

Coding Guidance
Hydrocele puncture aspiration is already included in hernia repairs and procedures involving the tunica vaginalis, scrotum, and vas deferens.

55000 Puncture aspiration of hydrocele, tunica vaginalis, with or without injection of medication ♂ P3 T

Coding Tip: *For a bilateral procedure - add modifier 50*

Mod	Non-Fac Total	Fac Total	Global Days	51	50	62	80	MUE
	3.34	2.44	000	2	1	0	1	1

Excisional Tunica Vaginalis Procedures

55040 Excision of hydrocele; unilateral ♂ A2 T

Mod	Non-Fac Total	Fac Total	Global Days	51	50	62	80	MUE
	9.69	9.69	090	2	0	0	1	1

AMA: Jun 08: 4

55041 Excision of hydrocele; bilateral ♂ A2 T

Mod	Non-Fac Total	Fac Total	Global Days	51	50	62	80	MUE
	14.65	14.65	090	2	2	0	1	1

● New ▲ Revised ✖ Deleted ⊙ Moderate Sedation ✚ Add-on Codes ⊖ High Risk Denial ⒶAge Edit ♀ Female ♂ Male **AMA** CPT® Assistant **MUE** Medically Unlikely Edit · ⊘ Modifier 51 Exempt ⊖ Modifier 63 Exempt ✗ Unlisted **Modifiers:** See Inside Back Cover Ⓜ Maternity A2–Z3 ASC Payment Indicators A–Y OPPS Status Indicators

516   CPT © 2015 American Medical Association. All Rights Reserved.   © 2016 DecisionHealth

Tunica Vaginalis Repair

55060 Repair of tunica vaginalis hydrocele (Bottle type)

♂ A 2 T

RVU			Global Days	Modifiers				
Mod	Non-Fac Total	Fac Total		51	50	62	80	MUE
	10.93	10.93	090	2	1	0	0	1

AMA: Nov 14: 14

Scrotal Procedures

Incisional Scrotal Procedures

55100 Drainage of scrotal wall abscess

♂ A 2 T

RVU			Global Days	Modifiers				
Mod	Non-Fac Total	Fac Total		51	50	62	80	MUE
	6.15	4.78	010	2	0	0	1	2

Drainage of scrotal wall abscess

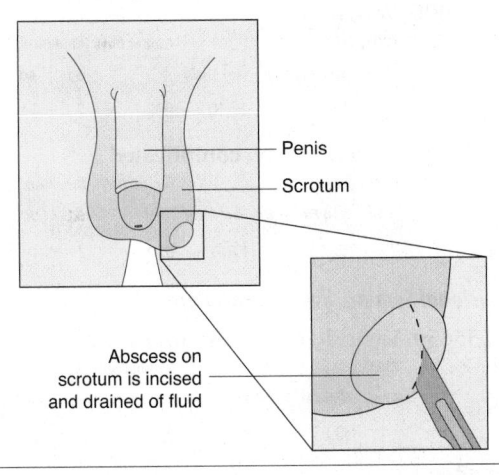

- Penis
- Scrotum

Abscess on scrotum is incised and drained of fluid

55110 Scrotal exploration

♂ A 2 T

RVU			Global Days	Modifiers				
Mod	Non-Fac Total	Fac Total		51	50	62	80	MUE
	11.14	11.14	090	2	0	0	1	1

55120 Removal of foreign body in scrotum

♂ A 2 T

Coding Tip: Do not code local anesthesia

Coding Tip: Closure is included. For scrotoplasty repair - 55175-55180

RVU			Global Days	Modifiers				
Mod	Non-Fac Total	Fac Total		51	50	62	80	MUE
	10.25	10.25	090	2	0	0	0	1

Excisional Scrotal Procedures

55150 Resection of scrotum

♂ A 2 T

RVU			Global Days	Modifiers				
Mod	Non-Fac Total	Fac Total		51	50	62	80	MUE
	14.13	14.13	090	2	0	1	2	1

Scrotal Repair

55175 Scrotoplasty; simple

♂ A 2 T

RVU			Global Days	Modifiers				
Mod	Non-Fac Total	Fac Total		51	50	62	80	MUE
	10.40	10.40	090	2	0	0	0	1

AMA: Dec 14: 16

55180 Scrotoplasty; complicated

♂ A 2 J 1

Documentation Finder: The documentation may have reference to a defective or damaged scrotum, but it also can be performed for gender reassignment surgery.

RVU			Global Days	Modifiers				
Mod	Non-Fac Total	Fac Total		51	50	62	80	MUE
	19.93	19.93	090	2	0	0	0	1

Vas Deferens Procedures

Incisional Vas Deferens Procedures

55200 Vasotomy, cannulization with or without incision of vas, unilateral or bilateral (separate procedure)

♂ A 2 T

RVU			Global Days	Modifiers				
Mod	Non-Fac Total	Fac Total		51	50	62	80	MUE
	12.37	7.98	090	2	2	0	0	1

Excisional Vas Deferens Procedures

55250 Vasectomy, unilateral or bilateral (separate procedure), including postoperative semen examination(s)

∞ ♂ A 2 T

Coding Tip: Vasectomy is often included as a component of a more complex procedure

Coding Tip: Report this procedure separately only when performed alone, or distinct from other procedures on the same day

RVU			Global Days	Modifiers				
Mod	Non-Fac Total	Fac Total		51	50	62	80	MUE
	10.89	6.51	090	2	2	0	1	1

AMA: Jun 98: 10, Jul 98: 10

Introduction Vas Deferens Procedures

55300 Vasotomy for vasograms, seminal vesiculograms, or epididymograms, unilateral or bilateral

∞ N 1 N

Coding Tip: Vasogram, vesiculogram, or epididymogram - 74440

RVU			Global Days	Modifiers				
Mod	Non-Fac Total	Fac Total		51	50	62	80	MUE
	5.39	5.39	000	2	2	0	0	1

Vas Deferens Repair

55400 Vasovasostomy, vasovasorrhaphy

♂ A 2 T

RVU			Global Days	Modifiers				
Mod	Non-Fac Total	Fac Total		51	50	62	80	MUE
	14.66	14.66	090	2	1	1	2	1

AMA: Nov 98: 16, Oct 01: 8, Jun 04: 11

● New   ▲ Revised   Deleted   ⊙ Moderate Sedation   ✚ Add-on Codes   ⊘ High Risk Denial   Ⓐ Age Edit   ♀ Female   ♂ Male   **AMA** *CPT Assistant*   **MUE** Medically Unlikely Edit
⊘ Modifier 51 Exempt   ⊖ Modifier 63 Exempt   ✗ Unlisted   **Modifiers:** *See Inside Back Cover*   Ⓜ Maternity   A 2 - Z 3 ASC Payment Indicators   A - Y OPPS Status Indicators

Surgical Procedures

55450 – 55706

Vas Deferens Ligation

55450 Ligation (percutaneous) of vas deferens, unilateral or bilateral (separate procedure) ⊘♂ P 3 T

Mod	RVU Non-Fac Total	Fac Total	Global Days	Modifiers 51	50	62	80	MUE
	10.20	7.38	010	2	2	0	0	1

Ligation (percutaneous) of vas deferens

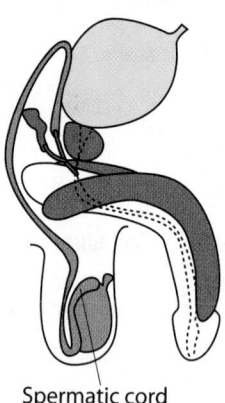

Spermatic cord

The physician ties off one or both of the vas deferens.

Spermatic Cord Procedures

Excisional Spermatic Cord Procedures

55500 Excision of hydrocele of spermatic cord, unilateral (separate procedure) ♂ A 2 T

Mod	RVU Non-Fac Total	Fac Total	Global Days	Modifiers 51	50	62	80	MUE
	11.35	11.35	090	2	1	0	0	1

AMA: Oct 01: 8

55520 Excision of lesion of spermatic cord (separate procedure) ♂ A 2 T

Mod	RVU Non-Fac Total	Fac Total	Global Days	Modifiers 51	50	62	80	MUE
	13.02	13.02	090	2	1	1	2	1

AMA: Sep 00: 10, Oct 01: 8

55530 Excision of varicocele or ligation of spermatic veins for varicocele; (separate procedure) ♂ A 2 T

Mod	RVU Non-Fac Total	Fac Total	Global Days	Modifiers 51	50	62	80	MUE
	10.08	10.08	090	2	1	1	1	1

AMA: Oct 01: 8

55535 Excision of varicocele or ligation of spermatic veins for varicocele; abdominal approach ♂ A 2 T

Mod	RVU Non-Fac Total	Fac Total	Global Days	Modifiers 51	50	62	80	MUE
	12.36	12.36	090	2	1	1	2	1

AMA: Oct 01: 8

55540 Excision of varicocele or ligation of spermatic veins for varicocele; with hernia repair ♂ A 2 T

Mod	RVU Non-Fac Total	Fac Total	Global Days	Modifiers 51	50	62	80	MUE
	15.65	15.65	090	2	1	1	1	1

AMA: Oct 01: 8

Laparoscopic Spermatic Cord Procedures

55550 Laparoscopy, surgical, with ligation of spermatic veins for varicocele ♂ A 2 J I

Mod	RVU Non-Fac Total	Fac Total	Global Days	Modifiers 51	50	62	80	MUE
	12.34	12.34	090	2	1	1	2	1

AMA: Nov 99: 27, Mar 00: 9, Oct 01: 8

55559 Unlisted laparoscopy procedure, spermatic cord ⊘♂ ✖ J I

Mod	RVU Non-Fac Total	Fac Total	Global Days	Modifiers 51	50	62	80	MUE
	0.00	0.00	YYY	2	1	1	2	

AMA: Nov 99: 27, Mar 00: 9

Seminal Vesicle Procedures

Incisional Seminal Vesicle Procedures

55600 Vesiculotomy ♂ R 2 T

Mod	RVU Non-Fac Total	Fac Total	Global Days	Modifiers 51	50	62	80	MUE
	12.10	12.10	090	2	1	0	0	1

55605 Vesiculotomy; complicated ⊘♂ C

Mod	RVU Non-Fac Total	Fac Total	Global Days	Modifiers 51	50	62	80	MUE
	15.79	15.79	090	2	1	0	0	1

Excisional Seminal Vesicle Procedures

55650 Vesiculectomy, any approach ♂ C

Mod	RVU Non-Fac Total	Fac Total	Global Days	Modifiers 51	50	62	80	MUE
	20.65	20.65	090	2	1	1	2	1

55680 Excision of Mullerian duct cyst ♂ A 2 T

Mod	RVU Non-Fac Total	Fac Total	Global Days	Modifiers 51	50	62	80	MUE
	10.21	10.21	090	2	1	0	0	1

Prostate Procedures

Incisional Prostate Procedures

55700 Biopsy, prostate; needle or punch, single or multiple, any approach ♂ A 2 T

Coding Tip: Ultrasound guidance for correct needle placement - 76942

Mod	RVU Non-Fac Total	Fac Total	Global Days	Modifiers 51	50	62	80	MUE
	6.18	4.01	000	2	0	0	1	1

AMA: May 96: 3, Nov 10: 5

55705 Biopsy, prostate; incisional, any approach ♂ A 2 T

Mod	RVU Non-Fac Total	Fac Total	Global Days	Modifiers 51	50	62	80	MUE
	7.63	7.63	010	2	0	1	1	1

55706 Biopsies, prostate, needle, transperineal, stereotactic template guided saturation sampling, including imaging guidance ♂ G 2 T

Mod	RVU Non-Fac Total	Fac Total	Global Days	Modifiers 51	50	62	80	MUE
	10.72	10.72	010	2	0	1	2	1

AMA: Nov 10: 5

● New   ▲ Revised   ✖ Deleted   ⊙ Moderate Sedation   ✚ Add-on Codes   ⊘ High Risk Denial   Ⓐ Age Edit   ♀ Female   ♂ Male   **AMA** *CPT® Assistant*   **MUE** Medically Unlikely Edit
⊙ Modifier 51 Exempt   ⊖ Modifier 63 Exempt   ✖ Unlisted   **Modifiers:** *See Inside Back Cover*   Ⓜ Maternity   A 2 – Z 3 ASC Payment Indicators   A – Y OPPS Status Indicators

CPT © 2015 American Medical Association. All Rights Reserved.   © 2016 DecisionHealth

55720 Prostatotomy, external drainage of prostatic abscess, any approach; simple ♂ A2 T

RVU			Global Days	Modifiers				
Mod	Non-Fac Total	Fac Total		51	50	62	80	MUE
	13.01	13.01	090	2	0	1	2	1

55725 Prostatotomy, external drainage of prostatic abscess, any approach; complicated ♂ A2 T

RVU			Global Days	Modifiers				
Mod	Non-Fac Total	Fac Total		51	50	62	80	MUE
	17.04	17.04	090	2	0	1	2	1

Excisional Prostate Procedures

Coding Guidance

Cystoplasty or cystourethroplasty is included in the standard of practice for prostatectomy procedures. Code 51800 should not be reported separately with CPT codes 55801-55845. Multiple methods of accomplishing a prostatectomy involving different approaches or procedures that are progressively more comprehensive cannot be reported at the same patient encounter. Prostatectomy codes are mutually exclusive of one another and only one method per given procedure should be reported. In the case of an initial approach failing and a second method being employed, report only the successful method or the last unsuccessful approach used.

55801 Prostatectomy, perineal, subtotal (including control of postoperative bleeding, vasectomy, meatotomy, urethral calibration and/or dilation, and internal urethrotomy) ♂ C

RVU			Global Days	Modifiers				
Mod	Non-Fac Total	Fac Total		51	50	62	80	MUE
	31.67	31.67	090	2	0	1	2	1

AMA: Jun 03: 6, 7

55810 Prostatectomy, perineal radical ♂ C

RVU			Global Days	Modifiers				
Mod	Non-Fac Total	Fac Total		51	50	62	80	MUE
	37.94	37.94	090	2	0	1	2	1

AMA: Jun 03: 7

Radical perineal prostatectomy

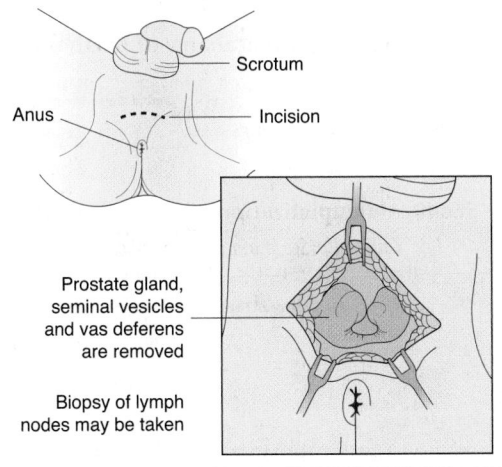

Scrotum
Anus
Incision
Prostate gland, seminal vesicles and vas deferens are removed
Biopsy of lymph nodes may be taken

55812 Prostatectomy, perineal radical; with lymph node biopsy(s) (limited pelvic lymphadenectomy) ♂ C

RVU			Global Days	Modifiers				
Mod	Non-Fac Total	Fac Total		51	50	62	80	MUE
	46.27	46.27	090	2	0	1	2	1

55815 Prostatectomy, perineal radical; with bilateral pelvic lymphadenectomy, including external iliac, hypogastric and obturator nodes ♂ C

RVU			Global Days	Modifiers				
Mod	Non-Fac Total	Fac Total		51	50	62	80	MUE
	50.94	50.94	090	2	2	1	2	1

55821 Prostatectomy (including control of postoperative bleeding, vasectomy, meatotomy, urethral calibration and/or dilation, and internal urethrotomy); suprapubic, subtotal, 1 or 2 stages ♂ C

RVU			Global Days	Modifiers				
Mod	Non-Fac Total	Fac Total		51	50	62	80	MUE
	25.11	25.11	090	2	0	1	2	1

AMA: Jun 03: 6

55831 Prostatectomy (including control of postoperative bleeding, vasectomy, meatotomy, urethral calibration and/or dilation, and internal urethrotomy); retropubic, subtotal ♂ C

RVU			Global Days	Modifiers				
Mod	Non-Fac Total	Fac Total		51	50	62	80	MUE
	27.17	27.17	090	2	0	1	2	1

AMA: Jun 03: 7

55840 Prostatectomy, retropubic radical, with or without nerve sparing ♂ C

RVU			Global Days	Modifiers				
Mod	Non-Fac Total	Fac Total		51	50	62	80	MUE
	33.72	33.72	090	2	0	1	2	1

AMA: Jun 03: 8

55842 Prostatectomy, retropubic radical, with or without nerve sparing; with lymph node biopsy(s) (limited pelvic lymphadenectomy) ♂ C

RVU			Global Days	Modifiers				
Mod	Non-Fac Total	Fac Total		51	50	62	80	MUE
	33.69	33.69	090	2	0	1	2	1

AMA: Jun 03: 8

55845 Prostatectomy, retropubic radical, with or without nerve sparing; with bilateral pelvic lymphadenectomy, including external iliac, hypogastric, and obturator nodes ♂ C

RVU			Global Days	Modifiers				
Mod	Non-Fac Total	Fac Total		51	50	62	80	MUE
	39.27	39.27	090	2	2	1	2	1

AMA: Jun 03: 8

Coding Guidance

Application of the radioactive elements into the tissue after exposure of the prostate is reported separately with 77776-77778.

55860 Exposure of prostate, any approach, for insertion of radioactive substance ♂ G2 T

RVU			Global Days	Modifiers				
Mod	Non-Fac Total	Fac Total		51	50	62	80	MUE
	25.15	25.15	090	2	0	1	1	1

● New　▲ Revised　Deleted　⊙ Moderate Sedation　✚ Add-on Codes　⊘ High Risk Denial　Ⓐ Age Edit　♀ Female　♂ Male　**AMA** *CPT® Assistant*　*MUE* Medically Unlikely Edit
⊗ Modifier 51 Exempt　⊖ Modifier 63 Exempt　✗ Unlisted　**Modifiers:** *See Inside Back Cover*　Ⓜ Maternity　A2–Z3 ASC Payment Indicators　A–Y OPPS Status Indicators

© 2016 DecisionHealth　　CPT © 2015 American Medical Association. All Rights Reserved.　　**519**

55862 Exposure of prostate, any approach, for insertion of radioactive substance; with lymph node biopsy(s) (limited pelvic lymphadenectomy) ♂C

RVU		Global Days	Modifiers				
Mod	Non-Fac Total	Fac Total		51	50	62	80	MUE
	33.17	33.17	090	2	0	1	2	1

55865 Exposure of prostate, any approach, for insertion of radioactive substance; with bilateral pelvic lymphadenectomy, including external iliac, hypogastric and obturator nodes ♂C

RVU		Global Days	Modifiers				
Mod	Non-Fac Total	Fac Total		51	50	62	80	MUE
	38.36	38.36	090	2	2	1	2	1

Laparoscopic Prostate Procedures

55866 Laparoscopy, surgical prostatectomy, retropubic radical, including nerve sparing, includes robotic assistance, when performed ♂C

RVU		Global Days	Modifiers				
Mod	Non-Fac Total	Fac Total		51	50	62	80	MUE
	40.28	40.28	090	2	0	1	2	1

AMA: Jun 03: 8, Mar 12: 10

Other Prostate Procedures

55870 Electroejaculation ♂P3T

RVU		Global Days	Modifiers				
Mod	Non-Fac Total	Fac Total		51	50	62	80	MUE
	5.01	4.09	000	2	0	1	1	1

55873 Cryosurgical ablation of the prostate (includes ultrasonic guidance and monitoring) ♂J8JI

RVU		Global Days	Modifiers				
Mod	Non-Fac Total	Fac Total		51	50	62	80	MUE
	200.30	22.07	090	2	0	0	1	1

AMA: Apr 01: 4, Sep 02: 9, Jun 03: 8, Feb 10: 7
Pub 100-04, 32, 180.2

55875 Transperineal placement of needles or catheters into prostate for interstitial radioelement application, with or without cystoscopy ♂A2Q3

Coding Tip: Subsequent placement of the interstitial radioactive sources is reported with 77776-77778; ultrasound guidance for the radioelement placement is reported with 76965.

RVU		Global Days	Modifiers				
Mod	Non-Fac Total	Fac Total		51	50	62	80	MUE
	21.92	21.92	090	2	0	0	0	1

AMA: May 07: 1, Apr 09: 3

55876 Placement of interstitial device(s) for radiation therapy guidance (eg, fiducial markers, dosimeter), prostate (via needle, any approach), single or multiple ♂P3S

Coding Tip: Radiological guidance for correct placement of devices - ultrasound 76942; fluoroscopy 77002; CT 77012; MRI 77021

RVU		Global Days	Modifiers				
Mod	Non-Fac Total	Fac Total		51	50	62	80	MUE
	3.86	2.89	000	2	0	1	1	1

AMA: May 07: 1, Oct 07: 1, Feb 10: 7, 12

55899 Unlisted procedure, male genital system ♂✗T

RVU		Global Days	Modifiers				
Mod	Non-Fac Total	Fac Total		51	50	62	80	MUE
	0.00	0.00	YYY	2	0	1	0	

AMA: Jun 03: 8, May 07: 11, Jun 15: 5

Reproductive System Procedures

55920 Placement of needles or catheters into pelvic organs and/or genitalia (except prostate) for subsequent interstitial radioelement application G2T

Coding Tip: Subsequent placement of the interstitial radioactive sources is reported with 77776-77778; ultrasound guidance for the radioelement application is reported with 76965.

RVU		Global Days	Modifiers				
Mod	Non-Fac Total	Fac Total		51	50	62	80	MUE
	12.89	12.89	000	2	0	0	0	1

AMA: Apr 09: 10

Intersex Procedures

55970 Intersex surgery; male to female ♂T

RVU		Global Days	Modifiers				
Mod	Non-Fac Total	Fac Total		51	50	62	80	MUE
	0.00	0.00	YYY	9	9	9	9	

55980 Intersex surgery; female to male ♀T

RVU		Global Days	Modifiers				
Mod	Non-Fac Total	Fac Total		51	50	62	80	MUE
	0.00	0.00	YYY	9	9	9	9	

Female Genital System

Vulvar/Perineum/Introitus Procedures

Incisional Vulvar/Perineum/Introitus Procedures

56405 Incision and drainage of vulva or perineal abscess ♀P3T

RVU		Global Days	Modifiers				
Mod	Non-Fac Total	Fac Total		51	50	62	80	MUE
	3.10	3.08	010	2	0	2	1	2

56420 Incision and drainage of Bartholin's gland abscess ♀P3T

RVU		Global Days	Modifiers				
Mod	Non-Fac Total	Fac Total		51	50	62	80	MUE
	3.45	2.59	010	2	0	0	1	1

56440 Marsupialization of Bartholin's gland cyst ♀A2T

Coding Tip: See also incision of Bartholin's gland abscess - 56420

RVU		Global Days	Modifiers				
Mod	Non-Fac Total	Fac Total		51	50	62	80	MUE
	5.18	5.18	010	2	0	0	1	1

CPT © 2015 American Medical Association. All Rights Reserved.

56441 Lysis of labial adhesions ♀ A2 T

Coding Tip: See also plastic repair of introitus - 56800

RVU			Global Days	Modifiers				
Mod	Non-Fac Total	Fac Total		51	50	62	80	MUE
	4.09	3.94	010	2	0	0	0	1

AMA: Winter 90: 7

Lysis of labial adhesions

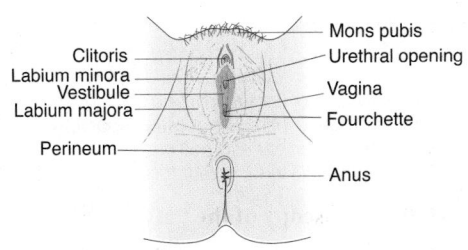

The physician fixes a condition in which the
two major lips of the vagina are stuck together.

56442 Hymenotomy, simple incision ♀ A2 T

Coding Tip: See also partial removal of the hymen or revision of hymenal ring - 56700

RVU			Global Days	Modifiers				
Mod	Non-Fac Total	Fac Total		51	50	62	80	MUE
	1.36	1.36	000	2	0	0	0	1

Destruction Vulvar/Perineum/Introitus Procedures

56501 Destruction of lesion(s), vulva; simple (eg, laser surgery, electrosurgery, cryosurgery, chemosurgery) ♀ P3 T

Coding Tip: Do not code local anesthesia

RVU			Global Days	Modifiers				
Mod	Non-Fac Total	Fac Total		51	50	62	80	MUE
	3.71	3.27	010	2	0	0	1	1

56515 Destruction of lesion(s), vulva; extensive (eg, laser surgery, electrosurgery, cryosurgery, chemosurgery) ♀ A2 T

RVU			Global Days	Modifiers				
Mod	Non-Fac Total	Fac Total		51	50	62	80	MUE
	6.43	5.75	010	2	0	0	1	1

Excisional Vulvar/Perineum/Introitus Procedures

56605 Biopsy of vulva or perineum (separate procedure); 1 lesion ♀ P3 T

Coding Tip: Code 99000 for specimen transfer from office setting to an outside laboratory

Coding Tip: Biopsy is usually included as a component of a more complex procedure, such as lesion excision

RVU			Global Days	Modifiers				
Mod	Non-Fac Total	Fac Total		51	50	62	80	MUE
	2.33	1.72	000	2	0	2	1	1

AMA: Sep 00: 9, Jun 08: 6

+ 56606 Biopsy of vulva or perineum (separate procedure); each separate additional lesion (List separately in addition to code for primary procedure) ♀ N N

RVU			Global Days	Modifiers				
Mod	Non-Fac Total	Fac Total		51	50	62	80	MUE
	1.08	0.85	ZZZ	0	0	2	1	6

56620 Vulvectomy simple; partial ♀ A2 T

RVU			Global Days	Modifiers				
Mod	Non-Fac Total	Fac Total		51	50	62	80	MUE
	14.91	14.91	090	2	0	1	2	1

AMA: Dec 13: 14

56625 Vulvectomy simple; complete ♀ A2 T

RVU			Global Days	Modifiers				
Mod	Non-Fac Total	Fac Total		51	50	62	80	MUE
	18.04	18.04	090	2	0	1	2	1

56630 Vulvectomy, radical, partial ♀ C

RVU			Global Days	Modifiers				
Mod	Non-Fac Total	Fac Total		51	50	62	80	MUE
	26.72	26.72	090	2	0	1	2	1

56631 Vulvectomy, radical, partial; with unilateral inguinofemoral lymphadenectomy ♀ C

RVU			Global Days	Modifiers				
Mod	Non-Fac Total	Fac Total		51	50	62	80	MUE
	34.10	34.10	090	2	0	2	2	1

56632 Vulvectomy, radical, partial; with bilateral inguinofemoral lymphadenectomy ♀ C

RVU			Global Days	Modifiers				
Mod	Non-Fac Total	Fac Total		51	50	62	80	MUE
	39.58	39.58	090	2	2	2	2	1

56633 Vulvectomy, radical, complete ♀ C

RVU			Global Days	Modifiers				
Mod	Non-Fac Total	Fac Total		51	50	62	80	MUE
	34.92	34.92	090	2	0	2	2	1

Vulvectomy radical, complete

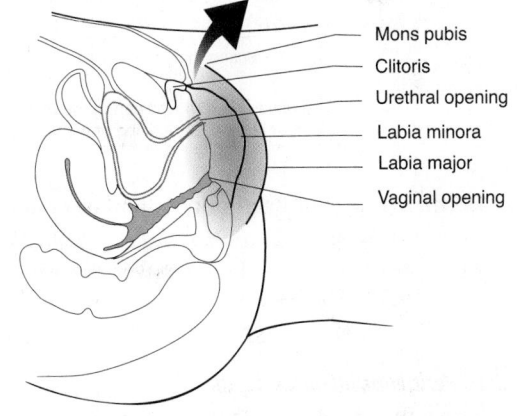

Complete (56633); with unilateral inguinofemeral
lymphadenectomy (56634); with bilateral inguinofemoral
lymphadenectomy (56637); with inguinofemoral, iliac,
and pelvic lymphadenectomy (56640)

● New ▲ Revised Deleted ⊙ Moderate Sedation ✚ Add-on Codes ⊘ High Risk Denial Ⓐ Age Edit ♀ Female ♂ Male **AMA** *CPT® Assistant* *MUE* Medically Unlikely Edit
⊘ Modifier 51 Exempt ⊖ Modifier 63 Exempt ✗ Unlisted **Modifiers:** *See Inside Back Cover* Ⓜ Maternity A2 – Z3 ASC Payment Indicators A – Y OPPS Status Indicators

56634 Vulvectomy, radical, complete; with unilateral inguinofemoral lymphadenectomy ♀C

RVU			Global Days	Modifiers				
Mod	Non-Fac Total	Fac Total		51	50	62	80	MUE
	37.80	37.80	090	2	0	2	2	1

56637 Vulvectomy, radical, complete; with bilateral inguinofemoral lymphadenectomy ♀C

RVU			Global Days	Modifiers				
Mod	Non-Fac Total	Fac Total		51	50	62	80	MUE
	43.43	43.43	090	2	0	2	2	1

56640 Vulvectomy, radical, complete, with inguinofemoral, iliac, and pelvic lymphadenectomy ♀C

RVU			Global Days	Modifiers				
Mod	Non-Fac Total	Fac Total		51	50	62	80	MUE
	43.84	43.84	090	2	1	1	2	1

56700 Partial hymenectomy or revision of hymenal ring ♀A 2 T

RVU			Global Days	Modifiers				
Mod	Non-Fac Total	Fac Total		51	50	62	80	MUE
	5.29	5.29	010	2	0	1	2	1

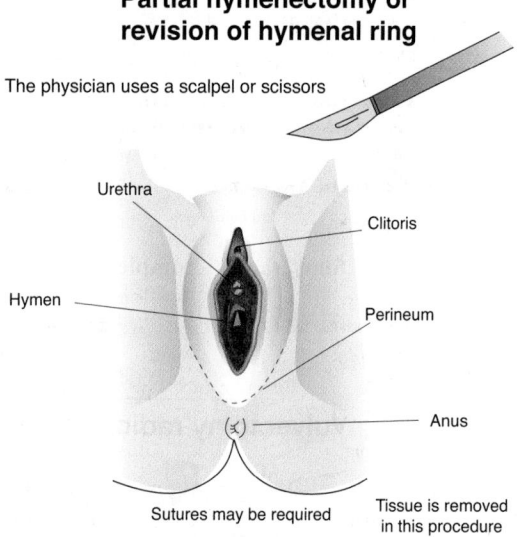

Partial hymenectomy or revision of hymenal ring

The physician uses a scalpel or scissors

Urethra

Clitoris

Hymen

Perineum

Anus

Sutures may be required

Tissue is removed in this procedure

The physician removes part of the membrane that covers the opening of the vagina.

56740 Excision of Bartholin's gland or cyst ♀A 2 T

Coding Tip: Marsupialization of Bartholin's gland cyst - 56440

RVU			Global Days	Modifiers				
Mod	Non-Fac Total	Fac Total		51	50	62	80	MUE
	8.57	8.57	010	2	1	0	1	1

Vulvar/Perineum/Introitus Repair

56800 Plastic repair of introitus ♀A 2 T

RVU			Global Days	Modifiers				
Mod	Non-Fac Total	Fac Total		51	50	62	80	MUE
	6.84	6.84	010	2	0	1	2	1

56805 Clitoroplasty for intersex state ♀G 2 T

RVU			Global Days	Modifiers				
Mod	Non-Fac Total	Fac Total		51	50	62	80	MUE
	33.17	33.17	090	2	0	1	2	1

56810 Perineoplasty, repair of perineum, nonobstetrical (separate procedure) ♀♂A 2 T

RVU			Global Days	Modifiers				
Mod	Non-Fac Total	Fac Total		51	50	62	80	MUE
	7.39	7.39	010	2	0	2	2	1

Endoscopic Vulvar/Perineum/Introitus Procedures

Coding Guidance

Diagnostic colposcopies should not be reported with other colposcopic procedures. Colposcopy code 56820 should not be reported when used to scout out the anatomy of the surgical field or to confirm a lesion or mass prior to a surgical procedure. When a diagnostic colposcopy is done separately and results in the decision to perform a noncolposcopic procedure, it may be reported with modifier 58 to show that the two are staged procedures.

56820 Colposcopy of the vulva ♀P 3 T

Coding Tip: Report 56820 when performed as a separate procedure alone or when performed independently, distinct from or unrelated to other procedures

Coding Tip: Colposcopies of multiple sites may be reported using modifier 51

RVU			Global Days	Modifiers				
Mod	Non-Fac Total	Fac Total		51	50	62	80	MUE
	3.20	2.48	000	2	0	0	1	1

AMA: Feb 03: 5

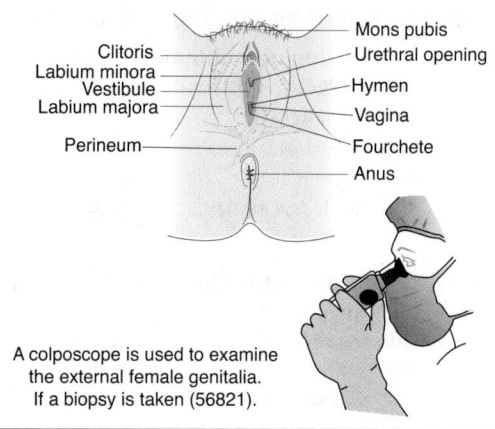

Colposcopy of the vulva

Mons pubis

Clitoris

Labium minora

Vestibule

Labium majora

Urethral opening

Hymen

Vagina

Perineum

Fourchete

Anus

A colposcope is used to examine the external female genitalia. If a biopsy is taken (56821).

56821 Colposcopy of the vulva; with biopsy(s) ♀P 3 T

RVU			Global Days	Modifiers				
Mod	Non-Fac Total	Fac Total		51	50	62	80	MUE
	4.21	3.31	000	2	0	0	1	1

AMA: Feb 03: 5, Jun 03: 11

Vaginal Procedures

Incisional Vaginal Procedures

Coding Guidance

A pelvic exam done in conjunction with a gynecological procedure, either to confirm the procedure or as a necessary part of it, is not reported separately. A diagnostic pelvic exam done to evaluate the need for a surgical procedure is included in the evaluation and management service at the time the decision to perform the procedure is made.

● New   ▲ Revised   ✖ Deleted   ⊙ Moderate Sedation   ✚ Add-on Codes   ⊗ High Risk Denial   Ⓐ Age Edit   ♀ Female   ♂ Male   **AMA** CPT® Assistant   **MUE** Medically Unlikely Edit
Ⓝ Modifier 51 Exempt   ⊖ Modifier 63 Exempt   ✗ Unlisted   **Modifiers:** See Inside Back Cover   Ⓜ Maternity   A 2 – Z 3 ASC Payment Indicators   A – Y OPPS Status Indicators

CPT © 2015 American Medical Association. All Rights Reserved.   © 2016 DecisionHealth

57000 Colpotomy; with exploration ♀ A 2 T

RVU			Global Days	Modifiers				
Mod	Non-Fac Total	Fac Total		51	50	62	80	MUE
	5.35	5.35	010	2	0	0	0	1

AMA: Nov 07: 1

Colpotomy

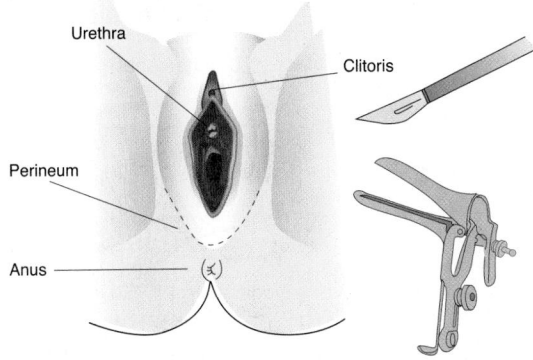

The physician makes an incision in the wall of the vagina, then examines the area around and behind the vagina for signs of disease or injury.

57010 Colpotomy; with drainage of pelvic abscess ♀ A 2 T

RVU			Global Days	Modifiers				
Mod	Non-Fac Total	Fac Total		51	50	62	80	MUE
	12.32	12.32	090	2	0	0	0	1

57020 Colpocentesis (separate procedure) ♀ A 2 T

RVU			Global Days	Modifiers				
Mod	Non-Fac Total	Fac Total		51	50	62	80	MUE
	2.64	2.30	000	2	0	0	0	1

57022 Incision and drainage of vaginal hematoma; obstetrical/postpartum ♀ R 2 T

RVU			Global Days	Modifiers				
Mod	Non-Fac Total	Fac Total		51	50	62	80	MUE
	4.82	4.82	010	2	0	0	0	1

57023 Incision and drainage of vaginal hematoma; non-obstetrical (eg, post-trauma, spontaneous bleeding) ♀ A 2 T

RVU			Global Days	Modifiers				
Mod	Non-Fac Total	Fac Total		51	50	62	80	MUE
	8.79	8.79	010	2	0	0	0	1

Vaginal Destruction Procedures

57061 Destruction of vaginal lesion(s); simple (eg, laser surgery, electrosurgery, cryosurgery, chemosurgery) ♀ P 3 T

Coding Tip: Do not code local anesthesia

RVU			Global Days	Modifiers				
Mod	Non-Fac Total	Fac Total		51	50	62	80	MUE
	3.22	2.79	010	2	0	0	1	1

AMA: Apr 96: 11

57065 Destruction of vaginal lesion(s); extensive (eg, laser surgery, electrosurgery, cryosurgery, chemosurgery) ♀ A 2 T

Coding Tip: Destruction of vulval lesions - 56501-56515

RVU			Global Days	Modifiers				
Mod	Non-Fac Total	Fac Total		51	50	62	80	MUE
	5.54	4.98	010	2	0	0	1	1

AMA: Apr 96: 11

Excisional Vaginal Procedures

57100 Biopsy of vaginal mucosa; simple (separate procedure) ♀ P 3 T

Coding Tip: Report this procedure separately only when performed alone, or distinct from other procedures on the same day

Coding Tip: Simple vaginal mucosal biopsy is usually included as a component of a more complex procedure

RVU			Global Days	Modifiers				
Mod	Non-Fac Total	Fac Total		51	50	62	80	MUE
	2.53	1.91	000	2	0	0	1	3

57105 Biopsy of vaginal mucosa; extensive, requiring suture (including cysts) ♀ A 2 T

Coding Tip: Code 99000 for specimen transfer from office setting to an outside laboratory

Coding Tip: Do not code separate closure of surgical wounds as suture is included in the extensive biopsy

RVU			Global Days	Modifiers				
Mod	Non-Fac Total	Fac Total		51	50	62	80	MUE
	3.88	3.60	010	2	0	0	1	2

57106 Vaginectomy, partial removal of vaginal wall ♀ T

RVU			Global Days	Modifiers				
Mod	Non-Fac Total	Fac Total		51	50	62	80	MUE
	14.21	14.21	090	2	0	1	2	1

AMA: Nov 98: 17, Oct 99: 5

57107 Vaginectomy, partial removal of vaginal wall; with removal of paravaginal tissue (radical vaginectomy) ♀ T

RVU			Global Days	Modifiers				
Mod	Non-Fac Total	Fac Total		51	50	62	80	MUE
	41.72	41.72	090	2	0	1	2	1

AMA: Nov 98: 17, Oct 99: 5

57109 Vaginectomy, partial removal of vaginal wall; with removal of paravaginal tissue (radical vaginectomy) with bilateral total pelvic lymphadenectomy and para-aortic lymph node sampling (biopsy) ♀ T

RVU			Global Days	Modifiers				
Mod	Non-Fac Total	Fac Total		51	50	62	80	MUE
	50.03	50.03	090	2	2	1	2	1

AMA: Nov 98: 17, Oct 99: 5

57110 Vaginectomy, complete removal of vaginal wall ♀ C

RVU			Global Days	Modifiers				
Mod	Non-Fac Total	Fac Total		51	50	62	80	MUE
	25.36	25.36	090	2	0	1	2	1

AMA: Nov 98: 17, Oct 99: 5

● New ▲ Revised Deleted ⊙ Moderate Sedation ✚ Add-on Codes ⊘ High Risk Denial Ⓐ Age Edit ♀ Female ♂ Male **AMA** CPT® Assistant **MUE** Medically Unlikely Edit
⊘ Modifier 51 Exempt ⊖ Modifier 63 Exempt ✗ Unlisted **Modifiers:** See Inside Back Cover Ⓜ Maternity A 2–Z 3 ASC Payment Indicators A–Y OPPS Status Indicators
© 2016 DecisionHealth | CPT © 2015 American Medical Association. All Rights Reserved.

57111 Vaginectomy, complete removal of vaginal wall; with removal of paravaginal tissue (radical vaginectomy) ♀C

RVU			Global Days	Modifiers				
Mod	Non-Fac Total	Fac Total		51	50	62	80	MUE
	45.86	45.86	090	2	2	1	2	1

AMA: Nov 98: 17, Oct 99: 5

57112 Vaginectomy, complete removal of vaginal wall; with removal of paravaginal tissue (radical vaginectomy) with bilateral total pelvic lymphadenectomy and para-aortic lymph node sampling (biopsy) ♂♀C

RVU			Global Days	Modifiers				
Mod	Non-Fac Total	Fac Total		51	50	62	80	MUE
	53.41	53.41	090	2	2	1	2	1

AMA: Nov 98: 17, Oct 99: 5

57120 Colpocleisis (Le Fort type) ♀G2 J I

RVU			Global Days	Modifiers				
Mod	Non-Fac Total	Fac Total		51	50	62	80	MUE
	14.47	14.47	090	2	0	1	2	1

57130 Excision of vaginal septum ♀A2 T

RVU			Global Days	Modifiers				
Mod	Non-Fac Total	Fac Total		51	50	62	80	MUE
	5.01	4.51	010	2	0	1	2	1

57135 Excision of vaginal cyst or tumor ♀A2 T

RVU			Global Days	Modifiers				
Mod	Non-Fac Total	Fac Total		51	50	62	80	MUE
	5.44	4.93	010	2	0	0	1	2

Introduction Vaginal Procedures

57150 Irrigation of vagina and/or application of medicament for treatment of bacterial, parasitic, or fungoid disease ♀N I Q I

Coding Tip: See also 57100 for simple biopsy of vaginal mucosa; 57180 for packing for spontaneous vaginal hemorrhage (nonobstetrical)

RVU			Global Days	Modifiers				
Mod	Non-Fac Total	Fac Total		51	50	62	80	MUE
	1.28	0.82	000	2	0	0	1	1

Coding Guidance

Codes 57155-57156 report the anatomical implantation of the brachytherapy delivery device. Subsequent insertion of intracavitary radioactive sources that are left in the patient is reported with 77761-77763. Subsequent high dose rate brachytherapy delivered through the channels of the implanted device for a specific amount of dwell time and then removed with no radiation left behind in the patient is reported with 77785-77787.

57155 ⊙ Insertion of uterine tandem and/or vaginal ovoids for clinical brachytherapy ♀A2 T

RVU			Global Days	Modifiers				
Mod	Non-Fac Total	Fac Total		51	50	62	80	MUE
	12.24	8.31	000	2	0	2	1	1

AMA: Feb 02: 8, Apr 09: 3

Insertion of uterine tandems/ vaginal ovoids

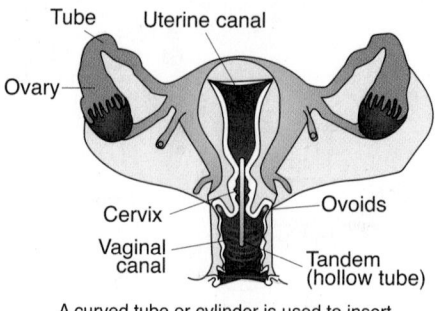

A curved tube or cylinder is used to insert radioactive material in the vagina

57156 Insertion of a vaginal radiation afterloading apparatus for clinical brachytherapy ♀G2 T

RVU			Global Days	Modifiers				
Mod	Non-Fac Total	Fac Total		51	50	62	80	MUE
	5.61	4.18	000	2	0	0	0	1

57160 Fitting and insertion of pessary or other intravaginal support device ♀P3 T

Coding Tip: Add supply of the new pessary or intravaginal device - 99070 or appropriate HCPCS code

Coding Tip: Use this code for the initial fitting and insertion. 57170 may also be coded when a new device is refit to the patient, requiring the physician to take new measurements. When the pessary is removed, cleansed, and reinserted, report the appropriate E&M code

RVU			Global Days	Modifiers				
Mod	Non-Fac Total	Fac Total		51	50	62	80	MUE
	2.16	1.34	000	2	0	0	1	1

AMA: Nov 96: 9, Oct 98: 11, Jun 00: 11, May 10: 10

57170 Diaphragm or cervical cap fitting with instructions ♂♀P3 T

Coding Tip: See also insertion of IUD - 58300

RVU			Global Days	Modifiers				
Mod	Non-Fac Total	Fac Total		51	50	62	80	MUE
	1.72	1.38	000	2	0	0	0	1

57180 Introduction of any hemostatic agent or pack for spontaneous or traumatic nonobstetrical vaginal hemorrhage (separate procedure) ♀A2 T

RVU			Global Days	Modifiers				
Mod	Non-Fac Total	Fac Total		51	50	62	80	MUE
	3.98	3.00	010	2	0	0	1	1

AMA: Nov 07: 1

● New   ▲ Revised   ✖ Deleted   ⊙ Moderate Sedation   ✚ Add-on Codes   ⊗ High Risk Denial   Ⓐ Age Edit   ♀ Female   ♂ Male   **AMA** CPT® Assistant   **MUE** Medically Unlikely Edit
⊗ Modifier 51 Exempt   ⊖ Modifier 63 Exempt   ✗ Unlisted   **Modifiers:** See Inside Back Cover   M Maternity   A2–Z3 ASC Payment Indicators   A–Y OPPS Status Indicators

524   CPT © 2015 American Medical Association. All Rights Reserved.   © 2016 DecisionHealth

Vaginal Repair

57200   Colporrhaphy, suture of injury of vagina (nonobstetrical)   ♀ A 2 T

Coding Tip: Vaginal suture repair in maternity care - 59300

RVU			Global Days	Modifiers				
Mod	Non-Fac Total	Fac Total		51	50	62	80	MUE
	8.55	8.55	090	2	0	1	2	1

57210   Colpoperineorrhaphy, suture of injury of vagina and/or perineum (nonobstetrical)   ♀ A 2 T

Coding Tip: Vaginal suture repair in maternity care - 59300

RVU			Global Days	Modifiers				
Mod	Non-Fac Total	Fac Total		51	50	62	80	MUE
	10.45	10.45	090	2	0	1	2	1

57220   Plastic operation on urethral sphincter, vaginal approach (eg, Kelly urethral plication)   ♀ A 2 J I

RVU			Global Days	Modifiers				
Mod	Non-Fac Total	Fac Total		51	50	62	80	MUE
	9.05	9.05	090	2	0	1	2	1

AMA: Winter 90: 7

57230   Plastic repair of urethrocele   ♀ A 2 T

RVU			Global Days	Modifiers				
Mod	Non-Fac Total	Fac Total		51	50	62	80	MUE
	11.22	11.22	090	2	0	1	2	1

AMA: Winter 90: 7

57240   Anterior colporrhaphy, repair of cystocele with or without repair of urethrocele   ♀ A 2 J I

RVU			Global Days	Modifiers				
Mod	Non-Fac Total	Fac Total		51	50	62	80	MUE
	19.08	19.08	090	2	0	1	2	1

AMA: Winter 90: 7, Jan 97: 3, Jun 02: 5, Jun 10: 6

57250   Posterior colporrhaphy, repair of rectocele with or without perineorrhaphy   ♀ A 2 J I

RVU			Global Days	Modifiers				
Mod	Non-Fac Total	Fac Total		51	50	62	80	MUE
	19.20	19.20	090	2	0	1	2	1

AMA: Winter 90: 7, Jun 02: 4, May 11: 9

57260   Combined anteroposterior colporrhaphy   ♀ A 2 J I

RVU			Global Days	Modifiers				
Mod	Non-Fac Total	Fac Total		51	50	62	80	MUE
	23.63	23.63	090	2	0	1	2	1

AMA: Jun 02: 5, Jun 10: 6

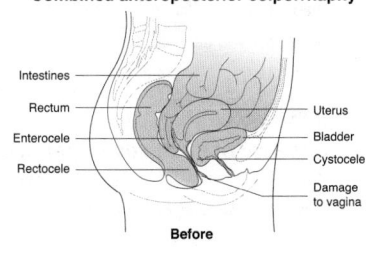
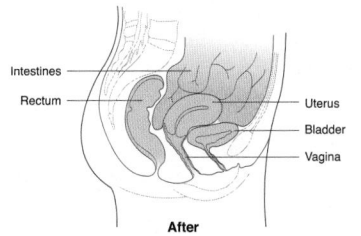

Combined anteroposterior colporrhaphy

Before

After

57265   Combined anteroposterior colporrhaphy; with enterocele repair   ♀ A 2 J I

RVU			Global Days	Modifiers				
Mod	Non-Fac Total	Fac Total		51	50	62	80	MUE
	25.89	25.89	090	2	0	1	2	1

AMA: Jun 02: 6, Jun 10: 6

+ 57267   Insertion of mesh or other prosthesis for repair of pelvic floor defect, each site (anterior, posterior compartment), vaginal approach (List separately in addition to code for primary procedure)   ♀ N I N

RVU			Global Days	Modifiers				
Mod	Non-Fac Total	Fac Total		51	50	62	80	MUE
	7.30	7.30	ZZZ	0	0	1	2	2

AMA: Jul 05: 16, May 11: 9, Jan 12: 10, Oct 13: 15

57268   Repair of enterocele, vaginal approach (separate procedure)   ♀ A 2 T

RVU			Global Days	Modifiers				
Mod	Non-Fac Total	Fac Total		51	50	62	80	MUE
	13.75	13.75	090	2	0	1	2	1

AMA: Jun 02: 6

57270   Repair of enterocele, abdominal approach (separate procedure)   ♀ C

RVU			Global Days	Modifiers				
Mod	Non-Fac Total	Fac Total		51	50	62	80	MUE
	22.67	22.67	090	2	0	1	2	1

AMA: Jun 02: 6

57280   Colpopexy, abdominal approach   ♀ C

RVU			Global Days	Modifiers				
Mod	Non-Fac Total	Fac Total		51	50	62	80	MUE
	27.08	27.08	090	2	0	1	2	1

AMA: Jan 97: 3, Jun 02: 6

Abdominal colpopexy

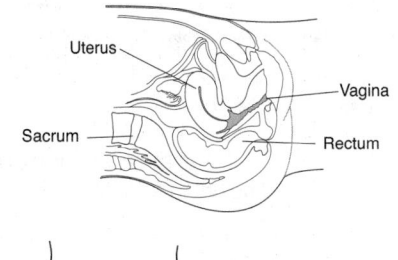

Uterus
Vagina
Sacrum
Rectum

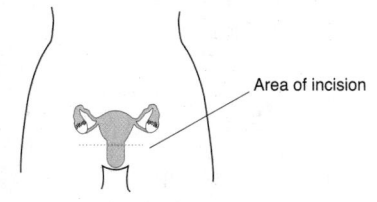

Area of incision

The physician fixes a displaced vagina by suturing it back to the abdominal wall

57282   Colpopexy, vaginal; extra-peritoneal approach (sacrospinous, iliococcygeus)   ♀ J I

RVU			Global Days	Modifiers				
Mod	Non-Fac Total	Fac Total		51	50	62	80	MUE
	14.23	14.23	090	2	0	1	2	1

AMA: Jan 97: 3, Jun 02: 6

● New   ▲ Revised   Deleted   ⊙ Moderate Sedation   ✚ Add-on Codes   ⊘ High Risk Denial   Ⓐ Age Edit   ♀ Female   ♂ Male   **AMA** *CPT® Assistant*   **MUE** Medically Unlikely Edit
⊘ Modifier 51 Exempt   ⊖ Modifier 63 Exempt   ▣ Unlisted   **Modifiers:** *See Inside Back Cover*   Ⓜ Maternity   A 2 – Z 3 ASC Payment Indicators   A – Y OPPS Status Indicators
© 2016 DecisionHealth   CPT © 2015 American Medical Association. All Rights Reserved.   **525**

57283 Colpopexy, vaginal; intra-peritoneal approach (uterosacral, levator myorrhaphy) ♀ J 1

RVU			Global Days	Modifiers				
Mod	Non-Fac Total	Fac Total		51	50	62	80	MUE
	19.56	19.56	090	2	0	1	2	1

AMA: May 11: 9

57284 Paravaginal defect repair (including repair of cystocele, if performed); open abdominal approach ♀ J 1

RVU			Global Days	Modifiers				
Mod	Non-Fac Total	Fac Total		51	50	62	80	MUE
	23.16	23.16	090	2	0	2	2	1

AMA: Jan 97: 1, Jun 02: 7, Jul 05: 16, Jun 10: 6

57285 Paravaginal defect repair (including repair of cystocele, if performed); vaginal approach ♀ J 1

RVU			Global Days	Modifiers				
Mod	Non-Fac Total	Fac Total		51	50	62	80	MUE
	19.09	19.09	090	2	0	2	2	1

AMA: Jun 10: 6

57287 Removal or revision of sling for stress incontinence (eg, fascia or synthetic) ♀ G 2 Q 2

RVU			Global Days	Modifiers				
Mod	Non-Fac Total	Fac Total		51	50	62	80	MUE
	19.36	19.36	090	2	0	1	2	1

AMA: Jun 02: 7, Nov 07: 9

57288 Sling operation for stress incontinence (eg, fascia or synthetic) ♀ A 2 J 1

RVU			Global Days	Modifiers				
Mod	Non-Fac Total	Fac Total		51	50	62	80	MUE
	20.33	20.33	090	2	0	1	2	1

AMA: Nov 99: 28, May 00: 4, Oct 00: 7, Apr 02: 18, Jun 02: 7

57289 Pereyra procedure, including anterior colporrhaphy ♀ A 2 J 1

RVU			Global Days	Modifiers				
Mod	Non-Fac Total	Fac Total		51	50	62	80	MUE
	20.91	20.91	090	2	0	1	2	1

AMA: Jan 97: 3, Jun 02: 7

Pereyra procedure
(including anterior colporrhaphy)

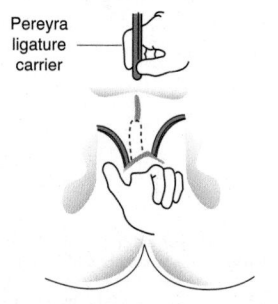
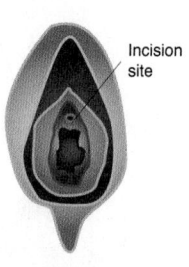

Pereyra ligature carrier

Incision site

The physician guides the ligaure with a finger inserted in the vagina

A cystocele is also repaired

The physician performs an operation to fix a condition in which the patient is unable to control the release of urine.

57291 Construction of artificial vagina; without graft ♀ A 2 T

RVU			Global Days	Modifiers				
Mod	Non-Fac Total	Fac Total		51	50	62	80	MUE
	17.53	17.53	090	2	0	0	2	1

57292 Construction of artificial vagina; with graft ♀ J 1

RVU			Global Days	Modifiers				
Mod	Non-Fac Total	Fac Total		51	50	62	80	MUE
	23.43	23.43	090	2	0	1	2	1

57295 Revision (including removal) of prosthetic vaginal graft; vaginal approach ♀ G 2 T

RVU			Global Days	Modifiers				
Mod	Non-Fac Total	Fac Total		51	50	62	80	MUE
	13.57	13.57	090	2	0	1	2	1

57296 Revision (including removal) of prosthetic vaginal graft; open abdominal approach ♀ C

RVU			Global Days	Modifiers				
Mod	Non-Fac Total	Fac Total		51	50	62	80	MUE
	26.91	26.91	090	2	0	1	2	1

57300 Closure of rectovaginal fistula; vaginal or transanal approach ♀ A 2 T

RVU			Global Days	Modifiers				
Mod	Non-Fac Total	Fac Total		51	50	62	80	MUE
	16.05	16.05	090	2	0	1	2	1

AMA: Nov 97: 21

57305 Closure of rectovaginal fistula; abdominal approach ♀ C

RVU			Global Days	Modifiers				
Mod	Non-Fac Total	Fac Total		51	50	62	80	MUE
	26.70	26.70	090	2	0	1	2	1

AMA: Nov 97: 21

57307 Closure of rectovaginal fistula; abdominal approach, with concomitant colostomy ♀ C

RVU			Global Days	Modifiers				
Mod	Non-Fac Total	Fac Total		51	50	62	80	MUE
	31.04	31.04	090	2	0	1	2	1

AMA: Nov 97: 21

57308 Closure of rectovaginal fistula; transperineal approach, with perineal body reconstruction, with or without levator plication ♀ C

RVU			Global Days	Modifiers				
Mod	Non-Fac Total	Fac Total		51	50	62	80	MUE
	18.82	18.82	090	2	0	1	2	1

AMA: Nov 97: 21

57310 Closure of urethrovaginal fistula ♀ G 2 J 1

RVU			Global Days	Modifiers				
Mod	Non-Fac Total	Fac Total		51	50	62	80	MUE
	13.21	13.21	090	2	0	1	2	1

● New ▲ Revised ✖ Deleted ⊙ Moderate Sedation ✚ Add-on Codes ⊘ High Risk Denial Ⓐ Age Edit ♀ Female ♂ Male **AMA** *CPT® Assistant* **MUE** Medically Unlikely Edit
⊘ Modifier 51 Exempt ⊖ Modifier 63 Exempt ✖ Unlisted **Modifiers:** *See Inside Back Cover* Ⓜ Maternity A 2 – Z 3 ASC Payment Indicators A – Y OPPS Status Indicators

CPT © 2015 American Medical Association. All Rights Reserved.   © 2016 DecisionHealth

57311 Closure of urethrovaginal fistula; with bulbocavernosus transplant ♀C

Mod	RVU Non-Fac Total	Fac Total	Global Days	51	50	62	80	MUE
	15.12	15.12	090	2	0	1	2	1

57320 Closure of vesicovaginal fistula; vaginal approach ♀G2 J 1

Mod	RVU Non-Fac Total	Fac Total	Global Days	51	50	62	80	MUE
	15.29	15.29	090	2	0	1	2	1

57330 Closure of vesicovaginal fistula; transvesical and vaginal approach ♀J 1

Mod	RVU Non-Fac Total	Fac Total	Global Days	51	50	62	80	MUE
	21.20	21.20	090	2	0	1	2	1

57335 Vaginoplasty for intersex state ⊗♀T

Mod	RVU Non-Fac Total	Fac Total	Global Days	51	50	62	80	MUE
	32.25	32.25	090	2	0	1	2	1

Vaginal Manipulation

Coding Guidance
Vaginal or cervical canal dilation that is done with a procedure using the vaginal approach is already included unless the code descriptor specifically states without cervical dilation.

57400 Dilation of vagina under anesthesia (other than local) ♀A2 T

Mod	RVU Non-Fac Total	Fac Total	Global Days	51	50	62	80	MUE
	3.86	3.86	000	2	0	0	0	1

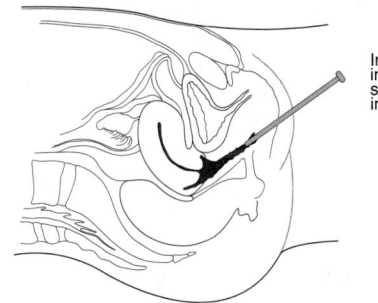

Dilation of vagina under anesthesia

Instruments of increasing size are inserted into the vagina

The physician puts the patient in an unconscious state with general anesthesia. Next, the physician inserts a device into the vagina to enlarge the vaginal passageway.

Coding Guidance
A pelvic exam under anesthesia done in conjunction with any major and most minor gynecological procedures is considered a routine evaluation of the surgical field already included in the service and is not reported separately.

57410 Pelvic examination under anesthesia (other than local) ♀A2 T

Mod	RVU Non-Fac Total	Fac Total	Global Days	51	50	62	80	MUE
	3.08	3.08	000	2	0	0	1	1

AMA: Spring 93: 34, Apr 06: 1, Nov 07: 1

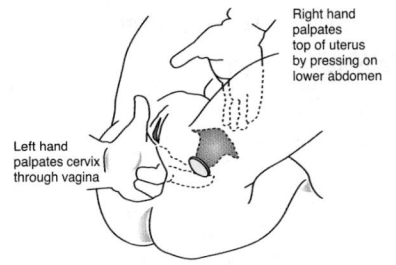

Pelvic examination under anesthesia

Right hand palpates top of uterus by pressing on lower abdomen

Left hand palpates cervix through vagina

The physician administers a nonlocal type of anesthesia and examines the female reproductive system through the vagina.

57415 Removal of impacted vaginal foreign body (separate procedure) under anesthesia (other than local) ♀A2 T

Mod	RVU Non-Fac Total	Fac Total	Global Days	51	50	62	80	MUE
	4.55	4.55	010	2	0	0	0	1

Endoscopic Vaginal Procedures

Coding Guidance
Diagnostic colposcopies should not be reported with other colposcopic procedures. Colposcopy code 57420 should not be reported when used to scout out the anatomy of the surgical field or to confirm a lesion or mass prior to a surgical procedure. When this diagnostic colposcopy is done separately and results in the decision to perform a noncolposcopic procedure, it may be reported with modifier 58 to show that the two are staged procedures.

57420 Colposcopy of the entire vagina, with cervix if present ♀P3 T

Coding Tip: *Report 57420 when performed as a separate procedure alone or when performed independently, distinct from or unrelated to other procedures*

Mod	RVU Non-Fac Total	Fac Total	Global Days	51	50	62	80	MUE
	3.35	2.63	000	2	0	0	1	1

AMA: Feb 03: 5

57421 Colposcopy of the entire vagina, with cervix if present; with biopsy(s) of vagina/cervix ♀P3 T

Mod	RVU Non-Fac Total	Fac Total	Global Days	51	50	62	80	MUE
	4.49	3.56	000	2	0	0	1	1

AMA: Feb 03: 5, Jun 03: 11, Jun 06: 16

57423 Paravaginal defect repair (including repair of cystocele, if performed), laparoscopic approach ♀J 1

Mod	RVU Non-Fac Total	Fac Total	Global Days	51	50	62	80	MUE
	25.89	25.89	090	2	0	2	2	1

AMA: Jun 10: 6

● New   ▲ Revised   Deleted   ⊙ Moderate Sedation   ✚ Add-on Codes   ⊗ High Risk Denial   Ⓐ Age Edit   ♀ Female   ♂ Male   **AMA** *CPT® Assistant*   **MUE** Medically Unlikely Edit
⊘ Modifier 51 Exempt   ⊖ Modifier 63 Exempt   ✗ Unlisted   **Modifiers:** *See Inside Back Cover*   Ⓜ Maternity   A2-Z3 ASC Payment Indicators   A-Y OPPS Status Indicators

Surgical Procedures

57425 – 57500

57425 Laparoscopy, surgical, colpopexy (suspension of vaginal apex) ♀ J I

RVU			Global Days	Modifiers				
Mod	Non-Fac Total	Fac Total		51	50	62	80	MUE
	27.52	27.52	090	2	0	1	2	1

57426 Revision (including removal) of prosthetic vaginal graft, laparoscopic approach ♀ G 2 J I

RVU			Global Days	Modifiers				
Mod	Non-Fac Total	Fac Total		51	50	62	80	MUE
	23.97	23.97	090	2	0	1	2	1

Cervical Procedures

Endoscopic Cervical Uteri Procedures

Coding Guidance

Diagnostic colposcopies should not be reported with other colposcopic procedures. Colposcopy code 57452 should not be reported when used to scout out the anatomy of the surgical field or to confirm a lesion or mass prior to a surgical procedure. When this diagnostic colposcopy is done separately and results in the decision to perform a noncolposcopic procedure, it may be reported with modifier 58 to show that the two are staged procedures. A pelvic exam done in conjunction with a gynecological procedure, either to confirm the procedure or as a necessary part of it, is not reported separately. A diagnostic pelvic exam done to evaluate the need for a surgical procedure is included in the evaluation and management service at the time the decision to perform the procedure is made.

57452 Colposcopy of the cervix including upper/adjacent vagina ♀ P 3 T

Coding Tip: Report 57452 when performed as a separate procedure alone or when performed independently, distinct from or unrelated to other procedures

RVU			Global Days	Modifiers				
Mod	Non-Fac Total	Fac Total		51	50	62	80	MUE
	3.10	2.63	000	2	0	0	1	1

AMA: Apr 00: 5, Feb 03: 5, Jun 03: 10

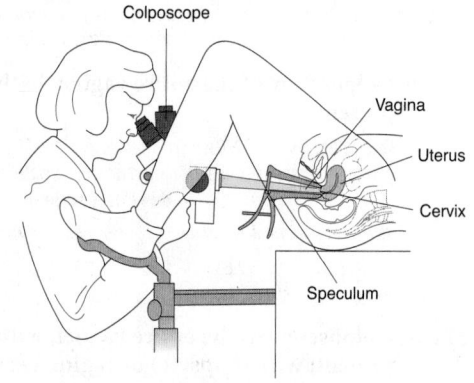

Colposcopy of the cervix including upper/adjacent vagina

Colposcopy (57452), with biopsy of cervix (57455), with endocervical curettage (57456), with cervix biopsy and endocervical curettage (57454)

57454 Colposcopy of the cervix including upper/adjacent vagina; with biopsy(s) of the cervix and endocervical curettage ♀ P 3 T

RVU			Global Days	Modifiers				
Mod	Non-Fac Total	Fac Total		51	50	62	80	MUE
	4.34	3.87	000	3	0	0	1	1

AMA: Apr 00: 5, Feb 03: 5, Jun 03: 10, Aug 11: 9

57455 Colposcopy of the cervix including upper/adjacent vagina; with biopsy(s) of the cervix ♀ P 3 T

RVU			Global Days	Modifiers				
Mod	Non-Fac Total	Fac Total		51	50	62	80	MUE
	4.05	3.16	000	3	0	0	1	1

AMA: Apr 00: 5, Feb 03: 5, Jun 03: 10

57456 Colposcopy of the cervix including upper/adjacent vagina; with endocervical curettage ♀ P 3 T

RVU			Global Days	Modifiers				
Mod	Non-Fac Total	Fac Total		51	50	62	80	MUE
	3.82	2.94	000	3	0	0	1	1

AMA: Apr 00: 5, Jan 03: 23, Feb 03: 5, Jun 03: 10

57460 Colposcopy of the cervix including upper/adjacent vagina; with loop electrode biopsy(s) of the cervix ♀ P 3 T

Coding Tip: Add endocervical curettage when performed - 57505

RVU			Global Days	Modifiers				
Mod	Non-Fac Total	Fac Total		51	50	62	80	MUE
	8.00	4.63	000	3	0	0	1	1

AMA: Apr 00: 5, Jan 03: 23, Feb 03: 5, Jun 03: 10, Jul 05: 15

57461 Colposcopy of the cervix including upper/adjacent vagina; with loop electrode conization of the cervix ♀ P 3 T

RVU			Global Days	Modifiers				
Mod	Non-Fac Total	Fac Total		51	50	62	80	MUE
	9.05	5.34	000	3	0	0	1	1

AMA: Jan 03: 23, Feb 03: 5, Jun 03: 10, Dec 06: 15

Excisional Cervical Procedures

57500 Biopsy of cervix, single or multiple, or local excision of lesion, with or without fulguration (separate procedure) ♀ P 3 T

Coding Tip: Report cervical biopsy when performed as a separate procedure alone or when performed independently, distinct from or unrelated to other procedures

Coding Tip: This code is reported once for any number of biopsies on the cervix; or when a local lesion excision is done; or when both lesion excision and biopsy(ies) are done

RVU			Global Days	Modifiers				
Mod	Non-Fac Total	Fac Total		51	50	62	80	MUE
	3.62	2.16	000	2	0	0	1	1

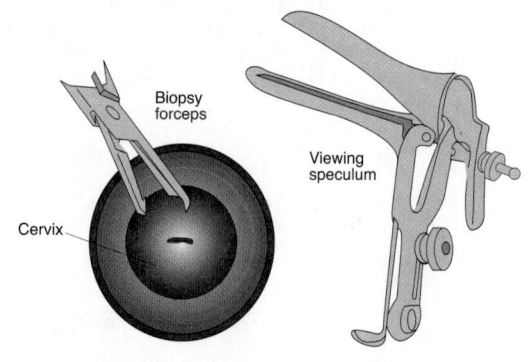

Biopsy of cervix, single or multiple, or local excision of lesion

● New   ▲ Revised   ✖ Deleted   ⊙ Moderate Sedation   ✚ Add-on Codes   ⊘ High Risk Denial   Ⓐ Age Edit   ♀ Female   ♂ Male   **AMA** *CPT® Assistant*   *MUE* Medically Unlikely Edit
⊘ Modifier 51 Exempt   ⊖ Modifier 63 Exempt   ✗ Unlisted   **Modifiers:** *See Inside Back Cover*   Ⓜ Maternity   A 2–Z 3 ASC Payment Indicators   A–Y OPPS Status Indicators

CPT © 2015 American Medical Association. All Rights Reserved.   © 2016 DecisionHealth

57505 Endocervical curettage (not done as part of a dilation and curettage) ♀ P 3 T

Coding Tip: Add loop electrode biopsy of cervix with colposcopy when performed - 57460

RVU			Global Days	Modifiers				
Mod	Non-Fac Total	Fac Total		51	50	62	80	MUE
	2.90	2.62	010	2	0	0	1	1

AMA: Jul 05: 15

57510 Cautery of cervix; electro or thermal ♀ P 3 T

RVU			Global Days	Modifiers				
Mod	Non-Fac Total	Fac Total		51	50	62	80	MUE
	3.72	3.28	010	2	0	0	1	1

57511 Cautery of cervix; cryocautery, initial or repeat ♀ P 3 T

RVU			Global Days	Modifiers				
Mod	Non-Fac Total	Fac Total		51	50	62	80	MUE
	4.10	3.75	010	2	0	0	1	1

57513 Cautery of cervix; laser ablation ♀ A 2 T

RVU			Global Days	Modifiers				
Mod	Non-Fac Total	Fac Total		51	50	62	80	MUE
	4.11	3.80	010	2	0	0	1	1

57520 Conization of cervix, with or without fulguration, with or without dilation and curettage, with or without repair; cold knife or laser ♀ A 2 T

Coding Tip: Report conization procedures by the technique used. Cold knife or laser excision of a cone-shaped section of endocervical tissue is a more complex procedure than conization by loop electrode excision

Coding Tip: Do not report any fulguration, repair, dilation, or currettage separately

RVU			Global Days	Modifiers				
Mod	Non-Fac Total	Fac Total		51	50	62	80	MUE
	8.72	7.83	090	2	0	0	1	1

AMA: Apr 00: 5

57522 Conization of cervix, with or without fulguration, with or without dilation and curettage, with or without repair; loop electrode excision ♀ A 2 T

Coding Tip: When the surgeon personally injects anesthetic into the paracervical uterine nerve before performing loop electrode conization of the cervix, add code 64435 to identify which nerve specifically was blocked, and append modifier 47 to the main surgical code (57522) to note that the physician personally performed the regional anesthesia

Coding Tip: Loop electrode excision with colposcopy - 57460

RVU			Global Days	Modifiers				
Mod	Non-Fac Total	Fac Total		51	50	62	80	MUE
	7.45	6.90	090	2	0	0	1	1

AMA: Apr 00: 5, Mar 03: 22, Jul 03: 15

57530 Trachelectomy (cervicectomy), amputation of cervix (separate procedure) ♀ A 2 T

RVU			Global Days	Modifiers				
Mod	Non-Fac Total	Fac Total		51	50	62	80	MUE
	9.89	9.89	090	2	0	1	2	1

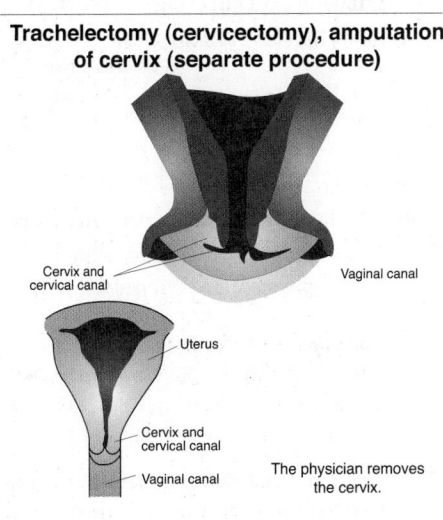

Trachelectomy (cervicectomy), amputation of cervix (separate procedure)

Cervix and cervical canal — Vaginal canal — Uterus — Cervix and cervical canal — Vaginal canal — The physician removes the cervix.

57531 Radical trachelectomy, with bilateral total pelvic lymphadenectomy and para-aortic lymph node sampling biopsy, with or without removal of tube(s), with or without removal of ovary(s) ♀ C

RVU			Global Days	Modifiers				
Mod	Non-Fac Total	Fac Total		51	50	62	80	MUE
	52.74	52.74	090	2	2	1	2	1

AMA: Nov 97: 21

57540 Excision of cervical stump, abdominal approach ♀ C

RVU			Global Days	Modifiers				
Mod	Non-Fac Total	Fac Total		51	50	62	80	MUE
	22.28	22.28	090	2	0	1	2	1

57545 Excision of cervical stump, abdominal approach; with pelvic floor repair ♀ C

RVU			Global Days	Modifiers				
Mod	Non-Fac Total	Fac Total		51	50	62	80	MUE
	24.07	24.07	090	2	0	1	2	1

57550 Excision of cervical stump, vaginal approach ♀ A 2 T

RVU			Global Days	Modifiers				
Mod	Non-Fac Total	Fac Total		51	50	62	80	MUE
	11.55	11.55	090	2	0	1	2	1

57555 Excision of cervical stump, vaginal approach; with anterior and/or posterior repair ♀ J 1

RVU			Global Days	Modifiers				
Mod	Non-Fac Total	Fac Total		51	50	62	80	MUE
	17.02	17.02	090	2	0	1	2	1

57556 Excision of cervical stump, vaginal approach; with repair of enterocele ♀ A 2 J 1

RVU			Global Days	Modifiers				
Mod	Non-Fac Total	Fac Total		51	50	62	80	MUE
	16.14	16.14	090	2	0	1	2	1

● New   ▲ Revised   Deleted   ⊙ Moderate Sedation   ✚ Add-on Codes   ⊘ High Risk Denial   Ⓐ Age Edit   ♀ Female   ♂ Male   AMA CPT® Assistant   MUE Medically Unlikely Edit
⊘ Modifier 51 Exempt   ⊖ Modifier 63 Exempt   ✗ Unlisted   Modifiers: See Inside Back Cover   Ⓜ Maternity   A 2–Z 3 ASC Payment Indicators   A –Y OPPS Status Indicators

Surgical Procedures

57558 Dilation and curettage of cervical stump ♀A2T

Coding Tip: Uterine dilation and currettage - 58120

RVU			Global Days	Modifiers				
Mod	Non-Fac Total	Fac Total		51	50	62	80	MUE
	3.53	3.22	010	2	0	0	1	1

Cervical Repair

57700 Cerclage of uterine cervix, nonobstetrical ♀A2T

Coding Tip: Use this code for tracheloplasty

Coding Tip: Cerclage to preserve pregnancy, vaginal - 59320; abdominal - 59325

Coding Tip: Removal of cerclage suture (obstetrical) under anesthesia - 59871

RVU			Global Days	Modifiers				
Mod	Non-Fac Total	Fac Total		51	50	62	80	MUE
	9.03	9.03	090	2	0	0	0	1

57720 Trachelorrhaphy, plastic repair of uterine cervix, vaginal approach ♀A2T

RVU			Global Days	Modifiers				
Mod	Non-Fac Total	Fac Total		51	50	62	80	MUE
	8.70	8.70	090	2	0	0	2	1

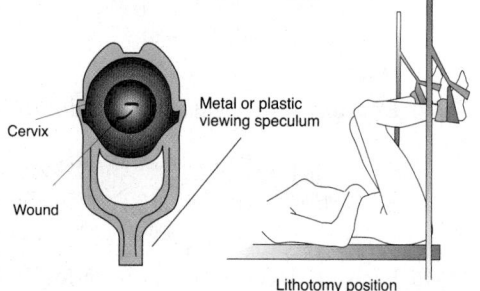

Trachelorrhaphy, plastic repair of uterine cervix, vaginal approach

Cervix

Metal or plastic viewing speculum

Wound

Lithotomy position

The physician sutures a wound on the cervix through the vagina.

Cervical Manipulation

57800 Dilation of cervical canal, instrumental (separate procedure) ⊙♀P3T

RVU			Global Days	Modifiers				
Mod	Non-Fac Total	Fac Total		51	50	62	80	MUE
	1.71	1.39	000	2	0	0	1	1

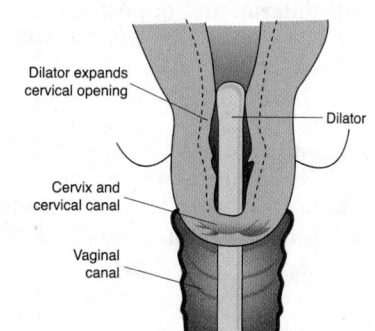

Dilation of cervical canal, instrumental

Dilator expands cervical opening

Dilator

Cervix and cervical canal

Vaginal canal

Dilators of increasing size are passed incrementally through the cervical canal.

Uterus Procedures

Excisional Uterus Procedures

58100 Endometrial sampling (biopsy) with or without endocervical sampling (biopsy), without cervical dilation, any method (separate procedure) ♀P3T

RVU			Global Days	Modifiers				
Mod	Non-Fac Total	Fac Total		51	50	62	80	MUE
	3.09	2.49	000	2	0	0	1	1

+ 58110 Endometrial sampling (biopsy) performed in conjunction with colposcopy (List separately in addition to code for primary procedure) ♀N1N

RVU			Global Days	Modifiers				
Mod	Non-Fac Total	Fac Total		51	50	62	80	MUE
	1.36	1.17	ZZZ	0	0	0	0	1

AMA: Jun 06: 17

58120 Dilation and curettage, diagnostic and/or therapeutic (nonobstetrical) ♀A2T

RVU			Global Days	Modifiers				
Mod	Non-Fac Total	Fac Total		51	50	62	80	MUE
	7.32	6.23	010	2	0	0	1	1

AMA: Fall 95: 16, Nov 97: 21, May 03: 19

58140 Myomectomy, excision of fibroid tumor(s) of uterus, 1 to 4 intramural myoma(s) with total weight of 250 g or less and/or removal of surface myomas; abdominal approach ♀C

RVU			Global Days	Modifiers				
Mod	Non-Fac Total	Fac Total		51	50	62	80	MUE
	26.22	26.22	090	2	0	1	2	1

AMA: Feb 03: 15, Jun 03: 5

58145 Myomectomy, excision of fibroid tumor(s) of uterus, 1 to 4 intramural myoma(s) with total weight of 250 g or less and/or removal of surface myomas; vaginal approach ♀A2T

RVU			Global Days	Modifiers				
Mod	Non-Fac Total	Fac Total		51	50	62	80	MUE
	15.61	15.61	090	2	0	1	2	1

58146 Myomectomy, excision of fibroid tumor(s) of uterus, 5 or more intramural myomas and/or intramural myomas with total weight greater than 250 g, abdominal approach ♀C

RVU			Global Days	Modifiers				
Mod	Non-Fac Total	Fac Total		51	50	62	80	MUE
	32.64	32.64	090	2	0	1	2	1

AMA: Feb 03: 15, Jun 03: 5

Hysterectomies

58150 Total abdominal hysterectomy (corpus and cervix), with or without removal of tube(s), with or without removal of ovary(s) ♀C

RVU			Global Days	Modifiers				
Mod	Non-Fac Total	Fac Total		51	50	62	80	MUE
	28.90	28.90	090	2	0	1	2	1

AMA: Dec 96: 10, Apr 97: 3, Nov 97: 21, Sep 00: 9, Aug 01: 11

● New   ▲ Revised   ✖ Deleted   ⊙ Moderate Sedation   ✚ Add-on Codes   ⊘ High Risk Denial   Ⓐ Age Edit   ♀ Female   ♂ Male   **AMA** *CPT® Assistant*   **MUE** Medically Unlikely Edit
⊘ Modifier 51 Exempt   ⊖ Modifier 63 Exempt   ✗ Unlisted   **Modifiers:** *See Inside Back Cover*   Ⓜ Maternity   A2–Z3 ASC Payment Indicators   A–Y OPPS Status Indicators

CPT © 2015 American Medical Association. All Rights Reserved.   © 2016 DecisionHealth

58152 Total abdominal hysterectomy (corpus and cervix), with or without removal of tube(s), with or without removal of ovary(s); with colpo-urethrocystopexy (eg, Marshall-Marchetti-Krantz, Burch) ♀Ⓒ

RVU		Global Days	Modifiers				
Mod	*Non-Fac Total* *Fac Total*		51	50	62	80	MUE
	35.52 35.52	090	2	0	1	2	1

AMA: Jan 97: 1, Nov 97: 22, Jun 10: 6

58180 Supracervical abdominal hysterectomy (subtotal hysterectomy), with or without removal of tube(s), with or without removal of ovary(s) ♀Ⓒ

RVU		Global Days	Modifiers				
Mod	*Non-Fac Total* *Fac Total*		51	50	62	80	MUE
	27.41 27.41	090	2	0	1	2	1

58200 Total abdominal hysterectomy, including partial vaginectomy, with para-aortic and pelvic lymph node sampling, with or without removal of tube(s), with or without removal of ovary(s) ♀Ⓒ

RVU		Global Days	Modifiers				
Mod	*Non-Fac Total* *Fac Total*		51	50	62	80	MUE
	39.28 39.28	090	2	0	1	2	1

58210 Radical abdominal hysterectomy, with bilateral total pelvic lymphadenectomy and para-aortic lymph node sampling (biopsy), with or without removal of tube(s), with or without removal of ovary(s) ♀Ⓒ

RVU		Global Days	Modifiers				
Mod	*Non-Fac Total* *Fac Total*		51	50	62	80	MUE
	52.99 52.99	090	2	2	1	2	1

AMA: Fall 92: 21, May 12: 14

58240 Pelvic exenteration for gynecologic malignancy, with total abdominal hysterectomy or cervicectomy, with or without removal of tube(s), with or without removal of ovary(s), with removal of bladder and ureteral transplantations, and/or abdominoperineal resection of rectum and colon and colostomy, or any combination thereof ♀Ⓒ

RVU		Global Days	Modifiers				
Mod	*Non-Fac Total* *Fac Total*		51	50	62	80	MUE
	83.67 83.67	090	2	0	1	2	1

Pelvic exenteration for gynecologic malignancy, with total abdominal hysterectomy or cervicectomy

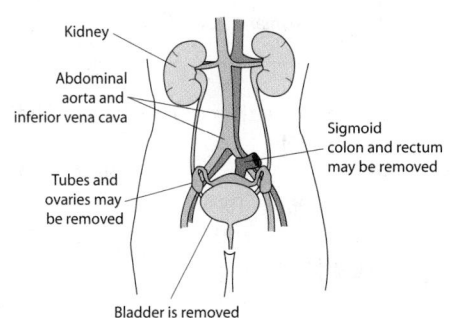

Kidney
Abdominal aorta and inferior vena cava
Sigmoid colon and rectum may be removed
Tubes and ovaries may be removed
Bladder is removed

The physician performs pelvic exenteration for gynecologic malignancy.

58260 Vaginal hysterectomy, for uterus 250 g or less ♀Ⓖ2ⒿⒾ

RVU		Global Days	Modifiers				
Mod	*Non-Fac Total* *Fac Total*		51	50	62	80	MUE
	23.43 23.43	090	2	0	1	2	1

AMA: May 11: 9

58262 Vaginal hysterectomy, for uterus 250 g or less; with removal of tube(s), and/or ovary(s) ♀Ⓖ2ⒿⒾ

RVU		Global Days	Modifiers				
Mod	*Non-Fac Total* *Fac Total*		51	50	62	80	MUE
	26.16 26.16	090	2	0	2	2	1

58263 Vaginal hysterectomy, for uterus 250 g or less; with removal of tube(s), and/or ovary(s), with repair of enterocele ♀ⒿⒾ

RVU		Global Days	Modifiers				
Mod	*Non-Fac Total* *Fac Total*		51	50	62	80	MUE
	28.06 28.06	090	2	0	2	2	1

58267 Vaginal hysterectomy, for uterus 250 g or less; with colpo-urethrocystopexy (Marshall-Marchetti-Krantz type, Pereyra type) with or without endoscopic control ♀Ⓒ

RVU		Global Days	Modifiers				
Mod	*Non-Fac Total* *Fac Total*		51	50	62	80	MUE
	29.92 29.92	090	2	0	1	2	1

AMA: Jun 10: 6

58270 Vaginal hysterectomy, for uterus 250 g or less; with repair of enterocele ♀ⒿⒾ

RVU		Global Days	Modifiers				
Mod	*Non-Fac Total* *Fac Total*		51	50	62	80	MUE
	25.00 25.00	090	2	0	1	2	1

58275 Vaginal hysterectomy, with total or partial vaginectomy ♀Ⓒ

RVU		Global Days	Modifiers				
Mod	*Non-Fac Total* *Fac Total*		51	50	62	80	MUE
	27.93 27.93	090	2	0	1	2	1

58280 Vaginal hysterectomy, with total or partial vaginectomy; with repair of enterocele ♀Ⓒ

RVU		Global Days	Modifiers				
Mod	*Non-Fac Total* *Fac Total*		51	50	62	80	MUE
	29.76 29.76	090	2	0	1	2	1

58285 Vaginal hysterectomy, radical (Schauta type operation) ♀Ⓒ

RVU		Global Days	Modifiers				
Mod	*Non-Fac Total* *Fac Total*		51	50	62	80	MUE
	38.33 38.33	090	2	0	1	2	1

AMA: Nov 07: 1

58290 Vaginal hysterectomy, for uterus greater than 250 g ♀ⒿⒾ

RVU		Global Days	Modifiers				
Mod	*Non-Fac Total* *Fac Total*		51	50	62	80	MUE
	32.65 32.65	090	2	0	1	2	1

● New ▲ Revised Deleted ⊙ Moderate Sedation ✚ Add-on Codes ⊘ High Risk Denial Ⓐ Age Edit ♀ Female ♂ Male **AMA** *CPT® Assistant* **MUE** Medically Unlikely Edit
⊘ Modifier 51 Exempt ⊖ Modifier 63 Exempt Ⓧ Unlisted **Modifiers:** *See Inside Back Cover* Ⓜ Maternity Ⓐ2–Ⓩ3 ASC Payment Indicators Ⓐ–Ⓨ OPPS Status Indicators

© 2016 DecisionHealth | CPT © 2015 American Medical Association. All Rights Reserved. | **531**

Surgical Procedures

58291 – 58350

58291 Vaginal hysterectomy, for uterus greater than 250 g; with removal of tube(s) and/or ovary(s) ♀ J 1

RVU			Global Days	Modifiers				
Mod	Non-Fac Total	Fac Total		51	50	62	80	MUE
	35.23	35.23	090	2	0	2	2	1

58292 Vaginal hysterectomy, for uterus greater than 250 g; with removal of tube(s) and/or ovary(s), with repair of enterocele ♀ J 1

RVU			Global Days	Modifiers				
Mod	Non-Fac Total	Fac Total		51	50	62	80	MUE
	37.21	37.21	090	2	0	2	2	1

58293 Vaginal hysterectomy, for uterus greater than 250 g; with colpo-urethrocystopexy (Marshall-Marchetti-Krantz type, Pereyra type) with or without endoscopic control ♀ C

RVU			Global Days	Modifiers				
Mod	Non-Fac Total	Fac Total		51	50	62	80	MUE
	38.68	38.68	090	2	0	1	2	1

58294 Vaginal hysterectomy, for uterus greater than 250 g; with repair of enterocele ♀ J 1

RVU			Global Days	Modifiers				
Mod	Non-Fac Total	Fac Total		51	50	62	80	MUE
	34.60	34.60	090	2	0	1	2	1

Introduction Uterus Procedures

58300 Insertion of intrauterine device (IUD) ♀♂ E

RVU			Global Days	Modifiers				
Mod	Non-Fac Total	Fac Total		51	50	62	80	MUE
	2.06	1.54	XXX	9	9	9	9	

AMA: Apr 98: 14

58301 Removal of intrauterine device (IUD) ♀♂ P 3 Q 2

Documentation Finder: Documentation should include a negative pregnancy test as well as the provider doing a bimanual exam of the uterus.

RVU			Global Days	Modifiers				
Mod	Non-Fac Total	Fac Total		51	50	62	80	MUE
	2.68	1.92	000	2	0	0	0	1

AMA: Apr 98: 14

58321 Artificial insemination; intra-cervical ♀ P 3 T

RVU			Global Days	Modifiers				
Mod	Non-Fac Total	Fac Total		51	50	62	80	MUE
	2.18	1.39	000	2	0	0	0	1

58322 Artificial insemination; intra-uterine ♀ P 3 T

RVU			Global Days	Modifiers				
Mod	Non-Fac Total	Fac Total		51	50	62	80	MUE
	2.43	1.66	000	2	0	0	0	1

58323 Sperm washing for artificial insemination ♀ P 3 T

RVU			Global Days	Modifiers				
Mod	Non-Fac Total	Fac Total		51	50	62	80	MUE
	0.43	0.34	000	2	0	0	0	1

AMA: Jan 98: 6

58340 Catheterization and introduction of saline or contrast material for saline infusion sonohysterography (SIS) or hysterosalpingography ♀ N 1 N

Coding Tip: Radiological portion of SIS - 76831

Coding Tip: Radiological portion of hysterosalpingography - 74740

RVU			Global Days	Modifiers				
Mod	Non-Fac Total	Fac Total		51	50	62	80	MUE
	3.36	1.66	000	2	0	0	1	1

AMA: Nov 97: 22, Jul 99: 8, Mar 09: 11

58345 Transcervical introduction of fallopian tube catheter for diagnosis and/or re-establishing patency (any method), with or without hysterosalpingography ♀ R 2 T

Coding Tip: Radiological guidance for transcervical fallopian tube catheterization - 74742

RVU			Global Days	Modifiers				
Mod	Non-Fac Total	Fac Total		51	50	62	80	MUE
	7.71	7.71	010	2	1	2	2	1

AMA: Nov 97: 22, Mar 09: 11

58346 Insertion of Heyman capsules for clinical brachytherapy ♀ A 2 T

Coding Tip: Report subsequent insertion of intracavitary radioactive sources that are left in the patient with 77761-77763.

Coding Tip: Report subsequent high dose rate brachytherapy delivered through the channel(s) of the implanted device with 77785-77787.

RVU			Global Days	Modifiers				
Mod	Non-Fac Total	Fac Total		51	50	62	80	MUE
	12.70	12.70	090	2	0	0	1	1

AMA: Feb 02: 8, Apr 09: 3

Insertion of Heyman capsules for clinical brachytherapy

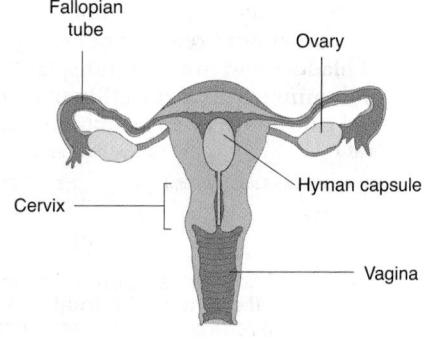

Heyman capsules are inserted into the uterus for clinical brachytherapy

58350 Chromotubation of oviduct, including materials ♀ A 2 J 1

RVU			Global Days	Modifiers				
Mod	Non-Fac Total	Fac Total		51	50	62	80	MUE
	2.72	2.22	010	2	1	0	1	1

AMA: May 02: 19, Dec 08: 7

● New   ▲ Revised   ✖ Deleted   ⊙ Moderate Sedation   ✚ Add-on Codes   ⊘ High Risk Denial   Ⓐ Age Edit   ♀ Female   ♂ Male   **AMA** *CPT® Assistant*   **MUE** Medically Unlikely Edit
⊘ Modifier 51 Exempt   ⊖ Modifier 63 Exempt   ⊠ Unlisted   **Modifiers:** *See Inside Back Cover*   Ⓜ Maternity   A 2 – Z 3 ASC Payment Indicators   A – Y OPPS Status Indicators

532   CPT © 2015 American Medical Association. All Rights Reserved.   © 2016 DecisionHealth

58353 Endometrial ablation, thermal, without hysteroscopic guidance ♀ A2 J 1

Mod	Non-Fac Total	Fac Total	Global Days	Modifiers 51	50	62	80	MUE
	28.40	6.21	010	2	0	2	1	1

AMA: Mar 02: 11, Apr 02: 19

58356 Endometrial cryoablation with ultrasonic guidance, including endometrial curettage, when performed ♀ P 3 J 1

Mod	Non-Fac Total	Fac Total	Global Days	Modifiers 51	50	62	80	MUE
	53.13	9.82	010	2	0	2	2	1

Endometrial cryoablation with ultrasonic guidance

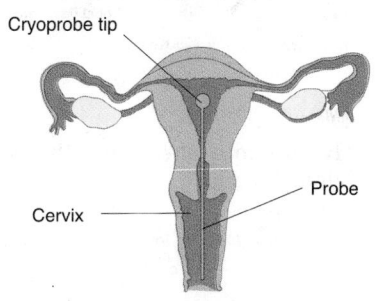

Cryoprobe tip

Probe

Cervix

The physician performs endometrial cryoablation using ultrasound guidance including endometrial curettage when performed

Uterus Repair

58400 Uterine suspension, with or without shortening of round ligaments, with or without shortening of sacrouterine ligaments; (separate procedure) ♀ C

Mod	Non-Fac Total	Fac Total	Global Days	Modifiers 51	50	62	80	MUE
	12.54	12.54	090	2	0	1	2	1

58410 Uterine suspension, with or without shortening of round ligaments, with or without shortening of sacrouterine ligaments; with presacral sympathectomy ♀ C

Mod	Non-Fac Total	Fac Total	Global Days	Modifiers 51	50	62	80	MUE
	23.31	23.31	090	2	0	1	2	1

AMA: Mar 07: 9

58520 Hysterorrhaphy, repair of ruptured uterus (nonobstetrical) ♀ C

Mod	Non-Fac Total	Fac Total	Global Days	Modifiers 51	50	62	80	MUE
	24.28	24.28	090	2	0	1	2	1

58540 Hysteroplasty, repair of uterine anomaly (Strassman type) ♀ C

Mod	Non-Fac Total	Fac Total	Global Days	Modifiers 51	50	62	80	MUE
	25.70	25.70	090	2	0	0	2	1

Laparoscopic/Hysteroscopic Uterus Procedures

58541 Laparoscopy, surgical, supracervical hysterectomy, for uterus 250 g or less ♀ G2 J 1

Mod	Non-Fac Total	Fac Total	Global Days	Modifiers 51	50	62	80	MUE
	20.34	20.34	090	3	0	2	2	1

AMA: Nov 07: 1

58542 Laparoscopy, surgical, supracervical hysterectomy, for uterus 250 g or less; with removal of tube(s) and/or ovary(s) ♀ G2 J 1

Mod	Non-Fac Total	Fac Total	Global Days	Modifiers 51	50	62	80	MUE
	23.26	23.26	090	2	0	2	2	1

AMA: Nov 07: 1

58543 Laparoscopy, surgical, supracervical hysterectomy, for uterus greater than 250 g ♀ G2 J 1

Mod	Non-Fac Total	Fac Total	Global Days	Modifiers 51	50	62	80	MUE
	23.51	23.51	090	2	0	2	2	1

AMA: Nov 07: 1

58544 Laparoscopy, surgical, supracervical hysterectomy, for uterus greater than 250 g; with removal of tube(s) and/or ovary(s) ♀ G2 J 1

Mod	Non-Fac Total	Fac Total	Global Days	Modifiers 51	50	62	80	MUE
	25.67	25.67	090	2	0	2	2	1

AMA: Nov 07: 1

58545 Laparoscopy, surgical, myomectomy, excision; 1 to 4 intramural myomas with total weight of 250 g or less and/or removal of surface myomas ♀ A2 J 1

Mod	Non-Fac Total	Fac Total	Global Days	Modifiers 51	50	62	80	MUE
	25.67	25.67	090	2	0	2	2	1

AMA: Jun 03: 5, 12

58546 Laparoscopy, surgical, myomectomy, excision; 5 or more intramural myomas and/or intramural myomas with total weight greater than 250 g ♀ A2 J 1

Mod	Non-Fac Total	Fac Total	Global Days	Modifiers 51	50	62	80	MUE
	31.84	31.84	090	2	0	2	2	1

AMA: Jun 03: 12, Jan 04: 26

58548 Laparoscopy, surgical, with radical hysterectomy, with bilateral total pelvic lymphadenectomy and para-aortic lymph node sampling (biopsy), with removal of tube(s) and ovary(s), if performed ♀ C

Mod	Non-Fac Total	Fac Total	Global Days	Modifiers 51	50	62	80	MUE
	54.55	54.55	090	2	2	2	2	1

AMA: Nov 07: 1

● New   ▲ Revised   Deleted   ⊙ Moderate Sedation   ✚ Add-on Codes   ⊘ High Risk Denial   Ⓐ Age Edit   ♀ Female   ♂ Male   **AMA** CPT® Assistant   **MUE** Medically Unlikely Edit
⦸ Modifier 51 Exempt   ⊖ Modifier 63 Exempt   Ⓧ Unlisted   **Modifiers:** See Inside Back Cover   Ⓜ Maternity   A2–Z3 ASC Payment Indicators   A–Y OPPS Status Indicators

58550 Laparoscopy, surgical, with vaginal hysterectomy, for uterus 250 g or less   ♀ A2 J I

RVU			Global Days	Modifiers				
Mod	*Non-Fac Total*	*Fac Total*		51	50	62	80	MUE
	25.01	25.01	090	3	0	2	2	1

AMA: Nov 99: 28, Mar 00: 9

Laparoscopy, surgical, with vaginal hysterectomy

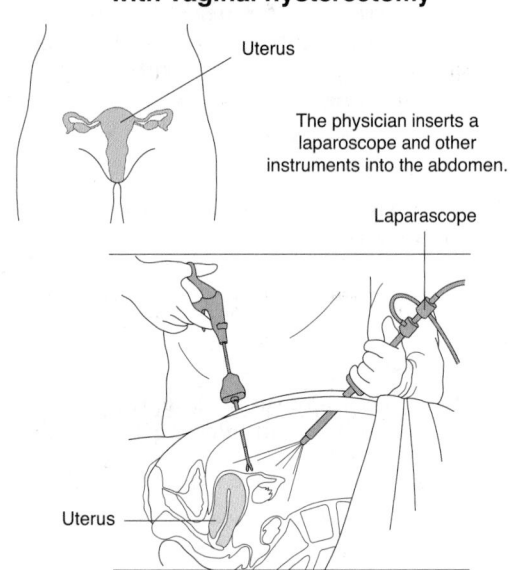

Uterus

The physician inserts a laparoscope and other instruments into the abdomen.

Laparascope

Uterus

58552 Laparoscopy, surgical, with vaginal hysterectomy, for uterus 250 g or less; with removal of tube(s) and/or ovary(s)   ♀ G2 J I

RVU			Global Days	Modifiers				
Mod	*Non-Fac Total*	*Fac Total*		51	50	62	80	MUE
	28.10	28.10	090	2	0	2	2	1

AMA: Nov 07: 1

58553 Laparoscopy, surgical, with vaginal hysterectomy, for uterus greater than 250 g   ♀ G2 J I

RVU			Global Days	Modifiers				
Mod	*Non-Fac Total*	*Fac Total*		51	50	62	80	MUE
	32.27	32.27	090	2	0	2	2	1

58554 Laparoscopy, surgical, with vaginal hysterectomy, for uterus greater than 250 g; with removal of tube(s) and/or ovary(s)   ♀ G2 J I

RVU			Global Days	Modifiers				
Mod	*Non-Fac Total*	*Fac Total*		51	50	62	80	MUE
	37.79	37.79	090	2	0	2	2	1

58555 Hysteroscopy, diagnostic (separate procedure)   ♀ A2 T

Coding Tip: Code 58555 is included in 58558-58565

RVU			Global Days	Modifiers				
Mod	*Non-Fac Total*	*Fac Total*		51	50	62	80	MUE
	8.81	5.38	000	2	0	2	0	1

AMA: Nov 99: 28, Mar 00: 10

58558 Hysteroscopy, surgical; with sampling (biopsy) of endometrium and/or polypectomy, with or without D & C   ♀ A2 T

RVU			Global Days	Modifiers				
Mod	*Non-Fac Total*	*Fac Total*		51	50	62	80	MUE
	11.46	7.58	000	3	0	2	1	1

AMA: Nov 99: 28, Mar 00: 10, Sep 02: 10, Jan 03: 7, May 03: 19

58559 Hysteroscopy, surgical; with lysis of intrauterine adhesions (any method)   ♀ A2 J I

RVU			Global Days	Modifiers				
Mod	*Non-Fac Total*	*Fac Total*		51	50	62	80	MUE
	9.70	9.70	000	3	0	2	1	1

AMA: Nov 99: 28, Mar 00: 10

58560 Hysteroscopy, surgical; with division or resection of intrauterine septum (any method)   ♀ A2 J I

RVU			Global Days	Modifiers				
Mod	*Non-Fac Total*	*Fac Total*		51	50	62	80	MUE
	10.93	10.93	000	3	0	2	2	1

AMA: Nov 99: 28, Mar 00: 10

58561 Hysteroscopy, surgical; with removal of leiomyomata   ♀ A2 J I

RVU			Global Days	Modifiers				
Mod	*Non-Fac Total*	*Fac Total*		51	50	62	80	MUE
	15.52	15.52	000	3	0	2	0	1

AMA: Nov 99: 28, Mar 00: 10, Jan 03: 7

Hysteroscopy, surgical; with removal of leiomyomata

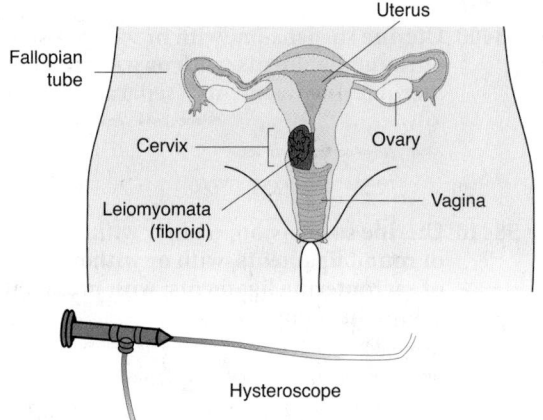

Fallopian tube

Uterus

Cervix

Ovary

Leiomyomata (fibroid)

Vagina

Hysteroscope

The physician inserts a hysteroscope into the uterus to check for injury or disease. Polyps/tissue sample may be removed. A tumor consisting of muscle fibers is removed.

58562 Hysteroscopy, surgical; with removal of impacted foreign body   ♀ A2 T

RVU			Global Days	Modifiers				
Mod	*Non-Fac Total*	*Fac Total*		51	50	62	80	MUE
	11.85	8.21	000	3	0	2	1	1

AMA: Nov 99: 28, Mar 00: 10

● New   ▲ Revised   ✖ Deleted   ⊙ Moderate Sedation   ✚ Add-on Codes   ⊘ High Risk Denial   Ⓐ Age Edit   ♀ Female   ♂ Male   **AMA** *CPT® Assistant*   **MUE** Medically Unlikely Edit
⊘ Modifier 51 Exempt   ⊖ Modifier 63 Exempt   ✗ Unlisted   **Modifiers:** *See Inside Back Cover*   Ⓜ Maternity   A2–Z3 ASC Payment Indicators   A–Y OPPS Status Indicators

CPT © 2015 American Medical Association. All Rights Reserved.   © 2016 DecisionHealth

58563   Hysteroscopy, surgical; with endometrial ablation (eg, endometrial resection, electrosurgical ablation, thermoablation) ♀ A2 J1

RVU			Global Days	Modifiers				
Mod	Non-Fac Total	Fac Total		51	50	62	80	MUE
	47.11	9.69	000	3	0	2	0	1

AMA: Nov 99: 28, Mar 00: 10, Mar 02: 11, Apr 02: 19, Jan 03: 7, Feb 12: 11, Jan 15: 14

58565   Hysteroscopy, surgical; with bilateral fallopian tube cannulation to induce occlusion by placement of permanent implants ♀♀ A2 J1

RVU			Global Days	Modifiers				
Mod	Non-Fac Total	Fac Total		51	50	62	80	MUE
	52.72	12.27	090	3	2	2	1	1

AMA: Feb 12: 11, Jan 11: 9

Hysteroscopy, surgical; with bilateral fallopian tube cannulation to induce occlusion by placement of permanent implants

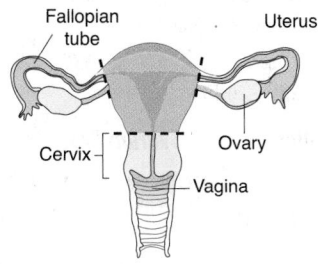

The physician performs a surgical hysteroscopy with bilateral fallopian tube cannulation and placement of permanent implants to occlude the fallopian tubes in an elective sterilization procedure.

58570   Laparoscopy, surgical, with total hysterectomy, for uterus 250 g or less ♀ G2 J1

RVU			Global Days	Modifiers				
Mod	Non-Fac Total	Fac Total		51	50	62	80	MUE
	22.11	22.11	090	2	0	2	2	1

58571   Laparoscopy, surgical, with total hysterectomy, for uterus 250 g or less; with removal of tube(s) and/or ovary(s) ♀ G2 J1

RVU			Global Days	Modifiers				
Mod	Non-Fac Total	Fac Total		51	50	62	80	MUE
	25.58	25.58	090	2	0	2	2	1

AMA: May 12: 14, Aug 12: 13

58572   Laparoscopy, surgical, with total hysterectomy, for uterus greater than 250 g ♀ J1

RVU			Global Days	Modifiers				
Mod	Non-Fac Total	Fac Total		51	50	62	80	MUE
	29.00	29.00	090	2	0	2	2	1

58573   Laparoscopy, surgical, with total hysterectomy, for uterus greater than 250 g; with removal of tube(s) and/or ovary(s) ♀ G2 J1

RVU			Global Days	Modifiers				
Mod	Non-Fac Total	Fac Total		51	50	62	80	MUE
	34.62	34.62	090	2	0	2	2	1

AMA: May 12: 14, Aug 12: 13

58578   Unlisted laparoscopy procedure, uterus ♀ ✗ J1

RVU			Global Days	Modifiers				
Mod	Non-Fac Total	Fac Total		51	50	62	80	MUE
	0.00	0.00	YYY	2	1	1	2	

AMA: Nov 99: 28, Mar 00: 10, Mar 07: 9

58579   Unlisted hysteroscopy procedure, uterus ♀ ✗ T

RVU			Global Days	Modifiers				
Mod	Non-Fac Total	Fac Total		51	50	62	80	MUE
	0.00	0.00	YYY	2	1	1	2	

AMA: Nov 99: 28, Mar 00: 10

Fallopian Tube/Ovarian Procedures

Incisional Fallopian Tube/Ovarian Procedures

58600   Ligation or transection of fallopian tube(s), abdominal or vaginal approach, unilateral or bilateral ♀♀ G2 T

RVU			Global Days	Modifiers				
Mod	Non-Fac Total	Fac Total		51	50	62	80	MUE
	10.31	10.31	090	2	2	1	2	1

AMA: Nov 99: 28

Ligation or transection of fallopian tube(s) when done at the time of cesarean delivery or intra-abdominal surgery

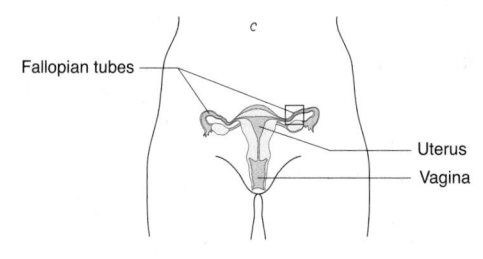

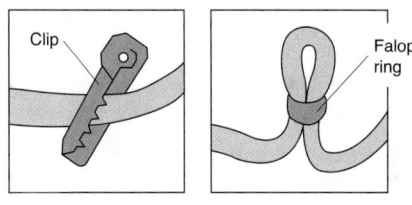

The physician ties off or severs one or both of the fallopian tubes through an abdominal incision or the vagina.

58605   Ligation or transection of fallopian tube(s), abdominal or vaginal approach, postpartum, unilateral or bilateral, during same hospitalization (separate procedure) ♀♀ C

RVU			Global Days	Modifiers				
Mod	Non-Fac Total	Fac Total		51	50	62	80	MUE
	9.31	9.31	090	2	2	0	2	1

AMA: Nov 99: 28

+ 58611   Ligation or transection of fallopian tube(s) when done at the time of cesarean delivery or intra-abdominal surgery (not a separate procedure) (List separately in addition to code for primary procedure) ♀♀ C

RVU			Global Days	Modifiers				
Mod	Non-Fac Total	Fac Total		51	50	62	80	MUE
	2.19	2.19	ZZZ	0	0	0	2	1

● New   ▲ Revised   Deleted   ⊙ Moderate Sedation   ✚ Add-on Codes   ⊘ High Risk Denial   Ⓐ Age Edit   ♀ Female   ♂ Male   **AMA** CPT® Assistant   **MUE** Medically Unlikely Edit
⊘ Modifier 51 Exempt   ⊖ Modifier 63 Exempt   ✗ Unlisted   **Modifiers:** See Inside Back Cover   Ⓜ Maternity   A2–Z3 ASC Payment Indicators   A–Y OPPS Status Indicators

58615 Occlusion of fallopian tube(s) by device (eg, band, clip, Falope ring) vaginal or suprapubic approach ♀⦶G2 T

RVU			Global Days	Modifiers				
Mod	Non-Fac Total	Fac Total		51	50	62	80	MUE
	6.88	6.88	010	2	0	0	2	1

AMA: Nov 99: 28

Laparoscopic Fallopian Tube/Ovarian Procedures

Coding Guidance

Lysis of adhesions should not be reported together with any other surgical laparoscopic procedure.

58660 Laparoscopy, surgical; with lysis of adhesions (salpingolysis, ovariolysis) (separate procedure) ♀A2 J I

RVU			Global Days	Modifiers				
Mod	Non-Fac Total	Fac Total		51	50	62	80	MUE
	19.17	19.17	090	3	0	2	2	1

AMA: Nov 99: 28, Mar 00: 10, Mar 03: 22, Dec 11: 16

58661 Laparoscopy, surgical; with removal of adnexal structures (partial or total oophorectomy and/or salpingectomy) ♀A2 J I

RVU			Global Days	Modifiers				
Mod	Non-Fac Total	Fac Total		51	50	62	80	MUE
	18.50	18.50	010	3	1	2	2	1

AMA: Nov 99: 28, Mar 00: 10, Jan 02: 11, Nov 07: 1, May 10: 10

58662 Laparoscopy, surgical; with fulguration or excision of lesions of the ovary, pelvic viscera, or peritoneal surface by any method ♀A2 J I

RVU			Global Days	Modifiers				
Mod	Non-Fac Total	Fac Total		51	50	62	80	MUE
	20.17	20.17	090	3	0	2	2	1

AMA: Nov 99: 28, Mar 00: 10

58670 Laparoscopy, surgical; with fulguration of oviducts (with or without transection) ♀⦶A2 J I

RVU			Global Days	Modifiers				
Mod	Non-Fac Total	Fac Total		51	50	62	80	MUE
	10.35	10.35	090	3	0	2	1	1

AMA: Nov 99: 29, Mar 00: 10, Nov 07: 2

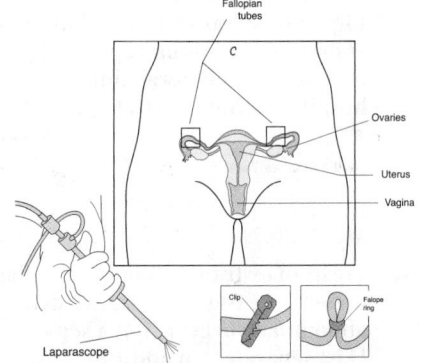

Laparoscopy, surgical; with fulguration of oviducts

Fallopian tubes

C

Ovaries

Uterus

Vagina

Clip

Falope ring

Laparoscope

The physician inserts a laparoscope and other instruments into the abdominal cavity. Next, the physician puts a device on the fallopian tubes to close them.

58671 Laparoscopy, surgical; with occlusion of oviducts by device (eg, band, clip, or Falope ring) ♀⦶A2 J I

RVU			Global Days	Modifiers				
Mod	Non-Fac Total	Fac Total		51	50	62	80	MUE
	10.34	10.34	090	3	0	2	1	1

AMA: Nov 99: 29, Mar 00: 10

58672 Laparoscopy, surgical; with fimbrioplasty ♀A2 J I

RVU			Global Days	Modifiers				
Mod	Non-Fac Total	Fac Total		51	50	62	80	MUE
	20.81	20.81	090	3	1	0	2	1

AMA: Nov 99: 29, Mar 00: 10

58673 Laparoscopy, surgical; with salpingostomy (salpingoneostomy) ♀A2 J I

RVU			Global Days	Modifiers				
Mod	Non-Fac Total	Fac Total		51	50	62	80	MUE
	22.61	22.61	090	3	1	0	2	1

AMA: Nov 99: 29, Mar 00: 10, May 02: 19

58679 Unlisted laparoscopy procedure, oviduct, ovary ♀⦶x J I

RVU			Global Days	Modifiers				
Mod	Non-Fac Total	Fac Total		51	50	62	80	MUE
	0.00	0.00	YYY	2	1	1	2	

AMA: Nov 99: 29, Mar 00: 10

Excisional Fallopian Tube/Ovarian Procedures

58700 Salpingectomy, complete or partial, unilateral or bilateral (separate procedure) ♀C

RVU			Global Days	Modifiers				
Mod	Non-Fac Total	Fac Total		51	50	62	80	MUE
	22.13	22.13	090	2	2	1	2	1

58720 Salpingo-oophorectomy, complete or partial, unilateral or bilateral (separate procedure) ♀C

RVU			Global Days	Modifiers				
Mod	Non-Fac Total	Fac Total		51	50	62	80	MUE
	21.00	21.00	090	2	2	1	2	1

AMA: Sep 00: 9, Jul 06: 19

Fallopian Tube/Ovarian Repair

58740 Lysis of adhesions (salpingolysis, ovariolysis) ♀⦶C

RVU			Global Days	Modifiers				
Mod	Non-Fac Total	Fac Total		51	50	62	80	MUE
	25.14	25.14	090	2	0	1	2	1

AMA: Sep 96: 9, Nov 99: 29

58750 Tubotubal anastomosis ♀⦶C

RVU			Global Days	Modifiers				
Mod	Non-Fac Total	Fac Total		51	50	62	80	MUE
	27.83	27.83	090	2	1	1	2	1

58752 Tubouterine implantation ♀⦶C

RVU			Global Days	Modifiers				
Mod	Non-Fac Total	Fac Total		51	50	62	80	MUE
	26.30	26.30	090	2	1	0	2	1

● New ▲ Revised ✖ Deleted ⊙ Moderate Sedation ✚ Add-on Codes ⊘ High Risk Denial Ⓐ Age Edit ♀ Female ♂ Male **AMA** *CPT® Assistant* **MUE** Medically Unlikely Edit
⦸ Modifier 51 Exempt ⊖ Modifier 63 Exempt ✗ Unlisted **Modifiers:** *See Inside Back Cover* Ⓜ Maternity A2–Z3 ASC Payment Indicators A–Y OPPS Status Indicators

CPT © 2015 American Medical Association. All Rights Reserved. | © 2016 DecisionHealth

58760   Fimbrioplasty   ♀⊘C

RVU			Global Days	Modifiers				
Mod	Non-Fac Total	Fac Total		51	50	62	80	MUE
	23.37	23.37	090	2	1	1	2	1

AMA: Nov 99: 29

58770   Salpingostomy (salpingoneostomy)   ♀T

RVU			Global Days	Modifiers				
Mod	Non-Fac Total	Fac Total		51	50	62	80	MUE
	26.39	26.39	090	2	1	0	2	1

AMA: Nov 99: 29

Ovarian Procedures

Incisional Ovarian Procedures

58800   Drainage of ovarian cyst(s), unilateral or bilateral (separate procedure); vaginal approach   ♀A2T

RVU			Global Days	Modifiers				
Mod	Non-Fac Total	Fac Total		51	50	62	80	MUE
	8.98	8.43	090	2	2	0	1	1

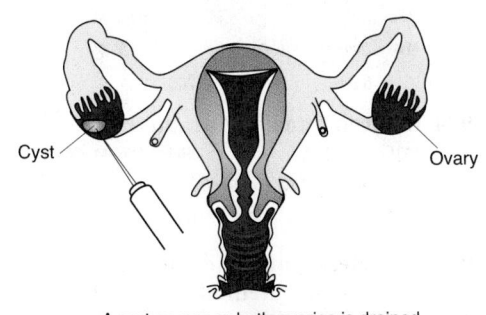

Drainage of ovarian cyst(s), unilateral or bilateral (separate procedure) vaginal/abdominal approach

A cyst on one or both ovaries is drained.
Vaginal (58800), or abdominal (58805) approach

58805   Drainage of ovarian cyst(s), unilateral or bilateral (separate procedure); abdominal approach   ♀G2T

RVU			Global Days	Modifiers				
Mod	Non-Fac Total	Fac Total		51	50	62	80	MUE
	11.44	11.44	090	2	2	1	2	1

58820   Drainage of ovarian abscess; vaginal approach, open   ♀A2T

RVU			Global Days	Modifiers				
Mod	Non-Fac Total	Fac Total		51	50	62	80	MUE
	8.83	8.83	090	2	1	0	2	1

AMA: Nov 97: 22

58822   Drainage of ovarian abscess; abdominal approach   ♀C

RVU			Global Days	Modifiers				
Mod	Non-Fac Total	Fac Total		51	50	62	80	MUE
	21.38	21.38	090	2	1	1	2	1

AMA: Nov 97: 22

58825   Transposition, ovary(s)   ♀C

RVU			Global Days	Modifiers				
Mod	Non-Fac Total	Fac Total		51	50	62	80	MUE
	19.83	19.83	090	2	0	1	2	1

Transposition, ovary(s)

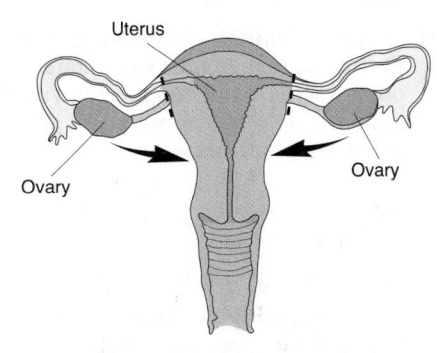

The ovaries are surgically accessed and positioned behind the uterus for the duration of pelvic radiation therapy.

Excisional Ovarian Procedures

58900   Biopsy of ovary, unilateral or bilateral (separate procedure)   ♀A2T

RVU			Global Days	Modifiers				
Mod	Non-Fac Total	Fac Total		51	50	62	80	MUE
	12.99	12.99	090	2	2	1	2	1

AMA: Nov 99: 29

58920   Wedge resection or bisection of ovary, unilateral or bilateral   ♀J1

RVU			Global Days	Modifiers				
Mod	Non-Fac Total	Fac Total		51	50	62	80	MUE
	21.77	21.77	090	2	2	1	2	1

58925   Ovarian cystectomy, unilateral or bilateral   ♀J1

RVU			Global Days	Modifiers				
Mod	Non-Fac Total	Fac Total		51	50	62	80	MUE
	21.24	21.24	090	2	2	1	2	1

58940   Oophorectomy, partial or total, unilateral or bilateral   ♀C

RVU			Global Days	Modifiers				
Mod	Non-Fac Total	Fac Total		51	50	62	80	MUE
	14.93	14.93	090	2	2	1	2	1

AMA: Mar 04: 3

58943   Oophorectomy, partial or total, unilateral or bilateral; for ovarian, tubal or primary peritoneal malignancy, with para-aortic and pelvic lymph node biopsies, peritoneal washings, peritoneal biopsies, diaphragmatic assessments, with or without salpingectomy(s), with or without omentectomy   ♀C

RVU			Global Days	Modifiers				
Mod	Non-Fac Total	Fac Total		51	50	62	80	MUE
	33.77	33.77	090	2	0	1	2	1

AMA: Oct 10: 16, Dec 10: 16

● New   ▲ Revised   Deleted   ⊙ Moderate Sedation   ✚ Add-on Codes   ⊘ High Risk Denial   Ⓐ Age Edit   ♀ Female   ♂ Male   **AMA** CPT® Assistant   **MUE** Medically Unlikely Edit
⊘ Modifier 51 Exempt   ⊖ Modifier 63 Exempt   ✗ Unlisted   **Modifiers:** See Inside Back Cover   Ⓜ Maternity   A2–Z3 ASC Payment Indicators   A–Y OPPS Status Indicators

© 2016 DecisionHealth   CPT © 2015 American Medical Association. All Rights Reserved.   **537**

Surgical Procedures

58760 – 58943

58950 Resection (initial) of ovarian, tubal or primary peritoneal malignancy with bilateral salpingo-oophorectomy and omentectomy ♀Ⓒ

RVU			Global Days	Modifiers				
Mod	Non-Fac Total	Fac Total		51	50	62	80	MUE
	32.47	32.47	090	2	2	1	2	1

AMA: Oct 10: 16, Dec 10: 16

58951 Resection (initial) of ovarian, tubal or primary peritoneal malignancy with bilateral salpingo-oophorectomy and omentectomy; with total abdominal hysterectomy, pelvic and limited para-aortic lymphadenectomy ♀Ⓒ

RVU			Global Days	Modifiers				
Mod	Non-Fac Total	Fac Total		51	50	62	80	MUE
	41.74	41.74	090	2	2	1	2	1

AMA: Aug 01: 11, Oct 10: 16, Dec 10: 16

58952 Resection (initial) of ovarian, tubal or primary peritoneal malignancy with bilateral salpingo-oophorectomy and omentectomy; with radical dissection for debulking (ie, radical excision or destruction, intra-abdominal or retroperitoneal tumors) ♀Ⓒ

RVU			Global Days	Modifiers				
Mod	Non-Fac Total	Fac Total		51	50	62	80	MUE
	47.18	47.18	090	2	2	1	2	1

AMA: Dec 96: 10, Aug 01: 11, Oct 10: 16, Dec 10: 16

58953 Bilateral salpingo-oophorectomy with omentectomy, total abdominal hysterectomy and radical dissection for debulking ♀Ⓒ

RVU			Global Days	Modifiers				
Mod	Non-Fac Total	Fac Total		51	50	62	80	MUE
	58.38	58.38	090	2	2	1	2	1

AMA: Feb 02: 8, Oct 10: 16, Dec 10: 16, May 14: 10

58954 Bilateral salpingo-oophorectomy with omentectomy, total abdominal hysterectomy and radical dissection for debulking; with pelvic lymphadenectomy and limited para-aortic lymphadenectomy ♀Ⓒ

RVU			Global Days	Modifiers				
Mod	Non-Fac Total	Fac Total		51	50	62	80	MUE
	63.36	63.36	090	2	2	1	2	1

AMA: Feb 02: 9, Oct 10: 16, Dec 10: 16

58956 Bilateral salpingo-oophorectomy with total omentectomy, total abdominal hysterectomy for malignancy ♀Ⓒ

RVU			Global Days	Modifiers				
Mod	Non-Fac Total	Fac Total		51	50	62	80	MUE
	39.67	39.67	090	2	2	1	2	1

AMA: May 14: 10

58957 Resection (tumor debulking) of recurrent ovarian, tubal, primary peritoneal, uterine malignancy (intra-abdominal, retroperitoneal tumors), with omentectomy, if performed ♀Ⓒ

RVU			Global Days	Modifiers				
Mod	Non-Fac Total	Fac Total		51	50	62	80	MUE
	45.66	45.66	090	2	2	1	2	1

58958 Resection (tumor debulking) of recurrent ovarian, tubal, primary peritoneal, uterine malignancy (intra-abdominal, retroperitoneal tumors), with omentectomy, if performed; with pelvic lymphadenectomy and limited para-aortic lymphadenectomy ♀Ⓒ

RVU			Global Days	Modifiers				
Mod	Non-Fac Total	Fac Total		51	50	62	80	MUE
	50.13	50.13	090	2	2	1	2	1

58960 Laparotomy, for staging or restaging of ovarian, tubal, or primary peritoneal malignancy (second look), with or without omentectomy, peritoneal washing, biopsy of abdominal and pelvic peritoneum, diaphragmatic assessment with pelvic and limited para-aortic lymphadenectomy ♀Ⓒ

RVU			Global Days	Modifiers				
Mod	Non-Fac Total	Fac Total		51	50	62	80	MUE
	27.98	27.98	090	2	0	1	2	1

In Vitro Fertilization Procedures

58970 Follicle puncture for oocyte retrieval, any method ♀ Ⓜ A2 T

Coding Tip: *Ultrasound guidance for follicle puncture - 76948*

RVU			Global Days	Modifiers				
Mod	Non-Fac Total	Fac Total		51	50	62	80	MUE
	6.30	5.69	000	2	0	0	0	1

58974 Embryo transfer, intrauterine ♀ Ⓜ A2 T

RVU			Global Days	Modifiers				
Mod	Non-Fac Total	Fac Total		51	50	62	80	MUE
	0.00	0.00	000	2	0	1	2	1

58976 Gamete, zygote, or embryo intrafallopian transfer, any method ♀ Ⓜ A2 T

RVU			Global Days	Modifiers				
Mod	Non-Fac Total	Fac Total		51	50	62	80	MUE
	7.18	6.23	000	2	0	1	2	2

AMA: Nov 99: 29

Other Female Genital System Procedures

58999 Unlisted procedure, female genital system (nonobstetrical) ♀ x T

RVU			Global Days	Modifiers				
Mod	Non-Fac Total	Fac Total		51	50	62	80	MUE
	0.00	0.00	YYY	2	0	1	1	

AMA: Apr 09: 9, 10

Maternity Care/Delivery Procedures

Antepartum Care

59000 Amniocentesis; diagnostic ♀ Ⓜ P3 T

Coding Tip: *Ultrasound guidance for amniocentesis - 76946*

RVU			Global Days	Modifiers				
Mod	Non-Fac Total	Fac Total		51	50	62	80	MUE
	3.60	2.34	000	2	0	0	1	1

AMA: Apr 97: 2, Feb 02: 7, Aug 02: 2, May 04: 2

CPT © 2015 American Medical Association. All Rights Reserved. © 2016 DecisionHealth

59001 Amniocentesis; therapeutic amniotic fluid reduction (includes ultrasound guidance) ♀ⓂR2T

RVU			Global Days	Modifiers				
Mod	Non-Fac Total	Fac Total		51	50	62	80	MUE
	5.23	5.23	000	2	0	0	1	1

AMA: Feb 02: 7, Aug 02: 2

Amniocentesis; therapeutic amniotic fluid reduction

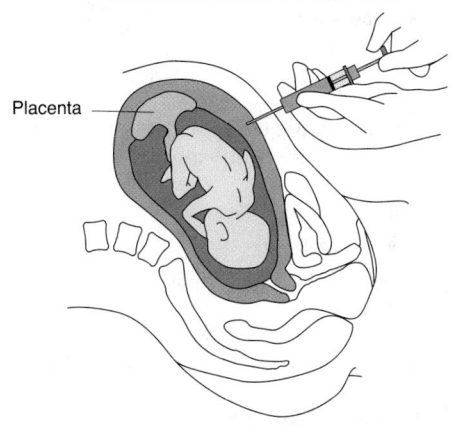

Placenta

Using ultrasonic guidance, amniotic fluid is aspirated for therapeutic purposes. As much as seven liters may be drained.

59012 Cordocentesis (intrauterine), any method ♀ⓂG2T

Coding Tip: Ultrasound guidance for sampling - 76945

RVU			Global Days	Modifiers				
Mod	Non-Fac Total	Fac Total		51	50	62	80	MUE
	5.90	5.90	000	2	0	0	0	1

AMA: Aug 02: 2

Cordocentesis (intrauterine), any method

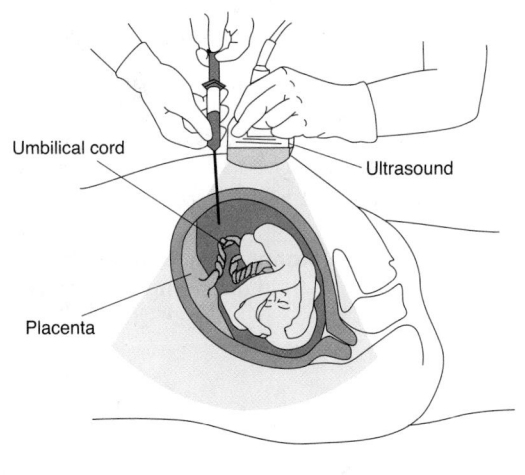

Umbilical cord

Ultrasound

Placenta

Fetal blood is aspirated using a transamniotic or transplacental approach.

59015 Chorionic villus sampling, any method ♀ⓂP3T

RVU			Global Days	Modifiers				
Mod	Non-Fac Total	Fac Total		51	50	62	80	MUE
	4.49	3.83	000	2	0	0	0	1

AMA: Apr 97: 2, Aug 02: 2

59020 Fetal contraction stress test ♀ⓂP3T

Coding Tip: Fetal monitoring during labor - 59050-59051

RVU			Global Days	Modifiers				
Mod	Non-Fac Total	Fac Total		51	50	62	80	MUE
	2.03	2.03	000	0	0	0	0	2
26	1.07	1.07	000	0	0	0	0	2
TC	0.96	0.96	000	0	0	0	0	2

AMA: Apr 97: 2, Aug 02: 2

59025 Fetal non-stress test ♀ⓂP3T

Coding Tip: Report 59025 when fetal heart rate acceleration only is evaluated. If the physician also evaluates other variables, such as fetal tone, diaphragmatic breathing, body movements, or amniotic fluid volume, report 76818

RVU			Global Days	Modifiers				
Mod	Non-Fac Total	Fac Total		51	50	62	80	MUE
	1.38	1.38	000	0	0	0	0	3
26	0.86	0.86	000	0	0	0	0	3
TC	0.52	0.52	000	0	0	0	0	3

AMA: Apr 97: 2, May 98: 10, Oct 04: 10, Dec 08: 8

59030 Fetal scalp blood sampling ♀ⓂT

RVU			Global Days	Modifiers				
Mod	Non-Fac Total	Fac Total		51	50	62	80	MUE
	2.89	2.89	000	2	0	0	0	4

AMA: Aug 02: 3

Coding Guidance
Fetal monitoring during labor is included in all delivery codes and is not reported separately.

59050 Fetal monitoring during labor by consulting physician (ie, non-attending physician) with written report; supervision and interpretation ⊗♀ⓂⓂ

Coding Tip: Fetal contraction stress test - 59020

RVU			Global Days	Modifiers				
Mod	Non-Fac Total	Fac Total		51	50	62	80	MUE
	1.47	1.47	XXX	0	0	0	0	1

AMA: Nov 97: 22

59051 Fetal monitoring during labor by consulting physician (ie, non-attending physician) with written report; interpretation only ♀ⓂB

RVU			Global Days	Modifiers				
Mod	Non-Fac Total	Fac Total		51	50	62	80	MUE
	1.22	1.22	XXX	0	0	0	0	1

AMA: Nov 97: 22

59070 Transabdominal amnioinfusion, including ultrasound guidance ♀ⓂG2T

RVU			Global Days	Modifiers				
Mod	Non-Fac Total	Fac Total		51	50	62	80	MUE
	11.46	8.74	000	2	0	0	2	2

AMA: May 04: 2, Jun 04: 11

● New   ▲ Revised   Deleted   ⊙ Moderate Sedation   ✚ Add-on Codes   ⊘ High Risk Denial   Ⓐ Age Edit   ♀ Female   ♂ Male   **AMA** *CPT® Assistant*   ***MUE*** Medically Unlikely Edit
⊘ Modifier 51 Exempt   ⊖ Modifier 63 Exempt   ✗ Unlisted   **Modifiers:** *See Inside Back Cover*   Ⓜ Maternity   A2–Z3 ASC Payment Indicators   A–Y OPPS Status Indicators

59072 **Fetal umbilical cord occlusion, including ultrasound guidance** ♀Ⓜ G2 T

RVU			Global Days	Modifiers				
Mod	Non-Fac Total	Fac Total		51	50	62	80	MUE
	13.50	13.50	000	2	0	0	1	2

AMA: May 04: 2, Jun 04: 11

59074 **Fetal fluid drainage (eg, vesicocentesis, thoracocentesis, paracentesis), including ultrasound guidance** ♀ⓂG2 T

RVU			Global Days	Modifiers				
Mod	Non-Fac Total	Fac Total		51	50	62	80	MUE
	10.97	8.64	000	2	0	0	2	1

AMA: May 04: 2, 4, Dec 04: 19, Jun 04: 11

59076 **Fetal shunt placement, including ultrasound guidance** ♀ⓂG2 T

RVU			Global Days	Modifiers				
Mod	Non-Fac Total	Fac Total		51	50	62	80	MUE
	13.50	13.50	000	2	0	0	2	1

AMA: May 04: 2, 4, Dec 04: 19, Jun 04: 11

Excisional Procedures

59100 **Hysterotomy, abdominal (eg, for hydatidiform mole, abortion)** ♀Ⓜ R2 T

RVU			Global Days	Modifiers				
Mod	Non-Fac Total	Fac Total		51	50	62	80	MUE
	22.82	22.82	090	2	0	1	2	1

59120 **Surgical treatment of ectopic pregnancy; tubal or ovarian, requiring salpingectomy and/or oophorectomy, abdominal or vaginal approach** ♀ⓂC

RVU			Global Days	Modifiers				
Mod	Non-Fac Total	Fac Total		51	50	62	80	MUE
	22.96	22.96	090	2	0	1	2	1

59121 **Surgical treatment of ectopic pregnancy; tubal or ovarian, without salpingectomy and/or oophorectomy** ⊘♀ⓂC

RVU			Global Days	Modifiers				
Mod	Non-Fac Total	Fac Total		51	50	62	80	MUE
	23.04	23.04	090	2	0	1	2	1

59130 **Surgical treatment of ectopic pregnancy; abdominal pregnancy** ♀ⓂC

RVU			Global Days	Modifiers				
Mod	Non-Fac Total	Fac Total		51	50	62	80	MUE
	26.91	26.91	090	2	0	0	0	1

59135 **Surgical treatment of ectopic pregnancy; interstitial, uterine pregnancy requiring total hysterectomy** ♀ⓂC

RVU			Global Days	Modifiers				
Mod	Non-Fac Total	Fac Total		51	50	62	80	MUE
	23.91	23.91	090	2	0	0	0	1

59136 **Surgical treatment of ectopic pregnancy; interstitial, uterine pregnancy with partial resection of uterus** ♀ⓂC

RVU			Global Days	Modifiers				
Mod	Non-Fac Total	Fac Total		51	50	62	80	MUE
	24.52	24.52	090	2	0	0	2	1

59140 **Surgical treatment of ectopic pregnancy; cervical, with evacuation** ♀ⓂC

RVU			Global Days	Modifiers				
Mod	Non-Fac Total	Fac Total		51	50	62	80	MUE
	11.50	11.50	090	2	0	0	2	1

59150 **Laparoscopic treatment of ectopic pregnancy; without salpingectomy and/or oophorectomy** ♀ⓂG2 J I

RVU			Global Days	Modifiers				
Mod	Non-Fac Total	Fac Total		51	50	62	80	MUE
	22.30	22.30	090	2	0	0	2	1

AMA: Sep 96: 9

59151 **Laparoscopic treatment of ectopic pregnancy; with salpingectomy and/or oophorectomy** ♀ⓂG2 J I

RVU			Global Days	Modifiers				
Mod	Non-Fac Total	Fac Total		51	50	62	80	MUE
	21.64	21.64	090	2	0	0	2	1

59160 **Curettage, postpartum** ♀Ⓜ A2 T

Coding Tip: Use 59160 for D&C of a retained placenta

RVU			Global Days	Modifiers				
Mod	Non-Fac Total	Fac Total		51	50	62	80	MUE
	5.87	5.02	010	2	0	0	0	1

AMA: Nov 97: 22, Sep 02: 11

Introduction Procedures

59200 **Insertion of cervical dilator (eg, laminaria, prostaglandin) (separate procedure)** ♀Ⓜ P3 T

RVU			Global Days	Modifiers				
Mod	Non-Fac Total	Fac Total		51	50	62	80	MUE
	2.06	1.29	000	2	0	0	1	1

AMA: Fall 93: 9, Apr 97: 3, Jul 05: 15

Maternity Care/Delivery Repair

Coding Guidance

Episiotomy is included in CPT codes for delivery.

59300 **Episiotomy or vaginal repair, by other than attending** ♀Ⓜ P3 T

RVU			Global Days	Modifiers				
Mod	Non-Fac Total	Fac Total		51	50	62	80	MUE
	5.55	4.31	000	2	0	0	0	1

Episiotomy or vaginal repair, by other than attending physician

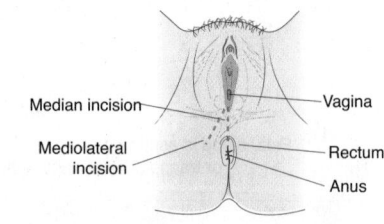

The physician repairs a perineal/vaginal tear that occurred during childbirth. The physician who performs these repairs is not the physician who delivered the baby.

● New   ▲ Revised   ✖ Deleted   ⊙ Moderate Sedation   ✚ Add-on Codes   ⊘ High Risk Denial   Ⓐ Age Edit   ♀ Female   ♂ Male   **AMA** *CPT® Assistant*   **MUE** Medically Unlikely Edit

⊘ Modifier 51 Exempt   ⊖ Modifier 63 Exempt   ✗ Unlisted   **Modifiers:** *See Inside Back Cover*   Ⓜ Maternity   A2 – Z3 ASC Payment Indicators   A – Y OPPS Status Indicators

540   CPT © 2015 American Medical Association. All Rights Reserved.   © 2016 DecisionHealth

59320 Cerclage of cervix, during pregnancy; vaginal
♀ⓂA2T

Coding Tip: Nonobstetrical cerclage of cervix - 57700

RVU			Global Days	Modifiers				
Mod	Non-Fac Total	Fac Total		51	50	62	80	MUE
	4.42	4.42	000	2	0	0	0	1

AMA: Aug 02: 2, Nov 06: 21, Feb 07: 10

59325 Cerclage of cervix, during pregnancy; abdominal
♀ⒸC

RVU			Global Days	Modifiers				
Mod	Non-Fac Total	Fac Total		51	50	62	80	MUE
	7.06	7.06	000	2	0	0	0	1

AMA: Aug 02: 2, Nov 06: 21, Feb 07: 10

59350 Hysterorrhaphy of ruptured uterus
♀ⒸC

RVU			Global Days	Modifiers				
Mod	Non-Fac Total	Fac Total		51	50	62	80	MUE
	7.52	7.52	000	2	0	0	2	1

AMA: Aug 02: 2

Antepartum/Postpartum Care, Vaginal Delivery

Coding Guidance
The total obstetrical package includes antepartum care, the type of delivery specified, and all postpartum care. Services such as ultrasound, amniocentesis, genetic screening, unrelated visits incidental to the pregnancy, and extra care due to high risk conditions are not included in the general obstetric care codes.

59400 Routine obstetric care including antepartum care, vaginal delivery (with or without episiotomy, and/or forceps) and postpartum care
♀ⒷB

RVU			Global Days	Modifiers				
Mod	Non-Fac Total	Fac Total		51	50	62	80	MUE
	60.31	60.31	MMM	2	0	0	1	1

AMA: Feb 96: 1, Mar 96: 11, Feb 97: 11, Apr 97: 3, Apr 98: 15, Jun 98: 10, Aug 02: 3, Feb 03: 15

59409 Vaginal delivery only (with or without episiotomy and/or forceps)
♀ⓉT

RVU			Global Days	Modifiers				
Mod	Non-Fac Total	Fac Total		51	50	62	80	MUE
	23.62	23.62	MMM	2	0	0	0	2

AMA: Feb 96: 1, Mar 96: 11, Jul 96: 11, Sep 96: 4, Feb 97: 11, Apr 97: 1, Aug 02: 3, Jun 09: 10, Dec 07: 13

59410 Vaginal delivery only (with or without episiotomy and/or forceps); including postpartum care
♀ⒷB

RVU			Global Days	Modifiers				
Mod	Non-Fac Total	Fac Total		51	50	62	80	MUE
	30.09	30.09	MMM	2	0	0	1	1

59412 External cephalic version, with or without tocolysis
♀ⓂG2T

RVU			Global Days	Modifiers				
Mod	Non-Fac Total	Fac Total		51	50	62	80	MUE
	3.00	3.00	MMM	0	0	0	0	1

AMA: Fall 94: 21, Feb 96: 1, Aug 02: 2, 3

59414 Delivery of placenta (separate procedure)
♀ⓂG2T

Coding Tip: Do not code 59414 in addition to a delivery service code
Coding Tip: Delivery of the placenta is reported in cases when the patient delivers vaginally before admission and the physician then subsequently delivers only the placenta

RVU			Global Days	Modifiers				
Mod	Non-Fac Total	Fac Total		51	50	62	80	MUE
	2.67	2.67	MMM	2	0	0	0	1

AMA: Jun 96: 10, Jun 98: 10, Aug 02: 3

Delivery of placenta (seperate procedure)

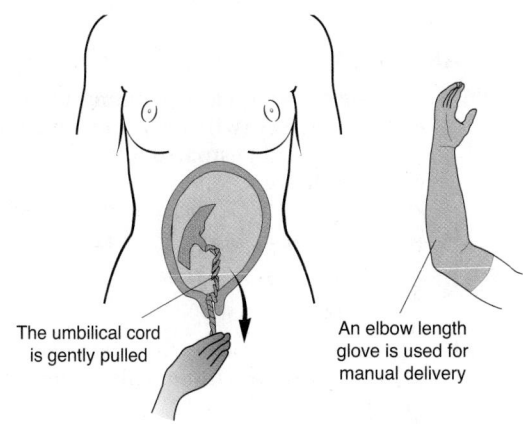

The umbilical cord is gently pulled

An elbow length glove is used for manual delivery

A nonexpelled placenta is removed following fetal delivery

59425 Antepartum care only; 4-6 visits
♀ⒷB

RVU			Global Days	Modifiers				
Mod	Non-Fac Total	Fac Total		51	50	62	80	MUE
	13.08	10.31	MMM	0	0	0	0	1

AMA: Fall 94: 21, Apr 97: 11, Aug 02: 3

59426 Antepartum care only; 7 or more visits
♀ⒷB

RVU			Global Days	Modifiers				
Mod	Non-Fac Total	Fac Total		51	50	62	80	MUE
	23.39	18.16	MMM	0	0	0	0	1

AMA: Fall 94: 21, Apr 97: 11, Aug 02: 3

59430 Postpartum care only (separate procedure)
♀ⒷB

RVU			Global Days	Modifiers				
Mod	Non-Fac Total	Fac Total		51	50	62	80	MUE
	5.30	4.02	MMM	2	0	0	1	1

AMA: Jun 96: 10, Aug 02: 3

Cesarean Delivery

59510 Routine obstetric care including antepartum care, cesarean delivery, and postpartum care
♀ⒷB

RVU			Global Days	Modifiers				
Mod	Non-Fac Total	Fac Total		51	50	62	80	MUE
	66.97	66.97	MMM	2	0	0	1	1

AMA: Jul 96: 11, Sep 96: 4, Oct 96: 10, Feb 97: 11, Apr 97: 2, Aug 02: 3, Mar 13: 13

59514 Cesarean delivery only
♀ⒸC

RVU			Global Days	Modifiers				
Mod	Non-Fac Total	Fac Total		51	50	62	80	MUE
	26.63	26.63	MMM	2	0	1	2	1

AMA: Oct 96: 10, Feb 97: 11, Mar 13: 13

● New ▲ Revised Deleted ⊙ Moderate Sedation ✚ Add-on Codes ⊘ High Risk Denial Ⓐ Age Edit ♀ Female ♂ Male **AMA** CPT® Assistant **MUE** Medically Unlikely Edit
⊘ Modifier 51 Exempt ⊖ Modifier 63 Exempt ✗ Unlisted **Modifiers:** See Inside Back Cover Ⓜ Maternity A2–Z3 ASC Payment Indicators A–Y OPPS Status Indicators

59515 Cesarean delivery only; including postpartum care ♀Ⓜ🄱

Mod	Non-Fac Total	Fac Total	Global Days	51	50	62	80	MUE
	36.61	36.61	MMM	2	0	0	1	1

AMA: Mar 13: 13

➕ 59525 Subtotal or total hysterectomy after cesarean delivery (List separately in addition to code for primary procedure) ♀Ⓜ🄲

Mod	Non-Fac Total	Fac Total	Global Days	51	50	62	80	MUE
	14.04	14.04	ZZZ	0	0	1	2	1

Vaginal Delivery After Previous Cesarean Delivery

59610 Routine obstetric care including antepartum care, vaginal delivery (with or without episiotomy, and/or forceps) and postpartum care, after previous cesarean delivery ♀Ⓜ🄱

Mod	Non-Fac Total	Fac Total	Global Days	51	50	62	80	MUE
	63.50	63.50	MMM	2	0	0	0	1

AMA: Feb 96: 2, Apr 97: 3, Aug 02: 3

59612 Vaginal delivery only, after previous cesarean delivery (with or without episiotomy and/or forceps) ♀Ⓜ🅃

Mod	Non-Fac Total	Fac Total	Global Days	51	50	62	80	MUE
	26.64	26.64	MMM	2	0	0	0	2

AMA: Feb 96: 2, Aug 02: 3

59614 Vaginal delivery only, after previous cesarean delivery (with or without episiotomy and/or forceps); including postpartum care ♀Ⓜ🄱

Mod	Non-Fac Total	Fac Total	Global Days	51	50	62	80	MUE
	33.13	33.13	MMM	2	0	0	0	1

AMA: Feb 96: 2

Cesarean Delivery After Previous Cesarean

59618 Routine obstetric care including antepartum care, cesarean delivery, and postpartum care, following attempted vaginal delivery after previous cesarean delivery ♀Ⓜ🄱

Mod	Non-Fac Total	Fac Total	Global Days	51	50	62	80	MUE
	67.87	67.87	MMM	2	0	0	0	1

AMA: Feb 96: 2, Aug 02: 4

Routine obstetric care following attempted vaginal delivery after previous cesarean delivery

Typical incision

After attempting to deliver a baby vaginally, the physician delivers the baby through an incision in the abdomen.

59620 Cesarean delivery only, following attempted vaginal delivery after previous cesarean delivery ♀Ⓜ🄲

Mod	Non-Fac Total	Fac Total	Global Days	51	50	62	80	MUE
	27.29	27.29	MMM	2	0	0	2	1

AMA: Feb 96: 2

59622 Cesarean delivery only, following attempted vaginal delivery after previous cesarean delivery; including postpartum care ♀Ⓜ🄱

Mod	Non-Fac Total	Fac Total	Global Days	51	50	62	80	MUE
	37.62	37.62	MMM	2	0	0	0	1

AMA: Feb 96: 2

Abortion Procedures

59812 Treatment of incomplete abortion, any trimester, completed surgically ♀Ⓜ🄰🄼🅃

Mod	Non-Fac Total	Fac Total	Global Days	51	50	62	80	MUE
	9.18	8.54	090	2	0	0	1	1

AMA: Fall 93: 9, Fall 95: 16

59820 Treatment of missed abortion, completed surgically; first trimester ♀Ⓜ🄰🄼🅃

Mod	Non-Fac Total	Fac Total	Global Days	51	50	62	80	MUE
	10.92	10.28	090	2	0	0	1	1

AMA: Fall 93: 9, Fall 95: 16, Feb 99: 10

59821 Treatment of missed abortion, completed surgically; second trimester ♀Ⓜ🄰🄼🅃

Mod	Non-Fac Total	Fac Total	Global Days	51	50	62	80	MUE
	11.02	10.32	090	2	0	0	0	1

AMA: Fall 93: 9, Fall 95: 16

59830 Treatment of septic abortion, completed surgically ♀Ⓜ🄲

Mod	Non-Fac Total	Fac Total	Global Days	51	50	62	80	MUE
	12.62	12.62	090	2	0	0	0	1

AMA: Fall 93: 9

59840 Induced abortion, by dilation and curettage ⊘♀Ⓜ🄰🄼🅃

Mod	Non-Fac Total	Fac Total	Global Days	51	50	62	80	MUE
	6.26	6.02	010	2	0	0	0	1

AMA: Fall 93: 9, Sep 03: 16

59841 Induced abortion, by dilation and evacuation ⊘♀Ⓜ🄰🄼🅃

Mod	Non-Fac Total	Fac Total	Global Days	51	50	62	80	MUE
	11.04	10.44	010	2	0	0	0	1

AMA: Fall 93: 9

59850 Induced abortion, by 1 or more intra-amniotic injections (amniocentesis-injections), including hospital admission and visits, delivery of fetus and secundines ♀Ⓜ🄲

Mod	Non-Fac Total	Fac Total	Global Days	51	50	62	80	MUE
	10.01	10.01	090	2	0	0	0	1

AMA: Fall 93: 10

● New   ▲ Revised   ✖ Deleted   ⊙ Moderate Sedation   ➕ Add-on Codes   ⊘ High Risk Denial   Ⓐ Age Edit   ♀ Female   ♂ Male   **AMA** *CPT® Assistant*   **MUE** Medically Unlikely Edit

⃠ Modifier 51 Exempt   ⊖ Modifier 63 Exempt   ⌧ Unlisted   **Modifiers:** *See Inside Back Cover*   Ⓜ Maternity   🄰🄼–🅉🄼 ASC Payment Indicators   🄰–🅈 OPPS Status Indicators

CPT © 2015 American Medical Association. All Rights Reserved.   © 2016 DecisionHealth

59851 Induced abortion, by 1 or more intra-amniotic injections (amniocentesis-injections), including hospital admission and visits, delivery of fetus and secundines; with dilation and curettage and/or evacuation ♀Ⓜ🄲

RVU			Global Days	Modifiers				
Mod	Non-Fac Total	Fac Total		51	50	62	80	MUE
	10.62	10.62	090	2	0	0	0	1

AMA: Fall 93: 10

59852 Induced abortion, by 1 or more intra-amniotic injections (amniocentesis-injections), including hospital admission and visits, delivery of fetus and secundines; with hysterotomy (failed intra-amniotic injection) ♀Ⓜ🄲

RVU			Global Days	Modifiers				
Mod	Non-Fac Total	Fac Total		51	50	62	80	MUE
	14.48	14.48	090	2	0	0	0	1

AMA: Fall 93: 10

59855 Induced abortion, by 1 or more vaginal suppositories (eg, prostaglandin) with or without cervical dilation (eg, laminaria), including hospital admission and visits, delivery of fetus and secundines ♀Ⓜ🄲

RVU			Global Days	Modifiers				
Mod	Non-Fac Total	Fac Total		51	50	62	80	MUE
	12.01	12.01	090	2	0	0	0	1

59856 Induced abortion, by 1 or more vaginal suppositories (eg, prostaglandin) with or without cervical dilation (eg, laminaria), including hospital admission and visits, delivery of fetus and secundines; with dilation and curettage and/or evacuation ♀Ⓜ🄲

RVU			Global Days	Modifiers				
Mod	Non-Fac Total	Fac Total		51	50	62	80	MUE
	14.12	14.12	090	2	0	0	0	1

59857 Induced abortion, by 1 or more vaginal suppositories (eg, prostaglandin) with or without cervical dilation (eg, laminaria), including hospital admission and visits, delivery of fetus and secundines; with hysterotomy (failed medical evacuation) ♀Ⓜ🄲

Coding Tip: The physician who performs the postoperative care only, should report the surgical code with modifier 55 appended

Coding Tip: The operating surgeon who performs the abortion only should report the surgical code with modifier 54

Coding Tip: If a single physician performs the preoperative care, abortion, and postoperative care submit code 59857 without a modifier

Coding Tip: The physician who performs the preoperative care only should report the surgical code with modifier 56

RVU			Global Days	Modifiers				
Mod	Non-Fac Total	Fac Total		51	50	62	80	MUE
	14.89	14.89	090	2	0	0	0	1

Other Maternity Care/Delivery Procedures

59866 Multifetal pregnancy reduction(s) (MPR) ♀Ⓜ🄶🄶🅃

RVU			Global Days	Modifiers				
Mod	Non-Fac Total	Fac Total		51	50	62	80	MUE
	6.23	6.23	000	2	0	1	2	1

59870 Uterine evacuation and curettage for hydatidiform mole ♀Ⓜ🄰🄰🅃

RVU			Global Days	Modifiers				
Mod	Non-Fac Total	Fac Total		51	50	62	80	MUE
	13.63	13.63	090	2	0	0	2	1

AMA: Feb 99: 10

Uterine evacuation and curettage for hydatidiform mole

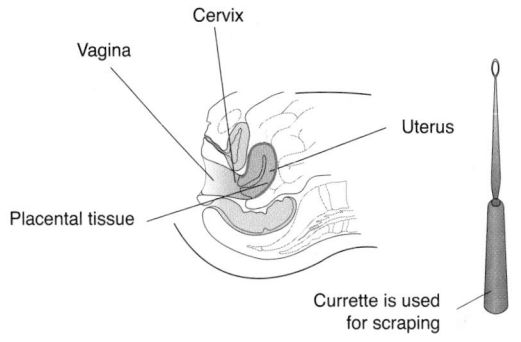

The uterus is suctioned and scraped to remove an abnormal mass of placental tissue/molar pregnancy

59871 Removal of cerclage suture under anesthesia (other than local) ♀Ⓜ🄰🄰🅀🅀

RVU			Global Days	Modifiers				
Mod	Non-Fac Total	Fac Total		51	50	62	80	MUE
	3.86	3.86	000	2	0	0	0	1

AMA: Nov 97: 22, Nov 06: 21, Feb 07: 10

Removal of cerclage suture under anesthesia (other than local)

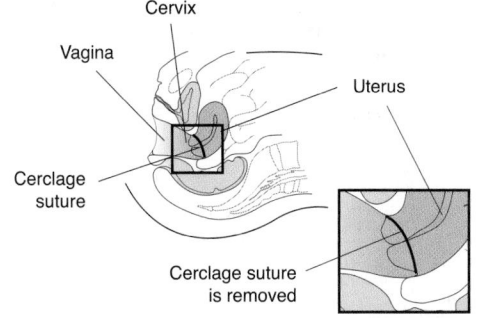

Under anesthesia, sutures are removed from around the cervix that were placed there to hold it closed during pregnancy.

● New   ▲ Revised   Deleted   ⊙ Moderate Sedation   ✚ Add-on Codes   ⊘ High Risk Denial   Ⓐ Age Edit   ♀ Female   ♂ Male   **AMA** *CPT® Assistant*   **MUE** Medically Unlikely Edit
⊘ Modifier 51 Exempt   ⊖ Modifier 63 Exempt   🅇 Unlisted   **Modifiers:** *See Inside Back Cover*   Ⓜ Maternity   🄰🄰-🅉🄱 ASC Payment Indicators   🄰-🅈 OPPS Status Indicators

59897   Unlisted fetal invasive procedure, including ultrasound guidance, when performed ⊗♀✗Ⓜ🅣

RVU Mod	Non-Fac Total	Fac Total	Global Days	Modifiers 51	50	62	80	MUE
	0.00	0.00	YYY	2	0	0		1

AMA: May 04: 5

59898   Unlisted laparoscopy procedure, maternity care and delivery ⊗♀✗🅙🅣

RVU Mod	Non-Fac Total	Fac Total	Global Days	Modifiers 51	50	62	80	MUE
	0.00	0.00	YYY	2	1	1		2

AMA: Nov 99: 29, Mar 00: 10

59899   Unlisted procedure, maternity care and delivery ⊗♀✗🅣

RVU Mod	Non-Fac Total	Fac Total	Global Days	Modifiers 51	50	62	80	MUE
	0.00	0.00	YYY	2	0	1		2

AMA: Jun 97: 10, May 04: 2, Oct 13: 3

● New   ▲ Revised   ✖ Deleted   ⊙ Moderate Sedation   ✚ Add-on Codes   ⊗ High Risk Denial   Ⓐ Age Edit   ♀ Female   ♂ Male   **AMA** *CPT® Assistant*   ***MUE*** Medically Unlikely Edit
⊘ Modifier 51 Exempt   ⊖ Modifier 63 Exempt   ✗ Unlisted   **Modifiers:** *See Inside Back Cover*   Ⓜ Maternity   Ⓐ2–Ⓩ3 ASC Payment Indicators   Ⓐ–Ⓨ OPPS Status Indicators

544   CPT © 2015 American Medical Association. All Rights Reserved.   © 2016 DecisionHealth

Endocrine System Procedures

Endocrine procedures are a small group of codes that encompass thyroid procedures, removal of the adrenal glands, parathyroid, and thymus gland, and carotid body tumor.

Thyroid Gland Procedures

Incisional Thyroid Gland Procedures

60000 Incision and drainage of thyroglossal duct cyst, infected   ⊗ A 2 T

Coding tip: Aspiration of thyroid cyst - 60300

RVU			Global Days	Modifiers				
Mod	Non-Fac Total	Fac Total		51	50	62	80	MUE
	4.90	4.41	010	2	0	0	0	1

Excisional Thyroid Gland Procedures

60100 Biopsy thyroid, percutaneous core needle   P 3 T

Coding tip: Radiological guidance for correct needle placement - ultrasound 76942; fluoroscopy 77002; CT 77012; MRI 77021

Coding tip: Report this procedure separately only when performed alone, or distinct from other procedures on the same day

Coding tip: Code 99000 for specimen transfer from office setting to outside laboratory

RVU			Global Days	Modifiers				
Mod	Non-Fac Total	Fac Total		51	50	62	80	MUE
	3.22	2.28	000	2	0	0	1	3

AMA: Jun 97: 5, Jun 07: 10

Percutaneous thyroid biopsy

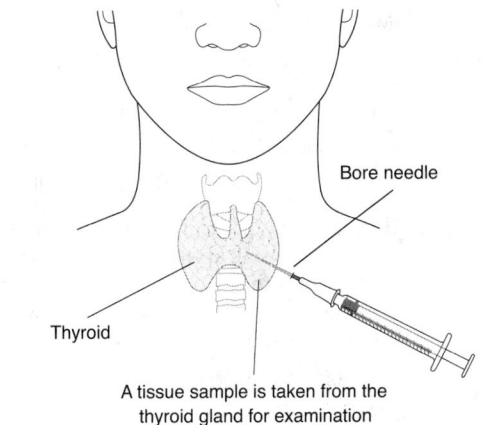

Bore needle

Thyroid

A tissue sample is taken from the thyroid gland for examination

60200 Excision of cyst or adenoma of thyroid, or transection of isthmus   A 2 J I

RVU			Global Days	Modifiers				
Mod	Non-Fac Total	Fac Total		51	50	62	80	MUE
	19.09	19.09	090	2	0	1	2	2

AMA: Aug 11: 10, Dec 12: 3

Excision of cyst or adenoma of thyroid

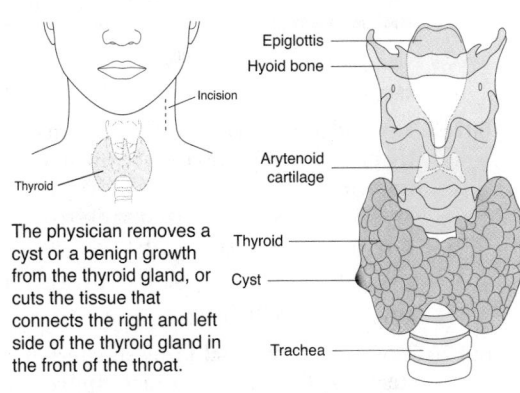

Epiglottis
Hyoid bone
Incision
Arytenoid cartilage
Thyroid
Thyroid
Cyst
Trachea

The physician removes a cyst or a benign growth from the thyroid gland, or cuts the tissue that connects the right and left side of the thyroid gland in the front of the throat.

60210 Partial thyroid lobectomy, unilateral; with or without isthmusectomy   G 2 J I

RVU			Global Days	Modifiers				
Mod	Non-Fac Total	Fac Total		51	50	62	80	MUE
	20.47	20.47	090	2	0	1	2	1

AMA: Aug 11: 9, Winter 94: 7, Dec 12: 3

60212 Partial thyroid lobectomy, unilateral; with contralateral subtotal lobectomy, including isthmusectomy   G 2 J I

RVU			Global Days	Modifiers				
Mod	Non-Fac Total	Fac Total		51	50	62	80	MUE
	29.12	29.12	090	2	0	1	2	1

AMA: Dec 12: 3

60220 Total thyroid lobectomy, unilateral; with or without isthmusectomy   G 2 J I

RVU			Global Days	Modifiers				
Mod	Non-Fac Total	Fac Total		51	50	62	80	MUE
	20.47	20.47	090	2	0	1	2	1

AMA: Aug 11: 10, Oct 10: 13, Dec 10: 13, Dec 12: 3

60225 Total thyroid lobectomy, unilateral; with contralateral subtotal lobectomy, including isthmusectomy   G 2 J I

RVU			Global Days	Modifiers				
Mod	Non-Fac Total	Fac Total		51	50	62	80	MUE
	26.99	26.99	090	2	0	1	2	1

AMA: Dec 12: 3

60240 Thyroidectomy, total or complete   G 2 J I

RVU			Global Days	Modifiers				
Mod	Non-Fac Total	Fac Total		51	50	62	80	MUE
	26.62	26.62	090	2	0	1	2	1

AMA: Dec 12: 3

60252 Thyroidectomy, total or subtotal for malignancy; with limited neck dissection   J1

RVU			Global Days	Modifiers				
Mod	Non-Fac Total	Fac Total		51	50	62	80	MUE
	38.28	38.28	090	2	0	1	2	1

AMA: Nov 00: 10, Dec 12: 3

60254 Thyroidectomy, total or subtotal for malignancy; with radical neck dissection   C

RVU			Global Days	Modifiers				
Mod	Non-Fac Total	Fac Total		51	50	62	80	MUE
	48.57	48.57	090	2	0	1	2	1

AMA: Nov 00: 10, Dec 12: 3

60260 Thyroidectomy, removal of all remaining thyroid tissue following previous removal of a portion of thyroid   J1

RVU			Global Days	Modifiers				
Mod	Non-Fac Total	Fac Total		51	50	62	80	MUE
	31.69	31.69	090	2	1	1	2	1

AMA: Oct 10: 13, Dec 10: 13, Dec 12: 3

60270 Thyroidectomy, including substernal thyroid; sternal split or transthoracic approach   C

RVU			Global Days	Modifiers				
Mod	Non-Fac Total	Fac Total		51	50	62	80	MUE
	39.68	39.68	090	2	0	1	2	1

AMA: Dec 12: 3

60271 Thyroidectomy, including substernal thyroid; cervical approach   J1

RVU			Global Days	Modifiers				
Mod	Non-Fac Total	Fac Total		51	50	62	80	MUE
	30.65	30.65	090	2	0	1	2	1

AMA: Dec 12: 3

60280 Excision of thyroglossal duct cyst or sinus   A2 J1

RVU			Global Days	Modifiers				
Mod	Non-Fac Total	Fac Total		51	50	62	80	MUE
	12.84	12.84	090	2	0	1	2	1

60281 Excision of thyroglossal duct cyst or sinus; recurrent   A2 J1

RVU			Global Days	Modifiers				
Mod	Non-Fac Total	Fac Total		51	50	62	80	MUE
	17.01	17.01	090	2	0	1	2	1

Thyroid Gland Removal Procedures

60300 Aspiration and/or injection, thyroid cyst   P3 T

Coding tip: *Radiological guidance for correct needle placement - ultrasound 76942; CT 77012*

RVU			Global Days	Modifiers				
Mod	Non-Fac Total	Fac Total		51	50	62	80	MUE
	3.37	1.44	000	2	0	0	1	2

Parathyroid/Thymus/Adrenal Glands, Pancreas, Carotid Body Procedures

Excisional Endocrine System Procedures

60500 Parathyroidectomy or exploration of parathyroid(s)   G2 J1

RVU			Global Days	Modifiers				
Mod	Non-Fac Total	Fac Total		51	50	62	80	MUE
	27.94	27.94	090	2	0	1	2	1

AMA: Dec 12: 3

60502 Parathyroidectomy or exploration of parathyroid(s); re-exploration   J1

RVU			Global Days	Modifiers				
Mod	Non-Fac Total	Fac Total		51	50	62	80	MUE
	37.27	37.27	090	2	0	1	2	1

AMA: Dec 12: 3

60505 Parathyroidectomy or exploration of parathyroid(s); with mediastinal exploration, sternal split or transthoracic approach   C

RVU			Global Days	Modifiers				
Mod	Non-Fac Total	Fac Total		51	50	62	80	MUE
	40.17	40.17	090	2	0	1	2	1

AMA: Dec 12: 3

+ 60512 Parathyroid autotransplantation (List separately in addition to code for primary procedure)   N

RVU			Global Days	Modifiers				
Mod	Non-Fac Total	Fac Total		51	50	62	80	MUE
	7.05	7.05	ZZZ	0	0	1	2	1

AMA: Aug 11: 9, Dec 12: 3

60520 Thymectomy, partial or total; transcervical approach (separate procedure)   J1

RVU			Global Days	Modifiers				
Mod	Non-Fac Total	Fac Total		51	50	62	80	MUE
	30.26	30.26	090	2	0	1	2	1

60521 Thymectomy, partial or total; sternal split or transthoracic approach, without radical mediastinal dissection (separate procedure)   C

RVU			Global Days	Modifiers				
Mod	Non-Fac Total	Fac Total		51	50	62	80	MUE
	32.58	32.58	090	2	0	1	2	1

AMA: Dec 07: 12

60522 Thymectomy, partial or total; sternal split or transthoracic approach, with radical mediastinal dissection (separate procedure)   C

RVU			Global Days	Modifiers				
Mod	Non-Fac Total	Fac Total		51	50	62	80	MUE
	39.48	39.48	090	2	0	1	2	1

60540 Adrenalectomy, partial or complete, or exploration of adrenal gland with or without biopsy, transabdominal, lumbar or dorsal (separate procedure)   C

RVU			Global Days	Modifiers				
Mod	Non-Fac Total	Fac Total		51	50	62	80	MUE
	30.68	30.68	090	2	1	1	2	1

AMA: Nov 98: 17

● New   ▲ Revised   ✘ Deleted   ⊙ Moderate Sedation   ✚ Add-on Codes   ⊘ High Risk Denial   Ⓐ Age Edit   ♀ Female   ♂ Male   **AMA** *CPT® Assistant*   **MUE** Medically Unlikely Edit
⊘ Modifier 51 Exempt   ⊖ Modifier 63 Exempt   ✗ Unlisted   **Modifiers:** *See Inside Back Cover*   Ⓜ Maternity   A2–Z3 ASC Payment Indicators   A–Y OPPS Status Indicators

CPT © 2015 American Medical Association. All Rights Reserved.   © 2016 DecisionHealth

60545 Adrenalectomy, partial or complete, or exploration of adrenal gland with or without biopsy, transabdominal, lumbar or dorsal (separate procedure); with excision of adjacent retroperitoneal tumor   **C**

Mod	Non-Fac Total	Fac Total	Global Days	51	50	62	80	MUE
RVU				Modifiers				
	35.21	35.21	090	2	1	1	2	1

AMA: Nov 98: 17

60600 Excision of carotid body tumor; without excision of carotid artery   **C**

Mod	Non-Fac Total	Fac Total	Global Days	51	50	62	80	MUE
RVU				Modifiers				
	40.46	40.46	090	2	0	1	2	1

Excision of carotid body tumor

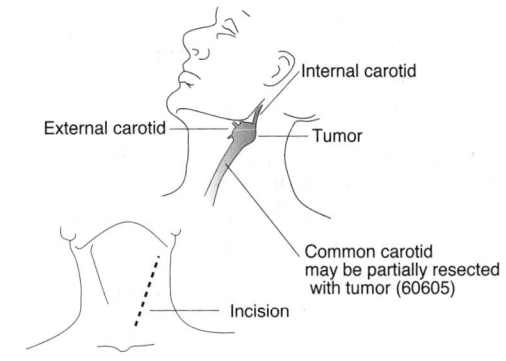

The physician removes a tumor from the common corotid artery

60605 Excision of carotid body tumor; with excision of carotid artery   **C**

Mod	Non-Fac Total	Fac Total	Global Days	51	50	62	80	MUE
RVU				Modifiers				
	49.96	49.96	090	2	0	1	2	1

Laparoscopic Endocrine System Procedures

60650 Laparoscopy, surgical, with adrenalectomy, partial or complete, or exploration of adrenal gland with or without biopsy, transabdominal, lumbar or dorsal   **C**

Mod	Non-Fac Total	Fac Total	Global Days	51	50	62	80	MUE
RVU				Modifiers				
	34.53	34.53	090	2	1	1	2	1

AMA: Nov 99: 30, Mar 00: 10, Nov 01: 8

60659 Unlisted laparoscopy procedure, endocrine system   **⚡ J 1**

Mod	Non-Fac Total	Fac Total	Global Days	51	50	62	80	MUE
RVU				Modifiers				
	0.00	0.00	YYY	2	1	0	2	

AMA: Nov 99: 30, Mar 00: 10

Other Endocrine Procedures

60699 Unlisted procedure, endocrine system   **⚡ J 1**

Mod	Non-Fac Total	Fac Total	Global Days	51	50	62	80	MUE
RVU				Modifiers				
	0.00	0.00	YYY	2	0	1	2	

AMA: Feb 06: 16, Dec 07: 12

Nervous System Procedures

Skull/Meninges/Brain Procedures

Injection/Drainage/Aspiration Procedures

Coding Guidance

Taps, punctures, or burr holes done with drainage of hematomas, abscesses, cysts, etc. and followed by other more comprehensive procedures are not reported separately, unless done as a planned or staged procedure. Biopsies done during surgery on the central nervous system are not reported separately. When different kinds of surgical services are done or performed in different surgical fields (i.e., opposite sides of the skull), modifier 59 should be used to identify distinct, separate services.

61000 Subdural tap through fontanelle, or suture, infant, unilateral or bilateral; initial   **⊘ Ⓐ R 2 T**

Coding tip: Do not code modifier 50

Mod	Non-Fac Total	Fac Total	Global Days	51	50	62	80	MUE
RVU				Modifiers				
	3.04	3.04	000	2	2	0	1	1

61001 Subdural tap through fontanelle, or suture, infant, unilateral or bilateral; subsequent taps   **⊘ Ⓐ R 2 T**

Coding tip: Do not code modifier 50

Mod	Non-Fac Total	Fac Total	Global Days	51	50	62	80	MUE
RVU				Modifiers				
	2.45	2.45	000	2	2	0	1	1

61020 Ventricular puncture through previous burr hole, fontanelle, suture, or implanted ventricular catheter/reservoir; without injection   **A 2 T**

Mod	Non-Fac Total	Fac Total	Global Days	51	50	62	80	MUE
RVU				Modifiers				
	2.94	2.94	000	2	0	0	1	2

61026 Ventricular puncture through previous burr hole, fontanelle, suture, or implanted ventricular catheter/reservoir; with injection of medication or other substance for diagnosis or treatment **A 2 T**

Mod	Non-Fac Total	Fac Total	Global Days	51	50	62	80	MUE
RVU				Modifiers				
	2.98	2.98	000	2	0	0	1	2

61050 Cisternal or lateral cervical (C1-C2) puncture; without injection (separate procedure)   **A 2 T**

Mod	Non-Fac Total	Fac Total	Global Days	51	50	62	80	MUE
RVU				Modifiers				
	2.47	2.47	000	2	0	0	0	1

61055 Cisternal or lateral cervical (C1-C2) puncture; with injection of medication or other substance for diagnosis or treatment   **A 2 T**

Coding tip: Myelography of cervical spine - 72240; thoracic spine - 72255; lumbosacral - 72265; two or more areas - 72270

Coding tip: CT of cervical spine - 72126 -72127; thoracic spine - 72129-72130; lumbar spine - 72132-72133

Coding tip: Use this code for contrast medium injection for diagnostic studies of the spine:

Mod	Non-Fac Total	Fac Total	Global Days	51	50	62	80	MUE
RVU				Modifiers				
	3.49	3.49	000	0	0	0	1	1

● New   ▲ Revised   Deleted   ⊙ Moderate Sedation   ✚ Add-on Codes   ⊗ High Risk Denial   Ⓐ Age Edit   ♀ Female   ♂ Male   **AMA** *CPT® Assistant*   **MUE** Medically Unlikely Edit
⊘ Modifier 51 Exempt   ⊖ Modifier 63 Exempt   ⚡ Unlisted   **Modifiers:** *See Inside Back Cover*   Ⓜ Maternity   **A 2 – Z 3** ASC Payment Indicators   **A – Y** OPPS Status Indicators

© 2016 DecisionHealth   CPT © 2015 American Medical Association. All Rights Reserved.   **547**

Surgical Procedures

60545 — 61055

Surgical Procedures

61070 – 61253

61070 Puncture of shunt tubing or reservoir for aspiration or injection procedure `A2T`

Coding tip: Shuntogram of indwelling (nonvascular) shunt - 75809

	RVU		Global Days	Modifiers				
Mod	Non-Fac Total	Fac Total		51	50	62	80	MUE
	1.67	1.67	000	2	0	0	1	2

Twist Drill/Burr Hole(s)/Trephine Procedures

61105 Twist drill hole for subdural or ventricular puncture `C`

	RVU		Global Days	Modifiers				
Mod	Non-Fac Total	Fac Total		51	50	62	80	MUE
	13.37	13.37	090	2	0	0	0	1

⊘ 61107 Twist drill hole(s) for subdural, intracerebral, or ventricular puncture; for implanting ventricular catheter, pressure recording device, or other intracerebral monitoring device `C`

	RVU		Global Days	Modifiers				
Mod	Non-Fac Total	Fac Total		51	50	62	80	MUE
	9.36	9.36	000	0	0	0	1	1

61108 Twist drill hole(s) for subdural, intracerebral, or ventricular puncture; for evacuation and/or drainage of subdural hematoma `C`

	RVU		Global Days	Modifiers				
Mod	Non-Fac Total	Fac Total		51	50	62	80	MUE
	26.72	26.72	090	2	0	0	1	1

Coding Guidance

Burr holes are often needed anticipatory to intracranial surgery to gain access to skull contents, alleviate pressure, or place an intracranial device, such as a pressure monitor. Burr holes integral to performing craniotomy or craniectomy are not reported at the same session. Burr holes that are done prior to a comprehensive procedure may be reported as staged with modifier 58.

61120 Burr hole(s) for ventricular puncture (including injection of gas, contrast media, dye, or radioactive material) `C`

	RVU		Global Days	Modifiers				
Mod	Non-Fac Total	Fac Total		51	50	62	80	MUE
	21.90	21.90	090	2	0	0	0	1

61140 Burr hole(s) or trephine; with biopsy of brain or intracranial lesion `C`

	RVU		Global Days	Modifiers				
Mod	Non-Fac Total	Fac Total		51	50	62	80	MUE
	37.26	37.26	090	2	0	0	2	1

Burr hole(s) or trephine

A burr drill or trephine is used to create a hole in the cranium

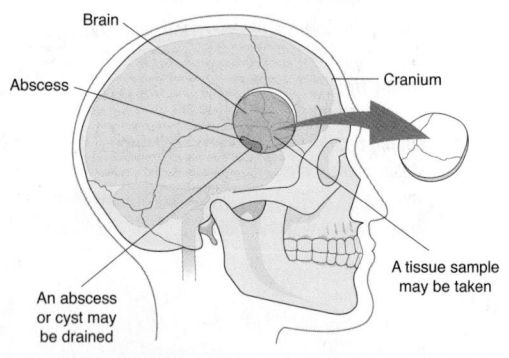

Brain

Abscess

A tissue sample may be taken

Cranium

An abscess or cyst may be drained

61150 Burr hole(s) or trephine; with drainage of brain abscess or cyst `C`

	RVU		Global Days	Modifiers				
Mod	Non-Fac Total	Fac Total		51	50	62	80	MUE
	39.58	39.58	090	2	0	1	1	1

61151 Burr hole(s) or trephine; with subsequent tapping (aspiration) of intracranial abscess or cyst `C`

	RVU		Global Days	Modifiers				
Mod	Non-Fac Total	Fac Total		51	50	62	80	MUE
	29.49	29.49	090	2	0	0	1	1

61154 Burr hole(s) with evacuation and/or drainage of hematoma, extradural or subdural `C`

	RVU		Global Days	Modifiers				
Mod	Non-Fac Total	Fac Total		51	50	62	80	MUE
	37.49	37.49	090	2	1	1	2	1

61156 Burr hole(s); with aspiration of hematoma or cyst, intracerebral `C`

	RVU		Global Days	Modifiers				
Mod	Non-Fac Total	Fac Total		51	50	62	80	MUE
	36.74	36.74	090	2	0	1	2	1

61210 Burr hole(s); for implanting ventricular catheter, reservoir, EEG electrode(s), pressure recording device, or other cerebral monitoring device (separate procedure) `C`

	RVU		Global Days	Modifiers				
Mod	Non-Fac Total	Fac Total		51	50	62	80	MUE
	10.97	10.97	000	2	0	0	1	1

61215 Insertion of subcutaneous reservoir, pump or continuous infusion system for connection to ventricular catheter `A2T`

	RVU		Global Days	Modifiers				
Mod	Non-Fac Total	Fac Total		51	50	62	80	MUE
	14.90	14.90	090	2	0	1	1	1

AMA: Spring 93: 13

61250 Burr hole(s) or trephine, supratentorial, exploratory, not followed by other surgery `C`

	RVU		Global Days	Modifiers				
Mod	Non-Fac Total	Fac Total		51	50	62	80	MUE
	23.81	23.81	090	2	1	1	2	1

61253 Burr hole(s) or trephine, infratentorial, unilateral or bilateral `C`

	RVU		Global Days	Modifiers				
Mod	Non-Fac Total	Fac Total		51	50	62	80	MUE
	23.70	23.70	090	2	2	0	2	1

AMA: Sep 02: 10

Craniectomies/Craniotomies

Coding Guidance

Intracranial procedures sometimes include bone grafting in the CPT descriptor and are inclusive in the main surgical procedure. General exploration of the surgical field accessible for surgery is included in craniectomies and craniotomies. Do not code 61304 or 61305 for an exploratory surgery when another surgery on intracranial contents is performed.

● New   ▲ Revised   ✖ Deleted   ⊙ Moderate Sedation   ✚ Add-on Codes   ⊘ High Risk Denial   ⒶAge Edit   ♀ Female   ♂ Male   **AMA** *CPT® Assistant*   **MUE** Medically Unlikely Edit
⊘ Modifier 51 Exempt   ⊖ Modifier 63 Exempt   ✗ Unlisted   **Modifiers:** *See Inside Back Cover*   Ⓜ Maternity   `A2`–`Z3` ASC Payment Indicators   `A`–`Y` OPPS Status Indicators

548   CPT © 2015 American Medical Association. All Rights Reserved.   © 2016 DecisionHealth

61304 Craniectomy or craniotomy, exploratory; supratentorial C

RVU		Global Days	Modifiers				
Mod	Non-Fac Total	Fac Total		51	50	62	80	MUE
	48.41	48.41	090	2	0	1	2	1

61305 Craniectomy or craniotomy, exploratory; infratentorial (posterior fossa) C

RVU		Global Days	Modifiers				
Mod	Non-Fac Total	Fac Total		51	50	62	80	MUE
	59.23	59.23	090	2	0	1	2	1

61312 Craniectomy or craniotomy for evacuation of hematoma, supratentorial; extradural or subdural C

RVU		Global Days	Modifiers				
Mod	Non-Fac Total	Fac Total		51	50	62	80	MUE
	61.35	61.35	090	2	0	1	2	2

61313 Craniectomy or craniotomy for evacuation of hematoma, supratentorial; intracerebral C

RVU		Global Days	Modifiers				
Mod	Non-Fac Total	Fac Total		51	50	62	80	MUE
	58.49	58.49	090	2	0	1	2	2

61314 Craniectomy or craniotomy for evacuation of hematoma, infratentorial; extradural or subdural C

RVU		Global Days	Modifiers				
Mod	Non-Fac Total	Fac Total		51	50	62	80	MUE
	53.55	53.55	090	2	0	1	2	2

61315 Craniectomy or craniotomy for evacuation of hematoma, infratentorial; intracerebellar C

RVU		Global Days	Modifiers				
Mod	Non-Fac Total	Fac Total		51	50	62	80	MUE
	60.82	60.82	090	2	0	1	2	1

+ 61316 Incision and subcutaneous placement of cranial bone graft (List separately in addition to code for primary procedure) C

RVU		Global Days	Modifiers				
Mod	Non-Fac Total	Fac Total		51	50	62	80	MUE
	2.61	2.61	ZZZ	0	0	0	1	1

61320 Craniectomy or craniotomy, drainage of intracranial abscess; supratentorial C

RVU		Global Days	Modifiers				
Mod	Non-Fac Total	Fac Total		51	50	62	80	MUE
	55.90	55.90	090	2	0	1	2	2

61321 Craniectomy or craniotomy, drainage of intracranial abscess; infratentorial C

RVU		Global Days	Modifiers				
Mod	Non-Fac Total	Fac Total		51	50	62	80	MUE
	62.08	62.08	090	2	0	1	2	1

61322 Craniectomy or craniotomy, decompressive, with or without duraplasty, for treatment of intracranial hypertension, without evacuation of associated intraparenchymal hematoma; without lobectomy C

RVU		Global Days	Modifiers				
Mod	Non-Fac Total	Fac Total		51	50	62	80	MUE
	70.27	70.27	090	2	0	1	2	1

61323 Craniectomy or craniotomy, decompressive, with or without duraplasty, for treatment of intracranial hypertension, without evacuation of associated intraparenchymal hematoma; with lobectomy C

RVU		Global Days	Modifiers				
Mod	Non-Fac Total	Fac Total		51	50	62	80	MUE
	71.20	71.20	090	2	0	1	1	1

61330 Decompression of orbit only, transcranial approach G2 J1

RVU		Global Days	Modifiers				
Mod	Non-Fac Total	Fac Total		51	50	62	80	MUE
	46.97	46.97	090	2	1	1	2	1

61332 Exploration of orbit (transcranial approach); with biopsy C

RVU		Global Days	Modifiers				
Mod	Non-Fac Total	Fac Total		51	50	62	80	MUE
	51.54	51.54	090	2	1	1	2	1

61333 Exploration of orbit (transcranial approach); with removal of lesion C

RVU		Global Days	Modifiers				
Mod	Non-Fac Total	Fac Total		51	50	62	80	MUE
	53.30	53.30	090	2	1	1	2	1

61340 Subtemporal cranial decompression (pseudotumor cerebri, slit ventricle syndrome) C

RVU		Global Days	Modifiers				
Mod	Non-Fac Total	Fac Total		51	50	62	80	MUE
	41.85	41.85	090	2	1	1	2	1

61343 Craniectomy, suboccipital with cervical laminectomy for decompression of medulla and spinal cord, with or without dural graft (eg, Arnold-Chiari malformation) C

RVU		Global Days	Modifiers				
Mod	Non-Fac Total	Fac Total		51	50	62	80	MUE
	64.47	64.47	090	2	0	1	2	1

61345 Other cranial decompression, posterior fossa C

RVU		Global Days	Modifiers				
Mod	Non-Fac Total	Fac Total		51	50	62	80	MUE
	60.09	60.09	090	2	0	1	2	1

61450 Craniectomy, subtemporal, for section, compression, or decompression of sensory root of gasserian ganglion C

RVU		Global Days	Modifiers				
Mod	Non-Fac Total	Fac Total		51	50	62	80	MUE
	56.87	56.87	090	2	0	1	2	1

● New   ▲ Revised   Deleted   ⊙ Moderate Sedation   ✚ Add-on Codes   ⊘ High Risk Denial   Ⓐ Age Edit   ♀ Female   ♂ Male   **AMA** *CPT® Assistant*   **MUE** Medically Unlikely Edit
⊘ Modifier 51 Exempt   ⊖ Modifier 63 Exempt   ✗ Unlisted   **Modifiers:** *See Inside Back Cover*   Ⓜ Maternity   A2–Z3 ASC Payment Indicators   A–Y OPPS Status Indicators

61458 Craniectomy, suboccipital; for exploration or decompression of cranial nerves C

RVU			Global Days	Modifiers				
Mod	Non-Fac Total	Fac Total		51	50	62	80	MUE
	58.94	58.94	090	2	0	1	2	1

61460 Craniectomy, suboccipital; for section of 1 or more cranial nerves C

RVU			Global Days	Modifiers				
Mod	Non-Fac Total	Fac Total		51	50	62	80	MUE
	62.54	62.54	090	2	0	2	2	1

61480 Craniectomy, suboccipital; for mesencephalic tractotomy or pedunculotomy C

RVU			Global Days	Modifiers				
Mod	Non-Fac Total	Fac Total		51	50	62	80	MUE
	46.74	46.74	090	2	0	1	2	1

61500 Craniectomy; with excision of tumor or other bone lesion of skull C

RVU			Global Days	Modifiers				
Mod	Non-Fac Total	Fac Total		51	50	62	80	MUE
	38.66	38.66	090	2	0	1	2	1

AMA: Jan 14: 9

61501 Craniectomy; for osteomyelitis C

RVU			Global Days	Modifiers				
Mod	Non-Fac Total	Fac Total		51	50	62	80	MUE
	33.85	33.85	090	2	0	1	2	1

AMA: Jan 14: 9

61510 Craniectomy, trephination, bone flap craniotomy; for excision of brain tumor, supratentorial, except meningioma C

RVU			Global Days	Modifiers				
Mod	Non-Fac Total	Fac Total		51	50	62	80	MUE
	64.16	64.16	090	2	0	1	2	1

61512 Craniectomy, trephination, bone flap craniotomy; for excision of meningioma, supratentorial C

RVU			Global Days	Modifiers				
Mod	Non-Fac Total	Fac Total		51	50	62	80	MUE
	74.73	74.73	090	2	0	1	2	1

61514 Craniectomy, trephination, bone flap craniotomy; for excision of brain abscess, supratentorial C

RVU			Global Days	Modifiers				
Mod	Non-Fac Total	Fac Total		51	50	62	80	MUE
	55.79	55.79	090	2	0	1	2	2

61516 Craniectomy, trephination, bone flap craniotomy; for excision or fenestration of cyst, supratentorial C

RVU			Global Days	Modifiers				
Mod	Non-Fac Total	Fac Total		51	50	62	80	MUE
	54.46	54.46	090	2	0	1	2	1

+ 61517 Implantation of brain intracavitary chemotherapy agent (List separately in addition to code for primary procedure) C

RVU			Global Days	Modifiers				
Mod	Non-Fac Total	Fac Total		51	50	62	80	MUE
	2.60	2.60	ZZZ	0	0	0	1	1

61518 Craniectomy for excision of brain tumor, infratentorial or posterior fossa; except meningioma, cerebellopontine angle tumor, or midline tumor at base of skull C

RVU			Global Days	Modifiers				
Mod	Non-Fac Total	Fac Total		51	50	62	80	MUE
	80.97	80.97	090	2	0	1	2	1

61519 Craniectomy for excision of brain tumor, infratentorial or posterior fossa; meningioma C

RVU			Global Days	Modifiers				
Mod	Non-Fac Total	Fac Total		51	50	62	80	MUE
	86.00	86.00	090	2	0	1	2	1

61520 Craniectomy for excision of brain tumor, infratentorial or posterior fossa; cerebellopontine angle tumor C

RVU			Global Days	Modifiers				
Mod	Non-Fac Total	Fac Total		51	50	62	80	MUE
	110.86	110.86	090	2	0	2	2	1

61521 Craniectomy for excision of brain tumor, infratentorial or posterior fossa; midline tumor at base of skull C

RVU			Global Days	Modifiers				
Mod	Non-Fac Total	Fac Total		51	50	62	80	MUE
	93.23	93.23	090	2	0	1	2	1

61522 Craniectomy, infratentorial or posterior fossa; for excision of brain abscess C

RVU			Global Days	Modifiers				
Mod	Non-Fac Total	Fac Total		51	50	62	80	MUE
	64.11	64.11	090	2	0	1	2	1

61524 Craniectomy, infratentorial or posterior fossa; for excision or fenestration of cyst C

RVU			Global Days	Modifiers				
Mod	Non-Fac Total	Fac Total		51	50	62	80	MUE
	61.19	61.19	090	2	0	1	2	2

61526 Craniectomy, bone flap craniotomy, transtemporal (mastoid) for excision of cerebellopontine angle tumor C

RVU			Global Days	Modifiers				
Mod	Non-Fac Total	Fac Total		51	50	62	80	MUE
	108.60	108.60	090	2	0	2	1	1

AMA: Summer 91: 8

61530 Craniectomy, bone flap craniotomy, transtemporal (mastoid) for excision of cerebellopontine angle tumor; combined with middle/posterior fossa craniotomy/craniectomy C

RVU			Global Days	Modifiers				
Mod	Non-Fac Total	Fac Total		51	50	62	80	MUE
	91.54	91.54	090	2	0	2	1	1

61531 Subdural implantation of strip electrodes through 1 or more burr or trephine hole(s) for long-term seizure monitoring C

RVU			Global Days	Modifiers				
Mod	Non-Fac Total	Fac Total		51	50	62	80	MUE
	36.01	36.01	090	2	0	2	2	1

● New   ▲ Revised   ✖ Deleted   ⊙ Moderate Sedation   ✚ Add-on Codes   ⊘ High Risk Denial   Ⓐ Age Edit   ♀ Female   ♂ Male   **AMA** CPT® Assistant   **MUE** Medically Unlikely Edit

⊘ Modifier 51 Exempt   ⊖ Modifier 63 Exempt   ✗ Unlisted   **Modifiers:** See Inside Back Cover   Ⓜ Maternity   A-2–Z-3 ASC Payment Indicators   A–Y OPPS Status Indicators

CPT © 2015 American Medical Association. All Rights Reserved.   © 2016 DecisionHealth

61533 Craniotomy with elevation of bone flap; for subdural implantation of an electrode array, for long-term seizure monitoring   C

Mod	RVU Non-Fac Total	Fac Total	Global Days	51	50	62	80	MUE
	44.79	44.79	090	2	0	1	2	2

Pub 100-04, 12, 40.1

61534 Craniotomy with elevation of bone flap; for excision of epileptogenic focus without electrocorticography during surgery   C

Mod	RVU Non-Fac Total	Fac Total	Global Days	51	50	62	80	MUE
	47.93	47.93	090	2	0	1	2	1

Pub 100-04, 12, 40.1

61535 Craniotomy with elevation of bone flap; for removal of epidural or subdural electrode array, without excision of cerebral tissue (separate procedure)   C

Mod	RVU Non-Fac Total	Fac Total	Global Days	51	50	62	80	MUE
	29.37	29.37	090	2	0	1	2	2

Pub 100-04, 12, 40.1

61536 Craniotomy with elevation of bone flap; for excision of cerebral epileptogenic focus, with electrocorticography during surgery (includes removal of electrode array)   C

Mod	RVU Non-Fac Total	Fac Total	Global Days	51	50	62	80	MUE
	76.69	76.69	090	2	0	1	2	1

Pub 100-04, 12, 40.1

61537 Craniotomy with elevation of bone flap; for lobectomy, temporal lobe, without electrocorticography during surgery   C

Mod	RVU Non-Fac Total	Fac Total	Global Days	51	50	62	80	MUE
	72.57	72.57	090	2	0	1	2	1

61538 Craniotomy with elevation of bone flap; for lobectomy, temporal lobe, with electrocorticography during surgery   C

Mod	RVU Non-Fac Total	Fac Total	Global Days	51	50	62	80	MUE
	79.23	79.23	090	2	0	1	2	1

61539 Craniotomy with elevation of bone flap; for lobectomy, other than temporal lobe, partial or total, with electrocorticography during surgery   C

Mod	RVU Non-Fac Total	Fac Total	Global Days	51	50	62	80	MUE
	69.39	69.39	090	2	0	1	2	1

Pub 100-04, 12, 40.1

61540 Craniotomy with elevation of bone flap; for lobectomy, other than temporal lobe, partial or total, without electrocorticography during surgery   C

Mod	RVU Non-Fac Total	Fac Total	Global Days	51	50	62	80	MUE
	64.88	64.88	090	2	0	1	2	1

61541 Craniotomy with elevation of bone flap; for transection of corpus callosum   C

Mod	RVU Non-Fac Total	Fac Total	Global Days	51	50	62	80	MUE
	63.87	63.87	090	2	0	1	2	1

Pub 100-04, 12, 40

61543 Craniotomy with elevation of bone flap; for partial or subtotal (functional) hemispherectomy   C

Mod	RVU Non-Fac Total	Fac Total	Global Days	51	50	62	80	MUE
	62.37	62.37	090	2	0	1	2	1

Pub 100-04, 12, 40.1

61544 Craniotomy with elevation of bone flap; for excision or coagulation of choroid plexus   C

Mod	RVU Non-Fac Total	Fac Total	Global Days	51	50	62	80	MUE
	56.52	56.52	090	2	0	0	2	1

61545 Craniotomy with elevation of bone flap; for excision of craniopharyngioma   C

Mod	RVU Non-Fac Total	Fac Total	Global Days	51	50	62	80	MUE
	94.69	94.69	090	2	0	1	2	1

61546 Craniotomy for hypophysectomy or excision of pituitary tumor, intracranial approach   C

Mod	RVU Non-Fac Total	Fac Total	Global Days	51	50	62	80	MUE
	68.59	68.59	090	2	0	1	2	1

61548 Hypophysectomy or excision of pituitary tumor, transnasal or transseptal approach, nonstereotactic   C

Mod	RVU Non-Fac Total	Fac Total	Global Days	51	50	62	80	MUE
	46.39	46.39	090	2	0	2	2	1

AMA: Nov 98: 17, Jul 11: 13

61550 Craniectomy for craniosynostosis; single cranial suture   C

Mod	RVU Non-Fac Total	Fac Total	Global Days	51	50	62	80	MUE
	27.96	27.96	090	2	0	1	2	1

AMA: Feb 12: 11

61552 Craniectomy for craniosynostosis; multiple cranial sutures   C

Mod	RVU Non-Fac Total	Fac Total	Global Days	51	50	62	80	MUE
	33.60	33.60	090	2	0	1	2	1

AMA: Feb 12: 11

61556 Craniotomy for craniosynostosis; frontal or parietal bone flap   C

Mod	RVU Non-Fac Total	Fac Total	Global Days	51	50	62	80	MUE
	44.86	44.86	090	2	0	0	2	1

● New   ▲ Revised   Deleted   ⊙ Moderate Sedation   ✚ Add-on Codes   ⊘ High Risk Denial   Ⓐ Age Edit   ♀ Female   ♂ Male   **AMA** *CPT® Assistant*   **MUE** Medically Unlikely Edit
⊘ Modifier 51 Exempt   ⊖ Modifier 63 Exempt   ✗ Unlisted   **Modifiers:** *See Inside Back Cover*   Ⓜ Maternity   A2-Z3 ASC Payment Indicators   A-Y OPPS Status Indicators

Surgical Procedures

61557 – 61582

61557 Craniotomy for craniosynostosis; bifrontal bone flap C

RVU			Global Days	Modifiers				
Mod	Non-Fac Total	Fac Total		51	50	62	80	MUE
	47.11	47.11	090	2	0	0	2	1

AMA: Feb 12: 11

61558 Extensive craniectomy for multiple cranial suture craniosynostosis (eg, cloverleaf skull); not requiring bone grafts C

RVU			Global Days	Modifiers				
Mod	Non-Fac Total	Fac Total		51	50	62	80	MUE
	51.48	51.48	090	2	0	0	2	1

AMA: Feb 12: 11

61559 Extensive craniectomy for multiple cranial suture craniosynostosis (eg, cloverleaf skull); recontouring with multiple osteotomies and bone autografts (eg, barrel-stave procedure) (includes obtaining grafts) C

RVU			Global Days	Modifiers				
Mod	Non-Fac Total	Fac Total		51	50	62	80	MUE
	60.71	60.71	090	2	0	1	2	1

AMA: Feb 12: 11

61563 Excision, intra and extracranial, benign tumor of cranial bone (eg, fibrous dysplasia); without optic nerve decompression C

RVU			Global Days	Modifiers				
Mod	Non-Fac Total	Fac Total		51	50	62	80	MUE
	56.31	56.31	090	2	0	1	2	2

61564 Excision, intra and extracranial, benign tumor of cranial bone (eg, fibrous dysplasia); with optic nerve decompression C

RVU			Global Days	Modifiers				
Mod	Non-Fac Total	Fac Total		51	50	62	80	MUE
	67.63	67.63	090	2	1	1	2	1

61566 Craniotomy with elevation of bone flap; for selective amygdalohippocampectomy C

RVU			Global Days	Modifiers				
Mod	Non-Fac Total	Fac Total		51	50	62	80	MUE
	66.46	66.46	090	2	0	1	2	1

61567 Craniotomy with elevation of bone flap; for multiple subpial transections, with electrocorticography during surgery C

RVU			Global Days	Modifiers				
Mod	Non-Fac Total	Fac Total		51	50	62	80	MUE
	76.16	76.16	090	2	0	1	2	1

61570 Craniectomy or craniotomy; with excision of foreign body from brain C

RVU			Global Days	Modifiers				
Mod	Non-Fac Total	Fac Total		51	50	62	80	MUE
	55.15	55.15	090	2	0	1	2	1

61571 Craniectomy or craniotomy; with treatment of penetrating wound of brain C

RVU			Global Days	Modifiers				
Mod	Non-Fac Total	Fac Total		51	50	62	80	MUE
	58.78	58.78	090	2	0	1	2	1

Coding Guidance

Do not report a separate tracheostomy code together with 61576 for transoral approach to the skull base, as a tracheostomy is included in the code descriptor.

61575 Transoral approach to skull base, brain stem or upper spinal cord for biopsy, decompression or excision of lesion C

RVU			Global Days	Modifiers				
Mod	Non-Fac Total	Fac Total		51	50	62	80	MUE
	62.48	62.48	090	2	0	1	2	1

61576 Transoral approach to skull base, brain stem or upper spinal cord for biopsy, decompression or excision of lesion; requiring splitting of tongue and/or mandible (including tracheostomy) C

RVU			Global Days	Modifiers				
Mod	Non-Fac Total	Fac Total		51	50	62	80	MUE
	105.67	105.67	090	2	0	1	2	1

Skull Base Procedures
Approach Procedures

61580 Craniofacial approach to anterior cranial fossa; extradural, including lateral rhinotomy, ethmoidectomy, sphenoidectomy, without maxillectomy or orbital exenteration C

RVU			Global Days	Modifiers				
Mod	Non-Fac Total	Fac Total		51	50	62	80	MUE
	72.83	72.83	090	2	1	1	1	1

AMA: Winter 93: 17, Spring 94: 11

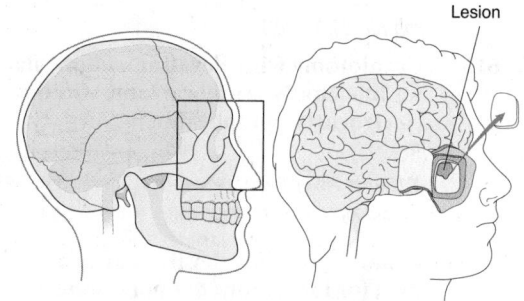

Craniofacial approach to anterior cranial fossa

Lesion

A lesion lying outside of the membrane that lines the skull is accessed through the face (61580), or through the lower sinus/eye socket (60581).

61581 Craniofacial approach to anterior cranial fossa; extradural, including lateral rhinotomy, orbital exenteration, ethmoidectomy, sphenoidectomy and/or maxillectomy C

RVU			Global Days	Modifiers				
Mod	Non-Fac Total	Fac Total		51	50	62	80	MUE
	77.18	77.18	090	2	1	2	1	1

AMA: Winter 93: 17, Spring 94: 11

61582 Craniofacial approach to anterior cranial fossa; extradural, including unilateral or bifrontal craniotomy, elevation of frontal lobe(s), osteotomy of base of anterior cranial fossa C

RVU			Global Days	Modifiers				
Mod	Non-Fac Total	Fac Total		51	50	62	80	MUE
	84.89	84.89	090	2	0	1	2	1

AMA: Winter 93: 17, Spring 94: 11

● New   ▲ Revised   ✖ Deleted   ⊙ Moderate Sedation   ✚ Add-on Codes   ⊘ High Risk Denial   Ⓐ Age Edit   ♀ Female   ♂ Male   **AMA** *CPT® Assistant*   **MUE** Medically Unlikely Edit
⊘ Modifier 51 Exempt   ⊖ Modifier 63 Exempt   ✗ Unlisted   **Modifiers:** *See Inside Back Cover*   Ⓜ Maternity   A2–Z3 ASC Payment Indicators   A–Y OPPS Status Indicators

CPT © 2015 American Medical Association. All Rights Reserved.   © 2016 DecisionHealth

61583 Craniofacial approach to anterior cranial fossa; intradural, including unilateral or bifrontal craniotomy, elevation or resection of frontal lobe, osteotomy of base of anterior cranial fossa ▣

RVU			Global Days	Modifiers				
Mod	Non-Fac Total	Fac Total		51	50	62	80	MUE
	85.12	85.12	090	2	0	1	2	1

AMA: Winter 93: 17, Spring 94: 11

61584 Orbitocranial approach to anterior cranial fossa, extradural, including supraorbital ridge osteotomy and elevation of frontal and/or temporal lobe(s); without orbital exenteration ▣

RVU			Global Days	Modifiers				
Mod	Non-Fac Total	Fac Total		51	50	62	80	MUE
	83.96	83.96	090	2	1	1	2	1

AMA: Winter 93: 18

61585 Orbitocranial approach to anterior cranial fossa, extradural, including supraorbital ridge osteotomy and elevation of frontal and/or temporal lobe(s); with orbital exenteration ▣

RVU			Global Days	Modifiers				
Mod	Non-Fac Total	Fac Total		51	50	62	80	MUE
	95.28	95.28	090	2	1	1	2	1

AMA: Winter 93: 18

61586 Bicoronal, transzygomatic and/or LeFort I osteotomy approach to anterior cranial fossa with or without internal fixation, without bone graft ▣

RVU			Global Days	Modifiers				
Mod	Non-Fac Total	Fac Total		51	50	62	80	MUE
	70.53	70.53	090	2	0	1	2	1

AMA: Winter 93: 18, Nov 96: 12

61590 Infratemporal pre-auricular approach to middle cranial fossa (parapharyngeal space, infratemporal and midline skull base, nasopharynx), with or without disarticulation of the mandible, including parotidectomy, craniotomy, decompression and/or mobilization of the facial nerve and/or petrous carotid artery ▣

RVU			Global Days	Modifiers				
Mod	Non-Fac Total	Fac Total		51	50	62	80	MUE
	88.24	88.24	090	2	1	1	2	1

AMA: Winter 93: 18

Infratemporal pre-auricular approach to middle cranial fossa

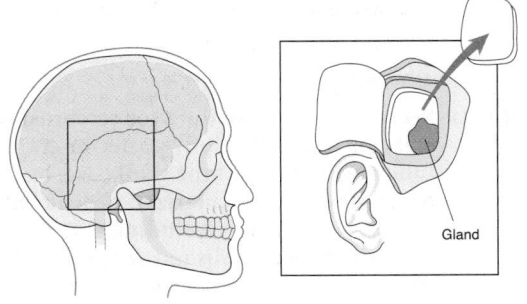

The middle of the head is accessed by removing the section of bone in front of and above the ear.

61591 Infratemporal post-auricular approach to middle cranial fossa (internal auditory meatus, petrous apex, tentorium, cavernous sinus, parasellar area, infratemporal fossa) including mastoidectomy, resection of sigmoid sinus, with or without decompression and/or mobilization of contents of auditory canal or petrous carotid artery ▣

RVU			Global Days	Modifiers				
Mod	Non-Fac Total	Fac Total		51	50	62	80	MUE
	90.29	90.29	090	2	1	1	2	1

AMA: Winter 93: 18

61592 Orbitocranial zygomatic approach to middle cranial fossa (cavernous sinus and carotid artery, clivus, basilar artery or petrous apex) including osteotomy of zygoma, craniotomy, extra- or intradural elevation of temporal lobe ▣

RVU			Global Days	Modifiers				
Mod	Non-Fac Total	Fac Total		51	50	62	80	MUE
	92.89	92.89	090	2	1	1	2	1

AMA: Winter 93: 18

61595 Transtemporal approach to posterior cranial fossa, jugular foramen or midline skull base, including mastoidectomy, decompression of sigmoid sinus and/or facial nerve, with or without mobilization ▣

RVU			Global Days	Modifiers				
Mod	Non-Fac Total	Fac Total		51	50	62	80	MUE
	68.02	68.02	090	2	1	1	1	1

AMA: Winter 93: 18

61596 Transcochlear approach to posterior cranial fossa, jugular foramen or midline skull base, including labyrinthectomy, decompression, with or without mobilization of facial nerve and/or petrous carotid artery ▣

RVU			Global Days	Modifiers				
Mod	Non-Fac Total	Fac Total		51	50	62	80	MUE
	70.73	70.73	090	2	1	1	2	1

AMA: Winter 93: 18

61597 Transcondylar (far lateral) approach to posterior cranial fossa, jugular foramen or midline skull base, including occipital condylectomy, mastoidectomy, resection of C1-C3 vertebral body(s), decompression of vertebral artery, with or without mobilization ▣

RVU			Global Days	Modifiers				
Mod	Non-Fac Total	Fac Total		51	50	62	80	MUE
	81.49	81.49	090	2	1	1	2	1

AMA: Winter 93: 18

61598 Transpetrosal approach to posterior cranial fossa, clivus or foramen magnum, including ligation of superior petrosal sinus and/or sigmoid sinus ▣

RVU			Global Days	Modifiers				
Mod	Non-Fac Total	Fac Total		51	50	62	80	MUE
	83.64	83.64	090	2	0	1	2	1

AMA: Winter 93: 18

● New   ▲ Revised   Deleted   ⊙ Moderate Sedation   ✚ Add-on Codes   ⊘ High Risk Denial   Ⓐ Age Edit   ♀ Female   ♂ Male   **AMA** CPT® Assistant   **MUE** Medically Unlikely Edit
⊘ Modifier 51 Exempt   ⊖ Modifier 63 Exempt   ☒ Unlisted   **Modifiers:** See Inside Back Cover   Ⓜ Maternity   A2-Z3 ASC Payment Indicators   A-Y OPPS Status Indicators

© 2016 DecisionHealth   CPT © 2015 American Medical Association. All Rights Reserved.   **553**

Surgical Procedures

61600 – 61619

Definitive Procedures

61600 Resection or excision of neoplastic, vascular or infectious lesion of base of anterior cranial fossa; extradural   C

Mod	RVU Non-Fac Total	Fac Total	Global Days	Modifiers 51	50	62	80	MUE
	61.53	61.53	090	2	0	1	2	1

AMA: Winter 93: 19, Spring 94: 12, Nov 96: 12

61601 Resection or excision of neoplastic, vascular or infectious lesion of base of anterior cranial fossa; intradural, including dural repair, with or without graft   C

Mod	RVU Non-Fac Total	Fac Total	Global Days	Modifiers 51	50	62	80	MUE
	70.51	70.51	090	2	0	1	2	1

AMA: Winter 93: 19, Spring 94: 12

61605 Resection or excision of neoplastic, vascular or infectious lesion of infratemporal fossa, parapharyngeal space, petrous apex; extradural   C

Mod	RVU Non-Fac Total	Fac Total	Global Days	Modifiers 51	50	62	80	MUE
	63.12	63.12	090	2	0	1	2	1

AMA: Winter 93: 19

61606 Resection or excision of neoplastic, vascular or infectious lesion of infratemporal fossa, parapharyngeal space, petrous apex; intradural, including dural repair, with or without graft   C

Mod	RVU Non-Fac Total	Fac Total	Global Days	Modifiers 51	50	62	80	MUE
	87.13	87.13	090	2	0	1	2	1

AMA: Winter 93: 20

61607 Resection or excision of neoplastic, vascular or infectious lesion of parasellar area, cavernous sinus, clivus or midline skull base; extradural   C

Mod	RVU Non-Fac Total	Fac Total	Global Days	Modifiers 51	50	62	80	MUE
	78.92	78.92	090	2	0	1	2	1

AMA: Winter 93: 20

61608 Resection or excision of neoplastic, vascular or infectious lesion of parasellar area, cavernous sinus, clivus or midline skull base; intradural, including dural repair, with or without graft   C

Mod	RVU Non-Fac Total	Fac Total	Global Days	Modifiers 51	50	62	80	MUE
	95.93	95.93	090	2	0	1	2	1

AMA: Winter 93: 20

+ 61610 Transection or ligation, carotid artery in cavernous sinus, with repair by anastomosis or graft (List separately in addition to code for primary procedure)   ⊘C

Mod	RVU Non-Fac Total	Fac Total	Global Days	Modifiers 51	50	62	80	MUE
	45.06	45.06	ZZZ	0	0	1	2	1

AMA: Winter 93: 20

+ 61611 Transection or ligation, carotid artery in petrous canal; without repair (List separately in addition to code for primary procedure)   C

Mod	RVU Non-Fac Total	Fac Total	Global Days	Modifiers 51	50	62	80	MUE
	11.27	11.27	ZZZ	0	0	1	2	1

AMA: Winter 93: 20

+ 61612 Transection or ligation, carotid artery in petrous canal; with repair by anastomosis or graft (List separately in addition to code for primary procedure)   ⊘C

Mod	RVU Non-Fac Total	Fac Total	Global Days	Modifiers 51	50	62	80	MUE
	42.35	42.35	ZZZ	0	0	1	2	1

AMA: Winter 93: 20

61613 Obliteration of carotid aneurysm, arteriovenous malformation, or carotid-cavernous fistula by dissection within cavernous sinus   C

Mod	RVU Non-Fac Total	Fac Total	Global Days	Modifiers 51	50	62	80	MUE
	95.07	95.07	090	2	1	1	2	1

AMA: Winter 93: 20

61615 Resection or excision of neoplastic, vascular or infectious lesion of base of posterior cranial fossa, jugular foramen, foramen magnum, or C1-C3 vertebral bodies; extradural   C

Mod	RVU Non-Fac Total	Fac Total	Global Days	Modifiers 51	50	62	80	MUE
	66.26	66.26	090	2	0	1	2	1

AMA: Winter 93: 20

61616 Resection or excision of neoplastic, vascular or infectious lesion of base of posterior cranial fossa, jugular foramen, foramen magnum, or C1-C3 vertebral bodies; intradural, including dural repair, with or without graft   C

Mod	RVU Non-Fac Total	Fac Total	Global Days	Modifiers 51	50	62	80	MUE
	98.10	98.10	090	2	0	1	2	1

Surgical Defects of Skull Base Repair and/or Reconstruction

61618 Secondary repair of dura for cerebrospinal fluid leak, anterior, middle or posterior cranial fossa following surgery of the skull base; by free tissue graft (eg, pericranium, fascia, tensor fascia lata, adipose tissue, homologous or synthetic grafts)   C

Mod	RVU Non-Fac Total	Fac Total	Global Days	Modifiers 51	50	62	80	MUE
	37.49	37.49	090	2	0	1	2	2

AMA: Winter 93: 20, Spring 94: 19, Mar 00: 11

61619 Secondary repair of dura for cerebrospinal fluid leak, anterior, middle or posterior cranial fossa following surgery of the skull base; by local or regionalized vascularized pedicle flap or myocutaneous flap (including galea, temporalis, frontalis or occipitalis muscle)   C

Mod	RVU Non-Fac Total	Fac Total	Global Days	Modifiers 51	50	62	80	MUE
	41.60	41.60	090	2	0	1	2	2

AMA: Winter 93: 20, Spring 94: 19, Mar 00: 11

● New   ▲ Revised   ✖ Deleted   ⊙ Moderate Sedation   ✚ Add-on Codes   ⊘ High Risk Denial   Ⓐ Age Edit   ♀ Female   ♂ Male   **AMA** CPT® Assistant   **MUE** Medically Unlikely Edit
⊘ Modifier 51 Exempt   ⊖ Modifier 63 Exempt   Ⓧ Unlisted   **Modifiers:** See Inside Back Cover   Ⓜ Maternity   A-2 – Z-3 ASC Payment Indicators   A-Y OPPS Status Indicators

CPT © 2015 American Medical Association. All Rights Reserved.   © 2016 DecisionHealth

Endovascular Procedures

61623 Endovascular temporary balloon arterial occlusion, head or neck (extracranial/intracranial) including selective catheterization of vessel to be occluded, positioning and inflation of occlusion balloon, concomitant neurological monitoring, and radiologic supervision and interpretation of all angiography required for balloon occlusion and to exclude vascular injury post occlusion   **J1**

RVU			Global Days	Modifiers				
Mod	Non-Fac Total	Fac Total		51	50	62	80	MUE
	16.58	16.58	000	2	0	0	1	2

Coding Guidance

The procedure described in code 61623 includes prolonged neurologic assessment and should not be used to report the temporary arterial occlusion component of the procedure inherent in code 61624.

61624 Transcatheter permanent occlusion or embolization (eg, for tumor destruction, to achieve hemostasis, to occlude a vascular malformation), percutaneous, any method; central nervous system (intracranial, spinal cord)   **C**

Coding tip: Radiological supervision for transcatheter embolization - 75894

RVU			Global Days	Modifiers				
Mod	Non-Fac Total	Fac Total		51	50	62	80	MUE
	33.34	33.34	000	2	0	0	1	2

AMA: Jun 99: 10, Nov 06: 8, Nov 13: 6

61626 Transcatheter permanent occlusion or embolization (eg, for tumor destruction, to achieve hemostasis, to occlude a vascular malformation), percutaneous, any method; non-central nervous system, head or neck (extracranial, brachiocephalic branch)   **J1**

RVU			Global Days	Modifiers				
Mod	Non-Fac Total	Fac Total		51	50	62	80	MUE
	24.99	24.99	000	2	0	0	1	2

AMA: Nov 13: 6

61630 Balloon angioplasty, intracranial (eg, atherosclerotic stenosis), percutaneous   ⊘**C**

RVU			Global Days	Modifiers				
Mod	Non-Fac Total	Fac Total		51	50	62	80	MUE
	38.79	38.79	XXX	2	0	1	2	1

61635 Transcatheter placement of intravascular stent(s), intracranial (eg, atherosclerotic stenosis), including balloon angioplasty, if performed   **C**

RVU			Global Days	Modifiers				
Mod	Non-Fac Total	Fac Total		51	50	62	80	MUE
	41.58	41.58	XXX	2	0	1	2	2

AMA: Mar 14: 8

61640 Balloon dilatation of intracranial vasospasm, percutaneous; initial vessel   ⊘**E**

RVU			Global Days	Modifiers				
Mod	Non-Fac Total	Fac Total		51	50	62	80	MUE
	18.74	18.74	000	9	9	9	9	

AMA: May 14: 10

+ 61641 Balloon dilatation of intracranial vasospasm, percutaneous; each additional vessel in same vascular family (List separately in addition to code for primary procedure)   ⊘**E**

RVU			Global Days	Modifiers				
Mod	Non-Fac Total	Fac Total		51	50	62	80	MUE
	6.58	6.58	ZZZ	9	9	9	9	

AMA: May 14: 10

+ 61642 Balloon dilatation of intracranial vasospasm, percutaneous; each additional vessel in different vascular family (List separately in addition to code for primary procedure)   ⊘**E**

RVU			Global Days	Modifiers				
Mod	Non-Fac Total	Fac Total		51	50	62	80	MUE
	13.17	13.17	ZZZ	9	9	9	9	

AMA: May 14: 10

● 61645 Percutaneous arterial transluminal mechanical thrombectomy and/or infusion for thrombolysis, intracranial, any method, including diagnostic angiography, fluoroscopic guidance, catheter placement, and intraprocedural pharmacological thrombolytic injection(s)   **E**

RVU			Global Days	Modifiers				
Mod	Non-Fac Total	Fac Total		51	50	62	80	MUE
	22.59	22.59	000	0	1	0	0	3

● 61650 Endovascular intracranial prolonged administration of pharmacologic agent(s) other than for thrombolysis, arterial, including catheter placement, diagnostic angiography, and imaging guidance; initial vascular territory   **C**

RVU			Global Days	Modifiers				
Mod	Non-Fac Total	Fac Total		51	50	62	80	MUE
	15.47	15.47	ZZZ	2	0	0	1	1

+● 61651 Endovascular intracranial prolonged administration of pharmacologic agent(s) other than for thrombolysis, arterial, including catheter placement, diagnostic angiography, and imaging guidance; each additional vascular territory (List separately in addition to code for primary procedure)   **C**

RVU			Global Days	Modifiers				
Mod	Non-Fac Total	Fac Total		51	50	62	80	MUE
	6.59	6.59	ZZZ	2	0	0	1	2

Aneursym/Arterious Malformation/Vascular Disease Procedures

61680 Surgery of intracranial arteriovenous malformation; supratentorial, simple   **C**

RVU			Global Days	Modifiers				
Mod	Non-Fac Total	Fac Total		51	50	62	80	MUE
	65.87	65.87	090	2	0	1	2	1

61682 Surgery of intracranial arteriovenous malformation; supratentorial, complex   **C**

RVU			Global Days	Modifiers				
Mod	Non-Fac Total	Fac Total		51	50	62	80	MUE
	122.60	122.60	090	2	0	1	2	1

AMA: Jun 13: 14

● New   ▲ Revised   Deleted   ⊙ Moderate Sedation   ✛ Add-on Codes   ⊘ High Risk Denial   Ⓐ Age Edit   ♀ Female   ♂ Male   **AMA** CPT® Assistant   **MUE** Medically Unlikely Edit
⊘ Modifier 51 Exempt   ⊖ Modifier 63 Exempt   ✗ Unlisted   **Modifiers:** See Inside Back Cover   Ⓜ Maternity   **A2–Z3** ASC Payment Indicators   **A–Y** OPPS Status Indicators

© 2016 DecisionHealth   CPT © 2015 American Medical Association. All Rights Reserved.   **555**

Surgical Procedures

61684 Surgery of intracranial arteriovenous malformation; infratentorial, simple   C

RVU			Global Days	Modifiers				
Mod	Non-Fac Total	Fac Total		51	50	62	80	MUE
	84.60	84.60	090	2	0	1	2	1

61686 Surgery of intracranial arteriovenous malformation; infratentorial, complex   C

RVU			Global Days	Modifiers				
Mod	Non-Fac Total	Fac Total		51	50	62	80	MUE
	132.85	132.85	090	2	0	1	2	1

AMA: Jun 13: 14

61690 Surgery of intracranial arteriovenous malformation; dural, simple   C

RVU			Global Days	Modifiers				
Mod	Non-Fac Total	Fac Total		51	50	62	80	MUE
	64.14	64.14	090	2	0	1	2	1

61692 Surgery of intracranial arteriovenous malformation; dural, complex   C

RVU			Global Days	Modifiers				
Mod	Non-Fac Total	Fac Total		51	50	62	80	MUE
	107.88	107.88	090	2	0	1	2	1

AMA: Jun 13: 14

61697 Surgery of complex intracranial aneurysm, intracranial approach; carotid circulation   C

RVU			Global Days	Modifiers				
Mod	Non-Fac Total	Fac Total		51	50	62	80	MUE
	124.88	124.88	090	2	0	1	2	2

61698 Surgery of complex intracranial aneurysm, intracranial approach; vertebrobasilar circulation   C

RVU			Global Days	Modifiers				
Mod	Non-Fac Total	Fac Total		51	50	62	80	MUE
	137.26	137.26	090	2	0	1	2	1

61700 Surgery of simple intracranial aneurysm, intracranial approach; carotid circulation   C

RVU			Global Days	Modifiers				
Mod	Non-Fac Total	Fac Total		51	50	62	80	MUE
	100.40	100.40	090	2	0	1	2	2

AMA: Jun 99: 11, Jul 99: 10

61702 Surgery of simple intracranial aneurysm, intracranial approach; vertebrobasilar circulation   C

RVU			Global Days	Modifiers				
Mod	Non-Fac Total	Fac Total		51	50	62	80	MUE
	118.85	118.85	090	2	0	1	2	1

61703 Surgery of intracranial aneurysm, cervical approach by application of occluding clamp to cervical carotid artery (Selverstone-Crutchfield type)   C

RVU			Global Days	Modifiers				
Mod	Non-Fac Total	Fac Total		51	50	62	80	MUE
	40.32	40.32	090	2	0	1	2	1

61705 Surgery of aneurysm, vascular malformation or carotid-cavernous fistula; by intracranial and cervical occlusion of carotid artery   C

RVU			Global Days	Modifiers				
Mod	Non-Fac Total	Fac Total		51	50	62	80	MUE
	75.82	75.82	090	2	0	1	2	1

61708 Surgery of aneurysm, vascular malformation or carotid-cavernous fistula; by intracranial electrothrombosis   C

RVU			Global Days	Modifiers				
Mod	Non-Fac Total	Fac Total		51	50	62	80	MUE
	61.35	61.35	090	2	0	0	2	1

61710 Surgery of aneurysm, vascular malformation or carotid-cavernous fistula; by intra-arterial embolization, injection procedure, or balloon catheter   C

RVU			Global Days	Modifiers				
Mod	Non-Fac Total	Fac Total		51	50	62	80	MUE
	63.96	63.96	090	2	0	0	0	1

AMA: Nov 13: 6

61711 Anastomosis, arterial, extracranial-intracranial (eg, middle cerebral/cortical) arteries   C

RVU			Global Days	Modifiers				
Mod	Non-Fac Total	Fac Total		51	50	62	80	MUE
	76.63	76.63	090	2	0	1	2	1

Skull/Brain Stereotaxis Procedures

61720 Creation of lesion by stereotactic method, including burr hole(s) and localizing and recording techniques, single or multiple stages; globus pallidus or thalamus   T

RVU			Global Days	Modifiers				
Mod	Non-Fac Total	Fac Total		51	50	62	80	MUE
	37.69	37.69	090	2	0	0	1	1

AMA: Jul 11: 12, Jul 14: 9

61735 Creation of lesion by stereotactic method, including burr hole(s) and localizing and recording techniques, single or multiple stages; subcortical structure(s) other than globus pallidus or thalamus   C

RVU			Global Days	Modifiers				
Mod	Non-Fac Total	Fac Total		51	50	62	80	MUE
	46.60	46.60	090	2	0	1	1	1

AMA: Jul 11: 12

61750 Stereotactic biopsy, aspiration, or excision, including burr hole(s), for intracranial lesion   C

RVU			Global Days	Modifiers				
Mod	Non-Fac Total	Fac Total		51	50	62	80	MUE
	41.59	41.59	090	2	0	1	1	2

AMA: Nov 99: 30

61751 Stereotactic biopsy, aspiration, or excision, including burr hole(s), for intracranial lesion; with computed tomography and/or magnetic resonance guidance   C

RVU			Global Days	Modifiers				
Mod	Non-Fac Total	Fac Total		51	50	62	80	MUE
	40.86	40.86	090	2	0	1	1	2

AMA: Jun 96: 10, Nov 99: 30, Dec 04: 20, Jul 11: 12

● New   ▲ Revised   ✖ Deleted   ⊙ Moderate Sedation   ➕ Add-on Codes   ⊘ High Risk Denial   Ⓐ Age Edit   ♀ Female   ♂ Male   **AMA** *CPT® Assistant*   **MUE** Medically Unlikely Edit
⊘ Modifier 51 Exempt   ⊖ Modifier 63 Exempt   ⓧ Unlisted   **Modifiers:** *See Inside Back Cover*   Ⓜ Maternity   A2–Z3 ASC Payment Indicators   A–Y OPPS Status Indicators

556   CPT © 2015 American Medical Association. All Rights Reserved.   © 2016 DecisionHealth

Surgical Procedures

61760 Stereotactic implantation of depth electrodes into the cerebrum for long-term seizure monitoring ◐

Mod	Non-Fac Total	Fac Total	Global Days	51	50	62	80	MUE
	46.95	46.95	090	2	0	2	1	1

AMA: Jul 11: 12

61770 Stereotactic localization, including burr hole(s), with insertion of catheter(s) or probe(s) for placement of radiation source G2T

Mod	Non-Fac Total	Fac Total	Global Days	51	50	62	80	MUE
	47.89	47.89	090	2	0	1	1	1

AMA: Jul 11: 12

+ 61781 Stereotactic computer-assisted (navigational) procedure; cranial, intradural (List separately in addition to code for primary procedure) N1N

Mod	Non-Fac Total	Fac Total	Global Days	51	50	62	80	MUE
	7.00	7.00	ZZZ	0	0	0	0	1

AMA: Jul 11: 12, Jul 14: 9, Sep 14: 14

+ 61782 Stereotactic computer-assisted (navigational) procedure; cranial, extradural (List separately in addition to code for primary procedure) N1N

Mod	Non-Fac Total	Fac Total	Global Days	51	50	62	80	MUE
	5.11	5.11	ZZZ	0	0	0	0	1

AMA: Jul 11: 12

+ 61783 Stereotactic computer-assisted (navigational) procedure; spinal (List separately in addition to code for primary procedure) ⊘N1N

Documentation Finder: Documentation should be clear that this navigational service is being performed on the spine. The documentation should reference a target selection, and physician work of image-based planning must be included when reporting this code.

Mod	Non-Fac Total	Fac Total	Global Days	51	50	62	80	MUE
	6.89	6.89	ZZZ	0	0	0	0	1

AMA: Jul 11: 12

61790 Creation of lesion by stereotactic method, percutaneous, by neurolytic agent (eg, alcohol, thermal, electrical, radiofrequency); gasserian ganglion A2T

Mod	Non-Fac Total	Fac Total	Global Days	51	50	62	80	MUE
	26.05	26.05	090	2	1	0	1	1

AMA: Jul 11: 12

61791 Creation of lesion by stereotactic method, percutaneous, by neurolytic agent (eg, alcohol, thermal, electrical, radiofrequency); trigeminal medullary tract A2T

Mod	Non-Fac Total	Fac Total	Global Days	51	50	62	80	MUE
	31.50	31.50	090	2	1	0	0	1

AMA: Jul 11: 12, Jul 14: 9

61796 Stereotactic radiosurgery (particle beam, gamma ray, or linear accelerator); 1 simple cranial lesion B

Mod	Non-Fac Total	Fac Total	Global Days	51	50	62	80	MUE
	30.01	30.01	090	0	0	0	2	1

AMA: Jul 11: 12, Apr 12: 11, Jul 14: 9, Jun 15: 6

+ 61797 Stereotactic radiosurgery (particle beam, gamma ray, or linear accelerator); each additional cranial lesion, simple (List separately in addition to code for primary procedure) B

Mod	Non-Fac Total	Fac Total	Global Days	51	50	62	80	MUE
	6.56	6.56	ZZZ	0	0	0	2	4

AMA: Jul 11: 12, Apr 12: 11, Jun 15: 6

61798 Stereotactic radiosurgery (particle beam, gamma ray, or linear accelerator); 1 complex cranial lesion B

Mod	Non-Fac Total	Fac Total	Global Days	51	50	62	80	MUE
	40.88	40.88	090	0	0	0	2	1

AMA: Jul 11: 12, Apr 12: 11, Jun 15: 6

+ 61799 Stereotactic radiosurgery (particle beam, gamma ray, or linear accelerator); each additional cranial lesion, complex (List separately in addition to code for primary procedure) B

Mod	Non-Fac Total	Fac Total	Global Days	51	50	62	80	MUE
	9.00	9.00	ZZZ	0	0	0	2	4

AMA: Jul 11: 12, Apr 12: 11, Jul 14: 9, Jun 15: 6

+ 61800 Application of stereotactic headframe for stereotactic radiosurgery (List separately in addition to code for primary procedure) B

Mod	Non-Fac Total	Fac Total	Global Days	51	50	62	80	MUE
	4.58	4.58	ZZZ	0	0	0	2	1

AMA: Apr 12: 11, Jun 15: 6

Intracranial Neurostimulator Insertion/Revision/Removal

61850 Twist drill or burr hole(s) for implantation of neurostimulator electrodes, cortical ⊘◐

Mod	Non-Fac Total	Fac Total	Global Days	51	50	62	80	MUE
	29.12	29.12	090	2	0	0	2	1

AMA: Sep 99: 5, Nov 99: 30

Coding Guidance
Craniectomy procedures described in this section include the twist drill hole, burr hole or other craniotomy required for access and these access procedures should not be reported separately.

61860 Craniectomy or craniotomy for implantation of neurostimulator electrodes, cerebral, cortical ◐

Coding tip: Twist drill hole or burr hole is included. Do not report 61850 with 61860.

Mod	Non-Fac Total	Fac Total	Global Days	51	50	62	80	MUE
	46.48	46.48	090	2	0	0	2	1

AMA: Sep 99: 5, Nov 99: 30

● New   ▲ Revised   Deleted   ⊙ Moderate Sedation   ✚ Add-on Codes   ⊘ High Risk Denial   Ⓐ Age Edit   ♀ Female   ♂ Male   **AMA** CPT® Assistant   **MUE** Medically Unlikely Edit
⊘ Modifier 51 Exempt   ⊖ Modifier 63 Exempt   ☒ Unlisted   **Modifiers:** See Inside Back Cover   Ⓜ Maternity   A2–Z3 ASC Payment Indicators   A–Y OPPS Status Indicators

© 2016 DecisionHealth   CPT © 2015 American Medical Association. All Rights Reserved.   **557**

Surgical Procedures

61863 – 62000

61863 Twist drill, burr hole, craniotomy, or craniectomy with stereotactic implantation of neurostimulator electrode array in subcortical site (eg, thalamus, globus pallidus, subthalamic nucleus, periventricular, periaqueductal gray), without use of intraoperative microelectrode recording; first array   Ⓒ

RVU			Global Days	Modifiers				
Mod	Non-Fac Total	Fac Total		51	50	62	80	MUE
	44.26	44.26	090	2	1	1	2	1

AMA: Sep 99: 5, Jul 11: 12, Oct 10: 10, Jul 14: 9

Twist drill, burr hole, craniotomy, or craniectomy

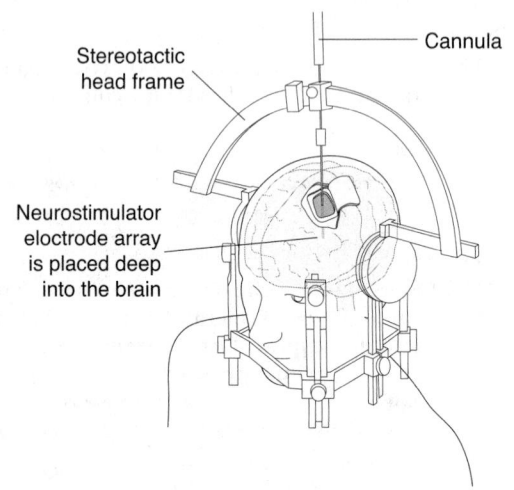

Cannula

Stereotactic head frame

Neurostimulator electrode array is placed deep into the brain

✚ 61864 Twist drill, burr hole, craniotomy, or craniectomy with stereotactic implantation of neurostimulator electrode array in subcortical site (eg, thalamus, globus pallidus, subthalamic nucleus, periventricular, periaqueductal gray), without use of intraoperative microelectrode recording; each additional array (List separately in addition to primary procedure)   Ⓒ

RVU			Global Days	Modifiers				
Mod	Non-Fac Total	Fac Total		51	50	62	80	MUE
	8.41	8.41	ZZZ	0	0	1	2	1

AMA: Sep 99: 5, Jul 11: 12

61867 Twist drill, burr hole, craniotomy, or craniectomy with stereotactic implantation of neurostimulator electrode array in subcortical site (eg, thalamus, globus pallidus, subthalamic nucleus, periventricular, periaqueductal gray), with use of intraoperative microelectrode recording; first array   Ⓒ

RVU			Global Days	Modifiers				
Mod	Non-Fac Total	Fac Total		51	50	62	80	MUE
	66.91	66.91	090	2	1	1	2	1

AMA: Jul 11: 12

✚ 61868 Twist drill, burr hole, craniotomy, or craniectomy with stereotactic implantation of neurostimulator electrode array in subcortical site (eg, thalamus, globus pallidus, subthalamic nucleus, periventricular, periaqueductal gray), with use of intraoperative microelectrode recording; each additional array (List separately in addition to primary procedure)   Ⓒ

RVU			Global Days	Modifiers				
Mod	Non-Fac Total	Fac Total		51	50	62	80	MUE
	14.64	14.64	ZZZ	0	0	1	2	2

AMA: Jul 11: 12, Jul 14: 9

61870 Craniectomy for implantation of neurostimulator electrodes, cerebellar, cortical   Ⓒ

RVU			Global Days	Modifiers				
Mod	Non-Fac Total	Fac Total		51	50	62	80	MUE
	33.80	33.80	090	2	0	1	2	1

61880 Revision or removal of intracranial neurostimulator electrodes   G2Q2

RVU			Global Days	Modifiers				
Mod	Non-Fac Total	Fac Total		51	50	62	80	MUE
	16.75	16.75	090	2	1	1	2	1

Pub 100-04, 32, 50.4.3

61885 Insertion or replacement of cranial neurostimulator pulse generator or receiver, direct or inductive coupling; with connection to a single electrode array   J8J1

RVU			Global Days	Modifiers				
Mod	Non-Fac Total	Fac Total		51	50	62	80	MUE
	15.13	15.13	090	2	1	0	0	1

AMA: Sep 99: 5, Nov 99: 30, Jun 00: 3, Apr 01: 8, Sep 03: 3, Sep 11: 8, Dec 10: 14, Feb 11: 5

Pub 100-04, 32, 50.4.3, 50.5

61886 Insertion or replacement of cranial neurostimulator pulse generator or receiver, direct or inductive coupling; with connection to 2 or more electrode arrays   J8J1

RVU			Global Days	Modifiers				
Mod	Non-Fac Total	Fac Total		51	50	62	80	MUE
	24.85	24.85	090	2	0	0	0	1

AMA: Nov 99: 30, Jun 00: 3, Apr 01: 8, Sep 11: 8, Feb 11: 5

Pub 100-04, 32, 50.4.3

61888 Revision or removal of cranial neurostimulator pulse generator or receiver   J8J1

RVU			Global Days	Modifiers				
Mod	Non-Fac Total	Fac Total		51	50	62	80	MUE
	11.64	11.64	010	2	1	0	1	1

AMA: Sep 11: 8

Pub 100-04, 32, 50.4.3, 50.5

Skull Repair Procedures

62000 Elevation of depressed skull fracture; simple, extradural   J1

RVU			Global Days	Modifiers				
Mod	Non-Fac Total	Fac Total		51	50	62	80	MUE
	30.55	30.55	090	2	0	0	1	1

● New   ▲ Revised   ✖ Deleted   ⊙ Moderate Sedation   ✚ Add-on Codes   ⊘ High Risk Denial   Ⓐ Age Edit   ♀ Female   ♂ Male   **AMA** *CPT® Assistant*   **MUE** Medically Unlikely Edit
⦸ Modifier 51 Exempt   ⊖ Modifier 63 Exempt   🗵 Unlisted   **Modifiers:** *See Inside Back Cover*   Ⓜ Maternity   A2–Z3 ASC Payment Indicators   A–Y OPPS Status Indicators

558   CPT © 2015 American Medical Association. All Rights Reserved.   © 2016 DecisionHealth

62005 Elevation of depressed skull fracture; compound or comminuted, extradural ⓒ

Mod	Non-Fac Total	Fac Total	Global Days	51	50	62	80	MUE
	36.60	36.60	090	2	0	1	2	1

62010 Elevation of depressed skull fracture; with repair of dura and/or debridement of brain ⓒ

Mod	Non-Fac Total	Fac Total	Global Days	51	50	62	80	MUE
	45.16	45.16	090	2	0	1	2	1

62100 Craniotomy for repair of dural/cerebrospinal fluid leak, including surgery for rhinorrhea/otorrhea ⓒ

Mod	Non-Fac Total	Fac Total	Global Days	51	50	62	80	MUE
	46.83	46.83	090	2	0	1	2	1

62115 Reduction of craniomegalic skull (eg, treated hydrocephalus); not requiring bone grafts or cranioplasty ⓒ

Mod	Non-Fac Total	Fac Total	Global Days	51	50	62	80	MUE
	37.89	37.89	090	2	0	1	2	1

62117 Reduction of craniomegalic skull (eg, treated hydrocephalus); requiring craniotomy and reconstruction with or without bone graft (includes obtaining grafts) ⓒ

Mod	Non-Fac Total	Fac Total	Global Days	51	50	62	80	MUE
	47.26	47.26	090	2	0	1	2	1

62120 Repair of encephalocele, skull vault, including cranioplasty ⓒ

Mod	Non-Fac Total	Fac Total	Global Days	51	50	62	80	MUE
	48.42	48.42	090	2	0	1	2	1

62121 Craniotomy for repair of encephalocele, skull base ⓒ

Mod	Non-Fac Total	Fac Total	Global Days	51	50	62	80	MUE
	46.60	46.60	090	2	0	1	2	1

62140 Cranioplasty for skull defect; up to 5 cm diameter ⓒ

Mod	Non-Fac Total	Fac Total	Global Days	51	50	62	80	MUE
	30.24	30.24	090	2	0	1	2	1

AMA: Jan 14: 9

62141 Cranioplasty for skull defect; larger than 5 cm diameter ⓒ

Mod	Non-Fac Total	Fac Total	Global Days	51	50	62	80	MUE
	33.33	33.33	090	2	0	1	2	1

AMA: Jan 14: 9

62142 Removal of bone flap or prosthetic plate of skull ⓒ

Mod	Non-Fac Total	Fac Total	Global Days	51	50	62	80	MUE
	26.06	26.06	090	2	0	0	2	2

AMA: Jan 14: 9

62143 Replacement of bone flap or prosthetic plate of skull ⓒ

Mod	Non-Fac Total	Fac Total	Global Days	51	50	62	80	MUE
	30.43	30.43	090	2	0	1	2	2

AMA: Jan 14: 9

62145 Cranioplasty for skull defect with reparative brain surgery ⓒ

Mod	Non-Fac Total	Fac Total	Global Days	51	50	62	80	MUE
	40.96	40.96	090	2	0	1	2	2

AMA: Jan 14: 9

62146 Cranioplasty with autograft (includes obtaining bone grafts); up to 5 cm diameter ⓒ

Mod	Non-Fac Total	Fac Total	Global Days	51	50	62	80	MUE
	36.62	36.62	090	2	0	1	2	2

AMA: Jan 14: 9

62147 Cranioplasty with autograft (includes obtaining bone grafts); larger than 5 cm diameter ⓒ

Mod	Non-Fac Total	Fac Total	Global Days	51	50	62	80	MUE
	41.73	41.73	090	2	0	1	2	1

AMA: Jan 14: 9

+ 62148 Incision and retrieval of subcutaneous cranial bone graft for cranioplasty (List separately in addition to code for primary procedure) ⓒ

Mod	Non-Fac Total	Fac Total	Global Days	51	50	62	80	MUE
	3.78	3.78	ZZZ	0	0	0	1	1

Neuroendoscopic Procedures

+ 62160 Neuroendoscopy, intracranial, for placement or replacement of ventricular catheter and attachment to shunt system or external drainage (List separately in addition to code for primary procedure) N1 N

Mod	Non-Fac Total	Fac Total	Global Days	51	50	62	80	MUE
	5.67	5.67	ZZZ	0	0	0	1	1

AMA: Jun 07: 11, Dec 12: 14

62161 Neuroendoscopy, intracranial; with dissection of adhesions, fenestration of septum pellucidum or intraventricular cysts (including placement, replacement, or removal of ventricular catheter) ⓒ

Mod	Non-Fac Total	Fac Total	Global Days	51	50	62	80	MUE
	44.88	44.88	090	2	0	1	2	1

62162 Neuroendoscopy, intracranial; with fenestration or excision of colloid cyst, including placement of external ventricular catheter for drainage ⓒ

Mod	Non-Fac Total	Fac Total	Global Days	51	50	62	80	MUE
	55.86	55.86	090	2	0	1	2	1

● New   ▲ Revised   Deleted   ⊙ Moderate Sedation   ✚ Add-on Codes   ⊘ High Risk Denial   Ⓐ Age Edit   ♀ Female   ♂ Male   **AMA** CPT® Assistant   **MUE** Medically Unlikely Edit
⊘ Modifier 51 Exempt   ⊖ Modifier 63 Exempt   ✗ Unlisted   **Modifiers:** See Inside Back Cover   Ⓜ Maternity   A2–Z3 ASC Payment Indicators   A–Y OPPS Status Indicators

© 2016 DecisionHealth   CPT © 2015 American Medical Association. All Rights Reserved.

62163 Neuroendoscopy, intracranial; with retrieval of foreign body 〇

Mod	Non-Fac Total	Fac Total	Global Days	51	50	62	80	MUE
	32.47	32.47	090	2	0	1	2	1

62164 Neuroendoscopy, intracranial; with excision of brain tumor, including placement of external ventricular catheter for drainage 〇

Mod	Non-Fac Total	Fac Total	Global Days	51	50	62	80	MUE
	61.41	61.41	090	2	0	1	2	1

62165 Neuroendoscopy, intracranial; with excision of pituitary tumor, transnasal or trans-sphenoidal approach 〇

Mod	Non-Fac Total	Fac Total	Global Days	51	50	62	80	MUE
	45.49	45.49	090	2	0	1	0	1

Cerebrospinal Fluid Shunt Procedures

62180 Ventriculocisternostomy (Torkildsen type operation) 〇

Mod	Non-Fac Total	Fac Total	Global Days	51	50	62	80	MUE
	47.14	47.14	090	2	0	0	2	1

62190 Creation of shunt; subarachnoid/subdural-atrial, -jugular, -auricular ⊘〇

Mod	Non-Fac Total	Fac Total	Global Days	51	50	62	80	MUE
	25.84	25.84	090	2	0	1	1	1

62192 Creation of shunt; subarachnoid/subdural-peritoneal, -pleural, other terminus 〇

Mod	Non-Fac Total	Fac Total	Global Days	51	50	62	80	MUE
	28.65	28.65	090	2	0	1	2	1

62194 Replacement or irrigation, subarachnoid/subdural catheter A2T

Mod	Non-Fac Total	Fac Total	Global Days	51	50	62	80	MUE
	13.57	13.57	010	2	0	0	0	1

AMA: Dec 11: 6

62200 Ventriculocisternostomy, third ventricle 〇

Mod	Non-Fac Total	Fac Total	Global Days	51	50	62	80	MUE
	40.70	40.70	090	2	0	1	2	1

62201 Ventriculocisternostomy, third ventricle; stereotactic, neuroendoscopic method 〇

Mod	Non-Fac Total	Fac Total	Global Days	51	50	62	80	MUE
	35.67	35.67	090	2	0	0	1	1

AMA: Aug 07: 15, Jul 11: 12, Jul 14: 9

62220 Creation of shunt; ventriculo-atrial, -jugular, -auricular 〇

Mod	Non-Fac Total	Fac Total	Global Days	51	50	62	80	MUE
	30.30	30.30	090	2	0	1	2	1

62223 Creation of shunt; ventriculo-peritoneal, -pleural, other terminus 〇

Mod	Non-Fac Total	Fac Total	Global Days	51	50	62	80	MUE
	30.92	30.92	090	2	0	1	2	1

62225 Replacement or irrigation, ventricular catheter A2T

Mod	Non-Fac Total	Fac Total	Global Days	51	50	62	80	MUE
	15.44	15.44	090	2	0	0	1	2

AMA: Dec 11: 6

62230 Replacement or revision of cerebrospinal fluid shunt, obstructed valve, or distal catheter in shunt system A2T

Mod	Non-Fac Total	Fac Total	Global Days	51	50	62	80	MUE
	24.80	24.80	090	2	0	1	2	2

AMA: Dec 11: 6, Dec 12: 14

62252 Reprogramming of programmable cerebrospinal shunt P3S

Mod	Non-Fac Total	Fac Total	Global Days	51	50	62	80	MUE
	2.47	2.47	XXX	0	0	0	0	2
26	1.37	1.37	XXX	0	0	0	0	2
TC	1.10	1.10	XXX	0	0	0	0	2

62256 Removal of complete cerebrospinal fluid shunt system; without replacement 〇

Mod	Non-Fac Total	Fac Total	Global Days	51	50	62	80	MUE
	17.58	17.58	090	2	0	0	2	1

62258 Removal of complete cerebrospinal fluid shunt system; with replacement by similar or other shunt at same operation 〇

Mod	Non-Fac Total	Fac Total	Global Days	51	50	62	80	MUE
	33.11	33.11	090	2	0	1	2	1

AMA: Dec 11: 6

Spine/Spinal Cord Procedures

Spinal Injection/Drainage/Aspiration Procedures

Coding Guidance

When spinal puncture is performed (62270-62272), the vascular access and any necessary monitoring, oximetry, and laboratory sample procurement are considered part of the spinal puncture procedure. Any necessary local anesthesia required for performing a spinal puncture is included in the procedure itself. Nerve or facet blocks reported separately are inappropriate when used for local anesthesia for spinal punctures. If cerebrospinal fluid is incidentally withdrawn while administering a nerve or other anesthetic block, only the nerve or other type of block is reported as the CSF was not acquired for diagnostic reasons.

● New ▲ Revised ✖ Deleted ⊙ Moderate Sedation ✚ Add-on Codes ⊘ High Risk Denial Ⓐ Age Edit ♀ Female ♂ Male **AMA** *CPT® Assistant* **MUE** Medically Unlikely Edit
⊘ Modifier 51 Exempt ⊖ Modifier 63 Exempt ✖ Unlisted **Modifiers:** *See Inside Back Cover* Ⓜ Maternity A2–Z3 ASC Payment Indicators A–Y OPPS Status Indicators

560 CPT © 2015 American Medical Association. All Rights Reserved. © 2016 DecisionHealth

62263 Percutaneous lysis of epidural adhesions using solution injection (eg, hypertonic saline, enzyme) or mechanical means (eg, catheter) including radiologic localization (includes contrast when administered), multiple adhesiolysis sessions; 2 or more days `A2T`

	RVU		Global Days	Modifiers				
Mod	Non-Fac Total	Fac Total		51	50	62	80	MUE
	18.70	9.81	010	2	0	0	1	1

AMA: Nov 99: 33, Dec 99: 11, Mar 02: 11, Dec 02: 10, Nov 05: 14, Jul 08: 9, Oct 09: 12, Nov 10: 3, Jun 12: 12, Jan 11: 8

Percutaneous lysis of epidural adhesions using solution injection

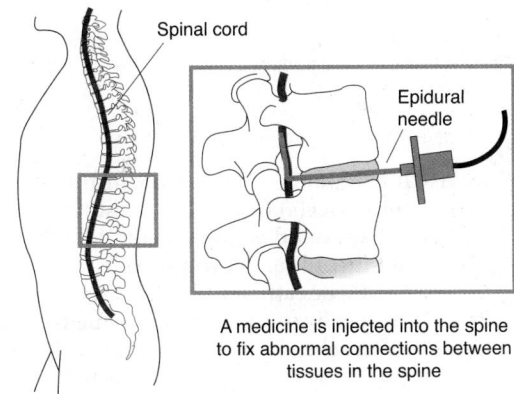

Spinal cord

Epidural needle

A medicine is injected into the spine to fix abnormal connections between tissues in the spine

Multiple adhesiolysis sessions, 2 or more days

62264 Percutaneous lysis of epidural adhesions using solution injection (eg, hypertonic saline, enzyme) or mechanical means (eg, catheter) including radiologic localization (includes contrast when administered), multiple adhesiolysis sessions; 1 day `A2T`

	RVU		Global Days	Modifiers				
Mod	Non-Fac Total	Fac Total		51	50	62	80	MUE
	12.20	6.94	010	2	0	0	1	1

AMA: Nov 05: 14, Jul 08: 9, Oct 09: 12, Nov 10: 3, Jun 12: 12, Jan 11: 8

62267 Percutaneous aspiration within the nucleus pulposus, intervertebral disc, or paravertebral tissue for diagnostic purposes `G2T`

	RVU		Global Days	Modifiers				
Mod	Non-Fac Total	Fac Total		51	50	62	80	MUE
	7.09	4.60	000	2	0	0	0	2

AMA: Nov 10: 3, Jul 12: 3, Jan 11: 8

62268 Percutaneous aspiration, spinal cord cyst or syrinx `A2T`

	RVU		Global Days	Modifiers				
Mod	Non-Fac Total	Fac Total		51	50	62	80	MUE
	7.51	7.51	000	2	0	0	1	1

62269 Biopsy of spinal cord, percutaneous needle `A2T`

	RVU		Global Days	Modifiers				
Mod	Non-Fac Total	Fac Total		51	50	62	80	MUE
	7.82	7.82	000	2	0	0	0	2

62270 Spinal puncture, lumbar, diagnostic `A2T`

	RVU		Global Days	Modifiers				
Mod	Non-Fac Total	Fac Total		51	50	62	80	MUE
	4.53	2.25	000	2	0	0	1	2

AMA: Nov 99: 32, 33, Oct 03: 2, Jul 06: 4, Jul 07: 1, Oct 09: 12, Nov 10: 3, Mar 12: 3, Jan 11: 8

62272 Spinal puncture, therapeutic, for drainage of cerebrospinal fluid (by needle or catheter) `A2T`

Coding tip: Therapeutic spinal puncture is not limited to the lumbar region

	RVU		Global Days	Modifiers				
Mod	Non-Fac Total	Fac Total		51	50	62	80	MUE
	5.79	2.43	000	2	0	0	1	1

AMA: Nov 99: 32, 33, Nov 10: 3, Dec 13: 14

62273 Injection, epidural, of blood or clot patch `A2T`

	RVU		Global Days	Modifiers				
Mod	Non-Fac Total	Fac Total		51	50	62	80	MUE
	5.00	3.31	000	2	0	0	1	2

AMA: Nov 99: 32, 34, Oct 09: 12, Nov 10: 3

62280 Injection/infusion of neurolytic substance (eg, alcohol, phenol, iced saline solutions), with or without other therapeutic substance; subarachnoid `A2T`

	RVU		Global Days	Modifiers				
Mod	Non-Fac Total	Fac Total		51	50	62	80	MUE
	8.80	4.69	010	2	0	0	1	1

AMA: Nov 99: 32, 34, Jan 00: 2, Jul 08: 9, Oct 09: 12, Feb 10: 11, Nov 10: 3, Jun 12: 12, Jan 11: 8

62281 Injection/infusion of neurolytic substance (eg, alcohol, phenol, iced saline solutions), with or without other therapeutic substance; epidural, cervical or thoracic `A2T`

	RVU		Global Days	Modifiers				
Mod	Non-Fac Total	Fac Total		51	50	62	80	MUE
	6.94	4.56	010	2	0	0	1	1

AMA: Apr 96: 11, Nov 99: 32, 34, Jan 00: 2, Jul 08: 9, Oct 09: 12, Feb 10: 11, May 10: 10, Nov 10: 3, Jun 12: 12, Jan 11: 8

62282 Injection/infusion of neurolytic substance (eg, alcohol, phenol, iced saline solutions), with or without other therapeutic substance; epidural, lumbar, sacral (caudal) `A2T`

	RVU		Global Days	Modifiers				
Mod	Non-Fac Total	Fac Total		51	50	62	80	MUE
	8.39	4.21	010	2	0	0	1	1

AMA: Apr 96: 11, Nov 99: 32, 34, Jan 00: 2, Jul 08: 9, Oct 09: 12, Feb 10: 11, Nov 10: 3, Jun 12: 12, Jan 11: 8

62284 Injection procedure for myelography and/or computed tomography, lumbar `N1N`

Coding tip: Computed tomography of cervical spine - 72126 -72127; thoracic spine - 72129-72130; lumbar spine - 72132-72133

Coding tip: Myelography of cervical spine - 72240; thoracic spine - 72255; lumbosacral - 72265; two or more areas - 72270

Documentation Finder: The operative report or procedure note may describe simple post-surgical care at the site of the intrathecal or epidural injection with the application of a dry sterile bandage.

	RVU		Global Days	Modifiers				
Mod	Non-Fac Total	Fac Total		51	50	62	80	MUE
	5.19	2.48	000	2	0	0	1	1

AMA: Fall 93: 13, Sep 04: 13

Surgical Procedures

62263 – 62284

● New   ▲ Revised   Deleted   ⊙ Moderate Sedation   ✚ Add-on Codes   ⊘ High Risk Denial   Ⓐ Age Edit   ♀ Female   ♂ Male   **AMA** CPT® Assistant   **MUE** Medically Unlikely Edit
⊘ Modifier 51 Exempt   ⊖ Modifier 63 Exempt   ✗ Unlisted   **Modifiers:** See Inside Back Cover   Ⓜ Maternity   A2-Z3 ASC Payment Indicators   A-Y OPPS Status Indicators

62287 Decompression procedure, percutaneous, of nucleus pulposus of intervertebral disc, any method utilizing needle based technique to remove disc material under fluoroscopic imaging or other form of indirect visualization, with the use of an endoscope, with discography and/or epidural injection(s) at the treated level(s), when performed, single or multiple levels, lumbar `A2T`

RVU			Global Days	Modifiers				
Mod	Non-Fac Total	Fac Total		51	50	62	80	MUE
	16.44	16.44	090	2	0	0	1	1

AMA: Nov 99: 34, Mar 02: 11, Oct 10: 9, Jul 12: 3, Oct 12: 14, Apr 14: 11, Mar 15: 10

62290 Injection procedure for discography, each level; lumbar `NIN`

RVU			Global Days	Modifiers				
Mod	Non-Fac Total	Fac Total		51	50	62	80	MUE
	9.58	5.00	000	2	0	0	1	5

AMA: Nov 99: 35, Apr 03: 27, Mar 11: 7, Jul 12: 3

62291 Injection procedure for discography, each level; cervical or thoracic `NIN`

RVU			Global Days	Modifiers				
Mod	Non-Fac Total	Fac Total		51	50	62	80	MUE
	9.48	4.94	000	2	0	0	1	4

AMA: Nov 99: 35, Mar 11: 7

62292 Injection procedure for chemonucleolysis, including discography, intervertebral disc, single or multiple levels, lumbar `R2T`

RVU			Global Days	Modifiers				
Mod	Non-Fac Total	Fac Total		51	50	62	80	MUE
	16.79	16.79	090	2	0	0	0	1

AMA: Oct 99: 10

62294 Injection procedure, arterial, for occlusion of arteriovenous malformation, spinal `⊘A2T`

RVU			Global Days	Modifiers				
Mod	Non-Fac Total	Fac Total		51	50	62	80	MUE
	22.68	22.68	090	2	0	0	1	1

62302 Myelography via lumbar injection, including radiological supervision and interpretation; cervical `NIQ2`

Documentation Finder: The operative report or procedure note may describe simple post-surgical care at the site of the intrathecal or epidural injection with the application of a dry sterile bandage.

RVU			Global Days	Modifiers				
Mod	Non-Fac Total	Fac Total		51	50	62	80	MUE
	6.87	3.54	000	2	0	0	1	1

62303 Myelography via lumbar injection, including radiological supervision and interpretation; thoracic `NIQ2`

RVU			Global Days	Modifiers				
Mod	Non-Fac Total	Fac Total		51	50	62	80	MUE
	7.14	3.59	000	2	0	0	1	1

62304 Myelography via lumbar injection, including radiological supervision and interpretation; lumbosacral `NIQ2`

RVU			Global Days	Modifiers				
Mod	Non-Fac Total	Fac Total		51	50	62	80	MUE
	6.80	3.49	000	2	0	0	1	1

62305 Myelography via lumbar injection, including radiological supervision and interpretation; 2 or more regions (eg, lumbar/thoracic, cervical/thoracic, lumbar/cervical, lumbar/thoracic/cervical) `NIQ2`

RVU			Global Days	Modifiers				
Mod	Non-Fac Total	Fac Total		51	50	62	80	MUE
	7.40	3.64	000	2	0	0	1	1

Coding Guidance

CPT bundles those procedures necessary for accomplishing a more comprehensive procedure into the major surgical service. Accordingly, the injection procedures described in codes 62310-62319 are included in those codes that report more extensive back procedures.

62310 Injection(s), of diagnostic or therapeutic substance(s) (including anesthetic, antispasmodic, opioid, steroid, other solution), not including neurolytic substances, including needle or catheter placement, includes contrast for localization when performed, epidural or subarachnoid; cervical or thoracic `A2T`

RVU			Global Days	Modifiers				
Mod	Non-Fac Total	Fac Total		51	50	62	80	MUE
	6.92	3.16	000	2	0	0	1	1

AMA: Nov 99: 32, 35, Jan 00: 2, Dec 00: 15, Sep 04: 5, Jul 08: 9, Nov 08: 11, May 10: 10, Nov 10: 3, Oct 09: 12, Feb 10: 12, Jan 11: 8, Jul 12: 4, 5, Feb 11: 4

62311 Injection(s), of diagnostic or therapeutic substance(s) (including anesthetic, antispasmodic, opioid, steroid, other solution), not including neurolytic substances, including needle or catheter placement, includes contrast for localization when performed, epidural or subarachnoid; lumbar or sacral (caudal) `A2T`

RVU			Global Days	Modifiers				
Mod	Non-Fac Total	Fac Total		51	50	62	80	MUE
	6.39	2.60	000	2	0	0	1	1

AMA: Dec 00: 15, Sep 04: 5, Jul 08: 9, Nov 99: 32, 35, Jul 12: 3, 4, 5, Jan 00: 1, Nov 08: 11, Oct 09: 12, Nov 10: 3, Jan 11: 8, Feb 11: 4

Coding Guidance

Codes 62318-62319 describe services that may be utilized for pain management purposes. Medicare global surgery rules block payment for postoperative pain management services provided by the same physician who performs the surgery. The services described by codes 62318-62319 may be reported by the physician performing the surgery only for purposes unrelated to the procedure, postoperative pain management, or anesthesia for the procedure.

● New ▲ Revised ✖ Deleted ⊙ Moderate Sedation ✚ Add-on Codes ⊘ High Risk Denial ⊛ Age Edit ♀ Female ♂ Male **AMA** *CPT® Assistant* **MUE** Medically Unlikely Edit
⊘ Modifier 51 Exempt ⊖ Modifier 63 Exempt ✗ Unlisted **Modifiers:** *See Inside Back Cover* Ⓜ Maternity `A2-Z3` ASC Payment Indicators `A-Y` OPPS Status Indicators

562 CPT © 2015 American Medical Association. All Rights Reserved. © 2016 DecisionHealth

62318 Injection(s), including indwelling catheter placement, continuous infusion or intermittent bolus, of diagnostic or therapeutic substance(s) (including anesthetic, antispasmodic, opioid, steroid, other solution), not including neurolytic substances, includes contrast for localization when performed, epidural or subarachnoid; cervical or thoracic   `A2 T`

RVU		Global Days	Modifiers				
Mod	Non-Fac Total	Fac Total		51	50	62	80	MUE
	6.81	2.92	000	2	0	0	1	1

AMA: Nov 99: 32, 35, Jan 00: 2, Dec 00: 15, Oct 01: 9, Jul 08: 9, Nov 08: 11, Oct 09: 12, Nov 10: 3, Jul 12: 4, 5, Jan 11: 8, Oct 12: 14

62319 Injection(s), including indwelling catheter placement, continuous infusion or intermittent bolus, of diagnostic or therapeutic substance(s) (including anesthetic, antispasmodic, opioid, steroid, other solution), not including neurolytic substances, includes contrast for localization when performed, epidural or subarachnoid; lumbar or sacral (caudal)   `A2 T`

RVU		Global Days	Modifiers				
Mod	Non-Fac Total	Fac Total		51	50	62	80	MUE
	4.91	2.81	000	2	0	0	1	1

AMA: Nov 99: 32, 35, Jan 00: 2, Dec 00: 15, Oct 01: 9, Jul 08: 9, Nov 08: 11, Oct 09: 12, Nov 10: 3, Jul 12: 4, 5, Jan 11: 8

Spinal Catheter Implantation

62350 Implantation, revision or repositioning of tunneled intrathecal or epidural catheter, for long-term medication administration via an external pump or implantable reservoir/infusion pump; without laminectomy   `A2 T`

RVU		Global Days	Modifiers				
Mod	Non-Fac Total	Fac Total		51	50	62	80	MUE
	11.70	11.70	010	2	0	1	1	1

AMA: Nov 99: 36

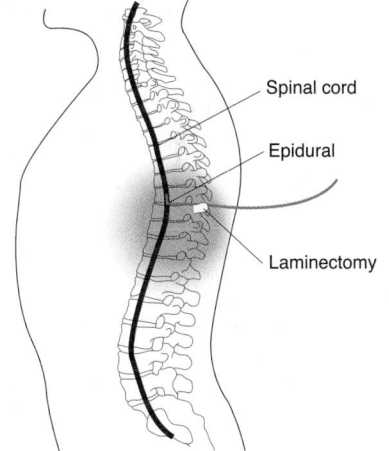

Implantation, revision or repositioning of tunneled intrathecal or epidural catheter,

Spinal cord

Epidural

Laminectomy

Without laminectomy (62350), with laminectomy (62351)

62351 Implantation, revision or repositioning of tunneled intrathecal or epidural catheter, for long-term medication administration via an external pump or implantable reservoir/infusion pump; with laminectomy   `J1`

RVU		Global Days	Modifiers				
Mod	Non-Fac Total	Fac Total		51	50	62	80	MUE
	25.47	25.47	090	2	0	2	2	1

AMA: Nov 99: 36

62355 Removal of previously implanted intrathecal or epidural catheter   `A2 Q2`

RVU		Global Days	Modifiers				
Mod	Non-Fac Total	Fac Total		51	50	62	80	MUE
	7.69	7.69	010	2	0	0	0	1

Spinal Reservoir/Pump Implantation

62360 Implantation or replacement of device for intrathecal or epidural drug infusion; subcutaneous reservoir   `J8 J1`

RVU		Global Days	Modifiers				
Mod	Non-Fac Total	Fac Total		51	50	62	80	MUE
	9.13	9.13	010	2	0	1	0	1

62361 Implantation or replacement of device for intrathecal or epidural drug infusion; nonprogrammable pump   `J8 J1`

RVU		Global Days	Modifiers				
Mod	Non-Fac Total	Fac Total		51	50	62	80	MUE
	10.54	10.54	010	2	0	1	0	1

62362 Implantation or replacement of device for intrathecal or epidural drug infusion; programmable pump, including preparation of pump, with or without programming   `J8 J1`

RVU		Global Days	Modifiers				
Mod	Non-Fac Total	Fac Total		51	50	62	80	MUE
	11.31	11.31	010	2	0	1	0	1

AMA: Mar 97: 11

62365 Removal of subcutaneous reservoir or pump, previously implanted for intrathecal or epidural infusion   `A2 Q2`

RVU		Global Days	Modifiers				
Mod	Non-Fac Total	Fac Total		51	50	62	80	MUE
	8.66	8.66	010	2	0	0	0	1

62367 Electronic analysis of programmable, implanted pump for intrathecal or epidural drug infusion (includes evaluation of reservoir status, alarm status, drug prescription status); without reprogramming or refill   `P3 S`

RVU		Global Days	Modifiers				
Mod	Non-Fac Total	Fac Total		51	50	62	80	MUE
	1.19	0.74	XXX	0	0	0	1	1

AMA: Jul 12: 5, 6, Aug 12: 10, 11, 12, 15

62368 Electronic analysis of programmable, implanted pump for intrathecal or epidural drug infusion (includes evaluation of reservoir status, alarm status, drug prescription status); with reprogramming   `P3 S`

RVU		Global Days	Modifiers				
Mod	Non-Fac Total	Fac Total		51	50	62	80	MUE
	1.63	1.02	XXX	0	0	0	1	1

AMA: Nov 02: 10, Jul 06: 1, Jul 12: 5, 6, Aug 12: 10, 11, 12, 15

● New   ▲ Revised   Deleted   ⊙ Moderate Sedation   ✚ Add-on Codes   ⊘ High Risk Denial   Ⓐ Age Edit   ♀ Female   ♂ Male   **AMA** *CPT® Assistant*   **MUE** Medically Unlikely Edit
⊘ Modifier 51 Exempt   ⊖ Modifier 63 Exempt   ☒ Unlisted   **Modifiers:** *See Inside Back Cover*   Ⓜ Maternity   `A2`–`Z3` ASC Payment Indicators   `A`–`Y` OPPS Status Indicators

Surgical Procedures

62318 — 62368

62369 **Electronic analysis of programmable, implanted pump for intrathecal or epidural drug infusion (includes evaluation of reservoir status, alarm status, drug prescription status); with reprogramming and refill**   `P 3 S`

RVU			Global Days	Modifiers				
Mod	Non-Fac Total	Fac Total		51	50	62	80	MUE
	3.45	1.04	XXX	0	0	0	1	1

AMA: Jul 12: 5, 6, Aug 12: 10, 11, 12, 15

62370 **Electronic analysis of programmable, implanted pump for intrathecal or epidural drug infusion (includes evaluation of reservoir status, alarm status, drug prescription status); with reprogramming and refill (requiring skill of a physician or other qualified health care professional)**   `P 3 S`

RVU			Global Days	Modifiers				
Mod	Non-Fac Total	Fac Total		51	50	62	80	MUE
	3.64	1.36	XXX	0	0	0	1	1

AMA: Jul 12: 5, 6, Aug 12: 10, 11, 12, 15

Laminotomy/Laminectomies for Decompression/Excision

Coding Guidance

CPT bundles those procedures necessary for accomplishing a more comprehensive procedure into the major surgical service. Accordingly, when done at the same site, laminotomy procedures are included in the laminectomy codes. Codes 22100-22116 for partial excision of vertebral components are distinct services and should not be reported together with laminotomy or laminectomy procedures unless those separate services are done as described in the codes.

63001 **Laminectomy with exploration and/or decompression of spinal cord and/or cauda equina, without facetectomy, foraminotomy or discectomy (eg, spinal stenosis), 1 or 2 vertebral segments; cervical**   `G2 J 1`

RVU			Global Days	Modifiers				
Mod	Non-Fac Total	Fac Total		51	50	62	80	MUE
	36.35	36.35	090	2	0	2	2	1

AMA: Jan 01: 12, Jun 07: 1, Jul 11: 13, Jul 12: 3, Jul 13: 3

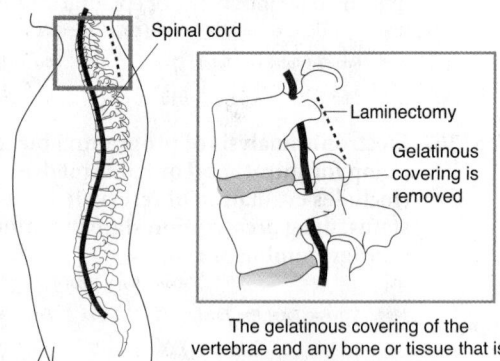

Laminectomy with exploration and/or decompression of spinal cord, cervical

Spinal cord

Laminectomy

Gelatinous covering is removed

The gelatinous covering of the vertebrae and any bone or tissue that is compressing the spinal cord is removed

63003 **Laminectomy with exploration and/or decompression of spinal cord and/or cauda equina, without facetectomy, foraminotomy or discectomy (eg, spinal stenosis), 1 or 2 vertebral segments; thoracic**   `G2 J 1`

RVU			Global Days	Modifiers				
Mod	Non-Fac Total	Fac Total		51	50	62	80	MUE
	36.12	36.12	090	2	0	2	2	1

AMA: Jan 01: 12, Jul 12: 3, Jul 13: 3

63005 **Laminectomy with exploration and/or decompression of spinal cord and/or cauda equina, without facetectomy, foraminotomy or discectomy (eg, spinal stenosis), 1 or 2 vertebral segments; lumbar, except for spondylolisthesis**   `G2 J 1`

RVU			Global Days	Modifiers				
Mod	Non-Fac Total	Fac Total		51	50	62	80	MUE
	34.37	34.37	090	2	0	2	2	1

AMA: Jan 01: 12, Jul 12: 3, Jul 13: 3, Dec 13: 17

63011 **Laminectomy with exploration and/or decompression of spinal cord and/or cauda equina, without facetectomy, foraminotomy or discectomy (eg, spinal stenosis), 1 or 2 vertebral segments; sacral**   `J 1`

RVU			Global Days	Modifiers				
Mod	Non-Fac Total	Fac Total		51	50	62	80	MUE
	31.59	31.59	090	2	0	2	2	1

AMA: Jan 01: 12, Jul 13: 3

63012 **Laminectomy with removal of abnormal facets and/or pars inter-articularis with decompression of cauda equina and nerve roots for spondylolisthesis, lumbar (Gill type procedure)**   `J 1`

RVU			Global Days	Modifiers				
Mod	Non-Fac Total	Fac Total		51	50	62	80	MUE
	34.43	34.43	090	2	0	2	2	1

AMA: Jan 01: 12, Jul 13: 3

63015 **Laminectomy with exploration and/or decompression of spinal cord and/or cauda equina, without facetectomy, foraminotomy or discectomy (eg, spinal stenosis), more than 2 vertebral segments; cervical**   `J 1`

RVU			Global Days	Modifiers				
Mod	Non-Fac Total	Fac Total		51	50	62	80	MUE
	43.42	43.42	090	2	0	2	2	1

AMA: Jan 01: 12, Jul 13: 3

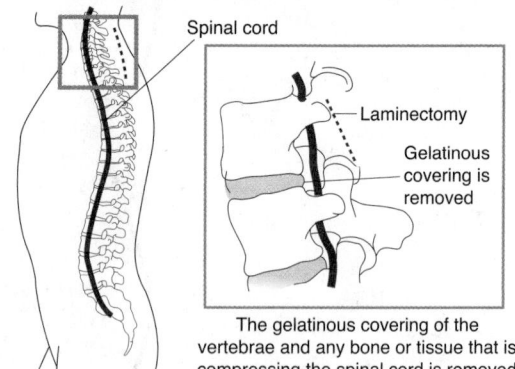

Laminectomy with exploration and/or decompression of spinal cord, more than two vertebral segments; cervical

Spinal cord

Laminectomy

Gelatinous covering is removed

The gelatinous covering of the vertebrae and any bone or tissue that is compressing the spinal cord is removed

---

● New   ▲ Revised   ✖ Deleted   ⊙ Moderate Sedation   ✚ Add-on Codes   ⊘ High Risk Denial   ⒶAge Edit   ♀ Female   ♂ Male   **AMA** *CPT® Assistant*   **MUE** Medically Unlikely Edit
⊘ Modifier 51 Exempt   ⊖ Modifier 63 Exempt   ☒ Unlisted   **Modifiers:** *See Inside Back Cover*   Ⓜ Maternity   `A2`–`Z3` ASC Payment Indicators   `A`–`Y` OPPS Status Indicators

CPT © 2015 American Medical Association. All Rights Reserved.   © 2016 DecisionHealth

63016 Laminectomy with exploration and/or decompression of spinal cord and/or cauda equina, without facetectomy, foraminotomy or discectomy (eg, spinal stenosis), more than 2 vertebral segments; thoracic J-1

RVU			Global Days	Modifiers				
Mod	Non-Fac Total	Fac Total		51	50	62	80	MUE
	44.55	44.55	090	2	0	2	2	1

AMA: Jan 01: 12, Jul 13: 3

63017 Laminectomy with exploration and/or decompression of spinal cord and/or cauda equina, without facetectomy, foraminotomy or discectomy (eg, spinal stenosis), more than 2 vertebral segments; lumbar J-1

RVU			Global Days	Modifiers				
Mod	Non-Fac Total	Fac Total		51	50	62	80	MUE
	36.50	36.50	090	2	0	2	2	1

AMA: Jan 01: 12, Jul 13: 3

63020 Laminotomy (hemilaminectomy), with decompression of nerve root(s), including partial facetectomy, foraminotomy and/or excision of herniated intervertebral disc; 1 interspace, cervical G2 J-1

RVU			Global Days	Modifiers				
Mod	Non-Fac Total	Fac Total		51	50	62	80	MUE
	33.88	33.88	090	2	1	2	2	1

AMA: Nov 99: 36, Jan 01: 12, Jul 12: 4, Dec 12: 13, Jul 13: 3

63030 Laminotomy (hemilaminectomy), with decompression of nerve root(s), including partial facetectomy, foraminotomy and/or excision of herniated intervertebral disc; 1 interspace, lumbar G2 J-1

RVU			Global Days	Modifiers				
Mod	Non-Fac Total	Fac Total		51	50	62	80	MUE
	28.21	28.21	090	2	1	2	2	1

AMA: Mar 96: 7, Nov 99: 36, Jan 01: 12, Feb 01: 10, Sep 02: 10, Oct 04: 12, Oct 08: 10, Oct 09: 9, Mar 11: 7, Jul 11: 13, Nov 10: 4, Jul 12: 3, 4, Dec 12: 13, Jul 13: 3, Dec 13: 17

+ **63035** Laminotomy (hemilaminectomy), with decompression of nerve root(s), including partial facetectomy, foraminotomy and/or excision of herniated intervertebral disc; each additional interspace, cervical or lumbar (List separately in addition to code for primary procedure) N

RVU			Global Days	Modifiers				
Mod	Non-Fac Total	Fac Total		51	50	62	80	MUE
	5.48	5.48	ZZZ	0	1	2	2	4

AMA: Fall 91: 8, Mar 96: 7, Nov 99: 36, Jan 01: 12, Feb 01: 10, Jul 12: 4

63040 Laminotomy (hemilaminectomy), with decompression of nerve root(s), including partial facetectomy, foraminotomy and/or excision of herniated intervertebral disc, reexploration, single interspace; cervical J-1

RVU			Global Days	Modifiers				
Mod	Non-Fac Total	Fac Total		51	50	62	80	MUE
	40.53	40.53	090	2	1	2	2	1

AMA: Jan 99: 11, Jan 01: 12, Jul 13: 3

63042 Laminotomy (hemilaminectomy), with decompression of nerve root(s), including partial facetectomy, foraminotomy and/or excision of herniated intervertebral disc, reexploration, single interspace; lumbar G2 J-1

RVU			Global Days	Modifiers				
Mod	Non-Fac Total	Fac Total		51	50	62	80	MUE
	37.69	37.69	090	2	1	2	2	1

AMA: Jan 99: 11, Jan 01: 12, Oct 08: 10, Oct 09: 9, Jul 11: 13, Jul 13: 3

+ **63043** Laminotomy (hemilaminectomy), with decompression of nerve root(s), including partial facetectomy, foraminotomy and/or excision of herniated intervertebral disc, reexploration, single interspace; each additional cervical interspace (List separately in addition to code for primary procedure) ⊙ N

RVU			Global Days	Modifiers				
Mod	Non-Fac Total	Fac Total		51	50	62	80	MUE
	0.00	0.00	ZZZ	0	1	2	2	4

+ **63044** Laminotomy (hemilaminectomy), with decompression of nerve root(s), including partial facetectomy, foraminotomy and/or excision of herniated intervertebral disc, reexploration, single interspace; each additional lumbar interspace (List separately in addition to code for primary procedure) N1 N

RVU			Global Days	Modifiers				
Mod	Non-Fac Total	Fac Total		51	50	62	80	MUE
	0.00	0.00	ZZZ	0	1	2	2	4

63045 Laminectomy, facetectomy and foraminotomy (unilateral or bilateral with decompression of spinal cord, cauda equina and/or nerve root[s], [eg, spinal or lateral recess stenosis]), single vertebral segment; cervical G2 J-1

RVU			Global Days	Modifiers				
Mod	Non-Fac Total	Fac Total		51	50	62	80	MUE
	37.53	37.53	090	2	2	2	2	1

AMA: Jan 01: 12, Dec 12: 13, Jul 13: 3

63046 Laminectomy, facetectomy and foraminotomy (unilateral or bilateral with decompression of spinal cord, cauda equina and/or nerve root[s], [eg, spinal or lateral recess stenosis]), single vertebral segment; thoracic G2 J-1

RVU			Global Days	Modifiers				
Mod	Non-Fac Total	Fac Total		51	50	62	80	MUE
	35.52	35.52	090	2	2	2	2	1

AMA: Jan 99: 11, Jan 01: 12, Dec 12: 13, Jul 13: 3

63047 Laminectomy, facetectomy and foraminotomy (unilateral or bilateral with decompression of spinal cord, cauda equina and/or nerve root[s], [eg, spinal or lateral recess stenosis]), single vertebral segment; lumbar G2 J-1

RVU			Global Days	Modifiers				
Mod	Non-Fac Total	Fac Total		51	50	62	80	MUE
	32.11	32.11	090	2	2	2	2	1

AMA: Jan 99: 11, Jan 01: 12, Feb 01: 10, Nov 02: 11, Apr 08: 11, Jul 08: 7, Oct 08: 10, Oct 09: 9, Jul 11: 13, Nov 10: 4, Dec 12: 13, Jul 13: 3, Dec 13: 17, Dec 14: 16

● New ▲ Revised Deleted ⊙ Moderate Sedation ✚ Add-on Codes ⊘ High Risk Denial Ⓐ Age Edit ♀ Female ♂ Male **AMA** CPT® Assistant **MUE** Medically Unlikely Edit
⊘ Modifier 51 Exempt ⊖ Modifier 63 Exempt ✕ Unlisted **Modifiers:** See Inside Back Cover Ⓜ Maternity A2–Z3 ASC Payment Indicators A–Y OPPS Status Indicators

© 2016 DecisionHealth · CPT © 2015 American Medical Association. All Rights Reserved. · **565**

✚ **63048** Laminectomy, facetectomy and foraminotomy (unilateral or bilateral with decompression of spinal cord, cauda equina and/or nerve root[s], [eg, spinal or lateral recess stenosis]), single vertebral segment; each additional segment, cervical, thoracic, or lumbar (List separately in addition to code for primary procedure) Ⓝ

RVU			Global Days	Modifiers				
Mod	Non-Fac Total	Fac Total		51	50	62	80	MUE
	6.03	6.03	ZZZ	0	0	2	2	5

AMA: Fall 91: 8, Jan 99: 11, Jan 01: 12, Dec 12: 13

63050 Laminoplasty, cervical, with decompression of the spinal cord, 2 or more vertebral segments Ⓒ

RVU			Global Days	Modifiers				
Mod	Non-Fac Total	Fac Total		51	50	62	80	MUE
	43.48	43.48	090	2	0	2	2	1

AMA: Jul 13: 3

63051 Laminoplasty, cervical, with decompression of the spinal cord, 2 or more vertebral segments; with reconstruction of the posterior bony elements (including the application of bridging bone graft and non-segmental fixation devices [eg, wire, suture, mini-plates], when performed)Ⓒ

RVU			Global Days	Modifiers				
Mod	Non-Fac Total	Fac Total		51	50	62	80	MUE
	49.74	49.74	090	2	0	2	2	1

AMA: Jul 11: 13, Jul 13: 3

Transpedicular/Costovertebral Approach for Exploration/Decompression

63055 Transpedicular approach with decompression of spinal cord, equina and/or nerve root(s) (eg, herniated intervertebral disc), single segment; thoracic Ⓖ②ⒿⓉ

RVU			Global Days	Modifiers				
Mod	Non-Fac Total	Fac Total		51	50	62	80	MUE
	47.48	47.48	090	2	0	1	2	1

AMA: Nov 99: 36, Jul 13: 3

63056 Transpedicular approach with decompression of spinal cord, equina and/or nerve root(s) (eg, herniated intervertebral disc), single segment; lumbar (including transfacet, or lateral extraforaminal approach) (eg, far lateral herniated intervertebral disc) Ⓖ②ⒿⓉ

RVU			Global Days	Modifiers				
Mod	Non-Fac Total	Fac Total		51	50	62	80	MUE
	42.98	42.98	090	2	0	1	2	1

AMA: Nov 99: 36, Oct 09: 9, Nov 11: 10, Jul 12: 3, Jul 13: 3, Jan 14: 9

✚ **63057** Transpedicular approach with decompression of spinal cord, equina and/or nerve root(s) (eg, herniated intervertebral disc), single segment; each additional segment, thoracic or lumbar (List separately in addition to code for primary procedure) Ⓝ

RVU			Global Days	Modifiers				
Mod	Non-Fac Total	Fac Total		51	50	62	80	MUE
	9.08	9.08	ZZZ	0	0	1	2	3

AMA: Nov 99: 36

63064 Costovertebral approach with decompression of spinal cord or nerve root(s) (eg, herniated intervertebral disc), thoracic; single segment ⒿⓉ

RVU			Global Days	Modifiers				
Mod	Non-Fac Total	Fac Total		51	50	62	80	MUE
	51.56	51.56	090	2	0	1	2	1

AMA: Fall 92: 19, Jul 13: 3

✚ **63066** Costovertebral approach with decompression of spinal cord or nerve root(s) (eg, herniated intervertebral disc), thoracic; each additional segment (List separately in addition to code for primary procedure) Ⓝ

RVU			Global Days	Modifiers				
Mod	Non-Fac Total	Fac Total		51	50	62	80	MUE
	6.18	6.18	ZZZ	0	0	1	2	1

Anterior/Anterolateral Approach for Exploration/Decompression

63075 Discectomy, anterior, with decompression of spinal cord and/or nerve root(s), including osteophytectomy; cervical, single interspace ⒿⓉ

RVU			Global Days	Modifiers				
Mod	Non-Fac Total	Fac Total		51	50	62	80	MUE
	39.53	39.53	090	2	0	2	2	1

AMA: Nov 98: 18, Jan 01: 12, Feb 02: 4, Jul 13: 3, Apr 15: 7

✚ **63076** Discectomy, anterior, with decompression of spinal cord and/or nerve root(s), including osteophytectomy; cervical, each additional interspace (List separately in addition to code for primary procedure) Ⓝ

RVU			Global Days	Modifiers				
Mod	Non-Fac Total	Fac Total		51	50	62	80	MUE
	7.08	7.08	ZZZ	0	0	2	2	3

AMA: Nov 98: 18, Jan 01: 12, Feb 02: 4

63077 Discectomy, anterior, with decompression of spinal cord and/or nerve root(s), including osteophytectomy; thoracic, single interspace Ⓒ

RVU			Global Days	Modifiers				
Mod	Non-Fac Total	Fac Total		51	50	62	80	MUE
	43.40	43.40	090	2	0	2	2	1

AMA: Nov 98: 18, Jan 01: 12, Feb 02: 4, Jul 13: 3

✚ **63078** Discectomy, anterior, with decompression of spinal cord and/or nerve root(s), including osteophytectomy; thoracic, each additional interspace (List separately in addition to code for primary procedure) Ⓒ

RVU			Global Days	Modifiers				
Mod	Non-Fac Total	Fac Total		51	50	62	80	MUE
	5.50	5.50	ZZZ	0	0	2	2	3

AMA: Nov 98: 18, Jan 01: 12, Feb 02: 4

63081 Vertebral corpectomy (vertebral body resection), partial or complete, anterior approach with decompression of spinal cord and/or nerve root(s); cervical, single segment Ⓒ

RVU			Global Days	Modifiers				
Mod	Non-Fac Total	Fac Total		51	50	62	80	MUE
	51.19	51.19	090	2	0	1	2	1

AMA: Spring 93: 37, Feb 02: 4, Jul 13: 3, Jun 15: 10

● New   ▲ Revised   ✖ Deleted   ⊙ Moderate Sedation   ✚ Add-on Codes   ⊘ High Risk Denial   Ⓐ Age Edit   ♀ Female   ♂ Male   **AMA** *CPT® Assistant*   *MUE* Medically Unlikely Edit
⊘ Modifier 51 Exempt   ⊖ Modifier 63 Exempt   Ⓧ Unlisted   **Modifiers:** *See Inside Back Cover*   Ⓜ Maternity   Ⓐ②–Ⓩ③ ASC Payment Indicators   Ⓐ–Ⓨ OPPS Status Indicators

CPT © 2015 American Medical Association. All Rights Reserved.   © 2016 DecisionHealth

✚ **63082** Vertebral corpectomy (vertebral body resection), partial or complete, anterior approach with decompression of spinal cord and/or nerve root(s); cervical, each additional segment (List separately in addition to code for primary procedure) **ⓒ**

RVU			Global Days	Modifiers				
Mod	Non-Fac Total	Fac Total		51	50	62	80	MUE
	7.58	7.58	ZZZ	0	0	1	2	6

AMA: Spring 93: 37, Feb 02: 4

63085 Vertebral corpectomy (vertebral body resection), partial or complete, transthoracic approach with decompression of spinal cord and/or nerve root(s); thoracic, single segment **ⓒ**

RVU			Global Days	Modifiers				
Mod	Non-Fac Total	Fac Total		51	50	62	80	MUE
	56.02	56.02	090	2	0	2	2	1

AMA: Spring 93: 37, Feb 02: 4, Jul 13: 3

✚ **63086** Vertebral corpectomy (vertebral body resection), partial or complete, transthoracic approach with decompression of spinal cord and/or nerve root(s); thoracic, each additional segment (List separately in addition to code for primary procedure) **ⓒ**

RVU			Global Days	Modifiers				
Mod	Non-Fac Total	Fac Total		51	50	62	80	MUE
	5.51	5.51	ZZZ	0	0	2	2	2

AMA: Spring 93: 37, Feb 02: 4

63087 Vertebral corpectomy (vertebral body resection), partial or complete, combined thoracolumbar approach with decompression of spinal cord, cauda equina or nerve root(s), lower thoracic or lumbar; single segment **ⓒ**

RVU			Global Days	Modifiers				
Mod	Non-Fac Total	Fac Total		51	50	62	80	MUE
	70.35	70.35	090	2	0	2	2	1

AMA: Spring 93: 37, Feb 02: 4, Jul 13: 3

✚ **63088** Vertebral corpectomy (vertebral body resection), partial or complete, combined thoracolumbar approach with decompression of spinal cord, cauda equina or nerve root(s), lower thoracic or lumbar; each additional segment (List separately in addition to code for primary procedure) **ⓒ**

RVU			Global Days	Modifiers				
Mod	Non-Fac Total	Fac Total		51	50	62	80	MUE
	7.50	7.50	ZZZ	0	0	2	2	4

AMA: Spring 93: 37, Feb 02: 4

63090 Vertebral corpectomy (vertebral body resection), partial or complete, transperitoneal or retroperitoneal approach with decompression of spinal cord, cauda equina or nerve root(s), lower thoracic, lumbar, or sacral; single segment **ⓒ**

RVU			Global Days	Modifiers				
Mod	Non-Fac Total	Fac Total		51	50	62	80	MUE
	56.81	56.81	090	2	0	2	2	1

AMA: Spring 93: 37, Mar 96: 6, Feb 02: 4, Jul 13: 3

✚ **63091** Vertebral corpectomy (vertebral body resection), partial or complete, transperitoneal or retroperitoneal approach with decompression of spinal cord, cauda equina or nerve root(s), lower thoracic, lumbar, or sacral; each additional segment (List separately in addition to code for primary procedure) **ⓒ**

RVU			Global Days	Modifiers				
Mod	Non-Fac Total	Fac Total		51	50	62	80	MUE
	5.02	5.02	ZZZ	0	0	2	2	3

AMA: Spring 93: 37, Mar 96: 6, Feb 02: 4

Lateral Extracavitary Approach for Exploration/Decompression

63101 Vertebral corpectomy (vertebral body resection), partial or complete, lateral extracavitary approach with decompression of spinal cord and/or nerve root(s) (eg, for tumor or retropulsed bone fragments); thoracic, single segment **ⓒ**

RVU			Global Days	Modifiers				
Mod	Non-Fac Total	Fac Total		51	50	62	80	MUE
	67.73	67.73	090	2	0	1	2	1

AMA: Jul 13: 3

63102 Vertebral corpectomy (vertebral body resection), partial or complete, lateral extracavitary approach with decompression of spinal cord and/or nerve root(s) (eg, for tumor or retropulsed bone fragments); lumbar, single segment **ⓒ**

RVU			Global Days	Modifiers				
Mod	Non-Fac Total	Fac Total		51	50	62	80	MUE
	66.11	66.11	090	2	0	1	2	1

AMA: Jul 13: 3

✚ **63103** Vertebral corpectomy (vertebral body resection), partial or complete, lateral extracavitary approach with decompression of spinal cord and/or nerve root(s) (eg, for tumor or retropulsed bone fragments); thoracic or lumbar, each additional segment (List separately in addition to code for primary procedure) **ⓒ**

RVU			Global Days	Modifiers				
Mod	Non-Fac Total	Fac Total		51	50	62	80	MUE
	8.40	8.40	ZZZ	0	0	1	2	3

Spinal Incision

63170 Laminectomy with myelotomy (eg, Bischof or DREZ type), cervical, thoracic, or thoracolumbar **ⓒ**

RVU			Global Days	Modifiers				
Mod	Non-Fac Total	Fac Total		51	50	62	80	MUE
	47.29	47.29	090	2	0	1	2	1

AMA: Jul 13: 3

63172 Laminectomy with drainage of intramedullary cyst/syrinx; to subarachnoid space **ⓒ**

RVU			Global Days	Modifiers				
Mod	Non-Fac Total	Fac Total		51	50	62	80	MUE
	40.65	40.65	090	2	0	1	2	1

AMA: Jul 13: 3

● New   ▲ Revised   Deleted   ⊙ Moderate Sedation   ✚ Add-on Codes   ⊘ High Risk Denial   Ⓐ Age Edit   ♀ Female   ♂ Male   **AMA** CPT® Assistant   **MUE** Medically Unlikely Edit
   ⊘ Modifier 51 Exempt   ⊖ Modifier 63 Exempt   ✗ Unlisted   **Modifiers:** See Inside Back Cover   Ⓜ Maternity   Ⓐ2–Ⓩ3 ASC Payment Indicators   Ⓐ–Ⓨ OPPS Status Indicators

Laminectomy with drainage of intramedullary cyst/syrinx

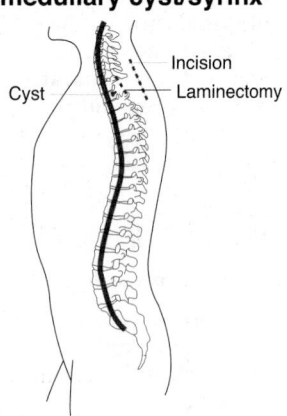

Incision
Cyst
Laminectomy

The lamina is removed from around a vertebra and a cyst is drained; into spinal cord (63172), into abdominal/chest cavity (63173)

63173 Laminectomy with drainage of intramedullary cyst/syrinx; to peritoneal or pleural space Ⓒ

RVU		Global Days	Modifiers				
Mod	Non-Fac Total	Fac Total		51	50	62	80	MUE
	50.61	50.61	090	2	0	1	2	1

AMA: Jul 13: 3

63180 Laminectomy and section of dentate ligaments, with or without dural graft, cervical; 1 or 2 segments ⊗Ⓒ

RVU		Global Days	Modifiers				
Mod	Non-Fac Total	Fac Total		51	50	62	80	MUE
	44.10	44.10	090	2	0	1	2	1

AMA: Jul 13: 3

63182 Laminectomy and section of dentate ligaments, with or without dural graft, cervical; more than 2 segments Ⓒ

RVU		Global Days	Modifiers				
Mod	Non-Fac Total	Fac Total		51	50	62	80	MUE
	40.05	40.05	090	2	0	1	2	1

AMA: Jul 13: 3

63185 Laminectomy with rhizotomy; 1 or 2 segments Ⓒ

RVU		Global Days	Modifiers				
Mod	Non-Fac Total	Fac Total		51	50	62	80	MUE
	33.01	33.01	090	2	0	1	2	1

AMA: Jul 13: 3

63190 Laminectomy with rhizotomy; more than 2 segments Ⓒ

RVU		Global Days	Modifiers				
Mod	Non-Fac Total	Fac Total		51	50	62	80	MUE
	36.45	36.45	090	2	0	1	2	1

AMA: Jul 13: 3

63191 Laminectomy with section of spinal accessory nerve Ⓒ

RVU		Global Days	Modifiers				
Mod	Non-Fac Total	Fac Total		51	50	62	80	MUE
	39.95	39.95	090	2	1	1	2	1

AMA: Jul 13: 3

63194 Laminectomy with cordotomy, with section of 1 spinothalamic tract, 1 stage; cervical Ⓒ

RVU		Global Days	Modifiers				
Mod	Non-Fac Total	Fac Total		51	50	62	80	MUE
	47.43	47.43	090	2	0	1	2	1

AMA: Jul 13: 3

63195 Laminectomy with cordotomy, with section of 1 spinothalamic tract, 1 stage; thoracic Ⓒ

RVU		Global Days	Modifiers				
Mod	Non-Fac Total	Fac Total		51	50	62	80	MUE
	45.65	45.65	090	2	0	1	2	1

AMA: Jul 13: 3

63196 Laminectomy with cordotomy, with section of both spinothalamic tracts, 1 stage; cervical ⊗Ⓒ

RVU		Global Days	Modifiers				
Mod	Non-Fac Total	Fac Total		51	50	62	80	MUE
	40.92	40.92	090	2	0	1	2	1

AMA: Jul 13: 3

63197 Laminectomy with cordotomy, with section of both spinothalamic tracts, 1 stage; thoracic Ⓒ

RVU		Global Days	Modifiers				
Mod	Non-Fac Total	Fac Total		51	50	62	80	MUE
	50.81	50.81	090	2	0	1	2	1

AMA: Jul 13: 3

63198 Laminectomy with cordotomy with section of both spinothalamic tracts, 2 stages within 14 days; cervical Ⓒ

RVU		Global Days	Modifiers				
Mod	Non-Fac Total	Fac Total		51	50	62	80	MUE
	48.18	48.18	090	2	0	1	2	1

AMA: Jul 13: 3

63199 Laminectomy with cordotomy with section of both spinothalamic tracts, 2 stages within 14 days; thoracic Ⓒ

RVU		Global Days	Modifiers				
Mod	Non-Fac Total	Fac Total		51	50	62	80	MUE
	50.58	50.58	090	2	0	1	2	1

AMA: Jul 13: 3

63200 Laminectomy, with release of tethered spinal cord, lumbar Ⓒ

RVU		Global Days	Modifiers				
Mod	Non-Fac Total	Fac Total		51	50	62	80	MUE
	45.06	45.06	090	2	0	0	2	1

AMA: Jul 13: 3

Lesion Laminectomy

63250 Laminectomy for excision or occlusion of arteriovenous malformation of spinal cord; cervical Ⓒ

RVU		Global Days	Modifiers				
Mod	Non-Fac Total	Fac Total		51	50	62	80	MUE
	82.81	82.81	090	2	0	1	2	1

AMA: Jul 13: 3

● New   ▲ Revised   ✖ Deleted   ⊙ Moderate Sedation   ✚ Add-on Codes   ⊗ High Risk Denial   Ⓐ Age Edit   ♀ Female   ♂ Male   **AMA** *CPT® Assistant*   **MUE** Medically Unlikely Edit
⊗ Modifier 51 Exempt   ⊖ Modifier 63 Exempt   ✖ Unlisted   **Modifiers:** *See Inside Back Cover*   Ⓜ Maternity   A2–Z3 ASC Payment Indicators   A–Y OPPS Status Indicators

63251 Laminectomy for excision or occlusion of arteriovenous malformation of spinal cord; thoracic Ⓒ

RVU			Global Days	Modifiers				
Mod	Non-Fac Total	Fac Total		51	50	62	80	MUE
	89.99	89.99	090	2	0	1	2	1

AMA: Jul 13: 3

63252 Laminectomy for excision or occlusion of arteriovenous malformation of spinal cord; thoracolumbar Ⓒ

RVU			Global Days	Modifiers				
Mod	Non-Fac Total	Fac Total		51	50	62	80	MUE
	89.88	89.88	090	2	0	1	2	1

AMA: Jul 13: 3

63265 Laminectomy for excision or evacuation of intraspinal lesion other than neoplasm, extradural; cervical Ⓒ

RVU			Global Days	Modifiers				
Mod	Non-Fac Total	Fac Total		51	50	62	80	MUE
	48.87	48.87	090	2	0	1	2	1

AMA: Jul 13: 3

63266 Laminectomy for excision or evacuation of intraspinal lesion other than neoplasm, extradural; thoracic Ⓒ

RVU			Global Days	Modifiers				
Mod	Non-Fac Total	Fac Total		51	50	62	80	MUE
	50.33	50.33	090	2	0	1	2	1

63267 Laminectomy for excision or evacuation of intraspinal lesion other than neoplasm, extradural; lumbar Ⓒ

RVU			Global Days	Modifiers				
Mod	Non-Fac Total	Fac Total		51	50	62	80	MUE
	39.79	39.79	090	2	0	1	2	1

AMA: Jul 13: 3

63268 Laminectomy for excision or evacuation of intraspinal lesion other than neoplasm, extradural; sacral Ⓒ

RVU			Global Days	Modifiers				
Mod	Non-Fac Total	Fac Total		51	50	62	80	MUE
	42.22	42.22	090	2	0	1	2	1

AMA: Jul 13: 3

63270 Laminectomy for excision of intraspinal lesion other than neoplasm, intradural; cervical Ⓒ

RVU			Global Days	Modifiers				
Mod	Non-Fac Total	Fac Total		51	50	62	80	MUE
	61.56	61.56	090	2	0	1	2	1

63271 Laminectomy for excision of intraspinal lesion other than neoplasm, intradural; thoracic Ⓒ

RVU			Global Days	Modifiers				
Mod	Non-Fac Total	Fac Total		51	50	62	80	MUE
	60.59	60.59	090	2	0	1	2	1

AMA: Jul 13: 3

63272 Laminectomy for excision of intraspinal lesion other than neoplasm, intradural; lumbar Ⓒ

RVU			Global Days	Modifiers				
Mod	Non-Fac Total	Fac Total		51	50	62	80	MUE
	55.22	55.22	090	2	0	1	2	1

AMA: Jul 13: 3

63273 Laminectomy for excision of intraspinal lesion other than neoplasm, intradural; sacral Ⓒ

RVU			Global Days	Modifiers				
Mod	Non-Fac Total	Fac Total		51	50	62	80	MUE
	55.06	55.06	090	2	0	0	2	1

AMA: Jul 13: 3

63275 Laminectomy for biopsy/excision of intraspinal neoplasm; extradural, cervical Ⓒ

RVU			Global Days	Modifiers				
Mod	Non-Fac Total	Fac Total		51	50	62	80	MUE
	52.71	52.71	090	2	0	1	2	1

AMA: Jul 13: 3

63276 Laminectomy for biopsy/excision of intraspinal neoplasm; extradural, thoracic Ⓒ

RVU			Global Days	Modifiers				
Mod	Non-Fac Total	Fac Total		51	50	62	80	MUE
	52.21	52.21	090	2	0	1	2	1

AMA: Jul 13: 3

63277 Laminectomy for biopsy/excision of intraspinal neoplasm; extradural, lumbar Ⓒ

RVU			Global Days	Modifiers				
Mod	Non-Fac Total	Fac Total		51	50	62	80	MUE
	45.11	45.11	090	2	0	1	2	1

AMA: Jul 13: 3

63278 Laminectomy for biopsy/excision of intraspinal neoplasm; extradural, sacral Ⓒ

RVU			Global Days	Modifiers				
Mod	Non-Fac Total	Fac Total		51	50	62	80	MUE
	47.16	47.16	090	2	0	1	2	1

AMA: Jul 13: 3

63280 Laminectomy for biopsy/excision of intraspinal neoplasm; intradural, extramedullary, cervical Ⓒ

RVU			Global Days	Modifiers				
Mod	Non-Fac Total	Fac Total		51	50	62	80	MUE
	61.85	61.85	090	2	0	1	2	1

AMA: Jul 13: 3

63281 Laminectomy for biopsy/excision of intraspinal neoplasm; intradural, extramedullary, thoracic Ⓒ

RVU			Global Days	Modifiers				
Mod	Non-Fac Total	Fac Total		51	50	62	80	MUE
	61.09	61.09	090	2	0	1	2	1

AMA: Jul 13: 3

63282 Laminectomy for biopsy/excision of intraspinal neoplasm; intradural, extramedullary, lumbar Ⓒ

RVU			Global Days	Modifiers				
Mod	Non-Fac Total	Fac Total		51	50	62	80	MUE
	57.35	57.35	090	2	0	1	2	1

AMA: Jul 13: 3

63283 Laminectomy for biopsy/excision of intraspinal neoplasm; intradural, sacral Ⓒ

RVU			Global Days	Modifiers				
Mod	Non-Fac Total	Fac Total		51	50	62	80	MUE
	55.82	55.82	090	2	0	1	2	1

AMA: Jul 13: 3

● New　▲ Revised　Deleted　⊙ Moderate Sedation　✛ Add-on Codes　⊘ High Risk Denial　Ⓐ Age Edit　♀ Female　♂ Male　**AMA** CPT® Assistant　**MUE** Medically Unlikely Edit
⊘ Modifier 51 Exempt　⊖ Modifier 63 Exempt　✗ Unlisted　**Modifiers:** See Inside Back Cover　Ⓜ Maternity　Ａ2–Ｚ3 ASC Payment Indicators　Ａ–Ｙ OPPS Status Indicators

Surgical Procedures

63285 – 63306

63285 Laminectomy for biopsy/excision of intraspinal neoplasm; intradural, intramedullary, cervical **C**

RVU			Global Days	Modifiers				
Mod	Non-Fac Total	Fac Total		51	50	62	80	MUE
	77.59	77.59	090	2	0	1	2	1

AMA: Jul 13: 3

63286 Laminectomy for biopsy/excision of intraspinal neoplasm; intradural, intramedullary, thoracic **C**

RVU			Global Days	Modifiers				
Mod	Non-Fac Total	Fac Total		51	50	62	80	MUE
	75.69	75.69	090	2	0	1	2	1

AMA: Jul 13: 3

63287 Laminectomy for biopsy/excision of intraspinal neoplasm; intradural, intramedullary, thoracolumbar **C**

RVU			Global Days	Modifiers				
Mod	Non-Fac Total	Fac Total		51	50	62	80	MUE
	81.64	81.64	090	2	0	1	2	1

AMA: Jul 13: 3

63290 Laminectomy for biopsy/excision of intraspinal neoplasm; combined extradural-intradural lesion, any level **C**

RVU			Global Days	Modifiers				
Mod	Non-Fac Total	Fac Total		51	50	62	80	MUE
	81.18	81.18	090	2	0	1	2	1

AMA: Jul 13: 3

+ 63295 Osteoplastic reconstruction of dorsal spinal elements, following primary intraspinal procedure (List separately in addition to code for primary procedure) **C**

RVU			Global Days	Modifiers				
Mod	Non-Fac Total	Fac Total		51	50	62	80	MUE
	9.89	9.89	ZZZ	0	2	2	2	1

Anterior/Anterolateral Approach, Intraspinal Lesion Excision

63300 Vertebral corpectomy (vertebral body resection), partial or complete, for excision of intraspinal lesion, single segment; extradural, cervical **C**

RVU			Global Days	Modifiers				
Mod	Non-Fac Total	Fac Total		51	50	62	80	MUE
	53.81	53.81	090	2	0	1	2	1

AMA: Feb 02: 4, Jul 13: 3

Vertebral corpectomy, partial or complete, for excision of intraspinal lesion, extradural

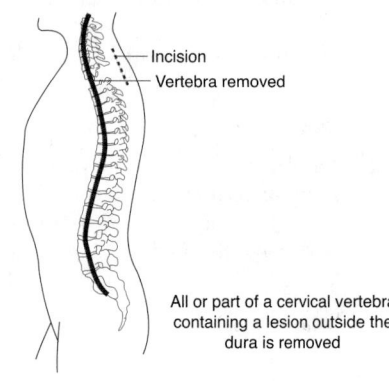

Incision
Vertebra removed

All or part of a cervical vertebra containing a lesion outside the dura is removed

63301 Vertebral corpectomy (vertebral body resection), partial or complete, for excision of intraspinal lesion, single segment; extradural, thoracic by transthoracic approach **C**

RVU			Global Days	Modifiers				
Mod	Non-Fac Total	Fac Total		51	50	62	80	MUE
	65.22	65.22	090	2	0	1	2	1

AMA: Feb 02: 4, Jul 13: 3

63302 Vertebral corpectomy (vertebral body resection), partial or complete, for excision of intraspinal lesion, single segment; extradural, thoracic by thoracolumbar approach **C**

RVU			Global Days	Modifiers				
Mod	Non-Fac Total	Fac Total		51	50	62	80	MUE
	64.11	64.11	090	2	0	1	2	1

AMA: Feb 02: 4, Jul 13: 3

63303 Vertebral corpectomy (vertebral body resection), partial or complete, for excision of intraspinal lesion, single segment; extradural, lumbar or sacral by transperitoneal or retroperitoneal approach **C**

RVU			Global Days	Modifiers				
Mod	Non-Fac Total	Fac Total		51	50	62	80	MUE
	68.31	68.31	090	2	0	1	2	1

AMA: Feb 02: 4, Jul 13: 3

63304 Vertebral corpectomy (vertebral body resection), partial or complete, for excision of intraspinal lesion, single segment; intradural, cervical **C**

RVU			Global Days	Modifiers				
Mod	Non-Fac Total	Fac Total		51	50	62	80	MUE
	68.94	68.94	090	2	0	1	2	1

AMA: Feb 02: 4, Jul 13: 3

63305 Vertebral corpectomy (vertebral body resection), partial or complete, for excision of intraspinal lesion, single segment; intradural, thoracic by transthoracic approach **C**

RVU			Global Days	Modifiers				
Mod	Non-Fac Total	Fac Total		51	50	62	80	MUE
	71.70	71.70	090	2	0	1	2	1

AMA: Feb 02: 4, Jul 13: 3

63306 Vertebral corpectomy (vertebral body resection), partial or complete, for excision of intraspinal lesion, single segment; intradural, thoracic by thoracolumbar approach **C**

RVU			Global Days	Modifiers				
Mod	Non-Fac Total	Fac Total		51	50	62	80	MUE
	67.73	67.73	090	2	0	1	2	1

AMA: Feb 02: 4, Jul 13: 3

● New   ▲ Revised   ✖ Deleted   ⊙ Moderate Sedation   ✚ Add-on Codes   ⊘ High Risk Denial   Ⓐ Age Edit   ♀ Female   ♂ Male   **AMA** CPT® Assistant   **MUE** Medically Unlikely Edit
⊘ Modifier 51 Exempt   ⊖ Modifier 63 Exempt   ✗ Unlisted   **Modifiers:** See Inside Back Cover   Ⓜ Maternity   A2–Z3 ASC Payment Indicators   A–Y OPPS Status Indicators

570   CPT © 2015 American Medical Association. All Rights Reserved.   © 2016 DecisionHealth

63307 Vertebral corpectomy (vertebral body resection), partial or complete, for excision of intraspinal lesion, single segment; intradural, lumbar or sacral by transperitoneal or retroperitoneal approach C

RVU			Global Days	Modifiers				
Mod	Non-Fac Total	Fac Total		51	50	62	80	MUE
	67.90	67.90	090	2	0	1	2	1

AMA: Feb 02: 4, Jul 13: 3

+ **63308** Vertebral corpectomy (vertebral body resection), partial or complete, for excision of intraspinal lesion, single segment; each additional segment (List separately in addition to codes for single segment) C

RVU			Global Days	Modifiers				
Mod	Non-Fac Total	Fac Total		51	50	62	80	MUE
	9.59	9.59	ZZZ	0	0	1	2	3

AMA: Feb 02: 4

Spinal Stereotaxis Procedures

63600 Creation of lesion of spinal cord by stereotactic method, percutaneous, any modality (including stimulation and/or recording) A2 T

RVU			Global Days	Modifiers				
Mod	Non-Fac Total	Fac Total		51	50	62	80	MUE
	26.24	26.24	090	2	0	0	0	2

63610 Stereotactic stimulation of spinal cord, percutaneous, separate procedure not followed by other surgery ⊘ A2 T

RVU			Global Days	Modifiers				
Mod	Non-Fac Total	Fac Total		51	50	62	80	MUE
	12.56	12.56	000	2	0	0	0	1

63615 Stereotactic biopsy, aspiration, or excision of lesion, spinal cord ⊘ R2 T

RVU			Global Days	Modifiers				
Mod	Non-Fac Total	Fac Total		51	50	62	80	MUE
	28.26	28.26	090	2	0	1	1	1

63620 Stereotactic radiosurgery (particle beam, gamma ray, or linear accelerator); 1 spinal lesion B

RVU			Global Days	Modifiers				
Mod	Non-Fac Total	Fac Total		51	50	62	80	MUE
	33.05	33.05	090	0	0	0	2	1

AMA: Jul 11: 12, Oct 10: 3, Jun 15: 6

+ **63621** Stereotactic radiosurgery (particle beam, gamma ray, or linear accelerator); each additional spinal lesion (List separately in addition to code for primary procedure) B

RVU			Global Days	Modifiers				
Mod	Non-Fac Total	Fac Total		51	50	62	80	MUE
	7.54	7.54	ZZZ	0	0	0	2	2

AMA: Jul 11: 12, Oct 10: 3, Jun 15: 6

Spinal Neurostimulators

63650 Percutaneous implantation of neurostimulator electrode array, epidural J8 J I

RVU			Global Days	Modifiers				
Mod	Non-Fac Total	Fac Total		51	50	62	80	MUE
	38.25	12.00	010	2	0	0	1	2

AMA: Jun 98: 3, 4, Nov 98: 18, Mar 99: 11, Apr 99: 10, Sep 99: 3, Dec 08: 8, Feb 10: 9, Apr 11: 10, Aug 10: 8, Dec 10: 14, Oct 13: 19

63655 Laminectomy for implantation of neurostimulator electrodes, plate/paddle, epidural J8 J I

RVU			Global Days	Modifiers				
Mod	Non-Fac Total	Fac Total		51	50	62	80	MUE
	24.00	24.00	090	2	0	1	2	1

AMA: Jun 98: 3, 4, Nov 98: 18, Sep 99: 3, 4, Dec 08: 8, Apr 11: 10, Aug 10: 8, Dec 10: 14

63661 Removal of spinal neurostimulator electrode percutaneous array(s), including fluoroscopy, when performed G2 Q2

RVU			Global Days	Modifiers				
Mod	Non-Fac Total	Fac Total		51	50	62	80	MUE
	16.64	9.30	010	2	0	1	2	1

AMA: Apr 11: 10, Aug 10: 8, Jan 11: 8, Feb 10: 9

63662 Removal of spinal neurostimulator electrode plate/paddle(s) placed via laminotomy or laminectomy, including fluoroscopy, when performed G2 Q2

RVU			Global Days	Modifiers				
Mod	Non-Fac Total	Fac Total		51	50	62	80	MUE
	24.34	24.34	090	2	0	1	2	1

AMA: Apr 11: 10, Aug 10: 8, Feb 10: 9

63663 Revision including replacement, when performed, of spinal neurostimulator electrode percutaneous array(s), including fluoroscopy, when performed J8 J I

RVU			Global Days	Modifiers				
Mod	Non-Fac Total	Fac Total		51	50	62	80	MUE
	22.84	13.17	010	2	0	1	2	1

AMA: Apr 11: 10, Aug 10: 8, Feb 10: 9

63664 Revision including replacement, when performed, of spinal neurostimulator electrode plate/paddle(s) placed via laminotomy or laminectomy, including fluoroscopy, when performed J8 J I

RVU			Global Days	Modifiers				
Mod	Non-Fac Total	Fac Total		51	50	62	80	MUE
	25.02	25.02	090	2	0	1	2	1

AMA: Apr 11: 10, Feb 10: 9, Aug 10: 8

63685 Insertion or replacement of spinal neurostimulator pulse generator or receiver, direct or inductive coupling J8 J I

RVU			Global Days	Modifiers				
Mod	Non-Fac Total	Fac Total		51	50	62	80	MUE
	10.64	10.64	010	2	0	1	2	1

AMA: Jun 98: 3, 4, Sep 99: 5, Feb 10: 9, Apr 11: 10, Oct 10: 14, Dec 10: 14

63688 Revision or removal of implanted spinal neurostimulator pulse generator or receiver A2 Q2

RVU			Global Days	Modifiers				
Mod	Non-Fac Total	Fac Total		51	50	62	80	MUE
	10.70	10.70	010	2	0	0	1	1

AMA: Jun 98: 3, 4, Sep 99: 5, Feb 10: 9, Apr 11: 11

● New   ▲ Revised   Deleted   ⊙ Moderate Sedation   + Add-on Codes   ⊘ High Risk Denial   ⊛ Age Edit   ♀ Female   ♂ Male   **AMA** CPT® Assistant   **MUE** Medically Unlikely Edit
⊘ Modifier 51 Exempt   ⊖ Modifier 63 Exempt   ⌧ Unlisted   **Modifiers:** See Inside Back Cover   Ⓜ Maternity   A2–Z3 ASC Payment Indicators   A–Y OPPS Status Indicators

© 2016 DecisionHealth | CPT © 2015 American Medical Association. All Rights Reserved.

Surgical Procedures

63700 – 64413

Spinal Repair

63700 Repair of meningocele; less than 5 cm diameter ⊖C

RVU			Global Days	Modifiers				
Mod	Non-Fac Total	Fac Total		51	50	62	80	MUE
	33.96	33.96	090	2	0	1	2	1

63702 Repair of meningocele; larger than 5 cm diameter ⊖C

RVU			Global Days	Modifiers				
Mod	Non-Fac Total	Fac Total		51	50	62	80	MUE
	37.04	37.04	090	2	0	1	2	1

63704 Repair of myelomeningocele; less than 5 cm diameter ⊖C

RVU			Global Days	Modifiers				
Mod	Non-Fac Total	Fac Total		51	50	62	80	MUE
	48.90	48.90	090	2	0	1	2	1

63706 Repair of myelomeningocele; larger than 5 cm diameter ⊖C

RVU			Global Days	Modifiers				
Mod	Non-Fac Total	Fac Total		51	50	62	80	MUE
	49.65	49.65	090	2	0	1	2	1

63707 Repair of dural/cerebrospinal fluid leak, not requiring laminectomy C

RVU			Global Days	Modifiers				
Mod	Non-Fac Total	Fac Total		51	50	62	80	MUE
	26.84	26.84	090	2	0	1	2	1

63709 Repair of dural/cerebrospinal fluid leak or pseudomeningocele, with laminectomy C

RVU			Global Days	Modifiers				
Mod	Non-Fac Total	Fac Total		51	50	62	80	MUE
	32.10	32.10	090	2	0	1	2	1

63710 Dural graft, spinal C

RVU			Global Days	Modifiers				
Mod	Non-Fac Total	Fac Total		51	50	62	80	MUE
	31.46	31.46	090	2	0	1	2	1

Shunting of Spinal Fluid

63740 Creation of shunt, lumbar, subarachnoid-peritoneal, -pleural, or other; including laminectomy C

RVU			Global Days	Modifiers				
Mod	Non-Fac Total	Fac Total		51	50	62	80	MUE
	27.64	27.64	090	2	0	1	2	1

AMA: Winter 90: 8

63741 Creation of shunt, lumbar, subarachnoid-peritoneal, -pleural, or other; percutaneous, not requiring laminectomy T

RVU			Global Days	Modifiers				
Mod	Non-Fac Total	Fac Total		51	50	62	80	MUE
	19.79	19.79	090	2	0	1	2	1

AMA: Winter 90: 8

63744 Replacement, irrigation or revision of lumbosubarachnoid shunt A2T

RVU			Global Days	Modifiers				
Mod	Non-Fac Total	Fac Total		51	50	62	80	MUE
	19.69	19.69	090	2	0	1	2	1

63746 Removal of entire lumbosubarachnoid shunt system without replacement A2Q2

RVU			Global Days	Modifiers				
Mod	Non-Fac Total	Fac Total		51	50	62	80	MUE
	17.73	17.73	090	2	0	0	0	1

Nerve Procedures

Nerve Block Introduction/Injection

Somatic Nerve Procedures

64400 Injection, anesthetic agent; trigeminal nerve, any division or branch P3T

RVU			Global Days	Modifiers				
Mod	Non-Fac Total	Fac Total		51	50	62	80	MUE
	3.65	2.05	000	2	1	0	1	4

AMA: Jul 98: 10, May 99: 8, Nov 99: 36, Apr 05: 13, Feb 10: 9, Jan 13: 13

64402 Injection, anesthetic agent; facial nerve N1Q1

RVU			Global Days	Modifiers				
Mod	Non-Fac Total	Fac Total		51	50	62	80	MUE
	3.73	2.27	000	2	1	0	1	1

AMA: Jul 98: 10, Apr 05: 13, Jan 13: 13

64405 Injection, anesthetic agent; greater occipital nerve P3T

RVU			Global Days	Modifiers				
Mod	Non-Fac Total	Fac Total		51	50	62	80	MUE
	2.89	1.82	000	2	1	0	1	1

AMA: Jul 98: 10, Apr 05: 13, Jan 13: 13

64408 Injection, anesthetic agent; vagus nerve P3T

RVU			Global Days	Modifiers				
Mod	Non-Fac Total	Fac Total		51	50	62	80	MUE
	3.00	2.19	000	2	1	0	0	1

AMA: Jul 98: 10, Apr 05: 13, Jan 13: 13

64410 Injection, anesthetic agent; phrenic nerve A2T

RVU			Global Days	Modifiers				
Mod	Non-Fac Total	Fac Total		51	50	62	80	MUE
	3.60	2.04	000	2	1	0	0	1

AMA: Jul 98: 10, Apr 05: 13, Jan 13: 13

✖ 64412 ~~Injection, anesthetic agent; spinal accessory nerve~~

64413 Injection, anesthetic agent; cervical plexus P3T

RVU			Global Days	Modifiers				
Mod	Non-Fac Total	Fac Total		51	50	62	80	MUE
	3.64	2.34	000	2	1	0	1	1

AMA: Jul 98: 10, Apr 05: 13, Jan 13: 13

Coding Guidance

Codes 64415-64417 describe services that may be utilized for pain management purposes. Medicare global surgery rules block payment for postoperative pain management services provided by the same physician who performs the surgery. The services described by codes 64415-64417 may be reported by the physician performing the surgery only for purposes unrelated to the procedure, postoperative pain management, or anesthesia for the procedure.

● New ▲ Revised ✖ Deleted ⊙ Moderate Sedation ➕ Add-on Codes ⊘ High Risk Denial ⊛ Age Edit ♀ Female ♂ Male **AMA** *CPT® Assistant* **MUE** Medically Unlikely Edit
⊘ Modifier 51 Exempt ⊖ Modifier 63 Exempt ⊠ Unlisted **Modifiers:** *See Inside Back Cover* Ⓜ Maternity A2–Z3 ASC Payment Indicators A–Y OPPS Status Indicators

572   CPT © 2015 American Medical Association. All Rights Reserved.   © 2016 DecisionHealth

64415 Injection, anesthetic agent; brachial plexus, single   A2 T

RVU			Global Days	Modifiers				
Mod	Non-Fac Total	Fac Total		51	50	62	80	MUE
	3.48	1.90	000	2	1	0	1	1

AMA: Fall 92: 17, Jul 98: 10, May 99: 8, Oct 01: 9, Feb 04: 7, Apr 05: 13, Nov 06: 23, Jan 13: 13

Brachial plexus injection, anesthetic agent

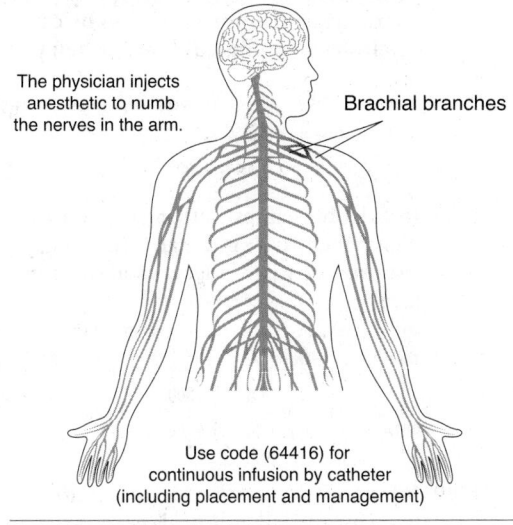

The physician injects anesthetic to numb the nerves in the arm.

Brachial branches

Use code (64416) for continuous infusion by catheter (including placement and management)

64416 Injection, anesthetic agent; brachial plexus, continuous infusion by catheter (including catheter placement)   G2 T

RVU			Global Days	Modifiers				
Mod	Non-Fac Total	Fac Total		51	50	62	80	MUE
	2.31	2.31	000	2	1	0	1	1

AMA: Feb 04: 7, Apr 05: 13, Jan 13: 13

64417 Injection, anesthetic agent; axillary nerve   A2 T

RVU			Global Days	Modifiers				
Mod	Non-Fac Total	Fac Total		51	50	62	80	MUE
	3.81	2.08	000	2	1	0	1	1

AMA: Jul 98: 10, Apr 05: 13, Jan 13: 13

64418 Injection, anesthetic agent; suprascapular nerve   P3 T

RVU			Global Days	Modifiers				
Mod	Non-Fac Total	Fac Total		51	50	62	80	MUE
	4.16	2.21	000	2	1	0	1	1

AMA: Jul 98: 10, Apr 05: 13, Aug 07: 15, Jan 13: 13

64420 Injection, anesthetic agent; intercostal nerve, single   A2 T

RVU			Global Days	Modifiers				
Mod	Non-Fac Total	Fac Total		51	50	62	80	MUE
	3.23	1.97	000	2	0	0	1	3

AMA: Jul 98: 10, Apr 05: 13, Aug 10: 12, Nov 10: 9, Jan 13: 13, Jun 15: 3

64421 Injection, anesthetic agent; intercostal nerves, multiple, regional block   A2 T

RVU			Global Days	Modifiers				
Mod	Non-Fac Total	Fac Total		51	50	62	80	MUE
	4.33	2.66	000	2	1	0	1	3

AMA: Jul 98: 10, Apr 05: 13, Aug 10: 12, Nov 10: 9, Jan 13: 13, Jun 15: 3

64425 Injection, anesthetic agent; ilioinguinal, iliohypogastric nerves   P3 T

RVU			Global Days	Modifiers				
Mod	Non-Fac Total	Fac Total		51	50	62	80	MUE
	3.81	2.71	000	2	1	0	1	1

AMA: Jul 98: 10, Apr 05: 13, Jan 13: 13, Jun 15: 3

64430 Injection, anesthetic agent; pudendal nerve ⊘A2 T

Coding tip: When a steroid agent is included, it does not change the basic application as an anesthetic nerve block and is included in the code

Documentation Finder: The documentation should note the approach – such as transvaginally, via the buttock locating the nerve using imaging guidance or through the rectum. It should also state what is being injected and the results of the injection. The documentation may reference the nerve in the Alcock's canal or to injecting at the ischial spine between the sacrotuberous and sacrospinous ligaments.

RVU			Global Days	Modifiers				
Mod	Non-Fac Total	Fac Total		51	50	62	80	MUE
	3.96	2.37	000	2	1	0	1	1

AMA: Jul 98: 10, Apr 05: 13, Jan 13: 13

64435 Injection, anesthetic agent; paracervical (uterine) nerve ⊘♀P3 T

Coding tip: When a steroid agent is included, it does not change the basic application as an anesthetic nerve block and is included in the code

RVU			Global Days	Modifiers				
Mod	Non-Fac Total	Fac Total		51	50	62	80	MUE
	3.88	2.39	000	2	1	0	1	1

AMA: Jul 98: 10, Mar 03: 22, Jul 03: 15, Apr 05: 13, Feb 12: 11, Jan 13: 13

64445 Injection, anesthetic agent; sciatic nerve, single   P3 T

RVU			Global Days	Modifiers				
Mod	Non-Fac Total	Fac Total		51	50	62	80	MUE
	3.93	2.10	000	2	1	0	1	1

AMA: Jul 98: 10, May 99: 8, Feb 04: 8, Apr 05: 13, Dec 11: 8, Apr 12: 19, Jan 13: 13

64446 Injection, anesthetic agent; sciatic nerve, continuous infusion by catheter (including catheter placement)   G2 T

RVU			Global Days	Modifiers				
Mod	Non-Fac Total	Fac Total		51	50	62	80	MUE
	2.31	2.31	000	2	1	0	1	1

AMA: Feb 04: 9, Apr 05: 13, Jan 13: 13

64447 Injection, anesthetic agent; femoral nerve, single   P3 T

RVU			Global Days	Modifiers				
Mod	Non-Fac Total	Fac Total		51	50	62	80	MUE
	3.53	1.93	000	2	1	0	1	1

AMA: Feb 04: 9, Apr 05: 13, Jan 13: 13, Nov 14: 14, Dec 14: 16

64448 Injection, anesthetic agent; femoral nerve, continuous infusion by catheter (including catheter placement)   G2 T

RVU			Global Days	Modifiers				
Mod	Non-Fac Total	Fac Total		51	50	62	80	MUE
	2.08	2.08	000	2	1	0	1	1

AMA: Feb 04: 10, Apr 05: 13, Jan 13: 13, Nov 14: 14, Dec 14: 16

● New   ▲ Revised   Deleted   ⊙ Moderate Sedation   ✚ Add-on Codes   ⊘ High Risk Denial   Ⓐ Age Edit   ♀ Female   ♂ Male   **AMA** CPT® Assistant   **MUE** Medically Unlikely Edit
⊘ Modifier 51 Exempt   ⊖ Modifier 63 Exempt   ✗ Unlisted   **Modifiers:** See Inside Back Cover   Ⓜ Maternity   A2–Z3 ASC Payment Indicators   A–Y OPPS Status Indicators

Surgical Procedures

64449 – 64484

64449 Injection, anesthetic agent; lumbar plexus, posterior approach, continuous infusion by catheter (including catheter placement) **G2T**

RVU			Global Days	Modifiers				
Mod	Non-Fac Total	Fac Total		51	50	62	80	MUE
	2.45	2.45	000	2	1	0	1	1

AMA: Apr 05: 13, Jan 13: 13

Coding Guidance

Codes 64450-64495 describe services that may be utilized for pain management purposes. Medicare global surgery rules do not allow additional payment for postoperative pain management services provided by the same physician who performs the surgery. The services described by codes 64450-64495 may be reported by the physician performing the surgery only for purposes unrelated to the procedure, postoperative pain management, or anesthesia for the procedure.

64450 Injection, anesthetic agent; other peripheral nerve or branch **P3T**

Coding tip: Injection for nerve destruction, other peripheral nerve or branch - 64620; paravertebral facet joint nerve with imaging guidance - 64633-64636; intercostal nerve - 64620

RVU			Global Days	Modifiers				
Mod	Non-Fac Total	Fac Total		51	50	62	80	MUE
	2.28	1.32	000	2	1	0	1	10

AMA: Jul 98: 10, Nov 99: 37, Dec 99: 7, Oct 01: 9, Aug 03: 6, Apr 05: 13, Jan 09: 6, Jan 13: 13

Injection, anesthetic agent; other peripheral nerve or branch

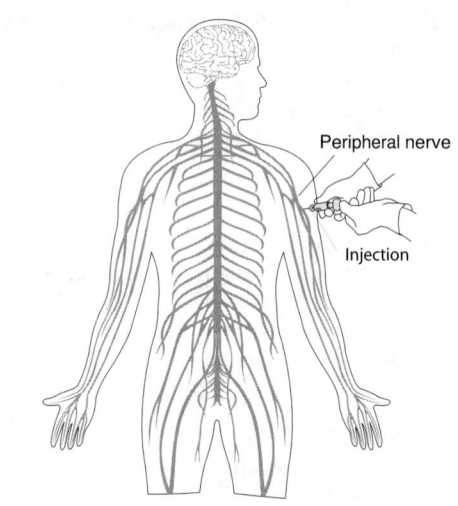

Peripheral nerve

Injection

64455 Injection(s), anesthetic agent and/or steroid, plantar common digital nerve(s) (eg, Morton's neuroma) **P3T**

RVU			Global Days	Modifiers				
Mod	Non-Fac Total	Fac Total		51	50	62	80	MUE
	1.36	1.00	000	2	1	0	0	1

AMA: Jan 13: 13

● **64461** Paravertebral block (PVB) (paraspinous block), thoracic; single injection site (includes imaging guidance, when performed) **P3T**

RVU			Global Days	Modifiers				
Mod	Non-Fac Total	Fac Total		51	50	62	80	MUE
	4.25	2.50	000	2	1	0	1	1

+● **64462** Paravertebral block (PVB) (paraspinous block), thoracic; second and any additional injection site(s) (includes imaging guidance, when performed) (List separately in addition to code for primary procedure) **NIN**

RVU			Global Days	Modifiers				
Mod	Non-Fac Total	Fac Total		51	50	62	80	MUE
	2.40	1.57	ZZZ	0	1	0	1	1

● **64463** Paravertebral block (PVB) (paraspinous block), thoracic; continuous infusion by catheter (includes imaging guidance, when performed) **P3T**

RVU			Global Days	Modifiers				
Mod	Non-Fac Total	Fac Total		51	50	62	80	MUE
	4.69	2.45	000	2	1	0	1	1

64479 Injection(s), anesthetic agent and/or steroid, transforaminal epidural, with imaging guidance (fluoroscopy or CT); cervical or thoracic, single level **A2T**

RVU			Global Days	Modifiers				
Mod	Non-Fac Total	Fac Total		51	50	62	80	MUE
	6.76	3.83	000	2	1	0	1	1

AMA: Nov 99: 33, 37, Feb 00: 4, Jul 08: 9, Nov 08: 11, Feb 10: 9, Jul 11: 16, Feb 11: 4, Jul 12: 5, Jan 11: 8

+ **64480** Injection(s), anesthetic agent and/or steroid, transforaminal epidural, with imaging guidance (fluoroscopy or CT); cervical or thoracic, each additional level (List separately in addition to code for primary procedure) **NIN**

RVU			Global Days	Modifiers				
Mod	Non-Fac Total	Fac Total		51	50	62	80	MUE
	3.24	1.83	ZZZ	0	1	0	1	4

AMA: Nov 99: 33, 37, Feb 00: 4, Feb 05: 14, Jul 08: 9, Feb 10: 9, Jul 11: 16, Feb 11: 4, Jul 12: 5, Jan 11: 8

64483 Injection(s), anesthetic agent and/or steroid, transforaminal epidural, with imaging guidance (fluoroscopy or CT); lumbar or sacral, single level **A2T**

RVU			Global Days	Modifiers				
Mod	Non-Fac Total	Fac Total		51	50	62	80	MUE
	6.29	3.26	000	2	1	0	1	1

AMA: Nov 99: 33, 37, Feb 00: 4, Jul 08: 9, Feb 10: 9, Jul 11: 16, Feb 11: 4, May 12: 14, Jul 12: 5, Jan 11: 8

+ **64484** Injection(s), anesthetic agent and/or steroid, transforaminal epidural, with imaging guidance (fluoroscopy or CT); lumbar or sacral, each additional level (List separately in addition to code for primary procedure) **NIN**

RVU			Global Days	Modifiers				
Mod	Non-Fac Total	Fac Total		51	50	62	80	MUE
	2.52	1.51	ZZZ	0	1	0	1	4

AMA: Nov 99: 33, 37, Feb 00: 4, Feb 05: 14, Jul 08: 9, Nov 08: 11, Feb 10: 9, Jul 11: 16, Feb 11: 4, Jul 12: 5

● New ▲ Revised ✖ Deleted ⊙ Moderate Sedation ✚ Add-on Codes ⊘ High Risk Denial Ⓐ Age Edit ♀ Female ♂ Male **AMA** *CPT® Assistant* **MUE** Medically Unlikely Edit
⊘ Modifier 51 Exempt ⊖ Modifier 63 Exempt ✗ Unlisted **Modifiers:** *See Inside Back Cover* Ⓜ Maternity **A2–Z3** ASC Payment Indicators **A–Y** OPPS Status Indicators

574 | CPT © 2015 American Medical Association. All Rights Reserved. | © 2016 DecisionHealth

64486 Transversus abdominis plane (TAP) block (abdominal plane block, rectus sheath block) unilateral; by injection(s) (includes imaging guidance, when performed) `NIN`

RVU			Global Days	Modifiers				
Mod	Non-Fac Total	Fac Total		51	50	62	80	MUE
	3.56	1.82	000	2	1	0	1	1

AMA: Jun 15: 3

64487 Transversus abdominis plane (TAP) block (abdominal plane block, rectus sheath block) unilateral; by continuous infusion(s) (includes imaging guidance, when performed) `NIN`

RVU			Global Days	Modifiers				
Mod	Non-Fac Total	Fac Total		51	50	62	80	MUE
	4.41	2.15	000	2	1	0	1	1

AMA: Jun 15: 3

64488 Transversus abdominis plane (TAP) block (abdominal plane block, rectus sheath block) bilateral; by injections (includes imaging guidance, when performed) `NIN`

RVU			Global Days	Modifiers				
Mod	Non-Fac Total	Fac Total		51	50	62	80	MUE
	4.39	2.31	000	2	2	0	1	1

AMA: Jun 15: 3

64489 Transversus abdominis plane (TAP) block (abdominal plane block, rectus sheath block) bilateral; by continuous infusions (includes imaging guidance, when performed) `NIN`

RVU			Global Days	Modifiers				
Mod	Non-Fac Total	Fac Total		51	50	62	80	MUE
	6.17	2.61	000	2	2	0	1	1

AMA: Jun 15: 3

64490 Injection(s), diagnostic or therapeutic agent, paravertebral facet (zygapophyseal) joint (or nerves innervating that joint) with image guidance (fluoroscopy or CT), cervical or thoracic; single level `G2T`

RVU			Global Days	Modifiers				
Mod	Non-Fac Total	Fac Total		51	50	62	80	MUE
	5.46	3.09	000	2	1	0	2	1

AMA: Aug 10: 12, Dec 10: 13, Jun 12: 10, Feb 10: 9, Jan 11: 8, Feb 11: 4, Oct 12: 15

+ 64491 Injection(s), diagnostic or therapeutic agent, paravertebral facet (zygapophyseal) joint (or nerves innervating that joint) with image guidance (fluoroscopy or CT), cervical or thoracic; second level (List separately in addition to code for primary procedure) `NIN`

RVU			Global Days	Modifiers				
Mod	Non-Fac Total	Fac Total		51	50	62	80	MUE
	2.69	1.75	ZZZ	0	1	0	2	1

AMA: Aug 10: 12, Jun 12: 10, Oct 12: 15

+ 64492 Injection(s), diagnostic or therapeutic agent, paravertebral facet (zygapophyseal) joint (or nerves innervating that joint) with image guidance (fluoroscopy or CT), cervical or thoracic; third and any additional level(s) (List separately in addition to code for primary procedure) `NIN`

RVU			Global Days	Modifiers				
Mod	Non-Fac Total	Fac Total		51	50	62	80	MUE
	2.71	1.77	ZZZ	0	1	0	2	1

AMA: Aug 10: 12, Jun 12: 10, Feb 10: 9, Jan 11: 8, Feb 11: 4, Oct 12: 15

64493 Injection(s), diagnostic or therapeutic agent, paravertebral facet (zygapophyseal) joint (or nerves innervating that joint) with image guidance (fluoroscopy or CT), lumbar or sacral; single level `G2T`

RVU			Global Days	Modifiers				
Mod	Non-Fac Total	Fac Total		51	50	62	80	MUE
	4.96	2.65	000	2	1	0	2	1

AMA: Feb 11: 4, Aug 10: 12, Jun 12: 10, Feb 10: 9, Jan 11: 8, Oct 12: 15

+ 64494 Injection(s), diagnostic or therapeutic agent, paravertebral facet (zygapophyseal) joint (or nerves innervating that joint) with image guidance (fluoroscopy or CT), lumbar or sacral; second level (List separately in addition to code for primary procedure) `NIN`

RVU			Global Days	Modifiers				
Mod	Non-Fac Total	Fac Total		51	50	62	80	MUE
	2.49	1.51	ZZZ	0	1	0	2	1

AMA: Aug 10: 12, Jun 12: 10, Feb 10: 9, Jan 11: 8, Feb 11: 4

+ 64495 Injection(s), diagnostic or therapeutic agent, paravertebral facet (zygapophyseal) joint (or nerves innervating that joint) with image guidance (fluoroscopy or CT), lumbar or sacral; third and any additional level(s) (List separately in addition to code for primary procedure) `NIN`

RVU			Global Days	Modifiers				
Mod	Non-Fac Total	Fac Total		51	50	62	80	MUE
	2.50	1.53	ZZZ	0	1	0	2	1

AMA: Aug 10: 12, Jun 12: 10, Feb 10: 9, Jan 11: 8, Feb 11: 4, Oct 12: 15

Sympathetic Nerve Procedures

64505 Injection, anesthetic agent; sphenopalatine ganglion `P3T`

Documentation Finder: *For this type of injection of anesthetic medication, the needle is inserted into the nose to access and inject the correct nerve. It also may be referred to in the documentation as a sphenopalatine ganglion block (SGB). The provider might reference the patient's condition as cluster or migraine headaches or facial pain.*

RVU			Global Days	Modifiers				
Mod	Non-Fac Total	Fac Total		51	50	62	80	MUE
	2.99	2.51	000	2	1	0	1	1

AMA: Jul 98: 10, Apr 05: 13, Jan 13: 13, Jun 13: 13, Jul 14: 8

64508 Injection, anesthetic agent; carotid sinus (separate procedure) `P3T`

RVU			Global Days	Modifiers				
Mod	Non-Fac Total	Fac Total		51	50	62	80	MUE
	1.78	2.11	000	2	1	0	0	1

AMA: Jul 98: 10, Apr 05: 13, Jan 13: 13

● New   ▲ Revised   Deleted   ⊙ Moderate Sedation   ✚ Add-on Codes   ⊘ High Risk Denial   Ⓐ Age Edit   ♀ Female   ♂ Male   **AMA** *CPT® Assistant*   ***MUE*** Medically Unlikely Edit
⊘ Modifier 51 Exempt   ⊖ Modifier 63 Exempt   ✗ Unlisted   **Modifiers:** *See Inside Back Cover*   Ⓜ Maternity   A2–Z3 ASC Payment Indicators   A–Y OPPS Status Indicators

© 2016 DecisionHealth   CPT © 2015 American Medical Association. All Rights Reserved.   **575**

Surgical Procedures

64510   64510 – 64566

64510   Injection, anesthetic agent; stellate ganglion (cervical sympathetic)   A 2 T

RVU			Global Days	Modifiers				
Mod	Non-Fac Total	Fac Total		51	50	62	80	MUE
	3.67	2.14	000	2	1	0	1	1

AMA: Jul 98: 10, Apr 05: 13, Jan 13: 13

64517   Injection, anesthetic agent; superior hypogastric plexus   A 2 T

RVU			Global Days	Modifiers				
Mod	Non-Fac Total	Fac Total		51	50	62	80	MUE
	5.25	3.56	000	2	0	0	1	1

AMA: Oct 04: 11, Apr 05: 13, Jan 13: 13

64520   Injection, anesthetic agent; lumbar or thoracic (paravertebral sympathetic)   A 2 T

RVU			Global Days	Modifiers				
Mod	Non-Fac Total	Fac Total		51	50	62	80	MUE
	5.36	2.35	000	2	1	0	1	1

AMA: Jul 98: 10, Apr 05: 13, Dec 10: 14, Jan 13: 13

64530   Injection, anesthetic agent; celiac plexus, with or without radiologic monitoring   A 2 T

RVU			Global Days	Modifiers				
Mod	Non-Fac Total	Fac Total		51	50	62	80	MUE
	5.49	2.68	000	2	0	0	1	1

AMA: Jul 98: 10, Apr 05: 13, Jan 13: 13

Peripheral Nerve Stimulators

Coding Guidance

Codes 64550-64595 are not appropriate for reporting electrical stimulation to aid in bone healing; use bone stimulation codes 20974-20975.

64550   Application of surface (transcutaneous) neurostimulator   A

Coding tip: *Use 64550 to report the initial application of a TENS unit before the patient leaves the office*

RVU			Global Days	Modifiers				
Mod	Non-Fac Total	Fac Total		51	50	62	80	MUE
	0.45	0.26	000	0	0	0	1	1

AMA: Jan 02: 11, Apr 02: 18

Application of surface (transcutaneous) neurostimulator

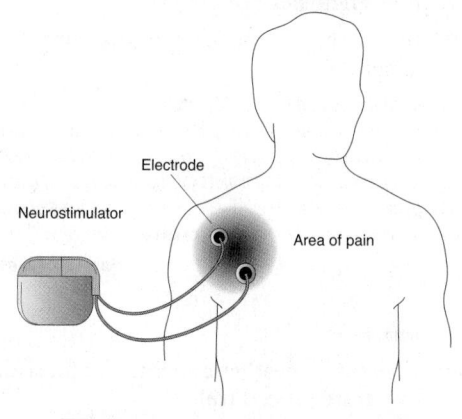

The physician places electrodes on an area outside the skin to stimulate nerve tissue and relieve pain.

64553   Percutaneous implantation of neurostimulator electrode array; cranial nerve   ⊘ J 8 J 1

RVU			Global Days	Modifiers				
Mod	Non-Fac Total	Fac Total		51	50	62	80	MUE
	5.99	4.51	010	2	0	0	0	1

AMA: Nov 99: 38, Apr 01: 9

Percutaneous implantation of neurostimulator electrode array; cranial nerve

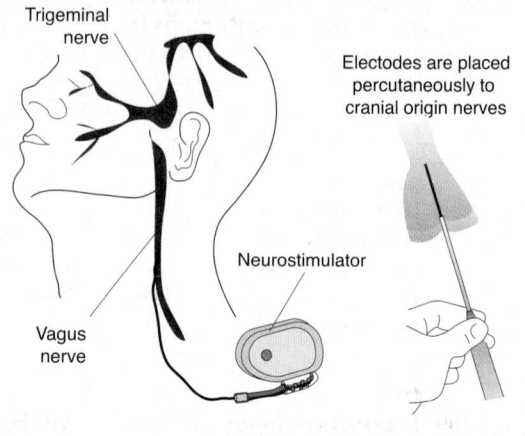

Electrodes are placed percutaneously to cranial origin nerves

64555   Percutaneous implantation of neurostimulator electrode array; peripheral nerve (excludes sacral nerve)   J 8 J 1

RVU			Global Days	Modifiers				
Mod	Non-Fac Total	Fac Total		51	50	62	80	MUE
	6.02	4.41	010	2	0	0	1	2

AMA: Jan 15: 14

64561   Percutaneous implantation of neurostimulator electrode array; sacral nerve (transforaminal placement) including image guidance, if performed   J 8 J 1

RVU			Global Days	Modifiers				
Mod	Non-Fac Total	Fac Total		51	50	62	80	MUE
	23.21	8.68	010	2	1	0	1	1

AMA: Dec 12: 14, Sep 14: 5

Pub 100-04, 32, 40.2

64565   Percutaneous implantation of neurostimulator electrode array; neuromuscular   J 8 J 1

RVU			Global Days	Modifiers				
Mod	Non-Fac Total	Fac Total		51	50	62	80	MUE
	5.37	3.77	010	2	0	0	1	2

AMA: Jul 00: 11, Dec 08: 8

64566   Posterior tibial neurostimulation, percutaneous needle electrode, single treatment, includes programming   P 3 T

RVU			Global Days	Modifiers				
Mod	Non-Fac Total	Fac Total		51	50	62	80	MUE
	3.59	0.88	000	2	0	0	0	1

AMA: Sep 11: 8, Feb 11: 5

● New   ▲ Revised   ✖ Deleted   ⊙ Moderate Sedation   ✚ Add-on Codes   ⊘ High Risk Denial   Ⓐ Age Edit   ♀ Female   ♂ Male   **AMA** *CPT® Assistant*   **MUE** Medically Unlikely Edit
⊘ Modifier 51 Exempt   ⊖ Modifier 63 Exempt   ✖ Unlisted   **Modifiers:** *See Inside Back Cover*   Ⓜ Maternity   A 2 – Z 3 ASC Payment Indicators   A – Y OPPS Status Indicators

CPT © 2015 American Medical Association. All Rights Reserved.   © 2016 DecisionHealth

64568 Incision for implantation of cranial nerve (eg, vagus nerve) neurostimulator electrode array and pulse generator `J 8 J I`

RVU			Global Days	Modifiers				
Mod	Non-Fac Total	Fac Total		51	50	62	80	MUE
	19.16	19.16	090	2	1	0	0	1

AMA: Sep 11: 8, 10, 12, Feb 11: 5

64569 Revision or replacement of cranial nerve (eg, vagus nerve) neurostimulator electrode array, including connection to existing pulse generator `J 8 J I`

RVU			Global Days	Modifiers				
Mod	Non-Fac Total	Fac Total		51	50	62	80	MUE
	22.92	22.92	090	2	1	1	0	1

AMA: Sep 11: 8, Feb 11: 5

64570 Removal of cranial nerve (eg, vagus nerve) neurostimulator electrode array and pulse generator `G 2 Q 2`

RVU			Global Days	Modifiers				
Mod	Non-Fac Total	Fac Total		51	50	62	80	MUE
	19.00	19.00	090	2	1	1	0	1

AMA: Sep 11: 10, Feb 11: 5

64575 Incision for implantation of neurostimulator electrode array; peripheral nerve (excludes sacral nerve) `J 8 J I`

RVU			Global Days	Modifiers				
Mod	Non-Fac Total	Fac Total		51	50	62	80	MUE
	9.29	9.29	090	2	0	0	1	2

64580 Incision for implantation of neurostimulator electrode array; neuromuscular `J 8 J I`

RVU			Global Days	Modifiers				
Mod	Non-Fac Total	Fac Total		51	50	62	80	MUE
	8.73	8.73	090	2	0	0	2	2

64581 Incision for implantation of neurostimulator electrode array; sacral nerve (transforaminal placement) `J 8 J I`

RVU			Global Days	Modifiers				
Mod	Non-Fac Total	Fac Total		51	50	62	80	MUE
	19.06	19.06	090	2	0	0	1	2

AMA: Dec 12: 14, Sep 14: 5

Pub 100-04, 32, 40.2

64585 Revision or removal of peripheral neurostimulator electrode array `A 2 Q 2`

RVU			Global Days	Modifiers				
Mod	Non-Fac Total	Fac Total		51	50	62	80	MUE
	6.96	4.12	010	2	0	0	1	2

Pub 100-04, 32, 40.2, 40.2.2

64590 Insertion or replacement of peripheral or gastric neurostimulator pulse generator or receiver, direct or inductive coupling `J 8 J I`

RVU			Global Days	Modifiers				
Mod	Non-Fac Total	Fac Total		51	50	62	80	MUE
	7.53	4.62	010	2	0	1	1	1

AMA: Sep 99: 4, Apr 01: 8, Mar 07: 4, Apr 07: 7, Sep 11: 9, Dec 12: 14, Jan 15: 14

Pub 100-04, 32, 40.2, 40.2.2

64595 Revision or removal of peripheral or gastric neurostimulator pulse generator or receiver `A 2 Q 2`

RVU			Global Days	Modifiers				
Mod	Non-Fac Total	Fac Total		51	50	62	80	MUE
	6.98	3.63	010	2	0	0	1	1

AMA: Sep 99: 3, Mar 07: 4, Jan 08: 8

Pub 100-04, 32, 40.2, 40.2.2

Nerve Destruction

Somatic Nerve Procedures

64600 Destruction by neurolytic agent, trigeminal nerve; supraorbital, infraorbital, mental, or inferior alveolar branch `A 2 T`

RVU			Global Days	Modifiers				
Mod	Non-Fac Total	Fac Total		51	50	62	80	MUE
	11.27	6.38	010	2	2	0	1	2

AMA: Aug 05: 13, Feb 10: 9, Sep 12: 14

64605 Destruction by neurolytic agent, trigeminal nerve; second and third division branches at foramen ovale `A 2 T`

RVU			Global Days	Modifiers				
Mod	Non-Fac Total	Fac Total		51	50	62	80	MUE
	21.58	12.00	010	2	1	0	0	1

AMA: Aug 05: 13, Feb 10: 9, Sep 12: 14

64610 Destruction by neurolytic agent, trigeminal nerve; second and third division branches at foramen ovale under radiologic monitoring `A 2 T`

RVU			Global Days	Modifiers				
Mod	Non-Fac Total	Fac Total		51	50	62	80	MUE
	21.49	14.30	010	2	1	0	1	1

AMA: Aug 05: 13, Feb 10: 9, Sep 12: 14

Coding Guidance

Muscle chemodenervation will occasionally require electrical stimulation (95873) or needle electromyography (EMG) (95874) guidance. When this is reasonable and necessary these codes may be reported in conjunction with codes 64611-64615. Codes 64611, and 64613-64615 are reported only once per session regardless of the number of injection sites. Code 64612 is a unilateral procedure; append modifier 50 if chemodenervation is performed bilaterally. Report 64612 only once with modifier 50 for bilateral procedures, regardless of the number of injection sites on each side.

64611 Chemodenervation of parotid and submandibular salivary glands, bilateral `P 3 T`

RVU			Global Days	Modifiers				
Mod	Non-Fac Total	Fac Total		51	50	62	80	MUE
	3.34	2.93	010	2	2	0	0	1

AMA: Feb 11: 10, Sep 12: 14

● New ▲ Revised ̶D̶e̶l̶e̶t̶e̶d̶ ⊙ Moderate Sedation ✚ Add-on Codes ⊘ High Risk Denial ⒶAge Edit ♀ Female ♂ Male **AMA** CPT® Assistant **MUE** Medically Unlikely Edit ⃠ Modifier 51 Exempt ⊖ Modifier 63 Exempt ⊠ Unlisted **Modifiers:** See Inside Back Cover Ⓜ Maternity `A 2`–`Z 3` ASC Payment Indicators `A`–`Y` OPPS Status Indicators

64612 Chemodenervation of muscle(s); muscle(s) innervated by facial nerve, unilateral (eg, for blepharospasm, hemifacial spasm) `P 3 T`

RVU		Global Days	Modifiers				
Mod	Non-Fac Total	Fac Total		51	50	62	80	MUE
	3.77	3.38	010	2	1	0	1	1

AMA: Oct 98: 10, Apr 01: 2, Aug 05: 13, Sep 06: 5, Dec 08: 9, Jan 09: 8, Feb 10: 9, 13, Dec 11: 19, Sep 12: 14, Apr 13: 5, Dec 13: 10, Jan 14: 6, May 14: 5

Chemodenervation of muscle(s)

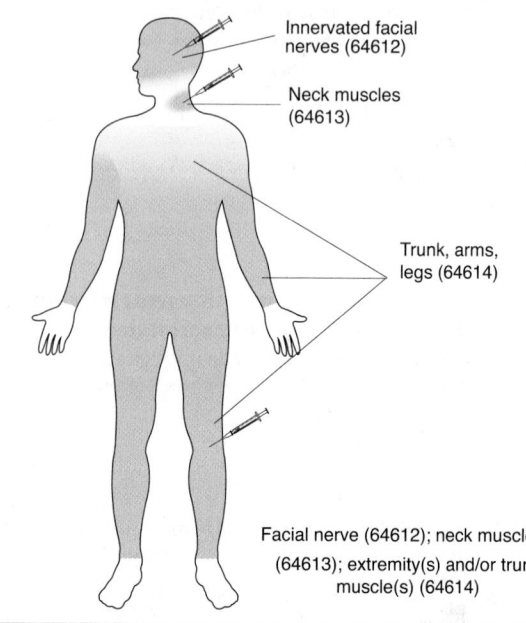

Innervated facial nerves (64612)

Neck muscles (64613)

Trunk, arms, legs (64614)

Facial nerve (64612); neck muscle(s) (64613); extremity(s) and/or trunk muscle(s) (64614)

64615 Chemodenervation of muscle(s); muscle(s) innervated by facial, trigeminal, cervical spinal and accessory nerves, bilateral (eg, for chronic migraine) `P 3 T`

RVU		Global Days	Modifiers				
Mod	Non-Fac Total	Fac Total		51	50	62	80	MUE
	4.14	3.60	010	2	2	0	1	1

AMA: Apr 13: 5, Jan 14: 6

64616 Chemodenervation of muscle(s); neck muscle(s), excluding muscles of the larynx, unilateral (eg, for cervical dystonia, spasmodic torticollis) `P 3 T`

RVU		Global Days	Modifiers				
Mod	Non-Fac Total	Fac Total		51	50	62	80	MUE
	3.62	3.15	010	2	1	0	1	1

AMA: Jan 14: 6, May 14: 5

64617 Chemodenervation of muscle(s); larynx, unilateral, percutaneous (eg, for spasmodic dysphonia), includes guidance by needle electromyography, when performed `P 3 T`

RVU		Global Days	Modifiers				
Mod	Non-Fac Total	Fac Total		51	50	62	80	MUE
	5.59	3.59	010	2	1	0	1	1

AMA: Jan 14: 6

64620 Destruction by neurolytic agent, intercostal nerve `A 2 T`

RVU		Global Days	Modifiers				
Mod	Non-Fac Total	Fac Total		51	50	62	80	MUE
	5.89	4.98	010	2	0	0	1	5

AMA: Nov 99: 38, Aug 05: 13, Sep 12: 14, Jan 14: 6

64630 Destruction by neurolytic agent; pudendal nerve `A 2 T`

RVU		Global Days	Modifiers				
Mod	Non-Fac Total	Fac Total		51	50	62	80	MUE
	6.67	5.57	010	2	0	0	0	1

AMA: Aug 05: 13, Feb 10: 9, Sep 12: 14

64632 Destruction by neurolytic agent; plantar common digital nerve `P 3 T`

RVU		Global Days	Modifiers				
Mod	Non-Fac Total	Fac Total		51	50	62	80	MUE
	2.44	1.97	010	2	1	0	0	1

AMA: Jan 09: 6, Sep 12: 14, Jan 13: 13, Jul 15: 11

64633 Destruction by neurolytic agent, paravertebral facet joint nerve(s), with imaging guidance (fluoroscopy or CT); cervical or thoracic, single facet joint `G 2 T`

RVU		Global Days	Modifiers				
Mod	Non-Fac Total	Fac Total		51	50	62	80	MUE
	12.14	6.57	010	2	1	0	1	1

AMA: Jun 12: 10, Jul 12: 6, Sep 12: 14, Apr 13: 10, Feb 15: 9

+ 64634 Destruction by neurolytic agent, paravertebral facet joint nerve(s), with imaging guidance (fluoroscopy or CT); cervical or thoracic, each additional facet joint (List separately in addition to code for primary procedure) `N I N`

RVU		Global Days	Modifiers				
Mod	Non-Fac Total	Fac Total		51	50	62	80	MUE
	5.46	1.99	ZZZ	0	1	0	1	4

AMA: Jun 12: 10, Jul 12: 6, Sep 12: 14, Apr 13: 10, Feb 15: 9

64635 Destruction by neurolytic agent, paravertebral facet joint nerve(s), with imaging guidance (fluoroscopy or CT); lumbar or sacral, single facet joint `G 2 T`

RVU		Global Days	Modifiers				
Mod	Non-Fac Total	Fac Total		51	50	62	80	MUE
	12.00	6.48	010	2	1	0	1	1

AMA: Jun 12: 10, Jul 12: 6, 14, Sep 12: 14, Apr 13: 10, Feb 15: 9

+ 64636 Destruction by neurolytic agent, paravertebral facet joint nerve(s), with imaging guidance (fluoroscopy or CT); lumbar or sacral, each additional facet joint (List separately in addition to code for primary procedure) `N I N`

RVU		Global Days	Modifiers				
Mod	Non-Fac Total	Fac Total		51	50	62	80	MUE
	4.96	1.74	ZZZ	0	1	0	1	4

AMA: Jun 12: 10, Jul 12: 6, 14, Sep 12: 14, Apr 13: 10, Feb 15: 9

● New   ▲ Revised   ✖ Deleted   ⊙ Moderate Sedation   ✚ Add-on Codes   ⊘ High Risk Denial   Ⓐ Age Edit   ♀ Female   ♂ Male   **AMA** *CPT® Assistant*   **MUE** Medically Unlikely Edit
⊘ Modifier 51 Exempt   ⊖ Modifier 63 Exempt   ✖ Unlisted   **Modifiers:** *See Inside Back Cover*   Ⓜ Maternity   `A 2`–`Z 3` ASC Payment Indicators   `A`–`Y` OPPS Status Indicators

CPT © 2015 American Medical Association. All Rights Reserved.   © 2016 DecisionHealth

64640 Destruction by neurolytic agent; other peripheral nerve or branch   P 3 T

RVU			Global Days	Modifiers				
Mod	Non-Fac Total	Fac Total		51	50	62	80	MUE
	3.80	2.68	010	2	1	0	1	5

AMA: Aug 05: 13, Feb 10: 9, Dec 09: 11, Jun 12: 15, Sep 12: 14

Destruction by neurolytic agent; other peripheral nerve or branch

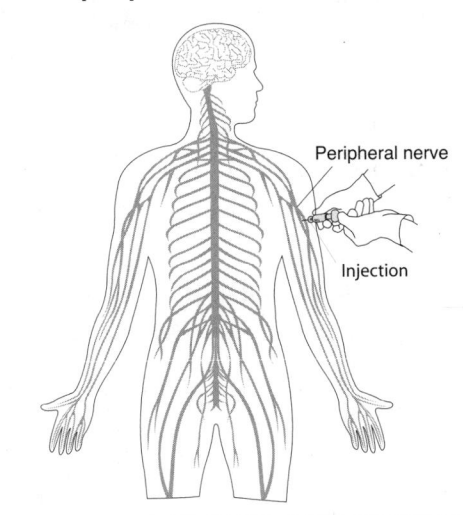

Peripheral nerve

Injection

64642 Chemodenervation of one extremity; 1-4 muscle(s)   P 3 T

RVU			Global Days	Modifiers				
Mod	Non-Fac Total	Fac Total		51	50	62	80	MUE
	4.06	3.14	000	2	0	0	1	1

AMA: Jan 14: 6, Oct 14: 15

+ 64643 Chemodenervation of one extremity; each additional extremity, 1-4 muscle(s) (List separately in addition to code for primary procedure)   N I N

RVU			Global Days	Modifiers				
Mod	Non-Fac Total	Fac Total		51	50	62	80	MUE
	2.66	2.09	ZZZ	0	0	0	1	3

AMA: Jan 14: 6, Oct 14: 15

64644 Chemodenervation of one extremity; 5 or more muscles   P 3 T

RVU			Global Days	Modifiers				
Mod	Non-Fac Total	Fac Total		51	50	62	80	MUE
	4.66	3.44	000	2	0	0	1	1

AMA: Jan 14: 6, Oct 14: 15

+ 64645 Chemodenervation of one extremity; each additional extremity, 5 or more muscles (List separately in addition to code for primary procedure)   N I N

RVU			Global Days	Modifiers				
Mod	Non-Fac Total	Fac Total		51	50	62	80	MUE
	3.28	2.41	ZZZ	0	0	0	1	3

AMA: Jan 14: 6, Oct 14: 15

64646 Chemodenervation of trunk muscle(s); 1-5 muscle(s)   P 3 T

RVU			Global Days	Modifiers				
Mod	Non-Fac Total	Fac Total		51	50	62	80	MUE
	4.31	3.38	000	2	0	0	1	1

AMA: Jan 14: 6

64647 Chemodenervation of trunk muscle(s); 6 or more muscles   P 3 T

RVU			Global Days	Modifiers				
Mod	Non-Fac Total	Fac Total		51	50	62	80	MUE
	5.08	3.95	000	2	0	0	1	1

AMA: Jan 14: 6

Sympathetic Nerve Procedures

64650 Chemodenervation of eccrine glands; both axillae   ⊝P 3 T

RVU			Global Days	Modifiers				
Mod	Non-Fac Total	Fac Total		51	50	62	80	MUE
	2.21	1.22	000	2	0	0	0	1

AMA: Jun 08: 9, Feb 10: 11, Sep 12: 14

64653 Chemodenervation of eccrine glands; other area(s) (eg, scalp, face, neck), per day   P 3 T

RVU			Global Days	Modifiers				
Mod	Non-Fac Total	Fac Total		51	50	62	80	MUE
	2.76	1.57	000	2	0	0	0	1

AMA: Jun 08: 9, Sep 12: 14

64680 Destruction by neurolytic agent, with or without radiologic monitoring; celiac plexus   A 2 T

RVU			Global Days	Modifiers				
Mod	Non-Fac Total	Fac Total		51	50	62	80	MUE
	8.87	4.80	010	2	0	0	1	1

AMA: Feb 99: 10, Aug 05: 13, Jun 08: 9, Sep 12: 14

64681 Destruction by neurolytic agent, with or without radiologic monitoring; superior hypogastric plexus   A 2 T

RVU			Global Days	Modifiers				
Mod	Non-Fac Total	Fac Total		51	50	62	80	MUE
	10.15	5.61	010	2	0	0	1	1

AMA: Aug 05: 13, Dec 07: 13, Sep 12: 14

Neuroplasty Procedures

64702 Neuroplasty; digital, 1 or both, same digit   A 2 T

RVU			Global Days	Modifiers				
Mod	Non-Fac Total	Fac Total		51	50	62	80	MUE
	14.39	14.39	090	2	0	0	1	2

AMA: Jun 01: 11

64704 Neuroplasty; nerve of hand or foot   A 2 T

RVU			Global Days	Modifiers				
Mod	Non-Fac Total	Fac Total		51	50	62	80	MUE
	9.13	9.13	090	2	0	1	2	4

AMA: Jun 01: 11

64708 Neuroplasty, major peripheral nerve, arm or leg, open; other than specified   G 2 T

RVU			Global Days	Modifiers				
Mod	Non-Fac Total	Fac Total		51	50	62	80	MUE
	14.36	14.36	090	2	0	1	2	3

AMA: Jun 01: 11, Jun 12: 12

● New   ▲ Revised   Deleted   ⊙ Moderate Sedation   ✚ Add-on Codes   ⊝ High Risk Denial   Ⓐ Age Edit   ♀ Female   ♂ Male   **AMA** CPT® Assistant   **MUE** Medically Unlikely Edit
⊗ Modifier 51 Exempt   ⊖ Modifier 63 Exempt   ✗ Unlisted   **Modifiers:** See Inside Back Cover   Ⓜ Maternity   A 2 – Z 3 ASC Payment Indicators   A – Y OPPS Status Indicators

Surgical Procedures

64712 – 64746

64712 Neuroplasty, major peripheral nerve, arm or leg, open; sciatic nerve G2 T

Mod	Non-Fac Total	Fac Total	Global Days	51	50	62	80	MUE
	16.52	16.52	090	2	1	1	2	1

AMA: Jun 01: 11, Jun 12: 12

64713 Neuroplasty, major peripheral nerve, arm or leg, open; brachial plexus G2 T

Mod	Non-Fac Total	Fac Total	Global Days	51	50	62	80	MUE
	21.02	21.02	090	2	1	1	2	1

AMA: Jun 01: 11, Jun 12: 12, May 13: 12

64714 Neuroplasty, major peripheral nerve, arm or leg, open; lumbar plexus G2 T

Mod	Non-Fac Total	Fac Total	Global Days	51	50	62	80	MUE
	18.60	18.60	090	2	1	1	2	1

AMA: Jun 97: 11, Sep 98: 16, Jun 01: 11, Jun 12: 12, Dec 13: 17

64716 Neuroplasty and/or transposition; cranial nerve (specify) A2 T

Mod	Non-Fac Total	Fac Total	Global Days	51	50	62	80	MUE
	15.55	15.55	090	2	0	1	2	2

AMA: Jun 01: 11

64718 Neuroplasty and/or transposition; ulnar nerve at elbow A2 T

Mod	Non-Fac Total	Fac Total	Global Days	51	50	62	80	MUE
	17.14	17.14	090	2	1	0	0	1

AMA: Jun 01: 11, Mar 09: 10

64719 Neuroplasty and/or transposition; ulnar nerve at wrist A2 T

Mod	Non-Fac Total	Fac Total	Global Days	51	50	62	80	MUE
	11.61	11.61	090	2	1	0	1	1

AMA: Jun 01: 11, Mar 09: 10

64721 Neuroplasty and/or transposition; median nerve at carpal tunnel A2 T

Coding tip: Code 64721 includes open release of the transverse carpal ligament

Coding tip: Do not report code 64721 with code 29848 for the same wrist at the same encounter. When an endoscopic release of the transverse carpal ligament is converted to an open release, only the open procedure may be reported.

Mod	Non-Fac Total	Fac Total	Global Days	51	50	62	80	MUE
	12.43	12.36	090	2	1	0	1	1

AMA: Fall 92: 17, Sep 97: 10, Jun 01: 11, Nov 06: 23, Aug 09: 11, Jun 12: 15, Sep 12: 16, Dec 13: 14, Jul 15: 10

64722 Decompression; unspecified nerve(s) (specify) A2 T

Mod	Non-Fac Total	Fac Total	Global Days	51	50	62	80	MUE
	10.63	10.63	090	2	0	1	2	4

AMA: Sep 98: 16, May 99: 11, Jun 01: 11, Oct 04: 12

64726 Decompression; plantar digital nerve A2 T

Mod	Non-Fac Total	Fac Total	Global Days	51	50	62	80	MUE
	7.83	7.83	090	2	0	0	1	2

AMA: Jun 01: 11

+ 64727 Internal neurolysis, requiring use of operating microscope (List separately in addition to code for neuroplasty) (Neuroplasty includes external neurolysis) N1 N

Mod	Non-Fac Total	Fac Total	Global Days	51	50	62	80	MUE
	5.37	5.37	ZZZ	0	0	0	1	2

AMA: Nov 98: 19, Jun 01: 11, Jun 12: 13

Nerve Transection/Avulsion

64732 Transection or avulsion of; supraorbital nerve A2 T

Mod	Non-Fac Total	Fac Total	Global Days	51	50	62	80	MUE
	10.85	10.85	090	2	1	0	2	1

AMA: Nov 99: 39

64734 Transection or avulsion of; infraorbital nerve A2 T

Mod	Non-Fac Total	Fac Total	Global Days	51	50	62	80	MUE
	11.87	11.87	090	2	1	0	0	1

64736 Transection or avulsion of; mental nerve A2 T

Mod	Non-Fac Total	Fac Total	Global Days	51	50	62	80	MUE
	11.48	11.48	090	2	1	0	2	1

64738 Transection or avulsion of; inferior alveolar nerve by osteotomy ⊘ A2 T

Mod	Non-Fac Total	Fac Total	Global Days	51	50	62	80	MUE
	12.19	12.19	090	2	1	0	1	1

64740 Transection or avulsion of; lingual nerve A2 T

Mod	Non-Fac Total	Fac Total	Global Days	51	50	62	80	MUE
	13.19	13.19	090	2	1	0	2	1

64742 Transection or avulsion of; facial nerve, differential or complete A2 T

Mod	Non-Fac Total	Fac Total	Global Days	51	50	62	80	MUE
	13.95	13.95	090	2	1	0	2	1

64744 Transection or avulsion of; greater occipital nerve A2 T

Mod	Non-Fac Total	Fac Total	Global Days	51	50	62	80	MUE
	14.35	14.35	090	2	1	0	0	1

64746 Transection or avulsion of; phrenic nerve A2 T

Mod	Non-Fac Total	Fac Total	Global Days	51	50	62	80	MUE
	13.29	13.29	090	2	1	1	2	1

● New   ▲ Revised   ✖ Deleted   ⊙ Moderate Sedation   ✚ Add-on Codes   ⊘ High Risk Denial   Ⓐ Age Edit   ♀ Female   ♂ Male   **AMA** CPT® Assistant   **MUE** Medically Unlikely Edit
⊘ Modifier 51 Exempt   ⊖ Modifier 63 Exempt   ✗ Unlisted   **Modifiers:** See Inside Back Cover   Ⓜ Maternity   A2–Z3 ASC Payment Indicators   A–Y OPPS Status Indicators

CPT © 2015 American Medical Association. All Rights Reserved.   © 2016 DecisionHealth

64755 Transection or avulsion of; vagus nerves limited to proximal stomach (selective proximal vagotomy, proximal gastric vagotomy, parietal cell vagotomy, supra- or highly selective vagotomy) `C`

Mod	Non-Fac Total	Fac Total	Global Days	51	50	62	80	MUE
	26.72	26.72	090	2	0	1	2	1

AMA: Nov 99: 39

64760 Transection or avulsion of; vagus nerve (vagotomy), abdominal `C`

Mod	Non-Fac Total	Fac Total	Global Days	51	50	62	80	MUE
	14.50	14.50	090	2	0	1	2	1

AMA: Nov 99: 39

64763 Transection or avulsion of obturator nerve, extrapelvic, with or without adductor tenotomy ⊘`G 2 T`

Mod	Non-Fac Total	Fac Total	Global Days	51	50	62	80	MUE
	14.58	14.58	090	2	1	1	2	1

Transection or avulsion of obturator nerve extrapelvic

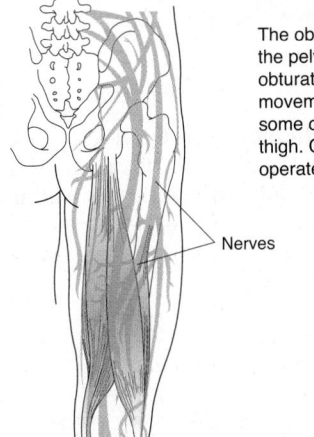

The obturator nerve outside of the pelvis is cut or removed. The obturator nerve provides movement and sensation to some of the muscles in the thigh. Code 64766 if the nerve is operated on inside of the pelvis.

Nerves

64766 Transection or avulsion of obturator nerve, intrapelvic, with or without adductor tenotomy `G 2 T`

Mod	Non-Fac Total	Fac Total	Global Days	51	50	62	80	MUE
	17.47	17.47	090	2	1	0	2	1

64771 Transection or avulsion of other cranial nerve, extradural `A 2 T`

Mod	Non-Fac Total	Fac Total	Global Days	51	50	62	80	MUE
	17.41	17.41	090	2	0	0	2	2

64772 Transection or avulsion of other spinal nerve, extradural `A 2 T`

Mod	Non-Fac Total	Fac Total	Global Days	51	50	62	80	MUE
	16.21	16.21	090	2	0	1	2	2

AMA: Apr 15: 10

Excisional Nerve Procedures

Somatic Nerve Procedures

64774 Excision of neuroma; cutaneous nerve, surgically identifiable `A 2 T`

Mod	Non-Fac Total	Fac Total	Global Days	51	50	62	80	MUE
	12.06	12.06	090	2	0	0	1	2

64776 Excision of neuroma; digital nerve, 1 or both, same digit `A 2 T`

Mod	Non-Fac Total	Fac Total	Global Days	51	50	62	80	MUE
	11.29	11.29	090	2	0	0	0	1

✚ **64778** Excision of neuroma; digital nerve, each additional digit (List separately in addition to code for primary procedure) ⊘`N 1 N`

Mod	Non-Fac Total	Fac Total	Global Days	51	50	62	80	MUE
	4.13	4.13	ZZZ	0	0	0	1	1

64782 Excision of neuroma; hand or foot, except digital nerve `A 2 T`

Mod	Non-Fac Total	Fac Total	Global Days	51	50	62	80	MUE
	12.99	12.99	090	2	0	1	1	2

✚ **64783** Excision of neuroma; hand or foot, each additional nerve, except same digit (List separately in addition to code for primary procedure) `N 1 N`

Mod	Non-Fac Total	Fac Total	Global Days	51	50	62	80	MUE
	6.48	6.48	ZZZ	0	0	0	1	1

64784 Excision of neuroma; major peripheral nerve, except sciatic `A 2 T`

Mod	Non-Fac Total	Fac Total	Global Days	51	50	62	80	MUE
	21.21	21.21	090	2	0	0	0	3

64786 Excision of neuroma; sciatic nerve `A 2 T`

Mod	Non-Fac Total	Fac Total	Global Days	51	50	62	80	MUE
	31.10	31.10	090	2	1	0	2	1

✚ **64787** Implantation of nerve end into bone or muscle (List separately in addition to neuroma excision) ⊘`N 1 N`

Mod	Non-Fac Total	Fac Total	Global Days	51	50	62	80	MUE
	7.08	7.08	ZZZ	0	0	0	0	4

64788 Excision of neurofibroma or neurolemmoma; cutaneous nerve `A 2 T`

Mod	Non-Fac Total	Fac Total	Global Days	51	50	62	80	MUE
	11.58	11.58	090	2	0	0	1	5

● New   ▲ Revised   Deleted   ⊙ Moderate Sedation   ✚ Add-on Codes   ⊘ High Risk Denial   Ⓐ Age Edit   ♀ Female   ♂ Male   **AMA** *CPT® Assistant*   **MUE** Medically Unlikely Edit
⊘ Modifier 51 Exempt   ⊖ Modifier 63 Exempt   ✗ Unlisted   **Modifiers:** *See Inside Back Cover*   Ⓜ Maternity   `A 2`–`Z 3` ASC Payment Indicators   `A`–`Y` OPPS Status Indicators

64790 Excision of neurofibroma or neurolemmoma; major peripheral nerve A2T

RVU			Global Days	Modifiers				
Mod	Non-Fac Total	Fac Total		51	50	62	80	MUE
	24.40	24.40	090	2	0	1	0	1

64792 Excision of neurofibroma or neurolemmoma; extensive (including malignant type) ⊘A2T

Documentation Finder: Documentation should indicate that the provider is excising a benign or malignant nerve sheath tumor. The documentation also may reference the tumor being Schwann cells or Schwannoma.

RVU			Global Days	Modifiers				
Mod	Non-Fac Total	Fac Total		51	50	62	80	MUE
	35.16	35.16	090	2	0	1	2	2

64795 Biopsy of nerve A2T

RVU			Global Days	Modifiers				
Mod	Non-Fac Total	Fac Total		51	50	62	80	MUE
	5.62	5.62	000	2	0	0	1	2

Sympathetic Nerve Procedures

64802 Sympathectomy, cervical A2T

RVU			Global Days	Modifiers				
Mod	Non-Fac Total	Fac Total		51	50	62	80	MUE
	19.24	19.24	090	2	1	1	2	1

64804 Sympathectomy, cervicothoracic T

RVU			Global Days	Modifiers				
Mod	Non-Fac Total	Fac Total		51	50	62	80	MUE
	29.17	29.17	090	2	1	1	2	1

64809 Sympathectomy, thoracolumbar C

RVU			Global Days	Modifiers				
Mod	Non-Fac Total	Fac Total		51	50	62	80	MUE
	29.62	29.62	090	2	1	1	2	1

64818 Sympathectomy, lumbar C

RVU			Global Days	Modifiers				
Mod	Non-Fac Total	Fac Total		51	50	62	80	MUE
	17.88	17.88	090	2	1	1	2	1

64820 Sympathectomy; digital arteries, each digit G2T

RVU			Global Days	Modifiers				
Mod	Non-Fac Total	Fac Total		51	50	62	80	MUE
	20.95	20.95	090	2	0	0	1	4

AMA: Jan 04: 27

64821 Sympathectomy; radial artery A2T

RVU			Global Days	Modifiers				
Mod	Non-Fac Total	Fac Total		51	50	62	80	MUE
	20.13	20.13	090	2	1	0	1	1

64822 Sympathectomy; ulnar artery G2T

RVU			Global Days	Modifiers				
Mod	Non-Fac Total	Fac Total		51	50	62	80	MUE
	20.13	20.13	090	2	1	0	1	1

64823 Sympathectomy; superficial palmar arch G2T

RVU			Global Days	Modifiers				
Mod	Non-Fac Total	Fac Total		51	50	62	80	MUE
	22.89	22.89	090	2	1	0	1	1

Nerve Suture Procedures

Coding Guidance

Neurorrhaphy includes suturing and anastomosis of nerves to repair traumatic injury or to connect proximally located nerves, such as facial-spinal or facial-hypoglossal.

64831 Suture of digital nerve, hand or foot; 1 nerve A2T

RVU			Global Days	Modifiers				
Mod	Non-Fac Total	Fac Total		51	50	62	80	MUE
	19.92	19.92	090	2	1	0	1	1

AMA: Apr 00: 6, Sep 14: 13

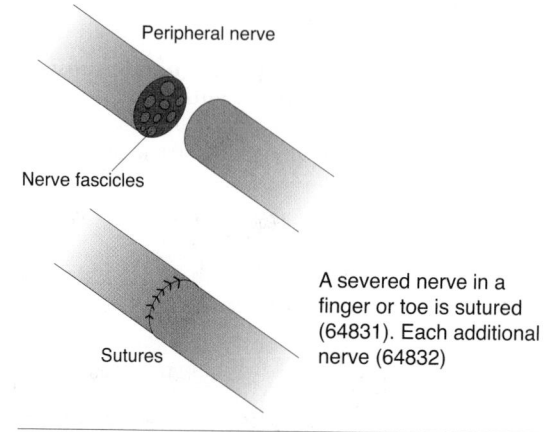

Suture of digital nerve hand or foot

Peripheral nerve

Nerve fascicles

Sutures

A severed nerve in a finger or toe is sutured (64831). Each additional nerve (64832)

+ 64832 Suture of digital nerve, hand or foot; each additional digital nerve (List separately in addition to code for primary procedure) NIN

RVU			Global Days	Modifiers				
Mod	Non-Fac Total	Fac Total		51	50	62	80	MUE
	9.87	9.87	ZZZ	0	0	0	0	3

AMA: Apr 00: 6

64834 Suture of 1 nerve; hand or foot, common sensory nerve A2T

RVU			Global Days	Modifiers				
Mod	Non-Fac Total	Fac Total		51	50	62	80	MUE
	21.53	21.53	090	2	1	0	0	1

64835 Suture of 1 nerve; median motor thenar A2T

RVU			Global Days	Modifiers				
Mod	Non-Fac Total	Fac Total		51	50	62	80	MUE
	23.38	23.38	090	2	1	0	2	1

64836 Suture of 1 nerve; ulnar motor A2T

RVU			Global Days	Modifiers				
Mod	Non-Fac Total	Fac Total		51	50	62	80	MUE
	23.45	23.45	090	2	1	0	2	1

+ 64837 Suture of each additional nerve, hand or foot (List separately in addition to code for primary procedure) NIN

RVU			Global Days	Modifiers				
Mod	Non-Fac Total	Fac Total		51	50	62	80	MUE
	10.93	10.93	ZZZ	0	0	0	2	2

● New   ▲ Revised   ✖ Deleted   ⊙ Moderate Sedation   ✚ Add-on Codes   ⊘ High Risk Denial   ⒶAge Edit   ♀ Female   ♂ Male   **AMA** CPT® Assistant   **MUE** Medically Unlikely Edit
⊘ Modifier 51 Exempt   ⊖ Modifier 63 Exempt   ✗ Unlisted   **Modifiers:** See Inside Back Cover   Ⓜ Maternity   A2–Z3 ASC Payment Indicators   A–Y OPPS Status Indicators

CPT © 2015 American Medical Association. All Rights Reserved.   © 2016 DecisionHealth

64840 Suture of posterior tibial nerve `A 2 T`

Mod	Non-Fac Total	Fac Total	Global Days	51	50	62	80	MUE
	29.47	29.47	090	2	1	0	2	1

64856 Suture of major peripheral nerve, arm or leg, except sciatic; including transposition `A 2 T`

Mod	Non-Fac Total	Fac Total	Global Days	51	50	62	80	MUE
	29.53	29.53	090	2	0	1	1	2

64857 Suture of major peripheral nerve, arm or leg, except sciatic; without transposition `A 2 T`

Mod	Non-Fac Total	Fac Total	Global Days	51	50	62	80	MUE
	30.68	30.68	090	2	0	1	2	2

64858 Suture of sciatic nerve `A 2 T`

Mod	Non-Fac Total	Fac Total	Global Days	51	50	62	80	MUE
	32.81	32.81	090	2	1	1	2	1

Suture of sciatic nerve

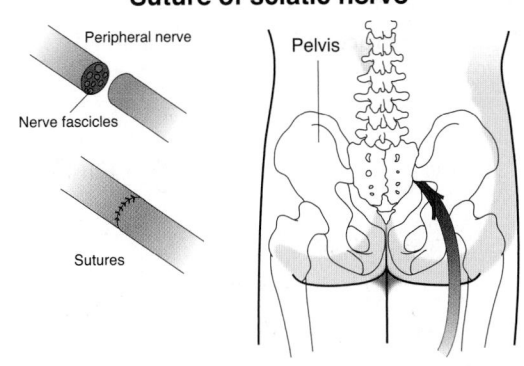

Peripheral nerve
Nerve fascicles
Sutures
Pelvis
Sciatic nerve

The sciatic nerve, which runs down the leg, is sutured together. Use code 64859 for each additional major peripheral nerve.

+ 64859 Suture of each additional major peripheral nerve (List separately in addition to code for primary procedure) `N I N`

Mod	Non-Fac Total	Fac Total	Global Days	51	50	62	80	MUE
	7.42	7.42	ZZZ	0	0	1	2	2

64861 Suture of; brachial plexus `A 2 T`

Mod	Non-Fac Total	Fac Total	Global Days	51	50	62	80	MUE
	38.35	38.35	090	2	1	1	2	1

64862 Suture of; lumbar plexus `A 2 T`

Mod	Non-Fac Total	Fac Total	Global Days	51	50	62	80	MUE
	45.15	45.15	090	2	1	0	2	1

64864 Suture of facial nerve; extracranial `A 2 T`

Mod	Non-Fac Total	Fac Total	Global Days	51	50	62	80	MUE
	25.63	25.63	090	2	0	1	2	2

64865 Suture of facial nerve; infratemporal, with or without grafting `A 2 T`

Mod	Non-Fac Total	Fac Total	Global Days	51	50	62	80	MUE
	32.65	32.65	090	2	0	1	2	1

64866 Anastomosis; facial-spinal accessory `C`

Mod	Non-Fac Total	Fac Total	Global Days	51	50	62	80	MUE
	33.32	33.32	090	2	0	1	2	1

64868 Anastomosis; facial-hypoglossal `C`

Mod	Non-Fac Total	Fac Total	Global Days	51	50	62	80	MUE
	29.39	29.39	090	2	0	1	2	1

+ 64872 Suture of nerve; requiring secondary or delayed suture (List separately in addition to code for primary neurorrhaphy) `N I N`

Mod	Non-Fac Total	Fac Total	Global Days	51	50	62	80	MUE
	3.54	3.54	ZZZ	0	0	1	2	1

+ 64874 Suture of nerve; requiring extensive mobilization, or transposition of nerve (List separately in addition to code for nerve suture) `⊘ N I N`

Mod	Non-Fac Total	Fac Total	Global Days	51	50	62	80	MUE
	4.98	4.98	ZZZ	0	0	1	2	1

+ 64876 Suture of nerve; requiring shortening of bone of extremity (List separately in addition to code for nerve suture) `N I N`

Mod	Non-Fac Total	Fac Total	Global Days	51	50	62	80	MUE
	5.12	5.12	ZZZ	0	0	1	2	1

Nerve Suture and Grafting/Conduit Procedures

Coding Guidance

Codes 64885-64907 report neurorrhaphies done with a nerve graft, for which a separate service is not reported for the primary nerve suture.

64885 Nerve graft (includes obtaining graft), head or neck; up to 4 cm in length `A 2 T`

Mod	Non-Fac Total	Fac Total	Global Days	51	50	62	80	MUE
	33.46	33.46	090	2	0	1	2	1

AMA: Nov 00: 11

64886 Nerve graft (includes obtaining graft), head or neck; more than 4 cm length `A 2 T`

Mod	Non-Fac Total	Fac Total	Global Days	51	50	62	80	MUE
	37.84	37.84	090	2	0	1	2	1

AMA: Nov 00: 11

64890 Nerve graft (includes obtaining graft), single strand, hand or foot; up to 4 cm length `A 2 T`

Mod	Non-Fac Total	Fac Total	Global Days	51	50	62	80	MUE
	31.81	31.81	090	2	0	0	2	2

AMA: Apr 15: 10, Aug 15: 8

● New   ▲ Revised   Deleted   ⊙ Moderate Sedation   ✚ Add-on Codes   ⊘ High Risk Denial   Ⓐ Age Edit   ♀ Female   ♂ Male   **AMA** *CPT® Assistant*   **MUE** Medically Unlikely Edit
⊗ Modifier 51 Exempt   ⊖ Modifier 63 Exempt   ☒ Unlisted   **Modifiers:** *See Inside Back Cover*   Ⓜ Maternity   A2 – Z3 ASC Payment Indicators   A – Y OPPS Status Indicators

Surgical Procedures

64840 – 64890

64891 Nerve graft (includes obtaining graft), single strand, hand or foot; more than 4 cm length `A2T`

Mod	Non-Fac Total	Fac Total	Global Days	51	50	62	80	MUE
	34.01	34.01	090	2	0	0	2	2

64892 Nerve graft (includes obtaining graft), single strand, arm or leg; up to 4 cm length `A2T`

Mod	Non-Fac Total	Fac Total	Global Days	51	50	62	80	MUE
	30.33	30.33	090	2	0	1	2	2

64893 Nerve graft (includes obtaining graft), single strand, arm or leg; more than 4 cm length `A2T`

Mod	Non-Fac Total	Fac Total	Global Days	51	50	62	80	MUE
	33.07	33.07	090	2	0	0	2	2

64895 Nerve graft (includes obtaining graft), multiple strands (cable), hand or foot; up to 4 cm length `A2T`

Mod	Non-Fac Total	Fac Total	Global Days	51	50	62	80	MUE
	39.13	39.13	090	2	0	1	2	2

AMA: Nov 00: 11

64896 Nerve graft (includes obtaining graft), multiple strands (cable), hand or foot; more than 4 cm length `A2T`

Mod	Non-Fac Total	Fac Total	Global Days	51	50	62	80	MUE
	42.12	42.12	090	2	0	1	2	2

AMA: Nov 00: 11

64897 Nerve graft (includes obtaining graft), multiple strands (cable), arm or leg; up to 4 cm length `A2T`

Mod	Non-Fac Total	Fac Total	Global Days	51	50	62	80	MUE
	36.22	36.22	090	2	0	0	2	2

AMA: Nov 00: 11

64898 Nerve graft (includes obtaining graft), multiple strands (cable), arm or leg; more than 4 cm length `A2T`

Mod	Non-Fac Total	Fac Total	Global Days	51	50	62	80	MUE
	39.65	39.65	090	2	0	1	2	2

AMA: Nov 00: 11

+ 64901 Nerve graft, each additional nerve; single strand (List separately in addition to code for primary procedure) `⊘N1N`

Mod	Non-Fac Total	Fac Total	Global Days	51	50	62	80	MUE
	16.22	16.22	ZZZ	0	0	1	2	2

AMA: Nov 00: 11

+ 64902 Nerve graft, each additional nerve; multiple strands (cable) (List separately in addition to code for primary procedure) `N1N`

Mod	Non-Fac Total	Fac Total	Global Days	51	50	62	80	MUE
	19.11	19.11	ZZZ	0	0	0	2	1

AMA: Nov 00: 11

64905 Nerve pedicle transfer; first stage `A2T`

Mod	Non-Fac Total	Fac Total	Global Days	51	50	62	80	MUE
	30.01	30.01	090	2	0	1	2	1

64907 Nerve pedicle transfer; second stage `⊘A2T`

Mod	Non-Fac Total	Fac Total	Global Days	51	50	62	80	MUE
	40.06	40.06	090	2	0	1	2	1

64910 Nerve repair; with synthetic conduit or vein allograft (eg, nerve tube), each nerve `G2T`

Mod	Non-Fac Total	Fac Total	Global Days	51	50	62	80	MUE
	23.98	23.98	090	2	0	1	2	3

AMA: Nov 07: 4, Apr 15: 10, Aug 15: 8

64911 Nerve repair; with autogenous vein graft (includes harvest of vein graft), each nerve `T`

Mod	Non-Fac Total	Fac Total	Global Days	51	50	62	80	MUE
	29.48	29.48	090	2	0	1	2	2

AMA: Nov 07: 4

Other Nervous System Procedures

64999 Unlisted procedure, nervous system `⊘xT`

Mod	Non-Fac Total	Fac Total	Global Days	51	50	62	80	MUE
	0.00	0.00	YYY	2	0	1	0	

AMA: Apr 96: 11, Sep 98: 16, Oct 98: 10, Jan 00: 10, Aug 00: 7, Sep 00: 10, Feb 02: 10, Nov 03: 5, Oct 04: 11, Apr 05: 13, Aug 05: 13, Sep 05: 9, Sep 07: 10, Nov 07: 4, Dec 07: 8, Jul 08: 9, Sep 08: 11, Aug 09: 8, Dec 09: 11, Apr 11: 12, Jul 11: 12, 16, 17, Sep 11: 12, Jan 12: 14, Feb 12: 11, Jun 10: 8, Sep 10: 10, Nov 10: 4, May 12: 14, Sep 12: 16, Oct 12: 14, Dec 12: 13, Apr 13: 5, 10, Jun 13: 13, Nov 13: 14, Dec 13: 14, Jan 14: 8, 9, Feb 14: 11, Jul 14: 8, Feb 15: 9, Apr 15: 10, Jul 15: 11, Aug 15: 8

Eye/Ocular Procedures

Eyeball Procedures

Eye Removal

65091 Evisceration of ocular contents; without implant `A2T`

Mod	Non-Fac Total	Fac Total	Global Days	51	50	62	80	MUE
	18.00	18.00	090	2	1	1	0	1

65093 Evisceration of ocular contents; with implant `A2T`

Mod	Non-Fac Total	Fac Total	Global Days	51	50	62	80	MUE
	17.80	17.80	090	2	1	1	1	1

65101 Enucleation of eye; without implant `A2T`

Mod	Non-Fac Total	Fac Total	Global Days	51	50	62	80	MUE
	20.90	20.90	090	2	1	0	1	1

65103 Enucleation of eye; with implant, muscles not attached to implant `A2T`

Mod	Non-Fac Total	Fac Total	Global Days	51	50	62	80	MUE
	21.82	21.82	090	2	1	1	1	1

● New   ▲ Revised   ✖ Deleted   ⊙ Moderate Sedation   ✚ Add-on Codes   ⊘ High Risk Denial   Ⓐ Age Edit   ♀ Female   ♂ Male   **AMA** CPT® Assistant   **MUE** Medically Unlikely Edit
⊘ Modifier 51 Exempt   ⊖ Modifier 63 Exempt   ✗ Unlisted   **Modifiers:** See Inside Back Cover   Ⓜ Maternity   `A2`–`Z3` ASC Payment Indicators   `A`–`Y` OPPS Status Indicators

CPT © 2015 American Medical Association. All Rights Reserved.   © 2016 DecisionHealth

65105 Enucleation of eye; with implant, muscles attached to implant `A2T`

RVU Mod	Non-Fac Total	Fac Total	Global Days	51	50	62	80	MUE
	24.08	24.08	090	2	1	1	2	1

65110 Exenteration of orbit (does not include skin graft), removal of orbital contents; only `A2T`

RVU Mod	Non-Fac Total	Fac Total	Global Days	51	50	62	80	MUE
	34.70	34.70	090	2	1	1	2	1

Exenteration of orbit (skin graft not included)

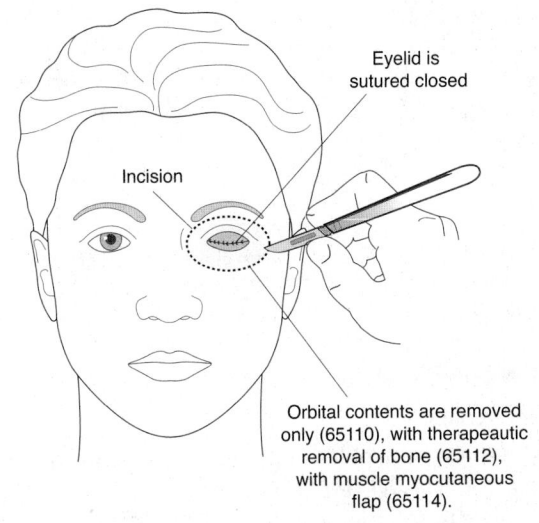

Eyelid is sutured closed

Incision

Orbital contents are removed only (65110), with therapeautic removal of bone (65112), with muscle myocutaneous flap (65114).

65112 Exenteration of orbit (does not include skin graft), removal of orbital contents; with therapeutic removal of bone `A2T`

RVU Mod	Non-Fac Total	Fac Total	Global Days	51	50	62	80	MUE
	40.36	40.36	090	2	1	1	2	1

65114 Exenteration of orbit (does not include skin graft), removal of orbital contents; with muscle or myocutaneous flap `A2T`

RVU Mod	Non-Fac Total	Fac Total	Global Days	51	50	62	80	MUE
	42.37	42.37	090	2	1	1	2	1

Secondary Eye Implant Procedures

65125 Modification of ocular implant with placement or replacement of pegs (eg, drilling receptacle for prosthesis appendage) (separate procedure) `G2T`

RVU Mod	Non-Fac Total	Fac Total	Global Days	51	50	62	80	MUE
	12.96	8.30	090	2	1	1	1	1

65130 Insertion of ocular implant secondary; after evisceration, in scleral shell `A2T`

RVU Mod	Non-Fac Total	Fac Total	Global Days	51	50	62	80	MUE
	20.74	20.74	090	2	1	1	1	1

65135 Insertion of ocular implant secondary; after enucleation, muscles not attached to implant `A2T`

RVU Mod	Non-Fac Total	Fac Total	Global Days	51	50	62	80	MUE
	21.04	21.04	090	2	1	0	1	1

65140 Insertion of ocular implant secondary; after enucleation, muscles attached to implant `A2T`

RVU Mod	Non-Fac Total	Fac Total	Global Days	51	50	62	80	MUE
	22.89	22.89	090	2	1	0	1	1

65150 Reinsertion of ocular implant; with or without conjunctival graft `A2T`

RVU Mod	Non-Fac Total	Fac Total	Global Days	51	50	62	80	MUE
	16.14	16.14	090	2	1	0	0	1

65155 Reinsertion of ocular implant; with use of foreign material for reinforcement and/or attachment of muscles to implant `A2T`

RVU Mod	Non-Fac Total	Fac Total	Global Days	51	50	62	80	MUE
	23.98	23.98	090	2	1	0	1	1

65175 Removal of ocular implant `A2T`

RVU Mod	Non-Fac Total	Fac Total	Global Days	51	50	62	80	MUE
	18.64	18.64	090	2	1	1	1	1

Foreign Body Removal

65205 Removal of foreign body, external eye; conjunctival superficial `NIQI`

RVU Mod	Non-Fac Total	Fac Total	Global Days	51	50	62	80	MUE
	1.58	1.25	000	2	1	0	1	1

AMA: Mar 05: 17, Oct 13: 19

65210 Removal of foreign body, external eye; conjunctival embedded (includes concretions), subconjunctival, or scleral nonperforating `NIQI`

RVU Mod	Non-Fac Total	Fac Total	Global Days	51	50	62	80	MUE
	1.93	1.50	000	2	1	0	1	1

65220 Removal of foreign body, external eye; corneal, without slit lamp `NIQI`

RVU Mod	Non-Fac Total	Fac Total	Global Days	51	50	62	80	MUE
	1.63	1.20	000	2	1	0	1	1

65222 Removal of foreign body, external eye; corneal, with slit lamp `NIQI`

RVU Mod	Non-Fac Total	Fac Total	Global Days	51	50	62	80	MUE
	1.88	1.47	000	2	1	0	1	1

65235 Removal of foreign body, intraocular; from anterior chamber of eye or lens `A2T`

RVU Mod	Non-Fac Total	Fac Total	Global Days	51	50	62	80	MUE
	20.18	20.18	090	2	1	0	0	1

● New ▲ Revised Deleted ⊙ Moderate Sedation ✚ Add-on Codes ⊘ High Risk Denial Ⓐ Age Edit ♀ Female ♂ Male **AMA** CPT® Assistant **MUE** Medically Unlikely Edit
⊘ Modifier 51 Exempt ⊖ Modifier 63 Exempt Ⓧ Unlisted **Modifiers**: See Inside Back Cover Ⓜ Maternity `A2`–`Z3` ASC Payment Indicators `A`–`Y` OPPS Status Indicators
© 2016 DecisionHealth — CPT © 2015 American Medical Association. All Rights Reserved.

65260 Removal of foreign body, intraocular; from posterior segment, magnetic extraction, anterior or posterior route   A 2 T

RVU		Global Days	Modifiers				
Mod	Non-Fac Total	Fac Total		51	50	62	80	MUE
	27.27	27.27	090	2	1	0	2	1

65265 Removal of foreign body, intraocular; from posterior segment, nonmagnetic extraction   A 2 T

RVU		Global Days	Modifiers				
Mod	Non-Fac Total	Fac Total		51	50	62	80	MUE
	30.74	30.74	090	2	1	1	2	1

Laceration Repair

65270 Repair of laceration; conjunctiva, with or without nonperforating laceration sclera, direct closure   A 2 T

RVU		Global Days	Modifiers				
Mod	Non-Fac Total	Fac Total		51	50	62	80	MUE
	7.54	4.00	010	2	1	0	0	1

AMA: Aug 12: 9

65272 Repair of laceration; conjunctiva, by mobilization and rearrangement, without hospitalization   A 2 T

RVU		Global Days	Modifiers				
Mod	Non-Fac Total	Fac Total		51	50	62	80	MUE
	14.23	9.97	090	2	1	0	1	1

65273 Repair of laceration; conjunctiva, by mobilization and rearrangement, with hospitalization   C

RVU		Global Days	Modifiers				
Mod	Non-Fac Total	Fac Total		51	50	62	80	MUE
	10.82	10.82	090	2	1	1	1	1

65275 Repair of laceration; cornea, nonperforating, with or without removal foreign body   A 2 T

RVU		Global Days	Modifiers				
Mod	Non-Fac Total	Fac Total		51	50	62	80	MUE
	16.39	13.13	090	2	1	0	0	1

65280 Repair of laceration; cornea and/or sclera, perforating, not involving uveal tissue   A 2 J I

RVU		Global Days	Modifiers				
Mod	Non-Fac Total	Fac Total		51	50	62	80	MUE
	19.07	19.07	090	2	1	0	0	1

AMA: Aug 12: 9

65285 Repair of laceration; cornea and/or sclera, perforating, with reposition or resection of uveal tissue   A 2 J I

RVU		Global Days	Modifiers				
Mod	Non-Fac Total	Fac Total		51	50	62	80	MUE
	31.50	31.50	090	2	1	0	1	1

AMA: Aug 12: 9

65286 Repair of laceration; application of tissue glue, wounds of cornea and/or sclera   P 3 T

RVU		Global Days	Modifiers				
Mod	Non-Fac Total	Fac Total		51	50	62	80	MUE
	19.94	14.08	090	2	1	0	1	1

AMA: May 99: 11, Apr 09: 5

65290 Repair of wound, extraocular muscle, tendon and/or Tenon's capsule   A 2 T

RVU		Global Days	Modifiers				
Mod	Non-Fac Total	Fac Total		51	50	62	80	MUE
	13.87	13.87	090	2	1	1	1	1

Repair of wound, extraocular muscle, tendon/Tenon's capsule

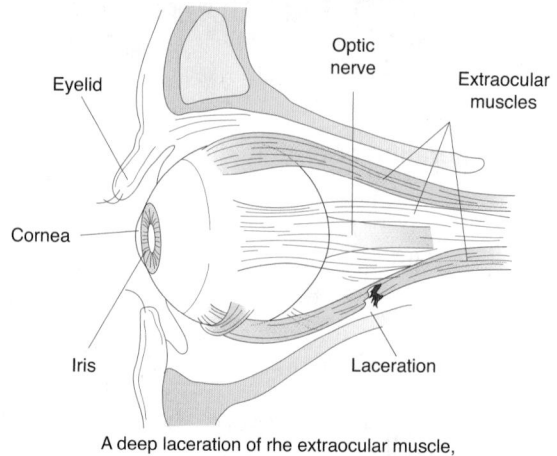

A deep laceration of rhe extraocular muscle, tendon/Tenon's capsule is repaired

Corneal Procedures

Corneal Excision

65400 Excision of lesion, cornea (keratectomy, lamellar, partial), except pterygium   A 2 T

RVU		Global Days	Modifiers				
Mod	Non-Fac Total	Fac Total		51	50	62	80	MUE
	19.27	17.13	090	2	1	0	1	1

Excision of lesion, cornea (keratectomy, lamellar, partial), except pterygium

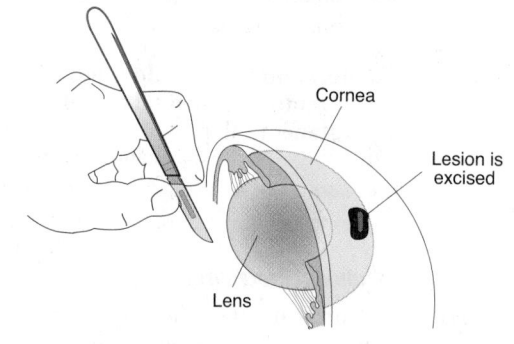

65410 Biopsy of cornea   A 2 T

RVU		Global Days	Modifiers				
Mod	Non-Fac Total	Fac Total		51	50	62	80	MUE
	4.04	2.97	000	2	1	0	0	1

65420 Excision or transposition of pterygium; without graft   A 2 T

RVU		Global Days	Modifiers				
Mod	Non-Fac Total	Fac Total		51	50	62	80	MUE
	14.62	10.72	090	2	1	0	1	1

AMA: Dec 07: 13

● New   ▲ Revised   ✖ Deleted   ⊙ Moderate Sedation   ✚ Add-on Codes   ⊘ High Risk Denial   Ⓐ Age Edit   ♀ Female   ♂ Male   **AMA** CPT® Assistant   **MUE** Medically Unlikely Edit
⊘ Modifier 51 Exempt   ⊖ Modifier 63 Exempt   ✗ Unlisted   **Modifiers:** See Inside Back Cover   Ⓜ Maternity   A 2 – Z 3 ASC Payment Indicators   A – Y OPPS Status Indicators

CPT © 2015 American Medical Association. All Rights Reserved.   © 2016 DecisionHealth

65426 Excision or transposition of pterygium; with graft

A 2 T

	RVU		Global Days	Modifiers				
Mod	Non-Fac Total	Fac Total		51	50	62	80	MUE
	18.46	13.58	090	2	1	0	1	1

Corneal Removal/Destruction

65430 Scraping of cornea, diagnostic, for smear and/or culture

N I Q I

	RVU		Global Days	Modifiers				
Mod	Non-Fac Total	Fac Total		51	50	62	80	MUE
	3.24	2.94	000	2	1	0	1	1

65435 Removal of corneal epithelium; with or without chemocauterization (abrasion, curettage)

P 3 T

	RVU		Global Days	Modifiers				
Mod	Non-Fac Total	Fac Total		51	50	62	80	MUE
	2.25	1.97	000	2	1	0	1	1

65436 Removal of corneal epithelium; with application of chelating agent (eg, EDTA)

P 3 T

	RVU		Global Days	Modifiers				
Mod	Non-Fac Total	Fac Total		51	50	62	80	MUE
	10.99	10.56	090	2	1	0	1	1

65450 Destruction of lesion of cornea by cryotherapy, photocoagulation or thermocauterization

G 2 T

	RVU		Global Days	Modifiers				
Mod	Non-Fac Total	Fac Total		51	50	62	80	MUE
	9.21	9.12	090	2	1	0	1	1

65600 Multiple punctures of anterior cornea (eg, for corneal erosion, tattoo)

P 3 T

	RVU		Global Days	Modifiers				
Mod	Non-Fac Total	Fac Total		51	50	62	80	MUE
	11.17	9.77	090	2	1	0	1	1

Keratoplasty

65710 Keratoplasty (corneal transplant); anterior lamellar

A 2 J 1

	RVU		Global Days	Modifiers				
Mod	Non-Fac Total	Fac Total		51	50	62	80	MUE
	31.44	31.44	090	2	1	1	2	1

AMA: Oct 02: 8, Apr 09: 5, Dec 09: 13, Aug 12: 15

65730 Keratoplasty (corneal transplant); penetrating (except in aphakia or pseudophakia)

A 2 J 1

	RVU		Global Days	Modifiers				
Mod	Non-Fac Total	Fac Total		51	50	62	80	MUE
	34.85	34.85	090	2	1	1	2	1

AMA: Oct 02: 8, Feb 06: 1, Apr 09: 5, Dec 09: 13, Aug 12: 15

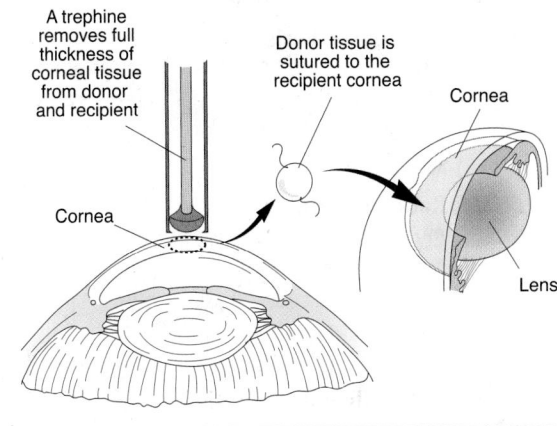

Keratoplasty (corneal transplant); penetrating (except in aphakia/pseudophakia)

A trephine removes full thickness of corneal tissue from donor and recipient

Donor tissue is sutured to the recipient cornea

Cornea

Cornea

Lens

65750 Keratoplasty (corneal transplant); penetrating (in aphakia)

A 2 J 1

	RVU		Global Days	Modifiers				
Mod	Non-Fac Total	Fac Total		51	50	62	80	MUE
	35.04	35.04	090	2	1	1	2	1

AMA: Oct 02: 8, Apr 09: 5, Dec 09: 13, Aug 12: 15

65755 Keratoplasty (corneal transplant); penetrating (in pseudophakia)

A 2 J 1

	RVU		Global Days	Modifiers				
Mod	Non-Fac Total	Fac Total		51	50	62	80	MUE
	34.85	34.85	090	2	1	1	2	1

AMA: Winter 90: 8, Oct 02: 9, Apr 09: 5, Dec 09: 13, Aug 12: 15

65756 Keratoplasty (corneal transplant); endothelial

G 2 J 1

	RVU		Global Days	Modifiers				
Mod	Non-Fac Total	Fac Total		51	50	62	80	MUE
	33.67	33.67	090	2	1	1	2	1

+ 65757 Backbench preparation of corneal endothelial allograft prior to transplantation (List separately in addition to code for primary procedure)

N I N

	RVU		Global Days	Modifiers				
Mod	Non-Fac Total	Fac Total		51	50	62	80	MUE
	0.00	0.00	ZZZ	0	0	0	0	1

AMA: Aug 14: 15

Other Corneal Procedures

65760 Keratomileusis

⊗ E

	RVU		Global Days	Modifiers				
Mod	Non-Fac Total	Fac Total		51	50	62	80	MUE
	0.00	0.00	XXX	9	9	9	9	

AMA: Oct 02: 9

65765 Keratophakia

⊗ E

	RVU		Global Days	Modifiers				
Mod	Non-Fac Total	Fac Total		51	50	62	80	MUE
	0.00	0.00	XXX	9	9	9	9	

AMA: Oct 02: 10

Surgical Procedures

65426 – 65765

● New   ▲ Revised   Deleted   ⊙ Moderate Sedation   ✚ Add-on Codes   ⊘ High Risk Denial   Ⓐ Age Edit   ♀ Female   ♂ Male   **AMA** CPT® Assistant   **MUE** Medically Unlikely Edit
⊘ Modifier 51 Exempt   ⊖ Modifier 63 Exempt   ✘ Unlisted   **Modifiers:** See Inside Back Cover   Ⓜ Maternity   A 2 – Z 3 ASC Payment Indicators   A – Y OPPS Status Indicators

© 2016 DecisionHealth | CPT © 2015 American Medical Association. All Rights Reserved. | **587**

65767 Epikeratoplasty ⊙E

RVU			Global Days	Modifiers				
Mod	Non-Fac Total	Fac Total		51	50	62	80	MUE
	0.00	0.00	XXX	9	9	9	9	

AMA: Winter 90: 8, Oct 02: 10

65770 Keratoprosthesis G2JI

RVU			Global Days	Modifiers				
Mod	Non-Fac Total	Fac Total		51	50	62	80	MUE
	39.88	39.88	090	2	1	0	2	1

AMA: Oct 02: 10

65771 Radial keratotomy ⊙E

RVU			Global Days	Modifiers				
Mod	Non-Fac Total	Fac Total		51	50	62	80	MUE
	0.00	0.00	XXX	9	9	9	9	

AMA: Winter 90: 8, Oct 02: 10

65772 Corneal relaxing incision for correction of surgically induced astigmatism A2T

RVU			Global Days	Modifiers				
Mod	Non-Fac Total	Fac Total		51	50	62	80	MUE
	12.78	11.55	090	2	1	0	1	1

AMA: Oct 02: 10, 12

65775 Corneal wedge resection for correction of surgically induced astigmatism A2T

RVU			Global Days	Modifiers				
Mod	Non-Fac Total	Fac Total		51	50	62	80	MUE
	15.65	15.65	090	2	1	0	1	1

AMA: Oct 02: 10, 12, Aug 12: 9

65778 Placement of amniotic membrane on the ocular surface; without sutures NIQ2

RVU			Global Days	Modifiers				
Mod	Non-Fac Total	Fac Total		51	50	62	80	MUE
	40.59	1.67	000	2	1	0	0	1

AMA: May 14: 5

65779 Placement of amniotic membrane on the ocular surface; single layer, sutured NIQ2

RVU			Global Days	Modifiers				
Mod	Non-Fac Total	Fac Total		51	50	62	80	MUE
	34.09	4.33	000	2	1	0	0	1

AMA: May 14: 5

65780 Ocular surface reconstruction; amniotic membrane transplantation, multiple layers A2T

RVU			Global Days	Modifiers				
Mod	Non-Fac Total	Fac Total		51	50	62	80	MUE
	20.34	20.34	090	2	1	1	1	1

AMA: May 04: 10, Jun 09: 9, May 14: 5

65781 Ocular surface reconstruction; limbal stem cell allograft (eg, cadaveric or living donor) A2JI

RVU			Global Days	Modifiers				
Mod	Non-Fac Total	Fac Total		51	50	62	80	MUE
	37.88	37.88	090	2	1	1	2	1

AMA: May 04: 10

65782 Ocular surface reconstruction; limbal conjunctival autograft (includes obtaining graft) A2T

RVU			Global Days	Modifiers				
Mod	Non-Fac Total	Fac Total		51	50	62	80	MUE
	32.68	32.68	090	2	1	1	1	1

AMA: Feb 04: 11, May 04: 10, Feb 05: 15, 16

● 65785 Implantation of intrastromal corneal ring segments R2JI

RVU			Global Days	Modifiers				
Mod	Non-Fac Total	Fac Total		51	50	62	80	MUE
	59.94	11.05	090	2	1	1	1	2

Anterior Chamber Procedures

Incisional Procedures

65800 Paracentesis of anterior chamber of eye (separate procedure); with removal of aqueous A2T

RVU			Global Days	Modifiers				
Mod	Non-Fac Total	Fac Total		51	50	62	80	MUE
	3.38	2.60	000	2	1	0	1	1

AMA: Nov 12: 10

65810 Paracentesis of anterior chamber of eye (separate procedure); with removal of vitreous and/or discission of anterior hyaloid membrane, with or without air injection A2T

RVU			Global Days	Modifiers				
Mod	Non-Fac Total	Fac Total		51	50	62	80	MUE
	13.22	13.22	090	2	1	0	1	1

AMA: Nov 12: 10

Paracentisis of anterior chamber of eye with removal of vitreous/discission of hyaloid membrane, with/without air injection

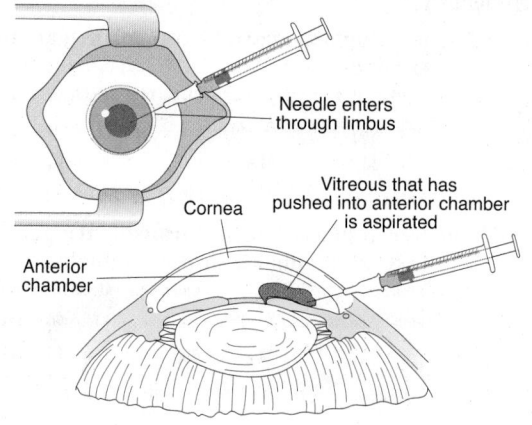

Needle enters through limbus

Vitreous that has pushed into anterior chamber is aspirated

Cornea

Anterior chamber

A laser may be used to destroy hyaloid membrane

65815 Paracentesis of anterior chamber of eye (separate procedure); with removal of blood, with or without irrigation and/or air injection A2T

RVU			Global Days	Modifiers				
Mod	Non-Fac Total	Fac Total		51	50	62	80	MUE
	18.08	13.56	090	2	1	0	1	1

AMA: Nov 12: 10

● New   ▲ Revised   ✖ Deleted   ⊙ Moderate Sedation   ✚ Add-on Codes   ⊘ High Risk Denial   Ⓐ Age Edit   ♀ Female   ♂ Male   **AMA** CPT® Assistant   **MUE** Medically Unlikely Edit
⊘ Modifier 51 Exempt   ⊖ Modifier 63 Exempt   ✖ Unlisted   **Modifiers:** See Inside Back Cover   Ⓜ Maternity   A2–Z3 ASC Payment Indicators   A–Y OPPS Status Indicators

CPT © 2015 American Medical Association. All Rights Reserved.   © 2016 DecisionHealth

65820 Goniotomy ⊖ A 2 J 1

RVU			Global Days	Modifiers				
Mod	Non-Fac Total	Fac Total		51	50	62	80	MUE
	21.25	21.25	090	2	1	0	0	1

AMA: Sep 05: 12

65850 Trabeculotomy ab externo A 2 T

RVU			Global Days	Modifiers				
Mod	Non-Fac Total	Fac Total		51	50	62	80	MUE
	23.84	23.84	090	2	1	1	1	1

▲ 65855 Trabeculoplasty by laser surgery P 3 T

RVU			Global Days	Modifiers				
Mod	Non-Fac Total	Fac Total		51	50	62	80	MUE
	7.73	6.80	010	2	2	1	1	1

AMA: Mar 98: 7, Mar 03: 23

65860 Severing adhesions of anterior segment, laser technique (separate procedure) P 3 T

RVU			Global Days	Modifiers				
Mod	Non-Fac Total	Fac Total		51	50	62	80	MUE
	8.75	7.19	090	2	1	0	0	1

65865 Severing adhesions of anterior segment of eye, incisional technique (with or without injection of air or liquid) (separate procedure); goniosynechiae A 2 T

RVU			Global Days	Modifiers				
Mod	Non-Fac Total	Fac Total		51	50	62	80	MUE
	13.42	13.42	090	2	1	1	1	1

65870 Severing adhesions of anterior segment of eye, incisional technique (with or without injection of air or liquid) (separate procedure); anterior synechiae, except goniosynechiae A 2 T

RVU			Global Days	Modifiers				
Mod	Non-Fac Total	Fac Total		51	50	62	80	MUE
	16.78	16.78	090	2	1	1	1	1

65875 Severing adhesions of anterior segment of eye, incisional technique (with or without injection of air or liquid) (separate procedure); posterior synechiae ⊗ A 2 T

RVU			Global Days	Modifiers				
Mod	Non-Fac Total	Fac Total		51	50	62	80	MUE
	17.89	17.89	090	2	1	1	1	1

AMA: Sep 05: 12

65880 Severing adhesions of anterior segment of eye, incisional technique (with or without injection of air or liquid) (separate procedure); corneovitreal adhesions A 2 T

RVU			Global Days	Modifiers				
Mod	Non-Fac Total	Fac Total		51	50	62	80	MUE
	18.80	18.80	090	2	1	0	1	1

Removal Procedures

65900 Removal of epithelial downgrowth, anterior chamber of eye A 2 T

RVU			Global Days	Modifiers				
Mod	Non-Fac Total	Fac Total		51	50	62	80	MUE
	27.24	27.24	090	2	1	0	2	1

65920 Removal of implanted material, anterior segment of eye A 2 T

RVU			Global Days	Modifiers				
Mod	Non-Fac Total	Fac Total		51	50	62	80	MUE
	22.40	22.40	090	2	1	1	1	1

AMA: Sep 05: 12

65930 Removal of blood clot, anterior segment of eye A 2 T

RVU			Global Days	Modifiers				
Mod	Non-Fac Total	Fac Total		51	50	62	80	MUE
	18.10	18.10	090	2	1	1	1	1

Anterior Chamber Injection Procedures

66020 Injection, anterior chamber of eye (separate procedure); air or liquid A 2 T

RVU			Global Days	Modifiers				
Mod	Non-Fac Total	Fac Total		51	50	62	80	MUE
	5.28	3.74	010	2	1	0	1	1

AMA: Nov 12: 10

Injection anterior chamber of eye air/liquid/medication

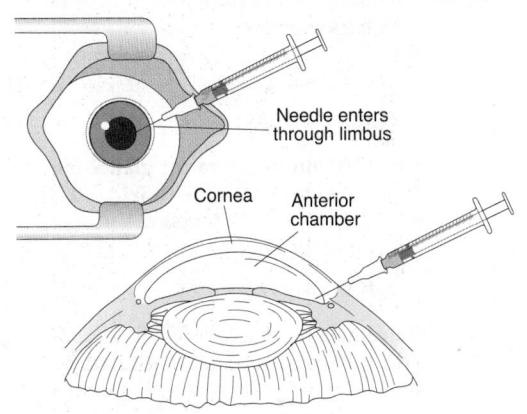

Needle enters through limbus

Cornea

Anterior chamber

A needle is inserted into the anterior chamber to inject air/liquid (66020), or medication (66030)

66030 Injection, anterior chamber of eye (separate procedure); medication A 2 T

RVU			Global Days	Modifiers				
Mod	Non-Fac Total	Fac Total		51	50	62	80	MUE
	4.69	3.15	010	2	1	0	1	1

AMA: Nov 12: 10

● New ▲ Revised Deleted ⊙ Moderate Sedation ✛ Add-on Codes ⊘ High Risk Denial ⒶAge Edit ♀ Female ♂ Male **AMA** CPT® Assistant **MUE** Medically Unlikely Edit
Ⓢ Modifier 51 Exempt ⊖ Modifier 63 Exempt ✗ Unlisted **Modifiers:** See Inside Back Cover Ⓜ Maternity A2–Z3 ASC Payment Indicators A–Y OPPS Status Indicators

Surgical Procedures

65820 – 66030

Anterior Scleral Procedures

Anterior Scleral Excision

66130 Excision of lesion, sclera `A 2 T`

RVU			Global Days	Modifiers				
Mod	Non-Fac Total	Fac Total		51	50	62	80	MUE
	19.72	16.14	090	2	1	0	0	1

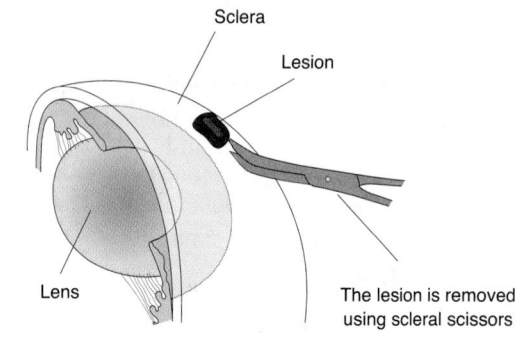

Excision of lesion, sclera

Sclera
Lesion
Lens
The lesion is removed using scleral scissors

66150 Fistulization of sclera for glaucoma; trephination with iridectomy `A 2 J I`

RVU			Global Days	Modifiers				
Mod	Non-Fac Total	Fac Total		51	50	62	80	MUE
	24.88	24.88	090	2	1	1	1	1

66155 Fistulization of sclera for glaucoma; thermocauterization with iridectomy `A 2 T`

RVU			Global Days	Modifiers				
Mod	Non-Fac Total	Fac Total		51	50	62	80	MUE
	24.87	24.87	090	2	1	0	1	1

66160 Fistulization of sclera for glaucoma; sclerectomy with punch or scissors, with iridectomy `A 2 T`

RVU			Global Days	Modifiers				
Mod	Non-Fac Total	Fac Total		51	50	62	80	MUE
	28.05	28.05	090	2	1	1	1	1

66170 Fistulization of sclera for glaucoma; trabeculectomy ab externo in absence of previous surgery `A 2 T`

RVU			Global Days	Modifiers				
Mod	Non-Fac Total	Fac Total		51	50	62	80	MUE
	27.46	27.46	090	2	1	1	2	1

AMA: Jul 03: 4, Nov 03: 10, Dec 12: 14

66172 Fistulization of sclera for glaucoma; trabeculectomy ab externo with scarring from previous ocular surgery or trauma (includes injection of antifibrotic agents) `A 2 T`

RVU			Global Days	Modifiers				
Mod	Non-Fac Total	Fac Total		51	50	62	80	MUE
	34.62	34.62	090	2	1	1	2	1

AMA: Jul 03: 4, Nov 03: 10, Dec 12: 14

66174 Transluminal dilation of aqueous outflow canal; without retention of device or stent `A 2 T`

RVU			Global Days	Modifiers				
Mod	Non-Fac Total	Fac Total		51	50	62	80	MUE
	26.91	26.91	090	2	1	1	2	1

66175 Transluminal dilation of aqueous outflow canal; with retention of device or stent `A 2 J I`

RVU			Global Days	Modifiers				
Mod	Non-Fac Total	Fac Total		51	50	62	80	MUE
	28.20	28.20	090	2	1	1	2	1

66179 Aqueous shunt to extraocular equatorial plate reservoir, external approach; without graft `G 2 J I`

RVU			Global Days	Modifiers				
Mod	Non-Fac Total	Fac Total		51	50	62	80	MUE
	30.61	30.61	090	2	1	0	2	1

AMA: Jan 15: 10

Aqueous Shunt Procedures

66180 Aqueous shunt to extraocular equatorial plate reservoir, external approach; with graft `A 2 J I`

RVU			Global Days	Modifiers				
Mod	Non-Fac Total	Fac Total		51	50	62	80	MUE
	32.31	32.31	090	2	1	0	2	1

AMA: Winter 90: 8, Aug 03: 9, Sep 03: 2, Jun 12: 15, Jan 15: 10

66183 Insertion of anterior segment aqueous drainage device, without extraocular reservoir, external approach `G 2 J I`

RVU			Global Days	Modifiers				
Mod	Non-Fac Total	Fac Total		51	50	62	80	MUE
	29.26	29.26	090	2	1	0	2	1

AMA: May 14: 5

66184 Revision of aqueous shunt to extraocular equatorial plate reservoir; without graft `G 2 T`

RVU			Global Days	Modifiers				
Mod	Non-Fac Total	Fac Total		51	50	62	80	MUE
	22.29	22.29	090	2	1	0	2	1

AMA: Jan 15: 10

66185 Revision of aqueous shunt to extraocular equatorial plate reservoir; with graft `A 2 T`

RVU			Global Days	Modifiers				
Mod	Non-Fac Total	Fac Total		51	50	62	80	MUE
	24.00	24.00	090	2	1	0	2	1

AMA: Winter 90: 8, Jan 15: 10

Anterior Scleral Repair/Revision Procedures

66220 Repair of scleral staphyloma; without graft `A 2 T`

RVU			Global Days	Modifiers				
Mod	Non-Fac Total	Fac Total		51	50	62	80	MUE
	21.19	21.19	090	2	1	1	2	1

66225 Repair of scleral staphyloma; with graft `A 2 T`

RVU			Global Days	Modifiers				
Mod	Non-Fac Total	Fac Total		51	50	62	80	MUE
	26.44	26.44	090	2	1	1	1	1

● New ▲ Revised ✖ Deleted ⊙ Moderate Sedation ✚ Add-on Codes ⊘ High Risk Denial ⓐ Age Edit ♀ Female ♂ Male **AMA** CPT® Assistant **MUE** Medically Unlikely Edit ⊘ Modifier 51 Exempt ⊖ Modifier 63 Exempt ✖ Unlisted **Modifiers:** See Inside Back Cover Ⓜ Maternity A2–Z3 ASC Payment Indicators A–Y OPPS Status Indicators

590 CPT © 2015 American Medical Association. All Rights Reserved. © 2016 DecisionHealth

66250 Revision or repair of operative wound of anterior segment, any type, early or late, major or minor procedure   A2 T

RVU			Global Days	Modifiers				
Mod	Non-Fac Total	Fac Total		51	50	62	80	MUE
	21.22	15.83	090	2	1	0	1	1

AMA: Oct 10: 15, Dec 10: 15

Iris/Ciliary Body Procedures

Iris Incisional Procedures

66500 Iridotomy by stab incision (separate procedure); except transfixion   A2 T

RVU			Global Days	Modifiers				
Mod	Non-Fac Total	Fac Total		51	50	62	80	MUE
	10.03	10.03	090	2	1	1	1	1

66505 Iridotomy by stab incision (separate procedure); with transfixion as for iris bombe   A2 T

RVU			Global Days	Modifiers				
Mod	Non-Fac Total	Fac Total		51	50	62	80	MUE
	11.01	11.01	090	2	1	0	1	1

Iris Excisional Procedures

66600 Iridectomy, with corneoscleral or corneal section; for removal of lesion   A2 T

RVU			Global Days	Modifiers				
Mod	Non-Fac Total	Fac Total		51	50	62	80	MUE
	23.60	23.60	090	2	1	0	1	1

66605 Iridectomy, with corneoscleral or corneal section; with cyclectomy   A2 T

RVU			Global Days	Modifiers				
Mod	Non-Fac Total	Fac Total		51	50	62	80	MUE
	30.01	30.01	090	2	1	0	1	1

66625 Iridectomy, with corneoscleral or corneal section; peripheral for glaucoma (separate procedure)   A2 T

RVU			Global Days	Modifiers				
Mod	Non-Fac Total	Fac Total		51	50	62	80	MUE
	12.19	12.19	090	2	1	0	1	1

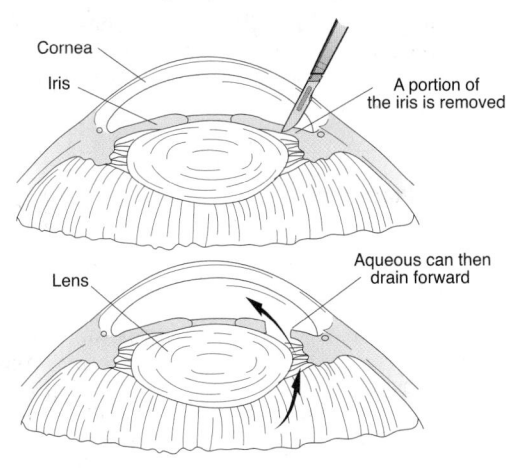

Iridectomy, with corneoscleral/corneal section; peripheral for glaucoma

Cornea

Iris

A portion of the iris is removed

Lens

Aqueous can then drain forward

66630 Iridectomy, with corneoscleral or corneal section; sector for glaucoma (separate procedure)   A2 T

RVU			Global Days	Modifiers				
Mod	Non-Fac Total	Fac Total		51	50	62	80	MUE
	16.16	16.16	090	2	1	0	1	1

66635 Iridectomy, with corneoscleral or corneal section; optical (separate procedure)   A2 T

RVU			Global Days	Modifiers				
Mod	Non-Fac Total	Fac Total		51	50	62	80	MUE
	16.32	16.32	090	2	1	0	1	1

Iris/Ciliary Body Repair

66680 Repair of iris, ciliary body (as for iridodialysis)   A2 T

RVU			Global Days	Modifiers				
Mod	Non-Fac Total	Fac Total		51	50	62	80	MUE
	14.68	14.68	090	2	1	1	1	1

66682 Suture of iris, ciliary body (separate procedure) with retrieval of suture through small incision (eg, McCannel suture)   A2 T

RVU			Global Days	Modifiers				
Mod	Non-Fac Total	Fac Total		51	50	62	80	MUE
	18.09	18.09	090	2	1	0	1	1

Iris/Ciliary Body Destruction Procedures

66700 Ciliary body destruction; diathermy   A2 T

RVU			Global Days	Modifiers				
Mod	Non-Fac Total	Fac Total		51	50	62	80	MUE
	12.75	11.17	090	2	1	0	0	1

66710 Ciliary body destruction; cyclophotocoagulation, transscleral   A2 T

RVU			Global Days	Modifiers				
Mod	Non-Fac Total	Fac Total		51	50	62	80	MUE
	12.47	11.16	090	2	1	0	1	1

AMA: Mar 05: 20, Sep 05: 5

66711 Ciliary body destruction; cyclophotocoagulation, endoscopic   A2 T

RVU			Global Days	Modifiers				
Mod	Non-Fac Total	Fac Total		51	50	62	80	MUE
	18.19	18.19	090	3	1	0	1	1

AMA: Mar 05: 20, Sep 05: 5, 12

⊙ **66720** Ciliary body destruction; cryotherapy   A2 T

RVU			Global Days	Modifiers				
Mod	Non-Fac Total	Fac Total		51	50	62	80	MUE
	13.43	12.02	090	2	1	0	1	1

● New   ▲ Revised   Deleted   ⊙ Moderate Sedation   ✚ Add-on Codes   ⊘ High Risk Denial   Ⓐ Age Edit   ♀ Female   ♂ Male   **AMA** CPT® Assistant   **MUE** Medically Unlikely Edit
⊘ Modifier 51 Exempt   ⊖ Modifier 63 Exempt   ✗ Unlisted   **Modifiers:** See Inside Back Cover   Ⓜ Maternity   A2–Z3 ASC Payment Indicators   A–Y OPPS Status Indicators

Surgical Procedures

66250 – 66720

Surgical Procedures

66740 – 66825

66740 Ciliary body destruction; cyclodialysis   `A2 T`

RVU		Global Days	Modifiers				
Mod	Non-Fac Total	Fac Total		51	50	62	80	MUE
	12.40	11.17	090	2	1	0	1	1

Ciliary body destruction; cyclodialysis

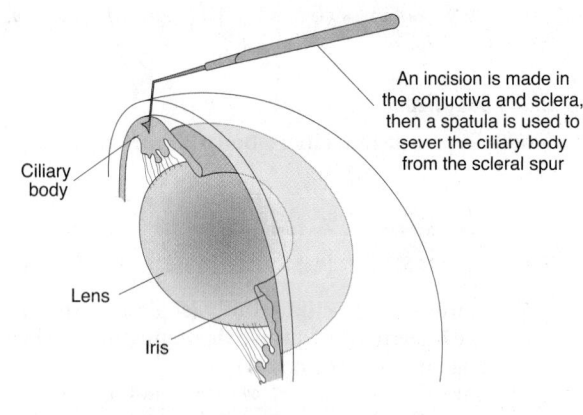

An incision is made in the conjuctiva and sclera, then a spatula is used to sever the ciliary body from the scleral spur

Ciliary body

Lens

Iris

66761 Iridotomy/iridectomy by laser surgery (eg, for glaucoma) (per session)   `P3 T`

RVU		Global Days	Modifiers				
Mod	Non-Fac Total	Fac Total		51	50	62	80	MUE
	8.39	6.69	010	2	1	0	1	1

AMA: Mar 98: 7

66762 Iridoplasty by photocoagulation (1 or more sessions) (eg, for improvement of vision, for widening of anterior chamber angle)   `P2 T`

RVU		Global Days	Modifiers				
Mod	Non-Fac Total	Fac Total		51	50	62	80	MUE
	13.46	12.11	090	2	1	0	1	1

AMA: Mar 98: 7

66770 Destruction of cyst or lesion iris or ciliary body (nonexcisional procedure)   `P2 T`

RVU		Global Days	Modifiers				
Mod	Non-Fac Total	Fac Total		51	50	62	80	MUE
	14.96	13.72	090	2	1	0	1	1

Lens Procedures

Incisional Lens Procedures

66820 Discission of secondary membranous cataract (opacified posterior lens capsule and/or anterior hyaloid); stab incision technique (Ziegler or Wheeler knife)   `G2 T`

RVU		Global Days	Modifiers				
Mod	Non-Fac Total	Fac Total		51	50	62	80	MUE
	11.06	11.06	090	2	1	0	1	1

Discission of secondary membranous cataract

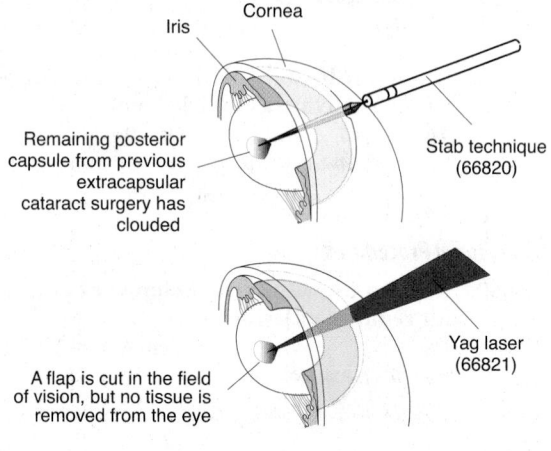

Iris

Cornea

Remaining posterior capsule from previous extracapsular cataract surgery has clouded

Stab technique (66820)

Yag laser (66821)

A flap is cut in the field of vision, but no tissue is removed from the eye

66821 Discission of secondary membranous cataract (opacified posterior lens capsule and/or anterior hyaloid); laser surgery (eg, YAG laser) (1 or more stages)   `A2 T`

Documentation Finder: *The documentation should indicate that the patient had a previous cataract extraction, usually more than three months ago to support this code. The provider must note that he or she is using a laser to perform the capsulotomies. If the scar issues need to be treated in more than one encounter, the provider should not have additional billing because this code represents one or more sessions.*

RVU		Global Days	Modifiers				
Mod	Non-Fac Total	Fac Total		51	50	62	80	MUE
	9.32	8.81	090	2	1	0	1	1

66825 Repositioning of intraocular lens prosthesis, requiring an incision (separate procedure)   `A2 T`

RVU		Global Days	Modifiers				
Mod	Non-Fac Total	Fac Total		51	50	62	80	MUE
	21.55	21.55	090	2	1	0	0	1

Removal Lens Procedures

Coding Guidance

The various techniques or approaches used for cataract removal are mutually exclusive of each other for the same eye. Only one type of extraction may be reported per eye. When cataracts are removed, an iridectomy, anterior vitrectomy, or trabeculectomy may also be done at the same operative session. An iridectomy done in order to accomplish the cataract extraction is integral to the procedure and cannot be reported. The normal, minimal amount of vitreous lost during routine cataract extraction does not constitute a vitrectomy. A vitrectomy may only be reported when it is medically necessary for a different diagnosis. If a trabeculectomy is necessary to control glaucoma at the same time as cataract extraction, it may be reported under the separate

● New   ▲ Revised   ✖ Deleted   ⊙ Moderate Sedation   ✚ Add-on Codes   ⊘ High Risk Denial   Ⓐ Age Edit   ♀ Female   ♂ Male   **AMA** *CPT® Assistant*   ***MUE*** Medically Unlikely Edit
⊘ Modifier 51 Exempt   ⊖ Modifier 63 Exempt   ✗ Unlisted   **Modifiers:** *See Inside Back Cover*   Ⓜ Maternity   `A2`–`Z3` ASC Payment Indicators   `A`–`Y` OPPS Status Indicators

592   CPT © 2015 American Medical Association. All Rights Reserved.   © 2016 DecisionHealth

diagnosis of glaucoma. A prophylactic trabeculectomy for prevention of expected postoperative increase in intraocular pressure occurring transiently, without other evidence of glaucoma, cannot be reported independently. When iridectomies, trabeculectomies, or anterior vitrectomies described by other codes are performed for a different diagnosis along with cataract removal, they may be billed as a separate service with modifier 59 to indicate a distinct service for a separate reason.

66830 Removal of secondary membranous cataract (opacified posterior lens capsule and/or anterior hyaloid) with corneo-scleral section, with or without iridectomy (iridocapsulotomy, iridocapsulectomy)   A 2 T

RVU Mod	Non-Fac Total	Fac Total	Global Days	Modifiers 51	50	62	80	MUE
	20.08	20.08	090	2	1	0	1	1

Removal of secondary membranous cataract with/without iridectomy

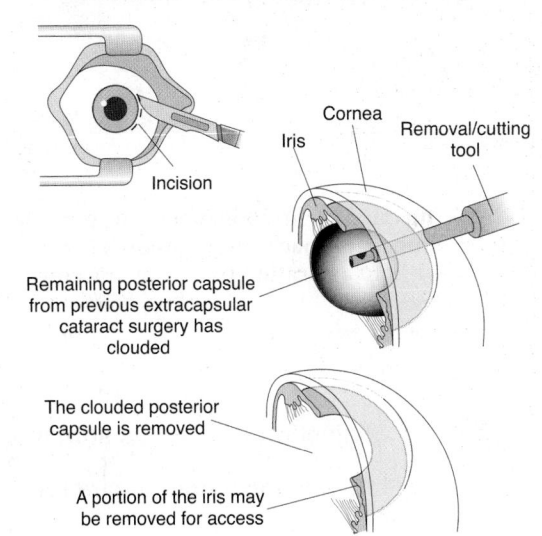

Incision

Iris — Cornea — Removal/cutting tool

Remaining posterior capsule from previous extracapsular cataract surgery has clouded

The clouded posterior capsule is removed

A portion of the iris may be removed for access

66840 Removal of lens material; aspiration technique, 1 or more stages   A 2 T

RVU Mod	Non-Fac Total	Fac Total	Global Days	Modifiers 51	50	62	80	MUE
	19.78	19.78	090	2	1	0	1	1

AMA: Fall 92: 4, Jan 09: 7, Apr 09: 9, Sep 09: 5

66850 Removal of lens material; phacofragmentation technique (mechanical or ultrasonic) (eg, phacoemulsification), with aspiration   A 2 T

RVU Mod	Non-Fac Total	Fac Total	Global Days	Modifiers 51	50	62	80	MUE
	22.50	22.50	090	2	1	0	1	1

AMA: Fall 92: 6, Jan 09: 7, Apr 09: 9, Sep 09: 5

66852 Removal of lens material; pars plana approach, with or without vitrectomy   A 2 J 1

RVU Mod	Non-Fac Total	Fac Total	Global Days	Modifiers 51	50	62	80	MUE
	23.99	23.99	090	2	1	1	0	1

AMA: Fall 92: 8, Jan 09: 7, Apr 09: 9, Sep 09: 5

66920 Removal of lens material; intracapsular   A 2 T

RVU Mod	Non-Fac Total	Fac Total	Global Days	Modifiers 51	50	62	80	MUE
	21.42	21.42	090	2	1	1	0	1

AMA: Fall 92: 8, Sep 09: 5

66930 Removal of lens material; intracapsular, for dislocated lens   A 2 J 1

RVU Mod	Non-Fac Total	Fac Total	Global Days	Modifiers 51	50	62	80	MUE
	24.34	24.34	090	2	1	0	0	1

AMA: Fall 92: 8, Sep 09: 5

66940 Removal of lens material; extracapsular (other than 66840, 66850, 66852)   A 2 T

RVU Mod	Non-Fac Total	Fac Total	Global Days	Modifiers 51	50	62	80	MUE
	22.23	22.23	090	2	1	1	0	1

AMA: Fall 92: 4, Jan 09: 7, Apr 09: 9, Sep 09: 5

Intraocular Lens Procedures

Coding Guidance

Laterality is required when reporting cataract removal with insertion of intraocular lens. Append modifier LT, RT or 50 to identify which eye(s) was treated. If intraocular lens power calculation is required at the time of insertion, the additional service may be reported with 66982-66985 using code 76519 for ultrasonic measurements or 92136 for optical lens measurements. Provision of the intraocular lens itself is not included and may be reported additionally with 99070 or HCPCS Level II codes Q1004-Q1005 or V2630-V2632 for supply of the lens.

66982 Extracapsular cataract removal with insertion of intraocular lens prosthesis (1-stage procedure), manual or mechanical technique (eg, irrigation and aspiration or phacoemulsification), complex, requiring devices or techniques not generally used in routine cataract surgery (eg, iris expansion device, suture support for intraocular lens, or primary posterior capsulorrhexis) or performed on patients in the amblyogenic developmental stage   A 2 T

RVU Mod	Non-Fac Total	Fac Total	Global Days	Modifiers 51	50	62	80	MUE
	22.48	22.48	090	2	1	0	1	1

AMA: Feb 01: 7, Nov 03: 10, Sep 09: 5, Mar 13: 6

Pub 100-04, 32, 120.2

66983 Intracapsular cataract extraction with insertion of intraocular lens prosthesis (1 stage procedure)   A 2 T

RVU Mod	Non-Fac Total	Fac Total	Global Days	Modifiers 51	50	62	80	MUE
	19.90	19.90	090	2	1	0	1	1

AMA: Fall 92: 5, 8, Nov 03: 10, Sep 09: 5, Mar 13: 6

Pub 100-04, 32, 120.2

● New   ▲ Revised   Deleted   ⊙ Moderate Sedation   ✚ Add-on Codes   ⊘ High Risk Denial   Ⓐ Age Edit   ♀ Female   ♂ Male   **AMA** *CPT® Assistant*   **MUE** Medically Unlikely Edit

⊘ Modifier 51 Exempt   ⊖ Modifier 63 Exempt   ⊠ Unlisted   **Modifiers:** *See Inside Back Cover*   Ⓜ Maternity   A 2 –Z 3 ASC Payment Indicators   A –Y OPPS Status Indicators

66984 Extracapsular cataract removal with insertion of intraocular lens prosthesis (1 stage procedure), manual or mechanical technique (eg, irrigation and aspiration or phacoemulsification) A 2 T

RVU			Global Days	Modifiers				
Mod	*Non-Fac Total*	*Fac Total*		51	50	62	80	MUE
	17.91	17.91	090	2	1	0	1	1

AMA: Fall 92: 5, 8, Feb 01: 7, Nov 03: 10, Mar 05: 11, Sep 09: 5, Mar 13: 6
Pub 100-04, 32, 120.2

66985 Insertion of intraocular lens prosthesis (secondary implant), not associated with concurrent cataract removal A 2 T

Coding tip: For implant of telescopic intraocular lens prosthesis for age-related macular degeneration, use Category III code 0308T. See HCPCS code C1840 for supply of the lens.

RVU			Global Days	Modifiers				
Mod	*Non-Fac Total*	*Fac Total*		51	50	62	80	MUE
	21.75	21.75	090	2	1	1	1	1

AMA: Sep 05: 12, Sep 09: 5, Dec 11: 16, Mar 13: 6
Pub 100-04, 32, 120.2

66986 Exchange of intraocular lens A 2 T

RVU			Global Days	Modifiers				
Mod	*Non-Fac Total*	*Fac Total*		51	50	62	80	MUE
	25.79	25.79	090	2	1	1	1	1

AMA: Sep 05: 12
Pub 100-04, 32, 120.2

Other Ophthalmic Procedures

✚ **66990** Use of ophthalmic endoscope (List separately in addition to code for primary procedure) ⊘N1N

RVU			Global Days	Modifiers				
Mod	*Non-Fac Total*	*Fac Total*		51	50	62	80	MUE
	2.57	2.57	ZZZ	0	0	0	1	1

AMA: Sep 05: 12, Oct 08: 3

66999 Unlisted procedure, anterior segment of eye ⊘x T

RVU			Global Days	Modifiers				
Mod	*Non-Fac Total*	*Fac Total*		51	50	62	80	MUE
	0.00	0.00	YYY	2	1	1	0	

Vitreous Procedures

67005 Removal of vitreous, anterior approach (open sky technique or limbal incision); partial removal A 2 T

RVU			Global Days	Modifiers				
Mod	*Non-Fac Total*	*Fac Total*		51	50	62	80	MUE
	13.40	13.40	090	2	1	1	1	1

AMA: Fall 92: 4

67010 Removal of vitreous, anterior approach (open sky technique or limbal incision); subtotal removal with mechanical vitrectomy A 2 T

RVU			Global Days	Modifiers				
Mod	*Non-Fac Total*	*Fac Total*		51	50	62	80	MUE
	15.40	15.40	090	2	1	1	1	1

AMA: Fall 92: 4

67015 Aspiration or release of vitreous, subretinal or choroidal fluid, pars plana approach (posterior sclerotomy) A 2 T

RVU			Global Days	Modifiers				
Mod	*Non-Fac Total*	*Fac Total*		51	50	62	80	MUE
	16.46	16.46	090	2	1	1	1	1

Aspiration or release of vitreous, subretinal or choroidal fluid, pars plana approach

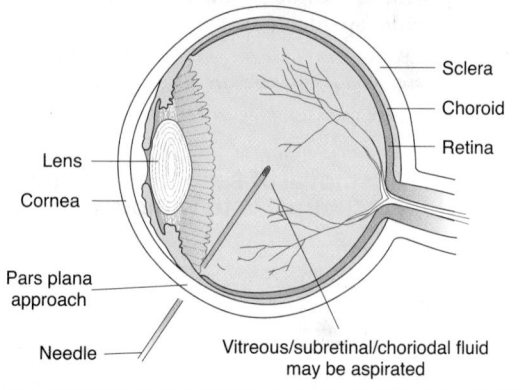

Sclera
Choroid
Retina
Lens
Cornea
Pars plana approach
Needle
Vitreous/subretinal/choroidal fluid may be aspirated

67025 Injection of vitreous substitute, pars plana or limbal approach (fluid-gas exchange), with or without aspiration (separate procedure) A 2 T

RVU			Global Days	Modifiers				
Mod	*Non-Fac Total*	*Fac Total*		51	50	62	80	MUE
	20.59	17.96	090	2	1	1	1	1

Injection of vitreous substitute, pars plana/limbal approach, with/without aspiration

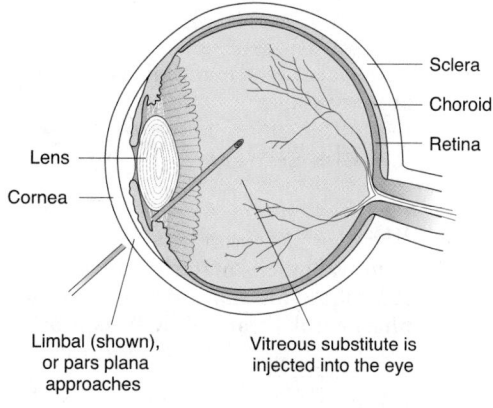

Sclera
Choroid
Retina
Lens
Cornea
Limbal (shown), or pars plana approaches
Vitreous substitute is injected into the eye

67027 Implantation of intravitreal drug delivery system (eg, ganciclovir implant), includes concomitant removal of vitreous A 2 J 1 1

RVU			Global Days	Modifiers				
Mod	*Non-Fac Total*	*Fac Total*		51	50	62	80	MUE
	24.22	24.22	090	2	1	1	2	1

AMA: Nov 97: 23, Nov 98: 1

● New   ▲ Revised   ✖ Deleted   ⊙ Moderate Sedation   ✚ Add-on Codes   ⊘ High Risk Denial   ⒶAge Edit   ♀ Female   ♂ Male   **AMA** *CPT® Assistant*   **MUE** Medically Unlikely Edit
⊘ Modifier 51 Exempt   ⊖ Modifier 63 Exempt   Ⓧ Unlisted   **Modifiers:** *See Inside Back Cover*   Ⓜ Maternity   A 2-Z 3 ASC Payment Indicators   A – Y OPPS Status Indicators

CPT © 2015 American Medical Association. All Rights Reserved.   © 2016 DecisionHealth

67028 Intravitreal injection of a pharmacologic agent (separate procedure) `P 3 S`

RVU		Global Days	Modifiers				
Mod	Non-Fac Total	Fac Total		51	50	62	80	MUE
	2.89	2.85	000	2	1	0	1	1

AMA: Winter 90: 9, Oct 12: 15

67030 Discission of vitreous strands (without removal), pars plana approach `A 2 T`

RVU		Global Days	Modifiers				
Mod	Non-Fac Total	Fac Total		51	50	62	80	MUE
	15.11	15.11	090	2	1	1	1	1

67031 Severing of vitreous strands, vitreous face adhesions, sheets, membranes or opacities, laser surgery (1 or more stages) `A 2 T`

RVU		Global Days	Modifiers				
Mod	Non-Fac Total	Fac Total		51	50	62	80	MUE
	11.02	10.13	090	2	1	0	1	1

67036 Vitrectomy, mechanical, pars plana approach `A 2 T`

RVU		Global Days	Modifiers				
Mod	Non-Fac Total	Fac Total		51	50	62	80	MUE
	25.61	25.61	090	2	1	1	2	1

AMA: Fall 92: 6, Oct 08: 3

67039 Vitrectomy, mechanical, pars plana approach; with focal endolaser photocoagulation `A 2 J 1`

RVU		Global Days	Modifiers				
Mod	Non-Fac Total	Fac Total		51	50	62	80	MUE
	27.44	27.44	090	2	1	1	2	1

AMA: Winter 90: 9, Sep 05: 12

67040 Vitrectomy, mechanical, pars plana approach; with endolaser panretinal photocoagulation `A 2 J 1`

RVU		Global Days	Modifiers				
Mod	Non-Fac Total	Fac Total		51	50	62	80	MUE
	29.65	29.65	090	2	1	1	2	1

AMA: Winter 90: 9, Sep 05: 12, Jul 07: 12

67041 Vitrectomy, mechanical, pars plana approach; with removal of preretinal cellular membrane (eg, macular pucker) `G 2 T`

RVU		Global Days	Modifiers				
Mod	Non-Fac Total	Fac Total		51	50	62	80	MUE
	32.76	32.76	090	2	1	1	2	1

67042 Vitrectomy, mechanical, pars plana approach; with removal of internal limiting membrane of retina (eg, for repair of macular hole, diabetic macular edema), includes, if performed, intraocular tamponade (ie, air, gas or silicone oil) `G 2 J 1`

RVU		Global Days	Modifiers				
Mod	Non-Fac Total	Fac Total		51	50	62	80	MUE
	32.76	32.76	090	2	1	1	2	1

67043 Vitrectomy, mechanical, pars plana approach; with removal of subretinal membrane (eg, choroidal neovascularization), includes, if performed, intraocular tamponade (ie, air, gas or silicone oil) and laser photocoagulation `G 2 J 1`

RVU		Global Days	Modifiers				
Mod	Non-Fac Total	Fac Total		51	50	62	80	MUE
	34.59	34.59	090	2	1	1	2	1

Retina/Choroid Procedures

Retina/Choroid Repair

Coding Guidance
Some retinal detachment repair codes include other vitreous procedures as part of the code descriptor. Some retinal detachment repair codes are mutually exclusive of anterior procedures, such as focal endolaser photocoagulation.

▲ 67101 Repair of retinal detachment, 1 or more sessions; cryotherapy or diathermy, including drainage of subretinal fluid, when performed `P 3 T`

RVU		Global Days	Modifiers				
Mod	Non-Fac Total	Fac Total		51	50	62	80	MUE
	22.22	19.15	090	2	1	0	1	1

AMA: Mar 98: 7

▲ 67105 Repair of retinal detachment, 1 or more sessions; photocoagulation, including drainage of subretinal fluid, when performed `P 2 T`

RVU		Global Days	Modifiers				
Mod	Non-Fac Total	Fac Total		51	50	62	80	MUE
	20.40	18.29	090	2	1	0	1	1

AMA: Mar 98: 7

▲ 67107 Repair of retinal detachment; scleral buckling (such as lamellar scleral dissection, imbrication or encircling procedure), including, when performed, implant, cryotherapy, photocoagulation, and drainage of subretinal fluid `G 2 J 1`

RVU		Global Days	Modifiers				
Mod	Non-Fac Total	Fac Total		51	50	62	80	MUE
	28.90	28.90	090	2	1	1	2	1

▲ 67108 Repair of retinal detachment; with vitrectomy, any method, including, when performed, air or gas tamponade, focal endolaser photocoagulation, cryotherapy, drainage of subretinal fluid, scleral buckling, and/or removal of lens by same technique `G 2 J 1`

Coding tip: Code 67108 includes 67015, 67025, 67028, 67031, 67036, 67039, and 67040.

RVU		Global Days	Modifiers				
Mod	Non-Fac Total	Fac Total		51	50	62	80	MUE
	30.83	30.83	090	2	1	1	2	1

AMA: Winter 90: 9, Mar 12: 9

67110 Repair of retinal detachment; by injection of air or other gas (eg, pneumatic retinopexy) `P 3 T`

Coding tip: Code 67108 is included in codes 67110 and 67112 and should not be reported separately.

RVU		Global Days	Modifiers				
Mod	Non-Fac Total	Fac Total		51	50	62	80	MUE
	21.56	19.79	090	2	1	0	1	1

AMA: Winter 90: 9

✗ ~~67112 Repair of retinal detachment; by scleral buckling or vitrectomy, on patient having previous ipsilateral retinal detachment repair(s) using scleral buckling or vitrectomy techniques~~

● New   ▲ Revised   Deleted   ⊙ Moderate Sedation   ✚ Add-on Codes   ⊘ High Risk Denial   Ⓐ Age Edit   ♀ Female   ♂ Male   **AMA** *CPT® Assistant*   **MUE** Medically Unlikely Edit
⊘ Modifier 51 Exempt   ⊖ Modifier 63 Exempt   ✗ Unlisted   **Modifiers:** *See Inside Back Cover*   Ⓜ Maternity   A2–Z3 ASC Payment Indicators   A–Y OPPS Status Indicators

Surgical Procedures

67113 – 67228

▲ **67113** Repair of complex retinal detachment (eg, proliferative vitreoretinopathy, stage C-1 or greater, diabetic traction retinal detachment, retinopathy of prematurity, retinal tear of greater than 90 degrees), with vitrectomy and membrane peeling, including, when performed, air, gas, or silicone oil tamponade, cryotherapy, endolaser photocoagulation, drainage of subretinal fluid, scleral buckling, and/or removal of lens G2 J I

RVU			Global Days	Modifiers				
Mod	Non-Fac Total	Fac Total		51	50	62	80	MUE
	38.09	38.09	090	2	1	1	2	1

67115 Release of encircling material (posterior segment) A 2 T

RVU			Global Days	Modifiers				
Mod	Non-Fac Total	Fac Total		51	50	62	80	MUE
	14.18	14.18	090	2	1	0	1	1

67120 Removal of implanted material, posterior segment; extraocular A 2 T

RVU			Global Days	Modifiers				
Mod	Non-Fac Total	Fac Total		51	50	62	80	MUE
	18.63	15.84	090	2	1	1	1	1

67121 Removal of implanted material, posterior segment; intraocular A 2 T

RVU			Global Days	Modifiers				
Mod	Non-Fac Total	Fac Total		51	50	62	80	MUE
	25.81	25.81	090	2	1	1	2	1

AMA: Nov 97: 23, Nov 98: 19

Retinal Detachment Prophylaxis

67141 Prophylaxis of retinal detachment (eg, retinal break, lattice degeneration) without drainage, 1 or more sessions; cryotherapy, diathermy A 2 T

RVU			Global Days	Modifiers				
Mod	Non-Fac Total	Fac Total		51	50	62	80	MUE
	14.85	13.85	090	2	1	0	1	1

AMA: Mar 98: 7, Oct 08: 3

67145 Prophylaxis of retinal detachment (eg, retinal break, lattice degeneration) without drainage, 1 or more sessions; photocoagulation (laser or xenon arc) P 2 T

RVU			Global Days	Modifiers				
Mod	Non-Fac Total	Fac Total		51	50	62	80	MUE
	14.94	14.13	090	2	1	0	1	1

AMA: Fall 92: 4, Mar 98: 7

Retina/Choroid Destruction

67208 Destruction of localized lesion of retina (eg, macular edema, tumors), 1 or more sessions; cryotherapy, diathermy P 2 T

RVU			Global Days	Modifiers				
Mod	Non-Fac Total	Fac Total		51	50	62	80	MUE
	17.01	16.42	090	2	1	0	1	1

AMA: Mar 98: 7, Nov 98: 19, Oct 08: 3

67210 Destruction of localized lesion of retina (eg, macular edema, tumors), 1 or more sessions; photocoagulation P 2 T

RVU			Global Days	Modifiers				
Mod	Non-Fac Total	Fac Total		51	50	62	80	MUE
	14.69	14.20	090	2	1	0	1	1

AMA: Mar 98: 7, Nov 98: 19, Oct 08: 3, Jan 12: 3

67218 Destruction of localized lesion of retina (eg, macular edema, tumors), 1 or more sessions; radiation by implantation of source (includes removal of source) A 2 T

RVU			Global Days	Modifiers				
Mod	Non-Fac Total	Fac Total		51	50	62	80	MUE
	39.32	39.32	090	2	1	0	1	1

AMA: Mar 98: 7, Oct 08: 3

67220 Destruction of localized lesion of choroid (eg, choroidal neovascularization); photocoagulation (eg, laser), 1 or more sessions P 2 T

RVU			Global Days	Modifiers				
Mod	Non-Fac Total	Fac Total		51	50	62	80	MUE
	15.15	14.20	090	2	1	0	1	1

AMA: Nov 98: 19, Nov 99: 39, Feb 01: 8, Oct 08: 3, Jan 12: 3

67221 Destruction of localized lesion of choroid (eg, choroidal neovascularization); photodynamic therapy (includes intravenous infusion) P 3 T

RVU			Global Days	Modifiers				
Mod	Non-Fac Total	Fac Total		51	50	62	80	MUE
	8.13	6.07	000	2	0	0	1	1

AMA: Feb 01: 8, Sep 01: 10, Jun 02: 10
Pub 100-04, 32, 300.1, 300.2

+ **67225** Destruction of localized lesion of choroid (eg, choroidal neovascularization); photodynamic therapy, second eye, at single session (List separately in addition to code for primary eye treatment) N I N

RVU			Global Days	Modifiers				
Mod	Non-Fac Total	Fac Total		51	50	62	80	MUE
	0.84	0.80	ZZZ	0	0	0	1	1

AMA: Jun 02: 10
Pub 100-04, 32, 300.1, 300.2

▲ **67227** Destruction of extensive or progressive retinopathy (eg, diabetic retinopathy), cryotherapy, diathermy G 2 T

RVU			Global Days	Modifiers				
Mod	Non-Fac Total	Fac Total		51	50	62	80	MUE
	8.21	7.29	090	2	1	0	1	1

AMA: Mar 98: 7, Oct 08: 3

▲ **67228** Treatment of extensive or progressive retinopathy (eg, diabetic retinopathy), photocoagulation P 3 T

RVU			Global Days	Modifiers				
Mod	Non-Fac Total	Fac Total		51	50	62	80	MUE
	9.67	8.72	090	2	1	0	1	1

AMA: Mar 98: 7, Oct 08: 3

● New   ▲ Revised   ✖ Deleted   ⊙ Moderate Sedation   ✚ Add-on Codes   ⊘ High Risk Denial   Ⓐ Age Edit   ♀ Female   ♂ Male   **AMA** *CPT® Assistant*   **MUE** Medically Unlikely Edit
⊘ Modifier 51 Exempt   ⊖ Modifier 63 Exempt   ✗ Unlisted   **Modifiers:** *See Inside Back Cover*   Ⓜ Maternity   A 2 – Z 3 ASC Payment Indicators   A – Y OPPS Status Indicators

596   CPT © 2015 American Medical Association. All Rights Reserved.   © 2016 DecisionHealth

67229 Treatment of extensive or progressive retinopathy, 1 or more sessions, preterm infant (less than 37 weeks gestation at birth), performed from birth up to 1 year of age (eg, retinopathy of prematurity), photocoagulation or cryotherapy   ⊗Ⓐ R 2 T

RVU			Global Days	Modifiers				
Mod	Non-Fac Total	Fac Total		51	50	62	80	MUE
	31.73	31.73	090	2	1	0	1	1

Posterior Scleral Procedures

Posterior Scleral Repair

67250 Scleral reinforcement (separate procedure); without graft   A 2 T

RVU			Global Days	Modifiers				
Mod	Non-Fac Total	Fac Total		51	50	62	80	MUE
	22.16	22.16	090	2	1	1	1	1

67255 Scleral reinforcement (separate procedure); with graft   A 2 T

RVU			Global Days	Modifiers				
Mod	Non-Fac Total	Fac Total		51	50	62	80	MUE
	19.40	19.40	090	2	1	1	2	1

AMA: Jun 12: 15, Jan 15: 10

Other Posterior Scleral Procedures

67299 Unlisted procedure, posterior segment   ✗ T

RVU			Global Days	Modifiers				
Mod	Non-Fac Total	Fac Total		51	50	62	80	MUE
	0.00	0.00	YYY	2	1	1	0	

Extraocular Muscle Procedures

67311 Strabismus surgery, recession or resection procedure; 1 horizontal muscle   A 2 T

RVU			Global Days	Modifiers				
Mod	Non-Fac Total	Fac Total		51	50	62	80	MUE
	16.99	16.99	090	2	1	0	1	1

AMA: Summer 93: 20, Mar 97: 5, Nov 98: 19, Sep 02: 10

67312 Strabismus surgery, recession or resection procedure; 2 horizontal muscles   A 2 T

RVU			Global Days	Modifiers				
Mod	Non-Fac Total	Fac Total		51	50	62	80	MUE
	20.24	20.24	090	2	1	1	1	1

AMA: Summer 93: 20, Mar 97: 5

67314 Strabismus surgery, recession or resection procedure; 1 vertical muscle (excluding superior oblique)   A 2 T

RVU			Global Days	Modifiers				
Mod	Non-Fac Total	Fac Total		51	50	62	80	MUE
	19.12	19.12	090	2	1	0	1	1

AMA: Summer 93: 20, Mar 97: 5

67316 Strabismus surgery, recession or resection procedure; 2 or more vertical muscles (excluding superior oblique)   A 2 T

RVU			Global Days	Modifiers				
Mod	Non-Fac Total	Fac Total		51	50	62	80	MUE
	22.77	22.77	090	2	1	0	0	1

AMA: Summer 93: 20, Mar 97: 5

67318 Strabismus surgery, any procedure, superior oblique muscle   A 2 T

RVU			Global Days	Modifiers				
Mod	Non-Fac Total	Fac Total		51	50	62	80	MUE
	19.99	19.99	090	2	1	1	1	1

AMA: Summer 93: 20, Mar 97: 5, Nov 98: 19

+ 67320 Transposition procedure (eg, for paretic extraocular muscle), any extraocular muscle (specify) (List separately in addition to code for primary procedure)   N I N

RVU			Global Days	Modifiers				
Mod	Non-Fac Total	Fac Total		51	50	62	80	MUE
	9.18	9.18	ZZZ	0	0	0	1	2

AMA: Summer 93: 20, Mar 97: 5

+ 67331 Strabismus surgery on patient with previous eye surgery or injury that did not involve the extraocular muscles (List separately in addition to code for primary procedure)   N I N

RVU			Global Days	Modifiers				
Mod	Non-Fac Total	Fac Total		51	50	62	80	MUE
	8.71	8.71	ZZZ	0	1	1	1	1

AMA: Summer 93: 20, Mar 97: 5

+ 67332 Strabismus surgery on patient with scarring of extraocular muscles (eg, prior ocular injury, strabismus or retinal detachment surgery) or restrictive myopathy (eg, dysthyroid ophthalmopathy) (List separately in addition to code for primary procedure)   N I N

RVU			Global Days	Modifiers				
Mod	Non-Fac Total	Fac Total		51	50	62	80	MUE
	9.46	9.46	ZZZ	0	1	1	1	1

AMA: Summer 93: 20, Mar 97: 5

+ 67334 Strabismus surgery by posterior fixation suture technique, with or without muscle recession (List separately in addition to code for primary procedure)   N I N

RVU			Global Days	Modifiers				
Mod	Non-Fac Total	Fac Total		51	50	62	80	MUE
	8.59	8.59	ZZZ	0	1	1	1	1

AMA: Summer 93: 20, Mar 97: 5

+ 67335 Placement of adjustable suture(s) during strabismus surgery, including postoperative adjustment(s) of suture(s) (List separately in addition to code for specific strabismus surgery)   N I N

RVU			Global Days	Modifiers				
Mod	Non-Fac Total	Fac Total		51	50	62	80	MUE
	4.24	4.24	ZZZ	0	1	1	1	1

AMA: Summer 93: 20, Mar 97: 5

● New   ▲ Revised   Deleted   ⊙ Moderate Sedation   ✚ Add-on Codes   ⊗ High Risk Denial   Ⓐ Age Edit   ♀ Female   ♂ Male   **AMA** CPT® Assistant   **MUE** Medically Unlikely Edit
⊘ Modifier 51 Exempt   ⊖ Modifier 63 Exempt   ✗ Unlisted   **Modifiers:** See Inside Back Cover   Ⓜ Maternity   A 2–Z 3 ASC Payment Indicators   A–Y OPPS Status Indicators

© 2016 DecisionHealth   CPT © 2015 American Medical Association. All Rights Reserved.   **597**

+ 67340 Strabismus surgery involving exploration and/ or repair of detached extraocular muscle(s) (List separately in addition to code for primary procedure) N1N

RVU			Global Days	Modifiers				
Mod	Non-Fac Total	Fac Total		51	50	62	80	MUE
	10.21	10.21	ZZZ	0	0	0	2	2

AMA: Summer 93: 20, Mar 97: 5

67343 Release of extensive scar tissue without detaching extraocular muscle (separate procedure) A2T

RVU			Global Days	Modifiers				
Mod	Non-Fac Total	Fac Total		51	50	62	80	MUE
	18.58	18.58	090	2	1	1	1	1

AMA: Summer 93: 20, Mar 97: 5

67345 Chemodenervation of extraocular muscle P3T

RVU			Global Days	Modifiers				
Mod	Non-Fac Total	Fac Total		51	50	62	80	MUE
	6.90	6.22	010	2	1	0	1	1

AMA: Summer 93: 20, Mar 97: 5, Apr 00: 2, Feb 10: 13, Dec 13: 10, May 14: 5

Chemodenervation of extraocular muscle

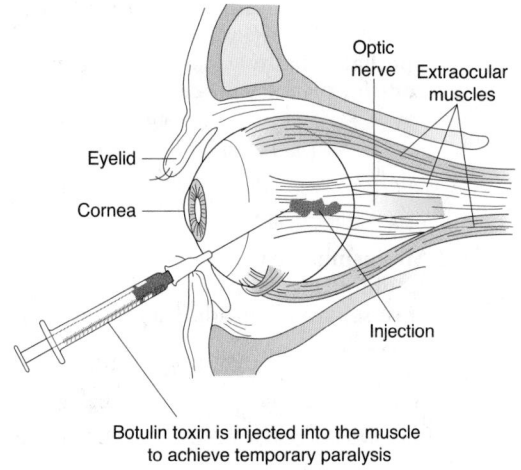

Botulin toxin is injected into the muscle to achieve temporary paralysis

67346 Biopsy of extraocular muscle A2T

RVU			Global Days	Modifiers				
Mod	Non-Fac Total	Fac Total		51	50	62	80	MUE
	5.50	5.50	000	2	1	0	0	1

Other Ocular Muscle Procedures

67399 Unlisted procedure, extraocular muscle ⊗x T

RVU			Global Days	Modifiers				
Mod	Non-Fac Total	Fac Total		51	50	62	80	MUE
	0.00	0.00	YYY	2	1	1	2	

Orbital Procedures

Orbital Exploration/Excision/Decompression Procedures

67400 Orbitotomy without bone flap (frontal or transconjunctival approach); for exploration, with or without biopsy A2T

RVU			Global Days	Modifiers				
Mod	Non-Fac Total	Fac Total		51	50	62	80	MUE
	26.40	26.40	090	2	1	1	1	1

Orbitotomy without bone flap (frontal/transconjuntival approach) exploration/biopsy/drainage

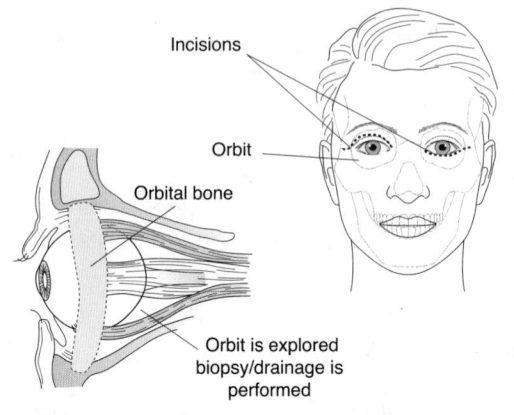

Incisions

Orbit

Orbital bone

Orbit is explored biopsy/drainage is performed

Exploration with/without biopsy use code (67400), for drainage only use code (67405)

67405 Orbitotomy without bone flap (frontal or transconjunctival approach); with drainage only A2T

RVU			Global Days	Modifiers				
Mod	Non-Fac Total	Fac Total		51	50	62	80	MUE
	22.56	22.56	090	2	1	0	1	1

67412 Orbitotomy without bone flap (frontal or transconjunctival approach); with removal of lesion A2T

RVU			Global Days	Modifiers				
Mod	Non-Fac Total	Fac Total		51	50	62	80	MUE
	24.16	24.16	090	2	1	1	1	1

67413 Orbitotomy without bone flap (frontal or transconjunctival approach); with removal of foreign body A2T

RVU			Global Days	Modifiers				
Mod	Non-Fac Total	Fac Total		51	50	62	80	MUE
	24.31	24.31	090	2	1	0	2	1

67414 Orbitotomy without bone flap (frontal or transconjunctival approach); with removal of bone for decompression G2T

RVU			Global Days	Modifiers				
Mod	Non-Fac Total	Fac Total		51	50	62	80	MUE
	37.63	37.63	090	2	1	1	2	1

AMA: Jul 99: 10

● New   ▲ Revised   ✖ Deleted   ⊙ Moderate Sedation   ✚ Add-on Codes   ⊘ High Risk Denial   Ⓐ Age Edit   ♀ Female   ♂ Male   **AMA** CPT® Assistant   **MUE** Medically Unlikely Edit
⊘ Modifier 51 Exempt   ⊖ Modifier 63 Exempt   ⊠ Unlisted   **Modifiers:** See Inside Back Cover   Ⓜ Maternity   A2–Z3 ASC Payment Indicators   A–Y OPPS Status Indicators

CPT © 2015 American Medical Association. All Rights Reserved.   © 2016 DecisionHealth

67415 Fine needle aspiration of orbital contents A 2 T

RVU			Global Days	Modifiers				
Mod	Non-Fac Total	Fac Total		51	50	62	80	MUE
	2.98	2.98	000	2	1	0	0	1

67420 Orbitotomy with bone flap or window, lateral approach (eg, Kroenlein); with removal of lesion A 2 T

RVU			Global Days	Modifiers				
Mod	Non-Fac Total	Fac Total		51	50	62	80	MUE
	45.96	45.96	090	2	1	1	2	1

67430 Orbitotomy with bone flap or window, lateral approach (eg, Kroenlein); with removal of foreign body A 2 T

RVU			Global Days	Modifiers				
Mod	Non-Fac Total	Fac Total		51	50	62	80	MUE
	35.18	35.18	090	2	1	0	2	1

67440 Orbitotomy with bone flap or window, lateral approach (eg, Kroenlein); with drainage A 2 T

RVU			Global Days	Modifiers				
Mod	Non-Fac Total	Fac Total		51	50	62	80	MUE
	34.17	34.17	090	2	1	1	2	1

67445 Orbitotomy with bone flap or window, lateral approach (eg, Kroenlein); with removal of bone for decompression A 2 T

RVU			Global Days	Modifiers				
Mod	Non-Fac Total	Fac Total		51	50	62	80	MUE
	39.80	39.80	090	2	1	1	2	1

67450 Orbitotomy with bone flap or window, lateral approach (eg, Kroenlein); for exploration, with or without biopsy A 2 T

RVU			Global Days	Modifiers				
Mod	Non-Fac Total	Fac Total		51	50	62	80	MUE
	35.64	35.64	090	2	1	1	2	1

Other Orbital Procedures

Coding Guidance

When it is medically necessary to inject a sclerosing agent during the same session as glaucoma surgery, the injection is included in the surgical service. Codes 67500, 67515, and 68200 for injection of the sclerosing agent should not be reported with other pressure-reducing or glaucoma procedures.

67500 Retrobulbar injection; medication (separate procedure, does not include supply of medication) G 2 T

RVU			Global Days	Modifiers				
Mod	Non-Fac Total	Fac Total		51	50	62	80	MUE
	2.25	2.07	000	2	1	0	1	1

AMA: Nov 12: 10

67505 Retrobulbar injection; alcohol P 3 T

RVU			Global Days	Modifiers				
Mod	Non-Fac Total	Fac Total		51	50	62	80	MUE
	2.53	2.31	000	2	1	0	1	1

67515 Injection of medication or other substance into Tenon's capsule P 3 T

RVU			Global Days	Modifiers				
Mod	Non-Fac Total	Fac Total		51	50	62	80	MUE
	2.75	2.54	000	2	1	0	1	1

AMA: Nov 12: 10

Injection of medication or other substance into Tenon's capsule

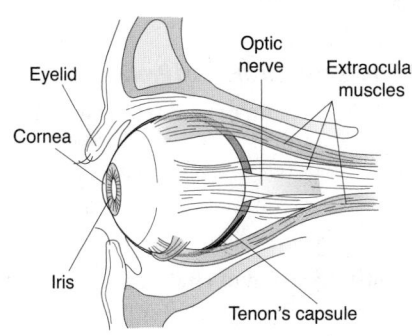

The physician injects medication or another substance into the the thin sac that surrounds the eye and allows it to move in the eye socket.

67550 Orbital implant (implant outside muscle cone); insertion A 2 T

RVU			Global Days	Modifiers				
Mod	Non-Fac Total	Fac Total		51	50	62	80	MUE
	27.38	27.38	090	2	1	1	1	1

67560 Orbital implant (implant outside muscle cone); removal or revision A 2 T

RVU			Global Days	Modifiers				
Mod	Non-Fac Total	Fac Total		51	50	62	80	MUE
	28.07	28.07	090	2	1	0	0	1

67570 Optic nerve decompression (eg, incision or fenestration of optic nerve sheath) A 2 T

RVU			Global Days	Modifiers				
Mod	Non-Fac Total	Fac Total		51	50	62	80	MUE
	32.95	32.95	090	2	1	1	2	1

67599 Unlisted procedure, orbit ⊘x T

RVU			Global Days	Modifiers				
Mod	Non-Fac Total	Fac Total		51	50	62	80	MUE
	0.00	0.00	YYY	2	1	1	2	

Eyelid Procedures

Incisional Eyelid Procedures

Coding Guidance

Incisional biopsy of eyelid skin including the lid margin (67810) is listed out of order under excision/destruction.

67700 Blepharotomy, drainage of abscess, eyelid P 2 T

RVU			Global Days	Modifiers				
Mod	Non-Fac Total	Fac Total		51	50	62	80	MUE
	7.58	3.31	010	2	1	0	1	2

AMA: Mar 13: 6

● New   ▲ Revised   Deleted   ⊙ Moderate Sedation   ✚ Add-on Codes   ⊘ High Risk Denial   Ⓐ Age Edit   ♀ Female   ♂ Male   **AMA** *CPT® Assistant*   **MUE** Medically Unlikely Edit
⊘ Modifier 51 Exempt   ⊖ Modifier 63 Exempt   🗙 Unlisted   **Modifiers:** *See Inside Back Cover*   Ⓜ Maternity   A 2 - Z 3 ASC Payment Indicators   A - Y OPPS Status Indicators

© 2016 DecisionHealth   CPT © 2015 American Medical Association. All Rights Reserved.   **599**

Surgical Procedures

67415 – 67700

Surgical Procedures

67710 – 67882

67710 Severing of tarsorrhaphy   P 3 T

RVU			Global Days	Modifiers				
Mod	Non-Fac Total	Fac Total		51	50	62	80	MUE
	6.32	2.77	010	2	1	0	1	1

AMA: Mar 13: 6

67715 Canthotomy (separate procedure)   A 2 T

RVU			Global Days	Modifiers				
Mod	Non-Fac Total	Fac Total		51	50	62	80	MUE
	6.77	3.08	010	2	1	0	1	1

AMA: Mar 13: 6

Excisional/Destruction Eyelid Procedures

67800 Excision of chalazion; single   P 3 T

RVU			Global Days	Modifiers				
Mod	Non-Fac Total	Fac Total		51	50	62	80	MUE
	3.60	2.94	010	2	0	0	1	1

AMA: Sep 99: 10

67801 Excision of chalazion; multiple, same lid   P 3 T

RVU			Global Days	Modifiers				
Mod	Non-Fac Total	Fac Total		51	50	62	80	MUE
	4.58	3.80	010	2	0	0	1	1

67805 Excision of chalazion; multiple, different lids   P 3 T

RVU			Global Days	Modifiers				
Mod	Non-Fac Total	Fac Total		51	50	62	80	MUE
	5.71	4.69	010	2	0	0	1	1

AMA: Sep 99: 10

67808 Excision of chalazion; under general anesthesia and/or requiring hospitalization, single or multiple   A 2 T

RVU			Global Days	Modifiers				
Mod	Non-Fac Total	Fac Total		51	50	62	80	MUE
	10.49	10.49	090	2	0	0	1	1

67810 Incisional biopsy of eyelid skin including lid margin   P 3 T

Coding tip: Code 67810 is listed out of numerical order in CPT. Related incision procedures - 67700-67715

RVU			Global Days	Modifiers				
Mod	Non-Fac Total	Fac Total		51	50	62	80	MUE
	4.87	2.05	000	2	1	0	1	2

AMA: Mar 13: 6, Dec 04: 19, Feb 13: 16

67820 Correction of trichiasis; epilation, by forceps only   N I Q I

RVU			Global Days	Modifiers				
Mod	Non-Fac Total	Fac Total		51	50	62	80	MUE
	1.41	1.50	000	2	1	0	1	1

AMA: Jul 98: 10

67825 Correction of trichiasis; epilation by other than forceps (eg, by electrosurgery, cryotherapy, laser surgery)   P 3 T

RVU			Global Days	Modifiers				
Mod	Non-Fac Total	Fac Total		51	50	62	80	MUE
	3.64	3.45	010	2	1	0	1	1

AMA: Jul 98: 10

67830 Correction of trichiasis; incision of lid margin   A 2 T

RVU			Global Days	Modifiers				
Mod	Non-Fac Total	Fac Total		51	50	62	80	MUE
	7.54	3.93	010	2	1	0	1	1

67835 Correction of trichiasis; incision of lid margin, with free mucous membrane graft   A 2 T

RVU			Global Days	Modifiers				
Mod	Non-Fac Total	Fac Total		51	50	62	80	MUE
	12.44	12.44	090	2	1	0	0	1

67840 Excision of lesion of eyelid (except chalazion) without closure or with simple direct closure   P 3 T

RVU			Global Days	Modifiers				
Mod	Non-Fac Total	Fac Total		51	50	62	80	MUE
	7.78	4.50	010	2	1	0	1	4

67850 Destruction of lesion of lid margin (up to 1 cm)   P 3 T

RVU			Global Days	Modifiers				
Mod	Non-Fac Total	Fac Total		51	50	62	80	MUE
	6.07	3.87	010	2	1	0	1	3

Eyelid Suture

67875 Temporary closure of eyelids by suture (eg, Frost suture)   G 2 T

RVU			Global Days	Modifiers				
Mod	Non-Fac Total	Fac Total		51	50	62	80	MUE
	4.85	2.77	000	2	1	0	1	1

AMA: Winter 90: 9

67880 Construction of intermarginal adhesions, median tarsorrhaphy, or canthorrhaphy   A 2 T

RVU			Global Days	Modifiers				
Mod	Non-Fac Total	Fac Total		51	50	62	80	MUE
	12.98	10.47	090	2	1	0	1	1

67882 Construction of intermarginal adhesions, median tarsorrhaphy, or canthorrhaphy; with transposition of tarsal plate   A 2 T

RVU			Global Days	Modifiers				
Mod	Non-Fac Total	Fac Total		51	50	62	80	MUE
	15.97	13.41	090	2	1	0	1	1

● New   ▲ Revised   ✖ Deleted   ⊙ Moderate Sedation   ✚ Add-on Codes   ⊘ High Risk Denial   Ⓐ Age Edit   ♀ Female   ♂ Male   **AMA** *CPT® Assistant*   **MUE** Medically Unlikely Edit
⊘ Modifier 51 Exempt   ⊖ Modifier 63 Exempt   ✖ Unlisted   **Modifiers:** *See Inside Back Cover*   Ⓜ Maternity   A 2 – Z 3 ASC Payment Indicators   A – Y OPPS Status Indicators

600   CPT © 2015 American Medical Association. All Rights Reserved.   © 2016 DecisionHealth

Surgical Procedures

Eyelid Repair

67900 Repair of brow ptosis (supraciliary, mid-forehead or coronal approach)   A 2 T

RVU			Global Days	Modifiers				
Mod	Non-Fac Total	Fac Total		51	50	62	80	MUE
	18.16	14.50	090	2	1	0	1	1

**Repair of brow ptosis
(supraciliary, mid-forehead/coronal**

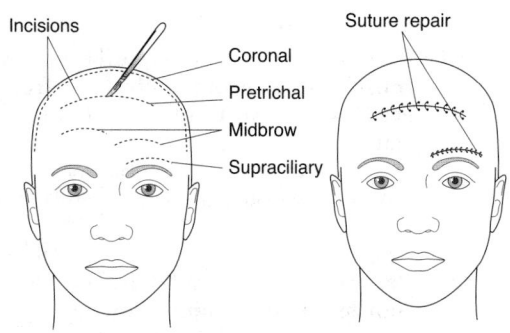

A droopy brow is repaired by making incisions and reapproximating its position

67901 Repair of blepharoptosis; frontalis muscle technique with suture or other material (eg, banked fascia)   ⊘ A 2 T

RVU			Global Days	Modifiers				
Mod	Non-Fac Total	Fac Total		51	50	62	80	MUE
	21.43	16.39	090	2	1	0	1	1

AMA: Sep 00: 7, Oct 06: 11

67902 Repair of blepharoptosis; frontalis muscle technique with autologous fascial sling (includes obtaining fascia)   A 2 T

RVU			Global Days	Modifiers				
Mod	Non-Fac Total	Fac Total		51	50	62	80	MUE
	20.58	20.58	090	2	1	1	1	1

AMA: Sep 00: 7, Oct 06: 11

67903 Repair of blepharoptosis; (tarso) levator resection or advancement, internal approach   A 2 T

RVU			Global Days	Modifiers				
Mod	Non-Fac Total	Fac Total		51	50	62	80	MUE
	16.81	13.75	090	2	1	1	1	1

AMA: Sep 00: 7, Oct 06: 11

67904 Repair of blepharoptosis; (tarso) levator resection or advancement, external approach   A 2 T

RVU			Global Days	Modifiers				
Mod	Non-Fac Total	Fac Total		51	50	62	80	MUE
	20.75	16.98	090	2	1	1	1	1

AMA: Sep 00: 7, Oct 06: 11, Aug 11: 8

67906 Repair of blepharoptosis; superior rectus technique with fascial sling (includes obtaining fascia)   A 2 T

RVU			Global Days	Modifiers				
Mod	Non-Fac Total	Fac Total		51	50	62	80	MUE
	14.40	14.40	090	2	1	0	1	1

AMA: Sep 00: 7, Oct 06: 11

67908 Repair of blepharoptosis; conjunctivo-tarso-Muller's muscle-levator resection (eg, Fasanella-Servat type)   A 2 T

RVU			Global Days	Modifiers				
Mod	Non-Fac Total	Fac Total		51	50	62	80	MUE
	13.97	12.06	090	2	1	0	1	1

AMA: Sep 00: 7, Oct 06: 11

67909 Reduction of overcorrection of ptosis   A 2 T

RVU			Global Days	Modifiers				
Mod	Non-Fac Total	Fac Total		51	50	62	80	MUE
	15.19	12.47	090	2	1	0	1	1

67911 Correction of lid retraction   A 2 T

Coding tip: A full-thickness graft is included as part of the total service for 67911; do not report code 15260 in addition to 67911

RVU			Global Days	Modifiers				
Mod	Non-Fac Total	Fac Total		51	50	62	80	MUE
	15.98	15.98	090	2	1	0	1	4

67912 Correction of lagophthalmos, with implantation of upper eyelid lid load (eg, gold weight)   A 2 T

RVU			Global Days	Modifiers				
Mod	Non-Fac Total	Fac Total		51	50	62	80	MUE
	25.02	13.99	090	2	1	0	1	1

AMA: May 04: 12, Aug 04: 10, Oct 06: 11

67914 Repair of ectropion; suture   A 2 T

RVU			Global Days	Modifiers				
Mod	Non-Fac Total	Fac Total		51	50	62	80	MUE
	13.29	9.30	090	2	1	0	1	1

67915 Repair of ectropion; thermocauterization   P 3 T

RVU			Global Days	Modifiers				
Mod	Non-Fac Total	Fac Total		51	50	62	80	MUE
	8.28	5.62	090	2	1	0	1	1

67916 Repair of ectropion; excision tarsal wedge   A 2 T

RVU			Global Days	Modifiers				
Mod	Non-Fac Total	Fac Total		51	50	62	80	MUE
	16.76	12.25	090	2	1	0	1	1

AMA: Feb 04: 11, May 04: 12, Feb 05: 16, Oct 06: 11

67917 Repair of ectropion; extensive (eg, tarsal strip operations)   A 2 T

Coding tip: Canthoplasty is included in blepharoplasties and some other repair/correction procedures. Do not report 67950 in addition to 67917.

RVU			Global Days	Modifiers				
Mod	Non-Fac Total	Fac Total		51	50	62	80	MUE
	17.07	13.02	090	2	1	0	1	1

AMA: Feb 04: 11, May 04: 12, Oct 06: 11

67921 Repair of entropion; suture   A 2 T

RVU			Global Days	Modifiers				
Mod	Non-Fac Total	Fac Total		51	50	62	80	MUE
	13.02	8.82	090	2	1	0	1	1

67922 Repair of entropion; thermocauterization   P 3 T

RVU			Global Days	Modifiers				
Mod	Non-Fac Total	Fac Total		51	50	62	80	MUE
	8.20	5.61	090	2	1	0	1	1

67900 – 67922

● New   ▲ Revised   Deleted   ⊙ Moderate Sedation   ✚ Add-on Codes   ⊘ High Risk Denial   ⓐ Age Edit   ♀ Female   ♂ Male   **AMA** CPT® Assistant   **MUE** Medically Unlikely Edit
⊘ Modifier 51 Exempt   ⊖ Modifier 63 Exempt   ✗ Unlisted   **Modifiers:** See Inside Back Cover   Ⓜ Maternity   A2–Z3 ASC Payment Indicators   A–Y OPPS Status Indicators

© 2016 DecisionHealth   CPT © 2015 American Medical Association. All Rights Reserved.

67923 Repair of entropion; excision tarsal wedge A 2 T

| RVU | | | Global Days | Modifiers | | | | |
Mod	Non-Fac Total	Fac Total		51	50	62	80	MUE
	16.74	12.24	090	2	1	0	1	1

AMA: May 04: 12, Oct 06: 11

67924 Repair of entropion; extensive (eg, tarsal strip or capsulopalpebral fascia repairs operation) A 2 T

Coding tip: *Canthoplasty is included in blepharoplasties and some other repair/correction procedures. Do not report 67950 in addition to 67924.*

| RVU | | | Global Days | Modifiers | | | | |
Mod	Non-Fac Total	Fac Total		51	50	62	80	MUE
	17.85	13.02	090	2	1	0	1	1

AMA: May 04: 12, Oct 06: 11

Eyelid Reconstruction

67930 Suture of recent wound, eyelid, involving lid margin, tarsus, and/or palpebral conjunctiva direct closure; partial thickness P 3 T

| RVU | | | Global Days | Modifiers | | | | |
Mod	Non-Fac Total	Fac Total		51	50	62	80	MUE
	10.29	6.82	010	2	1	0	1	2

67935 Suture of recent wound, eyelid, involving lid margin, tarsus, and/or palpebral conjunctiva direct closure; full thickness A 2 T

| RVU | | | Global Days | Modifiers | | | | |
Mod	Non-Fac Total	Fac Total		51	50	62	80	MUE
	16.84	12.59	090	2	1	0	1	2

67938 Removal of embedded foreign body, eyelid P 2 T

| RVU | | | Global Days | Modifiers | | | | |
Mod	Non-Fac Total	Fac Total		51	50	62	80	MUE
	6.79	3.26	010	2	1	0	1	2

AMA: May 14: 5

67950 Canthoplasty (reconstruction of canthus) A 2 T

Coding tip: *Canthoplasty is included in blepharoplasties and some other repair/correction procedures*

Coding tip: *Do not report 67950 in addition to 67917, 67924, 67961, or 67966*

| RVU | | | Global Days | Modifiers | | | | |
Mod	Non-Fac Total	Fac Total		51	50	62	80	MUE
	16.22	13.18	090	2	1	1	1	2

67961 Excision and repair of eyelid, involving lid margin, tarsus, conjunctiva, canthus, or full thickness, may include preparation for skin graft or pedicle flap with adjacent tissue transfer or rearrangement; up to one-fourth of lid margin A 2 T

Coding tip: *Canthoplasty is included in blepharoplasties and some other repair/correction procedures. Do not report 67950 in addition to 67961*

| RVU | | | Global Days | Modifiers | | | | |
Mod	Non-Fac Total	Fac Total		51	50	62	80	MUE
	16.28	12.93	090	2	1	0	0	4

67966 Excision and repair of eyelid, involving lid margin, tarsus, conjunctiva, canthus, or full thickness, may include preparation for skin graft or pedicle flap with adjacent tissue transfer or rearrangement; over one-fourth of lid margin A 2 T

Coding tip: *Canthoplasty is included in blepharoplasties and some other repair/correction procedures. Do not report 67950 in addition to 67966*

| RVU | | | Global Days | Modifiers | | | | |
Mod	Non-Fac Total	Fac Total		51	50	62	80	MUE
	21.80	18.71	090	2	1	0	1	4

AMA: Nov 12: 13

67971 Reconstruction of eyelid, full thickness by transfer of tarsoconjunctival flap from opposing eyelid; up to two-thirds of eyelid, 1 stage or first stage A 2 T

| RVU | | | Global Days | Modifiers | | | | |
Mod	Non-Fac Total	Fac Total		51	50	62	80	MUE
	20.58	20.58	090	2	1	1	1	1

67973 Reconstruction of eyelid, full thickness by transfer of tarsoconjunctival flap from opposing eyelid; total eyelid, lower, 1 stage or first stage A 2 T

| RVU | | | Global Days | Modifiers | | | | |
Mod	Non-Fac Total	Fac Total		51	50	62	80	MUE
	26.47	26.47	090	2	1	1	2	1

67974 Reconstruction of eyelid, full thickness by transfer of tarsoconjunctival flap from opposing eyelid; total eyelid, upper, 1 stage or first stage A 2 T

| RVU | | | Global Days | Modifiers | | | | |
Mod	Non-Fac Total	Fac Total		51	50	62	80	MUE
	26.41	26.41	090	2	1	1	2	1

67975 Reconstruction of eyelid, full thickness by transfer of tarsoconjunctival flap from opposing eyelid; second stage A 2 T

| RVU | | | Global Days | Modifiers | | | | |
Mod	Non-Fac Total	Fac Total		51	50	62	80	MUE
	19.47	19.47	090	2	1	0	1	1

Other Eyelid Procedures

67999 Unlisted procedure, eyelids ⊙ x T

| RVU | | | Global Days | Modifiers | | | | |
Mod	Non-Fac Total	Fac Total		51	50	62	80	MUE
	0.00	0.00	YYY	2	1	1	0	

● New   ▲ Revised   ✖ Deleted   ⊙ Moderate Sedation   ✚ Add-on Codes   ⊘ High Risk Denial   Ⓐ Age Edit   ♀ Female   ♂ Male   **AMA** *CPT® Assistant*   **MUE** Medically Unlikely Edit
⊘ Modifier 51 Exempt   ⊖ Modifier 63 Exempt   ✖ Unlisted   **Modifiers:** *See Inside Back Cover*   Ⓜ Maternity   A 2–Z 3 ASC Payment Indicators   A –Y OPPS Status Indicators

CPT © 2015 American Medical Association. All Rights Reserved.   © 2016 DecisionHealth

Conjunctival Procedures

Conjunctival Incision and Drainage

Coding Guidance

Codes 68020-68135 for incision, drainage, excision, and destruction on the conjunctiva are included in all conjunctivoplasties (68320-68362).

68020   Incision of conjunctiva, drainage of cyst   P 3 T

RVU			Global Days	Modifiers				
Mod	Non-Fac Total	Fac Total		51	50	62	80	MUE
	3.38	3.14	010	2	1	0	1	1

Incision/drainage conjuntival cyst

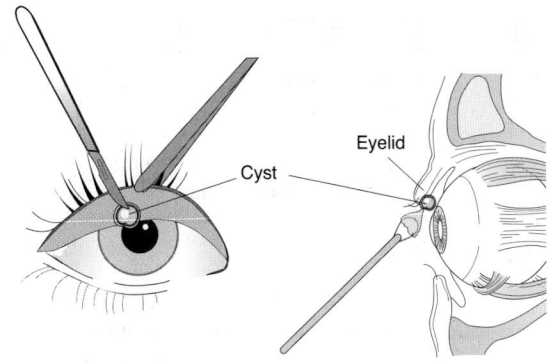

The cyst is incised and the contents drained using a cotton tipped probe or curette

68040   Expression of conjunctival follicles (eg, for trachoma)   P 3 T

RVU			Global Days	Modifiers				
Mod	Non-Fac Total	Fac Total		51	50	62	80	MUE
	1.77	1.44	000	2	1	0	1	1

AMA: May 14: 5

Expression of conjuntival follicles (eg, for trachoma)

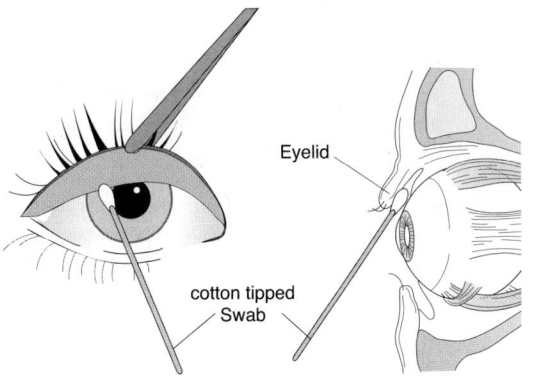

Granulations are removed using a cotton tipped swab or a curette

Conjunctival Excision and/or Destruction Procedures

68100   Biopsy of conjunctiva   P 3 T

RVU			Global Days	Modifiers				
Mod	Non-Fac Total	Fac Total		51	50	62	80	MUE
	4.80	2.77	000	2	1	0	1	1

68110   Excision of lesion, conjunctiva; up to 1 cm   P 3 T

RVU			Global Days	Modifiers				
Mod	Non-Fac Total	Fac Total		51	50	62	80	MUE
	6.37	4.23	010	2	1	0	1	1

68115   Excision of lesion, conjunctiva; over 1 cm   A 2 T

RVU			Global Days	Modifiers				
Mod	Non-Fac Total	Fac Total		51	50	62	80	MUE
	8.81	5.23	010	2	1	0	1	1

68130   Excision of lesion, conjunctiva; with adjacent sclera   A 2 T

RVU			Global Days	Modifiers				
Mod	Non-Fac Total	Fac Total		51	50	62	80	MUE
	15.25	11.71	090	2	1	0	1	1

68135   Destruction of lesion, conjunctiva   P 3 T

RVU			Global Days	Modifiers				
Mod	Non-Fac Total	Fac Total		51	50	62	80	MUE
	4.43	4.29	010	2	1	0	1	1

Conjunctival Injection

Coding Guidance

When a subconjunctival local anesthetic injection is performed as part of a more extensive peribulbar or retrobulbar block, it is considered a routine part of the more comprehensive anesthetic procedure and is not coded separately. When it is medically necessary to inject a sclerosing agent during the same session as glaucoma surgery, the injection is included in the surgical service. Codes 67500, 67515, and 68200 for injection of the sclerosing agent should not be reported with other pressure-reducing or glaucoma procedures.

68200   Subconjunctival injection   N I Q 1

RVU			Global Days	Modifiers				
Mod	Non-Fac Total	Fac Total		51	50	62	80	MUE
	1.17	0.99	000	2	1	0	1	1

AMA: Aug 03: 15, Nov 12: 10

Subconjunctival injection

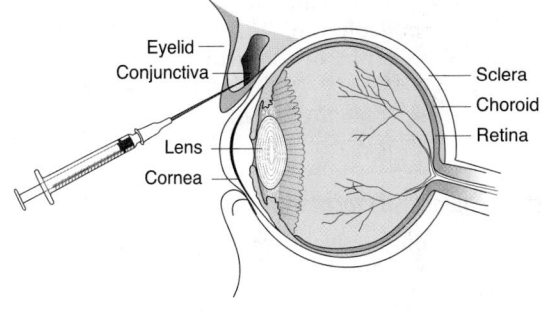

The physician injects a substance under the top layer of tissue on the inside of the eyelid.

● New   ▲ Revised   Deleted   ⊙ Moderate Sedation   ✚ Add-on Codes   ⊘ High Risk Denial   Ⓐ Age Edit   ♀ Female   ♂ Male   **AMA** CPT® Assistant   **MUE** Medically Unlikely Edit   ⊘ Modifier 51 Exempt   ⊖ Modifier 63 Exempt   🗷 Unlisted   **Modifiers:** See Inside Back Cover   Ⓜ Maternity   A 2 – Z 3 ASC Payment Indicators   A – Y OPPS Status Indicators

Surgical Procedures

68320 – 68525

Conjunctivoplasty Procedures

Coding Guidance

Conjunctivoplasties include the codes 68020-68135 for incision, drainage, excision, and destruction done on the conjunctiva .

68320 Conjunctivoplasty; with conjunctival graft or extensive rearrangement A 2 T

	RVU		Global Days	Modifiers				
Mod	Non-Fac Total	Fac Total		51	50	62	80	MUE
	20.51	15.31	090	2	1	1	1	1

AMA: Feb 04: 11

68325 Conjunctivoplasty; with buccal mucous membrane graft (includes obtaining graft) A 2 T

	RVU		Global Days	Modifiers				
Mod	Non-Fac Total	Fac Total		51	50	62	80	MUE
	18.74	18.74	090	2	1	1	1	1

68326 Conjunctivoplasty, reconstruction cul-de-sac; with conjunctival graft or extensive rearrangement A 2 T

	RVU		Global Days	Modifiers				
Mod	Non-Fac Total	Fac Total		51	50	62	80	MUE
	18.35	18.35	090	2	1	0	1	2

68328 Conjunctivoplasty, reconstruction cul-de-sac; with buccal mucous membrane graft (includes obtaining graft) A 2 T

	RVU		Global Days	Modifiers				
Mod	Non-Fac Total	Fac Total		51	50	62	80	MUE
	20.14	20.14	090	2	1	0	0	2

68330 Repair of symblepharon; conjunctivoplasty, without graft A 2 T

	RVU		Global Days	Modifiers				
Mod	Non-Fac Total	Fac Total		51	50	62	80	MUE
	17.11	13.11	090	2	1	0	0	1

68335 Repair of symblepharon; with free graft conjunctiva or buccal mucous membrane (includes obtaining graft) A 2 T

	RVU		Global Days	Modifiers				
Mod	Non-Fac Total	Fac Total		51	50	62	80	MUE
	18.40	18.40	090	2	1	1	1	1

68340 Repair of symblepharon; division of symblepharon, with or without insertion of conformer or contact lens A 2 T

	RVU		Global Days	Modifiers				
Mod	Non-Fac Total	Fac Total		51	50	62	80	MUE
	15.43	11.35	090	2	1	0	0	1

Other Conjunctival Procedures

68360 Conjunctival flap; bridge or partial (separate procedure) A 2 T

	RVU		Global Days	Modifiers				
Mod	Non-Fac Total	Fac Total		51	50	62	80	MUE
	15.09	11.74	090	2	1	0	1	1

68362 Conjunctival flap; total (such as Gunderson thin flap or purse string flap) A 2 T

	RVU		Global Days	Modifiers				
Mod	Non-Fac Total	Fac Total		51	50	62	80	MUE
	18.65	18.65	090	2	1	1	1	1

68371 Harvesting conjunctival allograft, living donor A 2 T

	RVU		Global Days	Modifiers				
Mod	Non-Fac Total	Fac Total		51	50	62	80	MUE
	11.73	11.73	010	2	1	0	1	1

AMA: May 04: 10

68399 Unlisted procedure, conjunctiva x T

	RVU		Global Days	Modifiers				
Mod	Non-Fac Total	Fac Total		51	50	62	80	MUE
	0.00	0.00	YYY	2	1	1	0	

Lacrimal System Procedures

Incisional Lacrimal System Procedures

68400 Incision, drainage of lacrimal gland P 3 T

	RVU		Global Days	Modifiers				
Mod	Non-Fac Total	Fac Total		51	50	62	80	MUE
	8.02	3.75	010	2	1	0	1	1

68420 Incision, drainage of lacrimal sac (dacryocystotomy or dacryocystostomy) P 3 T

	RVU		Global Days	Modifiers				
Mod	Non-Fac Total	Fac Total		51	50	62	80	MUE
	9.10	4.80	010	2	1	0	1	1

68440 Snip incision of lacrimal punctum P 3 T

	RVU		Global Days	Modifiers				
Mod	Non-Fac Total	Fac Total		51	50	62	80	MUE
	2.90	2.82	010	2	1	0	1	2

Excisional Lacrimal System Procedures

68500 Excision of lacrimal gland (dacryoadenectomy), except for tumor; total A 2 T

	RVU		Global Days	Modifiers				
Mod	Non-Fac Total	Fac Total		51	50	62	80	MUE
	27.71	27.71	090	2	1	0	1	1

68505 Excision of lacrimal gland (dacryoadenectomy), except for tumor; partial A 2 T

	RVU		Global Days	Modifiers				
Mod	Non-Fac Total	Fac Total		51	50	62	80	MUE
	27.55	27.55	090	2	1	0	1	1

68510 Biopsy of lacrimal gland A 2 T

	RVU		Global Days	Modifiers				
Mod	Non-Fac Total	Fac Total		51	50	62	80	MUE
	12.60	8.31	000	2	1	0	0	1

68520 Excision of lacrimal sac (dacryocystectomy) A 2 T

	RVU		Global Days	Modifiers				
Mod	Non-Fac Total	Fac Total		51	50	62	80	MUE
	19.57	19.57	090	2	1	0	0	1

68525 Biopsy of lacrimal sac A 2 T

	RVU		Global Days	Modifiers				
Mod	Non-Fac Total	Fac Total		51	50	62	80	MUE
	7.51	7.51	000	2	1	1	1	1

● New   ▲ Revised   ✖ Deleted   ⊙ Moderate Sedation   ✚ Add-on Codes   ⊘ High Risk Denial   Ⓐ Age Edit   ♀ Female   ♂ Male   **AMA** *CPT® Assistant*   *MUE* Medically Unlikely Edit   ⊘ Modifier 51 Exempt   ⊖ Modifier 63 Exempt   ⊠ Unlisted   **Modifiers:** *See Inside Back Cover*   Ⓜ Maternity   A2–Z3 ASC Payment Indicators   A–Y OPPS Status Indicators

CPT © 2015 American Medical Association. All Rights Reserved.   © 2016 DecisionHealth

68530 Removal of foreign body or dacryolith, lacrimal passages P 2 T

RVU			Global Days	Modifiers				
Mod	Non-Fac Total	Fac Total		51	50	62	80	MUE
	12.09	7.32	010	2	1	0	1	1

68540 Excision of lacrimal gland tumor; frontal approach ⊘ A 2 T

RVU			Global Days	Modifiers				
Mod	Non-Fac Total	Fac Total		51	50	62	80	MUE
	26.45	26.45	090	2	1	1	1	1

68550 Excision of lacrimal gland tumor; involving osteotomy A 2 T

RVU			Global Days	Modifiers				
Mod	Non-Fac Total	Fac Total		51	50	62	80	MUE
	31.45	31.45	090	2	1	0	1	1

Lacrimal System Repair

68700 Plastic repair of canaliculi A 2 T

RVU			Global Days	Modifiers				
Mod	Non-Fac Total	Fac Total		51	50	62	80	MUE
	17.15	17.15	090	2	1	0	1	1

68705 Correction of everted punctum, cautery P 2 T

RVU			Global Days	Modifiers				
Mod	Non-Fac Total	Fac Total		51	50	62	80	MUE
	6.69	4.72	010	2	1	0	1	2

68720 Dacryocystorhinostomy (fistulization of lacrimal sac to nasal cavity) A 2 T

RVU			Global Days	Modifiers				
Mod	Non-Fac Total	Fac Total		51	50	62	80	MUE
	21.50	21.50	090	2	1	1	2	1

AMA: Sep 01: 10, Jul 03: 15, Aug 03: 14, Aug 09: 11

68745 Conjunctivorhinostomy (fistulization of conjunctiva to nasal cavity); without tube A 2 T

RVU			Global Days	Modifiers				
Mod	Non-Fac Total	Fac Total		51	50	62	80	MUE
	21.59	21.59	090	2	1	1	2	1

68750 Conjunctivorhinostomy (fistulization of conjunctiva to nasal cavity); with insertion of tube or stent A 2 T

RVU			Global Days	Modifiers				
Mod	Non-Fac Total	Fac Total		51	50	62	80	MUE
	22.35	22.35	090	2	1	1	2	1

68760 Closure of the lacrimal punctum; by thermocauterization, ligation, or laser surgery P 3 T

RVU			Global Days	Modifiers				
Mod	Non-Fac Total	Fac Total		51	50	62	80	MUE
	5.69	4.16	010	2	1	0	1	4

68761 Closure of the lacrimal punctum; by plug, each P 3 T

RVU			Global Days	Modifiers				
Mod	Non-Fac Total	Fac Total		51	50	62	80	MUE
	4.15	3.37	010	2	1	0	0	4

AMA: Jun 96: 10, Jan 07: 28

68770 Closure of lacrimal fistula (separate procedure) A 2 T

RVU			Global Days	Modifiers				
Mod	Non-Fac Total	Fac Total		51	50	62	80	MUE
	17.85	17.85	090	2	1	0	0	1

Lacrimal Probing/Other Related Procedures

68801 Dilation of lacrimal punctum, with or without irrigation N I Q I

RVU			Global Days	Modifiers				
Mod	Non-Fac Total	Fac Total		51	50	62	80	MUE
	2.84	2.46	010	2	1	0	1	4

Dilation of lacrimal punctum

A plastic probe, catheter, or large suture is inserted into the lacrimal punctum to increase the size of the opening

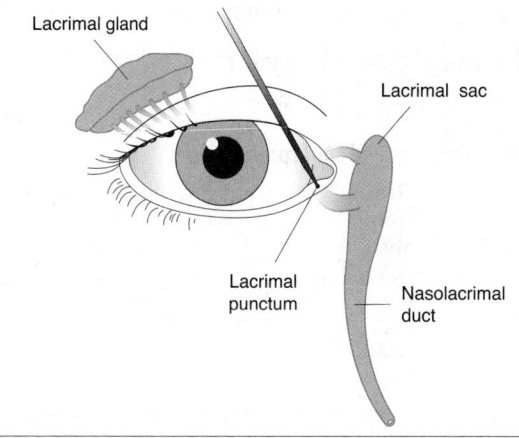

Lacrimal gland

Lacrimal sac

Lacrimal punctum

Nasolacrimal duct

68810 Probing of nasolacrimal duct, with or without irrigation A 2 T

RVU			Global Days	Modifiers				
Mod	Non-Fac Total	Fac Total		51	50	62	80	MUE
	5.51	4.30	010	2	1	0	1	1

AMA: Nov 02: 11, Oct 08: 3

68811 Probing of nasolacrimal duct, with or without irrigation; requiring general anesthesia A 2 T

RVU			Global Days	Modifiers				
Mod	Non-Fac Total	Fac Total		51	50	62	80	MUE
	4.72	4.72	010	2	1	0	1	1

AMA: Nov 02: 11, Oct 08: 3

68815 Probing of nasolacrimal duct, with or without irrigation; with insertion of tube or stent A 2 T

RVU			Global Days	Modifiers				
Mod	Non-Fac Total	Fac Total		51	50	62	80	MUE
	11.23	6.29	010	2	1	0	1	1

AMA: Nov 02: 11, Oct 08: 3, Aug 09: 11, Nov 10: 9

68816 Probing of nasolacrimal duct, with or without irrigation; with transluminal balloon catheter dilation G 2 T

RVU			Global Days	Modifiers				
Mod	Non-Fac Total	Fac Total		51	50	62	80	MUE
	18.26	5.73	010	2	1	0	1	1

● New   ▲ Revised   Deleted   ⊙ Moderate Sedation   ✚ Add-on Codes   ⊘ High Risk Denial   Ⓐ Age Edit   ♀ Female   ♂ Male   **AMA** CPT® Assistant   **MUE** Medically Unlikely Edit

⊘ Modifier 51 Exempt   ⊖ Modifier 63 Exempt   ✗ Unlisted   **Modifiers:** See Inside Back Cover   Ⓜ Maternity   A 2 – Z 3 ASC Payment Indicators   A – Y OPPS Status Indicators

68840 Probing of lacrimal canaliculi, with or without irrigation   P 3 T

Mod	RVU Non-Fac Total	Fac Total	Global Days	Modifiers 51	50	62	80	MUE
	3.62	3.32	010	2	1	0	1	1

68850 Injection of contrast medium for dacryocystography   N I N

Mod	RVU Non-Fac Total	Fac Total	Global Days	Modifiers 51	50	62	80	MUE
	1.73	1.59	000	2	1	0	1	1

AMA: Feb 01: 9

Other Lacrimal System Procedures

68899 Unlisted procedure, lacrimal system   ⊗ x T

Mod	RVU Non-Fac Total	Fac Total	Global Days	Modifiers 51	50	62	80	MUE
	0.00	0.00	YYY	2	1	1	0	

Auditory System Procedures

External Ear Procedures

Incisional External Ear Procedures

69000 Drainage external ear, abscess or hematoma; simple   P 2 T

Mod	RVU Non-Fac Total	Fac Total	Global Days	Modifiers 51	50	62	80	MUE
	5.34	3.42	010	2	1	0	1	1

AMA: Oct 97: 11, Oct 99: 10

Drainage, external ear, abscess/hematoma

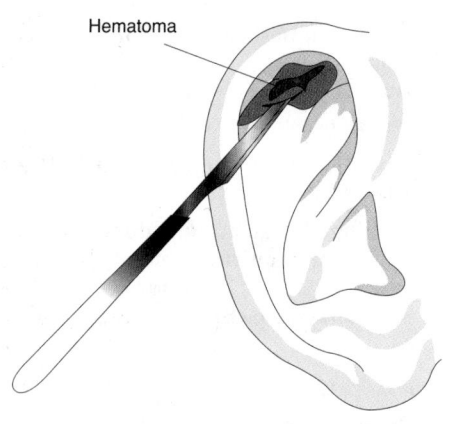

An abscess/hematoma of the pinna is drained.
Simple (69000), complex (69005)

69005 Drainage external ear, abscess or hematoma; complicated   P 3 T

Mod	RVU Non-Fac Total	Fac Total	Global Days	Modifiers 51	50	62	80	MUE
	6.16	4.53	010	2	1	0	1	1

69020 Drainage external auditory canal, abscess   P 2 T

Coding tip: Removal of foreign body from external auditory canal - 69200-69205

Mod	RVU Non-Fac Total	Fac Total	Global Days	Modifiers 51	50	62	80	MUE
	6.67	4.11	010	2	1	0	1	1

AMA: Oct 97: 11

69090 Ear piercing   ⊘ E

Mod	RVU Non-Fac Total	Fac Total	Global Days	Modifiers 51	50	62	80	MUE
	0.00	0.00	XXX	9	9	9	9	

Excisional External Ear Procedures

69100 Biopsy external ear   P 3 T

Coding tip: Code 99000 for specimen transfer from office setting to an outside laboratory

Coding tip: Report biopsy separately only when performed alone, or distinct from other procedures on the same day

Mod	RVU Non-Fac Total	Fac Total	Global Days	Modifiers 51	50	62	80	MUE
	2.86	1.41	000	2	0	0	1	3

Biopsy external ear

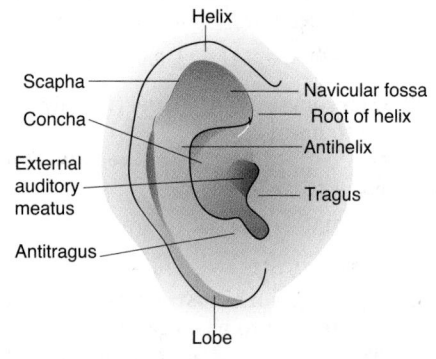

The physician takes a tissue sample from the external ear for examination and diagnosis

69105 Biopsy external auditory canal   P 3 T

Coding tip: Code 99000 for specimen transfer from office setting to an outside laboratory

Coding tip: Removal of entire lesion from external auditory canal - 69145

Mod	RVU Non-Fac Total	Fac Total	Global Days	Modifiers 51	50	62	80	MUE
	4.02	1.84	000	2	1	0	1	1

69110 Excision external ear; partial, simple repair   A 2 T

Mod	RVU Non-Fac Total	Fac Total	Global Days	Modifiers 51	50	62	80	MUE
	13.17	9.37	090	2	1	0	1	1

69120 Excision external ear; complete amputation   A 2 T

Mod	RVU Non-Fac Total	Fac Total	Global Days	Modifiers 51	50	62	80	MUE
	11.70	11.70	090	2	0	0	1	1

● New   ▲ Revised   ✖ Deleted   ⊙ Moderate Sedation   ✚ Add-on Codes   ⊘ High Risk Denial   Ⓐ Age Edit   ♀ Female   ♂ Male   **AMA** *CPT® Assistant*   **MUE** Medically Unlikely Edit
⊗ Modifier 51 Exempt   ⊖ Modifier 63 Exempt   ✗ Unlisted   **Modifiers:** *See Inside Back Cover*   Ⓜ Maternity   A 2 – Z 3 ASC Payment Indicators   A – Y OPPS Status Indicators

69140 Excision exostosis(es), external auditory canal

A 2 J 1

RVU			Global Days	Modifiers				
Mod	Non-Fac Total	Fac Total		51	50	62	80	MUE
	25.35	25.35	090	2	1	0	0	1

69145 Excision soft tissue lesion, external auditory canal

A 2 T

RVU			Global Days	Modifiers				
Mod	Non-Fac Total	Fac Total		51	50	62	80	MUE
	11.41	7.21	090	2	1	0	1	1

69150 Radical excision external auditory canal lesion; without neck dissection

A 2 T

RVU			Global Days	Modifiers				
Mod	Non-Fac Total	Fac Total		51	50	62	80	MUE
	30.34	30.34	090	2	0	1	1	1

69155 Radical excision external auditory canal lesion; with neck dissection

C

RVU			Global Days	Modifiers				
Mod	Non-Fac Total	Fac Total		51	50	62	80	MUE
	48.25	48.25	090	2	0	1	2	1

External Ear Removal Procedures

69200 Removal foreign body from external auditory canal; without general anesthesia

N I Q 1

RVU			Global Days	Modifiers				
Mod	Non-Fac Total	Fac Total		51	50	62	80	MUE
	2.83	1.36	000	2	1	0	1	1

69205 Removal foreign body from external auditory canal; with general anesthesia

A 2 T

RVU			Global Days	Modifiers				
Mod	Non-Fac Total	Fac Total		51	50	62	80	MUE
	2.93	2.93	010	2	1	0	1	1

AMA: Apr 13: 10

● **69209 Removal impacted cerumen using irrigation/lavage, unilateral**

N I Q 1

RVU			Global Days	Modifiers				
Mod	Non-Fac Total	Fac Total		51	50	62	80	MUE
	0.36	0.36	000	2	1	0	1	2

69210 Removal impacted cerumen requiring instrumentation, unilateral

N I Q 1

Documentation Finder: To support reporting this code, the provider must document tools or equipment used to remove wax from the patient's ear. The code represents a stand-alone procedure; if the provider had to remove the wax to evaluate the ear or perform a test on the ear, this code is not appropriate.

RVU			Global Days	Modifiers				
Mod	Non-Fac Total	Fac Total		51	50	62	80	MUE
	1.40	0.94	000	2	2	0	1	1

AMA: Apr 03: 9, Jul 05: 14, Oct 13: 14, Nov 14: 14

69220 Debridement, mastoidectomy cavity, simple (eg, routine cleaning)

N I Q 1

RVU			Global Days	Modifiers				
Mod	Non-Fac Total	Fac Total		51	50	62	80	MUE
	3.16	1.50	000	2	1	0	1	1

69222 Debridement, mastoidectomy cavity, complex (eg, with anesthesia or more than routine cleaning)

P 3 T

RVU			Global Days	Modifiers				
Mod	Non-Fac Total	Fac Total		51	50	62	80	MUE
	6.31	3.95	010	2	1	0	1	1

External Ear Repair

⊙ **69300 Otoplasty, protruding ear, with or without size reduction**

A 2 T

RVU			Global Days	Modifiers				
Mod	Non-Fac Total	Fac Total		51	50	62	80	MUE
	21.15	13.80	YYY	2	1	0	0	1

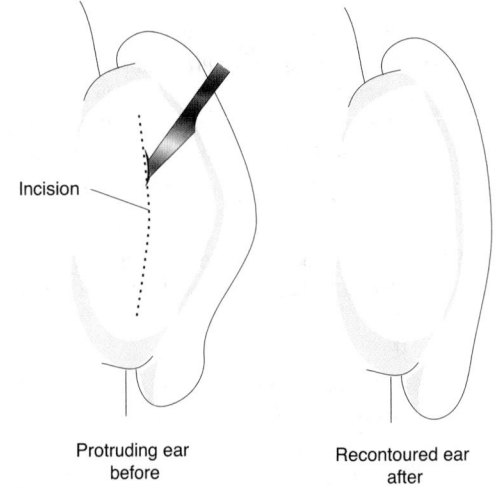

Otoplasty, protruding ear, with/without size reduction

Incision

Protruding ear before

Recontoured ear after

The protruding ear is corrected using contouring techniques

69310 Reconstruction of external auditory canal (meatoplasty) (eg, for stenosis due to injury, infection) (separate procedure)

A 2 J 1

RVU			Global Days	Modifiers				
Mod	Non-Fac Total	Fac Total		51	50	62	80	MUE
	31.55	31.55	090	2	1	0	1	1

AMA: Jan 14: 9, Jul 14: 9

69320 Reconstruction external auditory canal for congenital atresia, single stage

A 2 J 1

RVU			Global Days	Modifiers				
Mod	Non-Fac Total	Fac Total		51	50	62	80	MUE
	44.70	44.70	090	2	1	0	2	1

Other External Ear Procedures

69399 Unlisted procedure, external ear

x T

RVU			Global Days	Modifiers				
Mod	Non-Fac Total	Fac Total		51	50	62	80	MUE
	0.00	0.00	YYY	2	0	1	0	

● New   ▲ Revised   Deleted   ⊙ Moderate Sedation   ✚ Add-on Codes   ⊘ High Risk Denial   Ⓐ Age Edit   ♀ Female   ♂ Male   **AMA** *CPT® Assistant*   **MUE** Medically Unlikely Edit
⊘ Modifier 51 Exempt   ⊖ Modifier 63 Exempt   ✗ Unlisted   **Modifiers:** *See Inside Back Cover*   Ⓜ Maternity   A 2 – Z 3 ASC Payment Indicators   A – Y OPPS Status Indicators

Incisional Middle Ear Procedures

Coding Guidance

Myringotomies are included in tympanoplasty and tympanostomy surgical services.

69420 Myringotomy including aspiration and/or eustachian tube inflation `P 3 T`

RVU		Global Days	Modifiers				
Mod	Non-Fac Total	Fac Total		51	50	62	80	MUE
	5.50	3.49	010	2	1	0	1	1

AMA: May 11: 8

69421 Myringotomy including aspiration and/or eustachian tube inflation requiring general anesthesia `A 2 T`

RVU		Global Days	Modifiers				
Mod	Non-Fac Total	Fac Total		51	50	62	80	MUE
	4.31	4.31	010	2	1	0	1	1

AMA: May 11: 8

69424 Ventilating tube removal requiring general anesthesia `P 3 Q 2`

RVU		Global Days	Modifiers				
Mod	Non-Fac Total	Fac Total		51	50	62	80	MUE
	3.65	1.80	000	2	1	0	1	1

AMA: Mar 05: 17, Jun 10: 11, Nov 10: 9

69433 Tympanostomy (requiring insertion of ventilating tube), local or topical anesthesia `P 3 T`

RVU		Global Days	Modifiers				
Mod	Non-Fac Total	Fac Total		51	50	62	80	MUE
	5.82	3.83	010	2	1	0	1	1

AMA: May 11: 8

69436 Tympanostomy (requiring insertion of ventilating tube), general anesthesia `A 2 T`

RVU		Global Days	Modifiers				
Mod	Non-Fac Total	Fac Total		51	50	62	80	MUE
	4.64	4.64	010	2	1	0	1	1

AMA: May 11: 8, May 12: 14

69440 Middle ear exploration through postauricular or ear canal incision `A 2 J I`

RVU		Global Days	Modifiers				
Mod	Non-Fac Total	Fac Total		51	50	62	80	MUE
	19.96	19.96	090	2	1	0	1	1

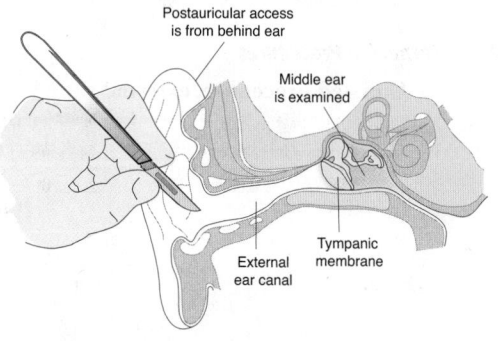

Middle ear exploration through postauricular or ear canal incision

Postauricular access is from behind ear

Middle ear is examined

External ear canal

Tympanic membrane

69450 Tympanolysis, transcanal `A 2 J I`

RVU		Global Days	Modifiers				
Mod	Non-Fac Total	Fac Total		51	50	62	80	MUE
	15.77	15.77	090	2	1	0	0	1

Excisional Middle Ear Procedures

69501 Transmastoid antrotomy (simple mastoidectomy) `A 2 J I`

RVU		Global Days	Modifiers				
Mod	Non-Fac Total	Fac Total		51	50	62	80	MUE
	21.25	21.25	090	2	1	0	1	1

69502 Mastoidectomy; complete `A 2 J I`

RVU		Global Days	Modifiers				
Mod	Non-Fac Total	Fac Total		51	50	62	80	MUE
	28.13	28.13	090	2	1	0	0	1

69505 Mastoidectomy; modified radical `A 2 J I`

RVU		Global Days	Modifiers				
Mod	Non-Fac Total	Fac Total		51	50	62	80	MUE
	34.79	34.79	090	2	1	0	0	1

69511 Mastoidectomy; radical `A 2 J I`

RVU		Global Days	Modifiers				
Mod	Non-Fac Total	Fac Total		51	50	62	80	MUE
	35.55	35.55	090	2	1	0	0	1

69530 Petrous apicectomy including radical mastoidectomy `A 2 J I`

Coding tip: *Mastoidectomy is included as part of the code descriptor for auditory procedure 69530; a separate mastoidectomy service code should not be reported.*

RVU		Global Days	Modifiers				
Mod	Non-Fac Total	Fac Total		51	50	62	80	MUE
	47.95	47.95	090	2	1	0	2	1

69535 Resection temporal bone, external approach `C`

RVU		Global Days	Modifiers				
Mod	Non-Fac Total	Fac Total		51	50	62	80	MUE
	77.73	77.73	090	2	1	1	1	1

69540 Excision aural polyp `P 3 T`

RVU		Global Days	Modifiers				
Mod	Non-Fac Total	Fac Total		51	50	62	80	MUE
	6.00	3.67	010	2	1	0	1	1

69550 Excision aural glomus tumor; transcanal `A 2 J I`

RVU		Global Days	Modifiers				
Mod	Non-Fac Total	Fac Total		51	50	62	80	MUE
	30.13	30.13	090	2	1	0	2	1

69552 Excision aural glomus tumor; transmastoid `A 2 J I`

RVU		Global Days	Modifiers				
Mod	Non-Fac Total	Fac Total		51	50	62	80	MUE
	45.25	45.25	090	2	1	0	2	1

69554 Excision aural glomus tumor; extended (extratemporal) `C`

RVU		Global Days	Modifiers				
Mod	Non-Fac Total	Fac Total		51	50	62	80	MUE
	70.46	70.46	090	2	1	1	2	1

● New ▲ Revised ✖ Deleted ⊙ Moderate Sedation ✚ Add-on Codes ⊗ High Risk Denial Ⓐ Age Edit ♀ Female ♂ Male **AMA** *CPT® Assistant* **MUE** Medically Unlikely Edit
⊘ Modifier 51 Exempt ⊖ Modifier 63 Exempt ✗ Unlisted **Modifiers:** *See Inside Back Cover* Ⓜ Maternity A 2 – Z 3 ASC Payment Indicators A – Y OPPS Status Indicators

CPT © 2015 American Medical Association. All Rights Reserved. © 2016 DecisionHealth

Middle Ear Repair

69601 Revision mastoidectomy; resulting in complete mastoidectomy   A 2 J 1

RVU			Global Days	Modifiers				
Mod	Non-Fac Total	Fac Total		51	50	62	80	MUE
	30.28	30.28	090	2	1	0	0	1

69602 Revision mastoidectomy; resulting in modified radical mastoidectomy   A 2 J 1

RVU			Global Days	Modifiers				
Mod	Non-Fac Total	Fac Total		51	50	62	80	MUE
	31.50	31.50	090	2	1	0	0	1

69603 Revision mastoidectomy; resulting in radical mastoidectomy   A 2 J 1

RVU			Global Days	Modifiers				
Mod	Non-Fac Total	Fac Total		51	50	62	80	MUE
	36.85	36.85	090	2	1	0	0	1

69604 Revision mastoidectomy; resulting in tympanoplasty   A 2 J 1

RVU			Global Days	Modifiers				
Mod	Non-Fac Total	Fac Total		51	50	62	80	MUE
	32.21	32.21	090	2	1	0	1	1

69605 Revision mastoidectomy; with apicectomy   A 2 J 1

RVU			Global Days	Modifiers				
Mod	Non-Fac Total	Fac Total		51	50	62	80	MUE
	45.17	45.17	090	2	1	0	2	1

69610 Tympanic membrane repair, with or without site preparation of perforation for closure, with or without patch   P 3 T

RVU			Global Days	Modifiers				
Mod	Non-Fac Total	Fac Total		51	50	62	80	MUE
	11.06	8.41	010	2	1	0	1	1

AMA: Mar 01: 10, Mar 03: 21, Aug 08: 4, Apr 15: 11, May 15: 11

69620 Myringoplasty (surgery confined to drumhead and donor area)   A 2 T

RVU			Global Days	Modifiers				
Mod	Non-Fac Total	Fac Total		51	50	62	80	MUE
	20.00	14.15	090	2	1	0	1	1

AMA: Mar 01: 10, Aug 08: 4, Apr 15: 11, May 15: 11

69631 Tympanoplasty without mastoidectomy (including canalplasty, atticotomy and/or middle ear surgery), initial or revision; without ossicular chain reconstruction   A 2 J 1

RVU			Global Days	Modifiers				
Mod	Non-Fac Total	Fac Total		51	50	62	80	MUE
	25.59	25.59	090	2	1	0	1	1

AMA: Jul 98: 11, Mar 01: 10, Mar 07: 9, Aug 08: 4, Dec 12: 11

69632 Tympanoplasty without mastoidectomy (including canalplasty, atticotomy and/or middle ear surgery), initial or revision; with ossicular chain reconstruction (eg, postfenestration)   A 2 J 1

RVU			Global Days	Modifiers				
Mod	Non-Fac Total	Fac Total		51	50	62	80	MUE
	31.15	31.15	090	2	1	0	1	1

69633 Tympanoplasty without mastoidectomy (including canalplasty, atticotomy and/or middle ear surgery), initial or revision; with ossicular chain reconstruction and synthetic prosthesis (eg, partial ossicular replacement prosthesis [PORP], total ossicular replacement prosthesis [TORP])   A 2 J 1

RVU			Global Days	Modifiers				
Mod	Non-Fac Total	Fac Total		51	50	62	80	MUE
	30.24	30.24	090	2	1	0	1	1

69635 Tympanoplasty with antrotomy or mastoidotomy (including canalplasty, atticotomy, middle ear surgery, and/or tympanic membrane repair); without ossicular chain reconstruction   A 2 J 1

RVU			Global Days	Modifiers				
Mod	Non-Fac Total	Fac Total		51	50	62	80	MUE
	35.79	35.79	090	2	1	0	1	1

69636 Tympanoplasty with antrotomy or mastoidotomy (including canalplasty, atticotomy, middle ear surgery, and/or tympanic membrane repair); with ossicular chain reconstruction   A 2 J 1

RVU			Global Days	Modifiers				
Mod	Non-Fac Total	Fac Total		51	50	62	80	MUE
	40.00	40.00	090	2	1	0	0	1

69637 Tympanoplasty with antrotomy or mastoidotomy (including canalplasty, atticotomy, middle ear surgery, and/or tympanic membrane repair); with ossicular chain reconstruction and synthetic prosthesis (eg, partial ossicular replacement prosthesis [PORP], total ossicular replacement prosthesis [TORP])   A 2 J 1

RVU			Global Days	Modifiers				
Mod	Non-Fac Total	Fac Total		51	50	62	80	MUE
	39.78	39.78	090	2	1	0	0	1

69641 Tympanoplasty with mastoidectomy (including canalplasty, middle ear surgery, tympanic membrane repair); without ossicular chain reconstruction   A 2 J 1

RVU			Global Days	Modifiers				
Mod	Non-Fac Total	Fac Total		51	50	62	80	MUE
	30.15	30.15	090	2	1	0	1	1

69642 Tympanoplasty with mastoidectomy (including canalplasty, middle ear surgery, tympanic membrane repair); with ossicular chain reconstruction   A 2 J 1

RVU			Global Days	Modifiers				
Mod	Non-Fac Total	Fac Total		51	50	62	80	MUE
	38.67	38.67	090	2	1	0	1	1

69643 Tympanoplasty with mastoidectomy (including canalplasty, middle ear surgery, tympanic membrane repair); with intact or reconstructed wall, without ossicular chain reconstruction   A 2 J 1

RVU			Global Days	Modifiers				
Mod	Non-Fac Total	Fac Total		51	50	62	80	MUE
	35.44	35.44	090	2	1	0	1	1

● New   ▲ Revised   Deleted   ⊙ Moderate Sedation   ✚ Add-on Codes   ⊘ High Risk Denial   Ⓐ Age Edit   ♀ Female   ♂ Male   **AMA** *CPT® Assistant*   **MUE** Medically Unlikely Edit
⊘ Modifier 51 Exempt   ⊖ Modifier 63 Exempt   ✗ Unlisted   **Modifiers:** *See Inside Back Cover*   Ⓜ Maternity   A 2 – Z 3 ASC Payment Indicators   A – Y OPPS Status Indicators

69644 Tympanoplasty with mastoidectomy (including canalplasty, middle ear surgery, tympanic membrane repair); with intact or reconstructed canal wall, with ossicular chain reconstruction A 2 J I

RVU			Global Days	Modifiers				
Mod	Non-Fac Total	Fac Total		51	50	62	80	MUE
	42.77	42.77	090	2	1	0	1	1

69645 Tympanoplasty with mastoidectomy (including canalplasty, middle ear surgery, tympanic membrane repair); radical or complete, without ossicular chain reconstruction A 2 J I

RVU			Global Days	Modifiers				
Mod	Non-Fac Total	Fac Total		51	50	62	80	MUE
	42.07	42.07	090	2	1	0	1	1

Tympanoplasty with mastoidectomy radical/complete with/without ossicular chain reconstruction

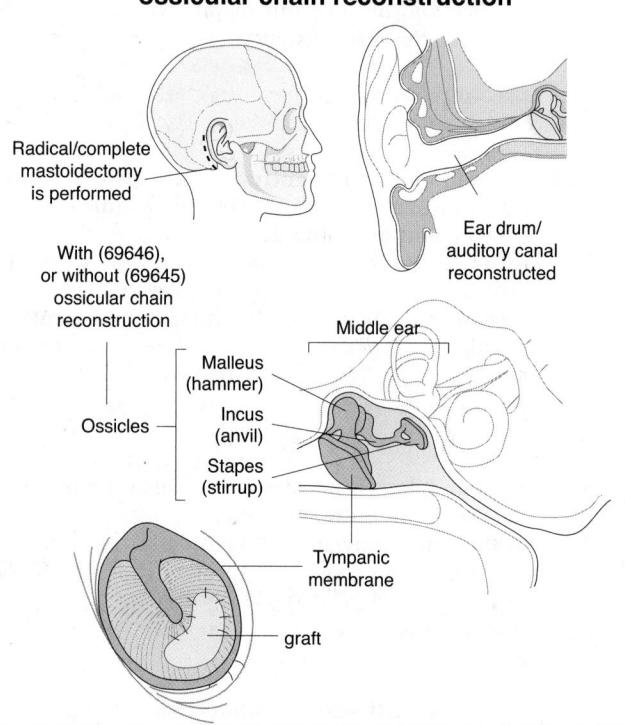

Radical/complete mastoidectomy is performed

With (69646), or without (69645) ossicular chain reconstruction

Ear drum/auditory canal reconstructed

Ossicles

Middle ear

Malleus (hammer)

Incus (anvil)

Stapes (stirrup)

Tympanic membrane

graft

69646 Tympanoplasty with mastoidectomy (including canalplasty, middle ear surgery, tympanic membrane repair); radical or complete, with ossicular chain reconstruction A 2 J I

RVU			Global Days	Modifiers				
Mod	Non-Fac Total	Fac Total		51	50	62	80	MUE
	44.70	44.70	090	2	1	0	0	1

69650 Stapes mobilization A 2 J I

RVU			Global Days	Modifiers				
Mod	Non-Fac Total	Fac Total		51	50	62	80	MUE
	23.34	23.34	090	2	1	0	1	1

69660 Stapedectomy or stapedotomy with reestablishment of ossicular continuity, with or without use of foreign material A 2 J I

RVU			Global Days	Modifiers				
Mod	Non-Fac Total	Fac Total		51	50	62	80	MUE
	26.85	26.85	090	2	1	0	1	1

69661 Stapedectomy or stapedotomy with reestablishment of ossicular continuity, with or without use of foreign material; with footplate drill out A 2 J I

RVU			Global Days	Modifiers				
Mod	Non-Fac Total	Fac Total		51	50	62	80	MUE
	35.00	35.00	090	2	1	0	0	1

69662 Revision of stapedectomy or stapedotomy A 2 J I

RVU			Global Days	Modifiers				
Mod	Non-Fac Total	Fac Total		51	50	62	80	MUE
	33.57	33.57	090	2	1	0	1	1

69666 Repair oval window fistula A 2 T

RVU			Global Days	Modifiers				
Mod	Non-Fac Total	Fac Total		51	50	62	80	MUE
	23.40	23.40	090	2	1	0	0	1

69667 Repair round window fistula A 2 T

RVU			Global Days	Modifiers				
Mod	Non-Fac Total	Fac Total		51	50	62	80	MUE
	23.42	23.42	090	2	1	0	0	1

69670 Mastoid obliteration (separate procedure) A 2 J I

RVU			Global Days	Modifiers				
Mod	Non-Fac Total	Fac Total		51	50	62	80	MUE
	27.44	27.44	090	2	1	0	2	1

Mastoid obliteration

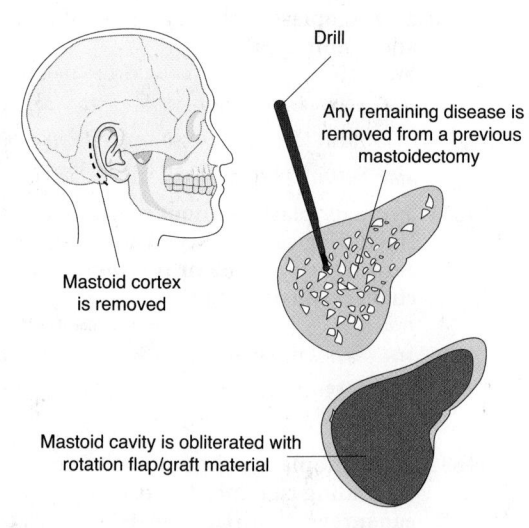

Drill

Any remaining disease is removed from a previous mastoidectomy

Mastoid cortex is removed

Mastoid cavity is obliterated with rotation flap/graft material

69676 Tympanic neurectomy A 2 T

RVU			Global Days	Modifiers				
Mod	Non-Fac Total	Fac Total		51	50	62	80	MUE
	24.05	24.05	090	2	1	0	1	1

● New   ▲ Revised   ✖ Deleted   ⊙ Moderate Sedation   ✚ Add-on Codes   ⊘ High Risk Denial   Ⓐ Age Edit   ♀ Female   ♂ Male   **AMA** *CPT® Assistant*   **MUE** Medically Unlikely Edit

⊘ Modifier 51 Exempt   ⊖ Modifier 63 Exempt   ☒ Unlisted   **Modifiers:** *See Inside Back Cover*   Ⓜ Maternity   A 2 – Z 3 ASC Payment Indicators   A – Y OPPS Status Indicators

CPT © 2015 American Medical Association. All Rights Reserved.   © 2016 DecisionHealth

Other Middle Ear Procedures

69700 Closure postauricular fistula, mastoid (separate procedure) `A2T`

RVU			Global Days	Modifiers				
Mod	Non-Fac Total	Fac Total		51	50	62	80	MUE
	19.84	19.84	090	2	1	0	1	1

Closure postauricular fistula, mastoid

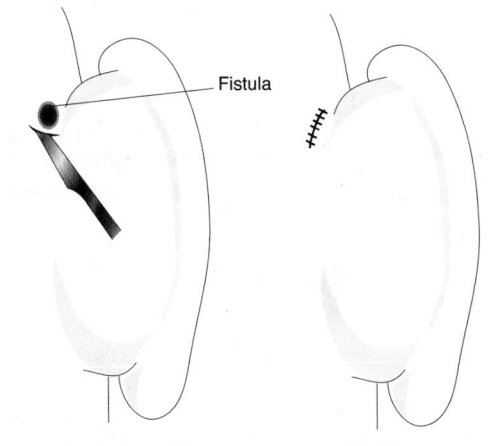

Fistula

The fistula tract is excised and repaired with sutures

69710 Implantation or replacement of electromagnetic bone conduction hearing device in temporal bone `⊗E`

RVU			Global Days	Modifiers				
Mod	Non-Fac Total	Fac Total		51	50	62	80	MUE
	0.00	0.00	XXX	9	9	9	9	

69711 Removal or repair of electromagnetic bone conduction hearing device in temporal bone `A2J I`

RVU			Global Days	Modifiers				
Mod	Non-Fac Total	Fac Total		51	50	62	80	MUE
	25.01	25.01	090	2	1	0	2	1

69714 Implantation, osseointegrated implant, temporal bone, with percutaneous attachment to external speech processor/cochlear stimulator; without mastoidectomy `J8J I`

RVU			Global Days	Modifiers				
Mod	Non-Fac Total	Fac Total		51	50	62	80	MUE
	31.20	31.20	090	2	1	0	1	1

AMA: Oct 13: 19

69715 Implantation, osseointegrated implant, temporal bone, with percutaneous attachment to external speech processor/cochlear stimulator; with mastoidectomy `J8J I`

RVU			Global Days	Modifiers				
Mod	Non-Fac Total	Fac Total		51	50	62	80	MUE
	38.49	38.49	090	2	1	0	1	1

69717 Replacement (including removal of existing device), osseointegrated implant, temporal bone, with percutaneous attachment to external speech processor/cochlear stimulator; without mastoidectomy `G2J I`

RVU			Global Days	Modifiers				
Mod	Non-Fac Total	Fac Total		51	50	62	80	MUE
	32.79	32.79	090	2	1	0	1	1

69718 Replacement (including removal of existing device), osseointegrated implant, temporal bone, with percutaneous attachment to external speech processor/cochlear stimulator; with mastoidectomy `G2J I`

RVU			Global Days	Modifiers				
Mod	Non-Fac Total	Fac Total		51	50	62	80	MUE
	38.89	38.89	090	2	1	0	1	1

69720 Decompression facial nerve, intratemporal; lateral to geniculate ganglion `A2J I`

RVU			Global Days	Modifiers				
Mod	Non-Fac Total	Fac Total		51	50	62	80	MUE
	35.27	35.27	090	2	1	1	0	1

69725 Decompression facial nerve, intratemporal; including medial to geniculate ganglion `J I`

RVU			Global Days	Modifiers				
Mod	Non-Fac Total	Fac Total		51	50	62	80	MUE
	54.48	54.48	090	2	1	0	2	1

69740 Suture facial nerve, intratemporal, with or without graft or decompression; lateral to geniculate ganglion `A2J I`

RVU			Global Days	Modifiers				
Mod	Non-Fac Total	Fac Total		51	50	62	80	MUE
	33.81	33.81	090	2	1	0	2	1

69745 Suture facial nerve, intratemporal, with or without graft or decompression; including medial to geniculate ganglion `A2J I`

RVU			Global Days	Modifiers				
Mod	Non-Fac Total	Fac Total		51	50	62	80	MUE
	40.91	40.91	090	2	1	0	2	1

69799 Unlisted procedure, middle ear `✗T`

RVU			Global Days	Modifiers				
Mod	Non-Fac Total	Fac Total		51	50	62	80	MUE
	0.00	0.00	YYY	2	1	1	0	

AMA: Oct 99: 10

Inner Ear Procedures

Incisional/Destruction Procedures

69801 Labyrinthotomy, with perfusion of vestibuloactive drug(s), transcanal `P3T`

RVU			Global Days	Modifiers				
Mod	Non-Fac Total	Fac Total		51	50	62	80	MUE
	5.63	3.65	000	2	1	0	0	1

AMA: Nov 96: 12, May 11: 8

● New   ▲ Revised   Deleted   ⊙ Moderate Sedation   ✚ Add-on Codes   ⊗ High Risk Denial   Ⓐ Age Edit   ♀ Female   ♂ Male   **AMA** CPT® Assistant   **MUE** Medically Unlikely Edit
⊘ Modifier 51 Exempt   ⊖ Modifier 63 Exempt   ✗ Unlisted   **Modifiers:** See Inside Back Cover   Ⓜ Maternity   A2–Z3 ASC Payment Indicators   A–Y OPPS Status Indicators

69805 Endolymphatic sac operation; without shunt `A2 J1`

RVU			Global Days	Modifiers				
Mod	Non-Fac Total	Fac Total		51	50	62	80	MUE
	30.55	30.55	090	2	1	0	2	1

69806 Endolymphatic sac operation; with shunt `A2 J1`

RVU			Global Days	Modifiers				
Mod	Non-Fac Total	Fac Total		51	50	62	80	MUE
	27.37	27.37	090	2	1	0	1	1

AMA: Nov 96: 12

69820 Fenestration semicircular canal `A2 J1`

RVU			Global Days	Modifiers				
Mod	Non-Fac Total	Fac Total		51	50	62	80	MUE
	24.80	24.80	090	2	1	0	2	1

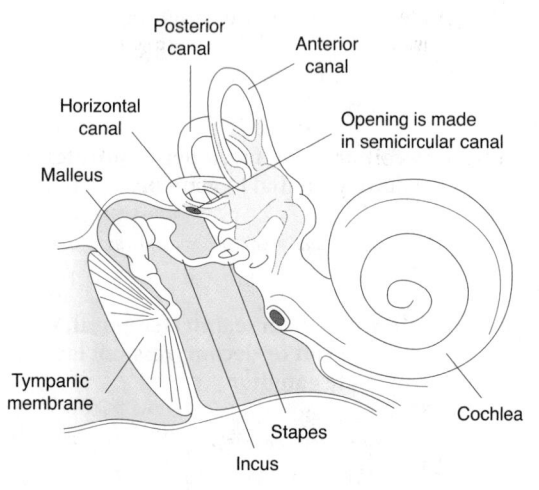

Semicircular canal fenestration

Primary fenestration (69820); fenestration revision (69840)

69840 Revision fenestration operation `A2 J1`

RVU			Global Days	Modifiers				
Mod	Non-Fac Total	Fac Total		51	50	62	80	MUE
	26.36	26.36	090	2	1	0	2	1

Excisional Inner Ear Procedures

69905 Labyrinthectomy; transcanal `A2 J1`

RVU			Global Days	Modifiers				
Mod	Non-Fac Total	Fac Total		51	50	62	80	MUE
	26.56	26.56	090	2	1	0	1	1

69910 Labyrinthectomy; with mastoidectomy `A2 J1`

Coding tip: *Mastoidectomy is included as part of the code descriptor for auditory procedure 69910; separate mastoidectomy service code should not be reported.*

RVU			Global Days	Modifiers				
Mod	Non-Fac Total	Fac Total		51	50	62	80	MUE
	29.45	29.45	090	2	1	0	0	1

69915 Vestibular nerve section, translabyrinthine approach `A2 J1`

RVU			Global Days	Modifiers				
Mod	Non-Fac Total	Fac Total		51	50	62	80	MUE
	44.58	44.58	090	2	1	1	2	1

Inner Ear Introduction Procedures

69930 Cochlear device implantation, with or without mastoidectomy `J8 J1`

RVU			Global Days	Modifiers				
Mod	Non-Fac Total	Fac Total		51	50	62	80	MUE
	35.48	35.48	090	2	1	0	0	1

Pub 100-04, 32, 100.4

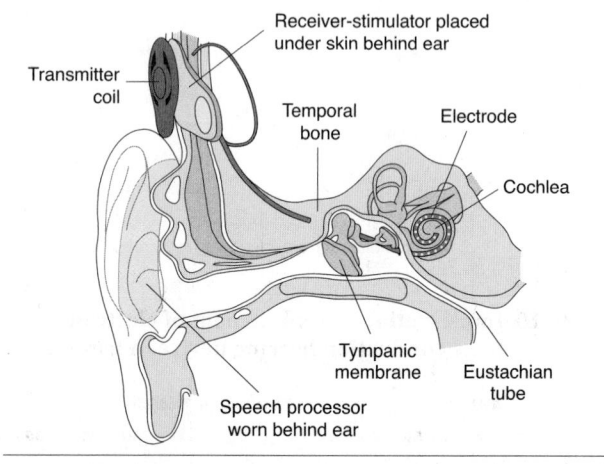

Cochlear device implantation

A device to aid hearing is inserted into the cochlea of the inner ear

Other Inner Ear Procedures

69949 Unlisted procedure, inner ear `X T`

RVU			Global Days	Modifiers				
Mod	Non-Fac Total	Fac Total		51	50	62	80	MUE
	0.00	0.00	YYY	2	1	1	0	

Temporal Bone/Middle Fossa Approach Procedures

69950 Vestibular nerve section, transcranial approach `C`

RVU			Global Days	Modifiers				
Mod	Non-Fac Total	Fac Total		51	50	62	80	MUE
	51.67	51.67	090	2	1	1	2	1

69955 Total facial nerve decompression and/or repair (may include graft) `J1`

RVU			Global Days	Modifiers				
Mod	Non-Fac Total	Fac Total		51	50	62	80	MUE
	57.82	57.82	090	2	1	1	2	1

69960 Decompression internal auditory canal `J1`

RVU			Global Days	Modifiers				
Mod	Non-Fac Total	Fac Total		51	50	62	80	MUE
	55.59	55.59	090	2	1	1	2	1

● New ▲ Revised ✖ Deleted ⊙ Moderate Sedation ✚ Add-on Codes ⊘ High Risk Denial Ⓐ Age Edit ♀ Female ♂ Male **AMA** CPT® Assistant **MUE** Medically Unlikely Edit
⊘ Modifier 51 Exempt ⊖ Modifier 63 Exempt ✗ Unlisted **Modifiers:** See Inside Back Cover Ⓜ Maternity `A2`–`Z3` ASC Payment Indicators `A`–`Y` OPPS Status Indicators

CPT © 2015 American Medical Association. All Rights Reserved. © 2016 DecisionHealth

69970 Removal of tumor, temporal bone

RVU			Global Days	Modifiers				
Mod	Non-Fac Total	Fac Total		51	50	62	80	MUE
	62.18	62.18	090	2	1	1	2	1

Removal of tumor, temporal bone

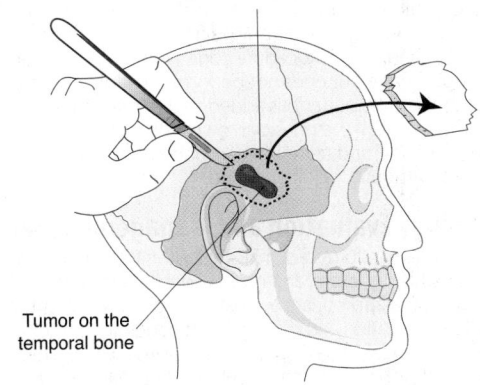

A section of the skull is removed with tumor

Tumor on the temporal bone

The physician isolates and removes the tumor

69979 Unlisted procedure, temporal bone, middle fossa approach

RVU			Global Days	Modifiers				
Mod	Non-Fac Total	Fac Total		51	50	62	80	MUE
	0.00	0.00	YYY	2	1	1	0	

AMA: Jan 07: 30, Sep 14: 14

Surgical Operating Microscope

Coding Guidance

CMS guidelines for reporting and payment of CPT code 69990 are different from those instructions found in the CPT Manual concerning this code. CMS allows payment for the use of an operating microscope with a list of specified procedures only. These procedures are identified in the Medicare Claims Processing Manual, Internet-Only Manuals (IOM). CMS bundles code 69990 into all other surgical procedures, and it should not be reported, even if used. Most edits do not allow modifier use.

+ 69990 Microsurgical techniques, requiring use of operating microscope (List separately in addition to code for primary procedure)

Documentation Finder: Documentation needs to show that a rather large operating microscope was brought into the surgical room and was used during a surgical procedure. The code is an add-on code and can't be reported on its own. This code is not appropriate if the surgeon documents using "loops" or "magnifying loops."

RVU			Global Days	Modifiers				
Mod	Non-Fac Total	Fac Total		51	50	62	80	MUE
	6.37	6.37	ZZZ	0	0	0	2	1

AMA: Nov 98: 20, Apr 99: 11, Jun 99: 11, Jul 99: 10, Oct 99: 10, Oct 00: 3, Oct 02: 8, Jan 04: 28, Mar 05: 11, Jul 05: 14, Aug 05: 1, Nov 07: 4, Sep 08: 10, Mar 09: 10, Dec 11: 14, Mar 12: 9, Jun 12: 17, Dec 12: 13, Oct 13: 14, Jan 14: 8, Apr 14: 10, Sep 14: 13, 14

● New ▲ Revised Deleted ⊙ Moderate Sedation ✚ Add-on Codes ⊘ High Risk Denial Ⓐ Age Edit ♀ Female ♂ Male **AMA** *CPT® Assistant* ***MUE*** Medically Unlikely Edit
⊘ Modifier 51 Exempt ⊖ Modifier 63 Exempt ✗ Unlisted **Modifiers:** *See Inside Back Cover* Ⓜ Maternity **A 2 – Z 3** ASC Payment Indicators **A – Y** OPPS Status Indicators

© 2016 DecisionHealth CPT © 2015 American Medical Association. All Rights Reserved. **613**

Radiology Procedures

Radiological Procedures

Introduction to Radiology

The codes in the Radiology Section of CPT (70010-79999) describe a broad spectrum of radiological imaging procedures, including standard radiographs with single or multiple views, contrast studies, ultrasound, mammography, computerized tomography (CT), magnetic resonance imaging (MRI), positron emission tomography (PET), and other radiological imaging services along with radiation oncology and nuclear medicine procedures. The diagnostic radiologic imaging subsection includes noninvasive procedures in addition to invasive, or interventional, procedures.

Diagnostic radiological imaging services are frequently performed by technicians under the supervision of a radiologist or other qualified health care professional, but a written, signed report by the interpreting physician or other qualified health care professional is an integral component of radiologic procedures.

The radiology CPT codes describe the type of service or modality, the anatomic site, and the use of any contrast material as well as various combinations of the number and/or type of radiographic views obtained. The code descriptors for many radiologic imaging services include a minimum number of views which may also include additional views when there isn't a more comprehensive code that includes those additional views. If additional views are necessary due to the patient's condition, separate reporting may sometimes be appropriate.

Use of Contrast Materials

Certain radiological studies are performed using contrast for image enhancement. Studies with contrast, without contrast, or both with and without contrast have separate codes describing all combinations of contrast usage. The phrase "with contrast" used in the code descriptors represents contrast material administered intravascularly, intraarticularly, or intrathecally. Oral and/or rectal contrast administration does not qualify as "with contrast." Injection of intravascular contrast material is considered part of the "with contrast" CT, CTA, MRI, and MRA procedures. Note that preliminary ""scout"" radiographs prior to contrast administration are not separately reportable.

Many interventional procedures require contrast injections for localization and/or guidance. The localization or guidance is considered integral to the interventional procedure and as such, is not separately reportable unless CPT specifically directs the user to report a specific code(s) for the localization or guidance.

Certain radiology services utilizing contrast include a procedural component and a radiologic supervision and interpretation component.

Radiologic Supervision and Interpretation

Many procedures include image guidance, which is stated in the code descriptor or guidelines and is not separately reportable. When imaging is not included in a procedure, the image guidance codes (codes labeled "radiological supervision and interpretation") may also be reported. Both services require image documentation. The radiological supervision, interpretation, and report services require a separate interpretation.

Radiological guidance procedures include all radiological services necessary to complete the procedure. Fluoroscopy is inherent in many radiological supervision and interpretation procedures including most spinal, endoscopic, and injection procedures and additional codes for fluoroscopic guidance should not be reported separately. Unless specifically noted, fluoroscopy is included in the radiologic procedure and should not be reported separately. There are however, separate fluoroscopic guidance codes which may be reported with some procedures.

Provision of Drugs/Radiopharmaceuticals

The nuclear medicine procedures in the Radiology Section involve the provision of drugs or radiopharmaceuticals, but the codes listed do not include the radiopharmaceutical or drug itself. Diagnostic and therapeutic radiopharmaceuticals and drugs supplied by the physician are reported separately using the appropriate supply code in addition to the nuclear medicine procedure code. The injection of a radiopharmaceutical is considered an integral component of a nuclear medicine procedure so codes for vascular access and injection of the radiopharmaceutical are not separately reportable.

Modifiers

Radiology procedures often require the use of modifiers such as modifier 50 Bilateral procedure, or the HCPCS Level II modifiers RT and LT. Radiologic imaging procedures such as chest X-rays are often repeated the same day; for example, for a patient with respiratory failure or chest trauma. To report these cases—and avoid duplicate claim denials—modifier 76 is appended to indicate a procedure or service was repeated by the same physician subsequent to the original service on the same day.

Radiology services differ from most other procedure codes in that they have professional and technical components. The professional component is the physician's services (supervising, interpreting, documenting) while the technical component represents the equipment, supplies, and staff used to perform the imaging. Modifier 26 (professional component) is added to a radiology procedure code when the physician interprets a radiologic image but does not perform the radiologic procedure. Modifier TC (technical component) is added to the imaging facility's radiology procedure code. If the physician owns the equipment and performs both the professional and technical components, the global service code is reported without a modifier added.

Radiology Evaluation and Management Services

If a radiologist performs a significant, separately identifiable service that includes a history, exam, and medical decision making distinct from the procedure, the appropriate evaluation and management service may be reported. Evaluation and management codes are not separately reportable in radiation oncology, except for an initial visit where a decision is made to proceed with the treatment. Subsequent evaluation and management services are included in the radiation treatment management CPT codes.

Diagnostic Radiology Procedures

Head/Neck Radiological Procedures

Coding Guidance

Non-invasive or non-interventional diagnostic imaging: This includes single or multiple view standard radiographs, computed tomography, magnetic resonance imaging, and some contrast studies. Because a combination of views is sometimes necessary to obtain the needed medical information, the code options should be reviewed for the most comprehensive code rather than billing multiple codes. If radiographs must be repeated due to substandard quality, only one unit of service may be billed. If the radiologist determines that additional views are necessary to render an interpretation after review of the initial films, the code that best describes the total service is reported, even if the patient was first released from the radiology department and returned for the additional views. The code descriptor may detail a minimum number of views. These services should be reported even if more than the minimum number was obtained to complete the series satisfactorily when there is no other more specific code available. When limited radiographic studies are done for comparison, such as following fracture reduction, catheter placement, intubation, etc., the comprehensive radiographic series should be reported with modifier 52 to indicate reduced services were provided. Fluoroscopy needed for obtaining permanent records and completing a procedure is included in the main service. Interventional or Invasive Diagnostic Imaging: When contrast required for an interventional or invasive diagnostic imaging procedure can be administered orally (for an upper GI), or rectally (a barium enema), the administration is part of the procedure. When contrast material is injected parenterally, the venous access and the administration are included in the main contrast study. When a contrast study requires that the timing be directly correlated with the contrast injection/administration and different providers are performing separate parts of the service, each provider would bill for the separate piece he/she rendered. The injection of contrast or radiopharmaceuticals is already inherent in radiological procedures. Codes 96372-96375 cannot be separately reported for inherent injection procedures with radiographic, CT, or MRI imaging codes. The procedural part of the service is coded from sections outside the radiology section. Radiographic supervision and interpretation portions of the service are coded from the 70000 series.

70010 Myelography, posterior fossa, radiological supervision and interpretation   N1 Q2

RVU				Global Days	Modifiers				
Mod	Non-Fac Total	Fac Total				51	50	62	80	MUE
	1.75	1.75	XXX			0	0	0	0	1

AMA: Mar 05: 11, Dec 07: 16

● New   ▲ Revised   ✖ Deleted   ⊙ Moderate Sedation   ✚ Add-on Codes   ⊖ High Risk Denial   ⒶAge Edit   ♀ Female   ♂ Male   **AMA** CPT® Assistant   **MUE** Medically Unlikely Edit
⊘ Modifier 51 Exempt   ⊖ Modifier 63 Exempt   ✗ Unlisted   **Modifiers:** See Inside Back Cover   Ⓜ Maternity   A2-Z3 ASC Payment Indicators   A-Y OPPS Status Indicators

Pub 100-04, 13, 30.1.3.4

70015 Cisternography, positive contrast, radiological supervision and interpretation N I Q2

Mod	Non-Fac Total	Fac Total	Global Days	51	50	62	80	MUE
	4.31	4.31	XXX	0	0	0	0	1
26	1.77	1.77	XXX	0	0	0	0	1
TC	2.54	2.54	XXX	0	0	0	0	1

Pub 100-04, 13, 30.1.3.5

70030 Radiologic examination, eye, for detection of foreign body N I Q1

Mod	Non-Fac Total	Fac Total	Global Days	51	50	62	80	MUE
	0.78	0.78	XXX	0	3	0	0	2
26	0.24	0.24	XXX	0	3	0	0	2
TC	0.54	0.54	XXX	0	3	0	0	2

70100 Radiologic examination, mandible; partial, less than 4 views N I Q1

Mod	Non-Fac Total	Fac Total	Global Days	51	50	62	80	MUE
	0.92	0.92	XXX	0	0	0	0	2
26	0.26	0.26	XXX	0	0	0	0	2
TC	0.66	0.66	XXX	0	0	0	0	2

70110 Radiologic examination, mandible; complete, minimum of 4 views N I Q1

Mod	Non-Fac Total	Fac Total	Global Days	51	50	62	80	MUE
	1.06	1.06	XXX	0	0	0	0	2
26	0.36	0.36	XXX	0	0	0	0	2
TC	0.70	0.70	XXX	0	0	0	0	2

70120 Radiologic examination, mastoids; less than 3 views per side N I Q1

Mod	Non-Fac Total	Fac Total	Global Days	51	50	62	80	MUE
	0.95	0.95	XXX	0	3	0	0	1
26	0.26	0.26	XXX	0	3	0	0	1
TC	0.69	0.69	XXX	0	3	0	0	1

70130 Radiologic examination, mastoids; complete, minimum of 3 views per side N I Q1

Mod	Non-Fac Total	Fac Total	Global Days	51	50	62	80	MUE
	1.53	1.53	XXX	0	3	0	0	1
26	0.49	0.49	XXX	0	3	0	0	1
TC	1.04	1.04	XXX	0	3	0	0	1

70134 Radiologic examination, internal auditory meati, complete N I Q1

Mod	Non-Fac Total	Fac Total	Global Days	51	50	62	80	MUE
	1.44	1.44	XXX	0	0	0	0	1
26	0.50	0.50	XXX	0	0	0	0	1
TC	0.94	0.94	XXX	0	0	0	0	1

70140 Radiologic examination, facial bones; less than 3 views N I Q1

Mod	Non-Fac Total	Fac Total	Global Days	51	50	62	80	MUE
	0.83	0.83	XXX	0	0	0	0	2
26	0.30	0.30	XXX	0	0	0	0	2
TC	0.53	0.53	XXX	0	0	0	0	2

70150 Radiologic examination, facial bones; complete, minimum of 3 views N I Q1

Mod	Non-Fac Total	Fac Total	Global Days	51	50	62	80	MUE
	1.16	1.16	XXX	0	0	0	0	1
26	0.38	0.38	XXX	0	0	0	0	1
TC	0.78	0.78	XXX	0	0	0	0	1

70160 Radiologic examination, nasal bones, complete, minimum of 3 views N I Q1

Mod	Non-Fac Total	Fac Total	Global Days	51	50	62	80	MUE
	0.91	0.91	XXX	0	0	0	0	1
26	0.25	0.25	XXX	0	0	0	0	1
TC	0.66	0.66	XXX	0	0	0	0	1

70170 Dacryocystography, nasolacrimal duct, radiological supervision and interpretation N I Q2

Mod	Non-Fac Total	Fac Total	Global Days	51	50	62	80	MUE
	0.00	0.00	XXX	0	0	0	0	2
26	0.43	0.43	XXX	0	0	0	0	2
TC	0.00	0.00	XXX	0	0	0	0	2

70190 Radiologic examination; optic foramina N I Q1

Mod	Non-Fac Total	Fac Total	Global Days	51	50	62	80	MUE
	1.00	1.00	XXX	0	3	0	0	1
26	0.32	0.32	XXX	0	3	0	0	1
TC	0.68	0.68	XXX	0	3	0	0	1

70200 Radiologic examination; orbits, complete, minimum of 4 views N I Q1

Mod	Non-Fac Total	Fac Total	Global Days	51	50	62	80	MUE
	1.18	1.18	XXX	0	0	0	0	2
26	0.40	0.40	XXX	0	0	0	0	2
TC	0.78	0.78	XXX	0	0	0	0	2

70210 Radiologic examination, sinuses, paranasal, less than 3 views N I Q1

Mod	Non-Fac Total	Fac Total	Global Days	51	50	62	80	MUE
	0.83	0.83	XXX	0	0	0	0	1
26	0.25	0.25	XXX	0	0	0	0	1
TC	0.58	0.58	XXX	0	0	0	0	1

70220 Radiologic examination, sinuses, paranasal, complete, minimum of 3 views N I Q1

Mod	Non-Fac Total	Fac Total	Global Days	51	50	62	80	MUE
	1.05	1.05	XXX	0	0	0	0	1
26	0.36	0.36	XXX	0	0	0	0	1
TC	0.69	0.69	XXX	0	0	0	0	1

70240 Radiologic examination, sella turcica N I Q1

Mod	Non-Fac Total	Fac Total	Global Days	51	50	62	80	MUE
	0.84	0.84	XXX	0	0	0	0	1
26	0.28	0.28	XXX	0	0	0	0	1
TC	0.56	0.56	XXX	0	0	0	0	1

● New ▲ Revised Deleted ⊙ Moderate Sedation ✚ Add-on Codes ⊘ High Risk Denial Ⓐ Age Edit ♀ Female ♂ Male **AMA** *CPT® Assistant* **MUE** Medically Unlikely Edit

Ⓢ Modifier 51 Exempt ⊖ Modifier 63 Exempt ⓧ Unlisted **Modifiers:** *See Inside Back Cover* Ⓜ Maternity A2–Z3 ASC Payment Indicators A–Y OPPS Status Indicators

© 2016 DecisionHealth | CPT © 2015 American Medical Association. All Rights Reserved. | 615

70250 Radiologic examination, skull; less than 4 views

N I Q 1

Mod	Non-Fac Total	Fac Total	Global Days	51	50	62	80	MUE
	1.01	1.01	XXX	0	0	0	0	2
26	0.36	0.36	XXX	0	0	0	0	2
TC	0.65	0.65	XXX	0	0	0	0	2

70260 Radiologic examination, skull; complete, minimum of 4 views

N I Q 1

Mod	Non-Fac Total	Fac Total	Global Days	51	50	62	80	MUE
	1.28	1.28	XXX	0	0	0	0	1
26	0.50	0.50	XXX	0	0	0	0	1
TC	0.78	0.78	XXX	0	0	0	0	1

70300 Radiologic examination, teeth; single view

C N I Q 1

Mod	Non-Fac Total	Fac Total	Global Days	51	50	62	80	MUE
	0.42	0.42	XXX	0	0	0	0	1
26	0.17	0.17	XXX	0	0	0	0	1
TC	0.25	0.25	XXX	0	0	0	0	1

70310 Radiologic examination, teeth; partial examination, less than full mouth

N I Q 1

Mod	Non-Fac Total	Fac Total	Global Days	51	50	62	80	MUE
	1.03	1.03	XXX	0	0	0	0	1
26	0.23	0.23	XXX	0	0	0	0	1
TC	0.80	0.80	XXX	0	0	0	0	1

70320 Radiologic examination, teeth; complete, full mouth

C N I Q 1

Mod	Non-Fac Total	Fac Total	Global Days	51	50	62	80	MUE
	1.47	1.47	XXX	0	0	0	0	1
26	0.34	0.34	XXX	0	0	0	0	1
TC	1.13	1.13	XXX	0	0	0	0	1

70328 Radiologic examination, temporomandibular joint, open and closed mouth; unilateral

N I Q 1

Mod	Non-Fac Total	Fac Total	Global Days	51	50	62	80	MUE
	0.86	0.86	XXX	0	0	0	0	1
26	0.26	0.26	XXX	0	0	0	0	1
TC	0.60	0.60	XXX	0	0	0	0	1

70330 Radiologic examination, temporomandibular joint, open and closed mouth; bilateral

N I Q 1

Mod	Non-Fac Total	Fac Total	Global Days	51	50	62	80	MUE
	1.32	1.32	XXX	0	2	0	0	1
26	0.36	0.36	XXX	0	2	0	0	1
TC	0.96	0.96	XXX	0	2	0	0	1

AMA: May 11: 10

70332 Temporomandibular joint arthrography, radiological supervision and interpretation

N I Q 2

Coding tip: Injection of temporomandibular joint - 21116

Mod	Non-Fac Total	Fac Total	Global Days	51	50	62	80	MUE
	2.29	2.29	XXX	0	3	0	0	2
26	0.89	0.89	XXX	0	3	0	0	2
TC	1.40	1.40	XXX	0	3	0	0	2

AMA: Feb 07: 11

70336 Magnetic resonance (eg, proton) imaging, temporomandibular joint(s)

Z 2 Q 3

Mod	Non-Fac Total	Fac Total	Global Days	51	50	62	80	MUE
	8.99	8.99	XXX	4	0	0	0	1
26	2.09	2.09	XXX	4	3	0	0	1
TC	6.90	6.90	XXX	4	0	0	0	1

AMA: Jul 99: 11, Jul 01: 7, Aug 15: 6

70350 Cephalogram, orthodontic

N I Q 1

Mod	Non-Fac Total	Fac Total	Global Days	51	50	62	80	MUE
	0.56	0.56	XXX	0	0	0	0	1
26	0.29	0.29	XXX	0	0	0	0	1
TC	0.27	0.27	XXX	0	0	0	0	1

AMA: Aug 12: 14

70355 Orthopantogram (eg, panoramic x-ray)

N I Q 1

Mod	Non-Fac Total	Fac Total	Global Days	51	50	62	80	MUE
	0.58	0.58	XXX	0	0	0	0	1
26	0.32	0.32	XXX	0	0	0	0	1
TC	0.26	0.26	XXX	0	0	0	0	1

70360 Radiologic examination; neck, soft tissue

N I Q 1

Mod	Non-Fac Total	Fac Total	Global Days	51	50	62	80	MUE
	0.79	0.79	XXX	0	0	0	0	2
26	0.24	0.24	XXX	0	0	0	0	2
TC	0.55	0.55	XXX	0	0	0	0	2

70370 Radiologic examination; pharynx or larynx, including fluoroscopy and/or magnification technique

N I Q 1

Coding tip: This code does not include any evaluation of dynamic motion. Report only for a diagnostic radiologic exam of the pharynx or larynx without contrast and without evaluation of movement.

Coding tip: Diagnostic radiologic exam of larynx with contrast - 70373

Mod	Non-Fac Total	Fac Total	Global Days	51	50	62	80	MUE
	2.20	2.20	XXX	0	0	0	0	1
26	0.46	0.46	XXX	0	0	0	0	1
TC	1.74	1.74	XXX	0	0	0	0	1

70371 Complex dynamic pharyngeal and speech evaluation by cine or video recording

N I Q 1

Mod	Non-Fac Total	Fac Total	Global Days	51	50	62	80	MUE
	2.57	2.57	XXX	0	0	0	0	1
26	1.22	1.22	XXX	0	0	0	0	1
TC	1.35	1.35	XXX	0	0	0	0	1

AMA: Dec 04: 17, Jul 14: 5

✖ ~~70373 Laryngography, contrast, radiological supervision and interpretation~~

70380 Radiologic examination, salivary gland for calculus

N I Q 1

Mod	Non-Fac Total	Fac Total	Global Days	51	50	62	80	MUE
	1.01	1.01	XXX	0	0	0	0	2
26	0.26	0.26	XXX	0	0	0	0	2
TC	0.75	0.75	XXX	0	0	0	0	2

● New   ▲ Revised   ✖ Deleted   ⊙ Moderate Sedation   ✚ Add-on Codes   ⊘ High Risk Denial   Ⓐ Age Edit   ♀ Female   ♂ Male   **AMA** *CPT® Assistant*   **MUE** Medically Unlikely Edit
⊘ Modifier 51 Exempt   ⊖ Modifier 63 Exempt   ✖ Unlisted   **Modifiers:** *See Inside Back Cover*   Ⓜ Maternity   A2–Z3 ASC Payment Indicators   A–Y OPPS Status Indicators

70390 Sialography, radiological supervision and interpretation N1Q2

RVU Mod	Non-Fac Total	Fac Total	Global Days	51	50	62	80	MUE
	2.64	2.64	XXX	0	0	0	0	2
26	0.54	0.54	XXX	0	0	0	0	2
TC	2.10	2.10	XXX	0	0	0	0	2

Coding Guidance
For supply of contrast material, refer to HCPCS Level II codes Q9951-Q9967.

70450 Computed tomography, head or brain; without contrast material Z2Q3

Documentation Finder: Documentation should state that they performed a CT or CAT scan image of the head or brain without contrast. No specific number of views is required. If CT imaging was taken without contrast and then followed with contrast, this is not the correct code.

RVU Mod	Non-Fac Total	Fac Total	Global Days	51	50	62	80	MUE
	3.25	3.25	XXX	4	0	0	0	3
26	1.21	1.21	XXX	4	0	0	0	3
TC	2.04	2.04	XXX	4	0	0	0	3

AMA: Apr 96: 11

70460 Computed tomography, head or brain; with contrast material(s) Z3Q3

RVU Mod	Non-Fac Total	Fac Total	Global Days	51	50	62	80	MUE
	4.54	4.54	XXX	4	0	0	0	1
26	1.61	1.61	XXX	4	0	0	0	1
TC	2.93	2.93	XXX	4	0	0	0	1

AMA: Apr 96: 11

70470 Computed tomography, head or brain; without contrast material, followed by contrast material(s) and further sections Z3Q3

RVU Mod	Non-Fac Total	Fac Total	Global Days	51	50	62	80	MUE
	5.37	5.37	XXX	4	0	0	0	2
26	1.81	1.81	XXX	4	0	0	0	2
TC	3.56	3.56	XXX	4	0	0	0	2

AMA: Apr 96: 11

70480 Computed tomography, orbit, sella, or posterior fossa or outer, middle, or inner ear; without contrast material Z2Q3

RVU Mod	Non-Fac Total	Fac Total	Global Days	51	50	62	80	MUE
	6.55	6.55	XXX	4	0	0	0	1
26	1.83	1.83	XXX	4	0	0	0	1
TC	4.72	4.72	XXX	4	0	0	0	1

70481 Computed tomography, orbit, sella, or posterior fossa or outer, middle, or inner ear; with contrast material(s) Z2Q3

RVU Mod	Non-Fac Total	Fac Total	Global Days	51	50	62	80	MUE
	7.75	7.75	XXX	4	0	0	0	1
26	1.97	1.97	XXX	4	0	0	0	1
TC	5.78	5.78	XXX	4	0	0	0	1

AMA: Apr 08: 11

70482 Computed tomography, orbit, sella, or posterior fossa or outer, middle, or inner ear; without contrast material, followed by contrast material(s) and further sections Z2Q3

RVU Mod	Non-Fac Total	Fac Total	Global Days	51	50	62	80	MUE
	8.46	8.46	XXX	4	0	0	0	1
26	2.06	2.06	XXX	4	0	0	0	1
TC	6.40	6.40	XXX	4	0	0	0	1

70486 Computed tomography, maxillofacial area; without contrast material Z2Q3

RVU Mod	Non-Fac Total	Fac Total	Global Days	51	50	62	80	MUE
	3.93	3.93	XXX	4	0	0	0	1
26	1.22	1.22	XXX	4	0	0	0	1
TC	2.71	2.71	XXX	4	0	0	0	1

AMA: Mar 02: 11

70487 Computed tomography, maxillofacial area; with contrast material(s) Z3Q3

RVU Mod	Non-Fac Total	Fac Total	Global Days	51	50	62	80	MUE
	4.72	4.72	XXX	4	0	0	0	1
26	1.61	1.61	XXX	4	0	0	0	1
TC	3.11	3.11	XXX	4	0	0	0	1

70488 Computed tomography, maxillofacial area; without contrast material, followed by contrast material(s) and further sections Z2Q3

RVU Mod	Non-Fac Total	Fac Total	Global Days	51	50	62	80	MUE
	5.76	5.76	XXX	4	0	0	0	1
26	1.81	1.81	XXX	4	0	0	0	1
TC	3.95	3.95	XXX	4	0	0	0	1

70490 Computed tomography, soft tissue neck; without contrast material Z2Q3

RVU Mod	Non-Fac Total	Fac Total	Global Days	51	50	62	80	MUE
	5.42	5.42	XXX	4	0	0	0	1
26	1.83	1.83	XXX	4	0	0	0	1
TC	3.59	3.59	XXX	4	0	0	0	1

70491 Computed tomography, soft tissue neck; with contrast material(s) Z2Q3

RVU Mod	Non-Fac Total	Fac Total	Global Days	51	50	62	80	MUE
	6.62	6.62	XXX	4	0	0	0	1
26	1.98	1.98	XXX	4	0	0	0	1
TC	4.64	4.64	XXX	4	0	0	0	1

70492 Computed tomography, soft tissue neck; without contrast material followed by contrast material(s) and further sections Z2Q3

RVU Mod	Non-Fac Total	Fac Total	Global Days	51	50	62	80	MUE
	7.79	7.79	XXX	4	0	0	0	1
26	2.06	2.06	XXX	4	0	0	0	1
TC	5.73	5.73	XXX	4	0	0	0	1

● New ▲ Revised Deleted ⊙ Moderate Sedation ✚ Add-on Codes ⊘ High Risk Denial Ⓐ Age Edit ♀ Female ♂ Male **AMA** *CPT® Assistant* **MUE** Medically Unlikely Edit
⊘ Modifier 51 Exempt ⊖ Modifier 63 Exempt ✗ Unlisted **Modifiers:** *See Inside Back Cover* Ⓜ Maternity A2–Z3 ASC Payment Indicators A–Y OPPS Status Indicators

70496 Computed tomographic angiography, head, with contrast material(s), including noncontrast images, if performed, and image postprocessing Z2Q3

RVU			Global Days	Modifiers				
Mod	Non-Fac Total	Fac Total		51	50	62	80	MUE
	8.27	8.27	XXX	4	0	0	0	2
26	2.49	2.49	XXX	4	0	0	0	2
TC	5.78	5.78	XXX	4	0	0	0	2

AMA: Jul 01: 4, Dec 05: 7, Jan 07: 31

70498 Computed tomographic angiography, neck, with contrast material(s), including noncontrast images, if performed, and image postprocessing Z2Q3

RVU			Global Days	Modifiers				
Mod	Non-Fac Total	Fac Total		51	50	62	80	MUE
	8.23	8.23	XXX	4	0	0	0	2
26	2.49	2.49	XXX	4	0	0	0	2
TC	5.74	5.74	XXX	4	0	0	0	2

AMA: Jul 01: 4, Dec 05: 7, Jan 07: 31

Coding Guidance

For supply of magnetic resonance contrast agent, refer to HCPCS Level II codes Q9953-Q9954.

Coding Guidance

MRI of the orbit, face, and/or neck (70540-70543) may only have one code reported per imaging session, regardless of whether only one, two, or all three areas are evaluated.

70540 Magnetic resonance (eg, proton) imaging, orbit, face, and/or neck; without contrast material(s) Z2Q3

RVU			Global Days	Modifiers				
Mod	Non-Fac Total	Fac Total		51	50	62	80	MUE
	10.07	10.07	XXX	4	0	0	0	1
26	1.92	1.92	XXX	4	0	0	0	1
TC	8.15	8.15	XXX	4	0	0	0	1

AMA: Jul 01: 6, Mar 07: 7, Sep 10: 10

70542 Magnetic resonance (eg, proton) imaging, orbit, face, and/or neck; with contrast material(s) Z2Q3

RVU			Global Days	Modifiers				
Mod	Non-Fac Total	Fac Total		51	50	62	80	MUE
	11.28	11.28	XXX	4	0	0	0	1
26	2.31	2.31	XXX	4	0	0	0	1
TC	8.97	8.97	XXX	4	0	0	0	1

AMA: Jul 01: 6, Sep 10: 10

70543 Magnetic resonance (eg, proton) imaging, orbit, face, and/or neck; without contrast material(s), followed by contrast material(s) and further sequences Z2Q3

RVU			Global Days	Modifiers				
Mod	Non-Fac Total	Fac Total		51	50	62	80	MUE
	13.80	13.80	XXX	4	0	0	0	1
26	3.05	3.05	XXX	4	0	0	0	1
TC	10.75	10.75	XXX	4	0	0	0	1

AMA: Jul 01: 6, Sep 10: 10

70544 Magnetic resonance angiography, head; without contrast material(s) Z2Q3

RVU			Global Days	Modifiers				
Mod	Non-Fac Total	Fac Total		51	50	62	80	MUE
	10.99	10.99	XXX	4	0	0	0	2
26	1.71	1.71	XXX	4	0	0	0	2
TC	9.28	9.28	XXX	4	0	0	0	2

AMA: Sep 01: 5, Dec 05: 7, Jan 07: 31

Pub 100-04, 13, 40.1.2

70545 Magnetic resonance angiography, head; with contrast material(s) Z2Q3

RVU			Global Days	Modifiers				
Mod	Non-Fac Total	Fac Total		51	50	62	80	MUE
	10.86	10.86	XXX	4	0	0	0	1
26	1.71	1.71	XXX	4	0	0	0	1
TC	9.15	9.15	XXX	4	0	0	0	1

AMA: Jul 01: 5, Dec 05: 7

Pub 100-04, 13, 40.1.2

70546 Magnetic resonance angiography, head; without contrast material(s), followed by contrast material(s) and further sequences Z2Q3

RVU			Global Days	Modifiers				
Mod	Non-Fac Total	Fac Total		51	50	62	80	MUE
	16.78	16.78	XXX	4	0	0	0	1
26	2.56	2.56	XXX	4	0	0	0	1
TC	14.22	14.22	XXX	4	0	0	0	1

AMA: Jul 01: 5, Dec 05: 7, Jan 07: 31

Pub 100-04, 13, 40.1.2

70547 Magnetic resonance angiography, neck; without contrast material(s) Z2Q3

RVU			Global Days	Modifiers				
Mod	Non-Fac Total	Fac Total		51	50	62	80	MUE
	11.04	11.04	XXX	4	0	0	0	1
26	1.72	1.72	XXX	4	0	0	0	1
TC	9.32	9.32	XXX	4	0	0	0	1

AMA: Sep 01: 5, Dec 05: 7, Jan 07: 31

Pub 100-04, 13, 40.1.2

70548 Magnetic resonance angiography, neck; with contrast material(s) Z2Q3

RVU			Global Days	Modifiers				
Mod	Non-Fac Total	Fac Total		51	50	62	80	MUE
	11.58	11.58	XXX	4	0	0	0	1
26	1.71	1.71	XXX	4	0	0	0	1
TC	9.87	9.87	XXX	4	0	0	0	1

AMA: Sep 01: 6, Dec 05: 7, Jan 07: 31

Pub 100-04, 13, 40.1.2

70549 Magnetic resonance angiography, neck; without contrast material(s), followed by contrast material(s) and further sequences Z2Q3

RVU			Global Days	Modifiers				
Mod	Non-Fac Total	Fac Total		51	50	62	80	MUE
	16.89	16.89	XXX	4	0	0	0	1
26	2.56	2.56	XXX	4	0	0	0	1
TC	14.33	14.33	XXX	4	0	0	0	1

AMA: Sep 01: 6, Dec 05: 7, Jan 07: 31

Pub 100-04, 13, 40.1.2

Coding Guidance

For supply of magnetic resonance contrast agent, refer to HCPCS Level II codes A9585 and Q9953-Q9954.

● New   ▲ Revised   ✖ Deleted   ⊙ Moderate Sedation   ✚ Add-on Codes   ⊘ High Risk Denial   Ⓐ Age Edit   ♀ Female   ♂ Male   **AMA** *CPT® Assistant*   **MUE** Medically Unlikely Edit
⊘ Modifier 51 Exempt   ⊖ Modifier 63 Exempt   🗶 Unlisted   **Modifiers:** *See Inside Back Cover*   Ⓜ Maternity   A2–Z3 ASC Payment Indicators   A–Y OPPS Status Indicators

618   CPT © 2015 American Medical Association. All Rights Reserved.   © 2016 DecisionHealth

Coding Guidance

Report MRI of the brain together with MRI of the orbit (70540-70543) only when both procedures are medically necessary and each is performed as a distinct service. An MRI of the orbit is not reportable with an MRI of the brain if an incidental orbital abnormality is identified during the brain study, as only one study service was performed.

70551 Magnetic resonance (eg, proton) imaging, brain (including brain stem); without contrast material `Z 2 Q 3`

Documentation Finder: Documentation should show that an MRI was performed without any injection of contrast for brain. This code should not be reported if they inject contrast after obtaining the initial MRI without contrast.

RVU			Global Days	Modifiers				
Mod	Non-Fac Total	Fac Total		51	50	62	80	MUE
	6.47	6.47	XXX	4	0	0	0	2
26	2.11	2.11	XXX	4	0	0	0	2
TC	4.36	4.36	XXX	4	0	0	0	2

AMA: May 98: 10, Mar 05: 20, Feb 07: 6

Pub 100-04, 13, 40

70552 Magnetic resonance (eg, proton) imaging, brain (including brain stem); with contrast material(s) `Z 3 Q 3`

RVU			Global Days	Modifiers				
Mod	Non-Fac Total	Fac Total		51	50	62	80	MUE
	8.97	8.97	XXX	4	0	0	0	2
26	2.54	2.54	XXX	4	0	0	0	2
TC	6.43	6.43	XXX	4	0	0	0	2

AMA: Jul 01: 6, Mar 05: 20, Feb 07: 6

70553 Magnetic resonance (eg, proton) imaging, brain (including brain stem); without contrast material, followed by contrast material(s) and further sequences `Z 2 Q 3`

Documentation Finder: Documentation should show that an MRI was performed without any injection of contrast for imaging of the brain. Then following the non-contrast imaging, an injection of contrast is given and further images of the brain are taken with contrast in place.

RVU			Global Days	Modifiers				
Mod	Non-Fac Total	Fac Total		51	50	62	80	MUE
	10.60	10.60	XXX	4	0	0	0	2
26	3.27	3.27	XXX	4	0	0	0	2
TC	7.33	7.33	XXX	4	0	0	0	2

AMA: Nov 97: 24, Jul 01: 6, Mar 05: 20, Feb 07: 6

Pub 100-04, 13, 40

70554 Magnetic resonance imaging, brain, functional MRI; including test selection and administration of repetitive body part movement and/or visual stimulation, not requiring physician or psychologist administration `Z 2 Q 3`

RVU			Global Days	Modifiers				
Mod	Non-Fac Total	Fac Total		51	50	62	80	MUE
	12.66	12.66	XXX	4	3	0	0	1
26	3.03	3.03	XXX	4	3	0	0	1
TC	9.63	9.63	XXX	4	3	0	0	1

AMA: Feb 07: 6, Mar 07: 7, Aug 08: 13

70555 Magnetic resonance imaging, brain, functional MRI; requiring physician or psychologist administration of entire neurofunctional testing `Z 2 S`

RVU			Global Days	Modifiers				
Mod	Non-Fac Total	Fac Total		51	50	62	80	MUE
	0.00	0.00	XXX	0	3	0	0	1
26	3.60	3.60	XXX	0	3	0	0	1
TC	0.00	0.00	XXX	0	3	0	0	1

AMA: Feb 07: 6, Mar 07: 7

70557 Magnetic resonance (eg, proton) imaging, brain (including brain stem and skull base), during open intracranial procedure (eg, to assess for residual tumor or residual vascular malformation); without contrast material `Z 2 S`

RVU			Global Days	Modifiers				
Mod	Non-Fac Total	Fac Total		51	50	62	80	MUE
	0.00	0.00	XXX	0	0	0	0	1
26	4.16	4.16	XXX	0	0	0	0	1
TC	0.00	0.00	XXX	0	0	0	0	1

70558 Magnetic resonance (eg, proton) imaging, brain (including brain stem and skull base), during open intracranial procedure (eg, to assess for residual tumor or residual vascular malformation); with contrast material(s) `Z 2 S`

RVU			Global Days	Modifiers				
Mod	Non-Fac Total	Fac Total		51	50	62	80	MUE
	0.00	0.00	XXX	0	0	0	0	1
26	4.58	4.58	XXX	0	0	0	0	1
TC	0.00	0.00	XXX	0	0	0	0	1

70559 Magnetic resonance (eg, proton) imaging, brain (including brain stem and skull base), during open intracranial procedure (eg, to assess for residual tumor or residual vascular malformation); without contrast material(s), followed by contrast material(s) and further sequences `Z 2 S`

RVU			Global Days	Modifiers				
Mod	Non-Fac Total	Fac Total		51	50	62	80	MUE
	0.00	0.00	XXX	0	0	0	0	1
26	4.61	4.61	XXX	0	0	0	0	1
TC	0.00	0.00	XXX	0	0	0	0	1

Chest Radiological Procedures

71010 Radiologic examination, chest; single view, frontal `Z 3 Q 3`

Documentation Finder: Documentation should state that only one frontal view of the chest was taken to support this code.

RVU			Global Days	Modifiers				
Mod	Non-Fac Total	Fac Total		51	50	62	80	MUE
	0.63	0.63	XXX	0	0	0	0	6
26	0.26	0.26	XXX	0	0	0	0	6
TC	0.37	0.37	XXX	0	0	0	0	6

AMA: Aug 00: 1, Feb 07: 10, Jul 07: 1, 6, Sep 13: 18, May 14: 4

Pub 100-04, 12, 30.6.12; 100-04, 13, 150; 100-04, 16, 120.2

● New   ▲ Revised   Deleted   ⊙ Moderate Sedation   ✚ Add-on Codes   ⊘ High Risk Denial   Ⓐ Age Edit   ♀ Female   ♂ Male   **AMA** *CPT® Assistant*   **MUE** Medically Unlikely Edit
⊘ Modifier 51 Exempt   ⊖ Modifier 63 Exempt   ✖ Unlisted   **Modifiers:** *See Inside Back Cover*   Ⓜ Maternity   A 2 – Z 3 ASC Payment Indicators   A – Y OPPS Status Indicators

71015 Radiologic examination, chest; stereo, frontal

`Z3Q3`

RVU Mod	Non-Fac Total	Fac Total	Global Days	Modifiers 51	50	62	80	MUE
	0.78	0.78	XXX	0	0	0	0	2
26	0.31	0.31	XXX	0	0	0	0	2
TC	0.47	0.47	XXX	0	0	0	0	2

AMA: Feb 07: 10, Jul 07: 1, May 14: 4

Pub 100-04, 12, 30.6.12; 100-04, 16, 120.2

71020 Radiologic examination, chest, 2 views, frontal and lateral

`Z3Q3`

Documentation Finder: Documentation should state clearly that frontal and lateral views of the chest were taken. This code should be reported only if the two views taken were identified as frontal and lateral views.

RVU Mod	Non-Fac Total	Fac Total	Global Days	Modifiers 51	50	62	80	MUE
	0.78	0.78	XXX	0	0	0	0	4
26	0.31	0.31	XXX	0	0	0	0	4
TC	0.47	0.47	XXX	0	0	0	0	4

AMA: Sep 03: 3, Mar 05: 11, Feb 07: 10, Jul 07: 1, 6, Dec 09: 14, Sep 10: 6, Sep 13: 18, May 14: 4, Jun 14: 14

Pub 100-04, 12, 30.6.12; 100-04, 16, 120.2

71021 Radiologic examination, chest, 2 views, frontal and lateral; with apical lordotic procedure

`NIQI`

RVU Mod	Non-Fac Total	Fac Total	Global Days	Modifiers 51	50	62	80	MUE
	0.95	0.95	XXX	0	0	0	0	1
26	0.39	0.39	XXX	0	0	0	0	1
TC	0.56	0.56	XXX	0	0	0	0	1

Pub 100-04, 16, 120.2

71022 Radiologic examination, chest, 2 views, frontal and lateral; with oblique projections

`NIQI`

RVU Mod	Non-Fac Total	Fac Total	Global Days	Modifiers 51	50	62	80	MUE
	1.17	1.17	XXX	0	0	0	0	1
26	0.47	0.47	XXX	0	0	0	0	1
TC	0.70	0.70	XXX	0	0	0	0	1

AMA: Jul 07: 6

Pub 100-04, 16, 120.2

71023 Radiologic examination, chest, 2 views, frontal and lateral; with fluoroscopy

`NIQI`

RVU Mod	Non-Fac Total	Fac Total	Global Days	Modifiers 51	50	62	80	MUE
	1.78	1.78	XXX	0	0	0	0	1
26	0.54	0.54	XXX	0	0	0	0	1
TC	1.24	1.24	XXX	0	0	0	0	1

AMA: Aug 03: 14, Dec 08: 7, Feb 13: 3, Mar 13: 10, Sep 13: 17, Sep 14: 5

71030 Radiologic examination, chest, complete, minimum of 4 views

`NIQI`

RVU Mod	Non-Fac Total	Fac Total	Global Days	Modifiers 51	50	62	80	MUE
	1.17	1.17	XXX	0	0	0	0	1
26	0.45	0.45	XXX	0	0	0	0	1
TC	0.72	0.72	XXX	0	0	0	0	1

AMA: Jul 07: 6, Dec 09: 14

Pub 100-04, 16, 120.2

71034 Radiologic examination, chest, complete, minimum of 4 views; with fluoroscopy

`NIQI`

RVU Mod	Non-Fac Total	Fac Total	Global Days	Modifiers 51	50	62	80	MUE
	2.33	2.33	XXX	0	0	0	0	1
26	0.66	0.66	XXX	0	0	0	0	1
TC	1.67	1.67	XXX	0	0	0	0	1

AMA: Aug 03: 14, Dec 08: 7, Feb 13: 3, Mar 13: 10, Sep 13: 17, Sep 14: 5

71035 Radiologic examination, chest, special views (eg, lateral decubitus, Bucky studies)

`NIQI`

RVU Mod	Non-Fac Total	Fac Total	Global Days	Modifiers 51	50	62	80	MUE
	0.92	0.92	XXX	0	0	0	0	3
26	0.26	0.26	XXX	0	0	0	0	3
TC	0.66	0.66	XXX	0	0	0	0	3

AMA: Sep 13: 18

Pub 100-04, 16, 120.2

71100 Radiologic examination, ribs, unilateral; 2 views

`NIQI`

RVU Mod	Non-Fac Total	Fac Total	Global Days	Modifiers 51	50	62	80	MUE
	0.92	0.92	XXX	0	0	0	0	2
26	0.32	0.32	XXX	0	0	0	0	2
TC	0.60	0.60	XXX	0	0	0	0	2

71101 Radiologic examination, ribs, unilateral; including posteroanterior chest, minimum of 3 views

`NIQI`

RVU Mod	Non-Fac Total	Fac Total	Global Days	Modifiers 51	50	62	80	MUE
	1.02	1.02	XXX	0	0	0	0	2
26	0.39	0.39	XXX	0	0	0	0	2
TC	0.63	0.63	XXX	0	0	0	0	2

71110 Radiologic examination, ribs, bilateral; 3 views

`NIQI`

RVU Mod	Non-Fac Total	Fac Total	Global Days	Modifiers 51	50	62	80	MUE
	1.05	1.05	XXX	0	2	0	0	1
26	0.39	0.39	XXX	0	2	0	0	1
TC	0.66	0.66	XXX	0	2	0	0	1

71111 Radiologic examination, ribs, bilateral; including posteroanterior chest, minimum of 4 views

`NIQI`

RVU Mod	Non-Fac Total	Fac Total	Global Days	Modifiers 51	50	62	80	MUE
	1.34	1.34	XXX	0	2	0	0	1
26	0.47	0.47	XXX	0	2	0	0	1
TC	0.87	0.87	XXX	0	2	0	0	1

71120 Radiologic examination; sternum, minimum of 2 views

`NIQI`

RVU Mod	Non-Fac Total	Fac Total	Global Days	Modifiers 51	50	62	80	MUE
	0.83	0.83	XXX	0	0	0	0	1
26	0.29	0.29	XXX	0	0	0	0	1
TC	0.54	0.54	XXX	0	0	0	0	1

● New   ▲ Revised   ✖ Deleted   ⊙ Moderate Sedation   ✚ Add-on Codes   ⊘ High Risk Denial   Ⓐ Age Edit   ♀ Female   ♂ Male   **AMA** *CPT® Assistant*   *MUE* Medically Unlikely Edit

⊘ Modifier 51 Exempt   ⊖ Modifier 63 Exempt   Ⓧ Unlisted   **Modifiers:** *See Inside Back Cover*   Ⓜ Maternity   `A2`–`Z3` ASC Payment Indicators   `A`–`Y` OPPS Status Indicators

CPT © 2015 American Medical Association. All Rights Reserved.   © 2016 DecisionHealth

71130 Radiologic examination; sternoclavicular joint or joints, minimum of 3 views N1 Q1

Mod	Non-Fac Total	Fac Total	Global Days	51	50	62	80	MUE
	1.01	1.01	XXX	0	0	0	0	1
26	0.32	0.32	XXX	0	0	0	0	1
TC	0.69	0.69	XXX	0	0	0	0	1

71250 Computed tomography, thorax; without contrast material Z2 Q3

Documentation Finder: Documentation should state that they performed a CT or (sometimes referred to as a CAT scan) scan image of the thorax without contrast. The code does not require a certain number of views. If CT imaging was taken without contrast then followed with contrast, this is not the correct code.

Mod	Non-Fac Total	Fac Total	Global Days	51	50	62	80	MUE
	5.06	5.06	XXX	4	0	0	0	2
26	1.46	1.46	XXX	4	0	0	0	2
TC	3.60	3.60	XXX	4	0	0	0	2

AMA: Jul 07: 13, Aug 11: 10

71260 Computed tomography, thorax; with contrast material(s) Z2 Q3

Documentation Finder: Documentation should state that contrast was injected and then CT imaging (or CAT scan) of the thorax was obtained. The code does not require a certain number of views. If CT imaging was taken without contrast then followed with contrast, this is not the correct code.

Mod	Non-Fac Total	Fac Total	Global Days	51	50	62	80	MUE
	6.44	6.44	XXX	4	0	0	0	2
26	1.78	1.78	XXX	4	0	0	0	2
TC	4.66	4.66	XXX	4	0	0	0	2

AMA: Jul 01: 4, Jun 09: 9

71270 Computed tomography, thorax; without contrast material, followed by contrast material(s) and further sections Z2 Q3

Mod	Non-Fac Total	Fac Total	Global Days	51	50	62	80	MUE
	7.72	7.72	XXX	4	0	0	0	1
26	1.97	1.97	XXX	4	0	0	0	1
TC	5.75	5.75	XXX	4	0	0	0	1

AMA: Jun 01: 10, Jul 07: 13

71275 Computed tomographic angiography, chest (noncoronary), with contrast material(s), including noncontrast images, if performed, and image postprocessing Z2 Q3

Documentation Finder: Documentation should show that a CTA of the chest was first performed without any contrast then after performing and taking these imagines, an injection of contrast is given and additional imagines (views) are taken. This chest CTA would not include the heart structures as this is a "noncoronary" study.

Mod	Non-Fac Total	Fac Total	Global Days	51	50	62	80	MUE
	8.41	8.41	XXX	4	0	0	0	1
26	2.59	2.59	XXX	4	0	0	0	1
TC	5.82	5.82	XXX	4	0	0	0	1

AMA: Jul 01: 4, Jun 05: 11, Dec 05: 7, Jan 07: 31, Mar 07: 7, Jun 09: 9, Aug 11: 10

71550 Magnetic resonance (eg, proton) imaging, chest (eg, for evaluation of hilar and mediastinal lymphadenopathy); without contrast material(s) Z2 Q3

Mod	Non-Fac Total	Fac Total	Global Days	51	50	62	80	MUE
	11.62	11.62	XXX	4	0	0	0	1
26	2.08	2.08	XXX	4	0	0	0	1
TC	9.54	9.54	XXX	4	0	0	0	1

AMA: Jul 01: 7, Apr 10: 10, Sep 10: 10

71551 Magnetic resonance (eg, proton) imaging, chest (eg, for evaluation of hilar and mediastinal lymphadenopathy); with contrast material(s) Z2 Q3

Mod	Non-Fac Total	Fac Total	Global Days	51	50	62	80	MUE
	12.86	12.86	XXX	4	0	0	0	1
26	2.46	2.46	XXX	4	0	0	0	1
TC	10.40	10.40	XXX	4	0	0	0	1

AMA: Jul 01: 7, Sep 10: 10

71552 Magnetic resonance (eg, proton) imaging, chest (eg, for evaluation of hilar and mediastinal lymphadenopathy); without contrast material(s), followed by contrast material(s) and further sequences Z2 Q3

Mod	Non-Fac Total	Fac Total	Global Days	51	50	62	80	MUE
	16.25	16.25	XXX	4	0	0	0	1
26	3.22	3.22	XXX	4	0	0	0	1
TC	13.03	13.03	XXX	4	0	0	0	1

AMA: Jul 01: 7, Apr 10: 10, Sep 10: 10

71555 Magnetic resonance angiography, chest (excluding myocardium), with or without contrast material(s) B

Coding tip: For OPPS codes for chest MRA, refer to HCPCS Level II codes C8909-C8911.

Mod	Non-Fac Total	Fac Total	Global Days	51	50	62	80	MUE
	11.15	11.15	XXX	4	0	0	0	1
26	2.55	2.55	XXX	4	0	0	0	1
TC	8.60	8.60	XXX	4	0	0	0	1

AMA: Fall 95: 2, Dec 05: 7, Jan 07: 31

Pub 100-04, 13, 40, 40.1.2

✖ 72010 ~~Radiologic examination, spine, entire, survey study, anteroposterior and lateral~~

72020 Radiologic examination, spine, single view, specify level N1 Q1

Mod	Non-Fac Total	Fac Total	Global Days	51	50	62	80	MUE
	0.62	0.62	XXX	0	0	0	0	4
26	0.22	0.22	XXX	0	0	0	0	4
TC	0.40	0.40	XXX	0	0	0	0	4

AMA: Jul 13: 10

● New ▲ Revised Deleted ⊙ Moderate Sedation ✚ Add-on Codes ⊗ High Risk Denial Ⓐ Age Edit ♀ Female ♂ Male **AMA** *CPT® Assistant* **MUE** Medically Unlikely Edit
⊘ Modifier 51 Exempt ⊖ Modifier 63 Exempt ✖ Unlisted **Modifiers:** *See Inside Back Cover* Ⓜ Maternity A2–Z3 ASC Payment Indicators A–Y OPPS Status Indicators

Coding Guidance

When initial AP and lateral views are taken in order to clear the spine in injury cases before moving the patient into oblique or extension positions for a complete cervical exam, they are also included and cannot be reported separately.

72040 Radiologic examination, spine, cervical; 2 or 3 views `N I Q I`

Documentation Finder: *Documentation should state clearly either the names of two or three views – such as anterior-posterior and lateral or oblique – or two views of the cervical spine were taken or three views of the cervical spine were taken.*

RVU Mod	Non-Fac Total	Fac Total	Global Days	Modifiers 51	50	62	80	MUE
	0.93	0.93	XXX	0	0	0	0	3
26	0.32	0.32	XXX	0	0	0	0	3
TC	0.61	0.61	XXX	0	0	0	0	3

AMA: Sep 01: 7, Jul 13: 10

72050 Radiologic examination, spine, cervical; 4 or 5 views `N I Q I`

RVU Mod	Non-Fac Total	Fac Total	Global Days	Modifiers 51	50	62	80	MUE
	1.26	1.26	XXX	0	0	0	0	1
26	0.45	0.45	XXX	0	0	0	0	1
TC	0.81	0.81	XXX	0	0	0	0	1

72052 Radiologic examination, spine, cervical; 6 or more views `N I Q I`

RVU Mod	Non-Fac Total	Fac Total	Global Days	Modifiers 51	50	62	80	MUE
	1.58	1.58	XXX	0	0	0	0	1
26	0.52	0.52	XXX	0	0	0	0	1
TC	1.06	1.06	XXX	0	0	0	0	1

✖ ~~72069 Radiologic examination, spine, thoracolumbar, standing (scoliosis)~~

72070 Radiologic examination, spine; thoracic, 2 views `N I Q I`

RVU Mod	Non-Fac Total	Fac Total	Global Days	Modifiers 51	50	62	80	MUE
	0.95	0.95	XXX	0	0	0	0	1
26	0.32	0.32	XXX	0	0	0	0	1
TC	0.63	0.63	XXX	0	0	0	0	1

AMA: Sep 01: 7

72072 Radiologic examination, spine; thoracic, 3 views `N I Q I`

RVU Mod	Non-Fac Total	Fac Total	Global Days	Modifiers 51	50	62	80	MUE
	0.97	0.97	XXX	0	0	0	0	1
26	0.31	0.31	XXX	0	0	0	0	1
TC	0.66	0.66	XXX	0	0	0	0	1

AMA: Sep 01: 7

72074 Radiologic examination, spine; thoracic, minimum of 4 views `N I Q I`

RVU Mod	Non-Fac Total	Fac Total	Global Days	Modifiers 51	50	62	80	MUE
	1.10	1.10	XXX	0	0	0	0	1
26	0.31	0.31	XXX	0	0	0	0	1
TC	0.79	0.79	XXX	0	0	0	0	1

AMA: Sep 01: 7

▲ 72080 Radiologic examination, spine; thoracolumbar junction, minimum of 2 views `N I Q I`

Coding tip: *Thoracolumbar views taken while standing to verify scoliosis curvature û 72069*

RVU Mod	Non-Fac Total	Fac Total	Global Days	Modifiers 51	50	62	80	MUE
	0.86	0.86	XXX	0	0	0	0	1
26	0.31	0.31	XXX	0	0	0	0	1
TC	0.55	0.55	XXX	0	0	0	0	1

AMA: Sep 01: 7

● 72081 Radiologic examination, spine, entire thoracic and lumbar, including skull, cervical and sacral spine if performed (eg, scoliosis evaluation); one view `Q I`

RVU Mod	Non-Fac Total	Fac Total	Global Days	Modifiers 51	50	62	80	MUE
	1.09	1.09	XXX	0	0	0	0	1
26	0.38	0.38	XXX	0	0	0	0	1
TC	0.71	0.71	XXX	0	0	0	0	1

● 72082 Radiologic examination, spine, entire thoracic and lumbar, including skull, cervical and sacral spine if performed (eg, scoliosis evaluation); 2 or 3 views `Q I`

RVU Mod	Non-Fac Total	Fac Total	Global Days	Modifiers 51	50	62	80	MUE
	1.75	1.75	XXX	0	0	0	0	1
26	0.46	0.46	XXX	0	0	0	0	1
TC	1.29	1.29	XXX	0	0	0	0	1

● 72083 Radiologic examination, spine, entire thoracic and lumbar, including skull, cervical and sacral spine if performed (eg, scoliosis evaluation); 4 or 5 views `Z 2 S`

RVU Mod	Non-Fac Total	Fac Total	Global Days	Modifiers 51	50	62	80	MUE
	1.90	1.90	XXX	0	0	0	0	1
26	0.50	0.50	XXX	0	0	0	0	1
TC	1.40	1.40	XXX	0	0	0	0	1

● 72084 Radiologic examination, spine, entire thoracic and lumbar, including skull, cervical and sacral spine if performed (eg, scoliosis evaluation); minimum of 6 views `Z 2 S`

RVU Mod	Non-Fac Total	Fac Total	Global Days	Modifiers 51	50	62	80	MUE
	2.26	2.26	XXX	0	0	0	0	1
26	0.58	0.58	XXX	0	0	0	0	1
TC	1.68	1.68	XXX	0	0	0	0	1

✖ ~~72090 Radiologic examination, spine; scoliosis study, including supine and erect studies~~

Coding Guidance

When initial AP and lateral views are taken in order to clear the spine in injury cases before moving the patient into oblique or bending positions for a complete lumbar exam, they are also included and cannot be reported separately.

● New ▲ Revised ✖ Deleted ⊙ Moderate Sedation ✚ Add-on Codes ⊘ High Risk Denial ⒶAge Edit ♀ Female ♂ Male **AMA** CPT® Assistant **MUE** Medically Unlikely Edit
⊘ Modifier 51 Exempt ⊖ Modifier 63 Exempt 🔀 Unlisted **Modifiers:** *See Inside Back Cover* Ⓜ Maternity A2–Z3 ASC Payment Indicators A–Y OPPS Status Indicators

72100 Radiologic examination, spine, lumbosacral; 2 or 3 views
`N I Q I`

Documentation Finder: *Documentation should state clearly either the names of two or three views – such as standing, anterior-posterior and lateral – or two views of the lumbosacral or LS spine were taken or three views of the lumbosacral spine were taken.*

RVU			Global Days	Modifiers				
Mod	Non-Fac Total	Fac Total		51	50	62	80	MUE
	0.98	0.98	XXX	0	0	0	0	2
26	0.32	0.32	XXX	0	0	0	0	2
TC	0.66	0.66	XXX	0	0	0	0	2

AMA: Sep 01: 7

72110 Radiologic examination, spine, lumbosacral; minimum of 4 views
`N I Q I`

Documentation Finder: *Documentation should state clearly either the names of at least four views – such as standing, AP, lateral and oblique – or four views of the lumbosacral or LS spine were taken. More than four views could be taken, but this code would be reported just once.*

RVU			Global Days	Modifiers				
Mod	Non-Fac Total	Fac Total		51	50	62	80	MUE
	1.37	1.37	XXX	0	0	0	0	1
26	0.45	0.45	XXX	0	0	0	0	1
TC	0.92	0.92	XXX	0	0	0	0	1

AMA: Sep 01: 7

72114 Radiologic examination, spine, lumbosacral; complete, including bending views, minimum of 6 views
`N I Q I`

RVU			Global Days	Modifiers				
Mod	Non-Fac Total	Fac Total		51	50	62	80	MUE
	1.75	1.75	XXX	0	0	0	0	1
26	0.47	0.47	XXX	0	0	0	0	1
TC	1.28	1.28	XXX	0	0	0	0	1

72120 Radiologic examination, spine, lumbosacral; bending views only, 2 or 3 views
`N I Q I`

RVU			Global Days	Modifiers				
Mod	Non-Fac Total	Fac Total		51	50	62	80	MUE
	1.13	1.13	XXX	0	0	0	0	1
26	0.32	0.32	XXX	0	0	0	0	1
TC	0.81	0.81	XXX	0	0	0	0	1

Coding Guidance

Intrathecal injection of contrast is reported separately for CT scans with contrast and without contrast followed by contrast materials. Report 61055 for intrathecal injection at C1-C2. Report 62284 for intrathecal injection at other levels. Intravenous administration of contrast is included and should not be reported separately. For supply of intravenous contrast material, refer to HCPCS Level II codes A9585 and Q9951-Q9967. Three-dimensional models of the spine can be created by stacking multiple, individual 2D slices together. When additional computer processing is used to create 3D images from CT scans of the spine, report 76376 or 76377 in addition to any injection procedure code and the radiological CT code.

72125 Computed tomography, cervical spine; without contrast material
`Z 2 Q 3`

RVU			Global Days	Modifiers				
Mod	Non-Fac Total	Fac Total		51	50	62	80	MUE
	5.18	5.18	XXX	4	0	0	0	1
26	1.53	1.53	XXX	4	0	0	0	1
TC	3.65	3.65	XXX	4	0	0	0	1

72126 Computed tomography, cervical spine; with contrast material
`Z 3 Q 3`

RVU			Global Days	Modifiers				
Mod	Non-Fac Total	Fac Total		51	50	62	80	MUE
	6.43	6.43	XXX	4	0	0	0	1
26	1.74	1.74	XXX	4	0	0	0	1
TC	4.69	4.69	XXX	4	0	0	0	1

AMA: Sep 14: 3

72127 Computed tomography, cervical spine; without contrast material, followed by contrast material(s) and further sections
`Z 2 Q 3`

RVU			Global Days	Modifiers				
Mod	Non-Fac Total	Fac Total		51	50	62	80	MUE
	7.60	7.60	XXX	4	0	0	0	1
26	1.81	1.81	XXX	4	0	0	0	1
TC	5.79	5.79	XXX	4	0	0	0	1

72128 Computed tomography, thoracic spine; without contrast material
`Z 2 Q 3`

RVU			Global Days	Modifiers				
Mod	Non-Fac Total	Fac Total		51	50	62	80	MUE
	5.06	5.06	XXX	4	0	0	0	1
26	1.43	1.43	XXX	4	0	0	0	1
TC	3.63	3.63	XXX	4	0	0	0	1

72129 Computed tomography, thoracic spine; with contrast material
`Z 2 Q 3`

RVU			Global Days	Modifiers				
Mod	Non-Fac Total	Fac Total		51	50	62	80	MUE
	6.44	6.44	XXX	4	0	0	0	1
26	1.74	1.74	XXX	4	0	0	0	1
TC	4.70	4.70	XXX	4	0	0	0	1

AMA: Sep 14: 3

72130 Computed tomography, thoracic spine; without contrast material, followed by contrast material(s) and further sections
`Z 2 Q 3`

RVU			Global Days	Modifiers				
Mod	Non-Fac Total	Fac Total		51	50	62	80	MUE
	7.65	7.65	XXX	4	0	0	0	1
26	1.81	1.81	XXX	4	0	0	0	1
TC	5.84	5.84	XXX	4	0	0	0	1

72131 Computed tomography, lumbar spine; without contrast material
`Z 2 Q 3`

RVU			Global Days	Modifiers				
Mod	Non-Fac Total	Fac Total		51	50	62	80	MUE
	5.04	5.04	XXX	4	0	0	0	1
26	1.43	1.43	XXX	4	0	0	0	1
TC	3.61	3.61	XXX	4	0	0	0	1

72132 Computed tomography, lumbar spine; with contrast material
`Z 3 Q 3`

RVU			Global Days	Modifiers				
Mod	Non-Fac Total	Fac Total		51	50	62	80	MUE
	6.41	6.41	XXX	4	0	0	0	1
26	1.74	1.74	XXX	4	0	0	0	1
TC	4.67	4.67	XXX	4	0	0	0	1

AMA: Sep 14: 3, Fall 93: 13

● New   ▲ Revised   Deleted   ⊙ Moderate Sedation   ✚ Add-on Codes   ⊘ High Risk Denial   Ⓐ Age Edit   ♀ Female   ♂ Male   **AMA** *CPT® Assistant*   ***MUE*** Medically Unlikely Edit

⊘ Modifier 51 Exempt   ⊖ Modifier 63 Exempt   ✗ Unlisted   **Modifiers:** *See Inside Back Cover*   Ⓜ Maternity   `A2–Z3` ASC Payment Indicators   `A –Y` OPPS Status Indicators

© 2016 DecisionHealth   CPT © 2015 American Medical Association. All Rights Reserved.   **623**

Radiology Procedures

72133 – 72159

72133 Computed tomography, lumbar spine; without contrast material, followed by contrast material(s) and further sections   Z2Q3

Mod	Non-Fac Total	Fac Total	Global Days	Modifiers 51	50	62	80	MUE
	7.59	7.59	XXX	4	0	0	0	1
26	1.81	1.81	XXX	4	0	0	0	1
TC	5.78	5.78	XXX	4	0	0	0	1

Coding Guidance

Intrathecal injection of contrast is reported separately for MRI with contrast and without contrast followed by contrast materials. Report 61055 for intrathecal injection at C1-C2. Report 62284 for intrathecal injection at other levels. Intravenous administration of contrast is included and should not be reported separately. For supply of intravenous contrast material, refer to HCPCS Level II codes Q9953-Q9954.

72141 Magnetic resonance (eg, proton) imaging, spinal canal and contents, cervical; without contrast material   Z3Q3

Mod	Non-Fac Total	Fac Total	Global Days	Modifiers 51	50	62	80	MUE
	6.28	6.28	XXX	4	0	0	0	1
26	2.12	2.12	XXX	4	0	0	0	1
TC	4.16	4.16	XXX	4	0	0	0	1

AMA: Apr 10: 10, Jun 14: 14

72142 Magnetic resonance (eg, proton) imaging, spinal canal and contents, cervical; with contrast material(s)   Z3Q3

Mod	Non-Fac Total	Fac Total	Global Days	Modifiers 51	50	62	80	MUE
	9.12	9.12	XXX	4	0	0	0	1
26	2.56	2.56	XXX	4	0	0	0	1
TC	6.56	6.56	XXX	4	0	0	0	1

AMA: Apr 10: 10

72146 Magnetic resonance (eg, proton) imaging, spinal canal and contents, thoracic; without contrast material   Z3Q3

Mod	Non-Fac Total	Fac Total	Global Days	Modifiers 51	50	62	80	MUE
	6.29	6.29	XXX	4	0	0	0	1
26	2.12	2.12	XXX	4	0	0	0	1
TC	4.17	4.17	XXX	4	0	0	0	1

AMA: May 99: 10, Apr 10: 10, Jun 14: 14

72147 Magnetic resonance (eg, proton) imaging, spinal canal and contents, thoracic; with contrast material(s)   Z3Q3

Mod	Non-Fac Total	Fac Total	Global Days	Modifiers 51	50	62	80	MUE
	9.02	9.02	XXX	4	0	0	0	1
26	2.54	2.54	XXX	4	0	0	0	1
TC	6.48	6.48	XXX	4	0	0	0	1

AMA: May 99: 10, Apr 10: 10

72148 Magnetic resonance (eg, proton) imaging, spinal canal and contents, lumbar; without contrast material   Z3Q3

Documentation Finder: *Documentation should be provided that shows that an MRI was performed without any injection of contrast for the lumbar, spinal area. This code should not be reported if they inject contrast after obtaining the initial MRI without contrast.*

Mod	Non-Fac Total	Fac Total	Global Days	Modifiers 51	50	62	80	MUE
	6.25	6.25	XXX	4	0	0	0	1
26	2.12	2.12	XXX	4	0	0	0	1
TC	4.13	4.13	XXX	4	0	0	0	1

AMA: Nov 05: 15, Jun 14: 14

72149 Magnetic resonance (eg, proton) imaging, spinal canal and contents, lumbar; with contrast material(s)   Z3Q3

Mod	Non-Fac Total	Fac Total	Global Days	Modifiers 51	50	62	80	MUE
	9.00	9.00	XXX	4	0	0	0	1
26	2.55	2.55	XXX	4	0	0	0	1
TC	6.45	6.45	XXX	4	0	0	0	1

72156 Magnetic resonance (eg, proton) imaging, spinal canal and contents, without contrast material, followed by contrast material(s) and further sequences; cervical   Z2Q3

Mod	Non-Fac Total	Fac Total	Global Days	Modifiers 51	50	62	80	MUE
	10.65	10.65	XXX	4	0	0	0	1
26	3.27	3.27	XXX	4	0	0	0	1
TC	7.38	7.38	XXX	4	0	0	0	1

Pub 100-04, 13, 40

72157 Magnetic resonance (eg, proton) imaging, spinal canal and contents, without contrast material, followed by contrast material(s) and further sequences; thoracic   Z2Q3

Mod	Non-Fac Total	Fac Total	Global Days	Modifiers 51	50	62	80	MUE
	10.66	10.66	XXX	4	0	0	0	1
26	3.27	3.27	XXX	4	0	0	0	1
TC	7.39	7.39	XXX	4	0	0	0	1

Pub 100-04, 13, 40

72158 Magnetic resonance (eg, proton) imaging, spinal canal and contents, without contrast material, followed by contrast material(s) and further sequences; lumbar   Z2Q3

Mod	Non-Fac Total	Fac Total	Global Days	Modifiers 51	50	62	80	MUE
	10.62	10.62	XXX	4	0	0	0	1
26	3.27	3.27	XXX	4	0	0	0	1
TC	7.35	7.35	XXX	4	0	0	0	1

Pub 100-04, 13, 40

72159 Magnetic resonance angiography, spinal canal and contents, with or without contrast material(s)   B

Mod	Non-Fac Total	Fac Total	Global Days	Modifiers 51	50	62	80	MUE
	11.69	11.69	XXX	4	0	0	0	
26	2.57	2.57	XXX	4	0	0	0	
TC	9.12	9.12	XXX	4	0	0	9	

AMA: Dec 05: 7, Jan 07: 31

● New   ▲ Revised   ✖ Deleted   ⊙ Moderate Sedation   ✚ Add-on Codes   ⊘ High Risk Denial   Ⓐ Age Edit   ♀ Female   ♂ Male   **AMA** *CPT® Assistant*   **MUE** Medically Unlikely Edit
⊘ Modifier 51 Exempt   ⊖ Modifier 63 Exempt   ✗ Unlisted   **Modifiers:** *See Inside Back Cover*   Ⓜ Maternity   A2–Z3 ASC Payment Indicators   A–Y OPPS Status Indicators

624   CPT © 2015 American Medical Association. All Rights Reserved.   © 2016 DecisionHealth

72170 Radiologic examination, pelvis; 1 or 2 views N1 Q1

Documentation Finder: Documentation must show that one or two views of the pelvis were taken, such as anterior-posterior and lateral pelvis. If additional hip views are taken, different coding would be reported.

RVU Mod	Non-Fac Total	Fac Total	Global Days	Modifiers 51	50	62	80	MUE
	0.89	0.89	XXX	0	0	0	0	2
26	0.25	0.25	XXX	0	0	0	0	2
TC	0.64	0.64	XXX	0	0	0	0	2

AMA: Sep 01: 7, Mar 03: 23

72190 Radiologic examination, pelvis; complete, minimum of 3 views N1 Q1

RVU Mod	Non-Fac Total	Fac Total	Global Days	Modifiers 51	50	62	80	MUE
	1.07	1.07	XXX	0	0	0	0	1
26	0.31	0.31	XXX	0	0	0	0	1
TC	0.76	0.76	XXX	0	0	0	0	1

Coding Guidance

Intravenous administration of contrast material is included in CTA and CT studies and should not be reported separately. For supply of intravenous contrast material, refer to HCPCS Level II codes Q9951-Q9967.

72191 Computed tomographic angiography, pelvis, with contrast material(s), including noncontrast images, if performed, and image postprocessing Z2 Q3

RVU Mod	Non-Fac Total	Fac Total	Global Days	Modifiers 51	50	62	80	MUE
	8.57	8.57	XXX	4	0	0	0	1
26	2.57	2.57	XXX	4	0	0	0	1
TC	6.00	6.00	XXX	4	0	0	0	1

AMA: Jul 01: 4, 6, Dec 05: 7, Jan 07: 31

72192 Computed tomography, pelvis; without contrast material Z2 Q3

RVU Mod	Non-Fac Total	Fac Total	Global Days	Modifiers 51	50	62	80	MUE
	4.09	4.09	XXX	4	0	0	0	1
26	1.55	1.55	XXX	4	0	0	0	1
TC	2.54	2.54	XXX	4	0	0	0	1

AMA: Mar 05: 1, 4, Mar 07: 10, Apr 10: 9, Nov 11: 6, Oct 12: 12

72193 Computed tomography, pelvis; with contrast material(s) Z2 Q3

RVU Mod	Non-Fac Total	Fac Total	Global Days	Modifiers 51	50	62	80	MUE
	6.34	6.34	XXX	4	0	0	0	1
26	1.66	1.66	XXX	4	0	0	0	1
TC	4.68	4.68	XXX	4	0	0	0	1

AMA: Mar 05: 1, 4, Mar 07: 10, Apr 10: 9, Nov 11: 6, Oct 12: 12

72194 Computed tomography, pelvis; without contrast material, followed by contrast material(s) and further sections Z2 Q3

RVU Mod	Non-Fac Total	Fac Total	Global Days	Modifiers 51	50	62	80	MUE
	7.30	7.30	XXX	4	0	0	0	1
26	1.73	1.73	XXX	4	0	0	0	1
TC	5.57	5.57	XXX	4	0	0	0	1

AMA: Mar 05: 1, 4, Mar 07: 10, Apr 10: 9, Nov 11: 6, Oct 12: 12

Coding Guidance

Intravenous administration of contrast is included in MRI studies and should not be reported separately. For supply of intravenous contrast material, refer to HCPCS Level II codes Q9953-Q9954.

72195 Magnetic resonance (eg, proton) imaging, pelvis; without contrast material(s) Z2 Q3

RVU Mod	Non-Fac Total	Fac Total	Global Days	Modifiers 51	50	62	80	MUE
	10.51	10.51	XXX	4	0	0	0	1
26	2.08	2.08	XXX	4	0	0	0	1
TC	8.43	8.43	XXX	4	0	0	0	1

AMA: Jul 01: 7, Jun 06: 17, Jun 14: 14

72196 Magnetic resonance (eg, proton) imaging, pelvis; with contrast material(s) Z2 Q3

RVU Mod	Non-Fac Total	Fac Total	Global Days	Modifiers 51	50	62	80	MUE
	11.54	11.54	XXX	4	0	0	0	1
26	2.47	2.47	XXX	4	0	0	0	1
TC	9.07	9.07	XXX	4	0	0	0	1

AMA: Jul 01: 7, Jun 06: 17

72197 Magnetic resonance (eg, proton) imaging, pelvis; without contrast material(s), followed by contrast material(s) and further sequences Z2 Q3

RVU Mod	Non-Fac Total	Fac Total	Global Days	Modifiers 51	50	62	80	MUE
	14.18	14.18	XXX	4	0	0	0	1
26	3.22	3.22	XXX	4	0	0	0	1
TC	10.96	10.96	XXX	4	0	0	0	1

AMA: Jul 01: 7

72198 Magnetic resonance angiography, pelvis, with or without contrast material(s) B

Coding tip: For OPPS codes for pelvic MRA, refer to HCPCS Level II codes C8918-C8920.

RVU Mod	Non-Fac Total	Fac Total	Global Days	Modifiers 51	50	62	80	MUE
	11.23	11.23	XXX	4	0	0	0	1
26	2.54	2.54	XXX	4	0	0	0	1
TC	8.69	8.69	XXX	4	0	0	0	1

AMA: Dec 05: 7, Jan 07: 31

Pub 100-04, 13, 40.1.2

72200 Radiologic examination, sacroiliac joints; less than 3 views N1 Q1

RVU Mod	Non-Fac Total	Fac Total	Global Days	Modifiers 51	50	62	80	MUE
	0.80	0.80	XXX	0	0	0	0	2
26	0.25	0.25	XXX	0	0	0	0	2
TC	0.55	0.55	XXX	0	0	0	0	2

72202 Radiologic examination, sacroiliac joints; 3 or more views N1 Q1

RVU Mod	Non-Fac Total	Fac Total	Global Days	Modifiers 51	50	62	80	MUE
	0.92	0.92	XXX	0	0	0	0	1
26	0.27	0.27	XXX	0	0	0	0	1
TC	0.65	0.65	XXX	0	0	0	0	1

● New ▲ Revised Deleted ⊙ Moderate Sedation ✚ Add-on Codes ⊗ High Risk Denial Ⓐ Age Edit ♀ Female ♂ Male **AMA** CPT® Assistant **MUE** Medically Unlikely Edit
⊘ Modifier 51 Exempt ⊖ Modifier 63 Exempt ✗ Unlisted **Modifiers:** See Inside Back Cover Ⓜ Maternity A2–Z3 ASC Payment Indicators A–Y OPPS Status Indicators

© 2016 DecisionHealth CPT © 2015 American Medical Association. All Rights Reserved. **625**

Radiology Procedures

72220 – 73030

72220 Radiologic examination, sacrum and coccyx, minimum of 2 views N I Q1

RVU Mod	Non-Fac Total	Fac Total	Global Days	Modifiers 51	50	62	80	MUE
	0.79	0.79	XXX	0	0	0	0	1
26	0.25	0.25	XXX	0	0	0	0	1
TC	0.54	0.54	XXX	0	0	0	0	1

Coding Guidance

The injection procedure for myelography is reported separately. Report code 61055 for injection of contrast agent at C1-C2 level. Report 62284 for injection of contrast agent at other levels of the spine.

72240 Myelography, cervical, radiological supervision and interpretation N I Q2

RVU Mod	Non-Fac Total	Fac Total	Global Days	Modifiers 51	50	62	80	MUE
	2.75	2.75	XXX	0	0	0	0	1
26	1.30	1.30	XXX	0	0	0	0	1
TC	1.45	1.45	XXX	0	0	0	0	1

AMA: Fall 93: 13, Sep 14: 3

Pub 100-04, 13, 30.1.3.6

72255 Myelography, thoracic, radiological supervision and interpretation N I Q2

RVU Mod	Non-Fac Total	Fac Total	Global Days	Modifiers 51	50	62	80	MUE
	2.74	2.74	XXX	0	0	0	0	1
26	1.32	1.32	XXX	0	0	0	0	1
TC	1.42	1.42	XXX	0	0	0	0	1

AMA: Sep 14: 3

Pub 100-04, 13, 30.1.3.7

72265 Myelography, lumbosacral, radiological supervision and interpretation N I Q2

RVU Mod	Non-Fac Total	Fac Total	Global Days	Modifiers 51	50	62	80	MUE
	2.59	2.59	XXX	0	0	0	0	1
26	1.19	1.19	XXX	0	0	0	0	1
TC	1.40	1.40	XXX	0	0	0	0	1

AMA: Fall 93: 13, Aug 00: 7, Sep 14: 3

Pub 100-04, 13, 30.1.3.8

72270 Myelography, 2 or more regions (eg, lumbar/thoracic, cervical/thoracic, lumbar/cervical, lumbar/thoracic/cervical), radiological supervision and interpretation N I Q2

RVU Mod	Non-Fac Total	Fac Total	Global Days	Modifiers 51	50	62	80	MUE
	3.58	3.58	XXX	0	0	0	0	1
26	1.91	1.91	XXX	0	0	0	0	1
TC	1.67	1.67	XXX	0	0	0	0	1

AMA: Sep 14: 3

Pub 100-04, 13, 30.1.3.9

72275 Epidurography, radiological supervision and interpretation N I N

Coding tip: Injection procedure for epiduragraphy - 62280-62282, 62310-62319, 64479-64484

RVU Mod	Non-Fac Total	Fac Total	Global Days	Modifiers 51	50	62	80	MUE
	3.26	3.26	XXX	9	9	9	9	3
26	1.12	1.12	XXX	9	9	9	9	3
TC	2.14	2.14	XXX	9	9	9	9	3

AMA: Nov 99: 40, Jan 00: 2, Aug 00: 7, Jul 08: 9, Oct 09: 12, Feb 10: 12, May 10: 10, Jun 12: 12, Jul 12: 5

72285 Discography, cervical or thoracic, radiological supervision and interpretation N I Q2

Coding tip: Injection procedure for cervical or thoracic discography - 62291

RVU Mod	Non-Fac Total	Fac Total	Global Days	Modifiers 51	50	62	80	MUE
	3.23	3.23	XXX	0	0	0	0	4
26	1.74	1.74	XXX	0	0	0	0	4
TC	1.49	1.49	XXX	0	0	0	0	4

AMA: Nov 99: 35, 40, Mar 11: 7

Pub 100-04, 13, 30.1.3.10

72295 Discography, lumbar, radiological supervision and interpretation N I Q2

Coding tip: Injection procedure for lumbar discography - 62290

RVU Mod	Non-Fac Total	Fac Total	Global Days	Modifiers 51	50	62	80	MUE
	2.79	2.79	XXX	0	0	0	0	5
26	1.24	1.24	XXX	0	0	0	0	5
TC	1.55	1.55	XXX	0	0	0	0	5

AMA: Apr 03: 27, Mar 11: 7, Jul 12: 3

Pub 100-04, 13, 30.1.3.11

Upper Extremity Radiological Procedures

73000 Radiologic examination; clavicle, complete N I Q1

RVU Mod	Non-Fac Total	Fac Total	Global Days	Modifiers 51	50	62	80	MUE
	0.77	0.77	XXX	0	3	0	0	2
26	0.24	0.24	XXX	0	3	0	0	2
TC	0.53	0.53	XXX	0	3	0	0	2

73010 Radiologic examination; scapula, complete N I Q1

RVU Mod	Non-Fac Total	Fac Total	Global Days	Modifiers 51	50	62	80	MUE
	0.84	0.84	XXX	0	3	0	0	2
26	0.26	0.26	XXX	0	3	0	0	2
TC	0.58	0.58	XXX	0	3	0	0	2

73020 Radiologic examination, shoulder; 1 view N I Q1

RVU Mod	Non-Fac Total	Fac Total	Global Days	Modifiers 51	50	62	80	MUE
	0.64	0.64	XXX	0	3	0	0	2
26	0.22	0.22	XXX	0	3	0	0	2
TC	0.42	0.42	XXX	0	3	0	0	2

73030 Radiologic examination, shoulder; complete, minimum of 2 views N I Q1

Documentation Finder: *Documentation should state clearly either the names of two views – such as anterior-posterior and lateral – or two views of the right or left shoulder were taken. More than two views could be taken but this code is reported only once per shoulder. This is a unilateral code.*

RVU Mod	Non-Fac Total	Fac Total	Global Days	Modifiers 51	50	62	80	MUE
	0.81	0.81	XXX	0	3	0	0	4
26	0.27	0.27	XXX	0	3	0	0	4
TC	0.54	0.54	XXX	0	3	0	0	4

● New   ▲ Revised   ✖ Deleted   ⊙ Moderate Sedation   ✚ Add-on Codes   ⊘ High Risk Denial   ⓐ Age Edit   ♀ Female   ♂ Male   **AMA** CPT® Assistant   **MUE** Medically Unlikely Edit
⊘ Modifier 51 Exempt   ⊖ Modifier 63 Exempt   ☒ Unlisted   **Modifiers:** See Inside Back Cover   Ⓜ Maternity   A2–Z3 ASC Payment Indicators   A–Y OPPS Status Indicators

626   CPT © 2015 American Medical Association. All Rights Reserved.   © 2016 DecisionHealth

73040 Radiologic examination, shoulder, arthrography, radiological supervision and interpretation N I Q 2

RVU Mod	Non-Fac Total	Fac Total	Global Days	Modifiers 51	50	62	80	MUE
	2.81	2.81	XXX	0	3	0	0	2
26	0.78	0.78	XXX	0	3	0	0	2
TC	2.03	2.03	XXX	0	3	0	0	2

AMA: Jul 01: 7, Feb 07: 11

73050 Radiologic examination; acromioclavicular joints, bilateral, with or without weighted distraction N I Q I

RVU Mod	Non-Fac Total	Fac Total	Global Days	Modifiers 51	50	62	80	MUE
	1.00	1.00	XXX	0	2	0	0	1
26	0.30	0.30	XXX	0	2	0	0	1
TC	0.70	0.70	XXX	0	2	0	0	1

73060 Radiologic examination; humerus, minimum of 2 views N I Q I

RVU Mod	Non-Fac Total	Fac Total	Global Days	Modifiers 51	50	62	80	MUE
	0.81	0.81	XXX	0	0	0	0	2
26	0.24	0.24	000	0	0	0	1	2
TC	0.57	0.57	000	0	0	0	1	2

73070 Radiologic examination, elbow; 2 views N I Q I

RVU Mod	Non-Fac Total	Fac Total	Global Days	Modifiers 51	50	62	80	MUE
	0.77	0.77	XXX	0	3	0	0	2
26	0.23	0.23	XXX	0	3	0	0	2
TC	0.54	0.54	XXX	0	3	0	0	2

AMA: Winter 90: 9, Sep 01: 8

73080 Radiologic examination, elbow; complete, minimum of 3 views N I Q I

RVU Mod	Non-Fac Total	Fac Total	Global Days	Modifiers 51	50	62	80	MUE
	0.87	0.87	XXX	0	3	0	0	2
26	0.25	0.25	XXX	0	3	0	0	2
TC	0.62	0.62	XXX	0	3	0	0	2

73085 Radiologic examination, elbow, arthrography, radiological supervision and interpretation N I Q 2

RVU Mod	Non-Fac Total	Fac Total	Global Days	Modifiers 51	50	62	80	MUE
	2.74	2.74	XXX	0	3	0	0	2
26	0.82	0.82	XXX	0	3	0	0	2
TC	1.92	1.92	XXX	0	3	0	0	2

AMA: Feb 07: 11

73090 Radiologic examination; forearm, 2 views N I Q I

RVU Mod	Non-Fac Total	Fac Total	Global Days	Modifiers 51	50	62	80	MUE
	0.72	0.72	XXX	0	3	0	0	2
26	0.24	0.24	XXX	0	3	0	0	2
TC	0.48	0.48	XXX	0	3	0	0	2

AMA: Sep 01: 8, Apr 02: 14

73092 Radiologic examination; upper extremity, infant, minimum of 2 views ⊘Ⓐ N I Q I

RVU Mod	Non-Fac Total	Fac Total	Global Days	Modifiers 51	50	62	80	MUE
	0.76	0.76	XXX	0	3	0	0	2
26	0.23	0.23	XXX	0	3	0	0	2
TC	0.53	0.53	XXX	0	3	0	0	2

73100 Radiologic examination, wrist; 2 views N I Q I

RVU Mod	Non-Fac Total	Fac Total	Global Days	Modifiers 51	50	62	80	MUE
	0.82	0.82	XXX	0	3	0	0	2
26	0.24	0.24	XXX	0	3	0	0	2
TC	0.58	0.58	XXX	0	3	0	0	2

AMA: Winter 90: 9, Sep 01: 8

● New ▲ Revised Deleted ⊙ Moderate Sedation ✚ Add-on Codes ⊗ High Risk Denial Ⓐ Age Edit ♀ Female ♂ Male **AMA** CPT® Assistant **MUE** Medically Unlikely Edit
⊘ Modifier 51 Exempt ⊖ Modifier 63 Exempt ✗ Unlisted **Modifiers:** See Inside Back Cover Ⓜ Maternity A2–Z3 ASC Payment Indicators A–Y OPPS Status Indicators

73110 Radiologic examination, wrist; complete, minimum of 3 views N1 Q1

Documentation Finder: *Documentation should state clearly either the names of three views – such as anterior-posterior, lateral and oblique – or three views of the right or left wrist were taken. More than three views could be taken but this code is reported only once per wrist. This is a unilateral code.*

RVU			Global Days	Modifiers				
Mod	Non-Fac Total	Fac Total		51	50	62	80	MUE
	0.99	0.99	XXX	0	3	0	0	3
26	0.25	0.25	XXX	0	3	0	0	3
TC	0.74	0.74	XXX	0	3	0	0	3

AMA: Mar 97: 10, Nov 06: 22

73115 Radiologic examination, wrist, arthrography, radiological supervision and interpretation N1 Q2

RVU			Global Days	Modifiers				
Mod	Non-Fac Total	Fac Total		51	50	62	80	MUE
	3.00	3.00	XXX	0	3	0	0	2
26	0.81	0.81	XXX	0	3	0	0	2
TC	2.19	2.19	XXX	0	3	0	0	2

AMA: Feb 07: 11

73120 Radiologic examination, hand; 2 views N1 Q1

RVU			Global Days	Modifiers				
Mod	Non-Fac Total	Fac Total		51	50	62	80	MUE
	0.73	0.73	XXX	0	3	0	0	3
26	0.24	0.24	XXX	0	3	0	0	3
TC	0.49	0.49	XXX	0	3	0	0	3

AMA: Winter 90: 9

Pub 100-04, 16, 120.2

73130 Radiologic examination, hand; minimum of 3 views N1 Q1

Documentation Finder: *Documentation should state clearly either the names of three views – such as anterior-posterior, lateral and oblique – or three views of the right or left hand were taken. More than three views could be taken but this code is reported only once per hand. This is a unilateral code.*

RVU			Global Days	Modifiers				
Mod	Non-Fac Total	Fac Total		51	50	62	80	MUE
	0.86	0.86	XXX	0	3	0	0	3
26	0.25	0.25	XXX	0	3	0	0	3
TC	0.61	0.61	XXX	0	3	0	0	3

73140 Radiologic examination, finger(s), minimum of 2 views N1 Q1

RVU			Global Days	Modifiers				
Mod	Non-Fac Total	Fac Total		51	50	62	80	MUE
	0.88	0.88	XXX	0	3	0	0	3
26	0.20	0.20	XXX	0	3	0	0	3
TC	0.68	0.68	XXX	0	3	0	0	3

AMA: Jan 07: 29

Coding Guidance

Enhanced CT may require fluoroscopic needle guidance for contrast injection. Report 77002 for fluoroscopic needle guidance in addition to the CT of the upper extremity, as well as the injection code for the procedure (e.g., shoulder arthrography). Intravenous injection of contrast material is not reported separately. For supply of intravenous contrast material, refer to HCPCS Level II codes Q9951-Q9967.

73200 Computed tomography, upper extremity; without contrast material Z2 Q3

RVU			Global Days	Modifiers				
Mod	Non-Fac Total	Fac Total		51	50	62	80	MUE
	5.02	5.02	XXX	4	3	0	0	2
26	1.43	1.43	XXX	4	3	0	0	2
TC	3.59	3.59	XXX	4	3	0	0	2

AMA: Jul 11: 17

73201 Computed tomography, upper extremity; with contrast material(s) Z3 Q3

RVU			Global Days	Modifiers				
Mod	Non-Fac Total	Fac Total		51	50	62	80	MUE
	6.25	6.25	XXX	4	3	0	0	2
26	1.66	1.66	XXX	4	3	0	0	2
TC	4.59	4.59	XXX	4	3	0	0	2

AMA: Jul 11: 17, Aug 15: 6

73202 Computed tomography, upper extremity; without contrast material, followed by contrast material(s) and further sections Z2 Q3

RVU			Global Days	Modifiers				
Mod	Non-Fac Total	Fac Total		51	50	62	80	MUE
	7.79	7.79	XXX	4	3	0	0	2
26	1.74	1.74	XXX	4	3	0	0	2
TC	6.05	6.05	XXX	4	3	0	0	2

73206 Computed tomographic angiography, upper extremity, with contrast material(s), including noncontrast images, if performed, and image postprocessing Z2 Q3

RVU			Global Days	Modifiers				
Mod	Non-Fac Total	Fac Total		51	50	62	80	MUE
	9.19	9.19	XXX	4	0	0	0	2
26	2.56	2.56	XXX	4	0	0	0	2
TC	6.63	6.63	XXX	4	0	0	0	2

AMA: Jul 01: 5, Dec 05: 7, Jan 07: 31

Coding Guidance

Intravenous injection of contrast is not reported separately. For supply of contrast material, refer to HCPCS Level II codes Q9953-Q9954.

73218 Magnetic resonance (eg, proton) imaging, upper extremity, other than joint; without contrast material(s) Z2 Q3

RVU			Global Days	Modifiers				
Mod	Non-Fac Total	Fac Total		51	50	62	80	MUE
	10.24	10.24	XXX	4	3	0	0	2
26	1.93	1.93	XXX	4	3	0	0	2
TC	8.31	8.31	XXX	4	3	0	0	2

AMA: Jul 01: 7, Sep 10: 10, Feb 11: 9

73219 Magnetic resonance (eg, proton) imaging, upper extremity, other than joint; with contrast material(s) Z2 Q3

RVU			Global Days	Modifiers				
Mod	Non-Fac Total	Fac Total		51	50	62	80	MUE
	11.34	11.34	XXX	4	3	0	0	2
26	2.31	2.31	XXX	4	3	0	0	2
TC	9.03	9.03	XXX	4	3	0	0	2

AMA: Jul 01: 7, Sep 10: 10

● New   ▲ Revised   ✖ Deleted   ⊙ Moderate Sedation   ✚ Add-on Codes   ⊗ High Risk Denial   Ⓐ Age Edit   ♀ Female   ♂ Male   **AMA** *CPT® Assistant*   **MUE** Medically Unlikely Edit
⊘ Modifier 51 Exempt   ⊖ Modifier 63 Exempt   Ⓧ Unlisted   **Modifiers:** *See Inside Back Cover*   Ⓜ Maternity   A2–Z3 ASC Payment Indicators   A–Y OPPS Status Indicators

628   CPT © 2015 American Medical Association. All Rights Reserved.   © 2016 DecisionHealth

73220 Magnetic resonance (eg, proton) imaging, upper extremity, other than joint; without contrast material(s), followed by contrast material(s) and further sequences Z2 Q3

RVU			Global Days	Modifiers				
Mod	Non-Fac Total	Fac Total		51	50	62	80	MUE
	14.03	14.03	XXX	4	3	0	0	2
26	3.07	3.07	XXX	4	3	0	0	2
TC	10.96	10.96	XXX	4	3	0	0	2

AMA: Jul 01: 7, Sep 10: 10

Coding Guidance

Contrast materials used for enhanced MRI may require fluoroscopic needle guidance for contrast injection. Report 77002 for fluoroscopic guidance in addition to 73222 or 73223, as well as the code for the injection procedure (e.g., shoulder arthrography).

73221 Magnetic resonance (eg, proton) imaging, any joint of upper extremity; without contrast material(s) Z2 Q3

RVU			Global Days	Modifiers				
Mod	Non-Fac Total	Fac Total		51	50	62	80	MUE
	6.63	6.63	XXX	4	3	0	0	2
26	1.94	1.94	XXX	4	3	0	0	2
TC	4.69	4.69	XXX	4	3	0	0	2

AMA: Jul 01: 7, Sep 10: 10, Feb 11: 9

73222 Magnetic resonance (eg, proton) imaging, any joint of upper extremity; with contrast material(s) Z2 Q3

RVU			Global Days	Modifiers				
Mod	Non-Fac Total	Fac Total		51	50	62	80	MUE
	10.61	10.61	XXX	4	3	0	0	2
26	2.32	2.32	XXX	4	3	0	0	2
TC	8.29	8.29	XXX	4	3	0	0	2

AMA: Jul 01: 7, Sep 10: 10, Aug 15: 6

73223 Magnetic resonance (eg, proton) imaging, any joint of upper extremity; without contrast material(s), followed by contrast material(s) and further sequences Z2 Q3

RVU			Global Days	Modifiers				
Mod	Non-Fac Total	Fac Total		51	50	62	80	MUE
	13.17	13.17	XXX	4	3	0	0	2
26	3.07	3.07	XXX	4	3	0	0	2
TC	10.10	10.10	XXX	4	3	0	0	2

AMA: Jul 01: 7, Sep 10: 10

73225 Magnetic resonance angiography, upper extremity, with or without contrast material(s) C B

RVU			Global Days	Modifiers				
Mod	Non-Fac Total	Fac Total		51	50	62	80	MUE
	11.37	11.37	XXX	4	0	0	0	
26	2.44	2.44	XXX	4	0	0	0	
TC	8.93	8.93	XXX	4	0	0	0	9

AMA: Dec 05: 7, Jan 07: 31

✖ ~~73500 Radiologic examination, hip, unilateral; 1 view~~

● **73501 Radiologic examination, hip, unilateral, with pelvis when performed; 1 view** Q1

RVU			Global Days	Modifiers				
Mod	Non-Fac Total	Fac Total		51	50	62	80	MUE
	0.84	0.84	XXX	0	0	0	0	2
26	0.27	0.27	XXX	0	0	0	0	2
TC	0.57	0.57	XXX	0	0	0	0	2

● **73502 Radiologic examination, hip, unilateral, with pelvis when performed; 2-3 views** Q1

RVU			Global Days	Modifiers				
Mod	Non-Fac Total	Fac Total		51	50	62	80	MUE
	1.16	1.16	XXX	0	0	0	0	2
26	0.32	0.32	XXX	0	0	0	0	2
TC	0.84	0.84	XXX	0	0	0	0	2

● **73503 Radiologic examination, hip, unilateral, with pelvis when performed; minimum of 4 views** Q1

RVU			Global Days	Modifiers				
Mod	Non-Fac Total	Fac Total		51	50	62	80	MUE
	1.45	1.45	XXX	0	0	0	0	2
26	0.41	0.41	XXX	0	0	0	0	2
TC	1.04	1.04	XXX	0	0	0	0	2

✖ ~~73510 Radiologic examination, hip, unilateral, complete, minimum of 2 views~~

✖ ~~73520 Radiologic examination, hips, bilateral, minimum of 2 views of each hip, including anteroposterior view of pelvis~~

● **73521 Radiologic examination, hips, bilateral, with pelvis when performed; 2 views** Q1

RVU			Global Days	Modifiers				
Mod	Non-Fac Total	Fac Total		51	50	62	80	MUE
	1.12	1.12	XXX	0	0	0	0	2
26	0.33	0.33	XXX	0	0	0	0	2
TC	0.79	0.79	XXX	0	0	0	0	2

● **73522 Radiologic examination, hips, bilateral, with pelvis when performed; 3-4 views** Q1

RVU			Global Days	Modifiers				
Mod	Non-Fac Total	Fac Total		51	50	62	80	MUE
	1.37	1.37	XXX	0	0	0	0	2
26	0.43	0.43	XXX	0	0	0	0	2
TC	0.94	0.94	XXX	0	0	0	0	2

● **73523 Radiologic examination, hips, bilateral, with pelvis when performed; minimum of 5 views** S

RVU			Global Days	Modifiers				
Mod	Non-Fac Total	Fac Total		51	50	62	80	MUE
	1.59	1.59	XXX	0	0	0	0	2
26	0.46	0.46	XXX	0	0	0	0	2
TC	1.13	1.13	XXX	0	0	0	0	2

73525 Radiologic examination, hip, arthrography, radiological supervision and interpretation N1 Q2

RVU			Global Days	Modifiers				
Mod	Non-Fac Total	Fac Total		51	50	62	80	MUE
	2.86	2.86	XXX	0	3	0	0	2
26	0.82	0.82	XXX	0	3	0	0	2
TC	2.04	2.04	XXX	0	3	0	0	2

AMA: Feb 07: 11, Jun 12: 14

✖ ~~73530 Radiologic examination, hip, during operative procedure~~

✖ ~~73540 Radiologic examination, pelvis and hips, infant or child, minimum of 2 views~~

✖ ~~73550 Radiologic examination, femur, 2 views~~

● New   ▲ Revised   Deleted   ⊙ Moderate Sedation   ✚ Add-on Codes   ⊗ High Risk Denial   Ⓐ Age Edit   ♀ Female   ♂ Male   **AMA** *CPT® Assistant*   **MUE** Medically Unlikely Edit   ⃠ Modifier 51 Exempt   ⊖ Modifier 63 Exempt   ✗ Unlisted   **Modifiers:** *See Inside Back Cover*   Ⓜ Maternity   A2–Z3 ASC Payment Indicators   A–Y OPPS Status Indicators

© 2016 DecisionHealth   CPT © 2015 American Medical Association. All Rights Reserved.   **629**

Radiology Procedures

73551 – 73620

● **73551 Radiologic examination, femur; 1 view** `QI`

Mod	Non-Fac Total	Fac Total	Global Days	51	50	62	80	MUE
	0.78	0.78	XXX	0	0	0	0	2
26	0.24	0.24	XXX	0	0	0	0	2
TC	0.54	0.54	XXX	0	0	0	0	2

● **73552 Radiologic examination, femur; minimum 2 views** `QI`

Mod	Non-Fac Total	Fac Total	Global Days	51	50	62	80	MUE
	0.91	0.91	XXX	0	0	0	0	2
26	0.27	0.27	XXX	0	3	0	0	2
TC	0.64	0.64	XXX	0	0	0	0	2

73560 Radiologic examination, knee; 1 or 2 views `NIQI`

Mod	Non-Fac Total	Fac Total	Global Days	51	50	62	80	MUE
	0.87	0.87	XXX	0	0	0	0	4
26	0.24	0.24	000	0	0	0	1	4
TC	0.63	0.63	XXX	0	3	0	0	4

AMA: Feb 15: 10, May 15: 10

73562 Radiologic examination, knee; 3 views `NIQI`

Documentation Finder: Documentation should state clearly either the names of three views – such as anterior-posterior, lateral and oblique – or three views of the right or left knee were taken. This is a unilateral code.

Mod	Non-Fac Total	Fac Total	Global Days	51	50	62	80	MUE
	1.00	1.00	XXX	0	3	0	0	4
26	0.27	0.27	XXX	0	3	0	0	4
TC	0.73	0.73	XXX	0	3	0	0	4

AMA: Apr 02: 15

73564 Radiologic examination, knee; complete, 4 or more views `NIQI`

Mod	Non-Fac Total	Fac Total	Global Days	51	50	62	80	MUE
	1.11	1.11	XXX	0	3	0	0	4
26	0.32	0.32	XXX	0	3	0	0	4
TC	0.79	0.79	XXX	0	3	0	0	4

AMA: Jun 98: 11, Nov 98: 21, Feb 15: 10, May 15: 10

73565 Radiologic examination, knee; both knees, standing, anteroposterior `NIQI`

Mod	Non-Fac Total	Fac Total	Global Days	51	50	62	80	MUE
	1.01	1.01	XXX	0	2	0	0	1
26	0.25	0.25	XXX	0	2	0	0	1
TC	0.76	0.76	XXX	0	2	0	0	1

AMA: Winter 90: 9, Feb 15: 10, May 15: 10

73580 Radiologic examination, knee, arthrography, radiological supervision and interpretation `NIQ2`

Mod	Non-Fac Total	Fac Total	Global Days	51	50	62	80	MUE
	3.24	3.24	XXX	0	3	0	0	2
26	0.81	0.81	XXX	0	3	0	0	2
TC	2.43	2.43	XXX	0	3	0	0	2

AMA: Feb 07: 11, Aug 15: 6

73590 Radiologic examination; tibia and fibula, 2 views `NIQI`

Mod	Non-Fac Total	Fac Total	Global Days	51	50	62	80	MUE
	0.80	0.80	XXX	0	3	0	0	3
26	0.24	0.24	XXX	0	3	0	0	3
TC	0.56	0.56	XXX	0	3	0	0	3

AMA: Sep 01: 8

73592 Radiologic examination; lower extremity, infant, minimum of 2 views `⊚A NIQI`

Mod	Non-Fac Total	Fac Total	Global Days	51	50	62	80	MUE
	0.78	0.78	XXX	0	3	0	0	2
26	0.23	0.23	XXX	0	3	0	0	2
TC	0.55	0.55	XXX	0	3	0	0	2

73600 Radiologic examination, ankle; 2 views `NIQI`

Mod	Non-Fac Total	Fac Total	Global Days	51	50	62	80	MUE
	0.84	0.84	XXX	0	3	0	0	3
26	0.24	0.24	XXX	0	3	0	0	3
TC	0.60	0.60	XXX	0	3	0	0	3

AMA: Sep 01: 8, Apr 02: 15, Mar 03: 9

73610 Radiologic examination, ankle; complete, minimum of 3 views `NIQI`

Documentation Finder: Documentation should state clearly either the names of three views – such as anterior-posterior, lateral and oblique – or three views of the right or left ankle were taken. More than three views could be taken but this code is reported only once per ankle.

Mod	Non-Fac Total	Fac Total	Global Days	51	50	62	80	MUE
	0.88	0.88	XXX	0	3	0	0	3
26	0.25	0.25	XXX	0	3	0	0	3
TC	0.63	0.63	XXX	0	3	0	0	3

AMA: Apr 02: 15, Mar 03: 9

73615 Radiologic examination, ankle, arthrography, radiological supervision and interpretation `NIQ2`

Mod	Non-Fac Total	Fac Total	Global Days	51	50	62	80	MUE
	2.96	2.96	XXX	0	3	0	0	2
26	0.82	0.82	XXX	0	3	0	0	2
TC	2.14	2.14	XXX	0	3	0	0	2

AMA: Feb 07: 11

73620 Radiologic examination, foot; 2 views `NIQI`

Documentation Finder: Documentation should state clearly either the names of two views – such as anterior-posterior, lateral or oblique – or two views of the right or left foot were taken. This is a unilateral code.

Mod	Non-Fac Total	Fac Total	Global Days	51	50	62	80	MUE
	0.73	0.73	XXX	0	3	0	0	3
26	0.22	0.22	XXX	0	3	0	0	3
TC	0.51	0.51	XXX	0	3	0	0	3

AMA: Sep 01: 8, Apr 02: 15, Mar 03: 9

● New   ▲ Revised   ✖ Deleted   ⊙ Moderate Sedation   ✚ Add-on Codes   ⊘ High Risk Denial   ⓐ Age Edit   ♀ Female   ♂ Male   **AMA** *CPT® Assistant*   **MUE** Medically Unlikely Edit
⊘ Modifier 51 Exempt   ⊖ Modifier 63 Exempt   ✗ Unlisted   **Modifiers:** *See Inside Back Cover*   Ⓜ Maternity   A2–Z3 ASC Payment Indicators   A–Y OPPS Status Indicators

630   CPT © 2015 American Medical Association. All Rights Reserved.   © 2016 DecisionHealth

73630 Radiologic examination, foot; complete, minimum of 3 views N1 Q1

Documentation Finder: *Documentation should state clearly either the names of three views – such as anterior-posterior, lateral and oblique – or three views of the right or left foot were taken. This is a unilateral code.*

Mod	Non-Fac Total	Fac Total	Global Days	51	50	62	80	MUE
	0.82	0.82	XXX	0	3	0	0	3
26	0.24	0.24	XXX	0	3	0	0	3
TC	0.58	0.58	XXX	0	3	0	0	3

73650 Radiologic examination; calcaneus, minimum of 2 views N1 Q1

Mod	Non-Fac Total	Fac Total	Global Days	51	50	62	80	MUE
	0.76	0.76	XXX	0	3	0	0	2
26	0.23	0.23	XXX	0	3	0	0	2
TC	0.53	0.53	XXX	0	3	0	0	2

73660 Radiologic examination; toe(s), minimum of 2 views N1 Q1

Mod	Non-Fac Total	Fac Total	Global Days	51	50	62	80	MUE
	0.79	0.79	XXX	0	3	0	0	2
26	0.19	0.19	XXX	0	3	0	0	2
TC	0.60	0.60	XXX	0	3	0	0	2

Coding Guidance

Enhanced CT may require fluoroscopic needle guidance for contrast injection. Report 77002 for fluoroscopic guidance in addition to the CT of the lower extremity, as well as the injection code for the procedure (e.g., hip arthrography). For supply of contrast material, refer to HCPCS Level II codes Q9951-Q9967.

Coding Guidance

Intravenous administration of contrast is not reported separately. For supply of contrast material, refer to HCPCS Level II codes Q9951-Q9967.

73700 Computed tomography, lower extremity; without contrast material Z2 Q3

Mod	Non-Fac Total	Fac Total	Global Days	51	50	62	80	MUE
	5.03	5.03	XXX	4	3	0	0	2
26	1.43	1.43	XXX	4	3	0	0	2
TC	3.60	3.60	XXX	4	3	0	0	2

AMA: Mar 07: 10, Jul 11: 17

73701 Computed tomography, lower extremity; with contrast material(s) Z2 Q3

Mod	Non-Fac Total	Fac Total	Global Days	51	50	62	80	MUE
	6.35	6.35	XXX	4	3	0	0	2
26	1.66	1.66	XXX	4	3	0	0	2
TC	4.69	4.69	XXX	4	3	0	0	2

AMA: Mar 07: 10, Jul 11: 17

73702 Computed tomography, lower extremity; without contrast material, followed by contrast material(s) and further sections Z2 Q3

Mod	Non-Fac Total	Fac Total	Global Days	51	50	62	80	MUE
	7.71	7.71	XXX	4	3	0	0	2
26	1.73	1.73	XXX	4	3	0	0	2
TC	5.98	5.98	XXX	4	3	0	0	2

AMA: Mar 07: 10, Jul 11: 17

73706 Computed tomographic angiography, lower extremity, with contrast material(s), including noncontrast images, if performed, and image postprocessing Z2 Q3

Mod	Non-Fac Total	Fac Total	Global Days	51	50	62	80	MUE
	9.87	9.87	XXX	4	3	0	0	2
26	2.69	2.69	XXX	4	3	0	0	2
TC	7.18	7.18	XXX	4	3	0	0	2

AMA: Jul 01: 5, 6, Dec 05: 7, Jan 07: 31, Apr 08: 11, Apr 11: 13

Coding Guidance

Intravenous administration of contrast material is not reported separately. For supply of magnetic resonance contrast agent, refer to HCPCS Level II codes Q9953-Q9954.

73718 Magnetic resonance (eg, proton) imaging, lower extremity other than joint; without contrast material(s) Z2 Q3

Mod	Non-Fac Total	Fac Total	Global Days	51	50	62	80	MUE
	10.24	10.24	XXX	4	3	0	0	2
26	1.93	1.93	XXX	4	3	0	0	2
TC	8.31	8.31	XXX	4	3	0	0	2

AMA: Jul 01: 3

73719 Magnetic resonance (eg, proton) imaging, lower extremity other than joint; with contrast material(s) Z2 Q3

Mod	Non-Fac Total	Fac Total	Global Days	51	50	62	80	MUE
	11.34	11.34	XXX	4	3	0	0	2
26	2.31	2.31	XXX	4	3	0	0	2
TC	9.03	9.03	XXX	4	3	0	0	2

AMA: Jul 01: 3

73720 Magnetic resonance (eg, proton) imaging, lower extremity other than joint; without contrast material(s), followed by contrast material(s) and further sequences Z2 Q3

Mod	Non-Fac Total	Fac Total	Global Days	51	50	62	80	MUE
	14.10	14.10	XXX	4	3	0	0	2
26	3.06	3.06	XXX	4	3	0	0	2
TC	11.04	11.04	XXX	4	3	0	0	2

AMA: Jul 01: 3

Coding Guidance

Contrast materials used for enhanced MRI may require fluoroscopic needle guidance for contrast injection. Report 77002 for fluoroscopic guidance in addition to 73722 or 73723, as well as the code for the injection procedure (e.g., hip arthrography). For supply of magnetic resonance contrast agent, refer to HCPCS Level II codes Q9953-Q9954.

73721 Magnetic resonance (eg, proton) imaging, any joint of lower extremity; without contrast material Z2 Q3

Mod	Non-Fac Total	Fac Total	Global Days	51	50	62	80	MUE
	6.64	6.64	XXX	4	3	0	0	3
26	1.94	1.94	XXX	4	3	0	0	3
TC	4.70	4.70	XXX	4	3	0	0	3

AMA: Jul 01: 3, Jun 06: 17

● New   ▲ Revised   Deleted   ⊙ Moderate Sedation   ✚ Add-on Codes   ⊘ High Risk Denial   Ⓐ Age Edit   ♀ Female   ♂ Male   **AMA** *CPT® Assistant*   ***MUE*** Medically Unlikely Edit   ⊘ Modifier 51 Exempt   ⊖ Modifier 63 Exempt   ✗ Unlisted   **Modifiers:** *See Inside Back Cover*   Ⓜ Maternity   A2–Z3 ASC Payment Indicators   A–Y OPPS Status Indicators

© 2016 DecisionHealth   CPT © 2015 American Medical Association. All Rights Reserved.   **631**

Radiology Procedures

73722 Magnetic resonance (eg, proton) imaging, any joint of lower extremity; with contrast material(s) Z 2 Q 3

Mod	RVU Non-Fac Total	Fac Total	Global Days	51	50	62	80	MUE
	10.72	10.72	XXX	4	3	0	0	2
26	2.32	2.32	XXX	4	3	0	0	2
TC	8.40	8.40	XXX	4	3	0	0	2

AMA: Jul 01: 3, Jun 06: 17, Aug 15: 6

73723 Magnetic resonance (eg, proton) imaging, any joint of lower extremity; without contrast material(s), followed by contrast material(s) and further sequences Z 2 Q 3

Mod	RVU Non-Fac Total	Fac Total	Global Days	51	50	62	80	MUE
	13.20	13.20	XXX	4	3	0	0	2
26	3.06	3.06	XXX	4	3	0	0	2
TC	10.14	10.14	XXX	4	3	0	0	2

AMA: Jul 01: 3

73725 Magnetic resonance angiography, lower extremity, with or without contrast material(s) B

Coding tip: For OPPS codes for lower extremity angiography, refer to HCPCS Level II codes C8912-C8914.

Mod	RVU Non-Fac Total	Fac Total	Global Days	51	50	62	80	MUE
	11.26	11.26	XXX	4	3	0	0	2
26	2.56	2.56	XXX	4	3	0	0	2
TC	8.70	8.70	XXX	4	3	0	0	2

AMA: Dec 05: 7, Jan 07: 31

Pub 100-04, 13, 40.1.2

Abdominal Radiological Procedures

74000 Radiologic examination, abdomen; single anteroposterior view N I Q I

Mod	RVU Non-Fac Total	Fac Total	Global Days	51	50	62	80	MUE
	0.66	0.66	XXX	0	0	0	0	4
26	0.26	0.26	XXX	0	0	0	0	4
TC	0.40	0.40	XXX	0	0	0	0	4

AMA: Nov 98: 21

74010 Radiologic examination, abdomen; anteroposterior and additional oblique and cone views N I Q I

Mod	RVU Non-Fac Total	Fac Total	Global Days	51	50	62	80	MUE
	0.99	0.99	XXX	0	0	0	0	2
26	0.33	0.33	XXX	0	0	0	0	2
TC	0.66	0.66	XXX	0	0	0	0	2

AMA: Jan 07: 29, Jun 14: 14

74020 Radiologic examination, abdomen; complete, including decubitus and/or erect views N I Q I

Documentation Finder: *The documentation should show that plain radiological images are being taken of the abdominal cavity from front to back, back to front or front to back with the patient lying on the side (lateral view) and/or standing (anterior-posterior view). You may see reference to looking for "free air under the diaphragms" when taking erect/decubitus views.*

Mod	RVU Non-Fac Total	Fac Total	Global Days	51	50	62	80	MUE
	1.05	1.05	XXX	0	0	0	0	2
26	0.39	0.39	XXX	0	0	0	0	2
TC	0.66	0.66	XXX	0	0	0	0	2

74022 Radiologic examination, abdomen; complete acute abdomen series, including supine, erect, and/or decubitus views, single view chest N I Q I

Mod	RVU Non-Fac Total	Fac Total	Global Days	51	50	62	80	MUE
	1.25	1.25	XXX	0	0	0	0	2
26	0.46	0.46	XXX	0	0	0	0	2
TC	0.79	0.79	XXX	0	0	0	0	2

Coding Guidance

Intravenous administration of contrast material is not reported separately. For supply of contrast material, refer to HCPCS Level II codes Q9951-Q9967.

74150 Computed tomography, abdomen; without contrast material Z 2 Q 3

Mod	RVU Non-Fac Total	Fac Total	Global Days	51	50	62	80	MUE
	4.20	4.20	XXX	4	0	0	0	1
26	1.70	1.70	XXX	4	0	0	0	1
TC	2.50	2.50	XXX	4	0	0	0	1

AMA: Oct 02: 12, Mar 05: 1, 4, Apr 10: 9, Nov 11: 6, Oct 12: 12

74160 Computed tomography, abdomen; with contrast material(s) Z 2 Q 3

Mod	RVU Non-Fac Total	Fac Total	Global Days	51	50	62	80	MUE
	6.47	6.47	XXX	4	0	0	0	1
26	1.81	1.81	XXX	4	0	0	0	1
TC	4.66	4.66	XXX	4	0	0	0	1

AMA: Mar 05: 1, 4, Apr 10: 9, Nov 11: 6, Oct 12: 12

74170 Computed tomography, abdomen; without contrast material, followed by contrast material(s) and further sections Z 2 Q 3

Mod	RVU Non-Fac Total	Fac Total	Global Days	51	50	62	80	MUE
	7.36	7.36	XXX	4	0	0	0	1
26	2.00	2.00	XXX	4	0	0	0	1
TC	5.36	5.36	XXX	4	0	0	0	1

AMA: Mar 05: 4, Apr 10: 9, Nov 11: 6, Oct 12: 12

74174 Computed tomographic angiography, abdomen and pelvis, with contrast material(s), including noncontrast images, if performed, and image postprocessing Z 2 S

Mod	RVU Non-Fac Total	Fac Total	Global Days	51	50	62	80	MUE
	10.90	10.90	XXX	4	0	0	0	1
26	3.12	3.12	XXX	4	0	0	0	1
TC	7.78	7.78	XXX	4	0	0	0	1

● New   ▲ Revised   ✖ Deleted   ⊙ Moderate Sedation   ✚ Add-on Codes   ⊘ High Risk Denial   Ⓐ Age Edit   ♀ Female   ♂ Male   **AMA** *CPT® Assistant*   **MUE** Medically Unlikely Edit
⊘ Modifier 51 Exempt   ⊖ Modifier 63 Exempt   Ⓧ Unlisted   **Modifiers:** *See Inside Back Cover*   Ⓜ Maternity   A 2 – Z 3 ASC Payment Indicators   A – Y OPPS Status Indicators

CPT © 2015 American Medical Association. All Rights Reserved.   © 2016 DecisionHealth

74175 Computed tomographic angiography, abdomen, with contrast material(s), including noncontrast images, if performed, and image postprocessing Z2Q3

Mod	RVU Non-Fac Total	Fac Total	Global Days	Modifiers 51	50	62	80	MUE
	8.61	8.61	XXX	4	0	0	0	1
26	2.58	2.58	XXX	4	0	0	0	1
TC	6.03	6.03	XXX	4	0	0	0	1

AMA: Jul 01: 6, Dec 05: 7, Jan 07: 31, Apr 11: 13

74176 Computed tomography, abdomen and pelvis; without contrast material Z2Q3

Documentation Finder: *Documentation should state that a CT scan (sometimes referred to as a CAT scan) is being performed on the abdomen and pelvis without contrast. It can be reported only once per CT abdomen and pelvis examination. This code should not be reported if the provider injects contrast after obtaining the initial the CT without contrast.*

Mod	RVU Non-Fac Total	Fac Total	Global Days	Modifiers 51	50	62	80	MUE
	5.61	5.61	XXX	4	0	0	9	2
26	2.48	2.48	XXX	4	0	0	9	2
TC	3.13	3.13	XXX	4	0	0	9	2

AMA: Nov 11: 6

74177 Computed tomography, abdomen and pelvis; with contrast material(s) Z2Q3

Mod	RVU Non-Fac Total	Fac Total	Global Days	Modifiers 51	50	62	80	MUE
	8.74	8.74	XXX	4	0	0	9	2
26	2.60	2.60	XXX	4	0	0	9	2
TC	6.14	6.14	XXX	4	0	0	9	2

AMA: Nov 11: 6

74178 Computed tomography, abdomen and pelvis; without contrast material in one or both body regions, followed by contrast material(s) and further sections in one or both body regions Z2Q3

Mod	RVU Non-Fac Total	Fac Total	Global Days	Modifiers 51	50	62	80	MUE
	9.90	9.90	XXX	4	0	0	9	1
26	2.86	2.86	XXX	4	0	0	9	1
TC	7.04	7.04	XXX	4	0	0	9	1

AMA: Nov 11: 6

74181 Magnetic resonance (eg, proton) imaging, abdomen; without contrast material(s) Z2Q3

Mod	RVU Non-Fac Total	Fac Total	Global Days	Modifiers 51	50	62	80	MUE
	9.34	9.34	XXX	4	0	0	0	1
26	2.08	2.08	XXX	4	0	0	0	1
TC	7.26	7.26	XXX	4	0	0	0	1

AMA: Jul 01: 3, Nov 07: 9, May 09: 9, Jul 09: 10

74182 Magnetic resonance (eg, proton) imaging, abdomen; with contrast material(s) Z2Q3

Mod	RVU Non-Fac Total	Fac Total	Global Days	Modifiers 51	50	62	80	MUE
	12.74	12.74	XXX	4	0	0	0	1
26	2.47	2.47	XXX	4	0	0	0	1
TC	10.27	10.27	XXX	4	0	0	0	1

AMA: Jul 01: 3, May 09: 9, Jul 09: 10

74183 Magnetic resonance (eg, proton) imaging, abdomen; without contrast material(s), followed by with contrast material(s) and further sequences Z2Q3

Mod	RVU Non-Fac Total	Fac Total	Global Days	Modifiers 51	50	62	80	MUE
	14.21	14.21	XXX	4	0	0	0	1
26	3.22	3.22	XXX	4	0	0	0	1
TC	10.99	10.99	XXX	4	0	0	0	1

AMA: Jul 01: 3, May 09: 9, Jul 09: 10

Coding Guidance
For OPPS codes for abdominal MRA, refer to HCPCS Level II codes C8900-C8902.

74185 Magnetic resonance angiography, abdomen, with or without contrast material(s) B

Mod	RVU Non-Fac Total	Fac Total	Global Days	Modifiers 51	50	62	80	MUE
	11.31	11.31	XXX	4	0	0	0	1
26	2.55	2.55	XXX	4	0	0	0	1
TC	8.76	8.76	XXX	4	0	0	0	1

AMA: Dec 05: 7, Jan 07: 31

Pub 100-04, 13, 40, 40.1.2

74190 Peritoneogram (eg, after injection of air or contrast), radiological supervision and interpretation N1Q2

Coding tip: *Injection procedure (air or contrast) - 49400*

Mod	RVU Non-Fac Total	Fac Total	Global Days	Modifiers 51	50	62	80	MUE
	0.00	0.00	XXX	0	0	0	0	1
26	0.67	0.67	XXX	0	0	0	0	1
TC	0.00	0.00	XXX	0	0	0	0	1

AMA: Dec 10: 13

Gastrointestinal Tract Radiological Procedures

74210 Radiologic examination; pharynx and/or cervical esophagus N1Q1

Mod	RVU Non-Fac Total	Fac Total	Global Days	Modifiers 51	50	62	80	MUE
	2.18	2.18	XXX	0	0	0	0	1
26	0.51	0.51	XXX	0	0	0	0	1
TC	1.67	1.67	XXX	0	0	0	0	1

74220 Radiologic examination; esophagus N1Q1

Mod	RVU Non-Fac Total	Fac Total	Global Days	Modifiers 51	50	62	80	MUE
	2.49	2.49	XXX	0	0	0	0	1
26	0.66	0.66	XXX	0	0	0	0	1
TC	1.83	1.83	XXX	0	0	0	0	1

74230 Swallowing function, with cineradiography/ videoradiography N1Q1

Mod	RVU Non-Fac Total	Fac Total	Global Days	Modifiers 51	50	62	80	MUE
	3.58	3.58	XXX	0	0	0	0	1
26	0.76	0.76	XXX	0	0	0	0	1
TC	2.82	2.82	XXX	0	0	0	0	1

AMA: Dec 04: 17, Jul 14: 5

● New   ▲ Revised   Deleted   ⊙ Moderate Sedation   ✚ Add-on Codes   ⊘ High Risk Denial   Ⓐ Age Edit   ♀ Female   ♂ Male   **AMA** *CPT® Assistant*   **MUE** Medically Unlikely Edit
⊘ Modifier 51 Exempt   ⊖ Modifier 63 Exempt   ✗ Unlisted   **Modifiers:** *See Inside Back Cover*   Ⓜ Maternity   A2-Z3 ASC Payment Indicators   A-Y OPPS Status Indicators

© 2016 DecisionHealth   CPT © 2015 American Medical Association. All Rights Reserved.   **633**

74235 Removal of foreign body(s), esophageal, with use of balloon catheter, radiological supervision and interpretation `N1N`

Coding tip: Endoscopic removal of foreign body by esophagoscopy - 43217; by upper gastrointestinal endoscopy - 43247

RVU			Global Days	Modifiers				
Mod	Non-Fac Total	Fac Total		51	50	62	80	MUE
	0.00	0.00	XXX	0	0	0	0	1
26	1.78	1.78	XXX	0	0	0	0	1
TC	0.00	0.00	XXX	0	0	0	0	1

▲ **74240 Radiologic examination, gastrointestinal tract, upper; with or without delayed images, without KUB** `Z2Q1`

RVU			Global Days	Modifiers				
Mod	Non-Fac Total	Fac Total		51	50	62	80	MUE
	3.18	3.18	XXX	0	0	0	0	2
26	0.99	0.99	XXX	0	0	0	0	2
TC	2.19	2.19	XXX	0	0	0	0	2

▲ **74241 Radiologic examination, gastrointestinal tract, upper; with or without delayed images, with KUB** `Z2Q1`

RVU			Global Days	Modifiers				
Mod	Non-Fac Total	Fac Total		51	50	62	80	MUE
	3.31	3.31	XXX	0	0	0	0	1
26	0.99	0.99	XXX	0	0	0	0	1
TC	2.32	2.32	XXX	0	0	0	0	1

▲ **74245 Radiologic examination, gastrointestinal tract, upper; with small intestine, includes multiple serial images** `Z2S`

RVU			Global Days	Modifiers				
Mod	Non-Fac Total	Fac Total		51	50	62	80	MUE
	4.81	4.81	XXX	0	0	0	0	1
26	1.30	1.30	XXX	0	0	0	0	1
TC	3.51	3.51	XXX	0	0	0	0	1

▲ **74246 Radiological examination, gastrointestinal tract, upper, air contrast, with specific high density barium, effervescent agent, with or without glucagon; with or without delayed images, without KUB** `Z2Q1`

RVU			Global Days	Modifiers				
Mod	Non-Fac Total	Fac Total		51	50	62	80	MUE
	3.56	3.56	XXX	0	0	0	0	1
26	0.98	0.98	XXX	0	0	0	0	1
TC	2.58	2.58	XXX	0	0	0	0	1

▲ **74247 Radiological examination, gastrointestinal tract, upper, air contrast, with specific high density barium, effervescent agent, with or without glucagon; with or without delayed images, with KUB** `Z2Q1`

RVU			Global Days	Modifiers				
Mod	Non-Fac Total	Fac Total		51	50	62	80	MUE
	3.95	3.95	XXX	0	0	0	0	1
26	0.99	0.99	XXX	0	0	0	0	1
TC	2.96	2.96	XXX	0	0	0	0	1

74249 Radiological examination, gastrointestinal tract, upper, air contrast, with specific high density barium, effervescent agent, with or without glucagon; with small intestine follow-through `Z2S`

RVU			Global Days	Modifiers				
Mod	Non-Fac Total	Fac Total		51	50	62	80	MUE
	5.16	5.16	XXX	0	0	0	0	1
26	1.30	1.30	XXX	0	0	0	0	1
TC	3.86	3.86	XXX	0	0	0	0	1

▲ **74250 Radiologic examination, small intestine, includes multiple serial images** `Z2Q1`

RVU			Global Days	Modifiers				
Mod	Non-Fac Total	Fac Total		51	50	62	80	MUE
	2.91	2.91	XXX	0	0	0	0	1
26	0.67	0.67	XXX	0	0	0	0	1
TC	2.24	2.24	XXX	0	0	0	0	1

▲ **74251 Radiologic examination, small intestine, includes multiple serial images; via enteroclysis tube** `Z2S`

RVU			Global Days	Modifiers				
Mod	Non-Fac Total	Fac Total		51	50	62	80	MUE
	11.74	11.74	XXX	0	0	0	0	1
26	0.99	0.99	XXX	0	0	0	0	1
TC	10.75	10.75	XXX	0	0	0	0	1

74260 Duodenography, hypotonic `N1Q1`

RVU			Global Days	Modifiers				
Mod	Non-Fac Total	Fac Total		51	50	62	80	MUE
	9.89	9.89	XXX	0	0	0	0	1
26	0.71	0.71	XXX	0	0	0	0	1
TC	9.18	9.18	XXX	0	0	0	0	1

74261 Computed tomographic (CT) colonography, diagnostic, including image postprocessing; without contrast material `Z2Q3`

RVU			Global Days	Modifiers				
Mod	Non-Fac Total	Fac Total		51	50	62	80	MUE
	13.63	13.63	XXX	4	0	0	0	1
26	3.43	3.43	XXX	4	0	0	0	1
TC	10.20	10.20	XXX	4	0	0	0	1

AMA: Apr 10: 9

Computed tomographic (CT) colonography diagnostic including image postprocessing

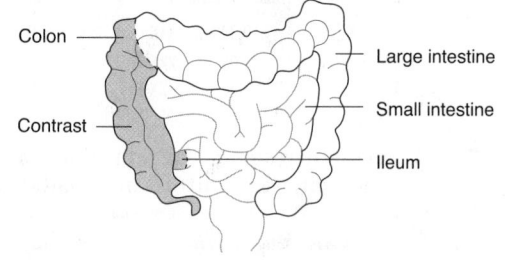

Colon — Large intestine — Small intestine

Contrast — Ileum

In 74261, non-contrast CT images of the abdomen and pelvis are obtained. In 74262, CT colonography is performed with contrast materials.

● New   ▲ Revised   ✖ Deleted   ⊙ Moderate Sedation   ✚ Add-on Codes   ⊘ High Risk Denial   Ⓐ Age Edit   ♀ Female   ♂ Male   **AMA** *CPT® Assistant*   **MUE** Medically Unlikely Edit
⊘ Modifier 51 Exempt   ⊖ Modifier 63 Exempt   🗷 Unlisted   **Modifiers:** *See Inside Back Cover*   Ⓜ Maternity   `A2`–`Z3` ASC Payment Indicators   `A`–`Y` OPPS Status Indicators

CPT © 2015 American Medical Association. All Rights Reserved.   © 2016 DecisionHealth

Radiology Procedures

74262 Computed tomographic (CT) colonography, diagnostic, including image postprocessing; with contrast material(s) including non-contrast images, if performed   Z2Q3

	RVU		Global Days	Modifiers				
Mod	Non-Fac Total	Fac Total		51	50	62	80	MUE
	15.17	15.17	XXX	4	0	0	0	1
26	3.57	3.57	XXX	4	0	0	0	1
TC	11.60	11.60	XXX	4	0	0	0	1

AMA: Apr 10: 9

74263 Computed tomographic (CT) colonography, screening, including image postprocessing   ⊘E

	RVU		Global Days	Modifiers				
Mod	Non-Fac Total	Fac Total		51	50	62	80	MUE
	21.22	21.22	XXX	9	9	9	9	
26	3.22	3.22	XXX	9	9	9	9	
TC	18.00	18.00	XXX	9	9	9	9	

AMA: Apr 10: 9

Computed tomographic (CT) colonography screening including image postprocessing

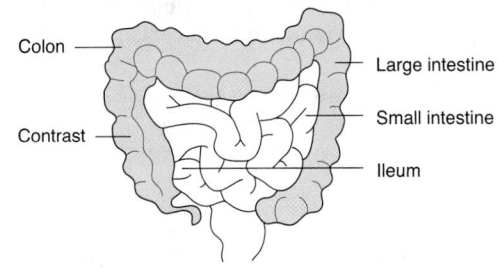

CT colonography, also referred to as virtual colonoscopy, is performed to screen for polyps or other masses or lesions in the colon. A bowel prep is performed the night before the procedure to clear the bowel of stool.

74270 Radiologic examination, colon; contrast (eg, barium) enema, with or without KUB   N I Q I

	RVU		Global Days	Modifiers				
Mod	Non-Fac Total	Fac Total		51	50	62	80	MUE
	4.21	4.21	XXX	0	0	0	0	1
26	0.99	0.99	XXX	0	0	0	0	1
TC	3.22	3.22	XXX	0	0	0	0	1

AMA: May 03: 19

74280 Radiologic examination, colon; air contrast with specific high density barium, with or without glucagon   Z2S

	RVU		Global Days	Modifiers				
Mod	Non-Fac Total	Fac Total		51	50	62	80	MUE
	5.97	5.97	XXX	0	0	0	0	1
26	1.42	1.42	XXX	0	0	0	0	1
TC	4.55	4.55	XXX	0	0	0	0	1

74283 Therapeutic enema, contrast or air, for reduction of intussusception or other intraluminal obstruction (eg, meconium ileus)   Z2S

	RVU		Global Days	Modifiers				
Mod	Non-Fac Total	Fac Total		51	50	62	80	MUE
	5.77	5.77	XXX	0	0	0	0	1
26	2.91	2.91	XXX	0	0	0	0	1
TC	2.86	2.86	XXX	0	0	0	0	1

AMA: Nov 97: 24

74290 Cholecystography, oral contrast   N I Q I

	RVU		Global Days	Modifiers				
Mod	Non-Fac Total	Fac Total		51	50	62	80	MUE
	1.97	1.97	XXX	0	0	0	0	1
26	0.46	0.46	XXX	0	0	0	0	1
TC	1.51	1.51	XXX	0	0	0	0	1

74300 Cholangiography and/or pancreatography; intraoperative, radiological supervision and interpretation   N I N

	RVU		Global Days	Modifiers				
Mod	Non-Fac Total	Fac Total		51	50	62	80	MUE
	0.00	0.00	XXX	0	0	0	0	1
26	0.52	0.52	XXX	0	0	0	0	1
TC	0.00	0.00	XXX	0	0	0	0	1

AMA: Nov 99: 41, Dec 00: 14

+ 74301 Cholangiography and/or pancreatography; additional set intraoperative, radiological supervision and interpretation (List separately in addition to code for primary procedure)   N I N

	RVU		Global Days	Modifiers				
Mod	Non-Fac Total	Fac Total		51	50	62	80	MUE
	0.00	0.00	ZZZ	0	0	0	0	1
26	0.30	0.30	ZZZ	0	0	0	0	1
TC	0.00	0.00	ZZZ	0	0	0	0	1

✖ 74305 ~~Cholangiography and/or pancreatography; through existing catheter, radiological supervision and interpretation~~

✖ 74320 ~~Cholangiography, percutaneous, transhepatic, radiological supervision and interpretation~~

✖ 74327 ~~Postoperative biliary duct calculus removal, percutaneous via T-tube tract, basket, or snare (eg, Burhenne technique), radiological supervision and interpretation~~

74328 Endoscopic catheterization of the biliary ductal system, radiological supervision and interpretation   N I N

	RVU		Global Days	Modifiers				
Mod	Non-Fac Total	Fac Total		51	50	62	80	MUE
	0.00	0.00	XXX	0	0	0	0	1
26	1.01	1.01	XXX	0	0	0	0	1
TC	0.00	0.00	XXX	0	0	0	0	1

74329 Endoscopic catheterization of the pancreatic ductal system, radiological supervision and interpretation   N I N

	RVU		Global Days	Modifiers				
Mod	Non-Fac Total	Fac Total		51	50	62	80	MUE
	0.00	0.00	XXX	0	0	0	0	1
26	1.02	1.02	XXX	0	0	0	0	1
TC	0.00	0.00	XXX	0	0	0	0	1

74330 Combined endoscopic catheterization of the biliary and pancreatic ductal systems, radiological supervision and interpretation   N I N

	RVU		Global Days	Modifiers				
Mod	Non-Fac Total	Fac Total		51	50	62	80	MUE
	0.00	0.00	XXX	0	0	0	0	1
26	1.29	1.29	XXX	0	0	0	0	1
TC	0.00	0.00	XXX	0	0	0	0	1

74262 – 74330

● New   ▲ Revised   Deleted   ⊙ Moderate Sedation   ✚ Add-on Codes   ⊘ High Risk Denial   Ⓐ Age Edit   ♀ Female   ♂ Male   **AMA** *CPT® Assistant*   **MUE** Medically Unlikely Edit
⊘ Modifier 51 Exempt   ⊖ Modifier 63 Exempt   ✗ Unlisted   **Modifiers:** *See Inside Back Cover*   Ⓜ Maternity   A2–Z3 ASC Payment Indicators   A –Y OPPS Status Indicators

© 2016 DecisionHealth   CPT © 2015 American Medical Association. All Rights Reserved.   **635**

Radiology Procedures

74340 – 74440

▲ **74340 Introduction of long gastrointestinal tube (eg, Miller-Abbott), including multiple fluoroscopies and images, radiological supervision and interpretation** N I N

Coding tip: Procedure for introduction of long GI tube - 44500

RVU			Global Days	Modifiers				
Mod	Non-Fac Total	Fac Total		51	50	62	80	MUE
	0.00	0.00	XXX	0	0	0	0	1
26	0.77	0.77	XXX	0	0	0	0	1
TC	0.00	0.00	XXX	0	0	0	0	1

74355 Percutaneous placement of enteroclysis tube, radiological supervision and interpretation N I N

RVU			Global Days	Modifiers				
Mod	Non-Fac Total	Fac Total		51	50	62	80	MUE
	0.00	0.00	XXX	0	0	0	0	1
26	1.10	1.10	XXX	0	0	0	0	1
TC	0.00	0.00	XXX	0	0	0	0	1

AMA: Feb 07: 11, Nov 10: 3, Jan 11: 8

74360 Intraluminal dilation of strictures and/or obstructions (eg, esophagus), radiological supervision and interpretation N I N

Coding tip: Esophageal dilation via esophagoscopy - 43220, 43226; via upper GI endoscopy - 43248-43249; with unguided sound or bougie - 43450; over guide wire - 43453; balloon dilation manipulation - 43456-43458

Coding tip: Intestinal dilation with rigid proctosigmoidoscopy - 45303; with flexible sigmoidoscopy - 45340; with colonoscopy - 45386

Coding tip: Dilation of gastric outlet - 43245

RVU			Global Days	Modifiers				
Mod	Non-Fac Total	Fac Total		51	50	62	80	MUE
	0.00	0.00	XXX	0	0	0	0	1
26	0.81	0.81	XXX	0	0	0	0	1
TC	0.00	0.00	XXX	0	0	0	0	1

AMA: Spring 94: 3, Oct 08: 6

74363 Percutaneous transhepatic dilation of biliary duct stricture with or without placement of stent, radiological supervision and interpretation N I N

RVU			Global Days	Modifiers				
Mod	Non-Fac Total	Fac Total		51	50	62	80	MUE
	0.00	0.00	XXX	0	0	0	0	2
26	1.22	1.22	XXX	0	0	0	0	2
TC	0.00	0.00	XXX	0	0	0	0	2

Urinary Tract Radiological Procedures

74400 Urography (pyelography), intravenous, with or without KUB, with or without tomography Z 2 S

RVU			Global Days	Modifiers				
Mod	Non-Fac Total	Fac Total		51	50	62	80	MUE
	3.07	3.07	XXX	0	0	0	0	1
26	0.70	0.70	XXX	0	0	0	0	1
TC	2.37	2.37	XXX	0	0	0	0	1

74410 Urography, infusion, drip technique and/or bolus technique Z 2 S

RVU			Global Days	Modifiers				
Mod	Non-Fac Total	Fac Total		51	50	62	80	MUE
	3.03	3.03	XXX	0	0	0	0	1
26	0.69	0.69	XXX	0	0	0	0	1
TC	2.34	2.34	XXX	0	0	0	0	1

74415 Urography, infusion, drip technique and/or bolus technique; with nephrotomography Z 2 S

RVU			Global Days	Modifiers				
Mod	Non-Fac Total	Fac Total		51	50	62	80	MUE
	3.83	3.83	XXX	0	0	0	0	1
26	0.70	0.70	XXX	0	0	0	0	1
TC	3.13	3.13	XXX	0	0	0	0	1

74420 Urography, retrograde, with or without KUB Z 2 S

RVU			Global Days	Modifiers				
Mod	Non-Fac Total	Fac Total		51	50	62	80	MUE
	0.00	0.00	XXX	0	0	0	0	2
26	0.50	0.50	XXX	0	0	0	0	2
TC	0.00	0.00	XXX	0	0	0	0	2

AMA: Sep 00: 11, Dec 10: 15

Coding Guidance

Procedures requiring the additional use of radiological supervision and interpretation code 74425 include percutaneous aspiration of renal cyst or pelvis, introduction of catheter into renal pelvis for drainage, injection for pyelography and manometric studies done through a nephrostomy, injection for ureterography through ureterostomy, and injection for visualization of ileal conduit.

74425 Urography, antegrade (pyelostogram, nephrostogram, loopogram), radiological supervision and interpretation N I Q 2

RVU			Global Days	Modifiers				
Mod	Non-Fac Total	Fac Total		51	50	62	80	MUE
	0.00	0.00	XXX	0	0	0	0	2
26	0.50	0.50	XXX	0	0	0	0	2
TC	0.00	0.00	XXX	0	0	0	0	2

AMA: Fall 93: 14, Dec 97: 7, Oct 05: 18

74430 Cystography, minimum of 3 views, radiological supervision and interpretation N I Q 2

Coding tip: Injection procedure and placement of chain for contrast/chain urethrocystography - 51605

Coding tip: Injection procedure for cystography - 51600

RVU			Global Days	Modifiers				
Mod	Non-Fac Total	Fac Total		51	50	62	80	MUE
	1.05	1.05	XXX	0	0	0	0	1
26	0.45	0.45	XXX	0	0	0	0	1
TC	0.60	0.60	XXX	0	0	0	0	1

74440 Vasography, vesiculography, or epididymography, radiological supervision and interpretation ♂ N I Q 2

Coding tip: Vasotomy or introduction for vasogram, vesiculogram, or epididymogram - 55300

Coding tip: Ejaculatory duct catheterization - 52010

RVU			Global Days	Modifiers				
Mod	Non-Fac Total	Fac Total		51	50	62	80	MUE
	2.28	2.28	XXX	0	0	0	0	1
26	0.52	0.52	XXX	0	0	0	0	1
TC	1.76	1.76	XXX	0	0	0	0	1

● New   ▲ Revised   ✖ Deleted   ⊙ Moderate Sedation   ✚ Add-on Codes   ⊖ High Risk Denial   Ⓐ Age Edit   ♀ Female   ♂ Male   **AMA** CPT® Assistant   **MUE** Medically Unlikely Edit   ⊘ Modifier 51 Exempt   ⊖ Modifier 63 Exempt   ⊠ Unlisted   **Modifiers:** See Inside Back Cover   Ⓜ Maternity   A 2 – Z 3 ASC Payment Indicators   A – Y OPPS Status Indicators

636   CPT © 2015 American Medical Association. All Rights Reserved.   © 2016 DecisionHealth

74445 Corpora cavernosography, radiological supervision and interpretation ♂ N I Q2

Coding tip: Injection procedure for corpora cavernosography - 54230

RVU			Global Days	Modifiers				
Mod	Non-Fac Total	Fac Total		51	50	62	80	MUE
	0.00	0.00	XXX	0	0	0	0	1
26	1.54	1.54	XXX	0	0	0	0	1
TC	0.00	0.00	XXX	0	0	0	0	1

AMA: Feb 07: 11, Nov 10: 3, Jan 11: 8

74450 Urethrocystography, retrograde, radiological supervision and interpretation N I Q2

Coding tip: Injection procedure for retrograde urethrocystography - 51610

RVU			Global Days	Modifiers				
Mod	Non-Fac Total	Fac Total		51	50	62	80	MUE
	0.00	0.00	XXX	0	0	0	0	1
26	0.47	0.47	XXX	0	0	0	0	1
TC	0.00	0.00	XXX	0	0	0	0	1

74455 Urethrocystography, voiding, radiological supervision and interpretation N I Q2

Coding tip: Injection procedure for voiding urethrocystography - 51600

RVU			Global Days	Modifiers				
Mod	Non-Fac Total	Fac Total		51	50	62	80	MUE
	2.29	2.29	XXX	0	0	0	0	1
26	0.47	0.47	XXX	0	0	0	0	1
TC	1.82	1.82	XXX	0	0	0	0	1

74470 Radiologic examination, renal cyst study, translumbar, contrast visualization, radiological supervision and interpretation N I Q2

RVU			Global Days	Modifiers				
Mod	Non-Fac Total	Fac Total		51	50	62	80	MUE
	0.00	0.00	XXX	0	0	0	0	2
26	0.75	0.75	XXX	0	0	0	0	2
TC	0.00	0.00	XXX	0	0	0	0	2

AMA: Oct 05: 18, Feb 07: 11, Nov 10: 3, Jan 11: 8

✗ ~~74475 Introduction of intracatheter or catheter into renal pelvis for drainage and/or injection, percutaneous, radiological supervision and interpretation~~

✗ ~~74480 Introduction of ureteral catheter or stent into ureter through renal pelvis for drainage and/or injection, percutaneous, radiological supervision and interpretation~~

74485 Dilation of nephrostomy, ureters, or urethra, radiological supervision and interpretation N I Q2

Coding tip: Urethral dilation, male - 53600-53621; female - 53660-53665

Coding tip: Dilation of ureter to establish nephrostomy - 50395

RVU			Global Days	Modifiers				
Mod	Non-Fac Total	Fac Total		51	50	62	80	MUE
	2.59	2.59	XXX	0	0	0	0	2
26	0.74	0.74	XXX	0	0	0	0	2
TC	1.85	1.85	XXX	0	0	0	0	2

AMA: Oct 05: 18, Dec 08: 7, Jan 09: 7

OB/GYN Radiological Procedures

74710 Pelvimetry, with or without placental localization ♀ N I Q1

RVU			Global Days	Modifiers				
Mod	Non-Fac Total	Fac Total		51	50	62	80	MUE
	1.03	1.03	XXX	0	0	0	0	1
26	0.49	0.49	XXX	0	0	0	0	1
TC	0.54	0.54	XXX	0	0	0	0	1

● ### 74712 Magnetic resonance (eg, proton) imaging, fetal, including placental and maternal pelvic imaging when performed; single or first gestation ♀ M Z2 S

RVU			Global Days	Modifiers				
Mod	Non-Fac Total	Fac Total		51	50	62	80	MUE
	13.53	13.53	XXX	4	0	0	0	1
26	4.29	4.29	XXX	4	0	0	0	1
TC	9.24	9.24	XXX	4	0	0	0	1

✚● ### 74713 Magnetic resonance (eg, proton) imaging, fetal, including placental and maternal pelvic imaging when performed; each additional gestation (List separately in addition to code for primary procedure) ♀ M N

RVU			Global Days	Modifiers				
Mod	Non-Fac Total	Fac Total		51	50	62	80	MUE
	6.50	6.50	ZZZ	0	0	0	0	2
26	2.54	2.54	ZZZ	0	0	0	0	2
TC	3.96	3.96	ZZZ	0	0	0	0	2

74740 Hysterosalpingography, radiological supervision and interpretation ♀ N I Q2

Coding tip: Introduction of contrast - 58340

RVU			Global Days	Modifiers				
Mod	Non-Fac Total	Fac Total		51	50	62	80	MUE
	2.10	2.10	XXX	0	0	0	0	1
26	0.54	0.54	XXX	0	0	0	0	1
TC	1.56	1.56	XXX	0	0	0	0	1

AMA: Nov 97: 24, Jul 99: 8, Mar 09: 11

74742 Transcervical catheterization of fallopian tube, radiological supervision and interpretation ♀ N I N

Coding tip: Introduction of fallopian tube catheter - 58345

RVU			Global Days	Modifiers				
Mod	Non-Fac Total	Fac Total		51	50	62	80	MUE
	0.00	0.00	XXX	0	0	0	0	2
26	0.84	0.84	XXX	0	0	0	0	2
TC	0.00	0.00	XXX	0	0	0	0	2

74775 Perineogram (eg, vaginogram, for sex determination or extent of anomalies) ♀ Z2 S

RVU			Global Days	Modifiers				
Mod	Non-Fac Total	Fac Total		51	50	62	80	MUE
	0.00	0.00	XXX	0	0	0	0	1
26	0.89	0.89	XXX	0	0	0	0	1
TC	0.00	0.00	XXX	0	0	0	0	1

Heart Radiological Procedures

75557 Cardiac magnetic resonance imaging for morphology and function without contrast material Z2 Q3

RVU			Global Days	Modifiers				
Mod	Non-Fac Total	Fac Total		51	50	62	80	MUE
	8.93	8.93	XXX	4	0	0	0	1
26	3.29	3.29	XXX	4	0	0	0	1
TC	5.64	5.64	XXX	4	0	0	0	1

AMA: Jul 10: 7

● New   ▲ Revised   Deleted   ⊙ Moderate Sedation   ✚ Add-on Codes   ⊘ High Risk Denial   Ⓐ Age Edit   ♀ Female   ♂ Male   **AMA** *CPT® Assistant*   **MUE** Medically Unlikely Edit
Ⓢ Modifier 51 Exempt   ⊖ Modifier 63 Exempt   ✗ Unlisted   **Modifiers:** *See Inside Back Cover*   M Maternity   A2–Z3 ASC Payment Indicators   A–Y OPPS Status Indicators

75559 Cardiac magnetic resonance imaging for morphology and function without contrast material; with stress imaging   Z 2 Q 3

Mod	RVU		Global Days	Modifiers				
	Non-Fac Total	Fac Total		51	50	62	80	MUE
	12.22	12.22	XXX	4	0	0	0	1
26	4.06	4.06	XXX	4	0	0	0	1
TC	8.16	8.16	XXX	4	0	0	0	1

AMA: Jul 10

75561 Cardiac magnetic resonance imaging for morphology and function without contrast material(s), followed by contrast material(s) and further sequences   Z 2 Q 3

Mod	RVU		Global Days	Modifiers				
	Non-Fac Total	Fac Total		51	50	62	80	MUE
	11.86	11.86	XXX	4	0	0	0	1
26	3.63	3.63	XXX	4	0	0	0	1
TC	8.23	8.23	XXX	4	0	0	0	1

AMA: Jul 10: 7

75563 Cardiac magnetic resonance imaging for morphology and function without contrast material(s), followed by contrast material(s) and further sequences; with stress imaging   Z 3 Q 3

Mod	RVU		Global Days	Modifiers				
	Non-Fac Total	Fac Total		51	50	62	80	MUE
	14.08	14.08	XXX	4	0	0	0	1
26	4.16	4.16	XXX	4	0	0	0	1
TC	9.92	9.92	XXX	4	0	0	0	1

AMA: Jul 10: 7

+ 75565 Cardiac magnetic resonance imaging for velocity flow mapping (List separately in addition to code for primary procedure)   N I N

Mod	RVU		Global Days	Modifiers				
	Non-Fac Total	Fac Total		51	50	62	80	MUE
	1.54	1.54	ZZZ	0	0	0	0	1
26	0.35	0.35	ZZZ	0	0	0	0	1
TC	1.19	1.19	ZZZ	0	0	0	0	1

AMA: Jul 10: 7

Cardiac magnetic resonance imaging for velocity flow mapping

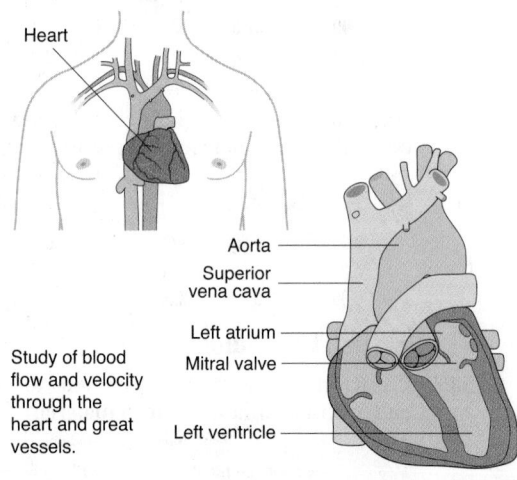

Study of blood flow and velocity through the heart and great vessels.

Heart
Aorta
Superior vena cava
Left atrium
Mitral valve
Left ventricle

Cross-section of heart

75571 Computed tomography, heart, without contrast material, with quantitative evaluation of coronary calcium   N I Q I

Documentation Finder: *The documentation should reference cardiac computed tomography (CT) and coronary computed tomographic angiography (CTA) and include any quantitative assessment during the same encounter. You may also see reference to 3D being performed, which would be considered inclusive in this code. Only one computed tomography heart service is reported per encounter.*

Mod	RVU		Global Days	Modifiers				
	Non-Fac Total	Fac Total		51	50	62	80	MUE
	2.82	2.82	XXX	4	0	0	0	1
26	0.82	0.82	XXX	4	0	0	0	1
TC	2.00	2.00	XXX	4	0	0	0	1

AMA: Jul 10: 7

Computed tomography, heart, without contrast material, with quantitative evaluation of coronary calcium

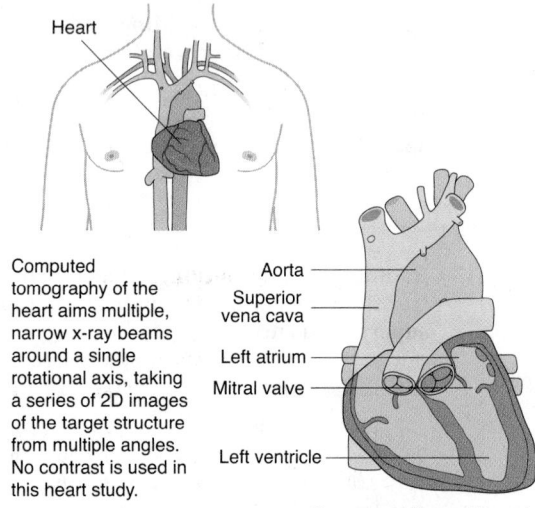

Heart

Computed tomography of the heart aims multiple, narrow x-ray beams around a single rotational axis, taking a series of 2D images of the target structure from multiple angles. No contrast is used in this heart study.

Aorta
Superior vena cava
Left atrium
Mitral valve
Left ventricle

Cross-section of heart

75572 Computed tomography, heart, with contrast material, for evaluation of cardiac structure and morphology (including 3D image postprocessing, assessment of cardiac function, and evaluation of venous structures, if performed)   Z 2 S

Mod	RVU		Global Days	Modifiers				
	Non-Fac Total	Fac Total		51	50	62	80	MUE
	7.96	7.96	XXX	4	0	0	0	1
26	2.46	2.46	XXX	4	0	0	0	1
TC	5.50	5.50	XXX	4	0	0	0	1

AMA: Jul 10: 7

75573 Computed tomography, heart, with contrast material, for evaluation of cardiac structure and morphology in the setting of congenital heart disease (including 3D image postprocessing, assessment of LV cardiac function, RV structure and function and evaluation of venous structures, if performed)   Z 2 S

Mod	RVU		Global Days	Modifiers				
	Non-Fac Total	Fac Total		51	50	62	80	MUE
	10.96	10.96	XXX	4	0	0	0	1
26	3.58	3.58	XXX	4	0	0	0	1
TC	7.38	7.38	XXX	4	0	0	0	1

AMA: Jul 10: 7

● New   ▲ Revised   ✖ Deleted   ⊙ Moderate Sedation   ✚ Add-on Codes   ⊗ High Risk Denial   Ⓐ Age Edit   ♀ Female   ♂ Male   **AMA** *CPT® Assistant*   ***MUE*** Medically Unlikely Edit
⊘ Modifier 51 Exempt   ⊖ Modifier 63 Exempt   ✄ Unlisted   **Modifiers:** *See Inside Back Cover*   Ⓜ Maternity   A 2 – Z 3 ASC Payment Indicators   A – Y OPPS Status Indicators

638   CPT © 2015 American Medical Association. All Rights Reserved.   © 2016 DecisionHealth

75574 **Computed tomographic angiography, heart, coronary arteries and bypass grafts (when present), with contrast material, including 3D image postprocessing (including evaluation of cardiac structure and morphology, assessment of cardiac function, and evaluation of venous structures, if performed)** `Z2 S`

Mod	RVU Non-Fac Total	Fac Total	Global Days	Modifiers 51	50	62	80	MUE
	11.75	11.75	XXX	4	0	0	0	1
26	3.36	3.36	XXX	4	0	0	0	1
TC	8.39	8.39	XXX	4	0	0	0	1

AMA: Jul 10: 7

Vascular Procedures

Aortic/Arterial Radiological Procedures

Coding Guidance

Diagnostic arteriograms done on the same day and encounter by the same provider as an intravascular interventional procedure may be reported separately if a previous catheter-based angiographic study is not available and the decision for the interventional procedure is based on the diagnostic study. If a diagnostic angiogram was done prior to the intravascular interventional procedure, a second, repeat diagnostic angiogram on the date of the interventional service may not be reported, unless it becomes medically necessary due to a change in the patient's condition regarding the clinical indications, or to further define anatomy and pathology from inadequate visualization, or a change during the procedure necessitates a new diagnostic evaluation outside the interventional target area. In these cases, the repeat diagnostic angiogram may be reported with modifier 59. If the previous diagnostic angiogram was complete, then a second angiogram for the dye injections necessary to complete the interventional procedure is not reported. Individual codes in the 70000 series will identify which is appropriate to use for the injection or administration for a given procedure. The injection of contrast or radiopharmaceuticals is already inherent in radiological procedures and should not be reported separately.

75600 **Aortography, thoracic, without serialography, radiological supervision and interpretation** `N1 Q2`

Mod	RVU Non-Fac Total	Fac Total	Global Days	Modifiers 51	50	62	80	MUE
	5.56	5.56	XXX	6	0	0	0	1
26	0.69	0.69	XXX	6	0	0	0	1
TC	4.87	4.87	XXX	6	0	0	0	1

75605 **Aortography, thoracic, by serialography, radiological supervision and interpretation** `N1 Q2`

Mod	RVU Non-Fac Total	Fac Total	Global Days	Modifiers 51	50	62	80	MUE
	3.92	3.92	XXX	6	0	0	0	1
26	1.59	1.59	XXX	6	0	0	0	1
TC	2.33	2.33	XXX	6	0	0	0	1

AMA: Spring 94: 29, Dec 98: 9, Jan 13: 6

Coding Guidance

Codes 74000-74022 are included in the total service for 75625. Any abdominal radiology procedure with a radiological supervision and interpretation code includes abdominal x-rays. Sometimes during cardiac catheterization, a small amount of dye may be injected upon catheter withdrawal to examine the aortiliac arteries. Abdominal aortography with or without iliofemoral angiography should not be reported unless a complete study is performed and interpreted, including the venous phase, just as it would normally be without the concomitant cardiac catheterization.

75625 **Aortography, abdominal, by serialography, radiological supervision and interpretation** `N1 Q2`

Mod	RVU Non-Fac Total	Fac Total	Global Days	Modifiers 51	50	62	80	MUE
	3.90	3.90	XXX	6	0	0	0	1
26	1.59	1.59	XXX	6	0	0	0	1
TC	2.31	2.31	XXX	6	0	0	0	1

AMA: Fall 93: 16, Jan 01: 14, Dec 07: 14, Apr 08: 11, Dec 09: 13, Jan 13: 6, Feb 13: 16

75630 **Aortography, abdominal plus bilateral iliofemoral lower extremity, catheter, by serialography, radiological supervision and interpretation** `N1 Q2`

Mod	RVU Non-Fac Total	Fac Total	Global Days	Modifiers 51	50	62	80	MUE
	4.82	4.82	XXX	6	0	0	0	1
26	2.51	2.51	XXX	6	0	0	0	1
TC	2.31	2.31	XXX	6	0	0	0	1

AMA: Fall 93: 16, Jan 01: 14, Apr 08: 11, Dec 09: 13

75635 **Computed tomographic angiography, abdominal aorta and bilateral iliofemoral lower extremity runoff, with contrast material(s), including noncontrast images, if performed, and image postprocessing** `N1 Q2`

Mod	RVU Non-Fac Total	Fac Total	Global Days	Modifiers 51	50	62	80	MUE
	10.67	10.67	XXX	4	0	0	0	1
26	3.39	3.39	XXX	4	0	0	0	1
TC	7.28	7.28	XXX	4	0	0	0	1

AMA: Jul 01: 4, 5, Dec 05: 7, Jan 07: 31, Apr 11: 13

75658 **Angiography, brachial, retrograde, radiological supervision and interpretation** `N1 Q2`

Mod	RVU Non-Fac Total	Fac Total	Global Days	Modifiers 51	50	62	80	MUE
	4.68	4.68	XXX	6	0	0	0	1
26	1.81	1.81	XXX	6	0	0	0	1
TC	2.87	2.87	XXX	6	0	0	0	1

75705 **Angiography, spinal, selective, radiological supervision and interpretation** `N1 Q2`

Mod	RVU Non-Fac Total	Fac Total	Global Days	Modifiers 51	50	62	80	MUE
	6.88	6.88	XXX	6	0	0	0	13
26	3.25	3.25	XXX	6	0	0	0	13
TC	3.63	3.63	XXX	6	0	0	0	13

75710 **Angiography, extremity, unilateral, radiological supervision and interpretation** `N1 Q2`

Mod	RVU Non-Fac Total	Fac Total	Global Days	Modifiers 51	50	62	80	MUE
	4.61	4.61	XXX	6	0	0	0	2
26	1.60	1.60	XXX	6	0	0	0	2
TC	3.01	3.01	XXX	6	0	0	0	2

AMA: Apr 99: 11, Jan 01: 14

Pub 100-04, 16, 120.2

● New   ▲ Revised   Deleted   ⊙ Moderate Sedation   ✚ Add-on Codes   ⊘ High Risk Denial   Ⓐ Age Edit   ♀ Female   ♂ Male   **AMA** *CPT® Assistant*   **MUE** Medically Unlikely Edit

⊘ Modifier 51 Exempt   ⊖ Modifier 63 Exempt   ✗ Unlisted   **Modifiers:** *See Inside Back Cover*   Ⓜ Maternity   `A2–Z3` ASC Payment Indicators   `A –Y` OPPS Status Indicators

© 2016 DecisionHealth   CPT © 2015 American Medical Association. All Rights Reserved.   **639**

75716 Angiography, extremity, bilateral, radiological supervision and interpretation ◼N◼1◼Q2

Mod	RVU Non-Fac Total	Fac Total	Global Days	51	50	62	80	MUE
	5.28	5.28	XXX	6	2	0	0	1
26	1.83	1.83	XXX	6	2	0	0	1
TC	3.45	3.45	XXX	6	2	0	0	1

AMA: Fall 93: 16, Jan 01: 14, Dec 07: 14, Apr 08: 11, Dec 09: 13

Pub 100-04, 16, 120.2

75726 Angiography, visceral, selective or supraselective (with or without flush aortogram), radiological supervision and interpretation ◼N◼1◼Q2

Mod	RVU Non-Fac Total	Fac Total	Global Days	51	50	62	80	MUE
	4.21	4.21	XXX	6	0	0	0	3
26	1.58	1.58	XXX	6	0	0	0	3
TC	2.63	2.63	XXX	6	0	0	0	3

75731 Angiography, adrenal, unilateral, selective, radiological supervision and interpretation ◼N◼1◼Q2

Mod	RVU Non-Fac Total	Fac Total	Global Days	51	50	62	80	MUE
	4.86	4.86	XXX	6	0	0	0	1
26	1.63	1.63	XXX	6	0	0	0	1
TC	3.23	3.23	XXX	6	0	0	0	1

75733 Angiography, adrenal, bilateral, selective, radiological supervision and interpretation ◼N◼1◼Q2

Mod	RVU Non-Fac Total	Fac Total	Global Days	51	50	62	80	MUE
	5.18	5.18	XXX	6	2	0	0	1
26	1.80	1.80	XXX	6	2	0	0	1
TC	3.38	3.38	XXX	6	2	0	0	1

75736 Angiography, pelvic, selective or supraselective, radiological supervision and interpretation ◼N◼1◼Q2

Mod	RVU Non-Fac Total	Fac Total	Global Days	51	50	62	80	MUE
	4.51	4.51	XXX	6	0	0	0	2
26	1.57	1.57	XXX	6	0	0	0	2
TC	2.94	2.94	XXX	6	0	0	0	2

75741 Angiography, pulmonary, unilateral, selective, radiological supervision and interpretation ◼N◼1◼Q2

Mod	RVU Non-Fac Total	Fac Total	Global Days	51	50	62	80	MUE
	4.26	4.26	XXX	6	0	0	0	1
26	1.81	1.81	XXX	6	0	0	0	1
TC	2.45	2.45	XXX	6	0	0	0	1

AMA: Mar 12: 10, Jan 13: 6

75743 Angiography, pulmonary, bilateral, selective, radiological supervision and interpretation ◼N◼1◼Q2

Mod	RVU Non-Fac Total	Fac Total	Global Days	51	50	62	80	MUE
	4.77	4.77	XXX	6	2	0	0	1
26	2.29	2.29	XXX	6	2	0	0	1
TC	2.48	2.48	XXX	6	2	0	0	1

AMA: Spring 94: 29, Apr 98: 7, Jan 13: 6

75746 Angiography, pulmonary, by nonselective catheter or venous injection, radiological supervision and interpretation ◼N◼1◼Q2

Mod	RVU Non-Fac Total	Fac Total	Global Days	51	50	62	80	MUE
	4.29	4.29	XXX	6	0	0	0	1
26	1.60	1.60	XXX	6	0	0	0	1
TC	2.69	2.69	XXX	6	0	0	0	1

75756 Angiography, internal mammary, radiological supervision and interpretation ◯◼N◼1◼Q2

Mod	RVU Non-Fac Total	Fac Total	Global Days	51	50	62	80	MUE
	4.69	4.69	XXX	6	0	0	0	2
26	1.60	1.60	XXX	6	0	0	0	2
TC	3.09	3.09	XXX	6	0	0	0	2

+ 75774 Angiography, selective, each additional vessel studied after basic examination, radiological supervision and interpretation (List separately in addition to code for primary procedure) ◼N◼1◼N

Mod	RVU Non-Fac Total	Fac Total	Global Days	51	50	62	80	MUE
	2.47	2.47	ZZZ	0	0	0	0	7
26	0.50	0.50	ZZZ	0	0	0	0	7
TC	1.97	1.97	ZZZ	0	0	0	0	7

AMA: Fall 93: 17, Spring 94: 29, Apr 11: 13, Feb 13: 17, Jun 13: 12, Oct 13: 18

Pub 100-04, 16, 120.2

75791 Angiography, arteriovenous shunt (eg, dialysis patient fistula/graft), complete evaluation of dialysis access, including fluoroscopy, image documentation and report (includes injections of contrast and all necessary imaging from the arterial anastomosis and adjacent artery through entire venous outflow including the inferior or superior vena cava), radiological supervision and interpretation ◼N◼1◼Q2

Mod	RVU Non-Fac Total	Fac Total	Global Days	51	50	62	80	MUE
	9.14	9.14	XXX	6	0	0	0	1
26	2.45	2.45	XXX	6	0	0	0	1
TC	6.69	6.69	XXX	6	0	0	0	1

AMA: Dec 11: 16

Angiography arteriovenous shunt

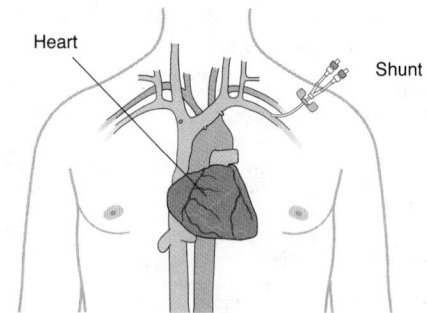

A radiological supervision and interpretation is performed during a separately reportable injection procedure for angiography of an arteriovenous shunt.

● New   ▲ Revised   ✖ Deleted   ⊙ Moderate Sedation   ✚ Add-on Codes   ⊘ High Risk Denial   Ⓐ Age Edit   ♀ Female   ♂ Male   **AMA** *CPT® Assistant*   **MUE** Medically Unlikely Edit

⊘ Modifier 51 Exempt   ⊖ Modifier 63 Exempt   ✗ Unlisted   **Modifiers:** *See Inside Back Cover*   Ⓜ Maternity   A 2 – Z 3 ASC Payment Indicators   A – Y OPPS Status Indicators

CPT © 2015 American Medical Association. All Rights Reserved.   © 2016 DecisionHealth

Vein/Lymphatic Radiological Procedures

Coding Guidance

For lymphangiography procedures, injection of dye into subcutaneous tissue is integral to the procedure. Do not report code 96372 separately for this injection of dye.

75801   Lymphangiography, extremity only, unilateral, radiological supervision and interpretation N1Q2

Mod	RVU Non-Fac Total	Fac Total	Global Days	Modifiers 51	50	62	80	MUE
	0.00	0.00	XXX	0	0	0	0	1
26	1.27	1.27	XXX	0	0	0	0	1
TC	0.00	0.00	XXX	0	0	0	0	1

75803   Lymphangiography, extremity only, bilateral, radiological supervision and interpretation N1Q2

Mod	RVU Non-Fac Total	Fac Total	Global Days	Modifiers 51	50	62	80	MUE
	0.00	0.00	XXX	0	2	0	0	1
26	1.67	1.67	XXX	0	2	0	0	1
TC	0.00	0.00	XXX	0	2	0	0	1

75805   Lymphangiography, pelvic/abdominal, unilateral, radiological supervision and interpretation N1Q2

Mod	RVU Non-Fac Total	Fac Total	Global Days	Modifiers 51	50	62	80	MUE
	0.00	0.00	XXX	0	0	0	0	1
26	1.16	1.16	XXX	0	0	0	0	1
TC	0.00	0.00	XXX	0	0	0	0	1

75807   Lymphangiography, pelvic/abdominal, bilateral, radiological supervision and interpretation N1Q2

Mod	RVU Non-Fac Total	Fac Total	Global Days	Modifiers 51	50	62	80	MUE
	0.00	0.00	XXX	0	2	0	0	1
26	1.68	1.68	XXX	0	2	0	0	1
TC	0.00	0.00	XXX	0	2	0	0	1

75809   Shuntogram for investigation of previously placed indwelling nonvascular shunt (eg, LeVeen shunt, ventriculoperitoneal shunt, indwelling infusion pump), radiological supervision and interpretation N1Q2

Coding tip: *Injection for evaluation of previously placed peritoneal-venous shunt - 49427*

Coding tip: *Puncture of shunt tubing for injection - 61070*

Mod	RVU Non-Fac Total	Fac Total	Global Days	Modifiers 51	50	62	80	MUE
	2.80	2.80	XXX	6	0	0	0	1
26	0.68	0.68	XXX	6	0	0	0	1
TC	2.12	2.12	XXX	6	0	0	0	1

AMA: Feb 07: 11, Jul 08: 13, Aug 08: 13, Sep 08: 10, Nov 10: 3, Jan 11: 8

75810   Splenoportography, radiological supervision and interpretation N1Q2

Coding tip: *Splenoportography injection procedure - 38200*

Mod	RVU Non-Fac Total	Fac Total	Global Days	Modifiers 51	50	62	80	MUE
	0.00	0.00	XXX	0	0	0	0	1
26	1.63	1.63	XXX	0	0	0	0	1
TC	0.00	0.00	XXX	0	0	0	0	1

AMA: Feb 07: 11, Nov 10: 3, Jan 11: 8

Coding Guidance

Diagnostic venograms done on the same day and encounter by the same provider as an intravascular interventional procedure may be reported separately if the previous catheter-based venographic study is not available and the decision for the interventional procedure is based on the diagnostic study. If a diagnostic venogram was done prior to the intravascular interventional procedure, a second, repeat diagnostic angiogram on the date of the interventional service may not be reported, unless it becomes medically necessary due to a change in the patient's condition regarding the clinical indications, or to further define anatomy and pathology from inadequate visualization, or a change during the procedure necessitates a new diagnostic evaluation outside the interventional target area. In these cases, the repeat diagnostic venogram may be reported with modifier 59. If the previous diagnostic venogram was complete, then a second venogram for the dye injections necessary to complete the interventional procedure is not reported. Codes in the 70000 series will identify which is appropriate to use for the injection or administration of a given procedure. The injection of contrast or radiopharmaceuticals is already inherent in radiological procedures and should not be reported separately except in the case of extremity venography. Use 36005 for the injection procedure for contrast extremity venography (75820, 75822).

75820   Venography, extremity, unilateral, radiological supervision and interpretation N1Q2

Mod	RVU Non-Fac Total	Fac Total	Global Days	Modifiers 51	50	62	80	MUE
	3.26	3.26	XXX	6	0	0	0	2
26	0.99	0.99	XXX	6	0	0	0	2
TC	2.27	2.27	XXX	6	0	0	0	2

AMA: Oct 97: 10, May 08: 14, May 15: 3

Pub 100-04, 16, 120.2

75822   Venography, extremity, bilateral, radiological supervision and interpretation N1Q2

Mod	RVU Non-Fac Total	Fac Total	Global Days	Modifiers 51	50	62	80	MUE
	3.88	3.88	XXX	6	2	0	0	1
26	1.49	1.49	XXX	6	2	0	0	1
TC	2.39	2.39	XXX	6	2	0	0	1

Pub 100-04, 16, 120.2

75825   Venography, caval, inferior, with serialography, radiological supervision and interpretation N1Q2

Mod	RVU Non-Fac Total	Fac Total	Global Days	Modifiers 51	50	62	80	MUE
	3.86	3.86	XXX	6	0	0	0	1
26	1.61	1.61	XXX	6	0	0	0	1
TC	2.25	2.25	XXX	6	0	0	0	1

75827   Venography, caval, superior, with serialography, radiological supervision and interpretation N1Q2

Mod	RVU Non-Fac Total	Fac Total	Global Days	Modifiers 51	50	62	80	MUE
	3.91	3.91	XXX	6	0	0	0	1
26	1.60	1.60	XXX	6	0	0	0	1
TC	2.31	2.31	XXX	6	0	0	0	1

AMA: Apr 98: 12

75831   Venography, renal, unilateral, selective, radiological supervision and interpretation N1Q2

Mod	RVU Non-Fac Total	Fac Total	Global Days	Modifiers 51	50	62	80	MUE
	3.96	3.96	XXX	6	0	0	0	1
26	1.57	1.57	XXX	6	0	0	0	1
TC	2.39	2.39	XXX	6	0	0	0	1

AMA: Sep 98: 7

● New   ▲ Revised   Deleted   ⊙ Moderate Sedation   ✚ Add-on Codes   ⊘ High Risk Denial   Ⓐ Age Edit   ♀ Female   ♂ Male   **AMA** *CPT® Assistant*   **MUE** Medically Unlikely Edit
⊘ Modifier 51 Exempt   ⊖ Modifier 63 Exempt   ✗ Unlisted   **Modifiers:** *See Inside Back Cover*   Ⓜ Maternity   A2–Z3 ASC Payment Indicators   A–Y OPPS Status Indicators

© 2016 DecisionHealth   CPT © 2015 American Medical Association. All Rights Reserved.

75833 Venography, renal, bilateral, selective, radiological supervision and interpretation N I Q2

RVU Mod	Non-Fac Total	Fac Total	Global Days	Modifiers 51	50	62	80	MUE
	4.64	4.64	XXX	6	2	0	0	1
26	2.06	2.06	XXX	6	2	0	0	1
TC	2.58	2.58	XXX	6	2	0	0	1

AMA: Sep 98: 7

75840 Venography, adrenal, unilateral, selective, radiological supervision and interpretation N I Q2

RVU Mod	Non-Fac Total	Fac Total	Global Days	Modifiers 51	50	62	80	MUE
	4.19	4.19	XXX	6	0	0	0	1
26	1.63	1.63	XXX	6	0	0	0	1
TC	2.56	2.56	XXX	6	0	0	0	1

75842 Venography, adrenal, bilateral, selective, radiological supervision and interpretation N I Q2

RVU Mod	Non-Fac Total	Fac Total	Global Days	Modifiers 51	50	62	80	MUE
	5.09	5.09	XXX	6	2	0	0	1
26	2.12	2.12	XXX	6	2	0	0	1
TC	2.97	2.97	XXX	6	2	0	0	1

75860 Venography, venous sinus (eg, petrosal and inferior sagittal) or jugular, catheter, radiological supervision and interpretation N I Q2

RVU Mod	Non-Fac Total	Fac Total	Global Days	Modifiers 51	50	62	80	MUE
	4.04	4.04	XXX	6	0	0	0	2
26	1.59	1.59	XXX	6	0	0	0	2
TC	2.45	2.45	XXX	6	0	0	0	2

75870 Venography, superior sagittal sinus, radiological supervision and interpretation N I Q2

RVU Mod	Non-Fac Total	Fac Total	Global Days	Modifiers 51	50	62	80	MUE
	4.17	4.17	XXX	6	0	0	0	1
26	1.63	1.63	XXX	6	0	0	0	1
TC	2.54	2.54	XXX	6	0	0	0	1

75872 Venography, epidural, radiological supervision and interpretation N I Q2

RVU Mod	Non-Fac Total	Fac Total	Global Days	Modifiers 51	50	62	80	MUE
	3.96	3.96	XXX	6	0	0	0	1
26	1.52	1.52	XXX	6	0	0	0	1
TC	2.44	2.44	XXX	6	0	0	0	1

75880 Venography, orbital, radiological supervision and interpretation N I Q2

RVU Mod	Non-Fac Total	Fac Total	Global Days	Modifiers 51	50	62	80	MUE
	4.03	4.03	XXX	6	0	0	0	1
26	1.03	1.03	XXX	6	0	0	0	1
TC	3.00	3.00	XXX	6	0	0	0	1

Coding Guidance
Use 36481 for the percutaneous portal vein catheterization.

75885 Percutaneous transhepatic portography with hemodynamic evaluation, radiological supervision and interpretation N I Q2

RVU Mod	Non-Fac Total	Fac Total	Global Days	Modifiers 51	50	62	80	MUE
	4.46	4.46	XXX	6	0	0	0	1
26	1.97	1.97	XXX	6	0	0	0	1
TC	2.49	2.49	XXX	6	0	0	0	1

AMA: Oct 96: 4, Mar 02: 10, Dec 03: 2, Feb 07: 11, Nov 10: 3, Jan 11: 8

75887 Percutaneous transhepatic portography without hemodynamic evaluation, radiological supervision and interpretation N I Q2

RVU Mod	Non-Fac Total	Fac Total	Global Days	Modifiers 51	50	62	80	MUE
	4.48	4.48	XXX	6	0	0	0	1
26	1.98	1.98	XXX	6	0	0	0	1
TC	2.50	2.50	XXX	6	0	0	0	1

AMA: Mar 02: 10, Dec 03: 2, Feb 07: 11, Jan 11: 8

75889 Hepatic venography, wedged or free, with hemodynamic evaluation, radiological supervision and interpretation N I Q2

RVU Mod	Non-Fac Total	Fac Total	Global Days	Modifiers 51	50	62	80	MUE
	4.06	4.06	XXX	6	0	0	0	1
26	1.57	1.57	XXX	6	0	0	0	1
TC	2.49	2.49	XXX	6	0	0	0	1

75891 Hepatic venography, wedged or free, without hemodynamic evaluation, radiological supervision and interpretation N I Q2

RVU Mod	Non-Fac Total	Fac Total	Global Days	Modifiers 51	50	62	80	MUE
	4.10	4.10	XXX	6	0	0	0	1
26	1.59	1.59	XXX	6	0	0	0	1
TC	2.51	2.51	XXX	6	0	0	0	1

Coding Guidance
Code 75893 may be reported for venous blood sampling through a catheter specifically placed for the sole purpose of obtaining the venous blood sample. When the catheter is placed for a purpose other than venous blood sampling, reporting 75893 or 36500 for venous blood sampling, in addition to the code for the other venous procedure is a misuse of this code. This code is not for blood sampling during an arterial procedure.

75893 Venous sampling through catheter, with or without angiography (eg, for parathyroid hormone, renin), radiological supervision and interpretation N I Q2

Coding tip: Venous catheterization for selective organ blood sampling - 36500

Coding tip: This code includes concomitant venography

RVU Mod	Non-Fac Total	Fac Total	Global Days	Modifiers 51	50	62	80	MUE
	3.33	3.33	XXX	6	0	0	0	2
26	0.77	0.77	XXX	6	0	0	0	2
TC	2.56	2.56	XXX	6	0	0	0	2

Pub 100-04, 16, 120.2

Transcatheter Procedures

Coding Guidance
Therapeutic transcatheter radiological interpretation codes include contrast injections, angiography and venography, fluoroscopic guidance, and vessel measurement. Unless the code descriptor specifically includes angiography, arteriograms and venograms done on the same day/encounter by the same

---

● New ▲ Revised ✖ Deleted ⊙ Moderate Sedation ✚ Add-on Codes ⊘ High Risk Denial Ⓐ Age Edit ♀ Female ♂ Male **AMA** CPT® Assistant **MUE** Medically Unlikely Edit
⊘ Modifier 51 Exempt ⊖ Modifier 63 Exempt ✗ Unlisted **Modifiers:** See Inside Back Cover Ⓜ Maternity A 2 – Z 3 ASC Payment Indicators A – Y OPPS Status Indicators

642 CPT © 2015 American Medical Association. All Rights Reserved. © 2016 DecisionHealth

provider as a therapeutic transcatheter procedure may be reported separately if there is no previous catheter-based, diagnostic angiographic/venographic study available of the target area; if it becomes medically necessary due to a change in the patient's condition regarding the clinical indications; or the previous study is inadequate for visualization.

75894 Transcatheter therapy, embolization, any method, radiological supervision and interpretation N I N

Coding tip: Procedure for uterine fibroid embolization - 37210 (includes radiological supervision and interpretation)

Coding tip: Transcatheter embolization therapy on CNS - 61624; on head or neck, non-CNS - 61626

Coding tip: Procedure for OB/GYN type embolization other than fibroids (e.g. postpartum hemorrhage) - 37204

RVU Mod	Non-Fac Total	Fac Total	Global Days	51	50	62	80	MUE
	0.00	0.00	XXX	0	0	0	0	2
26	1.89	1.89	XXX	0	0	0	0	2
TC	0.00	0.00	XXX	0	0	0	0	2

AMA: Sep 98: 7, Feb 08: 5, Apr 12: 5, Nov 13: 6, 7, 15, Oct 14: 6

Pub 100-04, 16, 120.2

✖ 75896 Transcatheter therapy, infusion, other than for thrombolysis, radiological supervision and interpretation

75898 Angiography through existing catheter for follow-up study for transcatheter therapy, embolization or infusion, other than for thrombolysis N I Q2

RVU Mod	Non-Fac Total	Fac Total	Global Days	51	50	62	80	MUE
	0.00	0.00	XXX	0	0	0	0	2
26	2.39	2.39	XXX	0	0	0	0	2
TC	0.00	0.00	XXX	0	0	0	0	2

AMA: Dec 07: 11, Nov 11: 11, Nov 13: 6, 15, Oct 14: 6

Pub 100-04, 16, 120.2

75901 Mechanical removal of pericatheter obstructive material (eg, fibrin sheath) from central venous device via separate venous access, radiologic supervision and interpretation N I N

Coding tip: Mechanical removal procedure - 36595

RVU Mod	Non-Fac Total	Fac Total	Global Days	51	50	62	80	MUE
	4.98	4.98	XXX	0	0	0	0	1
26	0.68	0.68	XXX	0	0	0	0	1
TC	4.30	4.30	XXX	0	0	0	0	1

AMA: Jul 03: 13, Dec 04: 12

Pub 100-04, 16, 120.2

75902 Mechanical removal of intraluminal (intracatheter) obstructive material from central venous device through device lumen, radiologic supervision and interpretation N I N

Coding tip: Mechanical removal procedure - 36596

RVU Mod	Non-Fac Total	Fac Total	Global Days	51	50	62	80	MUE
	2.02	2.02	XXX	0	0	0	0	2
26	0.54	0.54	XXX	0	0	0	0	2
TC	1.48	1.48	XXX	0	0	0	0	2

AMA: Jul 03: 13, Dec 04: 12

Pub 100-04, 16, 120.2

✖ 75945 Intravascular ultrasound (non-coronary vessel), radiological supervision and interpretation; initial vessel

✖ 75946 Intravascular ultrasound (non-coronary vessel), radiological supervision and interpretation; each additional non-coronary vessel (List separately in addition to code for primary procedure)

75952 Endovascular repair of infrarenal abdominal aortic aneurysm or dissection, radiological supervision and interpretation C

Coding tip: This code includes diagnostic angiography of the aorta and its branches before deployment of the endovascular device, fluoroscopic guidance for component delivery, and arterial angiography during the procedure to verify position, check endoleak, and evaluate runoff

RVU Mod	Non-Fac Total	Fac Total	Global Days	51	50	62	80	MUE
	0.00	0.00	XXX	0	0	0	0	1
26	6.41	6.41	XXX	0	0	0	0	1
TC	0.00	0.00	XXX	0	0	0	0	1

AMA: Apr 12: 3, Dec 13: 8

75953 Placement of proximal or distal extension prosthesis for endovascular repair of infrarenal aortic or iliac artery aneurysm, pseudoaneurysm, or dissection, radiological supervision and interpretation C

Coding tip: Report 75953 only for placement of extension prosthesis, not for placement of the original components a modular device.

Coding tip: This code includes diagnostic angiography before placement of an additional extension prosthesis, fluoroscopic guidance and arterial angiography during the procedure

RVU Mod	Non-Fac Total	Fac Total	Global Days	51	50	62	80	MUE
	0.00	0.00	XXX	0	0	0	0	4
26	1.94	1.94	XXX	0	0	0	0	4
TC	0.00	0.00	XXX	0	0	0	0	4

AMA: Feb 03: 3, Dec 13: 8

75954 Endovascular repair of iliac artery aneurysm, pseudoaneurysm, arteriovenous malformation, or trauma, using ilio-iliac tube endoprosthesis, radiological supervision and interpretation C

RVU Mod	Non-Fac Total	Fac Total	Global Days	51	50	62	80	MUE
	0.00	0.00	XXX	0	0	0	0	2
26	3.24	3.24	XXX	0	0	0	0	2
TC	0.00	0.00	XXX	0	0	0	0	2

AMA: Feb 03: 3

75956 Endovascular repair of descending thoracic aorta (eg, aneurysm, pseudoaneurysm, dissection, penetrating ulcer, intramural hematoma, or traumatic disruption); involving coverage of left subclavian artery origin, initial endoprosthesis plus descending thoracic aortic extension(s), if required, to level of celiac artery origin, radiological supervision and interpretation C

RVU Mod	Non-Fac Total	Fac Total	Global Days	51	50	62	80	MUE
	0.00	0.00	XXX	0	0	0	0	1
26	10.01	10.01	XXX	0	0	0	0	1
TC	0.00	0.00	XXX	0	0	0	0	1

● New ▲ Revised Deleted ⊙ Moderate Sedation ✚ Add-on Codes ⊘ High Risk Denial Ⓐ Age Edit ♀ Female ♂ Male **AMA** *CPT® Assistant* **MUE** Medically Unlikely Edit
⊘ Modifier 51 Exempt ⊖ Modifier 63 Exempt ✖ Unlisted **Modifiers:** *See Inside Back Cover* Ⓜ Maternity A2–Z3 ASC Payment Indicators A–Y OPPS Status Indicators

© 2016 DecisionHealth | CPT © 2015 American Medical Association. All Rights Reserved. | **643**

75957 Endovascular repair of descending thoracic aorta (eg, aneurysm, pseudoaneurysm, dissection, penetrating ulcer, intramural hematoma, or traumatic disruption); not involving coverage of left subclavian artery origin, initial endoprosthesis plus descending thoracic aortic extension(s), if required, to level of celiac artery origin, radiological supervision and interpretation   C

Mod	RVU Non-Fac Total	Fac Total	Global Days	Modifiers 51	50	62	80	MUE
	0.00	0.00	XXX	0	0	0	0	1
26	8.59	8.59	XXX	0	0	0	0	1
TC	0.00	0.00	XXX	0	0	0	0	1

75958 Placement of proximal extension prosthesis for endovascular repair of descending thoracic aorta (eg, aneurysm, pseudoaneurysm, dissection, penetrating ulcer, intramural hematoma, or traumatic disruption), radiological supervision and interpretation   C

Mod	RVU Non-Fac Total	Fac Total	Global Days	Modifiers 51	50	62	80	MUE
	0.00	0.00	XXX	0	0	0	0	2
26	5.70	5.70	XXX	0	0	0	0	2
TC	0.00	0.00	XXX	0	0	0	0	2

75959 Placement of distal extension prosthesis(s) (delayed) after endovascular repair of descending thoracic aorta, as needed, to level of celiac origin, radiological supervision and interpretation   C

Mod	RVU Non-Fac Total	Fac Total	Global Days	Modifiers 51	50	62	80	MUE
	0.00	0.00	XXX	0	0	0	0	1
26	4.97	4.97	XXX	0	0	0	0	1
TC	0.00	0.00	XXX	0	0	0	0	1

75962 Transluminal balloon angioplasty, peripheral artery other than renal, or other visceral artery, iliac or lower extremity, radiological supervision and interpretation   NIN

Coding tip: Transluminal ballooon angioplasty procedure, brachiocephalic trunk or branches - open 35458; percutaneous 35471

Mod	RVU Non-Fac Total	Fac Total	Global Days	Modifiers 51	50	62	80	MUE
	3.95	3.95	XXX	0	0	0	0	1
26	0.76	0.76	XXX	0	0	0	0	1
TC	3.19	3.19	XXX	0	0	0	0	1

AMA: Fall 93: 18, May 01: 4, Jul 11: 5, Apr 12: 6, Mar 14: 8

Pub 100-04, 16, 120.2

+ 75964 Transluminal balloon angioplasty, each additional peripheral artery other than renal or other visceral artery, iliac or lower extremity, radiological supervision and interpretation (List separately in addition to code for primary procedure)   NIN

Mod	RVU Non-Fac Total	Fac Total	Global Days	Modifiers 51	50	62	80	MUE
	2.49	2.49	ZZZ	0	0	0	0	2
26	0.51	0.51	ZZZ	0	0	0	0	2
TC	1.98	1.98	ZZZ	0	0	0	0	2

AMA: Dec 07: 10, Jul 11: 5, Apr 12: 9

Pub 100-04, 16, 120.2

75966 Transluminal balloon angioplasty, renal or other visceral artery, radiological supervision and interpretation   NIN

Coding tip: Transluminal balloon angioplasty procedure, renal/other visceral artery - open 35450; percutaneous 35471

Mod	RVU Non-Fac Total	Fac Total	Global Days	Modifiers 51	50	62	80	MUE
	4.83	4.83	XXX	0	0	0	0	1
26	1.83	1.83	XXX	0	0	0	0	1
TC	3.00	3.00	XXX	0	0	0	0	1

+ 75968 Transluminal balloon angioplasty, each additional visceral artery, radiological supervision and interpretation (List separately in addition to code for primary procedure)   NIN

Mod	RVU Non-Fac Total	Fac Total	Global Days	Modifiers 51	50	62	80	MUE
	2.47	2.47	ZZZ	0	0	0	0	2
26	0.51	0.51	ZZZ	0	0	0	0	2
TC	1.96	1.96	ZZZ	0	0	0	0	2

75970 Transcatheter biopsy, radiological supervision and interpretation   NIN

Coding tip: Transcatheter cardiovascular biopsy procedure - 37200

Mod	RVU Non-Fac Total	Fac Total	Global Days	Modifiers 51	50	62	80	MUE
	0.00	0.00	XXX	0	0	0	0	1
26	1.14	1.14	XXX	0	0	0	0	1
TC	0.00	0.00	XXX	0	0	0	0	1

75978 Transluminal balloon angioplasty, venous (eg, subclavian stenosis), radiological supervision and interpretation   NIN Q2

Mod	RVU Non-Fac Total	Fac Total	Global Days	Modifiers 51	50	62	80	MUE
	3.90	3.90	XXX	0	0	0	0	
26	0.76	0.76	XXX	0	0	0	0	
TC	3.14	3.14	XXX	0	0	0	0	

AMA: Oct 96: 4, Feb 97: 2, May 01: 4, Dec 03: 2, Dec 11: 16, Apr 12: 6

✖ 75980 ~~Percutaneous transhepatic biliary drainage with contrast monitoring, radiological supervision and interpretation~~

✖ 75982 ~~Percutaneous placement of drainage catheter for combined internal and external biliary drainage or of a drainage stent for internal biliary drainage in patients with an inoperable mechanical biliary obstruction, radiological supervision and interpretation~~

75984 Change of percutaneous tube or drainage catheter with contrast monitoring (eg, genitourinary system, abscess), radiological supervision and interpretation   NIN

Coding tip: Change of cystostomy tube - 51710; change of nephrostomy or pyelostomy tube - 50398; change of ureterostomy tube - 50688

Coding tip: Exchange of drainage catheter - 49423

Mod	RVU Non-Fac Total	Fac Total	Global Days	Modifiers 51	50	62	80	MUE
	3.00	3.00	XXX	0	0	0	0	2
26	1.00	1.00	XXX	0	0	0	0	2
TC	2.00	2.00	XXX	0	0	0	0	2

AMA: Nov 97: 24

● New   ▲ Revised   ✖ Deleted   ⊙ Moderate Sedation   ✚ Add-on Codes   ⊗ High Risk Denial   Ⓐ Age Edit   ♀ Female   ♂ Male   **AMA** CPT® Assistant   **MUE** Medically Unlikely Edit
⃠ Modifier 51 Exempt   ⊖ Modifier 63 Exempt   ⊠ Unlisted   **Modifiers:** See Inside Back Cover   Ⓜ Maternity   A2–Z3 ASC Payment Indicators   A–Y OPPS Status Indicators

CPT © 2015 American Medical Association. All Rights Reserved.   © 2016 DecisionHealth

75989 Radiological guidance (ie, fluoroscopy, ultrasound, or computed tomography), for percutaneous drainage (eg, abscess, specimen collection), with placement of catheter, radiological supervision and interpretation N I N

Coding tip: Percutaneous drainage via pneumonostomy ü 32201

Coding tip: Percutaneous drainage of pancreatic pseudocyst - 48511

Coding tip: Insertion of tunneled pleural catheter - 32550

Coding tip: Percutaneous drainage of appendiceal abscess - 44901; peritoneal abscess - 49021; subdiaphragmatic/subphrenic abscess - 49041; retroperitoneal abscess - 49061; pelvic abscess - 58823

Coding tip: Tube thoracostomy with seal - 32551

Coding tip: Percutaneous drainage of liver abscess - 47011; renal abscess - 50021

RVU			Global Days	Modifiers				
Mod	Non-Fac Total	Fac Total		51	50	62	80	MUE
	3.40	3.40	XXX	0	0	0	0	2
26	1.66	1.66	XXX	0	0	0	0	2
TC	1.74	1.74	XXX	0	0	0	0	2

AMA: Nov 97: 24, Mar 98: 8, Feb 07: 11, Apr 11: 12, Nov 10: 3, Nov 12: 3, Nov 13: 9, May 14: 9

Other Diagnostic Radiology Procedures

Coding Guidance

All the radiologic services necessary for the procedure are included in the radiologic supervision and interpretation codes for specific procedures. Do not report fluoroscopy in addition to these services.

76000 Fluoroscopy (separate procedure), up to 1 hour physician or other qualified health care professional time, other than 71023 or 71034 (eg, cardiac fluoroscopy) Z 3 S

Coding tip: When a gastric feeding tube is repositioned through the duodenum, it may require additional fluoroscopic guidance reported with 76000

RVU			Global Days	Modifiers				
Mod	Non-Fac Total	Fac Total		51	50	62	80	MUE
	1.33	1.33	XXX	0	0	0	0	3
26	0.25	0.25	XXX	0	0	0	0	3
TC	1.08	1.08	XXX	0	0	0	0	3

AMA: Apr 96: 11, Nov 99: 32, Dec 00: 14, Apr 03: 7, Jul 03: 16, Aug 03: 14, Jul 08: 9, Aug 08: 7, Dec 08: 7, 9, Jul 11: 5, Nov 11: 11, Aug 10: 8, Oct 10: 14, Nov 10: 3, Dec 10: 14, Feb 13: 3, Mar 13: 10, Sep 13: 17, Sep 14: 5, Oct 14: 6, May 15: 3

76001 Fluoroscopy, physician or other qualified health care professional time more than 1 hour, assisting a nonradiologic physician or other qualified health care professional (eg, nephrostolithotomy, ERCP, bronchoscopy, transbronchial biopsy) N I N

RVU			Global Days	Modifiers				
Mod	Non-Fac Total	Fac Total		51	50	62	80	MUE
	0.00	0.00	XXX	0	0	0	0	1
26	1.03	1.03	XXX	0	0	0	0	1
TC	0.00	0.00	XXX	0	0	0	0	1

AMA: Nov 11: 11, Nov 10: 3, Feb 13: 3, Mar 13: 10, Sep 14: 5, Oct 14: 6

76010 Radiologic examination from nose to rectum for foreign body, single view, child ⊙A N I Q I

RVU			Global Days	Modifiers				
Mod	Non-Fac Total	Fac Total		51	50	62	80	MUE
	0.73	0.73	XXX	0	0	0	0	2
26	0.26	0.26	XXX	0	0	0	0	2
TC	0.47	0.47	XXX	0	0	0	0	2

AMA: Feb 10: 12

76080 Radiologic examination, abscess, fistula or sinus tract study, radiological supervision and interpretation N I Q 2

Coding tip: Contrast injection into abscess via drainage tube - 49424

Coding tip: Contrast injection into sinus tract - 20501

RVU			Global Days	Modifiers				
Mod	Non-Fac Total	Fac Total		51	50	62	80	MUE
	1.55	1.55	XXX	0	0	0	0	3
26	0.75	0.75	XXX	0	0	0	0	3
TC	0.80	0.80	XXX	0	0	0	0	3

AMA: Nov 97: 24, Mar 98: 8, Nov 03: 14, Dec 06: 10, Jan 09: 8

Pub 100-04, 16, 120.2

76098 Radiological examination, surgical specimen N I Q 2

RVU			Global Days	Modifiers				
Mod	Non-Fac Total	Fac Total		51	50	62	80	MUE
	0.47	0.47	XXX	0	0	0	0	3
26	0.23	0.23	XXX	0	0	0	0	3
TC	0.24	0.24	XXX	0	0	0	0	3

76100 Radiologic examination, single plane body section (eg, tomography), other than with urography N I Q I

RVU			Global Days	Modifiers				
Mod	Non-Fac Total	Fac Total		51	50	62	80	MUE
	2.61	2.61	XXX	0	0	0	0	2
26	0.91	0.91	XXX	0	0	0	0	2
TC	1.70	1.70	XXX	0	0	0	0	2

76101 Radiologic examination, complex motion (ie, hypercycloidal) body section (eg, mastoid polytomography), other than with urography; unilateral Z 2 Q I

RVU			Global Days	Modifiers				
Mod	Non-Fac Total	Fac Total		51	50	62	80	MUE
	3.71	3.71	XXX	0	0	0	0	1
26	0.96	0.96	XXX	0	0	0	0	1
TC	2.75	2.75	XXX	0	0	0	0	1

76102 Radiologic examination, complex motion (ie, hypercycloidal) body section (eg, mastoid polytomography), other than with urography; bilateral Z 2 S

RVU			Global Days	Modifiers				
Mod	Non-Fac Total	Fac Total		51	50	62	80	MUE
	4.93	4.93	XXX	0	2	0	0	1
26	0.98	0.98	XXX	0	2	0	0	1
TC	3.95	3.95	XXX	0	2	0	0	1

76120 Cineradiography/videoradiography, except where specifically included N I Q I

RVU			Global Days	Modifiers				
Mod	Non-Fac Total	Fac Total		51	50	62	80	MUE
	2.35	2.35	XXX	0	0	0	0	1
26	0.55	0.55	XXX	0	0	0	0	1
TC	1.80	1.80	XXX	0	0	0	0	1

AMA: Sep 00: 4, Apr 04: 15, Apr 11: 13

● New ▲ Revised Deleted ⊙ Moderate Sedation ✚ Add-on Codes ⊘ High Risk Denial Ⓐ Age Edit ♀ Female ♂ Male **AMA** *CPT® Assistant* **MUE** Medically Unlikely Edit
⊘ Modifier 51 Exempt ⊖ Modifier 63 Exempt ✗ Unlisted **Modifiers:** *See Inside Back Cover* Ⓜ Maternity A 2 – Z 3 ASC Payment Indicators A – Y OPPS Status Indicators

© 2016 DecisionHealth | CPT © 2015 American Medical Association. All Rights Reserved.

+ 76125 Cineradiography/videoradiography to complement routine examination (List separately in addition to code for primary procedure) N1N

RVU			Global Days	Modifiers				
Mod	Non-Fac Total	Fac Total		51	50	62	80	MUE
	0.00	0.00	ZZZ	0	0	0	0	1
26	0.41	0.41	ZZZ	0	0	0	0	1
TC	0.00	0.00	ZZZ	0	0	0	0	1

AMA: Oct 97: 1, Sep 00: 4

76140 Consultation on X-ray examination made elsewhere, written report CE

RVU			Global Days	Modifiers				
Mod	Non-Fac Total	Fac Total		51	50	62	80	MUE
	0.00	0.00	XXX	9	9	9	9	

AMA: Summer 91: 13, Oct 97: 1

Coding Guidance

Codes 76376-76377 for 3-D rendering are not to be reported with nuclear medicine codes. 3-D rendering may be reported with modifier 59 on the same date of service as a nuclear medicine procedure when the 3-D rendering is provided in conjunction with a third, different procedure other than the nuclear medicine, for which 3-D can be appropriately billed.

76376 3D rendering with interpretation and reporting of computed tomography, magnetic resonance imaging, ultrasound, or other tomographic modality with image postprocessing under concurrent supervision; not requiring image postprocessing on an independent workstation N1N

Coding tip: Code with 70470, 70482, 70488, 70492, 71270, 72194, 73202, 73702, 74170

RVU			Global Days	Modifiers				
Mod	Non-Fac Total	Fac Total		51	50	62	80	MUE
	0.65	0.65	XXX	0	0	0	0	2
26	0.28	0.28	XXX	0	0	0	0	2
TC	0.37	0.37	XXX	0	0	0	0	2

AMA: May 13: 3, Dec 05: 1, 7, Jan 07: 31, Jul 08: 3, May 09: 9, Jun 09: 9, Jul 09: 10, Apr 10: 5, Jul 10: 7, Jun 13: 12

76377 3D rendering with interpretation and reporting of computed tomography, magnetic resonance imaging, ultrasound, or other tomographic modality with image postprocessing under concurrent supervision; requiring image postprocessing on an independent workstation N1N

Coding tip: Code with 70470, 70482, 70488, 70492, 71270, 72194, 73202, 73702, 74170

RVU			Global Days	Modifiers				
Mod	Non-Fac Total	Fac Total		51	50	62	80	MUE
	1.82	1.82	XXX	0	0	0	0	2
26	1.13	1.13	XXX	0	0	0	0	2
TC	0.69	0.69	XXX	0	0	0	0	2

AMA: May 13: 3, Dec 05: 1, Jan 07: 31, Jul 08: 3, May 09: 9, Jun 09: 9, Jul 09: 10, Apr 10: 5, 9, Dec 09: 13, Feb 10: 6, Jul 10: 7, Jun 13: 12

76380 Computed tomography, limited or localized follow-up study N1Q1

RVU			Global Days	Modifiers				
Mod	Non-Fac Total	Fac Total		51	50	62	80	MUE
	4.10	4.10	XXX	0	0	0	0	2
26	1.40	1.40	XXX	0	0	0	0	2
TC	2.70	2.70	XXX	0	0	0	0	2

AMA: Jul 07: 13

76390 Magnetic resonance spectroscopy CE

RVU			Global Days	Modifiers				
Mod	Non-Fac Total	Fac Total		51	50	62	80	MUE
	12.51	12.51	XXX	9	9	9	9	
26	1.98	1.98	XXX	9	9	9	9	
TC	10.53	10.53	XXX	9	9	9	9	

AMA: Nov 97: 25

76496 Unlisted fluoroscopic procedure (eg, diagnostic, interventional) QxN1Q1

RVU			Global Days	Modifiers				
Mod	Non-Fac Total	Fac Total		51	50	62	80	MUE
	0.00	0.00	XXX	0	0	0	0	
26	0.00	0.00	XXX	0	0	0	0	
TC	0.00	0.00	XXX	0	0	0	0	

76497 Unlisted computed tomography procedure (eg, diagnostic, interventional) QxN1Q1

RVU			Global Days	Modifiers				
Mod	Non-Fac Total	Fac Total		51	50	62	80	MUE
	0.00	0.00	XXX	0	0	0	0	
26	0.00	0.00	XXX	0	0	0	0	
TC	0.00	0.00	XXX	0	0	0	0	

AMA: Jun 05: 11

76498 Unlisted magnetic resonance procedure (eg, diagnostic, interventional) QxZ2S

RVU			Global Days	Modifiers				
Mod	Non-Fac Total	Fac Total		51	50	62	80	MUE
	0.00	0.00	XXX	0	0	0	0	
26	0.00	0.00	XXX	0	0	0	0	
TC	0.00	0.00	XXX	0	0	0	0	

AMA: Dec 11: 17

76499 Unlisted diagnostic radiographic procedure QxN1Q1

Coding tip: Radiological supervision and interpretation of bronchography, unilateral or bilateral, is reported with code 76499

RVU			Global Days	Modifiers				
Mod	Non-Fac Total	Fac Total		51	50	62	80	MUE
	0.00	0.00	XXX	0	0	0	0	
26	0.00	0.00	XXX	0	0	0	0	
TC	0.00	0.00	XXX	0	0	0	0	

AMA: Jul 99: 10, Sep 00: 4, Apr 04: 15, Nov 06: 22, Mar 08: 15, Dec 11: 17, Dec 13: 17

Pub 100-04, 13, 120

Diagnostic Ultrasound Procedures

Head/Neck Ultrasound Procedures

76506 Echoencephalography, real time with image documentation (gray scale) (for determination of ventricular size, delineation of cerebral contents, and detection of fluid masses or other intracranial abnormalities), including A-mode encephalography as secondary component where indicated N1Q1

RVU			Global Days	Modifiers				
Mod	Non-Fac Total	Fac Total		51	50	62	80	MUE
	3.34	3.34	XXX	0	0	0	0	1
26	0.92	0.92	XXX	0	0	0	0	1
TC	2.42	2.42	XXX	0	0	0	0	1

AMA: Mar 07: 7

● New   ▲ Revised   ✖ Deleted   ⊙ Moderate Sedation   ✚ Add-on Codes   ⊖ High Risk Denial   Ⓐ Age Edit   ♀ Female   ♂ Male   **AMA** CPT® Assistant   **MUE** Medically Unlikely Edit

⃠ Modifier 51 Exempt   ⊖ Modifier 63 Exempt   ✗ Unlisted   **Modifiers:** See Inside Back Cover   Ⓜ Maternity   A2–Z3 ASC Payment Indicators   A–Y OPPS Status Indicators

646   CPT © 2015 American Medical Association. All Rights Reserved.   © 2016 DecisionHealth

76510 Ophthalmic ultrasound, diagnostic; B-scan and quantitative A-scan performed during the same patient encounter N I Q I

Mod	Non-Fac Total	Fac Total	Global Days	51	50	62	80	MUE
	4.82	4.82	XXX	7	3	0	0	2
26	2.52	2.52	XXX	7	3	0	0	2
TC	2.30	2.30	XXX	7	3	0	0	2

AMA: Dec 05: 3

76511 Ophthalmic ultrasound, diagnostic; quantitative A-scan only N I Q I

Mod	Non-Fac Total	Fac Total	Global Days	51	50	62	80	MUE
	2.86	2.86	XXX	7	3	0	0	2
26	1.50	1.50	XXX	7	3	0	0	2
TC	1.36	1.36	XXX	7	3	0	0	2

AMA: Winter 93: 12, Oct 96: 9, Nov 99: 42, Jul 04: 12, Dec 05: 3

76512 Ophthalmic ultrasound, diagnostic; B-scan (with or without superimposed non-quantitative A-scan) N I Q I

Mod	Non-Fac Total	Fac Total	Global Days	51	50	62	80	MUE
	2.62	2.62	XXX	7	3	0	0	2
26	1.50	1.50	XXX	7	3	0	0	2
TC	1.12	1.12	XXX	7	3	0	0	2

AMA: Winter 93: 12, Oct 96: 9, Dec 05: 3

76513 Ophthalmic ultrasound, diagnostic; anterior segment ultrasound, immersion (water bath) B-scan or high resolution biomicroscopy N I Q I

Mod	Non-Fac Total	Fac Total	Global Days	51	50	62	80	MUE
	2.68	2.68	XXX	7	3	0	0	2
26	1.01	1.01	XXX	7	3	0	0	2
TC	1.67	1.67	XXX	7	3	0	0	2

AMA: Winter 93: 12, Nov 99: 42, Nov 09: 9, Apr 13: 7

76514 Ophthalmic ultrasound, diagnostic; corneal pachymetry, unilateral or bilateral (determination of corneal thickness) N I Q I

Mod	Non-Fac Total	Fac Total	Global Days	51	50	62	80	MUE
	0.43	0.43	XXX	7	2	0	0	1
26	0.28	0.28	XXX	7	2	0	0	1
TC	0.15	0.15	XXX	7	2	0	0	1

AMA: Jul 04: 12, 15, Feb 05: 13, Jun 05: 11, Dec 05: 3

76516 Ophthalmic biometry by ultrasound echography, A-scan N I Q I

Mod	Non-Fac Total	Fac Total	Global Days	51	50	62	80	MUE
	2.23	2.23	XXX	7	2	0	0	1
26	0.88	0.88	XXX	7	2	0	0	1
TC	1.35	1.35	XXX	7	2	0	0	1

AMA: Oct 03: 10, Dec 05: 3

76519 Ophthalmic biometry by ultrasound echography, A-scan; with intraocular lens power calculation N I Q I

Coding tip: Report 76519 in addition to cataract extraction with IOL insertion (66982-66984) when intraocular lens power calculation by ultrasound measurement is done at the time of insertion

Mod	Non-Fac Total	Fac Total	Global Days	51	50	62	80	MUE
	2.39	2.39	XXX	7	2	0	0	2
26	0.89	0.89	XXX	7	3	0	0	2
TC	1.50	1.50	XXX	7	2	0	0	2

AMA: Winter 93: 12, Oct 03: 10, Dec 05: 3, Sep 09: 5

76529 Ophthalmic ultrasonic foreign body localization N I Q I

Coding tip: By partial coherence interferometry - 92136

Mod	Non-Fac Total	Fac Total	Global Days	51	50	62	80	MUE
	2.24	2.24	XXX	0	3	0	0	2
26	0.92	0.92	XXX	0	3	0	0	2
TC	1.32	1.32	XXX	0	3	0	0	2

AMA: Winter 93: 12

76536 Ultrasound, soft tissues of head and neck (eg, thyroid, parathyroid, parotid), real time with image documentation N I Q I

Documentation Finder: This ultrasound imaging examination is performed to evaluate or examine a mass in the neck area to determine whether it is more than just a subcutaneous abnormality. Another term that in the documentation could be echography. This would also be the code if the provider needed to evaluate the patient's thyroid, and the documentation could state a thyroid ultrasonography is being performed.

Mod	Non-Fac Total	Fac Total	Global Days	51	50	62	80	MUE
	3.28	3.28	XXX	0	0	0	0	1
26	0.80	0.80	XXX	0	0	0	0	1
TC	2.48	2.48	XXX	0	0	0	0	1

AMA: Mar 07: 7, May 09: 7

Chest Ultrasound Procedures

76604 Ultrasound, chest (includes mediastinum), real time with image documentation N I Q I

Mod	Non-Fac Total	Fac Total	Global Days	51	50	62	80	MUE
	2.49	2.49	XXX	4	0	0	0	1
26	0.77	0.77	XXX	4	0	0	0	1
TC	1.72	1.72	XXX	4	0	0	0	1

AMA: Nov 12: 3

76641 Ultrasound, breast, unilateral, real time with image documentation, including axilla when performed; complete N I Q I

Mod	Non-Fac Total	Fac Total	Global Days	51	50	62	80	MUE
	3.04	3.04	XXX	0	1	0	0	2
26	1.04	1.04	XXX	0	1	0	0	2
TC	2.00	2.00	XXX	0	1	0	0	2

AMA: Aug 15: 11

● New   ▲ Revised   Deleted   ⊙ Moderate Sedation   ✚ Add-on Codes   ⊘ High Risk Denial   Ⓐ Age Edit   ♀ Female   ♂ Male   **AMA** *CPT® Assistant*   **MUE** Medically Unlikely Edit
⊘ Modifier 51 Exempt   ⊖ Modifier 63 Exempt   ✗ Unlisted   **Modifiers:** *See Inside Back Cover*   Ⓜ Maternity   A2–Z3 ASC Payment Indicators   A–Y OPPS Status Indicators

© 2016 DecisionHealth   CPT © 2015 American Medical Association. All Rights Reserved.   **647**

Radiology Procedures

76642 – 76805

76642 Ultrasound, breast, unilateral, real time with image documentation, including axilla when performed; limited   N I Q I

Mod	Non-Fac Total	Fac Total	Global Days	51	50	62	80	MUE
	2.50	2.50	XXX	0	1	0	0	2
26	0.97	0.97	XXX	0	1	0	0	2
TC	1.53	1.53	XXX	0	1	0	0	2

Abdominal/Retroperitoneal Ultrasound Procedures

Coding Guidance

Abdominal ultrasound and abdominal duplex exams (93975-93976) will generally be done for differing clinical scenarios, but some instances occur when both types of services may be necessary at the same time. When both services are necessary, report the ultrasound procedure with the appropriate modifier.

76700 Ultrasound, abdominal, real time with image documentation; complete   Z 3 Q 3

Coding tip: Ultrasound can only be reported separately when a thorough evaluation of the anatomic region is done with image documentation and written report

Mod	Non-Fac Total	Fac Total	Global Days	51	50	62	80	MUE
	3.47	3.47	XXX	4	0	0	0	1
26	1.15	1.15	XXX	4	0	0	0	1
TC	2.32	2.32	XXX	4	0	0	0	1

AMA: Fall 93: 13, Oct 01: 3, Dec 05: 3, Mar 07: 7

76705 Ultrasound, abdominal, real time with image documentation; limited (eg, single organ, quadrant, follow-up)   Z 3 Q 3

Mod	Non-Fac Total	Fac Total	Global Days	51	50	62	80	MUE
	2.58	2.58	XXX	4	0	0	0	2
26	0.84	0.84	XXX	4	0	0	0	2
TC	1.74	1.74	XXX	4	0	0	0	2

AMA: Fall 93: 13, Oct 01: 3, Apr 03: 27, Dec 05: 3, Feb 09: 22, May 09: 7, Mar 12: 10, Dec 12: 9

76770 Ultrasound, retroperitoneal (eg, renal, aorta, nodes), real time with image documentation; complete   Z 3 Q 3

Coding tip: Ultrasound can only be reported separately when a thorough evaluation of the anatomic region is done with image documentation and written report

Coding tip: Report 76857 when the urinary bladder alone is imaged

Mod	Non-Fac Total	Fac Total	Global Days	51	50	62	80	MUE
	3.20	3.20	XXX	4	0	0	0	1
26	1.05	1.05	XXX	4	0	0	0	1
TC	2.15	2.15	XXX	4	0	0	0	1

AMA: May 99: 10, Jun 99: 10, Mar 15: 10

76775 Ultrasound, retroperitoneal (eg, renal, aorta, nodes), real time with image documentation; limited   N I Q I

Mod	Non-Fac Total	Fac Total	Global Days	51	50	62	80	MUE
	1.64	1.64	XXX	4	0	0	0	2
26	0.82	0.82	XXX	4	0	0	0	2
TC	0.82	0.82	XXX	4	0	0	0	2

AMA: May 99: 10, Jun 99: 10, Dec 05: 3, Feb 09: 22, Mar 15: 10

76776 Ultrasound, transplanted kidney, real time and duplex Doppler with image documentation   Z 2 Q 3

Mod	Non-Fac Total	Fac Total	Global Days	51	50	62	80	MUE
	4.43	4.43	XXX	4	0	0	0	2
26	1.08	1.08	XXX	4	0	0	0	2
TC	3.35	3.35	XXX	4	0	0	0	2

AMA: Mar 07: 7

Spinal Canal Ultrasound Procedures

76800 Ultrasound, spinal canal and contents   N I Q I

Mod	Non-Fac Total	Fac Total	Global Days	51	50	62	80	MUE
	4.01	4.01	XXX	0	0	0	0	1
26	1.72	1.72	XXX	0	0	0	0	1
TC	2.29	2.29	XXX	0	0	0	0	1

AMA: Apr 98: 15

Pelvic Ultrasound Procedures

Obstetrical Procedures

76801 Ultrasound, pregnant uterus, real time with image documentation, fetal and maternal evaluation, first trimester (< 14 weeks 0 days), transabdominal approach; single or first gestation   ♀ M Z 3 S

Mod	Non-Fac Total	Fac Total	Global Days	51	50	62	80	MUE
	3.50	3.50	XXX	0	0	0	0	1
26	1.43	1.43	XXX	0	0	0	0	1
TC	2.07	2.07	XXX	0	0	0	0	1

AMA: Mar 03: 7, Nov 05: 15

+ 76802 Ultrasound, pregnant uterus, real time with image documentation, fetal and maternal evaluation, first trimester (< 14 weeks 0 days), transabdominal approach; each additional gestation (List separately in addition to code for primary procedure)   ♀ M N I N

Mod	Non-Fac Total	Fac Total	Global Days	51	50	62	80	MUE
	1.84	1.84	ZZZ	0	0	0	0	3
26	1.21	1.21	ZZZ	0	0	0	0	3
TC	0.63	0.63	ZZZ	0	0	0	0	3

AMA: Mar 03: 7, Nov 05: 15

76805 Ultrasound, pregnant uterus, real time with image documentation, fetal and maternal evaluation, after first trimester (> or = 14 weeks 0 days), transabdominal approach; single or first gestation   ♀ M Z 2 S

Mod	Non-Fac Total	Fac Total	Global Days	51	50	62	80	MUE
	4.02	4.02	XXX	0	0	0	0	1
26	1.44	1.44	XXX	0	0	0	0	1
TC	2.58	2.58	XXX	0	0	0	0	1

AMA: Apr 97: 2, Nov 97: 25, Oct 01: 3, Aug 02: 2, Mar 03: 7

● New   ▲ Revised   ✖ Deleted   ⊙ Moderate Sedation   ✚ Add-on Codes   ⊘ High Risk Denial   Ⓐ Age Edit   ♀ Female   ♂ Male   **AMA** *CPT® Assistant*   **MUE** Medically Unlikely Edit
⦸ Modifier 51 Exempt   ⊖ Modifier 63 Exempt   ✗ Unlisted   **Modifiers:** *See Inside Back Cover*   Ⓜ Maternity   A 2 – Z 3 ASC Payment Indicators   A – Y OPPS Status Indicators

CPT © 2015 American Medical Association. All Rights Reserved.   © 2016 DecisionHealth

✚ 76810 Ultrasound, pregnant uterus, real time with image documentation, fetal and maternal evaluation, after first trimester (> or = 14 weeks 0 days), transabdominal approach; each additional gestation (List separately in addition to code for primary procedure)   ♀ M N I N

RVU			Global Days	Modifiers				
Mod	Non-Fac Total	Fac Total		51	50	62	80	MUE
	2.66	2.66	ZZZ	0	0	0	0	3
26	1.43	1.43	ZZZ	0	0	0	0	3
TC	1.23	1.23	ZZZ	0	0	0	0	3

AMA: Apr 97: 2, Oct 01: 3, Aug 02: 2, Mar 03: 7

76811 Ultrasound, pregnant uterus, real time with image documentation, fetal and maternal evaluation plus detailed fetal anatomic examination, transabdominal approach; single or first gestation   ♀ M Z 3 S

RVU			Global Days	Modifiers				
Mod	Non-Fac Total	Fac Total		51	50	62	80	MUE
	5.18	5.18	XXX	0	0	0	0	1
26	2.80	2.80	XXX	0	0	0	0	1
TC	2.38	2.38	XXX	0	0	0	0	1

AMA: Mar 03: 7

✚ 76812 Ultrasound, pregnant uterus, real time with image documentation, fetal and maternal evaluation plus detailed fetal anatomic examination, transabdominal approach; each additional gestation (List separately in addition to code for primary procedure)   ♀ M N I N

RVU			Global Days	Modifiers				
Mod	Non-Fac Total	Fac Total		51	50	62	80	MUE
	5.87	5.87	ZZZ	0	0	0	0	3
26	2.63	2.63	ZZZ	0	0	0	0	3
TC	3.24	3.24	ZZZ	0	0	0	0	3

AMA: Mar 03: 7

76813 Ultrasound, pregnant uterus, real time with image documentation, first trimester fetal nuchal translucency measurement, transabdominal or transvaginal approach; single or first gestation   ♀ M N I Q I

RVU			Global Days	Modifiers				
Mod	Non-Fac Total	Fac Total		51	50	62	80	MUE
	3.45	3.45	XXX	0	0	0	0	1
26	1.74	1.74	XXX	0	0	0	0	1
TC	1.71	1.71	XXX	0	0	0	0	1

AMA: Mar 07: 7

✚ 76814 Ultrasound, pregnant uterus, real time with image documentation, first trimester fetal nuchal translucency measurement, transabdominal or transvaginal approach; each additional gestation (List separately in addition to code for primary procedure)   ♀ M N I N

RVU			Global Days	Modifiers				
Mod	Non-Fac Total	Fac Total		51	50	62	80	MUE
	2.32	2.32	XXX	0	0	0	0	3
26	1.47	1.47	XXX	0	0	0	0	3
TC	0.85	0.85	XXX	0	0	0	0	3

AMA: Mar 07: 7

76815 Ultrasound, pregnant uterus, real time with image documentation, limited (eg, fetal heart beat, placental location, fetal position and/or qualitative amniotic fluid volume), 1 or more fetuses   ♀ M N I Q I

RVU			Global Days	Modifiers				
Mod	Non-Fac Total	Fac Total		51	50	62	80	MUE
	2.39	2.39	XXX	0	0	0	0	1
26	0.93	0.93	XXX	0	0	0	0	1
TC	1.46	1.46	XXX	0	0	0	0	1

AMA: Apr 97: 2, Nov 97: 25, Oct 01: 3, Dec 01: 6, Aug 02: 2, Mar 03: 7, Nov 03: 14, May 10: 9

76816 Ultrasound, pregnant uterus, real time with image documentation, follow-up (eg, re-evaluation of fetal size by measuring standard growth parameters and amniotic fluid volume, re-evaluation of organ system(s) suspected or confirmed to be abnormal on a previous scan), transabdominal approach, per fetus   ♀ M N I Q I

RVU			Global Days	Modifiers				
Mod	Non-Fac Total	Fac Total		51	50	62	80	MUE
	3.27	3.27	XXX	0	0	0	
26	1.25	1.25	XXX	0	0	0	
TC	2.02	2.02	XXX	0	0	0	

AMA: Apr 97: 2, Oct 01: 3, Aug 02: 2, Mar 03: 7, Nov 11: 10, May 10: 9

76817 Ultrasound, pregnant uterus, real time with image documentation, transvaginal   ♀ M N I Q I

RVU			Global Days	Modifiers				
Mod	Non-Fac Total	Fac Total		51	50	62	80	MUE
	2.76	2.76	XXX	0	0	0	0	1
26	1.09	1.09	XXX	0	0	0	0	1
TC	1.67	1.67	XXX	0	0	0	0	1

AMA: Mar 03: 7, Nov 11: 10

76818 Fetal biophysical profile; with non-stress testing   ♀ M Z 3 S

Coding tip: Report 76815 when amniotic fluid index is done without non-stress testing

Coding tip: Report 59025 when fetal heart rate acceleration only is evaluated

RVU			Global Days	Modifiers				
Mod	Non-Fac Total	Fac Total		51	50	62	80	MUE
	3.46	3.46	XXX	0	0	0	
26	1.55	1.55	XXX	0	0	0	
TC	1.91	1.91	XXX	0	0	0	

AMA: Apr 97: 2, May 98: 10, Sep 01: 4, Oct 01: 3, Dec 01: 6, Nov 04: 10

76819 Fetal biophysical profile; without non-stress testing   ♀ M Z 3 S

RVU			Global Days	Modifiers				
Mod	Non-Fac Total	Fac Total		51	50	62	80	MUE
	2.53	2.53	XXX	0	0	0	
26	1.13	1.13	XXX	0	0	0	
TC	1.40	1.40	XXX	0	0	0	

AMA: Sep 01: 8, Dec 01: 6

76820 Doppler velocimetry, fetal; umbilical artery   M N I Q I

RVU			Global Days	Modifiers				
Mod	Non-Fac Total	Fac Total		51	50	62	80	MUE
	1.36	1.36	XXX	0	0	0	
26	0.74	0.74	XXX	0	0	0	
TC	0.62	0.62	XXX	0	0	0	

● New   ▲ Revised   Deleted   ⊙ Moderate Sedation   ✚ Add-on Codes   ⊘ High Risk Denial   Ⓐ Age Edit   ♀ Female   ♂ Male   **AMA** *CPT® Assistant*   **MUE** Medically Unlikely Edit
⊘ Modifier 51 Exempt   ⊖ Modifier 63 Exempt   ⓧ Unlisted   **Modifiers:** *See Inside Back Cover*   Ⓜ Maternity   A2–Z3 ASC Payment Indicators   A–Y OPPS Status Indicators

© 2016 DecisionHealth   CPT © 2015 American Medical Association. All Rights Reserved.   **649**

Radiology Procedures

76821 – 76881

AMA: Dec 05: 3

76821 Doppler velocimetry, fetal; middle cerebral artery ☒NIQI

Mod	Non-Fac Total	Fac Total	Global Days	51	50	62	80	MUE
	2.64	2.64	XXX	0	0	0	0	
26	1.03	1.03	XXX	0	0	0	0	
TC	1.61	1.61	XXX	0	0	0	0	

AMA: Dec 05: 3

76825 Echocardiography, fetal, cardiovascular system, real time with image documentation (2D), with or without M-mode recording ♀M Z3 S

Mod	Non-Fac Total	Fac Total	Global Days	51	50	62	80	MUE
	7.84	7.84	XXX	0	0	0	0	
26	2.39	2.39	XXX	0	0	0	0	
TC	5.45	5.45	XXX	0	0	0	0	

AMA: Apr 97: 2, Aug 02: 2

76826 Echocardiography, fetal, cardiovascular system, real time with image documentation (2D), with or without M-mode recording; follow-up or repeat study ♀M Z3 S

Mod	Non-Fac Total	Fac Total	Global Days	51	50	62	80	MUE
	4.63	4.63	XXX	0	0	0	0	
26	1.18	1.18	XXX	0	0	0	0	
TC	3.45	3.45	XXX	0	0	0	0	

AMA: Apr 97: 2, Aug 02: 2

76827 Doppler echocardiography, fetal, pulsed wave and/or continuous wave with spectral display; complete ♀M NIQI

Mod	Non-Fac Total	Fac Total	Global Days	51	50	62	80	MUE
	2.15	2.15	XXX	0	0	0	0	
26	0.82	0.82	XXX	0	0	0	0	
TC	1.33	1.33	XXX	0	0	0	0	

AMA: Apr 97: 2, Aug 02: 2, Dec 05: 3

76828 Doppler echocardiography, fetal, pulsed wave and/or continuous wave with spectral display; follow-up or repeat study ♀M NIQI

Mod	Non-Fac Total	Fac Total	Global Days	51	50	62	80	MUE
	1.52	1.52	XXX	0	0	0	0	
26	0.81	0.81	XXX	0	0	0	0	
TC	0.71	0.71	XXX	0	0	0	0	

AMA: Apr 97: 2, Aug 02: 2, Dec 05: 3

Non-obstetrical Procedures

76830 Ultrasound, transvaginal ♀Z2 S

Mod	Non-Fac Total	Fac Total	Global Days	51	50	62	80	MUE
	3.45	3.45	XXX	0	0	0	0	1
26	0.99	0.99	XXX	0	0	0	0	1
TC	2.46	2.46	XXX	0	0	0	0	1

AMA: Aug 96: 10, Jul 99: 8, Aug 02: 2, Mar 03: 7, Dec 05: 3, Feb 09: 22, Nov 11: 10

76831 Saline infusion sonohysterography (SIS), including color flow Doppler, when performed ♀Z3 Q3

Coding tip: Introduction of saline - 58340

Mod	Non-Fac Total	Fac Total	Global Days	51	50	62	80	MUE
	3.37	3.37	XXX	4	0	0	0	1
26	1.05	1.05	XXX	4	0	0	0	1
TC	2.32	2.32	XXX	4	0	0	0	1

AMA: Nov 97: 25, Jul 99: 8, Dec 05: 3, Mar 09: 11

76856 Ultrasound, pelvic (nonobstetric), real time with image documentation; complete Z3 Q3

Mod	Non-Fac Total	Fac Total	Global Days	51	50	62	80	MUE
	3.11	3.11	XXX	4	0	0	0	1
26	0.98	0.98	XXX	4	0	0	0	1
TC	2.13	2.13	XXX	4	0	0	0	1

AMA: Oct 01: 3, Dec 05: 3, Jan 06: 47, Mar 07: 7, Feb 09: 22

76857 Ultrasound, pelvic (nonobstetric), real time with image documentation; limited or follow-up (eg, for follicles) Z3 Q3

Mod	Non-Fac Total	Fac Total	Global Days	51	50	62	80	MUE
	1.34	1.34	XXX	4	0	0	0	1
26	0.70	0.70	XXX	4	0	0	0	1
TC	0.64	0.64	XXX	4	0	0	0	1

AMA: Jun 97: 10, Oct 01: 3, Dec 05: 3, Sep 07: 10, May 09: 7

Genitalia Ultrasound Procedures

76870 Ultrasound, scrotum and contents ♂NIQI

Mod	Non-Fac Total	Fac Total	Global Days	51	50	62	80	MUE
	1.91	1.91	XXX	4	0	0	0	1
26	0.91	0.91	XXX	4	0	0	0	1
TC	1.00	1.00	XXX	4	0	0	0	1

AMA: May 05: 3

76872 Ultrasound, transrectal Z3 S

Mod	Non-Fac Total	Fac Total	Global Days	51	50	62	80	MUE
	2.66	2.66	XXX	0	0	0	0	1
26	0.95	0.95	XXX	0	0	0	0	1
TC	1.71	1.71	XXX	0	0	0	0	1

AMA: May 96: 3, Nov 99: 42

76873 Ultrasound, transrectal; prostate volume study for brachytherapy treatment planning (separate procedure) ♂Z2 S

Mod	Non-Fac Total	Fac Total	Global Days	51	50	62	80	MUE
	4.74	4.74	XXX	9	9	9	9	1
26	2.21	2.21	XXX	9	9	9	9	1
TC	2.53	2.53	XXX	9	9	9	9	1

AMA: Nov 99: 42

Extremity Ultrasound Procedures

76881 Ultrasound, extremity, nonvascular, real-time with image documentation; complete Z3 S

Mod	Non-Fac Total	Fac Total	Global Days	51	50	62	80	MUE
	3.26	3.26	XXX	0	0	0	9	2
26	0.90	0.90	XXX	0	0	0	9	2
TC	2.36	2.36	XXX	0	0	0	9	2

● New   ▲ Revised   ✖ Deleted   ⊙ Moderate Sedation   ✚ Add-on Codes   ⊘ High Risk Denial   Ⓐ Age Edit   ♀ Female   ♂ Male   **AMA** CPT® Assistant   **MUE** Medically Unlikely Edit
⊘ Modifier 51 Exempt   ⊖ Modifier 63 Exempt   ✖ Unlisted   **Modifiers:** See Inside Back Cover   Ⓜ Maternity   A2–Z3 ASC Payment Indicators   A–Y OPPS Status Indicators

CPT © 2015 American Medical Association. All Rights Reserved.   © 2016 DecisionHealth

76882 **Ultrasound, extremity, nonvascular, real-time with image documentation; limited, anatomic specific** `N I Q I`

RVU			Global Days	Modifiers				
Mod	Non-Fac Total	Fac Total		51	50	62	80	MUE
	1.02	1.02	XXX	0	0	0	9	2
26	0.70	0.70	XXX	0	0	0	9	2
TC	0.32	0.32	XXX	0	0	0	9	2

76885 **Ultrasound, infant hips, real time with imaging documentation; dynamic (requiring physician or other qualified health care professional manipulation)** `⊙Ⓐ N I Q I`

RVU			Global Days	Modifiers				
Mod	Non-Fac Total	Fac Total		51	50	62	80	MUE
	4.12	4.12	XXX	0	0	0	0	1
26	1.06	1.06	XXX	0	0	0	0	1
TC	3.06	3.06	XXX	0	0	0	0	1

AMA: Nov 97: 25

76886 **Ultrasound, infant hips, real time with imaging documentation; limited, static (not requiring physician or other qualified health care professional manipulation)** `⊙Ⓐ N I Q I`

RVU			Global Days	Modifiers				
Mod	Non-Fac Total	Fac Total		51	50	62	80	MUE
	3.00	3.00	XXX	0	0	0	0	1
26	0.87	0.87	XXX	0	0	0	0	1
TC	2.13	2.13	XXX	0	0	0	0	1

AMA: Nov 97: 25

Ultrasonic Guidance

Coding Guidance

Ultrasonic guidance services of the heart and vascular system by themselves do not include diagnostic echography. Both ultrasound guidance and diagnostic echography can be reported when both procedures are done.

76930 **Ultrasonic guidance for pericardiocentesis, imaging supervision and interpretation** `N I N`

RVU			Global Days	Modifiers				
Mod	Non-Fac Total	Fac Total		51	50	62	80	MUE
	0.00	0.00	XXX	0	0	0	0	1
26	0.93	0.93	XXX	0	0	0	0	1
TC	0.00	0.00	XXX	0	0	0	0	1

76932 **Ultrasonic guidance for endomyocardial biopsy, imaging supervision and interpretation** `N I N`

RVU			Global Days	Modifiers				
Mod	Non-Fac Total	Fac Total		51	50	62	80	MUE
	0.00	0.00	YYY	0	0	0	0	1
26	0.92	0.92	XXX	0	0	0	0	1
TC	0.00	0.00	YYY	0	0	0	0	1

76936 **Ultrasound guided compression repair of arterial pseudoaneurysm or arteriovenous fistulae (includes diagnostic ultrasound evaluation, compression of lesion and imaging)** `Z 2 S`

RVU			Global Days	Modifiers				
Mod	Non-Fac Total	Fac Total		51	50	62	80	MUE
	7.68	7.68	XXX	0	0	0	0	2
26	2.80	2.80	XXX	0	0	0	0	2
TC	4.88	4.88	XXX	0	0	0	0	2

+ 76937 **Ultrasound guidance for vascular access requiring ultrasound evaluation of potential access sites, documentation of selected vessel patency, concurrent realtime ultrasound visualization of vascular needle entry, with permanent recording and reporting (List separately in addition to code for primary procedure)** `N I N`

Coding tip: *Insertion procedure for central venous access device/catheter - 36555-36571*

RVU			Global Days	Modifiers				
Mod	Non-Fac Total	Fac Total		51	50	62	80	MUE
	0.89	0.89	ZZZ	0	0	0	0	2
26	0.41	0.41	ZZZ	0	0	0	0	2
TC	0.48	0.48	ZZZ	0	0	0	0	2

AMA: May 13: 3, Dec 04: 13, Jan 09: 7, Jul 10: 6, Nov 10: 3, Jan 11: 8, Apr 12: 6, Feb 13: 3, Jun 13: 12, Sep 13: 18, Oct 14: 6, Jul 15: 10

76940 **Ultrasound guidance for, and monitoring of, parenchymal tissue ablation** `N I N`

Coding tip: *Renal tumor ablation - 50592-50593*
Coding tip: *Liver tumor ablation - 47370-47382*
Coding tip: *Pulmonary tumor ablation - 32998*

RVU			Global Days	Modifiers				
Mod	Non-Fac Total	Fac Total		51	50	62	80	MUE
	0.00	0.00	YYY	0	0	0	0	1
26	2.94	2.94	XXX	0	0	0	0	1
TC	0.00	0.00	YYY	0	0	0	0	1

AMA: Oct 02: 2, Mar 07: 7, Jul 15: 8

76941 **Ultrasonic guidance for intrauterine fetal transfusion or cordocentesis, imaging supervision and interpretation** `♀ M N I N`

Coding tip: *Cordocentesis procedure - 59012*
Coding tip: *Intrauterine fetal transfusion procedure - 36460*

RVU			Global Days	Modifiers				
Mod	Non-Fac Total	Fac Total		51	50	62	80	MUE
	0.00	0.00	XXX	0	0	0		
26	1.95	1.95	XXX	0	0	0		
TC	0.00	0.00	XXX	0	0	0		

Coding Guidance

All the radiologic services necessary for the procedure are included in the radiologic supervision and interpretation codes for specific procedures. Do not report ultrasound guidance in addition. Procedures that may require additional ultrasound guidance for needle placement include 10022, 10140-10160, 19000-19001, 20206, 20553, 20610, 20615, 32400, 38505, 42400-42405, 55700, and 60100.

76942 **Ultrasonic guidance for needle placement (eg, biopsy, aspiration, injection, localization device), imaging supervision and interpretation** `N I N`

RVU			Global Days	Modifiers				
Mod	Non-Fac Total	Fac Total		51	50	62	80	MUE
	1.73	1.73	XXX	0	0	0	0	1
26	0.95	0.95	XXX	0	0	0	0	1
TC	0.78	0.78	XXX	0	0	0	0	1

AMA: Fall 93: 12, Fall 94: 2, May 96: 3, Jun 97: 5, Oct 01: 2, May 04: 7, Dec 04: 12, Apr 05: 15, 16, Aug 08: 7, Mar 09: 8, Feb 10: 6, Mar 10: 9, Mar 11: 10, Apr 11: 12, Jul 10: 6, Feb 11: 4, Nov 12: 3, Dec 12: 9, Nov 13: 9, Oct 14: 6, Feb 15: 6, Aug 15: 8

● New   ▲ Revised   Deleted   ⊙ Moderate Sedation   ✚ Add-on Codes   ⊘ High Risk Denial   Ⓐ Age Edit   ♀ Female   ♂ Male   **AMA** *CPT® Assistant*   **MUE** Medically Unlikely Edit
⊘ Modifier 51 Exempt   ⊖ Modifier 63 Exempt   ✗ Unlisted   **Modifiers:** *See Inside Back Cover*   M Maternity   A2-Z3 ASC Payment Indicators   A-Y OPPS Status Indicators

Radiology Procedures

76945 – 77001

76945 Ultrasonic guidance for chorionic villus sampling, imaging supervision and interpretation ♀ M N I N

Coding tip: Chorionic villus sampling - 59015

RVU			Global Days	Modifiers				
Mod	Non-Fac Total	Fac Total		51	50	62	80	MUE
	0.00	0.00	XXX	0	0	0	0	1
26	0.99	0.99	XXX	0	0	0	0	1
TC	0.00	0.00	XXX	0	0	0	0	1

76946 Ultrasonic guidance for amniocentesis, imaging supervision and interpretation ♀ M N I N

Coding tip: Diagnostic amniocentesis procedure - 59000

RVU			Global Days	Modifiers				
Mod	Non-Fac Total	Fac Total		51	50	62	80	MUE
	0.93	0.93	XXX	0	0	0	0	1
26	0.56	0.56	XXX	0	0	0	0	1
TC	0.37	0.37	XXX	0	0	0	0	1

76948 Ultrasonic guidance for aspiration of ova, imaging supervision and interpretation ⊙♀ N I N

Coding tip: Follicle puncture for aspirating oocyte - 58970

RVU			Global Days	Modifiers				
Mod	Non-Fac Total	Fac Total		51	50	62	80	MUE
	2.10	2.10	XXX	0	0	0	0	1
26	0.98	0.98	XXX	0	0	0	0	1
TC	1.12	1.12	XXX	0	0	0	0	1

76965 Ultrasonic guidance for interstitial radioelement application N I N

Coding tip: Application of interstitial radiation source - 77776-77778

RVU			Global Days	Modifiers				
Mod	Non-Fac Total	Fac Total		51	50	62	80	MUE
	2.55	2.55	XXX	0	0	0	0	2
26	1.88	1.88	XXX	0	0	0	0	2
TC	0.67	0.67	XXX	0	0	0	0	2

Other Ultrasonic Procedures

76970 Ultrasound study follow-up (specify) N I Q 1

Coding tip: Do not report code 76970 with any other echocardiographic or ultrasound study for the same encounter

RVU			Global Days	Modifiers				
Mod	Non-Fac Total	Fac Total		51	50	62	80	MUE
	2.64	2.64	XXX	0	0	0	0	2
26	0.55	0.55	XXX	0	0	0	0	2
TC	2.09	2.09	XXX	0	0	0	0	2

76975 Gastrointestinal endoscopic ultrasound, supervision and interpretation ⊙ N I Q 2

RVU			Global Days	Modifiers				
Mod	Non-Fac Total	Fac Total		51	50	62	80	MUE
	0.00	0.00	XXX	0	0	0	0	1
26	1.21	1.21	XXX	0	0	0	0	1
TC	0.00	0.00	XXX	0	0	0	0	1

AMA: Spring 94: 5, May 04: 7, Mar 09: 8

Pub 100-04, 12, 30.1

76977 Ultrasound bone density measurement and interpretation, peripheral site(s), any method ⊙ Z 3 S

Documentation Finder: Documentation should show that they are doing bone density measurement using low-level ultrasound instead of ionizing radiation.

RVU			Global Days	Modifiers				
Mod	Non-Fac Total	Fac Total		51	50	62	80	MUE
	0.20	0.20	XXX	0	0	0	0	1
26	0.08	0.08	XXX	0	0	0	0	1
TC	0.12	0.12	XXX	0	0	0	0	1

AMA: Nov 98: 21

Pub 100-04, 13, 140.1; 100-04, 18, 1.2

Coding Guidance

All the radiologic services necessary for the procedure are included in the radiologic supervision and interpretation codes for specific procedures. Do not report ultrasound guidance in addition. Intraoperative ultrasound guidance may be used to report epi-aortic ultrasound during coronary artery bypass graft procedures using venous or combined grafts.

76998 Ultrasonic guidance, intraoperative N I N

RVU			Global Days	Modifiers				
Mod	Non-Fac Total	Fac Total		51	50	62	80	MUE
	0.00	0.00	XXX	0	0	0	0	1
26	1.81	1.81	XXX	0	0	0	0	1
TC	0.00	0.00	XXX	0	0	0	0	1

AMA: Mar 07: 7, Jul 10: 6, Jan 13: 6, Jan 14: 5, Oct 14: 6, Aug 15: 8

76999 Unlisted ultrasound procedure (eg, diagnostic, interventional) ⊙ X N I Q 1

RVU			Global Days	Modifiers				
Mod	Non-Fac Total	Fac Total		51	50	62	80	MUE
	0.00	0.00	XXX	0	0	0	0	
26	0.00	0.00	XXX	0	0	0	0	
TC	0.00	0.00	XXX	0	0	0	0	

Pub 100-04, 13, 120; 100-04, 32, 310.1, 310.2

Radiological Guidance

Fluoroscopic Guidance

+ **77001 Fluoroscopic guidance for central venous access device placement, replacement (catheter only or complete), or removal (includes fluoroscopic guidance for vascular access and catheter manipulation, any necessary contrast injections through access site or catheter with related venography radiologic supervision and interpretation, and radiographic documentation of final catheter position) (List separately in addition to code for primary procedure)** N I N

Coding tip: Central venous access device removal - 36589, 36590
Coding tip: Central venous access device insertion - 36555-36571
Coding tip: Central venous access device replacement - 36578-36585

RVU			Global Days	Modifiers				
Mod	Non-Fac Total	Fac Total		51	50	62	80	MUE
	1.98	1.98	ZZZ	0	0	0	9	2
26	0.54	0.54	ZZZ	0	0	0	9	2
TC	1.44	1.44	ZZZ	0	0	0	9	2

AMA: Mar 07: 7, Jul 08: 9, Nov 10: 3, Jan 11: 8

● New   ▲ Revised   ✖ Deleted   ⊙ Moderate Sedation   ✛ Add-on Codes   ⊘ High Risk Denial   Ⓐ Age Edit   ♀ Female   ♂ Male   **AMA** CPT® Assistant   **MUE** Medically Unlikely Edit

⊘ Modifier 51 Exempt   ⊖ Modifier 63 Exempt   ✗ Unlisted   **Modifiers:** See Inside Back Cover   M Maternity   A2–Z3 ASC Payment Indicators   A–Y OPPS Status Indicators

652   CPT © 2015 American Medical Association. All Rights Reserved.   © 2016 DecisionHealth

Coding Guidance

All the radiologic services necessary for the procedure are included in the radiologic supervision and interpretation codes for specific procedures. Do not report fluoroscopic guidance in addition. Procedures that may require additional fluoroscopic guidance for needle placement include 10022, 20225, 20553-20555, 20610, 32400, 32405, 36002, 41019, 42400-42405, 47000-47001, 48102, 49180, 50200, 50390, 51100-51102, 55876, and 60100.

77002 Fluoroscopic guidance for needle placement (eg, biopsy, aspiration, injection, localization device)

N I N

	RVU		Global Days	Modifiers				
Mod	Non-Fac Total	Fac Total		51	50	62	80	MUE
	2.62	2.62	XXX	0	0	0	9	1
26	0.80	0.80	XXX	0	0	0	9	1
TC	1.82	1.82	XXX	0	0	0	9	1

AMA: Feb 07: 11, Mar 07: 7, May 07: 1, Jun 07: 10, Jul 08: 9, Aug 08: 7, Dec 08: 9, Feb 10: 6, Dec 09: 12, Apr 11: 12, Feb 12: 11, Nov 10: 3, Jan 11: 8, Apr 12: 19, Jun 12: 14, Nov 12: 3, Dec 12: 9, Nov 13: 9, Jul 15: 8, Aug 15: 6

77003 Fluoroscopic guidance and localization of needle or catheter tip for spine or paraspinous diagnostic or therapeutic injection procedures (epidural or subarachnoid)

N I N

Documentation Finder: Documentation needs to show that fluoroscopic guidance was used when placing a needle or catheter tip into the spine region. This code represents only the imaging guidance; another code should be reported for the injection/catheter procedure.

	RVU		Global Days	Modifiers				
Mod	Non-Fac Total	Fac Total		51	50	62	80	MUE
	2.43	2.43	XXX	9	9	9	9	1
26	0.86	0.86	XXX	9	9	9	9	1
TC	1.57	1.57	XXX	9	9	9	9	1

AMA: Mar 07: 7, Jul 08: 9, Feb 10: 12, Mar 11: 7, Jul 11: 17, May 10: 10, Aug 10: 8, Oct 10: 14, Nov 10: 3, Dec 10: 14, Feb 11: 4, Jan 11: 8, Jun 12: 12, Jul 12: 3, 5, 6, Sep 12: 14, Nov 13: 9, Dec 13: 14

Computed Tomographic Guidance

77011 Computed tomography guidance for stereotactic localization

N I N

	RVU		Global Days	Modifiers				
Mod	Non-Fac Total	Fac Total		51	50	62	80	MUE
	6.27	6.27	XXX	0	0	0	9	1
26	1.78	1.78	XXX	0	0	0	9	1
TC	4.49	4.49	XXX	0	0	0	9	1

AMA: Mar 07: 7

77012 Computed tomography guidance for needle placement (eg, biopsy, aspiration, injection, localization device), radiological supervision and interpretation

N I N

	RVU		Global Days	Modifiers				
Mod	Non-Fac Total	Fac Total		51	50	62	80	MUE
	3.50	3.50	XXX	0	0	0	9	1
26	1.63	1.63	XXX	0	0	0	9	1
TC	1.87	1.87	XXX	0	0	0	9	1

AMA: Mar 07: 7, May 07: 1, Jun 07: 10, Aug 07: 8, Feb 10: 6, Apr 11: 12, Feb 11: 4, Jul 12: 3, 6, Sep 12: 14, Nov 12: 3, Dec 12: 9, Nov 13: 9, Feb 15: 6

77013 Computed tomography guidance for, and monitoring of, parenchymal tissue ablation

N I N

Coding tip: *Renal tumor ablation - 50592-50593*

Coding tip: *Pulmonary tumor ablation - 32998*

Coding tip: *Liver tumor ablation 47382*

	RVU		Global Days	Modifiers				
Mod	Non-Fac Total	Fac Total		51	50	62	80	MUE
	0.00	0.00	XXX	0	0	0	0	1
26	5.56	5.56	XXX	0	0	0	9	1
TC	0.00	0.00	XXX	0	0	0	0	1

AMA: Mar 07: 7, Jul 15: 8

Coding Guidance

Computerized tomographic guidance for radiation therapy field placement is mutually exclusive of ultrasonic guidance for radiation therapy field placement (76950).

77014 Computed tomography guidance for placement of radiation therapy fields

N I N

	RVU		Global Days	Modifiers				
Mod	Non-Fac Total	Fac Total		51	50	62	80	MUE
	3.32	3.32	XXX	0	0	0	9	2
26	1.24	1.24	XXX	0	0	0	9	2
TC	2.08	2.08	XXX	0	0	0	9	2

AMA: Mar 07: 7, Apr 15: 11

Magnetic Resonance Guidance

77021 Magnetic resonance guidance for needle placement (eg, for biopsy, needle aspiration, injection, or placement of localization device) radiological supervision and interpretation

N I N

	RVU		Global Days	Modifiers				
Mod	Non-Fac Total	Fac Total		51	50	62	80	MUE
	11.32	11.32	XXX	0	0	0	9	1
26	2.13	2.13	XXX	0	0	0	9	1
TC	9.19	9.19	XXX	0	0	0	9	1

AMA: Mar 07: 7, May 07: 1, Jun 07: 10, Aug 08: 7, Feb 10: 6, Apr 11: 12, Nov 12: 3, Dec 12: 9, Nov 13: 9, Feb 15: 6

77022 Magnetic resonance guidance for, and monitoring of, parenchymal tissue ablation

N I N

Coding tip: *Liver tumor ablation - 47382*

Coding tip: *Renal tumor ablation - 50592-50593*

Coding tip: *Pulmonary tumor ablation - 32998*

	RVU		Global Days	Modifiers				
Mod	Non-Fac Total	Fac Total		51	50	62	80	MUE
	0.00	0.00	XXX	0	0	0	0	1
26	6.04	6.04	XXX	0	0	0	9	1
TC	0.00	0.00	XXX	0	0	0	0	1

AMA: Mar 07: 7, Oct 14: 6, Jul 15: 8

● New   ▲ Revised   Deleted   ⊙ Moderate Sedation   ✚ Add-on Codes   ⊘ High Risk Denial   Ⓐ Age Edit   ♀ Female   ♂ Male   **AMA** *CPT® Assistant*   **MUE** Medically Unlikely Edit

⊘ Modifier 51 Exempt   ⊖ Modifier 63 Exempt   ✗ Unlisted   **Modifiers:** *See Inside Back Cover*   Ⓜ Maternity   A 2 – Z 3 ASC Payment Indicators   A – Y OPPS Status Indicators

© 2016 DecisionHealth   CPT © 2015 American Medical Association. All Rights Reserved.   **653**

Radiology Procedures

77051 – 77061

Mammographies/Breast Procedures

+ 77051 Computer-aided detection (computer algorithm analysis of digital image data for lesion detection) with further review for interpretation, with or without digitization of film radiographic images; diagnostic mammography (List separately in addition to code for primary procedure) 🅰

*Documentation Finder: Documentation often states "digital mammogram" for this service. This is an add-on code that should be reported with **77055** or **77056**. Medicare has its own G code for these services that other payers may want instead. Look for whether the service was performed in a facility; modifier **26** may need to be added for professional services only.*

RVU			Global Days	Modifiers				
Mod	Non-Fac Total	Fac Total		51	50	62	80	MUE
	0.23	0.23	ZZZ	0	0	0	9	2
26	0.08	0.08	ZZZ	0	0	0	9	2
TC	0.15	0.15	ZZZ	0	0	0	9	2

AMA: Mar 07: 7, Apr 07: 1, Jun 14: 14

Pub 100-04, 18, 20.2, 20.2.1, 20.2.1.1, 20.3.2.1, 20.3.2.2, 20.3.2.4, 20.4.1.2, 20.5.1.1

+ 77052 Computer-aided detection (computer algorithm analysis of digital image data for lesion detection) with further review for interpretation, with or without digitization of film radiographic images; screening mammography (List separately in addition to code for primary procedure) 🅰

RVU			Global Days	Modifiers				
Mod	Non-Fac Total	Fac Total		51	50	62	80	MUE
	0.23	0.23	ZZZ	0	0	0	9	1
26	0.08	0.08	ZZZ	0	0	0	9	1
TC	0.15	0.15	ZZZ	0	0	0	9	1

AMA: Mar 07: 7, Apr 07: 1, Jun 14: 14

Pub 100-04, 18, 1.2, 20.2, 20.2.1, 20.2.1.1, 20.3.2.1, 20.3.2.2, 20.3.2.3, 20.3.2.3.1, 20.3.2.4, 20.4.1.2, 20.4.2.1, 20.5.1.1

77053 Mammary ductogram or galactogram, single duct, radiological supervision and interpretation N Q2

RVU			Global Days	Modifiers				
Mod	Non-Fac Total	Fac Total		51	50	62	80	MUE
	1.64	1.64	XXX	0	0	0	9	2
26	0.51	0.51	XXX	0	0	0	9	2
TC	1.13	1.13	XXX	0	0	0	9	2

AMA: Mar 07: 7

77054 Mammary ductogram or galactogram, multiple ducts, radiological supervision and interpretation N Q2

RVU			Global Days	Modifiers				
Mod	Non-Fac Total	Fac Total		51	50	62	80	MUE
	2.16	2.16	XXX	0	0	0	9	2
26	0.65	0.65	XXX	0	0	0	9	2
TC	1.51	1.51	XXX	0	0	0	9	2

AMA: Mar 07: 7

77055 Mammography; unilateral 🅰

RVU			Global Days	Modifiers				
Mod	Non-Fac Total	Fac Total		51	50	62	80	MUE
	2.53	2.53	XXX	0	0	0	9	1
26	1.00	1.00	XXX	0	0	0	9	1
TC	1.53	1.53	XXX	0	0	0	9	1

AMA: Mar 07: 7, Jun 14: 14

Pub 100-04, 18, 20.2, 20.2.1, 20.2.1.1, 20.3.2.1, 20.3.2.2, 20.3.2.4, 20.4, 20.4.1.2, 20.5.1.1, 20.6, 20.7

77056 Mammography; bilateral 🅰

RVU			Global Days	Modifiers				
Mod	Non-Fac Total	Fac Total		51	50	62	80	MUE
	3.25	3.25	XXX	0	0	0	9	1
26	1.24	1.24	XXX	0	0	0	9	1
TC	2.01	2.01	XXX	0	0	0	9	1

AMA: Mar 07: 7

Pub 100-04, 18, 20.2, 20.2.1, 20.2.1.1, 20.3.1, 20.3.2.1, 20.3.2.2, 20.3.2.4, 20.4, 20.4.1.2, 20.5.1.1, 20.6, 20.7

▲ 77057 Screening mammography, bilateral (2-view study of each breast) ♀🅰

RVU			Global Days	Modifiers				
Mod	Non-Fac Total	Fac Total		51	50	62	80	MUE
	2.32	2.32	XXX	0	2	0	9	1
26	1.00	1.00	XXX	0	2	0	9	1
TC	1.32	1.32	XXX	0	2	0	9	1

AMA: Mar 07: 7, Jun 14: 14

Pub 100-04, 18, 1.2, 20.2, 20.2.1, 20.2.1.1, 20.3.1, 20.3.2, 20.3.2.1, 20.3.2.2, 20.3.2.3, 20.3.2.3.1, 20.3.2.4, 20.4, 20.4.1.2, 20.4.2, 20.4.2.1, 20.5.1.1, 20.7

77058 Magnetic resonance imaging, breast, without and/or with contrast material(s); unilateral 🅱

Coding tip: Add computer-aided lesion detection/characterization - 0159T

RVU			Global Days	Modifiers				
Mod	Non-Fac Total	Fac Total		51	50	62	80	MUE
	15.10	15.10	XXX	4	0	0	9	1
26	2.32	2.32	XXX	4	0	0	9	1
TC	12.78	12.78	XXX	4	0	0	9	1

AMA: Mar 07: 7

77059 Magnetic resonance imaging, breast, without and/or with contrast material(s); bilateral 🅱

Coding tip: Add computer-aided lesion detection/characterization - 0159T

RVU			Global Days	Modifiers				
Mod	Non-Fac Total	Fac Total		51	50	62	80	MUE
	15.03	15.03	XXX	4	2	0	9	1
26	2.32	2.32	XXX	4	2	0	9	1
TC	12.71	12.71	XXX	4	2	0	9	1

AMA: Mar 07: 7, Jul 07: 6

77061 Digital breast tomosynthesis; unilateral 🅴

RVU			Global Days	Modifiers				
Mod	Non-Fac Total	Fac Total		51	50	62	80	MUE
	0.00	0.00	XXX	0	0	0	9	
26	0.00	0.00	XXX	0	0	0	9	
TC	0.00	0.00	XXX	0	0	0	9	

● New   ▲ Revised   ✖ Deleted   ☉ Moderate Sedation   ✚ Add-on Codes   ⊘ High Risk Denial   Ⓐ Age Edit   ♀ Female   ♂ Male   **AMA** *CPT® Assistant*   **MUE** Medically Unlikely Edit
⊘ Modifier 51 Exempt   ⊖ Modifier 63 Exempt   ✗ Unlisted   **Modifiers:** *See Inside Back Cover*   Ⓜ Maternity   A2–Z3 ASC Payment Indicators   A–Y OPPS Status Indicators

654   CPT © 2015 American Medical Association. All Rights Reserved.   © 2016 DecisionHealth

77062 Digital breast tomosynthesis; bilateral 　E

RVU			Global Days	Modifiers				
Mod	Non-Fac Total	Fac Total		51	50	62	80	MUE
	0.00	0.00	XXX	0	0	0	9	
26	0.00	0.00	XXX	0	0	0	9	
TC	0.00	0.00	XXX	0	0	0	9	

+ 77063 Screening digital breast tomosynthesis, bilateral (List separately in addition to code for primary procedure) 　A

RVU			Global Days	Modifiers				
Mod	Non-Fac Total	Fac Total		51	50	62	80	MUE
	1.57	1.57	ZZZ	0	2	0	9	1
26	0.85	0.85	ZZZ	0	2	0	9	1
TC	0.72	0.72	ZZZ	0	2	0	9	1

Pub 100-04, 18, 1.2, 20.2, 20.2.3

Bone/Joint Studies

77071 Manual application of stress performed by physician or other qualified health care professional for joint radiography, including contralateral joint if indicated 　N I Q I

RVU			Global Days	Modifiers				
Mod	Non-Fac Total	Fac Total		51	50	62	80	MUE
	1.37	1.37	XXX	0	2	0	0	1

AMA: Mar 07: 7

Coding Guidance

Bone studies always require a series of radiographs. Billing for a bone study (77072-77076) together with codes for individual radiographs taking during the course of the study is incorrect coding.

77072 Bone age studies 　N I Q I

RVU			Global Days	Modifiers				
Mod	Non-Fac Total	Fac Total		51	50	62	80	MUE
	0.65	0.65	XXX	0	0	0	0	1
26	0.27	0.27	XXX	0	0	0	0	1
TC	0.38	0.38	XXX	0	0	0	0	1

AMA: Mar 07: 7

77073 Bone length studies (orthoroentgenogram, scanogram) 　N I Q I

Coding tip: *Do not code individual radiographs taken during the course of the study*

RVU			Global Days	Modifiers				
Mod	Non-Fac Total	Fac Total		51	50	62	80	MUE
	1.02	1.02	XXX	0	0	0	0	1
26	0.41	0.41	XXX	0	0	0	0	1
TC	0.61	0.61	XXX	0	0	0	0	1

AMA: Mar 07: 7

77074 Radiologic examination, osseous survey; limited (eg, for metastases) 　N I Q I

RVU			Global Days	Modifiers				
Mod	Non-Fac Total	Fac Total		51	50	62	80	MUE
	1.81	1.81	XXX	0	0	0	0	1
26	0.65	0.65	XXX	0	0	0	0	1
TC	1.16	1.16	XXX	0	0	0	0	1

AMA: Mar 07: 7

77075 Radiologic examination, osseous survey; complete (axial and appendicular skeleton) 　N I Q I

RVU			Global Days	Modifiers				
Mod	Non-Fac Total	Fac Total		51	50	62	80	MUE
	2.46	2.46	XXX	0	0	0	0	1
26	0.77	0.77	XXX	0	0	0	0	1
TC	1.69	1.69	XXX	0	0	0	0	1

AMA: Mar 07: 7

77076 Radiologic examination, osseous survey, infant 　○A N I Q I

RVU			Global Days	Modifiers				
Mod	Non-Fac Total	Fac Total		51	50	62	80	MUE
	2.70	2.70	XXX	0	0	0	0	1
26	1.00	1.00	XXX	0	0	0	0	1
TC	1.70	1.70	XXX	0	0	0	0	1

AMA: Mar 07: 7

77077 Joint survey, single view, 2 or more joints (specify) 　N I Q I

RVU			Global Days	Modifiers				
Mod	Non-Fac Total	Fac Total		51	50	62	80	MUE
	1.05	1.05	XXX	0	0	0	0	1
26	0.46	0.46	XXX	0	0	0	0	1
TC	0.59	0.59	XXX	0	0	0	0	1

AMA: Mar 07: 7

Coding Guidance

Sometimes it may be medically necessary to report both axial (77078, 77080) and peripheral (77081, 76977) bone density studies on the same date of service. However, edits will generally prevent reporting multiple axial or multiple peripheral site bone density studies on the same date of service.

77078 Computed tomography, bone mineral density study, 1 or more sites, axial skeleton (eg, hips, pelvis, spine) 　Z2 S

RVU			Global Days	Modifiers				
Mod	Non-Fac Total	Fac Total		51	50	62	80	MUE
	3.18	3.18	XXX	0	0	0	0	1
26	0.35	0.35	XXX	0	0	0	0	1
TC	2.83	2.83	XXX	0	0	0	0	1

AMA: Mar 07: 7

Pub 100-04, 13, 140.1; 100-04, 18, 1.2

77080 Dual-energy X-ray absorptiometry (DXA), bone density study, 1 or more sites; axial skeleton (eg, hips, pelvis, spine) 　Z3 S

RVU			Global Days	Modifiers				
Mod	Non-Fac Total	Fac Total		51	50	62	80	MUE
	1.16	1.16	XXX	0	0	0	0	1
26	0.29	0.29	XXX	0	0	0	0	1
TC	0.87	0.87	XXX	0	0	0	0	1

AMA: Mar 07: 7

Pub 100-04, 13, 140.1; 100-04, 18, 1.2

© 2016 DecisionHealth 　　CPT © 2015 American Medical Association. All Rights Reserved.

77081 Dual-energy X-ray absorptiometry (DXA), bone density study, 1 or more sites; appendicular skeleton (peripheral) (eg, radius, wrist, heel) ⊘Z3 S

Documentation Finder: *The documentation should make reference to the dexa scan being performed on the wrist, heel, ulna, etc. You may see this also referred to as bone mass density. Note: Payers including Medicare will have internal policies regarding diagnoses and utilization requirements.*

RVU			Global Days	Modifiers				
Mod	Non-Fac Total	Fac Total		51	50	62	80	MUE
	0.79	0.79	XXX	0	0	0	0	1
26	0.31	0.31	XXX	0	0	0	0	1
TC	0.48	0.48	XXX	0	0	0	0	1

AMA: Mar 07: 7

Pub 100-04, 13, 140.1; 100-04, 18, 1.2

77084 Magnetic resonance (eg, proton) imaging, bone marrow blood supply Z2 S

RVU			Global Days	Modifiers				
Mod	Non-Fac Total	Fac Total		51	50	62	80	MUE
	10.96	10.96	XXX	0	0	0	0	1
26	2.29	2.29	XXX	0	0	0	0	1
TC	8.67	8.67	XXX	0	0	0	0	1

AMA: Mar 07: 7

77085 Dual-energy X-ray absorptiometry (DXA), bone density study, 1 or more sites; axial skeleton (eg, hips, pelvis, spine), including vertebral fracture assessment N1 Q1

RVU			Global Days	Modifiers				
Mod	Non-Fac Total	Fac Total		51	50	62	80	MUE
	1.57	1.57	XXX	0	0	0	0	1
26	0.43	0.43	XXX	0	0	0	0	1
TC	1.14	1.14	XXX	0	0	0	0	1

77086 Vertebral fracture assessment via dual-energy X-ray absorptiometry (DXA) N1 Q1

RVU			Global Days	Modifiers				
Mod	Non-Fac Total	Fac Total		51	50	62	80	MUE
	1.00	1.00	XXX	0	0	0	0	1
26	0.25	0.25	XXX	0	0	0	0	1
TC	0.75	0.75	XXX	0	0	0	0	1

Radiation Oncology Services

Clinical Treatment Planning Services

Coding Guidance

Medicare's Internet Only Manuals (IOM) define services that cannot be reported with radiation oncology procedures. Edits based on these requirements bundle specific CPT codes for certain types of services into all radiation therapy procedures: tattooing, burn treatment, venipuncture or catheter introduction, urinary bladder catheterization, intravenous infusion, psychotherapy, pharmacologic management, medical nutrition therapy, anesthesia, moderate conscious sedation, regional hypothermia, evaluation and management.

77261 Therapeutic radiology treatment planning; simple B

RVU			Global Days	Modifiers				
Mod	Non-Fac Total	Fac Total		51	50	62	80	MUE
	2.14	2.14	XXX	0	0	0	0	1

AMA: Fall 91: 12, 15, Oct 97: 2, Oct 10: 3

77262 Therapeutic radiology treatment planning; intermediate B

RVU			Global Days	Modifiers				
Mod	Non-Fac Total	Fac Total		51	50	62	80	MUE
	3.20	3.20	XXX	0	0	0	0	1

AMA: Fall 91: 12, 15, Oct 97: 2, Apr 09: 3, Nov 09: 6, Oct 10: 3

77263 Therapeutic radiology treatment planning; complex B

RVU			Global Days	Modifiers				
Mod	Non-Fac Total	Fac Total		51	50	62	80	MUE
	4.68	4.68	XXX	0	0	0	0	1

AMA: Fall 91: 15, Oct 97: 2, Apr 09: 3, Nov 09: 6, Oct 10: 3

77280 Therapeutic radiology simulation-aided field setting; simple Z2 S

RVU			Global Days	Modifiers				
Mod	Non-Fac Total	Fac Total		51	50	62	80	MUE
	7.71	7.71	XXX	0	0	0	0	2
26	1.02	1.02	XXX	0	0	0	0	2
TC	6.69	6.69	XXX	0	0	0	0	2

AMA: Fall 91: 15, Oct 97: 2, Nov 97: 26, Apr 09: 10, Nov 09: 6, Oct 10: 3, Nov 13: 11, Apr 15: 11

77285 Therapeutic radiology simulation-aided field setting; intermediate Z2 S

RVU			Global Days	Modifiers				
Mod	Non-Fac Total	Fac Total		51	50	62	80	MUE
	12.16	12.16	XXX	0	0	0	0	1
26	1.54	1.54	XXX	0	0	0	0	1
TC	10.62	10.62	XXX	0	0	0	0	1

AMA: Fall 91: 15, Oct 97: 3, Nov 09: 6, Oct 10: 3, Apr 15: 11

77290 Therapeutic radiology simulation-aided field setting; complex Z2 S

RVU			Global Days	Modifiers				
Mod	Non-Fac Total	Fac Total		51	50	62	80	MUE
	14.52	14.52	XXX	0	0	0	0	1
26	2.28	2.28	XXX	0	0	0	0	1
TC	12.24	12.24	XXX	0	0	0	0	1

AMA: Fall 91: 12, 15, Oct 97: 3, Apr 09: 3, 10, Nov 09: 6, Oct 10: 3, Nov 13: 11, Apr 15: 11

+ 77293 Respiratory motion management simulation (List separately in addition to code for primary procedure) N

RVU			Global Days	Modifiers				
Mod	Non-Fac Total	Fac Total		51	50	62	80	MUE
	13.14	13.14	ZZZ	0	0	0	0	1
26	2.92	2.92	ZZZ	0	0	0	0	1
TC	10.22	10.22	ZZZ	0	0	0	0	1

AMA: Nov 13: 11

77295 3-dimensional radiotherapy plan, including dose-volume histograms Z3 S

Coding tip: *Code 77295 is listed out of numerical order in CPT. Related codes for medical radiation physics, dosimetry, treatment devices, and special services 77300-77370*

RVU			Global Days	Modifiers				
Mod	Non-Fac Total	Fac Total		51	50	62	80	MUE
	13.83	13.83	XXX	0	0	0	0	1
26	6.26	6.26	XXX	0	0	0	0	1
TC	7.57	7.57	XXX	0	0	0	0	1

AMA: Fall 91: 15, Oct 97: 3, Nov 97: 26, May 05: 7, Oct 07: 1, Nov 09: 3, Oct 10: 3, Nov 13: 11, Jun 15: 6

● New   ▲ Revised   ✖ Deleted   ⊙ Moderate Sedation   ✚ Add-on Codes   ⊘ High Risk Denial   ⒶAge Edit   ♀ Female   ♂ Male   **AMA** *CPT® Assistant*   ***MUE*** Medically Unlikely Edit
⊘ Modifier 51 Exempt   ⊖ Modifier 63 Exempt   ⊠ Unlisted   **Modifiers:** *See Inside Back Cover*   Ⓜ Maternity   A2–Z3 ASC Payment Indicators   A–Y OPPS Status Indicators

656   CPT © 2015 American Medical Association. All Rights Reserved.   © 2016 DecisionHealth

77299 Unlisted procedure, therapeutic radiology clinical treatment planning   ✗ Z 2 S

Mod	Non-Fac Total	Fac Total	Global Days	51	50	62	80	MUE
	0.00	0.00	XXX	0	0	0	0	
26	0.00	0.00	XXX	0	0	0	0	
TC	0.00	0.00	XXX	0	0	0	0	

AMA: Oct 10: 3

Pub 100-04, 13, 120

Radiation Physics/Dosimetry/Treatment Devices/Special Services

77300 Basic radiation dosimetry calculation, central axis depth dose calculation, TDF, NSD, gap calculation, off axis factor, tissue inhomogeneity factors, calculation of non-ionizing radiation surface and depth dose, as required during course of treatment, only when prescribed by the treating physician   Z 3 S

Mod	Non-Fac Total	Fac Total	Global Days	51	50	62	80	MUE
	1.88	1.88	XXX	0	0	0	0	10
26	0.91	0.91	XXX	0	0	0	0	10
TC	0.97	0.97	XXX	0	0	0	0	10

AMA: Fall 91: 14, Oct 97: 3, Dec 08: 9, Nov 09: 3, Oct 10: 3

Pub 100-04, 13, 70.5

77301 Intensity modulated radiotherapy plan, including dose-volume histograms for target and critical structure partial tolerance specifications   Z 2 S

Mod	Non-Fac Total	Fac Total	Global Days	51	50	62	80	MUE
	55.09	55.09	XXX	0	0	0	0	1
26	11.65	11.65	XXX	0	0	0	0	1
TC	43.44	43.44	XXX	0	0	0	0	1

AMA: Mar 05: 1, 6, May 05: 7, Oct 07: 1, Nov 09: 3, Oct 10: 3, Nov 13: 11

77306 Teletherapy isodose plan; simple (1 or 2 unmodified ports directed to a single area of interest), includes basic dosimetry calculation(s)   Z 3 S

Mod	Non-Fac Total	Fac Total	Global Days	51	50	62	80	MUE
	4.21	4.21	XXX	0	0	0	0	1
26	2.04	2.04	XXX	0	0	0	0	1
TC	2.17	2.17	XXX	0	0	0	0	1

77307 Teletherapy isodose plan; complex (multiple treatment areas, tangential ports, the use of wedges, blocking, rotational beam, or special beam considerations), includes basic dosimetry calculation(s)   Z 3 S

Mod	Non-Fac Total	Fac Total	Global Days	51	50	62	80	MUE
	8.14	8.14	XXX	0	0	0	0	1
26	4.23	4.23	XXX	0	0	0	0	1
TC	3.91	3.91	XXX	0	0	0	0	1

77316 Brachytherapy isodose plan; simple (calculation[s] made from 1 to 4 sources, or remote afterloading brachytherapy, 1 channel), includes basic dosimetry calculation(s)   Z 2 S

Mod	Non-Fac Total	Fac Total	Global Days	51	50	62	80	MUE
	5.32	5.32	XXX	0	0	0	0	1
26	2.05	2.05	XXX	0	0	0	0	1
TC	3.27	3.27	XXX	0	0	0	0	1

77317 Brachytherapy isodose plan; intermediate (calculation[s] made from 5 to 10 sources, or remote afterloading brachytherapy, 2-12 channels), includes basic dosimetry calculation(s)   Z 3 S

Mod	Non-Fac Total	Fac Total	Global Days	51	50	62	80	MUE
	6.92	6.92	XXX	0	0	0	0	1
26	2.67	2.67	XXX	0	0	0	0	1
TC	4.25	4.25	XXX	0	0	0	0	1

77318 Brachytherapy isodose plan; complex (calculation[s] made from over 10 sources, or remote afterloading brachytherapy, over 12 channels), includes basic dosimetry calculation(s)   Z 2 S

Mod	Non-Fac Total	Fac Total	Global Days	51	50	62	80	MUE
	10.00	10.00	XXX	0	0	0	0	1
26	4.23	4.23	XXX	0	0	0	0	1
TC	5.77	5.77	XXX	0	0	0	0	1

77321 Special teletherapy port plan, particles, hemibody, total body   Z 3 S

Mod	Non-Fac Total	Fac Total	Global Days	51	50	62	80	MUE
	2.62	2.62	XXX	0	0	0	0	1
26	1.39	1.39	XXX	0	0	0	0	1
TC	1.23	1.23	XXX	0	0	0	0	1

AMA: Fall 91: 14, Oct 97: 4, Oct 10: 3

77331 Special dosimetry (eg, TLD, microdosimetry) (specify), only when prescribed by the treating physician   Z 3 S

Mod	Non-Fac Total	Fac Total	Global Days	51	50	62	80	MUE
	1.80	1.80	XXX	0	0	0	0	3
26	1.27	1.27	XXX	0	0	0	0	3
TC	0.53	0.53	XXX	0	0	0	0	3

AMA: Fall 91: 13, Oct 97: 4, Jun 15: 6

77332 Treatment devices, design and construction; simple (simple block, simple bolus)   Z 3 S

Mod	Non-Fac Total	Fac Total	Global Days	51	50	62	80	MUE
	2.35	2.35	XXX	0	0	0	0	4
26	0.80	0.80	XXX	0	0	0	0	4
TC	1.55	1.55	XXX	0	0	0	0	4

AMA: Oct 97: 4, Oct 10: 3

● New   ▲ Revised   Deleted   ⊙ Moderate Sedation   ✚ Add-on Codes   ⊘ High Risk Denial   Ⓐ Age Edit   ♀ Female   ♂ Male   **AMA** *CPT® Assistant*   **MUE** Medically Unlikely Edit
⊘ Modifier 51 Exempt   ⊖ Modifier 63 Exempt   ✗ Unlisted   **Modifiers:** *See Inside Back Cover*   Ⓜ Maternity   A 2 – Z 3 ASC Payment Indicators   A – Y OPPS Status Indicators

© 2016 DecisionHealth   CPT © 2015 American Medical Association. All Rights Reserved.

Radiology Procedures

77333 – 77387

77333 Treatment devices, design and construction; intermediate (multiple blocks, stents, bite blocks, special bolus) Z3 S

Mod	Non-Fac Total	Fac Total	Global Days	51	50	62	80	MUE
TC	0.27	0.27	XXX	0	0	0	0	2
	1.50	1.50	XXX	0	0	0	0	2
26	1.23	1.23	XXX	0	0	0	0	2

AMA: Oct 97: 3, Oct 10: 3

77334 Treatment devices, design and construction; complex (irregular blocks, special shields, compensators, wedges, molds or casts) Z3 S

Mod	Non-Fac Total	Fac Total	Global Days	51	50	62	80	MUE
	4.30	4.30	XXX	0	0	0	0	10
26	1.81	1.81	XXX	0	0	0	0	10
TC	2.49	2.49	XXX	0	0	0	0	10

AMA: Fall 91: 14, Oct 97: 4, Dec 08: 9, Nov 09: 3, Oct 10: 3, Dec 10: 15

Coding Guidance

Continuing medical physics consultation may be reported after every 5 radiation treatments per week of therapy. Report 77336 even if less than 5 treatments are completed. Planning for therapeutic radiology treatment (77261-77334) is generally performed before treatment begins. Radiation planning procedures may sometimes need to be repeated during treatment. Modifier 59 can be appended to 77336 when the planning procedure and the continuing medical physics consultation are done on the same day.

77336 Continuing medical physics consultation, including assessment of treatment parameters, quality assurance of dose delivery, and review of patient treatment documentation in support of the radiation oncologist, reported per week of therapy Z2 S

Mod	Non-Fac Total	Fac Total	Global Days	51	50	62	80	MUE
	2.24	2.24	XXX	0	0	0	0	1

AMA: Fall 91: 15, Oct 97: 4, Nov 98: 21, Oct 10: 3

Pub 100-04, 13, 70.5

77338 Multi-leaf collimator (MLC) device(s) for intensity modulated radiation therapy (IMRT), design and construction per IMRT plan Z2 S

Mod	Non-Fac Total	Fac Total	Global Days	51	50	62	80	MUE
	14.32	14.32	XXX	0	0	0	0	1
26	6.26	6.26	XXX	0	0	0	0	1
TC	8.06	8.06	XXX	0	0	0	0	1

AMA: Oct 10: 3, Dec 10: 15

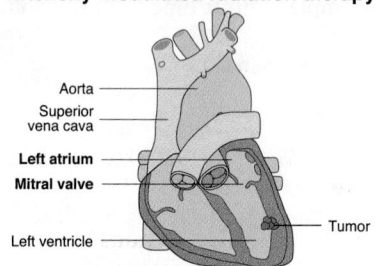

Multi-leaf collimator (MLC) device(s) for intensity modulated radiation therapy

Aorta
Superior vena cava
Left atrium
Mitral valve
Left ventricle
Tumor

Cross-section of heart

The multi-leaf collimator (MLC) device was originally used during radiation therapy as a replacement for conventional alloy block shaping to direct the radiation beam to the tumor and protect surrounding structures.

77370 Special medical radiation physics consultation Z2 S

Mod	Non-Fac Total	Fac Total	Global Days	51	50	62	80	MUE
	3.43	3.43	XXX	0	0	0	0	1

AMA: Fall 91: 14, Oct 97: 4, May 09: 8, Oct 10: 3, Jun 15: 6

Pub 100-04, 13, 70.5

Stereotactic Radiation Treatment

⊙ **77371** Radiation treatment delivery, stereotactic radiosurgery (SRS), complete course of treatment of cranial lesion(s) consisting of 1 session; multi-source Cobalt 60 based J1

Mod	Non-Fac Total	Fac Total	Global Days	51	50	62	80	MUE
	0.00	0.00	XXX	0	0	0	0	1

AMA: Mar 07: 7, Oct 07: 1, Jul 11: 12, Oct 10: 3, Jul 14: 9

77372 Radiation treatment delivery, stereotactic radiosurgery (SRS), complete course of treatment of cranial lesion(s) consisting of 1 session; linear accelerator based J1

Mod	Non-Fac Total	Fac Total	Global Days	51	50	62	80	MUE
	30.25	30.25	XXX	0	0	0	0	1

AMA: Mar 07: 7, Oct 07: 1, Jul 11: 12, Oct 10: 3

77373 Stereotactic body radiation therapy, treatment delivery, per fraction to 1 or more lesions, including image guidance, entire course not to exceed 5 fractions S

Mod	Non-Fac Total	Fac Total	Global Days	51	50	62	80	MUE
	38.44	38.44	XXX	0	0	0	0	1

AMA: Mar 07: 7, Oct 07: 1, Jul 11: 12, Oct 10: 3, Jul 14: 9, Jun 15: 6

77385 Intensity modulated radiation treatment delivery (IMRT), includes guidance and tracking, when performed; simple Z2 S

Mod	Non-Fac Total	Fac Total	Global Days	51	50	62	80	MUE
	0.00	0.00	XXX	0	0	0		

77386 Intensity modulated radiation treatment delivery (IMRT), includes guidance and tracking, when performed; complex Z2 S

Mod	Non-Fac Total	Fac Total	Global Days	51	50	62	80	MUE
	0.00	0.00	XXX	0	0	0		

77387 Guidance for localization of target volume for delivery of radiation treatment delivery, includes intrafraction tracking, when performed N1 N

Mod	Non-Fac Total	Fac Total	Global Days	51	50	62	80	MUE
	0.00	0.00	XXX	0	0	0		

● New   ▲ Revised   ✖ Deleted   ⊙ Moderate Sedation   ✚ Add-on Codes   ⊗ High Risk Denial   Ⓐ Age Edit   ♀ Female   ♂ Male   **AMA** *CPT® Assistant*   *MUE* Medically Unlikely Edit
⊘ Modifier 51 Exempt   ⊖ Modifier 63 Exempt   ✗ Unlisted   **Modifiers:** *See Inside Back Cover*   Ⓜ Maternity   A2–Z3 ASC Payment Indicators   A–Y OPPS Status Indicators

658   CPT © 2015 American Medical Association. All Rights Reserved.   © 2016 DecisionHealth

Other Radiation Physics/Dosimetry/Treatment Devices/Special Services Procedures

77399 Unlisted procedure, medical radiation physics, dosimetry and treatment devices, and special services ⊙✗Z2S

RVU			Global Days	Modifiers				
Mod	Non-Fac Total	Fac Total		51	50	62	80	MUE
	0.00	0.00	XXX	0	0	0	0	
26	0.00	0.00	XXX	0	0	0	0	
TC	0.00	0.00	XXX	0	0	0	0	

AMA: Nov 98: 21, Oct 10: 3
Pub 100-04, 13, 70.5, 120

Radiation Treatment Delivery

77401 Radiation treatment delivery, superficial and/or ortho voltage, per day Z3S

RVU			Global Days	Modifiers				
Mod	Non-Fac Total	Fac Total		51	50	62	80	MUE
	0.69	0.69	XXX	0	0	0	0	1

AMA: Apr 03: 14, Aug 03: 10, Oct 07: 1, Oct 10: 3
Pub 100-04, 13, 70.1, 70.3

77402 Radiation treatment delivery, >1 MeV; simple Z2S

RVU			Global Days	Modifiers				
Mod	Non-Fac Total	Fac Total		51	50	62	80	MUE
	0.00	0.00	XXX	0	0	0	0	2
	0.00	0.00	XXX	0	0	0	0	2

AMA: Apr 03: 14, Aug 03: 10, Oct 07: 1, Oct 10: 3
Pub 100-04, 13, 70.1, 70.3

77407 Radiation treatment delivery, >1 MeV; intermediate Z2S

RVU			Global Days	Modifiers				
Mod	Non-Fac Total	Fac Total		51	50	62	80	MUE
	0.00	0.00	XXX	0	0	0	0	2
	0.00	0.00	XXX	0	0	0	0	2

AMA: Apr 03: 14, Aug 03: 10, Oct 07: 1
Pub 100-04, 13, 70.1, 70.3

77412 Radiation treatment delivery, >1 MeV; complex Z2S

RVU			Global Days	Modifiers				
Mod	Non-Fac Total	Fac Total		51	50	62	80	MUE
	0.00	0.00	XXX	0	0	0	0	2

AMA: Apr 03: 14, Aug 03: 10, Oct 07: 1
Pub 100-04, 13, 70.3

▲ **77417** Therapeutic radiology port image(s) N1N

RVU			Global Days	Modifiers				
Mod	Non-Fac Total	Fac Total		51	50	62	80	MUE
	0.31	0.31	XXX	0	0	0	0	1

AMA: Fall 91: 14, Dec 97: 11, Feb 06: 14, Oct 07: 1
Pub 100-04, 13, 70.3

Neutron Beam Treatment Delivery

77422 High energy neutron radiation treatment delivery; single treatment area using a single port or parallel-opposed ports with no blocks or simple blocking Z3S

RVU			Global Days	Modifiers				
Mod	Non-Fac Total	Fac Total		51	50	62	80	MUE
	0.00	0.00	XXX	0	0	0	0	1

77423 High energy neutron radiation treatment delivery; 1 or more isocenter(s) with coplanar or non-coplanar geometry with blocking and/or wedge, and/or compensator(s) Z3S

RVU			Global Days	Modifiers				
Mod	Non-Fac Total	Fac Total		51	50	62	80	MUE
	0.00	0.00	XXX	0	0	0	0	1

77424 Intraoperative radiation treatment delivery, x-ray, single treatment session Z2J1

RVU			Global Days	Modifiers				
Mod	Non-Fac Total	Fac Total		51	50	62	80	MUE
	0.00	0.00	XXX	9	9	9	9	1

77425 Intraoperative radiation treatment delivery, electrons, single treatment session ⊙Z2J1

RVU			Global Days	Modifiers				
Mod	Non-Fac Total	Fac Total		51	50	62	80	MUE
	0.00	0.00	XXX	9	9	9	9	1

Pub 100-04, 13, 70.1

Radiation Treatment Management

77427 Radiation treatment management, 5 treatments B

RVU			Global Days	Modifiers				
Mod	Non-Fac Total	Fac Total		51	50	62	80	MUE
	5.24	5.24	XXX	9	9	9	9	1

AMA: Nov 99: 42, Feb 00: 7, Oct 07: 1, Nov 09: 6, Jun 15: 6
Pub 100-04, 12, 30; 100-04, 13, 70.1

77431 Radiation therapy management with complete course of therapy consisting of 1 or 2 fractions only B

RVU			Global Days	Modifiers				
Mod	Non-Fac Total	Fac Total		51	50	62	80	MUE
	2.88	2.88	XXX	0	0	0	0	1

AMA: Winter 90: 10, Oct 97: 4, Nov 09: 6
Pub 100-04, 13, 70.1

77432 Stereotactic radiation treatment management of cranial lesion(s) (complete course of treatment consisting of 1 session) B

RVU			Global Days	Modifiers				
Mod	Non-Fac Total	Fac Total		51	50	62	80	MUE
	11.79	11.79	XXX	0	0	0	0	1

AMA: Oct 97: 4, Nov 09: 6, Jul 11: 12, Jul 14: 9

77435 Stereotactic body radiation therapy, treatment management, per treatment course, to 1 or more lesions, including image guidance, entire course not to exceed 5 fractions N1N

RVU			Global Days	Modifiers				
Mod	Non-Fac Total	Fac Total		51	50	62	80	MUE
	17.79	17.79	XXX	0	0	0	0	1

AMA: Mar 07: 7, Oct 07: 1, Nov 09: 6, Jun 15: 6

● New   ▲ Revised   Deleted   ⊙ Moderate Sedation   ✚ Add-on Codes   ⊘ High Risk Denial   Ⓐ Age Edit   ♀ Female   ♂ Male   **AMA** *CPT® Assistant*   **MUE** Medically Unlikely Edit
⊘ Modifier 51 Exempt   ⊖ Modifier 63 Exempt   ✗ Unlisted   **Modifiers:** *See Inside Back Cover*   Ⓜ Maternity   A2–Z3 ASC Payment Indicators   A–Y OPPS Status Indicators

© 2016 DecisionHealth   CPT © 2015 American Medical Association. All Rights Reserved.   **659**

Radiology Procedures

77469 – 77762

77469 Intraoperative radiation treatment management   B

Mod	Non-Fac Total	Fac Total	Global Days	51	50	62	80	MUE
	9.09	9.09	XXX	0	0	0	0	1

77470 Special treatment procedure (eg, total body irradiation, hemibody radiation, per oral or endocavitary irradiation)   Z3 S

Mod	Non-Fac Total	Fac Total	Global Days	51	50	62	80	MUE
	4.41	4.41	XXX	0	0	0	0	1
26	3.05	3.05	XXX	0	0	0	0	1
TC	1.36	1.36	XXX	0	0	0	0	1

AMA: Winter 91: 22, Oct 97: 1, Apr 09: 3

77499 Unlisted procedure, therapeutic radiology treatment management   ⊘x B

Mod	Non-Fac Total	Fac Total	Global Days	51	50	62	80	MUE
	0.00	0.00	XXX	0	0	0	0	
26	0.00	0.00	XXX	0	0	0	0	
TC	0.00	0.00	XXX	0	0	0	0	

AMA: Nov 99: 42, Feb 00: 7, Nov 09: 6, Jun 15: 6

Pub 100-04, 13, 120

Proton Beam Treatment Delivery

77520 Proton treatment delivery; simple, without compensation   Z2 S

Mod	Non-Fac Total	Fac Total	Global Days	51	50	62	80	MUE
	0.00	0.00	XXX	0	0	0	0	1

AMA: Nov 99: 43

77522 Proton treatment delivery; simple, with compensation   Z2 S

Mod	Non-Fac Total	Fac Total	Global Days	51	50	62	80	MUE
	0.00	0.00	XXX	0	0	0	0	1

77523 Proton treatment delivery; intermediate   Z2 S

Mod	Non-Fac Total	Fac Total	Global Days	51	50	62	80	MUE
	0.00	0.00	XXX	0	0	0	0	1

AMA: Nov 99: 43

77525 Proton treatment delivery; complex   Z2 S

Mod	Non-Fac Total	Fac Total	Global Days	51	50	62	80	MUE
	0.00	0.00	XXX	0	0	0	0	1

Hyperthermia Procedures

⊙ 77600 Hyperthermia, externally generated; superficial (ie, heating to a depth of 4 cm or less)   Z2 S

Mod	Non-Fac Total	Fac Total	Global Days	51	50	62	80	MUE
	11.88	11.88	XXX	0	0	0	0	1
26	2.32	2.32	XXX	0	0	0	0	1
TC	9.56	9.56	XXX	0	0	0	0	1

AMA: Winter 91: 22, Dec 13: 17

⊙ 77605 Hyperthermia, externally generated; deep (ie, heating to depths greater than 4 cm)   Z2 S

Mod	Non-Fac Total	Fac Total	Global Days	51	50	62	80	MUE
	22.58	22.58	XXX	0	0	0	0	1
26	3.29	3.29	XXX	0	0	0	0	1
TC	19.29	19.29	XXX	0	0	0	0	1

AMA: Winter 91: 22, Dec 13: 17

⊙ 77610 Hyperthermia generated by interstitial probe(s); 5 or fewer interstitial applicators   Z2 S

Mod	Non-Fac Total	Fac Total	Global Days	51	50	62	80	MUE
	28.05	28.05	XXX	0	0	0	0	1
26	2.44	2.44	XXX	0	0	0	0	1
TC	25.61	25.61	XXX	0	0	0	0	1

AMA: Winter 91: 22

⊙ 77615 Hyperthermia generated by interstitial probe(s); more than 5 interstitial applicators   ⊘ Z2 S

Mod	Non-Fac Total	Fac Total	Global Days	51	50	62	80	MUE
	29.98	29.98	XXX	0	0	0	0	1
26	3.04	3.04	XXX	0	0	0	0	1
TC	26.94	26.94	XXX	0	0	0	0	1

AMA: Winter 91: 22

Intracavitary Hyperthermia Procedures

77620 Hyperthermia generated by intracavitary probe(s)   Z2 S

Mod	Non-Fac Total	Fac Total	Global Days	51	50	62	80	MUE
	10.82	10.82	XXX	0	0	0	0	1
26	2.28	2.28	XXX	0	0	0	0	1
TC	8.54	8.54	XXX	0	0	0	0	1

AMA: Winter 91: 22, Dec 13: 17

Brachytherapy Procedures

77750 Infusion or instillation of radioelement solution (includes 3-month follow-up care)   Z2 S

Mod	Non-Fac Total	Fac Total	Global Days	51	50	62	80	MUE
	10.47	10.47	090	0	0	0	0	1
26	7.28	7.28	090	0	0	0	0	1
TC	3.19	3.19	090	0	0	0	0	1

AMA: Sep 05: 1

77761 Intracavitary radiation source application; simple   Z3 S

Mod	Non-Fac Total	Fac Total	Global Days	51	50	62	80	MUE
	10.98	10.98	090	0	0	0	0	1
26	5.55	5.55	090	0	0	0	0	1
TC	5.43	5.43	090	0	0	0	0	1

AMA: Winter 91: 23, Jan 96: 7, Mar 99: 3, Feb 02: 7, Sep 05: 1

77762 Intracavitary radiation source application; intermediate   Z3 S

Mod	Non-Fac Total	Fac Total	Global Days	51	50	62	80	MUE
	14.61	14.61	090	0	0	0	0	1
26	8.38	8.38	090	0	0	0	0	1
TC	6.23	6.23	090	0	0	0	0	1

AMA: Winter 91: 23, Feb 02: 7, Sep 05: 1

● New   ▲ Revised   ✖ Deleted   ⊙ Moderate Sedation   ✚ Add-on Codes   ⊘ High Risk Denial   Ⓐ Age Edit   ♀ Female   ♂ Male   **AMA** *CPT® Assistant*   **MUE** Medically Unlikely Edit
⊘ Modifier 51 Exempt   ⊖ Modifier 63 Exempt   ✗ Unlisted   **Modifiers:** *See Inside Back Cover*   Ⓜ Maternity   A2–Z3 ASC Payment Indicators   A–Y OPPS Status Indicators

77763 Intracavitary radiation source application; complex `Z3 S`

Mod	Non-Fac Total	Fac Total	Global Days	51	50	62	80	MUE
	20.69	20.69	090	0	0	0	0	1
26	12.63	12.63	090	0	0	0	0	1
TC	8.06	8.06	090	0	0	0	0	1

AMA: Winter 91: 23, Mar 99: 3, Feb 02: 7, Sep 05: 1

● **77767 Remote afterloading high dose rate radionuclide skin surface brachytherapy, includes basic dosimetry, when performed; lesion diameter up to 2.0 cm or 1 channel** `Z2 S`

Mod	Non-Fac Total	Fac Total	Global Days	51	50	62	80	MUE
	6.34	6.34	XXX	0	0	0	0	2
26	1.54	1.54	XXX	0	0	0	0	2
TC	4.80	4.80	XXX	0	0	0	0	2

● **77768 Remote afterloading high dose rate radionuclide skin surface brachytherapy, includes basic dosimetry, when performed; lesion diameter over 2.0 cm and 2 or more channels, or multiple lesions** `Z2 S`

Mod	Non-Fac Total	Fac Total	Global Days	51	50	62	80	MUE
	9.93	9.93	XXX	0	0	0	0	2
26	2.04	2.04	XXX	0	0	0	0	2
TC	7.89	7.89	XXX	0	0	0	0	2

● **77770 Remote afterloading high dose rate radionuclide interstitial or intracavitary brachytherapy, includes basic dosimetry, when performed; 1 channel** `Z2 S`

Mod	Non-Fac Total	Fac Total	Global Days	51	50	62	80	MUE
	9.05	9.05	XXX	0	0	0	0	2
26	2.84	2.84	XXX	0	0	0	0	2
TC	6.21	6.21	XXX	0	0	0	0	2

● **77771 Remote afterloading high dose rate radionuclide interstitial or intracavitary brachytherapy, includes basic dosimetry, when performed; 2-12 channels** `Z2 S`

Mod	Non-Fac Total	Fac Total	Global Days	51	50	62	80	MUE
	16.86	16.86	XXX	0	0	0	0	2
26	5.55	5.55	XXX	0	0	0	0	2
TC	11.31	11.31	XXX	0	0	0	0	2

● **77772 Remote afterloading high dose rate radionuclide interstitial or intracavitary brachytherapy, includes basic dosimetry, when performed; over 12 channels** `Z2 S`

Mod	Non-Fac Total	Fac Total	Global Days	51	50	62	80	MUE
	25.72	25.72	XXX	0	0	0	0	2
26	7.87	7.87	XXX	0	0	0	0	2
TC	17.85	17.85	XXX	0	0	0	0	2

✖ 77776 Interstitial radiation source application; simple

✖ 77777 Interstitial radiation source application; intermediate

▲ **77778 Interstitial radiation source application, complex, includes supervision, handling, loading of radiation source, when performed** `Z3 Q3`

Mod	Non-Fac Total	Fac Total	Global Days	51	50	62	80	MUE
	22.01	22.01	000	0	0	0	0	1
26	11.63	11.63	000	0	0	0	0	1
TC	10.38	10.38	000	0	0	0	0	1

AMA: Winter 91: 23, Apr 04: 6, Sep 05: 1, May 07: 1

✖ 77785 Remote afterloading high dose rate radionuclide brachytherapy; 1 channel

✖ 77786 Remote afterloading high dose rate radionuclide brachytherapy; 2-12 channels

✖ 77787 Remote afterloading high dose rate radionuclide brachytherapy; over 12 channels

▲ **77789 Surface application of low dose rate radionuclide source** `Z3 S`

Mod	Non-Fac Total	Fac Total	Global Days	51	50	62	80	MUE
	3.39	3.39	000	0	0	0	0	2
26	1.68	1.68	000	0	0	0	0	2
TC	1.71	1.71	000	0	0	0	0	2

AMA: Sep 05: 1

Coding Guidance

Supervision, handling, and loading of the radiation source is inherent in all remote afterloading brachytherapy codes. Code 77790 is therefore not to be used in conjunction with 77785-77787.

77790 Supervision, handling, loading of radiation source `N IN`

Mod	Non-Fac Total	Fac Total	Global Days	51	50	62	80	MUE
	0.42	0.42	XXX	0	0	0	0	1

AMA: Sep 05: 1

77799 Unlisted procedure, clinical brachytherapy ⊗✖`Z2 S`

Mod	Non-Fac Total	Fac Total	Global Days	51	50	62	80	MUE
	0.00	0.00	XXX	0	0	0	0	
26	0.00	0.00	XXX	0	0	0	0	
TC	0.00	0.00	XXX	0	0	0	0	

AMA: Sep 05: 1
Pub 100-04, 13, 120

78012 Thyroid uptake, single or multiple quantitative measurement(s) (including stimulation, suppression, or discharge, when performed) `Z2 S`

Mod	Non-Fac Total	Fac Total	Global Days	51	50	62	80	MUE
	2.30	2.30	XXX	0	0	0	0	1
26	0.27	0.27	XXX	0	0	0	0	1
TC	2.03	2.03	XXX	0	0	0	0	1

AMA: Jun 13: 9

78013 Thyroid imaging (including vascular flow, when performed) `Z2 S`

Mod	Non-Fac Total	Fac Total	Global Days	51	50	62	80	MUE
	5.54	5.54	XXX	0	0	0	0	1
26	0.52	0.52	XXX	0	0	0	0	1
TC	5.02	5.02	XXX	0	0	0	0	1

AMA: Jun 13: 9

● New   ▲ Revised   Deleted   ⊙ Moderate Sedation   ✚ Add-on Codes   ⊗ High Risk Denial   ⒶAge Edit   ♀ Female   ♂ Male   **AMA** CPT® Assistant   **MUE** Medically Unlikely Edit
⊘ Modifier 51 Exempt   ⊖ Modifier 63 Exempt   ✖ Unlisted   **Modifiers:** See Inside Back Cover   Ⓜ Maternity   `A2`–`Z3` ASC Payment Indicators   `A`–`Y` OPPS Status Indicators

Radiology Procedures

78014 – 78075

78014 Thyroid imaging (including vascular flow, when performed); with single or multiple uptake(s) quantitative measurement(s) (including stimulation, suppression, or discharge, when performed) Z 2 S

	RVU		Global Days	Modifiers				
Mod	Non-Fac Total	Fac Total		51	50	62	80	MUE
	7.02	7.02	XXX	0	0	0	0	1
26	0.70	0.70	XXX	0	0	0	0	1
TC	6.32	6.32	XXX	0	0	0	0	1

AMA: Jun 13: 9

Coding Guidance
For supply of contrast material, refer to HCPCS Level II codes A9512, A9516, A9528-A9531.

78015 Thyroid carcinoma metastases imaging; limited area (eg, neck and chest only) Z 2 S

	RVU		Global Days	Modifiers				
Mod	Non-Fac Total	Fac Total		51	50	62	80	MUE
	6.40	6.40	XXX	0	0	0	0	1
26	0.93	0.93	XXX	0	0	0	0	1
TC	5.47	5.47	XXX	0	0	0	0	1

AMA: Nov 98: 21, Jan 07: 31

78016 Thyroid carcinoma metastases imaging; with additional studies (eg, urinary recovery) Z 2 S

	RVU		Global Days	Modifiers				
Mod	Non-Fac Total	Fac Total		51	50	62	80	MUE
	8.10	8.10	XXX	0	0	0	0	1
26	0.97	0.97	XXX	0	0	0	0	1
TC	7.13	7.13	XXX	0	0	0	0	1

AMA: Jan 07: 31

78018 Thyroid carcinoma metastases imaging; whole body Z 2 S

Coding tip: *Add uptake when performed - 78020*

	RVU		Global Days	Modifiers				
Mod	Non-Fac Total	Fac Total		51	50	62	80	MUE
	9.07	9.07	XXX	0	0	0	0	1
26	1.17	1.17	XXX	0	0	0	0	1
TC	7.90	7.90	XXX	0	0	0	0	1

AMA: Apr 99: 4, Jan 07: 31

+ 78020 Thyroid carcinoma metastases uptake (List separately in addition to code for primary procedure) N I N

	RVU		Global Days	Modifiers				
Mod	Non-Fac Total	Fac Total		51	50	62	80	MUE
TC	1.63	1.63	ZZZ	0	0	0	0	1
	2.42	2.42	ZZZ	0	0	0	0	1
26	0.79	0.79	ZZZ	0	0	0	0	1

AMA: Nov 98: 21, Apr 99: 4, Jan 07: 31

Coding Guidance
For supply of contrast material, refer to HCPCS Level II code A9505.

78070 Parathyroid planar imaging (including subtraction, when performed) Z 2 S

	RVU		Global Days	Modifiers				
Mod	Non-Fac Total	Fac Total		51	50	62	80	MUE
	8.70	8.70	XXX	0	0	0	0	1
26	1.11	1.11	XXX	0	0	0	0	1
TC	7.59	7.59	XXX	0	0	0	0	1

AMA: Jan 07: 31

Pub 100-04, 16, 120.2

78071 Parathyroid planar imaging (including subtraction, when performed); with tomographic (SPECT) Z 2 S

	RVU		Global Days	Modifiers				
Mod	Non-Fac Total	Fac Total		51	50	62	80	MUE
	10.40	10.40	XXX	0	0	0	0	1
26	1.66	1.66	XXX	0	0	0	0	1
TC	8.74	8.74	XXX	0	0	0	0	1

78072 Parathyroid planar imaging (including subtraction, when performed); with tomographic (SPECT), and concurrently acquired computed tomography (CT) for anatomical localization Z 2 S

	RVU		Global Days	Modifiers				
Mod	Non-Fac Total	Fac Total		51	50	62	80	MUE
	12.01	12.01	XXX	0	0	0	0	1
26	2.18	2.18	XXX	0	0	0	0	1
TC	9.83	9.83	XXX	0	0	0	0	1

Coding Guidance
For supply of contrast material, refer to HCPCS Level II code A9508.

78075 Adrenal imaging, cortex and/or medulla Z 2 S

	RVU		Global Days	Modifiers				
Mod	Non-Fac Total	Fac Total		51	50	62	80	MUE
	12.43	12.43	XXX	0	0	0	0	1
26	1.00	1.00	XXX	0	0	0	0	1
TC	11.43	11.43	XXX	0	0	0	0	1

AMA: Jan 07: 31, Feb 12: 9

● New   ▲ Revised   ✖ Deleted   ⊙ Moderate Sedation   ✚ Add-on Codes   ⊘ High Risk Denial   Ⓐ Age Edit   ♀ Female   ♂ Male   **AMA** *CPT® Assistant*   **MUE** Medically Unlikely Edit
⊘ Modifier 51 Exempt   ⊖ Modifier 63 Exempt   ✗ Unlisted   **Modifiers:** *See Inside Back Cover*   Ⓜ Maternity   A 2 – Z 3 ASC Payment Indicators   A – Y OPPS Status Indicators

662   CPT © 2015 American Medical Association. All Rights Reserved.   © 2016 DecisionHealth

78099 Unlisted endocrine procedure, diagnostic nuclear medicine ✗ Z 2 S

Mod	RVU Non-Fac Total	Fac Total	Global Days	Modifiers 51	50	62	80	MUE
TC	0.00	0.00	XXX	0	0	0	0	
	0.00	0.00	XXX	0	0	0	0	
26	0.00	0.00	XXX	0	0	0	0	

AMA: Dec 05: 7, Jan 07: 31

Pub 100-04, 13, 120

Hematopoietic/Reticuloendothelial/Lymphatic System Procedures

Coding Guidance

For supply of contrast material, refer to HCPCS Level II code A9541.

78102 Bone marrow imaging; limited area Z 2 S

Mod	RVU Non-Fac Total	Fac Total	Global Days	Modifiers 51	50	62	80	MUE
	4.92	4.92	XXX	0	0	0	0	1
26	0.75	0.75	XXX	0	0	0	0	1
TC	4.17	4.17	XXX	0	0	0	0	1

AMA: Dec 05: 7, Feb 12: 9

78103 Bone marrow imaging; multiple areas Z 2 S

Mod	RVU Non-Fac Total	Fac Total	Global Days	Modifiers 51	50	62	80	MUE
	6.46	6.46	XXX	0	0	0	0	1
26	1.03	1.03	XXX	0	0	0	0	1
TC	5.43	5.43	XXX	0	0	0	0	1

78104 Bone marrow imaging; whole body Z 2 S

Mod	RVU Non-Fac Total	Fac Total	Global Days	Modifiers 51	50	62	80	MUE
	7.12	7.12	XXX	0	0	0	0	1
26	1.09	1.09	XXX	0	0	0	0	1
TC	6.03	6.03	XXX	0	0	0	0	1

78110 Plasma volume, radiopharmaceutical volume-dilution technique (separate procedure); single sampling ⊘ Z 2 S

Mod	RVU Non-Fac Total	Fac Total	Global Days	Modifiers 51	50	62	80	MUE
	2.72	2.72	XXX	0	0	0	0	1
26	0.27	0.27	XXX	0	0	0	0	1
TC	2.45	2.45	XXX	0	0	0	0	1

78111 Plasma volume, radiopharmaceutical volume-dilution technique (separate procedure); multiple samplings Z 2 S

Mod	RVU Non-Fac Total	Fac Total	Global Days	Modifiers 51	50	62	80	MUE
	2.79	2.79	XXX	0	0	0	0	1
26	0.31	0.31	XXX	0	0	0	0	1
TC	2.48	2.48	XXX	0	0	0	0	1

Coding Guidance

For supply of contrast material, refer to HCPCS Level II codes A9532 and A9553.

78120 Red cell volume determination (separate procedure); single sampling ⊘ Z 2 S

Mod	RVU Non-Fac Total	Fac Total	Global Days	Modifiers 51	50	62	80	MUE
	2.72	2.72	XXX	0	0	0	0	1
26	0.33	0.33	XXX	0	0	0	0	1
TC	2.39	2.39	XXX	0	0	0	0	1

78121 Red cell volume determination (separate procedure); multiple samplings ⊘ Z 2 S

Mod	RVU Non-Fac Total	Fac Total	Global Days	Modifiers 51	50	62	80	MUE
	2.96	2.96	XXX	0	0	0	0	1
26	0.46	0.46	XXX	0	0	0	0	1
TC	2.50	2.50	XXX	0	0	0	0	1

78122 Whole blood volume determination, including separate measurement of plasma volume and red cell volume (radiopharmaceutical volume-dilution technique) Z 2 S

Mod	RVU Non-Fac Total	Fac Total	Global Days	Modifiers 51	50	62	80	MUE
	2.84	2.84	XXX	0	0	0	0	1
26	0.61	0.61	XXX	0	0	0	0	1
TC	2.23	2.23	XXX	0	0	0	0	1

78130 Red cell survival study Z 2 S

Mod	RVU Non-Fac Total	Fac Total	Global Days	Modifiers 51	50	62	80	MUE
	4.89	4.89	XXX	0	0	0	0	1
26	0.86	0.86	XXX	0	0	0	0	1
TC	4.03	4.03	XXX	0	0	0	0	1

78135 Red cell survival study; differential organ/tissue kinetics (eg, splenic and/or hepatic sequestration) Z 2 S

Mod	RVU Non-Fac Total	Fac Total	Global Days	Modifiers 51	50	62	80	MUE
	10.25	10.25	XXX	0	0	0	0	1
26	0.91	0.91	XXX	0	0	0	0	1
TC	9.34	9.34	XXX	0	0	0	0	1

78140 Labeled red cell sequestration, differential organ/tissue (eg, splenic and/or hepatic) Z 2 S

Mod	RVU Non-Fac Total	Fac Total	Global Days	Modifiers 51	50	62	80	MUE
	3.95	3.95	XXX	0	0	0	0	1
26	0.87	0.87	XXX	0	0	0	0	1
TC	3.08	3.08	XXX	0	0	0	0	1

78185 Spleen imaging only, with or without vascular flow Z 2 S

Mod	RVU Non-Fac Total	Fac Total	Global Days	Modifiers 51	50	62	80	MUE
	6.15	6.15	XXX	0	0	0	0	1
26	0.57	0.57	XXX	0	0	0	0	1
TC	5.58	5.58	XXX	0	0	0	0	1

78190 Kinetics, study of platelet survival, with or without differential organ/tissue localization Z 2 S

Mod	RVU Non-Fac Total	Fac Total	Global Days	Modifiers 51	50	62	80	MUE
	11.45	11.45	XXX	0	0	0	0	1
26	1.54	1.54	XXX	0	0	0	0	1
TC	9.91	9.91	XXX	0	0	0	0	1

● New ▲ Revised Deleted ⊙ Moderate Sedation ✚ Add-on Codes ⊗ High Risk Denial Ⓐ Age Edit ♀ Female ♂ Male **AMA** *CPT® Assistant* **MUE** Medically Unlikely Edit
⊘ Modifier 51 Exempt ⊖ Modifier 63 Exempt ✗ Unlisted **Modifiers:** *See Inside Back Cover* Ⓜ Maternity A 2–Z 3 ASC Payment Indicators A –Y OPPS Status Indicators

© 2016 DecisionHealth | CPT © 2015 American Medical Association. All Rights Reserved. | **663**

Coding Guidance

For supply of contrast material, refer to HCPCS Level II codes A9532 and A9553.

78191 Platelet survival study   ⊘Z2S

Mod	Non-Fac Total	Fac Total	Global Days	51	50	62	80	MUE
	4.89	4.89	XXX	0	0	0	0	1
26	0.86	0.86	XXX	0	0	0	0	1
TC	4.03	4.03	XXX	0	0	0	0	1

Coding Guidance

For supply of contrast material, refer to HCPCS Level II codes A9541 and A9556.

78195 Lymphatics and lymph nodes imaging   Z2S

Mod	Non-Fac Total	Fac Total	Global Days	51	50	62	80	MUE
	10.34	10.34	XXX	0	0	0	0	1
26	1.67	1.67	XXX	0	0	0	0	1
TC	8.67	8.67	XXX	0	0	0	0	1

AMA: Nov 98: 22, Jul 99: 6, Nov 99: 43, Dec 99: 8, Sep 08: 5, Feb 12: 9

78199 Unlisted hematopoietic, reticuloendothelial and lymphatic procedure, diagnostic nuclear medicine   ⊘xZ2S

Mod	Non-Fac Total	Fac Total	Global Days	51	50	62	80	MUE
	0.00	0.00	XXX	0	0	0	0	
26	0.00	0.00	XXX	0	0	0	0	
TC	0.00	0.00	XXX	0	0	0	0	

AMA: Dec 05: 7

Pub 100-04, 13, 120

Gastrointestinal System Procedures

Coding Guidance

For supply of contrast material, refer to HCPCS Level II codes A9510, A9537, and A9541.

78201 Liver imaging; static only   Z2S

Mod	Non-Fac Total	Fac Total	Global Days	51	50	62	80	MUE
	5.45	5.45	XXX	0	0	0	0	1
26	0.60	0.60	XXX	0	0	0	0	1
TC	4.85	4.85	XXX	0	0	0	0	1

AMA: Dec 05: 7, Feb 12: 9

78202 Liver imaging; with vascular flow   Z2S

Mod	Non-Fac Total	Fac Total	Global Days	51	50	62	80	MUE
	5.86	5.86	XXX	0	0	0	0	1
26	0.68	0.68	XXX	0	0	0	0	1
TC	5.18	5.18	XXX	0	0	0	0	1

AMA: Feb 12: 9

78205 Liver imaging (SPECT)   Z2S

Mod	Non-Fac Total	Fac Total	Global Days	51	50	62	80	MUE
	6.15	6.15	XXX	0	0	0	0	1
26	0.96	0.96	XXX	0	0	0	0	1
TC	5.19	5.19	XXX	0	0	0	0	1

AMA: Nov 98: 22

78206 Liver imaging (SPECT); with vascular flow   Z2S

Mod	Non-Fac Total	Fac Total	Global Days	51	50	62	80	MUE
	9.96	9.96	XXX	0	0	0	0	1
26	1.33	1.33	XXX	0	0	0	0	1
TC	8.63	8.63	XXX	0	0	0	0	1

AMA: Nov 98: 22

78215 Liver and spleen imaging; static only   Z2S

Mod	Non-Fac Total	Fac Total	Global Days	51	50	62	80	MUE
	5.66	5.66	XXX	0	0	0	0	1
26	0.69	0.69	XXX	0	0	0	0	1
TC	4.97	4.97	XXX	0	0	0	0	1

78216 Liver and spleen imaging; with vascular flow   Z2S

Mod	Non-Fac Total	Fac Total	Global Days	51	50	62	80	MUE
	3.64	3.64	XXX	0	0	0	0	1
26	0.78	0.78	XXX	0	0	0	0	1
TC	2.86	2.86	XXX	0	0	0	0	1

78226 Hepatobiliary system imaging, including gallbladder when present   Z2S

Mod	Non-Fac Total	Fac Total	Global Days	51	50	62	80	MUE
	9.64	9.64	XXX	0	0	0	0	1
26	1.04	1.04	XXX	0	0	0	0	1
TC	8.60	8.60	XXX	0	0	0	0	1

78227 Hepatobiliary system imaging, including gallbladder when present; with pharmacologic intervention, including quantitative measurement(s) when performed   Z2S

Mod	Non-Fac Total	Fac Total	Global Days	51	50	62	80	MUE
	13.10	13.10	XXX	0	0	0	0	1
26	1.27	1.27	XXX	0	0	0	0	1
TC	11.83	11.83	XXX	0	0	0	0	1

Coding Guidance

For supply of contrast material, refer to HCPCS Level II code A9512.

78230 Salivary gland imaging   Z2S

Mod	Non-Fac Total	Fac Total	Global Days	51	50	62	80	MUE
	4.09	4.09	XXX	0	0	0	0	1
26	0.54	0.54	XXX	0	0	0	0	1
TC	3.55	3.55	XXX	0	0	0	0	1

78231 Salivary gland imaging; with serial images   Z2S

Mod	Non-Fac Total	Fac Total	Global Days	51	50	62	80	MUE
	3.77	3.77	XXX	0	0	0	0	1
26	0.74	0.74	XXX	0	0	0	0	1
TC	3.03	3.03	XXX	0	0	0	0	1

78232 Salivary gland function study   Z2S

Mod	Non-Fac Total	Fac Total	Global Days	51	50	62	80	MUE
	2.86	2.86	XXX	0	0	0	0	1
26	0.56	0.56	XXX	0	0	0	0	1
TC	2.30	2.30	XXX	0	0	0	0	1

● New   ▲ Revised   ✖ Deleted   ⊙ Moderate Sedation   ✚ Add-on Codes   ⊘ High Risk Denial   Ⓐ Age Edit   ♀ Female   ♂ Male   **AMA** *CPT® Assistant*   **MUE** Medically Unlikely Edit

⊘ Modifier 51 Exempt   ⊖ Modifier 63 Exempt   🗶 Unlisted   **Modifiers:** *See Inside Back Cover*   Ⓜ Maternity   A2–Z3 ASC Payment Indicators   A–Y OPPS Status Indicators

664   CPT © 2015 American Medical Association. All Rights Reserved.   © 2016 DecisionHealth

Coding Guidance

For supply of contrast material, refer to HCPCS Level II codes A9542.

78258 Esophageal motility · Z 2 S

Mod	Non-Fac Total	Fac Total	Global Days	51	50	62	80	MUE
	6.44	6.44	XXX	0	0	0	0	1
26	1.04	1.04	XXX	0	0	0	0	1
TC	5.40	5.40	XXX	0	0	0	0	1

78261 Gastric mucosa imaging · Z 2 S

Mod	Non-Fac Total	Fac Total	Global Days	51	50	62	80	MUE
	7.22	7.22	XXX	0	0	0	0	1
26	0.97	0.97	XXX	0	0	0	0	1
TC	6.25	6.25	XXX	0	0	0	0	1

Coding Guidance

For supply of contrast material, refer to HCPCS Level II codes A9541.

78262 Gastroesophageal reflux study · Z 2 S

Mod	Non-Fac Total	Fac Total	Global Days	51	50	62	80	MUE
	7.10	7.10	XXX	0	0	0	0	1
26	0.94	0.94	XXX	0	0	0	0	1
TC	6.16	6.16	XXX	0	0	0	0	1

▲ 78264 Gastric emptying imaging study (eg, solid, liquid, or both) · Z 2 S

Mod	Non-Fac Total	Fac Total	Global Days	51	50	62	80	MUE
	9.73	9.73	XXX	0	0	0	0	1
26	1.04	1.04	XXX	0	0	0	1	1
TC	8.69	8.69	XXX	0	0	0	0	1

● 78265 Gastric emptying imaging study (eg, solid, liquid, or both); with small bowel transit · Z 2 S

Mod	Non-Fac Total	Fac Total	Global Days	51	50	62	80	MUE
	11.60	11.60	XXX	0	0	0	1	1
26	1.37	1.37	XXX	0	0	0	0	1
TC	10.23	10.23	XXX	0	0	0	1	1

● 78266 Gastric emptying imaging study (eg, solid, liquid, or both); with small bowel and colon transit, multiple days · Z 2 S

Mod	Non-Fac Total	Fac Total	Global Days	51	50	62	80	MUE
	13.76	13.76	XXX	0	0	0	1	1
26	1.52	1.52	XXX	0	0	0	0	1
TC	12.24	12.24	XXX	0	0	0	0	1

78267 Urea breath test, C-14 (isotopic); acquisition for analysis · A

Mod	Non-Fac Total	Fac Total	Global Days	51	50	62	80	MUE
	0.00	0.00	XXX	9	9	9	9	1

AMA: Nov 99: 43

78268 Urea breath test, C-14 (isotopic); analysis · A

Mod	Non-Fac Total	Fac Total	Global Days	51	50	62	80	MUE
	0.00	0.00	XXX	9	9	9	9	1

AMA: Nov 99: 43

Coding Guidance

For supply of contrast material, refer to HCPCS Level II codes A9546 and A9559.

78270 Vitamin B-12 absorption study (eg, Schilling test); without intrinsic factor · Z 2 S

Mod	Non-Fac Total	Fac Total	Global Days	51	50	62	80	MUE
	2.93	2.93	XXX	0	0	0	0	1
26	0.30	0.30	XXX	0	0	0	0	1
TC	2.63	2.63	XXX	0	0	0	0	1

78271 Vitamin B-12 absorption study (eg, Schilling test); with intrinsic factor · ⊘ Z 2 S

Mod	Non-Fac Total	Fac Total	Global Days	51	50	62	80	MUE
	2.63	2.63	XXX	0	0	0	0	1
26	0.29	0.29	XXX	0	0	0	0	1
TC	2.34	2.34	XXX	0	0	0	0	1

78272 Vitamin B-12 absorption studies combined, with and without intrinsic factor · ⊘ Z 2 S

Mod	Non-Fac Total	Fac Total	Global Days	51	50	62	80	MUE
TC	2.43	2.43	XXX	0	0	0	0	1
	2.81	2.81	XXX	0	0	0	0	1
26	0.38	0.38	XXX	0	0	0	0	1

Coding Guidance

For supply of contrast material, refer to HCPCS Level II code A9560.

78278 Acute gastrointestinal blood loss imaging · Z 2 S

Mod	Non-Fac Total	Fac Total	Global Days	51	50	62	80	MUE
	10.14	10.14	XXX	0	0	0	0	2
26	1.39	1.39	XXX	0	0	0	0	2
TC	8.75	8.75	XXX	0	0	0	0	2

78282 Gastrointestinal protein loss · Z 2 S

Mod	Non-Fac Total	Fac Total	Global Days	51	50	62	80	MUE
	0.00	0.00	XXX	0	0	0	0	1
26	0.54	0.54	XXX	0	0	0	0	1
TC	0.00	0.00	XXX	0	0	0	0	1

Coding Guidance

For supply of contrast material, refer to HCPCS Level II code A9538.

78290 Intestine imaging (eg, ectopic gastric mucosa, Meckel's localization, volvulus) · Z 2 S

Mod	Non-Fac Total	Fac Total	Global Days	51	50	62	80	MUE
	9.70	9.70	XXX	0	0	0	0	1
26	0.96	0.96	XXX	0	0	0	0	1
TC	8.74	8.74	XXX	0	0	0	0	1

78291 Peritoneal-venous shunt patency test (eg, for LeVeen, Denver shunt) · Z 2 S

Coding tip: *Injection for evaluation of previously placed peritoneal-venous shunt - 49427*

Mod	Non-Fac Total	Fac Total	Global Days	51	50	62	80	MUE
	7.32	7.32	XXX	0	0	0	0	1
26	1.20	1.20	XXX	0	0	0	0	1
TC	6.12	6.12	XXX	0	0	0	0	1

AMA: Feb 12: 9

● New ▲ Revised Deleted ⊙ Moderate Sedation ✚ Add-on Codes ⊘ High Risk Denial ⓐ Age Edit ♀ Female ♂ Male **AMA** *CPT® Assistant* **MUE** Medically Unlikely Edit
⊘ Modifier 51 Exempt ⊖ Modifier 63 Exempt ✗ Unlisted **Modifiers:** *See Inside Back Cover* Ⓜ Maternity A2–Z3 ASC Payment Indicators A–Y OPPS Status Indicators

78299 Unlisted gastrointestinal procedure, diagnostic nuclear medicine ⊗ x Z2 S

Mod	RVU Non-Fac Total	Fac Total	Global Days	Modifiers 51	50	62	80	MUE
	0.00	0.00	XXX	0	0	0	0	
26	0.00	0.00	XXX	0	0	0	0	
TC	0.00	0.00	XXX	0	0	0	0	

AMA: Dec 05: 7

Pub 100-04, 13, 120

Musculoskeletal System Procedures

Coding Guidance

For supply of contrast material, refer to HCPCS Level II codes A9503, A9538, and A9561.

78300 Bone and/or joint imaging; limited area Z2 S

Mod	RVU Non-Fac Total	Fac Total	Global Days	Modifiers 51	50	62	80	MUE
	5.26	5.26	XXX	0	0	0	0	1
26	0.89	0.89	XXX	0	0	0	0	1
TC	4.37	4.37	XXX	0	0	0	0	1

AMA: Mar 97: 11, Dec 05: 7, Feb 12: 9

78305 Bone and/or joint imaging; multiple areas Z2 S

Mod	RVU Non-Fac Total	Fac Total	Global Days	Modifiers 51	50	62	80	MUE
	6.72	6.72	XXX	0	0	0	0	1
26	1.17	1.17	XXX	0	0	0	0	1
TC	5.55	5.55	XXX	0	0	0	0	1

AMA: Mar 97: 11

78306 Bone and/or joint imaging; whole body Z2 S

Mod	RVU Non-Fac Total	Fac Total	Global Days	Modifiers 51	50	62	80	MUE
	7.34	7.34	XXX	2	0	0	0	1
26	1.21	1.21	XXX	2	0	0	0	1
TC	6.13	6.13	XXX	2	0	0	0	1

AMA: Mar 97: 11, Jan 02: 10, Jun 03: 11, Feb 12: 10

Pub 100-04, 13, 50.3

78315 Bone and/or joint imaging; 3 phase study Z2 S

Mod	RVU Non-Fac Total	Fac Total	Global Days	Modifiers 51	50	62	80	MUE
	10.08	10.08	XXX	0	0	0	0	1
26	1.42	1.42	XXX	0	0	0	0	1
TC	8.66	8.66	XXX	0	0	0	0	1

AMA: Jan 02: 10

78320 Bone and/or joint imaging; tomographic (SPECT) Z2 S

Mod	RVU Non-Fac Total	Fac Total	Global Days	Modifiers 51	50	62	80	MUE
	6.61	6.61	XXX	2	0	0	0	1
26	1.43	1.43	XXX	2	0	0	0	1
TC	5.18	5.18	XXX	2	0	0	0	1

AMA: Mar 97: 11, Jun 03: 11, Jan 08: 9

Pub 100-04, 13, 50.3

78350 Bone density (bone mineral content) study, 1 or more sites; single photon absorptiometry ⊙ E

Mod	RVU Non-Fac Total	Fac Total	Global Days	Modifiers 51	50	62	80	MUE
	0.93	0.93	XXX	9	9	9	9	
26	0.31	0.31	XXX	9	9	9	9	
TC	0.62	0.62	XXX	9	9	9	9	

AMA: Nov 97: 26

Pub 100-04, 13, 140.1

78351 Bone density (bone mineral content) study, 1 or more sites; dual photon absorptiometry, 1 or more sites ⊙ E

Mod	RVU Non-Fac Total	Fac Total	Global Days	Modifiers 51	50	62	80	MUE
	0.43	0.43	XXX	9	9	9	9	

AMA: Nov 97: 26, Feb 12: 9

Pub 100-04, 13, 140.1; 100-04, 16, 120.2

78399 Unlisted musculoskeletal procedure, diagnostic nuclear medicine ⊗ x Z2 S

Mod	RVU Non-Fac Total	Fac Total	Global Days	Modifiers 51	50	62	80	MUE
	0.00	0.00	XXX	0	0	0	0	
26	0.00	0.00	XXX	0	0	0	0	
TC	0.00	0.00	XXX	0	0	0	0	

AMA: Dec 05: 7

Pub 100-04, 13, 120

Cardiovascular System Procedures

78414 Determination of central c-v hemodynamics (non-imaging) (eg, ejection fraction with probe technique) with or without pharmacologic intervention or exercise, single or multiple determinations Z2 S

Mod	RVU Non-Fac Total	Fac Total	Global Days	Modifiers 51	50	62	80	MUE
	0.00	0.00	XXX	0	0	0	0	1
26	0.63	0.63	XXX	0	0	0	0	1
TC	0.00	0.00	XXX	0	0	0	0	1

AMA: Dec 05: 7, Feb 12: 9, May 10: 6

78428 Cardiac shunt detection Z2 S

Mod	RVU Non-Fac Total	Fac Total	Global Days	Modifiers 51	50	62	80	MUE
	5.23	5.23	XXX	6	0	0	0	1
26	1.07	1.07	XXX	6	0	0	0	1
TC	4.16	4.16	XXX	6	0	0	0	1

AMA: May 10: 6

78445 Non-cardiac vascular flow imaging (ie, angiography, venography) ⊙ Z2 S

Mod	RVU Non-Fac Total	Fac Total	Global Days	Modifiers 51	50	62	80	MUE
	5.08	5.08	XXX	6	0	0	0	1
26	0.66	0.66	XXX	6	0	0	0	1
TC	4.42	4.42	XXX	6	0	0	0	1

AMA: May 10: 6

● New   ▲ Revised   ✖ Deleted   ⊙ Moderate Sedation   ✚ Add-on Codes   ⊗ High Risk Denial   Ⓐ Age Edit   ♀ Female   ♂ Male   **AMA** CPT® Assistant   **MUE** Medically Unlikely Edit

⊘ Modifier 51 Exempt   ⊖ Modifier 63 Exempt   ✖ Unlisted   **Modifiers:** See Inside Back Cover   Ⓜ Maternity   A2–Z3 ASC Payment Indicators   A–Y OPPS Status Indicators

666

CPT © 2015 American Medical Association. All Rights Reserved.   © 2016 DecisionHealth

78451 Myocardial perfusion imaging, tomographic (SPECT) (including attenuation correction, qualitative or quantitative wall motion, ejection fraction by first pass or gated technique, additional quantification, when performed); single study, at rest or stress (exercise or pharmacologic) Z 2 S

	RVU			Global Days	Modifiers				
Mod	Non-Fac Total	Fac Total			51	50	62	80	MUE
	9.90	9.90	XXX		6	0	0	0	1
26	1.90	1.90	XXX		6	0	0	0	1
TC	8.00	8.00	XXX		6	0	0	0	1

AMA: Feb 12: 10, May 10: 5, Feb 11: 9

Myocardial perfusion imaging tomographic

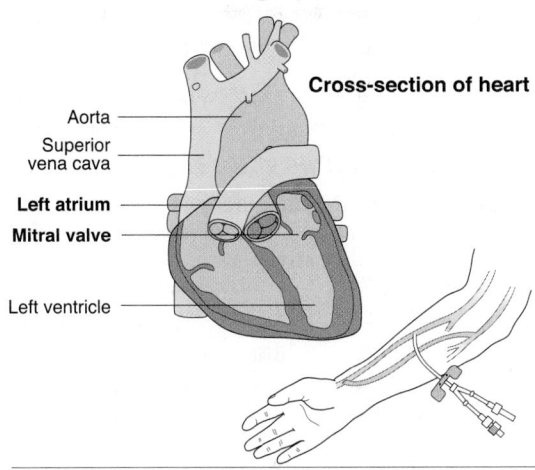

Cross-section of heart

Aorta
Superior vena cava
Left atrium
Mitral valve
Left ventricle

78452 Myocardial perfusion imaging, tomographic (SPECT) (including attenuation correction, qualitative or quantitative wall motion, ejection fraction by first pass or gated technique, additional quantification, when performed); multiple studies, at rest and/or stress (exercise or pharmacologic) and/or redistribution and/or rest reinjection Z 2 S

	RVU			Global Days	Modifiers				
Mod	Non-Fac Total	Fac Total			51	50	62	80	MUE
	13.74	13.74	XXX		6	0	0	0	1
26	2.24	2.24	XXX		6	0	0	0	1
TC	11.50	11.50	XXX		6	0	0	0	1

AMA: Feb 12: 9, May 10: 5, Feb 11: 9

78453 Myocardial perfusion imaging, planar (including qualitative or quantitative wall motion, ejection fraction by first pass or gated technique, additional quantification, when performed); single study, at rest or stress (exercise or pharmacologic) Z 2 S

	RVU			Global Days	Modifiers				
Mod	Non-Fac Total	Fac Total			51	50	62	80	MUE
	8.83	8.83	XXX		6	0	0	0	1
26	1.40	1.40	XXX		6	0	0	0	1
TC	7.43	7.43	XXX		6	0	0	0	1

AMA: May 10: 5

78454 Myocardial perfusion imaging, planar (including qualitative or quantitative wall motion, ejection fraction by first pass or gated technique, additional quantification, when performed); multiple studies, at rest and/or stress (exercise or pharmacologic) and/or redistribution and/or rest reinjection Z 2 S

	RVU			Global Days	Modifiers				
Mod	Non-Fac Total	Fac Total			51	50	62	80	MUE
	12.70	12.70	XXX		6	0	0	0	1
26	1.89	1.89	XXX		6	0	0	0	1
TC	10.81	10.81	XXX		6	0	0	0	1

AMA: May 10: 5

78456 Acute venous thrombosis imaging, peptide Z 2 S

	RVU			Global Days	Modifiers				
Mod	Non-Fac Total	Fac Total			51	50	62	80	MUE
	9.18	9.18	XXX		6	9	9	9	1
26	1.38	1.38	XXX		6	9	9	9	1
TC	7.80	7.80	XXX		6	9	9	9	1

AMA: Nov 99: 43, May 10: 6

78457 Venous thrombosis imaging, venogram; unilateral Z 2 S

	RVU			Global Days	Modifiers				
Mod	Non-Fac Total	Fac Total			51	50	62	80	MUE
	5.46	5.46	XXX		6	0	0	0	1
26	1.09	1.09	XXX		6	0	0	0	1
TC	4.37	4.37	XXX		6	0	0	0	1

AMA: Nov 99: 43

78458 Venous thrombosis imaging, venogram; bilateral Z 2 S

	RVU			Global Days	Modifiers				
Mod	Non-Fac Total	Fac Total			51	50	62	80	MUE
	4.85	4.85	XXX		6	2	0	0	1
26	1.07	1.07	XXX		6	2	0	0	1
TC	3.78	3.78	XXX		6	2	0	0	1

AMA: Nov 99: 43, May 10: 6

78459 Myocardial imaging, positron emission tomography (PET), metabolic evaluation Z 2 S

	RVU			Global Days	Modifiers				
Mod	Non-Fac Total	Fac Total			51	50	62	80	MUE
TC	0.00	0.00	XXX		0	0	0	0	1
	0.00	0.00	XXX		0	0	0	0	1
26	2.00	2.00	XXX		0	0	0	0	1

AMA: Jun 96: 5, Nov 97: 26, May 10: 6

Pub 100-04, 13, 60.3, 60.3.1, 60.3.2, 60.9

Coding Guidance

For supply of contrast material, refer to HCPCS Level II codes A9502, A9505, and A9538.

78466 Myocardial imaging, infarct avid, planar; qualitative or quantitative Z 2 S

	RVU			Global Days	Modifiers				
Mod	Non-Fac Total	Fac Total			51	50	62	80	MUE
	5.61	5.61	XXX		6	0	0	0	1
26	0.99	0.99	XXX		6	0	0	0	1
TC	4.62	4.62	XXX		6	0	0	0	1

AMA: May 10: 6

● New   ▲ Revised   Deleted   ⊙ Moderate Sedation   ✚ Add-on Codes   ⊘ High Risk Denial   Ⓐ Age Edit   ♀ Female   ♂ Male   **AMA** *CPT® Assistant*   **MUE** Medically Unlikely Edit
⊘ Modifier 51 Exempt   ⊖ Modifier 63 Exempt   ☒ Unlisted   **Modifiers:** *See Inside Back Cover*   Ⓜ Maternity   A2–Z3 ASC Payment Indicators   A–Y OPPS Status Indicators

© 2016 DecisionHealth   CPT © 2015 American Medical Association. All Rights Reserved.   **667**

Radiology Procedures

78468 – 78499

78468 Myocardial imaging, infarct avid, planar; with ejection fraction by first pass technique `Z2 S`

RVU Mod	Non-Fac Total	Fac Total	Global Days	Modifiers 51	50	62	80	MUE
	5.74	5.74	XXX	6	0	0	0	1
26	1.11	1.11	XXX	6	0	0	0	1
TC	4.63	4.63	XXX	6	0	0	0	1

AMA: May 10: 6

78469 Myocardial imaging, infarct avid, planar; tomographic SPECT with or without quantification `Z2 S`

RVU Mod	Non-Fac Total	Fac Total	Global Days	Modifiers 51	50	62	80	MUE
	6.60	6.60	XXX	6	0	0	0	1
26	1.29	1.29	XXX	6	0	0	0	1
TC	5.31	5.31	XXX	6	0	0	0	1

AMA: May 10: 6

78472 Cardiac blood pool imaging, gated equilibrium; planar, single study at rest or stress (exercise and/or pharmacologic), wall motion study plus ejection fraction, with or without additional quantitative processing `Z2 S`

RVU Mod	Non-Fac Total	Fac Total	Global Days	Modifiers 51	50	62	80	MUE
	6.67	6.67	XXX	6	0	0	0	1
26	1.36	1.36	XXX	6	0	0	0	1
TC	5.31	5.31	XXX	6	0	0	0	1

AMA: Nov 98: 22, Nov 99: 44, May 10: 6

78473 Cardiac blood pool imaging, gated equilibrium; multiple studies, wall motion study plus ejection fraction, at rest and stress (exercise and/or pharmacologic), with or without additional quantification `Z2 S`

RVU Mod	Non-Fac Total	Fac Total	Global Days	Modifiers 51	50	62	80	MUE
	8.39	8.39	XXX	6	0	0	0	1
26	2.02	2.02	XXX	6	0	0	0	1
TC	6.37	6.37	XXX	6	0	0	0	1

AMA: May 10: 6

78481 Cardiac blood pool imaging (planar), first pass technique; single study, at rest or with stress (exercise and/or pharmacologic), wall motion study plus ejection fraction, with or without quantification `Z2 S`

RVU Mod	Non-Fac Total	Fac Total	Global Days	Modifiers 51	50	62	80	MUE
	5.05	5.05	XXX	6	0	0	0	1
26	1.35	1.35	XXX	6	0	0	0	1
TC	3.70	3.70	XXX	6	0	0	0	1

AMA: May 10: 6
Pub 100-04, 13, 60.3

78483 Cardiac blood pool imaging (planar), first pass technique; multiple studies, at rest and with stress (exercise and/or pharmacologic), wall motion study plus ejection fraction, with or without quantification `Z2 S`

RVU Mod	Non-Fac Total	Fac Total	Global Days	Modifiers 51	50	62	80	MUE
	7.00	7.00	XXX	6	0	0	0	1
26	2.02	2.02	XXX	6	0	0	0	1
TC	4.98	4.98	XXX	6	0	0	0	1

AMA: May 10: 6
Pub 100-04, 13, 60.3

78491 Myocardial imaging, positron emission tomography (PET), perfusion; single study at rest or stress `Z2 S`

RVU Mod	Non-Fac Total	Fac Total	Global Days	Modifiers 51	50	62	80	MUE
	0.00	0.00	XXX	0	0	0	0	1
26	2.02	2.02	XXX	0	0	0	0	1
TC	0.00	0.00	XXX	0	0	0	0	1

AMA: Nov 97: 27, May 10: 6
Pub 100-04, 13, 60.3.1, 60.3.2

78492 Myocardial imaging, positron emission tomography (PET), perfusion; multiple studies at rest and/or stress `Z2 S`

RVU Mod	Non-Fac Total	Fac Total	Global Days	Modifiers 51	50	62	80	MUE
	0.00	0.00	XXX	0	0	0	0	1
26	2.54	2.54	XXX	0	0	0	0	1
TC	0.00	0.00	XXX	0	0	0	0	1

AMA: Nov 97: 27, May 10: 6
Pub 100-04, 13, 60.3.1, 60.3.2

78494 Cardiac blood pool imaging, gated equilibrium, SPECT, at rest, wall motion study plus ejection fraction, with or without quantitative processing `Z2 S`

RVU Mod	Non-Fac Total	Fac Total	Global Days	Modifiers 51	50	62	80	MUE
	6.51	6.51	XXX	6	0	0	0	1
26	1.64	1.64	XXX	6	0	0	0	1
TC	4.87	4.87	XXX	6	0	0	0	1

AMA: Nov 98: 22, Jun 99: 3, May 10: 6

+ 78496 Cardiac blood pool imaging, gated equilibrium, single study, at rest, with right ventricular ejection fraction by first pass technique (List separately in addition to code for primary procedure) `N N`

RVU Mod	Non-Fac Total	Fac Total	Global Days	Modifiers 51	50	62	80	MUE
	1.27	1.27	ZZZ	0	0	0	0	1
26	0.69	0.69	ZZZ	0	0	0	0	1
TC	0.58	0.58	ZZZ	0	0	0	0	1

AMA: Nov 98: 22, Jun 99: 3, 11, Feb 12: 9, May 10: 6

78499 Unlisted cardiovascular procedure, diagnostic nuclear medicine `⊘ x Z2 S`

RVU Mod	Non-Fac Total	Fac Total	Global Days	Modifiers 51	50	62	80	MUE
	0.00	0.00	XXX	0	0	0	0	
26	0.00	0.00	XXX	0	0	0	0	
TC	0.00	0.00	XXX	0	0	0	0	

AMA: Dec 05: 7, May 10: 6
Pub 100-04, 13, 120

● New ▲ Revised ✖ Deleted ⊙ Moderate Sedation ✚ Add-on Codes ⊘ High Risk Denial Ⓐ Age Edit ♀ Female ♂ Male **AMA** *CPT® Assistant* **MUE** Medically Unlikely Edit
⊘ Modifier 51 Exempt ⊖ Modifier 63 Exempt Ⓧ Unlisted **Modifiers:** *See Inside Back Cover* Ⓜ Maternity A2-Z3 ASC Payment Indicators A-Y OPPS Status Indicators

668
CPT © 2015 American Medical Association. All Rights Reserved.
© 2016 DecisionHealth

Respiratory System Procedures

78579 Pulmonary ventilation imaging (eg, aerosol or gas) Z2S

Mod	Non-Fac Total	Fac Total	Global Days	51	50	62	80	MUE
	5.42	5.42	XXX	0	0	0	0	1
26	0.67	0.67	XXX	0	0	0	0	1
TC	4.75	4.75	XXX	0	0	0	0	1

AMA: Feb 12: 9

78580 Pulmonary perfusion imaging (eg, particulate) Z2S

Mod	Non-Fac Total	Fac Total	Global Days	51	50	62	80	MUE
	6.96	6.96	XXX	0	0	0	0	1
26	1.04	1.04	XXX	0	0	0	0	1
TC	5.92	5.92	XXX	0	0	0	0	1

AMA: Mar 99: 4, Dec 05: 7, May 10: 6

78582 Pulmonary ventilation (eg, aerosol or gas) and perfusion imaging Z2S

Mod	Non-Fac Total	Fac Total	Global Days	51	50	62	80	MUE
	9.74	9.74	XXX	0	0	0	0	1
26	1.50	1.50	XXX	0	0	0	0	1
TC	8.24	8.24	XXX	0	0	0	0	1

78597 Quantitative differential pulmonary perfusion, including imaging when performed Z2S

Mod	Non-Fac Total	Fac Total	Global Days	51	50	62	80	MUE
	5.87	5.87	XXX	0	0	0	0	1
26	1.01	1.01	XXX	0	0	0	0	1
TC	4.86	4.86	XXX	0	0	0	0	1

78598 Quantitative differential pulmonary perfusion and ventilation (eg, aerosol or gas), including imaging when performed Z2S

Mod	Non-Fac Total	Fac Total	Global Days	51	50	62	80	MUE
	8.92	8.92	XXX	0	0	0	0	1
26	1.18	1.18	XXX	0	0	0	0	1
TC	7.74	7.74	XXX	0	0	0	0	1

AMA: Feb 12: 9

78599 Unlisted respiratory procedure, diagnostic nuclear medicine X Z2S

Mod	Non-Fac Total	Fac Total	Global Days	51	50	62	80	MUE
	0.00	0.00	XXX	0	0	0	0	
26	0.00	0.00	XXX	0	0	0	0	
TC	0.00	0.00	XXX	0	0	0	0	

AMA: Dec 05: 7

Pub 100-04, 13, 120

Nervous System Procedures

78600 Brain imaging, less than 4 static views Z2S

Mod	Non-Fac Total	Fac Total	Global Days	51	50	62	80	MUE
	5.37	5.37	XXX	0	0	0	0	1
26	0.63	0.63	XXX	0	0	0	0	1
TC	4.74	4.74	XXX	0	0	0	0	1

AMA: Dec 05: 7, Feb 12: 9

78601 Brain imaging, less than 4 static views; with vascular flow Z2S

Mod	Non-Fac Total	Fac Total	Global Days	51	50	62	80	MUE
	6.22	6.22	XXX	0	0	0	0	1
26	0.71	0.71	XXX	0	0	0	0	1
TC	5.51	5.51	XXX	0	0	0	0	1

78605 Brain imaging, minimum 4 static views Z2S

Mod	Non-Fac Total	Fac Total	Global Days	51	50	62	80	MUE
	5.79	5.79	XXX	0	0	0	0	1
26	0.76	0.76	XXX	0	0	0	0	1
TC	5.03	5.03	XXX	0	0	0	0	1

78606 Brain imaging, minimum 4 static views; with vascular flow Z2S

Mod	Non-Fac Total	Fac Total	Global Days	51	50	62	80	MUE
	9.62	9.62	XXX	0	0	0	0	1
26	0.89	0.89	XXX	0	0	0	0	1
TC	8.73	8.73	XXX	0	0	0	0	1

78607 Brain imaging, tomographic (SPECT) Z2S

Mod	Non-Fac Total	Fac Total	Global Days	51	50	62	80	MUE
	10.20	10.20	XXX	0	0	0	0	1
26	1.68	1.68	XXX	0	0	0	0	1
TC	8.52	8.52	XXX	0	0	0	0	1

78608 Brain imaging, positron emission tomography (PET); metabolic evaluation Z2S

Mod	Non-Fac Total	Fac Total	Global Days	51	50	62	80	MUE
	0.00	0.00	XXX	0	0	0	0	1
26	2.04	2.04	XXX	0	0	0	0	1
TC	0.00	0.00	XXX	0	0	0	0	1

Pub 100-04, 13, 60.16, 60.3.1, 60.3.2

78609 Brain imaging, positron emission tomography (PET); perfusion evaluation CE

Mod	Non-Fac Total	Fac Total	Global Days	51	50	62	80	MUE
	2.11	2.11	XXX	9	9	9	9	
26	2.11	2.11	XXX	9	9	9	9	
TC	0.00	0.00	XXX	9	9	9	9	

Pub 100-04, 13, 60.3.1, 60.3.2, 60.3.3, 60.3.4

78610 Brain imaging, vascular flow only Z2S

Mod	Non-Fac Total	Fac Total	Global Days	51	50	62	80	MUE
	5.08	5.08	XXX	0	0	0	0	1
26	0.43	0.43	XXX	0	0	0	0	1
TC	4.65	4.65	XXX	0	0	0	0	1

78630 Cerebrospinal fluid flow, imaging (not including introduction of material); cisternography Z2S

Mod	Non-Fac Total	Fac Total	Global Days	51	50	62	80	MUE
	9.85	9.85	XXX	0	0	0	0	1
26	0.96	0.96	XXX	0	0	0	0	1
TC	8.89	8.89	XXX	0	0	0	0	1

Radiology Procedures

78579 – 78630

● New ▲ Revised Deleted ⊙ Moderate Sedation ✚ Add-on Codes ⊘ High Risk Denial Ⓐ Age Edit ♀ Female ♂ Male **AMA** *CPT® Assistant* **MUE** Medically Unlikely Edit ⊘ Modifier 51 Exempt ⊖ Modifier 63 Exempt X Unlisted **Modifiers:** *See Inside Back Cover* Ⓜ Maternity A2–Z3 ASC Payment Indicators A–Y OPPS Status Indicators

© 2016 DecisionHealth | CPT © 2015 American Medical Association. All Rights Reserved. | **669**

78635 Cerebrospinal fluid flow, imaging (not including introduction of material); ventriculography Z2 S

Mod	RVU Non-Fac Total	Fac Total	Global Days	Modifiers 51	50	62	80	MUE
	9.86	9.86	XXX	0	0	0	0	1
26	0.87	0.87	XXX	0	0	0	0	1
TC	8.99	8.99	XXX	0	0	0	0	1

78645 Cerebrospinal fluid flow, imaging (not including introduction of material); shunt evaluation Z2 S

Mod	RVU Non-Fac Total	Fac Total	Global Days	Modifiers 51	50	62	80	MUE
	9.39	9.39	XXX	0	0	0	0	1
26	0.79	0.79	XXX	0	0	0	0	1
TC	8.60	8.60	XXX	0	0	0	0	1

78647 Cerebrospinal fluid flow, imaging (not including introduction of material); tomographic (SPECT) Z2 S

Mod	RVU Non-Fac Total	Fac Total	Global Days	Modifiers 51	50	62	80	MUE
	10.18	10.18	XXX	0	0	0	0	1
26	1.28	1.28	XXX	0	0	0	0	1
TC	8.90	8.90	XXX	0	0	0	0	1

Coding Guidance

For supply of contrast material, refer to HCPCS Level II code A9548.

78650 Cerebrospinal fluid leakage detection and localization Z2 S

Mod	RVU Non-Fac Total	Fac Total	Global Days	Modifiers 51	50	62	80	MUE
	9.58	9.58	XXX	0	0	0	0	1
26	0.85	0.85	XXX	0	0	0	0	1
TC	8.73	8.73	XXX	0	0	0	0	1

78660 Radiopharmaceutical dacryocystography Z2 S

Mod	RVU Non-Fac Total	Fac Total	Global Days	Modifiers 51	50	62	80	MUE
	5.24	5.24	XXX	0	0	0	0	1
26	0.76	0.76	XXX	0	0	0	0	1
TC	4.48	4.48	XXX	0	0	0	0	1

AMA: Feb 12: 9

78699 Unlisted nervous system procedure, diagnostic nuclear medicine ⊙ ✗ Z2 S

Mod	RVU Non-Fac Total	Fac Total	Global Days	Modifiers 51	50	62	80	MUE
	0.00	0.00	XXX	0	0	0		
26	0.00	0.00	XXX	0	0	0		
TC	0.00	0.00	XXX	0	0	0		

AMA: Dec 05: 7

Pub 100-04, 13, 120

Genitourinary System Procedures

78700 Kidney imaging morphology Z2 S

Mod	RVU Non-Fac Total	Fac Total	Global Days	Modifiers 51	50	62	80	MUE
	5.00	5.00	XXX	0	0	0	0	1
26	0.63	0.63	XXX	0	0	0	0	1
TC	4.37	4.37	XXX	0	0	0	0	1

AMA: Dec 05: 7, Mar 07: 7, Feb 12: 9

78701 Kidney imaging morphology; with vascular flow Z2 S

Mod	RVU Non-Fac Total	Fac Total	Global Days	Modifiers 51	50	62	80	MUE
	6.13	6.13	XXX	0	0	0	0	1
26	0.67	0.67	XXX	0	0	0	0	1
TC	5.46	5.46	XXX	0	0	0	0	1

78707 Kidney imaging morphology; with vascular flow and function, single study without pharmacological intervention Z2 S

Mod	RVU Non-Fac Total	Fac Total	Global Days	Modifiers 51	50	62	80	MUE
	6.75	6.75	XXX	0	0	0	0	1
26	1.33	1.33	XXX	0	0	0	0	1
TC	5.42	5.42	XXX	0	0	0	0	1

AMA: Nov 97: 27, Mar 07: 7

78708 Kidney imaging morphology; with vascular flow and function, single study, with pharmacological intervention (eg, angiotensin converting enzyme inhibitor and/or diuretic) Z2 S

Mod	RVU Non-Fac Total	Fac Total	Global Days	Modifiers 51	50	62	80	MUE
	5.04	5.04	XXX	0	0	0	0	1
26	1.68	1.68	XXX	0	0	0	0	1
TC	3.36	3.36	XXX	0	0	0	0	1

AMA: Nov 97: 27, Mar 07: 7

78709 Kidney imaging morphology; with vascular flow and function, multiple studies, with and without pharmacological intervention (eg, angiotensin converting enzyme inhibitor and/or diuretic) Z2 S

Mod	RVU Non-Fac Total	Fac Total	Global Days	Modifiers 51	50	62	80	MUE
	10.56	10.56	XXX	0	0	0	0	1
26	1.94	1.94	XXX	0	0	0	0	1
TC	8.62	8.62	XXX	0	0	0	0	1

AMA: Nov 97: 27, Mar 07: 7

78710 Kidney imaging morphology; tomographic (SPECT) Z2 S

Mod	RVU Non-Fac Total	Fac Total	Global Days	Modifiers 51	50	62	80	MUE
	5.81	5.81	XXX	0	0	0	0	1
26	0.87	0.87	XXX	0	0	0	0	1
TC	4.94	4.94	XXX	0	0	0	0	1

AMA: Nov 97: 27, Mar 07: 7

78725 Kidney function study, non-imaging radioisotopic study Z2 S

Mod	RVU Non-Fac Total	Fac Total	Global Days	Modifiers 51	50	62	80	MUE
	3.13	3.13	XXX	0	0	0	0	1
26	0.52	0.52	XXX	0	0	0	0	1
TC	2.61	2.61	XXX	0	0	0	0	1

AMA: Nov 98: 22

● New　　▲ Revised　　✖ Deleted　　⊙ Moderate Sedation　　✚ Add-on Codes　　⊘ High Risk Denial　　Ⓐ Age Edit　　♀ Female　　♂ Male　　**AMA** *CPT® Assistant*　　**MUE** Medically Unlikely Edit
⊘ Modifier 51 Exempt　　⊖ Modifier 63 Exempt　　✗ Unlisted　　**Modifiers:** *See Inside Back Cover*　　Ⓜ Maternity　　A2–Z3 ASC Payment Indicators　　A–Y OPPS Status Indicators

670　　　　CPT © 2015 American Medical Association. All Rights Reserved.　　　　© 2016 DecisionHealth

Coding Guidance

Procedure 78730 uses a radiopharmaceutical to determine residual urine in the bladder in conjunction with a radiopharmaceutical voiding cystogram and should not be used for a residual study by any other method, such as ultrasound.

✚ **78730 Urinary bladder residual study (List separately in addition to code for primary procedure)** ⓒ N1 N

RVU Mod	Non-Fac Total	Fac Total	Global Days	51	50	62	80	MUE
TC	2.00	2.00	ZZZ	0	0	0	0	1
	2.22	2.22	ZZZ	0	0	0	0	1
26	0.22	0.22	ZZZ	0	0	0	0	1

AMA: Mar 07: 7

78740 Ureteral reflux study (radiopharmaceutical voiding cystogram) Z2 S

RVU Mod	Non-Fac Total	Fac Total	Global Days	51	50	62	80	MUE
	6.33	6.33	XXX	0	0	0	0	1
26	0.78	0.78	XXX	0	0	0	0	1
TC	5.55	5.55	XXX	0	0	0	0	1

78761 Testicular imaging with vascular flow ♂ Z2 S

RVU Mod	Non-Fac Total	Fac Total	Global Days	51	50	62	80	MUE
	6.06	6.06	XXX	0	0	0	0	1
26	1.01	1.01	XXX	0	0	0	0	1
TC	5.05	5.05	XXX	0	0	0	0	1

AMA: Mar 07: 7, Feb 12: 9

78799 Unlisted genitourinary procedure, diagnostic nuclear medicine ✗ Z2 S

RVU Mod	Non-Fac Total	Fac Total	Global Days	51	50	62	80	MUE
	0.00	0.00	XXX	0	0	0	0	
26	0.00	0.00	XXX	0	0	0	0	
TC	0.00	0.00	XXX	0	0	0	0	

AMA: Dec 05: 7

Pub 100-04, 13, 120

Other Nuclear Medicine Diagnostic Procedures

78800 Radiopharmaceutical localization of tumor or distribution of radiopharmaceutical agent(s); limited area Z2 S

RVU Mod	Non-Fac Total	Fac Total	Global Days	51	50	62	80	MUE
	5.56	5.56	XXX	0	0	0	0	1
26	0.96	0.96	XXX	0	0	0	0	1
TC	4.60	4.60	XXX	0	0	0	0	1

AMA: Dec 05: 7, Dec 11: 17, Feb 12: 9

78801 Radiopharmaceutical localization of tumor or distribution of radiopharmaceutical agent(s); multiple areas Z2 S

RVU Mod	Non-Fac Total	Fac Total	Global Days	51	50	62	80	MUE
	7.59	7.59	XXX	0	0	0	0	1
26	1.14	1.14	XXX	0	0	0	0	1
TC	6.45	6.45	XXX	0	0	0	0	1

AMA: Dec 11: 17, Feb 12: 9

78802 Radiopharmaceutical localization of tumor or distribution of radiopharmaceutical agent(s); whole body, single day imaging Z2 S

RVU Mod	Non-Fac Total	Fac Total	Global Days	51	50	62	80	MUE
	9.45	9.45	XXX	2	0	0	0	1
26	1.19	1.19	XXX	2	0	0	0	1
TC	8.26	8.26	XXX	2	0	0	0	1

AMA: Jun 03: 11, Feb 12: 9

Pub 100-04, 13, 50.3

78803 Radiopharmaceutical localization of tumor or distribution of radiopharmaceutical agent(s); tomographic (SPECT) Z2 S

RVU Mod	Non-Fac Total	Fac Total	Global Days	51	50	62	80	MUE
	9.89	9.89	XXX	2	0	0	0	1
26	1.47	1.47	XXX	2	0	0	0	1
TC	8.42	8.42	XXX	2	0	0	0	1

AMA: Jun 03: 11, Feb 12: 9

Pub 100-04, 13, 50.3

78804 Radiopharmaceutical localization of tumor or distribution of radiopharmaceutical agent(s); whole body, requiring 2 or more days imaging Z2 S

RVU Mod	Non-Fac Total	Fac Total	Global Days	51	50	62	80	MUE
	16.48	16.48	XXX	0	0	0	0	1
26	1.47	1.47	XXX	0	0	0	0	1
TC	15.01	15.01	XXX	0	0	0	0	1

AMA: Feb 12: 9

78805 Radiopharmaceutical localization of inflammatory process; limited area Z2 S

RVU Mod	Non-Fac Total	Fac Total	Global Days	51	50	62	80	MUE
	5.29	5.29	XXX	0	0	0	0	1
26	1.02	1.02	XXX	0	0	0	0	1
TC	4.27	4.27	XXX	0	0	0	0	1

AMA: Nov 99: 44, Feb 12: 9

78806 Radiopharmaceutical localization of inflammatory process; whole body Z2 S

RVU Mod	Non-Fac Total	Fac Total	Global Days	51	50	62	80	MUE
	9.67	9.67	XXX	2	0	0	0	1
26	1.19	1.19	XXX	2	0	0	0	1
TC	8.48	8.48	XXX	2	0	0	0	1

AMA: Nov 99: 44, Jun 03: 11, Feb 12: 9

Pub 100-04, 13, 50.3

78807 Radiopharmaceutical localization of inflammatory process; tomographic (SPECT) Z2 S

RVU Mod	Non-Fac Total	Fac Total	Global Days	51	50	62	80	MUE
	9.88	9.88	XXX	2	0	0	0	1
26	1.47	1.47	XXX	2	0	0	0	1
TC	8.41	8.41	XXX	2	0	0	0	1

AMA: Jun 03: 11, Feb 12: 9

Pub 100-04, 13, 50.3

● New ▲ Revised Deleted ⊙ Moderate Sedation ✚ Add-on Codes ⊗ High Risk Denial Ⓐ Age Edit ♀ Female ♂ Male **AMA** *CPT® Assistant* **MUE** Medically Unlikely Edit
⊘ Modifier 51 Exempt ⊖ Modifier 63 Exempt ✗ Unlisted **Modifiers:** *See Inside Back Cover* Ⓜ Maternity A2 – Z3 ASC Payment Indicators A – Y OPPS Status Indicators

© 2016 DecisionHealth | CPT © 2015 American Medical Association. All Rights Reserved. | **671**

78808 Injection procedure for radiopharmaceutical localization by non-imaging probe study, intravenous (eg, parathyroid adenoma) ⊘N1Q1

RVU		Global Days	Modifiers				
Mod	Non-Fac Total	Fac Total		51	50	62	80	MUE
	1.31	1.31	XXX	0	0	0	0	1

AMA: Feb 12: 9

Coding Guidance

Positron emission tomography (PET) for tumor imaging is reported with 78811-78816. CPT codes 78814-78816 should be used when a concurrently acquired CT scan for attenuation or localization is done. Other, separate CT scans for localization should not be reported together with codes 78811-78816. A separate, diagnostic CT scan that is deemed necessary may be reported with an associated modifier.

78811 Positron emission tomography (PET) imaging; limited area (eg, chest, head/neck) Z2 S

RVU		Global Days	Modifiers				
Mod	Non-Fac Total	Fac Total		51	50	62	80	MUE
	0.00	0.00	XXX	0	0	0	0	1
26	2.19	2.19	XXX	0	0	0	0	1
TC	0.00	0.00	XXX	0	0	0	0	1

AMA: Dec 05: 7, Feb 12: 9

Pub 100-04, 13, 60.12, 60.16, 60.18, 60.3.1, 60.3.2; 100-04, 32, 60.12

78812 Positron emission tomography (PET) imaging; skull base to mid-thigh Z2 S

RVU		Global Days	Modifiers				
Mod	Non-Fac Total	Fac Total		51	50	62	80	MUE
	0.00	0.00	XXX	0	0	0	0	1
26	2.67	2.67	XXX	0	0	0	0	1
TC	0.00	0.00	XXX	0	0	0	0	1

AMA: Dec 05: 7, Feb 12: 9, Feb 13: 16

Pub 100-04, 13, 60.16, 60.18, 60.3.1, 60.3.2

78813 Positron emission tomography (PET) imaging; whole body Z2 S

RVU		Global Days	Modifiers				
Mod	Non-Fac Total	Fac Total		51	50	62	80	MUE
	0.00	0.00	XXX	0	0	0	0	1
26	2.78	2.78	XXX	0	0	0	0	1
TC	0.00	0.00	XXX	0	0	0	0	1

AMA: Dec 05: 7, Feb 12: 9, Feb 13: 16

Pub 100-04, 13, 60.16, 60.18, 60.3.1, 60.3.2

78814 Positron emission tomography (PET) with concurrently acquired computed tomography (CT) for attenuation correction and anatomical localization imaging; limited area (eg, chest, head/neck) Z2 S

RVU		Global Days	Modifiers				
Mod	Non-Fac Total	Fac Total		51	50	62	80	MUE
	0.00	0.00	XXX	0	0	0	0	1
26	3.08	3.08	XXX	0	0	0	0	1
TC	0.00	0.00	XXX	0	0	0	0	1

AMA: Feb 05: 13, Jun 05: 10, Dec 05: 7, Feb 12: 9, Feb 13: 16

Pub 100-04, 13, 60.12, 60.16, 60.18, 60.3.1, 60.3.2; 100-04, 32, 60.12

78815 Positron emission tomography (PET) with concurrently acquired computed tomography (CT) for attenuation correction and anatomical localization imaging; skull base to mid-thigh Z2 S

RVU		Global Days	Modifiers				
Mod	Non-Fac Total	Fac Total		51	50	62	80	MUE
	0.00	0.00	XXX	0	0	0	0	1
26	3.39	3.39	XXX	0	0	0	0	1
TC	0.00	0.00	XXX	0	0	0	0	1

AMA: Feb 05: 13, Jun 05: 10, Dec 05: 7, Feb 12: 9, Feb 13: 16

Pub 100-04, 13, 60.18, 60.3.1, 60.3.2,

78816 Positron emission tomography (PET) with concurrently acquired computed tomography (CT) for attenuation correction and anatomical localization imaging; whole body Z2 S

RVU		Global Days	Modifiers				
Mod	Non-Fac Total	Fac Total		51	50	62	80	MUE
	0.00	0.00	XXX	0	0	0	0	1
26	3.42	3.42	XXX	0	0	0	0	1
TC	0.00	0.00	XXX	0	0	0	0	1

AMA: Feb 05: 13, Jun 05: 10, Dec 05: 7, Feb 12: 9, Feb 13: 16

Pub 100-04, 13, 60.16, 60.18, 60.3.2

78999 Unlisted miscellaneous procedure, diagnostic nuclear medicine ⊘✗Z2 S

RVU		Global Days	Modifiers				
Mod	Non-Fac Total	Fac Total		51	50	62	80	MUE
	0.00	0.00	XXX	0	0	0	
26	0.00	0.00	XXX	0	0	0	
TC	0.00	0.00	XXX	0	0	0	

AMA: Dec 05: 7, Feb 12: 9

Pub 100-04, 13, 120

Radiopharmaceutical Therapy Procedures

79005 Radiopharmaceutical therapy, by oral administration Z3 S

RVU		Global Days	Modifiers				
Mod	Non-Fac Total	Fac Total		51	50	62	80	MUE
	3.88	3.88	XXX	0	0	0	0	1
26	2.49	2.49	XXX	0	0	0	0	1
TC	1.39	1.39	XXX	0	0	0	0	1

AMA: Sep 05: 1, Feb 12: 9

79101 Radiopharmaceutical therapy, by intravenous administration Z3 S

RVU		Global Days	Modifiers				
Mod	Non-Fac Total	Fac Total		51	50	62	80	MUE
	4.05	4.05	XXX	0	0	0	0	1
26	2.70	2.70	XXX	0	0	0	0	1
TC	1.35	1.35	XXX	0	0	0	0	1

AMA: Sep 05: 1, Feb 12: 9

79200 Radiopharmaceutical therapy, by intracavitary administration Z3 S

RVU		Global Days	Modifiers				
Mod	Non-Fac Total	Fac Total		51	50	62	80	MUE
	4.54	4.54	XXX	0	0	0	0	1
26	2.89	2.89	XXX	0	0	0	0	1
TC	1.65	1.65	XXX	0	0	0	0	1

AMA: Sep 05: 1, Feb 12: 9

● New ▲ Revised ✖ Deleted ⊙ Moderate Sedation ✚ Add-on Codes ⊘ High Risk Denial ⒶAge Edit ♀ Female ♂ Male **AMA** CPT® Assistant **MUE** Medically Unlikely Edit ⊘ Modifier 51 Exempt ⊖ Modifier 63 Exempt ✗ Unlisted **Modifiers:** See Inside Back Cover Ⓜ Maternity Ⓩ2 - Ⓩ3 ASC Payment Indicators Ⓐ - Ⓨ OPPS Status Indicators

CPT © 2015 American Medical Association. All Rights Reserved. © 2016 DecisionHealth

Radiology Procedures

79300   Radiopharmaceutical therapy, by interstitial radioactive colloid administration   Z 2 S

Mod	RVU Non-Fac Total	Fac Total	Global Days	Modifiers 51	50	62	80	MUE
	0.00	0.00	XXX	0	0	0	0	1
26	2.26	2.26	XXX	0	0	0	0	1
TC	0.00	0.00	XXX	0	0	0	0	1

AMA: Sep 05: 1, Feb 12: 9

79403   Radiopharmaceutical therapy, radiolabeled monoclonal antibody by intravenous infusion   Z 3 S

Mod	RVU Non-Fac Total	Fac Total	Global Days	Modifiers 51	50	62	80	MUE
	5.47	5.47	XXX	0	0	0	0	1
26	3.15	3.15	XXX	0	0	0	0	1
TC	2.32	2.32	XXX	0	0	0	0	1

AMA: Sep 05: 1, Feb 12: 9

79440   Radiopharmaceutical therapy, by intra-articular administration   Z 3 S

Mod	RVU Non-Fac Total	Fac Total	Global Days	Modifiers 51	50	62	80	MUE
	4.11	4.11	XXX	0	0	0	0	1
26	2.69	2.69	XXX	0	0	0	0	1
TC	1.42	1.42	XXX	0	0	0	0	1

AMA: Sep 05: 1, Feb 12: 9

79445   Radiopharmaceutical therapy, by intra-arterial particulate administration   Z 2 S

Mod	RVU Non-Fac Total	Fac Total	Global Days	Modifiers 51	50	62	80	MUE
	0.00	0.00	XXX	0	0	0	0	1
26	3.27	3.27	XXX	0	0	0	0	1
TC	0.00	0.00	XXX	0	0	0	0	1

AMA: Sep 05: 1, Dec 06: 10, Feb 12: 9, Nov 13: 6

79999   Radiopharmaceutical therapy, unlisted procedure   ⊘✗ Z 2 S

Mod	RVU Non-Fac Total	Fac Total	Global Days	Modifiers 51	50	62	80	MUE
	0.00	0.00	XXX	0	0	0	0	
26	0.00	0.00	XXX	0	0	0	0	
TC	0.00	0.00	XXX	0	0	0	0	

AMA: Mar 05: 11, Sep 05: 1, Jan 07: 30, Feb 12: 9

Pub 100-04, 13, 120

79300 – 79999

● New   ▲ Revised   Deleted   ⊙ Moderate Sedation   ✚ Add-on Codes   ⊗ High Risk Denial   Ⓐ Age Edit   ♀ Female   ♂ Male   **AMA** *CPT® Assistant*   ***MUE*** Medically Unlikely Edit
⊘ Modifier 51 Exempt   ⊖ Modifier 63 Exempt   ✗ Unlisted   **Modifiers:** *See Inside Back Cover*   Ⓜ Maternity   A 2 – Z 3 ASC Payment Indicators   A – Y OPPS Status Indicators

Laboratory/Pathology Services

Introduction to Laboratory/Pathology

Laboratory and pathology procedures, CPT codes 80047-89398, report services to assess specimens obtained from patients such tissue, blood, or other body fluids. These specimens are usually prepared, screened, or tested by laboratory technologists under the supervision of a pathologist with the exception of certain tests which are reviewed or interpreted personally by the pathologist.

During surgical procedures, tissue is removed and submitted for pathologic (gross and microscopic) examination. According to the CPT surgical pathology coding guidelines, a surgical pathology specimen is defined as tissue from a patient that is submitted for individual examination and pathologic diagnosis. Two or more specimens from the same patient that are submitted, separately examined, and pathologically diagnosed, may each be reported separately with an appropriate code that reflects the service provided.

Reporting Laboratory Panels

The Laboratory and Pathology Section includes codes that describe organ and disease specific panels of laboratory tests. If all tests included in one of these panels are performed, the CPT code for the panel of tests is reported. If one of the component tests is repeated as a medically necessary service on the same date of service, the CPT code corresponding to the repeated laboratory test may be reported with modifier 91.

Reporting Multiple Laboratory or Pathology Procedures

Multiple laboratory and pathology procedures are frequently rendered on the same date. Typically, it is appropriate to report these separately; however, if an additional related procedure is necessary to complete or verify the result, these are considered part of the initial test ordered. For example, if a patient has an abnormal test result and the test is repeated to verify the abnormal result, the test would be reported as one unit of service rather than two.

There are also certain laboratory tests that require additional, separate testing if results are positive because the positive result alone has limited clinical value without additional testing. For example, when a urine culture is positive, the laboratory performs specific organism identification testing which is separately reportable. This type of testing must be distinguished from additional testing performed on a test result that does have value clinically without the additional testing. In these cases, separate reporting of the additional testing would not be appropriate unless it was specifically ordered by the treating physician.

Qualitative Assays

Qualitative assays are laboratory tests performed to determine a numerical amount of a specific analyte or constituent in a specimen. CPT codes for quantitative drug testing are located in two different subsections of the Pathology and Laboratory Section—Therapeutic Drug Assays (80150-80299) and Chemistry (82000-84999). Codes specific to single or multiple sequential procedures were created in order to clarify reporting of qualitative testing for multiple drugs classes (e.g., qualitative analysis using a multiplexed method for 2-15 drugs or drug classes)

Molecular Pathology

Molecular pathology (MOPATH), or molecular diagnostics, is a new pathology discipline that studies and diagnoses disease through newly developed techniques for examining the molecular signatures of cells. Combining genomics (the study of genes in a cell) and proteomics (the study of proteins in a cell), molecular diagnostics determines how these genes and proteins are interacting within the cell. For example, molecular assays in, cancer, genetics, and histocompatibility are molecular based, rather than serology based. To identify and describe more accurately the new technology used in these services, a new subsection of CPT codes for reporting molecular pathology was added to the Pathology and Laboratory Section in 2012, including guidelines and definitions. Codes were also included for common analytes and multianalyte assays which utilize multiple testing derived from molecular pathology and other lab tests to derive a single result.

Pathologist Evaluation and Management Services

Although codes in this section do not normally involve patient contact or evaluation and management services rendered directly by the pathologist, if a pathologist does provide significant, separately identifiable face-to-face patient care services that satisfy the E/M criteria, he or she may report the appropriate evaluation and management code.

Unlisted Procedures and Special Reports

When a laboratory or pathology service or procedure is provided that does not have a distinct CPT code, the appropriate "unlisted procedure" code is used to indicate the service, identifying it by "special report". According to the guidelines for reporting a service that is unusual and requires a special report, providers should include a description of the nature, extent, and need for the procedure, along with the time, effort, and equipment necessary to provide the service.

Organ/Disease Panel Studies
Coding Guidance

Organ or disease-oriented panels consist of a group of tests. The panel code may be reported whether the test is ordered as the panel code or whether individual component tests ordered separately equal the same content as the panel code. Edits will pair a panel code with the separate CPT codes that correspond to each of the individual laboratory tests comprising the panel. Modifier 91 is allowed for bypassing these edits when one or more of the individual tests are repeated on the same patient and day of service. Modifier 91 is not allowed when repeat testing is performed to confirm the initial results due to specimen or equipment problems.

80047　**Basic metabolic panel (Calcium, ionized) This panel must include the following:**

Calcium, ionized (82330)

Carbon dioxide (bicarbonate) (82374)

Chloride (82435)

Creatinine (82565)

Glucose (82947)

Potassium (84132)

Sodium (84295)

Urea Nitrogen (BUN) (84520)　　　　Q4

Coding tip: For a CLIA-waived test, append modifier QW to 80047

RVU		Global Days	Modifiers				
Mod	Non-Fac Total　Fac Total		51	50	62	80	MUE
	0.00　　　　0.00	XXX	9	9	9	9	2

AMA: Apr 08: 5, Apr 13: 10

Pub 100-04, 16, 40.6.1, 100.6

80048　**Basic metabolic panel (Calcium, total)**

This panel must include the following:

Calcium, total (82310)

Carbon dioxide (bicarbonate) (82374)

Chloride (82435)

Creatinine (82565)

Glucose (82947)

Potassium (84132)

Sodium (84295)

Urea nitrogen (BUN) (84520)　　　　Q4

Coding tip: For a CLIA-waived test, append modifier QW to 80048

RVU		Global Days	Modifiers				
Mod	Non-Fac Total　Fac Total		51	50	62	80	MUE
	0.00　　　　0.00	XXX	9	9	9	9	2

AMA: Jan 98: 6, Sep 99: 11, Nov 99: 44, Jan 00: 7, Aug 05: 9

Pub 100-04, 16, 40.6.2, 100.6, 120.2

● New　▲ Revised　✖ Deleted　⊙ Moderate Sedation　✚ Add-on Codes　⊘ High Risk Denial　Ⓐ Age Edit　♀ Female　♂ Male　**AMA** *CPT® Assistant*　***MUE*** Medically Unlikely Edit
⊘ Modifier 51 Exempt　⊖ Modifier 63 Exempt　✗ Unlisted　**Modifiers:** *See Inside Back Cover*　Ⓜ Maternity　A 2 - Z 3 ASC Payment Indicators　A - Y OPPS Status Indicators

80050 General health panel

This panel must include the following:

Comprehensive metabolic panel (80053)

Blood count, complete (CBC), automated and automated differential WBC count (85025 or 85027 and 85004) OR Blood count, complete (CBC), automated (85027) and appropriate manual differential WBC count (85007 or 85009) Thyroid stimulating hormone (TSH) (84443) ⊗🄴

RVU			Global Days	Modifiers				
Mod	Non-Fac Total	Fac Total		51	50	62	80	MUE
	0.00	0.00	XXX	9	9	9	9	

AMA: Winter 92: 14, Summer 93: 14, Jun 97: 10, Nov 97: 28, Jan 98: 6, Sep 99: 11

80051 Electrolyte panel

This panel must include the following:

Carbon dioxide (bicarbonate) (82374)

Chloride (82435)

Potassium (84132)

Sodium (84295) 🇶4

RVU			Global Days	Modifiers				
Mod	Non-Fac Total	Fac Total		51	50	62	80	MUE
	0.00	0.00	XXX	9	9	9	9	2

AMA: Nov 97: 28, Jan 98: 7, Sep 99: 11

Pub 100-04, 16, 100.6, 120.2

80053 Comprehensive metabolic panel

This panel must include the following:

Albumin (82040)

Bilirubin, total (82247)

Calcium, total (82310)

Carbon dioxide (bicarbonate) (82374)

Chloride (82435)

Creatinine (82565)

Glucose (82947)

Phosphatase, alkaline (84075)

Potassium (84132)

Protein, total (84155)

Sodium (84295)

Transferase, alanine amino (ALT) (SGPT) (84460)

Transferase, aspartate amino (AST) (SGOT) (84450) Urea nitrogen (BUN) (84520) 🇶4

Coding tip: *For a CLIA-waived test, append modifier QW to 80053*

RVU			Global Days	Modifiers				
Mod	Non-Fac Total	Fac Total		51	50	62	80	MUE
	0.00	0.00	XXX	9	9	9	9	1

AMA: Jan 98: 6, Nov 98: 23, Sep 99: 11, Nov 99: 44, May 00: 11, Jan 05: 46, Apr 08: 5, Apr 10: 11, Apr 13: 10

Pub 100-04, 16, 40.6.3, 100.6, 120.2

80055 Obstetric panel

This panel must include the following:

Blood count, complete (CBC), automated and automated differential WBC count (85025 or 85027 and 85004) OR Blood count, complete (CBC), automated (85027) and appropriate manual differential WBC count (85007 or 85009)

Hepatitis B surface antigen (HBsAg) (87340)

Antibody, rubella (86762)

Syphilis test, non-treponemal antibody; qualitative (eg, VDRL, RPR, ART) (86592)

Antibody screen, RBC, each serum technique (86850)

Blood typing, ABO (86900) AND Blood typing, Rh (D) (86901) ⊗♀Ⓜ🄴

RVU			Global Days	Modifiers				
Mod	Non-Fac Total	Fac Total		51	50	62	80	MUE
	0.00	0.00	XXX	9	9	9	9	

AMA: Winter 92: 14, Summer 93: 14, Jun 97: 10, Apr 99: 6, Sep 99: 11

80061 Lipid panel

This panel must include the following:

Cholesterol, serum, total (82465)

Lipoprotein, direct measurement, high density cholesterol (HDL cholesterol) (83718)

Triglycerides (84478) 🄰

Coding tip: *Do not use 83721 to report a calculated LDL cholesterol. A direct measurement of LDL cholesterol with total cholesterol (82465) or lipid panel (80061) is sometimes done with high triglyceride levels greater than 400mg/dl, in order to measure the LDL cholesterol. In these cases, report 83721 with modifier 59.*

Coding tip: *For a CLIA-waived test, append modifier QW to 80061*

RVU			Global Days	Modifiers				
Mod	Non-Fac Total	Fac Total		51	50	62	80	MUE
	0.00	0.00	XXX	9	9	9	9	1

AMA: Winter 92: 14, Summer 93: 14, Jun 97: 10, Sep 99: 11, Mar 00: 11, Feb 05: 9

Pub 100-04, 12, 30; 100-04, 16, 40.6.4, 90.2, 100.5, 120.2; 100-04, 18, 1.2, 100.1, 100.2, 100.3, 100.5
NCD: 190.23B

80069 Renal function panel

This panel must include the following:

Albumin (82040)

Calcium, total (82310)

Carbon dioxide (bicarbonate) (82374)

Chloride (82435)

Creatinine (82565)

Glucose (82947)

Phosphorus inorganic (phosphate) (84100)

Potassium (84132)

Sodium (84295)

Urea nitrogen (BUN) (84520) 🇶4

Coding tip: *For a CLIA-waived test, append modifier QW to 80069*

RVU			Global Days	Modifiers				
Mod	Non-Fac Total	Fac Total		51	50	62	80	MUE
	0.00	0.00	XXX	9	9	9	9	1

AMA: Sep 99: 11, Nov 99: 44

Pub 100-04, 16, 40.6.5, 100.6, 120.2

● New   ▲ Revised   Deleted   ⊙ Moderate Sedation   ✛ Add-on Codes   ⊗ High Risk Denial   Ⓐ Age Edit   ♀ Female   ♂ Male   **AMA** *CPT® Assistant*   **MUE** Medically Unlikely Edit
⊘ Modifier 51 Exempt   ⊖ Modifier 63 Exempt   ✗ Unlisted   **Modifiers:** *See Inside Back Cover*   Ⓜ Maternity   🄰2–🅉3 ASC Payment Indicators   🄰–🅈 OPPS Status Indicators

© 2016 DecisionHealth   CPT © 2015 American Medical Association. All Rights Reserved.   **675**

80074 Acute hepatitis panel

This panel must include the following:

Hepatitis A antibody (HAAb), IgM antibody (86709)

Hepatitis B core antibody (HBcAb), IgM antibody (86705)

Hepatitis B surface antigen (HBsAg) (87340)

Hepatitis C antibody (86803) Q4

RVU			Global Days	Modifiers				
Mod	Non-Fac Total	Fac Total		51	50	62	80	MUE
	0.00	0.00	XXX	9	9	9	9	1

AMA: Sep 99: 11, Nov 99: 45

Pub 100-04, 16, 120.2
NCD: 190.33

80076 Hepatic function panel

This panel must include the following:

Albumin (82040)

Bilirubin, total (82247)

Bilirubin, direct (82248)

Phosphatase, alkaline (84075)

Protein, total (84155)

Transferase, alanine amino (ALT) (SGPT) (84460)

Transferase, aspartate amino (AST) (SGOT) (84450) Q4

RVU			Global Days	Modifiers				
Mod	Non-Fac Total	Fac Total		51	50	62	80	MUE
	0.00	0.00	XXX	9	9	9	9	1

AMA: Winter 92: 14, Summer 93: 14, Jun 97: 10, Jan 98: 6, Apr 99: 6, Sep 99: 11, Nov 99: 45, Jan 00: 7, Aug 05: 9

Pub 100-04, 16, 40.6.6, 100.6, 120.2

● **80081 Obstetric panel (includes HIV testing)**

This panel must include the following:

Blood count, complete (CBC), and automated differential WBC count (85025 or 85027 and 85004) OR Blood count, complete (CBC), automated (85027) and appropriate manual differential WBC count (85007 or 85009)

Hepatitis B surface antigen (HBsAg) (87340)

HIV-1 antigen(s), with HIV-1 and HIV-2 antibodies, single result (87389)

Antibody, rubella (86762)

Syphilis test, non-treponemal antibody; qualitative (eg, VDRL, RPR, ART) (86592)

Antibody screen, RBC, each serum technique (86850)

Blood typing, ABO (86900) AND Blood typing, Rh (D) (86901) ♀ⓂE

RVU			Global Days	Modifiers				
Mod	Non-Fac Total	Fac Total		51	50	62	80	MUE
	0.00	0.00	XXX	9	9	9	9	1

Quantitative Therapeutic Drug Testing

80150 Amikacin Q4

RVU			Global Days	Modifiers				
Mod	Non-Fac Total	Fac Total		51	50	62	80	MUE
	0.00	0.00	XXX	9	9	9	9	2

AMA: Aug 05: 9, Mar 11: 10, Oct 10: 7, Dec 10: 7, Apr 15: 3

80155 Caffeine Q4

RVU			Global Days	Modifiers				
Mod	Non-Fac Total	Fac Total		51	50	62	80	MUE
	0.00	0.00	XXX	9	9	9	9	1

80156 Carbamazepine; total Q4

RVU			Global Days	Modifiers				
Mod	Non-Fac Total	Fac Total		51	50	62	80	MUE
	0.00	0.00	XXX	9	9	9	9	2

AMA: Mar 11: 10, Oct 10: 7

80157 Carbamazepine; free Q4

RVU			Global Days	Modifiers				
Mod	Non-Fac Total	Fac Total		51	50	62	80	MUE
	0.00	0.00	XXX	9	9	9	9	2

AMA: Mar 11: 10, Oct 10: 7

80158 Cyclosporine Q4

RVU			Global Days	Modifiers				
Mod	Non-Fac Total	Fac Total		51	50	62	80	MUE
	0.00	0.00	XXX	9	9	9	9	2

AMA: Mar 11: 10, Oct 10: 7

80159 Clozapine Q4

RVU			Global Days	Modifiers				
Mod	Non-Fac Total	Fac Total		51	50	62	80	MUE
	0.00	0.00	XXX	9	9	9	9	2

80162 Digoxin; total Q4

RVU			Global Days	Modifiers				
Mod	Non-Fac Total	Fac Total		51	50	62	80	MUE
	0.00	0.00	XXX	9	9	9	9	2

AMA: Oct 10: 7, Mar 11: 10, Apr 15: 3
NCD: 190.24

80163 Digoxin; free Q4

RVU			Global Days	Modifiers				
Mod	Non-Fac Total	Fac Total		51	50	62	80	MUE
	0.00	0.00	XXX	9	9	9	9	2

AMA: Apr 15: 3

80164 Valproic acid (dipropylacetic acid); total Q4

RVU			Global Days	Modifiers				
Mod	Non-Fac Total	Fac Total		51	50	62	80	MUE
	0.00	0.00	XXX	9	9	9	9	2

AMA: Oct 10: 7, Mar 11: 10, Apr 15: 3

80165 Valproic acid (dipropylacetic acid); free Q4

RVU			Global Days	Modifiers				
Mod	Non-Fac Total	Fac Total		51	50	62	80	MUE
	0.00	0.00	XXX	9	9	9	9	2

AMA: Apr 15: 3

80168 Ethosuximide Q4

RVU			Global Days	Modifiers				
Mod	Non-Fac Total	Fac Total		51	50	62	80	MUE
	0.00	0.00	XXX	9	9	9	9	2

AMA: Oct 10: 7, Mar 11: 10

● New ▲ Revised ✖ Deleted ⊙ Moderate Sedation ✚ Add-on Codes ⊘ High Risk Denial Ⓐ Age Edit ♀ Female ♂ Male **AMA** CPT® Assistant **MUE** Medically Unlikely Edit
⊘ Modifier 51 Exempt ⊖ Modifier 63 Exempt ✗ Unlisted **Modifiers:** See Inside Back Cover Ⓜ Maternity A2–Z3 ASC Payment Indicators A–Y OPPS Status Indicators

676 CPT © 2015 American Medical Association. All Rights Reserved. © 2016 DecisionHealth

80169 Everolimus   ⊙4

Mod	Non-Fac Total	Fac Total	Global Days	51	50	62	80	MUE
	0.00	0.00	XXX	9	9	9	9	1

80170 Gentamicin   ⊙4

Mod	Non-Fac Total	Fac Total	Global Days	51	50	62	80	MUE
	0.00	0.00	XXX	9	9	9	9	2

AMA: Oct 10: 7, Mar 11: 10

80171 Gabapentin, whole blood, serum, or plasma   ⊙4

Mod	Non-Fac Total	Fac Total	Global Days	51	50	62	80	MUE
	0.00	0.00	XXX	9	9	9	9	1

AMA: Apr 15: 3

80173 Haloperidol   ⊙4

Mod	Non-Fac Total	Fac Total	Global Days	51	50	62	80	MUE
	0.00	0.00	XXX	9	9	9	9	2

AMA: Oct 10: 7, Mar 11: 10

80175 Lamotrigine   ⊙4

Mod	Non-Fac Total	Fac Total	Global Days	51	50	62	80	MUE
	0.00	0.00	XXX	9	9	9	9	1

80176 Lidocaine   ⊘⊙4

Mod	Non-Fac Total	Fac Total	Global Days	51	50	62	80	MUE
	0.00	0.00	XXX	9	9	9	9	1

AMA: Oct 10: 7, Mar 11: 10

80177 Levetiracetam   ⊙4

Mod	Non-Fac Total	Fac Total	Global Days	51	50	62	80	MUE
	0.00	0.00	XXX	9	9	9	9	1

80178 Lithium   ⊙4

Coding tip: For a CLIA-waived test, append modifier QW to 80178

Mod	Non-Fac Total	Fac Total	Global Days	51	50	62	80	MUE
	0.00	0.00	XXX	9	9	9	9	2

AMA: Oct 10: 7, Mar 11: 10

80180 Mycophenolate (mycophenolic acid)   ⊙4

Mod	Non-Fac Total	Fac Total	Global Days	51	50	62	80	MUE
	0.00	0.00	XXX	9	9	9	9	1

80183 Oxcarbazepine   ⊙4

Mod	Non-Fac Total	Fac Total	Global Days	51	50	62	80	MUE
	0.00	0.00	XXX	9	9	9	9	1

80184 Phenobarbital   ⊙4

Mod	Non-Fac Total	Fac Total	Global Days	51	50	62	80	MUE
	0.00	0.00	XXX	9	9	9	9	2

AMA: Oct 10: 7, Mar 11: 10

80185 Phenytoin; total   ⊙4

Mod	Non-Fac Total	Fac Total	Global Days	51	50	62	80	MUE
	0.00	0.00	XXX	9	9	9	9	2

AMA: Oct 10: 7, Mar 11: 10

80186 Phenytoin; free   ⊙4

Mod	Non-Fac Total	Fac Total	Global Days	51	50	62	80	MUE
	0.00	0.00	XXX	9	9	9	9	2

AMA: Oct 10: 7, Mar 11: 10

80188 Primidone   ⊙4

Mod	Non-Fac Total	Fac Total	Global Days	51	50	62	80	MUE
	0.00	0.00	XXX	9	9	9	9	2

AMA: Oct 10: 7, Mar 11: 10

80190 Procainamide   ⊘⊙4

Mod	Non-Fac Total	Fac Total	Global Days	51	50	62	80	MUE
	0.00	0.00	XXX	9	9	9	9	2

AMA: Oct 10: 7, Mar 11: 10

80192 Procainamide; with metabolites (eg, n-acetyl procainamide)   ⊙4

Mod	Non-Fac Total	Fac Total	Global Days	51	50	62	80	MUE
	0.00	0.00	XXX	9	9	9	9	2

AMA: Oct 10: 7, Mar 11: 10

80194 Quinidine   ⊘⊙4

Mod	Non-Fac Total	Fac Total	Global Days	51	50	62	80	MUE
	0.00	0.00	XXX	9	9	9	9	2

AMA: Oct 10: 7, Mar 11: 10

80195 Sirolimus   ⊙4

Mod	Non-Fac Total	Fac Total	Global Days	51	50	62	80	MUE
	0.00	0.00	XXX	9	9	9	9	2

AMA: Mar 06: 6, Oct 10: 7, Mar 11: 10

80197 Tacrolimus   ⊙4

Mod	Non-Fac Total	Fac Total	Global Days	51	50	62	80	MUE
	0.00	0.00	XXX	9	9	9	9	2

AMA: Oct 10: 7, Mar 11: 10
Pub 100-04, 16, 120.2

80198 Theophylline   ⊙4

Mod	Non-Fac Total	Fac Total	Global Days	51	50	62	80	MUE
	0.00	0.00	XXX	9	9	9	9	2

AMA: Oct 10: 7, Mar 11: 10

80199 Tiagabine   ⊙4

Mod	Non-Fac Total	Fac Total	Global Days	51	50	62	80	MUE
	0.00	0.00	XXX	9	9	9	9	1

● New   ▲ Revised   Deleted   ⊙ Moderate Sedation   ✚ Add-on Codes   ⊘ High Risk Denial   Ⓐ Age Edit   ♀ Female   ♂ Male   **AMA** *CPT® Assistant*   **MUE** Medically Unlikely Edit

⊗ Modifier 51 Exempt   ⊖ Modifier 63 Exempt   ✗ Unlisted   **Modifiers:** *See Inside Back Cover*   Ⓜ Maternity   A2–Z3 ASC Payment Indicators   A–Y OPPS Status Indicators

© 2016 DecisionHealth   CPT © 2015 American Medical Association. All Rights Reserved.

80200 Tobramycin ⊙4

Mod	Non-Fac Total	Fac Total	Global Days	Modifiers 51	50	62	80	MUE
	0.00	0.00	XXX	9	9	9	9	2

AMA: Oct 10: 7, Mar 11: 10

80201 Topiramate ⊙4

Mod	Non-Fac Total	Fac Total	Global Days	Modifiers 51	50	62	80	MUE
	0.00	0.00	XXX	9	9	9	9	2

AMA: Nov 97: 28, Oct 10: 7, Mar 11: 10

80202 Vancomycin ⊙4

Mod	Non-Fac Total	Fac Total	Global Days	Modifiers 51	50	62	80	MUE
	0.00	0.00	XXX	9	9	9	9	2

AMA: Mar 11: 10, Oct 10: 7, Apr 15: 3

80203 Zonisamide ⊙4

Mod	Non-Fac Total	Fac Total	Global Days	Modifiers 51	50	62	80	MUE
	0.00	0.00	XXX	9	9	9	9	1

80299 Quantitation of therapeutic drug, not elsewhere specified ✗⊙4

Mod	Non-Fac Total	Fac Total	Global Days	Modifiers 51	50	62	80	MUE
	0.00	0.00	XXX	9	9	9	9	3

AMA: Mar 00: 3, Oct 04: 14, Aug 05: 9, Mar 11: 10, Oct 10: 7, Dec 10: 3, Apr 15: 3

80300 Drug screen, any number of drug classes from Drug Class List A; any number of non-TLC devices or procedures, (eg, immunoassay) capable of being read by direct optical observation, including instrumented-assisted when performed (eg, dipsticks, cups, cards, cartridges), per date of service B

Mod	Non-Fac Total	Fac Total	Global Days	Modifiers 51	50	62	80	MUE
	0.00	0.00	XXX	9	9	9	9	

80301 Drug screen, any number of drug classes from Drug Class List A; single drug class method, by instrumented test systems (eg, discrete multichannel chemistry analyzers utilizing immunoassay or enzyme assay), per date of service B

Mod	Non-Fac Total	Fac Total	Global Days	Modifiers 51	50	62	80	MUE
	0.00	0.00	XXX	9	9	9	9	

80302 Drug screen, presumptive, single drug class from Drug Class List B, by immunoassay (eg, ELISA) or non-TLC chromatography without mass spectrometry (eg, GC, HPLC), each procedure B

Mod	Non-Fac Total	Fac Total	Global Days	Modifiers 51	50	62	80	MUE
	0.00	0.00	XXX	9	9	9	9	

80303 Drug screen, any number of drug classes, presumptive, single or multiple drug class method; thin layer chromatography procedure(s) (TLC) (eg, acid, neutral, alkaloid plate), per date of service B

Mod	Non-Fac Total	Fac Total	Global Days	Modifiers 51	50	62	80	MUE
	0.00	0.00	XXX	9	9	9	9	

80304 Drug screen, any number of drug classes, presumptive, single or multiple drug class method; not otherwise specified presumptive procedure (eg, TOF, MALDI, LDTD, DESI, DART), each procedure B

Mod	Non-Fac Total	Fac Total	Global Days	Modifiers 51	50	62	80	MUE
	0.00	0.00	XXX	9	9	9	9	

AMA: Jun 15: 10

80320 Alcohols B

Mod	Non-Fac Total	Fac Total	Global Days	Modifiers 51	50	62	80	MUE
	0.00	0.00	XXX	9	9	9	9	

AMA: Apr 15: 3

80321 Alcohol biomarkers; 1 or 2 B

Mod	Non-Fac Total	Fac Total	Global Days	Modifiers 51	50	62	80	MUE
	0.00	0.00	XXX	9	9	9	9	

80322 Alcohol biomarkers; 3 or more B

Mod	Non-Fac Total	Fac Total	Global Days	Modifiers 51	50	62	80	MUE
	0.00	0.00	XXX	9	9	9	9	

80323 Alkaloids, not otherwise specified B

Mod	Non-Fac Total	Fac Total	Global Days	Modifiers 51	50	62	80	MUE
	0.00	0.00	XXX	9	9	9	9	

80324 Amphetamines; 1 or 2 B

Mod	Non-Fac Total	Fac Total	Global Days	Modifiers 51	50	62	80	MUE
	0.00	0.00	XXX	9	9	9	9	

80325 Amphetamines; 3 or 4 B

Mod	Non-Fac Total	Fac Total	Global Days	Modifiers 51	50	62	80	MUE
	0.00	0.00	XXX	9	9	9	9	

80326 Amphetamines; 5 or more B

Mod	Non-Fac Total	Fac Total	Global Days	Modifiers 51	50	62	80	MUE
	0.00	0.00	XXX	9	9	9	9	

80327 Anabolic steroids; 1 or 2 B

Mod	Non-Fac Total	Fac Total	Global Days	Modifiers 51	50	62	80	MUE
	0.00	0.00	XXX	9	9	9	9	

AMA: Apr 15: 5

● New   ▲ Revised   ✖ Deleted   ⊙ Moderate Sedation   ✚ Add-on Codes   ⊘ High Risk Denial   Ⓐ Age Edit   ♀ Female   ♂ Male   **AMA** CPT® Assistant   **MUE** Medically Unlikely Edit
⊘ Modifier 51 Exempt   ⊖ Modifier 63 Exempt   ✗ Unlisted   **Modifiers:** See Inside Back Cover   Ⓜ Maternity   A2–Z3 ASC Payment Indicators   A–Y OPPS Status Indicators

CPT © 2015 American Medical Association. All Rights Reserved.   © 2016 DecisionHealth

80328 Anabolic steroids; 3 or more   [B]

RVU Mod	Non-Fac Total	Fac Total	Global Days	51	50	62	80	MUE
	0.00	0.00	XXX	9	9	9	9	

AMA: Apr 15: 5

80329 Analgesics, non-opioid; 1 or 2   [B]

RVU Mod	Non-Fac Total	Fac Total	Global Days	51	50	62	80	MUE
	0.00	0.00	XXX	9	9	9	9	

80330 Analgesics, non-opioid; 3-5   [B]

RVU Mod	Non-Fac Total	Fac Total	Global Days	51	50	62	80	MUE
	0.00	0.00	XXX	9	9	9	9	

80331 Analgesics, non-opioid; 6 or more   [B]

RVU Mod	Non-Fac Total	Fac Total	Global Days	51	50	62	80	MUE
	0.00	0.00	XXX	9	9	9	9	

80332 Antidepressants, serotonergic class; 1 or 2   [B]

RVU Mod	Non-Fac Total	Fac Total	Global Days	51	50	62	80	MUE
	0.00	0.00	XXX	9	9	9	9	

80333 Antidepressants, serotonergic class; 3-5   [B]

RVU Mod	Non-Fac Total	Fac Total	Global Days	51	50	62	80	MUE
	0.00	0.00	XXX	9	9	9	9	

80334 Antidepressants, serotonergic class; 6 or more   [B]

RVU Mod	Non-Fac Total	Fac Total	Global Days	51	50	62	80	MUE
	0.00	0.00	XXX	9	9	9	9	

80335 Antidepressants, tricyclic and other cyclicals; 1 or 2   [B]

RVU Mod	Non-Fac Total	Fac Total	Global Days	51	50	62	80	MUE
	0.00	0.00	XXX	9	9	9	9	

80336 Antidepressants, tricyclic and other cyclicals; 3-5   [B]

RVU Mod	Non-Fac Total	Fac Total	Global Days	51	50	62	80	MUE
	0.00	0.00	XXX	9	9	9	9	

80337 Antidepressants, tricyclic and other cyclicals; 6 or more   [B]

RVU Mod	Non-Fac Total	Fac Total	Global Days	51	50	62	80	MUE
	0.00	0.00	XXX	9	9	9	9	

80338 Antidepressants, not otherwise specified   [B]

RVU Mod	Non-Fac Total	Fac Total	Global Days	51	50	62	80	MUE
	0.00	0.00	XXX	9	9	9	9	

80339 Antiepileptics, not otherwise specified; 1-3   [B]

RVU Mod	Non-Fac Total	Fac Total	Global Days	51	50	62	80	MUE
	0.00	0.00	XXX	9	9	9	9	

80340 Antiepileptics, not otherwise specified; 4-6   [B]

RVU Mod	Non-Fac Total	Fac Total	Global Days	51	50	62	80	MUE
	0.00	0.00	XXX	9	9	9	9	

80341 Antiepileptics, not otherwise specified; 7 or more   [B]

RVU Mod	Non-Fac Total	Fac Total	Global Days	51	50	62	80	MUE
	0.00	0.00	XXX	9	9	9	9	

80342 Antipsychotics, not otherwise specified; 1-3   [B]

RVU Mod	Non-Fac Total	Fac Total	Global Days	51	50	62	80	MUE
	0.00	0.00	XXX	9	9	9	9	

80343 Antipsychotics, not otherwise specified; 4-6   [B]

RVU Mod	Non-Fac Total	Fac Total	Global Days	51	50	62	80	MUE
	0.00	0.00	XXX	9	9	9	9	

80344 Antipsychotics, not otherwise specified; 7 or more   [B]

RVU Mod	Non-Fac Total	Fac Total	Global Days	51	50	62	80	MUE
	0.00	0.00	XXX	9	9	9	9	

80345 Barbiturates   [B]

RVU Mod	Non-Fac Total	Fac Total	Global Days	51	50	62	80	MUE
	0.00	0.00	XXX	9	9	9	9	

80346 Benzodiazepines; 1-12   [B]

RVU Mod	Non-Fac Total	Fac Total	Global Days	51	50	62	80	MUE
	0.00	0.00	XXX	9	9	9	9	

80347 Benzodiazepines; 13 or more   [B]

RVU Mod	Non-Fac Total	Fac Total	Global Days	51	50	62	80	MUE
	0.00	0.00	XXX	9	9	9	9	

80348 Buprenorphine   [B]

RVU Mod	Non-Fac Total	Fac Total	Global Days	51	50	62	80	MUE
	0.00	0.00	XXX	9	9	9	9	

80349 Cannabinoids, natural   [B]

RVU Mod	Non-Fac Total	Fac Total	Global Days	51	50	62	80	MUE
	0.00	0.00	XXX	9	9	9	9	

80350 Cannabinoids, synthetic; 1-3   [B]

RVU Mod	Non-Fac Total	Fac Total	Global Days	51	50	62	80	MUE
	0.00	0.00	XXX	9	9	9	9	

80351 Cannabinoids, synthetic; 4-6   [B]

RVU Mod	Non-Fac Total	Fac Total	Global Days	51	50	62	80	MUE
	0.00	0.00	XXX	9	9	9	9	

● New   ▲ Revised   Deleted   ⊙ Moderate Sedation   ✚ Add-on Codes   ⊘ High Risk Denial   Ⓐ Age Edit   ♀ Female   ♂ Male   **AMA** *CPT® Assistant*   **MUE** Medically Unlikely Edit
⊘ Modifier 51 Exempt   ⊖ Modifier 63 Exempt   ☒ Unlisted   **Modifiers:** *See Inside Back Cover*   Ⓜ Maternity   A2–Z3 ASC Payment Indicators   A–Y OPPS Status Indicators

80352 Cannabinoids, synthetic; 7 or more   B

Mod	RVU Non-Fac Total	Fac Total	Global Days	Modifiers 51	50	62	80	MUE
	0.00	0.00	XXX	9	9	9	9	

80353 Cocaine   B

Mod	RVU Non-Fac Total	Fac Total	Global Days	Modifiers 51	50	62	80	MUE
	0.00	0.00	XXX	9	9	9	9	

80354 Fentanyl   B

Mod	RVU Non-Fac Total	Fac Total	Global Days	Modifiers 51	50	62	80	MUE
	0.00	0.00	XXX	9	9	9	9	

80355 Gabapentin, non-blood   B

Mod	RVU Non-Fac Total	Fac Total	Global Days	Modifiers 51	50	62	80	MUE
	0.00	0.00	XXX	9	9	9	9	

AMA: Apr 15: 3

80356 Heroin metabolite   B

Mod	RVU Non-Fac Total	Fac Total	Global Days	Modifiers 51	50	62	80	MUE
	0.00	0.00	XXX	9	9	9	9	

80357 Ketamine and norketamine   B

Mod	RVU Non-Fac Total	Fac Total	Global Days	Modifiers 51	50	62	80	MUE
	0.00	0.00	XXX	9	9	9	9	

80358 Methadone   B

Mod	RVU Non-Fac Total	Fac Total	Global Days	Modifiers 51	50	62	80	MUE
	0.00	0.00	XXX	9	9	9	9	

80359 Methylenedioxyamphetamines (MDA, MDEA, MDMA)   B

Mod	RVU Non-Fac Total	Fac Total	Global Days	Modifiers 51	50	62	80	MUE
	0.00	0.00	XXX	9	9	9	9	

80360 Methylphenidate   B

Mod	RVU Non-Fac Total	Fac Total	Global Days	Modifiers 51	50	62	80	MUE
	0.00	0.00	XXX	9	9	9	9	

80361 Opiates, 1 or more   B

Mod	RVU Non-Fac Total	Fac Total	Global Days	Modifiers 51	50	62	80	MUE
	0.00	0.00	XXX	9	9	9	9	

80362 Opioids and opiate analogs; 1 or 2   B

Mod	RVU Non-Fac Total	Fac Total	Global Days	Modifiers 51	50	62	80	MUE
	0.00	0.00	XXX	9	9	9	9	

80363 Opioids and Opiate analogs; 3 or 4   B

Mod	RVU Non-Fac Total	Fac Total	Global Days	Modifiers 51	50	62	80	MUE
	0.00	0.00	XXX	9	9	9	9	

80364 Opioids and Opiate analogs; 5 or more   B

Mod	RVU Non-Fac Total	Fac Total	Global Days	Modifiers 51	50	62	80	MUE
	0.00	0.00	XXX	9	9	9	9	

80365 Oxycodone   B

Mod	RVU Non-Fac Total	Fac Total	Global Days	Modifiers 51	50	62	80	MUE
	0.00	0.00	XXX	9	9	9	9	

80366 Pregabalin   B

Mod	RVU Non-Fac Total	Fac Total	Global Days	Modifiers 51	50	62	80	MUE
	0.00	0.00	XXX	9	9	9	9	

80367 Propoxyphene   B

Mod	RVU Non-Fac Total	Fac Total	Global Days	Modifiers 51	50	62	80	MUE
	0.00	0.00	XXX	9	9	9	9	

80368 Sedative hypnotics (non-benzodiazepines)   B

Mod	RVU Non-Fac Total	Fac Total	Global Days	Modifiers 51	50	62	80	MUE
	0.00	0.00	XXX	9	9	9	9	

80369 Skeletal muscle relaxants; 1 or 2   B

Mod	RVU Non-Fac Total	Fac Total	Global Days	Modifiers 51	50	62	80	MUE
	0.00	0.00	XXX	9	9	9	9	

80370 Skeletal muscle relaxants; 3 or more   B

Mod	RVU Non-Fac Total	Fac Total	Global Days	Modifiers 51	50	62	80	MUE
	0.00	0.00	XXX	9	9	9	9	

80371 Stimulants, synthetic   B

Mod	RVU Non-Fac Total	Fac Total	Global Days	Modifiers 51	50	62	80	MUE
	0.00	0.00	XXX	9	9	9	9	

80372 Tapentadol   B

Mod	RVU Non-Fac Total	Fac Total	Global Days	Modifiers 51	50	62	80	MUE
	0.00	0.00	XXX	9	9	9	9	

80373 Tramadol   B

Mod	RVU Non-Fac Total	Fac Total	Global Days	Modifiers 51	50	62	80	MUE
	0.00	0.00	XXX	9	9	9	9	

80374 Stereoisomer (enantiomer) analysis, single drug class   B

Mod	RVU Non-Fac Total	Fac Total	Global Days	Modifiers 51	50	62	80	MUE
	0.00	0.00	XXX	9	9	9	9	

80375 Drug(s) or substance(s), definitive, qualitative or quantitative, not otherwise specified; 1-3   B

Mod	RVU Non-Fac Total	Fac Total	Global Days	Modifiers 51	50	62	80	MUE
	0.00	0.00	XXX	9	9	9	9	

AMA: Apr 15: 3

● New   ▲ Revised   ✖ Deleted   ⊙ Moderate Sedation   ✚ Add-on Codes   ⊘ High Risk Denial   Ⓐ Age Edit   ♀ Female   ♂ Male   **AMA** *CPT® Assistant*   **MUE** Medically Unlikely Edit
⊘ Modifier 51 Exempt   ⊖ Modifier 63 Exempt   ✗ Unlisted   **Modifiers:** *See Inside Back Cover*   Ⓜ Maternity   A2–Z3 ASC Payment Indicators   A–Y OPPS Status Indicators

680

CPT © 2015 American Medical Association. All Rights Reserved.   © 2016 DecisionHealth

80376 Drug(s) or substance(s), definitive, qualitative or quantitative, not otherwise specified; 4-6 B

RVU			Global Days	Modifiers				
Mod	Non-Fac Total	Fac Total		51	50	62	80	MUE
	0.00	0.00	XXX	9	9	9	9	

AMA: Apr 15: 3

80377 Drug(s) or substance(s), definitive, qualitative or quantitative, not otherwise specified; 7 or more B

RVU			Global Days	Modifiers				
Mod	Non-Fac Total	Fac Total		51	50	62	80	MUE
	0.00	0.00	XXX	9	9	9	9	

AMA: Apr 15: 3

Evocative/Suppressive Tests

Coding Guidance

Evocative or suppression testing involves the use of agents administered to the patient to determine response to those agents. Codes 80400-80440 report the laboratory components for this kind of test. For the test that requires physician administration of the agent, codes 96360-96375 should be reported separately. When the agent is given by ancillary personnel and no physician attendance is required, these codes should not be reported. The service can be reported in the office setting if the physician gives direct supervision. Although the supplies necessary to complete the evocative/suppression testing are included, the actual drugs may be separately reported with the appropriate HCPCS Level II J code(s) for the diagnostic agents.

80400 ACTH stimulation panel; for adrenal insufficiency

This panel must include the following: Cortisol (82533 x 2)   Q4

RVU			Global Days	Modifiers				
Mod	Non-Fac Total	Fac Total		51	50	62	80	MUE
	0.00	0.00	XXX	9	9	9	9	1

AMA: Summer 94: 1, Fall 94: 10, Aug 05: 9

80402 ACTH stimulation panel; for 21 hydroxylase deficiency

This panel must include the following:

Cortisol (82533 x 2)

17 hydroxyprogesterone (83498 x 2)   Q4

RVU			Global Days	Modifiers				
Mod	Non-Fac Total	Fac Total		51	50	62	80	MUE
	0.00	0.00	XXX	9	9	9	9	1

AMA: Summer 94: 1, Fall 94: 10

80406 ACTH stimulation panel; for 3 beta-hydroxydehydrogenase deficiency

This panel must include the following:

Cortisol (82533 x 2)

17 hydroxypregnenolone (84143 x 2)   Q4

RVU			Global Days	Modifiers				
Mod	Non-Fac Total	Fac Total		51	50	62	80	MUE
	0.00	0.00	XXX	9	9	9	9	1

AMA: Summer 94: 1, Fall 94: 10

80408 Aldosterone suppression evaluation panel (eg, saline infusion)

This panel must include the following:

Aldosterone (82088 x 2)
Renin (84244 x 2)   Q4

RVU			Global Days	Modifiers				
Mod	Non-Fac Total	Fac Total		51	50	62	80	MUE
	0.00	0.00	XXX	9	9	9	9	1

AMA: Summer 94: 1, Fall 94: 10

80410 Calcitonin stimulation panel (eg, calcium, pentagastrin)

This panel must include the following: Calcitonin (82308 x 3)   ⊗Q4

RVU			Global Days	Modifiers				
Mod	Non-Fac Total	Fac Total		51	50	62	80	MUE
	0.00	0.00	XXX	9	9	9	9	1

AMA: Summer 94: 1, Fall 94: 11
Pub 100-04, 16, 120.2

80412 Corticotropic releasing hormone (CRH) stimulation panel

This panel must include the following:

Cortisol (82533 x 6)

Adrenocorticotropic hormone (ACTH) (82024 x 6)   ⊗Q4

RVU			Global Days	Modifiers				
Mod	Non-Fac Total	Fac Total		51	50	62	80	MUE
	0.00	0.00	XXX	9	9	9	9	1

AMA: Summer 94: 1, Fall 94: 11

80414 Chorionic gonadotropin stimulation panel; testosterone response

This panel must include the following: Testosterone (84403 x 2 on 3 pooled blood samples)   Q4

RVU			Global Days	Modifiers				
Mod	Non-Fac Total	Fac Total		51	50	62	80	MUE
	0.00	0.00	XXX	9	9	9	9	1

AMA: Summer 94: 1, Fall 94: 11

80415 Chorionic gonadotropin stimulation panel; estradiol response

This panel must include the following: Estradiol (82670 x 2 on 3 pooled blood samples)   Q4

RVU			Global Days	Modifiers				
Mod	Non-Fac Total	Fac Total		51	50	62	80	MUE
	0.00	0.00	XXX	9	9	9	9	1

AMA: Summer 94: 1, Fall 94: 11

+ 80416 Renal vein renin stimulation panel (eg, captopril)

This panel must include the following: Renin (84244 x 6)   Q4

RVU			Global Days	Modifiers				
Mod	Non-Fac Total	Fac Total		51	50	62	80	MUE
	0.00	0.00	XXX	9	9	9	9	1

AMA: Summer 94: 1

● New   ▲ Revised   Deleted   ⊙ Moderate Sedation   ✚ Add-on Codes   ⊘ High Risk Denial   Ⓐ Age Edit   ♀ Female   ♂ Male   **AMA** *CPT® Assistant*   **MUE** Medically Unlikely Edit
⊘ Modifier 51 Exempt   ⊖ Modifier 63 Exempt   Ⓧ Unlisted   **Modifiers:** *See Inside Back Cover*   Ⓜ Maternity   A2-Z3 ASC Payment Indicators   A-Y OPPS Status Indicators

© 2016 DecisionHealth   CPT © 2015 American Medical Association. All Rights Reserved.   **681**

80417 Peripheral vein renin stimulation panel (eg, captopril)

This panel must include the following: Renin (84244 x 2) ⊗◎4

| RVU | | | Global Days | Modifiers | | | | |
Mod	Non-Fac Total	Fac Total		51	50	62	80	MUE
	0.00	0.00	XXX	9	9	9	9	1

80418 Combined rapid anterior pituitary evaluation panel

This panel must include the following:

Adrenocorticotropic hormone (ACTH) (82024 x 4)

Luteinizing hormone (LH) (83002 x 4)

Follicle stimulating hormone (FSH) (83001 x 4)

Prolactin (84146 x 4)

Human growth hormone (HGH) (83003 x 4)

Cortisol (82533 x 4)

Thyroid stimulating hormone (TSH) (84443 x 4) ◎4

| RVU | | | Global Days | Modifiers | | | | |
Mod	Non-Fac Total	Fac Total		51	50	62	80	MUE
	0.00	0.00	XXX	9	9	9	9	1

AMA: Summer 94: 1, Fall 94: 13

80420 Dexamethasone suppression panel, 48 hour

This panel must include the following:

Free cortisol, urine (82530 x 2)

Cortisol (82533 x 2)

Volume measurement for timed collection (81050 x 2) ⊗◎4

| RVU | | | Global Days | Modifiers | | | | |
Mod	Non-Fac Total	Fac Total		51	50	62	80	MUE
	0.00	0.00	XXX	9	9	9	9	1

AMA: Fall 94: 13

80422 Glucagon tolerance panel; for insulinoma

This panel must include the following:

Glucose (82947 x 3)

Insulin (83525 x 3) ⊗◎4

| RVU | | | Global Days | Modifiers | | | | |
Mod	Non-Fac Total	Fac Total		51	50	62	80	MUE
	0.00	0.00	XXX	9	9	9	9	1

AMA: Summer 94: 1, Fall 94: 13

80424 Glucagon tolerance panel; for pheochromocytoma

This panel must include the following:
Catecholamines, fractionated (82384 x 2) ◎4

| RVU | | | Global Days | Modifiers | | | | |
Mod	Non-Fac Total	Fac Total		51	50	62	80	MUE
	0.00	0.00	XXX	9	9	9	9	1

AMA: Summer 94: 1, Fall 94: 14

80426 Gonadotropin releasing hormone stimulation panel

This panel must include the following:

Follicle stimulating hormone (FSH) (83001 x 4)

Luteinizing hormone (LH) (83002 x 4) ◎4

| RVU | | | Global Days | Modifiers | | | | |
Mod	Non-Fac Total	Fac Total		51	50	62	80	MUE
	0.00	0.00	XXX	9	9	9	9	1

AMA: Summer 94: 1, Fall 94: 14

80428 Growth hormone stimulation panel (eg, arginine infusion, l-dopa administration)

This panel must include the following: Human growth hormone (HGH) (83003 x 4) ⊗◎4

| RVU | | | Global Days | Modifiers | | | | |
Mod	Non-Fac Total	Fac Total		51	50	62	80	MUE
	0.00	0.00	XXX	9	9	9	9	1

AMA: Summer 94: 1, Fall 94: 14

80430 Growth hormone suppression panel (glucose administration)

This panel must include the following:

Glucose (82947 x 3)

Human growth hormone (HGH) (83003 x 4) ◎4

| RVU | | | Global Days | Modifiers | | | | |
Mod	Non-Fac Total	Fac Total		51	50	62	80	MUE
	0.00	0.00	XXX	9	9	9	9	1

AMA: Summer 94: 1, Fall 94: 14

80432 Insulin-induced C-peptide suppression panel

This panel must include the following:

Insulin (83525)

C-peptide (84681 x 5)

Glucose (82947 x 5) ◎4

| RVU | | | Global Days | Modifiers | | | | |
Mod	Non-Fac Total	Fac Total		51	50	62	80	MUE
	0.00	0.00	XXX	9	9	9	9	1

AMA: Summer 94: 1, Fall 94: 15

80434 Insulin tolerance panel; for ACTH insufficiency

This panel must include the following:

Cortisol (82533 x 5)

Glucose (82947 x 5) ◎4

| RVU | | | Global Days | Modifiers | | | | |
Mod	Non-Fac Total	Fac Total		51	50	62	80	MUE
	0.00	0.00	XXX	9	9	9	9	1

AMA: Summer 94: 1, Fall 94: 15

80435 Insulin tolerance panel; for growth hormone deficiency

This panel must include the following:

Glucose (82947 x 5)

Human growth hormone (HGH) (83003 x 5) ◎4

| RVU | | | Global Days | Modifiers | | | | |
Mod	Non-Fac Total	Fac Total		51	50	62	80	MUE
	0.00	0.00	XXX	9	9	9	9	1

AMA: Summer 94: 1, Fall 94: 15

● New   ▲ Revised   ✖ Deleted   ⊙ Moderate Sedation   ✚ Add-on Codes   ⊗ High Risk Denial   Ⓐ Age Edit   ♀ Female   ♂ Male   **AMA** *CPT® Assistant*   **MUE** Medically Unlikely Edit

⊘ Modifier 51 Exempt   ⊖ Modifier 63 Exempt   ✗ Unlisted   **Modifiers:** *See Inside Back Cover*   Ⓜ Maternity   A2–Z3 ASC Payment Indicators   A–Y OPPS Status Indicators

CPT © 2015 American Medical Association. All Rights Reserved.   © 2016 DecisionHealth

80436 Metyrapone panel

This panel must include the following:

Cortisol (82533 x 2)

11 deoxycortisol (82634 x 2)   ⊘◯4

RVU			Global Days	Modifiers				
Mod	Non-Fac Total	Fac Total		51	50	62	80	MUE
	0.00	0.00	XXX	9	9	9	9	1

AMA: Summer 94: 1, Fall 94: 16

80438 Thyrotropin releasing hormone (TRH) stimulation panel; 1 hour

This panel must include the following: Thyroid stimulating hormone (TSH) (84443 x 3)   ◯4

RVU			Global Days	Modifiers				
Mod	Non-Fac Total	Fac Total		51	50	62	80	MUE
	0.00	0.00	XXX	9	9	9	9	1

AMA: Summer 94: 1, Fall 94: 16

80439 Thyrotropin releasing hormone (TRH) stimulation panel; 2 hour

This panel must include the following: Thyroid stimulating hormone (TSH) (84443 x 4)   ◯4

RVU			Global Days	Modifiers				
Mod	Non-Fac Total	Fac Total		51	50	62	80	MUE
	0.00	0.00	XXX	9	9	9	9	1

AMA: Summer 94: 1, Fall 94: 16

Clinical Pathology Consultations

Coding Guidance

Codes 80500 and 80502 report that a pathologist has reviewed, interpreted, and supplied a subsequent written report for a clinical pathology test. Do not use 80500, 80502 with other pathology codes that also include a physician interpretation, such as clinical pathology. If the pathologist provides face-to-face evaluation and management services for the patient, the appropriate E&M code should be reported rather than the clinical pathology consultation, even if a test result review is done as part of the evaluation and management service.

80500 Clinical pathology consultation; limited, without review of patient's history and medical records ◯1

RVU			Global Days	Modifiers				
Mod	Non-Fac Total	Fac Total		51	50	62	80	MUE
	0.62	0.55	XXX	0	0	0	0	1

AMA: Apr 97: 9, Nov 02: 9, Aug 05: 9
Pub 100-04, 12, 60

80502 Clinical pathology consultation; comprehensive, for a complex diagnostic problem, with review of patient's history and medical records ◯1

RVU			Global Days	Modifiers				
Mod	Non-Fac Total	Fac Total		51	50	62	80	MUE
	2.02	1.94	XXX	0	0	0	0	1

AMA: Apr 97: 9, Nov 02: 9, Aug 05: 9
Pub 100-04, 12, 60

Urinalysis/Urine Tests

81000 Urinalysis, by dip stick or tablet reagent for bilirubin, glucose, hemoglobin, ketones, leukocytes, nitrite, pH, protein, specific gravity, urobilinogen, any number of these constituents; non-automated, with microscopy   ◯4

RVU			Global Days	Modifiers				
Mod	Non-Fac Total	Fac Total		51	50	62	80	MUE
	0.00	0.00	XXX	9	9	9	9	2

AMA: Aug 05: 9, Winter 91: 10, Fall 93: 25, Winter 90
Pub 100-04, 16, 70.6, 120.2

81001 Urinalysis, by dip stick or tablet reagent for bilirubin, glucose, hemoglobin, ketones, leukocytes, nitrite, pH, protein, specific gravity, urobilinogen, any number of these constituents; automated, with microscopy   ◯4

RVU			Global Days	Modifiers				
Mod	Non-Fac Total	Fac Total		51	50	62	80	MUE
	0.00	0.00	XXX	9	9	9	9	2

Pub 100-04, 16, 70.6, 120.2

81002 Urinalysis, by dip stick or tablet reagent for bilirubin, glucose, hemoglobin, ketones, leukocytes, nitrite, pH, protein, specific gravity, urobilinogen, any number of these constituents; non-automated, without microscopy   ◯4

Coding tip: This is a CLIA-waived test, but does not require the use of modifier QW to be recognized as such

RVU			Global Days	Modifiers				
Mod	Non-Fac Total	Fac Total		51	50	62	80	MUE
	0.00	0.00	XXX	9	9	9	9	2

AMA: Mar 98: 3, Apr 07: 1
Pub 100-04, 16, 120.2

81003 Urinalysis, by dip stick or tablet reagent for bilirubin, glucose, hemoglobin, ketones, leukocytes, nitrite, pH, protein, specific gravity, urobilinogen, any number of these constituents; automated, without microscopy   ◯4

Coding tip: For a CLIA-waived test, append modifier QW to 81003

RVU			Global Days	Modifiers				
Mod	Non-Fac Total	Fac Total		51	50	62	80	MUE
	0.00	0.00	XXX	9	9	9	9	2

AMA: Apr 07: 1
Pub 100-04, 16, 120.2

81005 Urinalysis; qualitative or semiquantitative, except immunoassays   ◯4

RVU			Global Days	Modifiers				
Mod	Non-Fac Total	Fac Total		51	50	62	80	MUE
	0.00	0.00	XXX	9	9	9	9	2

AMA: Winter 90, Winter 91: 10, Fall 93: 25
Pub 100-04, 16, 120.2

81007 Urinalysis; bacteriuria screen, except by culture or dipstick   ◯4

Coding tip: For a CLIA-waived test, append modifier QW to 81007

RVU			Global Days	Modifiers				
Mod	Non-Fac Total	Fac Total		51	50	62	80	MUE
	0.00	0.00	XXX	9	9	9	9	1

Pub 100-04, 16, 120.2

● New   ▲ Revised   Deleted   ⊙ Moderate Sedation   ✛ Add-on Codes   ⊘ High Risk Denial   Ⓐ Age Edit   ♀ Female   ♂ Male   **AMA** *CPT® Assistant*   **MUE** Medically Unlikely Edit
⊘ Modifier 51 Exempt   ⊖ Modifier 63 Exempt   ✗ Unlisted   **Modifiers:** *See Inside Back Cover*   Ⓜ Maternity   A2–Z3 ASC Payment Indicators   A–Y OPPS Status Indicators

81015 Urinalysis; microscopic only   Q4

Coding tip: *Use this code for the detection of sperm in urine*

RVU			Global Days	Modifiers				
Mod	Non-Fac Total	Fac Total		51	50	62	80	MUE
	0.00	0.00	XXX	9	9	9	9	2

Pub 100-04, 16, 70.6, 120.2

81020 Urinalysis; 2 or 3 glass test   Q4

RVU			Global Days	Modifiers				
Mod	Non-Fac Total	Fac Total		51	50	62	80	MUE
	0.00	0.00	XXX	9	9	9	9	1

AMA: Winter 90, Winter 91: 10

Pub 100-04, 16, 70.6

81025 Urine pregnancy test, by visual color comparison methods   ♀Q4

Coding tip: *This is a CLIA-waived test, but does not require the use of modifier QW to be recognized as such*

RVU			Global Days	Modifiers				
Mod	Non-Fac Total	Fac Total		51	50	62	80	MUE
	0.00	0.00	XXX	9	9	9	9	1

AMA: Mar 98: 3

81050 Volume measurement for timed collection, each   Q4

RVU			Global Days	Modifiers				
Mod	Non-Fac Total	Fac Total		51	50	62	80	MUE
	0.00	0.00	XXX	9	9	9	9	2

81099 Unlisted urinalysis procedure   ✗Q4

RVU			Global Days	Modifiers				
Mod	Non-Fac Total	Fac Total		51	50	62	80	MUE
	0.00	0.00	XXX	9	9	9	9	

AMA: Aug 05: 9

Pub 100-04, 16, 100.4

81161 DMD (dystrophin) (eg, Duchenne/Becker muscular dystrophy) deletion analysis, and duplication analysis, if performed   ⊗A

RVU			Global Days	Modifiers				
Mod	Non-Fac Total	Fac Total		51	50	62	80	MUE
	0.00	0.00	XXX	9	9	9	9	1

● 81162 BRCA1, BRCA2 (breast cancer 1 and 2) (eg, hereditary breast and ovarian cancer) gene analysis; full sequence analysis and full duplication/deletion analysis   A

RVU			Global Days	Modifiers				
Mod	Non-Fac Total	Fac Total		51	50	62	80	MUE
	0.00	0.00	XXX	9	9	9	9	1

● 81170 ABL1 (ABL proto-oncogene 1, non-receptor tyrosine kinase) (eg, acquired imatinib tyrosine kinase inhibitor resistance), gene analysis, variants in the kinase domain   A

RVU			Global Days	Modifiers				
Mod	Non-Fac Total	Fac Total		51	50	62	80	MUE
	0.00	0.00	XXX	9	9	9	9	1

Molecular Pathology

Tier 1 Procedures

81200 ASPA (aspartoacylase) (eg, Canavan disease) gene analysis, common variants (eg, E285A, Y231X)   ⊗A

RVU			Global Days	Modifiers				
Mod	Non-Fac Total	Fac Total		51	50	62	80	MUE
	0.00	0.00	XXX	9	9	9	9	1

AMA: May 12: 4

81201 APC (adenomatous polyposis coli) (eg, familial adenomatosis polyposis [FAP], attenuated FAP) gene analysis; full gene sequence   A

RVU			Global Days	Modifiers				
Mod	Non-Fac Total	Fac Total		51	50	62	80	MUE
	0.00	0.00	XXX	9	9	9	9	1

AMA: May 12: 4, Sep 13: 3

81202 APC (adenomatous polyposis coli) (eg, familial adenomatosis polyposis [FAP], attenuated FAP) gene analysis; known familial variants   ⊗A

RVU			Global Days	Modifiers				
Mod	Non-Fac Total	Fac Total		51	50	62	80	MUE
	0.00	0.00	XXX	9	9	9	9	1

AMA: May 12: 4, Sep 13: 3

81203 APC (adenomatous polyposis coli) (eg, familial adenomatosis polyposis [FAP], attenuated FAP) gene analysis; duplication/deletion variants   A

RVU			Global Days	Modifiers				
Mod	Non-Fac Total	Fac Total		51	50	62	80	MUE
	0.00	0.00	XXX	9	9	9	9	1

AMA: May 12: 4, Sep 13: 3

81205 BCKDHB (branched-chain keto acid dehydrogenase E1, beta polypeptide) (eg, maple syrup urine disease) gene analysis, common variants (eg, R183P, G278S, E422X)   ⊗A

RVU			Global Days	Modifiers				
Mod	Non-Fac Total	Fac Total		51	50	62	80	MUE
	0.00	0.00	XXX	9	9	9	9	1

AMA: May 12: 4

81206 BCR/ABL1 (t(9;22)) (eg, chronic myelogenous leukemia) translocation analysis; major breakpoint, qualitative or quantitative   A

RVU			Global Days	Modifiers				
Mod	Non-Fac Total	Fac Total		51	50	62	80	MUE
	0.00	0.00	XXX	9	9	9	9	1

AMA: May 12: 4

81207 BCR/ABL1 (t(9;22)) (eg, chronic myelogenous leukemia) translocation analysis; minor breakpoint, qualitative or quantitative   A

RVU			Global Days	Modifiers				
Mod	Non-Fac Total	Fac Total		51	50	62	80	MUE
	0.00	0.00	XXX	9	9	9	9	1

AMA: May 12: 4

● New   ▲ Revised   ✖ Deleted   ⊙ Moderate Sedation   ✚ Add-on Codes   ⊗ High Risk Denial   ⊛ Age Edit   ♀ Female   ♂ Male   **AMA** *CPT® Assistant*   *MUE* Medically Unlikely Edit

⊘ Modifier 51 Exempt   ⊖ Modifier 63 Exempt   ✗ Unlisted   **Modifiers:** *See Inside Back Cover*   M Maternity   A2-Z3 ASC Payment Indicators   A-Y OPPS Status Indicators

CPT © 2015 American Medical Association. All Rights Reserved.   © 2016 DecisionHealth

81208 BCR/ABL1 (t(9;22)) (eg, chronic myelogenous leukemia) translocation analysis; other breakpoint, qualitative or quantitative ▣

RVU			Global Days	Modifiers				
Mod	Non-Fac Total	Fac Total		51	50	62	80	MUE
	0.00	0.00	XXX	9	9	9	9	1

AMA: May 12: 4

81209 BLM (Bloom syndrome, RecQ helicase-like) (eg, Bloom syndrome) gene analysis, 2281del6ins7 variant ⊙▣

RVU			Global Days	Modifiers				
Mod	Non-Fac Total	Fac Total		51	50	62	80	MUE
	0.00	0.00	XXX	9	9	9	9	1

AMA: May 12: 4

▲ **81210** BRAF (B-Raf proto-oncogene, serine/threonine kinase) (eg, colon cancer, melanoma), gene analysis, V600 variant(s) ▣

RVU			Global Days	Modifiers				
Mod	Non-Fac Total	Fac Total		51	50	62	80	MUE
	0.00	0.00	XXX	9	9	9	9	1

AMA: May 12: 4

81211 BRCA1, BRCA2 (breast cancer 1 and 2) (eg, hereditary breast and ovarian cancer) gene analysis; full sequence analysis and common duplication/deletion variants in BRCA1 (ie, exon 13 del 3.835kb, exon 13 dup 6kb, exon 14-20 del 26kb, exon 22 del 510bp, exon 8-9 del 7.1kb) ▣

RVU			Global Days	Modifiers				
Mod	Non-Fac Total	Fac Total		51	50	62	80	MUE
	0.00	0.00	XXX	9	9	9	9	1

AMA: May 12: 4

81212 BRCA1, BRCA2 (breast cancer 1 and 2) (eg, hereditary breast and ovarian cancer) gene analysis; 185delAG, 5385insC, 6174delT variants ▣

RVU			Global Days	Modifiers				
Mod	Non-Fac Total	Fac Total		51	50	62	80	MUE
	0.00	0.00	XXX	9	9	9	9	1

AMA: May 12: 4

81213 BRCA1, BRCA2 (breast cancer 1 and 2) (eg, hereditary breast and ovarian cancer) gene analysis; uncommon duplication/deletion variants ▣

RVU			Global Days	Modifiers				
Mod	Non-Fac Total	Fac Total		51	50	62	80	MUE
	0.00	0.00	XXX	9	9	9	9	1

AMA: May 12: 4

81214 BRCA1 (breast cancer 1) (eg, hereditary breast and ovarian cancer) gene analysis; full sequence analysis and common duplication/deletion variants (ie, exon 13 del 3.835kb, exon 13 dup 6kb, exon 14-20 del 26kb, exon 22 del 510bp, exon 8-9 del 7.1kb) ▣

RVU			Global Days	Modifiers				
Mod	Non-Fac Total	Fac Total		51	50	62	80	MUE
	0.00	0.00	XXX	9	9	9	9	1

AMA: May 12: 4

81215 BRCA1 (breast cancer 1) (eg, hereditary breast and ovarian cancer) gene analysis; known familial variant ⊙▣

RVU			Global Days	Modifiers				
Mod	Non-Fac Total	Fac Total		51	50	62	80	MUE
	0.00	0.00	XXX	9	9	9	9	1

AMA: May 12: 4

81216 BRCA2 (breast cancer 2) (eg, hereditary breast and ovarian cancer) gene analysis; full sequence analysis ⊙▣

RVU			Global Days	Modifiers				
Mod	Non-Fac Total	Fac Total		51	50	62	80	MUE
	0.00	0.00	XXX	9	9	9	9	1

AMA: May 12: 4

81217 BRCA2 (breast cancer 2) (eg, hereditary breast and ovarian cancer) gene analysis; known familial variant ⊙▣

RVU			Global Days	Modifiers				
Mod	Non-Fac Total	Fac Total		51	50	62	80	MUE
	0.00	0.00	XXX	9	9	9	9	1

AMA: May 12: 4

● **81218** CEBPA (CCAAT/enhancer binding protein [C/EBP], alpha) (eg, acute myeloid leukemia), gene analysis, full gene sequence ▣

RVU			Global Days	Modifiers				
Mod	Non-Fac Total	Fac Total		51	50	62	80	MUE
	0.00	0.00	XXX	9	9	9	9	1

● **81219** CALR (calreticulin) (eg, myeloproliferative disorders), gene analysis, common variants in exon 9 ▣

RVU			Global Days	Modifiers				
Mod	Non-Fac Total	Fac Total		51	50	62	80	MUE
	0.00	0.00	XXX	9	9	9	9	1

81220 CFTR (cystic fibrosis transmembrane conductance regulator) (eg, cystic fibrosis) gene analysis; common variants (eg, ACMG/ACOG guidelines) ⊙▣

RVU			Global Days	Modifiers				
Mod	Non-Fac Total	Fac Total		51	50	62	80	MUE
	0.00	0.00	XXX	9	9	9	9	1

AMA: May 12: 4

81221 CFTR (cystic fibrosis transmembrane conductance regulator) (eg, cystic fibrosis) gene analysis; known familial variants ⊙▣

RVU			Global Days	Modifiers				
Mod	Non-Fac Total	Fac Total		51	50	62	80	MUE
	0.00	0.00	XXX	9	9	9	9	1

AMA: May 12: 4

81222 CFTR (cystic fibrosis transmembrane conductance regulator) (eg, cystic fibrosis) gene analysis; duplication/deletion variants ⊙▣

RVU			Global Days	Modifiers				
Mod	Non-Fac Total	Fac Total		51	50	62	80	MUE
	0.00	0.00	XXX	9	9	9	9	1

AMA: May 12: 4

● New   ▲ Revised   Deleted   ⊙ Moderate Sedation   ✚ Add-on Codes   ⊘ High Risk Denial   Ⓐ Age Edit   ♀ Female   ♂ Male   **AMA** *CPT® Assistant*   **MUE** Medically Unlikely Edit
⊘ Modifier 51 Exempt   ⊖ Modifier 63 Exempt   ☒ Unlisted   **Modifiers:** *See Inside Back Cover*   Ⓜ Maternity   A2–Z3 ASC Payment Indicators   A–Y OPPS Status Indicators

© 2016 DecisionHealth   CPT © 2015 American Medical Association. All Rights Reserved.   **685**

81223 CFTR (cystic fibrosis transmembrane conductance regulator) (eg, cystic fibrosis) gene analysis; full gene sequence ⊘🅰

RVU Mod	Non-Fac Total	Fac Total	Global Days	Modifiers 51	50	62	80	MUE
	0.00	0.00	XXX	9	9	9	9	1

AMA: May 12: 4

81224 CFTR (cystic fibrosis transmembrane conductance regulator) (eg, cystic fibrosis) gene analysis; intron 8 poly-T analysis (eg, male infertility) ⊘🅰

RVU Mod	Non-Fac Total	Fac Total	Global Days	Modifiers 51	50	62	80	MUE
	0.00	0.00	XXX	9	9	9	9	1

AMA: May 12: 4

81225 CYP2C19 (cytochrome P450, family 2, subfamily C, polypeptide 19) (eg, drug metabolism), gene analysis, common variants (eg, *2, *3, *4, *8, *17) 🅰

RVU Mod	Non-Fac Total	Fac Total	Global Days	Modifiers 51	50	62	80	MUE
	0.00	0.00	XXX	9	9	9	9	1

AMA: May 12: 4

81226 CYP2D6 (cytochrome P450, family 2, subfamily D, polypeptide 6) (eg, drug metabolism), gene analysis, common variants (eg, *2, *3, *4, *5, *6, *9, *10, *17, *19, *29, *35, *41, *1XN, *2XN, *4XN) 🅰

RVU Mod	Non-Fac Total	Fac Total	Global Days	Modifiers 51	50	62	80	MUE
	0.00	0.00	XXX	9	9	9	9	1

AMA: May 12: 4

81227 CYP2C9 (cytochrome P450, family 2, subfamily C, polypeptide 9) (eg, drug metabolism), gene analysis, common variants (eg, *2, *3, *5, *6) 🅰

RVU Mod	Non-Fac Total	Fac Total	Global Days	Modifiers 51	50	62	80	MUE
	0.00	0.00	XXX	9	9	9	9	1

AMA: May 12: 4

81228 Cytogenomic constitutional (genome-wide) microarray analysis; interrogation of genomic regions for copy number variants (eg, bacterial artificial chromosome [BAC] or oligo-based comparative genomic hybridization [CGH] microarray analysis) ⊘🅰

RVU Mod	Non-Fac Total	Fac Total	Global Days	Modifiers 51	50	62	80	MUE
	0.00	0.00	XXX	9	9	9	9	1

AMA: May 12: 4, Sep 13: 4, 6

81229 Cytogenomic constitutional (genome-wide) microarray analysis; interrogation of genomic regions for copy number and single nucleotide polymorphism (SNP) variants for chromosomal abnormalities ⊘🅰

RVU Mod	Non-Fac Total	Fac Total	Global Days	Modifiers 51	50	62	80	MUE
	0.00	0.00	XXX	9	9	9	9	1

AMA: May 12: 4, Sep 13: 4

81235 EGFR (epidermal growth factor receptor) (eg, non-small cell lung cancer) gene analysis, common variants (eg, exon 19 LREA deletion, L858R, T790M, G719A, G719S, L861Q) 🅰

RVU Mod	Non-Fac Total	Fac Total	Global Days	Modifiers 51	50	62	80	MUE
	0.00	0.00	XXX	9	9	9	9	1

AMA: Sep 13: 3

81240 F2 (prothrombin, coagulation factor II) (eg, hereditary hypercoagulability) gene analysis, 20210G>A variant 🅰

RVU Mod	Non-Fac Total	Fac Total	Global Days	Modifiers 51	50	62	80	MUE
	0.00	0.00	XXX	9	9	9	9	1

AMA: May 12: 4

81241 F5 (coagulation factor V) (eg, hereditary hypercoagulability) gene analysis, Leiden variant 🅰

RVU Mod	Non-Fac Total	Fac Total	Global Days	Modifiers 51	50	62	80	MUE
	0.00	0.00	XXX	9	9	9	9	1

AMA: May 12: 4

81242 FANCC (Fanconi anemia, complementation group C) (eg, Fanconi anemia, type C) gene analysis, common variant (eg, IVS4+4A>T) ⊘🅰

RVU Mod	Non-Fac Total	Fac Total	Global Days	Modifiers 51	50	62	80	MUE
	0.00	0.00	XXX	9	9	9	9	1

AMA: May 12: 4

81243 FMR1 (fragile X mental retardation 1) (eg, fragile X mental retardation) gene analysis; evaluation to detect abnormal (eg, expanded) alleles ⊘🅰

RVU Mod	Non-Fac Total	Fac Total	Global Days	Modifiers 51	50	62	80	MUE
	0.00	0.00	XXX	9	9	9	9	1

AMA: May 12: 4

81244 FMR1 (Fragile X mental retardation 1) (eg, fragile X mental retardation) gene analysis; characterization of alleles (eg, expanded size and methylation status) ⊘🅰

RVU Mod	Non-Fac Total	Fac Total	Global Days	Modifiers 51	50	62	80	MUE
	0.00	0.00	XXX	9	9	9	9	1

AMA: May 12: 4

81245 FLT3 (fms-related tyrosine kinase 3) (eg, acute myeloid leukemia), gene analysis; internal tandem duplication (ITD) variants (ie, exons 14, 15) 🅰

RVU Mod	Non-Fac Total	Fac Total	Global Days	Modifiers 51	50	62	80	MUE
	0.00	0.00	XXX	9	9	9	9	1

AMA: May 12: 4, Jan 15: 3

● New   ▲ Revised   ✖ Deleted   ⊙ Moderate Sedation   ✚ Add-on Codes   ⊘ High Risk Denial   ⒶAge Edit   ♀ Female   ♂ Male   **AMA** *CPT® Assistant*   **MUE** Medically Unlikely Edit
⃠ Modifier 51 Exempt   ⊖ Modifier 63 Exempt   ✗ Unlisted   **Modifiers:** *See Inside Back Cover*   Ⓜ Maternity   A2–Z3 ASC Payment Indicators   🅰–Y OPPS Status Indicators

CPT © 2015 American Medical Association. All Rights Reserved.   © 2016 DecisionHealth

81246 FLT3 (fms-related tyrosine kinase 3) (eg, acute myeloid leukemia), gene analysis; tyrosine kinase domain (TKD) variants (eg, D835, I836) A

Mod	Non-Fac Total	Fac Total	Global Days	51	50	62	80	MUE
	0.00	0.00	XXX	9	9	9	9	1

81250 G6PC (glucose-6-phosphatase, catalytic subunit) (eg, Glycogen storage disease, type 1a, von Gierke disease) gene analysis, common variants (eg, R83C, Q347X) ⊘A

Mod	Non-Fac Total	Fac Total	Global Days	51	50	62	80	MUE
	0.00	0.00	XXX	9	9	9	9	1

AMA: May 12: 4

81251 GBA (glucosidase, beta, acid) (eg, Gaucher disease) gene analysis, common variants (eg, N370S, 84GG, L444P, IVS2+1G>A) ⊘A

Mod	Non-Fac Total	Fac Total	Global Days	51	50	62	80	MUE
	0.00	0.00	XXX	9	9	9	9	1

AMA: May 12: 4

81252 GJB2 (gap junction protein, beta 2, 26kDa, connexin 26) (eg, nonsyndromic hearing loss) gene analysis; full gene sequence ⊘A

Mod	Non-Fac Total	Fac Total	Global Days	51	50	62	80	MUE
	0.00	0.00	XXX	9	9	9	9	1

AMA: Sep 13: 3

81253 GJB2 (gap junction protein, beta 2, 26kDa, connexin 26) (eg, nonsyndromic hearing loss) gene analysis; known familial variants A

Mod	Non-Fac Total	Fac Total	Global Days	51	50	62	80	MUE
	0.00	0.00	XXX	9	9	9	9	1

AMA: Sep 13: 3

81254 GJB6 (gap junction protein, beta 6, 30kDa, connexin 30) (eg, nonsyndromic hearing loss) gene analysis, common variants (eg, 309kb [del(GJB6-D13S1830)] and 232kb [del(GJB6-D13S1854)]) A

Mod	Non-Fac Total	Fac Total	Global Days	51	50	62	80	MUE
	0.00	0.00	XXX	9	9	9	9	1

AMA: Sep 13: 3

81255 HEXA (hexosaminidase A [alpha polypeptide]) (eg, Tay-Sachs disease) gene analysis, common variants (eg, 1278insTATC, 1421+1G>C, G269S) ⊘A

Mod	Non-Fac Total	Fac Total	Global Days	51	50	62	80	MUE
	0.00	0.00	XXX	9	9	9	9	1

AMA: May 12: 4

81256 HFE (hemochromatosis) (eg, hereditary hemochromatosis) gene analysis, common variants (eg, C282Y, H63D) A

Mod	Non-Fac Total	Fac Total	Global Days	51	50	62	80	MUE
	0.00	0.00	XXX	9	9	9	9	1

AMA: May 12: 4

81257 HBA1/HBA2 (alpha globin 1 and alpha globin 2) (eg, alpha thalassemia, Hb Bart hydrops fetalis syndrome, HbH disease), gene analysis, for common deletions or variant (eg, Southeast Asian, Thai, Filipino, Mediterranean, alpha3.7, alpha4.2, alpha20.5, and Constant Spring) ⊘A

Mod	Non-Fac Total	Fac Total	Global Days	51	50	62	80	MUE
	0.00	0.00	XXX	9	9	9	9	1

AMA: May 12: 4

81260 IKBKAP (inhibitor of kappa light polypeptide gene enhancer in B-cells, kinase complex-associated protein) (eg, familial dysautonomia) gene analysis, common variants (eg, 2507+6T>C, R696P) ⊘A

Mod	Non-Fac Total	Fac Total	Global Days	51	50	62	80	MUE
	0.00	0.00	XXX	9	9	9	9	1

AMA: May 12: 4

81261 IGH@ (Immunoglobulin heavy chain locus) (eg, leukemias and lymphomas, B-cell), gene rearrangement analysis to detect abnormal clonal population(s); amplified methodology (eg, polymerase chain reaction) A

Mod	Non-Fac Total	Fac Total	Global Days	51	50	62	80	MUE
	0.00	0.00	XXX	9	9	9	9	1

AMA: May 12: 4, Sep 13: 7

81262 IGH@ (Immunoglobulin heavy chain locus) (eg, leukemias and lymphomas, B-cell), gene rearrangement analysis to detect abnormal clonal population(s); direct probe methodology (eg, Southern blot) A

Mod	Non-Fac Total	Fac Total	Global Days	51	50	62	80	MUE
	0.00	0.00	XXX	9	9	9	9	1

AMA: May 12: 4

81263 IGH@ (Immunoglobulin heavy chain locus) (eg, leukemia and lymphoma, B-cell), variable region somatic mutation analysis A

Mod	Non-Fac Total	Fac Total	Global Days	51	50	62	80	MUE
	0.00	0.00	XXX	9	9	9	9	1

AMA: May 12: 4

81264 IGK@ (Immunoglobulin kappa light chain locus) (eg, leukemia and lymphoma, B-cell), gene rearrangement analysis, evaluation to detect abnormal clonal population(s) A

Mod	Non-Fac Total	Fac Total	Global Days	51	50	62	80	MUE
	0.00	0.00	XXX	9	9	9	9	1

AMA: May 12: 4

● New   ▲ Revised   Deleted   ⊙ Moderate Sedation   ✚ Add-on Codes   ⊘ High Risk Denial   ⒶAge Edit   ♀ Female   ♂ Male   **AMA** CPT® Assistant   **MUE** Medically Unlikely Edit
⊘ Modifier 51 Exempt   ⊖ Modifier 63 Exempt   ☒ Unlisted   **Modifiers:** See Inside Back Cover   Ⓜ Maternity   A2–Z3 ASC Payment Indicators   A–Y OPPS Status Indicators

© 2016 DecisionHealth   CPT © 2015 American Medical Association. All Rights Reserved.

Laboratory/Pathology Procedures

81265 – 81287

81265 Comparative analysis using Short Tandem Repeat (STR) markers; patient and comparative specimen (eg, pre-transplant recipient and donor germline testing, post-transplant non-hematopoietic recipient germline [eg, buccal swab or other germline tissue sample] and donor testing, twin zygosity testing, or maternal cell contamination of fetal cells) ⊘Ⓐ

RVU			Global Days	Modifiers				
Mod	Non-Fac Total	Fac Total		51	50	62	80	MUE
	0.00	0.00	XXX	9	9	9	9	1

AMA: May 12: 4

+ 81266 Comparative analysis using Short Tandem Repeat (STR) markers; each additional specimen (eg, additional cord blood donor, additional fetal samples from different cultures, or additional zygosity in multiple birth pregnancies) (List separately in addition to code for primary procedure) ♀Ⓐ

RVU			Global Days	Modifiers				
Mod	Non-Fac Total	Fac Total		51	50	62	80	MUE
	0.00	0.00	XXX	9	9	9	9	2

AMA: May 12: 4

81267 Chimerism (engraftment) analysis, post transplantation specimen (eg, hematopoietic stem cell), includes comparison to previously performed baseline analyses; without cell selection Ⓐ

RVU			Global Days	Modifiers				
Mod	Non-Fac Total	Fac Total		51	50	62	80	MUE
	0.00	0.00	XXX	9	9	9	9	1

AMA: May 12: 4

81268 Chimerism (engraftment) analysis, post transplantation specimen (eg, hematopoietic stem cell), includes comparison to previously performed baseline analyses; with cell selection (eg, CD3, CD33), each cell type Ⓐ

RVU			Global Days	Modifiers				
Mod	Non-Fac Total	Fac Total		51	50	62	80	MUE
	0.00	0.00	XXX	9	9	9	9	4

AMA: May 12: 4

81270 JAK2 (Janus kinase 2) (eg, myeloproliferative disorder) gene analysis, p.Val617Phe (V617F) variant Ⓐ

RVU			Global Days	Modifiers				
Mod	Non-Fac Total	Fac Total		51	50	62	80	MUE
	0.00	0.00	XXX	9	9	9	9	1

AMA: May 12: 4

● 81272 KIT (v-kit Hardy-Zuckerman 4 feline sarcoma viral oncogene homolog) (eg, gastrointestinal stromal tumor [GIST], acute myeloid leukemia, melanoma), gene analysis, targeted sequence analysis (eg, exons 8, 11, 13, 17, 18) Ⓐ

RVU			Global Days	Modifiers				
Mod	Non-Fac Total	Fac Total		51	50	62	80	MUE
	0.00	0.00	XXX	9	9	9	9	1

● 81273 KIT (v-kit Hardy-Zuckerman 4 feline sarcoma viral oncogene homolog) (eg, mastocytosis), gene analysis, D816 variant(s) Ⓐ

RVU			Global Days	Modifiers				
Mod	Non-Fac Total	Fac Total		51	50	62	80	MUE
	0.00	0.00	XXX	9	9	9	9	1

▲ 81275 KRAS (Kirsten rat sarcoma viral oncogene homolog) (eg, carcinoma) gene analysis; variants in exon 2 (eg, codons 12 and 13) Ⓐ

RVU			Global Days	Modifiers				
Mod	Non-Fac Total	Fac Total		51	50	62	80	MUE
	0.00	0.00	XXX	9	9	9	9	1

AMA: May 12: 4, Sep 13: 6

● 81276 KRAS (Kirsten rat sarcoma viral oncogene homolog) (eg, carcinoma) gene analysis; additional variant(s) (eg, codon 61, codon 146) Ⓐ

RVU			Global Days	Modifiers				
Mod	Non-Fac Total	Fac Total		51	50	62	80	MUE
	0.00	0.00	XXX	9	9	9	9	1

81280 Long QT syndrome gene analyses (eg, KCNQ1, KCNH2, SCN5A, KCNE1, KCNE2, KCNJ2, CACNA1C, CAV3, SCN4B, AKAP, SNTA1, and ANK2); full sequence analysis ⊘Ⓐ

RVU			Global Days	Modifiers				
Mod	Non-Fac Total	Fac Total		51	50	62	80	MUE
	0.00	0.00	XXX	9	9	9	9	1

AMA: May 12: 4

81281 Long QT syndrome gene analyses (eg, KCNQ1, KCNH2, SCN5A, KCNE1, KCNE2, KCNJ2, CACNA1C, CAV3, SCN4B, AKAP, SNTA1, and ANK2); known familial sequence variant ⊘Ⓐ

RVU			Global Days	Modifiers				
Mod	Non-Fac Total	Fac Total		51	50	62	80	MUE
	0.00	0.00	XXX	9	9	9	9	1

AMA: May 12: 4

81282 Long QT syndrome gene analyses (eg, KCNQ1, KCNH2, SCN5A, KCNE1, KCNE2, KCNJ2, CACNA1C, CAV3, SCN4B, AKAP, SNTA1, and ANK2); duplication/deletion variants ⊘Ⓐ

RVU			Global Days	Modifiers				
Mod	Non-Fac Total	Fac Total		51	50	62	80	MUE
	0.00	0.00	XXX	9	9	9	9	1

AMA: May 12: 4

81287 MGMT (O-6-methylguanine-DNA methyltransferase) (eg, glioblastoma multiforme), methylation analysis Ⓐ

Coding tip: *Code 81287 is listed out of numerical order in CPT. Related code for MCOLN1 gene analysis - 81290*

RVU			Global Days	Modifiers				
Mod	Non-Fac Total	Fac Total		51	50	62	80	MUE
	0.00	0.00	XXX	9	9	9	9	1

● New   ▲ Revised   ✖ Deleted   ⊙ Moderate Sedation   ✚ Add-on Codes   ⊘ High Risk Denial   Ⓐ Age Edit   ♀ Female   ♂ Male   **AMA** *CPT® Assistant*   **MUE** Medically Unlikely Edit
⊘ Modifier 51 Exempt   ⊖ Modifier 63 Exempt   ✗ Unlisted   **Modifiers:** *See Inside Back Cover*   Ⓜ Maternity   Ⓐ2–Z3 ASC Payment Indicators   Ⓐ–Y OPPS Status Indicators

688   CPT © 2015 American Medical Association. All Rights Reserved.   © 2016 DecisionHealth

81288 MLH1 (mutL homolog 1, colon cancer, nonpolyposis type 2) (eg, hereditary non-polyposis colorectal cancer, Lynch syndrome) gene analysis; promoter methylation analysis A

RVU			Global Days	Modifiers				
Mod	Non-Fac Total	Fac Total		51	50	62	80	MUE
	0.00	0.00	XXX	9	9	9	9	1

AMA: Jan 15: 3

81290 MCOLN1 (mucolipin 1) (eg, Mucolipidosis, type IV) gene analysis, common variants (eg, IVS3-2A>G, del6.4kb) ⊘A

Coding tip: Related code MGMT methylation analysis - 81287

RVU			Global Days	Modifiers				
Mod	Non-Fac Total	Fac Total		51	50	62	80	MUE
	0.00	0.00	XXX	9	9	9	9	1

AMA: May 12: 4

81291 MTHFR (5,10-methylenetetrahydrofolate reductase) (eg, hereditary hypercoagulability) gene analysis, common variants (eg, 677T, 1298C) A

RVU			Global Days	Modifiers				
Mod	Non-Fac Total	Fac Total		51	50	62	80	MUE
	0.00	0.00	XXX	9	9	9	9	1

AMA: May 12: 4

81292 MLH1 (mutL homolog 1, colon cancer, nonpolyposis type 2) (eg, hereditary non-polyposis colorectal cancer, Lynch syndrome) gene analysis; full sequence analysis A

RVU			Global Days	Modifiers				
Mod	Non-Fac Total	Fac Total		51	50	62	80	MUE
	0.00	0.00	XXX	9	9	9	9	1

AMA: May 12: 4, Jan 15: 3

81293 MLH1 (mutL homolog 1, colon cancer, nonpolyposis type 2) (eg, hereditary non-polyposis colorectal cancer, Lynch syndrome) gene analysis; known familial variants ⊘A

RVU			Global Days	Modifiers				
Mod	Non-Fac Total	Fac Total		51	50	62	80	MUE
	0.00	0.00	XXX	9	9	9	9	1

AMA: May 12: 4

81294 MLH1 (mutL homolog 1, colon cancer, nonpolyposis type 2) (eg, hereditary non-polyposis colorectal cancer, Lynch syndrome) gene analysis; duplication/deletion variants A

RVU			Global Days	Modifiers				
Mod	Non-Fac Total	Fac Total		51	50	62	80	MUE
	0.00	0.00	XXX	9	9	9	9	1

AMA: May 12: 4

81295 MSH2 (mutS homolog 2, colon cancer, nonpolyposis type 1) (eg, hereditary non-polyposis colorectal cancer, Lynch syndrome) gene analysis; full sequence analysis A

RVU			Global Days	Modifiers				
Mod	Non-Fac Total	Fac Total		51	50	62	80	MUE
	0.00	0.00	XXX	9	9	9	9	1

AMA: May 12: 4

81296 MSH2 (mutS homolog 2, colon cancer, nonpolyposis type 1) (eg, hereditary non-polyposis colorectal cancer, Lynch syndrome) gene analysis; known familial variants ⊘A

RVU			Global Days	Modifiers				
Mod	Non-Fac Total	Fac Total		51	50	62	80	MUE
	0.00	0.00	XXX	9	9	9	9	1

AMA: May 12: 3

81297 MSH2 (mutS homolog 2, colon cancer, nonpolyposis type 1) (eg, hereditary non-polyposis colorectal cancer, Lynch syndrome) gene analysis; duplication/deletion variants A

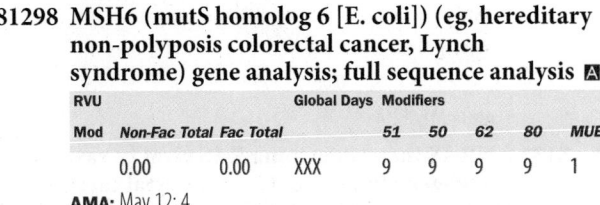

RVU			Global Days	Modifiers				
Mod	Non-Fac Total	Fac Total		51	50	62	80	MUE
	0.00	0.00	XXX	9	9	9	9	1

AMA: May 12: 4

81298 MSH6 (mutS homolog 6 [E. coli]) (eg, hereditary non-polyposis colorectal cancer, Lynch syndrome) gene analysis; full sequence analysis A

RVU			Global Days	Modifiers				
Mod	Non-Fac Total	Fac Total		51	50	62	80	MUE
	0.00	0.00	XXX	9	9	9	9	1

AMA: May 12: 4

81299 MSH6 (mutS homolog 6 [E. coli]) (eg, hereditary non-polyposis colorectal cancer, Lynch syndrome) gene analysis; known familial variants ⊘A

RVU			Global Days	Modifiers				
Mod	Non-Fac Total	Fac Total		51	50	62	80	MUE
	0.00	0.00	XXX	9	9	9	9	1

AMA: May 12: 4

81300 MSH6 (mutS homolog 6 [E. coli]) (eg, hereditary non-polyposis colorectal cancer, Lynch syndrome) gene analysis; duplication/deletion variants A

RVU			Global Days	Modifiers				
Mod	Non-Fac Total	Fac Total		51	50	62	80	MUE
	0.00	0.00	XXX	9	9	9	9	1

AMA: May 12: 4

81301 Microsatellite instability analysis (eg, hereditary non-polyposis colorectal cancer, Lynch syndrome) of markers for mismatch repair deficiency (eg, BAT25, BAT26), includes comparison of neoplastic and normal tissue, if performed A

RVU			Global Days	Modifiers				
Mod	Non-Fac Total	Fac Total		51	50	62	80	MUE
	0.00	0.00	XXX	9	9	9	9	1

AMA: May 12: 4

81302 MECP2 (methyl CpG binding protein 2) (eg, Rett syndrome) gene analysis; full sequence analysis ⊘A

RVU			Global Days	Modifiers				
Mod	Non-Fac Total	Fac Total		51	50	62	80	MUE
	0.00	0.00	XXX	9	9	9	9	1

AMA: May 12: 4

● New   ▲ Revised   Deleted   ⊙ Moderate Sedation   ✚ Add-on Codes   ⊘ High Risk Denial   Ⓐ Age Edit   ♀ Female   ♂ Male   **AMA** *CPT® Assistant*   **MUE** Medically Unlikely Edit
⦸ Modifier 51 Exempt   ⊖ Modifier 63 Exempt   ⊠ Unlisted   **Modifiers:** *See Inside Back Cover*   Ⓜ Maternity   A2-Z3 ASC Payment Indicators   A-Y OPPS Status Indicators

Laboratory/Pathology Procedures

81303 – 81323

81303 MECP2 (methyl CpG binding protein 2) (eg, Rett syndrome) gene analysis; known familial variant ⊗🅰

RVU			Global Days	Modifiers				
Mod	*Non-Fac Total*	*Fac Total*		51	50	62	80	MUE
	0.00	0.00	XXX	9	9	9	9	1

AMA: May 12: 4

81304 MECP2 (methyl CpG binding protein 2) (eg, Rett syndrome) gene analysis; duplication/deletion variants ⊗🅰

RVU			Global Days	Modifiers				
Mod	*Non-Fac Total*	*Fac Total*		51	50	62	80	MUE
	0.00	0.00	XXX	9	9	9	9	1

AMA: May 12: 4

81310 NPM1 (nucleophosmin) (eg, acute myeloid leukemia) gene analysis, exon 12 variants 🅰

RVU			Global Days	Modifiers				
Mod	*Non-Fac Total*	*Fac Total*		51	50	62	80	MUE
	0.00	0.00	XXX	9	9	9	9	1

AMA: May 12: 4

● **81311** NRAS (neuroblastoma RAS viral [v-ras] oncogene homolog) (eg, colorectal carcinoma), gene analysis, variants in exon 2 (eg, codons 12 and 13) and exon 3 (eg, codon 61) 🅰

RVU			Global Days	Modifiers				
Mod	*Non-Fac Total*	*Fac Total*		51	50	62	80	MUE
	0.00	0.00	XXX	9	9	9	9	1

81313 PCA3/KLK3 (prostate cancer antigen 3 [non-protein coding]/kallikrein-related peptidase 3 [prostate specific antigen]) ratio (eg, prostate cancer) 🅰

RVU			Global Days	Modifiers				
Mod	*Non-Fac Total*	*Fac Total*		51	50	62	80	MUE
	0.00	0.00	XXX	9	9	9	9	1

AMA: Jan 15: 3

● **81314** PDGFRA (platelet-derived growth factor receptor, alpha polypeptide) (eg, gastrointestinal stromal tumor [GIST]), gene analysis, targeted sequence analysis (eg, exons 12, 18) 🅰

RVU			Global Days	Modifiers				
Mod	*Non-Fac Total*	*Fac Total*		51	50	62	80	MUE
	0.00	0.00	XXX	9	9	9	9	1

81315 PML/RARalpha, (t(15;17)), (promyelocytic leukemia/retinoic acid receptor alpha) (eg, promyelocytic leukemia) translocation analysis; common breakpoints (eg, intron 3 and intron 6), qualitative or quantitative 🅰

RVU			Global Days	Modifiers				
Mod	*Non-Fac Total*	*Fac Total*		51	50	62	80	MUE
	0.00	0.00	XXX	9	9	9	9	1

AMA: May 12: 4

81316 PML/RARalpha, (t(15;17)), (promyelocytic leukemia/retinoic acid receptor alpha) (eg, promyelocytic leukemia) translocation analysis; single breakpoint (eg, intron 3, intron 6 or exon 6), qualitative or quantitative 🅰

RVU			Global Days	Modifiers				
Mod	*Non-Fac Total*	*Fac Total*		51	50	62	80	MUE
	0.00	0.00	XXX	9	9	9	9	1

AMA: May 12: 4

81317 PMS2 (postmeiotic segregation increased 2 [S. cerevisiae]) (eg, hereditary non-polyposis colorectal cancer, Lynch syndrome) gene analysis; full sequence analysis 🅰

RVU			Global Days	Modifiers				
Mod	*Non-Fac Total*	*Fac Total*		51	50	62	80	MUE
	0.00	0.00	XXX	9	9	9	9	1

AMA: May 12: 4

81318 PMS2 (postmeiotic segregation increased 2 [S. cerevisiae]) (eg, hereditary non-polyposis colorectal cancer, Lynch syndrome) gene analysis; known familial variants ⊗🅰

RVU			Global Days	Modifiers				
Mod	*Non-Fac Total*	*Fac Total*		51	50	62	80	MUE
	0.00	0.00	XXX	9	9	9	9	1

AMA: May 12: 4

81319 PMS2 (postmeiotic segregation increased 2 [S. cerevisiae]) (eg, hereditary non-polyposis colorectal cancer, Lynch syndrome) gene analysis; duplication/deletion variants 🅰

RVU			Global Days	Modifiers				
Mod	*Non-Fac Total*	*Fac Total*		51	50	62	80	MUE
	0.00	0.00	XXX	9	9	9	9	1

AMA: May 12: 4

81321 PTEN (phosphatase and tensin homolog) (eg, Cowden syndrome, PTEN hamartoma tumor syndrome) gene analysis; full sequence analysis ⊗🅰

RVU			Global Days	Modifiers				
Mod	*Non-Fac Total*	*Fac Total*		51	50	62	80	MUE
	0.00	0.00	XXX	9	9	9	9	1

AMA: Sep 13: 3

81322 PTEN (phosphatase and tensin homolog) (eg, Cowden syndrome, PTEN hamartoma tumor syndrome) gene analysis; known familial variant ⊗🅰

RVU			Global Days	Modifiers				
Mod	*Non-Fac Total*	*Fac Total*		51	50	62	80	MUE
	0.00	0.00	XXX	9	9	9	9	1

AMA: Sep 13: 3

81323 PTEN (phosphatase and tensin homolog) (eg, Cowden syndrome, PTEN hamartoma tumor syndrome) gene analysis; duplication/deletion variant 🅰

RVU			Global Days	Modifiers				
Mod	*Non-Fac Total*	*Fac Total*		51	50	62	80	MUE
	0.00	0.00	XXX	9	9	9	9	1

AMA: Sep 13: 3

● New   ▲ Revised   ✖ Deleted   ⊙ Moderate Sedation   ✚ Add-on Codes   ⊗ High Risk Denial   ⊛ Age Edit   ♀ Female   ♂ Male   **AMA** *CPT® Assistant*   **MUE** Medically Unlikely Edit
⊘ Modifier 51 Exempt   ⊖ Modifier 63 Exempt   ✖ Unlisted   **Modifiers:** *See Inside Back Cover*   Ⓜ Maternity   🄰 2 – 🅉 3 ASC Payment Indicators   🄰 –🆈 OPPS Status Indicators

CPT © 2015 American Medical Association. All Rights Reserved.   © 2016 DecisionHealth

81324 PMP22 (peripheral myelin protein 22) (eg, Charcot-Marie-Tooth, hereditary neuropathy with liability to pressure palsies) gene analysis; duplication/deletion analysis ⊘🅰

RVU			Global Days	Modifiers				
Mod	Non-Fac Total	Fac Total		51	50	62	80	MUE
	0.00	0.00	XXX	9	9	9	9	1

AMA: Sep 13: 3

81325 PMP22 (peripheral myelin protein 22) (eg, Charcot-Marie-Tooth, hereditary neuropathy with liability to pressure palsies) gene analysis; full sequence analysis ⊘🅰

RVU			Global Days	Modifiers				
Mod	Non-Fac Total	Fac Total		51	50	62	80	MUE
	0.00	0.00	XXX	9	9	9	9	1

AMA: Sep 13: 3

81326 PMP22 (peripheral myelin protein 22) (eg, Charcot-Marie-Tooth, hereditary neuropathy with liability to pressure palsies) gene analysis; known familial variant 🅰

RVU			Global Days	Modifiers				
Mod	Non-Fac Total	Fac Total		51	50	62	80	MUE
	0.00	0.00	XXX	9	9	9	9	1

AMA: Sep 13: 3

81330 SMPD1(sphingomyelin phosphodiesterase 1, acid lysosomal) (eg, Niemann-Pick disease, Type A) gene analysis, common variants (eg, R496L, L302P, fsP330) ⊘🅰

RVU			Global Days	Modifiers				
Mod	Non-Fac Total	Fac Total		51	50	62	80	MUE
	0.00	0.00	XXX	9	9	9	9	1

AMA: May 12: 4

81331 SNRPN/UBE3A (small nuclear ribonucleoprotein polypeptide N and ubiquitin protein ligase E3A) (eg, Prader-Willi syndrome and/or Angelman syndrome), methylation analysis ⊘🅰

RVU			Global Days	Modifiers				
Mod	Non-Fac Total	Fac Total		51	50	62	80	MUE
	0.00	0.00	XXX	9	9	9	9	1

AMA: May 12: 4

81332 SERPINA1 (serpin peptidase inhibitor, clade A, alpha-1 antiproteinase, antitrypsin, member 1) (eg, alpha-1-antitrypsin deficiency), gene analysis, common variants (eg, *S and *Z) 🅰

RVU			Global Days	Modifiers				
Mod	Non-Fac Total	Fac Total		51	50	62	80	MUE
	0.00	0.00	XXX	9	9	9	9	1

AMA: May 12: 4

81340 TRB@ (T cell antigen receptor, beta) (eg, leukemia and lymphoma), gene rearrangement analysis to detect abnormal clonal population(s); using amplification methodology (eg, polymerase chain reaction) 🅰

RVU			Global Days	Modifiers				
Mod	Non-Fac Total	Fac Total		51	50	62	80	MUE
	0.00	0.00	XXX	9	9	9	9	1

AMA: May 12: 4

81341 TRB@ (T cell antigen receptor, beta) (eg, leukemia and lymphoma), gene rearrangement analysis to detect abnormal clonal population(s); using direct probe methodology (eg, Southern blot) ⊘🅰

RVU			Global Days	Modifiers				
Mod	Non-Fac Total	Fac Total		51	50	62	80	MUE
	0.00	0.00	XXX	9	9	9	9	1

AMA: May 12: 4

81342 TRG@ (T cell antigen receptor, gamma) (eg, leukemia and lymphoma), gene rearrangement analysis, evaluation to detect abnormal clonal population(s) 🅰

RVU			Global Days	Modifiers				
Mod	Non-Fac Total	Fac Total		51	50	62	80	MUE
	0.00	0.00	XXX	9	9	9	9	1

AMA: May 12: 4

81350 UGT1A1 (UDP glucuronosyltransferase 1 family, polypeptide A1) (eg, irinotecan metabolism), gene analysis, common variants (eg, *28, *36, *37) 🅰

RVU			Global Days	Modifiers				
Mod	Non-Fac Total	Fac Total		51	50	62	80	MUE
	0.00	0.00	XXX	9	9	9	9	1

AMA: May 12: 4

▲ **81355** VKORC1 (vitamin K epoxide reductase complex, subunit 1) (eg, warfarin metabolism), gene analysis, common variant(s) (eg, -1639G>A, c.173+1000C>T) ⊘🅰

RVU			Global Days	Modifiers				
Mod	Non-Fac Total	Fac Total		51	50	62	80	MUE
	0.00	0.00	XXX	9	9	9	9	1

AMA: May 12: 4

81370 HLA Class I and II typing, low resolution (eg, antigen equivalents); HLA-A, -B, -C, -DRB1/3/4/5, and -DQB1 🅰

RVU			Global Days	Modifiers				
Mod	Non-Fac Total	Fac Total		51	50	62	80	MUE
	0.00	0.00	XXX	9	9	9	9	1

AMA: May 12: 4

81371 HLA Class I and II typing, low resolution (eg, antigen equivalents); HLA-A, -B, and -DRB1 (eg, verification typing) 🅰

RVU			Global Days	Modifiers				
Mod	Non-Fac Total	Fac Total		51	50	62	80	MUE
	0.00	0.00	XXX	9	9	9	9	1

AMA: May 12: 4

81372 HLA Class I typing, low resolution (eg, antigen equivalents); complete (ie, HLA-A, -B, and -C) 🅰

RVU			Global Days	Modifiers				
Mod	Non-Fac Total	Fac Total		51	50	62	80	MUE
	0.00	0.00	XXX	9	9	9	9	1

AMA: May 12: 4

● New   ▲ Revised   Deleted   ⊙ Moderate Sedation   ✚ Add-on Codes   ⊘ High Risk Denial   Ⓐ Age Edit   ♀ Female   ♂ Male   **AMA** *CPT® Assistant*   **MUE** Medically Unlikely Edit
Ⓢ Modifier 51 Exempt   ⊖ Modifier 63 Exempt   🅇 Unlisted   **Modifiers:** *See Inside Back Cover*   Ⓜ Maternity   🅰2–🆉3 ASC Payment Indicators   🅰–🆈 OPPS Status Indicators

81373 HLA Class I typing, low resolution (eg, antigen equivalents); one locus (eg, HLA-A, -B, or -C), each ⊘Ⓐ

RVU			Global Days	Modifiers				
Mod	Non-Fac Total	Fac Total		51	50	62	80	MUE
	0.00	0.00	XXX	9	9	9	9	2

AMA: May 12: 4, Jun 12: 16

81374 HLA Class I typing, low resolution (eg, antigen equivalents); one antigen equivalent (eg, B*27), each Ⓐ

RVU			Global Days	Modifiers				
Mod	Non-Fac Total	Fac Total		51	50	62	80	MUE
	0.00	0.00	XXX	9	9	9	9	1

AMA: May 12: 4, Jun 12: 16

81375 HLA Class II typing, low resolution (eg, antigen equivalents); HLA-DRB1/3/4/5 and -DQB1 Ⓐ

RVU			Global Days	Modifiers				
Mod	Non-Fac Total	Fac Total		51	50	62	80	MUE
	0.00	0.00	XXX	9	9	9	9	1

AMA: May 12: 4

81376 HLA Class II typing, low resolution (eg, antigen equivalents); one locus (eg, HLA-DRB1, -DRB3/4/5, -DQB1, -DQA1, -DPB1, or -DPA1), each ⊘Ⓐ

RVU			Global Days	Modifiers				
Mod	Non-Fac Total	Fac Total		51	50	62	80	MUE
	0.00	0.00	XXX	9	9	9	9	5

AMA: May 12: 4, Jun 12: 16

81377 HLA Class II typing, low resolution (eg, antigen equivalents); one antigen equivalent, each Ⓐ

RVU			Global Days	Modifiers				
Mod	Non-Fac Total	Fac Total		51	50	62	80	MUE
	0.00	0.00	XXX	9	9	9	9	2

AMA: May 12: 4, Jun 12: 16

81378 HLA Class I and II typing, high resolution (ie, alleles or allele groups), HLA-A, -B, -C, and -DRB1 Ⓐ

RVU			Global Days	Modifiers				
Mod	Non-Fac Total	Fac Total		51	50	62	80	MUE
	0.00	0.00	XXX	9	9	9	9	1

AMA: May 12: 4, Jun 12: 16

81379 HLA Class I typing, high resolution (ie, alleles or allele groups); complete (ie, HLA-A, -B, and -C) Ⓐ

RVU			Global Days	Modifiers				
Mod	Non-Fac Total	Fac Total		51	50	62	80	MUE
	0.00	0.00	XXX	9	9	9	9	1

AMA: May 12: 4

81380 HLA Class I typing, high resolution (ie, alleles or allele groups); one locus (eg, HLA-A, -B, or -C), each Ⓐ

RVU			Global Days	Modifiers				
Mod	Non-Fac Total	Fac Total		51	50	62	80	MUE
	0.00	0.00	XXX	9	9	9	9	2

AMA: May 12: 4, Jun 12: 16

81381 HLA Class I typing, high resolution (ie, alleles or allele groups); one allele or allele group (eg, B*57:01P), each Ⓐ

RVU			Global Days	Modifiers				
Mod	Non-Fac Total	Fac Total		51	50	62	80	MUE
	0.00	0.00	XXX	9	9	9	9	3

AMA: May 12: 4, Jun 12: 16

81382 HLA Class II typing, high resolution (ie, alleles or allele groups); one locus (eg, HLA-DRB1, -DRB3/4/5, -DQB1, -DQA1, -DPB1, or -DPA1), each Ⓐ

RVU			Global Days	Modifiers				
Mod	Non-Fac Total	Fac Total		51	50	62	80	MUE
	0.00	0.00	XXX	9	9	9	9	6

AMA: May 12: 4, Jun 12: 16

81383 HLA Class II typing, high resolution (ie, alleles or allele groups); one allele or allele group (eg, HLA-DQB1*06:02P), each Ⓐ

RVU			Global Days	Modifiers				
Mod	Non-Fac Total	Fac Total		51	50	62	80	MUE
	0.00	0.00	XXX	9	9	9	9	2

AMA: May 12: 4, Jun 12: 16

Tier 2 Procedures

81400 Molecular pathology procedure, Level 1 (eg, identification of single germline variant [eg, SNP] by techniques such as restriction enzyme digestion or melt curve analysis)

ACADM (acyl-CoA dehydrogenase, C-4 to C-12 straight chain, MCAD) (eg, medium chain acyl dehydrogenase deficiency), K304E variant

ACE (angiotensin converting enzyme) (eg, hereditary blood pressure regulation), insertion/deletion variant

AGTR1 (angiotensin II receptor, type 1) (eg, essential hypertension), 1166A>C variant

BCKDHA (branched chain keto acid dehydrogenase E1, alpha polypeptide) (eg, maple syrup urine disease, type 1A), Y438N variant

CCR5 (chemokine C-C motif receptor 5) (eg, HIV resistance), 32-bp deletion mutation/794 825del32 deletion

CLRN1 (clarin 1) (eg, Usher syndrome, type 3), N48K variant

DPYD (dihydropyrimidine dehydrogenase) (eg, 5-fluorouracil/5-FU and capecitabine drug metabolism), IVS14+1G>A variant

F2 (coagulation factor 2) (eg, hereditary hypercoagulability), 1199G>A variant

F5 (coagulation factor V) (eg, hereditary hypercoagulability), HR2 variant

F7 (coagulation factor VII [serum prothrombin conversion accelerator]) (eg, hereditary hypercoagulability), R353Q variant

F13B (coagulation factor XIII, B polypeptide) (eg, hereditary hypercoagulability), V34L variant

FGB (fibrinogen beta chain) (eg, hereditary ischemic heart disease), -455G>A variant

---

● New   ▲ Revised   ✖ Deleted   ⊙ Moderate Sedation   ✚ Add-on Codes   ⊘ High Risk Denial   Ⓐ Age Edit   ♀ Female   ♂ Male   **AMA** *CPT® Assistant*   *MUE* Medically Unlikely Edit
⊘ Modifier 51 Exempt   ⊖ Modifier 63 Exempt   Ⓧ Unlisted   **Modifiers:** *See Inside Back Cover*   Ⓜ Maternity   Ⓐ2–Ⓩ3 ASC Payment Indicators   Ⓐ–Ⓨ OPPS Status Indicators

   CPT © 2015 American Medical Association. All Rights Reserved.   © 2016 DecisionHealth

FGFR1 (fibroblast growth factor receptor 1) (eg, Pfeiffer syndrome type 1, craniosynostosis), P252R variant

FGFR3 (fibroblast growth factor receptor 3) (eg, Muenke syndrome), P250R variant

FKTN (fukutin) (eg, Fukuyama congenital muscular dystrophy), retrotransposon insertion variant

GNE (glucosamine [UDP-N-acetyl]-2-epimerase/N-acetylmannosamine kinase) (eg, inclusion body myopathy 2 [IBM2], Nonaka myopathy), M712T variant

Human Platelet Antigen 1 genotyping (HPA-1), ITGB3 (integrin, beta 3 [platelet glycoprotein IIIa], antigen CD61 [GPIIIa]) (eg, neonatal alloimmune thrombocytopenia [NAIT], post-transfusion purpura), HPA-1a/b (L33P)

Human Platelet Antigen 2 genotyping (HPA-2), GP1BA (glycoprotein Ib [platelet], alpha polypeptide [GPIba]) (eg, neonatal alloimmune thrombocytopenia [NAIT], post-transfusion purpura), HPA-2a/b (T145M)

Human Platelet Antigen 3 genotyping (HPA-3), ITGA2B (integrin, alpha 2b [platelet glycoprotein IIb of IIb/IIIa complex], antigen CD41 [GPIIb]) (eg, neonatal alloimmune thrombocytopenia [NAIT], post-transfusion purpura), HPA-3a/b (I843S)

Human Platelet Antigen 4 genotyping (HPA-4), ITGB3 (integrin, beta 3 [platelet glycoprotein IIIa], antigen CD61 [GPIIIa]) (eg, neonatal alloimmune thrombocytopenia [NAIT], post-transfusion purpura), HPA-4a/b (R143Q)

Human Platelet Antigen 5 genotyping (HPA-5), ITGA2 (integrin, alpha 2 [CD49B, alpha 2 subunit of VLA-2 receptor] [GPIa]) (eg, neonatal alloimmune thrombocytopenia [NAIT], post-transfusion purpura), HPA-5a/b (K505E)

Human Platelet Antigen 6 genotyping (HPA-6w), ITGB3 (integrin, beta 3 [platelet glycoprotein IIIa, antigen CD61] [GPIIIa]) (eg, neonatal alloimmune thrombocytopenia [NAIT], post-transfusion purpura), HPA-6a/b (R489Q)

Human Platelet Antigen 9 genotyping (HPA-9w), ITGA2B (integrin, alpha 2b [platelet glycoprotein IIb of IIb/IIIa complex, antigen CD41] [GPIIb]) (eg, neonatal alloimmune thrombocytopenia [NAIT], post-transfusion purpura), HPA-9a/b (V837M)

Human Platelet Antigen 15 genotyping (HPA-15), CD109 (CD109 molecule) (eg, neonatal alloimmune thrombocytopenia [NAIT], post-transfusion purpura), HPA-15a/b (S682Y) IL28B (interleukin 28B [interferon, lambda 3]) (eg, drug response), rs12979860 variant

IVD (isovaleryl-CoA dehydrogenase) (eg, isovaleric acidemia), A282V variant

LCT (lactase-phlorizin hydrolase) (eg, lactose intolerance), 13910 C>T variant

NEB (nebulin) (eg, nemaline myopathy 2), exon 55 deletion variant

PCDH15 (protocadherin-related 15) (eg, Usher syndrome type 1F), R245X variant

SERPINE1 (serpine peptidase inhibitor clade E, member 1, plasminogen activator inhibitor -1, PAI-1) (eg, thrombophilia), 4G variant

SHOC2 (soc-2 suppressor of clear homolog) (eg, Noonan-like syndrome with loose anagen hair), S2G variant

SLCO1B1 (solute carrier organic anion transporter family, member 1B1) (eg, adverse drug reaction), V174A variant

SMN1 (survival of motor neuron 1, telomeric) (eg, spinal muscular atrophy), exon 7 deletion

SRY (sex determining region Y) (eg, 46,XX testicular disorder of sex development, gonadal dysgenesis), gene analysis

TOR1A (torsin family 1, member A [torsin A]) (eg, early-onset primary dystonia [DYT1]), 907_909delGAG (904_906delGAG) variant ⊘🅰

RVU				Global Days	Modifiers			
Mod	Non-Fac Total	Fac Total			51	50	62	80	MUE
	0.00	0.00	XXX		9	9	9	9	2

AMA: May 12: 4, Jul 13: 12, Sep 13: 4, 5, 8, Jan 15: 3

▲ **81401 Molecular pathology procedure, Level 2 (eg, 2-10 SNPs, 1 methylated variant, or 1 somatic variant [typically using nonsequencing target variant analysis], or detection of a dynamic mutation disorder/triplet repeat)**

ABCC8 (ATP-binding cassette, sub-family C [CFTR/MRP], member 8) (eg, familial hyperinsulinism), common variants (eg, c.3898-9G>A [c.3992-9G>A], F1388del)

ABL (c-abl oncogene 1, receptor tyrosine kinase) (eg, acquired imatinib resistance), T315I variant

ACADM (acyl-CoA dehydrogenase, C-4 to C-12 straight chain, MCAD) (eg, medium chain acyl dehydrogenase deficiency), commons variants (eg, K304E, Y42H) ADRB2 (adrenergic beta-2 receptor surface) (eg, drug metabolism), common variants (eg, G16R, Q27E)

AFF2 (AF4/FMR2 family, member 2 [FMR2]) (eg, fragile X mental retardation 2 [FRAXE]), evaluation to detect abnormal (eg, expanded) alleles

APOB (apolipoprotein B) (eg, familial hypercholesterolemia type B), common variants (eg, R3500Q, R3500W)

APOE (apolipoprotein E) (eg, hyperlipoproteinemia type III, cardiovascular disease, Alzheimer disease), common variants (eg, *2, *3, *4)

AR (androgen receptor) (eg, spinal and bulbar muscular atrophy, Kennedy disease, X chromosome inactivation), characterization of alleles (eg, expanded size or methylation status)

ATN1 (atrophin 1) (eg, dentatorubral-pallidoluysian atrophy), evaluation to detect abnormal (eg, expanded) alleles

ATXN1 (ataxin 1) (eg, spinocerebellar ataxia), evaluation to detect abnormal (eg, expanded) alleles

© 2016 DecisionHealth | CPT © 2015 American Medical Association. All Rights Reserved.

ATXN2 (ataxin 2) (eg, spinocerebellar ataxia), evaluation to detect abnormal (eg, expanded) alleles

ATXN3 (ataxin 3) (eg, spinocerebellar ataxia, Machado-Joseph disease), evaluation to detect abnormal (eg, expanded) alleles

ATXN7 (ataxin 7) (eg, spinocerebellar ataxia), evaluation to detect abnormal (eg, expanded) alleles

ATXN8OS (ATXN8 opposite strand [non-protein coding]) (eg, spinocerebellar ataxia), evaluation to detect abnormal (eg, expanded) alleles

ATXN10 (ataxin 10) (eg, spinocerebellar ataxia), evaluation to detect abnormal (eg, expanded) alleles

CACNA1A (calcium channel, voltage-dependent, P/Q type, alpha 1A subunit) (eg, spinocerebellar ataxia), evaluation to detect abnormal (eg, expanded) alleles

CBFB/MYH11 (inv(16)) (eg, acute myeloid leukemia), qualitative, and quantitative, if performed

CBS (cystathionine-beta-synthase) (eg, homocystinuria, cystathionine beta-synthase deficiency), common variants (eg, I278T, G307S)

CCND1/IGH (BCL1/IgH, t(11;14)) (eg, mantle cell lymphoma) translocation analysis, major breakpoint, qualitative, and quantitative, if performed

CFH/ARMS2 (complement factor H/age-related maculopathy susceptibility 2) (eg, macular degeneration), common variants (eg, Y402H [CFH], A69S [ARMS2])

CNBP (CCHC-type zinc finger, nucleic acid binding protein) (eg, myotonic dystrophy type 2), evaluation to detect abnormal (eg, expanded) alleles

CSTB (cystatin B [stefin B]) (eg, Unverricht-Lundborg disease), evaluation to detect abnormal (eg, expanded) alleles

CYP3A4 (cytochrome P450, family 3, subfamily A, polypeptide 4) (eg, drug metabolism), common variants (eg, *2, *3, *4, *5, *6)

CYP3A5 (cytochrome P450, family 3, subfamily A, polypeptide 5) (eg, drug metabolism), common variants (eg, *2, *3, *4, *5, *6)

DMPK (dystrophia myotonica-protein kinase) (eg, myotonic dystrophy, type 1), evaluation to detect abnormal (eg, expanded) alleles

E2A/PBX1 (t(1;19)) (eg, acute lymphocytic leukemia), translocation analysis, qualitative, and quantitative, if performed

EML4/ALK (inv(2)) (eg, non-small cell lung cancer), translocation or inversion analysis

ETV6/NTRK3 (t(12;15)) (eg, congenital/infantile fibrosarcoma), translocation analysis, qualitative, and quantitative, if performed

ETV6/RUNX1 (t(12;21)) (eg, acute lymphocytic leukemia), translocation analysis, qualitative, and quantitative, if performed

EWSR1/ATF1 (t(12;22)) (eg, clear cell sarcoma), translocation analysis, qualitative, and quantitative, if performed

EWSR1/ERG (t(21;22)) (eg, Ewing sarcoma/peripheral neuroectodermal tumor), translocation analysis, qualitative, and quantitative, if performed

EWSR1/FLI1 (t(11;22)) (eg, Ewing sarcoma/peripheral neuroectodermal tumor), translocation analysis, qualitative, and quantitative, if performed

EWSR1/WT1 (t(11;22)) (eg, desmoplastic small round cell tumor), translocation analysis, qualitative, and quantitative, if performed

F11 (coagulation factor XI) (eg, coagulation disorder), common variants (eg, E117X [Type II], F283L [Type III], IVS14del14, and IVS14+1G>A [Type I])

FGFR3 (fibroblast growth factor receptor 3) (eg, achondroplasia, hypochondroplasia), common variants (eg, 1138G>A, 1138G>C, 1620C>A, 1620C>G)

FIP1L1/PDGFRA (del[4q12]) (eg, imatinib-sensitive chronic eosinophilic leukemia), qualitative, and quantitative, if performed

FLG (filaggrin) (eg, icthyosis vulgaris), common variants (eg, R501X, 2282del4, R2447X, S3247X, 3702delG)

FOXO1/PAX3 (t(2;13)) (eg, alveolar rhabdomyosarcoma), translocation analysis, qualitative, and quantitative, if performed

FOXO1/PAX7 (t(1;13)) (eg, alveolar rhabdomyosarcoma), translocation analysis, qualitative, and quantitative, if performed

FUS/DDIT3 (t(12;16)) (eg, myxoid liposarcoma), translocation analysis, qualitative, and quantitative, if performed

FXN (frataxin) (eg, Friedreich ataxia), evaluation to detect abnormal (expanded) alleles

GALC (galactosylceramidase) (eg, Krabbe disease), common variants (eg, c.857G>A, 30-kb deletion)

GALT (galactose-1-phosphate uridylyltransferase) (eg, galactosemia), common variants (eg, Q188R, S135L, K285N, T138M, L195P, Y209C, IVS2-2A>G, P171S, del5kb, N314D, L218L/N314D)

H19 (imprinted maternally expressed transcript [non-protein coding]) (eg, Beckwith-Wiedemann syndrome), methylation analysis

HBB (hemoglobin, beta) (eg, sickle cell anemia, hemoglobin C, hemoglobin E), common variants (eg, HbS, HbC, HbE)

HTT (huntingtin) (eg, Huntington disease), evaluation to detect abnormal (eg, expanded) alleles

KCNQ1OT1 (KCNQ1 overlapping transcript 1 [non-protein coding]) (eg, Beckwith-Wiedemann syndrome), methylation analysis

LRRK2 (leucine-rich repeat kinase 2) (eg, Parkinson disease), common variants (eg, R1441G, G2019S, I2020T)

● New   ▲ Revised   ✖ Deleted   ⊙ Moderate Sedation   ✚ Add-on Codes   ⊘ High Risk Denial   Ⓐ Age Edit   ♀ Female   ♂ Male   AMA *CPT® Assistant*   *MUE* Medically Unlikely Edit
⦸ Modifier 51 Exempt   ⊖ Modifier 63 Exempt   ⓧ Unlisted   Modifiers: *See Inside Back Cover*   Ⓜ Maternity   A2-Z3 ASC Payment Indicators   A-Y OPPS Status Indicators

    CPT © 2015 American Medical Association. All Rights Reserved.   © 2016 DecisionHealth

MED12 (mediator complex subunit 12) (eg, FG syndrome type 1, Lujan syndrome), common variants (eg, R961W, N1007S)

MEG3/DLK1 (maternally expressed 3 [non-protein coding]/delta-like 1 homolog [Drosophila]) (eg, intrauterine growth retardation), methylation analysis MLL/AFF1 (t(4;11)) (eg, acute lymphoblastic leukemia), translocation analysis, qualitative, and quantitative, if performed

MLL/MLLT3 (t(9;11)) (eg, acute myeloid leukemia), translocation analysis, qualitative, and quantitative, if performed

MT-ATP6 (mitochondrially encoded ATP synthase 6) (eg, neuropathy with ataxia and retinitis pigmentosa [NARP], Leigh syndrome), common variants (eg, m.8993T>G, m.8993T>C)

MT-ND4, MT-ND6 (mitochondrially encoded NADH dehydrogenase 4, mitochondrially encoded NADH dehydrogenase 6) (eg, Leber hereditary optic neuropathy [LHON]), common variants (eg, m.11778G>A, m.3460G>A, m.14484T>C)

MT-RNR1 (mitochondrially encoded 12S RNA) (eg, nonsyndromic hearing loss), common variants (eg, m.1555A>G, m.1494C>T)

MT-TK (mitochondrially encoded tRNA lysine) (eg, myoclonic epilepsy with ragged-red fibers [MERRF]), common variants (eg, m.8344A>G, m.8356T>C)

MT-TL1 (mitochondrially encoded tRNA leucine 1 [UUA/G]) (eg, diabetes and hearing loss), common variants (eg, m.3243A>G, m.14709 T>C)

MT-TL1 MT-ND5 (mitochondrially encoded tRNA leucine 1 [UUA/G], mitochondrially encoded NADH dehydrogenase 5) (eg, mitochondrial encephalopathy with lactic acidosis and stroke-like episodes [MELAS]), common variants (eg, m.3243A>G, m.3271T>C, m.3252A>G, m.13513G>A)

MT-TS1, MT-RNR1 (mitochondrially encoded tRNA serine 1 [UCN], mitochondrially encoded 12S RNA) (eg, nonsyndromic sensorineural deafness [including aminoglycoside-induced nonsyndromic deafness]), common variants (eg, m.7445A>G, m.1555A>G)

MUTYH (mutY homolog [E. coli]) (eg, MYH-associated polyposis), common variants (eg, Y165C, G382D)

NOD2 (nucleotide-binding oligomerization domain containing 2) (eg, Crohn's disease, Blau syndrome), common variants (eg, SNP 8, SNP 12, SNP 13)

NPM1/ALK (t(2;5)) (eg, anaplastic large cell lymphoma), translocation analysis

PABPN1 (poly[A] binding protein, nuclear 1) (eg, oculopharyngeal muscular dystrophy), evaluation to detect abnormal (eg, expanded) alleles

PAX8/PPARG (t(2;3) (q13;p25)) (eg, follicular thyroid carcinoma), translocation analysis

PPP2R2B (protein phosphatase 2, regulatory subunit B, beta) (eg, spinocerebellar ataxia), evaluation to detect abnormal (eg, expanded) alleles

PRSS1 (protease, serine, 1 [trypsin 1]) (eg, hereditary pancreatitis), common variants (eg, N29I, A16V, R122H)

PYGM (phosphorylase, glycogen, muscle) (eg, glycogen storage disease type V, McArdle disease), common variants (eg, R50X, G205S)

RUNX1/RUNX1T1 (t(8;21)) (eg, acute myeloid leukemia) translocation analysis, qualitative, and quantitative, if performed

SEPT9 (septin 9) (eg, colon cancer), methylation analysis

SMN1/SMN2 (survival of motor neuron 1, telomeric/survival of motor neuron 2, centromeric) (eg, spinal muscular atrophy), dosage analysis (eg, carrier testing) (For duplication/deletion analysis of SMN1/SMN2, use 81401)

SS18/SSX1 (t(X;18)) (eg, synovial sarcoma), translocation analysis, qualitative, and quantitative, if performed

SS18/SSX2 (t(X;18)) (eg, synovial sarcoma), translocation analysis, qualitative, and quantitative, if performed

TBP (TATA box binding protein) (eg, spinocerebellar ataxia), evaluation to detect abnormal (eg, expanded) alleles

TPMT (thiopurine S-methyltransferase) (eg, drug metabolism), common variants (eg, *2, *3)

TYMS (thymidylate synthetase) (eg, 5-fluorouracil/5-FU drug metabolism), tandem repeat variant

VWF (von Willebrand factor) (eg, von Willebrand disease type 2N), common variants (eg, T791M, R816W, R854Q) ⊙Ⓐ

RVU			Global Days	Modifiers				
Mod	Non-Fac Total	Fac Total		51	50	62	80	MUE
	0.00	0.00	XXX	9	9	9	9	2

AMA: May 12: 4, Jul 13: 12, Sep 13: 5, Jan 15: 3

▲ **81402** **Molecular pathology procedure, Level 3 (eg, >10 SNPs, 2-10 methylated variants, or 2-10 somatic variants [typically using non-sequencing target variant analysis], immunoglobulin and T-cell receptor gene rearrangements, duplication/deletion variants of 1 exon, loss of heterozygosity [LOH], uniparental disomy [UPD])**

Chromosome 1p-/19q- (eg, glial tumors), deletion analysis

Chromosome 18q- (eg, D18S55, D18S58, D18S61, D18S64, and D18S69) (eg, colon cancer), allelic imbalance assessment (ie, loss of heterozygosity)

COL1A1/PDGFB (t(17;22)) (eg, dermatofibrosarcoma protuberans), translocation analysis, multiple breakpoints, qualitative, and quantitative, if performed

CYP21A2 (cytochrome P450, family 21, subfamily A, polypeptide 2) (eg, congenital adrenal hyperplasia, 21-hydroxylase deficiency), common variants (eg, IVS2-13G, P30L, I172N, exon 6 mutation cluster [I235N, V236E, M238K], V281L, L307FfsX6, Q318X, R356W, P453S, G110VfsX21, 30-kb deletion variant)

● New   ▲ Revised   Deleted   ⊙ Moderate Sedation   ✚ Add-on Codes   ⊘ High Risk Denial   Ⓐ Age Edit   ♀ Female   ♂ Male   **AMA** CPT® Assistant   **MUE** Medically Unlikely Edit
⊘ Modifier 51 Exempt   ⊖ Modifier 63 Exempt   ⊠ Unlisted   **Modifiers:** See Inside Back Cover   Ⓜ Maternity   Ⓐ2-Ⓩ3 ASC Payment Indicators   Ⓐ-Ⓨ OPPS Status Indicators

ESR1/PGR (receptor 1/progesterone receptor) ratio (eg, breast cancer)

IGH@/BCL2 (t(14;18)) (eg, follicular lymphoma), translocation analysis; major breakpoint region (MBR) and minor cluster region (mcr) breakpoints, qualitative or quantitative

MEFV (Mediterranean fever) (eg, familial Mediterranean fever), common variants (eg, E148Q, P369S, F479L, M680I, I692del, M694V, M694I, K695R, V726A, A744S, R761H)

MPL (myeloproliferative leukemia virus oncogene, thrombopoietin receptor, TPOR) (eg, myeloproliferative disorder), common variants (eg, W515A, W515K, W515L, W515R)

TRD@ (T cell antigen receptor, delta) (eg, leukemia and lymphoma), gene rearrangement analysis, evaluation to detect abnormal clonal population

Uniparental disomy (UPD) (eg, Russell-Silver syndrome, Prader-Willi/Angelman syndrome), short tandem repeat (STR) analysis ⊘🅰

RVU			Global Days	Modifiers				
Mod	Non-Fac Total	Fac Total		51	50	62	80	MUE
	0.00	0.00	XXX	9	9	9	9	1

AMA: May 12: 4, Jul 13: 12, Sep 13: 5, 9, Jan 15: 3

▲ **81403 Molecular pathology procedure, Level 4 (eg, analysis of single exon by DNA sequence analysis, analysis of >10 amplicons using multiplex PCR in 2 or more independent reactions, mutation scanning or duplication/deletion variants of 2-5 exons)**

ANG (angiogenin, ribonuclease, RNase A family, 5) (eg, amyotrophic lateral sclerosis), full gene sequence

ARX (aristaless-related homeobox) (eg, X-linked lissencephaly with ambiguous genitalia, X-linked mental retardation), duplication/deletion analysis

CEL (carboxyl ester lipase [bile salt-stimulated lipase]) (eg, maturity-onset diabetes of the young [MODY]), targeted sequence analysis of exon 11 (eg, c.1785delC, c.1686delT)

CTNNB1 (catenin [cadherin-associated protein], beta 1, 88kDa) (eg, desmoid tumors), targeted sequence analysis (eg, exon 3)

DAZ/SRY (deleted in azoospermia and sex determining region Y) (eg, male infertility), common deletions (eg, AZFa, AZFb, AZFc, AZFd)

DNMT3A (DNA [cytosine-5-]-methyltransferase 3 alpha) (eg, acute myeloid leukemia), targeted sequence analysis (eg, exon 23)

EPCAM (epithelial cell adhesion molecule) (eg, Lynch syndrome), duplication/deletion analysis
F8 (coagulation factor VIII) (eg, hemophilia A), inversion analysis, intron 1 and intron 22A

F12 (coagulation factor XII [Hageman factor]) (eg, angioedema, hereditary, type III; factor XII deficiency), targeted sequence analysis of exon 9

FGFR3 (fibroblast growth factor receptor 3) (eg, isolated craniosynostosis), targeted sequence analysis (eg, exon 7) (For targeted sequence analysis of multiple FGFR3 exons, use 81404)

GJB1 (gap junction protein, beta 1) (eg, Charcot-Marie-Tooth X-linked), full gene sequence

GNAQ (guanine nucleotide-binding protein G[q] subunit alpha) (eg, uveal melanoma), common variants (eg, R183, Q209)

HBB (hemoglobin, beta, beta-globin) (eg, beta thalassemia), duplication/deletion analysis

Human erythrocyte antigen gene analyses (eg, SLC14A1 [Kidd blood group], BCAM [Lutheran blood group], ICAM4 [Landsteiner-Wiener blood group], SLC4A1 [Diego blood group], AQP1 [Colton blood group], ERMAP [Scianna blood group], RHCE [Rh blood group, CcEe antigens], KEL [Kell blood group], DARC [Duffy blood group], GYPA, GYPB, GYPE [MNS blood group], ART4 [Dombrock blood group]) (eg, sickle-cell disease, thalassemia, hemolytic transfusion reactions, hemolytic disease of the fetus or newborn), common variants

HRAS (v-Ha-ras Harvey rat sarcoma viral oncogene homolog) (eg, Costello syndrome), exon 2 sequence
IDH1 (isocitrate dehydrogenase 1 [NADP+], soluble) (eg, glioma), common exon 4 variants (eg, R132H, R132C)

IDH2 (isocitrate dehydrogenase 2 [NADP+], mitochondrial) (eg, glioma), common exon 4 variants (eg, R140W, R172M)

JAK2 (Janus kinase 2) (eg, myeloproliferative disorder), exon 12 sequence and exon 13 sequence, if performed

KCNC3 (potassium voltage-gated channel, Shaw-related subfamily, member 3) (eg, spinocerebellar ataxia), targeted sequence analysis (eg, exon 2)

KCNJ2 (potassium inwardly-rectifying channel, subfamily J, member 2) (eg, Andersen-Tawil syndrome), full gene sequence

KCNJ11 (potassium inwardly-rectifying channel, subfamily J, member 11) (eg, familial hyperinsulinism), full gene sequence

Killer cell immunoglobulin-like receptor (KIR) gene family (eg, hematopoietic stem cell transplantation), genotyping of KIR family genes

Known familial variant not otherwise specified, for gene listed in Tier 1 or Tier 2, DNA sequence analysis, each variant exon (For a known familial variant that is considered a common variant, use specific common variant Tier 1 or Tier 2 code)

MC4R (melanocortin 4 receptor) (eg, obesity), full gene sequence

MICA (MHC class I polypeptide-related sequence A) (eg, solid organ transplantation), common variants (eg, *001, *002)

MPL (myeloproliferative leukemia virus oncogene, thrombopoietin receptor, TPOR) (eg, myeloproliferative disorder), exon 10 sequence

● New   ▲ Revised   ✖ Deleted   ⊙ Moderate Sedation   ✚ Add-on Codes   ⊘ High Risk Denial   ⒶAge Edit   ♀ Female   ♂ Male   **AMA** *CPT® Assistant*   **MUE** Medically Unlikely Edit
⊘ Modifier 51 Exempt   ⊖ Modifier 63 Exempt   🆇 Unlisted   **Modifiers:** *See Inside Back Cover*   Ⓜ Maternity   🅰2–🆉3 ASC Payment Indicators   🅰–🆈 OPPS Status Indicators

CPT © 2015 American Medical Association. All Rights Reserved.   © 2016 DecisionHealth

MT-RNR1 (mitochondrially encoded 12S RNA) (eg, nonsyndromic hearing loss), full gene sequence

MT-TS1 (mitochondrially encoded tRNA serine 1) (eg, nonsyndromic hearing loss), full gene sequence

NDP (Norrie disease [pseudoglioma]) (eg, Norrie disease), duplication/deletion analysis

NHLRC1 (NHL repeat containing 1) (eg, progressive myoclonus epilepsy), full gene sequence

PHOX2B (paired-like homeobox 2b) (eg, congenital central hypoventilation syndrome), duplication/deletion analysis

PLN (phospholamban) (eg, dilated cardiomyopathy, hypertrophic cardiomyopathy), full gene sequence

RHD (Rh blood group, D antigen) (eg, hemolytic disease of the fetus and newborn, Rh maternal/fetal compatibility), deletion analysis (eg, exons 4, 5, and 7, pseudogene)

RHD (Rh blood group, D antigen) (eg, hemolytic disease of the fetus and newborn, Rh maternal/fetal compatibility), deletion analysis (eg, exons 4, 5, and 7, pseudogene), performed on cell-free fetal DNA in maternal blood (For human erythrocyte gene analysis of RHD, use a separate unit of 81403)

SH2D1A (SH2 domain containing 1A) (eg, X-linked lymphoproliferative syndrome), duplication/deletion analysis

SMN1 (survival of motor neuron 1, telomeric) (eg, spinal muscular atrophy), known familial sequence variant(s)

TWIST1 (twist homolog 1 [Drosophila]) (eg, Saethre-Chotzen syndrome), duplication/deletion analysis UBA1 (ubiquitin-like modifier activating enzyme 1) (eg, spinal muscular atrophy, X-linked), targeted sequence analysis (eg, exon 15)

VHL (von Hippel-Lindau tumor suppressor) (eg, von Hippel-Lindau familial cancer syndrome), deletion/duplication analysis

VWF (von Willebrand factor) (eg, von Willebrand disease types 2A, 2B, 2M), targeted sequence analysis (eg, exon 28)   ⊗🅰

RVU			Global Days	Modifiers				
Mod	Non-Fac Total	Fac Total		51	50	62	80	MUE
	0.00	0.00	XXX	9	9	9	9	4

AMA: May 12: 4, Jul 13: 12, Sep 13: 3, Jan 15: 3

▲ 81404 **Molecular pathology procedure, Level 5 (eg, analysis of 2-5 exons by DNA sequence analysis, mutation scanning or duplication/deletion variants of 6-10 exons, or characterization of a dynamic mutation disorder/triplet repeat by Southern blot analysis)**

ACADS (acyl-CoA dehydrogenase, C-2 to C-3 short chain) (eg, short chain acyl-CoA dehydrogenase deficiency), targeted sequence analysis (eg, exons 5 and 6)

AFF2 (AF4/FMR2 family, member 2 [FMR2]) (eg, fragile X mental retardation 2 [FRAXE]), characterization of alleles (eg, expanded size and methylation status)

AQP2 (aquaporin 2 [collecting duct]) (eg, nephrogenic diabetes insipidus), full gene sequence

ARX (aristaless related homeobox) (eg, X-linked lissencephaly with ambiguous genitalia, X-linked mental retardation), full gene sequence

AVPR2 (arginine vasopressin receptor 2) (eg, nephrogenic diabetes insipidus), full gene sequence

BBS10 (Bardet-Biedl syndrome 10) (eg, Bardet-Biedl syndrome), full gene sequence

BTD (biotinidase) (eg, biotinidase deficiency), full gene sequence

C10orf2 (chromosome 10 open reading frame 2) (eg, mitochondrial DNA depletion syndrome), full gene sequence

CAV3 (caveolin 3) (eg, CAV3-related distal myopathy, limb-girdle muscular dystrophy type 1C), full gene sequence

CD40LG (CD40 ligand) (eg, X-linked hyper IgM syndrome), full gene sequence

CDKN2A (cyclin-dependent kinase inhibitor 2A) (eg, CDKN2A-related cutaneous malignant melanoma, familial atypical mole-malignant melanoma syndrome), full gene sequence

CLRN1 (clarin 1) (eg, Usher syndrome, type 3), full gene sequence

COX6B1 (cytochrome c oxidase subunit VIb polypeptide 1) (eg, mitochondrial respiratory chain complex IV deficiency), full gene sequence

CPT2 (carnitine palmitoyltransferase 2) (eg, carnitine palmitoyltransferase II deficiency), full gene sequence

CRX (cone-rod homeobox) (eg, cone-rod dystrophy 2, Leber congenital amaurosis), full gene sequence

CSTB (cystatin B [stefin B]) (eg, Unverricht-Lundborg disease), full gene sequence

CYP1B1 (cytochrome P450, family 1, subfamily B, polypeptide 1) (eg, primary congenital glaucoma), full gene sequence

DMPK (dystrophia myotonica-protein kinase) (eg, myotonic dystrophy type 1), characterization of abnormal (eg, expanded) alleles

EGR2 (early growth response 2) (eg, Charcot-Marie-Tooth), full gene sequence

EMD (emerin) (eg, Emery-Dreifuss muscular dystrophy), duplication/deletion analysis

EPM2A (epilepsy, progressive myoclonus type 2A, Lafora disease [laforin]) (eg, progressive myoclonus epilepsy), full gene sequence

FGF23 (fibroblast growth factor 23) (eg, hypophosphatemic rickets), full gene sequence

FGFR2 (fibroblast growth factor receptor 2) (eg, craniosynostosis, Apert syndrome, Crouzon syndrome), targeted sequence analysis (eg, exons 8, 10)

FGFR3 (fibroblast growth factor receptor 3) (eg, achondroplasia, hypochondroplasia), targeted sequence analysis (eg, exons 8, 11, 12, 13)

© 2016 DecisionHealth   CPT © 2015 American Medical Association. All Rights Reserved.   **697**

FHL1 (four and a half LIM domains 1) (eg, Emery-Dreifuss muscular dystrophy), full gene sequence

FKRP (fukutin related protein) (eg, congenital muscular dystrophy type 1C [MDC1C], limb-girdle muscular dystrophy [LGMD] type 2I), full gene sequence

FOXG1 (forkhead box G1) (eg, Rett syndrome), full gene sequence

FSHMD1A (facioscapulohumeral muscular dystrophy 1A) (eg, facioscapulohumeral muscular dystrophy), evaluation to detect abnormal (eg, deleted) alleles

FSHMD1A (facioscapulohumeral muscular dystrophy 1A) (eg, facioscapulohumeral muscular dystrophy), characterization of haplotype(s) (ie, chromosome 4A and 4B haplotypes)

FXN (frataxin) (eg, Friedreich ataxia), full gene sequence GH1 (growth hormone 1) (eg, growth hormone deficiency), full gene sequence

GP1BB (glycoprotein Ib [platelet], beta polypeptide) (eg, Bernard-Soulier syndrome type B), full gene sequence

HBA1/HBA2 (alpha globin 1 and alpha globin 2) (eg, alpha thalassemia), duplication/deletion analysis (For common deletion variants of alpha globin 1 and alpha globin 2 genes, use 81257)

HBB (hemoglobin, beta, Beta-Globin) (eg, thalassemia), full gene sequence

HNF1B (HNF1 homeobox B) (eg, maturity-onset diabetes of the young [MODY]), duplication/deletion analysis

HRAS (v-Ha-ras Harvey rat sarcoma viral oncogene homolog) (eg, Costello syndrome), full gene sequence

HSD3B2 (hydroxy-delta-5-steroid dehydrogenase, 3 beta- and steroid delta-isomerase 2) (eg, 3-beta-hydroxysteroid dehydrogenase type II deficiency), full gene sequence

HSD11B2 (hydroxysteroid [11-beta] dehydrogenase 2) (eg, mineralocorticoid excess syndrome), full gene sequence

HSPB1 (heat shock 27kDa protein 1) (eg, Charcot-Marie-Tooth disease), full gene sequence

INS (insulin) (eg, diabetes mellitus), full gene sequence

KCNJ1 (potassium inwardly-rectifying channel, subfamily J, member 1) (eg, Bartter syndrome), full gene sequence

KCNJ10 (potassium inwardly-rectifying channel, subfamily J, member 10) (eg, SeSAME syndrome, EAST syndrome, sensorineural hearing loss), full gene sequence

KIT (C-kit) (v-kit Hardy-Zuckerman 4 feline sarcoma viral oncogene homolog) (eg, GIST, acute myeloid leukemia, melanoma), targeted gene analysis (eg, exons 8, 11, 13, 17, 18)

LITAF (lipopolysaccharide-induced TNF factor) (eg, Charcot-Marie-Tooth), full gene sequence

MEFV (Mediterranean fever) (eg, familial Mediterranean fever), full gene sequence

MEN1 (multiple endocrine neoplasia I) (eg, multiple endocrine neoplasia type 1, Wermer syndrome), duplication/deletion analysis

MMACHC (methylmalonic aciduria [cobalamin deficiency] cblC type, with homocystinuria) (eg, methylmalonic acidemia and homocystinuria), full gene sequence

NDP (Norrie disease [pseudoglioma]) (eg, Norrie disease), full gene sequence

NDUFA1 (NADH dehydrogenase [ubiquinone] 1 alpha subcomplex, 1, 7.5kDa) (eg, Leigh syndrome, mitochondrial complex I deficiency), full gene sequence

NDUFAF2 (NADH dehydrogenase [ubiquinone] 1 alpha subcomplex, assembly factor 2) (eg, Leigh syndrome, mitochondrial complex I deficiency), full gene sequence

NDUFS4 (NADH dehydrogenase [ubiquinone] Fe-S protein 4, 18kDa [NADH-coenzyme Q reductase]) (eg, Leigh syndrome, mitochondrial complex I deficiency), full gene sequence

NIPA1 (non-imprinted in Prader-Willi/Angelman syndrome 1) (eg, spastic paraplegia), full gene sequence

NLGN4X (neuroligin 4, X-linked) (eg, autism spectrum disorders), duplication/deletion analysis

NPC2 (Niemann-Pick disease, type C2 [epididymal secretory protein E1]) (eg, Niemann-Pick disease type C2), full gene sequence

NR0B1 (nuclear receptor subfamily 0, group B, member 1) (eg, congenital adrenal hypoplasia), full gene sequence

NRAS (neuroblastoma RAS viral oncogene homolog) (eg, colorectal carcinoma), exon 1 and exon 2 sequences

PDGFRA (platelet-derived growth factor receptor alpha polypeptide) (eg, gastrointestinal stromal tumor), targeted sequence analysis (eg, exons 12, 18)

PDX1 (pancreatic and duodenal homeobox 1) (eg, maturity-onset diabetes of the young [MODY]), full gene sequence

PHOX2B (paired-like homeobox 2b) (eg, congenital central hypoventilation syndrome), full gene sequence

PLP1 (proteolipid protein 1) (eg, Pelizaeus-Merzbacher disease, spastic paraplegia), duplication/deletion analysis

PQBP1 (polyglutamine binding protein 1) (eg, Renpenning syndrome), duplication/deletion analysis PRNP (prion protein) (eg, genetic prion disease), full gene sequence

PROP1 (PROP paired-like homeobox 1) (eg, combined pituitary hormone deficiency), full gene sequence

PRPH2 (peripherin 2 [retinal degeneration, slow]) (eg, retinitis pigmentosa), full gene sequence

---

● New   ▲ Revised   ✖ Deleted   ⊙ Moderate Sedation   ✚ Add-on Codes   ⊘ High Risk Denial   Ⓐ Age Edit   ♀ Female   ♂ Male   **AMA** *CPT® Assistant*   **MUE** Medically Unlikely Edit
◌ Modifier 51 Exempt   ⊖ Modifier 63 Exempt   🄫 Unlisted   **Modifiers:** *See Inside Back Cover*   Ⓜ Maternity   **A2–Z3** ASC Payment Indicators   **A–Y** OPPS Status Indicators

698   CPT © 2015 American Medical Association. All Rights Reserved.   © 2016 DecisionHealth

PRSS1 (protease, serine, 1 [trypsin 1]) (eg, hereditary pancreatitis), full gene sequence

RAF1 (v-raf-1 murine leukemia viral oncogene homolog 1) (eg, LEOPARD syndrome), targeted sequence analysis (eg, exons 7, 12, 14, 17)

RET (ret proto-oncogene) (eg, multiple endocrine neoplasia, type 2B and familial medullary thyroid carcinoma), common variants (eg, M918T, 2647_2648delinsTT, A883F)

RHO (rhodopsin) (eg, retinitis pigmentosa), full gene sequence

RP1 (retinitis pigmentosa 1) (eg, retinitis pigmentosa), full gene sequence

SCN1B (sodium channel, voltage-gated, type I, beta) (eg, Brugada syndrome), full gene sequence

SCO2 (SCO cytochrome oxidase deficient homolog 2 [SCO1L]) (eg, mitochondrial respiratory chain complex IV deficiency), full gene sequence

SDHC (succinate dehydrogenase complex, subunit C, integral membrane protein, 15kDa) (eg, hereditary paraganglioma-pheochromocytoma syndrome), duplication/deletion analysis

SDHD (succinate dehydrogenase complex, subunit D, integral membrane protein) (eg, hereditary paraganglioma), full gene sequence

SGCG (sarcoglycan, gamma [35kDa dystrophin-associated glycoprotein]) (eg, limb-girdle muscular dystrophy), duplication/deletion analysis

SH2D1A (SH2 domain containing 1A) (eg, X-linked lymphoproliferative syndrome), full gene sequence

SLC16A2 (solute carrier family 16, member 2 [thyroid hormone transporter]) (eg, specific thyroid hormone cell transporter deficiency, Allan-Herndon-Dudley syndrome), duplication/deletion analysis

SLC25A20 (solute carrier family 25 [carnitine/acylcarnitine translocase], member 20) (eg, carnitine-acylcarnitine translocase deficiency), duplication/deletion analysis

SLC25A4 (solute carrier family 25 [mitochondrial carrier; adenine nucleotide translocator], member 4) (eg, progressive external ophthalmoplegia), full gene sequence

SOD1 (superoxide dismutase 1, soluble) (eg, amyotrophic lateral sclerosis), full gene sequence

SPINK1 (serine peptidase inhibitor, Kazal type 1) (eg, hereditary pancreatitis), full gene sequence

STK11 (serine/threonine kinase 11) (eg, Peutz-Jeghers syndrome), duplication/deletion analysis

TACO1 (translational activator of mitochondrial encoded cytochrome c oxidase I) (eg, mitochondrial respiratory chain complex IV deficiency), full gene sequence

THAP1 (THAP domain containing, apoptosis associated protein 1) (eg, torsion dystonia), full gene sequence

TOR1A (torsin family 1, member A [torsin A]) (eg, torsion dystonia), full gene sequence

TP53 (tumor protein 53) (eg, tumor samples), targeted sequence analysis of 2-5 exons

TTPA (tocopherol [alpha] transfer protein) (eg, ataxia), full gene sequence

TTR (transthyretin) (eg, familial transthyretin amyloidosis), full gene sequence

TWIST1 (twist homolog 1 [Drosophila]) (eg, Saethre-Chotzen syndrome), full gene sequence

TYR (tyrosinase [oculocutaneous albinism IA]) (eg, oculocutaneous albinism IA), full gene sequence

USH1G (Usher syndrome 1G [autosomal recessive]) (eg, Usher syndrome, type 1), full gene sequence

VHL (von Hippel-Lindau tumor suppressor) (eg, von Hippel-Lindau familial cancer syndrome), full gene sequence

VWF (von Willebrand factor) (eg, von Willebrand disease type 1C), targeted sequence analysis (eg, exons 26, 27, 37)

ZEB2 (zinc finger E-box binding homeobox 2) (eg, Mowat-Wilson syndrome), duplication/deletion analysis

ZNF41 (zinc finger protein 41) (eg, X-linked mental retardation 89), full gene sequence   Ⓐ

RVU			Global Days	Modifiers				
Mod	Non-Fac Total	Fac Total		51	50	62	80	MUE
	0.00	0.00	XXX	9	9	9	9	5

AMA: May 12: 4, Jul 13: 12, Sep 13: 6, 7, 9, Jan 15: 3

▲ **81405** **Molecular pathology procedure, Level 6 (eg, analysis of 6-10 exons by DNA sequence analysis, mutation scanning or duplication/deletion variants of 11-25 exons), regionally targeted cytogenomic array analysis**

ABCD1 (ATP-binding cassette, sub-family D [ALD], member 1) (eg, adrenoleukodystrophy), full gene sequence

ACADS (acyl-CoA dehydrogenase, C-2 to C-3 short chain) (eg, short chain acyl-CoA dehydrogenase deficiency), full gene sequence

ACTA2 (actin, alpha 2, smooth muscle, aorta) (eg, thoracic aortic aneurysms and aortic dissections), full gene sequence

ACTC1 (actin, alpha, cardiac muscle 1) (eg, familial hypertrophic cardiomyopathy), full gene sequence

ANKRD1 (ankyrin repeat domain 1) (eg, dilated cardiomyopathy), full gene sequence

APTX (aprataxin) (eg, ataxia with oculomotor apraxia 1), full gene sequence

AR (androgen receptor) (eg, androgen insensitivity syndrome), full gene sequence

ARSA (arylsulfatase A) (eg, arylsulfatase A deficiency), full gene sequence

BCKDHA (branched chain keto acid dehydrogenase E1, alpha polypeptide) (eg, maple syrup urine disease, type 1A), full gene sequence

● New   ▲ Revised   Deleted   ⊙ Moderate Sedation   ✚ Add-on Codes   ⊘ High Risk Denial   Ⓐ Age Edit   ♀ Female   ♂ Male   **AMA** CPT® Assistant   **MUE** Medically Unlikely Edit
⊘ Modifier 51 Exempt   ⊖ Modifier 63 Exempt   ✖ Unlisted   **Modifiers:** See Inside Back Cover   Ⓜ Maternity   Ⓐ2–Ⓩ3 ASC Payment Indicators   Ⓐ–Ⓨ OPPS Status Indicators

BCS1L (BCS1-like [S. cerevisiae]) (eg, Leigh syndrome, mitochondrial complex III deficiency, GRACILE syndrome), full gene sequence

BMPR2 (bone morphogenetic protein receptor, type II [serine/threonine kinase]) (eg, heritable pulmonary arterial hypertension), duplication/deletion analysis

CASQ2 (calsequestrin 2 [cardiac muscle]) (eg, catecholaminergic polymorphic ventricular tachycardia), full gene sequence

CASR (calcium-sensing receptor) (eg, hypocalcemia), full gene sequence

CDKL5 (cyclin-dependent kinase-like 5) (eg, early infantile epileptic encephalopathy), duplication/deletion analysis

CHRNA4 (cholinergic receptor, nicotinic, alpha 4) (eg, nocturnal frontal lobe epilepsy), full gene sequence

CHRNB2 (cholinergic receptor, nicotinic, beta 2 [neuronal]) (eg, nocturnal frontal lobe epilepsy), full gene sequence

COX10 (COX10 homolog, cytochrome c oxidase assembly protein) (eg, mitochondrial respiratory chain complex IV deficiency), full gene sequence

COX15 (COX15 homolog, cytochrome c oxidase assembly protein) (eg, mitochondrial respiratory chain complex IV deficiency), full gene sequence

CYP11B1 (cytochrome P450, family 11, subfamily B, polypeptide 1) (eg, congenital adrenal hyperplasia), full gene sequence

CYP17A1 (cytochrome P450, family 17, subfamily A, polypeptide 1) (eg, congenital adrenal hyperplasia), full gene sequence

CYP21A2 (cytochrome P450, family 21, subfamily A, polypeptide2) (eg, steroid 21-hydroxylase isoform, congenital adrenal hyperplasia), full gene sequence

Cytogenomic constitutional targeted microarray analysis of the X chromosome by interrogation of genomic regions for copy number and single nucleotide polymorphism (SNP) variants for chromosomal abnormalities (When performing genome-wide cytogenomic constitutional microarray analysis, see 81228, (Do not report analyte-specific molecular pathology procedures separately when the specific analytes are included as part of the microarray analysis of the X chromosome) (Do not report 88271 when performing cytogenomic microarray analysis) Cytogenomic constitutional targeted microarray analysis of chromosome 22q13 by interrogation of genomic regions for copy number and single nucleotide polymorphism (SNP) variants for chromosomal abnormalities (When performing genome-wide cytogenomic constitutional microarray analysis, see 81228, (Do not report analyte-specific molecular pathology procedures separately when the specific analytes are included as part of the microarray analysis of chromosome 22q13) (Do not report 88271 when performing cytogenomic microarray analysis)

DBT (dihydrolipoamide branched chain transacylase E2) (eg, maple syrup urine disease, type 2), duplication/deletion analysis

DCX (doublecortin) (eg, X-linked lissencephaly), full gene sequence

DES (desmin) (eg, myofibrillar myopathy), full gene sequence

DFNB59 (deafness, autosomal recessive 59) (eg, autosomal recessive nonsyndromic hearing impairment), full gene sequence

DGUOK (deoxyguanosine kinase) (eg, hepatocerebral mitochondrial DNA depletion syndrome), full gene sequence

DHCR7 (7-dehydrocholesterol reductase) (eg, Smith-Lemli-Opitz syndrome), full gene sequence

EIF2B2 (eukaryotic translation initiation factor 2B, subunit 2 beta, 39kDa) (eg, leukoencephalopathy with vanishing white matter), full gene sequence

EMD (emerin) (eg, Emery-Dreifuss muscular dystrophy), full gene sequence

ENG (endoglin) (eg, hereditary hemorrhagic telangiectasia, type 1), duplication/deletion analysis

EYA1 (eyes absent homolog 1 [Drosophila]) (eg, branchio-oto-renal [BOR] spectrum disorders), duplication/deletion analysis

F9 (coagulation factor IX) (eg, hemophilia B), full gene sequence

FGFR1 (fibroblast growth factor receptor 1) (eg, Kallmann syndrome 2), full gene sequence

FH (fumarate hydratase) (eg, fumarate hydratase deficiency, hereditary leiomyomatosis with renal cell cancer), full gene sequence

FKTN (fukutin) (eg, limb-girdle muscular dystrophy [LGMD] type 2M or 2L), full gene sequence

FTSJ1 (FtsJ RNA methyltransferase homolog 1 [E. coli]) (eg, X-linked mental retardation 9), duplication/deletion analysis

GABRG2 (gamma-aminobutyric acid [GABA] A receptor, gamma 2) (eg, generalized epilepsy with febrile seizures), full gene sequence

GCH1 (GTP cyclohydrolase 1) (eg, autosomal dominant dopa-responsive dystonia), full gene sequence

GDAP1 (ganglioside-induced differentiation-associated protein 1) (eg, Charcot-Marie-Tooth disease), full gene sequence

GFAP (glial fibrillary acidic protein) (eg, Alexander disease), full gene sequence

GHR (growth hormone receptor) (eg, Laron syndrome), full gene sequence

GHRHR (growth hormone releasing hormone receptor) (eg, growth hormone deficiency), full gene sequence

GLA (galactosidase, alpha) (eg, Fabry disease), full gene sequence

● New   ▲ Revised   ✖ Deleted   ⊙ Moderate Sedation   ✚ Add-on Codes   ⊘ High Risk Denial   Ⓐ Age Edit   ♀ Female   ♂ Male   **AMA** *CPT® Assistant*   **MUE** Medically Unlikely Edit
⊘ Modifier 51 Exempt   ⊖ Modifier 63 Exempt   ✗ Unlisted   **Modifiers:** *See Inside Back Cover*   Ⓜ Maternity   A2–Z3 ASC Payment Indicators   A–Y OPPS Status Indicators

700   CPT © 2015 American Medical Association. All Rights Reserved.   © 2016 DecisionHealth

HBA1/HBA2 (alpha globin 1 and alpha globin 2) (eg, thalassemia), full gene sequence

HNF1A (HNF1 homeobox A) (eg, maturity-onset diabetes of the young [MODY]), full gene sequence

HNF1B (HNF1 homeobox B) (eg, maturity-onset diabetes of the young [MODY]), full gene sequence

HTRA1 (HtrA serine peptidase 1) (eg, macular degeneration), full gene sequence

IDS (iduronate 2-sulfatase) (eg, mucopolysacchridosis, type II), full gene sequence

IL2RG (interleukin 2 receptor, gamma) (eg, X-linked severe combined immunodeficiency), full gene sequence

ISPD (isoprenoid synthase domain containing) (eg, muscle-eye-brain disease, Walker-Warburg syndrome), full gene sequence

KRAS (v-Ki-ras2 Kirsten rat sarcoma viral oncogene homolog) (eg, Noonan syndrome), full gene sequence

LAMP2 (lysosomal-associated membrane protein 2) (eg, Danon disease), full gene sequence

LDLR (low density lipoprotein receptor) (eg, familial hypercholesterolemia), duplication/deletion analysis

MEN1 (multiple endocrine neoplasia I) (eg, multiple endocrine neoplasia type 1, Wermer syndrome), full gene sequence

Mitochondrial genome deletions (eg, Kearns-Sayre syndrome [KSS], chronic progressive external ophthalmoplegia [CPEO], Pearson syndrome), deletion analysis, and duplication analysis, if performed

MMAA (methylmalonic aciduria [cobalamine deficiency] type A) (eg, MMAA-related methylmalonic acidemia), full gene sequence

MMAB (methylmalonic aciduria [cobalamine deficiency] type B) (eg, MMAA-related methylmalonic acidemia), full gene sequence

MPI (mannose phosphate isomerase) (eg, congenital disorder of glycosylation 1b), full gene sequence

MPV17 (MpV17 mitochondrial inner membrane protein) (eg, mitochondrial DNA depletion syndrome), full gene sequence

MPZ (myelin protein zero) (eg, Charcot-Marie-Tooth), full gene sequence

MTM1 (myotubularin 1) (eg, X-linked centronuclear myopathy), duplication/deletion analysis

MYL2 (myosin, light chain 2, regulatory, cardiac, slow) (eg, familial hypertrophic cardiomyopathy), full gene sequence

MYL3 (myosin, light chain 3, alkali, ventricular, skeletal, slow) (eg, familial hypertrophic cardiomyopathy), full gene sequence

MYOT (myotilin) (eg, limb-girdle muscular dystrophy), full gene sequence

NDUFS7 (NADH dehydrogenase [ubiquinone] Fe-S protein 7, 20kDa [NADH-coenzyme Q reductase]) (eg, Leigh syndrome, mitochondrial complex I deficiency), full gene sequence

NDUFS8 (NADH dehydrogenase [ubiquinone] Fe-S protein 8, 23kDa [NADH-coenzyme Q reductase]) (eg, Leigh syndrome, mitochondrial complex I deficiency), full gene sequence

NDUFV1 (NADH dehydrogenase [ubiquinone] flavoprotein 1, 51kDa) (eg, Leigh syndrome, mitochondrial complex I deficiency), full gene sequence

NEFL (neurofilament, light polypeptide) (eg, Charcot-Marie-Tooth), full gene sequence

NF2 (neurofibromin 2 [merlin]) (eg, neurofibromatosis, type 2), duplication/deletion analysis

NLGN3 (neuroligin 3) (eg, autism spectrum disorders), full gene sequence

NLGN4X (neuroligin 4, X-linked) (eg, autism spectrum disorders), full gene sequence

NPHP1 (nephronophthisis 1 [juvenile]) (eg, Joubert syndrome), deletion analysis, and duplication analysis, if performed

NPHS2 (nephrosis 2, idiopathic, steroid-resistant [podocin]) (eg, steroid-resistant nephrotic syndrome), full gene sequence

NSD1 (nuclear receptor binding SET domain protein 1) (eg, Sotos syndrome), duplication/deletion analysis

OTC (ornithine carbamoyltransferase) (eg, ornithine transcarbamylase deficiency), full gene sequence

PAFAH1B1 (platelet-activating factor acetylhydrolase 1b, regulatory subunit 1 [45kDa]) (eg, lissencephaly, Miller-Dieker syndrome), duplication/deletion analysis

PARK2 (Parkinson protein 2, E3 ubiquitin protein ligase [parkin]) (eg, Parkinson disease), duplication/deletion analysis

PCCA (propionyl CoA carboxylase, alpha polypeptide) (eg, propionic acidemia, type 1), duplication/deletion analysis

PCDH19 (protocadherin 19) (eg, epileptic encephalopathy), full gene sequence

PDHA1 (pyruvate dehydrogenase [lipoamide] alpha 1) (eg, lactic acidosis), duplication/deletion analysis

PDHB (pyruvate dehydrogenase [lipoamide] beta) (eg, lactic acidosis), full gene sequence

PINK1 (PTEN induced putative kinase 1) (eg, Parkinson disease), full gene sequence

PLP1 (proteolipid protein 1) (eg, Pelizaeus-Merzbacher disease, spastic paraplegia), full gene sequence

POU1F1 (POU class 1 homeobox 1) (eg, combined pituitary hormone deficiency), full gene sequence

PRX (periaxin) (eg, Charcot-Marie-Tooth disease), full gene sequence

● New   ▲ Revised   Deleted   ⊙ Moderate Sedation   ✚ Add-on Codes   ⊘ High Risk Denial   Ⓐ Age Edit   ♀ Female   ♂ Male   **AMA** *CPT® Assistant*   **MUE** Medically Unlikely Edit
⊘ Modifier 51 Exempt   ⊖ Modifier 63 Exempt   ✗ Unlisted   **Modifiers:** *See Inside Back Cover*   Ⓜ Maternity   **A2–Z3** ASC Payment Indicators   **A–Y** OPPS Status Indicators

© 2016 DecisionHealth   CPT © 2015 American Medical Association. All Rights Reserved.

PQBP1 (polyglutamine binding protein 1) (eg, Renpenning syndrome), full gene sequence

PSEN1 (presenilin 1) (eg, Alzheimer disease), full gene sequence

RAB7A (RAB7A, member RAS oncogene family) (eg, Charcot-Marie-Tooth disease), full gene sequence

RAI1 (retinoic acid induced 1) (eg, Smith-Magenis syndrome), full gene sequence

REEP1 (receptor accessory protein 1) (eg, spastic paraplegia), full gene sequence

RET (ret proto-oncogene) (eg, multiple endocrine neoplasia, type 2A and familial medullary thyroid carcinoma), targeted sequence analysis (eg, exons 10, 11, 13-16)

RPS19 (ribosomal protein S19) (eg, Diamond-Blackfan anemia), full gene sequence

RRM2B (ribonucleotide reductase M2 B [TP53 inducible]) (eg, mitochondrial DNA depletion), full gene sequence

SCO1 (SCO cytochrome oxidase deficient homolog 1) (eg, mitochondrial respiratory chain complex IV deficiency), full gene sequence

SDHB (succinate dehydrogenase complex, subunit B, iron sulfur) (eg, hereditary paraganglioma), full gene sequence

SDHC (succinate dehydrogenase complex, subunit C, integral membrane protein, 15kDa) (eg, hereditary paraganglioma-pheochromocytoma syndrome), full gene sequence

SGCA (sarcoglycan, alpha [50kDa dystrophin-associated glycoprotein]) (eg, limb-girdle muscular dystrophy), full gene sequence

SGCB (sarcoglycan, beta [43kDa dystrophin-associated glycoprotein]) (eg, limb-girdle muscular dystrophy), full gene sequence

SGCD (sarcoglycan, delta [35kDa dystrophin-associated glycoprotein]) (eg, limb-girdle muscular dystrophy), full gene sequence

SGCE (sarcoglycan, epsilon) (eg, myoclonic dystonia), duplication/deletion analysis

SGCG (sarcoglycan, gamma [35kDa dystrophin-associated glycoprotein]) (eg, limb-girdle muscular dystrophy), full gene sequence

SHOC2 (soc-2 suppressor of clear homolog) (eg, Noonan-like syndrome with loose anagen hair), full gene sequence

SHOX (short stature homeobox) (eg, Langer mesomelic dysplasia), full gene sequence

SIL1 (SIL1 homolog, endoplasmic reticulum chaperone [S. cerevisiae]) (eg, ataxia), full gene sequence

SLC2A1 (solute carrier family 2 [facilitated glucose transporter], member 1) (eg, glucose transporter type 1 [GLUT 1] deficiency syndrome), full gene sequence

SLC16A2 (solute carrier family 16, member 2 [thyroid hormone transporter]) (eg, specific thyroid hormone cell transporter deficiency, Allan-Herndon-Dudley syndrome), full gene sequence

SLC22A5 (solute carrier family 22 [organic cation/carnitine transporter], member 5) (eg, systemic primary carnitine deficiency), full gene sequence

SLC25A20 (solute carrier family 25 [carnitine/acylcarnitine translocase], member 20) (eg, carnitine-acylcarnitine translocase deficiency), full gene sequence

SMAD4 (SMAD family member 4) (eg, hemorrhagic telangiectasia syndrome, juvenile polyposis), duplication/deletion analysis

SMN1 (survival of motor neuron 1, telomeric) (eg, spinal muscular atrophy), full gene sequence

SPAST (spastin) (eg, spastic paraplegia), duplication/deletion analysis

SPG7 (spastic paraplegia 7 [pure and complicated autosomal recessive]) (eg, spastic paraplegia), duplication/deletion analysis

SPRED1 (sprouty-related, EVH1 domain containing 1) (eg, Legius syndrome), full gene sequence

STAT3 (signal transducer and activator of transcription 3 [acute-phase response factor]) (eg, autosomal dominant hyper-IgE syndrome), targeted sequence analysis (eg, exons 12, 13, 14, 16, 17, 20, 21)

STK11 (serine/threonine kinase 11) (eg, Peutz-Jeghers syndrome), full gene sequence

SURF1 (surfeit 1) (eg, mitochondrial respiratory chain complex IV deficiency), full gene sequence

TARDBP (TAR DNA binding protein) (eg, amyotrophic lateral sclerosis), full gene sequence

TBX5 (T-box 5) (eg, Holt-Oram syndrome), full gene sequence

TCF4 (transcription factor 4) (eg, Pitt-Hopkins syndrome), duplication/deletion analysis

TGFBR1 (transforming growth factor, beta receptor 1) (eg, Marfan syndrome), full gene sequence

TGFBR2 (transforming growth factor, beta receptor 2) (eg, Marfan syndrome), full gene sequence

THRB (thyroid hormone receptor, beta) (eg, thyroid hormone resistance, thyroid hormone beta receptor deficiency), full gene sequence or targeted sequence analysis of >5 exons

TK2 (thymidine kinase 2, mitochondrial) (eg, mitochondrial DNA depletion syndrome), full gene sequence

TNNC1 (troponin C type 1 [slow]) (eg, hypertrophic cardiomyopathy or dilated cardiomyopathy), full gene sequence

TNNI3 (troponin I, type 3 [cardiac]) (eg, familial hypertrophic cardiomyopathy), full gene sequence

TP53 (tumor protein 53) (eg, Li-Fraumeni syndrome, tumor samples), full gene sequence or targeted sequence analysis of >5 exons

TPM1 (tropomyosin 1 [alpha]) (eg, familial hypertrophic cardiomyopathy), full gene sequence

TSC1 (tuberous sclerosis 1) (eg, tuberous sclerosis), duplication/deletion analysis

TYMP (thymidine phosphorylase) (eg, mitochondrial DNA depletion syndrome), full gene sequence

VWF (von Willebrand factor) (eg, von Willebrand disease type 2N), targeted sequence analysis (eg, exons 18-20, 23-25)

WT1 (Wilms tumor 1) (eg, Denys-Drash syndrome, familial Wilms tumor), full gene sequence

ZEB2 (zinc finger E-box binding homeobox 2) (eg, Mowat-Wilson syndrome), full gene sequence ⊘🅰

RVU			Global Days	Modifiers				
Mod	Non-Fac Total	Fac Total		51	50	62	80	MUE
	0.00	0.00	XXX	9	9	9	9	2

AMA: May 12: 4, Jul 13: 12, Sep 13: 8, 10, Jan 15: 3

▲ 81406 **Molecular pathology procedure, Level 7 (eg, analysis of 11-25 exons by DNA sequence analysis, mutation scanning or duplication/deletion variants of 26-50 exons, cytogenomic array analysis for neoplasia)**

ACADVL (acyl-CoA dehydrogenase, very long chain) (eg, very long chain acyl-coenzyme A dehydrogenase deficiency), full gene sequence

ACTN4 (actinin, alpha 4) (eg, focal segmental glomerulosclerosis), full gene sequence

AFG3L2 (AFG3 ATPase family gene 3-like 2 [S. cerevisiae]) (eg, spinocerebellar ataxia), full gene sequence

AIRE (autoimmune regulator) (eg, autoimmune polyendocrinopathy syndrome type 1), full gene sequence

ALDH7A1 (aldehyde dehydrogenase 7 family, member A1) (eg, pyridoxine-dependent epilepsy), full gene sequence

ANO5 (anoctamin 5) (eg, limb-girdle muscular dystrophy), full gene sequence

APP (amyloid beta [A4] precursor protein) (eg, Alzheimer disease), full gene sequence

ASS1 (argininosuccinate synthase 1) (eg, citrullinemia type I), full gene sequence

ATL1 (atlastin GTPase 1) (eg, spastic paraplegia), full gene sequence

ATP1A2 (ATPase, Na+/K+ transporting, alpha 2 polypeptide) (eg, familial hemiplegic migraine), full gene sequence

ATP7B (ATPase, Cu++ transporting, beta polypeptide) (eg, Wilson disease), full gene sequence

BBS1 (Bardet-Biedl syndrome 1) (eg, Bardet-Biedl syndrome), full gene sequence

BBS2 (Bardet-Biedl syndrome 2) (eg, Bardet-Biedl syndrome), full gene sequence

BCKDHB (branched-chain keto acid dehydrogenase E1, beta polypeptide) (eg, maple syrup urine disease, type 1B), full gene sequence

BEST1 (bestrophin 1) (eg, vitelliform macular dystrophy), full gene sequence

BMPR2 (bone morphogenetic protein receptor, type II [serine/threonine kinase]) (eg, heritable pulmonary arterial hypertension), full gene sequence

BRAF (v-raf murine sarcoma viral oncogene homolog B1) (eg, Noonan syndrome), full gene sequence

BSCL2 (Berardinelli-Seip congenital lipodystrophy 2 [seipin]) (eg, Berardinelli-Seip congenital lipodystrophy), full gene sequence

BTK (Bruton agammaglobulinemia tyrosine kinase) (eg, X-linked agammaglobulinemia), full gene sequence

CACNB2 (calcium channel, voltage-dependent, beta 2 subunit) (eg, Brugada syndrome), full gene sequence

CAPN3 (calpain 3) (eg, limb-girdle muscular dystrophy [LGMD] type 2A, calpainopathy), full gene sequence

CBS (cystathionine-beta-synthase) (eg, homocystinuria, cystathionine beta-synthase deficiency), full gene sequence

CDH1 (cadherin 1, type 1, E-cadherin [epithelial]) (eg, hereditary diffuse gastric cancer), full gene sequence

CDKL5 (cyclin-dependent kinase-like 5) (eg, early infantile epileptic encephalopathy), full gene sequence

CLCN1 (chloride channel 1, skeletal muscle) (eg, myotonia congenita), full gene sequence

CLCNKB (chloride channel, voltage-sensitive Kb) (eg, Bartter syndrome 3 and 4b), full gene sequence

CNTNAP2 (contactin-associated protein-like 2) (eg, Pitt-Hopkins-like syndrome 1), full gene sequence

COL6A2 (collagen, type VI, alpha 2) (eg, collagen type VI-related disorders), duplication/deletion analysis

CPT1A (carnitine palmitoyltransferase 1A [liver]) (eg, carnitine palmitoyltransferase 1A [CPT1A] deficiency), full gene sequence

CRB1 (crumbs homolog 1 [Drosophila]) (eg, Leber congenital amaurosis), full gene sequence

CREBBP (CREB binding protein) (eg, Rubinstein-Taybi syndrome), duplication/deletion analysis

● New ▲ Revised Deleted ⊙ Moderate Sedation ✚ Add-on Codes ⊘ High Risk Denial Ⓐ Age Edit ♀ Female ♂ Male AMA CPT® Assistant MUE Medically Unlikely Edit Ⓢ Modifier 51 Exempt ⊖ Modifier 63 Exempt 🅧 Unlisted Modifiers: See Inside Back Cover Ⓜ Maternity 🅰2-🅩3 ASC Payment Indicators 🅰-🅨 OPPS Status Indicators

© 2016 DecisionHealth   CPT © 2015 American Medical Association. All Rights Reserved.   703

Cytogenomic microarray analysis, neoplasia (eg, interrogation of copy number, and loss-of-heterozygosity via single nucleotide polymorphism [SNP]-based comparative genomic hybridization [CGH] microarray analysis) (Do not report analyte-specific molecular pathology procedures separately when the specific analytes are included as part of the cytogenomic microarray analysis for neoplasia) (Do not report 88271 when performing cytogenomic microarray analysis)

DBT (dihydrolipoamide branched chain transacylase E2) (eg, maple syrup urine disease, type 2), full gene sequence

DLAT (dihydrolipoamide S-acetyltransferase) (eg, pyruvate dehydrogenase E2 deficiency), full gene sequence

DLD (dihydrolipoamide dehydrogenase) (eg, maple syrup urine disease, type III), full gene sequence

DSC2 (desmocollin) (eg, arrhythmogenic right ventricular dysplasia/cardiomyopathy 11), full gene sequence

DSG2 (desmoglein 2) (eg, arrhythmogenic right ventricular dysplasia/cardiomyopathy 10), full gene sequence

DSP (desmoplakin) (eg, arrhythmogenic right ventricular dysplasia/cardiomyopathy 8), full gene sequence

EFHC1 (EF-hand domain [C-terminal] containing 1) (eg, juvenile myoclonic epilepsy), full gene sequence

EIF2B3 (eukaryotic translation initiation factor 2B, subunit 3 gamma, 58kDa) (eg, leukoencephalopathy with vanishing white matter), full gene sequence

EIF2B4 (eukaryotic translation initiation factor 2B, subunit 4 delta, 67kDa) (eg, leukoencephalopathy with vanishing white matter), full gene sequence

EIF2B5 (eukaryotic translation initiation factor 2B, subunit 5 epsilon, 82kDa) (eg, childhood ataxia with central nervous system hypomyelination/vanishing white matter), full gene sequence

ENG (endoglin) (eg, hereditary hemorrhagic telangiectasia, type 1), full gene sequence

EYA1 (eyes absent homolog 1 [Drosophila]) (eg, branchio-oto-renal [BOR] spectrum disorders), full gene sequence

F8 (coagulation factor VIII) (eg, hemophilia A), duplication/deletion analysis

FAH (fumarylacetoacetate hydrolase [fumarylacetoacetase]) (eg, tyrosinemia, type 1), full gene sequence

FASTKD2 (FAST kinase domains 2) (eg, mitochondrial respiratory chain complex IV deficiency), full gene sequence

FIG4 (FIG4 homolog, SAC1 lipid phosphatase domain containing [S. cerevisiae]) (eg, Charcot-Marie-Tooth disease), full gene sequence

FTSJ1 (FtsJ RNA methyltransferase homolog 1 [E. coli]) (eg, X-linked mental retardation 9), full gene sequence

FUS (fused in sarcoma) (eg, amyotrophic lateral sclerosis), full gene sequence

GAA (glucosidase, alpha; acid) (eg, glycogen storage disease type II [Pompe disease]), full gene sequence

GALC (galactosylceramidase) (eg, Krabbe disease), full gene sequence

GALT (galactose-1-phosphate uridylyltransferase) (eg, galactosemia), full gene sequence

GARS (glycyl-tRNA synthetase) (eg, Charcot-Marie-Tooth disease), full gene sequence

GCDH (glutaryl-CoA dehydrogenase) (eg, glutaricacidemia type 1), full gene sequence

GCK (glucokinase [hexokinase 4]) (eg, maturity-onset diabetes of the young [MODY]), full gene sequence

GLUD1 (glutamate dehydrogenase 1) (eg, familial hyperinsulinism), full gene sequence

GNE (glucosamine [UDP-N-acetyl]-2-epimerase/N-acetylmannosamine kinase) (eg, inclusion body myopathy 2 [IBM2], Nonaka myopathy), full gene sequence

GRN (granulin) (eg, frontotemporal dementia), full gene sequence

HADHA (hydroxyacyl-CoA dehydrogenase/3-ketoacyl-CoA thiolase/enoyl-CoA hydratase [trifunctional protein] alpha subunit) (eg, long chain acyl-coenzyme A dehydrogenase deficiency), full gene sequence

HADHB (hydroxyacyl-CoA dehydrogenase/3-ketoacyl-CoA thiolase/enoyl-CoA hydratase [trifunctional protein], beta subunit) (eg, trifunctional protein deficiency), full gene sequence

HEXA (hexosaminidase A, alpha polypeptide) (eg, Tay-Sachs disease), full gene sequence

HLCS (HLCS holocarboxylase synthetase) (eg, holocarboxylase synthetase deficiency), full gene sequence

HNF4A (hepatocyte nuclear factor 4, alpha) (eg, maturity-onset diabetes of the young [MODY]), full gene sequence

IDUA (iduronidase, alpha-L-) (eg, mucopolysaccharidosis type I), full gene sequence

INF2 (inverted formin, FH2 and WH2 domain containing) (eg, focal segmental glomerulosclerosis), full gene sequence

IVD (isovaleryl-CoA dehydrogenase) (eg, isovaleric acidemia), full gene sequence

JAG1 (jagged 1) (eg, Alagille syndrome), duplication/deletion analysis

JUP (junction plakoglobin) (eg, arrhythmogenic right ventricular dysplasia/cardiomyopathy 11), full gene sequence

KAL1 (Kallmann syndrome 1 sequence) (eg, Kallmann syndrome), full gene sequence

● New   ▲ Revised   ✖ Deleted   ⊙ Moderate Sedation   ✚ Add-on Codes   ⊘ High Risk Denial   Ⓐ Age Edit   ♀ Female   ♂ Male   **AMA** *CPT® Assistant*   **MUE** Medically Unlikely Edit
⊘ Modifier 51 Exempt   ⊖ Modifier 63 Exempt   ✗ Unlisted   **Modifiers:** *See Inside Back Cover*   Ⓜ Maternity   A 2 – Z 3 ASC Payment Indicators   A – Y OPPS Status Indicators

704   CPT © 2015 American Medical Association. All Rights Reserved.   © 2016 DecisionHealth

KCNH2 (potassium voltage-gated channel, subfamily H [eag-related], member 2) (eg, short QT syndrome, long QT syndrome), full gene sequence (Do not report 81406 for KCNH2 full gene sequence in conjunction with 81280)

KCNQ1 (potassium voltage-gated channel, KQT-like subfamily, member 1) (eg, short QT syndrome, long QT syndrome), full gene sequence (Do not report 81406 for KCNQ1 full gene sequence with 81280)

KCNQ2 (potassium voltage-gated channel, KQT-like subfamily, member 2) (eg, epileptic encephalopathy), full gene sequence LDB3 (LIM domain binding 3) (eg, familial dilated cardiomyopathy, myofibrillar myopathy), full gene sequence

LDLR (low density lipoprotein receptor) (eg, familial hypercholesterolemia), full gene sequence

LEPR (leptin receptor) (eg, obesity with hypogonadism), full gene sequence

LHCGR (luteinizing hormone/choriogonadotropin receptor) (eg, precocious male puberty), full gene sequence

LMNA (lamin A/C) (eg, Emery-Dreifuss muscular dystrophy [EDMD1, 2 and 3] limb-girdle muscular dystrophy [LGMD] type 1B, dilated cardiomyopathy [CMD1A], familial partial lipodystrophy [FPLD2]), full gene sequence

LRP5 (low density lipoprotein receptor-related protein 5) (eg, osteopetrosis), full gene sequence MAP2K1 (mitogen-activated protein kinase 1) (eg, cardiofaciocutaneous syndrome), full gene sequence

MAP2K2 (mitogen-activated protein kinase 2) (eg, cardiofaciocutaneous syndrome), full gene sequence

MAPT (microtubule-associated protein tau) (eg, frontotemporal dementia), full gene sequence

MCCC1 (methylcrotonoyl-CoA carboxylase 1 [alpha]) (eg, 3-methylcrotonyl-CoA carboxylase deficiency), full gene sequence

MCCC2 (methylcrotonoyl-CoA carboxylase 2 [beta]) (eg, 3-methylcrotonyl carboxylase deficiency), full gene sequence

MFN2 (mitofusin 2) (eg, Charcot-Marie-Tooth disease), full gene sequence

MTM1 (myotubularin 1) (eg, X-linked centronuclear myopathy), full gene sequence

MUT (methylmalonyl CoA mutase) (eg, methylmalonic acidemia), full gene sequence

MUTYH (mutY homolog [E. coli]) (eg, MYH-associated polyposis), full gene sequence

NDUFS1 (NADH dehydrogenase [ubiquinone] Fe-S protein 1, 75kDa [NADH-coenzyme Q reductase]) (eg, Leigh syndrome, mitochondrial complex I deficiency), full gene sequence

NF2 (neurofibromin 2 [merlin]) (eg, neurofibromatosis, type 2), full gene sequence

NOTCH3 (notch 3) (eg, cerebral autosomal dominant arteriopathy with subcortical infarcts and leukoencephalopathy [CADASIL]), targeted sequence analysis (eg, exons 1-23)

NPC1 (Niemann-Pick disease, type C1) (eg, Niemann-Pick disease), full gene sequence

NPHP1 (nephronophthisis 1 [juvenile]) (eg, Joubert syndrome), full gene sequence

NSD1 (nuclear receptor binding SET domain protein 1) (eg, Sotos syndrome), full gene sequence

OPA1 (optic atrophy 1) (eg, optic atrophy), duplication/deletion analysis OPTN (optineurin) (eg, amyotrophic lateral sclerosis), full gene sequence

PAFAH1B1 (platelet-activating factor acetylhydrolase 1b, regulatory subunit 1 [45kDa]) (eg, lissencephaly, Miller-Dieker syndrome), full gene sequence

PAH (phenylalanine hydroxylase) (eg, phenylketonuria), full gene sequence

PALB2 (partner and localizer of BRCA2) (eg, breast and pancreatic cancer), full gene sequence

PARK2 (Parkinson protein 2, E3 ubiquitin protein ligase [parkin]) (eg, Parkinson disease), full gene sequence

PAX2 (paired box 2) (eg, renal coloboma syndrome), full gene sequence

PC (pyruvate carboxylase) (eg, pyruvate carboxylase deficiency), full gene sequence

PCCA (propionyl CoA carboxylase, alpha polypeptide) (eg, propionic acidemia, type 1), full gene sequence

PCCB (propionyl CoA carboxylase, beta polypeptide) (eg, propionic acidemia), full gene sequence

PCDH15 (protocadherin-related 15) (eg, Usher syndrome type 1F), duplication/deletion analysis

PDHA1 (pyruvate dehydrogenase [lipoamide] alpha 1) (eg, lactic acidosis), full gene sequence

PDHX (pyruvate dehydrogenase complex, component X) (eg, lactic acidosis), full gene sequence

PHEX (phosphate-regulating endopeptidase homolog, X-linked) (eg, hypophosphatemic rickets), full gene sequence

PKD2 (polycystic kidney disease 2 [autosomal dominant]) (eg, polycystic kidney disease), full gene sequence

PKP2 (plakophilin 2) (eg, arrhythmogenic right ventricular dysplasia/cardiomyopathy 9), full gene sequence

PNKD (eg, paroxysmal nonkinesigenic dyskinesia) (eg, paroxysmal nonkinesigenic dyskinesia), full gene sequence

POLG (polymerase [DNA directed], gamma) (eg, Alpers-Huttenlocher syndrome, autosomal dominant progressive external ophthalmoplegia), full gene sequence

---

● New   ▲ Revised   Deleted   ⊙ Moderate Sedation   ✚ Add-on Codes   ⊘ High Risk Denial   Ⓐ Age Edit   ♀ Female   ♂ Male   **AMA** CPT® Assistant   **MUE** Medically Unlikely Edit
⊘ Modifier 51 Exempt   ⊖ Modifier 63 Exempt   ✗ Unlisted   **Modifiers:** See Inside Back Cover   Ⓜ Maternity   A2–Z3 ASC Payment Indicators   A–Y OPPS Status Indicators

© 2016 DecisionHealth   CPT © 2015 American Medical Association. All Rights Reserved.   **705**

POMGNT1 (protein O-linked mannose beta1,2-N acetylglucosaminyltransferase) (eg, muscle-eye-brain disease, Walker-Warburg syndrome), full gene sequence

POMT1 (protein-O-mannosyltransferase 1) (eg, limb-girdle muscular dystrophy [LGMD] type 2K, Walker-Warburg syndrome), full gene sequence

POMT2 (protein-O-mannosyltransferase 2) (eg, limb-girdle muscular dystrophy [LGMD] type 2N, Walker-Warburg syndrome), full gene sequence

PRKAG2 (protein kinase, AMP-activated, gamma 2 non-catalytic subunit) (eg, familial hypertrophic cardiomyopathy with Wolff-Parkinson-White syndrome, lethal congenital glycogen storage disease of heart), full gene sequence

PRKCG (protein kinase C, gamma) (eg, spinocerebellar ataxia), full gene sequence

PSEN2 (presenilin 2 [Alzheimer disease 4]) (eg, Alzheimer disease), full gene sequence

PTPN11 (protein tyrosine phosphatase, non-receptor type 11) (eg, Noonan syndrome, LEOPARD syndrome), full gene sequence

PYGM (phosphorylase, glycogen, muscle) (eg, glycogen storage disease type V, McArdle disease), full gene sequence

RAF1 (v-raf-1 murine leukemia viral oncogene homolog 1) (eg, LEOPARD syndrome), full gene sequence

RET (ret proto-oncogene) (eg, Hirschsprung disease), full gene sequence

RPE65 (retinal pigment epithelium-specific protein 65kDa) (eg, retinitis pigmentosa, Leber congenital amaurosis), full gene sequence

RYR1 (ryanodine receptor 1, skeletal) (eg, malignant hyperthermia), targeted sequence analysis of exons with functionally-confirmed mutations

SCN4A (sodium channel, voltage-gated, type IV, alpha subunit) (eg, hyperkalemic periodic paralysis), full gene sequence

SCNN1A (sodium channel, nonvoltage-gated 1 alpha) (eg, pseudohypoaldosteronism), full gene sequence

SCNN1B (sodium channel, nonvoltage-gated 1, beta) (eg, Liddle syndrome, pseudohypoaldosteronism), full gene sequence

SCNN1G (sodium channel, nonvoltage-gated 1, gamma) (eg, Liddle syndrome, pseudohypoaldosteronism), full gene sequence

SDHA (succinate dehydrogenase complex, subunit A, flavoprotein [Fp]) (eg, Leigh syndrome, mitochondrial complex II deficiency), full gene sequence

SETX (senataxin) (eg, ataxia), full gene sequence

SGCE (sarcoglycan, epsilon) (eg, myoclonic dystonia), full gene sequence

SH3TC2 (SH3 domain and tetratricopeptide repeats 2) (eg, Charcot-Marie-Tooth disease), full gene sequence

SLC9A6 (solute carrier family 9 [sodium/hydrogen exchanger], member 6) (eg, Christianson syndrome), full gene sequence

SLC26A4 (solute carrier family 26, member 4) (eg, Pendred syndrome), full gene sequence

SLC37A4 (solute carrier family 37 [glucose-6-phosphate transporter], member 4) (eg, glycogen storage disease type Ib), full gene sequence

SMAD4 (SMAD family member 4) (eg, hemorrhagic telangiectasia syndrome, juvenile polyposis), full gene sequence

SOS1 (son of sevenless homolog 1) (eg, Noonan syndrome, gingival fibromatosis), full gene sequence

SPAST (spastin) (eg, spastic paraplegia), full gene sequence

SPG7 (spastic paraplegia 7 [pure and complicated autosomal recessive]) (eg, spastic paraplegia), full gene sequence

STXBP1 (syntaxin-binding protein 1) (eg, epileptic encephalopathy), full gene sequence

TAZ (tafazzin) (eg, methylglutaconic aciduria type 2, Barth syndrome), full gene sequence

TCF4 (transcription factor 4) (eg, Pitt-Hopkins syndrome), full gene sequence

TH (tyrosine hydroxylase) (eg, Segawa syndrome), full gene sequence

TMEM43 (transmembrane protein 43) (eg, arrhythmogenic right ventricular cardiomyopathy), full gene sequence

TNNT2 (troponin T, type 2 [cardiac]) (eg, familial hypertrophic cardiomyopathy), full gene sequence

TRPC6 (transient receptor potential cation channel, subfamily C, member 6) (eg, focal segmental glomerulosclerosis), full gene sequence

TSC1 (tuberous sclerosis 1) (eg, tuberous sclerosis), full gene sequence

TSC2 (tuberous sclerosis 2) (eg, tuberous sclerosis), duplication/deletion analysis

UBE3A (ubiquitin protein ligase E3A) (eg, Angelman syndrome), full gene sequence

UMOD (uromodulin) (eg, glomerulocystic kidney disease with hyperuricemia and isosthenuria), full gene sequence

VWF (von Willebrand factor) (von Willebrand disease type 2A), extended targeted sequence analysis (eg, exons 11-16, 24-26, 51, 52)

WAS (Wiskott-Aldrich syndrome [eczema-thrombocytopenia]) (eg, Wiskott-Aldrich syndrome), full gene sequence ⊗🅰

RVU			Global Days	Modifiers				
Mod	Non-Fac Total	Fac Total			51	50	62	80	MUE
	0.00	0.00	XXX		9	9	9	9	2

AMA: May 12: 4, Jul 13: 12, Sep 13: 5, 6, 8, 11, Jan 15: 3

● New   ▲ Revised   ✖ Deleted   ⊙ Moderate Sedation   ✚ Add-on Codes   ⊘ High Risk Denial   Ⓐ Age Edit   ♀ Female   ♂ Male   **AMA** CPT® Assistant   **MUE** Medically Unlikely Edit
⊘ Modifier 51 Exempt   ⊖ Modifier 63 Exempt   🗵 Unlisted   **Modifiers:** See Inside Back Cover   Ⓜ Maternity   🄰2–🅉3 ASC Payment Indicators   🅰–Ⓨ OPPS Status Indicators

81407 **Molecular pathology procedure, Level 8 (eg, analysis of 26-50 exons by DNA sequence analysis, mutation scanning or duplication/deletion variants of >50 exons, sequence analysis of multiple genes on one platform)**

ABCC8 (ATP-binding cassette, sub-family C [CFTR/MRP], member 8) (eg, familial hyperinsulinism), full gene sequence

AGL (amylo-alpha-1, 6-glucosidase, 4-alpha-glucanotransferase) (eg, glycogen storage disease type III), full gene sequence

AHI1 (Abelson helper integration site 1) (eg, Joubert syndrome), full gene sequence

ASPM (asp [abnormal spindle] homolog, microcephaly associated [Drosophila]) (eg, primary microcephaly), full gene sequence

CACNA1A (calcium channel, voltage-dependent, P/Q type, alpha 1A subunit) (eg, familial hemiplegic migraine), full gene sequence

CHD7 (chromodomain helicase DNA binding protein 7) (eg, CHARGE syndrome), full gene sequence

COL4A4 (collagen, type IV, alpha 4) (eg, Alport syndrome), full gene sequence

COL4A5 (collagen, type IV, alpha 5) (eg, Alport syndrome), duplication/deletion analysis

COL6A1 (collagen, type VI, alpha 1) (eg, collagen type VI-related disorders), full gene sequence

COL6A2 (collagen, type VI, alpha 2) (eg, collagen type VI-related disorders), full gene sequence

COL6A3 (collagen, type VI, alpha 3) (eg, collagen type VI-related disorders), full gene sequence

CREBBP (CREB binding protein) (eg, Rubinstein-Taybi syndrome), full gene sequence

F8 (coagulation factor VIII) (eg, hemophilia A), full gene sequence

JAG1 (jagged 1) (eg, Alagille syndrome), full gene sequence

KDM5C (lysine [K]-specific demethylase 5C) (eg, X-linked mental retardation), full gene sequence

KIAA0196 (KIAA0196) (eg, spastic paraplegia), full gene sequence

L1CAM (L1 cell adhesion molecule) (eg, MASA syndrome, X-linked hydrocephaly), full gene sequence

LAMB2 (laminin, beta 2 [laminin S]) (eg, Pierson syndrome), full gene sequence

MYBPC3 (myosin binding protein C, cardiac) (eg, familial hypertrophic cardiomyopathy), full gene sequence

MYH6 (myosin, heavy chain 6, cardiac muscle, alpha) (eg, familial dilated cardiomyopathy), full gene sequence

MYH7 (myosin, heavy chain 7, cardiac muscle, beta) (eg, familial hypertrophic cardiomyopathy, Liang distal myopathy), full gene sequence

MYO7A (myosin VIIA) (eg, Usher syndrome, type 1), full gene sequence

NOTCH1 (notch 1) (eg, aortic valve disease), full gene sequence

NPHS1 (nephrosis 1, congenital, Finnish type [nephrin]) (eg, congenital Finnish nephrosis), full gene sequence

OPA1 (optic atrophy 1) (eg, optic atrophy), full gene sequence

PCDH15 (protocadherin-related 15) (eg, Usher syndrome, type 1), full gene sequence

PKD1 (polycystic kidney disease 1 [autosomal dominant]) (eg, polycystic kidney disease), full gene sequence

PLCE1 (phospholipase C, epsilon 1) (eg, nephrotic syndrome type 3), full gene sequence

SCN1A (sodium channel, voltage-gated, type 1, alpha subunit) (eg, generalized epilepsy with febrile seizures), full gene sequence

SCN5A (sodium channel, voltage-gated, type V, alpha subunit) (eg, familial dilated cardiomyopathy), full gene sequence

SLC12A1 (solute carrier family 12 [sodium/potassium/chloride transporters], member 1) (eg, Bartter syndrome), full gene sequence

SLC12A3 (solute carrier family 12 [sodium/chloride transporters], member 3) (eg, Gitelman syndrome), full gene sequence

SPG11 (spastic paraplegia 11 [autosomal recessive]) (eg, spastic paraplegia), full gene sequence

SPTBN2 (spectrin, beta, non-erythrocytic 2) (eg, spinocerebellar ataxia), full gene sequence

TMEM67 (transmembrane protein 67) (eg, Joubert syndrome), full gene sequence

TSC2 (tuberous sclerosis 2) (eg, tuberous sclerosis), full gene sequence

USH1C (Usher syndrome 1C [autosomal recessive, severe]) (eg, Usher syndrome, type 1), full gene sequence

VPS13B (vacuolar protein sorting 13 homolog B [yeast]) (eg, Cohen syndrome), duplication/deletion analysis

WDR62 (WD repeat domain 62) (eg, primary autosomal recessive microcephaly), full gene sequence ⊙🅐

RVU			Global Days	Modifiers				
Mod	Non-Fac Total	Fac Total		51	50	62	80	MUE
	0.00	0.00	XXX	9	9	9	9	1

AMA: May 12: 4, Jul 13: 12, Sep 13: 14, Jan 15: 3

© 2016 DecisionHealth   CPT © 2015 American Medical Association. All Rights Reserved.   **707**

81408 Molecular pathology procedure, Level 9 (eg, analysis of >50 exons in a single gene by DNA sequence analysis)

ABCA4 (ATP-binding cassette, sub-family A [ABC1], member 4) (eg, Stargardt disease, age-related macular degeneration), full gene sequence

ATM (ataxia telangiectasia mutated) (eg, ataxia telangiectasia), full gene sequence

CDH23 (cadherin-related 23) (eg, Usher syndrome, type 1), full gene sequence

CEP290 (centrosomal protein 290kDa) (eg, Joubert syndrome), full gene sequence

COL1A1 (collagen, type I, alpha 1) (eg, osteogenesis imperfecta, type I), full gene sequence

COL1A2 (collagen, type I, alpha 2) (eg, osteogenesis imperfecta, type I), full gene sequence

COL4A1 (collagen, type IV, alpha 1) (eg, brain small-vessel disease with hemorrhage), full gene sequence

COL4A3 (collagen, type IV, alpha 3 [Goodpasture antigen]) (eg, Alport syndrome), full gene sequence

COL4A5 (collagen, type IV, alpha 5) (eg, Alport syndrome), full gene sequence

DMD (dystrophin) (eg, Duchenne/Becker muscular dystrophy), full gene sequence

DYSF (dysferlin, limb girdle muscular dystrophy 2B [autosomal recessive]) (eg, limb-girdle muscular dystrophy), full gene sequence

FBN1 (fibrillin 1) (eg, Marfan syndrome), full gene sequence

ITPR1 (inositol 1,4,5-trisphosphate receptor, type 1) (eg, spinocerebellar ataxia), full gene sequence

LAMA2 (laminin, alpha 2) (eg, congenital muscular dystrophy), full gene sequence

LRRK2 (leucine-rich repeat kinase 2) (eg, Parkinson disease), full gene sequence

MYH11 (myosin, heavy chain 11, smooth muscle) (eg, thoracic aortic aneurysms and aortic dissections), full gene sequence

NEB (nebulin) (eg, nemaline myopathy 2), full gene sequence

NF1 (neurofibromin 1) (eg, neurofibromatosis, type 1), full gene sequence

PKHD1 (polycystic kidney and hepatic disease 1) (eg, autosomal recessive polycystic kidney disease), full gene sequence

RYR1 (ryanodine receptor 1, skeletal) (eg, malignant hyperthermia), full gene sequence

RYR2 (ryanodine receptor 2 [cardiac]) (eg, catecholaminergic polymorphic ventricular tachycardia, arrhythmogenic right ventricular dysplasia), full gene sequence or targeted sequence analysis of > 50 exons

USH2A (Usher syndrome 2A [autosomal recessive, mild]) (eg, Usher syndrome, type 2), full gene sequence

VPS13B (vacuolar protein sorting 13 homolog B [yeast]) (eg, Cohen syndrome), full gene sequence

VWF (von Willebrand factor) (eg, von Willebrand disease types 1 and 3), full gene sequence ⊘🅰

RVU			Global Days	Modifiers				
Mod	Non-Fac Total	Fac Total		51	50	62	80	MUE
	0.00	0.00	XXX	9	9	9	9	2

AMA: May 12: 4, Jul 13: 12, Sep 13: 4, 5, 14, Jan 15: 3

81410 Aortic dysfunction or dilation (eg, Marfan syndrome, Loeys Dietz syndrome, Ehler Danlos syndrome type IV, arterial tortuosity syndrome); genomic sequence analysis panel, must include sequencing of at least 9 genes, including FBN1, TGFBR1, TGFBR2, COL3A1, MYH11, ACTA2, SLC2A10, SMAD3, and MYLK 🅰

RVU			Global Days	Modifiers				
Mod	Non-Fac Total	Fac Total		51	50	62	80	MUE
	0.00	0.00	XXX	9	9	9	9	1

AMA: Jan 15: 3

81411 Aortic dysfunction or dilation (eg, Marfan syndrome, Loeys Dietz syndrome, Ehler Danlos syndrome type IV, arterial tortuosity syndrome); duplication/deletion analysis panel, must include analyses for TGFBR1, TGFBR2, MYH11, and COL3A1 🅰

RVU			Global Days	Modifiers				
Mod	Non-Fac Total	Fac Total		51	50	62	80	MUE
	0.00	0.00	XXX	9	9	9	9	1

● **81412 Ashkenazi Jewish associated disorders (eg, Bloom syndrome, Canavan disease, cystic fibrosis, familial dysautonomia, Fanconi anemia group C, Gaucher disease, Tay-Sachs disease), genomic sequence analysis panel, must include sequencing of at least 9 genes, including ASPA, BLM, CFTR, FANCC, GBA, HEXA, IKBKAP, MCOLN1, and SMPD1** 🅰

RVU			Global Days	Modifiers				
Mod	Non-Fac Total	Fac Total		51	50	62	80	MUE
	0.00	0.00	XXX	9	9	9	9	1

81415 Exome (eg, unexplained constitutional or heritable disorder or syndrome); sequence analysis 🅰

RVU			Global Days	Modifiers				
Mod	Non-Fac Total	Fac Total		51	50	62	80	MUE
	0.00	0.00	XXX	9	9	9	9	1

AMA: Jan 15: 3

✚ **81416 Exome (eg, unexplained constitutional or heritable disorder or syndrome); sequence analysis, each comparator exome (eg, parents, siblings) (List separately in addition to code for primary procedure)** 🅰

RVU			Global Days	Modifiers				
Mod	Non-Fac Total	Fac Total		51	50	62	80	MUE
	0.00	0.00	XXX	9	9	9	9	2

AMA: Jan 15: 3

CPT © 2015 American Medical Association. All Rights Reserved.   © 2016 DecisionHealth

81417 Exome (eg, unexplained constitutional or heritable disorder or syndrome); re-evaluation of previously obtained exome sequence (eg, updated knowledge or unrelated condition/syndrome) Ⓐ

Mod	Non-Fac Total	Fac Total	Global Days	51	50	62	80	MUE
	0.00	0.00	XXX	9	9	9	9	1

81420 Fetal chromosomal aneuploidy (eg, trisomy 21, monosomy X) genomic sequence analysis panel, circulating cell-free fetal DNA in maternal blood, must include analysis of chromosomes 13, 18, and 21 Ⓐ

Mod	Non-Fac Total	Fac Total	Global Days	51	50	62	80	MUE
	0.00	0.00	XXX	9	9	9	9	1

AMA: Jan 15: 3

81425 Genome (eg, unexplained constitutional or heritable disorder or syndrome); sequence analysis Ⓐ

Mod	Non-Fac Total	Fac Total	Global Days	51	50	62	80	MUE
	0.00	0.00	XXX	9	9	9	9	1

+ 81426 Genome (eg, unexplained constitutional or heritable disorder or syndrome); sequence analysis, each comparator genome (eg, parents, siblings) (List separately in addition to code for primary procedure) Ⓐ

Mod	Non-Fac Total	Fac Total	Global Days	51	50	62	80	MUE
	0.00	0.00	XXX	9	9	9	9	2

AMA: Jan 15: 3

81427 Genome (eg, unexplained constitutional or heritable disorder or syndrome); re-evaluation of previously obtained genome sequence (eg, updated knowledge or unrelated condition/syndrome) Ⓐ

Mod	Non-Fac Total	Fac Total	Global Days	51	50	62	80	MUE
	0.00	0.00	XXX	9	9	9	9	1

AMA: Jan 15: 3

81430 Hearing loss (eg, nonsyndromic hearing loss, Usher syndrome, Pendred syndrome); genomic sequence analysis panel, must include sequencing of at least 60 genes, including CDH23, CLRN1, GJB2, GPR98, MTRNR1, MYO7A, MYO15A, PCDH15, OTOF, SLC26A4, TMC1, TMPRSS3, USH1C, USH1G, USH2A, and WFS1 Ⓐ

Mod	Non-Fac Total	Fac Total	Global Days	51	50	62	80	MUE
	0.00	0.00	XXX	9	9	9	9	1

81431 Hearing loss (eg, nonsyndromic hearing loss, Usher syndrome, Pendred syndrome); duplication/deletion analysis panel, must include copy number analyses for STRC and DFNB1 deletions in GJB2 and GJB6 genes Ⓐ

Mod	Non-Fac Total	Fac Total	Global Days	51	50	62	80	MUE
	0.00	0.00	XXX	9	9	9	9	1

81432 Hereditary breast cancer-related disorders (eg, hereditary breast cancer, hereditary ovarian cancer, hereditary endometrial cancer); genomic sequence analysis panel, must include sequencing of at least 14 genes, including ATM, BRCA1, BRCA2, BRIP1, CDH1, MLH1, MSH2, MSH6, NBN, PALB2, PTEN, RAD51C, STK11, and TP53 Ⓐ

Mod	Non-Fac Total	Fac Total	Global Days	51	50	62	80	MUE
	0.00	0.00	XXX	9	9	9	9	1

81433 Hereditary breast cancer-related disorders (eg, hereditary breast cancer, hereditary ovarian cancer, hereditary endometrial cancer); duplication/deletion analysis panel, must include analyses for BRCA1, BRCA2, MLH1, MSH2, and STK11 Ⓐ

Mod	Non-Fac Total	Fac Total	Global Days	51	50	62	80	MUE
	0.00	0.00	XXX	9	9	9	9	1

81434 Hereditary retinal disorders (eg, retinitis pigmentosa, Leber congenital amaurosis, cone-rod dystrophy), genomic sequence analysis panel, must include sequencing of at least 15 genes, including ABCA4, CNGA1, CRB1, EYS, PDE6A, PDE6B, PRPF31, PRPH2, RDH12, RHO, RP1, RP2, RPE65, RPGR, and USH2A Ⓐ

Mod	Non-Fac Total	Fac Total	Global Days	51	50	62	80	MUE
	0.00	0.00	XXX	9	9	9	9	1

▲ 81435 Hereditary colon cancer disorders (eg, Lynch syndrome, PTEN hamartoma syndrome, Cowden syndrome, familial adenomatosis polyposis); genomic sequence analysis panel, must include sequencing of at least 10 genes, including APC, BMPR1A, CDH1, MLH1, MSH2, MSH6, MUTYH, PTEN, SMAD4, and STK11 Ⓐ

Mod	Non-Fac Total	Fac Total	Global Days	51	50	62	80	MUE
	0.00	0.00	XXX	9	9	9	9	1

AMA: Jan 15: 3

▲ 81436 Hereditary colon cancer disorders (eg, Lynch syndrome, PTEN hamartoma syndrome, Cowden syndrome, familial adenomatosis polyposis); duplication/deletion analysis panel, must include analysis of at least 5 genes, including MLH1, MSH2, EPCAM, SMAD4, and STK11 Ⓐ

Mod	Non-Fac Total	Fac Total	Global Days	51	50	62	80	MUE
	0.00	0.00	XXX	9	9	9	9	1

● New ▲ Revised Deleted ⊙ Moderate Sedation ✚ Add-on Codes ⊘ High Risk Denial Ⓐ Age Edit ♀ Female ♂ Male **AMA** *CPT® Assistant* **MUE** Medically Unlikely Edit
⊘ Modifier 51 Exempt ⊖ Modifier 63 Exempt Ⓧ Unlisted **Modifiers:** *See Inside Back Cover* Ⓜ Maternity A2–Z3 ASC Payment Indicators Ⓐ–Ⓨ OPPS Status Indicators

© 2016 DecisionHealth — CPT © 2015 American Medical Association. All Rights Reserved. — **709**

● **81437** Hereditary neuroendocrine tumor disorders (eg, medullary thyroid carcinoma, parathyroid carcinoma, malignant pheochromocytoma or paraganglioma); genomic sequence analysis panel, must include sequencing of at least 6 genes, including MAX, SDHB, SDHC, SDHD, TMEM127, and VHL 🅰

RVU			Global Days	Modifiers				
Mod	Non-Fac Total	Fac Total		51	50	62	80	MUE
	0.00	0.00	XXX	9	9	9	9	1

● **81438** Hereditary neuroendocrine tumor disorders (eg, medullary thyroid carcinoma, parathyroid carcinoma, malignant pheochromocytoma or paraganglioma); duplication/deletion analysis panel, must include analyses for SDHB, SDHC, SDHD, and VHL 🅰

RVU			Global Days	Modifiers				
Mod	Non-Fac Total	Fac Total		51	50	62	80	MUE
	0.00	0.00	XXX	9	9	9	9	1

81440 Nuclear encoded mitochondrial genes (eg, neurologic or myopathic phenotypes), genomic sequence panel, must include analysis of at least 100 genes, including BCS1L, C10orf2, COQ2, COX10, DGUOK, MPV17, OPA1, PDSS2, POLG, POLG2, RRM2B, SCO1, SCO2, SLC25A4, SUCLA2, SUCLG1, TAZ, TK2, and TYMP 🅰

RVU			Global Days	Modifiers				
Mod	Non-Fac Total	Fac Total		51	50	62	80	MUE
	0.00	0.00	XXX	9	9	9	9	1

AMA: Jan 15: 3

● **81442** Noonan spectrum disorders (eg, Noonan syndrome, cardio-facio-cutaneous syndrome, Costello syndrome, LEOPARD syndrome, Noonan-like syndrome), genomic sequence analysis panel, must include sequencing of at least 12 genes, including BRAF, CBL, HRAS, KRAS, MAP2K1, MAP2K2, NRAS, PTPN11, RAF1, RIT1, SHOC2, and SOS1 🅰

RVU			Global Days	Modifiers				
Mod	Non-Fac Total	Fac Total		51	50	62	80	MUE
	0.00	0.00	XXX	9	9	9	9	1

▲ **81445** Targeted genomic sequence analysis panel, solid organ neoplasm, DNA analysis, and RNA analysis when performed, 5-50 genes (eg, ALK, BRAF, CDKN2A, EGFR, ERBB2, KIT, KRAS, NRAS, MET, PDGFRA, PDGFRB, PGR, PIK3CA, PTEN, RET), interrogation for sequence variants and copy number variants or rearrangements, if performed 🅰

RVU			Global Days	Modifiers				
Mod	Non-Fac Total	Fac Total		51	50	62	80	MUE
	0.00	0.00	XXX	9	9	9	9	1

AMA: Jan 15: 3

▲ **81450** Targeted genomic sequence analysis panel, hematolymphoid neoplasm or disorder, DNA analysis, and RNA analysis when performed, 5-50 genes (eg, BRAF, CEBPA, DNMT3A, EZH2, FLT3, IDH1, IDH2, JAK2, KRAS, KIT, MLL, NRAS, NPM1, NOTCH1), interrogation for sequence variants, and copy number variants or rearrangements, or isoform expression or mRNA expression levels, if performed 🅰

RVU			Global Days	Modifiers				
Mod	Non-Fac Total	Fac Total		51	50	62	80	MUE
	0.00	0.00	XXX	9	9	9	9	1

▲ **81455** Targeted genomic sequence analysis panel, solid organ or hematolymphoid neoplasm, DNA analysis, and RNA analysis when performed, 51 or greater genes (eg, ALK, BRAF, CDKN2A, CEBPA, DNMT3A, EGFR, ERBB2, EZH2, FLT3, IDH1, IDH2, JAK2, KIT, KRAS, MLL, NPM1, NRAS, MET, NOTCH1, PDGFRA, PDGFRB, PGR, PIK3CA, PTEN, RET), interrogation for sequence variants and copy number variants or rearrangements, if performed 🅰

RVU			Global Days	Modifiers				
Mod	Non-Fac Total	Fac Total		51	50	62	80	MUE
	0.00	0.00	XXX	9	9	9	9	1

81460 Whole mitochondrial genome (eg, Leigh syndrome, mitochondrial encephalomyopathy, lactic acidosis, and stroke-like episodes [MELAS], myoclonic epilepsy with ragged-red fibers [MERFF], neuropathy, ataxia, and retinitis pigmentosa [NARP], Leber hereditary optic neuropathy [LHON]), genomic sequence, must include sequence analysis of entire mitochondrial genome with heteroplasmy detection 🅰

RVU			Global Days	Modifiers				
Mod	Non-Fac Total	Fac Total		51	50	62	80	MUE
	0.00	0.00	XXX	9	9	9	9	1

81465 Whole mitochondrial genome large deletion analysis panel (eg, Kearns-Sayre syndrome, chronic progressive external ophthalmoplegia), including heteroplasmy detection, if performed 🅰

RVU			Global Days	Modifiers				
Mod	Non-Fac Total	Fac Total		51	50	62	80	MUE
	0.00	0.00	XXX	9	9	9	9	1

AMA: Jan 15: 3

81470 X-linked intellectual disability (XLID) (eg, syndromic and non-syndromic XLID); genomic sequence analysis panel, must include sequencing of at least 60 genes, including ARX, ATRX, CDKL5, FGD1, FMR1, HUWE1, IL1RAPL, KDM5C, L1CAM, MECP2, MED12, MID1, OCRL, RPS6KA3, and SLC16A2 🅰

RVU			Global Days	Modifiers				
Mod	Non-Fac Total	Fac Total		51	50	62	80	MUE
	0.00	0.00	XXX	9	9	9	9	1

● New   ▲ Revised   ✖ Deleted   ⊙ Moderate Sedation   ✚ Add-on Codes   ⊗ High Risk Denial   Ⓐ Age Edit   ♀ Female   ♂ Male   **AMA** CPT® Assistant   **MUE** Medically Unlikely Edit
⊘ Modifier 51 Exempt   ⊖ Modifier 63 Exempt   ⊠ Unlisted   **Modifiers:** See Inside Back Cover   Ⓜ Maternity   🅰2–🆉3 ASC Payment Indicators   🅰–🆈 OPPS Status Indicators

CPT © 2015 American Medical Association. All Rights Reserved.   © 2016 DecisionHealth

81471 X-linked intellectual disability (XLID) (eg, syndromic and non-syndromic XLID); duplication/deletion gene analysis, must include analysis of at least 60 genes, including ARX, ATRX, CDKL5, FGD1, FMR1, HUWE1, IL1RAPL, KDM5C, L1CAM, MECP2, MED12, MID1, OCRL, RPS6KA3, and SLC16A2　　🅐

RVU			Global Days	Modifiers				
Mod	Non-Fac Total	Fac Total		51	50	62	80	MUE
	0.00	0.00	XXX	9	9	9	9	1

81479 Unlisted molecular pathology procedure　　⊘🅧🅐

RVU			Global Days	Modifiers				
Mod	Non-Fac Total	Fac Total		51	50	62	80	MUE
	0.00	0.00	XXX	9	9	9	9	

AMA: Jul 13: 12, Sep 13: 4, 8, Jan 15: 3

● **81490** Autoimmune (rheumatoid arthritis), analysis of 12 biomarkers using immunoassays, utilizing serum, prognostic algorithm reported as a disease activity score　　🅠4

RVU			Global Days	Modifiers				
Mod	Non-Fac Total	Fac Total		51	50	62	80	MUE
	0.00	0.00	XXX	9	9	9	9	1

● **81493** Coronary artery disease, mRNA, gene expression profiling by real-time RT-PCR of 23 genes, utilizing whole peripheral blood, algorithm reported as a risk score　　🅐

RVU			Global Days	Modifiers				
Mod	Non-Fac Total	Fac Total		51	50	62	80	MUE
	0.00	0.00	XXX	9	9	9	9	1

Multianalyte Assays with Algorithmic Analyses

81500 Oncology (ovarian), biochemical assays of two proteins (CA-125 and HE4), utilizing serum, with menopausal status, algorithm reported as a risk score　　♀🅔

RVU			Global Days	Modifiers				
Mod	Non-Fac Total	Fac Total		51	50	62	80	MUE
	0.00	0.00	XXX	9	9	9	9	1

81503 Oncology (ovarian), biochemical assays of five proteins (CA-125, apolipoprotein A1, beta-2 microglobulin, transferrin, and pre-albumin), utilizing serum, algorithm reported as a risk score　　⊘♀🅔

RVU			Global Days	Modifiers				
Mod	Non-Fac Total	Fac Total		51	50	62	80	MUE
	0.00	0.00	XXX	9	9	9	9	1

81504 Oncology (tissue of origin), microarray gene expression profiling of > 2000 genes, utilizing formalin-fixed paraffin-embedded tissue, algorithm reported as tissue similarity scores　　🅐

RVU			Global Days	Modifiers				
Mod	Non-Fac Total	Fac Total		51	50	62	80	MUE
	0.00	0.00	XXX	9	9	9	9	1

81506 Endocrinology (type 2 diabetes), biochemical assays of seven analytes (glucose, HbA1c, insulin, hs-CRP, adiponectin, ferritin, interleukin 2-receptor alpha), utilizing serum or plasma, algorithm reporting a risk score　　🅔

RVU			Global Days	Modifiers				
Mod	Non-Fac Total	Fac Total		51	50	62	80	MUE
	0.00	0.00	XXX	9	9	9	9	1

81507 Fetal aneuploidy (trisomy 21, 18, and 13) DNA sequence analysis of selected regions using maternal plasma, algorithm reported as a risk score for each trisomy　　⊘♀🅐

RVU			Global Days	Modifiers				
Mod	Non-Fac Total	Fac Total		51	50	62	80	MUE
	0.00	0.00	XXX	9	9	9	9	1

81508 Fetal congenital abnormalities, biochemical assays of two proteins (PAPP-A, hCG [any form]), utilizing maternal serum, algorithm reported as a risk score　　⊘♀🅔

RVU			Global Days	Modifiers				
Mod	Non-Fac Total	Fac Total		51	50	62	80	MUE
	0.00	0.00	XXX	9	9	9	9	1

81509 Fetal congenital abnormalities, biochemical assays of three proteins (PAPP-A, hCG [any form], DIA), utilizing maternal serum, algorithm reported as a risk score　　♀🅔

RVU			Global Days	Modifiers				
Mod	Non-Fac Total	Fac Total		51	50	62	80	MUE
	0.00	0.00	XXX	9	9	9	9	1

81510 Fetal congenital abnormalities, biochemical assays of three analytes (AFP, uE3, hCG [any form]), utilizing maternal serum, algorithm reported as a risk score　　♀🅔

RVU			Global Days	Modifiers				
Mod	Non-Fac Total	Fac Total		51	50	62	80	MUE
	0.00	0.00	XXX	9	9	9	9	1

81511 Fetal congenital abnormalities, biochemical assays of four analytes (AFP, uE3, hCG [any form], DIA) utilizing maternal serum, algorithm reported as a risk score (may include additional results from previous biochemical testing)　　⊘♀🅔

RVU			Global Days	Modifiers				
Mod	Non-Fac Total	Fac Total		51	50	62	80	MUE
	0.00	0.00	XXX	9	9	9	9	1

81512 Fetal congenital abnormalities, biochemical assays of five analytes (AFP, uE3, total hCG, hyperglycosylated hCG, DIA) utilizing maternal serum, algorithm reported as a risk score　　♀🅔

RVU			Global Days	Modifiers				
Mod	Non-Fac Total	Fac Total		51	50	62	80	MUE
	0.00	0.00	XXX	9	9	9	9	1

● New　▲ Revised　Deleted　⊙ Moderate Sedation　➕ Add-on Codes　⊘ High Risk Denial　🅐 Age Edit　♀ Female　♂ Male　**AMA** *CPT® Assistant*　*MUE* Medically Unlikely Edit
⊗ Modifier 51 Exempt　⊖ Modifier 63 Exempt　🅧 Unlisted　**Modifiers:** *See Inside Back Cover*　Ⓜ Maternity　🅐2–🅩3 ASC Payment Indicators　🅐–🅨 OPPS Status Indicators

© 2016 DecisionHealth　　　CPT © 2015 American Medical Association. All Rights Reserved.

Laboratory/Pathology Procedures

81519 – 82016

● **81519** Oncology (breast), mRNA, gene expression profiling by real-time RT-PCR of 21 genes, utilizing formalin-fixed paraffin embedded tissue, algorithm reported as recurrence score ▲

RVU			Global Days	Modifiers				
Mod	Non-Fac Total	Fac Total		51	50	62	80	MUE
	0.00	0.00	XXX	9	9	9	9	1

AMA: Jan 15: 3

● **81525** Oncology (colon), mRNA, gene expression profiling by real-time RT-PCR of 12 genes (7 content and 5 housekeeping), utilizing formalin-fixed paraffin-embedded tissue, algorithm reported as a recurrence score ▲

RVU			Global Days	Modifiers				
Mod	Non-Fac Total	Fac Total		51	50	62	80	MUE
	0.00	0.00	XXX	9	9	9	9	1

● **81528** Oncology (colorectal) screening, quantitative real-time target and signal amplification of 10 DNA markers (KRAS mutations, promoter methylation of NDRG4 and BMP3) and fecal hemoglobin, utilizing stool, algorithm reported as a positive or negative result ▲

RVU			Global Days	Modifiers				
Mod	Non-Fac Total	Fac Total		51	50	62	80	MUE
	0.00	0.00	XXX	9	9	9	9	1

● **81535** Oncology (gynecologic), live tumor cell culture and chemotherapeutic response by DAPI stain and morphology, predictive algorithm reported as a drug response score; first single drug or drug combination ♀◎4

RVU			Global Days	Modifiers				
Mod	Non-Fac Total	Fac Total		51	50	62	80	MUE
	0.00	0.00	XXX	9	9	9	9	1

+● **81536** Oncology (gynecologic), live tumor cell culture and chemotherapeutic response by DAPI stain and morphology, predictive algorithm reported as a drug response score; each additional single drug or drug combination (List separately in addition to code for primary procedure) ♀◎4

RVU			Global Days	Modifiers				
Mod	Non-Fac Total	Fac Total		51	50	62	80	MUE
	0.00	0.00	XXX	9	9	9	9	

● **81538** Oncology (lung), mass spectrometric 8-protein signature, including amyloid A, utilizing serum, prognostic and predictive algorithm reported as good versus poor overall survival ◎4

RVU			Global Days	Modifiers				
Mod	Non-Fac Total	Fac Total		51	50	62	80	MUE
	0.00	0.00	XXX	9	9	9	9	1

● **81540** Oncology (tumor of unknown origin), mRNA, gene expression profiling by real-time RT-PCR of 92 genes (87 content and 5 housekeeping) to classify tumor into main cancer type and subtype, utilizing formalin-fixed paraffin-embedded tissue, algorithm reported as a probability of a predicted main cancer type and subtype ▲

RVU			Global Days	Modifiers				
Mod	Non-Fac Total	Fac Total		51	50	62	80	MUE
	0.00	0.00	XXX	9	9	9	9	1

● **81545** Oncology (thyroid), gene expression analysis of 142 genes, utilizing fine needle aspirate, algorithm reported as a categorical result (eg, benign or suspicious) ▲

RVU			Global Days	Modifiers				
Mod	Non-Fac Total	Fac Total		51	50	62	80	MUE
	0.00	0.00	XXX	9	9	9	9	1

● **81595** Cardiology (heart transplant), mRNA, gene expression profiling by real-time quantitative PCR of 20 genes (11 content and 9 housekeeping), utilizing subfraction of peripheral blood, algorithm reported as a rejection risk score ▲

RVU			Global Days	Modifiers				
Mod	Non-Fac Total	Fac Total		51	50	62	80	MUE
	0.00	0.00	XXX	9	9	9	9	1

81599 Unlisted multianalyte assay with algorithmic analysis ⊗✗E

RVU			Global Days	Modifiers				
Mod	Non-Fac Total	Fac Total		51	50	62	80	MUE
	0.00	0.00	XXX	9	9	9	9	

82009 Ketone body(s) (eg, acetone, acetoacetic acid, beta-hydroxybutyrate); qualitative ◎4

RVU			Global Days	Modifiers				
Mod	Non-Fac Total	Fac Total		51	50	62	80	MUE
	0.00	0.00	XXX	9	9	9	9	1

AMA: Oct 11: 11, Jun 15: 10
Pub 100-04, 16, 120.2

82010 Ketone body(s) (eg, acetone, acetoacetic acid, beta-hydroxybutyrate); quantitative ◎4

Coding tip: *For a CLIA-waived test, append modifier QW to 82010*

RVU			Global Days	Modifiers				
Mod	Non-Fac Total	Fac Total		51	50	62	80	MUE
	0.00	0.00	XXX	9	9	9	9	1

AMA: Oct 11: 11
Pub 100-04, 16, 120.2

82013 Acetylcholinesterase ◎4

RVU			Global Days	Modifiers				
Mod	Non-Fac Total	Fac Total		51	50	62	80	MUE
	0.00	0.00	XXX	9	9	9	9	1

82016 Acylcarnitines; qualitative, each specimen ⊗◎4

RVU			Global Days	Modifiers				
Mod	Non-Fac Total	Fac Total		51	50	62	80	MUE
	0.00	0.00	XXX	9	9	9	9	1

AMA: Nov 98: 23

● New   ▲ Revised   ✖ Deleted   ⊙ Moderate Sedation   ✚ Add-on Codes   ⊗ High Risk Denial   Ⓐ Age Edit   ♀ Female   ♂ Male   **AMA** *CPT® Assistant*   **MUE** Medically Unlikely Edit
⊘ Modifier 51 Exempt   ⊖ Modifier 63 Exempt   ✗ Unlisted   **Modifiers:** *See Inside Back Cover*   Ⓜ Maternity   A2–Z3 ASC Payment Indicators   A–Y OPPS Status Indicators

CPT © 2015 American Medical Association. All Rights Reserved.   © 2016 DecisionHealth

82017 Acylcarnitines; quantitative, each specimen ⊙◉4

Mod	Non-Fac Total	Fac Total	Global Days	51	50	62	80	MUE
	0.00	0.00	XXX	9	9	9	9	1

AMA: Nov 98: 23

Pub 100-04, 16, 120.2

82024 Adrenocorticotropic hormone (ACTH) ◉4

Mod	Non-Fac Total	Fac Total	Global Days	51	50	62	80	MUE
	0.00	0.00	XXX	9	9	9	9	4

82030 Adenosine, 5-monophosphate, cyclic (cyclic AMP) ◉4

Mod	Non-Fac Total	Fac Total	Global Days	51	50	62	80	MUE
	0.00	0.00	XXX	9	9	9	9	1

82040 Albumin; serum, plasma or whole blood ◉4

Coding tip: For a CLIA-waived test, append modifier QW to 82040

Mod	Non-Fac Total	Fac Total	Global Days	51	50	62	80	MUE
	0.00	0.00	XXX	9	9	9	9	1

AMA: Dec 99: 2

Pub 100-04, 16, 90.2, 120.2

82042 Albumin; urine or other source, quantitative, each specimen ◉4

Mod	Non-Fac Total	Fac Total	Global Days	51	50	62	80	MUE
	0.00	0.00	XXX	9	9	9	9	2

Pub 100-04, 16, 120.2

82043 Albumin; urine, microalbumin, quantitative ◉4

Coding tip: For a CLIA-waived test, append modifier QW to 82043

Mod	Non-Fac Total	Fac Total	Global Days	51	50	62	80	MUE
	0.00	0.00	XXX	9	9	9	9	1

AMA: Summer 94: 2

82044 Albumin; urine, microalbumin, semiquantitative (eg, reagent strip assay) ◉4

Coding tip: For a CLIA-waived test, append modifier QW to 82044

Mod	Non-Fac Total	Fac Total	Global Days	51	50	62	80	MUE
	0.00	0.00	XXX	9	9	9	9	1

AMA: Summer 94: 2, Mar 98: 3, Sep 02: 10

82045 Albumin; ischemia modified ◉4

Mod	Non-Fac Total	Fac Total	Global Days	51	50	62	80	MUE
	0.00	0.00	XXX	9	9	9	9	1

82075 Alcohol (ethanol), breath ◉4

Mod	Non-Fac Total	Fac Total	Global Days	51	50	62	80	MUE
	0.00	0.00	XXX	9	9	9	9	2

82085 Aldolase ◉4

Mod	Non-Fac Total	Fac Total	Global Days	51	50	62	80	MUE
	0.00	0.00	XXX	9	9	9	9	1

82088 Aldosterone ◉4

Mod	Non-Fac Total	Fac Total	Global Days	51	50	62	80	MUE
	0.00	0.00	XXX	9	9	9	9	2

AMA: Oct 10: 7

82103 Alpha-1-antitrypsin; total ◉4

Mod	Non-Fac Total	Fac Total	Global Days	51	50	62	80	MUE
	0.00	0.00	XXX	9	9	9	9	1

82104 Alpha-1-antitrypsin; phenotype ◉4

Mod	Non-Fac Total	Fac Total	Global Days	51	50	62	80	MUE
	0.00	0.00	XXX	9	9	9	9	1

82105 Alpha-fetoprotein (AFP); serum ◉4

Mod	Non-Fac Total	Fac Total	Global Days	51	50	62	80	MUE
	0.00	0.00	XXX	9	9	9	9	1

NCD: 190.25

82106 Alpha-fetoprotein (AFP); amniotic fluid Ⓜ◉4

Mod	Non-Fac Total	Fac Total	Global Days	51	50	62	80	MUE
	0.00	0.00	XXX	9	9	9	9	2

82107 Alpha-fetoprotein (AFP); AFP-L3 fraction isoform and total AFP (including ratio) ◉4

Mod	Non-Fac Total	Fac Total	Global Days	51	50	62	80	MUE
	0.00	0.00	XXX	9	9	9	9	1

82108 Aluminum ◉4

Mod	Non-Fac Total	Fac Total	Global Days	51	50	62	80	MUE
	0.00	0.00	XXX	9	9	9	9	1

Pub 100-04, 16, 120.2

82120 Amines, vaginal fluid, qualitative ♀◉4

Coding tip: For a CLIA-waived test, append modifier QW to 82120

Mod	Non-Fac Total	Fac Total	Global Days	51	50	62	80	MUE
	0.00	0.00	XXX	9	9	9	9	1

AMA: Nov 99: 45

82127 Amino acids; single, qualitative, each specimen ◉4

Mod	Non-Fac Total	Fac Total	Global Days	51	50	62	80	MUE
	0.00	0.00	XXX	9	9	9	9	1

AMA: Nov 98: 24

82128 Amino acids; multiple, qualitative, each specimen ◉4

Mod	Non-Fac Total	Fac Total	Global Days	51	50	62	80	MUE
	0.00	0.00	XXX	9	9	9	9	2

AMA: Nov 98: 24

● New   ▲ Revised   Deleted   ⊙ Moderate Sedation   ✚ Add-on Codes   ⊘ High Risk Denial   Ⓐ Age Edit   ♀ Female   ♂ Male   **AMA** *CPT® Assistant*   **MUE** Medically Unlikely Edit
⊘ Modifier 51 Exempt   ⊖ Modifier 63 Exempt   ✗ Unlisted   **Modifiers:** *See Inside Back Cover*   Ⓜ Maternity   Ⓐ2–Z3 ASC Payment Indicators   Ⓐ–Y OPPS Status Indicators

© 2016 DecisionHealth   CPT © 2015 American Medical Association. All Rights Reserved.

Laboratory/Pathology Procedures

82131 – 82252

82131 Amino acids; single, quantitative, each specimen Q4

RVU Mod	Non-Fac Total	Fac Total	Global Days	Modifiers 51	50	62	80	MUE
	0.00	0.00	XXX	9	9	9	9	2

AMA: May 98: 11, Nov 98: 24

82135 Aminolevulinic acid, delta (ALA) Q4

RVU Mod	Non-Fac Total	Fac Total	Global Days	Modifiers 51	50	62	80	MUE
	0.00	0.00	XXX	9	9	9	9	1

82136 Amino acids, 2 to 5 amino acids, quantitative, each specimen Q4

RVU Mod	Non-Fac Total	Fac Total	Global Days	Modifiers 51	50	62	80	MUE
	0.00	0.00	XXX	9	9	9	9	2

AMA: Nov 98: 24

82139 Amino acids, 6 or more amino acids, quantitative, each specimen Q4

RVU Mod	Non-Fac Total	Fac Total	Global Days	Modifiers 51	50	62	80	MUE
	0.00	0.00	XXX	9	9	9	9	2

AMA: Nov 98: 24

82140 Ammonia Q4

RVU Mod	Non-Fac Total	Fac Total	Global Days	Modifiers 51	50	62	80	MUE
	0.00	0.00	XXX	9	9	9	9	2

82143 Amniotic fluid scan (spectrophotometric) ♀ Q4

RVU Mod	Non-Fac Total	Fac Total	Global Days	Modifiers 51	50	62	80	MUE
	0.00	0.00	XXX	9	9	9	9	2

82150 Amylase Q4

Coding tip: *For a CLIA-waived test, append modifier QW to 82150*

RVU Mod	Non-Fac Total	Fac Total	Global Days	Modifiers 51	50	62	80	MUE
	0.00	0.00	XXX	9	9	9	9	2

82154 Androstanediol glucuronide Q4

RVU Mod	Non-Fac Total	Fac Total	Global Days	Modifiers 51	50	62	80	MUE
	0.00	0.00	XXX	9	9	9	9	1

AMA: Summer 94: 5

82157 Androstenedione Q4

RVU Mod	Non-Fac Total	Fac Total	Global Days	Modifiers 51	50	62	80	MUE
	0.00	0.00	XXX	9	9	9	9	1

82160 Androsterone Q4

RVU Mod	Non-Fac Total	Fac Total	Global Days	Modifiers 51	50	62	80	MUE
	0.00	0.00	XXX	9	9	9	9	1

82163 Angiotensin II Q4

RVU Mod	Non-Fac Total	Fac Total	Global Days	Modifiers 51	50	62	80	MUE
	0.00	0.00	XXX	9	9	9	9	1

82164 Angiotensin I - converting enzyme (ACE) Q4

RVU Mod	Non-Fac Total	Fac Total	Global Days	Modifiers 51	50	62	80	MUE
	0.00	0.00	XXX	9	9	9	9	1

82172 Apolipoprotein, each Q4

RVU Mod	Non-Fac Total	Fac Total	Global Days	Modifiers 51	50	62	80	MUE
	0.00	0.00	XXX	9	9	9	9	3

82175 Arsenic Q4

RVU Mod	Non-Fac Total	Fac Total	Global Days	Modifiers 51	50	62	80	MUE
	0.00	0.00	XXX	9	9	9	9	2

82180 Ascorbic acid (Vitamin C), blood Q4

RVU Mod	Non-Fac Total	Fac Total	Global Days	Modifiers 51	50	62	80	MUE
	0.00	0.00	XXX	9	9	9	9	1

82190 Atomic absorption spectroscopy, each analyte Q4

RVU Mod	Non-Fac Total	Fac Total	Global Days	Modifiers 51	50	62	80	MUE
	0.00	0.00	XXX	9	9	9	9	2

AMA: Oct 10: 7

82232 Beta-2 microglobulin Q4

RVU Mod	Non-Fac Total	Fac Total	Global Days	Modifiers 51	50	62	80	MUE
	0.00	0.00	XXX	9	9	9	9	2

Pub 100-04, 16, 120.2

82239 Bile acids; total Q4

RVU Mod	Non-Fac Total	Fac Total	Global Days	Modifiers 51	50	62	80	MUE
	0.00	0.00	XXX	9	9	9	9	1

82240 Bile acids; cholylglycine Q4

RVU Mod	Non-Fac Total	Fac Total	Global Days	Modifiers 51	50	62	80	MUE
	0.00	0.00	XXX	9	9	9	9	1

82247 Bilirubin; total Q4

Coding tip: *For a CLIA-waived test, append modifier QW to 82247*

RVU Mod	Non-Fac Total	Fac Total	Global Days	Modifiers 51	50	62	80	MUE
	0.00	0.00	XXX	9	9	9	9	2

AMA: Nov 98: 24, Apr 99: 6, Dec 99: 1, Jan 00: 7, Dec 08: 5, Apr 10: 11
Pub 100-04, 16, 90.2, 120.2

82248 Bilirubin; direct Q4

RVU Mod	Non-Fac Total	Fac Total	Global Days	Modifiers 51	50	62	80	MUE
	0.00	0.00	XXX	9	9	9	9	2

AMA: Nov 98: 24, Apr 99: 6, Dec 99: 1, Apr 10: 11
Pub 100-04, 16, 90.2, 120.2

82252 Bilirubin; feces, qualitative ⊗ Q4

RVU Mod	Non-Fac Total	Fac Total	Global Days	Modifiers 51	50	62	80	MUE
	0.00	0.00	XXX	9	9	9	9	1

● New   ▲ Revised   ✖ Deleted   ⊙ Moderate Sedation   ✚ Add-on Codes   ⊘ High Risk Denial   Ⓐ Age Edit   ♀ Female   ♂ Male   **AMA** *CPT® Assistant*   ***MUE*** Medically Unlikely Edit
⊘ Modifier 51 Exempt   ⊖ Modifier 63 Exempt   ✗ Unlisted   **Modifiers:** *See Inside Back Cover*   Ⓜ Maternity   A-2–Z-3 ASC Payment Indicators   A–Y OPPS Status Indicators

CPT © 2015 American Medical Association. All Rights Reserved.   © 2016 DecisionHealth

82261 Biotinidase, each specimen ⊗ Q4

RVU			Global Days	Modifiers				
Mod	Non-Fac Total	Fac Total		51	50	62	80	MUE
	0.00	0.00	XXX	9	9	9	9	1

AMA: Nov 98: 24

82270 Blood, occult, by peroxidase activity (eg, guaiac), qualitative; feces, consecutive collected specimens with single determination, for colorectal neoplasm screening (ie, patient was provided 3 cards or single triple card for consecutive collection) A

Coding tip: This is a CLIA-waived test, but does not require the use of modifier QW to be recognized as such

RVU			Global Days	Modifiers				
Mod	Non-Fac Total	Fac Total		51	50	62	80	MUE
	0.00	0.00	XXX	9	9	9	9	1

AMA: Sep 03: 15, Feb 06: 7, Apr 08: 5

Pub 100-02, 15, 280.2.2; 100-04, 18, 1.2, 60.2, 60.2.1, 60.6, 60.7

82271 Blood, occult, by peroxidase activity (eg, guaiac), qualitative; other sources Q4

Coding tip: For a CLIA-waived test, append modifier QW to 82271

RVU			Global Days	Modifiers				
Mod	Non-Fac Total	Fac Total		51	50	62	80	MUE
	0.00	0.00	XXX	9	9	9	9	1

AMA: Feb 06: 7

82272 Blood, occult, by peroxidase activity (eg, guaiac), qualitative, feces, 1-3 simultaneous determinations, performed for other than colorectal neoplasm screening Q4

Coding tip: This is a CLIA-waived test, but does not require the use of modifier QW to be recognized as such

RVU			Global Days	Modifiers				
Mod	Non-Fac Total	Fac Total		51	50	62	80	MUE
	0.00	0.00	XXX	9	9	9	9	1

AMA: Feb 06: 7, Apr 08: 5, Jun 09: 10
NCD: 190.34

82274 Blood, occult, by fecal hemoglobin determination by immunoassay, qualitative, feces, 1-3 simultaneous determinations Q4

Coding tip: For a CLIA-waived test, append modifier QW to 82274

RVU			Global Days	Modifiers				
Mod	Non-Fac Total	Fac Total		51	50	62	80	MUE
	0.00	0.00	XXX	9	9	9	9	1

82286 Bradykinin Q4

RVU			Global Days	Modifiers				
Mod	Non-Fac Total	Fac Total		51	50	62	80	MUE
	0.00	0.00	XXX	9	9	9	9	1

AMA: Oct 10: 7

82300 Cadmium Q4

RVU			Global Days	Modifiers				
Mod	Non-Fac Total	Fac Total		51	50	62	80	MUE
	0.00	0.00	XXX	9	9	9	9	1

AMA: Aug 05: 9, Oct 10: 7

82306 Vitamin D; 25 hydroxy, includes fraction(s), if performed Q4

Coding tip: Vitamin D 1,25 dihydroxy - 82652

RVU			Global Days	Modifiers				
Mod	Non-Fac Total	Fac Total		51	50	62	80	MUE
	0.00	0.00	XXX	9	9	9	9	1

Pub 100-04, 16, 120.2

82308 Calcitonin Q4

RVU			Global Days	Modifiers				
Mod	Non-Fac Total	Fac Total		51	50	62	80	MUE
	0.00	0.00	XXX	9	9	9	9	1

82310 Calcium; total Q4

Coding tip: For a CLIA-waived test, append modifier QW to 82310

RVU			Global Days	Modifiers				
Mod	Non-Fac Total	Fac Total		51	50	62	80	MUE
	0.00	0.00	XXX	9	9	9	9	2

AMA: Dec 99: 2
Pub 100-04, 16, 90.2, 120.2

82330 Calcium; ionized Q4

Coding tip: For a CLIA-waived test, append modifier QW to 82330

RVU			Global Days	Modifiers				
Mod	Non-Fac Total	Fac Total		51	50	62	80	MUE
	0.00	0.00	XXX	9	9	9	9	2

AMA: Apr 13: 10
Pub 100-04, 16, 90.2, 120.2

82331 Calcium; after calcium infusion test Q4

RVU			Global Days	Modifiers				
Mod	Non-Fac Total	Fac Total		51	50	62	80	MUE
	0.00	0.00	XXX	9	9	9	9	1

82340 Calcium; urine quantitative, timed specimen Q4

RVU			Global Days	Modifiers				
Mod	Non-Fac Total	Fac Total		51	50	62	80	MUE
	0.00	0.00	XXX	9	9	9	9	1

82355 Calculus; qualitative analysis Q4

RVU			Global Days	Modifiers				
Mod	Non-Fac Total	Fac Total		51	50	62	80	MUE
	0.00	0.00	XXX	9	9	9	9	2

82360 Calculus; quantitative analysis, chemical Q4

RVU			Global Days	Modifiers				
Mod	Non-Fac Total	Fac Total		51	50	62	80	MUE
	0.00	0.00	XXX	9	9	9	9	2

82365 Calculus; infrared spectroscopy Q4

RVU			Global Days	Modifiers				
Mod	Non-Fac Total	Fac Total		51	50	62	80	MUE
	0.00	0.00	XXX	9	9	9	9	2

82370 Calculus; X-ray diffraction Q4

RVU			Global Days	Modifiers				
Mod	Non-Fac Total	Fac Total		51	50	62	80	MUE
	0.00	0.00	XXX	9	9	9	9	2

● New ▲ Revised Deleted ⊙ Moderate Sedation ✚ Add-on Codes ⊗ High Risk Denial Ⓐ Age Edit ♀ Female ♂ Male **AMA** CPT® Assistant **MUE** Medically Unlikely Edit
⊝ Modifier 51 Exempt ⊖ Modifier 63 Exempt ✖ Unlisted **Modifiers:** See Inside Back Cover Ⓜ Maternity A 2 – Z 3 ASC Payment Indicators A – Y OPPS Status Indicators

© 2016 DecisionHealth CPT © 2015 American Medical Association. All Rights Reserved. **715**

82373 Carbohydrate deficient transferrin ◨4

RVU Mod	Non-Fac Total	Fac Total	Global Days	51	50	62	80	MUE
	0.00	0.00	XXX	9	9	9	9	1

82374 Carbon dioxide (bicarbonate) ◨4

Coding tip: See also blood gases - 82803-82805

Coding tip: For a CLIA-waived test, append modifier QW to 82374

RVU Mod	Non-Fac Total	Fac Total	Global Days	51	50	62	80	MUE
	0.00	0.00	XXX	9	9	9	9	2

AMA: Dec 99: 2, Apr 13: 10

Pub 100-04, 16, 90.2, 120.2

82375 Carboxyhemoglobin; quantitative ◨4

RVU Mod	Non-Fac Total	Fac Total	Global Days	51	50	62	80	MUE
	0.00	0.00	XXX	9	9	9	9	1

82376 Carboxyhemoglobin; qualitative ◨4

RVU Mod	Non-Fac Total	Fac Total	Global Days	51	50	62	80	MUE
	0.00	0.00	XXX	9	9	9	9	1

82378 Carcinoembryonic antigen (CEA) ◨4

RVU Mod	Non-Fac Total	Fac Total	Global Days	51	50	62	80	MUE
	0.00	0.00	XXX	9	9	9	9	1

AMA: Fall 93: 25, Aug 96: 11
NCD: 190.26

82379 Carnitine (total and free), quantitative, each specimen ⊗◨4

RVU Mod	Non-Fac Total	Fac Total	Global Days	51	50	62	80	MUE
	0.00	0.00	XXX	9	9	9	9	1

AMA: Nov 98: 24

Pub 100-04, 16, 120.2

82380 Carotene ◨4

RVU Mod	Non-Fac Total	Fac Total	Global Days	51	50	62	80	MUE
	0.00	0.00	XXX	9	9	9	9	1

82382 Catecholamines; total urine ◨4

RVU Mod	Non-Fac Total	Fac Total	Global Days	51	50	62	80	MUE
	0.00	0.00	XXX	9	9	9	9	1

82383 Catecholamines; blood ◨4

RVU Mod	Non-Fac Total	Fac Total	Global Days	51	50	62	80	MUE
	0.00	0.00	XXX	9	9	9	9	1

82384 Catecholamines; fractionated ◨4

RVU Mod	Non-Fac Total	Fac Total	Global Days	51	50	62	80	MUE
	0.00	0.00	XXX	9	9	9	9	2

82387 Cathepsin-D ◨4

RVU Mod	Non-Fac Total	Fac Total	Global Days	51	50	62	80	MUE
	0.00	0.00	XXX	9	9	9	9	1

82390 Ceruloplasmin ◨4

RVU Mod	Non-Fac Total	Fac Total	Global Days	51	50	62	80	MUE
	0.00	0.00	XXX	9	9	9	9	1

82397 Chemiluminescent assay ◨4

RVU Mod	Non-Fac Total	Fac Total	Global Days	51	50	62	80	MUE
	0.00	0.00	XXX	9	9	9	9	3

AMA: Fall 93: 25, Oct 10: 7

82415 Chloramphenicol ◨4

RVU Mod	Non-Fac Total	Fac Total	Global Days	51	50	62	80	MUE
	0.00	0.00	XXX	9	9	9	9	1

AMA: Aug 05: 9, Oct 10: 7

82435 Chloride; blood ◨4

Coding tip: For a CLIA-waived test, append modifier QW to 82435

RVU Mod	Non-Fac Total	Fac Total	Global Days	51	50	62	80	MUE
	0.00	0.00	XXX	9	9	9	9	2

AMA: Dec 99: 2, Apr 13: 10

Pub 100-04, 16, 90.2, 120.2

82436 Chloride; urine ◨4

RVU Mod	Non-Fac Total	Fac Total	Global Days	51	50	62	80	MUE
	0.00	0.00	XXX	9	9	9	9	1

82438 Chloride; other source ◨4

RVU Mod	Non-Fac Total	Fac Total	Global Days	51	50	62	80	MUE
	0.00	0.00	XXX	9	9	9	9	1

AMA: Jul 03: 7

82441 Chlorinated hydrocarbons, screen ◨4

RVU Mod	Non-Fac Total	Fac Total	Global Days	51	50	62	80	MUE
	0.00	0.00	XXX	9	9	9	9	1

Coding Guidance

Do not use 83721 to report a calculated LDL cholesterol. A direct measurement of LDL cholesterol with total cholesterol (82465) or lipid panel (80061) is sometimes done with high triglyceride levels greater than 400mg/dl, in order to measure the LDL cholesterol. In these cases, report 83721 with modifier 59.

82465 Cholesterol, serum or whole blood, total 🅰

Coding tip: For a CLIA-waived test, append modifier QW to 82465

RVU Mod	Non-Fac Total	Fac Total	Global Days	51	50	62	80	MUE
	0.00	0.00	XXX	9	9	9	9	1

AMA: Dec 99: 2, Mar 00: 11, Feb 05: 9

Pub 100-04, 16, 90.2, 120.2; 100-04, 18, 1.2, 100.1, 100.2, 100.3, 100.5

82480 Cholinesterase; serum ◨4

RVU Mod	Non-Fac Total	Fac Total	Global Days	51	50	62	80	MUE
	0.00	0.00	XXX	9	9	9	9	2

● New ▲ Revised ✖ Deleted ⊙ Moderate Sedation ✚ Add-on Codes ⊗ High Risk Denial Ⓐ Age Edit ♀ Female ♂ Male **AMA** CPT® Assistant **MUE** Medically Unlikely Edit
⊘ Modifier 51 Exempt ⊖ Modifier 63 Exempt ✗ Unlisted **Modifiers:** See Inside Back Cover Ⓜ Maternity A2–Z3 ASC Payment Indicators A–Y OPPS Status Indicators

CPT © 2015 American Medical Association. All Rights Reserved.   © 2016 DecisionHealth

82482 Cholinesterase; RBC [Q4]

Mod	Non-Fac Total	Fac Total	Global Days	51	50	62	80	MUE
	0.00	0.00	XXX	9	9	9	9	1

82485 Chondroitin B sulfate, quantitative ⊘[Q4]

Mod	Non-Fac Total	Fac Total	Global Days	51	50	62	80	MUE
	0.00	0.00	XXX	9	9	9	9	1

✗ ~~82486 Chromatography, qualitative; column (eg, gas liquid or HPLC), analyte not elsewhere specified~~

✗ ~~82487 Chromatography, qualitative; paper, 1-dimensional, analyte not elsewhere specified~~

✗ ~~82488 Chromatography, qualitative; paper, 2-dimensional, analyte not elsewhere specified~~

✗ ~~82489 Chromatography, qualitative; thin layer, analyte not elsewhere specified~~

✗ ~~82491 Chromatography, quantitative, column (eg, gas liquid or HPLC); single analyte not elsewhere specified, single stationary and mobile phase~~

✗ ~~82492 Chromatography, quantitative, column (eg, gas liquid or HPLC); multiple analytes, single stationary and mobile phase~~

82495 Chromium [Q4]

Mod	Non-Fac Total	Fac Total	Global Days	51	50	62	80	MUE
	0.00	0.00	XXX	9	9	9	9	1

AMA: Oct 10: 7

82507 Citrate [Q4]

Mod	Non-Fac Total	Fac Total	Global Days	51	50	62	80	MUE
	0.00	0.00	XXX	9	9	9	9	1

AMA: Aug 05: 9, Oct 10: 7

82523 Collagen cross links, any method [Q4]

Coding tip: For a CLIA-waived test, append modifier QW to 82523

Mod	Non-Fac Total	Fac Total	Global Days	51	50	62	80	MUE
	0.00	0.00	XXX	9	9	9	9	1

NCD: 190.19

82525 Copper [Q4]

Mod	Non-Fac Total	Fac Total	Global Days	51	50	62	80	MUE
	0.00	0.00	XXX	9	9	9	9	2

82528 Corticosterone [Q4]

Mod	Non-Fac Total	Fac Total	Global Days	51	50	62	80	MUE
	0.00	0.00	XXX	9	9	9	9	1

82530 Cortisol; free [Q4]

Mod	Non-Fac Total	Fac Total	Global Days	51	50	62	80	MUE
	0.00	0.00	XXX	9	9	9	9	4

AMA: Summer 94: 3

82533 Cortisol; total [Q4]

Mod	Non-Fac Total	Fac Total	Global Days	51	50	62	80	MUE
	0.00	0.00	XXX	9	9	9	9	5

AMA: Summer 94: 3

82540 Creatine [Q4]

Mod	Non-Fac Total	Fac Total	Global Days	51	50	62	80	MUE
	0.00	0.00	XXX	9	9	9	9	1

✗ ~~82541 Column chromatography/mass spectrometry (eg, GC/MS, or HPLC/MS), non-drug analyte not elsewhere specified; qualitative, single stationary and mobile phase~~

▲ 82542 Column chromatography, includes mass spectrometry, if performed (eg, HPLC, LC, LC/MS, LC/MS-MS, GC, GC/MS-MS, GC/MS, HPLC/MS), non-drug analyte(s) not elsewhere specified, qualitative or quantitative, each specimen [Q4]

Mod	Non-Fac Total	Fac Total	Global Days	51	50	62	80	MUE
	0.00	0.00	XXX	9	9	9	9	6

AMA: Nov 98: 24, 25, Apr 15: 3

✗ ~~82543 Column chromatography/mass spectrometry (eg, GC/MS, or HPLC/MS), non-drug analyte not elsewhere specified; stable isotope dilution, single analyte, quantitative, single stationary and mobile phase~~

✗ ~~82544 Column chromatography/mass spectrometry (eg, GC/MS, or HPLC/MS), non-drug analyte not elsewhere specified; stable isotope dilution, multiple analytes, quantitative, single stationary and mobile phase~~

82550 Creatine kinase (CK), (CPK); total [Q4]

Coding tip: For a CLIA-waived test, append modifier QW to 82550

Mod	Non-Fac Total	Fac Total	Global Days	51	50	62	80	MUE
	0.00	0.00	XXX	9	9	9	9	3

AMA: Feb 98: 1, Dec 99: 2
Pub 100-04, 16, 90.2, 120.2

82552 Creatine kinase (CK), (CPK); isoenzymes [Q4]

Mod	Non-Fac Total	Fac Total	Global Days	51	50	62	80	MUE
	0.00	0.00	XXX	9	9	9	9	3

AMA: Feb 98: 1

82553 Creatine kinase (CK), (CPK); MB fraction only [Q4]

Mod	Non-Fac Total	Fac Total	Global Days	51	50	62	80	MUE
	0.00	0.00	XXX	9	9	9	9	3

AMA: Feb 98: 1

82554 Creatine kinase (CK), (CPK); isoforms [Q4]

Mod	Non-Fac Total	Fac Total	Global Days	51	50	62	80	MUE
	0.00	0.00	XXX	9	9	9	9	1

AMA: Feb 98: 1

● New ▲ Revised Deleted ⊙ Moderate Sedation ✚ Add-on Codes ⊘ High Risk Denial Ⓐ Age Edit ♀ Female ♂ Male **AMA** CPT® Assistant **MUE** Medically Unlikely Edit
Ⓢ Modifier 51 Exempt ⊖ Modifier 63 Exempt ✗ Unlisted **Modifiers:** See Inside Back Cover Ⓜ Maternity A-2–Z-3 ASC Payment Indicators A–Y OPPS Status Indicators

© 2016 DecisionHealth | CPT © 2015 American Medical Association. All Rights Reserved. | **717**

Laboratory/Pathology Procedures

82482 – 82554

82565 Creatinine; blood   Q4

Coding tip: For a CLIA-waived test, append modifier QW to 82565

RVU			Global Days	Modifiers				
Mod	Non-Fac Total	Fac Total		51	50	62	80	MUE
	0.00	0.00	XXX	9	9	9	9	2

AMA: Dec 99: 2, Apr 13: 10

Pub 100-04, 16, 90.2

82570 Creatinine; other source   Q4

Coding tip: For a CLIA-waived test, append modifier QW to 82570

RVU			Global Days	Modifiers				
Mod	Non-Fac Total	Fac Total		51	50	62	80	MUE
	0.00	0.00	XXX	9	9	9	9	3

Pub 100-04, 16, 120.2

82575 Creatinine; clearance   Q4

RVU			Global Days	Modifiers				
Mod	Non-Fac Total	Fac Total		51	50	62	80	MUE
	0.00	0.00	XXX	9	9	9	9	1

Pub 100-04, 16, 120.2

82585 Cryofibrinogen   Q4

RVU			Global Days	Modifiers				
Mod	Non-Fac Total	Fac Total		51	50	62	80	MUE
	0.00	0.00	XXX	9	9	9	9	1

82595 Cryoglobulin, qualitative or semi-quantitative (eg, cryocrit)   Q4

RVU			Global Days	Modifiers				
Mod	Non-Fac Total	Fac Total		51	50	62	80	MUE
	0.00	0.00	XXX	9	9	9	9	1

AMA: Oct 10: 7

82600 Cyanide   Q4

RVU			Global Days	Modifiers				
Mod	Non-Fac Total	Fac Total		51	50	62	80	MUE
	0.00	0.00	XXX	9	9	9	9	1

AMA: Aug 05: 9, Oct 10: 7

82607 Cyanocobalamin (Vitamin B-12)   Q4

RVU			Global Days	Modifiers				
Mod	Non-Fac Total	Fac Total		51	50	62	80	MUE
	0.00	0.00	XXX	9	9	9	9	1

Pub 100-04, 16, 120.2

82608 Cyanocobalamin (Vitamin B-12); unsaturated binding capacity   Q4

RVU			Global Days	Modifiers				
Mod	Non-Fac Total	Fac Total		51	50	62	80	MUE
	0.00	0.00	XXX	9	9	9	9	1

82610 Cystatin C   Q4

RVU			Global Days	Modifiers				
Mod	Non-Fac Total	Fac Total		51	50	62	80	MUE
	0.00	0.00	XXX	9	9	9	9	1

AMA: Apr 08: 5, Aug 08: 13

82615 Cystine and homocystine, urine, qualitative   Q4

RVU			Global Days	Modifiers				
Mod	Non-Fac Total	Fac Total		51	50	62	80	MUE
	0.00	0.00	XXX	9	9	9	9	1

82626 Dehydroepiandrosterone (DHEA)   Q4

RVU			Global Days	Modifiers				
Mod	Non-Fac Total	Fac Total		51	50	62	80	MUE
	0.00	0.00	XXX	9	9	9	9	1

AMA: Summer 94: 4

82627 Dehydroepiandrosterone-sulfate (DHEA-S)   Q4

RVU			Global Days	Modifiers				
Mod	Non-Fac Total	Fac Total		51	50	62	80	MUE
	0.00	0.00	XXX	9	9	9	9	1

AMA: Summer 94: 4

82633 Desoxycorticosterone, 11-   Q4

RVU			Global Days	Modifiers				
Mod	Non-Fac Total	Fac Total		51	50	62	80	MUE
	0.00	0.00	XXX	9	9	9	9	1

82634 Deoxycortisol, 11-   Q4

RVU			Global Days	Modifiers				
Mod	Non-Fac Total	Fac Total		51	50	62	80	MUE
	0.00	0.00	XXX	9	9	9	9	1

82638 Dibucaine number   Q4

RVU			Global Days	Modifiers				
Mod	Non-Fac Total	Fac Total		51	50	62	80	MUE
	0.00	0.00	XXX	9	9	9	9	1

82652 Vitamin D; 1, 25 dihydroxy, includes fraction(s), if performed   Q4

Coding tip: Code 82652 is listed out of numerical order in CPT. Related laboratory procedure code vitamin D, 25 hydroxy - 82306

RVU			Global Days	Modifiers				
Mod	Non-Fac Total	Fac Total		51	50	62	80	MUE
	0.00	0.00	XXX	9	9	9	9	1

82656 Elastase, pancreatic (EL-1), fecal, qualitative or semi-quantitative   Q4

RVU			Global Days	Modifiers				
Mod	Non-Fac Total	Fac Total		51	50	62	80	MUE
	0.00	0.00	XXX	9	9	9	9	1

AMA: Sep 05: 9

82657 Enzyme activity in blood cells, cultured cells, or tissue, not elsewhere specified; nonradioactive substrate, each specimen   Q4

RVU			Global Days	Modifiers				
Mod	Non-Fac Total	Fac Total		51	50	62	80	MUE
	0.00	0.00	XXX	9	9	9	9	3

AMA: Nov 98: 25

82658 Enzyme activity in blood cells, cultured cells, or tissue, not elsewhere specified; radioactive substrate, each specimen   Q4

RVU			Global Days	Modifiers				
Mod	Non-Fac Total	Fac Total		51	50	62	80	MUE
	0.00	0.00	XXX	9	9	9	9	2

AMA: Nov 98: 25

82664 Electrophoretic technique, not elsewhere specified   Q4

RVU			Global Days	Modifiers				
Mod	Non-Fac Total	Fac Total		51	50	62	80	MUE
	0.00	0.00	XXX	9	9	9	9	2

● New   ▲ Revised   ✖ Deleted   ⊙ Moderate Sedation   ✚ Add-on Codes   ⊖ High Risk Denial   Ⓐ Age Edit   ♀ Female   ♂ Male   **AMA** CPT® Assistant   **MUE** Medically Unlikely Edit

⊘ Modifier 51 Exempt   ⊖ Modifier 63 Exempt   ✗ Unlisted   **Modifiers:** See Inside Back Cover   Ⓜ Maternity   A2–Z3 ASC Payment Indicators   A–Y OPPS Status Indicators

CPT © 2015 American Medical Association. All Rights Reserved.   © 2016 DecisionHealth

82668 Erythropoietin ▣4

RVU Mod	Non-Fac Total	Fac Total	Global Days	51	50	62	80	MUE
	0.00	0.00	XXX	9	9	9	9	1

82670 Estradiol ▣4

RVU Mod	Non-Fac Total	Fac Total	Global Days	51	50	62	80	MUE
	0.00	0.00	XXX	9	9	9	9	2

82671 Estrogens; fractionated ▣4

RVU Mod	Non-Fac Total	Fac Total	Global Days	51	50	62	80	MUE
	0.00	0.00	XXX	9	9	9	9	1

82672 Estrogens; total ▣4

RVU Mod	Non-Fac Total	Fac Total	Global Days	51	50	62	80	MUE
	0.00	0.00	XXX	9	9	9	9	1

82677 Estriol ▣4

RVU Mod	Non-Fac Total	Fac Total	Global Days	51	50	62	80	MUE
	0.00	0.00	XXX	9	9	9	9	1

82679 Estrone ▣4

Coding tip: For a CLIA-waived test, append modifier QW to 82679

RVU Mod	Non-Fac Total	Fac Total	Global Days	51	50	62	80	MUE
	0.00	0.00	XXX	9	9	9	9	1

82693 Ethylene glycol ▣4

RVU Mod	Non-Fac Total	Fac Total	Global Days	51	50	62	80	MUE
	0.00	0.00	XXX	9	9	9	9	2

82696 Etiocholanolone ▣4

RVU Mod	Non-Fac Total	Fac Total	Global Days	51	50	62	80	MUE
	0.00	0.00	XXX	9	9	9	9	1

AMA: Oct 10: 7

82705 Fat or lipids, feces; qualitative ▣4

RVU Mod	Non-Fac Total	Fac Total	Global Days	51	50	62	80	MUE
	0.00	0.00	XXX	9	9	9	9	1

AMA: Aug 05: 9, Oct 10: 7

82710 Fat or lipids, feces; quantitative ▣4

RVU Mod	Non-Fac Total	Fac Total	Global Days	51	50	62	80	MUE
	0.00	0.00	XXX	9	9	9	9	1

82715 Fat differential, feces, quantitative ▣4

RVU Mod	Non-Fac Total	Fac Total	Global Days	51	50	62	80	MUE
	0.00	0.00	XXX	9	9	9	9	3

82725 Fatty acids, nonesterified ▣4

RVU Mod	Non-Fac Total	Fac Total	Global Days	51	50	62	80	MUE
	0.00	0.00	XXX	9	9	9	9	1

82726 Very long chain fatty acids ▣4

RVU Mod	Non-Fac Total	Fac Total	Global Days	51	50	62	80	MUE
	0.00	0.00	XXX	9	9	9	9	1

AMA: Nov 98: 25

82728 Ferritin ▣4

RVU Mod	Non-Fac Total	Fac Total	Global Days	51	50	62	80	MUE
	0.00	0.00	XXX	9	9	9	9	1

Pub 100-04, 16, 120.2
NCD: 190.18

82731 Fetal fibronectin, cervicovaginal secretions, semi-quantitative ♀Ⓜ▣4

RVU Mod	Non-Fac Total	Fac Total	Global Days	51	50	62	80	MUE
	0.00	0.00	XXX	9	9	9	9	1

AMA: Nov 98: 25

82735 Fluoride ▣4

RVU Mod	Non-Fac Total	Fac Total	Global Days	51	50	62	80	MUE
	0.00	0.00	XXX	9	9	9	9	1

82746 Folic acid; serum ▣4

RVU Mod	Non-Fac Total	Fac Total	Global Days	51	50	62	80	MUE
	0.00	0.00	XXX	9	9	9	9	1

Pub 100-04, 16, 120.2

82747 Folic acid; RBC ▣4

RVU Mod	Non-Fac Total	Fac Total	Global Days	51	50	62	80	MUE
	0.00	0.00	XXX	9	9	9	9	1

Pub 100-04, 16, 120.2

82757 Fructose, semen ▣4

RVU Mod	Non-Fac Total	Fac Total	Global Days	51	50	62	80	MUE
	0.00	0.00	XXX	9	9	9	9	1

82759 Galactokinase, RBC ▣4

RVU Mod	Non-Fac Total	Fac Total	Global Days	51	50	62	80	MUE
	0.00	0.00	XXX	9	9	9	9	1

82760 Galactose ▣4

RVU Mod	Non-Fac Total	Fac Total	Global Days	51	50	62	80	MUE
	0.00	0.00	XXX	9	9	9	9	1

82775 Galactose-1-phosphate uridyl transferase; quantitative ⊘▣4

RVU Mod	Non-Fac Total	Fac Total	Global Days	51	50	62	80	MUE
	0.00	0.00	XXX	9	9	9	9	1

82776 Galactose-1-phosphate uridyl transferase; screen ⊘▣4

RVU Mod	Non-Fac Total	Fac Total	Global Days	51	50	62	80	MUE
	0.00	0.00	XXX	9	9	9	9	1

● New ▲ Revised Deleted ⊙ Moderate Sedation ✚ Add-on Codes ⊘ High Risk Denial ⒶAge Edit ♀ Female ♂ Male **AMA** *CPT® Assistant* **MUE** Medically Unlikely Edit
⃠ Modifier 51 Exempt ⊖ Modifier 63 Exempt ✗ Unlisted **Modifiers:** *See Inside Back Cover* Ⓜ Maternity Ａ2–Ｚ3 ASC Payment Indicators Ａ–Ｙ OPPS Status Indicators

Laboratory/Pathology Procedures

82777 – 82948

82777 Galectin-3 [Q4]

	RVU			Global Days	Modifiers				
Mod	Non-Fac Total	Fac Total			51	50	62	80	MUE
	0.00	0.00	XXX		9	9	9	9	1

82784 Gammaglobulin (immunoglobulin); IgA, IgD, IgG, IgM, each [Q4]

	RVU			Global Days	Modifiers				
Mod	Non-Fac Total	Fac Total			51	50	62	80	MUE
	0.00	0.00	XXX		9	9	9	9	6

AMA: Spring 94: 31, Aug 00: 11

82785 Gammaglobulin (immunoglobulin); IgE [Q4]

	RVU			Global Days	Modifiers				
Mod	Non-Fac Total	Fac Total			51	50	62	80	MUE
	0.00	0.00	XXX		9	9	9	9	1

AMA: Spring 94: 31

82787 Gammaglobulin (immunoglobulin); immunoglobulin subclasses (eg, IgG1, 2, 3, or 4), each [Q4]

	RVU			Global Days	Modifiers				
Mod	Non-Fac Total	Fac Total			51	50	62	80	MUE
	0.00	0.00	XXX		9	9	9	9	4

AMA: Oct 10: 7

82800 Gases, blood, pH only [Q4]

	RVU			Global Days	Modifiers				
Mod	Non-Fac Total	Fac Total			51	50	62	80	MUE
	0.00	0.00	XXX		9	9	9	9	1

AMA: Aug 05: 9, Oct 10: 7
Pub 100-04, 16, 120.2

82803 Gases, blood, any combination of pH, pCO2, pO2, CO2, HCO3 (including calculated O2 saturation) [Q4]

	RVU			Global Days	Modifiers				
Mod	Non-Fac Total	Fac Total			51	50	62	80	MUE
	0.00	0.00	XXX		9	9	9	9	

Pub 100-04, 16, 120.2

82805 Gases, blood, any combination of pH, pCO2, pO2, CO2, HCO3 (including calculated O2 saturation); with O2 saturation, by direct measurement, except pulse oximetry [Q4]

Coding tip: If only a single analyte from the listed blood gas analytes is tested, refer to the code for the specific analyte

	RVU			Global Days	Modifiers				
Mod	Non-Fac Total	Fac Total			51	50	62	80	MUE
	0.00	0.00	XXX		9	9	9	9	2

Pub 100-04, 16, 120.2

82810 Gases, blood, O2 saturation only, by direct measurement, except pulse oximetry [Q4]

	RVU			Global Days	Modifiers				
Mod	Non-Fac Total	Fac Total			51	50	62	80	MUE
	0.00	0.00	XXX		9	9	9	9	2

Pub 100-04, 16, 120.2

82820 Hemoglobin-oxygen affinity (pO2 for 50% hemoglobin saturation with oxygen) [Q4]

Coding tip: Gas liquid chromatography [GLC] - 82486

	RVU			Global Days	Modifiers				
Mod	Non-Fac Total	Fac Total			51	50	62	80	MUE
	0.00	0.00	XXX		9	9	9	9	1

AMA: Oct 10: 7

82930 Gastric acid analysis, includes pH if performed, each specimen [⊘][Q4]

	RVU			Global Days	Modifiers				
Mod	Non-Fac Total	Fac Total			51	50	62	80	MUE
	0.00	0.00	XXX		9	9	9	9	1

AMA: Sep 11: 3, Oct 10: 7, Dec 10: 7

82938 Gastrin after secretin stimulation [Q4]

	RVU			Global Days	Modifiers				
Mod	Non-Fac Total	Fac Total			51	50	62	80	MUE
	0.00	0.00	XXX		9	9	9	9	1

82941 Gastrin [Q4]

	RVU			Global Days	Modifiers				
Mod	Non-Fac Total	Fac Total			51	50	62	80	MUE
	0.00	0.00	XXX		9	9	9	9	1

AMA: Aug 05: 9

82943 Glucagon [⊘][Q4]

	RVU			Global Days	Modifiers				
Mod	Non-Fac Total	Fac Total			51	50	62	80	MUE
	0.00	0.00	XXX		9	9	9	9	1

82945 Glucose, body fluid, other than blood [Q4]

	RVU			Global Days	Modifiers				
Mod	Non-Fac Total	Fac Total			51	50	62	80	MUE
	0.00	0.00	XXX		9	9	9	9	4

Pub 100-04, 16, 120.2

82946 Glucagon tolerance test [Q4]

	RVU			Global Days	Modifiers				
Mod	Non-Fac Total	Fac Total			51	50	62	80	MUE
	0.00	0.00	XXX		9	9	9	9	1

82947 Glucose; quantitative, blood (except reagent strip) [A]

Coding tip: For a CLIA-waived test, append modifier QW to 82947

	RVU			Global Days	Modifiers				
Mod	Non-Fac Total	Fac Total			51	50	62	80	MUE
	0.00	0.00	XXX		9	9	9	9	5

AMA: Summer 93: 14, Summer 94: 5, Sep 99: 10, Dec 99: 2, Jun 02: 3, Feb 05: 9, Apr 13: 10
Pub 100-04, 16, 120.2
NCD: 190.20B

82948 Glucose; blood, reagent strip [Q4]

	RVU			Global Days	Modifiers				
Mod	Non-Fac Total	Fac Total			51	50	62	80	MUE
	0.00	0.00	XXX		9	9	9	9	

AMA: Summer 94: 5, Jan 99: 10, Oct 11: 8, Nov 10: 10
Pub 100-04, 16, 120.2
NCD: 190.20A

● New   ▲ Revised   ✖ Deleted   ⊙ Moderate Sedation   ✚ Add-on Codes   ⊘ High Risk Denial   Ⓐ Age Edit   ♀ Female   ♂ Male   **AMA** *CPT® Assistant*   **MUE** Medically Unlikely Edit
⊘ Modifier 51 Exempt   ⊖ Modifier 63 Exempt   🅧 Unlisted   **Modifiers:** *See Inside Back Cover*   Ⓜ Maternity   A2–Z3 ASC Payment Indicators   A–Y OPPS Status Indicators

720   CPT © 2015 American Medical Association. All Rights Reserved.   © 2016 DecisionHealth

82950 Glucose; post glucose dose (includes glucose) [A]

Coding tip: For a CLIA-waived test, append modifier QW to 82950

RVU			Global Days	Modifiers				
Mod	Non-Fac Total	Fac Total		51	50	62	80	MUE
	0.00	0.00	XXX	9	9	9	9	3

AMA: Sep 99: 10, Jun 02: 3, Feb 05: 9

Pub 100-04, 18, 1.2, 90.1, 90.2, 90.2.1, 90.3, 90.5

82951 Glucose; tolerance test (GTT), 3 specimens (includes glucose) [A]

Coding tip: For a CLIA-waived test, append modifier QW to 82951

RVU			Global Days	Modifiers				
Mod	Non-Fac Total	Fac Total		51	50	62	80	MUE
	0.00	0.00	XXX	9	9	9	9	1

AMA: Feb 01: 10, Feb 05: 9, Oct 10: 7

Pub 100-04, 18, 1.2, 90.1, 90.2, 90.2.1, 90.3, 90.5

+ 82952 Glucose; tolerance test, each additional beyond 3 specimens (List separately in addition to code for primary procedure) [Q4]

Coding tip: For a CLIA-waived test, append modifier QW to 82952

RVU			Global Days	Modifiers				
Mod	Non-Fac Total	Fac Total		51	50	62	80	MUE
	0.00	0.00	XXX	9	9	9	9	3

AMA: Feb 01: 10, Oct 10: 7, Dec 10: 7

82955 Glucose-6-phosphate dehydrogenase (G6PD); quantitative [Q4]

RVU			Global Days	Modifiers				
Mod	Non-Fac Total	Fac Total		51	50	62	80	MUE
	0.00	0.00	XXX	9	9	9	9	1

82960 Glucose-6-phosphate dehydrogenase (G6PD); screen [Q4]

RVU			Global Days	Modifiers				
Mod	Non-Fac Total	Fac Total		51	50	62	80	MUE
	0.00	0.00	XXX	9	9	9	9	1

82962 Glucose, blood by glucose monitoring device(s) cleared by the FDA specifically for home use [Q4]

Coding tip: This is a CLIA-waived test, but does not require the use of modifier QW to be recognized as such

RVU			Global Days	Modifiers				
Mod	Non-Fac Total	Fac Total		51	50	62	80	MUE
	0.00	0.00	XXX	9	9	9	9	

AMA: Summer 94: 4, Jan 99: 10, Oct 11: 8, Nov 10: 10

82963 Glucosidase, beta [⊗Q4]

RVU			Global Days	Modifiers				
Mod	Non-Fac Total	Fac Total		51	50	62	80	MUE
	0.00	0.00	XXX	9	9	9	9	1

82965 Glutamate dehydrogenase [Q4]

RVU			Global Days	Modifiers				
Mod	Non-Fac Total	Fac Total		51	50	62	80	MUE
	0.00	0.00	XXX	9	9	9	9	1

82977 Glutamyltransferase, gamma (GGT) [Q4]

Coding tip: For a CLIA-waived test, append modifier QW to 82977

RVU			Global Days	Modifiers				
Mod	Non-Fac Total	Fac Total		51	50	62	80	MUE
	0.00	0.00	XXX	9	9	9	9	1

AMA: Dec 99: 1

Pub 100-04, 16, 90.2
NCD: 190.32

82978 Glutathione [Q4]

RVU			Global Days	Modifiers				
Mod	Non-Fac Total	Fac Total		51	50	62	80	MUE
	0.00	0.00	XXX	9	9	9	9	1

82979 Glutathione reductase, RBC [Q4]

RVU			Global Days	Modifiers				
Mod	Non-Fac Total	Fac Total		51	50	62	80	MUE
	0.00	0.00	XXX	9	9	9	9	1

82985 Glycated protein [Q4]

Coding tip: For a CLIA-waived test, append modifier QW to 82985

RVU			Global Days	Modifiers				
Mod	Non-Fac Total	Fac Total		51	50	62	80	MUE
	0.00	0.00	XXX	9	9	9	9	1

AMA: Summer 94: 2, Oct 10: 7
NCD: 190.21

83001 Gonadotropin; follicle stimulating hormone (FSH) [Q4]

Coding tip: For a CLIA-waived test, append modifier QW to 83001

RVU			Global Days	Modifiers				
Mod	Non-Fac Total	Fac Total		51	50	62	80	MUE
	0.00	0.00	XXX	9	9	9	9	1

AMA: Aug 05: 9, Oct 10: 7

83002 Gonadotropin; luteinizing hormone (LH) [Q4]

Coding tip: For a CLIA-waived test, append modifier QW to 83002

RVU			Global Days	Modifiers				
Mod	Non-Fac Total	Fac Total		51	50	62	80	MUE
	0.00	0.00	XXX	9	9	9	9	1

83003 Growth hormone, human (HGH) (somatotropin) [Q4]

RVU			Global Days	Modifiers				
Mod	Non-Fac Total	Fac Total		51	50	62	80	MUE
	0.00	0.00	XXX	9	9	9	9	5

83006 Growth stimulation expressed gene 2 (ST2, Interleukin 1 receptor like-1) [Q4]

RVU			Global Days	Modifiers				
Mod	Non-Fac Total	Fac Total		51	50	62	80	MUE
	0.00	0.00	XXX	9	9	9	9	1

83009 Helicobacter pylori, blood test analysis for urease activity, non-radioactive isotope (eg, C-13) [Q4]

RVU			Global Days	Modifiers				
Mod	Non-Fac Total	Fac Total		51	50	62	80	MUE
	0.00	0.00	XXX	9	9	9	9	1

83010 Haptoglobin; quantitative [Q4]

RVU			Global Days	Modifiers				
Mod	Non-Fac Total	Fac Total		51	50	62	80	MUE
	0.00	0.00	XXX	9	9	9	9	1

● New ▲ Revised Deleted ⊙ Moderate Sedation + Add-on Codes ⊘ High Risk Denial Ⓐ Age Edit ♀ Female ♂ Male **AMA** *CPT® Assistant* **MUE** Medically Unlikely Edit
⊘ Modifier 51 Exempt ⊖ Modifier 63 Exempt ✗ Unlisted **Modifiers:** *See Inside Back Cover* Ⓜ Maternity Ⓐ2–Ⓩ3 ASC Payment Indicators Ⓐ–Ⓨ OPPS Status Indicators

© 2016 DecisionHealth
CPT © 2015 American Medical Association. All Rights Reserved.

83012 Haptoglobin; phenotypes   Q4

Mod	Non-Fac Total	Fac Total	Global Days	51	50	62	80	MUE
	0.00	0.00	XXX	9	9	9	9	1

83013 Helicobacter pylori; breath test analysis for urease activity, non-radioactive isotope (eg, C-13)   Q4

Mod	Non-Fac Total	Fac Total	Global Days	51	50	62	80	MUE
	0.00	0.00	XXX	9	9	9	9	1

AMA: Nov 98: 25, Feb 99: 8, Nov 99: 45

83014 Helicobacter pylori; drug administration   Q4

Mod	Non-Fac Total	Fac Total	Global Days	51	50	62	80	MUE
	0.00	0.00	XXX	9	9	9	9	1

AMA: Nov 98: 25, Feb 99: 8, Nov 99: 45

83015 Heavy metal (eg, arsenic, barium, beryllium, bismuth, antimony, mercury); screen   Q4

Mod	Non-Fac Total	Fac Total	Global Days	51	50	62	80	MUE
	0.00	0.00	XXX	9	9	9	9	1

83018 Heavy metal (eg, arsenic, barium, beryllium, bismuth, antimony, mercury); quantitative, each   Q4

Mod	Non-Fac Total	Fac Total	Global Days	51	50	62	80	MUE
	0.00	0.00	XXX	9	9	9	9	4

83020 Hemoglobin fractionation and quantitation; electrophoresis (eg, A2, S, C, and/or F)   Q4

Mod	Non-Fac Total	Fac Total	Global Days	51	50	62	80	MUE
	0.00	0.00	XXX	9	9	9	9	2
26	0.52	0.52	XXX	0	0	0	0	2

AMA: Nov 98: 25

83021 Hemoglobin fractionation and quantitation; chromatography (eg, A2, S, C, and/or F)   Q4

Mod	Non-Fac Total	Fac Total	Global Days	51	50	62	80	MUE
	0.00	0.00	XXX	9	9	9	9	2

AMA: Nov 98: 25, Dec 99: 7

83026 Hemoglobin; by copper sulfate method, non-automated   Q4

Coding tip: This is a CLIA-waived test, but does not require the use of modifier QW to be recognized as such

Mod	Non-Fac Total	Fac Total	Global Days	51	50	62	80	MUE
	0.00	0.00	XXX	9	9	9	9	1

83030 Hemoglobin; F (fetal), chemical   M Q4

Mod	Non-Fac Total	Fac Total	Global Days	51	50	62	80	MUE
	0.00	0.00	XXX	9	9	9	9	1

83033 Hemoglobin; F (fetal), qualitative   M Q4

Mod	Non-Fac Total	Fac Total	Global Days	51	50	62	80	MUE
	0.00	0.00	XXX	9	9	9	9	1

83036 Hemoglobin; glycosylated (A1C)   Q4

Coding tip: For a CLIA-waived test, append modifier QW to 83036

Mod	Non-Fac Total	Fac Total	Global Days	51	50	62	80	MUE
	0.00	0.00	XXX	9	9	9	9	1

AMA: Summer 94: 2, Feb 06: 7, Oct 06: 15

83037 Hemoglobin; glycosylated (A1C) by device cleared by FDA for home use   Q4

Coding tip: For a CLIA-waived test, append modifier QW to 83037

Mod	Non-Fac Total	Fac Total	Global Days	51	50	62	80	MUE
	0.00	0.00	XXX	9	9	9	9	1

AMA: Feb 06: 7, Oct 06: 15

83045 Hemoglobin; methemoglobin, qualitative   Q4

Mod	Non-Fac Total	Fac Total	Global Days	51	50	62	80	MUE
	0.00	0.00	XXX	9	9	9	9	1

83050 Hemoglobin; methemoglobin, quantitative   Q4

Mod	Non-Fac Total	Fac Total	Global Days	51	50	62	80	MUE
	0.00	0.00	XXX	9	9	9	9	1

83051 Hemoglobin; plasma   Q4

Mod	Non-Fac Total	Fac Total	Global Days	51	50	62	80	MUE
	0.00	0.00	XXX	9	9	9	9	1

83060 Hemoglobin; sulfhemoglobin, quantitative   Q4

Mod	Non-Fac Total	Fac Total	Global Days	51	50	62	80	MUE
	0.00	0.00	XXX	9	9	9	9	1

83065 Hemoglobin; thermolabile   Q4

Mod	Non-Fac Total	Fac Total	Global Days	51	50	62	80	MUE
	0.00	0.00	XXX	9	9	9	9	1

83068 Hemoglobin; unstable, screen   Q4

Mod	Non-Fac Total	Fac Total	Global Days	51	50	62	80	MUE
	0.00	0.00	XXX	9	9	9	9	1

83069 Hemoglobin; urine   Q4

Mod	Non-Fac Total	Fac Total	Global Days	51	50	62	80	MUE
	0.00	0.00	XXX	9	9	9	9	1

83070 Hemosiderin, qualitative   Q4

Mod	Non-Fac Total	Fac Total	Global Days	51	50	62	80	MUE
	0.00	0.00	XXX	9	9	9	9	1

83080 b-Hexosaminidase, each assay   Q4

Mod	Non-Fac Total	Fac Total	Global Days	51	50	62	80	MUE
	0.00	0.00	XXX	9	9	9	9	2

AMA: Nov 98: 25

● New   ▲ Revised   ✖ Deleted   ⊙ Moderate Sedation   ✚ Add-on Codes   ⊗ High Risk Denial   Ⓐ Age Edit   ♀ Female   ♂ Male   **AMA** *CPT® Assistant*   **MUE** Medically Unlikely Edit

⊘ Modifier 51 Exempt   ⊖ Modifier 63 Exempt   ✗ Unlisted   **Modifiers:** *See Inside Back Cover*   Ⓜ Maternity   A2–Z3 ASC Payment Indicators   A–Y OPPS Status Indicators

722   CPT © 2015 American Medical Association. All Rights Reserved.   © 2016 DecisionHealth

83088 Histamine Q4

RVU			Global Days	Modifiers				
Mod	Non-Fac Total	Fac Total		51	50	62	80	MUE
	0.00	0.00	XXX	9	9	9	9	1

83090 Homocysteine Q4

RVU			Global Days	Modifiers				
Mod	Non-Fac Total	Fac Total		51	50	62	80	MUE
	0.00	0.00	XXX	9	9	9	9	2

AMA: Jan 01: 13, Oct 10: 7

83150 Homovanillic acid (HVA) Q4

RVU			Global Days	Modifiers				
Mod	Non-Fac Total	Fac Total		51	50	62	80	MUE
	0.00	0.00	XXX	9	9	9	9	1

AMA: Aug 05: 9, Oct 10: 7

83491 Hydroxycorticosteroids, 17- (17-OHCS) Q4

RVU			Global Days	Modifiers				
Mod	Non-Fac Total	Fac Total		51	50	62	80	MUE
	0.00	0.00	XXX	9	9	9	9	1

AMA: Aug 05: 9, Oct 10: 7

83497 Hydroxyindolacetic acid, 5-(HIAA) Q4

RVU			Global Days	Modifiers				
Mod	Non-Fac Total	Fac Total		51	50	62	80	MUE
	0.00	0.00	XXX	9	9	9	9	1

83498 Hydroxyprogesterone, 17-d Q4

RVU			Global Days	Modifiers				
Mod	Non-Fac Total	Fac Total		51	50	62	80	MUE
	0.00	0.00	XXX	9	9	9	9	2

83499 Hydroxyprogesterone, 20- Q4

RVU			Global Days	Modifiers				
Mod	Non-Fac Total	Fac Total		51	50	62	80	MUE
	0.00	0.00	XXX	9	9	9	9	1

AMA: Oct 10: 7

83500 Hydroxyproline; free Q4

RVU			Global Days	Modifiers				
Mod	Non-Fac Total	Fac Total		51	50	62	80	MUE
	0.00	0.00	XXX	9	9	9	9	1

AMA: Aug 05: 9, Oct 10: 7

83505 Hydroxyproline; total Q4

RVU			Global Days	Modifiers				
Mod	Non-Fac Total	Fac Total		51	50	62	80	MUE
	0.00	0.00	XXX	9	9	9	9	1

83516 Immunoassay for analyte other than infectious agent antibody or infectious agent antigen; qualitative or semiquantitative, multiple step method Q4

RVU			Global Days	Modifiers				
Mod	Non-Fac Total	Fac Total		51	50	62	80	MUE
	0.00	0.00	XXX	9	9	9	9	4

AMA: Nov 98: 25

83518 Immunoassay for analyte other than infectious agent antibody or infectious agent antigen; qualitative or semiquantitative, single step method (eg, reagent strip) Q4

RVU			Global Days	Modifiers				
Mod	Non-Fac Total	Fac Total		51	50	62	80	MUE
	0.00	0.00	XXX	9	9	9	9	1

AMA: Fall 93: 26

83519 Immunoassay for analyte other than infectious agent antibody or infectious agent antigen; quantitative, by radioimmunoassay (eg, RIA) Q4

RVU			Global Days	Modifiers				
Mod	Non-Fac Total	Fac Total		51	50	62	80	MUE
	0.00	0.00	XXX	9	9	9	9	5

AMA: Fall 93: 26, Summer 94: 2

83520 Immunoassay for analyte other than infectious agent antibody or infectious agent antigen; quantitative, not otherwise specified Q4

RVU			Global Days	Modifiers				
Mod	Non-Fac Total	Fac Total		51	50	62	80	MUE
	0.00	0.00	XXX	9	9	9	9	8

AMA: Fall 93: 26

83525 Insulin; total Q4

RVU			Global Days	Modifiers				
Mod	Non-Fac Total	Fac Total		51	50	62	80	MUE
	0.00	0.00	XXX	9	9	9	9	4

83527 Insulin; free Q4

RVU			Global Days	Modifiers				
Mod	Non-Fac Total	Fac Total		51	50	62	80	MUE
	0.00	0.00	XXX	9	9	9	9	1

AMA: Summer 94: 5

83528 Intrinsic factor Q4

RVU			Global Days	Modifiers				
Mod	Non-Fac Total	Fac Total		51	50	62	80	MUE
	0.00	0.00	XXX	9	9	9	9	1

83540 Iron Q4

RVU			Global Days	Modifiers				
Mod	Non-Fac Total	Fac Total		51	50	62	80	MUE
	0.00	0.00	XXX	9	9	9	9	2

AMA: Fall 93: 25

83550 Iron binding capacity Q4

RVU			Global Days	Modifiers				
Mod	Non-Fac Total	Fac Total		51	50	62	80	MUE
	0.00	0.00	XXX	9	9	9	9	1

Pub 100-04, 16, 120.2

83570 Isocitric dehydrogenase (IDH) Q4

RVU			Global Days	Modifiers				
Mod	Non-Fac Total	Fac Total		51	50	62	80	MUE
	0.00	0.00	XXX	9	9	9	9	1

83582 Ketogenic steroids, fractionation Q4

RVU			Global Days	Modifiers				
Mod	Non-Fac Total	Fac Total		51	50	62	80	MUE
	0.00	0.00	XXX	9	9	9	9	1

● New ▲ Revised Deleted ⊙ Moderate Sedation ✚ Add-on Codes ⊘ High Risk Denial Ⓐ Age Edit ♀ Female ♂ Male **AMA** *CPT® Assistant* **MUE** Medically Unlikely Edit
⊘ Modifier 51 Exempt ⊝ Modifier 63 Exempt Ⓧ Unlisted **Modifiers:** *See Inside Back Cover* Ⓜ Maternity A2–Z3 ASC Payment Indicators A–Y OPPS Status Indicators
© 2016 DecisionHealth CPT © 2015 American Medical Association. All Rights Reserved.

83586 Ketosteroids, 17- (17-KS); total �Q4

RVU			Global Days	Modifiers				
Mod	Non-Fac Total	Fac Total		51	50	62	80	MUE
	0.00	0.00	XXX	9	9	9	9	1

83593 Ketosteroids, 17- (17-KS); fractionation ⊘Q4

RVU			Global Days	Modifiers				
Mod	Non-Fac Total	Fac Total		51	50	62	80	MUE
	0.00	0.00	XXX	9	9	9	9	1

AMA: Oct 10: 7

83605 Lactate (lactic acid) Q4

Coding tip: For a CLIA-waived test, add modifier QW to 83605

RVU			Global Days	Modifiers				
Mod	Non-Fac Total	Fac Total		51	50	62	80	MUE
	0.00	0.00	XXX	9	9	9	9	3

AMA: Aug 05: 9, Oct 10: 7

83615 Lactate dehydrogenase (LD), (LDH) Q4

RVU			Global Days	Modifiers				
Mod	Non-Fac Total	Fac Total		51	50	62	80	MUE
	0.00	0.00	XXX	9	9	9	9	2

AMA: Fall 93: 25, Feb 98: 1, Dec 99: 2

83625 Lactate dehydrogenase (LD), (LDH); isoenzymes, separation and quantitation Q4

RVU			Global Days	Modifiers				
Mod	Non-Fac Total	Fac Total		51	50	62	80	MUE
	0.00	0.00	XXX	9	9	9	9	1

AMA: Fall 93: 25, Feb 98: 1

83630 Lactoferrin, fecal; qualitative Q4

RVU			Global Days	Modifiers				
Mod	Non-Fac Total	Fac Total		51	50	62	80	MUE
	0.00	0.00	XXX	9	9	9	9	1

AMA: Feb 06: 7

83631 Lactoferrin, fecal; quantitative Q4

RVU			Global Days	Modifiers				
Mod	Non-Fac Total	Fac Total		51	50	62	80	MUE
	0.00	0.00	XXX	9	9	9	9	1

AMA: Feb 06: 7, Jan 07: 29

83632 Lactogen, human placental (HPL) human chorionic somatomammotropin Q4

RVU			Global Days	Modifiers				
Mod	Non-Fac Total	Fac Total		51	50	62	80	MUE
	0.00	0.00	XXX	9	9	9	9	1

83633 Lactose, urine, qualitative Q4

RVU			Global Days	Modifiers				
Mod	Non-Fac Total	Fac Total		51	50	62	80	MUE
	0.00	0.00	XXX	9	9	9	9	1

83655 Lead Q4

Coding tip: For a CLIA-waived test, append modifier QW to 83655

RVU			Global Days	Modifiers				
Mod	Non-Fac Total	Fac Total		51	50	62	80	MUE
	0.00	0.00	XXX	9	9	9	9	2

83661 Fetal lung maturity assessment; lecithin sphingomyelin (L/S) ratio Ⓜ Q4

RVU			Global Days	Modifiers				
Mod	Non-Fac Total	Fac Total		51	50	62	80	MUE
	0.00	0.00	XXX	9	9	9	9	3

83662 Fetal lung maturity assessment; foam stability test Q4

RVU			Global Days	Modifiers				
Mod	Non-Fac Total	Fac Total		51	50	62	80	MUE
	0.00	0.00	XXX	9	9	9	9	4

83663 Fetal lung maturity assessment; fluorescence polarization Ⓜ Q4

RVU			Global Days	Modifiers				
Mod	Non-Fac Total	Fac Total		51	50	62	80	MUE
	0.00	0.00	XXX	9	9	9	9	3

83664 Fetal lung maturity assessment; lamellar body density ⊘Q4

RVU			Global Days	Modifiers				
Mod	Non-Fac Total	Fac Total		51	50	62	80	MUE
	0.00	0.00	XXX	9	9	9	9	3

83670 Leucine aminopeptidase (LAP) Q4

RVU			Global Days	Modifiers				
Mod	Non-Fac Total	Fac Total		51	50	62	80	MUE
	0.00	0.00	XXX	9	9	9	9	1

83690 Lipase Q4

RVU			Global Days	Modifiers				
Mod	Non-Fac Total	Fac Total		51	50	62	80	MUE
	0.00	0.00	XXX	9	9	9	9	2

83695 Lipoprotein (a) Q4

RVU			Global Days	Modifiers				
Mod	Non-Fac Total	Fac Total		51	50	62	80	MUE
	0.00	0.00	XXX	9	9	9	9	1

AMA: Feb 06: 7

83698 Lipoprotein-associated phospholipase A2 (Lp-PLA2) Q4

RVU			Global Days	Modifiers				
Mod	Non-Fac Total	Fac Total		51	50	62	80	MUE
	0.00	0.00	XXX	9	9	9	9	1

AMA: Oct 10: 7

83700 Lipoprotein, blood; electrophoretic separation and quantitation Q4

RVU			Global Days	Modifiers				
Mod	Non-Fac Total	Fac Total		51	50	62	80	MUE
	0.00	0.00	XXX	9	9	9	9	1

AMA: Feb 06: 7, Oct 10: 7
NCD: 190.23A

83701 Lipoprotein, blood; high resolution fractionation and quantitation of lipoproteins including lipoprotein subclasses when performed (eg, electrophoresis, ultracentrifugation) ⊘Q4

RVU			Global Days	Modifiers				
Mod	Non-Fac Total	Fac Total		51	50	62	80	MUE
	0.00	0.00	XXX	9	9	9	9	1

AMA: Feb 06: 7

● New ▲ Revised ✖ Deleted ⊙ Moderate Sedation ✚ Add-on Codes ⊘ High Risk Denial Ⓐ Age Edit ♀ Female ♂ Male **AMA** *CPT® Assistant* **MUE** Medically Unlikely Edit
⊘ Modifier 51 Exempt ⊖ Modifier 63 Exempt ✖ Unlisted **Modifiers:** *See Inside Back Cover* Ⓜ Maternity A2–Z3 ASC Payment Indicators A–Y OPPS Status Indicators

724 | CPT © 2015 American Medical Association. All Rights Reserved. | © 2016 DecisionHealth

83704 Lipoprotein, blood; quantitation of lipoprotein particle numbers and lipoprotein particle subclasses (eg, by nuclear magnetic resonance spectroscopy) Q4

RVU			Global Days	Modifiers				
Mod	Non-Fac Total	Fac Total		51	50	62	80	MUE
	0.00	0.00	XXX	9	9	9	9	1

AMA: Feb 06: 7

83718 Lipoprotein, direct measurement; high density cholesterol (HDL cholesterol) A

Coding tip: For a CLIA-waived test, append modifier QW to 83718

RVU			Global Days	Modifiers				
Mod	Non-Fac Total	Fac Total		51	50	62	80	MUE
	0.00	0.00	XXX	9	9	9	9	1

AMA: Oct 99: 11, Mar 00: 11, Feb 05: 9

Pub 100-04, 16, 90.2; 100-04, 18, 1.2, 100.1, 100.2, 100.3, 100.5

83719 Lipoprotein, direct measurement; VLDL cholesterol Q4

RVU			Global Days	Modifiers				
Mod	Non-Fac Total	Fac Total		51	50	62	80	MUE
	0.00	0.00	XXX	9	9	9	9	1

AMA: Oct 99: 11

83721 Lipoprotein, direct measurement; LDL cholesterol Q4

Coding tip: For a CLIA-waived test, append modifier QW to 83721

RVU			Global Days	Modifiers				
Mod	Non-Fac Total	Fac Total		51	50	62	80	MUE
	0.00	0.00	XXX	9	9	9	9	1

AMA: Nov 98: 25, Oct 99: 11

83727 Luteinizing releasing factor (LRH) Q4

RVU			Global Days	Modifiers				
Mod	Non-Fac Total	Fac Total		51	50	62	80	MUE
	0.00	0.00	XXX	9	9	9	9	1

83735 Magnesium Q4

RVU			Global Days	Modifiers				
Mod	Non-Fac Total	Fac Total		51	50	62	80	MUE
	0.00	0.00	XXX	9	9	9	9	4

Pub 100-04, 16, 120.2

83775 Malate dehydrogenase Q4

RVU			Global Days	Modifiers				
Mod	Non-Fac Total	Fac Total		51	50	62	80	MUE
	0.00	0.00	XXX	9	9	9	9	1

83785 Manganese Q4

RVU			Global Days	Modifiers				
Mod	Non-Fac Total	Fac Total		51	50	62	80	MUE
	0.00	0.00	XXX	9	9	9	9	1

✖ ~~83788 Mass spectrometry and tandem mass spectrometry (MS, MS/MS), analyte not elsewhere specified; qualitative, each specimen~~

▲ **83789 Mass spectrometry and tandem mass spectrometry (eg, MS, MS/MS, MALDI, MS-TOF, QTOF), non-drug analyte(s) not elsewhere specified, qualitative or quantitative, each specimen** Q4

RVU			Global Days	Modifiers				
Mod	Non-Fac Total	Fac Total		51	50	62	80	MUE
	0.00	0.00	XXX	9	9	9	9	4

AMA: Nov 98: 26, Oct 10: 7

83825 Mercury, quantitative Q4

RVU			Global Days	Modifiers				
Mod	Non-Fac Total	Fac Total		51	50	62	80	MUE
	0.00	0.00	XXX	9	9	9	9	2

83835 Metanephrines Q4

RVU			Global Days	Modifiers				
Mod	Non-Fac Total	Fac Total		51	50	62	80	MUE
	0.00	0.00	XXX	9	9	9	9	2

83857 Methemalbumin Q4

RVU			Global Days	Modifiers				
Mod	Non-Fac Total	Fac Total		51	50	62	80	MUE
	0.00	0.00	XXX	9	9	9	9	1

83861 Microfluidic analysis utilizing an integrated collection and analysis device, tear osmolarity Q4

Coding tip: For a CLIA-waived test, add modifier QW to 83861

RVU			Global Days	Modifiers				
Mod	Non-Fac Total	Fac Total		51	50	62	80	MUE
	0.00	0.00	XXX	9	9	9	9	2

AMA: Dec 10: 7

83864 Mucopolysaccharides, acid, quantitative Q4

RVU			Global Days	Modifiers				
Mod	Non-Fac Total	Fac Total		51	50	62	80	MUE
	0.00	0.00	XXX	9	9	9	9	1

83872 Mucin, synovial fluid (Ropes test) Q4

RVU			Global Days	Modifiers				
Mod	Non-Fac Total	Fac Total		51	50	62	80	MUE
	0.00	0.00	XXX	9	9	9	9	2

83873 Myelin basic protein, cerebrospinal fluid Q4

RVU			Global Days	Modifiers				
Mod	Non-Fac Total	Fac Total		51	50	62	80	MUE
	0.00	0.00	XXX	9	9	9	9	1

83874 Myoglobin Q4

RVU			Global Days	Modifiers				
Mod	Non-Fac Total	Fac Total		51	50	62	80	MUE
	0.00	0.00	XXX	9	9	9	9	2

AMA: Feb 98: 1

83876 Myeloperoxidase (MPO) Q4

RVU			Global Days	Modifiers				
Mod	Non-Fac Total	Fac Total		51	50	62	80	MUE
	0.00	0.00	XXX	9	9	9	9	1

83880 Natriuretic peptide Q4

Coding tip: For a CLIA-waived test, append modifier QW to 83880

RVU			Global Days	Modifiers				
Mod	Non-Fac Total	Fac Total		51	50	62	80	MUE
	0.00	0.00	XXX	9	9	9	9	1

● New   ▲ Revised   Deleted   ⊙ Moderate Sedation   ✚ Add-on Codes   ⊘ High Risk Denial   Ⓐ Age Edit   ♀ Female   ♂ Male   **AMA** CPT® Assistant   **MUE** Medically Unlikely Edit
⊘ Modifier 51 Exempt   ⊖ Modifier 63 Exempt   ✗ Unlisted   **Modifiers:** See Inside Back Cover   Ⓜ Maternity   A2–Z3 ASC Payment Indicators   A –Y OPPS Status Indicators

© 2016 DecisionHealth   CPT © 2015 American Medical Association. All Rights Reserved.   **725**

AMA: Jul 03: 7

83883 Nephelometry, each analyte not elsewhere specified ▣4

Mod	Non-Fac Total	Fac Total	Global Days	51	50	62	80	MUE
	0.00	0.00	XXX	9	9	9	9	6

83885 Nickel ▣4

Mod	Non-Fac Total	Fac Total	Global Days	51	50	62	80	MUE
	0.00	0.00	XXX	9	9	9	9	2

83915 Nucleotidase 5'- ▣4

Mod	Non-Fac Total	Fac Total	Global Days	51	50	62	80	MUE
	0.00	0.00	XXX	9	9	9	9	1

83916 Oligoclonal immune (oligoclonal bands) ▣4

Mod	Non-Fac Total	Fac Total	Global Days	51	50	62	80	MUE
	0.00	0.00	XXX	9	9	9	9	2

83918 Organic acids; total, quantitative, each specimen ▣4

Mod	Non-Fac Total	Fac Total	Global Days	51	50	62	80	MUE
	0.00	0.00	XXX	9	9	9	9	2

AMA: Mar 96: 11, Nov 98: 26

83919 Organic acids; qualitative, each specimen ▣4

Mod	Non-Fac Total	Fac Total	Global Days	51	50	62	80	MUE
	0.00	0.00	XXX	9	9	9	9	1

AMA: Nov 98: 26

83921 Organic acid, single, quantitative ▣4

Mod	Non-Fac Total	Fac Total	Global Days	51	50	62	80	MUE
	0.00	0.00	XXX	9	9	9	9	2

83930 Osmolality; blood ▣4

Mod	Non-Fac Total	Fac Total	Global Days	51	50	62	80	MUE
	0.00	0.00	XXX	9	9	9	9	2

83935 Osmolality; urine ▣4

Mod	Non-Fac Total	Fac Total	Global Days	51	50	62	80	MUE
	0.00	0.00	XXX	9	9	9	9	2

83937 Osteocalcin (bone g1a protein) ▣4

Mod	Non-Fac Total	Fac Total	Global Days	51	50	62	80	MUE
	0.00	0.00	XXX	9	9	9	9	1

AMA: Summer 94: 5
Pub 100-04, 16, 120.2

83945 Oxalate ▣4

Mod	Non-Fac Total	Fac Total	Global Days	51	50	62	80	MUE
	0.00	0.00	XXX	9	9	9	9	2

83950 Oncoprotein; HER-2/neu ▣4

Mod	Non-Fac Total	Fac Total	Global Days	51	50	62	80	MUE
	0.00	0.00	XXX	9	9	9	9	1

83951 Oncoprotein; des-gamma-carboxy-prothrombin (DCP) ▣4

Mod	Non-Fac Total	Fac Total	Global Days	51	50	62	80	MUE
	0.00	0.00	XXX	9	9	9	9	1

83970 Parathormone (parathyroid hormone) ▣4

Mod	Non-Fac Total	Fac Total	Global Days	51	50	62	80	MUE
	0.00	0.00	XXX	9	9	9	9	2

Pub 100-04, 16, 120.2

83986 pH; body fluid, not otherwise specified ▣4

Coding tip: *For a CLIA-waived test, append modifier QW to 83986*

Mod	Non-Fac Total	Fac Total	Global Days	51	50	62	80	MUE
	0.00	0.00	XXX	9	9	9	9	2

AMA: Sep 13: 13
Pub 100-04, 16, 120.2

83987 pH; exhaled breath condensate ▣4

Mod	Non-Fac Total	Fac Total	Global Days	51	50	62	80	MUE
	0.00	0.00	XXX	9	9	9	9	1

83992 Phencyclidine (PCP) ▣4

Mod	Non-Fac Total	Fac Total	Global Days	51	50	62	80	MUE
	0.00	0.00	XXX	9	9	9	9	2

AMA: Apr 15: 3

83993 Calprotectin, fecal ▣4

Mod	Non-Fac Total	Fac Total	Global Days	51	50	62	80	MUE
	0.00	0.00	XXX	9	9	9	9	1

AMA: Apr 08: 5, Oct 10: 7

84030 Phenylalanine (PKU), blood ▣4

Mod	Non-Fac Total	Fac Total	Global Days	51	50	62	80	MUE
	0.00	0.00	XXX	9	9	9	9	1

84035 Phenylketones, qualitative ⊘▣4

Mod	Non-Fac Total	Fac Total	Global Days	51	50	62	80	MUE
	0.00	0.00	XXX	9	9	9	9	1

84060 Phosphatase, acid; total ▣4

Mod	Non-Fac Total	Fac Total	Global Days	51	50	62	80	MUE
	0.00	0.00	XXX	9	9	9	9	1

84061 Phosphatase, acid; forensic examination ▣4

Mod	Non-Fac Total	Fac Total	Global Days	51	50	62	80	MUE
	0.00	0.00	XXX	9	9	9	9	1

● New   ▲ Revised   ✖ Deleted   ⊙ Moderate Sedation   ✚ Add-on Codes   ⊗ High Risk Denial   Ⓐ Age Edit   ♀ Female   ♂ Male   **AMA** *CPT® Assistant*   **MUE** Medically Unlikely Edit
⊘ Modifier 51 Exempt   ⊖ Modifier 63 Exempt   ✖ Unlisted   **Modifiers:** *See Inside Back Cover*   Ⓜ Maternity   A2–Z3 ASC Payment Indicators   A–Y OPPS Status Indicators

84066 Phosphatase, acid; prostatic Q4

Mod	Non-Fac Total	Fac Total	Global Days	51	50	62	80	MUE
	0.00	0.00	XXX	9	9	9	9	1

84075 Phosphatase, alkaline Q4

Coding tip: For a CLIA-waived test, append modifier QW to 84075

Mod	Non-Fac Total	Fac Total	Global Days	51	50	62	80	MUE
	0.00	0.00	XXX	9	9	9	9	2

AMA: Dec 99: 2

Pub 100-04, 16, 90.2, 120.2

84078 Phosphatase, alkaline; heat stable (total not included) Q4

Mod	Non-Fac Total	Fac Total	Global Days	51	50	62	80	MUE
	0.00	0.00	XXX	9	9	9	9	1

84080 Phosphatase, alkaline; isoenzymes Q4

Mod	Non-Fac Total	Fac Total	Global Days	51	50	62	80	MUE
	0.00	0.00	XXX	9	9	9	9	1

84081 Phosphatidylglycerol Q4

Mod	Non-Fac Total	Fac Total	Global Days	51	50	62	80	MUE
	0.00	0.00	XXX	9	9	9	9	1

84085 Phosphogluconate, 6-, dehydrogenase, RBC Q4

Mod	Non-Fac Total	Fac Total	Global Days	51	50	62	80	MUE
	0.00	0.00	XXX	9	9	9	9	1

84087 Phosphohexose isomerase Q4

Mod	Non-Fac Total	Fac Total	Global Days	51	50	62	80	MUE
	0.00	0.00	XXX	9	9	9	9	1

AMA: Oct 10: 7

84100 Phosphorus inorganic (phosphate) Q4

Mod	Non-Fac Total	Fac Total	Global Days	51	50	62	80	MUE
	0.00	0.00	XXX	9	9	9	9	2

AMA: Dec 99: 2, Aug 05: 9, Oct 10: 7

Pub 100-04, 16, 120.2

84105 Phosphorus inorganic (phosphate); urine Q4

Mod	Non-Fac Total	Fac Total	Global Days	51	50	62	80	MUE
	0.00	0.00	XXX	9	9	9	9	1

Pub 100-04, 16, 120.2

84106 Porphobilinogen, urine; qualitative Q4

Mod	Non-Fac Total	Fac Total	Global Days	51	50	62	80	MUE
	0.00	0.00	XXX	9	9	9	9	1

84110 Porphobilinogen, urine; quantitative Q4

Mod	Non-Fac Total	Fac Total	Global Days	51	50	62	80	MUE
	0.00	0.00	XXX	9	9	9	9	1

84112 Evaluation of cervicovaginal fluid for specific amniotic fluid protein(s) (eg, placental alpha microglobulin-1 [PAMG-1], placental protein 12 [PP12], alpha-fetoprotein), qualitative, each specimen ♀Q4

Mod	Non-Fac Total	Fac Total	Global Days	51	50	62	80	MUE
	0.00	0.00	XXX	9	9	9	9	1

AMA: Oct 10: 8, Dec 10: 8

84119 Porphyrins, urine; qualitative Q4

Mod	Non-Fac Total	Fac Total	Global Days	51	50	62	80	MUE
	0.00	0.00	XXX	9	9	9	9	1

84120 Porphyrins, urine; quantitation and fractionation Q4

Mod	Non-Fac Total	Fac Total	Global Days	51	50	62	80	MUE
	0.00	0.00	XXX	9	9	9	9	1

84126 Porphyrins, feces, quantitative Q4

Mod	Non-Fac Total	Fac Total	Global Days	51	50	62	80	MUE
	0.00	0.00	XXX	9	9	9	9	1

84132 Potassium; serum, plasma or whole blood Q4

Coding tip: For a CLIA-waived test, append modifier QW to 84132

Mod	Non-Fac Total	Fac Total	Global Days	51	50	62	80	MUE
	0.00	0.00	XXX	9	9	9	9	2

AMA: Dec 99: 2, Jun 02: 3, Apr 13: 10

Pub 100-04, 16, 120.2

84133 Potassium; urine Q4

Mod	Non-Fac Total	Fac Total	Global Days	51	50	62	80	MUE
	0.00	0.00	XXX	9	9	9	9	2

Pub 100-04, 16, 120.2

84134 Prealbumin Q4

Mod	Non-Fac Total	Fac Total	Global Days	51	50	62	80	MUE
	0.00	0.00	XXX	9	9	9	9	1

Pub 100-04, 16, 120.2

84135 Pregnanediol ♀Q4

Mod	Non-Fac Total	Fac Total	Global Days	51	50	62	80	MUE
	0.00	0.00	XXX	9	9	9	9	1

84138 Pregnanetriol ♀Q4

Mod	Non-Fac Total	Fac Total	Global Days	51	50	62	80	MUE
	0.00	0.00	XXX	9	9	9	9	1

84140 Pregnenolone Q4

Mod	Non-Fac Total	Fac Total	Global Days	51	50	62	80	MUE
	0.00	0.00	XXX	9	9	9	9	1

AMA: Summer 94: 6

● New ▲ Revised Deleted ⊙ Moderate Sedation ✛ Add-on Codes ⊘ High Risk Denial Ⓐ Age Edit ♀ Female ♂ Male **AMA** *CPT® Assistant* ***MUE*** Medically Unlikely Edit
⊘ Modifier 51 Exempt ⊖ Modifier 63 Exempt ✗ Unlisted **Modifiers:** *See Inside Back Cover* Ⓜ Maternity Ⓐ2–Ⓩ3 ASC Payment Indicators Ⓐ–Ⓨ OPPS Status Indicators

84143 17-hydroxypregnenolone   Q4

Mod	Non-Fac Total	Fac Total	Global Days	51	50	62	80	MUE
	0.00	0.00	XXX	9	9	9	9	2

AMA: Summer 94: 6

84144 Progesterone   Q4

Mod	Non-Fac Total	Fac Total	Global Days	51	50	62	80	MUE
	0.00	0.00	XXX	9	9	9	9	1

84145 Procalcitonin (PCT)   Q4

Mod	Non-Fac Total	Fac Total	Global Days	51	50	62	80	MUE
	0.00	0.00	XXX	9	9	9	9	1

84146 Prolactin   Q4

Mod	Non-Fac Total	Fac Total	Global Days	51	50	62	80	MUE
	0.00	0.00	XXX	9	9	9	9	3

84150 Prostaglandin, each   Q4

Mod	Non-Fac Total	Fac Total	Global Days	51	50	62	80	MUE
	0.00	0.00	XXX	9	9	9	9	2

84152 Prostate specific antigen (PSA); complexed (direct measurement)   ♂ Q4

Mod	Non-Fac Total	Fac Total	Global Days	51	50	62	80	MUE
	0.00	0.00	XXX	9	9	9	9	1

84153 Prostate specific antigen (PSA); total   ♂ Q4

Mod	Non-Fac Total	Fac Total	Global Days	51	50	62	80	MUE
	0.00	0.00	XXX	9	9	9	9	1

AMA: Fall 93: 26, May 96: 10, Aug 96: 10, Jan 97: 10, Nov 98: 26, Aug 99: 5, Dec 99: 10

Pub 100-04, 18, 50.3
NCD: 190.31

84154 Prostate specific antigen (PSA); free   ♂ Q4

Mod	Non-Fac Total	Fac Total	Global Days	51	50	62	80	MUE
	0.00	0.00	XXX	9	9	9	9	1

AMA: Nov 98: 26, Aug 99: 5, Dec 99: 10

84155 Protein, total, except by refractometry; serum, plasma or whole blood   Q4

Coding tip: For a CLIA-waived test, append modifier QW to 84155

Mod	Non-Fac Total	Fac Total	Global Days	51	50	62	80	MUE
	0.00	0.00	XXX	9	9	9	9	1

AMA: Dec 99: 2, Jan 00: 7

Pub 100-04, 16, 120.2

84156 Protein, total, except by refractometry; urine   Q4

Mod	Non-Fac Total	Fac Total	Global Days	51	50	62	80	MUE
	0.00	0.00	XXX	9	9	9	9	1

84157 Protein, total, except by refractometry; other source (eg, synovial fluid, cerebrospinal fluid)   Q4

Mod	Non-Fac Total	Fac Total	Global Days	51	50	62	80	MUE
	0.00	0.00	XXX	9	9	9	9	2

84160 Protein, total, by refractometry, any source   Q4

Mod	Non-Fac Total	Fac Total	Global Days	51	50	62	80	MUE
	0.00	0.00	XXX	9	9	9	9	2

Pub 100-04, 16, 120.2

84163 Pregnancy-associated plasma protein-A (PAPP-A)   ♀ M Q4

Mod	Non-Fac Total	Fac Total	Global Days	51	50	62	80	MUE
	0.00	0.00	XXX	9	9	9	9	1

84165 Protein; electrophoretic fractionation and quantitation, serum   Q4

Mod	Non-Fac Total	Fac Total	Global Days	51	50	62	80	MUE
	0.00	0.00	XXX	9	9	9	9	1
26	0.52	0.52	XXX	0	0	0	0	1

84166 Protein; electrophoretic fractionation and quantitation, other fluids with concentration (eg, urine, CSF)   Q4

Mod	Non-Fac Total	Fac Total	Global Days	51	50	62	80	MUE
	0.00	0.00	XXX	9	9	9	9	2
26	0.52	0.52	XXX	0	0	0	0	2

84181 Protein; Western Blot, with interpretation and report, blood or other body fluid   Q4

Mod	Non-Fac Total	Fac Total	Global Days	51	50	62	80	MUE
	0.00	0.00	XXX	9	9	9	9	3
26	0.52	0.52	XXX	0	0	0	0	3

84182 Protein; Western Blot, with interpretation and report, blood or other body fluid, immunological probe for band identification, each   Q4

Mod	Non-Fac Total	Fac Total	Global Days	51	50	62	80	MUE
	0.00	0.00	XXX	9	9	9	9	6
26	0.52	0.52	XXX	0	0	0	0	6

AMA: Oct 10: 7

84202 Protoporphyrin, RBC; quantitative   Q4

Mod	Non-Fac Total	Fac Total	Global Days	51	50	62	80	MUE
	0.00	0.00	XXX	9	9	9	9	1

AMA: Aug 05: 9, Oct 10: 7

84203 Protoporphyrin, RBC; screen   Q4

Mod	Non-Fac Total	Fac Total	Global Days	51	50	62	80	MUE
	0.00	0.00	XXX	9	9	9	9	1

84206 Proinsulin   Q4

Mod	Non-Fac Total	Fac Total	Global Days	51	50	62	80	MUE
	0.00	0.00	XXX	9	9	9	9	1

● New   ▲ Revised   ✖ Deleted   ⊙ Moderate Sedation   ✚ Add-on Codes   ⊘ High Risk Denial   Ⓐ Age Edit   ♀ Female   ♂ Male   **AMA** *CPT® Assistant*   **MUE** Medically Unlikely Edit
⊘ Modifier 51 Exempt   ⊖ Modifier 63 Exempt   ✖ Unlisted   **Modifiers:** *See Inside Back Cover*   M Maternity   A2–Z3 ASC Payment Indicators   A–Y OPPS Status Indicators

CPT © 2015 American Medical Association. All Rights Reserved.   © 2016 DecisionHealth

84207 Pyridoxal phosphate (Vitamin B-6) Q4

RVU Mod	Non-Fac Total	Fac Total	Global Days	Modifiers 51	50	62	80	MUE
	0.00	0.00	XXX	9	9	9	9	1

84210 Pyruvate Q4

RVU Mod	Non-Fac Total	Fac Total	Global Days	Modifiers 51	50	62	80	MUE
	0.00	0.00	XXX	9	9	9	9	1

84220 Pyruvate kinase Q4

RVU Mod	Non-Fac Total	Fac Total	Global Days	Modifiers 51	50	62	80	MUE
	0.00	0.00	XXX	9	9	9	9	1

84228 Quinine Q4

RVU Mod	Non-Fac Total	Fac Total	Global Days	Modifiers 51	50	62	80	MUE
	0.00	0.00	XXX	9	9	9	9	1

AMA: Apr 15: 3

84233 Receptor assay; estrogen Q4

RVU Mod	Non-Fac Total	Fac Total	Global Days	Modifiers 51	50	62	80	MUE
	0.00	0.00	XXX	9	9	9	9	1

84234 Receptor assay; progesterone Q4

RVU Mod	Non-Fac Total	Fac Total	Global Days	Modifiers 51	50	62	80	MUE
	0.00	0.00	XXX	9	9	9	9	1

84235 Receptor assay; endocrine, other than estrogen or progesterone (specify hormone) Q4

RVU Mod	Non-Fac Total	Fac Total	Global Days	Modifiers 51	50	62	80	MUE
	0.00	0.00	XXX	9	9	9	9	1

84238 Receptor assay; non-endocrine (specify receptor) Q4

RVU Mod	Non-Fac Total	Fac Total	Global Days	Modifiers 51	50	62	80	MUE
	0.00	0.00	XXX	9	9	9	9	3

AMA: Nov 05: 14

84244 Renin Q4

RVU Mod	Non-Fac Total	Fac Total	Global Days	Modifiers 51	50	62	80	MUE
	0.00	0.00	XXX	9	9	9	9	2

84252 Riboflavin (Vitamin B-2) Q4

RVU Mod	Non-Fac Total	Fac Total	Global Days	Modifiers 51	50	62	80	MUE
	0.00	0.00	XXX	9	9	9	9	1

84255 Selenium Q4

RVU Mod	Non-Fac Total	Fac Total	Global Days	Modifiers 51	50	62	80	MUE
	0.00	0.00	XXX	9	9	9	9	2

84260 Serotonin Q4

RVU Mod	Non-Fac Total	Fac Total	Global Days	Modifiers 51	50	62	80	MUE
	0.00	0.00	XXX	9	9	9	9	1

84270 Sex hormone binding globulin (SHBG) Q4

RVU Mod	Non-Fac Total	Fac Total	Global Days	Modifiers 51	50	62	80	MUE
	0.00	0.00	XXX	9	9	9	9	1

AMA: Summer 94: 4

84275 Sialic acid Q4

RVU Mod	Non-Fac Total	Fac Total	Global Days	Modifiers 51	50	62	80	MUE
	0.00	0.00	XXX	9	9	9	9	1

84285 Silica Q4

RVU Mod	Non-Fac Total	Fac Total	Global Days	Modifiers 51	50	62	80	MUE
	0.00	0.00	XXX	9	9	9	9	1

84295 Sodium; serum, plasma or whole blood Q4

Coding tip: *For a CLIA-waived test, append modifier QW to 84295*

RVU Mod	Non-Fac Total	Fac Total	Global Days	Modifiers 51	50	62	80	MUE
	0.00	0.00	XXX	9	9	9	9	3

AMA: Dec 99: 2, Oct 10: 7, Apr 13: 10

Pub 100-04, 16, 120.2

84300 Sodium; urine Q4

RVU Mod	Non-Fac Total	Fac Total	Global Days	Modifiers 51	50	62	80	MUE
	0.00	0.00	XXX	9	9	9	9	2

AMA: Aug 05: 9, Oct 10: 7

84302 Sodium; other source Q4

RVU Mod	Non-Fac Total	Fac Total	Global Days	Modifiers 51	50	62	80	MUE
	0.00	0.00	XXX	9	9	9	9	1

AMA: Jul 03: 7

84305 Somatomedin Q4

RVU Mod	Non-Fac Total	Fac Total	Global Days	Modifiers 51	50	62	80	MUE
	0.00	0.00	XXX	9	9	9	9	1

AMA: Summer 94: 4

84307 Somatostatin Q4

RVU Mod	Non-Fac Total	Fac Total	Global Days	Modifiers 51	50	62	80	MUE
	0.00	0.00	XXX	9	9	9	9	1

AMA: Summer 94: 4

84311 Spectrophotometry, analyte not elsewhere specified Q4

RVU Mod	Non-Fac Total	Fac Total	Global Days	Modifiers 51	50	62	80	MUE
	0.00	0.00	XXX	9	9	9	9	2

84315 Specific gravity (except urine) Q4

RVU Mod	Non-Fac Total	Fac Total	Global Days	Modifiers 51	50	62	80	MUE
	0.00	0.00	XXX	9	9	9	9	1

Pub 100-04, 16, 120.2

● New   ▲ Revised   Deleted   ⊙ Moderate Sedation   ✚ Add-on Codes   ⊘ High Risk Denial   Ⓐ Age Edit   ♀ Female   ♂ Male   **AMA** *CPT® Assistant*   **MUE** Medically Unlikely Edit
⊘ Modifier 51 Exempt   ⊖ Modifier 63 Exempt   ✗ Unlisted   **Modifiers:** *See Inside Back Cover*   Ⓜ Maternity   Ⓐ2–Ⓩ3 ASC Payment Indicators   Ⓐ–Ⓨ OPPS Status Indicators

© 2016 DecisionHealth   CPT © 2015 American Medical Association. All Rights Reserved.   **729**

84375 Sugars, chromatographic, TLC or paper chromatography ◘4

Mod	Non-Fac Total	Fac Total	Global Days	51	50	62	80	MUE
	0.00	0.00	XXX	9	9	9	9	1

84376 Sugars (mono-, di-, and oligosaccharides); single qualitative, each specimen ◘4

Mod	Non-Fac Total	Fac Total	Global Days	51	50	62	80	MUE
	0.00	0.00	XXX	9	9	9	9	1

AMA: Nov 98: 26, 27, Dec 99: 7

84377 Sugars (mono-, di-, and oligosaccharides); multiple qualitative, each specimen ◘4

Mod	Non-Fac Total	Fac Total	Global Days	51	50	62	80	MUE
	0.00	0.00	XXX	9	9	9	9	1

AMA: Nov 98: 26, 27, Jul 03: 7

84378 Sugars (mono-, di-, and oligosaccharides); single quantitative, each specimen ◘4

Mod	Non-Fac Total	Fac Total	Global Days	51	50	62	80	MUE
	0.00	0.00	XXX	9	9	9	9	2

AMA: Nov 98: 26, 27

84379 Sugars (mono-, di-, and oligosaccharides); multiple quantitative, each specimen ◘4

Mod	Non-Fac Total	Fac Total	Global Days	51	50	62	80	MUE
	0.00	0.00	XXX	9	9	9	9	1

AMA: Nov 98: 26, 27, Dec 99: 7, Jul 03: 7

84392 Sulfate, urine ◘4

Mod	Non-Fac Total	Fac Total	Global Days	51	50	62	80	MUE
	0.00	0.00	XXX	9	9	9	9	1

AMA: Oct 10: 7

84402 Testosterone; free ◘4

Mod	Non-Fac Total	Fac Total	Global Days	51	50	62	80	MUE
	0.00	0.00	XXX	9	9	9	9	1

AMA: Aug 05: 9, Oct 10: 7

84403 Testosterone; total ◘4

Mod	Non-Fac Total	Fac Total	Global Days	51	50	62	80	MUE
	0.00	0.00	XXX	9	9	9	9	2

84425 Thiamine (Vitamin B-1) ◘4

Mod	Non-Fac Total	Fac Total	Global Days	51	50	62	80	MUE
	0.00	0.00	XXX	9	9	9	9	1

84430 Thiocyanate ◘4

Mod	Non-Fac Total	Fac Total	Global Days	51	50	62	80	MUE
	0.00	0.00	XXX	9	9	9	9	1

84431 Thromboxane metabolite(s), including thromboxane if performed, urine ◘4

Mod	Non-Fac Total	Fac Total	Global Days	51	50	62	80	MUE
	0.00	0.00	XXX	9	9	9	9	1

84432 Thyroglobulin ◘4

Mod	Non-Fac Total	Fac Total	Global Days	51	50	62	80	MUE
	0.00	0.00	XXX	9	9	9	9	1

AMA: Summer 94: 2

84436 Thyroxine; total ◘4

Mod	Non-Fac Total	Fac Total	Global Days	51	50	62	80	MUE
	0.00	0.00	XXX	9	9	9	9	1

AMA: Fall 93: 25, Summer 94: 3
NCD: 190.22

84437 Thyroxine; requiring elution (eg, neonatal) ◘4

Mod	Non-Fac Total	Fac Total	Global Days	51	50	62	80	MUE
	0.00	0.00	XXX	9	9	9	9	1

84439 Thyroxine; free ◘4

Mod	Non-Fac Total	Fac Total	Global Days	51	50	62	80	MUE
	0.00	0.00	XXX	9	9	9	9	1

84442 Thyroxine binding globulin (TBG) ◘4

Mod	Non-Fac Total	Fac Total	Global Days	51	50	62	80	MUE
	0.00	0.00	XXX	9	9	9	9	1

84443 Thyroid stimulating hormone (TSH) ◘4

Coding tip: Thyroid hormone uptake or thyroid hormone binding ratio - 84479

Coding tip: For a CLIA-waived test, append modifier QW to 84443

Mod	Non-Fac Total	Fac Total	Global Days	51	50	62	80	MUE
	0.00	0.00	XXX	9	9	9	9	4

AMA: Summer 94: 3

84445 Thyroid stimulating immune globulins (TSI) ◘4

Mod	Non-Fac Total	Fac Total	Global Days	51	50	62	80	MUE
	0.00	0.00	XXX	9	9	9	9	1

AMA: Summer 94: 3

84446 Tocopherol alpha (Vitamin E) ◘4

Mod	Non-Fac Total	Fac Total	Global Days	51	50	62	80	MUE
	0.00	0.00	XXX	9	9	9	9	1

84449 Transcortin (cortisol binding globulin) ◘4

Mod	Non-Fac Total	Fac Total	Global Days	51	50	62	80	MUE
	0.00	0.00	XXX	9	9	9	9	1

AMA: Summer 94: 6

● New   ▲ Revised   ✖ Deleted   ⊙ Moderate Sedation   ✚ Add-on Codes   ⊘ High Risk Denial   Ⓐ Age Edit   ♀ Female   ♂ Male   **AMA** CPT® Assistant   **MUE** Medically Unlikely Edit
⊘ Modifier 51 Exempt   ⊖ Modifier 63 Exempt   ✗ Unlisted   **Modifiers:** See Inside Back Cover   Ⓜ Maternity   A2–Z3 ASC Payment Indicators   A–Y OPPS Status Indicators

730   CPT © 2015 American Medical Association. All Rights Reserved.   © 2016 DecisionHealth

84450 Transferase; aspartate amino (AST) (SGOT)   Q4

Coding tip: For a CLIA-waived test, append modifier QW to 84450

RVU			Global Days	Modifiers				
Mod	Non-Fac Total	Fac Total		51	50	62	80	MUE
	0.00	0.00	XXX	9	9	9	9	1

AMA: Dec 99: 2

Pub 100-04, 16, 90.2, 120.2

84460 Transferase; alanine amino (ALT) (SGPT)   Q4

Coding tip: For a CLIA-waived test, append modifier QW to 84460

RVU			Global Days	Modifiers				
Mod	Non-Fac Total	Fac Total		51	50	62	80	MUE
	0.00	0.00	XXX	9	9	9	9	1

AMA: Dec 99: 2

Pub 100-04, 16, 90.2, 120.2

84466 Transferrin   Q4

RVU			Global Days	Modifiers				
Mod	Non-Fac Total	Fac Total		51	50	62	80	MUE
	0.00	0.00	XXX	9	9	9	9	1

AMA: Summer 94: 4

Pub 100-04, 16, 120.2

84478 Triglycerides   A

Coding tip: For a CLIA-waived test, append modifier QW to 84478

RVU			Global Days	Modifiers				
Mod	Non-Fac Total	Fac Total		51	50	62	80	MUE
	0.00	0.00	XXX	9	9	9	9	1

AMA: Dec 99: 2, Mar 00: 11, Feb 05: 9

Pub 100-04, 18, 1.2, 100.1, 100.2, 100.3, 100.5

84479 Thyroid hormone (T3 or T4) uptake or thyroid hormone binding ratio (THBR)   Q4

Coding tip: This is a CLIA-waived test, but does not require the use of modifier QW to be recognized as such

RVU			Global Days	Modifiers				
Mod	Non-Fac Total	Fac Total		51	50	62	80	MUE
	0.00	0.00	XXX	9	9	9	9	1

AMA: Fall 93: 25, Summer 94: 3

84480 Triiodothyronine T3; total (TT-3)   Q4

RVU			Global Days	Modifiers				
Mod	Non-Fac Total	Fac Total		51	50	62	80	MUE
	0.00	0.00	XXX	9	9	9	9	1

84481 Triiodothyronine T3; free   Q4

RVU			Global Days	Modifiers				
Mod	Non-Fac Total	Fac Total		51	50	62	80	MUE
	0.00	0.00	XXX	9	9	9	9	1

84482 Triiodothyronine T3; reverse   Q4

RVU			Global Days	Modifiers				
Mod	Non-Fac Total	Fac Total		51	50	62	80	MUE
	0.00	0.00	XXX	9	9	9	9	1

AMA: Summer 94: 2

84484 Troponin, quantitative   Q4

RVU			Global Days	Modifiers				
Mod	Non-Fac Total	Fac Total		51	50	62	80	MUE
	0.00	0.00	XXX	9	9	9	9	2

AMA: Nov 97: 29, Jan 98: 6, Feb 98: 1

84485 Trypsin; duodenal fluid   Q4

RVU			Global Days	Modifiers				
Mod	Non-Fac Total	Fac Total		51	50	62	80	MUE
	0.00	0.00	XXX	9	9	9	9	1

84488 Trypsin; feces, qualitative   Q4

RVU			Global Days	Modifiers				
Mod	Non-Fac Total	Fac Total		51	50	62	80	MUE
	0.00	0.00	XXX	9	9	9	9	1

84490 Trypsin; feces, quantitative, 24-hour collection   Q4

RVU			Global Days	Modifiers				
Mod	Non-Fac Total	Fac Total		51	50	62	80	MUE
	0.00	0.00	XXX	9	9	9	9	1

AMA: Oct 10: 7

84510 Tyrosine   Q4

RVU			Global Days	Modifiers				
Mod	Non-Fac Total	Fac Total		51	50	62	80	MUE
	0.00	0.00	XXX	9	9	9	9	1

AMA: Oct 10: 7

84512 Troponin, qualitative   Q4

RVU			Global Days	Modifiers				
Mod	Non-Fac Total	Fac Total		51	50	62	80	MUE
	0.00	0.00	XXX	9	9	9	9	1

AMA: Nov 97: 29, Jan 98: 6, Feb 98: 1

84520 Urea nitrogen; quantitative   Q4

Coding tip: For a CLIA-waived test, append modifier QW to 84520

RVU			Global Days	Modifiers				
Mod	Non-Fac Total	Fac Total		51	50	62	80	MUE
	0.00	0.00	XXX	9	9	9	9	4

AMA: Dec 99: 2, Apr 13: 10

Pub 100-04, 16, 120.2

84525 Urea nitrogen; semiquantitative (eg, reagent strip test)   Q4

RVU			Global Days	Modifiers				
Mod	Non-Fac Total	Fac Total		51	50	62	80	MUE
	0.00	0.00	XXX	9	9	9	9	1

AMA: Mar 98: 3

84540 Urea nitrogen, urine   Q4

RVU			Global Days	Modifiers				
Mod	Non-Fac Total	Fac Total		51	50	62	80	MUE
	0.00	0.00	XXX	9	9	9	9	2

Pub 100-04, 16, 120.2

84545 Urea nitrogen, clearance   Q4

RVU			Global Days	Modifiers				
Mod	Non-Fac Total	Fac Total		51	50	62	80	MUE
	0.00	0.00	XXX	9	9	9	9	1

Pub 100-04, 16, 120.2

84550 Uric acid; blood   Q4

Coding tip: For a CLIA-waived test, append modifier QW to 84550

RVU			Global Days	Modifiers				
Mod	Non-Fac Total	Fac Total		51	50	62	80	MUE
	0.00	0.00	XXX	9	9	9	9	1

AMA: Dec 99: 2

● New   ▲ Revised   Deleted   ⊙ Moderate Sedation   ✚ Add-on Codes   ⊘ High Risk Denial   Ⓐ Age Edit   ♀ Female   ♂ Male   **AMA** *CPT® Assistant*   **MUE** Medically Unlikely Edit
Ⓢ Modifier 51 Exempt   ⊖ Modifier 63 Exempt   ✘ Unlisted   **Modifiers:** *See Inside Back Cover*   Ⓜ Maternity   **A 2 – Z 3** ASC Payment Indicators   **A – Y** OPPS Status Indicators

© 2016 DecisionHealth   CPT © 2015 American Medical Association. All Rights Reserved.

84560 Uric acid; other source   Q4

Mod	Non-Fac Total	Fac Total	Global Days	51	50	62	80	MUE
	0.00	0.00	XXX	9	9	9	9	2

84577 Urobilinogen, feces, quantitative   Q4

Mod	Non-Fac Total	Fac Total	Global Days	51	50	62	80	MUE
	0.00	0.00	XXX	9	9	9	9	1

84578 Urobilinogen, urine; qualitative   Q4

Mod	Non-Fac Total	Fac Total	Global Days	51	50	62	80	MUE
	0.00	0.00	XXX	9	9	9	9	1

84580 Urobilinogen, urine; quantitative, timed specimen   Q4

Mod	Non-Fac Total	Fac Total	Global Days	51	50	62	80	MUE
	0.00	0.00	XXX	9	9	9	9	1

84583 Urobilinogen, urine; semiquantitative   Q4

Mod	Non-Fac Total	Fac Total	Global Days	51	50	62	80	MUE
	0.00	0.00	XXX	9	9	9	9	1

84585 Vanillylmandelic acid (VMA), urine   Q4

Mod	Non-Fac Total	Fac Total	Global Days	51	50	62	80	MUE
	0.00	0.00	XXX	9	9	9	9	1

84586 Vasoactive intestinal peptide (VIP)   Q4

Mod	Non-Fac Total	Fac Total	Global Days	51	50	62	80	MUE
	0.00	0.00	XXX	9	9	9	9	1

AMA: Summer 94: 6

84588 Vasopressin (antidiuretic hormone, ADH)   Q4

Mod	Non-Fac Total	Fac Total	Global Days	51	50	62	80	MUE
	0.00	0.00	XXX	9	9	9	9	1

84590 Vitamin A   Q4

Mod	Non-Fac Total	Fac Total	Global Days	51	50	62	80	MUE
	0.00	0.00	XXX	9	9	9	9	1

AMA: Aug 05: 9

84591 Vitamin, not otherwise specified   Q4

Mod	Non-Fac Total	Fac Total	Global Days	51	50	62	80	MUE
	0.00	0.00	XXX	9	9	9	9	1

84597 Vitamin K   Q4

Mod	Non-Fac Total	Fac Total	Global Days	51	50	62	80	MUE
	0.00	0.00	XXX	9	9	9	9	1

AMA: Oct 10: 7

84600 Volatiles (eg, acetic anhydride, diethylether)   Q4

Mod	Non-Fac Total	Fac Total	Global Days	51	50	62	80	MUE
	0.00	0.00	XXX	9	9	9	9	2

AMA: Aug 05: 9, Oct 10: 7

84620 Xylose absorption test, blood and/or urine   Q4

Mod	Non-Fac Total	Fac Total	Global Days	51	50	62	80	MUE
	0.00	0.00	XXX	9	9	9	9	1

84630 Zinc   Q4

Mod	Non-Fac Total	Fac Total	Global Days	51	50	62	80	MUE
	0.00	0.00	XXX	9	9	9	9	2

Pub 100-04, 16, 120.2

84681 C-peptide   Q4

Mod	Non-Fac Total	Fac Total	Global Days	51	50	62	80	MUE
	0.00	0.00	XXX	9	9	9	9	1

AMA: Oct 10: 7

84702 Gonadotropin, chorionic (hCG); quantitative   Q4

Mod	Non-Fac Total	Fac Total	Global Days	51	50	62	80	MUE
	0.00	0.00	XXX	9	9	9	9	2

AMA: Oct 10: 7
NCD: 190.27

84703 Gonadotropin, chorionic (hCG); qualitative   Q4

Coding tip: For a CLIA-waived test, append modifier QW to 84703

Mod	Non-Fac Total	Fac Total	Global Days	51	50	62	80	MUE
	0.00	0.00	XXX	9	9	9	9	1

84704 Gonadotropin, chorionic (hCG); free beta chain   Q4

Mod	Non-Fac Total	Fac Total	Global Days	51	50	62	80	MUE
	0.00	0.00	XXX	9	9	9	9	1

AMA: Apr 08: 5, Aug 08: 13, Oct 10: 7

84830 Ovulation tests, by visual color comparison methods for human luteinizing hormone   ♀Q4

Coding tip: This is a CLIA-waived test, but does not require the use of modifier QW to be recognized as such

Mod	Non-Fac Total	Fac Total	Global Days	51	50	62	80	MUE
	0.00	0.00	XXX	9	9	9	9	1

AMA: Oct 10: 7, Jun 15: 10

84999 Unlisted chemistry procedure   ✗Q4

Coding tip: Use 84999 to report direct measurement of intermediate density lipoproteins [IDL], also referred to as remnant lipoproteins

Mod	Non-Fac Total	Fac Total	Global Days	51	50	62	80	MUE
	0.00	0.00	XXX	9	9	9	9	

AMA: Oct 00: 24, Aug 05: 9, Oct 10: 7, Dec 10: 7, Apr 15: 3
Pub 100-04, 16, 100.4

Hematology/Coagulation Testing

85002 Bleeding time   Q4

Mod	Non-Fac Total	Fac Total	Global Days	51	50	62	80	MUE
	0.00	0.00	XXX	9	9	9	9	1

AMA: Aug 05: 9
Pub 100-04, 16, 120.2

● New   ▲ Revised   ✖ Deleted   ⊙ Moderate Sedation   ✚ Add-on Codes   ⊘ High Risk Denial   Ⓐ Age Edit   ♀ Female   ♂ Male   **AMA** CPT® Assistant   **MUE** Medically Unlikely Edit
⊘ Modifier 51 Exempt   ⊖ Modifier 63 Exempt   ✗ Unlisted   **Modifiers:** See Inside Back Cover   Ⓜ Maternity   A2–Z3 ASC Payment Indicators   A–Y OPPS Status Indicators

CPT © 2015 American Medical Association. All Rights Reserved.   © 2016 DecisionHealth

85004 Blood count; automated differential WBC count
Q4

RVU			Global Days	Modifiers				
Mod	Non-Fac Total	Fac Total		51	50	62	80	MUE
	0.00	0.00	XXX	9	9	9	9	1

AMA: Jan 04: 26
Pub 100-04, 16, 120.2
NCD: 190.15

85007 Blood count; blood smear, microscopic examination with manual differential WBC count
Q4

RVU			Global Days	Modifiers				
Mod	Non-Fac Total	Fac Total		51	50	62	80	MUE
	0.00	0.00	XXX	9	9	9	9	1

AMA: Jul 03: 7, Jan 04: 26
Pub 100-04, 16, 120.2

85008 Blood count; blood smear, microscopic examination without manual differential WBC count
Q4

RVU			Global Days	Modifiers				
Mod	Non-Fac Total	Fac Total		51	50	62	80	MUE
	0.00	0.00	XXX	9	9	9	9	1

AMA: Jul 03: 8, Jan 04: 26
Pub 100-04, 16, 120.2

85009 Blood count; manual differential WBC count, buffy coat
Q4

RVU			Global Days	Modifiers				
Mod	Non-Fac Total	Fac Total		51	50	62	80	MUE
	0.00	0.00	XXX	9	9	9	9	1

AMA: Jul 03: 7, Jan 04: 26
Pub 100-04, 16, 120.2

85013 Blood count; spun microhematocrit
Q4

Coding tip: *This is a CLIA-waived test, but does not require the use of modifier QW to be recognized as such*

RVU			Global Days	Modifiers				
Mod	Non-Fac Total	Fac Total		51	50	62	80	MUE
	0.00	0.00	XXX	9	9	9	9	1

Pub 100-04, 16, 120.2

85014 Blood count; hematocrit (Hct)
Q4

Coding tip: *For a CLIA-waived test, append modifier QW to 85014*

RVU			Global Days	Modifiers				
Mod	Non-Fac Total	Fac Total		51	50	62	80	MUE
	0.00	0.00	XXX	9	9	9	9	2

AMA: Jul 03: 7
Pub 100-04, 16, 120.2

85018 Blood count; hemoglobin (Hgb)
Q4

Coding tip: *For a CLIA-waived test, append modifier QW to 85018*

RVU			Global Days	Modifiers				
Mod	Non-Fac Total	Fac Total		51	50	62	80	MUE
	0.00	0.00	XXX	9	9	9	9	2

AMA: Jul 03: 8
Pub 100-04, 16, 120.2

85025 Blood count; complete (CBC), automated (Hgb, Hct, RBC, WBC and platelet count) and automated differential WBC count
Q4

RVU			Global Days	Modifiers				
Mod	Non-Fac Total	Fac Total		51	50	62	80	MUE
	0.00	0.00	XXX	9	9	9	9	2

AMA: Jul 00: 11, Jul 03: 7, Jan 04: 26, Jul 11: 16
Pub 100-04, 16, 120.2

85027 Blood count; complete (CBC), automated (Hgb, Hct, RBC, WBC and platelet count)
Q4

RVU			Global Days	Modifiers				
Mod	Non-Fac Total	Fac Total		51	50	62	80	MUE
	0.00	0.00	XXX	9	9	9	9	2

AMA: Jul 03: 8, Jan 04: 26
Pub 100-04, 16, 120.2

85032 Blood count; manual cell count (erythrocyte, leukocyte, or platelet) each
Q4

RVU			Global Days	Modifiers				
Mod	Non-Fac Total	Fac Total		51	50	62	80	MUE
	0.00	0.00	XXX	9	9	9	9	1

AMA: Jul 03: 8, Nov 03: 15
Pub 100-04, 16, 120.2

85041 Blood count; red blood cell (RBC), automated
Q4

RVU			Global Days	Modifiers				
Mod	Non-Fac Total	Fac Total		51	50	62	80	MUE
	0.00	0.00	XXX	9	9	9	9	1

AMA: Jul 03: 8
Pub 100-04, 16, 120.2

85044 Blood count; reticulocyte, manual
Q4

RVU			Global Days	Modifiers				
Mod	Non-Fac Total	Fac Total		51	50	62	80	MUE
	0.00	0.00	XXX	9	9	9	9	1

AMA: Jul 03: 8
Pub 100-04, 16, 120.2

85045 Blood count; reticulocyte, automated
Q4

RVU			Global Days	Modifiers				
Mod	Non-Fac Total	Fac Total		51	50	62	80	MUE
	0.00	0.00	XXX	9	9	9	9	1

AMA: Jul 03: 8
Pub 100-04, 16, 120.2

85046 Blood count; reticulocytes, automated, including 1 or more cellular parameters (eg, reticulocyte hemoglobin content [CHr], immature reticulocyte fraction [IRF], reticulocyte volume [MRV], RNA content), direct measurement
Q4

RVU			Global Days	Modifiers				
Mod	Non-Fac Total	Fac Total		51	50	62	80	MUE
	0.00	0.00	XXX	9	9	9	9	1

AMA: Nov 98: 27
Pub 100-04, 16, 120.2

85048 Blood count; leukocyte (WBC), automated
Q4

RVU			Global Days	Modifiers				
Mod	Non-Fac Total	Fac Total		51	50	62	80	MUE
	0.00	0.00	XXX	9	9	9	9	2

AMA: Jul 03: 8
Pub 100-04, 16, 120.2

● New   ▲ Revised   Deleted   ⊙ Moderate Sedation   ✚ Add-on Codes   ⊘ High Risk Denial   Ⓐ Age Edit   ♀ Female   ♂ Male   **AMA** *CPT® Assistant*   **MUE** Medically Unlikely Edit
⊘ Modifier 51 Exempt   ⊖ Modifier 63 Exempt   ☒ Unlisted   **Modifiers:** *See Inside Back Cover*   Ⓜ Maternity   A2–Z3 ASC Payment Indicators   A–Y OPPS Status Indicators

85049 Blood count; platelet, automated   ◎4

Mod	Non-Fac Total	Fac Total	Global Days	51	50	62	80	MUE
	0.00	0.00	XXX	9	9	9	9	2

Pub 100-04, 16, 120.2

85055 Reticulated platelet assay   ◎4

Mod	Non-Fac Total	Fac Total	Global Days	51	50	62	80	MUE
	0.00	0.00	XXX	9	9	9	9	1

85060 Blood smear, peripheral, interpretation by physician with written report   B

Mod	Non-Fac Total	Fac Total	Global Days	51	50	62	80	MUE
	0.70	0.70	XXX	0	0	0	0	1

Pub 100-04, 12, 60; 100-04, 16, 80.2

Coding Guidance

Use code 38220 for the bone marrow aspiration procedure. Code 85097 is reported when the only laboratory service provided is the bone marrow smear interpretation. The pathological interpretation codes 88300-88309 are not reported additionally, unless the processing of separate specimens is done.

85097 Bone marrow, smear interpretation   ◎2

Mod	Non-Fac Total	Fac Total	Global Days	51	50	62	80	MUE
	2.54	1.42	XXX	0	0	0	0	2

AMA: Winter 92: 17, Jul 98: 4, Mar 03: 22

Pub 100-04, 12, 60

85130 Chromogenic substrate assay   ⊘◎4

Mod	Non-Fac Total	Fac Total	Global Days	51	50	62	80	MUE
	0.00	0.00	XXX	9	9	9	9	1

AMA: Aug 05: 9

85170 Clot retraction   ◎4

Mod	Non-Fac Total	Fac Total	Global Days	51	50	62	80	MUE
	0.00	0.00	XXX	9	9	9	9	1

85175 Clot lysis time, whole blood dilution   ⊘◎4

Mod	Non-Fac Total	Fac Total	Global Days	51	50	62	80	MUE
	0.00	0.00	XXX	9	9	9	9	1

85210 Clotting; factor II, prothrombin, specific   ◎4

Mod	Non-Fac Total	Fac Total	Global Days	51	50	62	80	MUE
	0.00	0.00	XXX	9	9	9	9	2

AMA: Aug 05: 9

85220 Clotting; factor V (AcG or proaccelerin), labile factor   ◎4

Mod	Non-Fac Total	Fac Total	Global Days	51	50	62	80	MUE
	0.00	0.00	XXX	9	9	9	9	2

85230 Clotting; factor VII (proconvertin, stable factor)   ◎4

Mod	Non-Fac Total	Fac Total	Global Days	51	50	62	80	MUE
	0.00	0.00	XXX	9	9	9	9	2

85240 Clotting; factor VIII (AHG), 1-stage   ◎4

Mod	Non-Fac Total	Fac Total	Global Days	51	50	62	80	MUE
	0.00	0.00	XXX	9	9	9	9	2

85244 Clotting; factor VIII related antigen   ◎4

Mod	Non-Fac Total	Fac Total	Global Days	51	50	62	80	MUE
	0.00	0.00	XXX	9	9	9	9	1

85245 Clotting; factor VIII, VW factor, ristocetin cofactor   ◎4

Mod	Non-Fac Total	Fac Total	Global Days	51	50	62	80	MUE
	0.00	0.00	XXX	9	9	9	9	2

85246 Clotting; factor VIII, VW factor antigen   ◎4

Mod	Non-Fac Total	Fac Total	Global Days	51	50	62	80	MUE
	0.00	0.00	XXX	9	9	9	9	2

85247 Clotting; factor VIII, von Willebrand factor, multimetric analysis   ◎4

Mod	Non-Fac Total	Fac Total	Global Days	51	50	62	80	MUE
	0.00	0.00	XXX	9	9	9	9	2

85250 Clotting; factor IX (PTC or Christmas)   ◎4

Mod	Non-Fac Total	Fac Total	Global Days	51	50	62	80	MUE
	0.00	0.00	XXX	9	9	9	9	2

85260 Clotting; factor X (Stuart-Prower)   ◎4

Mod	Non-Fac Total	Fac Total	Global Days	51	50	62	80	MUE
	0.00	0.00	XXX	9	9	9	9	2

85270 Clotting; factor XI (PTA)   ◎4

Mod	Non-Fac Total	Fac Total	Global Days	51	50	62	80	MUE
	0.00	0.00	XXX	9	9	9	9	2

85280 Clotting; factor XII (Hageman)   ◎4

Mod	Non-Fac Total	Fac Total	Global Days	51	50	62	80	MUE
	0.00	0.00	XXX	9	9	9	9	2

85290 Clotting; factor XIII (fibrin stabilizing)   ◎4

Mod	Non-Fac Total	Fac Total	Global Days	51	50	62	80	MUE
	0.00	0.00	XXX	9	9	9	9	2

85291 Clotting; factor XIII (fibrin stabilizing), screen solubility   ◎4

Mod	Non-Fac Total	Fac Total	Global Days	51	50	62	80	MUE
	0.00	0.00	XXX	9	9	9	9	1

85292 Clotting; prekallikrein assay (Fletcher factor assay)   ◎4

Mod	Non-Fac Total	Fac Total	Global Days	51	50	62	80	MUE
	0.00	0.00	XXX	9	9	9	9	1

● New   ▲ Revised   ✖ Deleted   ⊙ Moderate Sedation   ✚ Add-on Codes   ⊘ High Risk Denial   Ⓐ Age Edit   ♀ Female   ♂ Male   **AMA** CPT® Assistant   **MUE** Medically Unlikely Edit

⊘ Modifier 51 Exempt   ⊖ Modifier 63 Exempt   🗷 Unlisted   **Modifiers:** See Inside Back Cover   Ⓜ Maternity   A2–Z3 ASC Payment Indicators   A–Y OPPS Status Indicators

CPT © 2015 American Medical Association. All Rights Reserved.   © 2016 DecisionHealth

85293 Clotting; high molecular weight kininogen assay (Fitzgerald factor assay) ◘4

Mod	Non-Fac Total	Fac Total	Global Days	51	50	62	80	MUE
	0.00	0.00	XXX	9	9	9	9	1

85300 Clotting inhibitors or anticoagulants; antithrombin III, activity ◘4

Mod	Non-Fac Total	Fac Total	Global Days	51	50	62	80	MUE
	0.00	0.00	XXX	9	9	9	9	2

AMA: Aug 05: 9

85301 Clotting inhibitors or anticoagulants; antithrombin III, antigen assay ◘4

Mod	Non-Fac Total	Fac Total	Global Days	51	50	62	80	MUE
	0.00	0.00	XXX	9	9	9	9	1

85302 Clotting inhibitors or anticoagulants; protein C, antigen ◘4

Mod	Non-Fac Total	Fac Total	Global Days	51	50	62	80	MUE
	0.00	0.00	XXX	9	9	9	9	1

85303 Clotting inhibitors or anticoagulants; protein C, activity ◘4

Mod	Non-Fac Total	Fac Total	Global Days	51	50	62	80	MUE
	0.00	0.00	XXX	9	9	9	9	2

85305 Clotting inhibitors or anticoagulants; protein S, total ◘4

Mod	Non-Fac Total	Fac Total	Global Days	51	50	62	80	MUE
	0.00	0.00	XXX	9	9	9	9	2

85306 Clotting inhibitors or anticoagulants; protein S, free ◘4

Mod	Non-Fac Total	Fac Total	Global Days	51	50	62	80	MUE
	0.00	0.00	XXX	9	9	9	9	2

85307 Activated Protein C (APC) resistance assay ◘4

Mod	Non-Fac Total	Fac Total	Global Days	51	50	62	80	MUE
	0.00	0.00	XXX	9	9	9	9	2

85335 Factor inhibitor test ◘4

Mod	Non-Fac Total	Fac Total	Global Days	51	50	62	80	MUE
	0.00	0.00	XXX	9	9	9	9	2

85337 Thrombomodulin ◘4

Mod	Non-Fac Total	Fac Total	Global Days	51	50	62	80	MUE
	0.00	0.00	XXX	9	9	9	9	1

85345 Coagulation time; Lee and White ◘4

Mod	Non-Fac Total	Fac Total	Global Days	51	50	62	80	MUE
	0.00	0.00	XXX	9	9	9	9	1

Pub 100-04, 16, 120.2

85347 Coagulation time; activated ◘4

Mod	Non-Fac Total	Fac Total	Global Days	51	50	62	80	MUE
	0.00	0.00	XXX	9	9	9	9	5

Pub 100-04, 16, 120.2

85348 Coagulation time; other methods ◘4

Mod	Non-Fac Total	Fac Total	Global Days	51	50	62	80	MUE
	0.00	0.00	XXX	9	9	9	9	1

Pub 100-04, 16, 120.2

85360 Euglobulin lysis ◘4

Mod	Non-Fac Total	Fac Total	Global Days	51	50	62	80	MUE
	0.00	0.00	XXX	9	9	9	9	1

85362 Fibrin(ogen) degradation (split) products (FDP) (FSP); agglutination slide, semiquantitative ◘4

Mod	Non-Fac Total	Fac Total	Global Days	51	50	62	80	MUE
	0.00	0.00	XXX	9	9	9	9	2

85366 Fibrin(ogen) degradation (split) products (FDP) (FSP); paracoagulation ◘4

Mod	Non-Fac Total	Fac Total	Global Days	51	50	62	80	MUE
	0.00	0.00	XXX	9	9	9	9	1

85370 Fibrin(ogen) degradation (split) products (FDP) (FSP); quantitative ◘4

Mod	Non-Fac Total	Fac Total	Global Days	51	50	62	80	MUE
	0.00	0.00	XXX	9	9	9	9	1

85378 Fibrin degradation products, D-dimer; qualitative or semiquantitative ◘4

Mod	Non-Fac Total	Fac Total	Global Days	51	50	62	80	MUE
	0.00	0.00	XXX	9	9	9	9	1

AMA: Jul 03: 8

85379 Fibrin degradation products, D-dimer; quantitative ◘4

Mod	Non-Fac Total	Fac Total	Global Days	51	50	62	80	MUE
	0.00	0.00	XXX	9	9	9	9	2

85380 Fibrin degradation products, D-dimer; ultrasensitive (eg, for evaluation for venous thromboembolism), qualitative or semiquantitative ◘4

Mod	Non-Fac Total	Fac Total	Global Days	51	50	62	80	MUE
	0.00	0.00	XXX	9	9	9	9	1

AMA: Jul 03: 8

85384 Fibrinogen; activity ◘4

Mod	Non-Fac Total	Fac Total	Global Days	51	50	62	80	MUE
	0.00	0.00	XXX	9	9	9	9	2

● New ▲ Revised Deleted ⊙ Moderate Sedation ✚ Add-on Codes ⊘ High Risk Denial Ⓐ Age Edit ♀ Female ♂ Male **AMA** *CPT® Assistant* **MUE** Medically Unlikely Edit
⊘ Modifier 51 Exempt ⊖ Modifier 63 Exempt ✗ Unlisted **Modifiers:** *See Inside Back Cover* Ⓜ Maternity A2–Z3 ASC Payment Indicators A–Y OPPS Status Indicators
© 2016 DecisionHealth   CPT © 2015 American Medical Association. All Rights Reserved.

85385 Fibrinogen; antigen Q4

RVU			Global Days	Modifiers				
Mod	Non-Fac Total	Fac Total		51	50	62	80	MUE
	0.00	0.00	XXX	9	9	9	9	1

85390 Fibrinolysins or coagulopathy screen, interpretation and report Q4

RVU			Global Days	Modifiers				
Mod	Non-Fac Total	Fac Total		51	50	62	80	MUE
	0.00	0.00	XXX	9	9	9	9	3
26	0.52	0.52	XXX	0	0	0	0	3

85396 Coagulation/fibrinolysis assay, whole blood (eg, viscoelastic clot assessment), including use of any pharmacologic additive(s), as indicated, including interpretation and written report, per day Q4

RVU			Global Days	Modifiers				
Mod	Non-Fac Total	Fac Total		51	50	62	80	MUE
	0.59	0.59	XXX	0	0	0	0	1

85397 Coagulation and fibrinolysis, functional activity, not otherwise specified (eg, ADAMTS-13), each analyte Q4

RVU			Global Days	Modifiers				
Mod	Non-Fac Total	Fac Total		51	50	62	80	MUE
	0.00	0.00	XXX	9	9	9	9	3

85400 Fibrinolytic factors and inhibitors; plasmin Q4

RVU			Global Days	Modifiers				
Mod	Non-Fac Total	Fac Total		51	50	62	80	MUE
	0.00	0.00	XXX	9	9	9	9	1

AMA: Aug 05: 9

85410 Fibrinolytic factors and inhibitors; alpha-2 antiplasmin Q4

RVU			Global Days	Modifiers				
Mod	Non-Fac Total	Fac Total		51	50	62	80	MUE
	0.00	0.00	XXX	9	9	9	9	1

85415 Fibrinolytic factors and inhibitors; plasminogen activator Q4

RVU			Global Days	Modifiers				
Mod	Non-Fac Total	Fac Total		51	50	62	80	MUE
	0.00	0.00	XXX	9	9	9	9	2

85420 Fibrinolytic factors and inhibitors; plasminogen, except antigenic assay Q4

RVU			Global Days	Modifiers				
Mod	Non-Fac Total	Fac Total		51	50	62	80	MUE
	0.00	0.00	XXX	9	9	9	9	2

85421 Fibrinolytic factors and inhibitors; plasminogen, antigenic assay Q4

RVU			Global Days	Modifiers				
Mod	Non-Fac Total	Fac Total		51	50	62	80	MUE
	0.00	0.00	XXX	9	9	9	9	1

85441 Heinz bodies; direct Q4

RVU			Global Days	Modifiers				
Mod	Non-Fac Total	Fac Total		51	50	62	80	MUE
	0.00	0.00	XXX	9	9	9	9	1

85445 Heinz bodies; induced, acetyl phenylhydrazine Q4

RVU			Global Days	Modifiers				
Mod	Non-Fac Total	Fac Total		51	50	62	80	MUE
	0.00	0.00	XXX	9	9	9	9	1

85460 Hemoglobin or RBCs, fetal, for fetomaternal hemorrhage; differential lysis (Kleihauer-Betke) ♀ M Q4

RVU			Global Days	Modifiers				
Mod	Non-Fac Total	Fac Total		51	50	62	80	MUE
	0.00	0.00	XXX	9	9	9	9	1

AMA: Fall 93: 25

85461 Hemoglobin or RBCs, fetal, for fetomaternal hemorrhage; rosette ♀ M Q4

RVU			Global Days	Modifiers				
Mod	Non-Fac Total	Fac Total		51	50	62	80	MUE
	0.00	0.00	XXX	9	9	9	9	1

85475 Hemolysin, acid Q4

RVU			Global Days	Modifiers				
Mod	Non-Fac Total	Fac Total		51	50	62	80	MUE
	0.00	0.00	XXX	9	9	9	9	1

85520 Heparin assay Q4

RVU			Global Days	Modifiers				
Mod	Non-Fac Total	Fac Total		51	50	62	80	MUE
	0.00	0.00	XXX	9	9	9	9	1

AMA: Aug 05: 9
Pub 100-04, 16, 120.2

85525 Heparin neutralization Q4

RVU			Global Days	Modifiers				
Mod	Non-Fac Total	Fac Total		51	50	62	80	MUE
	0.00	0.00	XXX	9	9	9	9	2

85530 Heparin-protamine tolerance test Q4

RVU			Global Days	Modifiers				
Mod	Non-Fac Total	Fac Total		51	50	62	80	MUE
	0.00	0.00	XXX	9	9	9	9	1

85536 Iron stain, peripheral blood Q4

RVU			Global Days	Modifiers				
Mod	Non-Fac Total	Fac Total		51	50	62	80	MUE
	0.00	0.00	XXX	9	9	9	9	1

85540 Leukocyte alkaline phosphatase with count Q4

RVU			Global Days	Modifiers				
Mod	Non-Fac Total	Fac Total		51	50	62	80	MUE
	0.00	0.00	XXX	9	9	9	9	1

85547 Mechanical fragility, RBC Q4

RVU			Global Days	Modifiers				
Mod	Non-Fac Total	Fac Total		51	50	62	80	MUE
	0.00	0.00	XXX	9	9	9	9	1

85549 Muramidase Q4

RVU			Global Days	Modifiers				
Mod	Non-Fac Total	Fac Total		51	50	62	80	MUE
	0.00	0.00	XXX	9	9	9	9	1

● New ▲ Revised ✖ Deleted ⊙ Moderate Sedation ✚ Add-on Codes ⊘ High Risk Denial Ⓐ Age Edit ♀ Female ♂ Male AMA CPT® Assistant MUE Medically Unlikely Edit
⊘ Modifier 51 Exempt ⊖ Modifier 63 Exempt Ⓧ Unlisted Modifiers: See Inside Back Cover M Maternity A2–Z3 ASC Payment Indicators A–Y OPPS Status Indicators
CPT © 2015 American Medical Association. All Rights Reserved. © 2016 DecisionHealth

85555 Osmotic fragility, RBC; unincubated   Q4

RVU Mod	Non-Fac Total	Fac Total	Global Days	51	50	62	80	MUE
	0.00	0.00	XXX	9	9	9	9	1

85557 Osmotic fragility, RBC; incubated   Q4

RVU Mod	Non-Fac Total	Fac Total	Global Days	51	50	62	80	MUE
	0.00	0.00	XXX	9	9	9	9	1

85576 Platelet, aggregation (in vitro), each agent   Q4

Coding tip: For a CLIA-waived test, append modifier QW to 85576

RVU Mod	Non-Fac Total	Fac Total	Global Days	51	50	62	80	MUE
	0.00	0.00	XXX	9	9	9	9	7
26	0.52	0.52	XXX	0	0	0	0	7

AMA: Jul 96: 10

85597 Phospholipid neutralization; platelet   Q4

RVU Mod	Non-Fac Total	Fac Total	Global Days	51	50	62	80	MUE
	0.00	0.00	XXX	9	9	9	9	1

AMA: Apr 11: 9, Oct 10: 8, Dec 10: 8

85598 Phospholipid neutralization; hexagonal phospholipid   Q4

RVU Mod	Non-Fac Total	Fac Total	Global Days	51	50	62	80	MUE
	0.00	0.00	XXX	9	9	9	9	1

AMA: Apr 11: 9, Oct 10: 8, Dec 10: 8

85610 Prothrombin time   Q4

Coding tip: For a CLIA-waived test, append modifier QW to 85610

RVU Mod	Non-Fac Total	Fac Total	Global Days	51	50	62	80	MUE
	0.00	0.00	XXX	9	9	9	9	4

AMA: Aug 05: 9

Pub 100-04, 16, 120.2
NCD: 190.17

85611 Prothrombin time; substitution, plasma fractions, each   Q4

RVU Mod	Non-Fac Total	Fac Total	Global Days	51	50	62	80	MUE
	0.00	0.00	XXX	9	9	9	9	2

Pub 100-04, 16, 120.2

85612 Russell viper venom time (includes venom); undiluted   Q4

RVU Mod	Non-Fac Total	Fac Total	Global Days	51	50	62	80	MUE
	0.00	0.00	XXX	9	9	9	9	1

85613 Russell viper venom time (includes venom); diluted   Q4

RVU Mod	Non-Fac Total	Fac Total	Global Days	51	50	62	80	MUE
	0.00	0.00	XXX	9	9	9	9	1

85635 Reptilase test   Q4

RVU Mod	Non-Fac Total	Fac Total	Global Days	51	50	62	80	MUE
	0.00	0.00	XXX	9	9	9	9	1

85651 Sedimentation rate, erythrocyte; non-automated   Q4

Coding tip: This is a CLIA-waived test, but does not require the use of modifier QW to be recognized as such

RVU Mod	Non-Fac Total	Fac Total	Global Days	51	50	62	80	MUE
	0.00	0.00	XXX	9	9	9	9	1

Pub 100-04, 16, 120.2

85652 Sedimentation rate, erythrocyte; automated   Q4

RVU Mod	Non-Fac Total	Fac Total	Global Days	51	50	62	80	MUE
	0.00	0.00	XXX	9	9	9	9	1

Pub 100-04, 16, 120.2

85660 Sickling of RBC, reduction   Q4

RVU Mod	Non-Fac Total	Fac Total	Global Days	51	50	62	80	MUE
	0.00	0.00	XXX	9	9	9	9	1

85670 Thrombin time; plasma   Q4

RVU Mod	Non-Fac Total	Fac Total	Global Days	51	50	62	80	MUE
	0.00	0.00	XXX	9	9	9	9	2

85675 Thrombin time; titer   Q4

RVU Mod	Non-Fac Total	Fac Total	Global Days	51	50	62	80	MUE
	0.00	0.00	XXX	9	9	9	9	1

85705 Thromboplastin inhibition, tissue   Q4

RVU Mod	Non-Fac Total	Fac Total	Global Days	51	50	62	80	MUE
	0.00	0.00	XXX	9	9	9	9	1

AMA: Aug 05: 9

85730 Thromboplastin time, partial (PTT); plasma or whole blood   Q4

RVU Mod	Non-Fac Total	Fac Total	Global Days	51	50	62	80	MUE
	0.00	0.00	XXX	9	9	9	9	4

Pub 100-04, 16, 120.2
NCD: 190.16

85732 Thromboplastin time, partial (PTT); substitution, plasma fractions, each   Q4

RVU Mod	Non-Fac Total	Fac Total	Global Days	51	50	62	80	MUE
	0.00	0.00	XXX	9	9	9	9	4

AMA: Apr 11: 9

85810 Viscosity   Q4

RVU Mod	Non-Fac Total	Fac Total	Global Days	51	50	62	80	MUE
	0.00	0.00	XXX	9	9	9	9	2

85999 Unlisted hematology and coagulation procedure   ✗ Q4

RVU Mod	Non-Fac Total	Fac Total	Global Days	51	50	62	80	MUE
	0.00	0.00	XXX	9	9	9	9	

AMA: Aug 05: 9, Oct 09: 12
Pub 100-04, 16, 100.4

● New   ▲ Revised   Deleted   ⊙ Moderate Sedation   ✚ Add-on Codes   ⊘ High Risk Denial   Ⓐ Age Edit   ♀ Female   ♂ Male   AMA CPT® Assistant   MUE Medically Unlikely Edit
⊘ Modifier 51 Exempt   ⊖ Modifier 63 Exempt   ✗ Unlisted   Modifiers: See Inside Back Cover   Ⓜ Maternity   A2–Z3 ASC Payment Indicators   A–Y OPPS Status Indicators

Immunological Testing

86000 Agglutinins, febrile (eg, Brucella, Francisella, Murine typhus, Q fever, Rocky Mountain spotted fever, scrub typhus), each antigen Q4

RVU			Global Days	Modifiers				
Mod	Non-Fac Total	Fac Total		51	50	62	80	MUE
	0.00	0.00	XXX	9	9	9	9	6

AMA: Aug 05: 9

86001 Allergen specific IgG quantitative or semiquantitative, each allergen Q4

RVU			Global Days	Modifiers				
Mod	Non-Fac Total	Fac Total		51	50	62	80	MUE
	0.00	0.00	XXX	9	9	9	9	

86003 Allergen specific IgE; quantitative or semiquantitative, each allergen Q4

RVU			Global Days	Modifiers				
Mod	Non-Fac Total	Fac Total		51	50	62	80	MUE
	0.00	0.00	XXX	9	9	9	9	

AMA: Spring 94: 31

86005 Allergen specific IgE; qualitative, multiallergen screen (dipstick, paddle, or disk) Q4

RVU			Global Days	Modifiers				
Mod	Non-Fac Total	Fac Total		51	50	62	80	MUE
	0.00	0.00	XXX	9	9	9	9	2

AMA: Spring 94: 31

86021 Antibody identification; leukocyte antibodies Q4

RVU			Global Days	Modifiers				
Mod	Non-Fac Total	Fac Total		51	50	62	80	MUE
	0.00	0.00	XXX	9	9	9	9	1

86022 Antibody identification; platelet antibodies Q4

RVU			Global Days	Modifiers				
Mod	Non-Fac Total	Fac Total		51	50	62	80	MUE
	0.00	0.00	XXX	9	9	9	9	1

86023 Antibody identification; platelet associated immunoglobulin assay Q4

RVU			Global Days	Modifiers				
Mod	Non-Fac Total	Fac Total		51	50	62	80	MUE
	0.00	0.00	XXX	9	9	9	9	3

86038 Antinuclear antibodies (ANA) Q4

RVU			Global Days	Modifiers				
Mod	Non-Fac Total	Fac Total		51	50	62	80	MUE
	0.00	0.00	XXX	9	9	9	9	1

86039 Antinuclear antibodies (ANA); titer Q4

RVU			Global Days	Modifiers				
Mod	Non-Fac Total	Fac Total		51	50	62	80	MUE
	0.00	0.00	XXX	9	9	9	9	1

86060 Antistreptolysin 0; titer Q4

RVU			Global Days	Modifiers				
Mod	Non-Fac Total	Fac Total		51	50	62	80	MUE
	0.00	0.00	XXX	9	9	9	9	1

86063 Antistreptolysin 0; screen Q4

RVU			Global Days	Modifiers				
Mod	Non-Fac Total	Fac Total		51	50	62	80	MUE
	0.00	0.00	XXX	9	9	9	9	1

86077 Blood bank physician services; difficult cross match and/or evaluation of irregular antibody(s), interpretation and written report Q1

RVU			Global Days	Modifiers				
Mod	Non-Fac Total	Fac Total		51	50	62	80	MUE
	1.59	1.48	XXX	0	0	0	0	1

Pub 100-04, 12, 60

86078 Blood bank physician services; investigation of transfusion reaction including suspicion of transmissible disease, interpretation and written report Q1

RVU			Global Days	Modifiers				
Mod	Non-Fac Total	Fac Total		51	50	62	80	MUE
	1.59	1.48	XXX	0	0	0	0	1

Pub 100-04, 12, 60

86079 Blood bank physician services; authorization for deviation from standard blood banking procedures (eg, use of outdated blood, transfusion of Rh incompatible units), with written report Q1

RVU			Global Days	Modifiers				
Mod	Non-Fac Total	Fac Total		51	50	62	80	MUE
	1.57	1.46	XXX	0	0	0	0	1

Pub 100-04, 12, 60

86140 C-reactive protein Q4

RVU			Global Days	Modifiers				
Mod	Non-Fac Total	Fac Total		51	50	62	80	MUE
	0.00	0.00	XXX	9	9	9	9	1

AMA: Aug 05: 9

86141 C-reactive protein; high sensitivity (hsCRP) Q4

RVU			Global Days	Modifiers				
Mod	Non-Fac Total	Fac Total		51	50	62	80	MUE
	0.00	0.00	XXX	9	9	9	9	1

86146 Beta 2 Glycoprotein I antibody, each Q4

RVU			Global Days	Modifiers				
Mod	Non-Fac Total	Fac Total		51	50	62	80	MUE
	0.00	0.00	XXX	9	9	9	9	3

86147 Cardiolipin (phospholipid) antibody, each Ig class Q4

RVU			Global Days	Modifiers				
Mod	Non-Fac Total	Fac Total		51	50	62	80	MUE
	0.00	0.00	XXX	9	9	9	9	4

86148 Anti-phosphatidylserine (phospholipid) antibody Q4

RVU			Global Days	Modifiers				
Mod	Non-Fac Total	Fac Total		51	50	62	80	MUE
	0.00	0.00	XXX	9	9	9	9	3

AMA: Nov 97: 30, Jul 03: 8, Nov 03: 5

86152 Cell enumeration using immunologic selection and identification in fluid specimen (eg, circulating tumor cells in blood) Q4

RVU			Global Days	Modifiers				
Mod	Non-Fac Total	Fac Total		51	50	62	80	MUE
	0.00	0.00	XXX	9	9	9	9	1

● New ▲ Revised ✖ Deleted ⊙ Moderate Sedation ✚ Add-on Codes ⊘ High Risk Denial Ⓐ Age Edit ♀ Female ♂ Male **AMA** CPT® Assistant **MUE** Medically Unlikely Edit

⊘ Modifier 51 Exempt ⊖ Modifier 63 Exempt ☒ Unlisted **Modifiers:** See Inside Back Cover Ⓜ Maternity A2–Z3 ASC Payment Indicators A–Y OPPS Status Indicators

CPT © 2015 American Medical Association. All Rights Reserved. © 2016 DecisionHealth

86153 Cell enumeration using immunologic selection and identification in fluid specimen (eg, circulating tumor cells in blood); physician interpretation and report, when required ⓒⒷ

Mod	Non-Fac Total	Fac Total	Global Days	51	50	62	80	MUE
26	0.97	0.97	XXX	0	0	0	0	1

86155 Chemotaxis assay, specify method ⓒⓆ4

Mod	Non-Fac Total	Fac Total	Global Days	51	50	62	80	MUE
	0.00	0.00	XXX	9	9	9	9	1

86156 Cold agglutinin; screen Ⓠ4

Mod	Non-Fac Total	Fac Total	Global Days	51	50	62	80	MUE
	0.00	0.00	XXX	9	9	9	9	1

86157 Cold agglutinin; titer Ⓠ4

Mod	Non-Fac Total	Fac Total	Global Days	51	50	62	80	MUE
	0.00	0.00	XXX	9	9	9	9	1

86160 Complement; antigen, each component Ⓠ4

Mod	Non-Fac Total	Fac Total	Global Days	51	50	62	80	MUE
	0.00	0.00	XXX	9	9	9	9	4

86161 Complement; functional activity, each component Ⓠ4

Mod	Non-Fac Total	Fac Total	Global Days	51	50	62	80	MUE
	0.00	0.00	XXX	9	9	9	9	2

86162 Complement; total hemolytic (CH50) Ⓠ4

Mod	Non-Fac Total	Fac Total	Global Days	51	50	62	80	MUE
	0.00	0.00	XXX	9	9	9	9	1

86171 Complement fixation tests, each antigen Ⓠ4

Mod	Non-Fac Total	Fac Total	Global Days	51	50	62	80	MUE
	0.00	0.00	XXX	9	9	9	9	2

86185 Counterimmunoelectrophoresis, each antigen Ⓠ4

Mod	Non-Fac Total	Fac Total	Global Days	51	50	62	80	MUE
	0.00	0.00	XXX	9	9	9	9	1

86200 Cyclic citrullinated peptide (CCP), antibody Ⓠ4

Mod	Non-Fac Total	Fac Total	Global Days	51	50	62	80	MUE
	0.00	0.00	XXX	9	9	9	9	1

AMA: Mar 06: 6

86215 Deoxyribonuclease, antibody Ⓠ4

Mod	Non-Fac Total	Fac Total	Global Days	51	50	62	80	MUE
	0.00	0.00	XXX	9	9	9	9	1

AMA: Aug 05: 9

86225 Deoxyribonucleic acid (DNA) antibody; native or double stranded Ⓠ4

Mod	Non-Fac Total	Fac Total	Global Days	51	50	62	80	MUE
	0.00	0.00	XXX	9	9	9	9	1

86226 Deoxyribonucleic acid (DNA) antibody; single stranded Ⓠ4

Mod	Non-Fac Total	Fac Total	Global Days	51	50	62	80	MUE
	0.00	0.00	XXX	9	9	9	9	1

86235 Extractable nuclear antigen, antibody to, any method (eg, nRNP, SS-A, SS-B, Sm, RNP, Sc170, J01), each antibody Ⓠ4

Mod	Non-Fac Total	Fac Total	Global Days	51	50	62	80	MUE
	0.00	0.00	XXX	9	9	9	9	10

86243 Fc receptor Ⓠ4

Mod	Non-Fac Total	Fac Total	Global Days	51	50	62	80	MUE
	0.00	0.00	XXX	9	9	9	9	1

86255 Fluorescent noninfectious agent antibody; screen, each antibody Ⓠ4

Mod	Non-Fac Total	Fac Total	Global Days	51	50	62	80	MUE
	0.00	0.00	XXX	9	9	9	9	5
26	0.52	0.52	XXX	0	0	0	0	5

AMA: Nov 98: 27

86256 Fluorescent noninfectious agent antibody; titer, each antibody Ⓠ4

Mod	Non-Fac Total	Fac Total	Global Days	51	50	62	80	MUE
	0.00	0.00	XXX	9	9	9	9	9
26	0.52	0.52	XXX	0	0	0	0	9

86277 Growth hormone, human (HGH), antibody Ⓠ4

Mod	Non-Fac Total	Fac Total	Global Days	51	50	62	80	MUE
	0.00	0.00	XXX	9	9	9	9	1

86280 Hemagglutination inhibition test (HAI) Ⓠ4

Mod	Non-Fac Total	Fac Total	Global Days	51	50	62	80	MUE
	0.00	0.00	XXX	9	9	9	9	1

86294 Immunoassay for tumor antigen, qualitative or semiquantitative (eg, bladder tumor antigen) Ⓠ4

Coding tip: For a CLIA-waived test, append modifier QW to 86294

Mod	Non-Fac Total	Fac Total	Global Days	51	50	62	80	MUE
	0.00	0.00	XXX	9	9	9	9	1

86300 Immunoassay for tumor antigen, quantitative; CA 15-3 (27.29) Ⓠ4

Mod	Non-Fac Total	Fac Total	Global Days	51	50	62	80	MUE
	0.00	0.00	XXX	9	9	9	9	2

AMA: Aug 05: 9
NCD: 190.29

● New ▲ Revised Deleted ⊙ Moderate Sedation ✚ Add-on Codes ⊘ High Risk Denial Ⓐ Age Edit ♀ Female ♂ Male **AMA** CPT® Assistant **MUE** Medically Unlikely Edit ⊘ Modifier 51 Exempt ⊖ Modifier 63 Exempt Ⓧ Unlisted **Modifiers:** See Inside Back Cover Ⓜ Maternity Ⓐ2–Ⓩ3 ASC Payment Indicators Ⓐ–Ⓨ OPPS Status Indicators

86301 Immunoassay for tumor antigen, quantitative; CA 19-9 [Q4]

Mod	Non-Fac Total	Fac Total	Global Days	51	50	62	80	MUE
	0.00	0.00	XXX	9	9	9	9	1

NCD: 190.30

86304 Immunoassay for tumor antigen, quantitative; CA 125 [Q4]

Mod	Non-Fac Total	Fac Total	Global Days	51	50	62	80	MUE
	0.00	0.00	XXX	9	9	9	9	1

NCD: 190.28

86305 Human epididymis protein 4 (HE4) [Q4]

Mod	Non-Fac Total	Fac Total	Global Days	51	50	62	80	MUE
	0.00	0.00	XXX	9	9	9	9	1

86308 Heterophile antibodies; screening [Q4]

Coding tip: For a CLIA-waived test, append modifier QW to 86308

Mod	Non-Fac Total	Fac Total	Global Days	51	50	62	80	MUE
	0.00	0.00	XXX	9	9	9	9	1

86309 Heterophile antibodies; titer [Q4]

Mod	Non-Fac Total	Fac Total	Global Days	51	50	62	80	MUE
	0.00	0.00	XXX	9	9	9	9	1

86310 Heterophile antibodies; titers after absorption with beef cells and guinea pig kidney [Q4]

Mod	Non-Fac Total	Fac Total	Global Days	51	50	62	80	MUE
	0.00	0.00	XXX	9	9	9	9	1

86316 Immunoassay for tumor antigen, other antigen, quantitative (eg, CA 50, 72-4, 549), each [Q4]

Mod	Non-Fac Total	Fac Total	Global Days	51	50	62	80	MUE
	0.00	0.00	XXX	9	9	9	9	2

AMA: May 96: 11, Aug 96: 11, Apr 98: 15, Aug 99: 5, Dec 99: 10
Pub 100-04, 18, 50.3

86317 Immunoassay for infectious agent antibody, quantitative, not otherwise specified [⊘Q4]

Mod	Non-Fac Total	Fac Total	Global Days	51	50	62	80	MUE
	0.00	0.00	XXX	9	9	9	9	

AMA: Nov 97: 30, 31

86318 Immunoassay for infectious agent antibody, qualitative or semiquantitative, single step method (eg, reagent strip) [Q4]

Coding tip: For a CLIA-waived test, append modifier QW to 86318

Mod	Non-Fac Total	Fac Total	Global Days	51	50	62	80	MUE
	0.00	0.00	XXX	9	9	9	9	2

AMA: Mar 07: 10

86320 Immunoelectrophoresis; serum [Q4]

Mod	Non-Fac Total	Fac Total	Global Days	51	50	62	80	MUE
	0.00	0.00	XXX	9	9	9	9	1
26	0.52	0.52	XXX	0	0	0	0	1

86325 Immunoelectrophoresis; other fluids (eg, urine, cerebrospinal fluid) with concentration [Q4]

Mod	Non-Fac Total	Fac Total	Global Days	51	50	62	80	MUE
	0.00	0.00	XXX	9	9	9	9	2
26	0.52	0.52	XXX	0	0	0	0	2

86327 Immunoelectrophoresis; crossed (2-dimensional assay) [Q4]

Mod	Non-Fac Total	Fac Total	Global Days	51	50	62	80	MUE
	0.00	0.00	XXX	9	9	9	9	1
26	0.59	0.59	XXX	0	0	0	0	1

86329 Immunodiffusion; not elsewhere specified [Q4]

Mod	Non-Fac Total	Fac Total	Global Days	51	50	62	80	MUE
	0.00	0.00	XXX	9	9	9	9	3

AMA: Aug 00: 11

86331 Immunodiffusion; gel diffusion, qualitative (Ouchterlony), each antigen or antibody [Q4]

Mod	Non-Fac Total	Fac Total	Global Days	51	50	62	80	MUE
	0.00	0.00	XXX	9	9	9	9	12

86332 Immune complex assay [Q4]

Mod	Non-Fac Total	Fac Total	Global Days	51	50	62	80	MUE
	0.00	0.00	XXX	9	9	9	9	1

86334 Immunofixation electrophoresis; serum [Q4]

Mod	Non-Fac Total	Fac Total	Global Days	51	50	62	80	MUE
	0.00	0.00	XXX	9	9	9	9	1
26	0.52	0.52	XXX	0	0	0	0	1

86335 Immunofixation electrophoresis; other fluids with concentration (eg, urine, CSF) [Q4]

Mod	Non-Fac Total	Fac Total	Global Days	51	50	62	80	MUE
	0.00	0.00	XXX	9	9	9	9	2
26	0.52	0.52	XXX	0	0	0	0	2

86336 Inhibin A [Q4]

Mod	Non-Fac Total	Fac Total	Global Days	51	50	62	80	MUE
	0.00	0.00	XXX	9	9	9	9	1

86337 Insulin antibodies [Q4]

Mod	Non-Fac Total	Fac Total	Global Days	51	50	62	80	MUE
	0.00	0.00	XXX	9	9	9	9	1

86340 Intrinsic factor antibodies [Q4]

Mod	Non-Fac Total	Fac Total	Global Days	51	50	62	80	MUE
	0.00	0.00	XXX	9	9	9	9	1

● New ▲ Revised ✖ Deleted ⊙ Moderate Sedation ✚ Add-on Codes ⊘ High Risk Denial Ⓐ Age Edit ♀ Female ♂ Male **AMA** CPT® Assistant **MUE** Medically Unlikely Edit
⊘ Modifier 51 Exempt ⊖ Modifier 63 Exempt ✗ Unlisted **Modifiers:** See Inside Back Cover Ⓜ Maternity A2–Z3 ASC Payment Indicators A–Y OPPS Status Indicators

740   CPT © 2015 American Medical Association. All Rights Reserved.   © 2016 DecisionHealth

86341 Islet cell antibody   Q4

Mod	Non-Fac Total	Fac Total	Global Days	51	50	62	80	MUE
	0.00	0.00	XXX	9	9	9	9	1

AMA: Summer 94: 6

86343 Leukocyte histamine release test (LHR)   Q4

Mod	Non-Fac Total	Fac Total	Global Days	51	50	62	80	MUE
	0.00	0.00	XXX	9	9	9	9	1

86344 Leukocyte phagocytosis   Q4

Mod	Non-Fac Total	Fac Total	Global Days	51	50	62	80	MUE
	0.00	0.00	XXX	9	9	9	9	1

86352 Cellular function assay involving stimulation (eg, mitogen or antigen) and detection of biomarker (eg, ATP)   Q4

Mod	Non-Fac Total	Fac Total	Global Days	51	50	62	80	MUE
	0.00	0.00	XXX	9	9	9	9	1

86353 Lymphocyte transformation, mitogen (phytomitogen) or antigen induced blastogenesis   Q4

Mod	Non-Fac Total	Fac Total	Global Days	51	50	62	80	MUE
	0.00	0.00	XXX	9	9	9	9	7

Coding Guidance

There is no interpretive service for quantitative cell counts. Do not report flow cytometry interpretation codes 88187-88189 together with 86355-86367.

86355 B cells, total count   Q4

Mod	Non-Fac Total	Fac Total	Global Days	51	50	62	80	MUE
	0.00	0.00	XXX	9	9	9	9	1

AMA: Mar 06: 6, Apr 08: 5

86356 Mononuclear cell antigen, quantitative (eg, flow cytometry), not otherwise specified, each antigen   Q4

Mod	Non-Fac Total	Fac Total	Global Days	51	50	62	80	MUE
	0.00	0.00	XXX	9	9	9	9	7

AMA: Apr 08: 5

86357 Natural killer (NK) cells, total count   Q4

Mod	Non-Fac Total	Fac Total	Global Days	51	50	62	80	MUE
	0.00	0.00	XXX	9	9	9	9	1

AMA: Mar 06: 6, Apr 08: 5

86359 T cells; total count   Q4

Mod	Non-Fac Total	Fac Total	Global Days	51	50	62	80	MUE
	0.00	0.00	XXX	9	9	9	9	1

AMA: Nov 97: 30, Apr 08: 5

86360 T cells; absolute CD4 and CD8 count, including ratio   Q4

Mod	Non-Fac Total	Fac Total	Global Days	51	50	62	80	MUE
	0.00	0.00	XXX	9	9	9	9	1

AMA: Nov 97: 30, Jan 07: 29, Apr 08: 5

86361 T cells; absolute CD4 count   Q4

Mod	Non-Fac Total	Fac Total	Global Days	51	50	62	80	MUE
	0.00	0.00	XXX	9	9	9	9	1

AMA: Nov 97: 30, Apr 08: 5

86367 Stem cells (ie, CD34), total count   Q4

Mod	Non-Fac Total	Fac Total	Global Days	51	50	62	80	MUE
	0.00	0.00	XXX	9	9	9	9	1

AMA: Mar 06: 6, Apr 08: 5, Oct 13: 3

86376 Microsomal antibodies (eg, thyroid or liver-kidney), each   Q4

Mod	Non-Fac Total	Fac Total	Global Days	51	50	62	80	MUE
	0.00	0.00	XXX	9	9	9	9	2

86378 Migration inhibitory factor test (MIF)   Q4

Mod	Non-Fac Total	Fac Total	Global Days	51	50	62	80	MUE
	0.00	0.00	XXX	9	9	9	9	1

86382 Neutralization test, viral   Q4

Mod	Non-Fac Total	Fac Total	Global Days	51	50	62	80	MUE
	0.00	0.00	XXX	9	9	9	9	3

86384 Nitroblue tetrazolium dye test (NTD)   Q4

Mod	Non-Fac Total	Fac Total	Global Days	51	50	62	80	MUE
	0.00	0.00	XXX	9	9	9	9	1

86386 Nuclear Matrix Protein 22 (NMP22), qualitative   Q4

Mod	Non-Fac Total	Fac Total	Global Days	51	50	62	80	MUE
	0.00	0.00	XXX	9	9	9	9	1

86403 Particle agglutination; screen, each antibody   Q4

Mod	Non-Fac Total	Fac Total	Global Days	51	50	62	80	MUE
	0.00	0.00	XXX	9	9	9		

AMA: Aug 05: 9

86406 Particle agglutination; titer, each antibody   Q4

Mod	Non-Fac Total	Fac Total	Global Days	51	50	62	80	MUE
	0.00	0.00	XXX	9	9	9	9	2

86430 Rheumatoid factor; qualitative   Q4

Mod	Non-Fac Total	Fac Total	Global Days	51	50	62	80	MUE
	0.00	0.00	XXX	9	9	9	9	2

● New   ▲ Revised   Deleted   ⊙ Moderate Sedation   ✚ Add-on Codes   ⊘ High Risk Denial   Ⓐ Age Edit   ♀ Female   ♂ Male   **AMA** *CPT® Assistant*   **MUE** Medically Unlikely Edit

⊘ Modifier 51 Exempt   ⊖ Modifier 63 Exempt   ✗ Unlisted   **Modifiers:** *See Inside Back Cover*   Ⓜ Maternity   A2–Z3 ASC Payment Indicators   A–Y OPPS Status Indicators

© 2016 DecisionHealth   CPT © 2015 American Medical Association. All Rights Reserved.

86431 Rheumatoid factor; quantitative ⊙4

RVU		Global Days	Modifiers				
Mod	Non-Fac Total	Fac Total		51	50	62	80	MUE
	0.00	0.00	XXX	9	9	9	9	2

86480 Tuberculosis test, cell mediated immunity antigen response measurement; gamma interferon ⊙4

RVU		Global Days	Modifiers				
Mod	Non-Fac Total	Fac Total		51	50	62	80	MUE
	0.00	0.00	XXX	9	9	9	9	1

AMA: Mar 06: 6, Oct 10: 7, Dec 10: 8

86481 Tuberculosis test, cell mediated immunity antigen response measurement; enumeration of gamma interferon-producing T-cells in cell suspension ⊙4

RVU		Global Days	Modifiers				
Mod	Non-Fac Total	Fac Total		51	50	62	80	MUE
	0.00	0.00	XXX	9	9	9	9	1

AMA: Oct 10: 8, Dec 10: 8

86485 Skin test; candida ⊙1

RVU		Global Days	Modifiers				
Mod	Non-Fac Total	Fac Total		51	50	62	80	MUE
	0.00	0.00	XXX	0	0	0	0	1

86486 Skin test; unlisted antigen, each ⊙1

RVU		Global Days	Modifiers				
Mod	Non-Fac Total	Fac Total		51	50	62	80	MUE
	0.14	0.14	XXX	0	0	0	0	2

86490 Skin test; coccidioidomycosis ⊙1

RVU		Global Days	Modifiers				
Mod	Non-Fac Total	Fac Total		51	50	62	80	MUE
	1.97	1.97	XXX	0	0	0	0	1

86510 Skin test; histoplasmosis ⊙1

RVU		Global Days	Modifiers				
Mod	Non-Fac Total	Fac Total		51	50	62	80	MUE
	0.17	0.17	XXX	0	0	0	0	1

AMA: Aug 05: 9

86580 Skin test; tuberculosis, intradermal ⊙1

RVU		Global Days	Modifiers				
Mod	Non-Fac Total	Fac Total		51	50	62	80	MUE
	0.22	0.22	XXX	0	0	0	0	1

86590 Streptokinase, antibody ⊙4

RVU		Global Days	Modifiers				
Mod	Non-Fac Total	Fac Total		51	50	62	80	MUE
	0.00	0.00	XXX	9	9	9	9	1

Pub 100-04, 16, 120.2

86592 Syphilis test, non-treponemal antibody; qualitative (eg, VDRL, RPR, ART) Ⓐ

RVU		Global Days	Modifiers				
Mod	Non-Fac Total	Fac Total		51	50	62	80	MUE
	0.00	0.00	XXX	9	9	9	9	2

Pub 100-04, 18, 170.1

86593 Syphilis test, non-treponemal antibody; quantitative Ⓐ

RVU		Global Days	Modifiers				
Mod	Non-Fac Total	Fac Total		51	50	62	80	MUE
	0.00	0.00	XXX	9	9	9	9	2

Pub 100-04, 18, 170.1

Coding Guidance
Examples of other antibody testing coded elsewhere include: leukocyte, platelet, microsomal, and RBC.

86602 Antibody; actinomyces ⊙4

RVU		Global Days	Modifiers				
Mod	Non-Fac Total	Fac Total		51	50	62	80	MUE
	0.00	0.00	XXX	9	9	9	9	3

AMA: Aug 05: 9

86603 Antibody; adenovirus ⊙4

RVU		Global Days	Modifiers				
Mod	Non-Fac Total	Fac Total		51	50	62	80	MUE
	0.00	0.00	XXX	9	9	9	9	2

86606 Antibody; Aspergillus ⊙4

RVU		Global Days	Modifiers				
Mod	Non-Fac Total	Fac Total		51	50	62	80	MUE
	0.00	0.00	XXX	9	9	9	9	

86609 Antibody; bacterium, not elsewhere specified ⊙4

RVU		Global Days	Modifiers				
Mod	Non-Fac Total	Fac Total		51	50	62	80	MUE
	0.00	0.00	XXX	9	9	9	9	14

86611 Antibody; Bartonella ⊙4

RVU		Global Days	Modifiers				
Mod	Non-Fac Total	Fac Total		51	50	62	80	MUE
	0.00	0.00	XXX	9	9	9	9	4

86612 Antibody; Blastomyces ⊙4

RVU		Global Days	Modifiers				
Mod	Non-Fac Total	Fac Total		51	50	62	80	MUE
	0.00	0.00	XXX	9	9	9	9	2

86615 Antibody; Bordetella ⊙4

RVU		Global Days	Modifiers				
Mod	Non-Fac Total	Fac Total		51	50	62	80	MUE
	0.00	0.00	XXX	9	9	9	9	6

86617 Antibody; Borrelia burgdorferi (Lyme disease) confirmatory test (eg, Western Blot or immunoblot) ⊙4

RVU		Global Days	Modifiers				
Mod	Non-Fac Total	Fac Total		51	50	62	80	MUE
	0.00	0.00	XXX	9	9	9	9	2

86618 Antibody; Borrelia burgdorferi (Lyme disease) ⊙4

Coding tip: For a CLIA-waived test, append modifier QW to 86618

RVU		Global Days	Modifiers				
Mod	Non-Fac Total	Fac Total		51	50	62	80	MUE
	0.00	0.00	XXX	9	9	9	9	2

86619 Antibody; Borrelia (relapsing fever) ⊙4

RVU		Global Days	Modifiers				
Mod	Non-Fac Total	Fac Total		51	50	62	80	MUE
	0.00	0.00	XXX	9	9	9	9	2

● New   ▲ Revised   ✖ Deleted   ⊙ Moderate Sedation   ✚ Add-on Codes   ⊘ High Risk Denial   Ⓐ Age Edit   ♀ Female   ♂ Male   **AMA** *CPT® Assistant*   **MUE** Medically Unlikely Edit
⊘ Modifier 51 Exempt   ⊖ Modifier 63 Exempt   ✗ Unlisted   **Modifiers:** *See Inside Back Cover*   Ⓜ Maternity   A2–Z3 ASC Payment Indicators   A–Y OPPS Status Indicators

742   CPT © 2015 American Medical Association. All Rights Reserved.   © 2016 DecisionHealth

86622 Antibody; Brucella   Q4

RVU			Global Days	Modifiers				
Mod	Non-Fac Total	Fac Total		51	50	62	80	MUE
	0.00	0.00	XXX	9	9	9	9	2

86625 Antibody; Campylobacter   Q4

RVU			Global Days	Modifiers				
Mod	Non-Fac Total	Fac Total		51	50	62	80	MUE
	0.00	0.00	XXX	9	9	9	9	1

86628 Antibody; Candida   Q4

RVU			Global Days	Modifiers				
Mod	Non-Fac Total	Fac Total		51	50	62	80	MUE
	0.00	0.00	XXX	9	9	9	9	3

86631 Antibody; Chlamydia   A

RVU			Global Days	Modifiers				
Mod	Non-Fac Total	Fac Total		51	50	62	80	MUE
	0.00	0.00	XXX	9	9	9	9	6

Pub 100-04, 18, 170.1

86632 Antibody; Chlamydia, IgM   A

RVU			Global Days	Modifiers				
Mod	Non-Fac Total	Fac Total		51	50	62	80	MUE
	0.00	0.00	XXX	9	9	9	9	3

AMA: Nov 97: 31
Pub 100-04, 18, 170.1

86635 Antibody; Coccidioides   Q4

RVU			Global Days	Modifiers				
Mod	Non-Fac Total	Fac Total		51	50	62	80	MUE
	0.00	0.00	XXX	9	9	9	9	4

86638 Antibody; Coxiella burnetii (Q fever)   Q4

RVU			Global Days	Modifiers				
Mod	Non-Fac Total	Fac Total		51	50	62	80	MUE
	0.00	0.00	XXX	9	9	9	9	6

86641 Antibody; Cryptococcus   Q4

RVU			Global Days	Modifiers				
Mod	Non-Fac Total	Fac Total		51	50	62	80	MUE
	0.00	0.00	XXX	9	9	9	9	2

86644 Antibody; cytomegalovirus (CMV)   Q4

RVU			Global Days	Modifiers				
Mod	Non-Fac Total	Fac Total		51	50	62	80	MUE
	0.00	0.00	XXX	9	9	9	9	2

Pub 100-04, 16, 120.2

86645 Antibody; cytomegalovirus (CMV), IgM   Q4

RVU			Global Days	Modifiers				
Mod	Non-Fac Total	Fac Total		51	50	62	80	MUE
	0.00	0.00	XXX	9	9	9	9	1

AMA: Jul 03: 7
Pub 100-04, 16, 120.2

86648 Antibody; Diphtheria   Q4

RVU			Global Days	Modifiers				
Mod	Non-Fac Total	Fac Total		51	50	62	80	MUE
	0.00	0.00	XXX	9	9	9	9	2

86651 Antibody; encephalitis, California (La Crosse)   Q4

RVU			Global Days	Modifiers				
Mod	Non-Fac Total	Fac Total		51	50	62	80	MUE
	0.00	0.00	XXX	9	9	9	9	2

86652 Antibody; encephalitis, Eastern equine   Q4

RVU			Global Days	Modifiers				
Mod	Non-Fac Total	Fac Total		51	50	62	80	MUE
	0.00	0.00	XXX	9	9	9	9	2

86653 Antibody; encephalitis, St. Louis   Q4

RVU			Global Days	Modifiers				
Mod	Non-Fac Total	Fac Total		51	50	62	80	MUE
	0.00	0.00	XXX	9	9	9	9	2

86654 Antibody; encephalitis, Western equine   Q4

RVU			Global Days	Modifiers				
Mod	Non-Fac Total	Fac Total		51	50	62	80	MUE
	0.00	0.00	XXX	9	9	9	9	2

86658 Antibody; enterovirus (eg, coxsackie, echo, polio)   Q4

RVU			Global Days	Modifiers				
Mod	Non-Fac Total	Fac Total		51	50	62	80	MUE
	0.00	0.00	XXX	9	9	9	9	12

86663 Antibody; Epstein-Barr (EB) virus, early antigen (EA)   Q4

RVU			Global Days	Modifiers				
Mod	Non-Fac Total	Fac Total		51	50	62	80	MUE
	0.00	0.00	XXX	9	9	9	9	2

86664 Antibody; Epstein-Barr (EB) virus, nuclear antigen (EBNA)   Q4

RVU			Global Days	Modifiers				
Mod	Non-Fac Total	Fac Total		51	50	62	80	MUE
	0.00	0.00	XXX	9	9	9	9	2

86665 Antibody; Epstein-Barr (EB) virus, viral capsid (VCA)   Q4

RVU			Global Days	Modifiers				
Mod	Non-Fac Total	Fac Total		51	50	62	80	MUE
	0.00	0.00	XXX	9	9	9	9	2

86666 Antibody; Ehrlichia   Q4

RVU			Global Days	Modifiers				
Mod	Non-Fac Total	Fac Total		51	50	62	80	MUE
	0.00	0.00	XXX	9	9	9	9	4

86668 Antibody; Francisella tularensis   Q4

RVU			Global Days	Modifiers				
Mod	Non-Fac Total	Fac Total		51	50	62	80	MUE
	0.00	0.00	XXX	9	9	9	9	2

86671 Antibody; fungus, not elsewhere specified   Q4

RVU			Global Days	Modifiers				
Mod	Non-Fac Total	Fac Total		51	50	62	80	MUE
	0.00	0.00	XXX	9	9	9	9	3

86674 Antibody; Giardia lamblia   Q4

RVU			Global Days	Modifiers				
Mod	Non-Fac Total	Fac Total		51	50	62	80	MUE
	0.00	0.00	XXX	9	9	9	9	3

● New   ▲ Revised   Deleted   ⊙ Moderate Sedation   ✚ Add-on Codes   ⊘ High Risk Denial   Ⓐ Age Edit   ♀ Female   ♂ Male   **AMA** CPT® Assistant   **MUE** Medically Unlikely Edit
⊘ Modifier 51 Exempt   ⊖ Modifier 63 Exempt   ✗ Unlisted   **Modifiers:** See Inside Back Cover   Ⓜ Maternity   A2–Z3 ASC Payment Indicators   A–Y OPPS Status Indicators

© 2016 DecisionHealth   CPT © 2015 American Medical Association. All Rights Reserved.

86677 Antibody; Helicobacter pylori ▣4

	RVU		Global Days	Modifiers				
Mod	Non-Fac Total	Fac Total		51	50	62	80	MUE
	0.00	0.00	XXX	9	9	9	9	3

AMA: Jan 98: 6

86682 Antibody; helminth, not elsewhere specified ▣4

	RVU		Global Days	Modifiers				
Mod	Non-Fac Total	Fac Total		51	50	62	80	MUE
	0.00	0.00	XXX	9	9	9	9	2

86684 Antibody; Haemophilus influenza ▣4

	RVU		Global Days	Modifiers				
Mod	Non-Fac Total	Fac Total		51	50	62	80	MUE
	0.00	0.00	XXX	9	9	9	9	2

86687 Antibody; HTLV-I ▣4

	RVU		Global Days	Modifiers				
Mod	Non-Fac Total	Fac Total		51	50	62	80	MUE
	0.00	0.00	XXX	9	9	9	9	1

Pub 100-04, 16, 120.2

86688 Antibody; HTLV-II ▣4

	RVU		Global Days	Modifiers				
Mod	Non-Fac Total	Fac Total		51	50	62	80	MUE
	0.00	0.00	XXX	9	9	9	9	1

Pub 100-04, 16, 120.2

86689 Antibody; HTLV or HIV antibody, confirmatory test (eg, Western Blot) ▣4

	RVU		Global Days	Modifiers				
Mod	Non-Fac Total	Fac Total		51	50	62	80	MUE
	0.00	0.00	XXX	9	9	9	9	2

AMA: Mar 08: 3
Pub 100-04, 16, 120.2
NCD: 190.14

86692 Antibody; hepatitis, delta agent ▣4

	RVU		Global Days	Modifiers				
Mod	Non-Fac Total	Fac Total		51	50	62	80	MUE
	0.00	0.00	XXX	9	9	9	9	2

AMA: Nov 97: 31
Pub 100-04, 16, 120.2

86694 Antibody; herpes simplex, non-specific type test ▣4

	RVU		Global Days	Modifiers				
Mod	Non-Fac Total	Fac Total		51	50	62	80	MUE
	0.00	0.00	XXX	9	9	9	9	2

86695 Antibody; herpes simplex, type 1 ▣4

	RVU		Global Days	Modifiers				
Mod	Non-Fac Total	Fac Total		51	50	62	80	MUE
	0.00	0.00	XXX	9	9	9	9	2

86696 Antibody; herpes simplex, type 2 ▣4

	RVU		Global Days	Modifiers				
Mod	Non-Fac Total	Fac Total		51	50	62	80	MUE
	0.00	0.00	XXX	9	9	9	9	2

86698 Antibody; histoplasma ▣4

	RVU		Global Days	Modifiers				
Mod	Non-Fac Total	Fac Total		51	50	62	80	MUE
	0.00	0.00	XXX	9	9	9	9	3

86701 Antibody; HIV-1 ▣4

Coding tip: For a CLIA-waived test, append modifier QW to 86701

	RVU		Global Days	Modifiers				
Mod	Non-Fac Total	Fac Total		51	50	62	80	MUE
	0.00	0.00	XXX	9	9	9	9	1

AMA: Aug 05: 9, Mar 08: 3, Apr 08: 5
Pub 100-04, 16, 120.2
NCD: 190.14

86702 Antibody; HIV-2 ▣4

	RVU		Global Days	Modifiers				
Mod	Non-Fac Total	Fac Total		51	50	62	80	MUE
	0.00	0.00	XXX	9	9	9	9	2

AMA: Mar 08: 3, Apr 08: 5
Pub 100-04, 16, 120.2
NCD: 190.14

86703 Antibody; HIV-1 and HIV-2, single result ⊙▣4

	RVU		Global Days	Modifiers				
Mod	Non-Fac Total	Fac Total		51	50	62	80	MUE
	0.00	0.00	XXX	9	9	9	9	1

AMA: Nov 97: 31, Mar 08: 3, Apr 08: 5
Pub 100-04, 16, 120.2
NCD: 190.14

86704 Hepatitis B core antibody (HBcAb); total ▣4

	RVU		Global Days	Modifiers				
Mod	Non-Fac Total	Fac Total		51	50	62	80	MUE
	0.00	0.00	XXX	9	9	9	9	1

AMA: Nov 97: 31, 32
Pub 100-04, 16, 120.2

86705 Hepatitis B core antibody (HBcAb); IgM antibody ▣4

	RVU		Global Days	Modifiers				
Mod	Non-Fac Total	Fac Total		51	50	62	80	MUE
	0.00	0.00	XXX	9	9	9	9	1

AMA: Nov 97: 31, 32
Pub 100-04, 16, 120.2

86706 Hepatitis B surface antibody (HBsAb) ▣4

	RVU		Global Days	Modifiers				
Mod	Non-Fac Total	Fac Total		51	50	62	80	MUE
	0.00	0.00	XXX	9	9	9	9	2

AMA: Nov 97: 31, 32
Pub 100-04, 16, 120.2

86707 Hepatitis Be antibody (HBeAb) ▣4

	RVU		Global Days	Modifiers				
Mod	Non-Fac Total	Fac Total		51	50	62	80	MUE
	0.00	0.00	XXX	9	9	9	9	1

AMA: Nov 97: 31, 32
Pub 100-04, 16, 120.2

▲ 86708 Hepatitis A antibody (HAAb) ▣4

	RVU		Global Days	Modifiers				
Mod	Non-Fac Total	Fac Total		51	50	62	80	MUE
	0.00	0.00	XXX	9	9	9	9	1

AMA: Nov 97: 31, 32, Jun 00: 11

● New ▲ Revised ✖ Deleted ⊙ Moderate Sedation ✚ Add-on Codes ⊘ High Risk Denial ⊛ Age Edit ♀ Female ♂ Male **AMA** *CPT® Assistant* **MUE** Medically Unlikely Edit
⊘ Modifier 51 Exempt ⊖ Modifier 63 Exempt ⊠ Unlisted **Modifiers:** *See Inside Back Cover* Ⓜ Maternity A2–Z3 ASC Payment Indicators A–Y OPPS Status Indicators

CPT © 2015 American Medical Association. All Rights Reserved.   © 2016 DecisionHealth

86709 Hepatitis A antibody (HAAb), IgM antibody ▲ ☑4

Mod	RVU Non-Fac Total	Fac Total	Global Days	51	50	62	80	MUE
	0.00	0.00	XXX	9	9	9	9	1

AMA: Nov 97: 31, 32, Jun 00: 11
Pub 100-04, 16, 120.2

86710 Antibody; influenza virus ☑4

Mod	RVU Non-Fac Total	Fac Total	Global Days	51	50	62	80	MUE
	0.00	0.00	XXX	9	9	9	9	4

86711 Antibody; JC (John Cunningham) virus ☑4

Mod	RVU Non-Fac Total	Fac Total	Global Days	51	50	62	80	MUE
	0.00	0.00	XXX	9	9	9	9	2

86713 Antibody; Legionella ☑4

Mod	RVU Non-Fac Total	Fac Total	Global Days	51	50	62	80	MUE
	0.00	0.00	XXX	9	9	9	9	3

86717 Antibody; Leishmania ☑4

Mod	RVU Non-Fac Total	Fac Total	Global Days	51	50	62	80	MUE
	0.00	0.00	XXX	9	9	9	9	8

86720 Antibody; Leptospira ☑4

Mod	RVU Non-Fac Total	Fac Total	Global Days	51	50	62	80	MUE
	0.00	0.00	XXX	9	9	9	9	2

86723 Antibody; Listeria monocytogenes ☑4

Mod	RVU Non-Fac Total	Fac Total	Global Days	51	50	62	80	MUE
	0.00	0.00	XXX	9	9	9	9	2

86727 Antibody; lymphocytic choriomeningitis ☑4

Mod	RVU Non-Fac Total	Fac Total	Global Days	51	50	62	80	MUE
	0.00	0.00	XXX	9	9	9	9	2

86729 Antibody; lymphogranuloma venereum ☑4

Mod	RVU Non-Fac Total	Fac Total	Global Days	51	50	62	80	MUE
	0.00	0.00	XXX	9	9	9	9	0

86732 Antibody; mucormycosis ☑4

Mod	RVU Non-Fac Total	Fac Total	Global Days	51	50	62	80	MUE
	0.00	0.00	XXX	9	9	9	9	2

86735 Antibody; mumps ☑4

Mod	RVU Non-Fac Total	Fac Total	Global Days	51	50	62	80	MUE
	0.00	0.00	XXX	9	9	9	9	2

86738 Antibody; mycoplasma ☑4

Mod	RVU Non-Fac Total	Fac Total	Global Days	51	50	62	80	MUE
	0.00	0.00	XXX	9	9	9	9	2

86741 Antibody; Neisseria meningitidis ☑4

Mod	RVU Non-Fac Total	Fac Total	Global Days	51	50	62	80	MUE
	0.00	0.00	XXX	9	9	9	9	2

86744 Antibody; Nocardia ☑4

Mod	RVU Non-Fac Total	Fac Total	Global Days	51	50	62	80	MUE
	0.00	0.00	XXX	9	9	9	9	2

86747 Antibody; parvovirus ☑4

Mod	RVU Non-Fac Total	Fac Total	Global Days	51	50	62	80	MUE
	0.00	0.00	XXX	9	9	9	9	2

86750 Antibody; Plasmodium (malaria) ☑4

Mod	RVU Non-Fac Total	Fac Total	Global Days	51	50	62	80	MUE
	0.00	0.00	XXX	9	9	9	9	4

86753 Antibody; protozoa, not elsewhere specified ☑4

Mod	RVU Non-Fac Total	Fac Total	Global Days	51	50	62	80	MUE
	0.00	0.00	XXX	9	9	9	9	3

86756 Antibody; respiratory syncytial virus ☑4

Mod	RVU Non-Fac Total	Fac Total	Global Days	51	50	62	80	MUE
	0.00	0.00	XXX	9	9	9	9	2

86757 Antibody; Rickettsia ☑4

Mod	RVU Non-Fac Total	Fac Total	Global Days	51	50	62	80	MUE
	0.00	0.00	XXX	9	9	9	9	6

86759 Antibody; rotavirus ☑4

Mod	RVU Non-Fac Total	Fac Total	Global Days	51	50	62	80	MUE
	0.00	0.00	XXX	9	9	9	9	2

86762 Antibody; rubella ☑4

Mod	RVU Non-Fac Total	Fac Total	Global Days	51	50	62	80	MUE
	0.00	0.00	XXX	9	9	9	9	2

86765 Antibody; rubeola ☑4

Mod	RVU Non-Fac Total	Fac Total	Global Days	51	50	62	80	MUE
	0.00	0.00	XXX	9	9	9	9	2

86768 Antibody; Salmonella ☑4

Mod	RVU Non-Fac Total	Fac Total	Global Days	51	50	62	80	MUE
	0.00	0.00	XXX	9	9	9	9	5

86771 Antibody; Shigella ☑4

Mod	RVU Non-Fac Total	Fac Total	Global Days	51	50	62	80	MUE
	0.00	0.00	XXX	9	9	9	9	2

86774 Antibody; tetanus ☑4

Mod	RVU Non-Fac Total	Fac Total	Global Days	51	50	62	80	MUE
	0.00	0.00	XXX	9	9	9	9	2

● New   ▲ Revised   Deleted   ☉ Moderate Sedation   ✚ Add-on Codes   ⊘ High Risk Denial   Ⓐ Age Edit   ♀ Female   ♂ Male   AMA *CPT® Assistant*   MUE Medically Unlikely Edit
⊘ Modifier 51 Exempt   ⊖ Modifier 63 Exempt   ✗ Unlisted   Modifiers: *See Inside Back Cover*   Ⓜ Maternity   A2–Z3 ASC Payment Indicators   A–Y OPPS Status Indicators

86777 Antibody; Toxoplasma   Q4

RVU			Global Days	Modifiers				
Mod	Non-Fac Total	Fac Total		51	50	62	80	MUE
	0.00	0.00	XXX	9	9	9	9	2

86778 Antibody; Toxoplasma, IgM   Q4

RVU			Global Days	Modifiers				
Mod	Non-Fac Total	Fac Total		51	50	62	80	MUE
	0.00	0.00	XXX	9	9	9	9	2

86780 Antibody; Treponema pallidum   Q4

RVU			Global Days	Modifiers				
Mod	Non-Fac Total	Fac Total		51	50	62	80	MUE
	0.00	0.00	XXX	9	9	9	9	2

Pub 100-04, 18, 170.1

86784 Antibody; Trichinella   Q4

RVU			Global Days	Modifiers				
Mod	Non-Fac Total	Fac Total		51	50	62	80	MUE
	0.00	0.00	XXX	9	9	9	9	1

86787 Antibody; varicella-zoster   Q4

RVU			Global Days	Modifiers				
Mod	Non-Fac Total	Fac Total		51	50	62	80	MUE
	0.00	0.00	XXX	9	9	9	9	2

86788 Antibody; West Nile virus, IgM   Q4

RVU			Global Days	Modifiers				
Mod	Non-Fac Total	Fac Total		51	50	62	80	MUE
	0.00	0.00	XXX	9	9	9	9	2

86789 Antibody; West Nile virus   Q4

RVU			Global Days	Modifiers				
Mod	Non-Fac Total	Fac Total		51	50	62	80	MUE
	0.00	0.00	XXX	9	9	9	9	2

86790 Antibody; virus, not elsewhere specified   Q4

RVU			Global Days	Modifiers				
Mod	Non-Fac Total	Fac Total		51	50	62	80	MUE
	0.00	0.00	XXX	9	9	9	9	4

86793 Antibody; Yersinia   Q4

RVU			Global Days	Modifiers				
Mod	Non-Fac Total	Fac Total		51	50	62	80	MUE
	0.00	0.00	XXX	9	9	9	9	2

86800 Thyroglobulin antibody   Q4

RVU			Global Days	Modifiers				
Mod	Non-Fac Total	Fac Total		51	50	62	80	MUE
	0.00	0.00	XXX	9	9	9	9	1

AMA: Aug 05: 9

86803 Hepatitis C antibody   Q4

RVU			Global Days	Modifiers				
Mod	Non-Fac Total	Fac Total		51	50	62	80	MUE
	0.00	0.00	XXX	9	9	9	9	1

AMA: Nov 97: 31, 32
Pub 100-04, 16, 120.2

86804 Hepatitis C antibody; confirmatory test (eg, immunoblot)   Q4

RVU			Global Days	Modifiers				
Mod	Non-Fac Total	Fac Total		51	50	62	80	MUE
	0.00	0.00	XXX	9	9	9	9	1

AMA: Nov 97: 31, 32
Pub 100-04, 16, 120.2

Tissue Type Testing

86805 Lymphocytotoxicity assay, visual crossmatch; with titration   Q4

RVU			Global Days	Modifiers				
Mod	Non-Fac Total	Fac Total		51	50	62	80	MUE
	0.00	0.00	XXX	9	9	9	9	2

86806 Lymphocytotoxicity assay, visual crossmatch; without titration   Q4

RVU			Global Days	Modifiers				
Mod	Non-Fac Total	Fac Total		51	50	62	80	MUE
	0.00	0.00	XXX	9	9	9	9	

86807 Serum screening for cytotoxic percent reactive antibody (PRA); standard method   Q4

RVU			Global Days	Modifiers				
Mod	Non-Fac Total	Fac Total		51	50	62	80	MUE
	0.00	0.00	XXX	9	9	9	9	2

AMA: Jun 01: 11

86808 Serum screening for cytotoxic percent reactive antibody (PRA); quick method   Q4

RVU			Global Days	Modifiers				
Mod	Non-Fac Total	Fac Total		51	50	62	80	MUE
	0.00	0.00	XXX	9	9	9	9	1

AMA: Jun 01: 11

86812 HLA typing; A, B, or C (eg, A10, B7, B27), single antigen   Q4

RVU			Global Days	Modifiers				
Mod	Non-Fac Total	Fac Total		51	50	62	80	MUE
	0.00	0.00	XXX	9	9	9	9	1

AMA: Mar 03: 23, Jun 06: 17
Pub 100-04, 16, 120.2

86813 HLA typing; A, B, or C, multiple antigens   Q4

RVU			Global Days	Modifiers				
Mod	Non-Fac Total	Fac Total		51	50	62	80	MUE
	0.00	0.00	XXX	9	9	9	9	1

AMA: Mar 03: 23, Jun 06: 17
Pub 100-04, 16, 120.2

86816 HLA typing; DR/DQ, single antigen   Q4

RVU			Global Days	Modifiers				
Mod	Non-Fac Total	Fac Total		51	50	62	80	MUE
	0.00	0.00	XXX	9	9	9	9	1

AMA: Mar 03: 23
Pub 100-04, 16, 120.2

86817 HLA typing; DR/DQ, multiple antigens   Q4

RVU			Global Days	Modifiers				
Mod	Non-Fac Total	Fac Total		51	50	62	80	MUE
	0.00	0.00	XXX	9	9	9	9	1

AMA: Mar 03: 23
Pub 100-04, 16, 120.2

● New   ▲ Revised   ✖ Deleted   ⊙ Moderate Sedation   ✚ Add-on Codes   ⊘ High Risk Denial   Ⓐ Age Edit   ♀ Female   ♂ Male   **AMA** *CPT® Assistant*   **MUE** Medically Unlikely Edit

⊘ Modifier 51 Exempt   ⊖ Modifier 63 Exempt   ✗ Unlisted   **Modifiers:** *See Inside Back Cover*   Ⓜ Maternity   A2–Z3 ASC Payment Indicators   A–Y OPPS Status Indicators

CPT © 2015 American Medical Association. All Rights Reserved.   © 2016 DecisionHealth

86821 HLA typing; lymphocyte culture, mixed (MLC) ○4

RVU			Global Days	Modifiers				
Mod	Non-Fac Total	Fac Total		51	50	62	80	MUE
	0.00	0.00	XXX	9	9	9	9	1

AMA: Mar 03: 23

86822 HLA typing; lymphocyte culture, primed (PLC) ○4

RVU			Global Days	Modifiers				
Mod	Non-Fac Total	Fac Total		51	50	62	80	MUE
	0.00	0.00	XXX	9	9	9	9	1

AMA: Mar 03: 23

86825 Human leukocyte antigen (HLA) crossmatch, non-cytotoxic (eg, using flow cytometry); first serum sample or dilution ⊘○4

RVU			Global Days	Modifiers				
Mod	Non-Fac Total	Fac Total		51	50	62	80	MUE
	0.00	0.00	XXX	9	9	9	9	1

+ **86826 Human leukocyte antigen (HLA) crossmatch, non-cytotoxic (eg, using flow cytometry); each additional serum sample or sample dilution (List separately in addition to primary procedure)** ⊘○4

RVU			Global Days	Modifiers				
Mod	Non-Fac Total	Fac Total		51	50	62	80	MUE
	0.00	0.00	XXX	9	9	9	9	2

86828 Antibody to human leukocyte antigens (HLA), solid phase assays (eg, microspheres or beads, ELISA, flow cytometry); qualitative assessment of the presence or absence of antibody(ies) to HLA Class I and Class II HLA antigens ○4

RVU			Global Days	Modifiers				
Mod	Non-Fac Total	Fac Total		51	50	62	80	MUE
	0.00	0.00	XXX	9	9	9	9	1

86829 Antibody to human leukocyte antigens (HLA), solid phase assays (eg, microspheres or beads, ELISA, Flow cytometry); qualitative assessment of the presence or absence of antibody(ies) to HLA Class I or Class II HLA antigens ○4

RVU			Global Days	Modifiers				
Mod	Non-Fac Total	Fac Total		51	50	62	80	MUE
	0.00	0.00	XXX	9	9	9	9	1

86830 Antibody to human leukocyte antigens (HLA), solid phase assays (eg, microspheres or beads, ELISA, Flow cytometry); antibody identification by qualitative panel using complete HLA phenotypes, HLA Class I ○4

RVU			Global Days	Modifiers				
Mod	Non-Fac Total	Fac Total		51	50	62	80	MUE
	0.00	0.00	XXX	9	9	9	9	2

86831 Antibody to human leukocyte antigens (HLA), solid phase assays (eg, microspheres or beads, ELISA, Flow cytometry); antibody identification by qualitative panel using complete HLA phenotypes, HLA Class II ○4

RVU			Global Days	Modifiers				
Mod	Non-Fac Total	Fac Total		51	50	62	80	MUE
	0.00	0.00	XXX	9	9	9	9	2

86832 Antibody to human leukocyte antigens (HLA), solid phase assays (eg, microspheres or beads, ELISA, Flow cytometry); high definition qualitative panel for identification of antibody specificities (eg, individual antigen per bead methodology), HLA Class I ○4

RVU			Global Days	Modifiers				
Mod	Non-Fac Total	Fac Total		51	50	62	80	MUE
	0.00	0.00	XXX	9	9	9	9	2

86833 Antibody to human leukocyte antigens (HLA), solid phase assays (eg, microspheres or beads, ELISA, Flow cytometry); high definition qualitative panel for identification of antibody specificities (eg, individual antigen per bead methodology), HLA Class II ○4

RVU			Global Days	Modifiers				
Mod	Non-Fac Total	Fac Total		51	50	62	80	MUE
	0.00	0.00	XXX	9	9	9	9	1

86834 Antibody to human leukocyte antigens (HLA), solid phase assays (eg, microspheres or beads, ELISA, Flow cytometry); semi-quantitative panel (eg, titer), HLA Class I ○4

RVU			Global Days	Modifiers				
Mod	Non-Fac Total	Fac Total		51	50	62	80	MUE
	0.00	0.00	XXX	9	9	9	9	1

86835 Antibody to human leukocyte antigens (HLA), solid phase assays (eg, microspheres or beads, ELISA, Flow cytometry); semi-quantitative panel (eg, titer), HLA Class II ○4

RVU			Global Days	Modifiers				
Mod	Non-Fac Total	Fac Total		51	50	62	80	MUE
	0.00	0.00	XXX	9	9	9	9	1

86849 Unlisted immunology procedure ⋇N

RVU			Global Days	Modifiers				
Mod	Non-Fac Total	Fac Total		51	50	62	80	MUE
	0.00	0.00	XXX	9	9	9	9	

AMA: Mar 98: 10

Transfusion-Related Procedures

86850 Antibody screen, RBC, each serum technique ○1

RVU			Global Days	Modifiers				
Mod	Non-Fac Total	Fac Total		51	50	62	80	MUE
	0.00	0.00	XXX	9	9	9	9	3

AMA: Fall 93: 25, Aug 05: 9, Apr 08: 5

86860 Antibody elution (RBC), each elution ○1

RVU			Global Days	Modifiers				
Mod	Non-Fac Total	Fac Total		51	50	62	80	MUE
	0.00	0.00	XXX	9	9	9	9	2

86870 Antibody identification, RBC antibodies, each panel for each serum technique ○2

RVU			Global Days	Modifiers				
Mod	Non-Fac Total	Fac Total		51	50	62	80	MUE
	0.00	0.00	XXX	9	9	9	9	2

AMA: Fall 93: 25, Mar 01: 10

Pub 100-04, 16, 90.2

● New ▲ Revised   Deleted   ⊙ Moderate Sedation   ✚ Add-on Codes   ⊘ High Risk Denial   Ⓐ Age Edit   ♀ Female   ♂ Male   **AMA** *CPT® Assistant*   **MUE** Medically Unlikely Edit
⊘ Modifier 51 Exempt   ⊖ Modifier 63 Exempt   ⋇ Unlisted   **Modifiers:** *See Inside Back Cover*   Ⓜ Maternity   A2–Z3 ASC Payment Indicators   A–Y OPPS Status Indicators

© 2016 DecisionHealth   CPT © 2015 American Medical Association. All Rights Reserved.   **747**

Laboratory/Pathology Procedures

86880 – 86923

86880 Antihuman globulin test (Coombs test); direct, each antiserum

Mod	Non-Fac Total	Fac Total	Global Days	51	50	62	80	MUE
	0.00	0.00	XXX	9	9	9	9	4

Pub 100-04, 16, 90.2

86885 Antihuman globulin test (Coombs test); indirect, qualitative, each reagent red cell

Mod	Non-Fac Total	Fac Total	Global Days	51	50	62	80	MUE
	0.00	0.00	XXX	9	9	9	9	2

AMA: Apr 08: 5

Pub 100-04, 16, 90.2

86886 Antihuman globulin test (Coombs test); indirect, each antibody titer

Mod	Non-Fac Total	Fac Total	Global Days	51	50	62	80	MUE
	0.00	0.00	XXX	9	9	9	9	3

AMA: Apr 08: 5

Pub 100-04, 16, 90.2

86890 Autologous blood or component, collection processing and storage; predeposited

Mod	Non-Fac Total	Fac Total	Global Days	51	50	62	80	MUE
	0.00	0.00	XXX	9	9	9	9	1

AMA: Apr 96: 2

Pub 100-04, 16, 90.2

86891 Autologous blood or component, collection processing and storage; intra- or postoperative salvage

Mod	Non-Fac Total	Fac Total	Global Days	51	50	62	80	MUE
	0.00	0.00	XXX	9	9	9	9	1

Pub 100-04, 16, 90.2

86900 Blood typing, serologic; ABO

Mod	Non-Fac Total	Fac Total	Global Days	51	50	62	80	MUE
	0.00	0.00	XXX	9	9	9	9	1

AMA: Aug 05: 9

Pub 100-04, 16, 120.2

86901 Blood typing, serologic; Rh (D)

Mod	Non-Fac Total	Fac Total	Global Days	51	50	62	80	MUE
	0.00	0.00	XXX	9	9	9	9	1

AMA: Fall 93: 25

Pub 100-04, 16, 90.2, 120.2

86902 Blood typing, serologic; antigen testing of donor blood using reagent serum, each antigen test

Mod	Non-Fac Total	Fac Total	Global Days	51	50	62	80	MUE
	0.00	0.00	XXX	9	9	9	9	6

AMA: Oct 10: 8, Dec 10: 8

86904 Blood typing, serologic; antigen screening for compatible unit using patient serum, per unit screened

Mod	Non-Fac Total	Fac Total	Global Days	51	50	62	80	MUE
	0.00	0.00	XXX	9	9	9	9	2

Pub 100-04, 16, 120.2

86905 Blood typing, serologic; RBC antigens, other than ABO or Rh (D), each

Mod	Non-Fac Total	Fac Total	Global Days	51	50	62	80	MUE
	0.00	0.00	XXX	9	9	9	9	8

Pub 100-04, 16, 90.2, 120.2

86906 Blood typing, serologic; Rh phenotyping, complete

Mod	Non-Fac Total	Fac Total	Global Days	51	50	62	80	MUE
	0.00	0.00	XXX	9	9	9	9	1

Pub 100-04, 16, 120.2

86910 Blood typing, for paternity testing, per individual; ABO, Rh and MN

Mod	Non-Fac Total	Fac Total	Global Days	51	50	62	80	MUE
	0.00	0.00	XXX	9	9	9	9	

86911 Blood typing, for paternity testing, per individual; each additional antigen system

Mod	Non-Fac Total	Fac Total	Global Days	51	50	62	80	MUE
	0.00	0.00	XXX	9	9	9	9	

86920 Compatibility test each unit; immediate spin technique

Mod	Non-Fac Total	Fac Total	Global Days	51	50	62	80	MUE
	0.00	0.00	XXX	9	9	9	9	

AMA: Mar 06: 6

Pub 100-04, 16, 90.2

86921 Compatibility test each unit; incubation technique

Mod	Non-Fac Total	Fac Total	Global Days	51	50	62	80	MUE
	0.00	0.00	XXX	9	9	9	9	2

AMA: Mar 06: 6

86922 Compatibility test each unit; antiglobulin technique

Mod	Non-Fac Total	Fac Total	Global Days	51	50	62	80	MUE
	0.00	0.00	XXX	9	9	9	9	5

AMA: Mar 06: 6

Pub 100-04, 16, 90.2

86923 Compatibility test each unit; electronic

Mod	Non-Fac Total	Fac Total	Global Days	51	50	62	80	MUE
	0.00	0.00	XXX	9	9	9	9	10

AMA: Mar 06: 6

● New   ▲ Revised   ✖ Deleted   ⊙ Moderate Sedation   ✚ Add-on Codes   ⊗ High Risk Denial   Ⓐ Age Edit   ♀ Female   ♂ Male   **AMA** *CPT® Assistant*   **MUE** Medically Unlikely Edit
⊘ Modifier 51 Exempt   ⊖ Modifier 63 Exempt   ✗ Unlisted   **Modifiers:** *See Inside Back Cover*   Ⓜ Maternity   A2–Z3 ASC Payment Indicators   A–Y OPPS Status Indicators

CPT © 2015 American Medical Association. All Rights Reserved.   © 2016 DecisionHealth

86927 Fresh frozen plasma, thawing, each unit   **S**

Mod	Non-Fac Total	Fac Total	Global Days	51	50	62	80	MUE
	0.00	0.00	XXX	9	9	9	9	2

86930 Frozen blood, each unit; freezing (includes preparation)   **Q1**

Mod	Non-Fac Total	Fac Total	Global Days	51	50	62	80	MUE
	0.00	0.00	XXX	9	9	9	9	0

AMA: Apr 96: 2, Jul 03: 8
Pub 100-04, 16, 90.2

86931 Frozen blood, each unit; thawing   **Q1**

Mod	Non-Fac Total	Fac Total	Global Days	51	50	62	80	MUE
	0.00	0.00	XXX	9	9	9	9	1

AMA: Jul 03: 8
Pub 100-04, 16, 90.2

86932 Frozen blood, each unit; freezing (includes preparation) and thawing   **Q1**

Mod	Non-Fac Total	Fac Total	Global Days	51	50	62	80	MUE
	0.00	0.00	XXX	9	9	9	9	2

AMA: Jul 03: 8
Pub 100-04, 16, 90.2

86940 Hemolysins and agglutinins; auto, screen, each **Q4**

Mod	Non-Fac Total	Fac Total	Global Days	51	50	62	80	MUE
	0.00	0.00	XXX	9	9	9	9	1

86941 Hemolysins and agglutinins; incubated   **Q4**

Mod	Non-Fac Total	Fac Total	Global Days	51	50	62	80	MUE
	0.00	0.00	XXX	9	9	9	9	1

86945 Irradiation of blood product, each unit   **Q1**

Mod	Non-Fac Total	Fac Total	Global Days	51	50	62	80	MUE
	0.00	0.00	XXX	9	9	9	9	2

AMA: Dec 07: 14

86950 Leukocyte transfusion   **Q1**

Mod	Non-Fac Total	Fac Total	Global Days	51	50	62	80	MUE
	0.00	0.00	XXX	9	9	9	9	1

AMA: Oct 13: 3

86960 Volume reduction of blood or blood product (eg, red blood cells or platelets), each unit   **Q1**

Mod	Non-Fac Total	Fac Total	Global Days	51	50	62	80	MUE
	0.00	0.00	XXX	9	9	9	9	1

AMA: Mar 06: 6

86965 Pooling of platelets or other blood products   **Q1**

Mod	Non-Fac Total	Fac Total	Global Days	51	50	62	80	MUE
	0.00	0.00	XXX	9	9	9	9	1

AMA: Oct 10: 8, Dec 10: 8

86970 Pretreatment of RBCs for use in RBC antibody detection, identification, and/or compatibility testing; incubation with chemical agents or drugs, each   **Q1**

Mod	Non-Fac Total	Fac Total	Global Days	51	50	62	80	MUE
	0.00	0.00	XXX	9	9	9	9	1

86971 Pretreatment of RBCs for use in RBC antibody detection, identification, and/or compatibility testing; incubation with enzymes, each   **Q1**

Mod	Non-Fac Total	Fac Total	Global Days	51	50	62	80	MUE
	0.00	0.00	XXX	9	9	9	9	1

Pub 100-04, 16, 90.2

86972 Pretreatment of RBCs for use in RBC antibody detection, identification, and/or compatibility testing; by density gradient separation   **Q1**

Mod	Non-Fac Total	Fac Total	Global Days	51	50	62	80	MUE
	0.00	0.00	XXX	9	9	9	9	1

86975 Pretreatment of serum for use in RBC antibody identification; incubation with drugs, each   **Q1**

Mod	Non-Fac Total	Fac Total	Global Days	51	50	62	80	MUE
	0.00	0.00	XXX	9	9	9	9	1

86976 Pretreatment of serum for use in RBC antibody identification; by dilution   **Q1**

Mod	Non-Fac Total	Fac Total	Global Days	51	50	62	80	MUE
	0.00	0.00	XXX	9	9	9	9	1

86977 Pretreatment of serum for use in RBC antibody identification; incubation with inhibitors, each   **Q1**

Mod	Non-Fac Total	Fac Total	Global Days	51	50	62	80	MUE
	0.00	0.00	XXX	9	9	9	9	1

86978 Pretreatment of serum for use in RBC antibody identification; by differential red cell absorption using patient RBCs or RBCs of known phenotype, each absorption   **Q1**

Mod	Non-Fac Total	Fac Total	Global Days	51	50	62	80	MUE
	0.00	0.00	XXX	9	9	9	9	1

86985 Splitting of blood or blood products, each unit   **Q1**

Mod	Non-Fac Total	Fac Total	Global Days	51	50	62	80	MUE
	0.00	0.00	XXX	9	9	9	9	1

AMA: Apr 96: 2, May 12: 11

86999 Unlisted transfusion medicine procedure   **⊗x Q1**

Mod	Non-Fac Total	Fac Total	Global Days	51	50	62	80	MUE
	0.00	0.00	XXX	9	9	9	9	

AMA: Aug 05: 9, Nov 05: 14, Mar 09: 10, Apr 09: 9, May 12: 11
Pub 100-04, 16, 100.4

● New   ▲ Revised   Deleted   ⊙ Moderate Sedation   ✚ Add-on Codes   ⊘ High Risk Denial   Ⓐ Age Edit   ♀ Female   ♂ Male   **AMA** *CPT® Assistant*   ***MUE*** Medically Unlikely Edit
⊘ Modifier 51 Exempt   ⊖ Modifier 63 Exempt   ⊠ Unlisted   **Modifiers:** *See Inside Back Cover*   Ⓜ Maternity   A2–Z3 ASC Payment Indicators   A–Y OPPS Status Indicators
© 2016 DecisionHealth   CPT © 2015 American Medical Association. All Rights Reserved.   **749**

87003 Animal inoculation, small animal, with observation and dissection ⊘Q4

Mod	Non-Fac Total	Fac Total	Global Days	51	50	62	80	MUE
	0.00	0.00	XXX	9	9	9	9	1

87015 Concentration (any type), for infectious agents Q4

Mod	Non-Fac Total	Fac Total	Global Days	51	50	62	80	MUE
	0.00	0.00	XXX	9	9	9	9	4

Coding Guidance

Codes 87040-87158 are for microbial culture studies. Report the type of culture by coding to the highest level of specificity for the source or type. When commercial kits are used, report the test to the highest specific level. Since a screening culture and a definitive identification culture are not performed on the same day on the same specimen, they cannot be reported together.

87040 Culture, bacterial; blood, aerobic, with isolation and presumptive identification of isolates (includes anaerobic culture, if appropriate) Q4

Mod	Non-Fac Total	Fac Total	Global Days	51	50	62	80	MUE
	0.00	0.00	XXX	9	9	9	9	2

AMA: Aug 97: 18, Jun 02: 2, Oct 10: 17, Dec 10: 17
Pub 100-04, 16, 120.2

87045 Culture, bacterial; stool, aerobic, with isolation and preliminary examination (eg, KIA, LIA), Salmonella and Shigella species Q4

Mod	Non-Fac Total	Fac Total	Global Days	51	50	62	80	MUE
	0.00	0.00	XXX	9	9	9	9	3

87046 Culture, bacterial; stool, aerobic, additional pathogens, isolation and presumptive identification of isolates, each plate Q4

Mod	Non-Fac Total	Fac Total	Global Days	51	50	62	80	MUE
	0.00	0.00	XXX	9	9	9	9	6

87070 Culture, bacterial; any other source except urine, blood or stool, aerobic, with isolation and presumptive identification of isolates Q4

Mod	Non-Fac Total	Fac Total	Global Days	51	50	62	80	MUE
	0.00	0.00	XXX	9	9	9	9	3

AMA: Aug 97: 18, Nov 01: 10, Oct 03: 10, Nov 11: 11
Pub 100-04, 16, 120.2

87071 Culture, bacterial; quantitative, aerobic with isolation and presumptive identification of isolates, any source except urine, blood or stool Q4

Mod	Non-Fac Total	Fac Total	Global Days	51	50	62	80	MUE
	0.00	0.00	XXX	9	9	9	9	4

AMA: Jun 02: 3, Sep 03: 3
Pub 100-04, 16, 120.2

87073 Culture, bacterial; quantitative, anaerobic with isolation and presumptive identification of isolates, any source except urine, blood or stool Q4

Mod	Non-Fac Total	Fac Total	Global Days	51	50	62	80	MUE
	0.00	0.00	XXX	9	9	9	9	3

AMA: Jun 02: 3
Pub 100-04, 16, 120.2

87075 Culture, bacterial; any source, except blood, anaerobic with isolation and presumptive identification of isolates Q4

Mod	Non-Fac Total	Fac Total	Global Days	51	50	62	80	MUE
	0.00	0.00	XXX	9	9	9	9	6

Pub 100-04, 16, 120.2

87076 Culture, bacterial; anaerobic isolate, additional methods required for definitive identification, each isolate Q4

Coding tip: Add additional gas liquid chromatography studies - 87143

Mod	Non-Fac Total	Fac Total	Global Days	51	50	62	80	MUE
	0.00	0.00	XXX	9	9	9	9	6

Pub 100-04, 16, 120.2

87077 Culture, bacterial; aerobic isolate, additional methods required for definitive identification, each isolate Q4

Coding tip: Add additional gas liquid chromatography studies - 87143
Coding tip: For a CLIA-waived test, append modifier QW to 87077

Mod	Non-Fac Total	Fac Total	Global Days	51	50	62	80	MUE
	0.00	0.00	XXX	9	9	9	9	10

AMA: Nov 01: 10, Nov 11: 10
Pub 100-04, 16, 120.2

87081 Culture, presumptive, pathogenic organisms, screening only Q4

Mod	Non-Fac Total	Fac Total	Global Days	51	50	62	80	MUE
	0.00	0.00	XXX	9	9	9	9	6

AMA: Nov 01: 10
Pub 100-04, 16, 120.2

87084 Culture, presumptive, pathogenic organisms, screening only; with colony estimation from density chart Q4

Mod	Non-Fac Total	Fac Total	Global Days	51	50	62	80	MUE
	0.00	0.00	XXX	9	9	9	9	1

Pub 100-04, 16, 120.2

87086 Culture, bacterial; quantitative colony count, urine Q4

Mod	Non-Fac Total	Fac Total	Global Days	51	50	62	80	MUE
	0.00	0.00	XXX	9	9	9	9	3

AMA: Nov 11: 10
Pub 100-03, 3, 190.12; 100-04, 16, 120.2
NCD: 190.12

● New   ▲ Revised   ✖ Deleted   ⊙ Moderate Sedation   ✚ Add-on Codes   ⊘ High Risk Denial   Ⓐ Age Edit   ♀ Female   ♂ Male   **AMA** *CPT® Assistant*   ***MUE*** Medically Unlikely Edit
⊘ Modifier 51 Exempt   ⊖ Modifier 63 Exempt   Ⓧ Unlisted   **Modifiers:** *See Inside Back Cover*   Ⓜ Maternity   A2–Z3 ASC Payment Indicators   A–Y OPPS Status Indicators

750   CPT © 2015 American Medical Association. All Rights Reserved.   © 2016 DecisionHealth

87088   Culture, bacterial; with isolation and presumptive identification of each isolate, urine   Q4

Mod	Non-Fac Total	Fac Total	Global Days	51	50	62	80	MUE
	0.00	0.00	XXX	9	9	9	9	6

AMA: Nov 11: 10

Pub 100-03, 3, 190.12; 100-04, 16, 120.2
NCD: 190.12

87101   Culture, fungi (mold or yeast) isolation, with presumptive identification of isolates; skin, hair, or nail   Q4

Coding tip: *Add definitive identification, each organism - 87106, 87107*

Mod	Non-Fac Total	Fac Total	Global Days	51	50	62	80	MUE
	0.00	0.00	XXX	9	9	9	9	4

AMA: Sep 99: 10, Aug 05: 9

87102   Culture, fungi (mold or yeast) isolation, with presumptive identification of isolates; other source (except blood)   Q4

Mod	Non-Fac Total	Fac Total	Global Days	51	50	62	80	MUE
	0.00	0.00	XXX	9	9	9	9	4

87103   Culture, fungi (mold or yeast) isolation, with presumptive identification of isolates; blood   Q4

Mod	Non-Fac Total	Fac Total	Global Days	51	50	62	80	MUE
	0.00	0.00	XXX	9	9	9	9	2

87106   Culture, fungi, definitive identification, each organism; yeast   Q4

Mod	Non-Fac Total	Fac Total	Global Days	51	50	62	80	MUE
	0.00	0.00	XXX	9	9	9	9	4

87107   Culture, fungi, definitive identification, each organism; mold   Q4

Mod	Non-Fac Total	Fac Total	Global Days	51	50	62	80	MUE
	0.00	0.00	XXX	9	9	9	9	4

87109   Culture, mycoplasma, any source   Q4

Mod	Non-Fac Total	Fac Total	Global Days	51	50	62	80	MUE
	0.00	0.00	XXX	9	9	9	9	2

87110   Culture, chlamydia, any source   A

Mod	Non-Fac Total	Fac Total	Global Days	51	50	62	80	MUE
	0.00	0.00	XXX	9	9	9	9	2

Pub 100-04, 18, 170.1

87116   Culture, tubercle or other acid-fast bacilli (eg, TB, AFB, mycobacteria) any source, with isolation and presumptive identification of isolates   Q4

Mod	Non-Fac Total	Fac Total	Global Days	51	50	62	80	MUE
	0.00	0.00	XXX	9	9	9	9	2

87118   Culture, mycobacterial, definitive identification, each isolate   Q4

Coding tip: *Add additional identification studies by molecular probe - 87149; by liquid chromatography - 87143*

Mod	Non-Fac Total	Fac Total	Global Days	51	50	62	80	MUE
	0.00	0.00	XXX	9	9	9	9	3

87140   Culture, typing; immunofluorescent method, each antiserum   Q4

Mod	Non-Fac Total	Fac Total	Global Days	51	50	62	80	MUE
	0.00	0.00	XXX	9	9	9	9	3

AMA: Nov 01: 10, Sep 03: 3

87143   Culture, typing; gas liquid chromatography (GLC) or high pressure liquid chromatography (HPLC) method   Q4

Mod	Non-Fac Total	Fac Total	Global Days	51	50	62	80	MUE
	0.00	0.00	XXX	9	9	9	9	2

87147   Culture, typing; immunologic method, other than immunofluoresence (eg, agglutination grouping), per antiserum   Q4

Mod	Non-Fac Total	Fac Total	Global Days	51	50	62	80	MUE
	0.00	0.00	XXX	9	9	9		

AMA: Apr 02: 18, Oct 03: 10

87149   Culture, typing; identification by nucleic acid (DNA or RNA) probe, direct probe technique, per culture or isolate, each organism probed   Q4

Mod	Non-Fac Total	Fac Total	Global Days	51	50	62	80	MUE
	0.00	0.00	XXX	9	9	9	9	4

AMA: Nov 01: 10, May 12: 5, Sep 13: 3

87150   Culture, typing; identification by nucleic acid (DNA or RNA) probe, amplified probe technique, per culture or isolate, each organism probed   Q4

Mod	Non-Fac Total	Fac Total	Global Days	51	50	62	80	MUE
	0.00	0.00	XXX	9	9	9	9	12

AMA: May 12: 5, Sep 13: 3

87152   Culture, typing; identification by pulse field gel typing   Q4

Mod	Non-Fac Total	Fac Total	Global Days	51	50	62	80	MUE
	0.00	0.00	XXX	9	9	9	9	1

AMA: May 12: 5, Sep 13: 3

87153   Culture, typing; identification by nucleic acid sequencing method, each isolate (eg, sequencing of the 16S rRNA gene)   Q4

Mod	Non-Fac Total	Fac Total	Global Days	51	50	62	80	MUE
	0.00	0.00	XXX	9	9	9	9	3

AMA: May 12: 5, Sep 13: 3

87158   Culture, typing; other methods   Q4

Mod	Non-Fac Total	Fac Total	Global Days	51	50	62	80	MUE
	0.00	0.00	XXX	9	9	9	9	1

AMA: Nov 01: 10, Sep 03: 3

● New   ▲ Revised   Deleted   ☉ Moderate Sedation   ✚ Add-on Codes   ⊘ High Risk Denial   Ⓐ Age Edit   ♀ Female   ♂ Male   **AMA** *CPT® Assistant*   **MUE** Medically Unlikely Edit

⊘ Modifier 51 Exempt   ⊖ Modifier 63 Exempt   ✗ Unlisted   **Modifiers:** *See Inside Back Cover*   Ⓜ Maternity   A2–Z3 ASC Payment Indicators   A–Y OPPS Status Indicators

© 2016 DecisionHealth   CPT © 2015 American Medical Association. All Rights Reserved.

87164 Dark field examination, any source (eg, penile, vaginal, oral, skin); includes specimen collection ◯4

Mod	Non-Fac Total	Fac Total	Global Days	51	50	62	80	MUE
	0.00	0.00	XXX	9	9	9	9	2
26	0.52	0.52	XXX	0	0	0	0	2

87166 Dark field examination, any source (eg, penile, vaginal, oral, skin); without collection ◯4

Mod	Non-Fac Total	Fac Total	Global Days	51	50	62	80	MUE
	0.00	0.00	XXX	9	9	9	9	2

87168 Macroscopic examination; arthropod ◯4

Mod	Non-Fac Total	Fac Total	Global Days	51	50	62	80	MUE
	0.00	0.00	XXX	9	9	9	9	2

87169 Macroscopic examination; parasite ◯4

Mod	Non-Fac Total	Fac Total	Global Days	51	50	62	80	MUE
	0.00	0.00	XXX	9	9	9	9	2

87172 Pinworm exam (eg, cellophane tape prep) ◯4

Mod	Non-Fac Total	Fac Total	Global Days	51	50	62	80	MUE
	0.00	0.00	XXX	9	9	9	9	1

87176 Homogenization, tissue, for culture ◯4

Mod	Non-Fac Total	Fac Total	Global Days	51	50	62	80	MUE
	0.00	0.00	XXX	9	9	9	9	2

87177 Ova and parasites, direct smears, concentration and identification ◯4

Mod	Non-Fac Total	Fac Total	Global Days	51	50	62	80	MUE
	0.00	0.00	XXX	9	9	9	9	3

AMA: Jul 03: 8, Nov 03: 15, Mar 06: 6

87181 Susceptibility studies, antimicrobial agent; agar dilution method, per agent (eg, antibiotic gradient strip) ◯4

Mod	Non-Fac Total	Fac Total	Global Days	51	50	62	80	MUE
	0.00	0.00	XXX	9	9	9	9	12

AMA: Nov 01: 10
Pub 100-04, 16, 120.2

87184 Susceptibility studies, antimicrobial agent; disk method, per plate (12 or fewer agents) ◯4

Mod	Non-Fac Total	Fac Total	Global Days	51	50	62	80	MUE
	0.00	0.00	XXX	9	9	9	9	8

AMA: Nov 01: 10
Pub 100-03, 3, 190.12; 100-04, 16, 120.2

87185 Susceptibility studies, antimicrobial agent; enzyme detection (eg, beta lactamase), per enzyme ◯4

Mod	Non-Fac Total	Fac Total	Global Days	51	50	62	80	MUE
	0.00	0.00	XXX	9	9	9	9	4

AMA: Nov 01: 10
Pub 100-04, 16, 120.2

87186 Susceptibility studies, antimicrobial agent; microdilution or agar dilution (minimum inhibitory concentration [MIC] or breakpoint), each multi-antimicrobial, per plate ◯4

Mod	Non-Fac Total	Fac Total	Global Days	51	50	62	80	MUE
	0.00	0.00	XXX	9	9	9	9	12

AMA: Nov 01: 10
Pub 100-03, 3, 190.12; 100-04, 16, 120.2

+ **87187** Susceptibility studies, antimicrobial agent; microdilution or agar dilution, minimum lethal concentration (MLC), each plate (List separately in addition to code for primary procedure) ◯4

Mod	Non-Fac Total	Fac Total	Global Days	51	50	62	80	MUE
	0.00	0.00	XXX	9	9	9	9	3

AMA: Nov 01: 10
Pub 100-04, 16, 120.2

87188 Susceptibility studies, antimicrobial agent; macrobroth dilution method, each agent ◯4

Mod	Non-Fac Total	Fac Total	Global Days	51	50	62	80	MUE
	0.00	0.00	XXX	9	9	9	9	6

AMA: Nov 01: 10
Pub 100-04, 16, 120.2

87190 Susceptibility studies, antimicrobial agent; mycobacteria, proportion method, each agent ◯4

Mod	Non-Fac Total	Fac Total	Global Days	51	50	62	80	MUE
	0.00	0.00	XXX	9	9	9	9	9

Pub 100-04, 16, 120.2

87197 Serum bactericidal titer (Schlicter test) ◯4

Mod	Non-Fac Total	Fac Total	Global Days	51	50	62	80	MUE
	0.00	0.00	XXX	9	9	9	9	1

Pub 100-04, 16, 120.2

87205 Smear, primary source with interpretation; Gram or Giemsa stain for bacteria, fungi, or cell types ◯4

Mod	Non-Fac Total	Fac Total	Global Days	51	50	62	80	MUE
	0.00	0.00	XXX	9	9	9	9	3

AMA: Aug 05: 9, Oct 09: 12
Pub 100-04, 16, 120.2

87206 Smear, primary source with interpretation; fluorescent and/or acid fast stain for bacteria, fungi, parasites, viruses or cell types ◯4

Mod	Non-Fac Total	Fac Total	Global Days	51	50	62	80	MUE
	0.00	0.00	XXX	9	9	9	9	6

● New   ▲ Revised   ✖ Deleted   ⊙ Moderate Sedation   ✚ Add-on Codes   ⊖ High Risk Denial   Ⓐ Age Edit   ♀ Female   ♂ Male   **AMA** *CPT® Assistant*   **MUE** Medically Unlikely Edit
⊘ Modifier 51 Exempt   ⊖ Modifier 63 Exempt   ✗ Unlisted   **Modifiers:** *See Inside Back Cover*   Ⓜ Maternity   Ⓐ2–Ⓩ3 ASC Payment Indicators   Ⓐ–Ⓨ OPPS Status Indicators

CPT © 2015 American Medical Association. All Rights Reserved.   © 2016 DecisionHealth

87207 Smear, primary source with interpretation; special stain for inclusion bodies or parasites (eg, malaria, coccidia, microsporidia, trypanosomes, herpes viruses) ◻4

Mod	Non-Fac Total	Fac Total	Global Days	51	50	62	80	MUE
	0.00	0.00	XXX	9	9	9	9	3
26	0.52	0.52	XXX	0	0	0	0	3

AMA: Jul 03: 8, Mar 06: 6

87209 Smear, primary source with interpretation; complex special stain (eg, trichrome, iron hemotoxylin) for ova and parasites ◻4

Mod	Non-Fac Total	Fac Total	Global Days	51	50	62	80	MUE
	0.00	0.00	XXX	9	9	9	9	4

AMA: Mar 06: 6

87210 Smear, primary source with interpretation; wet mount for infectious agents (eg, saline, India ink, KOH preps) ◻4

Coding tip: For a CLIA-waived test, append modifier QW to 87210

Mod	Non-Fac Total	Fac Total	Global Days	51	50	62	80	MUE
	0.00	0.00	XXX	9	9	9	9	4

87220 Tissue examination by KOH slide of samples from skin, hair, or nails for fungi or ectoparasite ova or mites (eg, scabies) ◻4

Mod	Non-Fac Total	Fac Total	Global Days	51	50	62	80	MUE
	0.00	0.00	XXX	9	9	9	9	3

87230 Toxin or antitoxin assay, tissue culture (eg, Clostridium difficile toxin) ◻4

Mod	Non-Fac Total	Fac Total	Global Days	51	50	62	80	MUE
	0.00	0.00	XXX	9	9	9	9	3

87250 Virus isolation; inoculation of embryonated eggs, or small animal, includes observation and dissection ◻4

Mod	Non-Fac Total	Fac Total	Global Days	51	50	62	80	MUE
	0.00	0.00	XXX	9	9	9	9	1

87252 Virus isolation; tissue culture inoculation, observation, and presumptive identification by cytopathic effect ◻4

Mod	Non-Fac Total	Fac Total	Global Days	51	50	62	80	MUE
	0.00	0.00	XXX	9	9	9	9	2

87253 Virus isolation; tissue culture, additional studies or definitive identification (eg, hemabsorption, neutralization, immunofluoresence stain), each isolate ◻4

Mod	Non-Fac Total	Fac Total	Global Days	51	50	62	80	MUE
	0.00	0.00	XXX	9	9	9	9	2

87254 Virus isolation; centrifuge enhanced (shell vial) technique, includes identification with immunofluorescence stain, each virus ◻4

Mod	Non-Fac Total	Fac Total	Global Days	51	50	62	80	MUE
	0.00	0.00	XXX	9	9	9	9	7

AMA: Jul 03: 8

87255 Virus isolation; including identification by non-immunologic method, other than by cytopathic effect (eg, virus specific enzymatic activity) ◻4

Mod	Non-Fac Total	Fac Total	Global Days	51	50	62	80	MUE
	0.00	0.00	XXX	9	9	9	9	2

AMA: Jul 03: 9

Coding Guidance

Multiple tests/different techniques should not be reported for identifying the same analyte, marker, or infectious agent. For instance, both a direct probe and an amplified probe technique test should not be reported for the same infectious agent.

87260 Infectious agent antigen detection by immunofluorescent technique; adenovirus ◻4

Mod	Non-Fac Total	Fac Total	Global Days	51	50	62	80	MUE
	0.00	0.00	XXX	9	9	9	9	1

AMA: Nov 97: 32

87265 Infectious agent antigen detection by immunofluorescent technique; Bordetella pertussis/parapertussis ◻4

Mod	Non-Fac Total	Fac Total	Global Days	51	50	62	80	MUE
	0.00	0.00	XXX	9	9	9	9	1

AMA: Nov 97: 32

87267 Infectious agent antigen detection by immunofluorescent technique; Enterovirus, direct fluorescent antibody (DFA) ◻4

Mod	Non-Fac Total	Fac Total	Global Days	51	50	62	80	MUE
	0.00	0.00	XXX	9	9	9	9	1

AMA: Jul 03: 8

87269 Infectious agent antigen detection by immunofluorescent technique; giardia ◻4

Mod	Non-Fac Total	Fac Total	Global Days	51	50	62	80	MUE
	0.00	0.00	XXX	9	9	9	9	1

87270 Infectious agent antigen detection by immunofluorescent technique; Chlamydia trachomatis ◻A

Mod	Non-Fac Total	Fac Total	Global Days	51	50	62	80	MUE
	0.00	0.00	XXX	9	9	9	9	1

AMA: Nov 97: 32
Pub 100-04, 18, 170.1

● New   ▲ Revised   Deleted   ⊙ Moderate Sedation   ✚ Add-on Codes   ⊘ High Risk Denial   Ⓐ Age Edit   ♀ Female   ♂ Male   **AMA** *CPT® Assistant*   **MUE** Medically Unlikely Edit
⊘ Modifier 51 Exempt   ⊖ Modifier 63 Exempt   ⬚ Unlisted   **Modifiers:** *See Inside Back Cover*   Ⓜ Maternity   A2-Z3 ASC Payment Indicators   A-Y OPPS Status Indicators

© 2016 DecisionHealth   CPT © 2015 American Medical Association. All Rights Reserved.   **753**

87271 Infectious agent antigen detection by immunofluorescent technique; Cytomegalovirus, direct fluorescent antibody (DFA)   ▣4

RVU			Global Days	Modifiers				
Mod	Non-Fac Total	Fac Total		51	50	62	80	MUE
	0.00	0.00	XXX	9	9	9	9	1

AMA: Jul 03: 7

Pub 100-04, 16, 120.2

87272 Infectious agent antigen detection by immunofluorescent technique; cryptosporidium   ▣4

RVU			Global Days	Modifiers				
Mod	Non-Fac Total	Fac Total		51	50	62	80	MUE
	0.00	0.00	XXX	9	9	9	9	1

AMA: Nov 97: 32

87273 Infectious agent antigen detection by immunofluorescent technique; Herpes simplex virus type 2   ▣4

RVU			Global Days	Modifiers				
Mod	Non-Fac Total	Fac Total		51	50	62	80	MUE
	0.00	0.00	XXX	9	9	9	9	1

87274 Infectious agent antigen detection by immunofluorescent technique; Herpes simplex virus type 1   ▣4

RVU			Global Days	Modifiers				
Mod	Non-Fac Total	Fac Total		51	50	62	80	MUE
	0.00	0.00	XXX	9	9	9	9	1

AMA: Nov 97: 32

87275 Infectious agent antigen detection by immunofluorescent technique; influenza B virus   ▣4

RVU			Global Days	Modifiers				
Mod	Non-Fac Total	Fac Total		51	50	62	80	MUE
	0.00	0.00	XXX	9	9	9	9	1

87276 Infectious agent antigen detection by immunofluorescent technique; influenza A virus   ▣4

RVU			Global Days	Modifiers				
Mod	Non-Fac Total	Fac Total		51	50	62	80	MUE
	0.00	0.00	XXX	9	9	9	9	1

AMA: Nov 97: 32, May 09: 6

87277 Infectious agent antigen detection by immunofluorescent technique; Legionella micdadei   ▣4

RVU			Global Days	Modifiers				
Mod	Non-Fac Total	Fac Total		51	50	62	80	MUE
	0.00	0.00	XXX	9	9	9	9	1

87278 Infectious agent antigen detection by immunofluorescent technique; Legionella pneumophila   ▣4

RVU			Global Days	Modifiers				
Mod	Non-Fac Total	Fac Total		51	50	62	80	MUE
	0.00	0.00	XXX	9	9	9	9	1

AMA: Nov 97: 32

87279 Infectious agent antigen detection by immunofluorescent technique; Parainfluenza virus, each type   ⊘▣4

RVU			Global Days	Modifiers				
Mod	Non-Fac Total	Fac Total		51	50	62	80	MUE
	0.00	0.00	XXX	9	9	9	9	1

87280 Infectious agent antigen detection by immunofluorescent technique; respiratory syncytial virus   ▣4

RVU			Global Days	Modifiers				
Mod	Non-Fac Total	Fac Total		51	50	62	80	MUE
	0.00	0.00	XXX	9	9	9	9	1

AMA: Nov 97: 32

87281 Infectious agent antigen detection by immunofluorescent technique; Pneumocystis carinii   ▣4

RVU			Global Days	Modifiers				
Mod	Non-Fac Total	Fac Total		51	50	62	80	MUE
	0.00	0.00	XXX	9	9	9	9	1

87283 Infectious agent antigen detection by immunofluorescent technique; Rubeola   ▣4

RVU			Global Days	Modifiers				
Mod	Non-Fac Total	Fac Total		51	50	62	80	MUE
	0.00	0.00	XXX	9	9	9	9	1

87285 Infectious agent antigen detection by immunofluorescent technique; Treponema pallidum   ▣4

RVU			Global Days	Modifiers				
Mod	Non-Fac Total	Fac Total		51	50	62	80	MUE
	0.00	0.00	XXX	9	9	9	9	1

AMA: Nov 97: 32

87290 Infectious agent antigen detection by immunofluorescent technique; Varicella zoster virus   ▣4

RVU			Global Days	Modifiers				
Mod	Non-Fac Total	Fac Total		51	50	62	80	MUE
	0.00	0.00	XXX	9	9	9	9	1

AMA: Nov 97: 32

87299 Infectious agent antigen detection by immunofluorescent technique; not otherwise specified, each organism   ▣4

RVU			Global Days	Modifiers				
Mod	Non-Fac Total	Fac Total		51	50	62	80	MUE
	0.00	0.00	XXX	9	9	9	9	1

AMA: Nov 97: 32, Nov 01: 10

87300 Infectious agent antigen detection by immunofluorescent technique, polyvalent for multiple organisms, each polyvalent antiserum   ▣4

RVU			Global Days	Modifiers				
Mod	Non-Fac Total	Fac Total		51	50	62	80	MUE
	0.00	0.00	XXX	9	9	9	9	2

AMA: Aug 05: 9

● New   ▲ Revised   ✖ Deleted   ⊙ Moderate Sedation   ✚ Add-on Codes   ⊘ High Risk Denial   Ⓐ Age Edit   ♀ Female   ♂ Male   **AMA** *CPT® Assistant*   **MUE** Medically Unlikely Edit
⊘ Modifier 51 Exempt   ⊖ Modifier 63 Exempt   ✗ Unlisted   **Modifiers:** *See Inside Back Cover*   Ⓜ Maternity   A-2 – Z-3 ASC Payment Indicators   A – Y OPPS Status Indicators

CPT © 2015 American Medical Association. All Rights Reserved.   © 2016 DecisionHealth

▲ 87301 Infectious agent antigen detection by immunoassay technique, (eg, enzyme immunoassay [EIA], enzyme-linked immunosorbent assay [ELISA], immunochemiluminometric assay [IMCA]) qualitative or semiquantitative, multiple-step method; adenovirus enteric types 40/41 **Q4**

RVU			Global Days	Modifiers				
Mod	Non-Fac Total	Fac Total		51	50	62	80	MUE
	0.00	0.00	XXX	9	9	9	9	1

AMA: Nov 97: 32, Nov 99: 46

▲ 87305 Infectious agent antigen detection by immunoassay technique, (eg, enzyme immunoassay [EIA], enzyme-linked immunosorbent assay [ELISA], immunochemiluminometric assay [IMCA]) qualitative or semiquantitative, multiple-step method; Aspergillus **Q4**

RVU			Global Days	Modifiers				
Mod	Non-Fac Total	Fac Total		51	50	62	80	MUE
	0.00	0.00	XXX	9	9	9	9	1

▲ 87320 Infectious agent antigen detection by immunoassay technique, (eg, enzyme immunoassay [EIA], enzyme-linked immunosorbent assay [ELISA], immunochemiluminometric assay [IMCA]) qualitative or semiquantitative, multiple-step method; Chlamydia trachomatis **A**

RVU			Global Days	Modifiers				
Mod	Non-Fac Total	Fac Total		51	50	62	80	MUE
	0.00	0.00	XXX	9	9	9	9	1

AMA: Nov 97: 32
Pub 100-04, 18, 170.1

▲ 87324 Infectious agent antigen detection by immunoassay technique, (eg, enzyme immunoassay [EIA], enzyme-linked immunosorbent assay [ELISA], immunochemiluminometric assay [IMCA]) qualitative or semiquantitative, multiple-step method; Clostridium difficile toxin(s) **Q4**

RVU			Global Days	Modifiers				
Mod	Non-Fac Total	Fac Total		51	50	62	80	MUE
	0.00	0.00	XXX	9	9	9	9	2

AMA: Nov 97: 32

▲ 87327 Infectious agent antigen detection by immunoassay technique, (eg, enzyme immunoassay [EIA], enzyme-linked immunosorbent assay [ELISA], immunochemiluminometric assay [IMCA]) qualitative or semiquantitative, multiple-step method; Cryptococcus neoformans **Q4**

RVU			Global Days	Modifiers				
Mod	Non-Fac Total	Fac Total		51	50	62	80	MUE
	0.00	0.00	XXX	9	9	9	9	1

▲ 87328 Infectious agent antigen detection by immunoassay technique, (eg, enzyme immunoassay [EIA], enzyme-linked immunosorbent assay [ELISA], immunochemiluminometric assay [IMCA]) qualitative or semiquantitative, multiple-step method; cryptosporidium **Q4**

RVU			Global Days	Modifiers				
Mod	Non-Fac Total	Fac Total		51	50	62	80	MUE
	0.00	0.00	XXX	9	9	9	9	2

AMA: Nov 97: 32

▲ 87329 Infectious agent antigen detection by immunoassay technique, (eg, enzyme immunoassay [EIA], enzyme-linked immunosorbent assay [ELISA], immunochemiluminometric assay [IMCA]) qualitative or semiquantitative, multiple-step method; giardia **Q4**

RVU			Global Days	Modifiers				
Mod	Non-Fac Total	Fac Total		51	50	62	80	MUE
	0.00	0.00	XXX	9	9	9	9	2

▲ 87332 Infectious agent antigen detection by immunoassay technique, (eg, enzyme immunoassay [EIA], enzyme-linked immunosorbent assay [ELISA], immunochemiluminometric assay [IMCA]) qualitative or semiquantitative, multiple-step method; cytomegalovirus **Q4**

RVU			Global Days	Modifiers				
Mod	Non-Fac Total	Fac Total		51	50	62	80	MUE
	0.00	0.00	XXX	9	9	9	9	1

AMA: Nov 97: 32

▲ 87335 Infectious agent antigen detection by immunoassay technique, (eg, enzyme immunoassay [EIA], enzyme-linked immunosorbent assay [ELISA], immunochemiluminometric assay [IMCA]) qualitative or semiquantitative, multiple-step method; Escherichia coli 0157 **Q4**

RVU			Global Days	Modifiers				
Mod	Non-Fac Total	Fac Total		51	50	62	80	MUE
	0.00	0.00	XXX	9	9	9	9	1

AMA: Nov 97: 32

▲ 87336 Infectious agent antigen detection by immunoassay technique, (eg, enzyme immunoassay [EIA], enzyme-linked immunosorbent assay [ELISA], immunochemiluminometric assay [IMCA]) qualitative or semiquantitative, multiple-step method; Entamoeba histolytica dispar group **Q4**

RVU			Global Days	Modifiers				
Mod	Non-Fac Total	Fac Total		51	50	62	80	MUE
	0.00	0.00	XXX	9	9	9	9	1

● New　▲ Revised　Deleted　⊙ Moderate Sedation　✚ Add-on Codes　⊘ High Risk Denial　Ⓐ Age Edit　♀ Female　♂ Male　**AMA** CPT® Assistant　**MUE** Medically Unlikely Edit
⊘ Modifier 51 Exempt　⊖ Modifier 63 Exempt　Ⓧ Unlisted　**Modifiers:** See Inside Back Cover　Ⓜ Maternity　A2–Z3 ASC Payment Indicators　A–Y OPPS Status Indicators

© 2016 DecisionHealth　CPT © 2015 American Medical Association. All Rights Reserved.　755

Laboratory/Pathology Procedures

87337 – 87390

▲ **87337** Infectious agent antigen detection by immunoassay technique, (eg, enzyme immunoassay [EIA], enzyme-linked immunosorbent assay [ELISA], immunochemiluminometric assay [IMCA]) qualitative or semiquantitative, multiple-step method; Entamoeba histolytica group   Q4

RVU			Global Days	Modifiers				
Mod	Non-Fac Total	Fac Total		51	50	62	80	MUE
	0.00	0.00	XXX	9	9	9	9	1

▲ **87338** Infectious agent antigen detection by immunoassay technique, (eg, enzyme immunoassay [EIA], enzyme-linked immunosorbent assay [ELISA], immunochemiluminometric assay [IMCA]) qualitative or semiquantitative, multiple-step method; Helicobacter pylori, stool   Q4

RVU			Global Days	Modifiers				
Mod	Non-Fac Total	Fac Total		51	50	62	80	MUE
	0.00	0.00	XXX	9	9	9	9	1

AMA: Nov 99: 46

▲ **87339** Infectious agent antigen detection by immunoassay technique, (eg, enzyme immunoassay [EIA], enzyme-linked immunosorbent assay [ELISA], immunochemiluminometric assay [IMCA]) qualitative or semiquantitative, multiple-step method; Helicobacter pylori   Q4

RVU			Global Days	Modifiers				
Mod	Non-Fac Total	Fac Total		51	50	62	80	MUE
	0.00	0.00	XXX	9	9	9	9	1

▲ **87340** Infectious agent antigen detection by immunoassay technique, (eg, enzyme immunoassay [EIA], enzyme-linked immunosorbent assay [ELISA], immunochemiluminometric assay [IMCA]) qualitative or semiquantitative, multiple-step method; hepatitis B surface antigen (HBsAg)   Q4

RVU			Global Days	Modifiers				
Mod	Non-Fac Total	Fac Total		51	50	62	80	MUE
	0.00	0.00	XXX	9	9	9	9	1

AMA: Nov 97: 32, Jan 00: 11
Pub 100-04, 16, 120.2; 100-04, 18, 170.1

▲ **87341** Infectious agent antigen detection by immunoassay technique, (eg, enzyme immunoassay [EIA], enzyme-linked immunosorbent assay [ELISA], immunochemiluminometric assay [IMCA]) qualitative or semiquantitative, multiple-step method; hepatitis B surface antigen (HBsAg) neutralization   A

RVU			Global Days	Modifiers				
Mod	Non-Fac Total	Fac Total		51	50	62	80	MUE
	0.00	0.00	XXX	9	9	9	9	1

Pub 100-04, 16, 120.2; 100-04, 18, 170.1

▲ **87350** Infectious agent antigen detection by immunoassay technique, (eg, enzyme immunoassay [EIA], enzyme-linked immunosorbent assay [ELISA], immunochemiluminometric assay [IMCA]) qualitative or semiquantitative, multiple-step method; hepatitis Be antigen (HBeAg)   Q4

RVU			Global Days	Modifiers				
Mod	Non-Fac Total	Fac Total		51	50	62	80	MUE
	0.00	0.00	XXX	9	9	9	9	1

AMA: Nov 97: 32
Pub 100-04, 16, 120.2

▲ **87380** Infectious agent antigen detection by immunoassay technique, (eg, enzyme immunoassay [EIA], enzyme-linked immunosorbent assay [ELISA], immunochemiluminometric assay [IMCA]) qualitative or semiquantitative, multiple-step method; hepatitis, delta agent   Q4

RVU			Global Days	Modifiers				
Mod	Non-Fac Total	Fac Total		51	50	62	80	MUE
	0.00	0.00	XXX	9	9	9	9	1

AMA: Nov 97: 32

▲ **87385** Infectious agent antigen detection by immunoassay technique, (eg, enzyme immunoassay [EIA], enzyme-linked immunosorbent assay [ELISA], immunochemiluminometric assay [IMCA]) qualitative or semiquantitative, multiple-step method; Histoplasma capsulatum   Q4

RVU			Global Days	Modifiers				
Mod	Non-Fac Total	Fac Total		51	50	62	80	MUE
	0.00	0.00	XXX	9	9	9	9	2

AMA: Nov 97: 32

▲ **87389** Infectious agent antigen detection by immunoassay technique, (eg, enzyme immunoassay [EIA], enzyme-linked immunosorbent assay [ELISA], immunochemiluminometric assay [IMCA]) qualitative or semiquantitative, multiple-step method; HIV-1 antigen(s), with HIV-1 and HIV-2 antibodies, single result   Q4

RVU			Global Days	Modifiers				
Mod	Non-Fac Total	Fac Total		51	50	62	80	MUE
	0.00	0.00	XXX	9	9	9	9	1

▲ **87390** Infectious agent antigen detection by immunoassay technique, (eg, enzyme immunoassay [EIA], enzyme-linked immunosorbent assay [ELISA], immunochemiluminometric assay [IMCA]) qualitative or semiquantitative, multiple-step method; HIV-1   Q4

RVU			Global Days	Modifiers				
Mod	Non-Fac Total	Fac Total		51	50	62	80	MUE
	0.00	0.00	XXX	9	9	9	9	1

AMA: Nov 97: 32
Pub 100-04, 16, 120.2
NCD: 190.14

● New   ▲ Revised   ✖ Deleted   ⊙ Moderate Sedation   ✚ Add-on Codes   ⊘ High Risk Denial   Ⓐ Age Edit   ♀ Female   ♂ Male   **AMA** *CPT® Assistant*   **MUE** Medically Unlikely Edit
⊘ Modifier 51 Exempt   ⊖ Modifier 63 Exempt   ⊠ Unlisted   **Modifiers:** *See Inside Back Cover*   Ⓜ Maternity   A2 – Z3 ASC Payment Indicators   A – Y OPPS Status Indicators

756   CPT © 2015 American Medical Association. All Rights Reserved.   © 2016 DecisionHealth

▲ **87391** Infectious agent antigen detection by immunoassay technique, (eg, enzyme immunoassay [EIA], enzyme-linked immunosorbent assay [ELISA], immunochemiluminometric assay [IMCA]) qualitative or semiquantitative, multiple-step method; HIV-2 ⊗Q4

RVU			Global Days	Modifiers				
Mod	Non-Fac Total	Fac Total		51	50	62	80	MUE
	0.00	0.00	XXX	9	9	9	9	1

AMA: Nov 97: 32

Pub 100-04, 16, 120.2
NCD: 190.14

▲ **87400** Infectious agent antigen detection by immunoassay technique, (eg, enzyme immunoassay [EIA], enzyme-linked immunosorbent assay [ELISA], immunochemiluminometric assay [IMCA]) qualitative or semiquantitative, multiple-step method; Influenza, A or B, each Q4

RVU			Global Days	Modifiers				
Mod	Non-Fac Total	Fac Total		51	50	62	80	MUE
	0.00	0.00	XXX	9	9	9	9	2

AMA: Jun 01: 11, Dec 01: 6, Aug 05: 9, May 09: 6

▲ **87420** Infectious agent antigen detection by immunoassay technique, (eg, enzyme immunoassay [EIA], enzyme-linked immunosorbent assay [ELISA], immunochemiluminometric assay [IMCA]) qualitative or semiquantitative, multiple-step method; respiratory syncytial virus Q4

RVU			Global Days	Modifiers				
Mod	Non-Fac Total	Fac Total		51	50	62	80	MUE
	0.00	0.00	XXX	9	9	9	9	1

AMA: Nov 97: 32

▲ **87425** Infectious agent antigen detection by immunoassay technique, (eg, enzyme immunoassay [EIA], enzyme-linked immunosorbent assay [ELISA], immunochemiluminometric assay [IMCA]) qualitative or semiquantitative, multiple-step method; rotavirus Q4

RVU			Global Days	Modifiers				
Mod	Non-Fac Total	Fac Total		51	50	62	80	MUE
	0.00	0.00	XXX	9	9	9	9	1

AMA: Nov 97: 32

▲ **87427** Infectious agent antigen detection by immunoassay technique, (eg, enzyme immunoassay [EIA], enzyme-linked immunosorbent assay [ELISA], immunochemiluminometric assay [IMCA]) qualitative or semiquantitative, multiple-step method; Shiga-like toxin Q4

RVU			Global Days	Modifiers				
Mod	Non-Fac Total	Fac Total		51	50	62	80	MUE
	0.00	0.00	XXX	9	9	9	9	2

▲ **87430** Infectious agent antigen detection by immunoassay technique, (eg, enzyme immunoassay [EIA], enzyme-linked immunosorbent assay [ELISA], immunochemiluminometric assay [IMCA]) qualitative or semiquantitative, multiple-step method; Streptococcus, group A Q4

RVU			Global Days	Modifiers				
Mod	Non-Fac Total	Fac Total		51	50	62	80	MUE
	0.00	0.00	XXX	9	9	9	9	1

AMA: Nov 97: 32

▲ **87449** Infectious agent antigen detection by immunoassay technique, (eg, enzyme immunoassay [EIA], enzyme-linked immunosorbent assay [ELISA], immunochemiluminometric assay [IMCA]), qualitative or semiquantitative; multiple-step method, not otherwise specified, each organism Q4

Coding tip: For a CLIA-waived test, append modifier QW to 87449
Coding tip: Use for CLIA-waived ZymeTx Zstatflu(R) Test - Qualitative test for influenza Type A and B that does not differentiate between the two types

RVU			Global Days	Modifiers				
Mod	Non-Fac Total	Fac Total		51	50	62	80	MUE
	0.00	0.00	XXX	9	9	9	9	3

AMA: Nov 97: 32, Jan 00: 11, Nov 01: 10

▲ **87450** Infectious agent antigen detection by immunoassay technique, (eg, enzyme immunoassay [EIA], enzyme-linked immunosorbent assay [ELISA], immunochemiluminometric assay [IMCA]), qualitative or semiquantitative; single step method, not otherwise specified, each organism ⊗Q4

RVU			Global Days	Modifiers				
Mod	Non-Fac Total	Fac Total		51	50	62	80	MUE
	0.00	0.00	XXX	9	9	9	9	2

AMA: Nov 97: 33

▲ **87451** Infectious agent antigen detection by immunoassay technique, (eg, enzyme immunoassay [EIA], enzyme-linked immunosorbent assay [ELISA], immunochemiluminometric assay [IMCA]), qualitative or semiquantitative; multiple step method, polyvalent for multiple organisms, each polyvalent antiserum Q4

RVU			Global Days	Modifiers				
Mod	Non-Fac Total	Fac Total		51	50	62	80	MUE
	0.00	0.00	XXX	9	9	9	9	2

Coding Guidance
Infectious agent molecular diagnostic testing utilizing nucleic acid probes is reported with CPT codes 87470-87801, 87901-87906, 87910, 87912.

87470 Infectious agent detection by nucleic acid (DNA or RNA); Bartonella henselae and Bartonella quintana, direct probe technique Q4

RVU			Global Days	Modifiers				
Mod	Non-Fac Total	Fac Total		51	50	62	80	MUE
	0.00	0.00	XXX	9	9	9	9	1

AMA: Nov 97: 33, 34, May 12: 5, Sep 13: 3

● New ▲ Revised Deleted ⊙ Moderate Sedation ✚ Add-on Codes ⊘ High Risk Denial Ⓐ Age Edit ♀ Female ♂ Male **AMA** *CPT® Assistant* **MUE** Medically Unlikely Edit
⊘ Modifier 51 Exempt ⊖ Modifier 63 Exempt 🗵 Unlisted **Modifiers:** *See Inside Back Cover* Ⓜ Maternity A 2–Z 3 ASC Payment Indicators A –Y OPPS Status Indicators

© 2016 DecisionHealth CPT © 2015 American Medical Association. All Rights Reserved. **757**

87471 Infectious agent detection by nucleic acid (DNA or RNA); Bartonella henselae and Bartonella quintana, amplified probe technique ◎4

Mod	Non-Fac Total	Fac Total	Global Days	Modifiers 51	50	62	80	MUE
	0.00	0.00	XXX	9	9	9	9	1

AMA: May 12: 5, Sep 13: 3

87472 Infectious agent detection by nucleic acid (DNA or RNA); Bartonella henselae and Bartonella quintana, quantification ◎◎4

Mod	Non-Fac Total	Fac Total	Global Days	Modifiers 51	50	62	80	MUE
	0.00	0.00	XXX	9	9	9	9	1

AMA: Sep 13: 3

87475 Infectious agent detection by nucleic acid (DNA or RNA); Borrelia burgdorferi, direct probe technique ◎◎4

Mod	Non-Fac Total	Fac Total	Global Days	Modifiers 51	50	62	80	MUE
	0.00	0.00	XXX	9	9	9	9	1

AMA: May 12: 5, Sep 13: 3

87476 Infectious agent detection by nucleic acid (DNA or RNA); Borrelia burgdorferi, amplified probe technique ◎4

Mod	Non-Fac Total	Fac Total	Global Days	Modifiers 51	50	62	80	MUE
	0.00	0.00	XXX	9	9	9	9	1

AMA: Sep 13: 3

87477 Infectious agent detection by nucleic acid (DNA or RNA); Borrelia burgdorferi, quantification ◎4

Mod	Non-Fac Total	Fac Total	Global Days	Modifiers 51	50	62	80	MUE
	0.00	0.00	XXX	9	9	9	9	1

AMA: Sep 13: 3

87480 Infectious agent detection by nucleic acid (DNA or RNA); Candida species, direct probe technique ◎4

Mod	Non-Fac Total	Fac Total	Global Days	Modifiers 51	50	62	80	MUE
	0.00	0.00	XXX	9	9	9	9	1

AMA: May 12: 5, Sep 13: 3

87481 Infectious agent detection by nucleic acid (DNA or RNA); Candida species, amplified probe technique ◎4

Mod	Non-Fac Total	Fac Total	Global Days	Modifiers 51	50	62	80	MUE
	0.00	0.00	XXX	9	9	9	9	1

AMA: Sep 13: 3

87482 Infectious agent detection by nucleic acid (DNA or RNA); Candida species, quantification ◎4

Mod	Non-Fac Total	Fac Total	Global Days	Modifiers 51	50	62	80	MUE
	0.00	0.00	XXX	9	9	9	9	1

AMA: Sep 13: 3

87485 Infectious agent detection by nucleic acid (DNA or RNA); Chlamydia pneumoniae, direct probe technique ◎◎4

Mod	Non-Fac Total	Fac Total	Global Days	Modifiers 51	50	62	80	MUE
	0.00	0.00	XXX	9	9	9	9	1

AMA: May 12: 5, Sep 13: 3

87486 Infectious agent detection by nucleic acid (DNA or RNA); Chlamydia pneumoniae, amplified probe technique ◎4

Mod	Non-Fac Total	Fac Total	Global Days	Modifiers 51	50	62	80	MUE
	0.00	0.00	XXX	9	9	9	9	1

AMA: Sep 13: 3

87487 Infectious agent detection by nucleic acid (DNA or RNA); Chlamydia pneumoniae, quantification ◎4

Mod	Non-Fac Total	Fac Total	Global Days	Modifiers 51	50	62	80	MUE
	0.00	0.00	XXX	9	9	9	9	1

AMA: Sep 13: 3

87490 Infectious agent detection by nucleic acid (DNA or RNA); Chlamydia trachomatis, direct probe technique Ⓐ

Mod	Non-Fac Total	Fac Total	Global Days	Modifiers 51	50	62	80	MUE
	0.00	0.00	XXX	9	9	9	9	1

AMA: Sep 13: 3
Pub 100-04, 18, 170.1

87491 Infectious agent detection by nucleic acid (DNA or RNA); Chlamydia trachomatis, amplified probe technique Ⓐ

Mod	Non-Fac Total	Fac Total	Global Days	Modifiers 51	50	62	80	MUE
	0.00	0.00	XXX	9	9	9	9	2

AMA: Jun 13: 14, Sep 13: 3
Pub 100-04, 18, 170.1

87492 Infectious agent detection by nucleic acid (DNA or RNA); Chlamydia trachomatis, quantification ◎◎4

Mod	Non-Fac Total	Fac Total	Global Days	Modifiers 51	50	62	80	MUE
	0.00	0.00	XXX	9	9	9	9	1

AMA: Sep 13: 3

87493 Infectious agent detection by nucleic acid (DNA or RNA); Clostridium difficile, toxin gene(s), amplified probe technique ◎4

Mod	Non-Fac Total	Fac Total	Global Days	Modifiers 51	50	62	80	MUE
	0.00	0.00	XXX	9	9	9	9	2

AMA: Sep 10: 8, May 12: 5, Sep 13: 3

87495 Infectious agent detection by nucleic acid (DNA or RNA); cytomegalovirus, direct probe technique ◎4

Mod	Non-Fac Total	Fac Total	Global Days	Modifiers 51	50	62	80	MUE
	0.00	0.00	XXX	9	9	9	9	1

● New   ▲ Revised   ✖ Deleted   ⊙ Moderate Sedation   ✚ Add-on Codes   ⊘ High Risk Denial   Ⓐ Age Edit   ♀ Female   ♂ Male   **AMA** *CPT® Assistant*   **MUE** Medically Unlikely Edit
⊘ Modifier 51 Exempt   ⊖ Modifier 63 Exempt   ✗ Unlisted   **Modifiers:** *See Inside Back Cover*   Ⓜ Maternity   A2–Z3 ASC Payment Indicators   A–Y OPPS Status Indicators

CPT © 2015 American Medical Association. All Rights Reserved.   © 2016 DecisionHealth

AMA: May 12: 5, Sep 13: 3

87496 Infectious agent detection by nucleic acid (DNA or RNA); cytomegalovirus, amplified probe technique   Q4

RVU			Global Days	Modifiers				
Mod	Non-Fac Total	Fac Total		51	50	62	80	MUE
	0.00	0.00	XXX	9	9	9	9	1

AMA: Sep 13: 3

87497 Infectious agent detection by nucleic acid (DNA or RNA); cytomegalovirus, quantification   Q4

RVU			Global Days	Modifiers				
Mod	Non-Fac Total	Fac Total		51	50	62	80	MUE
	0.00	0.00	XXX	9	9	9	9	2

AMA: Sep 13: 3

87498 Infectious agent detection by nucleic acid (DNA or RNA); enterovirus, amplified probe technique, includes reverse transcription when performed   Q4

RVU			Global Days	Modifiers				
Mod	Non-Fac Total	Fac Total		51	50	62	80	MUE
	0.00	0.00	XXX	9	9	9	9	1

AMA: May 12: 5, Sep 13: 3

87500 Infectious agent detection by nucleic acid (DNA or RNA); vancomycin resistance (eg, enterococcus species van A, van B), amplified probe technique   Q4

RVU			Global Days	Modifiers				
Mod	Non-Fac Total	Fac Total		51	50	62	80	MUE
	0.00	0.00	XXX	9	9	9	9	1

AMA: Apr 08: 5, May 12: 5, Sep 13: 3

87501 Infectious agent detection by nucleic acid (DNA or RNA); influenza virus, includes reverse transcription, when performed, and amplified probe technique, each type or subtype   ⊘Q4

RVU			Global Days	Modifiers				
Mod	Non-Fac Total	Fac Total		51	50	62	80	MUE
	0.00	0.00	XXX	9	9	9	9	1

AMA: Oct 10: 8, Dec 10: 8, May 12: 5, Sep 13: 3

▲ **87502** Infectious agent detection by nucleic acid (DNA or RNA); influenza virus, for multiple types or sub-types, includes multiplex reverse transcription, when performed, and multiplex amplified probe technique, first 2 types or sub-types   Q4

RVU			Global Days	Modifiers				
Mod	Non-Fac Total	Fac Total		51	50	62	80	MUE
	0.00	0.00	XXX	9	9	9	9	1

AMA: Oct 10: 8, Dec 10: 8, Sep 13: 3

✚▲ **87503** Infectious agent detection by nucleic acid (DNA or RNA); influenza virus, for multiple types or sub-types, includes multiplex reverse transcription, when performed, and multiplex amplified probe technique, each additional influenza virus type or sub-type beyond 2 (List separately in addition to code for primary procedure)   Q4

RVU			Global Days	Modifiers				
Mod	Non-Fac Total	Fac Total		51	50	62	80	MUE
	0.00	0.00	XXX	9	9	9	9	1

AMA: Oct 10: 8, Dec 10: 8, Sep 13: 3

87505 Infectious agent detection by nucleic acid (DNA or RNA); gastrointestinal pathogen (eg, Clostridium difficile, E. coli, Salmonella, Shigella, norovirus, Giardia), includes multiplex reverse transcription, when performed, and multiplex amplified probe technique, multiple types or subtypes, 3-5 targets   Q4

RVU			Global Days	Modifiers				
Mod	Non-Fac Total	Fac Total		51	50	62	80	MUE
	0.00	0.00	XXX	9	9	9	9	1

87506 Infectious agent detection by nucleic acid (DNA or RNA); gastrointestinal pathogen (eg, Clostridium difficile, E. coli, Salmonella, Shigella, norovirus, Giardia), includes multiplex reverse transcription, when performed, and multiplex amplified probe technique, multiple types or subtypes, 6-11 targets   Q4

RVU			Global Days	Modifiers				
Mod	Non-Fac Total	Fac Total		51	50	62	80	MUE
	0.00	0.00	XXX	9	9	9	9	1

87507 Infectious agent detection by nucleic acid (DNA or RNA); gastrointestinal pathogen (eg, Clostridium difficile, E. coli, Salmonella, Shigella, norovirus, Giardia), includes multiplex reverse transcription, when performed, and multiplex amplified probe technique, multiple types or subtypes, 12-25 targets   Q4

RVU			Global Days	Modifiers				
Mod	Non-Fac Total	Fac Total		51	50	62	80	MUE
	0.00	0.00	XXX	9	9	9	9	1

87510 Infectious agent detection by nucleic acid (DNA or RNA); Gardnerella vaginalis, direct probe technique   Q4

RVU			Global Days	Modifiers				
Mod	Non-Fac Total	Fac Total		51	50	62	80	MUE
	0.00	0.00	XXX	9	9	9	9	1

AMA: Aug 05: 9, May 12: 5, Sep 13: 3

87511 Infectious agent detection by nucleic acid (DNA or RNA); Gardnerella vaginalis, amplified probe technique   Q4

RVU			Global Days	Modifiers				
Mod	Non-Fac Total	Fac Total		51	50	62	80	MUE
	0.00	0.00	XXX	9	9	9	9	1

AMA: May 12: 5, Sep 13: 3

87512 Infectious agent detection by nucleic acid (DNA or RNA); Gardnerella vaginalis, quantification   Q4

RVU			Global Days	Modifiers				
Mod	Non-Fac Total	Fac Total		51	50	62	80	MUE
	0.00	0.00	XXX	9	9	9	9	1

AMA: Sep 13: 3

87515 Infectious agent detection by nucleic acid (DNA or RNA); hepatitis B virus, direct probe technique   Q4

RVU			Global Days	Modifiers				
Mod	Non-Fac Total	Fac Total		51	50	62	80	MUE
	0.00	0.00	XXX	9	9	9	9	1

AMA: May 12: 5, Sep 13: 3

Pub 100-04, 16, 120.2

● New   ▲ Revised   Deleted   ⊙ Moderate Sedation   ✚ Add-on Codes   ⊘ High Risk Denial   Ⓐ Age Edit   ♀ Female   ♂ Male   **AMA** *CPT® Assistant*   *MUE* Medically Unlikely Edit
⊘ Modifier 51 Exempt   ⊖ Modifier 63 Exempt   ⓧ Unlisted   **Modifiers:** *See Inside Back Cover*   Ⓜ Maternity   A2–Z3 ASC Payment Indicators   A–Y OPPS Status Indicators

87516 Infectious agent detection by nucleic acid (DNA or RNA); hepatitis B virus, amplified probe technique ◎4

RVU Mod	Non-Fac Total	Fac Total	Global Days	51	50	62	80	MUE
	0.00	0.00	XXX	9	9	9	9	1

AMA: Sep 13: 3
Pub 100-04, 16, 120.2

87517 Infectious agent detection by nucleic acid (DNA or RNA); hepatitis B virus, quantification ◎4

RVU Mod	Non-Fac Total	Fac Total	Global Days	51	50	62	80	MUE
	0.00	0.00	XXX	9	9	9	9	1

AMA: Sep 13: 3
Pub 100-04, 16, 120.2

87520 Infectious agent detection by nucleic acid (DNA or RNA); hepatitis C, direct probe technique ◎4

RVU Mod	Non-Fac Total	Fac Total	Global Days	51	50	62	80	MUE
	0.00	0.00	XXX	9	9	9	9	1

AMA: Sep 13: 3
Pub 100-04, 16, 120.2

87521 Infectious agent detection by nucleic acid (DNA or RNA); hepatitis C, amplified probe technique, includes reverse transcription when performed ◎4

RVU Mod	Non-Fac Total	Fac Total	Global Days	51	50	62	80	MUE
	0.00	0.00	XXX	9	9	9	9	1

AMA: Sep 13: 3
Pub 100-04, 16, 120.2

87522 Infectious agent detection by nucleic acid (DNA or RNA); hepatitis C, quantification, includes reverse transcription when performed ◎4

RVU Mod	Non-Fac Total	Fac Total	Global Days	51	50	62	80	MUE
	0.00	0.00	XXX	9	9	9	9	1

AMA: Sep 13: 3
Pub 100-04, 16, 120.2

87525 Infectious agent detection by nucleic acid (DNA or RNA); hepatitis G, direct probe technique ⊘◎4

RVU Mod	Non-Fac Total	Fac Total	Global Days	51	50	62	80	MUE
	0.00	0.00	XXX	9	9	9	9	1

AMA: Sep 13: 3
Pub 100-04, 16, 120.2

87526 Infectious agent detection by nucleic acid (DNA or RNA); hepatitis G, amplified probe technique ◎4

RVU Mod	Non-Fac Total	Fac Total	Global Days	51	50	62	80	MUE
	0.00	0.00	XXX	9	9	9	9	1

AMA: Sep 13: 3
Pub 100-04, 16, 120.2

87527 Infectious agent detection by nucleic acid (DNA or RNA); hepatitis G, quantification ◎4

RVU Mod	Non-Fac Total	Fac Total	Global Days	51	50	62	80	MUE
	0.00	0.00	XXX	9	9	9	9	1

AMA: Sep 13: 3
Pub 100-04, 16, 120.2

87528 Infectious agent detection by nucleic acid (DNA or RNA); Herpes simplex virus, direct probe technique ◎4

RVU Mod	Non-Fac Total	Fac Total	Global Days	51	50	62	80	MUE
	0.00	0.00	XXX	9	9	9	9	1

AMA: May 12: 5, Sep 13: 3

87529 Infectious agent detection by nucleic acid (DNA or RNA); Herpes simplex virus, amplified probe technique ◎4

RVU Mod	Non-Fac Total	Fac Total	Global Days	51	50	62	80	MUE
	0.00	0.00	XXX	9	9	9	9	2

AMA: Sep 13: 3

87530 Infectious agent detection by nucleic acid (DNA or RNA); Herpes simplex virus, quantification ⊘◎4

RVU Mod	Non-Fac Total	Fac Total	Global Days	51	50	62	80	MUE
	0.00	0.00	XXX	9	9	9	9	2

AMA: Sep 13: 3

87531 Infectious agent detection by nucleic acid (DNA or RNA); Herpes virus-6, direct probe technique ◎4

RVU Mod	Non-Fac Total	Fac Total	Global Days	51	50	62	80	MUE
	0.00	0.00	XXX	9	9	9	9	1

AMA: Sep 13: 3

87532 Infectious agent detection by nucleic acid (DNA or RNA); Herpes virus-6, amplified probe technique ◎4

RVU Mod	Non-Fac Total	Fac Total	Global Days	51	50	62	80	MUE
	0.00	0.00	XXX	9	9	9	9	1

AMA: Sep 13: 3
Pub 100-04, 16, 120.2

87533 Infectious agent detection by nucleic acid (DNA or RNA); Herpes virus-6, quantification ◎4

RVU Mod	Non-Fac Total	Fac Total	Global Days	51	50	62	80	MUE
	0.00	0.00	XXX	9	9	9	9	1

AMA: Sep 13: 3

87534 Infectious agent detection by nucleic acid (DNA or RNA); HIV-1, direct probe technique ◎4

RVU Mod	Non-Fac Total	Fac Total	Global Days	51	50	62	80	MUE
	0.00	0.00	XXX	9	9	9	9	1

AMA: May 12: 5, Sep 13: 3
NCD: 190.14

● New   ▲ Revised   ✖ Deleted   ⊙ Moderate Sedation   ✚ Add-on Codes   ⊗ High Risk Denial   Ⓐ Age Edit   ♀ Female   ♂ Male   **AMA** *CPT® Assistant*   **MUE** Medically Unlikely Edit
⊘ Modifier 51 Exempt   ⊖ Modifier 63 Exempt   ✗ Unlisted   **Modifiers:** *See Inside Back Cover*   Ⓜ Maternity   A2–Z3 ASC Payment Indicators   A–Y OPPS Status Indicators

CPT © 2015 American Medical Association. All Rights Reserved.   © 2016 DecisionHealth

87535 Infectious agent detection by nucleic acid (DNA or RNA); HIV-1, amplified probe technique, includes reverse transcription when performed ⊘Q4

RVU			Global Days	Modifiers				
Mod	Non-Fac Total	Fac Total		51	50	62	80	MUE
	0.00	0.00	XXX	9	9	9	9	1

AMA: Mar 08: 3, Sep 13: 3
NCD: 190.14

87536 Infectious agent detection by nucleic acid (DNA or RNA); HIV-1, quantification, includes reverse transcription when performed Q4

RVU			Global Days	Modifiers				
Mod	Non-Fac Total	Fac Total		51	50	62	80	MUE
	0.00	0.00	XXX	9	9	9	9	1

AMA: Sep 13: 3
NCD: 190.13

87537 Infectious agent detection by nucleic acid (DNA or RNA); HIV-2, direct probe technique ⊘Q4

RVU			Global Days	Modifiers				
Mod	Non-Fac Total	Fac Total		51	50	62	80	MUE
	0.00	0.00	XXX	9	9	9	9	1

AMA: Sep 13: 3
NCD: 190.13

87538 Infectious agent detection by nucleic acid (DNA or RNA); HIV-2, amplified probe technique, includes reverse transcription when performed Q4

RVU			Global Days	Modifiers				
Mod	Non-Fac Total	Fac Total		51	50	62	80	MUE
	0.00	0.00	XXX	9	9	9	9	1

AMA: Sep 13: 3
NCD: 190.14

87539 Infectious agent detection by nucleic acid (DNA or RNA); HIV-2, quantification, includes reverse transcription when performed ⊘Q4

RVU			Global Days	Modifiers				
Mod	Non-Fac Total	Fac Total		51	50	62	80	MUE
	0.00	0.00	XXX	9	9	9	9	1

AMA: Sep 13: 3
NCD: 190.14

87540 Infectious agent detection by nucleic acid (DNA or RNA); Legionella pneumophila, direct probe technique ⊘Q4

RVU			Global Days	Modifiers				
Mod	Non-Fac Total	Fac Total		51	50	62	80	MUE
	0.00	0.00	XXX	9	9	9	9	1

AMA: May 12: 5, Sep 13: 3

87541 Infectious agent detection by nucleic acid (DNA or RNA); Legionella pneumophila, amplified probe technique Q4

RVU			Global Days	Modifiers				
Mod	Non-Fac Total	Fac Total		51	50	62	80	MUE
	0.00	0.00	XXX	9	9	9	9	1

AMA: Sep 13: 3

87542 Infectious agent detection by nucleic acid (DNA or RNA); Legionella pneumophila, quantification ⊘Q4

RVU			Global Days	Modifiers				
Mod	Non-Fac Total	Fac Total		51	50	62	80	MUE
	0.00	0.00	XXX	9	9	9	9	1

AMA: Sep 13: 3

87550 Infectious agent detection by nucleic acid (DNA or RNA); Mycobacteria species, direct probe technique Q4

RVU			Global Days	Modifiers				
Mod	Non-Fac Total	Fac Total		51	50	62	80	MUE
	0.00	0.00	XXX	9	9	9	9	1

AMA: May 12: 5, Sep 13: 3

87551 Infectious agent detection by nucleic acid (DNA or RNA); Mycobacteria species, amplified probe technique Q4

RVU			Global Days	Modifiers				
Mod	Non-Fac Total	Fac Total		51	50	62	80	MUE
	0.00	0.00	XXX	9	9	9	9	2

AMA: Sep 13: 3

87552 Infectious agent detection by nucleic acid (DNA or RNA); Mycobacteria species, quantification Q4

RVU			Global Days	Modifiers				
Mod	Non-Fac Total	Fac Total		51	50	62	80	MUE
	0.00	0.00	XXX	9	9	9	9	1

AMA: Sep 13: 3

87555 Infectious agent detection by nucleic acid (DNA or RNA); Mycobacteria tuberculosis, direct probe technique Q4

RVU			Global Days	Modifiers				
Mod	Non-Fac Total	Fac Total		51	50	62	80	MUE
	0.00	0.00	XXX	9	9	9	9	1

AMA: Sep 13: 3

87556 Infectious agent detection by nucleic acid (DNA or RNA); Mycobacteria tuberculosis, amplified probe technique Q4

RVU			Global Days	Modifiers				
Mod	Non-Fac Total	Fac Total		51	50	62	80	MUE
	0.00	0.00	XXX	9	9	9	9	1

AMA: Sep 13: 3

87557 Infectious agent detection by nucleic acid (DNA or RNA); Mycobacteria tuberculosis, quantification Q4

RVU			Global Days	Modifiers				
Mod	Non-Fac Total	Fac Total		51	50	62	80	MUE
	0.00	0.00	XXX	9	9	9	9	1

AMA: Sep 13: 3

87560 Infectious agent detection by nucleic acid (DNA or RNA); Mycobacteria avium-intracellulare, direct probe technique Q4

RVU			Global Days	Modifiers				
Mod	Non-Fac Total	Fac Total		51	50	62	80	MUE
	0.00	0.00	XXX	9	9	9	9	1

AMA: Sep 13: 3

● New   ▲ Revised   Deleted   ⊙ Moderate Sedation   ✚ Add-on Codes   ⊘ High Risk Denial   Ⓐ Age Edit   ♀ Female   ♂ Male   **AMA** *CPT® Assistant*   **MUE** Medically Unlikely Edit
⊘ Modifier 51 Exempt   ⊖ Modifier 63 Exempt   ✗ Unlisted   **Modifiers:** *See Inside Back Cover*   Ⓜ Maternity   Ａ2–Ｚ3 ASC Payment Indicators   Ａ–Ｙ OPPS Status Indicators

87561 Infectious agent detection by nucleic acid (DNA or RNA); Mycobacteria avium-intracellulare, amplified probe technique ⊘Q4

RVU			Global Days	Modifiers				
Mod	Non-Fac Total	Fac Total		51	50	62	80	MUE
	0.00	0.00	XXX	9	9	9	9	1

AMA: Sep 13: 3

87562 Infectious agent detection by nucleic acid (DNA or RNA); Mycobacteria avium-intracellulare, quantification Q4

RVU			Global Days	Modifiers				
Mod	Non-Fac Total	Fac Total		51	50	62	80	MUE
	0.00	0.00	XXX	9	9	9	9	1

AMA: Sep 13: 3

87580 Infectious agent detection by nucleic acid (DNA or RNA); Mycoplasma pneumoniae, direct probe technique ⊘Q4

RVU			Global Days	Modifiers				
Mod	Non-Fac Total	Fac Total		51	50	62	80	MUE
	0.00	0.00	XXX	9	9	9	9	1

AMA: Sep 13: 3

87581 Infectious agent detection by nucleic acid (DNA or RNA); Mycoplasma pneumoniae, amplified probe technique Q4

RVU			Global Days	Modifiers				
Mod	Non-Fac Total	Fac Total		51	50	62	80	MUE
	0.00	0.00	XXX	9	9	9	9	1

AMA: Sep 13: 3

87582 Infectious agent detection by nucleic acid (DNA or RNA); Mycoplasma pneumoniae, quantification ⊘Q4

RVU			Global Days	Modifiers				
Mod	Non-Fac Total	Fac Total		51	50	62	80	MUE
	0.00	0.00	XXX	9	9	9	9	1

AMA: Sep 13: 3

87590 Infectious agent detection by nucleic acid (DNA or RNA); Neisseria gonorrhoeae, direct probe technique A

RVU			Global Days	Modifiers				
Mod	Non-Fac Total	Fac Total		51	50	62	80	MUE
	0.00	0.00	XXX	9	9	9	9	1

AMA: May 12: 5, Sep 13: 3
Pub 100-04, 18, 170.1

87591 Infectious agent detection by nucleic acid (DNA or RNA); Neisseria gonorrhoeae, amplified probe technique ⊘A

RVU			Global Days	Modifiers				
Mod	Non-Fac Total	Fac Total		51	50	62	80	MUE
	0.00	0.00	XXX	9	9	9	9	2

AMA: Jun 13: 14, Sep 13: 3
Pub 100-04, 18, 170.1

87592 Infectious agent detection by nucleic acid (DNA or RNA); Neisseria gonorrhoeae, quantification Q4

RVU			Global Days	Modifiers				
Mod	Non-Fac Total	Fac Total		51	50	62	80	MUE
	0.00	0.00	XXX	9	9	9	9	1

AMA: Sep 13: 3

87623 Infectious agent detection by nucleic acid (DNA or RNA); Human Papillomavirus (HPV), low-risk types (eg, 6, 11, 42, 43, 44) Q4

RVU			Global Days	Modifiers				
Mod	Non-Fac Total	Fac Total		51	50	62	80	MUE
	0.00	0.00	XXX	9	9	9	9	1

87624 Infectious agent detection by nucleic acid (DNA or RNA); Human Papillomavirus (HPV), high-risk types (eg, 16, 18, 31, 33, 35, 39, 45, 51, 52, 56, 58, 59, 68) Q4

RVU			Global Days	Modifiers				
Mod	Non-Fac Total	Fac Total		51	50	62	80	MUE
	0.00	0.00	XXX	9	9	9	9	1

87625 Infectious agent detection by nucleic acid (DNA or RNA); Human Papillomavirus (HPV), types 16 and 18 only, includes type 45, if performed Q4

RVU			Global Days	Modifiers				
Mod	Non-Fac Total	Fac Total		51	50	62	80	MUE
	0.00	0.00	XXX	9	9	9	9	1

AMA: Jun 15: 10

87631 Infectious agent detection by nucleic acid (DNA or RNA); respiratory virus (eg, adenovirus, influenza virus, coronavirus, metapneumovirus, parainfluenza virus, respiratory syncytial virus, rhinovirus), includes multiplex reverse transcription, when performed, and multiplex amplified probe technique, multiple types or subtypes, 3-5 targets Q4

RVU			Global Days	Modifiers				
Mod	Non-Fac Total	Fac Total		51	50	62	80	MUE
	0.00	0.00	XXX	9	9	9	9	1

AMA: Sep 13: 3

87632 Infectious agent detection by nucleic acid (DNA or RNA); respiratory virus (eg, adenovirus, influenza virus, coronavirus, metapneumovirus, parainfluenza virus, respiratory syncytial virus, rhinovirus), includes multiplex reverse transcription, when performed, and multiplex amplified probe technique, multiple types or subtypes, 6-11 targets Q4

RVU			Global Days	Modifiers				
Mod	Non-Fac Total	Fac Total		51	50	62	80	MUE
	0.00	0.00	XXX	9	9	9	9	1

AMA: Sep 13: 3

● New   ▲ Revised   ✖ Deleted   ⊙ Moderate Sedation   ✚ Add-on Codes   ⊘ High Risk Denial   Ⓐ Age Edit   ♀ Female   ♂ Male   **AMA** *CPT® Assistant*   **MUE** Medically Unlikely Edit
Ⓢ Modifier 51 Exempt   ⊖ Modifier 63 Exempt   ✗ Unlisted   **Modifiers:** *See Inside Back Cover*   Ⓜ Maternity   A2–Z3 ASC Payment Indicators   A–Y OPPS Status Indicators

CPT © 2015 American Medical Association. All Rights Reserved.   © 2016 DecisionHealth

87633 Infectious agent detection by nucleic acid (DNA or RNA); respiratory virus (eg, adenovirus, influenza virus, coronavirus, metapneumovirus, parainfluenza virus, respiratory syncytial virus, rhinovirus), includes multiplex reverse transcription, when performed, and multiplex amplified probe technique, multiple types or subtypes, 12-25 targets   Q4

RVU			Global Days	Modifiers				
Mod	Non-Fac Total	Fac Total		51	50	62	80	MUE
	0.00	0.00	XXX	9	9	9	9	1

AMA: Sep 13: 3

87640 Infectious agent detection by nucleic acid (DNA or RNA); Staphylococcus aureus, amplified probe technique   Q4

RVU			Global Days	Modifiers				
Mod	Non-Fac Total	Fac Total		51	50	62	80	MUE
	0.00	0.00	XXX	9	9	9	9	1

AMA: Aug 07: 7, May 12: 5, Sep 13: 3

87641 Infectious agent detection by nucleic acid (DNA or RNA); Staphylococcus aureus, methicillin resistant, amplified probe technique   Q4

RVU			Global Days	Modifiers				
Mod	Non-Fac Total	Fac Total		51	50	62	80	MUE
	0.00	0.00	XXX	9	9	9	9	1

AMA: Aug 07: 7, Sep 13: 3

87650 Infectious agent detection by nucleic acid (DNA or RNA); Streptococcus, group A, direct probe technique   Q4

RVU			Global Days	Modifiers				
Mod	Non-Fac Total	Fac Total		51	50	62	80	MUE
	0.00	0.00	XXX	9	9	9	9	1

AMA: Sep 13: 4

87651 Infectious agent detection by nucleic acid (DNA or RNA); Streptococcus, group A, amplified probe technique   Q4

RVU			Global Days	Modifiers				
Mod	Non-Fac Total	Fac Total		51	50	62	80	MUE
	0.00	0.00	XXX	9	9	9	9	1

AMA: Sep 13: 4

87652 Infectious agent detection by nucleic acid (DNA or RNA); Streptococcus, group A, quantification   Q4

RVU			Global Days	Modifiers				
Mod	Non-Fac Total	Fac Total		51	50	62	80	MUE
	0.00	0.00	XXX	9	9	9	9	1

AMA: Sep 13: 4

87653 Infectious agent detection by nucleic acid (DNA or RNA); Streptococcus, group B, amplified probe technique   Q4

RVU			Global Days	Modifiers				
Mod	Non-Fac Total	Fac Total		51	50	62	80	MUE
	0.00	0.00	XXX	9	9	9	9	1

AMA: Aug 07: 7, Sep 13: 3

87660 Infectious agent detection by nucleic acid (DNA or RNA); Trichomonas vaginalis, direct probe technique   Q4

RVU			Global Days	Modifiers				
Mod	Non-Fac Total	Fac Total		51	50	62	80	MUE
	0.00	0.00	XXX	9	9	9	9	1

AMA: May 12: 5, Sep 13: 3

87661 Infectious agent detection by nucleic acid (DNA or RNA); Trichomonas vaginalis, amplified probe technique   Q4

RVU			Global Days	Modifiers				
Mod	Non-Fac Total	Fac Total		51	50	62	80	MUE
	0.00	0.00	XXX	9	9	9	9	1

87797 Infectious agent detection by nucleic acid (DNA or RNA), not otherwise specified; direct probe technique, each organism   Q4

RVU			Global Days	Modifiers				
Mod	Non-Fac Total	Fac Total		51	50	62	80	MUE
	0.00	0.00	XXX	9	9	9	9	3

AMA: Nov 97: 34, Nov 01: 10, Aug 05: 9, May 12: 5, Sep 13: 3

87798 Infectious agent detection by nucleic acid (DNA or RNA), not otherwise specified; amplified probe technique, each organism   Q4

RVU			Global Days	Modifiers				
Mod	Non-Fac Total	Fac Total		51	50	62	80	MUE
	0.00	0.00	XXX	9	9	9	9	13

AMA: Nov 97: 34, Nov 01: 10, Aug 07: 7, Sep 13: 3

87799 Infectious agent detection by nucleic acid (DNA or RNA), not otherwise specified; quantification, each organism   Q4

RVU			Global Days	Modifiers				
Mod	Non-Fac Total	Fac Total		51	50	62	80	MUE
	0.00	0.00	XXX	9	9	9	9	3

AMA: Nov 97: 34, Sep 13: 3

87800 Infectious agent detection by nucleic acid (DNA or RNA), multiple organisms; direct probe(s) technique   A

RVU			Global Days	Modifiers				
Mod	Non-Fac Total	Fac Total		51	50	62	80	MUE
	0.00	0.00	XXX	9	9	9	9	2

AMA: Aug 05: 9, May 12: 5, Sep 13: 3
Pub 100-04, 18, 170.1

87801 Infectious agent detection by nucleic acid (DNA or RNA), multiple organisms; amplified probe(s) technique   Q4

RVU			Global Days	Modifiers				
Mod	Non-Fac Total	Fac Total		51	50	62	80	MUE
	0.00	0.00	XXX	9	9	9	9	3

AMA: May 12: 5, Jun 13: 14, Sep 13: 3

87802 Infectious agent antigen detection by immunoassay with direct optical observation; Streptococcus, group B   Q4

RVU			Global Days	Modifiers				
Mod	Non-Fac Total	Fac Total		51	50	62	80	MUE
	0.00	0.00	XXX	9	9	9	9	2

AMA: Jun 03: 12

● New   ▲ Revised   Deleted   ⊙ Moderate Sedation   ✚ Add-on Codes   ⊘ High Risk Denial   Ⓐ Age Edit   ♀ Female   ♂ Male   **AMA** *CPT® Assistant*   *MUE* Medically Unlikely Edit
⦸ Modifier 51 Exempt   ⊖ Modifier 63 Exempt   ⊠ Unlisted   **Modifiers:** *See Inside Back Cover*   Ⓜ Maternity   A2–Z3 ASC Payment Indicators   A–Y OPPS Status Indicators

© 2016 DecisionHealth   CPT © 2015 American Medical Association. All Rights Reserved.   **763**

87803 Infectious agent antigen detection by immunoassay with direct optical observation; Clostridium difficile toxin A   Q4

RVU			Global Days	Modifiers				
Mod	Non-Fac Total	Fac Total		51	50	62	80	MUE
	0.00	0.00	XXX	9	9	9	9	3

AMA: Jun 03: 12

87804 Infectious agent antigen detection by immunoassay with direct optical observation; Influenza   Q4

Coding tip: For a CLIA-waived test, append modifier QW to 87804

RVU			Global Days	Modifiers				
Mod	Non-Fac Total	Fac Total		51	50	62	80	MUE
	0.00	0.00	XXX	9	9	9	9	3

AMA: Jun 03: 11, 12, May 09: 6

87806 Infectious agent antigen detection by immunoassay with direct optical observation; HIV-1 antigen(s), with HIV-1 and HIV-2 antibodies   Q4

RVU			Global Days	Modifiers				
Mod	Non-Fac Total	Fac Total		51	50	62	80	MUE
	0.00	0.00	XXX	9	9	9	9	1

87807 Infectious agent antigen detection by immunoassay with direct optical observation; respiratory syncytial virus   Q4

Coding tip: For a CLIA-waived test, append modifier QW to 87807

RVU			Global Days	Modifiers				
Mod	Non-Fac Total	Fac Total		51	50	62	80	MUE
	0.00	0.00	XXX	9	9	9	9	2

87808 Infectious agent antigen detection by immunoassay with direct optical observation; Trichomonas vaginalis   Q4

Coding tip: For a CLIA-waived test, append modifier QW to 87808

RVU			Global Days	Modifiers				
Mod	Non-Fac Total	Fac Total		51	50	62	80	MUE
	0.00	0.00	XXX	9	9	9	9	1

87809 Infectious agent antigen detection by immunoassay with direct optical observation; adenovirus   Q4

Coding tip: For a CLIA-waived test, append modifier QW to 87809

RVU			Global Days	Modifiers				
Mod	Non-Fac Total	Fac Total		51	50	62	80	MUE
	0.00	0.00	XXX	9	9	9	9	2

AMA: Apr 08: 5

87810 Infectious agent antigen detection by immunoassay with direct optical observation; Chlamydia trachomatis   A

RVU			Global Days	Modifiers				
Mod	Non-Fac Total	Fac Total		51	50	62	80	MUE
	0.00	0.00	XXX	9	9	9	9	2

AMA: Nov 97: 34, Jan 98: 6
Pub 100-04, 18, 170.1

87850 Infectious agent antigen detection by immunoassay with direct optical observation; Neisseria gonorrhoeae   A

RVU			Global Days	Modifiers				
Mod	Non-Fac Total	Fac Total		51	50	62	80	MUE
	0.00	0.00	XXX	9	9	9	9	1

AMA: Nov 97: 34, Jan 98: 6
Pub 100-04, 18, 170.1

87880 Infectious agent antigen detection by immunoassay with direct optical observation; Streptococcus, group A   Q4

Coding tip: For a CLIA-waived test, add modifier QW to 87880

RVU			Global Days	Modifiers				
Mod	Non-Fac Total	Fac Total		51	50	62	80	MUE
	0.00	0.00	XXX	9	9	9	9	2

AMA: Nov 97: 34, Jan 98: 6, Dec 98: 8

87899 Infectious agent antigen detection by immunoassay with direct optical observation; not otherwise specified   Q4

Coding tip: For a CLIA-waived test, add modifier QW to 87899

RVU			Global Days	Modifiers				
Mod	Non-Fac Total	Fac Total		51	50	62	80	MUE
	0.00	0.00	XXX	9	9	9	9	4

AMA: Jan 98: 6, Jun 01: 11

87900 Infectious agent drug susceptibility phenotype prediction using regularly updated genotypic bioinformatics   Q4

RVU			Global Days	Modifiers				
Mod	Non-Fac Total	Fac Total		51	50	62	80	MUE
	0.00	0.00	XXX	9	9	9	9	1

AMA: Mar 06: 6, May 12: 5, Sep 13: 3

87901 Infectious agent genotype analysis by nucleic acid (DNA or RNA); HIV-1, reverse transcriptase and protease regions   Q4

RVU			Global Days	Modifiers				
Mod	Non-Fac Total	Fac Total		51	50	62	80	MUE
	0.00	0.00	XXX	9	9	9	9	1

AMA: Aug 05: 9, Mar 06: 6, Oct 10: 9, Dec 10: 9, May 12: 5, Sep 13: 3

87902 Infectious agent genotype analysis by nucleic acid (DNA or RNA); Hepatitis C virus   Q4

RVU			Global Days	Modifiers				
Mod	Non-Fac Total	Fac Total		51	50	62	80	MUE
	0.00	0.00	XXX	9	9	9	9	1

AMA: May 12: 5, Sep 13: 3

87903 Infectious agent phenotype analysis by nucleic acid (DNA or RNA) with drug resistance tissue culture analysis, HIV 1; first through 10 drugs tested   Q4

RVU			Global Days	Modifiers				
Mod	Non-Fac Total	Fac Total		51	50	62	80	MUE
	0.00	0.00	XXX	9	9	9	9	1

AMA: Apr 04: 15, Mar 06: 6, May 12: 3, Sep 13: 3

● New   ▲ Revised   ✖ Deleted   ⊙ Moderate Sedation   ✚ Add-on Codes   ⊘ High Risk Denial   Ⓐ Age Edit   ♀ Female   ♂ Male   **AMA** *CPT® Assistant*   **MUE** Medically Unlikely Edit
⊘ Modifier 51 Exempt   ⊖ Modifier 63 Exempt   🗷 Unlisted   **Modifiers:** *See Inside Back Cover*   Ⓜ Maternity   A2–Z3 ASC Payment Indicators   A–Y OPPS Status Indicators

+ 87904 Infectious agent phenotype analysis by nucleic acid (DNA or RNA) with drug resistance tissue culture analysis, HIV 1; each additional drug tested (List separately in addition to code for primary procedure) ⊘Q4

RVU			Global Days	Modifiers				
Mod	Non-Fac Total	Fac Total		51	50	62	80	MUE
	0.00	0.00	XXX	9	9	9	9	14

AMA: Apr 04: 15, Mar 06: 6, May 12: 3, Sep 13: 3

87905 Infectious agent enzymatic activity other than virus (eg, sialidase activity in vaginal fluid) Q4

Coding tip: For a CLIA-waived test, add modifier QW to 87905

RVU			Global Days	Modifiers				
Mod	Non-Fac Total	Fac Total		51	50	62	80	MUE
	0.00	0.00	XXX	9	9	9	9	2

87906 Infectious agent genotype analysis by nucleic acid (DNA or RNA); HIV-1, other region (eg, integrase, fusion) Q4

Coding tip: Code 87906 is listed out of numerical order in CPT. Related laboratory procedures for infectious agent genotype analysis: HIV-1 - 87901; hepatitis C virus - 87902; cytomegalovirus - 87910; hepatitis B virus (HBV) - 87912

RVU			Global Days	Modifiers				
Mod	Non-Fac Total	Fac Total		51	50	62	80	MUE
	0.00	0.00	XXX	9	9	9	9	2

AMA: Oct 10: 8, Dec 10: 8, Sep 13: 3

87910 Infectious agent genotype analysis by nucleic acid (DNA or RNA); cytomegalovirus Q4

Coding tip: Code 87910 is listed out of numerical order in CPT. Related laboratory procedures for infectious agent genotype analysis: HIV-1 - 87901, 87906; hepatitis C virus - 87902; hepatitis B virus (HBV) - 87912

RVU			Global Days	Modifiers				
Mod	Non-Fac Total	Fac Total		51	50	62	80	MUE
	0.00	0.00	XXX	9	9	9	9	1

AMA: Sep 13: 3

87912 Infectious agent genotype analysis by nucleic acid (DNA or RNA); Hepatitis B virus Q4

Coding tip: Code 87912 is listed out of numerical order in CPT. Related laboratory procedures for infectious agent genotype analysis: HIV-1 - 87901, 87906; hepatitis C virus - 87902; cytomegalovirus (CMV) 87910

RVU			Global Days	Modifiers				
Mod	Non-Fac Total	Fac Total		51	50	62	80	MUE
	0.00	0.00	XXX	9	9	9	9	1

AMA: Sep 13: 3

87999 Unlisted microbiology procedure ⊘✕N

RVU			Global Days	Modifiers				
Mod	Non-Fac Total	Fac Total		51	50	62	80	MUE
	0.00	0.00	XXX	9	9	9	9	

AMA: Aug 05: 9
Pub 100-04, 16, 100.4

Anatomical Pathology (Necropsy)

Postmortem Exam

88000 Necropsy (autopsy), gross examination only; without CNS ⊘E

RVU			Global Days	Modifiers				
Mod	Non-Fac Total	Fac Total		51	50	62	80	MUE
	0.00	0.00	XXX	9	9	9	9	

AMA: Aug 05: 9

88005 Necropsy (autopsy), gross examination only; with brain ⊘E

RVU			Global Days	Modifiers				
Mod	Non-Fac Total	Fac Total		51	50	62	80	MUE
	0.00	0.00	XXX	9	9	9	9	

88007 Necropsy (autopsy), gross examination only; with brain and spinal cord ⊘E

RVU			Global Days	Modifiers				
Mod	Non-Fac Total	Fac Total		51	50	62	80	MUE
	0.00	0.00	XXX	9	9	9	9	

88012 Necropsy (autopsy), gross examination only; infant with brain ⊘AE

RVU			Global Days	Modifiers				
Mod	Non-Fac Total	Fac Total		51	50	62	80	MUE
	0.00	0.00	XXX	9	9	9	9	

88014 Necropsy (autopsy), gross examination only; stillborn or newborn with brain ⊘AE

RVU			Global Days	Modifiers				
Mod	Non-Fac Total	Fac Total		51	50	62	80	MUE
	0.00	0.00	XXX	9	9	9	9	

88016 Necropsy (autopsy), gross examination only; macerated stillborn AE

RVU			Global Days	Modifiers				
Mod	Non-Fac Total	Fac Total		51	50	62	80	MUE
	0.00	0.00	XXX	9	9	9	9	

88020 Necropsy (autopsy), gross and microscopic; without CNS ⊘E

RVU			Global Days	Modifiers				
Mod	Non-Fac Total	Fac Total		51	50	62	80	MUE
	0.00	0.00	XXX	9	9	9	9	

88025 Necropsy (autopsy), gross and microscopic; with brain ⊘E

RVU			Global Days	Modifiers				
Mod	Non-Fac Total	Fac Total		51	50	62	80	MUE
	0.00	0.00	XXX	9	9	9	9	

88027 Necropsy (autopsy), gross and microscopic; with brain and spinal cord ⊘E

RVU			Global Days	Modifiers				
Mod	Non-Fac Total	Fac Total		51	50	62	80	MUE
	0.00	0.00	XXX	9	9	9	9	

88028 Necropsy (autopsy), gross and microscopic; infant with brain AE

RVU			Global Days	Modifiers				
Mod	Non-Fac Total	Fac Total		51	50	62	80	MUE
	0.00	0.00	XXX	9	9	9	9	

● New   ▲ Revised   Deleted   ⊙ Moderate Sedation   ✚ Add-on Codes   ⊘ High Risk Denial   Ⓐ Age Edit   ♀ Female   ♂ Male   **AMA** *CPT® Assistant*   **MUE** Medically Unlikely Edit

⃠ Modifier 51 Exempt   ⊖ Modifier 63 Exempt   ✕ Unlisted   **Modifiers:** *See Inside Back Cover*   Ⓜ Maternity   A2–Z3 ASC Payment Indicators   A–Y OPPS Status Indicators

88029 Necropsy (autopsy), gross and microscopic; stillborn or newborn with brain ⒜🅔

RVU			Global Days	Modifiers				
Mod	Non-Fac Total	Fac Total		51	50	62	80	MUE
	0.00	0.00	XXX	9	9	9	9	

88036 Necropsy (autopsy), limited, gross and/or microscopic; regional ⒞🅔

RVU			Global Days	Modifiers				
Mod	Non-Fac Total	Fac Total		51	50	62	80	MUE
	0.00	0.00	XXX	9	9	9	9	

88037 Necropsy (autopsy), limited, gross and/or microscopic; single organ ⒞🅔

RVU			Global Days	Modifiers				
Mod	Non-Fac Total	Fac Total		51	50	62	80	MUE
	0.00	0.00	XXX	9	9	9	9	

88040 Necropsy (autopsy); forensic examination ⒞🅔

RVU			Global Days	Modifiers				
Mod	Non-Fac Total	Fac Total		51	50	62	80	MUE
	0.00	0.00	XXX	9	9	9	9	

88045 Necropsy (autopsy); coroner's call 🅔

RVU			Global Days	Modifiers				
Mod	Non-Fac Total	Fac Total		51	50	62	80	MUE
	0.00	0.00	XXX	9	9	9	9	

88099 Unlisted necropsy (autopsy) procedure 🅧🅔

RVU			Global Days	Modifiers				
Mod	Non-Fac Total	Fac Total		51	50	62	80	MUE
	0.00	0.00	XXX	9	9	9	9	

Cytopathology Testing

Coding Guidance

Appropriate billing for cytopathology codes requires that the highest level of specificity that most accurately describes the services done is reported. For any given specimen, only one code from a related group of service codes that could be performed for the same end result may be reported. A modifier must be used to identify when different levels of service were provided on multiple specimens from different anatomic locations. It is not appropriate to use codes 88160-88162 for smears in addition to the cytopathology codes 88104-88112, since smears are already included in preparation from fluids, washings, or brushings.

88104 Cytopathology, fluids, washings or brushings, except cervical or vaginal; smears with interpretation 🅠1

RVU			Global Days	Modifiers				
Mod	Non-Fac Total	Fac Total		51	50	62	80	MUE
	2.14	2.14	XXX	0	0	0	0	5
26	0.84	0.84	XXX	0	0	0	0	5
TC	1.30	1.30	XXX	0	0	0	0	5

AMA: Spring 91: 6, Fall 94: 3, Aug 05: 9

88106 Cytopathology, fluids, washings or brushings, except cervical or vaginal; simple filter method with interpretation 🅠1

RVU			Global Days	Modifiers				
Mod	Non-Fac Total	Fac Total		51	50	62	80	MUE
	2.11	2.11	XXX	0	0	0	0	5
26	0.57	0.57	XXX	0	0	0	0	5
TC	1.54	1.54	XXX	0	0	0	0	5

AMA: Fall 94: 3

88108 Cytopathology, concentration technique, smears and interpretation (eg, Saccomanno technique) 🅠1

RVU			Global Days	Modifiers				
Mod	Non-Fac Total	Fac Total		51	50	62	80	MUE
	2.04	2.04	XXX	0	0	0	0	6
26	0.66	0.66	XXX	0	0	0	0	6
TC	1.38	1.38	XXX	0	0	0	0	6

AMA: Fall 94: 3, Nov 97: 34, Jan 98: 6

88112 Cytopathology, selective cellular enhancement technique with interpretation (eg, liquid based slide preparation method), except cervical or vaginal 🅠1

RVU			Global Days	Modifiers				
Mod	Non-Fac Total	Fac Total		51	50	62	80	MUE
	2.02	2.02	XXX	0	0	0	0	6
26	0.81	0.81	XXX	0	0	0	0	6
TC	1.21	1.21	XXX	0	0	0	0	6

88120 Cytopathology, in situ hybridization (eg, FISH), urinary tract specimen with morphometric analysis, 3-5 molecular probes, each specimen; manual 🅠2

RVU			Global Days	Modifiers				
Mod	Non-Fac Total	Fac Total		51	50	62	80	MUE
	17.86	17.86	XXX	0	0	0	0	2
26	1.68	1.68	XXX	0	0	0	0	2
TC	16.18	16.18	XXX	0	0	0	0	2

AMA: Oct 10: 9, Dec 10: 9

88121 Cytopathology, in situ hybridization (eg, FISH), urinary tract specimen with morphometric analysis, 3-5 molecular probes, each specimen; using computer-assisted technology 🅠1

RVU			Global Days	Modifiers				
Mod	Non-Fac Total	Fac Total		51	50	62	80	MUE
	15.58	15.58	XXX	0	0	0	0	2
26	1.45	1.45	XXX	0	0	0	0	2
TC	14.13	14.13	XXX	0	0	0	0	2

AMA: Oct 10: 9, Dec 10: 9

88125 Cytopathology, forensic (eg, sperm) 🅠1

RVU			Global Days	Modifiers				
Mod	Non-Fac Total	Fac Total		51	50	62	80	MUE
	0.66	0.66	XXX	0	0	0	0	1
26	0.39	0.39	XXX	0	0	0	0	1
TC	0.27	0.27	XXX	0	0	0	0	1

88130 Sex chromatin identification; Barr bodies ⒞🅠4

RVU			Global Days	Modifiers				
Mod	Non-Fac Total	Fac Total		51	50	62	80	MUE
	0.00	0.00	XXX	9	9	9	9	1

88140 Sex chromatin identification; peripheral blood smear, polymorphonuclear drumsticks ⒞🅠4

RVU			Global Days	Modifiers				
Mod	Non-Fac Total	Fac Total		51	50	62	80	MUE
	0.00	0.00	XXX	9	9	9	9	1

AMA: Nov 98: 27, 28, Mar 06: 6

● New   ▲ Revised   ✖ Deleted   ⊙ Moderate Sedation   ✚ Add-on Codes   ⊘ High Risk Denial   ⒜ Age Edit   ♀ Female   ♂ Male   **AMA** *CPT® Assistant*   **MUE** Medically Unlikely Edit
⊘ Modifier 51 Exempt   ⊖ Modifier 63 Exempt   🅧 Unlisted   **Modifiers:** *See Inside Back Cover*   Ⓜ Maternity   🄰2–🅉3 ASC Payment Indicators   🄰–🅈 OPPS Status Indicators

88141 Cytopathology, cervical or vaginal (any reporting system), requiring interpretation by physician ♀⊙4

RVU			Global Days	Modifiers				
Mod	Non-Fac Total	Fac Total		51	50	62	80	MUE
	0.91	0.91	XXX	0	0	0	0	1

AMA: Nov 97: 35, Jan 98: 6, Jan 99: 11, May 99: 6, Nov 99: 46, Mar 04: 6, Mar 05: 16, May 11: 10, Dec 11: 17

88142 Cytopathology, cervical or vaginal (any reporting system), collected in preservative fluid, automated thin layer preparation; manual screening under physician supervision ♀⊙4

RVU			Global Days	Modifiers				
Mod	Non-Fac Total	Fac Total		51	50	62	80	MUE
	0.00	0.00	XXX	9	9	9	9	1

AMA: Nov 97: 34, 35, Jan 98: 6, Nov 98: 28, May 99: 6, Jul 03: 7, Mar 04: 4
Pub 100-04, 16, 80.3

88143 Cytopathology, cervical or vaginal (any reporting system), collected in preservative fluid, automated thin layer preparation; with manual screening and rescreening under physician supervision ♀⊙4

RVU			Global Days	Modifiers				
Mod	Non-Fac Total	Fac Total		51	50	62	80	MUE
	0.00	0.00	XXX	9	9	9	9	1

AMA: Nov 97: 34, 35, Nov 98: 28, May 99: 6, Jul 03: 7, Mar 04: 4, Mar 05: 16
Pub 100-04, 16, 80.3

88147 Cytopathology smears, cervical or vaginal; screening by automated system under physician supervision ⊙♀⊙4

RVU			Global Days	Modifiers				
Mod	Non-Fac Total	Fac Total		51	50	62	80	MUE
	0.00	0.00	XXX	9	9	9	9	1

AMA: Nov 97: 35, Nov 98: 28, Jan 99: 11, May 99: 6, Nov 99: 46, Mar 04: 6
Pub 100-04, 16, 80.3

88148 Cytopathology smears, cervical or vaginal; screening by automated system with manual rescreening under physician supervision ♀⊙4

RVU			Global Days	Modifiers				
Mod	Non-Fac Total	Fac Total		51	50	62	80	MUE
	0.00	0.00	XXX	9	9	9	9	1

AMA: Jan 99: 1, May 99: 6, Nov 99: 46, Mar 04: 6
Pub 100-04, 16, 80.3

88150 Cytopathology, slides, cervical or vaginal; manual screening under physician supervision ⊙♀⊙4

RVU			Global Days	Modifiers				
Mod	Non-Fac Total	Fac Total		51	50	62	80	MUE
	0.00	0.00	XXX	9	9	9	9	1

AMA: Winter 91: 19, Nov 97: 34, 35, Nov 98: 28, May 99: 6, Mar 04: 5
Pub 100-04, 16, 80.2, 80.3

88152 Cytopathology, slides, cervical or vaginal; with manual screening and computer-assisted rescreening under physician supervision ⊙⊙4

RVU			Global Days	Modifiers				
Mod	Non-Fac Total	Fac Total		51	50	62	80	MUE
	0.00	0.00	XXX	9	9	9	9	1

AMA: Nov 97: 35, Jan 98: 6, May 99: 6, Mar 04: 5
Pub 100-04, 16, 80.3

88153 Cytopathology, slides, cervical or vaginal; with manual screening and rescreening under physician supervision ⊙♀⊙4

RVU			Global Days	Modifiers				
Mod	Non-Fac Total	Fac Total		51	50	62	80	MUE
	0.00	0.00	XXX	9	9	9	9	1

AMA: Nov 97: 34, 35, Nov 98: 28, May 99: 6, Mar 04: 5, Mar 05: 16

88154 Cytopathology, slides, cervical or vaginal; with manual screening and computer-assisted rescreening using cell selection and review under physician supervision ♀⊙4

RVU			Global Days	Modifiers				
Mod	Non-Fac Total	Fac Total		51	50	62	80	MUE
	0.00	0.00	XXX	9	9	9	9	1

AMA: Nov 97: 34, 35, Nov 98: 28, May 99: 6, Mar 04: 5
Pub 100-04, 16, 80.3

✚ **88155** Cytopathology, slides, cervical or vaginal, definitive hormonal evaluation (eg, maturation index, karyopyknotic index, estrogenic index) (List separately in addition to code[s] for other technical and interpretation services) ♀⊙4

RVU			Global Days	Modifiers				
Mod	Non-Fac Total	Fac Total		51	50	62	80	MUE
	0.00	0.00	XXX	9	9	9	9	1

AMA: Nov 97: 35, Nov 98: 28, May 99: 6, Nov 99: 46, Mar 04: 5, May 11: 10

Coding Guidance

It is not appropriate to use codes 88160-88162 for smears in addition to the cytopathology codes 88104-88112, since smears are already included in preparation from fluids, washings, or brushings. Codes 88160-88162 specify æany other source' in the code descriptor, which excludes fluids, brushings, and washings.

88160 Cytopathology, smears, any other source; screening and interpretation ⊙1

Coding tip: *Use 88160-88162 to report Tzanck smear*

RVU			Global Days	Modifiers				
Mod	Non-Fac Total	Fac Total		51	50	62	80	MUE
	2.04	2.04	XXX	0	0	0	0	4
26	0.76	0.76	XXX	0	0	0	0	4
TC	1.28	1.28	XXX	0	0	0	0	4

AMA: Jan 98: 6

88161 Cytopathology, smears, any other source; preparation, screening and interpretation ⊙1

RVU			Global Days	Modifiers				
Mod	Non-Fac Total	Fac Total		51	50	62	80	MUE
	1.83	1.83	XXX	0	0	0	0	4
26	0.73	0.73	XXX	0	0	0	0	4
TC	1.10	1.10	XXX	0	0	0	0	4

AMA: Aug 97: 18, Jan 98: 6

88162 Cytopathology, smears, any other source; extended study involving over 5 slides and/or multiple stains ⊙1

RVU			Global Days	Modifiers				
Mod	Non-Fac Total	Fac Total		51	50	62	80	MUE
	2.95	2.95	XXX	0	0	0	0	3
26	1.15	1.15	XXX	0	0	0	0	3
TC	1.80	1.80	XXX	0	0	0	0	3

● New   ▲ Revised   Deleted   ⊙ Moderate Sedation   ✚ Add-on Codes   ⊘ High Risk Denial   Ⓐ Age Edit   ♀ Female   ♂ Male   **AMA** *CPT® Assistant*   **MUE** Medically Unlikely Edit
⊘ Modifier 51 Exempt   ⊖ Modifier 63 Exempt   Ⓧ Unlisted   **Modifiers:** *See Inside Back Cover*   Ⓜ Maternity   A2-Z3 ASC Payment Indicators   A-Y OPPS Status Indicators

© 2016 DecisionHealth   CPT © 2015 American Medical Association. All Rights Reserved.   **767**

88164 Cytopathology, slides, cervical or vaginal (the Bethesda System); manual screening under physician supervision ♀ Q4

RVU			Global Days	Modifiers				
Mod	Non-Fac Total	Fac Total		51	50	62	80	MUE
	0.00	0.00	XXX	9	9	9	9	1

AMA: Nov 98: 28, May 99: 6, Mar 04: 5

Pub 100-04, 16, 80.3

88165 Cytopathology, slides, cervical or vaginal (the Bethesda System); with manual screening and rescreening under physician supervision ⊘♀Q4

RVU			Global Days	Modifiers				
Mod	Non-Fac Total	Fac Total		51	50	62	80	MUE
	0.00	0.00	XXX	9	9	9	9	1

AMA: Nov 98: 28, May 99: 6, Mar 04: 5, Mar 05: 16

Pub 100-04, 16, 80.3

88166 Cytopathology, slides, cervical or vaginal (the Bethesda System); with manual screening and computer-assisted rescreening under physician supervision ⊘♀Q4

RVU			Global Days	Modifiers				
Mod	Non-Fac Total	Fac Total		51	50	62	80	MUE
	0.00	0.00	XXX	9	9	9	9	1

AMA: Nov 98: 28, May 99: 6, Mar 04: 5

88167 Cytopathology, slides, cervical or vaginal (the Bethesda System); with manual screening and computer-assisted rescreening using cell selection and review under physician supervision ⊘♀Q4

RVU			Global Days	Modifiers				
Mod	Non-Fac Total	Fac Total		51	50	62	80	MUE
	0.00	0.00	XXX	9	9	9	9	1

AMA: Nov 98: 28, May 99: 6, Jul 03: 7, Mar 04: 5

Pub 100-04, 16, 80.3

88172 Cytopathology, evaluation of fine needle aspirate; immediate cytohistologic study to determine adequacy for diagnosis, first evaluation episode, each site Q1

RVU			Global Days	Modifiers				
Mod	Non-Fac Total	Fac Total		51	50	62	80	MUE
	1.62	1.62	XXX	0	0	0	0	5
26	1.06	1.06	XXX	0	0	0	0	5
TC	0.56	0.56	XXX	0	0	0	0	5

AMA: Fall 93: 26, Fall 94: 2, Dec 98: 8, Aug 07: 15, Oct 10: 9, Dec 10: 9

88173 Cytopathology, evaluation of fine needle aspirate; interpretation and report Q1

RVU			Global Days	Modifiers				
Mod	Non-Fac Total	Fac Total		51	50	62	80	MUE
	4.34	4.34	XXX	0	0	0	0	5
26	2.07	2.07	XXX	0	0	0	0	5
TC	2.27	2.27	XXX	0	0	0	0	5

AMA: Fall 93: 26, Fall 94: 2, Dec 98: 8, Oct 10: 9, Dec 10: 9

88174 Cytopathology, cervical or vaginal (any reporting system), collected in preservative fluid, automated thin layer preparation; screening by automated system, under physician supervision ♀ N

RVU			Global Days	Modifiers				
Mod	Non-Fac Total	Fac Total		51	50	62	80	MUE
	0.00	0.00	XXX	9	9	9	9	1

AMA: Jul 03: 9, Mar 04: 4

88175 Cytopathology, cervical or vaginal (any reporting system), collected in preservative fluid, automated thin layer preparation; with screening by automated system and manual rescreening or review, under physician supervision ♀ N

RVU			Global Days	Modifiers				
Mod	Non-Fac Total	Fac Total		51	50	62	80	MUE
	0.00	0.00	XXX	9	9	9	9	1

AMA: Jul 03: 9, Mar 04: 4, Mar 06: 6, May 11: 10

+ 88177 Cytopathology, evaluation of fine needle aspirate; immediate cytohistologic study to determine adequacy for diagnosis, each separate additional evaluation episode, same site (List separately in addition to code for primary procedure) N

Coding tip: Code 88177 is listed out of numerical order in CPT. Cytopathology testing, evaluation of fine needle aspirate - 88172

RVU			Global Days	Modifiers				
Mod	Non-Fac Total	Fac Total		51	50	62	80	MUE
	0.85	0.85	ZZZ	0	0	0	0	6
26	0.64	0.64	ZZZ	0	0	0	0	6
TC	0.21	0.21	ZZZ	0	0	0	0	6

AMA: Oct 10: 9, Dec 10: 9

88182 Flow cytometry, cell cycle or DNA analysis Q2

RVU			Global Days	Modifiers				
Mod	Non-Fac Total	Fac Total		51	50	62	80	MUE
	3.17	3.17	XXX	0	0	0	0	2
26	1.05	1.05	XXX	0	0	0	0	2
TC	2.12	2.12	XXX	0	0	0	0	2

AMA: Oct 13: 3

Coding Guidance

Code 88342 should generally not be reported together with flow cytometry codes (88184-88189) for the same or similar specimens. Similar specimens include: blood and bone marrow; bone marrow aspiration and bone marrow biopsy; two separate lymph nodes; or lymph node and other tissue with lymphoid infiltrate. The diagnosis should be established using one of these methods. Medicare and other payers do not pay for duplicate testing. The provider may report codes for both methods, using the appropriate modifier, if both were required due to the initial method being non-diagnostic or failing to explain all the light microscopy findings.

88184 Flow cytometry, cell surface, cytoplasmic, or nuclear marker, technical component only; first marker Q2

RVU			Global Days	Modifiers				
Mod	Non-Fac Total	Fac Total		51	50	62	80	MUE
	2.13	2.13	XXX	0	0	0	0	2

AMA: Dec 07: 14, Oct 13: 3

● New   ▲ Revised   ✖ Deleted   ⊙ Moderate Sedation   ✚ Add-on Codes   ⊘ High Risk Denial   Ⓐ Age Edit   ♀ Female   ♂ Male   **AMA** *CPT® Assistant*   **MUE** Medically Unlikely Edit
⊘ Modifier 51 Exempt   ⊖ Modifier 63 Exempt   ✖ Unlisted   **Modifiers:** *See Inside Back Cover*   Ⓜ Maternity   A2–Z3 ASC Payment Indicators   A–Y OPPS Status Indicators

768   CPT © 2015 American Medical Association. All Rights Reserved.   © 2016 DecisionHealth

+ 88185 Flow cytometry, cell surface, cytoplasmic, or nuclear marker, technical component only; each additional marker (List separately in addition to code for first marker) N

RVU			Global Days	Modifiers				
Mod	Non-Fac Total	Fac Total		51	50	62	80	MUE
	1.29	1.29	ZZZ	0	0	0	0	

AMA: Dec 07: 14, Oct 13: 3

88187 Flow cytometry, interpretation; 2 to 8 markers B

RVU			Global Days	Modifiers				
Mod	Non-Fac Total	Fac Total		51	50	62	80	MUE
	2.04	2.04	XXX	0	0	0	0	2

AMA: Apr 05: 14, Oct 13: 3

88188 Flow cytometry, interpretation; 9 to 15 markers B

RVU			Global Days	Modifiers				
Mod	Non-Fac Total	Fac Total		51	50	62	80	MUE
	2.59	2.59	XXX	0	0	0	0	2

AMA: Apr 05: 14, Oct 13: 3

88189 Flow cytometry, interpretation; 16 or more markers B

RVU			Global Days	Modifiers				
Mod	Non-Fac Total	Fac Total		51	50	62	80	MUE
	3.19	3.19	XXX	0	0	0	0	2

AMA: Apr 05: 14, Oct 13: 3

88199 Unlisted cytopathology procedure ⊗✗Q1

RVU			Global Days	Modifiers				
Mod	Non-Fac Total	Fac Total		51	50	62	80	MUE
	0.00	0.00	XXX	0	0	0	0	
26	0.00	0.00	XXX	0	0	0	0	
TC	0.00	0.00	XXX	0	0	0	0	

Cytogenic Testing

88230 Tissue culture for non-neoplastic disorders; lymphocyte Q4

RVU			Global Days	Modifiers				
Mod	Non-Fac Total	Fac Total		51	50	62	80	MUE
	0.00	0.00	XXX	9	9	9	9	2

AMA: Nov 98: 29, Oct 99: 2, Aug 05: 9, May 08: 5

88233 Tissue culture for non-neoplastic disorders; skin or other solid tissue biopsy ⊗Q4

RVU			Global Days	Modifiers				
Mod	Non-Fac Total	Fac Total		51	50	62	80	MUE
	0.00	0.00	XXX	9	9	9	9	2

AMA: Nov 98: 29, Oct 99: 2, May 08: 5

88235 Tissue culture for non-neoplastic disorders; amniotic fluid or chorionic villus cells M Q4

RVU			Global Days	Modifiers				
Mod	Non-Fac Total	Fac Total		51	50	62	80	MUE
	0.00	0.00	XXX	9	9	9	9	2

AMA: Nov 98: 29, Oct 99: 2, May 08: 5

88237 Tissue culture for neoplastic disorders; bone marrow, blood cells Q4

RVU			Global Days	Modifiers				
Mod	Non-Fac Total	Fac Total		51	50	62	80	MUE
	0.00	0.00	XXX	9	9	9	9	4

AMA: Nov 98: 29, Oct 99: 2, May 08: 5

88239 Tissue culture for neoplastic disorders; solid tumor ⊗Q4

RVU			Global Days	Modifiers				
Mod	Non-Fac Total	Fac Total		51	50	62	80	MUE
	0.00	0.00	XXX	9	9	9	9	3

AMA: Nov 98: 29, Oct 99: 2, May 08: 5

88240 Cryopreservation, freezing and storage of cells, each cell line Q4

RVU			Global Days	Modifiers				
Mod	Non-Fac Total	Fac Total		51	50	62	80	MUE
	0.00	0.00	XXX	9	9	9	9	1

AMA: Nov 98: 29, Oct 99: 2, Jul 03: 9, May 08: 5, Oct 13: 3

88241 Thawing and expansion of frozen cells, each aliquot ⊗Q4

RVU			Global Days	Modifiers				
Mod	Non-Fac Total	Fac Total		51	50	62	80	MUE
	0.00	0.00	XXX	9	9	9	9	3

AMA: Nov 98: 29, Oct 99: 2, Jul 03: 9, May 08: 5, Oct 13: 3

88245 Chromosome analysis for breakage syndromes; baseline Sister Chromatid Exchange (SCE), 20-25 cells ⊗Q4

RVU			Global Days	Modifiers				
Mod	Non-Fac Total	Fac Total		51	50	62	80	MUE
	0.00	0.00	XXX	9	9	9	9	1

AMA: Nov 98: 29, Oct 99: 2, Jul 05: 1, May 08: 5

88248 Chromosome analysis for breakage syndromes; baseline breakage, score 50-100 cells, count 20 cells, 2 karyotypes (eg, for ataxia telangiectasia, Fanconi anemia, fragile X) Q4

RVU			Global Days	Modifiers				
Mod	Non-Fac Total	Fac Total		51	50	62	80	MUE
	0.00	0.00	XXX	9	9	9	9	1

AMA: Nov 98: 29, Oct 99: 2, Jul 05: 1, May 08: 5

88249 Chromosome analysis for breakage syndromes; score 100 cells, clastogen stress (eg, diepoxybutane, mitomycin C, ionizing radiation, UV radiation) Q4

RVU			Global Days	Modifiers				
Mod	Non-Fac Total	Fac Total		51	50	62	80	MUE
	0.00	0.00	XXX	9	9	9	9	1

AMA: Nov 98: 29, Oct 99: 2, Jul 05: 1, May 08: 5

88261 Chromosome analysis; count 5 cells, 1 karyotype, with banding Q4

RVU			Global Days	Modifiers				
Mod	Non-Fac Total	Fac Total		51	50	62	80	MUE
	0.00	0.00	XXX	9	9	9	9	2

AMA: Nov 98: 29, Oct 99: 2, Jul 05: 1, May 08: 5

88262 Chromosome analysis; count 15-20 cells, 2 karyotypes, with banding Q4

RVU			Global Days	Modifiers				
Mod	Non-Fac Total	Fac Total		51	50	62	80	MUE
	0.00	0.00	XXX	9	9	9	9	2

AMA: Nov 98: 29, Oct 99: 2, May 08: 5, May 11: 10

● New   ▲ Revised   Deleted   ⊙ Moderate Sedation   ✚ Add-on Codes   ⊘ High Risk Denial   Ⓐ Age Edit   ♀ Female   ♂ Male   **AMA** CPT® Assistant   **MUE** Medically Unlikely Edit
⊘ Modifier 51 Exempt   ⊖ Modifier 63 Exempt   ✗ Unlisted   **Modifiers:** See Inside Back Cover   M Maternity   A2–Z3 ASC Payment Indicators   A–Y OPPS Status Indicators

88263 Chromosome analysis; count 45 cells for mosaicism, 2 karyotypes, with banding ◎4

RVU		Global Days	Modifiers				
Mod	Non-Fac Total	Fac Total		51	50	62	80	MUE
	0.00	0.00	XXX	9	9	9	9	1

AMA: Nov 98: 29, Oct 99: 2, Jul 05: 1, May 08: 5

88264 Chromosome analysis; analyze 20-25 cells ◎4

RVU		Global Days	Modifiers				
Mod	Non-Fac Total	Fac Total		51	50	62	80	MUE
	0.00	0.00	XXX	9	9	9	9	2

AMA: Nov 98: 29, Oct 99: 2, Jul 05: 1, May 08: 5

88267 Chromosome analysis, amniotic fluid or chorionic villus, count 15 cells, 1 karyotype, with banding ♀ Ⓜ ◎4

RVU		Global Days	Modifiers				
Mod	Non-Fac Total	Fac Total		51	50	62	80	MUE
	0.00	0.00	XXX	9	9	9	9	2

AMA: Jul 05: 1

88269 Chromosome analysis, in situ for amniotic fluid cells, count cells from 6-12 colonies, 1 karyotype, with banding ♀ Ⓜ ◎4

RVU		Global Days	Modifiers				
Mod	Non-Fac Total	Fac Total		51	50	62	80	MUE
	0.00	0.00	XXX	9	9	9	9	2

AMA: Jul 05: 1

88271 Molecular cytogenetics; DNA probe, each (eg, FISH) Ⓜ ◎4

RVU		Global Days	Modifiers				
Mod	Non-Fac Total	Fac Total		51	50	62	80	MUE
	0.00	0.00	XXX	9	9	9	9	16

AMA: Nov 98: 29, Mar 99: 10, Oct 99: 3, Jun 02: 11, Jul 05: 1, May 08: 5, May 12: 5, Sep 13: 3

88272 Molecular cytogenetics; chromosomal in situ hybridization, analyze 3-5 cells (eg, for derivatives and markers) ◎4

RVU		Global Days	Modifiers				
Mod	Non-Fac Total	Fac Total		51	50	62	80	MUE
	0.00	0.00	XXX	9	9	9	9	12

AMA: Nov 98: 29, Mar 99: 10, Oct 99: 3, Jun 02: 11, Jul 05: 1, May 08: 5, May 12: 5, Sep 13: 3

88273 Molecular cytogenetics; chromosomal in situ hybridization, analyze 10-30 cells (eg, for microdeletions) ◎4

RVU		Global Days	Modifiers				
Mod	Non-Fac Total	Fac Total		51	50	62	80	MUE
	0.00	0.00	XXX	9	9	9	9	3

AMA: Nov 98: 29, Mar 99: 10, Oct 99: 3, Jun 02: 11, Jul 05: 1, May 08: 5, May 12: 5, Sep 13: 3

88274 Molecular cytogenetics; interphase in situ hybridization, analyze 25-99 cells ◎4

RVU		Global Days	Modifiers				
Mod	Non-Fac Total	Fac Total		51	50	62	80	MUE
	0.00	0.00	XXX	9	9	9	9	5

AMA: Nov 98: 29, Mar 99: 10, Oct 99: 3, Jun 02: 11, Jul 05: 1, May 08: 5, May 12: 5, Sep 13: 3

88275 Molecular cytogenetics; interphase in situ hybridization, analyze 100-300 cells ◎4

RVU		Global Days	Modifiers				
Mod	Non-Fac Total	Fac Total		51	50	62	80	MUE
	0.00	0.00	XXX	9	9	9	9	12

AMA: Nov 98: 29, Mar 99: 10, Oct 99: 3, Jun 02: 11, Jul 05: 1, May 08: 5, May 12: 5, Sep 13: 3

88280 Chromosome analysis; additional karyotypes, each study ◎4

RVU		Global Days	Modifiers				
Mod	Non-Fac Total	Fac Total		51	50	62	80	MUE
	0.00	0.00	XXX	9	9	9	9	8

AMA: Jul 05: 1, May 08: 5

88283 Chromosome analysis; additional specialized banding technique (eg, NOR, C-banding) ◎4

RVU		Global Days	Modifiers				
Mod	Non-Fac Total	Fac Total		51	50	62	80	MUE
	0.00	0.00	XXX	9	9	9	9	5

AMA: Jul 05: 1, May 08: 5

88285 Chromosome analysis; additional cells counted, each study ◎4

RVU		Global Days	Modifiers				
Mod	Non-Fac Total	Fac Total		51	50	62	80	MUE
	0.00	0.00	XXX	9	9	9	9	10

AMA: Jul 05: 1, Dec 07: 14, May 08: 5, May 11: 10

88289 Chromosome analysis; additional high resolution study ◎4

RVU		Global Days	Modifiers				
Mod	Non-Fac Total	Fac Total		51	50	62	80	MUE
	0.00	0.00	XXX	9	9	9	9	1

AMA: Oct 99: 3, Jul 05: 1

88291 Cytogenetics and molecular cytogenetics, interpretation and report Ⓜ

RVU		Global Days	Modifiers				
Mod	Non-Fac Total	Fac Total		51	50	62	80	MUE
	0.90	0.90	XXX	0	0	0	0	1

AMA: Nov 98: 29, Oct 99: 3, Jul 05: 1, May 08: 5

88299 Unlisted cytogenetic study ⊘Ⓧ◎1

RVU		Global Days	Modifiers				
Mod	Non-Fac Total	Fac Total		51	50	62	80	MUE
	0.00	0.00	XXX	0	0	0	0	

AMA: Oct 99: 3

Pub 100-04, 16, 100.4

Surgical Pathology Specimen Testing

Coding Guidance

If it is necessary to submit multiple lesion specimens for separate pathological evaluation, documentation must precisely identify the location of each lesion. If multiple lesion specimens are submitted as a collective whole without documentation of specific lesion sites, the surgical pathology code should be submitted for only one specimen, i.e., one unit of service, even if the specimens are later separated. Lesions or the marginal areas of lesions obtained using Moh's Micrographic surgical technique are not reported under surgical pathology codes. Surgical pathology service is included in the definition of the Moh's Micrographic Surgery codes. Codes for surgical pathology (88000-88309) are not reported additionally with 85097 for an interpretation of a bone marrow smear unless separate specimens are processed.

● New   ▲ Revised   ✖ Deleted   ⊙ Moderate Sedation   ✚ Add-on Codes   ⊘ High Risk Denial   Ⓐ Age Edit   ♀ Female   ♂ Male   **AMA** *CPT® Assistant*   **MUE** Medically Unlikely Edit
⊘ Modifier 51 Exempt   ⊖ Modifier 63 Exempt   Ⓧ Unlisted   **Modifiers:** *See Inside Back Cover*   Ⓜ Maternity   A2–Z3 ASC Payment Indicators   A–Y OPPS Status Indicators

770   CPT © 2015 American Medical Association. All Rights Reserved.   © 2016 DecisionHealth

88300 Level I - Surgical pathology, gross examination only   Q1

Mod	Non-Fac Total	Fac Total	Global Days	51	50	62	80	MUE
	0.43	0.43	XXX	0	0	0	0	4
26	0.13	0.13	XXX	0	0	0	0	4
TC	0.30	0.30	XXX	0	0	0	0	4

AMA: Winter 91: 18, Sep 00: 10, Aug 05: 9

Coding Guidance
Use 88307 for the surgical pathology evaluation of bone matrix structure and 20220 for the biopsy procedure.

88302 Level II - Surgical pathology, gross and microscopic examination Appendix, incidental Fallopian tube, sterilization Fingers/toes, amputation, traumatic Foreskin, newborn Hernia sac, any location Hydrocele sac Nerve Skin, plastic repair Sympathetic ganglion Testis, castration Vaginal mucosa, incidental Vas deferens, sterilization   Q1

Mod	Non-Fac Total	Fac Total	Global Days	51	50	62	80	MUE
	0.92	0.92	XXX	0	0	0	0	4
26	0.21	0.21	XXX	0	0	0	0	4
TC	0.71	0.71	XXX	0	0	0	0	4

AMA: Winter 91: 18, Sep 00: 10, Nov 06: 1, Jan 07: 29, Dec 11: 17, Feb 14: 10

88304 Level III - Surgical pathology, gross and microscopic examination

Abortion, induced

Abscess Aneurysm - arterial/ventricular

Anus, tag

Appendix, other than incidental

Artery, atheromatous plaque

Bartholin's gland cyst

Bone fragment(s), other than pathologic fracture

Bursa/synovial cyst

Carpal tunnel tissue

Cartilage, shavings

Cholesteatoma

Colon, colostomy stoma

Conjunctiva - biopsy/pterygium

Cornea

Diverticulum - esophagus/small intestine

Dupuytren's contracture tissue

Femoral head, other than fracture

Fissure/fistula

Foreskin, other than newborn

Gallbladder

Ganglion cyst

Hematoma

Hemorrhoids

Hydatid of Morgagni

Intervertebral disc

Joint, loose body

Meniscus

Mucocele, salivary

Neuroma - Morton's/traumatic

Pilonidal cyst/sinus

Polyps, inflammatory - nasal/sinusoidal

Skin - cyst/tag/debridement

Soft tissue, debridement

Soft tissue, lipoma

Spermatocele

Tendon/tendon sheath

Testicular appendage

Thrombus or embolus

Tonsil and/or adenoids

Varicocele

Vas deferens, other than sterilization

Vein, varicosity   Q1

Mod	Non-Fac Total	Fac Total	Global Days	51	50	62	80	MUE
	1.29	1.29	XXX	0	0	0	0	5
26	0.33	0.33	XXX	0	0	0	0	5
TC	0.96	0.96	XXX	0	0	0	0	5

AMA: Winter 91: 18, Spring 91: 2, Aug 97: 18, Sep 00: 10, Jan 07: 29, Dec 11: 17

88305 Level IV - Surgical pathology, gross and microscopic examination

Abortion - spontaneous/missed

Artery, biopsy

Bone marrow, biopsy

Bone exostosis

Brain/meninges, other than for tumor resection

Breast, biopsy, not requiring microscopic evaluation of surgical margins

Breast, reduction mammoplasty

Bronchus, biopsy

Cell block, any source

Cervix, biopsy

Colon, biopsy

Duodenum, biopsy

Endocervix, curettings/biopsy

Endometrium, curettings/biopsy

Esophagus, biopsy

Extremity, amputation, traumatic

Fallopian tube, biopsy

Fallopian tube, ectopic pregnancy

Femoral head, fracture

Fingers/toes, amputation, non-traumatic

Gingiva/oral mucosa, biopsy

Heart valve

Joint, resection

Kidney, biopsy

● New   ▲ Revised   Deleted   ⊙ Moderate Sedation   ✚ Add-on Codes   ⊘ High Risk Denial   Ⓐ Age Edit   ♀ Female   ♂ Male   **AMA** *CPT® Assistant*   **MUE** Medically Unlikely Edit
⊘ Modifier 51 Exempt   ⊖ Modifier 63 Exempt   ✗ Unlisted   **Modifiers:** *See Inside Back Cover*   Ⓜ Maternity   A2-Z3 ASC Payment Indicators   A-Y OPPS Status Indicators

© 2016 DecisionHealth   CPT © 2015 American Medical Association. All Rights Reserved.   **771**

Larynx, biopsy

Leiomyoma(s), uterine myomectomy - without uterus

Lip, biopsy/wedge resection

Lung, transbronchial biopsy

Lymph node, biopsy

Muscle, biopsy

Nasal mucosa, biopsy

Nasopharynx/oropharynx, biopsy

Nerve, biopsy

Odontogenic/dental cyst

Omentum, biopsy

Ovary with or without tube, non-neoplastic

Ovary, biopsy/wedge resection

Parathyroid gland

Peritoneum, biopsy

Pituitary tumor

Placenta, other than third trimester

Pleura/pericardium - biopsy/tissue

Polyp, cervical/endometrial

Polyp, colorectal

Polyp, stomach/small intestine

Prostate, needle biopsy

Prostate, TUR

Salivary gland, biopsy

Sinus, paranasal biopsy

Skin, other than cyst/tag/debridement/plastic repair

Small intestine, biopsy

Soft tissue, other than tumor/mass/lipoma/debridement

Spleen

Stomach, biopsy

Synovium

Testis, other than tumor/biopsy/castration

Thyroglossal duct/brachial cleft cyst

Tongue, biopsy

Tonsil, biopsy

Trachea, biopsy

Ureter, biopsy

Urethra, biopsy

Urinary bladder, biopsy

Uterus, with or without tubes and ovaries, for prolapse

Vagina, biopsy

Vulva/labia, biopsy   Q1

RVU			Global Days	Modifiers				
Mod	Non-Fac Total	Fac Total		51	50	62	80	MUE
	2.07	2.07	XXX	0	0	0	0	16
26	1.11	1.11	XXX	0	0	0	0	16
TC	0.96	0.96	XXX	0	0	0	0	16

AMA: Winter 90: 2, Winter 91: 18, Spring 91: 6, Winter 92: 17, Aug 97: 18, Jul 98: 4, Nov 98: 29, 30, Jul 00: 4, Sep 00: 10, Dec 00: 15, Jul 05: 13, Nov 06: 1, Jan 07: 29, Dec 11: 17

88307 Level V - Surgical pathology, gross and microscopic examination

Adrenal, resection

Bone - biopsy/curettings

Bone fragment(s), pathologic fracture

Brain, biopsy

Brain/meninges, tumor resection

Breast, excision of lesion, requiring microscopic evaluation of surgical margins

Breast, mastectomy - partial/simple

Cervix, conization

Colon, segmental resection, other than for tumor

Extremity, amputation, non-traumatic

Eye, enucleation

Kidney, partial/total nephrectomy

Larynx, partial/total resection

Liver, biopsy - needle/wedge

Liver, partial resection

Lung, wedge biopsy

Lymph nodes, regional resection

Mediastinum, mass

Myocardium, biopsy

Odontogenic tumor

Ovary with or without tube, neoplastic

Pancreas, biopsy

Placenta, third trimester

Prostate, except radical resection

Salivary gland

Sentinel lymph node

Small intestine, resection, other than for tumor

Soft tissue mass (except lipoma) - biopsy/simple excision

Stomach - subtotal/total resection, other than for tumor

Testis, biopsy

Thymus, tumor

Thyroid, total/lobe

Ureter, resection

Urinary bladder, TUR

Uterus, with or without tubes and ovaries, other than neoplastic/prolapse   Q2

RVU			Global Days	Modifiers				
Mod	Non-Fac Total	Fac Total		51	50	62	80	MUE
	8.71	8.71	XXX	0	0	0	0	8
26	2.44	2.44	XXX	0	0	0	0	8
TC	6.27	6.27	XXX	0	0	0	0	8

AMA: Winter 91: 18, Winter 92: 18, Jul 98: 4, Nov 98: 29, 30, Jul 00: 4, Sep 00: 10, Dec 00: 15, Dec 03: 11, Nov 06: 1, Jan 07: 29, Dec 11: 17

● New   ▲ Revised   ✖ Deleted   ⊙ Moderate Sedation   ✚ Add-on Codes   ⊘ High Risk Denial   Ⓐ Age Edit   ♀ Female   ♂ Male   **AMA** CPT® Assistant   **MUE** Medically Unlikely Edit
⊘ Modifier 51 Exempt   ⊖ Modifier 63 Exempt   ✘ Unlisted   **Modifiers:** See Inside Back Cover   Ⓜ Maternity   A2–Z3 ASC Payment Indicators   A–Y OPPS Status Indicators

772   CPT © 2015 American Medical Association. All Rights Reserved.   © 2016 DecisionHealth

88309 Level VI - Surgical pathology, gross and microscopic examination

Bone resection

Breast, mastectomy - with regional lymph nodes

Colon, segmental resection for tumor

Colon, total resection

Esophagus, partial/total resection

Extremity, disarticulation

Fetus, with dissection

Larynx, partial/total resection - with regional lymph nodes

Lung - total/lobe/segment resection

Pancreas, total/subtotal resection

Prostate, radical resection

Small intestine, resection for tumor

Soft tissue tumor, extensive resection

Stomach - subtotal/total resection for tumor

Testis, tumor

Tongue/tonsil -resection for tumor

Urinary bladder, partial/total resection

Uterus, with or without tubes and ovaries, neoplastic

Vulva, total/subtotal resection

RVU			Global Days	Modifiers				
Mod	Non-Fac Total	Fac Total		51	50	62	80	MUE
	13.21	13.21	XXX	0	0	0	0	3
26	4.31	4.31	XXX	0	0	0	0	3
TC	8.90	8.90	XXX	0	0	0	0	3

AMA: Winter 91: 18, Spring 91: 2, Fall 93: 2, 26, Jul 00: 4, Sep 00: 10, Dec 03: 11, Nov 06: 1, Jan 07: 29, Dec 11: 18, Feb 14: 10

+ 88311 Decalcification procedure (List separately in addition to code for surgical pathology examination)

RVU			Global Days	Modifiers				
Mod	Non-Fac Total	Fac Total		51	50	62	80	MUE
	0.61	0.61	XXX	0	0	0	0	4
26	0.37	0.37	XXX	0	0	0	0	4
TC	0.24	0.24	XXX	0	0	0	0	4

AMA: Winter 92: 18, Jul 98: 4, Jun 02: 11, Nov 02: 7, Nov 06: 1, Dec 11: 18

88312 Special stain including interpretation and report; Group I for microorganisms (eg, acid fast, methenamine silver)

RVU			Global Days	Modifiers				
Mod	Non-Fac Total	Fac Total		51	50	62	80	MUE
	2.76	2.76	XXX	0	0	0	0	9
26	0.79	0.79	XXX	0	0	0	0	9
TC	1.97	1.97	XXX	0	0	0	0	9

AMA: Winter 91: 19, Jun 02: 11, Nov 02: 7, Nov 06: 1, Dec 11: 18

88313 Special stain including interpretation and report; Group II, all other (eg, iron, trichrome), except stain for microorganisms, stains for enzyme constituents, or immunocytochemistry and immunohistochemistry

RVU			Global Days	Modifiers				
Mod	Non-Fac Total	Fac Total		51	50	62	80	MUE
	1.93	1.93	XXX	0	0	0	0	8
26	0.35	0.35	XXX	0	0	0	0	8
TC	1.58	1.58	XXX	0	0	0	0	8

AMA: Jun 02: 11, Nov 02: 7, Mar 03: 22, Nov 03: 15, Jun 06: 17, Nov 06: 1, Dec 11: 18

+ 88314 Special stain including interpretation and report; histochemical stain on frozen tissue block (List separately in addition to code for primary procedure)

RVU			Global Days	Modifiers				
Mod	Non-Fac Total	Fac Total		51	50	62	80	MUE
	2.18	2.18	XXX	0	0	0	0	6
26	0.65	0.65	XXX	0	0	0	0	6
TC	1.53	1.53	XXX	0	0	0	0	6

AMA: Nov 02: 7, Nov 06: 1, Dec 11: 18

88319 Special stain including interpretation and report; Group III, for enzyme constituents

RVU			Global Days	Modifiers				
Mod	Non-Fac Total	Fac Total		51	50	62	80	MUE
	2.49	2.49	XXX	0	0	0	0	11
26	0.78	0.78	XXX	0	0	0	0	11
TC	1.71	1.71	XXX	0	0	0	0	11

AMA: Dec 11: 18

Coding Guidance

Codes 88321-88325 are used for a second opinion review of slides, tissues, or other samples obtained and prepared at a different location. The pathologist who provides the second opinion must not be another pathologist within the same provider group. Medicare and other payers will generally not allow payment for two interpretations of a given technical service. These codes are reported with only one unit of service regardless of the number of slides, specimens, paraffin blocks, etc. Other pathology codes for interpretation of stains, slides, or other material previously interpreted, such as 88187-88189, 88312-88313, 88342, should not be reported together with 88321-88325. When the provider interprets stains anew, or fresh again from the beginning, then codes 88312-88314, and 88342 may be reported together with 88323. When a physician provides a face-to-face service to the patient and, in the course of the evaluation and management, specimens that were obtained elsewhere are reviewed as well, only the E&M code may be reported. Codes 88321-88325 should not be reported separately.

88321 Consultation and report on referred slides prepared elsewhere

RVU			Global Days	Modifiers				
Mod	Non-Fac Total	Fac Total		51	50	62	80	MUE
	2.89	2.45	XXX	0	0	0	0	1

AMA: Winter 91: 19, Apr 97: 9, Oct 00: 7, Dec 02: 10, Jan 10: 11, Dec 11: 18, Jun 13: 15

88323 Consultation and report on referred material requiring preparation of slides

RVU			Global Days	Modifiers				
Mod	Non-Fac Total	Fac Total		51	50	62	80	MUE
	3.93	3.93	XXX	0	0	0	0	1
26	2.51	2.51	XXX	0	0	0	0	1
TC	1.42	1.42	XXX	0	0	0	0	1

AMA: Winter 91: 19, Apr 97: 9, Oct 00: 7, Dec 02: 10, Dec 11: 18, Jun 13: 15

● New ▲ Revised Deleted ⊙ Moderate Sedation ✚ Add-on Codes ⊘ High Risk Denial Ⓐ Age Edit ♀ Female ♂ Male **AMA** *CPT® Assistant* **MUE** Medically Unlikely Edit
⊘ Modifier 51 Exempt ⊖ Modifier 63 Exempt ✖ Unlisted **Modifiers:** *See Inside Back Cover* Ⓜ Maternity A2–Z3 ASC Payment Indicators A–Y OPPS Status Indicators

© 2016 DecisionHealth CPT © 2015 American Medical Association. All Rights Reserved.

Laboratory/Pathology Procedures

88325 – 88350

88325 Consultation, comprehensive, with review of records and specimens, with report on referred material ◐❶

Mod	Non-Fac Total	Fac Total	Global Days	51	50	62	80	MUE
	4.88	3.86	XXX	0	0	0	0	1

AMA: Winter 91: 19, Apr 97: 9, Dec 02: 10, Dec 11: 18, Jun 13: 15

88329 Pathology consultation during surgery ◐❶

Mod	Non-Fac Total	Fac Total	Global Days	51	50	62	80	MUE
	1.42	1.06	XXX	0	0	0	0	2

AMA: Winter 91: 19, Apr 97: 12, Aug 97: 18, Jan 07: 29, Dec 11: 18

88331 Pathology consultation during surgery; first tissue block, with frozen section(s), single specimen ◐❶

Mod	Non-Fac Total	Fac Total	Global Days	51	50	62	80	MUE
	2.71	2.71	XXX	0	0	0	0	11
26	1.83	1.83	XXX	0	0	0	0	11
TC	0.88	0.88	XXX	0	0	0	0	11

AMA: Winter 91: 19, Spring 91: 2, Apr 97: 12, Aug 97: 18, Jul 00: 4, Nov 02: 7, Mar 06: 6, Nov 06: 1, Jan 07: 29, Oct 10: 9, Dec 10: 9, Dec 11: 18

+ 88332 Pathology consultation during surgery; each additional tissue block with frozen section(s) (List separately in addition to code for primary procedure) Ⓝ

Mod	Non-Fac Total	Fac Total	Global Days	51	50	62	80	MUE
	1.43	1.43	XXX	0	0	0	0	13
26	0.90	0.90	XXX	0	0	0	0	13
TC	0.53	0.53	XXX	0	0	0	0	13

AMA: Winter 91: 19, Apr 97: 12, Aug 97: 18, Jul 00: 4, Mar 06: 6, Jan 07: 29, Oct 10: 9, Dec 10: 9, Dec 11: 18

88333 Pathology consultation during surgery; cytologic examination (eg, touch prep, squash prep), initial site ◐❷

Mod	Non-Fac Total	Fac Total	Global Days	51	50	62	80	MUE
	2.84	2.84	XXX	0	0	0	0	4
26	1.84	1.84	XXX	0	0	0	0	4
TC	1.00	1.00	XXX	0	0	0	0	4

AMA: Mar 06: 6, Jan 07: 29, Jun 08: 15, Dec 10: 9, Dec 11: 18

+ 88334 Pathology consultation during surgery; cytologic examination (eg, touch prep, squash prep), each additional site (List separately in addition to code for primary procedure) Ⓝ

Mod	Non-Fac Total	Fac Total	Global Days	51	50	62	80	MUE
	1.74	1.74	XXX	0	0	0	0	5
26	1.13	1.13	XXX	0	0	0	0	5
TC	0.61	0.61	XXX	0	0	0	0	5

AMA: Mar 06: 6, Jan 07: 29, Oct 10: 9, Dec 11: 18

Coding Guidance

Code 88342 should generally not be reported together with flow cytometry codes (88184-88189) for the same or morphologically similar specimens. Similar specimens include: blood and bone marrow; bone marrow aspiration and bone marrow biopsy; two separate lymph nodes; or lymph node and other tissue with lymphoid infiltrate. The diagnosis should be established using one of these methods. Medicare and other payers do not pay for duplicate testing. The provider may report codes for both methods, using the appropriate

modifier, if both were required due to the initial method being non-diagnostic or failing to explain all the light microscopy findings.

+ 88341 Immunohistochemistry or immunocytochemistry, per specimen; each additional single antibody stain procedure (List separately in addition to code for primary procedure) Ⓝ

Mod	Non-Fac Total	Fac Total	Global Days	51	50	62	80	MUE
	2.53	2.53	ZZZ	0	0	0	0	
26	0.78	0.78	ZZZ	0	0	0	0	
TC	1.75	1.75	ZZZ	0	0	0	0	

AMA: Jun 15: 11

88342 Immunohistochemistry or immunocytochemistry, per specimen; initial single antibody stain procedure ◐◐❷

Mod	Non-Fac Total	Fac Total	Global Days	51	50	62	80	MUE
	3.00	3.00	XXX	0	0	0	0	3
26	1.04	1.04	XXX	0	0	0	0	3
TC	1.96	1.96	XXX	0	0	0	0	3

AMA: Winter 91: 17, Jul 00: 10, Nov 02: 6, 7, Nov 06: 1, Dec 11: 18, Jun 14: 15, Jun 15: 11

88344 Immunohistochemistry or immunocytochemistry, per specimen; each multiplex antibody stain procedure ◐❶

Mod	Non-Fac Total	Fac Total	Global Days	51	50	62	80	MUE
26	1.14	1.14	XXX	0	0	0	0	1
TC	3.71	3.71	XXX	0	0	0	0	1
	4.85	4.85	XXX	0	0	0	0	1

AMA: Jun 15: 11

▲ 88346 Immunofluorescence, per specimen; initial single antibody stain procedure ◐❷

Mod	Non-Fac Total	Fac Total	Global Days	51	50	62	80	MUE
	2.62	2.62	XXX	0	0	0	0	
26	1.07	1.07	XXX	0	0	0	0	
TC	1.55	1.55	XXX	0	0	0	0	

AMA: Dec 11: 18

✖ 88347 Immunofluorescent study, each antibody; indirect method

88348 Electron microscopy, diagnostic ◐❷

Mod	Non-Fac Total	Fac Total	Global Days	51	50	62	80	MUE
	9.72	9.72	XXX	0	0	0	0	1
26	2.21	2.21	XXX	0	0	0	0	1
TC	7.51	7.51	XXX	0	0	0	0	1

AMA: Dec 11: 18

+● 88350 Immunofluorescence, per specimen; each additional single antibody stain procedure (List separately in addition to code for primary procedure) Ⓝ

Mod	Non-Fac Total	Fac Total	Global Days	51	50	62	80	MUE
	2.02	2.02	ZZZ	0	0	0	0	
26	0.80	0.80	ZZZ	0	0	0	0	
TC	1.22	1.22	ZZZ	0	0	0	0	

● New   ▲ Revised   ✖ Deleted   ⊙ Moderate Sedation   ✚ Add-on Codes   ⊖ High Risk Denial   ⒶAge Edit   ♀ Female   ♂ Male   **AMA** CPT® Assistant   **MUE** Medically Unlikely Edit
⊘ Modifier 51 Exempt   ⊖ Modifier 63 Exempt   ⊠ Unlisted   **Modifiers:** See Inside Back Cover   Ⓜ Maternity   A2–Z3 ASC Payment Indicators   A–Y OPPS Status Indicators

CPT © 2015 American Medical Association. All Rights Reserved.   © 2016 DecisionHealth

88355 Morphometric analysis; skeletal muscle   Q1

Mod	Non-Fac Total	Fac Total	Global Days	51	50	62	80	MUE
	4.42	4.42	XXX	0	0	0	0	1
26	2.35	2.35	XXX	0	0	0	0	1
TC	2.07	2.07	XXX	0	0	0	0	1

AMA: Dec 11: 18

88356 Morphometric analysis; nerve   Q1

Mod	Non-Fac Total	Fac Total	Global Days	51	50	62	80	MUE
	5.79	5.79	XXX	0	0	0	0	1
26	3.45	3.45	XXX	0	0	0	0	1
TC	2.34	2.34	XXX	0	0	0	0	1

AMA: Dec 11: 18, Jun 14: 15

Coding Guidance

Code 88358 should not be reported for any service other than DNA ploidy and S-phase tumor analysis by digital cellular imaging techniques. One unit of service includes both DNA ploidy and the S-phase analysis.

88358 Morphometric analysis; tumor (eg, DNA ploidy)   Q2

Mod	Non-Fac Total	Fac Total	Global Days	51	50	62	80	MUE
	2.40	2.40	XXX	0	0	0	0	2
26	1.29	1.29	XXX	0	0	0	0	2
TC	1.11	1.11	XXX	0	0	0	0	2

AMA: Jul 98: 4, Jul 99: 11, Jun 02: 11, Jun 06: 17, Dec 11: 18

Coding Guidance

Quantitative or semiquantitative tumor immunohistochemistry using computer-assisted technology, or digital cellular imaging, includes computer software analysis of stained microscopic slides. Report immunohistochemistry with qualitative grading, such as 1+ to 4+ with 88342.

88360 Morphometric analysis, tumor immunohistochemistry (eg, Her-2/neu, estrogen receptor/progesterone receptor), quantitative or semiquantitative, per specimen, each single antibody stain procedure; manual   Q2

Mod	Non-Fac Total	Fac Total	Global Days	51	50	62	80	MUE
	3.40	3.40	XXX	0	0	0	0	6
26	1.58	1.58	XXX	0	0	0	0	6
TC	1.82	1.82	XXX	0	0	0	0	6

AMA: Dec 11: 18, Jun 14: 15

88361 Morphometric analysis, tumor immunohistochemistry (eg, Her-2/neu, estrogen receptor/progesterone receptor), quantitative or semiquantitative, per specimen, each single antibody stain procedure; using computer-assisted technology   Q2

Mod	Non-Fac Total	Fac Total	Global Days	51	50	62	80	MUE
	4.17	4.17	XXX	0	0	0	0	6
26	1.70	1.70	XXX	0	0	0	0	6
TC	2.47	2.47	XXX	0	0	0	0	6

AMA: Dec 11: 18, Jun 14: 15

88362 Nerve teasing preparations   Q2

Mod	Non-Fac Total	Fac Total	Global Days	51	50	62	80	MUE
	7.30	7.30	XXX	0	0	0	0	1
26	3.15	3.15	XXX	0	0	0	0	1
TC	4.15	4.15	XXX	0	0	0	0	1

AMA: Dec 11: 18

88363 Examination and selection of retrieved archival (ie, previously diagnosed) tissue(s) for molecular analysis (eg, KRAS mutational analysis)   Q1

Mod	Non-Fac Total	Fac Total	Global Days	51	50	62	80	MUE
	0.65	0.56	XXX	0	0	0	0	2

AMA: Oct 10: 10, Dec 10: 10, Dec 11: 18

Coding Guidance

The work reported by these codes requires that a physician (MD or DO) read, quantitate, or interpret the cells stained with the probe. Only when a physician reports the professional component (modifier 26), may the laboratory or a hospital reporting an outpatient laboratory test report the technical component. When the work is done by a non-physician, such as a laboratory technician or scientist, the appropriate codes from range 88271-88275 should be reported instead. Codes from both ranges should not be reported together. Do not report 88365 together with codes 88367 or 88368 for the same probe. For codes 88365-88368, only one unit of service may be reported for each probe.

+ 88364 In situ hybridization (eg, FISH), per specimen; each additional single probe stain procedure (List separately in addition to code for primary procedure)   N

Mod	Non-Fac Total	Fac Total	Global Days	51	50	62	80	MUE
	3.77	3.77	ZZZ	0	0	0	0	3
26	0.98	0.98	ZZZ	0	0	0	0	3
TC	2.79	2.79	ZZZ	0	0	0	0	3

88365 In situ hybridization (eg, FISH), per specimen; initial single probe stain procedure   Q1

Mod	Non-Fac Total	Fac Total	Global Days	51	50	62	80	MUE
	4.98	4.98	XXX	0	0	0	0	4
26	1.28	1.28	XXX	0	0	0	0	4
TC	3.70	3.70	XXX	0	0	0	0	4

AMA: Jun 02: 11, Mar 05: 16, May 12: 3, Dec 11: 18, Sep 13: 3

88366 In situ hybridization (eg, FISH), per specimen; each multiplex probe stain procedure   Q1

Mod	Non-Fac Total	Fac Total	Global Days	51	50	62	80	MUE
26	1.80	1.80	XXX	0	0	0	0	2
TC	5.53	5.53	XXX	0	0	0	0	2
	7.33	7.33	XXX	0	0	0	0	2

88367 Morphometric analysis, in situ hybridization (quantitative or semi-quantitative), using computer-assisted technology, per specimen; initial single probe stain procedure   Q2

Mod	Non-Fac Total	Fac Total	Global Days	51	50	62	80	MUE
	3.00	3.00	XXX	0	0	0	0	2
26	1.00	1.00	XXX	0	0	0	0	2
TC	2.00	2.00	XXX	0	0	0	0	2

AMA: Mar 05: 16, Oct 10: 9, Dec 11: 18, May 12: 5, Sep 13: 3

● New   ▲ Revised   Deleted   ⊙ Moderate Sedation   ✚ Add-on Codes   ⊘ High Risk Denial   Ⓐ Age Edit   ♀ Female   ♂ Male   **AMA** *CPT® Assistant*   **MUE** Medically Unlikely Edit
⊘ Modifier 51 Exempt   ⊖ Modifier 63 Exempt   ✗ Unlisted   **Modifiers:** *See Inside Back Cover*   Ⓜ Maternity   A2–Z3 ASC Payment Indicators   A–Y OPPS Status Indicators

Laboratory/Pathology Procedures

88368 – 88388

88368 Morphometric analysis, in situ hybridization (quantitative or semi-quantitative), manual, per specimen; initial single probe stain procedure ◨2

RVU			Global Days	Modifiers				
Mod	Non-Fac Total	Fac Total		51	50	62	80	MUE
	3.21	3.21	XXX	0	0	0	0	2
26	1.15	1.15	XXX	0	0	0	0	2
TC	2.06	2.06	XXX	0	0	0	0	2

AMA: Mar 05: 16, Oct 10: 9, May 12: 5, Dec 11: 18, Sep 13: 3

+ 88369 Morphometric analysis, in situ hybridization (quantitative or semi-quantitative), manual, per specimen; each additional single probe stain procedure (List separately in addition to code for primary procedure) N

RVU			Global Days	Modifiers				
Mod	Non-Fac Total	Fac Total		51	50	62	80	MUE
	3.03	3.03	ZZZ	0	0	0	0	3
26	0.89	0.89	ZZZ	0	0	0	0	3
TC	2.14	2.14	ZZZ	0	0	0	0	3

88371 Protein analysis of tissue by Western Blot, with interpretation and report N

RVU			Global Days	Modifiers				
Mod	Non-Fac Total	Fac Total		51	50	62	80	MUE
	0.00	0.00	XXX	9	9	9	9	1
26	0.52	0.52	XXX	0	0	0	0	1

AMA: Dec 11: 18

88372 Protein analysis of tissue by Western Blot, with interpretation and report; immunological probe for band identification, each ⊘N

RVU			Global Days	Modifiers				
Mod	Non-Fac Total	Fac Total		51	50	62	80	MUE
	0.00	0.00	XXX	9	9	9	9	1
26	0.52	0.52	XXX	0	0	0	0	1

AMA: Dec 11: 8

+ 88373 Morphometric analysis, in situ hybridization (quantitative or semi-quantitative), using computer-assisted technology, per specimen; each additional single probe stain procedure (List separately in addition to code for primary procedure) N

RVU			Global Days	Modifiers				
Mod	Non-Fac Total	Fac Total		51	50	62	80	MUE
	2.10	2.10	ZZZ	0	0	0	0	3
26	0.60	0.60	ZZZ	0	0	0	0	3
TC	1.50	1.50	ZZZ	0	0	0	0	3

88374 Morphometric analysis, in situ hybridization (quantitative or semi-quantitative), using computer-assisted technology, per specimen; each multiplex probe stain procedure ◨1

RVU			Global Days	Modifiers				
Mod	Non-Fac Total	Fac Total		51	50	62	80	MUE
	9.66	9.66	XXX	0	0	0	0	5
26	1.29	1.29	XXX	0	0	0	0	5
TC	8.37	8.37	XXX	0	0	0	0	5

88375 Optical endomicroscopic image(s), interpretation and report, real-time or referred, each endoscopic session B

RVU			Global Days	Modifiers				
Mod	Non-Fac Total	Fac Total		51	50	62	80	MUE
	1.40	1.40	XXX	0	0	0	0	1

AMA: Aug 13: 5

88377 Morphometric analysis, in situ hybridization (quantitative or semi-quantitative), manual, per specimen; each multiplex probe stain procedure ◨1

RVU			Global Days	Modifiers				
Mod	Non-Fac Total	Fac Total		51	50	62	80	MUE
	11.50	11.50	XXX	0	0	0	0	5
26	1.85	1.85	XXX	0	0	0	0	5
TC	9.65	9.65	XXX	0	0	0	0	5

88380 Microdissection (ie, sample preparation of microscopically identified target); laser capture N

RVU			Global Days	Modifiers				
Mod	Non-Fac Total	Fac Total		51	50	62	80	MUE
	4.06	4.06	XXX	0	0	0	0	1
26	1.64	1.64	XXX	0	0	0	0	1
TC	2.42	2.42	XXX	0	0	0	0	1

AMA: Apr 02: 17, Apr 08: 5, May 12: 8, 10, Dec 11: 18, Sep 13: 3

88381 Microdissection (ie, sample preparation of microscopically identified target); manual N

RVU			Global Days	Modifiers				
Mod	Non-Fac Total	Fac Total		51	50	62	80	MUE
	3.29	3.29	XXX	0	0	0	0	1
26	0.72	0.72	XXX	0	0	0	0	1
TC	2.57	2.57	XXX	0	0	0	0	1

AMA: Apr 08: 5, May 12: 8, 10, Dec 11: 18, Sep 13: 3

88387 Macroscopic examination, dissection, and preparation of tissue for non-microscopic analytical studies (eg, nucleic acid-based molecular studies); each tissue preparation (eg, a single lymph node) ⊘N

RVU			Global Days	Modifiers				
Mod	Non-Fac Total	Fac Total		51	50	62	80	MUE
	1.19	1.19	XXX	0	0	0	0	2
26	0.93	0.93	XXX	0	0	0	0	2
TC	0.26	0.26	XXX	0	0	0	0	2

AMA: Dec 11: 18

+ 88388 Macroscopic examination, dissection, and preparation of tissue for non-microscopic analytical studies (eg, nucleic acid-based molecular studies); in conjunction with a touch imprint, intraoperative consultation, or frozen section, each tissue preparation (eg, a single lymph node) (List separately in addition to code for primary procedure) N

RVU			Global Days	Modifiers				
Mod	Non-Fac Total	Fac Total		51	50	62	80	MUE
	0.98	0.98	XXX	0	0	0	0	1
26	0.70	0.70	XXX	0	0	0	0	1
TC	0.28	0.28	XXX	0	0	0	0	1

AMA: Dec 11: 18

● New   ▲ Revised   ✖ Deleted   ⊙ Moderate Sedation   ✚ Add-on Codes   ⊘ High Risk Denial   Ⓐ Age Edit   ♀ Female   ♂ Male   **AMA** CPT® Assistant   **MUE** Medically Unlikely Edit
⦸ Modifier 51 Exempt   ⊖ Modifier 63 Exempt   ✗ Unlisted   **Modifiers:** See Inside Back Cover   Ⓜ Maternity   A2–Z3 ASC Payment Indicators   A–Y OPPS Status Indicators

88399 Unlisted surgical pathology procedure ⊗ⓧ◯❶

Mod	Non-Fac Total	Fac Total	Global Days	51	50	62	80	MUE
	0.00	0.00	XXX	0	0	0	0	
26	0.00	0.00	XXX	0	0	0	0	
TC	0.00	0.00	XXX	0	0	0	0	

AMA: Jun 14: 15

In Vivo Measurements

88720 Bilirubin, total, transcutaneous ⊗◯❹

Mod	Non-Fac Total	Fac Total	Global Days	51	50	62	80	MUE
	0.00	0.00	XXX	9	9	9	9	1

AMA: Dec 10: 10

88738 Hemoglobin (Hgb), quantitative, transcutaneous ◯❹

Mod	Non-Fac Total	Fac Total	Global Days	51	50	62	80	MUE
	0.00	0.00	XXX	9	9	9	9	1

88740 Hemoglobin, quantitative, transcutaneous, per day; carboxyhemoglobin ◯❹

Mod	Non-Fac Total	Fac Total	Global Days	51	50	62	80	MUE
	0.00	0.00	XXX	9	9	9	9	1

88741 Hemoglobin, quantitative, transcutaneous, per day; methemoglobin ◯❹

Mod	Non-Fac Total	Fac Total	Global Days	51	50	62	80	MUE
	0.00	0.00	XXX	9	9	9	9	1

88749 Unlisted in vivo (eg, transcutaneous) laboratory service �◯❹

Mod	Non-Fac Total	Fac Total	Global Days	51	50	62	80	MUE
	0.00	0.00	XXX	9	9	9	9	

AMA: Oct 10: 10, Dec 10: 10

Other Laboratory/Pathology Procedures

89049 Caffeine halothane contracture test (CHCT) for malignant hyperthermia susceptibility, including interpretation and report ⊗◯❶

Mod	Non-Fac Total	Fac Total	Global Days	51	50	62	80	MUE
	7.56	1.88	XXX	0	0	0	0	1

AMA: Mar 06: 6, May 06: 19, Sep 11: 4

89050 Cell count, miscellaneous body fluids (eg, cerebrospinal fluid, joint fluid), except blood ◯❹

Mod	Non-Fac Total	Fac Total	Global Days	51	50	62	80	MUE
	0.00	0.00	XXX	9	9	9	9	2

AMA: Aug 05: 9, Sep 11: 4
Pub 100-04, 16, 120.2

89051 Cell count, miscellaneous body fluids (eg, cerebrospinal fluid, joint fluid), except blood; with differential count ◯❹

Mod	Non-Fac Total	Fac Total	Global Days	51	50	62	80	MUE
	0.00	0.00	XXX	9	9	9	9	2

AMA: Sep 11: 4
Pub 100-04, 16, 120.2

89055 Leukocyte assessment, fecal, qualitative or semiquantitative ◯❹

Mod	Non-Fac Total	Fac Total	Global Days	51	50	62	80	MUE
	0.00	0.00	XXX	9	9	9	9	2

AMA: Jul 03: 9, Sep 11: 4

89060 Crystal identification by light microscopy with or without polarizing lens analysis, tissue or any body fluid (except urine) ◯❹

Mod	Non-Fac Total	Fac Total	Global Days	51	50	62	80	MUE
	0.00	0.00	XXX	9	9	9	9	2
26	0.52	0.52	XXX	0	0	0	0	2

AMA: Sep 11: 4

89125 Fat stain, feces, urine, or respiratory secretions ◯❹

Mod	Non-Fac Total	Fac Total	Global Days	51	50	62	80	MUE
	0.00	0.00	XXX	9	9	9	9	2

AMA: Sep 11: 4

89160 Meat fibers, feces ◯❹

Mod	Non-Fac Total	Fac Total	Global Days	51	50	62	80	MUE
	0.00	0.00	XXX	9	9	9	9	1

AMA: Sep 11: 4

89190 Nasal smear for eosinophils ◯❹

Mod	Non-Fac Total	Fac Total	Global Days	51	50	62	80	MUE
	0.00	0.00	XXX	9	9	9	9	1

AMA: Sep 11: 4

89220 Sputum, obtaining specimen, aerosol induced technique (separate procedure) ◯❶

Mod	Non-Fac Total	Fac Total	Global Days	51	50	62	80	MUE
	0.46	0.46	XXX	0	0	0	0	1

AMA: Aug 05: 9, Sep 11: 4

89230 Sweat collection by iontophoresis ◯❶

Mod	Non-Fac Total	Fac Total	Global Days	51	50	62	80	MUE
	0.15	0.15	XXX	0	0	0	0	1

AMA: Sep 11: 4

89240 Unlisted miscellaneous pathology test ⓧ◯❶

Mod	Non-Fac Total	Fac Total	Global Days	51	50	62	80	MUE
	0.00	0.00	XXX	0	0	0	0	

AMA: Nov 05: 14, Jan 07: 30, Sep 11: 4

● New   ▲ Revised   Deleted   ⊙ Moderate Sedation   ✚ Add-on Codes   ⊗ High Risk Denial   Ⓐ Age Edit   ♀ Female   ♂ Male   **AMA** *CPT® Assistant*   **MUE** Medically Unlikely Edit
⊘ Modifier 51 Exempt   ⊖ Modifier 63 Exempt   ⓧ Unlisted   **Modifiers:** *See Inside Back Cover*   Ⓜ Maternity   Ⓐ❷–❼ ASC Payment Indicators   Ⓐ–Ⓨ OPPS Status Indicators

Reproductive Medicine Procedures/Testing

89250 Culture of oocyte(s)/embryo(s), less than 4 days

RVU			Global Days	Modifiers				
Mod	Non-Fac Total	Fac Total		51	50	62	80	MUE
	0.00	0.00	XXX	9	9	9	9	1

AMA: Nov 97: 35, 36, Jan 98: 6, Oct 98: 1, Apr 04: 2, May 04: 16, Jun 04: 9, Sep 11: 4

89251 Culture of oocyte(s)/embryo(s), less than 4 days; with co-culture of oocyte(s)/embryos

RVU			Global Days	Modifiers				
Mod	Non-Fac Total	Fac Total		51	50	62	80	MUE
	0.00	0.00	XXX	9	9	9	9	1

AMA: Nov 97: 35, 36, Jan 98: 6, Oct 98: 1, Apr 04: 2

89253 Assisted embryo hatching, microtechniques (any method)

RVU			Global Days	Modifiers				
Mod	Non-Fac Total	Fac Total		51	50	62	80	MUE
	0.00	0.00	XXX	9	9	9	9	1

AMA: Nov 97: 35, 36, Jan 98: 6, Oct 98: 1, Apr 04: 2, May 04: 16, Jun 04: 9

89254 Oocyte identification from follicular fluid

RVU			Global Days	Modifiers				
Mod	Non-Fac Total	Fac Total		51	50	62	80	MUE
	0.00	0.00	XXX	9	9	9	9	1

AMA: Nov 97: 35, 36, Jan 98: 6, Oct 98: 1, Apr 04: 2, May 04: 16, Jun 04: 9

89255 Preparation of embryo for transfer (any method)

RVU			Global Days	Modifiers				
Mod	Non-Fac Total	Fac Total		51	50	62	80	MUE
	0.00	0.00	XXX	9	9	9	9	1

AMA: Nov 97: 35, 36, Jan 98: 6, Oct 98: 1, Apr 04: 2, May 04: 16, Jun 04: 9

89257 Sperm identification from aspiration (other than seminal fluid)

RVU			Global Days	Modifiers				
Mod	Non-Fac Total	Fac Total		51	50	62	80	MUE
	0.00	0.00	XXX	9	9	9	9	1

AMA: Nov 97: 35, 36, Jan 98: 6, Oct 98: 1, Nov 98: 30, Apr 04: 2

89258 Cryopreservation; embryo(s)

RVU			Global Days	Modifiers				
Mod	Non-Fac Total	Fac Total		51	50	62	80	MUE
	0.00	0.00	XXX	9	9	9	9	1

AMA: Nov 97: 36, Jan 98: 6, Oct 98: 1, Apr 04: 2, 4

89259 Cryopreservation; sperm

RVU			Global Days	Modifiers				
Mod	Non-Fac Total	Fac Total		51	50	62	80	MUE
	0.00	0.00	XXX	9	9	9	9	1

AMA: Nov 97: 36, Jan 98: 6, Oct 98: 1, Apr 04: 2, 4

89260 Sperm isolation; simple prep (eg, sperm wash and swim-up) for insemination or diagnosis with semen analysis

RVU			Global Days	Modifiers				
Mod	Non-Fac Total	Fac Total		51	50	62	80	MUE
	0.00	0.00	XXX	9	9	9	9	1

AMA: Nov 97: 36, Jan 98: 6, Oct 98: 1, Apr 04: 3, 4

89261 Sperm isolation; complex prep (eg, Percoll gradient, albumin gradient) for insemination or diagnosis with semen analysis

RVU			Global Days	Modifiers				
Mod	Non-Fac Total	Fac Total		51	50	62	80	MUE
	0.00	0.00	XXX	9	9	9	9	1

AMA: Nov 97: 36, Jan 98: 6, Oct 98: 1, Apr 04: 3, 4

89264 Sperm identification from testis tissue, fresh or cryopreserved

RVU			Global Days	Modifiers				
Mod	Non-Fac Total	Fac Total		51	50	62	80	MUE
	0.00	0.00	XXX	9	9	9	9	1

AMA: Nov 98: 30, Apr 04: 3, 4

89268 Insemination of oocytes

RVU			Global Days	Modifiers				
Mod	Non-Fac Total	Fac Total		51	50	62	80	MUE
	0.00	0.00	XXX	9	9	9	9	1

AMA: Apr 04: 3, 4

89272 Extended culture of oocyte(s)/embryo(s), 4-7 days

RVU			Global Days	Modifiers				
Mod	Non-Fac Total	Fac Total		51	50	62	80	MUE
	0.00	0.00	XXX	9	9	9	9	1

AMA: Apr 04: 3, 4

89280 Assisted oocyte fertilization, microtechnique; less than or equal to 10 oocytes

RVU			Global Days	Modifiers				
Mod	Non-Fac Total	Fac Total		51	50	62	80	MUE
	0.00	0.00	XXX	9	9	9	9	1

AMA: Apr 04: 3, 4

89281 Assisted oocyte fertilization, microtechnique; greater than 10 oocytes

RVU			Global Days	Modifiers				
Mod	Non-Fac Total	Fac Total		51	50	62	80	MUE
	0.00	0.00	XXX	9	9	9	9	1

AMA: Apr 04: 3, 4

89290 Biopsy, oocyte polar body or embryo blastomere, microtechnique (for pre-implantation genetic diagnosis); less than or equal to 5 embryos

RVU			Global Days	Modifiers				
Mod	Non-Fac Total	Fac Total		51	50	62	80	MUE
	0.00	0.00	XXX	9	9	9	9	1

AMA: Apr 04: 5

89291 Biopsy, oocyte polar body or embryo blastomere, microtechnique (for pre-implantation genetic diagnosis); greater than 5 embryos

RVU			Global Days	Modifiers				
Mod	Non-Fac Total	Fac Total		51	50	62	80	MUE
	0.00	0.00	XXX	9	9	9	9	1

AMA: Apr 04: 3, 5

89300 Semen analysis; presence and/or motility of sperm including Huhner test (post coital)

Coding tip: For a CLIA-waived test, add modifier QW to 89300

RVU			Global Days	Modifiers				
Mod	Non-Fac Total	Fac Total		51	50	62	80	MUE
	0.00	0.00	XXX	9	9	9	9	1

● New   ▲ Revised   ✖ Deleted   ⊙ Moderate Sedation   ✚ Add-on Codes   ⊘ High Risk Denial   Ⓐ Age Edit   ♀ Female   ♂ Male   **AMA** CPT® Assistant   **MUE** Medically Unlikely Edit   ⊗ Modifier 51 Exempt   ⊖ Modifier 63 Exempt   🅇 Unlisted   **Modifiers:** See Inside Back Cover   Ⓜ Maternity   A2–Z3 ASC Payment Indicators   A–Y OPPS Status Indicators

CPT © 2015 American Medical Association. All Rights Reserved.   © 2016 DecisionHealth

AMA: Nov 97: 36, Jul 98: 10, Oct 98: 4, Apr 04: 3, Aug 05: 9

89310 Semen analysis; motility and count (not including Huhner test) ⚭♂ Q4

RVU			Global Days	Modifiers				
Mod	Non-Fac Total	Fac Total		51	50	62	80	MUE
	0.00	0.00	XXX	9	9	9	9	1

AMA: Jul 03: 9, Apr 04: 3

89320 Semen analysis; volume, count, motility, and differential ♂ Q4

RVU			Global Days	Modifiers				
Mod	Non-Fac Total	Fac Total		51	50	62	80	MUE
	0.00	0.00	XXX	9	9	9	9	1

AMA: Apr 04: 3, Apr 08: 5

89321 Semen analysis; sperm presence and motility of sperm, if performed ⚭♂ Q4

Coding tip: For a CLIA-waived test, add modifier QW to 89321

RVU			Global Days	Modifiers				
Mod	Non-Fac Total	Fac Total		51	50	62	80	MUE
	0.00	0.00	XXX	9	9	9	9	1

89322 Semen analysis; volume, count, motility, and differential using strict morphologic criteria (eg, Kruger) ♂ Q4

RVU			Global Days	Modifiers				
Mod	Non-Fac Total	Fac Total		51	50	62	80	MUE
	0.00	0.00	XXX	9	9	9	9	1

AMA: Apr 08: 5

89325 Sperm antibodies ⚭♂ Q4

RVU			Global Days	Modifiers				
Mod	Non-Fac Total	Fac Total		51	50	62	80	MUE
	0.00	0.00	XXX	9	9	9	9	1

89329 Sperm evaluation; hamster penetration test ⚭♂ Q4

RVU			Global Days	Modifiers				
Mod	Non-Fac Total	Fac Total		51	50	62	80	MUE
	0.00	0.00	XXX	9	9	9	9	1

89330 Sperm evaluation; cervical mucus penetration test, with or without spinnbarkeit test ⚭♂ Q4

RVU			Global Days	Modifiers				
Mod	Non-Fac Total	Fac Total		51	50	62	80	MUE
	0.00	0.00	XXX	9	9	9	9	1

AMA: Nov 05: 14

89331 Sperm evaluation, for retrograde ejaculation, urine (sperm concentration, motility, and morphology, as indicated) ♂ Q4

RVU			Global Days	Modifiers				
Mod	Non-Fac Total	Fac Total		51	50	62	80	MUE
	0.00	0.00	XXX	9	9	9	9	1

AMA: Apr 08: 5

89335 Cryopreservation, reproductive tissue, testicular Q1

RVU			Global Days	Modifiers				
Mod	Non-Fac Total	Fac Total		51	50	62	80	MUE
	0.00	0.00	XXX	9	9	9	9	1

AMA: Apr 04: 5

89337 Cryopreservation, mature oocyte(s) Q1

RVU			Global Days	Modifiers				
Mod	Non-Fac Total	Fac Total		51	50	62	80	MUE
	0.00	0.00	XXX	9	9	9	9	1

89342 Storage (per year); embryo(s) ⚭ Q1

RVU			Global Days	Modifiers				
Mod	Non-Fac Total	Fac Total		51	50	62	80	MUE
	0.00	0.00	XXX	9	9	9	9	1

AMA: Apr 04: 5

89343 Storage (per year); sperm/semen ⚭ Q1

RVU			Global Days	Modifiers				
Mod	Non-Fac Total	Fac Total		51	50	62	80	MUE
	0.00	0.00	XXX	9	9	9	9	1

AMA: Apr 04: 5

89344 Storage (per year); reproductive tissue, testicular/ovarian Q1

RVU			Global Days	Modifiers				
Mod	Non-Fac Total	Fac Total		51	50	62	80	MUE
	0.00	0.00	XXX	9	9	9	9	1

AMA: Apr 04: 5

89346 Storage (per year); oocyte(s) Q2

RVU			Global Days	Modifiers				
Mod	Non-Fac Total	Fac Total		51	50	62	80	MUE
	0.00	0.00	XXX	9	9	9	9	1

AMA: Apr 04: 5

89352 Thawing of cryopreserved; embryo(s) ⚭ Q1

RVU			Global Days	Modifiers				
Mod	Non-Fac Total	Fac Total		51	50	62	80	MUE
	0.00	0.00	XXX	9	9	9	9	1

AMA: Apr 04: 5

89353 Thawing of cryopreserved; sperm/semen, each aliquot ⚭ Q1

RVU			Global Days	Modifiers				
Mod	Non-Fac Total	Fac Total		51	50	62	80	MUE
	0.00	0.00	XXX	9	9	9	9	1

AMA: Apr 04: 5

89354 Thawing of cryopreserved; reproductive tissue, testicular/ovarian Q1

RVU			Global Days	Modifiers				
Mod	Non-Fac Total	Fac Total		51	50	62	80	MUE
	0.00	0.00	XXX	9	9	9	9	1

AMA: Apr 04: 5

89356 Thawing of cryopreserved; oocytes, each aliquot Q1

RVU			Global Days	Modifiers				
Mod	Non-Fac Total	Fac Total		51	50	62	80	MUE
	0.00	0.00	XXX	9	9	9	9	2

AMA: Apr 04: 5, Aug 05: 9

89398 Unlisted reproductive medicine laboratory procedure ⊗x Q1

RVU			Global Days	Modifiers				
Mod	Non-Fac Total	Fac Total		51	50	62	80	MUE
	0.00	0.00	XXX	9	9	9	

● New ▲ Revised   Deleted ⊙ Moderate Sedation ✚ Add-on Codes ⊗ High Risk Denial Ⓐ Age Edit ♀ Female ♂ Male **AMA** *CPT® Assistant* **MUE** Medically Unlikely Edit
⊘ Modifier 51 Exempt ⊖ Modifier 63 Exempt ☒ Unlisted **Modifiers:** *See Inside Back Cover* Ⓜ Maternity A2–Z3 ASC Payment Indicators A–Y OPPS Status Indicators

Medicine Procedures/Services

Introduction to Medicine Procedures/Services

The Medicine Section (90281-99199, 99500-99607) of CPT classifies a multitude of diagnostic, therapeutic, and miscellaneous procedures that are not included in other sections. Many of the codes in this section apply to specific medical specialties, such as services provided by a psychiatrist or a physical therapist, and codes for ophthalmology and otorhinolaryngology. Although many procedures in this section refer to a specific specialty such as cardiology or gastroenterology, the codes are not limited to use by these specialists.

The Medicine section includes codes for specialty services (e.g., cardiology, gastroenterology) as well as codes for noninvasive or minimally invasive (e.g., percutaneous access) procedures such as therapeutic or diagnostic infusions, injections, and immunizations. Specific rules and guidelines apply to these services so coding guidance and tips appear throughout the Medicine section to assist users in appropriate application of the codes.

Add-on Codes and Separate Procedures

Some of the procedures in the Medicine Section are typically performed in addition to a primary procedure rather than as stand-alone procedures; these are designated as "add-on" codes. All add-on codes are exempt from the multiple procedure concept and use of modifier 51. Add-on codes are identified by code descriptors which include "each additional" or "list separately in addition to primary procedure."

Other procedures or services in CPT are usually performed as an integral component of a total procedure; these are identified with the term "separate procedure." Codes designated as separate procedures are not reported in addition to the code for the total procedure. If a designated separate procedure is distinct, unrelated to, and/or performed independently from another procedure, it may be reported by itself or in addition to other procedures/services with modifier 59.

Unlisted Procedures and Special Reports

When a medicine service or procedure is provided that does not have a distinct CPT code, the appropriate "unlisted procedure" code is used to indicate the service. The guidelines for reporting an unusual service require a "special report" and direct the provider to include a description of the nature, extent, and need for the procedure, along with the time, effort, and equipment necessary to provide the service.

Serum/Recombinant Immune Globulin Products

90281   Immune globulin (Ig), human, for intramuscular use   ⊘E

RVU			Global Days	Modifiers				
Mod	Non-Fac Total	Fac Total		51	50	62	80	MUE
	0.00	0.00	XXX	9	9	9	9	

AMA: Nov 98: 30, Jan 99: 3, Sep 99: 10

90283   Immune globulin (IgIV), human, for intravenous use   ⊘E

RVU			Global Days	Modifiers				
Mod	Non-Fac Total	Fac Total		51	50	62	80	MUE
	0.00	0.00	XXX	9	9	9	9	

AMA: Nov 98: 30, Jan 99: 3

90284   Immune globulin (SCIg), human, for use in subcutaneous infusions, 100 mg, each   ⊘E

RVU			Global Days	Modifiers				
Mod	Non-Fac Total	Fac Total		51	50	62	80	MUE
	0.00	0.00	XXX	9	9	9	9	1

90287   Botulinum antitoxin, equine, any route   E

RVU			Global Days	Modifiers				
Mod	Non-Fac Total	Fac Total		51	50	62	80	MUE
	0.00	0.00	XXX	9	9	9	9	

AMA: Nov 98: 30, Jan 99: 3

90288   Botulism immune globulin, human, for intravenous use   E

RVU			Global Days	Modifiers				
Mod	Non-Fac Total	Fac Total		51	50	62	80	MUE
	0.00	0.00	XXX	9	9	9	9	

AMA: Nov 98: 30, Jan 99: 3

90291   Cytomegalovirus immune globulin (CMV-IgIV), human, for intravenous use   ⊘E

RVU			Global Days	Modifiers				
Mod	Non-Fac Total	Fac Total		51	50	62	80	MUE
	0.00	0.00	XXX	9	9	9	9	

AMA: Nov 98: 30, Jan 99: 3

90296   Diphtheria antitoxin, equine, any route   ⊘E

RVU			Global Days	Modifiers				
Mod	Non-Fac Total	Fac Total		51	50	62	80	MUE
	0.00	0.00	XXX	9	9	9	9	1

AMA: Nov 98: 30, Jan 99: 3

90371   Hepatitis B immune globulin (HBIg), human, for intramuscular use   K 2K

RVU			Global Days	Modifiers				
Mod	Non-Fac Total	Fac Total		51	50	62	80	MUE
	0.00	0.00	XXX	9	9	9	9	

AMA: Nov 98: 30, Jan 99: 3

90375   Rabies immune globulin (RIg), human, for intramuscular and/or subcutaneous use   K 2K

RVU			Global Days	Modifiers				
Mod	Non-Fac Total	Fac Total		51	50	62	80	MUE
	0.00	0.00	XXX	9	9	9	9	20

AMA: Nov 98: 30, Jan 99: 3

90376   Rabies immune globulin, heat-treated (RIg-HT), human, for intramuscular and/or subcutaneous use   K 2K

RVU			Global Days	Modifiers				
Mod	Non-Fac Total	Fac Total		51	50	62	80	MUE
	0.00	0.00	XXX	9	9	9	9	20

AMA: Nov 98: 30, Jan 99: 3

90378   Respiratory syncytial virus, monoclonal antibody, recombinant, for intramuscular use, 50 mg, each   ⊘K 2K

RVU			Global Days	Modifiers				
Mod	Non-Fac Total	Fac Total		51	50	62	80	MUE
	0.00	0.00	XXX	9	9	9	9	

AMA: Jan 99: 3, Nov 99: 47, Jun 00: 10

90384   Rho(D) immune globulin (RhIg), human, full-dose, for intramuscular use   ⊘E

RVU			Global Days	Modifiers				
Mod	Non-Fac Total	Fac Total		51	50	62	80	MUE
	0.00	0.00	XXX	9	9	9	9	

AMA: Nov 98: 30, Jan 99: 3

90385   Rho(D) immune globulin (RhIg), human, mini-dose, for intramuscular use   ⊘N 1N

RVU			Global Days	Modifiers				
Mod	Non-Fac Total	Fac Total		51	50	62	80	MUE
	0.00	0.00	XXX	9	9	9	9	1

AMA: Nov 98: 30, Jan 99: 3

● New   ▲ Revised   ✖ Deleted   ⊙ Moderate Sedation   ✚ Add-on Codes   ⊘ High Risk Denial   Ⓐ Age Edit   ♀ Female   ♂ Male   **AMA** CPT® Assistant   **MUE** Medically Unlikely Edit
⊘ Modifier 51 Exempt   ⊖ Modifier 63 Exempt   ✗ Unlisted   **Modifiers:** See Inside Back Cover   Ⓜ Maternity   A2–Z3 ASC Payment Indicators   A–Y OPPS Status Indicators

780   CPT © 2015 American Medical Association. All Rights Reserved.   © 2016 DecisionHealth

90386 Rho(D) immune globulin (RhIgIV), human, for intravenous use ⊖E

RVU		Global Days	Modifiers				
Mod	Non-Fac Total	Fac Total		51	50	62	80	MUE
	0.00	0.00	XXX	9	9	9	9	

AMA: Nov 98: 30, Jan 99: 3

90389 Tetanus immune globulin (TIg), human, for intramuscular use ⊖E

RVU		Global Days	Modifiers				
Mod	Non-Fac Total	Fac Total		51	50	62	80	MUE
	0.00	0.00	XXX	9	9	9	9	

AMA: Nov 98: 30, Jan 99: 3

90393 Vaccinia immune globulin, human, for intramuscular use ⊖N

RVU		Global Days	Modifiers				
Mod	Non-Fac Total	Fac Total		51	50	62	80	MUE
	0.00	0.00	XXX	9	9	9	9	1

AMA: Nov 98: 30, Jan 99: 3

90396 Varicella-zoster immune globulin, human, for intramuscular use ⊖K 2 K

RVU		Global Days	Modifiers				
Mod	Non-Fac Total	Fac Total		51	50	62	80	MUE
	0.00	0.00	XXX	9	9	9	9	1

AMA: Nov 98: 30, Jan 99: 3

90399 Unlisted immune globulin ⊖xE

RVU		Global Days	Modifiers				
Mod	Non-Fac Total	Fac Total		51	50	62	80	MUE
	0.00	0.00	XXX	9	9	9	9	

AMA: Nov 98: 30, Jan 99: 3, Feb 99: 11, Sep 99: 10

Vaccine/Toxoid Immunization Administration

90460 Immunization administration through 18 years of age via any route of administration, with counseling by physician or other qualified health care professional; first or only component of each vaccine or toxoid administered ⊙Ⓐ℻

Documentation Finder: The documentation must show that the vaccination was administered to a patient 18 years or younger and that the physician or non-physician practitioner clearly gave counseling about risk and complications regarding the vaccinations that the patient will be having.

RVU		Global Days	Modifiers				
Mod	Non-Fac Total	Fac Total		51	50	62	80	MUE
	0.71	0.71	XXX	0	0	0	0	6

AMA: Apr 15: 9, 11, Mar 11: 3, Jul 12: 7, Jun 11: 14, Jan 12: 43, Aug 13: 10, Mar 14: 10, May 15: 6

+ 90461 Immunization administration through 18 years of age via any route of administration, with counseling by physician or other qualified health care professional; each additional vaccine or toxoid component administered (List separately in addition to code for primary procedure) ⊙Ⓐ℻

RVU		Global Days	Modifiers				
Mod	Non-Fac Total	Fac Total		51	50	62	80	MUE
	0.35	0.35	ZZZ	0	0	0	0	

AMA: Mar 11: 3, Jul 12: 7, Jun 11: 14, Jan 12: 43, Aug 13: 10, Mar 14: 10, Apr 15: 4, May 15: 6

90471 Immunization administration (includes percutaneous, intradermal, subcutaneous, or intramuscular injections); 1 vaccine (single or combination vaccine/toxoid) ⊖S

Documentation Finder: The documentation must reflect how the vaccination was administered: percutaneous, intradermal, subcutaneous or intramuscular (IM).

RVU		Global Days	Modifiers				
Mod	Non-Fac Total	Fac Total		51	50	62	80	MUE
	0.71	0.71	XXX	0	0	0	0	1

AMA: Apr 15: 9, 11, Mar 11: 3, Nov 98: 31, Jan 99: 2, Apr 99: 10, Oct 99: 9, Nov 99: 47, 48, Nov 00: 10, Feb 01: 5, Jul 01: 2, Nov 02: 11, Mar 04: 11, Apr 04: 14, Apr 05: 1, 3, 5, Nov 05: 1, Jan 09: 8, Jul 09: 7, Aug 09: 9, Sep 09: 7, Oct 09: 3, Jul 12: 7, Jun 11: 14, Aug 13: 10, Mar 14: 10, May 15: 6

Pub 100-04, 18, 10.2.1, 10.2.2.1, 10.3.1

+ 90472 Immunization administration (includes percutaneous, intradermal, subcutaneous, or intramuscular injections); each additional vaccine (single or combination vaccine/toxoid) (List separately in addition to code for primary procedure) ⊖N

Documentation Finder: In the documentation, you should see reference to the route (how) they performed this vaccination: words such as percutaneous, subcutaneous, intramuscular (IM) or intradermal. This add-on code reflects that more than one injection/vaccination was performed and must be reported with 90471.

RVU		Global Days	Modifiers				
Mod	Non-Fac Total	Fac Total		51	50	62	80	MUE
	0.35	0.35	ZZZ	0	0	0	0	4

AMA: Apr 15: 9, 11, Mar 11: 3, Nov 98: 31, Jan 99: 2, Apr 99: 10, Oct 99: 9, Nov 99: 47, 48, Nov 00: 10, Feb 01: 5, Jul 01: 2, Nov 02: 11, Mar 04: 11, Apr 04: 14, Apr 05: 1, 3, Nov 05: 1, Jan 09: 3, 8, Jul 09: 7, Aug 09: 9, Sep 09: 7, Oct 09: 3, Jul 12: 7, Jun 11: 14, Aug 13: 10, Mar 14: 10, May 15: 6

Pub 100-04, 18, 10.2.1

90473 Immunization administration by intranasal or oral route; 1 vaccine (single or combination vaccine/toxoid) ⊖S

RVU		Global Days	Modifiers				
Mod	Non-Fac Total	Fac Total		51	50	62	80	MUE
	0.71	0.71	XXX	0	0	0	0	1

AMA: Mar 11: 3, Feb 01: 5, Nov 02: 11, Apr 04: 14, Apr 05: 1, 3, Jan 09: 3, 8, Jul 09: 7, Aug 09: 9, Oct 09: 3, Jul 12: 7, Jun 11: 14, Aug 13: 10, Mar 14: 10, Apr 15: 9, May 15: 6

+ 90474 Immunization administration by intranasal or oral route; each additional vaccine (single or combination vaccine/toxoid) (List separately in addition to code for primary procedure) ⊖N

RVU		Global Days	Modifiers				
Mod	Non-Fac Total	Fac Total		51	50	62	80	MUE
	0.35	0.35	ZZZ	0	0	0	0	1

AMA: Mar 11: 3, Feb 01: 5, Nov 02: 11, Apr 04: 14, Apr 05: 1, 3, Jan 09: 3, 8, Jul 09: 7, Aug 09: 9, Oct 09: 3, Jul 12: 7, Jun 11: 14, Aug 13: 10, Mar 14: 10, Apr 15: 9, May 15: 6

Vaccine/Toxoid Supply

90476 Adenovirus vaccine, type 4, live, for oral use ⊖N 1 N

RVU		Global Days	Modifiers				
Mod	Non-Fac Total	Fac Total		51	50	62	80	MUE
	0.00	0.00	XXX	9	9	9	9	1

AMA: Mar 11: 4, Nov 98: 31, 33, Jan 99: 2, Sep 99: 10, Oct 99: 9, Nov 99: 48, Aug 13: 10, May 15: 6

● New ▲ Revised Deleted ⊙ Moderate Sedation ✚ Add-on Codes ⊗ High Risk Denial Ⓐ Age Edit ♀ Female ♂ Male **AMA** *CPT® Assistant* **MUE** Medically Unlikely Edit
⊘ Modifier 51 Exempt ⊖ Modifier 63 Exempt ✗ Unlisted **Modifiers:** *See Inside Back Cover* Ⓜ Maternity A 2–Z 3 ASC Payment Indicators A –Y OPPS Status Indicators

© 2016 DecisionHealth   CPT © 2015 American Medical Association. All Rights Reserved.   **781**

90477 Adenovirus vaccine, type 7, live, for oral use ⊙E

RVU			Global Days	Modifiers				
Mod	Non-Fac Total	Fac Total		51	50	62	80	MUE
	0.00	0.00	XXX	9	9	9	9	1

AMA: Mar 11: 4, Nov 98: 31, 33, Jan 99: 2, Oct 99: 9, Aug 13: 10

90581 Anthrax vaccine, for subcutaneous or intramuscular use ⊙N I N

Coding tip: Brand name(s): BioThrax

RVU			Global Days	Modifiers				
Mod	Non-Fac Total	Fac Total		51	50	62	80	MUE
	0.00	0.00	XXX	9	9	9	9	1

AMA: Mar 11: 4, Nov 98: 31, 33, Jan 99: 2, Oct 99: 9, Aug 13: 10

90585 Bacillus Calmette-Guerin vaccine (BCG) for tuberculosis, live, for percutaneous use ⊙K 2 K

RVU			Global Days	Modifiers				
Mod	Non-Fac Total	Fac Total		51	50	62	80	MUE
	0.00	0.00	XXX	9	9	9	9	1

AMA: Nov 98: 31, 33, Jan 99: 2, Oct 99: 9, Mar 11: 4, Aug 13: 10

90586 Bacillus Calmette-Guerin vaccine (BCG) for bladder cancer, live, for intravesical use ⊙B

Coding tip: Intravesical administration (instillation) BCG vaccine - 51720

RVU			Global Days	Modifiers				
Mod	Non-Fac Total	Fac Total		51	50	62	80	MUE
	0.00	0.00	XXX	9	9	9	9	1

AMA: Nov 98: 31, 33, Jan 99: 2, Oct 99: 9, Nov 02: 11, Mar 11: 4, Aug 13: 10

● **90620 Meningococcal recombinant protein and outer membrane vesicle vaccine, serogroup B (MenB), 2 dose schedule, for intramuscular use** K 2 K

RVU			Global Days	Modifiers				
Mod	Non-Fac Total	Fac Total		51	50	62	80	MUE
	0.00	0.00	XXX	9	9	9	9	1

● **90621 Meningococcal recombinant lipoprotein vaccine, serogroup B (MenB), 3 dose schedule, for intramuscular use** K 2 K

RVU			Global Days	Modifiers				
Mod	Non-Fac Total	Fac Total		51	50	62	80	MUE
	0.00	0.00	XXX	9	9	9	9	1

⚹● **90625 Cholera vaccine, live, adult dosage, 1 dose schedule, for oral use** E

RVU			Global Days	Modifiers				
Mod	Non-Fac Total	Fac Total		51	50	62	80	MUE
	0.00	0.00	XXX	9	9	9	9	1

90630 Influenza virus vaccine, quadrivalent (IIV4), split virus, preservative free, for intradermal use L I L

RVU			Global Days	Modifiers				
Mod	Non-Fac Total	Fac Total		51	50	62	80	MUE
	0.00	0.00	XXX	9	9	9	9	1

AMA: May 15: 6

▲ **90632 Hepatitis A vaccine (HepA), adult dosage, for intramuscular use** ⊙ⒶN I N

Coding tip: Brand name(s): Havrix, Vaqta

Documentation Finder: Make sure of the patient's age and that the documentation states Hepatitis A to support this CPT code.

RVU			Global Days	Modifiers				
Mod	Non-Fac Total	Fac Total		51	50	62	80	MUE

| | 0.00 | 0.00 | XXX | 9 | 9 | 9 | 9 | 1 |

AMA: Nov 98: 31, 33, Jan 99: 2, Oct 99: 9, Mar 11: 4, Aug 13: 10

▲ **90633 Hepatitis A vaccine (HepA), pediatric/adolescent dosage-2 dose schedule, for intramuscular use** ⊙ⒶN I N

Coding tip: Brand name(s): Havrix, Vaqta

RVU			Global Days	Modifiers				
Mod	Non-Fac Total	Fac Total		51	50	62	80	MUE
	0.00	0.00	XXX	9	9	9	9	1

AMA: Nov 98: 31, 33, Jan 99: 2, Oct 99: 9, Mar 11: 4, Aug 13: 10

▲ **90634 Hepatitis A vaccine (HepA), pediatric/adolescent dosage-3 dose schedule, for intramuscular use** ⊙ⒶN I N

Coding tip: Brand name(s): Havrix, Vaqta

RVU			Global Days	Modifiers				
Mod	Non-Fac Total	Fac Total		51	50	62	80	MUE
	0.00	0.00	XXX	9	9	9	9	1

AMA: Nov 98: 31, 33, Jan 99: 2, Oct 99: 9, Mar 11: 4, Aug 13: 10

90636 Hepatitis A and hepatitis B vaccine (HepA-HepB), adult dosage, for intramuscular use ⊙ⒶN I N

Coding tip: Brand name(s):Twinrix

RVU			Global Days	Modifiers				
Mod	Non-Fac Total	Fac Total		51	50	62	80	MUE
	0.00	0.00	XXX	9	9	9	9	1

AMA: Nov 98: 31, 33, Jan 99: 2, Oct 99: 9, Mar 11: 4, Aug 13: 10

▲ **90644 Meningococcal conjugate vaccine, serogroups C & Y and Haemophilus influenzae type b vaccine (Hib-MenCY), 4 dose schedule, when administered to children 2-18 months of age, for intramuscular use** ⊙ⒶN I E

RVU			Global Days	Modifiers				
Mod	Non-Fac Total	Fac Total		51	50	62	80	MUE
	0.00	0.00	XXX	9	9	9	9	1

AMA: Mar 11: 4, Aug 13: 10

⚹ ~~90645 Hemophilus influenza b vaccine (Hib), HbOC conjugate (4 dose schedule), for intramuscular use~~

⚹ ~~90646 Hemophilus influenza b vaccine (Hib), PRP-D conjugate, for booster use only, intramuscular use~~

▲ **90647 Haemophilus influenzae type b vaccine (Hib), PRP-OMP conjugate, 3 dose schedule, for intramuscular use** ⊙N I N

Coding tip: Brand name(s): ActHIB

RVU			Global Days	Modifiers				
Mod	Non-Fac Total	Fac Total		51	50	62	80	MUE
	0.00	0.00	XXX	9	9	9	9	1

AMA: Nov 98: 31, 33, Jan 99: 2, Oct 99: 9, Mar 11: 4, Aug 13: 10

▲ **90648 Haemophilus influenzae type b vaccine (Hib), PRP-T conjugate, 4 dose schedule, for intramuscular use** ⊙N I N

Coding tip: Brand name(s): PedvaxHIB

RVU			Global Days	Modifiers				
Mod	Non-Fac Total	Fac Total		51	50	62	80	MUE
	0.00	0.00	XXX	9	9	9	9	1

AMA: Nov 98: 31, 33, Jan 99: 2, Oct 99: 9, Sep 09: 7, Mar 11: 4, Aug 13: 10

● New   ▲ Revised   ⚹ Deleted   ⊙ Moderate Sedation   ✚ Add-on Codes   ⊘ High Risk Denial   Ⓐ Age Edit   ♀ Female   ♂ Male   **AMA** *CPT® Assistant*   **MUE** Medically Unlikely Edit
⊘ Modifier 51 Exempt   ⊖ Modifier 63 Exempt   ⊠ Unlisted   **Modifiers:** *See Inside Back Cover*   Ⓜ Maternity   A2–Z3 ASC Payment Indicators   A–Y OPPS Status Indicators

CPT © 2015 American Medical Association. All Rights Reserved.   © 2016 DecisionHealth

▲ **90649** **Human Papillomavirus vaccine, types 6, 11, 16, 18, quadrivalent (4vHPV), 3 dose schedule, for intramuscular use** ⊗M

RVU			Global Days	Modifiers				
Mod	Non-Fac Total	Fac Total		51	50	62	80	MUE
	0.00	0.00	XXX	9	9	9	9	1

AMA: Dec 05: 9, Jun 06: 8, Sep 06: 14, Jul 07: 13, Mar 11: 4, Aug 13: 10

▲ **90650** **Human Papillomavirus vaccine, types 16, 18, bivalent (2vHPV), 3 dose schedule, for intramuscular use** ⊗M

Coding tip: Brand name(s): Cervarix

RVU			Global Days	Modifiers				
Mod	Non-Fac Total	Fac Total		51	50	62	80	MUE
	0.00	0.00	XXX	9	9	9	9	1

AMA: Mar 11: 4, Aug 13: 10

▲ **90651** **Human Papillomavirus vaccine types 6, 11, 16, 18, 31, 33, 45, 52, 58, nonavalent (9vHPV), 3 dose schedule, for intramuscular use** E

RVU			Global Days	Modifiers				
Mod	Non-Fac Total	Fac Total		51	50	62	80	MUE
	0.00	0.00	XXX	9	9	9	9	1

AMA: May 15: 6

✐▲**90653** **Influenza vaccine, inactivated (IIV), subunit, adjuvanted, for intramuscular use** ⊗E

RVU			Global Days	Modifiers				
Mod	Non-Fac Total	Fac Total		51	50	62	80	MUE
	0.00	0.00	XXX	9	9	9	9	1

AMA: Aug 13: 10
Pub 100-04, 18, 1.2, 10.2.1, 10.4.1, 10.4.2, 10.4.3

90654 **Influenza virus vaccine, trivalent (IIV3), split virus, preservative-free, for intradermal use** LIL

RVU			Global Days	Modifiers				
Mod	Non-Fac Total	Fac Total		51	50	62	80	MUE
	0.00	0.00	XXX	9	9	9	9	1

AMA: Aug 13: 10, Apr 15: 9, May 15: 6
Pub 100-04, 18, 1.2, 10.2.1, 10.4.1, 10.4.2, 10.4.3

▲ **90655** **Influenza virus vaccine, trivalent (IIV3), split virus, preservative free, when administered to children 6-35 months of age, for intramuscular use** ⊗Ⓐ LIL

Coding tip: Brand name(s): Fluzone

RVU			Global Days	Modifiers				
Mod	Non-Fac Total	Fac Total		51	50	62	80	MUE
	0.00	0.00	XXX	9	9	9	9	1

AMA: Oct 99: 9, Feb 04: 2, Apr 07: 12, Apr 08: 8, Oct 09: 3, Mar 11: 4, Aug 13: 10
Pub 100-04, 18, 1.2, 10.2.1, 10.4.1, 10.4.2, 10.4.3

▲ **90656** **Influenza virus vaccine, trivalent (IIV3), split virus, preservative free, when administered to individuals 3 years and older, for intramuscular use** LIL

Coding tip: Brand name(s): Fluvirin, Fluzone

RVU			Global Days	Modifiers				
Mod	Non-Fac Total	Fac Total		51	50	62	80	MUE
	0.00	0.00	XXX	9	9	9	9	1

AMA: Apr 08: 8, Oct 09: 3, Mar 11: 4, Aug 13: 10
Pub 100-04, 18, 1.2, 10.2.2, 10.4.1, 10.4.2, 10.4.3

▲ **90657** **Influenza virus vaccine, trivalent (IIV3), split virus, when administered to children 6-35 months of age, for intramuscular use** ⊗Ⓐ LIL

Coding tip: Brand name(s): Afluria

RVU			Global Days	Modifiers				
Mod	Non-Fac Total	Fac Total		51	50	62	80	MUE
	0.00	0.00	XXX	9	9	9	9	1

AMA: Nov 98: 31, 33, Jan 99: 2, Oct 99: 9, Feb 02: 10, Feb 04: 2, Apr 05: 5, Apr 08: 8, Oct 09: 3, Mar 11: 4, Aug 13: 10
Pub 100-04, 18, 1.2, 10.2.3, 10.4.1, 10.4.2, 10.4.3

▲ **90658** **Influenza virus vaccine, trivalent (IIV3), split virus, when administered to individuals 3 years of age and older, for intramuscular use** ⊗E

Coding tip: Brand name(s): Agriflu, Fluarix, FluLaval, Fluvirin, Fluzone

RVU			Global Days	Modifiers				
Mod	Non-Fac Total	Fac Total		51	50	62	80	MUE
	0.00	0.00	XXX	9	9	9	9	1

AMA: Nov 98: 31, 33, Jan 99: 2, Oct 99: 9, Feb 04: 2, Apr 07: 12, Apr 08: 8, Oct 09: 3, Mar 11: 4, Aug 13: 10

▲ **90660** **Influenza virus vaccine, trivalent, live (LAIV3), for intranasal use** LIL

Coding tip: Brand name(s): FluMist

Coding tip: Influenza vaccine, quadravalent, live, for intranasal use - 90672

RVU			Global Days	Modifiers				
Mod	Non-Fac Total	Fac Total		51	50	62	80	MUE
	0.00	0.00	XXX	9	9	9	9	1

AMA: Nov 98: 31, 33, Jan 99: 2, Oct 99: 9, Mar 04: 11, Apr 04: 14, Oct 09: 3, Mar 11: 4, Aug 13: 10
Pub 100-04, 18, 1.2, 10.2.1, 10.4.1, 10.4.2, 10.4.3

▲ **90661** **Influenza virus vaccine (ccIIV3), derived from cell cultures, subunit, preservative and antibiotic free, for intramuscular use** LIL

Coding tip: Influenza vaccine, trivalent, derived from DNA (RIV3), HA protein, for intramuscular use - 90673

RVU			Global Days	Modifiers				
Mod	Non-Fac Total	Fac Total		51	50	62	80	MUE
	0.00	0.00	XXX	9	9	9	9	1

AMA: Apr 08: 8, Oct 09: 3, Mar 11: 4, Aug 13: 10
Pub 100-04, 18, 1.2, 10.2.1, 10.4.1, 10.4.2, 10.4.3

▲ **90662** **Influenza virus vaccine (IIV), split virus, preservative free, enhanced immunogenicity via increased antigen content, for intramuscular use** LIL

RVU			Global Days	Modifiers				
Mod	Non-Fac Total	Fac Total		51	50	62	80	MUE
	0.00	0.00	XXX	9	9	9	9	1

AMA: Apr 08: 8, Oct 09: 3, 6, Mar 11: 4, Aug 13: 10
Pub 100-04, 18, 1.2, 10.2.1, 10.4.1, 10.4.2, 10.4.3

▲ **90664** **Influenza virus vaccine, live (LAIV), pandemic formulation, for intranasal use** ⊗E

RVU			Global Days	Modifiers				
Mod	Non-Fac Total	Fac Total		51	50	62	80	MUE
	0.00	0.00	XXX	9	9	9	9	1

AMA: Mar 11: 4, Aug 13: 10

● New   ▲ Revised   Deleted   ⊙ Moderate Sedation   ✚ Add-on Codes   ⊗ High Risk Denial   Ⓐ Age Edit   ♀ Female   ♂ Male   **AMA** *CPT® Assistant*   **MUE** Medically Unlikely Edit
⊘ Modifier 51 Exempt   ⊖ Modifier 63 Exempt   ⊠ Unlisted   **Modifiers:** *See Inside Back Cover*   Ⓜ Maternity   A2–Z3 ASC Payment Indicators   A–Y OPPS Status Indicators

© 2016 DecisionHealth   CPT © 2015 American Medical Association. All Rights Reserved.   **783**

⌀▲90666 Influenza virus vaccine (IIV), pandemic formulation, split virus, preservative free, for intramuscular use   ⓒE

RVU			Global Days	Modifiers				
Mod	Non-Fac Total	Fac Total		51	50	62	80	MUE
	0.00	0.00	XXX	9	9	9	9	1

AMA: May 11: 4, Aug 13: 10

⌀▲90667 Influenza virus vaccine (IIV), pandemic formulation, split virus, adjuvanted, for intramuscular use   ⓒE

RVU			Global Days	Modifiers				
Mod	Non-Fac Total	Fac Total		51	50	62	80	MUE
	0.00	0.00	XXX	9	9	9	9	1

AMA: Mar 11: 4, Aug 13: 10

⌀▲90668 Influenza virus vaccine (IIV), pandemic formulation, split virus, for intramuscular use   ⓒE

RVU			Global Days	Modifiers				
Mod	Non-Fac Total	Fac Total		51	50	62	80	MUE
	0.00	0.00	XXX	9	9	9	9	1

AMA: Mar 11: 4, Aug 13: 10

✖ 90669 ~~Pneumococcal conjugate vaccine, 7 valent, for intramuscular use~~

▲ 90670 Pneumococcal conjugate vaccine, 13 valent (PCV13), for intramuscular use   L I L

Coding tip: Brand name(s): Prevnar 13

RVU			Global Days	Modifiers				
Mod	Non-Fac Total	Fac Total		51	50	62	80	MUE
	0.00	0.00	XXX	9	9	9	9	1

AMA: Mar 11: 4, Aug 13: 10

Pub 100-04, 18, 1.2, 10.2.1, 10.4.1, 10.4.2, 10.4.3

▲ 90672 Influenza virus vaccine, quadrivalent, live (LAIV4), for intranasal use   L I L

Coding tip: Code 90672 is listed out of numerical order in CPT. Related influenza vaccine product code, trivalent, live, for intranasal use - 90660

RVU			Global Days	Modifiers				
Mod	Non-Fac Total	Fac Total		51	50	62	80	MUE
	0.00	0.00	XXX	9	9	9	9	1

AMA: Aug 13: 10

Pub 100-04, 18, 1.2, 10.2.1, 10.4.1, 10.4.2, 10.4.3

▲ 90673 Influenza virus vaccine, trivalent (RIV3), derived from recombinant DNA, hemagglutinin (HA) protein only, preservative and antibiotic free, for intramuscular use   L I L

Coding tip: Code 90673 is listed out of numerical order in CPT. Related code for influenza virus vaccine, derived from cell cultures û 90661. Related codes for influenza virus vaccine, trivalent û 90655-90658, 90660

RVU			Global Days	Modifiers				
Mod	Non-Fac Total	Fac Total		51	50	62	80	MUE
	0.00	0.00	XXX	9	9	9	9	1

AMA: Mar 14: 10

Pub 100-04, 18, 1.2, 10.2.1, 10.4.1, 10.4.2, 10.4.3

90675 Rabies vaccine, for intramuscular use   ⓒK 2 K

Coding tip: Brand name(s): Imovax Rabies, RabAvert

RVU			Global Days	Modifiers				
Mod	Non-Fac Total	Fac Total		51	50	62	80	MUE
	0.00	0.00	XXX	9	9	9	9	1

AMA: Nov 98: 31, 33, Jan 99: 2, Oct 99: 9, Mar 11: 4, Aug 13: 10

90676 Rabies vaccine, for intradermal use   ⓒK 2 K

RVU			Global Days	Modifiers				
Mod	Non-Fac Total	Fac Total		51	50	62	80	MUE
	0.00	0.00	XXX	9	9	9	9	1

AMA: Nov 98: 31, 33, Jan 99: 2, Oct 99: 9, Mar 11: 4, Jul 12: 7, Aug 13: 10

▲ 90680 Rotavirus vaccine, pentavalent (RV5), 3 dose schedule, live, for oral use   ⓒN I N

Coding tip: Brand name(s): Rota Teq, Rotarix

RVU			Global Days	Modifiers				
Mod	Non-Fac Total	Fac Total		51	50	62	80	MUE
	0.00	0.00	XXX	9	9	9	9	1

AMA: Nov 98: 31, 33, Jan 99: 2, Oct 99: 9, Jun 05: 6, Dec 05: 9, Jun 06: 8, Mar 11: 4, Aug 13: 10

▲ 90681 Rotavirus vaccine, human, attenuated (RV1), 2 dose schedule, live, for oral use   ⓒK 2 E

RVU			Global Days	Modifiers				
Mod	Non-Fac Total	Fac Total		51	50	62	80	MUE
	0.00	0.00	XXX	9	9	9	9	1

AMA: Mar 11: 4, Jul 12: 7, Aug 13: 10

▲ 90685 Influenza virus vaccine, quadrivalent (IIV4), split virus, preservative free, when administered to children 6-35 months of age, for intramuscular use   ⓒL I L

RVU			Global Days	Modifiers				
Mod	Non-Fac Total	Fac Total		51	50	62	80	MUE
	0.00	0.00	XXX	9	9	9	9	1

AMA: Mar 14: 10

Pub 100-04, 18, 1.2, 10.2.1, 10.4.1, 10.4.2, 10.4.3

▲ 90686 Influenza virus vaccine, quadrivalent (IIV4), split virus, preservative free, when administered to individuals 3 years of age and older, for intramuscular use   L I L

RVU			Global Days	Modifiers				
Mod	Non-Fac Total	Fac Total		51	50	62	80	MUE
	0.00	0.00	XXX	9	9	9	9	1

AMA: Mar 14: 10

Pub 100-04, 18, 1.2, 10.2.1, 10.4.1, 10.4.2, 10.4.3

▲ 90687 Influenza virus vaccine, quadrivalent (IIV4), split virus, when administered to children 6-35 months of age, for intramuscular use   ⓒL I L

RVU			Global Days	Modifiers				
Mod	Non-Fac Total	Fac Total		51	50	62	80	MUE
	0.00	0.00	XXX	9	9	9	9	1

AMA: Mar 14: 10

Pub 100-04, 18, 1.2, 10.2.1, 10.4.1, 10.4.2, 10.4.3

▲ 90688 Influenza virus vaccine, quadrivalent (IIV4), split virus, when administered to individuals 3 years of age and older, for intramuscular use   L I L

RVU			Global Days	Modifiers				
Mod	Non-Fac Total	Fac Total		51	50	62	80	MUE
	0.00	0.00	XXX	9	9	9	9	1

AMA: Mar 14: 10

Pub 100-04, 18, 1.2, 10.2.1, 10.4.1, 10.4.2, 10.4.3

● New   ▲ Revised   ✖ Deleted   ⊙ Moderate Sedation   ✚ Add-on Codes   ⊘ High Risk Denial   Ⓐ Age Edit   ♀ Female   ♂ Male   **AMA** *CPT® Assistant*   **MUE** Medically Unlikely Edit
⊘ Modifier 51 Exempt   ⊖ Modifier 63 Exempt   ✄ Unlisted   **Modifiers:** *See Inside Back Cover*   Ⓜ Maternity   A 2 – Z 3 ASC Payment Indicators   A – Y OPPS Status Indicators

CPT © 2015 American Medical Association. All Rights Reserved.   © 2016 DecisionHealth

90690 Typhoid vaccine, live, oral   Ⓝ Ⓘ Ⓝ

	RVU		Global Days	Modifiers				
Mod	Non-Fac Total	Fac Total		51	50	62	80	MUE
	0.00	0.00	XXX	9	9	9	9	1

AMA: Nov 98: 31, 33, Jan 99: 2, Oct 99: 9, Mar 11: 4, Aug 13: 10

90691 Typhoid vaccine, Vi capsular polysaccharide (ViCPs), for intramuscular use   Ⓝ Ⓘ Ⓝ

Coding tip: *Brand name(s): Typhim Vi*

Documentation Finder: *The documentation should support that they are injecting/vaccinating a patient with the following toxoids: Typhoid and Vi capsular polysaccharide (ViCPS). CPT guidelines state that the documentation must clearly support the description of a given CPT code. Make sure there is reference to the actual name of two toxoids being injected.*

	RVU		Global Days	Modifiers				
Mod	Non-Fac Total	Fac Total		51	50	62	80	MUE
	0.00	0.00	XXX	9	9	9	9	1

AMA: Nov 98: 31, 33, Jan 99: 2, Oct 99: 9, Mar 11: 4, Aug 13: 10

✖ 90692 ~~Typhoid vaccine, heat- and phenol-inactivated (H-P), for subcutaneous or intradermal use~~

✖ 90693 ~~Typhoid vaccine, acetone-killed, dried (AKD), for subcutaneous use (U.S. military)~~

▲ 90696 Diphtheria, tetanus toxoids, acellular pertussis vaccine and inactivated poliovirus vaccine (DTaP-IPV), when administered to children 4 through 6 years of age, for intramuscular use   Ⓐ Ⓝ Ⓘ Ⓝ

	RVU		Global Days	Modifiers				
Mod	Non-Fac Total	Fac Total		51	50	62	80	MUE
	0.00	0.00	XXX	9	9	9	9	1

AMA: Mar 11: 4, Aug 13: 10

↗ ● 90697 Diphtheria, tetanus toxoids, acellular pertussis vaccine, inactivated poliovirus vaccine, Haemophilus influenzae type b PRP-OMP conjugate vaccine, and hepatitis B vaccine (DTaP-IPV-Hib-HepB), for intramuscular use   Ⓔ

	RVU		Global Days	Modifiers				
Mod	Non-Fac Total	Fac Total		51	50	62	80	MUE
	0.00	0.00	XXX	9	9	9	9	1

▲ 90698 Diphtheria, tetanus toxoids, acellular pertussis vaccine, haemophilus influenzae type b, and inactivated poliovirus vaccine, (DTap-IPV/Hib), for intramuscular use   Ⓝ Ⓘ Ⓝ

Coding tip: *Brand name(s): Pentacel*

	RVU		Global Days	Modifiers				
Mod	Non-Fac Total	Fac Total		51	50	62	80	MUE
	0.00	0.00	XXX	9	9	9	9	1

AMA: Oct 99: 9, Dec 05: 9, Jun 06: 8, Mar 11: 4, Aug 13: 10

90700 Diphtheria, tetanus toxoids, and acellular pertussis vaccine (DTaP), when administered to individuals younger than 7 years, for intramuscular use   Ⓐ Ⓝ Ⓘ Ⓝ

Coding tip: *Brand name(s): Daptacel, Infanrix, Tripedia*

	RVU		Global Days	Modifiers				
Mod	Non-Fac Total	Fac Total		51	50	62	80	MUE
	0.00	0.00	XXX	9	9	9	9	1

AMA: Jan 96: 5, Apr 97: 10, Nov 98: 31, 33, Jan 99: 2, Oct 99: 9, Nov 03: 13, Mar 11: 4, Jul 12: 7, Aug 13: 10

▲ 90702 Diphtheria and tetanus toxoids adsorbed (DT) when administered to individuals younger than 7 years, for intramuscular use   Ⓐ Ⓝ Ⓘ Ⓝ

	RVU		Global Days	Modifiers				
Mod	Non-Fac Total	Fac Total		51	50	62	80	MUE
	0.00	0.00	XXX	9	9	9	9	1

AMA: Jan 96: 6, Aug 96: 10, Apr 97: 10, Nov 98: 31, 33, Jan 99: 2, Sep 99: 10, Oct 99: 9, Jun 00: 10, Feb 07: 11, Mar 11: 4, Aug 13: 10

✖ 90703 ~~Tetanus toxoid adsorbed, for intramuscular use~~

✖ 90704 ~~Mumps virus vaccine, live, for subcutaneous use~~

✖ 90705 ~~Measles virus vaccine, live, for subcutaneous use~~

✖ 90706 ~~Rubella virus vaccine, live, for subcutaneous use~~

90707 Measles, mumps and rubella virus vaccine (MMR), live, for subcutaneous use   Ⓝ Ⓘ Ⓝ

Coding tip: *Brand name(s): M-M-R II*

	RVU		Global Days	Modifiers				
Mod	Non-Fac Total	Fac Total		51	50	62	80	MUE
	0.00	0.00	XXX	9	9	9	9	1

AMA: Jan 96: 6, May 96: 10, Apr 97: 10, Nov 98: 31, 33, Jan 99: 2, Oct 99: 9, Apr 05: 1, 5, Mar 11: 4, Jul 12: 7, Aug 13: 10

✖ 90708 ~~Measles and rubella virus vaccine, live, for subcutaneous use~~

90710 Measles, mumps, rubella, and varicella vaccine (MMRV), live, for subcutaneous use   Ⓝ Ⓘ Ⓝ

	RVU		Global Days	Modifiers				
Mod	Non-Fac Total	Fac Total		51	50	62	80	MUE
	0.00	0.00	XXX	9	9	9	9	1

AMA: May 96: 10, Apr 97: 10, Nov 98: 31, 33, Jan 99: 2, Oct 99: 9, Dec 05: 9, Jun 06: 8, Mar 11: 4, Aug 13: 10

✖ 90712 ~~Poliovirus vaccine, (any type[s]) (OPV), live, for oral use~~

90713 Poliovirus vaccine, inactivated (IPV), for subcutaneous or intramuscular use   Ⓝ Ⓘ Ⓝ

Coding tip: *Brand name(s): Ipol*

	RVU		Global Days	Modifiers				
Mod	Non-Fac Total	Fac Total		51	50	62	80	MUE
	0.00	0.00	XXX	9	9	9	9	1

AMA: Apr 97: 10, Nov 98: 31, 33, Jan 99: 2, Oct 99: 9, Jun 05: 6, Mar 11: 4, Aug 13: 10

▲ 90714 Tetanus and diphtheria toxoids adsorbed (Td), preservative free, when administered to individuals 7 years or older, for intramuscular use   Ⓝ Ⓘ Ⓝ

Coding tip: *Brand name(s): Decavac*

Documentation Finder: *You will find in the documentation the reference to Td being injected into a patient (vaccination) who is 7 years old or older. This code is for specific combination of toxoids, Tetanus and diphtheria toxoids adsorbed, preservative free.*

	RVU		Global Days	Modifiers				
Mod	Non-Fac Total	Fac Total		51	50	62	80	MUE
	0.00	0.00	XXX	9	9	9	9	1

AMA: Jun 05: 6, Mar 11: 4, Aug 13: 10

● New   ▲ Revised   Deleted   ⊙ Moderate Sedation   ✚ Add-on Codes   ⊗ High Risk Denial   Ⓐ Age Edit   ♀ Female   ♂ Male   **AMA** *CPT® Assistant*   **MUE** Medically Unlikely Edit
Ⓢ Modifier 51 Exempt   ⊖ Modifier 63 Exempt   Ⓧ Unlisted   **Modifiers:** *See Inside Back Cover*   Ⓜ Maternity   A2–Z3 ASC Payment Indicators   A–Y OPPS Status Indicators

90715 Tetanus, diphtheria toxoids and acellular pertussis vaccine (Tdap), when administered to individuals 7 years or older, for intramuscular use ⊘N I N

Coding tip: Brand name(s): Adacel

Documentation Finder: The documentation will reference an injection or vaccination of Tdap into a patient who is 7 years old or older. This code is for specific combination of toxoids, Tetanus, diphtheria toxoids and acellular pertussis.

RVU			Global Days	Modifiers				
Mod	*Non-Fac Total*	*Fac Total*		51	50	62	80	MUE
	0.00	0.00	XXX	9	9	9	9	1

AMA: Oct 99: 9, Jun 05: 6, Dec 05: 9, Jun 06: 8, Mar 11: 4, Aug 13: 10

▲ **90716 Varicella virus vaccine (VAR), live, for subcutaneous use** ⊘M

Coding tip: Brand name(s): Varivax

RVU			Global Days	Modifiers				
Mod	*Non-Fac Total*	*Fac Total*		51	50	62	80	MUE
	0.00	0.00	XXX	9	9	9	9	1

AMA: Jan 96: 6, May 96: 10, Apr 97: 10, Nov 98: 31, 33, Jan 99: 2, Oct 99: 9, Mar 11: 4, Aug 13: 10

90717 Yellow fever vaccine, live, for subcutaneous use ⊘N I N

Coding tip: Brand name(s): YF-Vax

RVU			Global Days	Modifiers				
Mod	*Non-Fac Total*	*Fac Total*		51	50	62	80	MUE
	0.00	0.00	XXX	9	9	9	9	1

AMA: Apr 97: 10, Nov 98: 31, 33, Jan 99: 2, Oct 99: 9, Mar 11: 4, Aug 13: 10

✖ ~~90719 Diphtheria toxoid, for intramuscular use~~

✖ ~~90720 Diphtheria, tetanus toxoids, and whole cell pertussis vaccine and Hemophilus influenza B vaccine (DTP-Hib), for intramuscular use~~

✖ ~~90721 Diphtheria, tetanus toxoids, and acellular pertussis vaccine and Hemophilus influenza B vaccine (DTaP/Hib), for intramuscular use~~

90723 Diphtheria, tetanus toxoids, acellular pertussis vaccine, hepatitis B, and inactivated poliovirus vaccine (DTaP-HepB-IPV), for intramuscular use ⊘E

Coding tip: Brand name(s): Pediarix

RVU			Global Days	Modifiers				
Mod	*Non-Fac Total*	*Fac Total*		51	50	62	80	MUE
	0.00	0.00	XXX	9	9	9	9	

AMA: Apr 97: 10, Oct 99: 9, Mar 11: 4, Aug 13: 10, May 15: 6

✖ ~~90725 Cholera vaccine for injectable use~~

✖ ~~90727 Plague vaccine, for intramuscular use~~

▲ **90732 Pneumococcal polysaccharide vaccine, 23-valent (PPSV23), adult or immunosuppressed patient dosage, when administered to individuals 2 years or older, for subcutaneous or intramuscular use** L I L

Coding tip: Brand name(s): Pneumovax 23

RVU			Global Days	Modifiers				
Mod	*Non-Fac Total*	*Fac Total*		51	50	62	80	MUE
	0.00	0.00	XXX	9	9	9	9	1

AMA: Apr 97: 10, Nov 98: 31, 33, Jan 99: 2, Oct 99: 9, Mar 11: 4, Aug 13: 10
Pub 100-04, 18, 1.2, 10.2.1, 10.4.1, 10.4.2, 10.4.3

▲ **90733 Meningococcal polysaccharide vaccine, serogroups A, C, Y, W-135, quadrivalent (MPSV4), for subcutaneous use** ⊘K 2 K

Coding tip: Brand name(s): Menomune

RVU			Global Days	Modifiers				
Mod	*Non-Fac Total*	*Fac Total*		51	50	62	80	MUE
	0.00	0.00	XXX	9	9	9	9	1

AMA: Apr 97: 10, Nov 98: 31, 33, Jan 99: 2, Oct 99: 9, Dec 99: 7, Mar 11: 4, Aug 13: 10

▲ **90734 Meningococcal conjugate vaccine, serogroups A, C, Y and W-135, quadrivalent (MenACWY), for intramuscular use** ⊘K 2 K

Coding tip: Brand name(s): Menactra, Menveo

RVU			Global Days	Modifiers				
Mod	*Non-Fac Total*	*Fac Total*		51	50	62	80	MUE
	0.00	0.00	XXX	9	9	9	9	1

AMA: Oct 99: 9, Mar 11: 4, Aug 13: 10, May 15: 6

✖ ~~90735 Japanese encephalitis virus vaccine, for subcutaneous use~~

▲ **90736 Zoster (shingles) vaccine (HZV), live, for subcutaneous injection** ⊘M

Coding tip: Brand name(s): Zostavax

RVU			Global Days	Modifiers				
Mod	*Non-Fac Total*	*Fac Total*		51	50	62	80	MUE
	0.00	0.00	XXX	9	9	9	9	1

AMA: Dec 05: 9, Jun 06: 8, Jul 07: 13, Mar 11: 4, Aug 13: 10

90738 Japanese encephalitis virus vaccine, inactivated, for intramuscular use ⊘M

RVU			Global Days	Modifiers				
Mod	*Non-Fac Total*	*Fac Total*		51	50	62	80	MUE
	0.00	0.00	XXX	9	9	9	9	1

AMA: Mar 11: 4, Aug 13: 10

↗▲ **90739 Hepatitis B vaccine (HepB), adult dosage, 2 dose schedule, for intramuscular use** ⊘E

RVU			Global Days	Modifiers				
Mod	*Non-Fac Total*	*Fac Total*		51	50	62	80	MUE
	0.00	0.00	XXX	9	9	9	9	1

AMA: Aug 13: 10
Pub 100-04, 18, 1.2, 10.2.1

▲ **90740 Hepatitis B vaccine (HepB), dialysis or immunosuppressed patient dosage, 3 dose schedule, for intramuscular use** F 4 F

RVU			Global Days	Modifiers				
Mod	*Non-Fac Total*	*Fac Total*		51	50	62	80	MUE
	0.00	0.00	XXX	9	9	9	9	1

AMA: Apr 97: 10, Oct 99: 9, Apr 01: 10, Mar 11: 4, Aug 13: 10
Pub 100-04, 18, 1.2, 10.2.1

▲ **90743 Hepatitis B vaccine (HepB), adolescent, 2 dose schedule, for intramuscular use** F 4 F

RVU			Global Days	Modifiers				
Mod	*Non-Fac Total*	*Fac Total*		51	50	62	80	MUE
	0.00	0.00	XXX	9	9	9	9	1

AMA: Apr 97: 10, Oct 99: 9, Mar 11: 4, Aug 13: 10
Pub 100-04, 18, 1.2, 10.2.1

● New   ▲ Revised   ✖ Deleted   ⊙ Moderate Sedation   ✚ Add-on Codes   ⊘ High Risk Denial   ⒶAge Edit   ♀ Female   ♂ Male   **AMA** *CPT® Assistant*   **MUE** Medically Unlikely Edit
⊘ Modifier 51 Exempt   ⊖ Modifier 63 Exempt   ⊠ Unlisted   **Modifiers:** *See Inside Back Cover*   Ⓜ Maternity   A 2–Z 3 ASC Payment Indicators   A –Y OPPS Status Indicators

CPT © 2015 American Medical Association. All Rights Reserved.   © 2016 DecisionHealth

▲ **90744 Hepatitis B vaccine (HepB), pediatric/adolescent dosage, 3 dose schedule, for intramuscular use** ⒸF 4 F

RVU			Global Days	Modifiers				
Mod	Non-Fac Total	Fac Total		51	50	62	80	MUE
	0.00	0.00	XXX	9	9	9	9	1

AMA: Jan 96: 5, Apr 97: 10, Jun 97: 10, Nov 98: 31, 33, Jan 99: 2, Oct 99: 9, Nov 99: 48, 49, Jun 00: 10, Mar 11: 4, Aug 13: 10

Pub 100-04, 18, 1.2, 10.2.1

▲ **90746 Hepatitis B vaccine (HepB), adult dosage, 3 dose schedule, for intramuscular use** F 4 F

RVU			Global Days	Modifiers				
Mod	Non-Fac Total	Fac Total		51	50	62	80	MUE
	0.00	0.00	XXX	9	9	9	9	1

AMA: Jan 96: 5, Apr 97: 10, Nov 98: 31, 33, Jan 99: 2, Oct 99: 9, Mar 11: 4, Aug 13: 10

Pub 100-04, 18, 1.2, 10.2.1

▲ **90747 Hepatitis B vaccine (HepB), dialysis or immunosuppressed patient dosage, 4 dose schedule, for intramuscular use** F 4 F

RVU			Global Days	Modifiers				
Mod	Non-Fac Total	Fac Total		51	50	62	80	MUE
	0.00	0.00	XXX	9	9	9	9	1

AMA: Jan 96: 5, Apr 97: 10, Jun 97: 10, Nov 98: 31, 33, Jan 99: 2, Oct 99: 9, Jun 00: 10, Apr 01: 10, Mar 11: 4, Aug 13: 10

Pub 100-04, 18, 1.2, 10.2.1

▲ **90748 Hepatitis B and Haemophilus influenzae type b vaccine (Hib-HepB), for intramuscular use** ⒸE

Coding tip: Brand name(s): Comvax

RVU			Global Days	Modifiers				
Mod	Non-Fac Total	Fac Total		51	50	62	80	MUE
	0.00	0.00	XXX	9	9	9		

AMA: Apr 97: 10, Nov 97: 37, Nov 98: 31, 33, Jan 99: 2, Sep 99: 10, Oct 99: 9, Mar 11: 4, Jul 12: 7, Aug 13: 10

90749 Unlisted vaccine/toxoid Ⓢ✗N I N

RVU			Global Days	Modifiers				
Mod	Non-Fac Total	Fac Total		51	50	62	80	MUE
	0.00	0.00	XXX	9	9	9	9	

AMA: Jan 96: 6, Apr 97: 10, Jun 97: 10, Nov 98: 31, 33, Jan 99: 2, Oct 99: 9, Nov 02: 11, Mar 11: 4, May 15: 6

Interactive Complexity

Coding Guidance

Interactive complexity is an additional service that should be reported for services that require additional work due to specific communication factors that complicate psychiatric diagnostic procedures (90791, 90792), psychotherapy with or without evaluation and management services (90832-90838), evaluation and management services (99201-99255, 99304-99337, 99341-99350) and group psychotherapy (90853).

✚ **90785 Interactive complexity (List separately in addition to the code for primary procedure)** N

RVU			Global Days	Modifiers				
Mod	Non-Fac Total	Fac Total		51	50	62	80	MUE
	0.39	0.39	ZZZ	0	0	0	9	1

AMA: Apr 14: 6, May 13: 12, Jun 13: 3

Psychiatric Diagnostic Evaluation

Coding Guidance

Report psychiatric diagnostic evaluation codes 99791 and 99792 for the initial diagnostic assessment and subsequent reassessments when medically necessary. These codes are reported only when no psychotherapy services are performed on the same date of service. For ongoing diagnostic assessments performed with psychotherapy services, refer to codes 90832-90938, 90839-90840.

90791 Psychiatric diagnostic evaluation Ⓠ3

RVU			Global Days	Modifiers				
Mod	Non-Fac Total	Fac Total		51	50	62	80	MUE
	3.69	3.58	XXX	0	0	0	9	1

AMA: May 13: 12, Jun 13: 3, Dec 13: 18, Jun 14: 3

Pub 100-04, 12, 190.3

90792 Psychiatric diagnostic evaluation with medical services Ⓠ3

RVU			Global Days	Modifiers				
Mod	Non-Fac Total	Fac Total		51	50	62	80	MUE
	4.09	3.97	XXX	0	0	0	9	1

AMA: Jun 13: 3, Dec 13: 18, Jun 14: 3

Pub 100-04, 12, 190.3

Psychotherapy

Coding Guidance

Psychotherapy services are reported based on the actual face-to-face time spent with the patient and/or family. Psychotherapy codes 99832-99838 can only be reported when the patient is present for a portion of the service. If the patient is not present, refer to code 90846. When psychotherapy is provided in conjunction with a significant, separately identifiable evaluation and management service, the evaluation and management service (99201-99255, 99304-99337, 99341-99350) is reported as the primary service and an additional code is reported for the psychotherapy service (90833, 90836, 90838) based on the face-to-face time spent providing psychotherapy services.

90832 Psychotherapy, 30 minutes with patient and/or family member Ⓠ3

RVU			Global Days	Modifiers				
Mod	Non-Fac Total	Fac Total		51	50	62	80	MUE
	1.79	1.77	XXX	0	0	0	9	1

AMA: Jan 13: 3, May 13: 12, Jun 13: 3, Aug 13: 14, Feb 14: 3, Aug 14: 5

Pub 100-04, 12, 190.3

✚ **90833 Psychotherapy, 30 minutes with patient and/or family member when performed with an evaluation and management service (List separately in addition to the code for primary procedure)** N

RVU			Global Days	Modifiers				
Mod	Non-Fac Total	Fac Total		51	50	62	80	MUE
	1.85	1.83	ZZZ	0	0	0	9	1

AMA: Jan 13: 3, May 13: 12, Jun 13: 3, Aug 13: 14, Aug 14: 5

90834 Psychotherapy, 45 minutes with patient and/or family member Ⓠ3

RVU			Global Days	Modifiers				
Mod	Non-Fac Total	Fac Total		51	50	62	80	MUE
	2.38	2.36	XXX	0	0	0	9	1

AMA: Jan 13: 3, May 13: 12, Jun 13: 3, Aug 13: 14, Jun 14: 3

Pub 100-04, 12, 190.3

● New ▲ Revised Deleted ⊙ Moderate Sedation ✚ Add-on Codes ⊗ High Risk Denial Ⓐ Age Edit ♀ Female ♂ Male **AMA** *CPT® Assistant* **MUE** Medically Unlikely Edit ⊘ Modifier 51 Exempt ⊖ Modifier 63 Exempt ✗ Unlisted **Modifiers:** *See Inside Back Cover* Ⓜ Maternity Ⓐ2–Ⓩ3 ASC Payment Indicators Ⓐ–Ⓨ OPPS Status Indicators

© 2016 DecisionHealth | CPT © 2015 American Medical Association. All Rights Reserved. | **787**

Medicine Procedures

90836 – 90867

✚ **90836** Psychotherapy, 45 minutes with patient and/or family member when performed with an evaluation and management service (List separately in addition to the code for primary procedure) 🅽

Mod	RVU Non-Fac Total	Fac Total	Global Days	Modifiers 51	50	62	80	MUE
	2.35	2.33	ZZZ	0	0	0	9	1

AMA: Jan 13: 3, May 13: 12, Jun 13: 3, Aug 13: 14

Pub 100-04, 12, 190.3

90837 Psychotherapy, 60 minutes with patient and/or family member ⓠ3

Mod	RVU Non-Fac Total	Fac Total	Global Days	Modifiers 51	50	62	80	MUE
	3.57	3.55	XXX	0	0	0	9	1

AMA: Jan 13: 3, May 13: 12, Jun 13: 3, Aug 13: 14, Apr 14: 6

✚ **90838** Psychotherapy, 60 minutes with patient and/or family member when performed with an evaluation and management service (List separately in addition to the code for primary procedure) 🅽

Mod	RVU Non-Fac Total	Fac Total	Global Days	Modifiers 51	50	62	80	MUE
	3.10	3.08	ZZZ	0	0	0	9	1

AMA: Jan 13: 3, May 13: 12, Jun 13: 3, Aug 13: 14, Apr 14: 6, Feb 14: 3

Pub 100-04, 12, 190.3

Coding Guidance

Codes for psychotherapy for crises should be reported for patients in severe distress requiring immediate care often for a life-threatening situation. Psychotherapy for crisis is reported based on total face-to-face time spent with the patient and/or family.

90839 Psychotherapy for crisis; first 60 minutes ⓠ3

Mod	RVU Non-Fac Total	Fac Total	Global Days	Modifiers 51	50	62	80	MUE
	3.73	3.70	XXX	0	0	0	0	1

AMA: Jun 13: 3, Aug 14: 5

✚ **90840** Psychotherapy for crisis; each additional 30 minutes (List separately in addition to code for primary service) 🅒🅝

Documentation Finder: *If the documentation states that at least 77 minutes was spent providing psychotherapy, this add-on code would be supported with **90839** (Psychotherapy for crisis; first 60 minutes).*

Mod	RVU Non-Fac Total	Fac Total	Global Days	Modifiers 51	50	62	80	MUE
	1.78	1.77	ZZZ	0	0	0	0	

AMA: Jun 13: 3, Aug 14: 5

90845 Psychoanalysis ⓠ3

Mod	RVU Non-Fac Total	Fac Total	Global Days	Modifiers 51	50	62	80	MUE
	2.57	2.56	XXX	0	0	0	0	1

AMA: Summer 92: 15, Nov 97: 40, 41, Mar 01: 8, Mar 02: 4, May 05: 1, Feb 06: 15, Mar 10: 6

90846 Family psychotherapy (without the patient present) ⓠ3

Mod	RVU Non-Fac Total	Fac Total	Global Days	Modifiers 51	50	62	80	MUE
	2.89	2.87	XXX	0	0	0	0	1

AMA: Summer 92: 15, Nov 97: 40, 41, Mar 01: 8, Mar 02: 4, May 05: 1, Mar 10: 6, Sep 09: 11, Jun 13: 3, Dec 13: 18

90847 Family psychotherapy (conjoint psychotherapy) (with patient present) ⓠ3

Mod	RVU Non-Fac Total	Fac Total	Global Days	Modifiers 51	50	62	80	MUE
	2.99	2.97	XXX	0	0	0	0	1

AMA: Summer 92: 15, Nov 97: 40, 41, Mar 01: 5, Mar 02: 4, May 05: 1, Mar 10: 6, Jun 13: 3, Dec 13: 18

Pub 100-04, 13, 70.2

90849 Multiple-family group psychotherapy ⓠ3

Mod	RVU Non-Fac Total	Fac Total	Global Days	Modifiers 51	50	62	80	MUE
	0.96	0.86	XXX	0	0	0	0	1

AMA: Summer 92: 15, Nov 97: 40, 41, Mar 01: 5, Mar 02: 4, May 05: 1, Mar 10: 6, Aug 14: 15

90853 Group psychotherapy (other than of a multiple-family group) ⓠ3

Mod	RVU Non-Fac Total	Fac Total	Global Days	Modifiers 51	50	62	80	MUE
	0.72	0.71	XXX	0	0	0	0	1

AMA: Summer 92: 15, Nov 97: 40, 41, Mar 01: 8, Mar 02: 4, May 05: 1, Mar 10: 6, Jun 13: 3, Jun 14: 3, Aug 14: 15

Coding Guidance

Report code 90863 for pharmocologic management only when provided in conjunction with a psychotherapy service that does not have an evaluation and management component (90832, 90834, 90837). When evaluation and management services are provided on the same date of service, pharmcologic managment is included in the evaluation and management service and is not reported additionally.

✚ **90863** Pharmacologic management, including prescription and review of medication, when performed with psychotherapy services (List separately in addition to the code for primary procedure) 🅒🅔

Mod	RVU Non-Fac Total	Fac Total	Global Days	Modifiers 51	50	62	80	MUE
	0.00	0.00	XXX	9	9	9	9	1

AMA: Jun 13: 3

90865 Narcosynthesis for psychiatric diagnostic and therapeutic purposes (eg, sodium amobarbital (Amytal) interview) ⓠ3

Mod	RVU Non-Fac Total	Fac Total	Global Days	Modifiers 51	50	62	80	MUE
	4.69	3.63	XXX	0	0	0	0	1

AMA: Nov 97: 41, Mar 01: 5, Mar 02: 4, May 05: 1

90867 Therapeutic repetitive transcranial magnetic stimulation (TMS) treatment; initial, including cortical mapping, motor threshold determination, delivery and management 🆂

Mod	RVU Non-Fac Total	Fac Total	Global Days	Modifiers 51	50	62	80	MUE
	0.00	0.00	000	0	0	0	1	1

● New   ▲ Revised   ✖ Deleted   ⊙ Moderate Sedation   ✚ Add-on Codes   ⊘ High Risk Denial   ⓐ Age Edit   ♀ Female   ♂ Male   **AMA** *CPT® Assistant*   **MUE** Medically Unlikely Edit
⊘ Modifier 51 Exempt   ⊖ Modifier 63 Exempt   🛇 Unlisted   **Modifiers:** *See Inside Back Cover*   Ⓜ Maternity   Ⓐ2–Ⓩ3 ASC Payment Indicators   Ⓐ–Ⓨ OPPS Status Indicators

CPT © 2015 American Medical Association. All Rights Reserved.   © 2016 DecisionHealth

90868 Therapeutic repetitive transcranial magnetic stimulation (TMS) treatment; subsequent delivery and management, per session [S]

RVU			Global Days	Modifiers				
Mod	Non-Fac Total	Fac Total		51	50	62	80	MUE
	0.00	0.00	000	0	0	0	1	1

90869 Therapeutic repetitive transcranial magnetic stimulation (TMS) treatment; subsequent motor threshold re-determination with delivery and management [S]

RVU			Global Days	Modifiers				
Mod	Non-Fac Total	Fac Total		51	50	62	80	MUE
	0.00	0.00	000	0	0	0	1	1

90870 Electroconvulsive therapy (includes necessary monitoring) [S]

RVU			Global Days	Modifiers				
Mod	Non-Fac Total	Fac Total		51	50	62	80	MUE
	4.99	3.12	000	0	0	0	0	2

AMA: Summer 92: 16, Mar 01: 5, Mar 02: 4, May 05: 1, Mar 10: 6, Feb 13: 3

90875 Individual psychophysiological therapy incorporating biofeedback training by any modality (face-to-face with the patient), with psychotherapy (eg, insight oriented, behavior modifying or supportive psychotherapy); 30 minutes [CE]

RVU			Global Days	Modifiers				
Mod	Non-Fac Total	Fac Total		51	50	62	80	MUE
	1.73	1.73	XXX	9	9	9	9	

AMA: Nov 96: 15, Sep 97: 11, Nov 97: 41, Apr 98: 14, Jun 99: 5, Mar 01: 5, Mar 02: 4, Mar 05: 16, May 05: 1

90876 Individual psychophysiological therapy incorporating biofeedback training by any modality (face-to-face with the patient), with psychotherapy (eg, insight oriented, behavior modifying or supportive psychotherapy); 45 minutes [CE]

RVU			Global Days	Modifiers				
Mod	Non-Fac Total	Fac Total		51	50	62	80	MUE
	3.05	2.74	XXX	9	9	9	9	

AMA: Nov 96: 15, Sep 97: 11, Nov 97: 41, Jun 99: 5, Mar 01: 5, Mar 05: 16, May 05: 1

90880 Hypnotherapy [Q3]

RVU			Global Days	Modifiers				
Mod	Non-Fac Total	Fac Total		51	50	62	80	MUE
	2.85	2.64	XXX	0	0	0	0	1

AMA: Summer 92: 16, Nov 97: 41, Mar 01: 5, Mar 02: 4, May 05: 1

90882 Environmental intervention for medical management purposes on a psychiatric patient's behalf with agencies, employers, or institutions [CE]

RVU			Global Days	Modifiers				
Mod	Non-Fac Total	Fac Total		51	50	62	80	MUE
	0.00	0.00	XXX	9	9	9	9	

AMA: Summer 92: 16, Mar 01: 5, Mar 02: 4, May 05: 1

90885 Psychiatric evaluation of hospital records, other psychiatric reports, psychometric and/or projective tests, and other accumulated data for medical diagnostic purposes [CN]

RVU			Global Days	Modifiers				
Mod	Non-Fac Total	Fac Total		51	50	62	80	MUE
	1.40	1.40	XXX	9	9	9	9	0

AMA: Nov 97: 41, Mar 01: 5, Mar 02: 4, Oct 04: 10, May 05: 1

90887 Interpretation or explanation of results of psychiatric, other medical examinations and procedures, or other accumulated data to family or other responsible persons, or advising them how to assist patient [CN]

RVU			Global Days	Modifiers				
Mod	Non-Fac Total	Fac Total		51	50	62	80	MUE
	2.49	2.14	XXX	9	9	9	9	0

AMA: Summer 92: 17, Mar 01: 5, Mar 02: 4, Oct 02: 11, May 05: 1

90889 Preparation of report of patient's psychiatric status, history, treatment, or progress (other than for legal or consultative purposes) for other individuals, agencies, or insurance carriers [CN]

RVU			Global Days	Modifiers				
Mod	Non-Fac Total	Fac Total		51	50	62	80	MUE
	0.00	0.00	XXX	9	9	9	9	0

AMA: Summer 92: 17, Mar 01: 5, Mar 02: 4, May 05: 1

90899 Unlisted psychiatric service or procedure [⊘x Q3]

RVU			Global Days	Modifiers				
Mod	Non-Fac Total	Fac Total		51	50	62	80	MUE
	0.00	0.00	XXX	0	0	0	0	

AMA: Mar 01: 5, Mar 02: 4, May 05: 1, Jan 10: 11, Apr 14: 6

Biofeedback Services

90901 Biofeedback training by any modality [A]

Documentation Finder: You should not find reference in the documentation to using psychophysiological therapy to determine the biofeedback. You should see reference to helping the patient gain voluntary control over his or her body functions. One example of documentation for code 90901 could be a patient that is being monitored with surface EMG electrodes placed over muscles that are causing ongoing tension. A session can last as short as 30 minutes to even longer.

RVU			Global Days	Modifiers				
Mod	Non-Fac Total	Fac Total		51	50	62	80	MUE
	1.08	0.56	000	0	0	0	0	1

AMA: Sep 97: 11, Apr 98: 14, Jun 98: 10, Jun 99: 5, May 02: 18, Sep 04: 13, Mar 05: 16

90911 Biofeedback training, perineal muscles, anorectal or urethral sphincter, including EMG and/or manometry [S]

RVU			Global Days	Modifiers				
Mod	Non-Fac Total	Fac Total		51	50	62	80	MUE
	2.37	1.26	000	0	0	0	0	1

AMA: Sep 97: 11, Nov 97: 41, Jun 98: 10, Jun 99: 5, Sep 14: 14

● New   ▲ Revised   Deleted   ⊙ Moderate Sedation   ✚ Add-on Codes   ⊘ High Risk Denial   Ⓐ Age Edit   ♀ Female   ♂ Male   **AMA** CPT® Assistant   **MUE** Medically Unlikely Edit
⊘ Modifier 51 Exempt   ⊖ Modifier 63 Exempt   ⊠ Unlisted   **Modifiers:** See Inside Back Cover   Ⓜ Maternity   [A2]–[Z3] ASC Payment Indicators   [A]–[Y] OPPS Status Indicators

© 2016 DecisionHealth   CPT © 2015 American Medical Association. All Rights Reserved.   **789**

Medicine Procedures

90935 – 90956

Hemodialysis Services/Procedures

90935 Hemodialysis procedure with single evaluation by a physician or other qualified health care professional ⓢ

RVU			Global Days	Modifiers				
Mod	Non-Fac Total	Fac Total		51	50	62	80	MUE
	2.04	2.04	000	0	0	0	0	1

AMA: Fall 93: 2, May 02: 17, Jan 03: 22

90937 Hemodialysis procedure requiring repeated evaluation(s) with or without substantial revision of dialysis prescription ⓑ

RVU			Global Days	Modifiers				
Mod	Non-Fac Total	Fac Total		51	50	62	80	MUE
	2.93	2.93	000	0	0	0	0	1

AMA: Fall 93: 2, May 02: 17, Jan 03: 22

90940 Hemodialysis access flow study to determine blood flow in grafts and arteriovenous fistulae by an indicator method ⊘ⓝ

RVU			Global Days	Modifiers				
Mod	Non-Fac Total	Fac Total		51	50	62	80	MUE
	0.00	0.00	XXX	9	9	9	9	2

AMA: Jan 03: 22, May 06: 18

Miscellaneous Dialysis Services/Procedures

90945 Dialysis procedure other than hemodialysis (eg, peritoneal dialysis, hemofiltration, or other continuous renal replacement therapies), with single evaluation by a physician or other qualified health care professional ⓥ

RVU			Global Days	Modifiers				
Mod	Non-Fac Total	Fac Total		51	50	62	80	MUE
	2.42	2.42	000	0	0	0	0	1

AMA: Fall 93: 2, Nov 97: 41, Jul 98: 10, Oct 01: 11, Jan 03: 22

90947 Dialysis procedure other than hemodialysis (eg, peritoneal dialysis, hemofiltration, or other continuous renal replacement therapies) requiring repeated evaluations by a physician or other qualified health care professional, with or without substantial revision of dialysis prescription ⓑ

RVU			Global Days	Modifiers				
Mod	Non-Fac Total	Fac Total		51	50	62	80	MUE
	3.50	3.50	000	0	0	0	0	1

AMA: Fall 93: 2, Nov 97: 41, Jul 98: 10, Oct 01: 11, Jan 03: 22

ESRD-Related Services

90951 End-stage renal disease (ESRD) related services monthly, for patients younger than 2 years of age to include monitoring for the adequacy of nutrition, assessment of growth and development, and counseling of parents; with 4 or more face-to-face visits by a physician or other qualified health care professional per month ⒶⓂ

RVU			Global Days	Modifiers				
Mod	Non-Fac Total	Fac Total		51	50	62	80	MUE
	26.62	26.62	XXX	0	0	0	0	1

AMA: Apr 13: 3, Nov 13: 3, Oct 14: 3
Pub 100-04, 12, 190.3

90952 End-stage renal disease (ESRD) related services monthly, for patients younger than 2 years of age to include monitoring for the adequacy of nutrition, assessment of growth and development, and counseling of parents; with 2-3 face-to-face visits by a physician or other qualified health care professional per month ⊘ⒶⓂ

RVU			Global Days	Modifiers				
Mod	Non-Fac Total	Fac Total		51	50	62	80	MUE
	0.00	0.00	XXX	0	0	0	0	1

AMA: Apr 13: 3
Pub 100-04, 12, 190.3

90953 End-stage renal disease (ESRD) related services monthly, for patients younger than 2 years of age to include monitoring for the adequacy of nutrition, assessment of growth and development, and counseling of parents; with 1 face-to-face visit by a physician or other qualified health care professional per month ⒶⓂ

RVU			Global Days	Modifiers				
Mod	Non-Fac Total	Fac Total		51	50	62	80	MUE
	0.00	0.00	XXX	0	0	0	0	1

AMA: Apr 13: 3

90954 End-stage renal disease (ESRD) related services monthly, for patients 2-11 years of age to include monitoring for the adequacy of nutrition, assessment of growth and development, and counseling of parents; with 4 or more face-to-face visits by a physician or other qualified health care professional per month ⒶⓂ

RVU			Global Days	Modifiers				
Mod	Non-Fac Total	Fac Total		51	50	62	80	MUE
	23.01	23.01	XXX	0	0	0	0	1

AMA: Apr 13: 3
Pub 100-04, 12, 190.3

90955 End-stage renal disease (ESRD) related services monthly, for patients 2-11 years of age to include monitoring for the adequacy of nutrition, assessment of growth and development, and counseling of parents; with 2-3 face-to-face visits by a physician or other qualified health care professional per month ⒶⓂ

RVU			Global Days	Modifiers				
Mod	Non-Fac Total	Fac Total		51	50	62	80	MUE
	12.88	12.88	XXX	0	0	0	0	1

AMA: Apr 13: 3
Pub 100-04, 12, 190.3

90956 End-stage renal disease (ESRD) related services monthly, for patients 2-11 years of age to include monitoring for the adequacy of nutrition, assessment of growth and development, and counseling of parents; with 1 face-to-face visit by a physician or other qualified health care professional per month ⒶⓂ

RVU			Global Days	Modifiers				
Mod	Non-Fac Total	Fac Total		51	50	62	80	MUE
	8.98	8.98	XXX	0	0	0	0	1

AMA: Apr 13: 3

● New ▲ Revised ✖ Deleted ⊙ Moderate Sedation ✚ Add-on Codes ⊘ High Risk Denial Ⓐ Age Edit ♀ Female ♂ Male **AMA** *CPT® Assistant* **MUE** Medically Unlikely Edit
⊘ Modifier 51 Exempt ⊖ Modifier 63 Exempt ⓧ Unlisted **Modifiers:** *See Inside Back Cover* Ⓜ Maternity Ⓐ2–Ⓩ3 ASC Payment Indicators Ⓐ–Ⓨ OPPS Status Indicators

CPT © 2015 American Medical Association. All Rights Reserved. | © 2016 DecisionHealth

90957 End-stage renal disease (ESRD) related services monthly, for patients 12-19 years of age to include monitoring for the adequacy of nutrition, assessment of growth and development, and counseling of parents; with 4 or more face-to-face visits by a physician or other qualified health care professional per month   Ⓜ

RVU			Global Days	Modifiers				
Mod	Non-Fac Total	Fac Total		51	50	62	80	MUE
	18.19	18.19	XXX	0	0	0	0	1

AMA: Apr 13: 3
Pub 100-04, 12, 190.3

90958 End-stage renal disease (ESRD) related services monthly, for patients 12-19 years of age to include monitoring for the adequacy of nutrition, assessment of growth and development, and counseling of parents; with 2-3 face-to-face visits by a physician or other qualified health care professional per month   Ⓜ

RVU			Global Days	Modifiers				
Mod	Non-Fac Total	Fac Total		51	50	62	80	MUE
	12.28	12.28	XXX	0	0	0	0	1

AMA: Apr 13: 3
Pub 100-04, 12, 190.3

90959 End-stage renal disease (ESRD) related services monthly, for patients 12-19 years of age to include monitoring for the adequacy of nutrition, assessment of growth and development, and counseling of parents; with 1 face-to-face visit by a physician or other qualified health care professional per month   Ⓜ

RVU			Global Days	Modifiers				
Mod	Non-Fac Total	Fac Total		51	50	62	80	MUE
	8.34	8.34	XXX	0	0	0	0	1

AMA: Apr 13: 3

90960 End-stage renal disease (ESRD) related services monthly, for patients 20 years of age and older; with 4 or more face-to-face visits by a physician or other qualified health care professional per month   ⒶⓂ

RVU			Global Days	Modifiers				
Mod	Non-Fac Total	Fac Total		51	50	62	80	MUE
	7.99	7.99	XXX	0	0	0	0	1

AMA: Apr 13: 3
Pub 100-04, 12, 190.3

90961 End-stage renal disease (ESRD) related services monthly, for patients 20 years of age and older; with 2-3 face-to-face visits by a physician or other qualified health care professional per month   ⒶⓂ

RVU			Global Days	Modifiers				
Mod	Non-Fac Total	Fac Total		51	50	62	80	MUE
	6.72	6.72	XXX	0	0	0	0	1

AMA: Apr 13: 3
Pub 100-04, 12, 190.3

90962 End-stage renal disease (ESRD) related services monthly, for patients 20 years of age and older; with 1 face-to-face visit by a physician or other qualified health care professional per month   ⒶⓂ

RVU			Global Days	Modifiers				
Mod	Non-Fac Total	Fac Total		51	50	62	80	MUE
	5.18	5.18	XXX	0	0	0	0	1

AMA: Apr 13: 3

90963 End-stage renal disease (ESRD) related services for home dialysis per full month, for patients younger than 2 years of age to include monitoring for the adequacy of nutrition, assessment of growth and development, and counseling of parents   ⒶⓂ

RVU			Global Days	Modifiers				
Mod	Non-Fac Total	Fac Total		51	50	62	80	MUE
	15.34	15.34	XXX	0	0	0	0	1

AMA: Apr 13: 3

90964 End-stage renal disease (ESRD) related services for home dialysis per full month, for patients 2-11 years of age to include monitoring for the adequacy of nutrition, assessment of growth and development, and counseling of parents   ⒶⓂ

RVU			Global Days	Modifiers				
Mod	Non-Fac Total	Fac Total		51	50	62	80	MUE
	13.41	13.41	XXX	0	0	0	0	1

AMA: Apr 13: 3

90965 End-stage renal disease (ESRD) related services for home dialysis per full month, for patients 12-19 years of age to include monitoring for the adequacy of nutrition, assessment of growth and development, and counseling of parents   Ⓜ

RVU			Global Days	Modifiers				
Mod	Non-Fac Total	Fac Total		51	50	62	80	MUE
	12.76	12.76	XXX	0	0	0	0	1

AMA: Apr 13: 3

90966 End-stage renal disease (ESRD) related services for home dialysis per full month, for patients 20 years of age and older   ⒶⓂ

RVU			Global Days	Modifiers				
Mod	Non-Fac Total	Fac Total		51	50	62	80	MUE
	6.70	6.70	XXX	0	0	0	0	1

AMA: Apr 13: 3

90967 End-stage renal disease (ESRD) related services for dialysis less than a full month of service, per day; for patients younger than 2 years of age   ⒶⓂ

RVU			Global Days	Modifiers				
Mod	Non-Fac Total	Fac Total		51	50	62	80	MUE
	0.51	0.51	XXX	0	0	0	0	1

AMA: Apr 13: 3

90968 End-stage renal disease (ESRD) related services for dialysis less than a full month of service, per day; for patients 2-11 years of age   ⒶⓂ

RVU			Global Days	Modifiers				
Mod	Non-Fac Total	Fac Total		51	50	62	80	MUE
	0.44	0.44	XXX	0	0	0	0	1

AMA: Apr 13: 3

● New   ▲ Revised   Deleted   ⊙ Moderate Sedation   ✚ Add-on Codes   ⊘ High Risk Denial   Ⓐ Age Edit   ♀ Female   ♂ Male   **AMA** *CPT® Assistant*   **MUE** Medically Unlikely Edit
⊘ Modifier 51 Exempt   ⊖ Modifier 63 Exempt   ☒ Unlisted   **Modifiers:** *See Inside Back Cover*   Ⓜ Maternity   Ⓐ2–Z3 ASC Payment Indicators   Ⓐ–Ⓨ OPPS Status Indicators

Medicine Procedures

90969 – 91037

90969 End-stage renal disease (ESRD) related services for dialysis less than a full month of service, per day; for patients 12-19 years of age   M

RVU			Global Days	Modifiers				
Mod	Non-Fac Total	Fac Total		51	50	62	80	MUE
	0.43	0.43	XXX	0	0	0	0	1

AMA: Apr 13: 3

90970 End-stage renal disease (ESRD) related services for dialysis less than a full month of service, per day; for patients 20 years of age and older   Ⓐ M

RVU			Global Days	Modifiers				
Mod	Non-Fac Total	Fac Total		51	50	62	80	MUE
	0.22	0.22	XXX	0	0	0	0	1

AMA: Apr 13: 3, Nov 13: 3, Oct 14: 3

Dialysis Training/Hemoperfusion

90989 Dialysis training, patient, including helper where applicable, any mode, completed course   B

RVU			Global Days	Modifiers				
Mod	Non-Fac Total	Fac Total		51	50	62	80	MUE
	0.00	0.00	XXX	9	9	9	9	1

AMA: Fall 93: 5, Jun 01: 10

90993 Dialysis training, patient, including helper where applicable, any mode, course not completed, per training session   B

RVU			Global Days	Modifiers				
Mod	Non-Fac Total	Fac Total		51	50	62	80	MUE
	0.00	0.00	XXX	9	9	9	9	1

AMA: Winter 90: 11, Fall 93: 5, Jun 01: 10

90997 Hemoperfusion (eg, with activated charcoal or resin)   B

RVU			Global Days	Modifiers				
Mod	Non-Fac Total	Fac Total		51	50	62	80	MUE
	2.64	2.64	000	0	0	0	0	1

90999 Unlisted dialysis procedure, inpatient or outpatient   ⊘✗B

RVU			Global Days	Modifiers				
Mod	Non-Fac Total	Fac Total		51	50	62	80	MUE
	0.00	0.00	XXX	0	0	0	0	

Gastroenterology Procedures

Coding Guidance

Many of the gastroenterologic tests described in this section are often complementary to endoscopic procedures and should not be separately reported when performed with an endoscopic procedure from the digestive system chapter.

91010 Esophageal motility (manometric study of the esophagus and/or gastroesophageal junction) study with interpretation and report   S

RVU			Global Days	Modifiers				
Mod	Non-Fac Total	Fac Total		51	50	62	80	MUE
	4.97	4.97	000	0	0	0	0	1
26	1.91	1.91	000	0	0	0	0	1
TC	3.06	3.06	000	0	0	0	0	1

AMA: Nov 97: 42

＋ 91013 Esophageal motility (manometric study of the esophagus and/or gastroesophageal junction) study with interpretation and report; with stimulation or perfusion (eg, stimulant, acid or alkali perfusion) (List separately in addition to code for primary procedure)   N

RVU			Global Days	Modifiers				
Mod	Non-Fac Total	Fac Total		51	50	62	80	MUE
	0.66	0.66	ZZZ	0	0	0	0	1
26	0.27	0.27	ZZZ	0	0	0	0	1
TC	0.39	0.39	ZZZ	0	0	0	0	1

91020 Gastric motility (manometric) studies   S

RVU			Global Days	Modifiers				
Mod	Non-Fac Total	Fac Total		51	50	62	80	MUE
	6.61	6.61	000	0	0	0	0	1
26	2.14	2.14	000	0	0	0	0	1
TC	4.47	4.47	000	0	0	0	0	1

AMA: Nov 97: 42, Sep 13: 13

91022 Duodenal motility (manometric) study   S

RVU			Global Days	Modifiers				
Mod	Non-Fac Total	Fac Total		51	50	62	80	MUE
	4.73	4.73	000	0	0	0	0	1
26	2.14	2.14	000	0	0	0	0	1
TC	2.59	2.59	000	0	0	0	0	1

AMA: Sep 13: 13

91030 Esophagus, acid perfusion (Bernstein) test for esophagitis   ⊘S

RVU			Global Days	Modifiers				
Mod	Non-Fac Total	Fac Total		51	50	62	80	MUE
	3.84	3.84	000	0	0	0	0	1
26	1.34	1.34	000	0	0	0	0	1
TC	2.50	2.50	000	0	0	0	0	1

91034 Esophagus, gastroesophageal reflux test; with nasal catheter pH electrode(s) placement, recording, analysis and interpretation   S

RVU			Global Days	Modifiers				
Mod	Non-Fac Total	Fac Total		51	50	62	80	MUE
	5.35	5.35	000	0	0	0	0	1
26	1.46	1.46	000	0	0	0	0	1
TC	3.89	3.89	000	0	0	0	0	1

AMA: May 05: 3, Feb 14: 11

91035 Esophagus, gastroesophageal reflux test; with mucosal attached telemetry pH electrode placement, recording, analysis and interpretation   Z2 S

RVU			Global Days	Modifiers				
Mod	Non-Fac Total	Fac Total		51	50	62	80	MUE
	13.57	13.57	000	0	0	0	0	1
26	2.39	2.39	000	0	0	0	0	1
TC	11.18	11.18	000	0	0	0	0	1

AMA: May 05: 3, Feb 14: 11

91037 Esophageal function test, gastroesophageal reflux test with nasal catheter intraluminal impedance electrode(s) placement, recording, analysis and interpretation   S

RVU			Global Days	Modifiers				
Mod	Non-Fac Total	Fac Total		51	50	62	80	MUE
	4.52	4.52	000	0	0	0	0	1
26	1.44	1.44	000	0	0	0	0	1
TC	3.08	3.08	000	0	0	0	0	1

AMA: May 05: 3

● New   ▲ Revised   ✖ Deleted   ⊙ Moderate Sedation   ＋ Add-on Codes   ⊘ High Risk Denial   Ⓐ Age Edit   ♀ Female   ♂ Male   **AMA** *CPT® Assistant*   **MUE** Medically Unlikely Edit
⊘ Modifier 51 Exempt   ⊖ Modifier 63 Exempt   ✗ Unlisted   **Modifiers:** *See Inside Back Cover*   M Maternity   A2–Z3 ASC Payment Indicators   A –Y OPPS Status Indicators

CPT © 2015 American Medical Association. All Rights Reserved.   © 2016 DecisionHealth

91038 Esophageal function test, gastroesophageal reflux test with nasal catheter intraluminal impedance electrode(s) placement, recording, analysis and interpretation; prolonged (greater than 1 hour, up to 24 hours) 🅂

Mod	Non-Fac Total	Fac Total	Global Days	51	50	62	80	MUE
	12.70	12.70	000	0	0	0	0	1
26	1.64	1.64	000	0	0	0	0	1
TC	11.06	11.06	000	0	0	0	0	1

AMA: May 05: 3, Feb 14: 11

▲ **91040** Esophageal balloon distension study, diagnostic, with provocation when performed 🅂

Mod	Non-Fac Total	Fac Total	Global Days	51	50	62	80	MUE
	12.25	12.25	000	0	0	0	0	1
26	1.42	1.42	000	0	0	0	0	1
TC	10.83	10.83	000	0	0	0	0	1

AMA: May 05: 3

91065 Breath hydrogen or methane test (eg, for detection of lactase deficiency, fructose intolerance, bacterial overgrowth, or oro-cecal gastrointestinal transit) 🅂

Mod	Non-Fac Total	Fac Total	Global Days	51	50	62	80	MUE
	2.21	2.21	000	0	0	0	0	2
26	0.29	0.29	000	0	0	0	0	2
TC	1.92	1.92	000	0	0	0	0	2

AMA: May 05: 3

91110 Gastrointestinal tract imaging, intraluminal (eg, capsule endoscopy), esophagus through ileum, with interpretation and report 🆃

Mod	Non-Fac Total	Fac Total	Global Days	51	50	62	80	MUE
	24.92	24.92	XXX	0	0	0	0	1
26	5.41	5.41	XXX	0	0	0	0	1
TC	19.51	19.51	XXX	0	0	0	0	1

AMA: Oct 04: 15, Aug 05: 14, May 09: 8, Sep 13: 13

91111 Gastrointestinal tract imaging, intraluminal (eg, capsule endoscopy), esophagus with interpretation and report 🆃

Mod	Non-Fac Total	Fac Total	Global Days	51	50	62	80	MUE
	20.45	20.45	XXX	0	0	0	0	1
26	1.49	1.49	XXX	0	0	0	0	1
TC	18.96	18.96	XXX	0	0	0	0	1

AMA: Sep 13: 13

91112 Gastrointestinal transit and pressure measurement, stomach through colon, wireless capsule, with interpretation and report 🆃

Mod	Non-Fac Total	Fac Total	Global Days	51	50	62	80	MUE
	30.51	30.51	XXX	0	0	0	0	1
26	3.12	3.12	XXX	0	0	0	0	1
TC	27.39	27.39	XXX	0	0	0	0	1

AMA: Sep 13: 13

91117 Colon motility (manometric) study, minimum 6 hours continuous recording (including provocation tests, eg, meal, intracolonic balloon distension, pharmacologic agents, if performed), with interpretation and report 🆃

Mod	Non-Fac Total	Fac Total	Global Days	51	50	62	80	MUE
	3.94	3.94	000	0	0	0	0	1

AMA: Sep 13: 13

91120 Rectal sensation, tone, and compliance test (ie, response to graded balloon distention) 🅂

Mod	Non-Fac Total	Fac Total	Global Days	51	50	62	80	MUE
	12.01	12.01	XXX	0	0	0	0	1
26	1.43	1.43	XXX	0	0	0	0	1
TC	10.58	10.58	XXX	0	0	0	0	1

AMA: May 05: 3

91122 Anorectal manometry 🆃

Mod	Non-Fac Total	Fac Total	Global Days	51	50	62	80	MUE
	6.41	6.41	000	0	0	0	0	1
26	2.57	2.57	000	0	0	0	0	1
TC	3.84	3.84	000	0	0	0	0	1

Gastric Physiology Procedures

91132 Electrogastrography, diagnostic, transcutaneous 🅲🅂

Mod	Non-Fac Total	Fac Total	Global Days	51	50	62	80	MUE
	4.36	4.36	XXX	0	0	0	0	1
26	0.80	0.80	XXX	0	0	0	0	1
TC	3.56	3.56	XXX	0	0	0	0	1

91133 Electrogastrography, diagnostic, transcutaneous; with provocative testing 🆀🅸

Mod	Non-Fac Total	Fac Total	Global Days	51	50	62	80	MUE
	4.85	4.85	XXX	0	0	0	0	1
26	0.98	0.98	XXX	0	0	0	0	1
TC	3.87	3.87	XXX	0	0	0	0	1

91200 Liver elastography, mechanically induced shear wave (eg, vibration), without imaging, with interpretation and report 🅽🅸🅂

Mod	Non-Fac Total	Fac Total	Global Days	51	50	62	80	MUE
	0.80	0.80	XXX	0	0	0	0	1
26	0.37	0.37	XXX	0	0	0	0	1
TC	0.43	0.43	XXX	0	0	0	0	1

Other Gastroenterology Procedures

91299 Unlisted diagnostic gastroenterology procedure ⊗🆇🅂

Mod	Non-Fac Total	Fac Total	Global Days	51	50	62	80	MUE
	0.00	0.00	XXX	0	0	0	0	
26	0.00	0.00	XXX	0	0	0	0	
TC	0.00	0.00	XXX	0	0	0	0	

AMA: Aug 05: 14
Pub 100-04, 13, 120

Ophthalmology Services/Procedures

General Opthalmological Examination

New Patient

Coding Guidance

General ophthalmological services cannot be reported together with evaluation and management codes as both ranges would represent the same services. If the E/M code more accurately reflects the services provided, it should be reported instead. The use of slit lamp, routine ophthalmoscopy, biomicroscopy, tonometry, keratometry, retinoscopy, and mydriasis to facilitate routine ophthalmoscopy are included in intermediate and comprehensive ophthalmology services. Gross visual field and visual acuity testing as well as corneal topography are also included in the general ophthalmological service codes. When an extended ophthalmoscopy is performed as described in 92225-92226, it may be reported in addition to the general ophthalmology service code.

92002 Ophthalmological services: medical examination and evaluation with initiation of diagnostic and treatment program; intermediate, new patient ☑

RVU			Global Days	Modifiers				
Mod	Non-Fac Total	Fac Total		51	50	62	80	MUE
	2.27	1.35	XXX	0	2	0	0	1

AMA: Feb 97: 6, Aug 98: 3, Jun 05: 11, Dec 05: 10, Jan 07: 30, Jan 08: 1, Sep 08: 7, Feb 11: 10, Aug 12: 9, Oct 12: 9

92004 Ophthalmological services: medical examination and evaluation with initiation of diagnostic and treatment program; comprehensive, new patient, 1 or more visits ☑

RVU			Global Days	Modifiers				
Mod	Non-Fac Total	Fac Total		51	50	62	80	MUE
	4.16	2.80	XXX	0	2	0	0	1

AMA: Feb 97: 6, Aug 98: 3, Jun 05: 11, Dec 05: 10, Jan 07: 30, Jan 08: 1, Sep 08: 7, Nov 10: 8, Feb 11: 10, Jan 11: 9, Aug 12: 9

Established Patient

92012 Ophthalmological services: medical examination and evaluation, with initiation or continuation of diagnostic and treatment program; intermediate, established patient ☑

RVU			Global Days	Modifiers				
Mod	Non-Fac Total	Fac Total		51	50	62	80	MUE
	2.40	1.49	XXX	0	2	0	0	1

AMA: Feb 97: 6, Aug 98: 3, Jun 05: 11, Dec 05: 10, Jan 07: 30, Jan 08: 1, Sep 08: 7, Feb 11: 10, Aug 12: 9

92014 Ophthalmological services: medical examination and evaluation, with initiation or continuation of diagnostic and treatment program; comprehensive, established patient, 1 or more visits ☑

RVU			Global Days	Modifiers				
Mod	Non-Fac Total	Fac Total		51	50	62	80	MUE
	3.48	2.26	XXX	0	2	0	0	1

AMA: Feb 97: 6, Aug 98: 3, Dec 99: 10, Jun 05: 11, Dec 05: 10, Jan 07: 30, Jan 08: 1, Sep 08: 7, Nov 10: 8, Feb 11: 10, Jan 11: 9, Aug 12: 9, Oct 12: 9

Special Ophthalmological Services/Procedures

Coding Guidance

Special ophthalmological services are specific services beyond a general or routine exam. These codes are recognized as distinct and separate services and may be reported in addition to general ophthalmological services and E/M codes when they are also provided.

92015 Determination of refractive state ⒼE

Coding tip: *Prescription of lenses is included in determining the refractive state*

RVU			Global Days	Modifiers				
Mod	Non-Fac Total	Fac Total		51	50	62	80	MUE
	0.56	0.55	XXX	9	9	9	9	

AMA: Mar 13: 6, Mar 96: 11, Feb 97: 6, Aug 98: 3, Aug 06: 11

Coding Guidance

When 92018 or 92019 is performed on one eye only, add reduced services modifier 52.

92018 Ophthalmological examination and evaluation, under general anesthesia, with or without manipulation of globe for passive range of motion or other manipulation to facilitate diagnostic examination; complete 🆃

RVU			Global Days	Modifiers				
Mod	Non-Fac Total	Fac Total		51	50	62	80	MUE
	4.12	4.12	XXX	0	0	0	0	1

AMA: Feb 97: 6, Aug 98: 3

92019 Ophthalmological examination and evaluation, under general anesthesia, with or without manipulation of globe for passive range of motion or other manipulation to facilitate diagnostic examination; limited 🆃

RVU			Global Days	Modifiers				
Mod	Non-Fac Total	Fac Total		51	50	62	80	MUE
	2.03	2.03	XXX	0	0	0	0	1

AMA: Feb 97: 6, Aug 98: 3

92020 Gonioscopy (separate procedure) Ⓠ1

RVU			Global Days	Modifiers				
Mod	Non-Fac Total	Fac Total		51	50	62	80	MUE
	0.75	0.59	XXX	0	2	0	0	1

AMA: Feb 97: 6, Aug 98: 3

92025 Computerized corneal topography, unilateral or bilateral, with interpretation and report Ⓠ1

RVU			Global Days	Modifiers				
Mod	Non-Fac Total	Fac Total		51	50	62	80	MUE
	1.07	1.07	XXX	7	2	0	0	1
26	0.57	0.57	XXX	7	2	0	0	1
TC	0.50	0.50	XXX	7	2	0	0	1

AMA: Oct 10: 10, Oct 12: 9

92060 Sensorimotor examination with multiple measurements of ocular deviation (eg, restrictive or paretic muscle with diplopia) with interpretation and report (separate procedure) Ⓠ1

RVU			Global Days	Modifiers				
Mod	Non-Fac Total	Fac Total		51	50	62	80	MUE
	1.83	1.83	XXX	7	2	0	0	1
26	1.08	1.08	XXX	7	2	0	0	1
TC	0.75	0.75	XXX	7	2	0	0	1

AMA: Feb 97: 6, Aug 98: 3

92065 Orthoptic and/or pleoptic training, with continuing medical direction and evaluation Ⓠ1

RVU			Global Days	Modifiers				
Mod	Non-Fac Total	Fac Total		51	50	62	80	MUE
	1.46	1.46	XXX	0	2	0	0	1
26	0.50	0.50	XXX	0	2	0	0	1
TC	0.96	0.96	XXX	0	2	0	0	1

AMA: Feb 97: 6, Jun 98: 10, Aug 98: 3

● New   ▲ Revised   ✖ Deleted   ⊙ Moderate Sedation   ➕ Add-on Codes   ⊘ High Risk Denial   Ⓐ Age Edit   ♀ Female   ♂ Male   **AMA** *CPT® Assistant*   **MUE** Medically Unlikely Edit

⊘ Modifier 51 Exempt   ⊖ Modifier 63 Exempt   ☒ Unlisted   **Modifiers:** *See Inside Back Cover*   Ⓜ Maternity   Ⓐ2–Ⓩ3 ASC Payment Indicators   Ⓐ–Ⓨ OPPS Status Indicators

794   CPT © 2015 American Medical Association. All Rights Reserved.   © 2016 DecisionHealth

92071 Fitting of contact lens for treatment of ocular surface disease `N I N`

Coding tip: This is a unilateral code. When both eyes are treated, report the code twice with LT and RT modifiers or add bilateral modifier 50, depending on the payer.

Coding tip: Supply of the lens should be reported with a HCPCS Level II supply code or CPT code 99070.

Coding tip: Use this code for the application of bandage soft contact lenses for healing a diseased or injured cornea; do not report 92071 for lens fitting for vision correction.

RVU			Global Days	Modifiers				
Mod	Non-Fac Total	Fac Total		51	50	62	80	MUE
	1.06	0.95	XXX	0	1	0	0	2

AMA: Aug 12: 9

92072 Fitting of contact lens for management of keratoconus, initial fitting `N I N`

Coding tip: Use this code for the application of bandage soft contact lenses for healing a diseased or injured cornea; do not report 92072 for lens fitting for vision correction.

Coding tip: Supply of the lens should be reported with a HCPCS Level II supply code or CPT code 99070.

Coding tip: This is a unilateral code. When both eyes are treated, report the code twice with LT and RT modifiers or add bilateral modifier 50, depending on the payer.

RVU			Global Days	Modifiers				
Mod	Non-Fac Total	Fac Total		51	50	62	80	MUE
	3.77	2.90	XXX	0	2	0	0	1

AMA: Aug 12: 9

92081 Visual field examination, unilateral or bilateral, with interpretation and report; limited examination (eg, tangent screen, Autoplot, arc perimeter, or single stimulus level automated test, such as Octopus 3 or 7 equivalent) `Q1`

RVU			Global Days	Modifiers				
Mod	Non-Fac Total	Fac Total		51	50	62	80	MUE
	0.95	0.95	XXX	7	2	0	0	1
26	0.46	0.46	XXX	7	2	0	0	1
TC	0.49	0.49	XXX	7	2	0	0	1

AMA: Feb 97: 6, Aug 98: 3, Sep 10: 10, Oct 12: 9

92082 Visual field examination, unilateral or bilateral, with interpretation and report; intermediate examination (eg, at least 2 isopters on Goldmann perimeter, or semiquantitative, automated suprathreshold screening program, Humphrey suprathreshold automatic diagnostic test, Octopus program 33) `Q1`

RVU			Global Days	Modifiers				
Mod	Non-Fac Total	Fac Total		51	50	62	80	MUE
	1.34	1.34	XXX	7	2	0	0	1
26	0.61	0.61	XXX	7	2	0	0	1
TC	0.73	0.73	XXX	7	2	0	0	1

AMA: Feb 97: 6, Aug 98: 3, Oct 12: 9

92083 Visual field examination, unilateral or bilateral, with interpretation and report; extended examination (eg, Goldmann visual fields with at least 3 isopters plotted and static determination within the central 30°, or quantitative, automated threshold perimetry, Octopus program G-1, 32 or 42, Humphrey visual field analyzer full threshold programs 30-2, 24-2, or 30/60-2) `Q1`

RVU			Global Days	Modifiers				
Mod	Non-Fac Total	Fac Total		51	50	62	80	MUE
	1.81	1.81	XXX	7	2	0	0	1
26	0.79	0.79	XXX	7	2	0	0	1
TC	1.02	1.02	XXX	7	2	0	0	1

AMA: Feb 97: 6, Aug 98: 3, Oct 12: 9

92100 Serial tonometry (separate procedure) with multiple measurements of intraocular pressure over an extended time period with interpretation and report, same day (eg, diurnal curve or medical treatment of acute elevation of intraocular pressure) `N`

RVU			Global Days	Modifiers				
Mod	Non-Fac Total	Fac Total		51	50	62	80	MUE
	2.25	0.96	XXX	0	2	0	0	1

AMA: Feb 97: 6, Jun 98: 10, Aug 98: 3, Aug 12: 9, 15, Oct 12: 9, May 14: 5

92132 Scanning computerized ophthalmic diagnostic imaging, anterior segment, with interpretation and report, unilateral or bilateral `Q1`

Coding tip: Use this code for anterior segment imaging with optical coherence tomography

Coding tip: This procedure is used for patients with certain kinds of macular abnormalities and glaucoma and has replaced category III code 0187T

Coding tip: Similar diagnostic anterior segment imaging done with ultrasound instead of light is reported with 76513

RVU			Global Days	Modifiers				
Mod	Non-Fac Total	Fac Total		51	50	62	80	MUE
	0.98	0.98	XXX	7	2	0	0	1
26	0.54	0.54	XXX	7	2	0	0	1
TC	0.44	0.44	XXX	7	2	0	0	1

AMA: Mar 13: 6, Feb 11: 6, Oct 12: 9, Apr 13: 7, May 14: 5

92133 Scanning computerized ophthalmic diagnostic imaging, posterior segment, with interpretation and report, unilateral or bilateral; optic nerve `Q1`

RVU			Global Days	Modifiers				
Mod	Non-Fac Total	Fac Total		51	50	62	80	MUE
	1.24	1.24	XXX	7	2	0	0	1
26	0.79	0.79	XXX	7	2	0	0	1
TC	0.45	0.45	XXX	7	2	0	0	1

AMA: Feb 11: 6, Oct 12: 9, Nov 14: 10

Pub 100-04, 32, 300.2

92134 Scanning computerized ophthalmic diagnostic imaging, posterior segment, with interpretation and report, unilateral or bilateral; retina `Q1`

RVU			Global Days	Modifiers				
Mod	Non-Fac Total	Fac Total		51	50	62	80	MUE
	1.27	1.27	XXX	7	2	0	0	1
26	0.81	0.81	XXX	7	2	0	0	1
TC	0.46	0.46	XXX	7	2	0	0	1

AMA: Feb 11: 6, Oct 12: 9, Nov 14: 10

Pub 100-04, 32, 300.2

● New   ▲ Revised   Deleted   ⊙ Moderate Sedation   ✚ Add-on Codes   ⊘ High Risk Denial   ⓐ Age Edit   ♀ Female   ♂ Male   **AMA** CPT® Assistant   **MUE** Medically Unlikely Edit
⊘ Modifier 51 Exempt   ⊖ Modifier 63 Exempt   ☒ Unlisted   **Modifiers:** See Inside Back Cover   Ⓜ Maternity   A2–Z3 ASC Payment Indicators   A–Y OPPS Status Indicators

© 2016 DecisionHealth   CPT © 2015 American Medical Association. All Rights Reserved.

92136 Ophthalmic biometry by partial coherence interferometry with intraocular lens power calculation   ◨▮

Coding tip: Report 92136 in addition to cataract extraction with IOL insertion (66982-66984) when intraocular lens power calculation by optical lens measurement is done at the time of insertion

RVU Mod	Non-Fac Total	Fac Total	Global Days	Modifiers 51	50	62	80	MUE
	2.55	2.55	XXX	7	2	0	0	2
26	0.89	0.89	XXX	7	3	0	0	2
TC	1.66	1.66	XXX	7	2	0	0	2

AMA: Aug 98: 3, Apr 02: 18, Sep 09: 5, May 14: 5

92140 Provocative tests for glaucoma, with interpretation and report, without tonography ◨▮

RVU Mod	Non-Fac Total	Fac Total	Global Days	Modifiers 51	50	62	80	MUE
	1.78	0.76	XXX	0	2	0	0	1

AMA: Feb 97: 6, Aug 98: 3, Oct 12: 9

92145 Corneal hysteresis determination, by air impulse stimulation, unilateral or bilateral, with interpretation and report   ◨▮

RVU Mod	Non-Fac Total	Fac Total	Global Days	Modifiers 51	50	62	80	MUE
	0.44	0.44	XXX	7	2	0	0	1
26	0.25	0.25	XXX	7	2	0	0	1
TC	0.19	0.19	XXX	7	2	0	0	1

Ophthalmoscopic Procedures

Coding Guidance

When an extended ophthalmoscopy is performed as described in 92225-92226, then it may be reported in addition to the general ophthalmology service codes 92002-92014. Extended ophthalmoscopy is done for severe posterior segment pathology. The drawing must be labeled, use standard color, and include detail of extent of detachment, location of holes, areas of traction, vitreous opacities, hemorrhaging, lesions, and other appropriate documentation for specific conditions, such as glaucoma (in which cupping, disc rim, pallor, slope, and pathology around the optic nerve should be identified). Reimbursement also requires an interpretation accompany the drawing that contains pertinent conclusions, findings, and impressions. Extended ophthalmoscopy with retinal drawing may be reported for each eye, if done bilaterally.

92225 Ophthalmoscopy, extended, with retinal drawing (eg, for retinal detachment, melanoma), with interpretation and report; initial   ◨▮

Coding tip: Use 92225 for the initial evaluation of a disease. This code may be reported more than once per eye when another initial extended exam is done that specifically focuses on a different condition.

RVU Mod	Non-Fac Total	Fac Total	Global Days	Modifiers 51	50	62	80	MUE
	0.76	0.60	XXX	0	3	0	0	2

AMA: Feb 97: 6, Aug 98: 2, Dec 99: 10, Feb 11: 6, Oct 12: 9

92226 Ophthalmoscopy, extended, with retinal drawing (eg, for retinal detachment, melanoma), with interpretation and report; subsequent   ◨▮

Coding tip: Use 92226 for a repeat evaluation of an established problem that is worsening or complicated by other pathology

RVU Mod	Non-Fac Total	Fac Total	Global Days	Modifiers 51	50	62	80	MUE
	0.70	0.54	XXX	0	3	0	0	2

AMA: Feb 97: 6, Aug 98: 2, Feb 11: 6

92227 Remote imaging for detection of retinal disease (eg, retinopathy in a patient with diabetes) with analysis and report under physician supervision, unilateral or bilateral   ◨▮

RVU Mod	Non-Fac Total	Fac Total	Global Days	Modifiers 51	50	62	80	MUE
	0.41	0.41	XXX	0	2	0	0	1

AMA: May 11: 9, Feb 11: 7, Oct 12: 9

92228 Remote imaging for monitoring and management of active retinal disease (eg, diabetic retinopathy) with physician review, interpretation and report, unilateral or bilateral   ◨▮

RVU Mod	Non-Fac Total	Fac Total	Global Days	Modifiers 51	50	62	80	MUE
	0.97	0.97	XXX	7	2	0	0	1
26	0.59	0.59	XXX	7	2	0	0	1
TC	0.38	0.38	XXX	7	2	0	0	1

AMA: May 11: 9, Feb 11: 7, Oct 12: 9

92230 Fluorescein angioscopy with interpretation and report   ◨▮

RVU Mod	Non-Fac Total	Fac Total	Global Days	Modifiers 51	50	62	80	MUE
	1.64	0.95	XXX	0	3	0	0	2

AMA: Feb 97: 6, Feb 11: 6

92235 Fluorescein angiography (includes multiframe imaging) with interpretation and report   Ⓢ

RVU Mod	Non-Fac Total	Fac Total	Global Days	Modifiers 51	50	62	80	MUE
	3.10	3.10	XXX	7	3	0	0	2
26	1.33	1.33	XXX	7	3	0	0	2
TC	1.77	1.77	XXX	7	3	0	0	2

AMA: Feb 97: 6, Feb 11: 6

Pub 100-04, 32, 300.2

92240 Indocyanine-green angiography (includes multiframe imaging) with interpretation and report   Ⓢ

RVU Mod	Non-Fac Total	Fac Total	Global Days	Modifiers 51	50	62	80	MUE
	7.21	7.21	XXX	7	3	0	0	2
26	1.81	1.81	XXX	7	3	0	0	2
TC	5.40	5.40	XXX	7	3	0	0	2

AMA: Feb 11: 6, Oct 12: 9

92250 Fundus photography with interpretation and report   ◨▮

RVU Mod	Non-Fac Total	Fac Total	Global Days	Modifiers 51	50	62	80	MUE
	2.20	2.20	XXX	7	2	0	0	1
26	0.67	0.67	XXX	7	2	0	0	1
TC	1.53	1.53	XXX	7	2	0	0	1

AMA: Feb 97: 6, Apr 99: 10, Feb 11: 6, Oct 12: 9, Nov 14: 10, Dec 14: 17, May 15: 9

92260 Ophthalmodynamometry   ◨▮

RVU Mod	Non-Fac Total	Fac Total	Global Days	Modifiers 51	50	62	80	MUE
	0.52	0.31	XXX	0	2	0	0	1

AMA: Feb 97: 6, Feb 11: 6

● New   ▲ Revised   ✖ Deleted   ⊙ Moderate Sedation   ✚ Add-on Codes   ⊘ High Risk Denial   Ⓐ Age Edit   ♀ Female   ♂ Male   **AMA** *CPT® Assistant*   *MUE* Medically Unlikely Edit
⊘ Modifier 51 Exempt   ⊖ Modifier 63 Exempt   Ⓧ Unlisted   **Modifiers:** *See Inside Back Cover*   Ⓜ Maternity   A2-Z3 ASC Payment Indicators   A-Y OPPS Status Indicators

CPT © 2015 American Medical Association. All Rights Reserved.   © 2016 DecisionHealth

Other Specialized Ophthalmological Services/Procedures

92265 Needle oculoelectromyography, 1 or more extraocular muscles, 1 or both eyes, with interpretation and report ▣▣

Mod	Non-Fac Total	Fac Total	Global Days	51	50	62	80	MUE
	2.21	2.21	XXX	7	2	0	0	1
26	1.21	1.21	XXX	7	2	0	0	1
TC	1.00	1.00	XXX	7	2	0	0	1

AMA: Feb 97: 6, Oct 12: 9

92270 Electro-oculography with interpretation and report ▣▣

Mod	Non-Fac Total	Fac Total	Global Days	51	50	62	80	MUE
	2.58	2.58	XXX	7	2	0	0	1
26	1.17	1.17	XXX	7	2	0	0	1
TC	1.41	1.41	XXX	7	2	0	0	1

AMA: Feb 97: 6, Aug 08: 12, May 09: 9, Oct 12: 9

92275 Electroretinography with interpretation and report ▣

Mod	Non-Fac Total	Fac Total	Global Days	51	50	62	80	MUE
	4.14	4.14	XXX	7	2	0	0	1
26	1.52	1.52	XXX	7	2	0	0	1
TC	2.62	2.62	XXX	7	2	0	0	1

AMA: Feb 97: 6, Oct 12: 9

92283 Color vision examination, extended, eg, anomaloscope or equivalent ▣▣

Mod	Non-Fac Total	Fac Total	Global Days	51	50	62	80	MUE
	1.55	1.55	XXX	7	2	0	0	1
26	0.26	0.26	XXX	7	2	0	0	1
TC	1.29	1.29	XXX	7	2	0	0	1

AMA: Feb 97: 6, Oct 12: 9

92284 Dark adaptation examination with interpretation and report ▣▣

Mod	Non-Fac Total	Fac Total	Global Days	51	50	62	80	MUE
	1.70	1.70	XXX	7	2	0	0	1
26	0.35	0.35	XXX	7	2	0	0	1
TC	1.35	1.35	XXX	7	2	0	0	1

AMA: Feb 97: 6, Oct 12: 9

92285 External ocular photography with interpretation and report for documentation of medical progress (eg, close-up photography, slit lamp photography, goniophotography, stereo-photography) ▣▣

Mod	Non-Fac Total	Fac Total	Global Days	51	50	62	80	MUE
	0.58	0.58	XXX	7	2	0	0	1
26	0.09	0.09	XXX	7	2	0	0	1
TC	0.49	0.49	XXX	7	2	0	0	1

AMA: Feb 97: 6, Sep 97: 10, Oct 12: 9, May 14: 5

92286 Anterior segment imaging with interpretation and report; with specular microscopy and endothelial cell analysis ▣▣

Mod	Non-Fac Total	Fac Total	Global Days	51	50	62	80	MUE
	1.07	1.07	XXX	7	2	0	0	1
26	0.62	0.62	XXX	7	2	0	0	1
TC	0.45	0.45	XXX	7	2	0	0	1

AMA: Mar 13: 6, Feb 97: 6, Oct 12: 9

92287 Anterior segment imaging with interpretation and report; with fluorescein angiography ▣▣

Mod	Non-Fac Total	Fac Total	Global Days	51	50	62	80	MUE
	3.90	3.90	XXX	0	2	0	0	1
26	1.33	1.33	XXX	0	2	0	0	1
TC	2.57	2.57	XXX	0	2	0	0	1

AMA: Mar 13: 6, Feb 97: 6

Contact Lens

92310 Prescription of optical and physical characteristics of and fitting of contact lens, with medical supervision of adaptation; corneal lens, both eyes, except for aphakia ▣▣

Mod	Non-Fac Total	Fac Total	Global Days	51	50	62	80	MUE
	2.71	1.69	XXX	9	9	9	9	

AMA: Feb 97: 6, Oct 12: 9

92311 Prescription of optical and physical characteristics of and fitting of contact lens, with medical supervision of adaptation; corneal lens for aphakia, 1 eye ▣▣

Mod	Non-Fac Total	Fac Total	Global Days	51	50	62	80	MUE
	2.82	1.56	XXX	0	0	0	0	1

AMA: Feb 97: 6, Oct 12: 9

92312 Prescription of optical and physical characteristics of and fitting of contact lens, with medical supervision of adaptation; corneal lens for aphakia, both eyes ▣▣

Mod	Non-Fac Total	Fac Total	Global Days	51	50	62	80	MUE
	3.23	1.78	XXX	0	2	0	0	1

AMA: Feb 97: 6, Oct 12: 9

92313 Prescription of optical and physical characteristics of and fitting of contact lens, with medical supervision of adaptation; corneoscleral lens ▣▣

Mod	Non-Fac Total	Fac Total	Global Days	51	50	62	80	MUE
	2.69	1.33	XXX	0	0	0	0	1

AMA: Feb 97: 7, Mar 03: 1

● New   ▲ Revised   Deleted   ⊙ Moderate Services   ✚ Add-on Codes   ⊘ High Risk Denial   Ⓐ Age Edit   ♀ Female   ♂ Male   **AMA** CPT® Assistant   **MUE** Medically Unlikely Edit

⊘ Modifier 51 Exempt   ⊖ Modifier 63 Exempt   ☒ Unlisted   **Modifiers:** See Inside Back Cover   Ⓜ Maternity   A2–Z3 ASC Payment Indicators   A–Y OPPS Status Indicators

Medicine Procedures

92265 – 92313

Medicine Procedures

92314 – 92371

92314 Prescription of optical and physical characteristics of contact lens, with medical supervision of adaptation and direction of fitting by independent technician; corneal lens, both eyes except for aphakia   ⊘Ε

RVU			Global Days	Modifiers				
Mod	Non-Fac Total	Fac Total		51	50	62	80	MUE
	2.25	0.99	XXX	9	9	9	9	

AMA: Feb 97: 7, Oct 12: 9

92315 Prescription of optical and physical characteristics of contact lens, with medical supervision of adaptation and direction of fitting by independent technician; corneal lens for aphakia, 1 eye   ⊘⊘1

RVU			Global Days	Modifiers				
Mod	Non-Fac Total	Fac Total		51	50	62	80	MUE
	2.00	0.61	XXX	0	0	0	0	1

AMA: Feb 97: 7, Oct 12: 9

92316 Prescription of optical and physical characteristics of contact lens, with medical supervision of adaptation and direction of fitting by independent technician; corneal lens for aphakia, both eyes   ⊘1

RVU			Global Days	Modifiers				
Mod	Non-Fac Total	Fac Total		51	50	62	80	MUE
	2.51	0.92	XXX	0	2	0	0	1

AMA: Feb 97: 7, Oct 12: 9

92317 Prescription of optical and physical characteristics of contact lens, with medical supervision of adaptation and direction of fitting by independent technician; corneoscleral lens ⊘⊘1

RVU			Global Days	Modifiers				
Mod	Non-Fac Total	Fac Total		51	50	62	80	MUE
	2.11	0.62	XXX	0	0	0	0	1

AMA: Feb 97: 7

92325 Modification of contact lens (separate procedure), with medical supervision of adaptation   ⊘⊘1

RVU			Global Days	Modifiers				
Mod	Non-Fac Total	Fac Total		51	50	62	80	MUE
	1.17	1.17	XXX	0	0	0	0	1

AMA: Feb 97: 7, Oct 12: 9

92326 Replacement of contact lens   ⊘⊘1

RVU			Global Days	Modifiers				
Mod	Non-Fac Total	Fac Total		51	50	62	80	MUE
	0.99	0.99	XXX	0	0	0	0	2

AMA: Feb 97: 7

Spectacle Services

92340 Fitting of spectacles, except for aphakia; monofocal   ⊘Ε

RVU			Global Days	Modifiers				
Mod	Non-Fac Total	Fac Total		51	50	62	80	MUE
	1.00	0.53	XXX	9	9	9	9	

AMA: Mar 13: 6, Feb 97: 7, Aug 98: 4

92341 Fitting of spectacles, except for aphakia; bifocal   ⊘Ε

RVU			Global Days	Modifiers				
Mod	Non-Fac Total	Fac Total		51	50	62	80	MUE
	1.15	0.68	XXX	9	9	9	9	

AMA: Mar 13: 6, Feb 97: 7, Aug 98: 4

92342 Fitting of spectacles, except for aphakia; multifocal, other than bifocal   ⊘Ε

RVU			Global Days	Modifiers				
Mod	Non-Fac Total	Fac Total		51	50	62	80	MUE
	1.23	0.76	XXX	9	9	9	9	

AMA: Mar 13: 6, Feb 97: 7, Aug 98: 4

92352 Fitting of spectacle prosthesis for aphakia; monofocal   ⊘⊘1

RVU			Global Days	Modifiers				
Mod	Non-Fac Total	Fac Total		51	50	62	80	MUE
	1.14	0.53	XXX	9	9	9	9	0

AMA: Mar 13: 6, Feb 97: 7, Aug 98: 4

92353 Fitting of spectacle prosthesis for aphakia; multifocal   ⊘⊘1

RVU			Global Days	Modifiers				
Mod	Non-Fac Total	Fac Total		51	50	62	80	MUE
	1.33	0.72	XXX	9	9	9	9	0

AMA: Mar 13: 6, Feb 97: 7, Aug 98: 4

92354 Fitting of spectacle mounted low vision aid; single element system   ⊘⊘1

RVU			Global Days	Modifiers				
Mod	Non-Fac Total	Fac Total		51	50	62	80	MUE
	0.38	0.38	XXX	9	9	9	9	0

AMA: Mar 13: 6, Feb 97: 7, Aug 98: 4

92355 Fitting of spectacle mounted low vision aid; telescopic or other compound lens system   ⊘⊘1

RVU			Global Days	Modifiers				
Mod	Non-Fac Total	Fac Total		51	50	62	80	MUE
	0.59	0.59	XXX	9	9	9	9	0

AMA: Mar 13: 6, Feb 97: 7, Aug 98: 4

92358 Prosthesis service for aphakia, temporary (disposable or loan, including materials)   ⊘⊘1

RVU			Global Days	Modifiers				
Mod	Non-Fac Total	Fac Total		51	50	62	80	MUE
	0.32	0.32	XXX	9	9	9	9	0

AMA: Mar 13: 6, Feb 97: 7, Aug 98: 4

92370 Repair and refitting spectacles; except for aphakia   ⊘Ε

RVU			Global Days	Modifiers				
Mod	Non-Fac Total	Fac Total		51	50	62	80	MUE
	0.87	0.46	XXX	9	9	9	9	

AMA: Mar 13: 6, Feb 97: 7

92371 Repair and refitting spectacles; spectacle prosthesis for aphakia   ⊘⊘1

RVU			Global Days	Modifiers				
Mod	Non-Fac Total	Fac Total		51	50	62	80	MUE
	0.33	0.33	XXX	9	9	9	9	0

AMA: Feb 97: 7, Aug 98: 4, Mar 13: 6

● New   ▲ Revised   ✖ Deleted   ⊙ Moderate Sedation   ✚ Add-on Codes   ⊘ High Risk Denial   Ⓐ Age Edit   ♀ Female   ♂ Male   **AMA** *CPT® Assistant*   ***MUE*** Medically Unlikely Edit
⊘ Modifier 51 Exempt   ⊖ Modifier 63 Exempt   ✗ Unlisted   **Modifiers:** *See Inside Back Cover*   Ⓜ Maternity   A2–Z3 ASC Payment Indicators   A–Y OPPS Status Indicators

798   CPT © 2015 American Medical Association. All Rights Reserved.   © 2016 DecisionHealth

Other Ophthalmological Services/Procedures

92499 Unlisted ophthalmological service or procedure

x̶ Q1

RVU			Global Days	Modifiers				
Mod	Non-Fac Total	Fac Total		51	50	62	80	MUE
	0.00	0.00	XXX	0	0	0	0	
26	0.00	0.00	XXX	0	0	0	0	
TC	0.00	0.00	XXX	0	0	0	0	

AMA: Feb 97: 7

Otorhinolaryngological Services

92502 Otolaryngologic examination under general anesthesia

T

RVU			Global Days	Modifiers				
Mod	Non-Fac Total	Fac Total		51	50	62	80	MUE
	2.77	2.77	000	0	0	0	0	1

92504 Binocular microscopy (separate diagnostic procedure)

N

RVU			Global Days	Modifiers				
Mod	Non-Fac Total	Fac Total		51	50	62	80	MUE
	0.85	0.27	XXX	0	0	0	0	1

AMA: Jul 05: 14, Oct 11: 10, Oct 13: 14

Coding Guidance
Services described by CPT codes 92507, 92508 may be performed by speech language pathologists.

92507 Treatment of speech, language, voice, communication, and/or auditory processing disorder; individual

A

RVU			Global Days	Modifiers				
Mod	Non-Fac Total	Fac Total		51	50	62	80	MUE
	2.23	2.23	XXX	5	0	0	0	1

AMA: Dec 04: 14, Jan 06: 7, Oct 13: 7
Pub 100-04, 12, 30.3; 100-04, 32, 100.4

92508 Treatment of speech, language, voice, communication, and/or auditory processing disorder; group, 2 or more individuals

A

RVU			Global Days	Modifiers				
Mod	Non-Fac Total	Fac Total		51	50	62	80	MUE
	0.65	0.65	XXX	5	0	0	0	1

AMA: Dec 04: 14, Oct 13: 7
Pub 100-04, 12, 30.3

92511 Nasopharyngoscopy with endoscope (separate procedure)

T

Coding tip: *Nasopharyngoscopy with endoscope is not considered a distinct service when it is done as a precursory inspection for another endoscopic procedure on the respiratory system*

RVU			Global Days	Modifiers				
Mod	Non-Fac Total	Fac Total		51	50	62	80	MUE
	3.18	1.12	000	0	0	0	0	1

92512 Nasal function studies (eg, rhinomanometry)

S

RVU			Global Days	Modifiers				
Mod	Non-Fac Total	Fac Total		51	50	62	80	MUE
	1.73	0.82	XXX	0	0	0	0	1

92516 Facial nerve function studies (eg, electroneuronography)

S

RVU			Global Days	Modifiers				
Mod	Non-Fac Total	Fac Total		51	50	62	80	MUE
	2.00	0.66	XXX	0	0	0	0	1

92520 Laryngeal function studies (ie, aerodynamic testing and acoustic testing)

Q1

RVU			Global Days	Modifiers				
Mod	Non-Fac Total	Fac Total		51	50	62	80	MUE
	2.14	1.19	XXX	0	0	0	0	1

AMA: Dec 04: 17, Jan 06: 7

92521 Evaluation of speech fluency (eg, stuttering, cluttering)

A

RVU			Global Days	Modifiers				
Mod	Non-Fac Total	Fac Total		51	50	62	80	MUE
	3.13	3.13	XXX	5	0	0	0	1

AMA: Jun 14: 3

92522 Evaluation of speech sound production (eg, articulation, phonological process, apraxia, dysarthria)

A

RVU			Global Days	Modifiers				
Mod	Non-Fac Total	Fac Total		51	50	62	80	MUE
	2.61	2.61	XXX	5	0	0	0	1

AMA: Jun 14: 3

92523 Evaluation of speech sound production (eg, articulation, phonological process, apraxia, dysarthria); with evaluation of language comprehension and expression (eg, receptive and expressive language)

A

RVU			Global Days	Modifiers				
Mod	Non-Fac Total	Fac Total		51	50	62	80	MUE
	5.47	5.47	XXX	5	0	0	0	1

AMA: Jun 14: 3

92524 Behavioral and qualitative analysis of voice and resonance

A

RVU			Global Days	Modifiers				
Mod	Non-Fac Total	Fac Total		51	50	62	80	MUE
	2.52	2.52	XXX	5	0	0	0	1

AMA: Jun 14: 3

92526 Treatment of swallowing dysfunction and/or oral function for feeding

A

RVU			Global Days	Modifiers				
Mod	Non-Fac Total	Fac Total		51	50	62	80	MUE
	2.42	2.42	XXX	5	0	0	0	1

Vestibular Function Testing

92531 Spontaneous nystagmus, including gaze

N

RVU			Global Days	Modifiers				
Mod	Non-Fac Total	Fac Total		51	50	62	80	MUE
	0.00	0.00	XXX	9	9	9	9	0

92532 Positional nystagmus test

N

RVU			Global Days	Modifiers				
Mod	Non-Fac Total	Fac Total		51	50	62	80	MUE
	0.00	0.00	XXX	9	9	9	9	0

● New   ▲ Revised   Deleted   ⊙ Moderate Sedation   ✚ Add-on Codes   ⊘ High Risk Denial   Ⓐ Age Edit   ♀ Female   ♂ Male   **AMA** *CPT® Assistant*   **MUE** Medically Unlikely Edit
⊘ Modifier 51 Exempt   ⊖ Modifier 63 Exempt   ✗ Unlisted   **Modifiers:** *See Inside Back Cover*   Ⓜ Maternity   A2–Z3 ASC Payment Indicators   A–Y OPPS Status Indicators

© 2016 DecisionHealth   CPT © 2015 American Medical Association. All Rights Reserved.   **799**

92533 Caloric vestibular test, each irrigation (binaural, bithermal stimulation constitutes 4 tests) ⊗N

Mod	Non-Fac Total	Fac Total	Global Days	51	50	62	80	MUE
	0.00	0.00	XXX	9	9	9	9	

AMA: May 96: 5

92534 Optokinetic nystagmus test ⊗N

Mod	Non-Fac Total	Fac Total	Global Days	51	50	62	80	MUE
	0.00	0.00	XXX	9	9	9	9	0

● **92537** Caloric vestibular test with recording, bilateral; bithermal (ie, one warm and one cool irrigation in each ear for a total of four irrigations) S

Mod	Non-Fac Total	Fac Total	Global Days	51	50	62	80	MUE
	1.14	1.14	XXX	0	1	0	0	1
26	0.90	0.90	XXX	0	0	0	0	1
TC	0.24	0.24	XXX	0	0	0	0	1

● **92538** Caloric vestibular test with recording, bilateral; monothermal (ie, one irrigation in each ear for a total of two irrigations) S

Mod	Non-Fac Total	Fac Total	Global Days	51	50	62	80	MUE
26	0.45	0.45	XXX	0	0	0	0	1
TC	0.13	0.13	XXX	0	0	0	0	1
	0.58	0.58	XXX	0	0	0	0	1

92540 Basic vestibular evaluation, includes spontaneous nystagmus test with eccentric gaze fixation nystagmus, with recording, positional nystagmus test, minimum of 4 positions, with recording, optokinetic nystagmus test, bidirectional foveal and peripheral stimulation, with recording, and oscillating tracking test, with recording S

Mod	Non-Fac Total	Fac Total	Global Days	51	50	62	80	MUE
	2.87	2.87	XXX	0	0	0	0	1
26	2.25	2.25	XXX	0	0	0	0	1
TC	0.62	0.62	XXX	0	0	0	0	1

92541 Spontaneous nystagmus test, including gaze and fixation nystagmus, with recording ⊗1

Mod	Non-Fac Total	Fac Total	Global Days	51	50	62	80	MUE
	0.68	0.68	XXX	0	0	0	0	1
26	0.59	0.59	XXX	0	0	0	0	1
TC	0.09	0.09	XXX	0	0	0	0	1

AMA: Feb 05: 13, Aug 08: 12, May 11: 10

92542 Positional nystagmus test, minimum of 4 positions, with recording ⊗1

Mod	Non-Fac Total	Fac Total	Global Days	51	50	62	80	MUE
	0.79	0.79	XXX	0	0	0	0	1
26	0.71	0.71	XXX	0	0	0	0	1
TC	0.08	0.08	XXX	0	0	0	0	1

AMA: Feb 05: 13, Aug 08: 12, Sep 10: 9

✖ 92543 Caloric vestibular test, each irrigation (binaural, bithermal stimulation constitutes 4 tests), with recording

92544 Optokinetic nystagmus test, bidirectional, foveal or peripheral stimulation, with recording S

Mod	Non-Fac Total	Fac Total	Global Days	51	50	62	80	MUE
	0.47	0.47	XXX	0	0	0	0	1
26	0.40	0.40	XXX	0	0	0	0	1
TC	0.07	0.07	XXX	0	0	0	0	1

AMA: Feb 05: 13, Aug 08: 12

92545 Oscillating tracking test, with recording S

Mod	Non-Fac Total	Fac Total	Global Days	51	50	62	80	MUE
	0.43	0.43	XXX	0	0	0	0	1
26	0.37	0.37	XXX	0	0	0	0	1
TC	0.06	0.06	XXX	0	0	0	0	1

AMA: Feb 05: 13, Aug 08: 12, May 11: 10

92546 Sinusoidal vertical axis rotational testing S

Mod	Non-Fac Total	Fac Total	Global Days	51	50	62	80	MUE
	2.90	2.90	XXX	0	0	0	0	1
26	0.42	0.42	XXX	0	0	0	0	1
TC	2.48	2.48	XXX	0	0	0	0	1

AMA: Sep 04: 13, Feb 05: 13, Aug 08: 12, May 11: 10, Jun 13: 14

+ **92547** Use of vertical electrodes (List separately in addition to code for primary procedure) N

Mod	Non-Fac Total	Fac Total	Global Days	51	50	62	80	MUE
	0.17	0.17	ZZZ	0	0	0	0	1

AMA: May 04: 14, Feb 05: 13, Aug 08: 12

92548 Computerized dynamic posturography ⊗1

Mod	Non-Fac Total	Fac Total	Global Days	51	50	62	80	MUE
	2.88	2.88	XXX	0	0	0	0	1
26	0.74	0.74	XXX	0	0	0	0	1
TC	2.14	2.14	XXX	0	0	0	0	1

AMA: May 11: 10

92550 Tympanometry and reflex threshold measurements ⊗1

Mod	Non-Fac Total	Fac Total	Global Days	51	50	62	80	MUE
	0.60	0.60	XXX	0	2	0	0	1

AMA: Aug 14: 3

Audiological Function Testing

92551 Screening test, pure tone, air only ⊗E

Mod	Non-Fac Total	Fac Total	Global Days	51	50	62	80	MUE
	0.34	0.34	XXX	9	9	9	9	

AMA: Aug 14: 3

Coding Guidance
Codes 92552-92557 are only to be used when calibrated electronic equipment is used. Qualitative estimation is part of the phyisician's E&M service.

92552 Pure tone audiometry (threshold); air only ⊗1

Mod	Non-Fac Total	Fac Total	Global Days	51	50	62	80	MUE
	0.88	0.88	XXX	0	2	0	0	1

AMA: Aug 14: 3

● New ▲ Revised ✖ Deleted ⊙ Moderate Sedation ✚ Add-on Codes ⊘ High Risk Denial Ⓐ Age Edit ♀ Female ♂ Male **AMA** CPT® Assistant **MUE** Medically Unlikely Edit ⊘ Modifier 51 Exempt ⊖ Modifier 63 Exempt ✗ Unlisted **Modifiers:** See Inside Back Cover Ⓜ Maternity A2–Z3 ASC Payment Indicators A–Y OPPS Status Indicators

CPT © 2015 American Medical Association. All Rights Reserved.   © 2016 DecisionHealth

92553 Pure tone audiometry (threshold); air and bone ⚫Ⅰ

RVU			Global Days	Modifiers				
Mod	Non-Fac Total	Fac Total		51	50	62	80	MUE
	1.05	1.05	XXX	0	2	0	0	1

AMA: Mar 11: 8, Aug 14: 3

92555 Speech audiometry threshold ⚫Ⅰ

RVU			Global Days	Modifiers				
Mod	Non-Fac Total	Fac Total		51	50	62	80	MUE
	0.65	0.65	XXX	0	2	0	0	1

AMA: Aug 14: 3

92556 Speech audiometry threshold; with speech recognition ⚫Ⅰ

RVU			Global Days	Modifiers				
Mod	Non-Fac Total	Fac Total		51	50	62	80	MUE
	1.05	1.05	XXX	0	2	0	0	1

AMA: Mar 11: 8, Aug 14: 3

92557 Comprehensive audiometry threshold evaluation and speech recognition (92553 and 92556 combined) ⚫Ⅰ

RVU			Global Days	Modifiers				
Mod	Non-Fac Total	Fac Total		51	50	62	80	MUE
	1.06	0.92	XXX	0	2	0	0	1

AMA: Sep 07: 11, Mar 11: 8, Aug 14: 3

92558 Evoked otoacoustic emissions, screening (qualitative measurement of distortion product or transient evoked otoacoustic emissions), automated analysis ⚫E

RVU			Global Days	Modifiers				
Mod	Non-Fac Total	Fac Total		51	50	62	80	MUE
	0.00	0.00	XXX	9	9	9	9	0

AMA: Aug 14: 3

92559 Audiometric testing of groups ⚫E

RVU			Global Days	Modifiers				
Mod	Non-Fac Total	Fac Total		51	50	62	80	MUE
	0.00	0.00	XXX	9	9	9	9	

AMA: Aug 14: 3

Coding Guidance

Codes 92561-92588 are only to be used when calibrated electronic equipment is used. Qualitative estimation is part of the phyisician's E&M service.

92560 Bekesy audiometry; screening ⚫E

RVU			Global Days	Modifiers				
Mod	Non-Fac Total	Fac Total		51	50	62	80	MUE
	0.00	0.00	XXX	9	9	9	9	

AMA: Aug 14: 3

92561 Bekesy audiometry; diagnostic ⚫Ⅰ

RVU			Global Days	Modifiers				
Mod	Non-Fac Total	Fac Total		51	50	62	80	MUE
	1.07	1.07	XXX	0	2	0	0	1

AMA: Aug 14: 3

92562 Loudness balance test, alternate binaural or monaural ⚫Ⅰ

RVU			Global Days	Modifiers				
Mod	Non-Fac Total	Fac Total		51	50	62	80	MUE
	1.31	1.31	XXX	0	2	0	0	1

AMA: Mar 05: 7, 9, Aug 14: 3

92563 Tone decay test ⚫Ⅰ

RVU			Global Days	Modifiers				
Mod	Non-Fac Total	Fac Total		51	50	62	80	MUE
	0.87	0.87	XXX	0	2	0	0	1

AMA: Aug 14: 3

92564 Short increment sensitivity index (SISI) ⚫Ⅰ

RVU			Global Days	Modifiers				
Mod	Non-Fac Total	Fac Total		51	50	62	80	MUE
	0.79	0.79	XXX	0	2	0	0	1

AMA: Oct 96: 9, Aug 14: 3

92565 Stenger test, pure tone ⚫Ⅰ

RVU			Global Days	Modifiers				
Mod	Non-Fac Total	Fac Total		51	50	62	80	MUE
	0.45	0.45	XXX	0	2	0	0	1

AMA: Aug 14: 3
Pub 100-04, 16, 120.2

92567 Tympanometry (impedance testing) ⚫Ⅰ

RVU			Global Days	Modifiers				
Mod	Non-Fac Total	Fac Total		51	50	62	80	MUE
	0.41	0.31	XXX	0	2	0	0	1

AMA: Winter 90: 11, Aug 14: 3

92568 Acoustic reflex testing, threshold ⚫Ⅰ

RVU			Global Days	Modifiers				
Mod	Non-Fac Total	Fac Total		51	50	62	80	MUE
	0.45	0.44	XXX	0	2	0	0	1

AMA: Jan 06: 7, Sep 07: 11, Jun 09: 10, Aug 14: 3

92570 Acoustic immittance testing, includes tympanometry (impedance testing), acoustic reflex threshold testing, and acoustic reflex decay testing ⚫Ⅰ

RVU			Global Days	Modifiers				
Mod	Non-Fac Total	Fac Total		51	50	62	80	MUE
	0.91	0.85	XXX	0	2	0	0	1

AMA: Aug 14: 3

92571 Filtered speech test ⚫Ⅰ

RVU			Global Days	Modifiers				
Mod	Non-Fac Total	Fac Total		51	50	62	80	MUE
	0.76	0.76	XXX	0	2	0	0	1

AMA: Mar 05: 7, Aug 14: 3

92572 Staggered spondaic word test ⚫Ⅰ

Coding tip: For Lombard test - 92700

RVU			Global Days	Modifiers				
Mod	Non-Fac Total	Fac Total		51	50	62	80	MUE
	1.01	1.01	XXX	0	2	0	0	1

AMA: Mar 05: 7, Aug 14: 3

92575 Sensorineural acuity level test ⚫Ⅰ

RVU			Global Days	Modifiers				
Mod	Non-Fac Total	Fac Total		51	50	62	80	MUE
	2.04	2.04	XXX	0	2	0	0	1

AMA: Aug 14: 3

92576 Synthetic sentence identification test ⚫Ⅰ

RVU			Global Days	Modifiers				
Mod	Non-Fac Total	Fac Total		51	50	62	80	MUE
	1.01	1.01	XXX	0	2	0	0	1

AMA: Mar 05: 7, Aug 14: 3

● New ▲ Revised Deleted ⊙ Moderate Sedation ✚ Add-on Codes ⊘ High Risk Denial Ⓐ Age Edit ♀ Female ♂ Male **AMA** *CPT® Assistant* **MUE** Medically Unlikely Edit
⊘ Modifier 51 Exempt ⊖ Modifier 63 Exempt ✗ Unlisted **Modifiers:** *See Inside Back Cover* Ⓜ Maternity Ⓐ2-Z3 ASC Payment Indicators Ⓐ-Y OPPS Status Indicators
© 2016 DecisionHealth CPT © 2015 American Medical Association. All Rights Reserved. **801**

Medicine Procedures

92577 Stenger test, speech ⊙Ⅰ

Mod	Non-Fac Total	Fac Total	Global Days	51	50	62	80	MUE
	0.47	0.47	XXX	0	2	0	0	1

AMA: Aug 14: 3

92579 Visual reinforcement audiometry (VRA) ⊙Ⅰ

Mod	Non-Fac Total	Fac Total	Global Days	51	50	62	80	MUE
	1.19	1.07	XXX	0	2	0	0	1

AMA: Aug 14: 3

92582 Conditioning play audiometry ⊙Ⅰ

Mod	Non-Fac Total	Fac Total	Global Days	51	50	62	80	MUE
	1.91	1.91	XXX	0	2	0	0	1

AMA: Aug 14: 3

92583 Select picture audiometry ⊙Ⅰ

Mod	Non-Fac Total	Fac Total	Global Days	51	50	62	80	MUE
	1.47	1.47	XXX	0	2	0	0	1

92584 Electrocochleography S

Mod	Non-Fac Total	Fac Total	Global Days	51	50	62	80	MUE
	2.07	2.07	XXX	0	2	0	0	1

AMA: Jul 11: 17, Aug 14: 3

92585 Auditory evoked potentials for evoked response audiometry and/or testing of the central nervous system; comprehensive S

Mod	Non-Fac Total	Fac Total	Global Days	51	50	62	80	MUE
	3.82	3.82	XXX	0	2	0	0	1
26	0.76	0.76	XXX	0	2	0	0	1
TC	3.06	3.06	XXX	0	2	0	0	1

AMA: May 13: 8, Winter 90: 11, Aug 14: 3

92586 Auditory evoked potentials for evoked response audiometry and/or testing of the central nervous system; limited S

Mod	Non-Fac Total	Fac Total	Global Days	51	50	62	80	MUE
	2.40	2.40	XXX	0	2	0	0	1

AMA: Aug 14: 3

92587 Distortion product evoked otoacoustic emissions; limited evaluation (to confirm the presence or absence of hearing disorder, 3-6 frequencies) or transient evoked otoacoustic emissions, with interpretation and report S

Mod	Non-Fac Total	Fac Total	Global Days	51	50	62	80	MUE
	0.61	0.61	XXX	0	2	0	0	1
26	0.52	0.52	XXX	0	2	0	0	1
TC	0.09	0.09	XXX	0	2	0	0	1

AMA: Sep 07: 11

92588 Distortion product evoked otoacoustic emissions; comprehensive diagnostic evaluation (quantitative analysis of outer hair cell function by cochlear mapping, minimum of 12 frequencies), with interpretation and report S

Mod	Non-Fac Total	Fac Total	Global Days	51	50	62	80	MUE
	0.93	0.93	XXX	0	2	0	0	1
26	0.82	0.82	XXX	0	2	0	0	1
TC	0.11	0.11	XXX	0	2	0	0	1

AMA: Aug 14: 3

92590 Hearing aid examination and selection; monaural ⊘E

Mod	Non-Fac Total	Fac Total	Global Days	51	50	62	80	MUE
	0.00	0.00	XXX	9	9	9	9	

AMA: Jul 14: 4, Aug 14: 3

92591 Hearing aid examination and selection; binaural ⊘E

Mod	Non-Fac Total	Fac Total	Global Days	51	50	62	80	MUE
	0.00	0.00	XXX	9	9	9	9	

92592 Hearing aid check; monaural ⊘E

Mod	Non-Fac Total	Fac Total	Global Days	51	50	62	80	MUE
	0.00	0.00	XXX	9	9	9	9	

92593 Hearing aid check; binaural ⊘E

Mod	Non-Fac Total	Fac Total	Global Days	51	50	62	80	MUE
	0.00	0.00	XXX	9	9	9	9	

92594 Electroacoustic evaluation for hearing aid; monaural ⊘E

Mod	Non-Fac Total	Fac Total	Global Days	51	50	62	80	MUE
	0.00	0.00	XXX	9	9	9	9	

92595 Electroacoustic evaluation for hearing aid; binaural ⊘E

Mod	Non-Fac Total	Fac Total	Global Days	51	50	62	80	MUE
	0.00	0.00	XXX	9	9	9	9	

AMA: Aug 14: 3

92596 Ear protector attenuation measurements ⊘⊙Ⅰ

Mod	Non-Fac Total	Fac Total	Global Days	51	50	62	80	MUE
	1.19	1.19	XXX	0	2	0	0	1

AMA: Aug 14: 3

92597 Evaluation for use and/or fitting of voice prosthetic device to supplement oral speech A

Mod	Non-Fac Total	Fac Total	Global Days	51	50	62	80	MUE
	2.04	2.04	XXX	5	0	0	0	

● New ▲ Revised ✖ Deleted ⊙ Moderate Sedation ✚ Add-on Codes ⊘ High Risk Denial Ⓐ Age Edit ♀ Female ♂ Male **AMA** CPT® Assistant **MUE** Medically Unlikely Edit
⊘ Modifier 51 Exempt ⊖ Modifier 63 Exempt ✗ Unlisted **Modifiers:** See Inside Back Cover Ⓜ Maternity Ⓐ2–Ⓩ3 ASC Payment Indicators Ⓐ–Ⓨ OPPS Status Indicators

802 CPT © 2015 American Medical Association. All Rights Reserved. © 2016 DecisionHealth

Evaluation/Therapeutic Services/Procedures

92601 Diagnostic analysis of cochlear implant, patient younger than 7 years of age; with programming ⊘Ⓐ🅂

RVU			Global Days	Modifiers				
Mod	Non-Fac Total	Fac Total		51	50	62	80	MUE
	4.00	3.40	XXX	0	0	0	0	1

AMA: Mar 03: 1, Jan 06: 7, Jul 11: 17, Oct 13: 7, Jul 14: 4
Pub 100-04, 12, 30.3; 100-04, 32, 100.3, 100.1.2, 100.4

92602 Diagnostic analysis of cochlear implant, patient younger than 7 years of age; subsequent reprogramming ⊘Ⓐ🅂

RVU			Global Days	Modifiers				
Mod	Non-Fac Total	Fac Total		51	50	62	80	MUE
	2.53	1.97	XXX	0	0	0	0	1

AMA: Mar 03: 1, 21, Jan 06: 7, Oct 13: 7
Pub 100-04, 12, 30.3; 100-04, 32, 100.3, 100.4

92603 Diagnostic analysis of cochlear implant, age 7 years or older; with programming 🅂

RVU			Global Days	Modifiers				
Mod	Non-Fac Total	Fac Total		51	50	62	80	MUE
	4.28	3.47	XXX	0	0	0	0	1

AMA: Mar 03: 2, 4, Jan 06: 7, Jul 11: 17, Oct 13: 7
Pub 100-04, 12, 30.3; 100-04, 32, 100.3, 100.1.2, 100.4

92604 Diagnostic analysis of cochlear implant, age 7 years or older; subsequent reprogramming 🅂

RVU			Global Days	Modifiers				
Mod	Non-Fac Total	Fac Total		51	50	62	80	MUE
	2.52	1.92	XXX	0	0	0	0	1

AMA: Mar 03: 2, 21, Jan 06: 7, Jul 11: 17, Oct 13: 7, Jul 14: 4
Pub 100-04, 12, 30.3; 100-04, 32, 100.3, 100.4

92605 Evaluation for prescription of non-speech-generating augmentative and alternative communication device, face-to-face with the patient; first hour ⊘Ⓐ

RVU			Global Days	Modifiers				
Mod	Non-Fac Total	Fac Total		51	50	62	80	MUE
	2.64	2.52	XXX	9	9	9	9	0

AMA: Mar 03: 2, 4, Oct 13: 7

92606 Therapeutic service(s) for the use of non-speech-generating device, including programming and modification ⊘Ⓐ

RVU			Global Days	Modifiers				
Mod	Non-Fac Total	Fac Total		51	50	62	80	MUE
	2.35	2.02	XXX	9	9	9	9	

AMA: Mar 03: 2, 4

92607 Evaluation for prescription for speech-generating augmentative and alternative communication device, face-to-face with the patient; first hour Ⓐ

RVU			Global Days	Modifiers				
Mod	Non-Fac Total	Fac Total		51	50	62	80	MUE
	3.56	3.56	XXX	5	0	0	0	

AMA: Mar 03: 2, 4, Dec 04: 16, Oct 13: 7

+ 92608 Evaluation for prescription for speech-generating augmentative and alternative communication device, face-to-face with the patient; each additional 30 minutes (List separately in addition to code for primary procedure) ⊘Ⓐ

RVU			Global Days	Modifiers				
Mod	Non-Fac Total	Fac Total		51	50	62	80	MUE
	1.49	1.49	ZZZ	0	0	0	0	

AMA: Mar 03: 2, 5, Dec 04: 16, Oct 13: 7

92609 Therapeutic services for the use of speech-generating device, including programming and modification Ⓐ

RVU			Global Days	Modifiers				
Mod	Non-Fac Total	Fac Total		51	50	62	80	MUE
	3.12	3.12	XXX	5	0	0	0	1

AMA: Mar 03: 2, 4, Dec 04: 16

92610 Evaluation of oral and pharyngeal swallowing function Ⓐ

RVU			Global Days	Modifiers				
Mod	Non-Fac Total	Fac Total		51	50	62	80	MUE
	2.41	2.06	XXX	0	0	0	0	1

AMA: Mar 03: 2, 5, Dec 04: 17

92611 Motion fluoroscopic evaluation of swallowing function by cine or video recording Ⓐ

RVU			Global Days	Modifiers				
Mod	Non-Fac Total	Fac Total		51	50	62	80	MUE
	2.46	2.46	XXX	0	0	0		

AMA: Mar 03: 2, 5, Dec 04: 17, Jan 06: 7, Jul 14: 5

92612 Flexible fiberoptic endoscopic evaluation of swallowing by cine or video recording Ⓐ

RVU			Global Days	Modifiers				
Mod	Non-Fac Total	Fac Total		51	50	62	80	MUE
	5.27	1.94	XXX	0	0	0		

AMA: Mar 03: 6, Jan 06: 7

92613 Flexible fiberoptic endoscopic evaluation of swallowing by cine or video recording; interpretation and report only Ⓑ

RVU			Global Days	Modifiers				
Mod	Non-Fac Total	Fac Total		51	50	62	80	MUE
	1.09	1.09	XXX	0	0	0	0	1

AMA: Jan 06: 7

92614 Flexible fiberoptic endoscopic evaluation, laryngeal sensory testing by cine or video recording Ⓐ

RVU			Global Days	Modifiers				
Mod	Non-Fac Total	Fac Total		51	50	62	80	MUE
	4.13	1.93	XXX	0	0	0		

AMA: Mar 03: 6, Jan 06: 7

92615 Flexible fiberoptic endoscopic evaluation, laryngeal sensory testing by cine or video recording; interpretation and report only Ⓔ

RVU			Global Days	Modifiers				
Mod	Non-Fac Total	Fac Total		51	50	62	80	MUE
	0.96	0.95	XXX	0	0	0	0	1

AMA: Mar 03: 6, Jan 06: 7

● New   ▲ Revised   Deleted   ⊙ Moderate Sedation   ✚ Add-on Codes   ⊘ High Risk Denial   Ⓐ Age Edit   ♀ Female   ♂ Male   **AMA** *CPT® Assistant*   **MUE** Medically Unlikely Edit
⊘ Modifier 51 Exempt   ⊖ Modifier 63 Exempt   ☒ Unlisted   **Modifiers:** *See Inside Back Cover*   Ⓜ Maternity   Ⓐ2–Ⓩ3 ASC Payment Indicators   Ⓐ–Ⓨ OPPS Status Indicators

92616 Flexible fiberoptic endoscopic evaluation of swallowing and laryngeal sensory testing by cine or video recording   **A**

RVU			Global Days	Modifiers				
Mod	Non-Fac Total	Fac Total		51	50	62	80	MUE
	5.90	2.88	XXX	0	0	0	0	

AMA: Mar 03: 6, Jan 06: 7

92617 Flexible fiberoptic endoscopic evaluation of swallowing and laryngeal sensory testing by cine or video recording; interpretation and report only   **E**

RVU			Global Days	Modifiers				
Mod	Non-Fac Total	Fac Total		51	50	62	80	MUE
	1.19	1.19	XXX	0	0	0	0	1

AMA: Mar 03: 6, Jan 06: 7

+ 92618 Evaluation for prescription of non-speech-generating augmentative and alternative communication device, face-to-face with the patient; each additional 30 minutes (List separately in addition to code for primary procedure)   **A**

RVU			Global Days	Modifiers				
Mod	Non-Fac Total	Fac Total		51	50	62	80	MUE
	0.96	0.94	ZZZ	9	9	9	9	0

92620 Evaluation of central auditory function, with report; initial 60 minutes   **Q1**

RVU			Global Days	Modifiers				
Mod	Non-Fac Total	Fac Total		51	50	62	80	MUE
	2.66	2.34	XXX	0	2	0	0	1

AMA: Mar 05: 7, 8, Aug 14: 3
Pub 100-04, 12, 30.3

+ 92621 Evaluation of central auditory function, with report; each additional 15 minutes (List separately in addition to code for primary procedure)   **N**

RVU			Global Days	Modifiers				
Mod	Non-Fac Total	Fac Total		51	50	62	80	MUE
	0.63	0.54	ZZZ	0	0	0	0	

AMA: Mar 05: 7, Aug 14: 3
Pub 100-04, 12, 30.3

92625 Assessment of tinnitus (includes pitch, loudness matching, and masking)   **Q1**

RVU			Global Days	Modifiers				
Mod	Non-Fac Total	Fac Total		51	50	62	80	MUE
	1.98	1.77	XXX	0	2	0	0	1

AMA: Mar 05: 7, 10, Aug 14: 3

Coding Guidance
When calculating time increments for 92626 and 92627, use face-to-face time with the patient and/or family.

92626 Evaluation of auditory rehabilitation status; first hour   **Q1**

RVU			Global Days	Modifiers				
Mod	Non-Fac Total	Fac Total		51	50	62	80	MUE
	2.53	2.16	XXX	0	2	0	0	1

AMA: Jan 06: 7, May 14: 10, Jul 14: 4
Pub 100-04, 12, 30.3

+ 92627 Evaluation of auditory rehabilitation status; each additional 15 minutes (List separately in addition to code for primary procedure)   **N**

Documentation Finder: *Look for documentation of more than an hour to support 92626 (Evaluation of auditory rehabilitation status; first hour) plus this add-on code. If the evaluation continues past the first hour, this code is reported for each addition 15 minutes.*

RVU			Global Days	Modifiers				
Mod	Non-Fac Total	Fac Total		51	50	62	80	MUE
	0.62	0.51	ZZZ	0	0	0	0	

AMA: Jan 06: 7, Jul 14: 4
Pub 100-04, 12, 30.3

92630 Auditory rehabilitation; prelingual hearing loss   **E**

RVU			Global Days	Modifiers				
Mod	Non-Fac Total	Fac Total		51	50	62	80	MUE
	0.00	0.00	XXX	9	9	9	9	

AMA: Jan 06: 7, Oct 13: 7

92633 Auditory rehabilitation; postlingual hearing loss   **E**

RVU			Global Days	Modifiers				
Mod	Non-Fac Total	Fac Total		51	50	62	80	MUE
	0.00	0.00	XXX	9	9	9	9	

AMA: Jan 06: 7, Oct 13: 7

Special Diagnostic Otorhinolaryngological Services

92640 Diagnostic analysis with programming of auditory brainstem implant, per hour   **S**

RVU			Global Days	Modifiers				
Mod	Non-Fac Total	Fac Total		51	50	62	80	MUE
	3.20	2.71	XXX	0	2	0	0	

Other Otorhinolaryngological Services

92700 Unlisted otorhinolaryngological service or procedure   **x Q1**

RVU			Global Days	Modifiers				
Mod	Non-Fac Total	Fac Total		51	50	62	80	MUE
	0.00	0.00	XXX	0	0	0	0	

AMA: Sep 04: 14, Oct 04: 10, Jan 06: 7, Sep 06: 13, Sep 07: 11, Mar 11: 10, Jul 11: 17, May 14: 10
Pub 100-04, 12, 30.3

Coronary Therapeutic Services/Procedures

Coding Guidance
When percutaneous coronary artery interventions are performed (stent placement, atherectomy, balloon angioplasty), the provider should report the code that describes the interventional procedure or combination of interventional procedures performed (angioplasty, atherectomy, stent placement). Percutaneous interventional procedures are also specific to native coronary arteries or branches (92920-92934), revascularization of or through coronary artery bypass grafts (92937-92938), revascularization of acute total or subtotal occlusion during an acute myocardial infarction (92941), revascularization of chronic total occlusion (92943-92944). When percutaneous interventions are performed on the major coronary arteries or branches, the first procedure reported with a primary code should correspond to the most complex service. The procedure(s) done in each additional branch of the target major coronary artery are then reported with the CPT add-on codes 92921, 92925, 92929. When a percutaneous coronary intervention is performed on a second major coronary artery or its branches, a second primary code is reported along with add-on codes for each additional branch of the second target artery that is treated. When revascularization is performed on or through a coronary artery bypass graft, codes 92937-92938 include any combination of intracoronary stent, atherectomy and angioplasty. Codes

● New   ▲ Revised   ✖ Deleted   ⊙ Moderate Sedation   ✚ Add-on Codes   ⊖ High Risk Denial   Ⓐ Age Edit   ♀ Female   ♂ Male   **AMA** *CPT® Assistant*   **MUE** Medically Unlikely Edit
⊘ Modifier 51 Exempt   ⊖ Modifier 63 Exempt   ✗ Unlisted   **Modifiers:** *See Inside Back Cover*   Ⓜ Maternity   **A2**-**Z3** ASC Payment Indicators   **A**-**Y** OPPS Status Indicators

804   CPT © 2015 American Medical Association. All Rights Reserved.   © 2016 DecisionHealth

92920-92944 for coronary therapeutic procedures are listed out of numerical order in CPT. For additional coronary therapeutic procedures, refer to 92973-92979.

⊙ **92920** Percutaneous transluminal coronary angioplasty; single major coronary artery or branch **J1**

RVU			Global Days	Modifiers				
Mod	Non-Fac Total	Fac Total		51	50	62	80	MUE
	15.87	15.87	000	2	0	0	0	1

AMA: Jan 13: 3, Dec 14: 6

⊙+**92921** Percutaneous transluminal coronary angioplasty; each additional branch of a major coronary artery (List separately in addition to code for primary procedure) **N**

RVU			Global Days	Modifiers				
Mod	Non-Fac Total	Fac Total		51	50	62	80	MUE
	0.00	0.00	ZZZ	9	9	9	9	

AMA: Jan 13: 3, Sep 14: 14, Dec 14: 6

⊙ **92924** Percutaneous transluminal coronary atherectomy, with coronary angioplasty when performed; single major coronary artery or branch **J1**

RVU			Global Days	Modifiers				
Mod	Non-Fac Total	Fac Total		51	50	62	80	MUE
	18.84	18.84	000	2	0	0	0	1

AMA: Jan 13: 3, Dec 14: 6

⊙+**92925** Percutaneous transluminal coronary atherectomy, with coronary angioplasty when performed; each additional branch of a major coronary artery (List separately in addition to code for primary procedure) **N**

RVU			Global Days	Modifiers				
Mod	Non-Fac Total	Fac Total		51	50	62	80	MUE
	0.00	0.00	ZZZ	9	9	9	9	

AMA: Jan 13: 3, Sep 14: 14, Dec 14: 6

⊙ **92928** Percutaneous transcatheter placement of intracoronary stent(s), with coronary angioplasty when performed; single major coronary artery or branch **J1**

RVU			Global Days	Modifiers				
Mod	Non-Fac Total	Fac Total		51	50	62	80	MUE
	17.62	17.62	000	2	0	0	0	1

AMA: Jan 13: 3, Jan 14: 3, Mar 14: 14, Sep 14: 14, Dec 14: 6

⊙+**92929** Percutaneous transcatheter placement of intracoronary stent(s), with coronary angioplasty when performed; each additional branch of a major coronary artery (List separately in addition to code for primary procedure) **N**

RVU			Global Days	Modifiers				
Mod	Non-Fac Total	Fac Total		51	50	62	80	MUE
	0.00	0.00	ZZZ	9	9	9	9	

AMA: Jan 13: 3, Sep 14: 14, Dec 14: 6

⊙ **92933** Percutaneous transluminal coronary atherectomy, with intracoronary stent, with coronary angioplasty when performed; single major coronary artery or branch **J1**

RVU			Global Days	Modifiers				
Mod	Non-Fac Total	Fac Total		51	50	62	80	MUE
	19.71	19.71	000	2	0	0	0	1

AMA: Jan 13: 3, Dec 14: 6

⊙+**92934** Percutaneous transluminal coronary atherectomy, with intracoronary stent, with coronary angioplasty when performed; each additional branch of a major coronary artery (List separately in addition to code for primary procedure) **N**

RVU			Global Days	Modifiers				
Mod	Non-Fac Total	Fac Total		51	50	62	80	MUE
	0.00	0.00	ZZZ	9	9	9	9	

AMA: Jan 13: 3, Sep 14: 14, Dec 14: 6

⊙ **92937** Percutaneous transluminal revascularization of or through coronary artery bypass graft (internal mammary, free arterial, venous), any combination of intracoronary stent, atherectomy and angioplasty, including distal protection when performed; single vessel **J1**

RVU			Global Days	Modifiers				
Mod	Non-Fac Total	Fac Total		51	50	62	80	MUE
	17.60	17.60	000	2	0	0	0	3

AMA: Jan 13: 3, Mar 14: 14, Dec 14: 6

⊙+**92938** Percutaneous transluminal revascularization of or through coronary artery bypass graft (internal mammary, free arterial, venous), any combination of intracoronary stent, atherectomy and angioplasty, including distal protection when performed; each additional branch subtended by the bypass graft (List separately in addition to code for primary procedure) **N**

RVU			Global Days	Modifiers				
Mod	Non-Fac Total	Fac Total		51	50	62	80	MUE
	0.00	0.00	ZZZ	9	9	9	9	3

AMA: Jan 13: 3, Mar 14: 14, Sep 14: 14, Dec 14: 6

⊙ **92941** Percutaneous transluminal revascularization of acute total/subtotal occlusion during acute myocardial infarction, coronary artery or coronary artery bypass graft, any combination of intracoronary stent, atherectomy and angioplasty, including aspiration thrombectomy when performed, single vessel **J1**

RVU			Global Days	Modifiers				
Mod	Non-Fac Total	Fac Total		51	50	62	80	MUE
	19.75	19.75	000	2	0	0	0	1

AMA: Jan 13: 3, Jan 14: 3, Mar 14: 14, Dec 14: 6

⊙ **92943** Percutaneous transluminal revascularization of chronic total occlusion, coronary artery, coronary artery branch, or coronary artery bypass graft, any combination of intracoronary stent, atherectomy and angioplasty; single vessel **J1**

RVU			Global Days	Modifiers				
Mod	Non-Fac Total	Fac Total		51	50	62	80	MUE
	19.74	19.74	000	2	0	0	0	1

AMA: Jan 13: 3, Dec 14: 6

● New ▲ Revised Deleted ⊙ Moderate Sedation ✚ Add-on Codes ⊘ High Risk Denial Ⓐ Age Edit ♀ Female ♂ Male **AMA** *CPT® Assistant* **MUE** Medically Unlikely Edit
⊘ Modifier 51 Exempt ⊖ Modifier 63 Exempt ✗ Unlisted **Modifiers:** *See Inside Back Cover* Ⓜ Maternity **A2-Z3** ASC Payment Indicators **A-Y** OPPS Status Indicators

© 2016 DecisionHealth | CPT © 2015 American Medical Association. All Rights Reserved. | **805**

Medicine Procedures

92944 – 92978

⊙**+92944** Percutaneous transluminal revascularization of chronic total occlusion, coronary artery, coronary artery branch, or coronary artery bypass graft, any combination of intracoronary stent, atherectomy and angioplasty; each additional coronary artery, coronary artery branch, or bypass graft (List separately in addition to code for primary procedure) ⊙N

RVU			Global Days	Modifiers				
Mod	Non-Fac Total	Fac Total		51	50	62	80	MUE
	0.00	0.00	ZZZ	9	9	9	9	1

AMA: Jan 13: 3, Sep 14: 14, Dec 14: 6

Cardiovascular Services/Procedures

Cardiovascular Therapeutic Services/Procedures

92950 Cardiopulmonary resuscitation (eg, in cardiac arrest) S

Coding tip: The time required to perform cardiopulmonary resuscitation is not included in any critical care or other timed E&M services

RVU			Global Days	Modifiers				
Mod	Non-Fac Total	Fac Total		51	50	62	80	MUE
	8.60	5.33	000	0	0	0	0	3

AMA: Jan 96: 7, Oct 04: 14, Nov 07: 5, Jul 12: 13, Sep 12: 17

⊙ 92953 Temporary transcutaneous pacing Q3

RVU			Global Days	Modifiers				
Mod	Non-Fac Total	Fac Total		51	50	62	80	MUE
	0.32	0.32	000	0	0	0	0	2

AMA: Nov 99: 49, Feb 07: 10, Jul 07: 1, May 14: 4

Pub 100-04, 12, 30.6.12

⊙ 92960 Cardioversion, elective, electrical conversion of arrhythmia; external S

RVU			Global Days	Modifiers				
Mod	Non-Fac Total	Fac Total		51	50	62	80	MUE
	5.81	3.47	000	0	0	0	0	2

AMA: Summer 93: 13, Nov 99: 49, Jun 00: 5, Nov 00: 9, Jul 01: 11, Jan 12: 13

⊙ 92961 Cardioversion, elective, electrical conversion of arrhythmia; internal (separate procedure) S

RVU			Global Days	Modifiers				
Mod	Non-Fac Total	Fac Total		51	50	62	80	MUE
	7.56	7.56	000	9	9	9	9	1

AMA: Summer 93: 13, Nov 99: 49, Jun 00: 5, Jul 00: 5, Nov 00: 9, Feb 15: 3

92970 Cardioassist-method of circulatory assist; internal C

RVU			Global Days	Modifiers				
Mod	Non-Fac Total	Fac Total		51	50	62	80	MUE
	5.40	5.40	000	0	0	0	0	1

92971 Cardioassist-method of circulatory assist; external C

RVU			Global Days	Modifiers				
Mod	Non-Fac Total	Fac Total		51	50	62	80	MUE
	2.92	2.92	000	0	0	0	0	1

Pub 100-04, 32, 130.1

Coding Guidance

Codes 92973-92979 for coronary therapeutic procedures are listed out of numerical order in CPT. For additional coronary therapeutic procedures, refer to 92920-92944.

⊙**+92973** Percutaneous transluminal coronary thrombectomy mechanical (List separately in addition to code for primary procedure) N

RVU			Global Days	Modifiers				
Mod	Non-Fac Total	Fac Total		51	50	62	80	MUE
	5.15	5.15	ZZZ	0	0	0	0	2

AMA: Mar 02: 2, 10, Mar 04: 10, Dec 14: 6

Percutaneous transluminal coronary thrombectomy

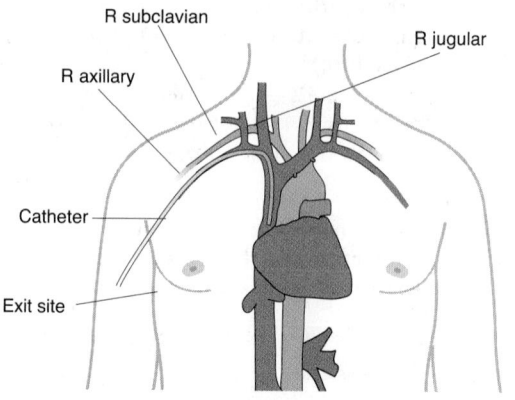

A blood clot is cleared by inserting a double-lumen catheter to the site, flushing the clot with a high-pressure saline wash and suctioning the debris.

⊙**+92974** Transcatheter placement of radiation delivery device for subsequent coronary intravascular brachytherapy (List separately in addition to code for primary procedure) N

RVU			Global Days	Modifiers				
Mod	Non-Fac Total	Fac Total		51	50	62	80	MUE
	4.71	4.71	ZZZ	0	0	0	0	1

AMA: Mar 02: 2, Dec 14: 6

⊙ 92975 Thrombolysis, coronary; by intracoronary infusion, including selective coronary angiography C

RVU			Global Days	Modifiers				
Mod	Non-Fac Total	Fac Total		51	50	62	80	MUE
	11.35	11.35	000	2	0	0	0	1

92977 Thrombolysis, coronary; by intravenous infusion ⊙T

RVU			Global Days	Modifiers				
Mod	Non-Fac Total	Fac Total		51	50	62	80	MUE
	1.75	1.75	XXX	0	0	0	0	1

⊙**+92978** Intravascular ultrasound (coronary vessel or graft) during diagnostic evaluation and/or therapeutic intervention including imaging supervision, interpretation and report; initial vessel (List separately in addition to code for primary procedure) N

RVU			Global Days	Modifiers				
Mod	Non-Fac Total	Fac Total		51	50	62	80	MUE
	0.00	0.00	ZZZ	0	0	0	0	1
26	2.77	2.77	ZZZ	0	0	0	0	1
TC	0.00	0.00	ZZZ	0	0	0	0	1

AMA: Nov 97: 43, 44, Nov 99: 49, Dec 13: 18, Dec 14: 6

● New　▲ Revised　✖ Deleted　⊙ Moderate Sedation　✚ Add-on Codes　⊘ High Risk Denial　Ⓐ Age Edit　♀ Female　♂ Male　**AMA** *CPT® Assistant*　*MUE* Medically Unlikely Edit
⊘ Modifier 51 Exempt　⊖ Modifier 63 Exempt　✖ Unlisted　**Modifiers:** *See Inside Back Cover*　Ⓜ Maternity　A2–Z3 ASC Payment Indicators　A–Y OPPS Status Indicators

CPT © 2015 American Medical Association. All Rights Reserved.　© 2016 DecisionHealth

⊙+92979 **Intravascular ultrasound (coronary vessel or graft) during diagnostic evaluation and/or therapeutic intervention including imaging supervision, interpretation and report; each additional vessel (List separately in addition to code for primary procedure)** N

RVU			Global Days	Modifiers				
Mod	Non-Fac Total	Fac Total		51	50	62	80	MUE
	0.00	0.00	ZZZ	0	0	0	0	2
26	2.22	2.22	ZZZ	0	0	0	0	2
TC	0.00	0.00	ZZZ	0	0	0	0	2

AMA: Nov 97: 43, 44, Nov 99: 49, Dec 13: 18, Dec 14: 6

⊙ 92986 **Percutaneous balloon valvuloplasty; aortic valve** J1

RVU			Global Days	Modifiers				
Mod	Non-Fac Total	Fac Total		51	50	62	80	MUE
	38.72	38.72	090	2	0	0	0	1

AMA: Jan 13: 6, Feb 15: 3

⊙ 92987 **Percutaneous balloon valvuloplasty; mitral valve** J1

RVU			Global Days	Modifiers				
Mod	Non-Fac Total	Fac Total		51	50	62	80	MUE
	39.92	39.92	090	2	0	0	0	1

AMA: Feb 15: 3

92990 **Percutaneous balloon valvuloplasty; pulmonary valve** J1

RVU			Global Days	Modifiers				
Mod	Non-Fac Total	Fac Total		51	50	62	80	MUE
	31.51	31.51	090	2	0	0	0	1

AMA: Winter 91: 3, Feb 15: 3, Jul 15: 11

92992 **Atrial septectomy or septostomy; transvenous method, balloon (eg, Rashkind type) (includes cardiac catheterization)** ⊙C

RVU			Global Days	Modifiers				
Mod	Non-Fac Total	Fac Total		51	50	62	80	MUE
	0.00	0.00	090	2	0	0	2	1

AMA: Nov 97: 44, Apr 98: 3, 10, Nov 07: 9

92993 **Atrial septectomy or septostomy; blade method (Park septostomy) (includes cardiac catheterization)** C

RVU			Global Days	Modifiers				
Mod	Non-Fac Total	Fac Total		51	50	62	80	MUE
	0.00	0.00	090	2	0	0	2	1

AMA: Apr 98: 10

92997 **Percutaneous transluminal pulmonary artery balloon angioplasty; single vessel** J1

RVU			Global Days	Modifiers				
Mod	Non-Fac Total	Fac Total		51	50	62	80	MUE
	19.06	19.06	000	2	0	0	0	1

AMA: Nov 97: 44, Feb 15: 3

✚ 92998 **Percutaneous transluminal pulmonary artery balloon angioplasty; each additional vessel (List separately in addition to code for primary procedure)** ⊙N

RVU			Global Days	Modifiers				
Mod	Non-Fac Total	Fac Total		51	50	62	80	MUE
	9.39	9.39	ZZZ	0	0	0	0	2

AMA: Nov 97: 44, Feb 15: 3

Cardiography Procedures

93000 **Electrocardiogram, routine ECG with at least 12 leads; with interpretation and report** M

RVU			Global Days	Modifiers				
Mod	Non-Fac Total	Fac Total		51	50	62	80	MUE
	0.48	0.48	XXX	6	0	0	0	3

AMA: Aug 97: 9, Feb 05: 9, Mar 05: 1, 11, Jul 08: 3

Pub 100-04, 12, 20.3; 100-04, 13, 60.3; 100-04, 16, 120.2; 100-04, 18, 80.2

93005 **Electrocardiogram, routine ECG with at least 12 leads; tracing only, without interpretation and report** Q1

RVU			Global Days	Modifiers				
Mod	Non-Fac Total	Fac Total		51	50	62	80	MUE
	0.24	0.24	XXX	6	0	0	0	3

AMA: Aug 97: 9, Mar 05: 1

Pub 100-04, 12, 20.3; 100-04, 16, 120.2

93010 **Electrocardiogram, routine ECG with at least 12 leads; interpretation and report only** B

RVU			Global Days	Modifiers				
Mod	Non-Fac Total	Fac Total		51	50	62	80	MUE
	0.24	0.24	XXX	0	0	0	0	

AMA: Aug 97: 9, Mar 05: 1, Apr 07: 1

Pub 100-04, 16, 120.2

93015 **Cardiovascular stress test using maximal or submaximal treadmill or bicycle exercise, continuous electrocardiographic monitoring, and/or pharmacological stress; with supervision, interpretation and report** B

RVU			Global Days	Modifiers				
Mod	Non-Fac Total	Fac Total		51	50	62	80	MUE
	2.13	2.13	XXX	6	0	0	0	1

AMA: Apr 96: 11, Jun 96: 10, Aug 02: 10, Jul 08: 3, Jan 10: 8, May 10: 6

Pub 100-04, 12, 90.4.5; 100-04, 13, 60.3

93016 **Cardiovascular stress test using maximal or submaximal treadmill or bicycle exercise, continuous electrocardiographic monitoring, and/or pharmacological stress; supervision only, without interpretation and report** B

RVU			Global Days	Modifiers				
Mod	Non-Fac Total	Fac Total		51	50	62	80	MUE
	0.62	0.62	XXX	0	0	0	0	1

AMA: Apr 96: 11, Aug 02: 10, Jul 08: 3, Jan 10: 8, May 10: 6

93017 **Cardiovascular stress test using maximal or submaximal treadmill or bicycle exercise, continuous electrocardiographic monitoring, and/or pharmacological stress; tracing only, without interpretation and report** Q1

RVU			Global Days	Modifiers				
Mod	Non-Fac Total	Fac Total		51	50	62	80	MUE
	1.10	1.10	XXX	6	0	0	0	1

AMA: Aug 02: 10, Jul 08: 3, Jan 10: 8, May 10: 6

● New   ▲ Revised   Deleted   ⊙ Moderate Sedation   ✚ Add-on Codes   ⊘ High Risk Denial   Ⓐ Age Edit   ♀ Female   ♂ Male   **AMA** CPT® Assistant   **MUE** Medically Unlikely Edit
⊘ Modifier 51 Exempt   ⊖ Modifier 63 Exempt   ⊠ Unlisted   **Modifiers:** See Inside Back Cover   M Maternity   A2–Z3 ASC Payment Indicators   A–Y OPPS Status Indicators

93018 Cardiovascular stress test using maximal or submaximal treadmill or bicycle exercise, continuous electrocardiographic monitoring, and/or pharmacological stress; interpretation and report only   B

RVU			Global Days	Modifiers				
Mod	Non-Fac Total	Fac Total		51	50	62	80	MUE
	0.41	0.41	XXX	0	0	0	0	1

AMA: Apr 96: 11, Jun 96: 10, Jul 08: 3, Jan 10: 8, May 10: 6

93024 Ergonovine provocation test   Q1

RVU			Global Days	Modifiers				
Mod	Non-Fac Total	Fac Total		51	50	62	80	MUE
	3.15	3.15	XXX	6	0	0	0	1
26	1.61	1.61	XXX	6	0	0	0	1
TC	1.54	1.54	XXX	6	0	0	0	1

93025 Microvolt T-wave alternans for assessment of ventricular arrhythmias   S

RVU			Global Days	Modifiers				
Mod	Non-Fac Total	Fac Total		51	50	62	80	MUE
	4.49	4.49	XXX	6	0	0	0	1
26	1.04	1.04	XXX	6	0	0	0	1
TC	3.45	3.45	XXX	6	0	0	0	1

AMA: Mar 02: 3

Pub 100-04, 32, 370.1

Coding Guidance

Diagnostic rhythm ECG testing is not to be reported for cardiac rhythm monitoring. Reporting ECG rhythm strips with critical care evaluation and management services is inappropriate, as routine monitoring of ECG rhythm strips is included in those services.

93040 Rhythm ECG, 1-3 leads; with interpretation and report   B

RVU			Global Days	Modifiers				
Mod	Non-Fac Total	Fac Total		51	50	62	80	MUE
	0.36	0.36	XXX	6	0	0	0	3

AMA: Apr 04: 8, Oct 10: 10, Nov 12: 6

Pub 100-04, 12, 20.3; 100-04, 16, 120.2; 100-04, 32, 130.1

93041 Rhythm ECG, 1-3 leads; tracing only without interpretation and report   Q1

Documentation Finder: *Providers may refer to a "rhythm strip" in the documentation, which would be one clue that this is the correct code. Additional documentation should identify how many leads are being placed. This code requires one to three leads.*

RVU			Global Days	Modifiers				
Mod	Non-Fac Total	Fac Total		51	50	62	80	MUE
	0.16	0.16	XXX	6	0	0	0	2

AMA: Apr 04: 8, Oct 10: 10

Pub 100-04, 12, 20.3; 100-04, 16, 120.2; 100-04, 32, 130.1

93042 Rhythm ECG, 1-3 leads; interpretation and report only   B

RVU			Global Days	Modifiers				
Mod	Non-Fac Total	Fac Total		51	50	62	80	MUE
	0.20	0.20	XXX	0	0	0	0	3

AMA: Apr 04: 8, Oct 11: 7, Oct 10: 10

Pub 100-04, 16, 120.2

● ### 93050 Arterial pressure waveform analysis for assessment of central arterial pressures, includes obtaining waveform(s), digitization and application of nonlinear mathematical transformations to determine central arterial pressures and augmentation index, with interpretation and report, upper extremity artery, non-invasive   Q1

RVU			Global Days	Modifiers				
Mod	Non-Fac Total	Fac Total		51	50	62	80	MUE
	0.50	0.50	XXX	6	2	0	0	1
26	0.25	0.25	XXX	6	2	0	0	1
TC	0.25	0.25	XXX	6	2	0	0	1

93224 External electrocardiographic recording up to 48 hours by continuous rhythm recording and storage; includes recording, scanning analysis with report, review and interpretation by a physician or other qualified health care professional   M

RVU			Global Days	Modifiers				
Mod	Non-Fac Total	Fac Total		51	50	62	80	MUE
	2.57	2.57	XXX	6	0	0	0	1

AMA: Oct 05: 14, Apr 07: 3, Mar 08: 4, Mar 09: 5, Oct 11: 5, Nov 11: 11

93225 External electrocardiographic recording up to 48 hours by continuous rhythm recording and storage; recording (includes connection, recording, and disconnection)   Q1

RVU			Global Days	Modifiers				
Mod	Non-Fac Total	Fac Total		51	50	62	80	MUE
	0.75	0.75	XXX	6	0	0	0	1

AMA: Oct 05: 14, Apr 07: 3, Mar 09: 5, Oct 11: 5

93226 External electrocardiographic recording up to 48 hours by continuous rhythm recording and storage; scanning analysis with report   Q1

RVU			Global Days	Modifiers				
Mod	Non-Fac Total	Fac Total		51	50	62	80	MUE
	1.07	1.07	XXX	6	0	0	0	1

AMA: Oct 05: 14, Apr 07: 3, Mar 09: 5, Oct 11: 5

93227 External electrocardiographic recording up to 48 hours by continuous rhythm recording and storage; review and interpretation by a physician or other qualified health care professional   M

RVU			Global Days	Modifiers				
Mod	Non-Fac Total	Fac Total		51	50	62	80	MUE
	0.75	0.75	XXX	0	0	0	0	1

AMA: Apr 07: 3, Mar 09: 5, Apr 09: 7, Oct 11: 5

93228 External mobile cardiovascular telemetry with electrocardiographic recording, concurrent computerized real time data analysis and greater than 24 hours of accessible ECG data storage (retrievable with query) with ECG triggered and patient selected events transmitted to a remote attended surveillance center for up to 30 days; review and interpretation with report by a physician or other qualified health care professional   M

RVU			Global Days	Modifiers				
Mod	Non-Fac Total	Fac Total		51	50	62	80	MUE
	0.74	0.74	XXX	0	0	0	0	1

AMA: Oct 11: 5

● New   ▲ Revised   ✖ Deleted   ⊙ Moderate Sedation   ✚ Add-on Codes   ⊘ High Risk Denial   Ⓐ Age Edit   ♀ Female   ♂ Male   **AMA** *CPT® Assistant*   **MUE** Medically Unlikely Edit
⊘ Modifier 51 Exempt   ⊖ Modifier 63 Exempt   ⊠ Unlisted   **Modifiers:** *See Inside Back Cover*   Ⓜ Maternity   A2–Z3 ASC Payment Indicators   A–Y OPPS Status Indicators

CPT © 2015 American Medical Association. All Rights Reserved.   © 2016 DecisionHealth

93229 External mobile cardiovascular telemetry with electrocardiographic recording, concurrent computerized real time data analysis and greater than 24 hours of accessible ECG data storage (retrievable with query) with ECG triggered and patient selected events transmitted to a remote attended surveillance center for up to 30 days; technical support for connection and patient instructions for use, attended surveillance, analysis and transmission of daily and emergent data reports as prescribed by a physician or other qualified health care professional **S**

RVU			Global Days	Modifiers				
Mod	Non-Fac Total	Fac Total		51	50	62	80	MUE
	20.45	20.45	XXX	6	0	0	0	1

AMA: Oct 11: 5

93260 Programming device evaluation (in person) with iterative adjustment of the implantable device to test the function of the device and select optimal permanent programmed values with analysis, review and report by a physician or other qualified health care professional; implantable subcutaneous lead defibrillator system **Q1**

RVU			Global Days	Modifiers				
Mod	Non-Fac Total	Fac Total		51	50	62	80	MUE
	1.89	1.89	XXX	6	0	0	0	1
26	1.27	1.27	XXX	6	0	0	0	1
TC	0.62	0.62	XXX	6	0	0	0	1

AMA: Nov 14: 5

93261 Interrogation device evaluation (in person) with analysis, review and report by a physician or other qualified health care professional, includes connection, recording and disconnection per patient encounter; implantable subcutaneous lead defibrillator system **Q1**

RVU			Global Days	Modifiers				
Mod	Non-Fac Total	Fac Total		51	50	62	80	MUE
	1.71	1.71	XXX	6	0	0	0	1
26	1.09	1.09	XXX	6	0	0	0	1
TC	0.62	0.62	XXX	6	0	0	0	1

AMA: Nov 14: 5

93268 External patient and, when performed, auto activated electrocardiographic rhythm derived event recording with symptom-related memory loop with remote download capability up to 30 days, 24-hour attended monitoring; includes transmission, review and interpretation by a physician or other qualified health care professional **M**

RVU			Global Days	Modifiers				
Mod	Non-Fac Total	Fac Total		51	50	62	80	MUE
	5.77	5.77	XXX	6	0	0	0	1

AMA: Jun 96: 2, Nov 99: 49, 50, Oct 05: 14, Apr 07: 3, Mar 08: 4, Mar 09: 5, Oct 11: 5

93270 External patient and, when performed, auto activated electrocardiographic rhythm derived event recording with symptom-related memory loop with remote download capability up to 30 days, 24-hour attended monitoring; recording (includes connection, recording, and disconnection) **Q1**

RVU			Global Days	Modifiers				
Mod	Non-Fac Total	Fac Total		51	50	62	80	MUE
	0.26	0.26	XXX	6	0	0	0	1

AMA: Jun 96: 2, Oct 05: 14, Apr 07: 3, Mar 09: 5, Oct 11: 5, Aug 10: 13

93271 External patient and, when performed, auto activated electrocardiographic rhythm derived event recording with symptom-related memory loop with remote download capability up to 30 days, 24-hour attended monitoring; transmission and analysis **S**

RVU			Global Days	Modifiers				
Mod	Non-Fac Total	Fac Total		51	50	62	80	MUE
	4.79	4.79	XXX	6	0	0	0	1

AMA: Jun 96: 2, Oct 05: 14, Apr 07: 3, Mar 09: 5, Oct 11: 5

93272 External patient and, when performed, auto activated electrocardiographic rhythm derived event recording with symptom-related memory loop with remote download capability up to 30 days, 24-hour attended monitoring; review and interpretation by a physician or other qualified health care professional **M**

RVU			Global Days	Modifiers				
Mod	Non-Fac Total	Fac Total		51	50	62	80	MUE
	0.72	0.72	XXX	0	0	0	0	1

AMA: Jun 96: 2, Apr 98: 14, Nov 99: 49, 50, Oct 05: 14, Apr 07: 3, Mar 09: 5, Apr 09: 7, Oct 11: 5

93278 Signal-averaged electrocardiography (SAECG), with or without ECG **Q1**

RVU			Global Days	Modifiers				
Mod	Non-Fac Total	Fac Total		51	50	62	80	MUE
	0.85	0.85	XXX	6	0	0	0	1
26	0.35	0.35	XXX	6	0	0	0	1
TC	0.50	0.50	XXX	6	0	0	0	1

AMA: Oct 11: 5

Cardiac Device Evaluation Services

93279 Programming device evaluation (in person) with iterative adjustment of the implantable device to test the function of the device and select optimal permanent programmed values with analysis, review and report by a physician or other qualified health care professional; single lead pacemaker system **Q1**

RVU			Global Days	Modifiers				
Mod	Non-Fac Total	Fac Total		51	50	62	80	MUE
	1.40	1.40	XXX	6	0	0	0	1
26	0.91	0.91	XXX	6	0	0	0	1
TC	0.49	0.49	XXX	6	0	0	0	1

AMA: Jun 12: 4, Jul 13: 7, Apr 14: 3, Jun 13: 6, Jul 14: 3, Nov 14: 5

● New ▲ Revised Deleted ⊙ Moderate Sedation ✚ Add-on Codes ⊘ High Risk Denial Ⓐ Age Edit ♀ Female ♂ Male **AMA** *CPT® Assistant* **MUE** Medically Unlikely Edit
⊘ Modifier 51 Exempt ⊖ Modifier 63 Exempt ⊠ Unlisted **Modifiers:** *See Inside Back Cover* Ⓜ Maternity A2-Z3 ASC Payment Indicators A-Y OPPS Status Indicators

© 2016 DecisionHealth | CPT © 2015 American Medical Association. All Rights Reserved. | **809**

93280 Programming device evaluation (in person) with iterative adjustment of the implantable device to test the function of the device and select optimal permanent programmed values with analysis, review and report by a physician or other qualified health care professional; dual lead pacemaker system   ◘1

RVU			Global Days	Modifiers				
Mod	Non-Fac Total	Fac Total		51	50	62	80	MUE
	1.63	1.63	XXX	6	0	0	0	1
26	1.08	1.08	XXX	6	0	0	0	1
TC	0.55	0.55	XXX	6	0	0	0	1

AMA: Jun 12: 4, Jul 13: 7, Jun 13: 6, Apr 14: 3

93281 Programming device evaluation (in person) with iterative adjustment of the implantable device to test the function of the device and select optimal permanent programmed values with analysis, review and report by a physician or other qualified health care professional; multiple lead pacemaker system   ◘1

RVU			Global Days	Modifiers				
Mod	Non-Fac Total	Fac Total		51	50	62	80	MUE
	1.92	1.92	XXX	6	0	0	0	1
26	1.27	1.27	XXX	6	0	0	0	1
TC	0.65	0.65	XXX	6	0	0	0	1

AMA: Jun 12: 4, Jul 13: 7, Jun 13: 6, Apr 14: 3

93282 Programming device evaluation (in person) with iterative adjustment of the implantable device to test the function of the device and select optimal permanent programmed values with analysis, review and report by a physician or other qualified health care professional; single lead transvenous implantable defibrillator system   ◘1

RVU			Global Days	Modifiers				
Mod	Non-Fac Total	Fac Total		51	50	62	80	MUE
	1.77	1.77	XXX	6	0	0	0	1
26	1.20	1.20	XXX	6	0	0	0	1
TC	0.57	0.57	XXX	6	0	0	0	1

AMA: Jul 13: 7, Jun 13: 6, Apr 14: 3

93283 Programming device evaluation (in person) with iterative adjustment of the implantable device to test the function of the device and select optimal permanent programmed values with analysis, review and report by a physician or other qualified health care professional; dual lead transvenous implantable defibrillator system   ◘1

RVU			Global Days	Modifiers				
Mod	Non-Fac Total	Fac Total		51	50	62	80	MUE
	2.30	2.30	XXX	6	0	0	0	1
26	1.63	1.63	XXX	6	0	0	0	1
TC	0.67	0.67	XXX	6	0	0	0	1

AMA: Jul 13: 7, Jun 13: 6, Apr 14: 3

93284 Programming device evaluation (in person) with iterative adjustment of the implantable device to test the function of the device and select optimal permanent programmed values with analysis, review and report by a physician or other qualified health care professional; multiple lead transvenous implantable defibrillator system   ◘1

RVU			Global Days	Modifiers				
Mod	Non-Fac Total	Fac Total		51	50	62	80	MUE
	2.54	2.54	XXX	6	0	0	0	1
26	1.78	1.78	XXX	6	0	0	0	1
TC	0.76	0.76	XXX	6	0	0	0	1

AMA: Jul 13: 7, Jun 13: 6, Apr 14: 3

93285 Programming device evaluation (in person) with iterative adjustment of the implantable device to test the function of the device and select optimal permanent programmed values with analysis, review and report by a physician or other qualified health care professional; implantable loop recorder system   ◘1

RVU			Global Days	Modifiers				
Mod	Non-Fac Total	Fac Total		51	50	62	80	MUE
	1.19	1.19	XXX	6	0	0	0	1
26	0.74	0.74	XXX	6	0	0	0	1
TC	0.45	0.45	XXX	6	0	0	0	1

93286 Peri-procedural device evaluation (in person) and programming of device system parameters before or after a surgery, procedure, or test with analysis, review and report by a physician or other qualified health care professional; single, dual, or multiple lead pacemaker system   N

RVU			Global Days	Modifiers				
Mod	Non-Fac Total	Fac Total		51	50	62	80	MUE
	0.77	0.77	XXX	6	0	0	0	2
26	0.43	0.43	XXX	6	0	0	0	2
TC	0.34	0.34	XXX	6	0	0	0	2

AMA: Jul 13: 7, Jun 13: 6, Apr 14: 3

93287 Peri-procedural device evaluation (in person) and programming of device system parameters before or after a surgery, procedure, or test with analysis, review and report by a physician or other qualified health care professional; single, dual, or multiple lead implantable defibrillator system   N

RVU			Global Days	Modifiers				
Mod	Non-Fac Total	Fac Total		51	50	62	80	MUE
	1.02	1.02	XXX	6	0	0	0	2
26	0.65	0.65	XXX	6	0	0	0	2
TC	0.37	0.37	XXX	6	0	0	0	2

AMA: Jul 13: 7, Jun 13: 6, Apr 14: 3, Jul 14: 3

93288 Interrogation device evaluation (in person) with analysis, review and report by a physician or other qualified health care professional, includes connection, recording and disconnection per patient encounter; single, dual, or multiple lead pacemaker system   ◘1

RVU			Global Days	Modifiers				
Mod	Non-Fac Total	Fac Total		51	50	62	80	MUE
	1.04	1.04	XXX	6	0	0	0	1
26	0.60	0.60	XXX	6	0	0	0	1
TC	0.44	0.44	XXX	6	0	0	0	1

AMA: Jun 12: 4, Jul 13: 7, Jun 13: 6, Apr 14: 3

● New   ▲ Revised   ✖ Deleted   ⊙ Moderate Sedation   ➕ Add-on Codes   ⊘ High Risk Denial   Ⓐ Age Edit   ♀ Female   ♂ Male   **AMA** CPT® Assistant   **MUE** Medically Unlikely Edit
⊘ Modifier 51 Exempt   ⊖ Modifier 63 Exempt   ✗ Unlisted   **Modifiers:** See Inside Back Cover   Ⓜ Maternity   A2–Z3 ASC Payment Indicators   A–Y OPPS Status Indicators

CPT © 2015 American Medical Association. All Rights Reserved.

© 2016 DecisionHealth

93289 Interrogation device evaluation (in person) with analysis, review and report by a physician or other qualified health care professional, includes connection, recording and disconnection per patient encounter; single, dual, or multiple lead transvenous implantable defibrillator system, including analysis of heart rhythm derived data elements ⊡

RVU			Global Days	Modifiers				
Mod	Non-Fac Total	Fac Total		51	50	62	80	MUE
	1.84	1.84	XXX	6	0	0	0	1
26	1.29	1.29	XXX	6	0	0	0	1
TC	0.55	0.55	XXX	6	0	0	0	1

AMA: Jul 13: 7, Jun 13: 6, Apr 14: 3

93290 Interrogation device evaluation (in person) with analysis, review and report by a physician or other qualified health care professional, includes connection, recording and disconnection per patient encounter; implantable cardiovascular monitor system, including analysis of 1 or more recorded physiologic cardiovascular data elements from all internal and external sensors ⊡

RVU			Global Days	Modifiers				
Mod	Non-Fac Total	Fac Total		51	50	62	80	MUE
	0.88	0.88	XXX	6	0	0	0	1
26	0.61	0.61	XXX	6	0	0	0	1
TC	0.27	0.27	XXX	6	0	0	0	1

AMA: Feb 10: 13, Apr 13: 11

93291 Interrogation device evaluation (in person) with analysis, review and report by a physician or other qualified health care professional, includes connection, recording and disconnection per patient encounter; implantable loop recorder system, including heart rhythm derived data analysis ⊡

RVU			Global Days	Modifiers				
Mod	Non-Fac Total	Fac Total		51	50	62	80	MUE
	1.02	1.02	XXX	6	0	0	0	1
26	0.61	0.61	XXX	6	0	0	0	1
TC	0.41	0.41	XXX	6	0	0	0	1

93292 Interrogation device evaluation (in person) with analysis, review and report by a physician or other qualified health care professional, includes connection, recording and disconnection per patient encounter; wearable defibrillator system ⊡

RVU			Global Days	Modifiers				
Mod	Non-Fac Total	Fac Total		51	50	62	80	MUE
	0.91	0.91	XXX	6	0	0	0	1
26	0.60	0.60	XXX	6	0	0	0	1
TC	0.31	0.31	XXX	6	0	0	0	1

93293 Transtelephonic rhythm strip pacemaker evaluation(s) single, dual, or multiple lead pacemaker system, includes recording with and without magnet application with analysis, review and report(s) by a physician or other qualified health care professional, up to 90 days ⊡

RVU			Global Days	Modifiers				
Mod	Non-Fac Total	Fac Total		51	50	62	80	MUE
	1.50	1.50	XXX	0	0	0	0	1
26	0.44	0.44	XXX	0	0	0	0	1
TC	1.06	1.06	XXX	0	0	0	0	1

93294 Interrogation device evaluation(s) (remote), up to 90 days; single, dual, or multiple lead pacemaker system with interim analysis, review(s) and report(s) by a physician or other qualified health care professional Ⓜ

RVU			Global Days	Modifiers				
Mod	Non-Fac Total	Fac Total		51	50	62	80	MUE
	0.96	0.96	XXX	0	0	0	0	1

AMA: Jun 12: 4

93295 Interrogation device evaluation(s) (remote), up to 90 days; single, dual, or multiple lead implantable defibrillator system with interim analysis, review(s) and report(s) by a physician or other qualified health care professional Ⓜ

RVU			Global Days	Modifiers				
Mod	Non-Fac Total	Fac Total		51	50	62	80	MUE
	1.90	1.90	XXX	0	0	0	0	1

93296 Interrogation device evaluation(s) (remote), up to 90 days; single, dual, or multiple lead pacemaker system or implantable defibrillator system, remote data acquisition(s), receipt of transmissions and technician review, technical support and distribution of results ⊡

RVU			Global Days	Modifiers				
Mod	Non-Fac Total	Fac Total		51	50	62	80	MUE
	0.73	0.73	XXX	0	0	0	0	1

93297 Interrogation device evaluation(s), (remote) up to 30 days; implantable cardiovascular monitor system, including analysis of 1 or more recorded physiologic cardiovascular data elements from all internal and external sensors, analysis, review(s) and report(s) by a physician or other qualified health care professional Ⓜ

RVU			Global Days	Modifiers				
Mod	Non-Fac Total	Fac Total		51	50	62	80	MUE
	0.75	0.75	XXX	0	0	0	0	1

AMA: Apr 13: 11, Feb 09: 9, 12

93298 Interrogation device evaluation(s), (remote) up to 30 days; implantable loop recorder system, including analysis of recorded heart rhythm data, analysis, review(s) and report(s) by a physician or other qualified health care professional Ⓜ

RVU			Global Days	Modifiers				
Mod	Non-Fac Total	Fac Total		51	50	62	80	MUE
	0.75	0.75	XXX	0	0	0	0	1

AMA: Feb 09: 9, 12

93299 Interrogation device evaluation(s), (remote) up to 30 days; implantable cardiovascular monitor system or implantable loop recorder system, remote data acquisition(s), receipt of transmissions and technician review, technical support and distribution of results [QI]

RVU			Global Days	Modifiers				
Mod	Non-Fac Total	Fac Total		51	50	62	80	MUE
	0.00	0.00	XXX	0	0	0	0	1

AMA: Apr 13: 11, Feb 09: 9, 12, Jul 14: 3, Nov 14: 5

Echocardiographies

93303 Transthoracic echocardiography for congenital cardiac anomalies; complete [S]

RVU			Global Days	Modifiers				
Mod	Non-Fac Total	Fac Total		51	50	62	80	MUE
	6.72	6.72	XXX	6	0	0	0	1
26	1.81	1.81	XXX	6	0	0	0	1
TC	4.91	4.91	XXX	6	0	0	0	1

AMA: Nov 97: 44, Dec 97: 5, Sep 05: 10, 11, Mar 08: 4, Oct 10: 17, Dec 10: 17, Aug 13: 3, Dec 13: 15, May 15: 10

93304 Transthoracic echocardiography for congenital cardiac anomalies; follow-up or limited study [S]

RVU			Global Days	Modifiers				
Mod	Non-Fac Total	Fac Total		51	50	62	80	MUE
	4.39	4.39	XXX	6	0	0	0	1
26	1.04	1.04	XXX	6	0	0	0	1
TC	3.35	3.35	XXX	6	0	0	0	1

AMA: Nov 97: 44, Dec 97: 5, Jan 10: 8, Oct 10: 17, Dec 10: 17, Aug 13: 3, Dec 13: 15, May 15: 10

93306 Echocardiography, transthoracic, real-time with image documentation (2D), includes M-mode recording, when performed, complete, with spectral Doppler echocardiography, and with color flow Doppler echocardiography [S]

RVU			Global Days	Modifiers				
Mod	Non-Fac Total	Fac Total		51	50	62	80	MUE
	6.42	6.42	XXX	6	0	0	0	1
26	1.80	1.80	XXX	6	0	0	0	1
TC	4.62	4.62	XXX	6	0	0	0	1

AMA: Oct 10: 17, Dec 10: 17, Aug 13: 3, May 15: 10

93307 Echocardiography, transthoracic, real-time with image documentation (2D), includes M-mode recording, when performed, complete, without spectral or color Doppler echocardiography [S]

RVU			Global Days	Modifiers				
Mod	Non-Fac Total	Fac Total		51	50	62	80	MUE
	3.67	3.67	XXX	6	0	0	0	1
26	1.28	1.28	XXX	6	0	0	0	1
TC	2.39	2.39	XXX	6	0	0	0	1

AMA: Dec 97: 5, Sep 05: 11, Oct 10: 17, Dec 10: 17, Aug 13: 3, May 15: 10
Pub 100-04, 16, 120.2

93308 Echocardiography, transthoracic, real-time with image documentation (2D), includes M-mode recording, when performed, follow-up or limited study [S]

RVU			Global Days	Modifiers				
Mod	Non-Fac Total	Fac Total		51	50	62	80	MUE
	3.51	3.51	XXX	6	0	0	0	1
26	0.73	0.73	XXX	6	0	0	0	1
TC	2.78	2.78	XXX	6	0	0	0	1

AMA: Dec 97: 5, Sep 05: 11, Jan 10: 8, Oct 10: 17, Mar 12: 10, Dec 10: 17, Aug 13: 3, May 15: 10
Pub 100-04, 16, 120.2

⊙ **93312** Echocardiography, transesophageal, real-time with image documentation (2D) (with or without M-mode recording); including probe placement, image acquisition, interpretation and report [S]

RVU			Global Days	Modifiers				
Mod	Non-Fac Total	Fac Total		51	50	62	80	MUE
	8.67	8.67	XXX	6	0	0	0	1
26	3.45	3.45	XXX	6	0	0	0	1
TC	5.22	5.22	XXX	6	0	0	0	1

AMA: Dec 97: 5, Jan 00: 10, Jan 10: 8, Oct 12: 15, Aug 13: 3, Jul 14: 9

⊙ **93313** Echocardiography, transesophageal, real-time with image documentation (2D) (with or without M-mode recording); placement of transesophageal probe only [S]

RVU			Global Days	Modifiers				
Mod	Non-Fac Total	Fac Total		51	50	62	80	MUE
	0.65	0.65	XXX	0	0	0	0	1

AMA: Dec 97: 5, Mar 08: 4, Jan 10: 8, Aug 13: 3

⊙ **93314** Echocardiography, transesophageal, real-time with image documentation (2D) (with or without M-mode recording); image acquisition, interpretation and report only [N]

RVU			Global Days	Modifiers				
Mod	Non-Fac Total	Fac Total		51	50	62	80	MUE
	8.47	8.47	XXX	6	0	0	0	1
26	2.95	2.95	XXX	6	0	0	0	1
TC	5.52	5.52	XXX	6	0	0	0	1

AMA: Dec 97: 5, Jan 00: 10, Jan 10: 8, Aug 13: 3

⊙ **93315** Transesophageal echocardiography for congenital cardiac anomalies; including probe placement, image acquisition, interpretation and report [S]

RVU			Global Days	Modifiers				
Mod	Non-Fac Total	Fac Total		51	50	62	80	MUE
	0.00	0.00	XXX	0	0	0	0	1
26	4.03	4.03	XXX	0	0	0	0	1
TC	0.00	0.00	XXX	0	0	0	0	1

AMA: Nov 97: 44, Dec 97: 5, Jan 10: 8, Aug 13: 3, Dec 13: 15, Jul 14: 9

⊙ **93316** Transesophageal echocardiography for congenital cardiac anomalies; placement of transesophageal probe only [S]

RVU			Global Days	Modifiers				
Mod	Non-Fac Total	Fac Total		51	50	62	80	MUE
	1.10	1.10	XXX	0	0	0	0	1

AMA: Nov 97: 44, Dec 97: 5, Jan 10: 8, Aug 13: 3

● New ▲ Revised ✖ Deleted ⊙ Moderate Sedation ✚ Add-on Codes ⊗ High Risk Denial ⊛ Age Edit ♀ Female ♂ Male **AMA** CPT® Assistant **MUE** Medically Unlikely Edit
⊘ Modifier 51 Exempt ⊖ Modifier 63 Exempt ✗ Unlisted **Modifiers:** See Inside Back Cover Ⓜ Maternity A2–Z3 ASC Payment Indicators A–Y OPPS Status Indicators

812 CPT © 2015 American Medical Association. All Rights Reserved. © 2016 DecisionHealth

⊙ **93317 Transesophageal echocardiography for congenital cardiac anomalies; image acquisition, interpretation and report only** Ⓝ

RVU			Global Days	Modifiers				
Mod	Non-Fac Total	Fac Total		51	50	62	80	MUE
	0.00	0.00	XXX	0	0	0	0	1
26	3.01	3.01	XXX	0	0	0	0	1
TC	0.00	0.00	XXX	0	0	0	0	1

AMA: Nov 97: 44, Dec 97: 5, Jan 10: 8, Aug 13: 3, Dec 13: 15

⊙ **93318 Echocardiography, transesophageal (TEE) for monitoring purposes, including probe placement, real time 2-dimensional image acquisition and interpretation leading to ongoing (continuous) assessment of (dynamically changing) cardiac pumping function and to therapeutic measures on an immediate time basis** ⊙Ⓢ

Documentation Finder: In the documentation, you should see reference to placing the ultrasound transducer in the esophagus achieving closer proximity to the anatomical structures of the heart and great vessels for improved image quality. If the provider documents the use of moderate (conscious) sedation, it would be included in this code.

RVU			Global Days	Modifiers				
Mod	Non-Fac Total	Fac Total		51	50	62	80	MUE
	0.00	0.00	XXX	6	0	0	0	1
26	3.32	3.32	XXX	6	0	0	0	1
TC	0.00	0.00	XXX	6	0	0	0	1

AMA: Jan 10: 8, Apr 10: 6, Aug 13: 3

✚ **93320 Doppler echocardiography, pulsed wave and/or continuous wave with spectral display (List separately in addition to codes for echocardiographic imaging); complete** Ⓝ

RVU			Global Days	Modifiers				
Mod	Non-Fac Total	Fac Total		51	50	62	80	MUE
	1.53	1.53	ZZZ	0	0	0	0	1
26	0.52	0.52	ZZZ	0	0	0	0	1
TC	1.01	1.01	ZZZ	0	0	0	0	1

AMA: Nov 97: 44, Dec 97: 5, Aug 13: 3

✚ **93321 Doppler echocardiography, pulsed wave and/or continuous wave with spectral display (List separately in addition to codes for echocardiographic imaging); follow-up or limited study (List separately in addition to codes for echocardiographic imaging)** Ⓝ

RVU			Global Days	Modifiers				
Mod	Non-Fac Total	Fac Total		51	50	62	80	MUE
	0.77	0.77	ZZZ	0	0	0	0	1
26	0.21	0.21	ZZZ	0	0	0	0	1
TC	0.56	0.56	ZZZ	0	0	0	0	1

AMA: Nov 97: 44, Dec 97: 5, Jan 10: 8, Aug 13: 3

✚ **93325 Doppler echocardiography color flow velocity mapping (List separately in addition to codes for echocardiography)** Ⓝ

RVU			Global Days	Modifiers				
Mod	Non-Fac Total	Fac Total		51	50	62	80	MUE
	0.72	0.72	ZZZ	0	0	0	0	1
26	0.09	0.09	ZZZ	0	0	0	0	1
TC	0.63	0.63	ZZZ	0	0	0	0	1

AMA: Nov 97: 44, Dec 97: 5, Aug 13: 3

93350 Echocardiography, transthoracic, real-time with image documentation (2D), includes M-mode recording, when performed, during rest and cardiovascular stress test using treadmill, bicycle exercise and/or pharmacologically induced stress, with interpretation and report Ⓢ

RVU			Global Days	Modifiers				
Mod	Non-Fac Total	Fac Total		51	50	62	80	MUE
	6.78	6.78	XXX	6	0	0	0	1
26	2.01	2.01	XXX	6	0	0	0	1
TC	4.77	4.77	XXX	6	0	0	0	1

AMA: Aug 02: 11, Jan 10: 8, Oct 10: 17, Dec 10: 17, Aug 13: 3, Jul 14: 9
Pub 100-04, 13, 60.3

93351 Echocardiography, transthoracic, real-time with image documentation (2D), includes M-mode recording, when performed, during rest and cardiovascular stress test using treadmill, bicycle exercise and/or pharmacologically induced stress, with interpretation and report; including performance of continuous electrocardiographic monitoring, with supervision by a physician or other qualified health care professional Ⓢ

RVU			Global Days	Modifiers				
Mod	Non-Fac Total	Fac Total		51	50	62	80	MUE
	7.63	7.63	XXX	6	0	9	9	1
26	2.41	2.41	XXX	6	0	9	9	1
TC	5.22	5.22	XXX	6	0	9	9	1

AMA: Oct 10: 17, Dec 10: 17, Jan 10: 8, Aug 13: 3, Jul 14: 9

✚ **93352 Use of echocardiographic contrast agent during stress echocardiography (List separately in addition to code for primary procedure)** Ⓜ

RVU			Global Days	Modifiers				
Mod	Non-Fac Total	Fac Total		51	50	62	80	MUE
	0.96	0.96	ZZZ	0	0	0	0	1

AMA: Oct 10: 17, Dec 10: 17, Jan 10: 8, Aug 13: 3

93355 Echocardiography, transesophageal (TEE) for guidance of a transcatheter intracardiac or great vessel(s) structural intervention(s) (eg, TAVR, transcathether pulmonary valve replacement, mitral valve repair, paravalvular regurgitation repair, left atrial appendage occlusion/closure, ventricular septal defect closure) (peri-and intra-procedural), real-time image acquisition and documentation, guidance with quantitative measurements, probe manipulation, interpretation, and report, including diagnostic transesophageal echocardiography and, when performed, administration of ultrasound contrast, Doppler, color flow, and 3D Ⓝ

RVU			Global Days	Modifiers				
Mod	Non-Fac Total	Fac Total		51	50	62	80	MUE
	6.44	6.44	XXX	6	0	0	0	1

● New ▲ Revised Deleted ⊙ Moderate Sedation ✚ Add-on Codes ⊘ High Risk Denial ⒶAge Edit ♀ Female ♂ Male **AMA** *CPT® Assistant* **MUE** Medically Unlikely Edit
⊘ Modifier 51 Exempt ⊖ Modifier 63 Exempt ⓧ Unlisted **Modifiers:** *See Inside Back Cover* Ⓜ Maternity A2–Z3 ASC Payment Indicators Ⓐ–Ⓨ OPPS Status Indicators

© 2016 DecisionHealth | CPT © 2015 American Medical Association. All Rights Reserved. | **813**

Cardiac Catheterizations

⊙⊘**93451** Right heart catheterization including measurement(s) of oxygen saturation and cardiac output, when performed ⏕

Mod	Non-Fac Total	Fac Total	Global Days	51	50	62	80	MUE
	22.15	22.15	000	2	0	0	0	1
26	4.16	4.16	000	2	0	0	0	1
TC	17.99	17.99	000	0	0	0	0	1

AMA: Aug 11: 5, Mar 12: 10, May 13: 12, Jul 14: 3

⊙ **93452** Left heart catheterization including intraprocedural injection(s) for left ventriculography, imaging supervision and interpretation, when performed ⏕

Mod	Non-Fac Total	Fac Total	Global Days	51	50	62	80	MUE
	25.02	25.02	000	2	0	0	0	1
26	7.30	7.30	000	2	0	0	0	1
TC	17.72	17.72	000	0	0	0	0	1

AMA: Mar 12: 10, Aug 11: 3, May 13: 12, Jan 13: 6

⊙ **93453** Combined right and left heart catheterization including intraprocedural injection(s) for left ventriculography, imaging supervision and interpretation, when performed ⏕

Mod	Non-Fac Total	Fac Total	Global Days	51	50	62	80	MUE
26	9.64	9.64	000	2	0	0	0	1
TC	22.58	22.58	000	0	0	0	0	1
	32.22	32.22	000	2	0	0	0	1

AMA: Aug 11: 3, Mar 12: 10, May 13: 12, Jan 13: 6

⊙ **93454** Catheter placement in coronary artery(s) for coronary angiography, including intraprocedural injection(s) for coronary angiography, imaging supervision and interpretation ⏕

Mod	Non-Fac Total	Fac Total	Global Days	51	50	62	80	MUE
TC	17.96	17.96	000	0	0	0	0	1
	25.36	25.36	000	2	0	0	0	1
26	7.40	7.40	000	2	0	0	0	1

AMA: Aug 11: 3, Mar 12: 10, May 13: 12, Dec 14: 6

⊙ **93455** Catheter placement in coronary artery(s) for coronary angiography, including intraprocedural injection(s) for coronary angiography, imaging supervision and interpretation; with catheter placement(s) in bypass graft(s) (internal mammary, free arterial, venous grafts) including intraprocedural injection(s) for bypass graft angiography ⏕

Mod	Non-Fac Total	Fac Total	Global Days	51	50	62	80	MUE
	29.54	29.54	000	2	0	0	0	1
26	8.55	8.55	000	2	0	0	0	1
TC	20.99	20.99	000	0	0	0	0	1

AMA: Aug 11: 3, Mar 12: 10, Dec 11: 9, May 13: 12

⊙⊘**93456** Catheter placement in coronary artery(s) for coronary angiography, including intraprocedural injection(s) for coronary angiography, imaging supervision and interpretation; with right heart catheterization ⏕

Mod	Non-Fac Total	Fac Total	Global Days	51	50	62	80	MUE
	31.78	31.78	000	2	0	0	0	1
26	9.49	9.49	000	2	0	0	0	1
TC	22.29	22.29	000	0	0	0	0	1

AMA: Aug 11: 3, Mar 12: 10, May 13: 12

⊙ **93457** Catheter placement in coronary artery(s) for coronary angiography, including intraprocedural injection(s) for coronary angiography, imaging supervision and interpretation; with catheter placement(s) in bypass graft(s) (internal mammary, free arterial, venous grafts) including intraprocedural injection(s) for bypass graft angiography and right heart catheterization ⏕

Mod	Non-Fac Total	Fac Total	Global Days	51	50	62	80	MUE
	35.94	35.94	000	2	0	0	0	1
26	10.64	10.64	000	2	0	0	0	1
TC	25.30	25.30	000	0	0	0	0	1

AMA: Aug 11: 3, Mar 12: 10, Dec 11: 9, May 13: 12

⊙ **93458** Catheter placement in coronary artery(s) for coronary angiography, including intraprocedural injection(s) for coronary angiography, imaging supervision and interpretation; with left heart catheterization including intraprocedural injection(s) for left ventriculography, when performed ⏕

Mod	Non-Fac Total	Fac Total	Global Days	51	50	62	80	MUE
	30.44	30.44	000	2	0	0	0	1
26	9.04	9.04	000	2	0	0	0	1
TC	21.40	21.40	000	0	0	0	0	1

AMA: Aug 11: 3, Mar 12: 10, May 13: 12, Jan 13: 6

⊙ **93459** Catheter placement in coronary artery(s) for coronary angiography, including intraprocedural injection(s) for coronary angiography, imaging supervision and interpretation; with left heart catheterization including intraprocedural injection(s) for left ventriculography, when performed, catheter placement(s) in bypass graft(s) (internal mammary, free arterial, venous grafts) with bypass graft angiography ⏕

Mod	Non-Fac Total	Fac Total	Global Days	51	50	62	80	MUE
	33.63	33.63	000	2	0	0	0	1
26	10.19	10.19	000	2	0	0	0	1
TC	23.44	23.44	000	0	0	0	0	1

AMA: Dec 11: 11, Aug 11: 3, Mar 12: 10, Jan 13: 6, May 13: 12

● New ▲ Revised ✖ Deleted ⊙ Moderate Sedation ✚ Add-on Codes ⊘ High Risk Denial ⒶAge Edit ♀ Female ♂ Male **AMA** *CPT® Assistant* **MUE** Medically Unlikely Edit
⊘ Modifier 51 Exempt ⊖ Modifier 63 Exempt ☒ Unlisted **Modifiers:** *See Inside Back Cover* Ⓜ Maternity 🄰2–🅉3 ASC Payment Indicators 🄰–🅈 OPPS Status Indicators

814 CPT © 2015 American Medical Association. All Rights Reserved. © 2016 DecisionHealth

⊙ **93460** **Catheter placement in coronary artery(s) for coronary angiography, including intraprocedural injection(s) for coronary angiography, imaging supervision and interpretation; with right and left heart catheterization including intraprocedural injection(s) for left ventriculography, when performed** 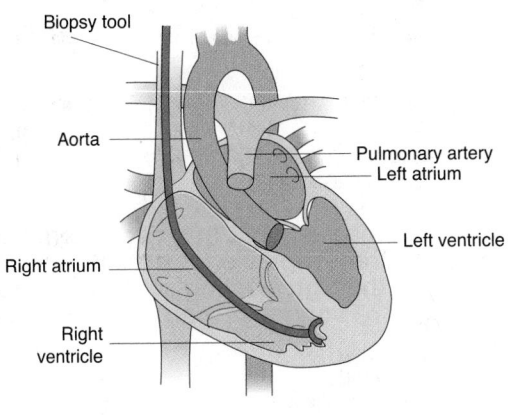T

Mod	RVU Non-Fac Total	Fac Total	Global Days	Modifiers 51	50	62	80	MUE
	36.07	36.07	000	2	0	0	0	1
26	11.34	11.34	000	2	0	0	0	1
TC	24.73	24.73	000	0	0	0	0	1

AMA: Aug 11: 3, Mar 12: 10, Jan 13: 6, May 13: 12

⊙ **93461** **Catheter placement in coronary artery(s) for coronary angiography, including intraprocedural injection(s) for coronary angiography, imaging supervision and interpretation; with right and left heart catheterization including intraprocedural injection(s) for left ventriculography, when performed, catheter placement(s) in bypass graft(s) (internal mammary, free arterial, venous grafts) with bypass graft angiography** T

Mod	RVU Non-Fac Total	Fac Total	Global Days	Modifiers 51	50	62	80	MUE
	41.25	41.25	000	2	0	0	0	1
26	12.50	12.50	000	2	0	0	0	1
TC	28.75	28.75	000	0	0	0	0	1

AMA: Aug 11: 3, Mar 12: 10, Dec 11: 9, Jan 13: 6, May 13: 12, Jul 14: 3, Dec 14: 6

⊙+**93462** **Left heart catheterization by transseptal puncture through intact septum or by transapical puncture (List separately in addition to code for primary procedure)** N

Mod	RVU Non-Fac Total	Fac Total	Global Days	Modifiers 51	50	62	80	MUE
	6.07	6.07	ZZZ	0	0	0	0	1

AMA: Aug 11: 3, Mar 12: 10, May 13: 12, Jun 13: 6, Jul 14: 3

⊙+**93463** **Pharmacologic agent administration (eg, inhaled nitric oxide, intravenous infusion of nitroprusside, dobutamine, milrinone, or other agent) including assessing hemodynamic measurements before, during, after and repeat pharmacologic agent administration, when performed (List separately in addition to code for primary procedure)** N

Mod	RVU Non-Fac Total	Fac Total	Global Days	Modifiers 51	50	62	80	MUE
	2.81	2.81	ZZZ	0	0	0	0	1

AMA: Aug 11: 3, Mar 12: 10, Dec 14: 6

⊙+**93464** **Physiologic exercise study (eg, bicycle or arm ergometry) including assessing hemodynamic measurements before and after (List separately in addition to code for primary procedure)** N

Mod	RVU Non-Fac Total	Fac Total	Global Days	Modifiers 51	50	62	80	MUE
	7.74	7.74	ZZZ	0	0	0	0	1
26	2.48	2.48	ZZZ	0	0	0	0	1
TC	5.26	5.26	ZZZ	0	0	0	0	1

AMA: Aug 11: 3, Mar 12: 10, Jul 14: 3

⊘ **93503** **Insertion and placement of flow directed catheter (eg, Swan-Ganz) for monitoring purposes** T

Mod	RVU Non-Fac Total	Fac Total	Global Days	Modifiers 51	50	62	80	MUE
	3.76	3.76	000	0	0	0	0	2

AMA: Winter 91: 3, Fall 95: 8, Feb 97: 5, Apr 98: 2, Mar 08: 4, Dec 11: 18, Aug 11: 3

Pub 100-04, 12, 30.6.12

⊙ **93505** **Endomyocardial biopsy** T

Mod	RVU Non-Fac Total	Fac Total	Global Days	Modifiers 51	50	62	80	MUE
	21.62	21.62	000	2	0	0	0	1
26	6.74	6.74	000	2	0	0	0	1
TC	14.88	14.88	000	0	0	0	0	1

AMA: Apr 98: 2, Apr 00: 10, Aug 11: 3

Endomyocardial biopsy

Biopsy tool
Aorta
Pulmonary artery
Left atrium
Right atrium
Left ventricle
Right ventricle

A sample of muscle tissue is obtained from inside the heart

⊙ **93530** **Right heart catheterization, for congenital cardiac anomalies** T

Mod	RVU Non-Fac Total	Fac Total	Global Days	Modifiers 51	50	62	80	MUE
	0.00	0.00	000	2	0	0	0	1
26	6.37	6.37	000	2	0	0	0	1
TC	0.00	0.00	000	0	0	0	0	1

AMA: Nov 97: 45, Jan 98: 11, Mar 98: 11, Apr 98: 3, 6, 7, Dec 11: 11, Aug 11: 3, Mar 12: 10, May 13: 12, Jul 14: 3

93531 **Combined right heart catheterization and retrograde left heart catheterization, for congenital cardiac anomalies** T

Mod	RVU Non-Fac Total	Fac Total	Global Days	Modifiers 51	50	62	80	MUE
	0.00	0.00	000	2	0	0	0	1
26	12.44	12.44	000	2	0	0	0	1
TC	0.00	0.00	000	0	0	0	0	1

AMA: Nov 97: 45, Jan 98: 11, Mar 98: 11, Apr 98: 8, 10, 11, Dec 11: 11, Aug 11: 3, Mar 12: 10

● New ▲ Revised Deleted ⊙ Moderate Sedation ✚ Add-on Codes ⊘ High Risk Denial Ⓐ Age Edit ♀ Female ♂ Male **AMA** *CPT® Assistant* **MUE** Medically Unlikely Edit
⊗ Modifier 51 Exempt ⊖ Modifier 63 Exempt ✗ Unlisted **Modifiers:** *See Inside Back Cover* Ⓜ Maternity A2–Z3 ASC Payment Indicators A–Y OPPS Status Indicators

© 2016 DecisionHealth — CPT © 2015 American Medical Association. All Rights Reserved. — **815**

93532 Combined right heart catheterization and transseptal left heart catheterization through intact septum with or without retrograde left heart catheterization, for congenital cardiac anomalies ⒼⓉ

Coding tip: Add intracardiac echocardiography - 93662

RVU Mod	Non-Fac Total	Fac Total	Global Days	51	50	62	80	MUE
	0.00	0.00	000	2	0	0	0	1
26	15.44	15.44	000	2	0	0	0	1
TC	0.00	0.00	000	0	0	0	0	1

AMA: Nov 97: 45, Jan 98: 11, Mar 98: 11, Apr 98: 10, 11, Dec 11: 11, Aug 11: 3, Mar 12: 10

93533 Combined right heart catheterization and transseptal left heart catheterization through existing septal opening, with or without retrograde left heart catheterization, for congenital cardiac anomalies Ⓣ

RVU Mod	Non-Fac Total	Fac Total	Global Days	51	50	62	80	MUE
	0.00	0.00	000	2	0	0	0	1
26	10.31	10.31	000	2	0	0	0	1
TC	0.00	0.00	000	0	0	0	0	1

AMA: Nov 97: 45, Jan 98: 11, Mar 98: 11, Apr 98: 12, 13, Dec 11: 11, Mar 12: 10, Aug 11: 3, Jul 14: 3

Combined right heart catheterization and transseptal left heart catheterization through existing septal opening, for congenital cardiac anomalies

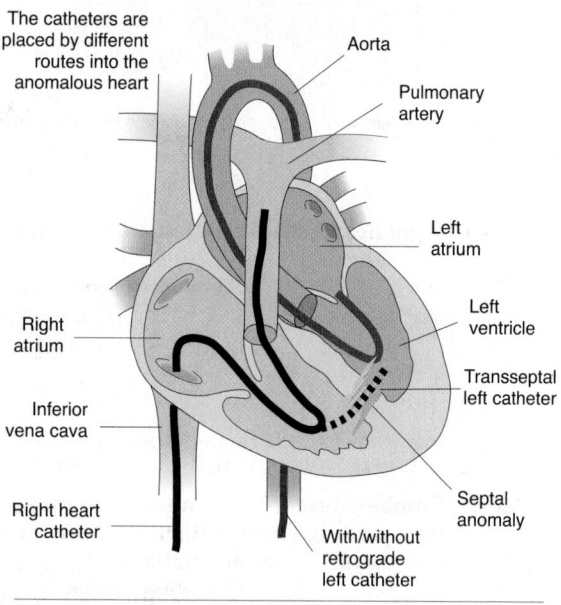

The catheters are placed by different routes into the anomalous heart

Aorta

Pulmonary artery

Left atrium

Left ventricle

Transseptal left catheter

Right atrium

Inferior vena cava

Right heart catheter

Septal anomaly

With/without retrograde left catheter

Cardiac Injection Procedures

Coding Guidance

Cardiac output measurement is a routine part of cardiac catheterization procedures. Do not report codes 93561-93562 with cardiac catheterization. Reporting cardiac output measurements with critical care evaluation and management services is inappropriate, as routine cardiac output review is included in those services.

⊙ 93561 Indicator dilution studies such as dye or thermodilution, including arterial and/or venous catheterization; with cardiac output measurement (separate procedure) Ⓝ

RVU Mod	Non-Fac Total	Fac Total	Global Days	51	50	62	80	MUE
	0.00	0.00	000	0	0	0	0	1
26	0.73	0.73	000	0	0	0	0	1
TC	0.00	0.00	000	0	0	0	0	1

AMA: Winter 91: 25, Summer 95: 2, Aug 00: 2, Feb 07: 10, Jul 07: 1, Aug 11: 3, Jul 14: 3

Pub 100-04, 12, 30.6.12

⊙ 93562 Indicator dilution studies such as dye or thermodilution, including arterial and/or venous catheterization; subsequent measurement of cardiac output Ⓝ

RVU Mod	Non-Fac Total	Fac Total	Global Days	51	50	62	80	MUE
	0.00	0.00	000	0	0	0	0	1
26	0.23	0.23	000	0	0	0	0	1
TC	0.00	0.00	000	0	0	0	0	1

AMA: Winter 91: 25, Summer 95: 2, Aug 00: 2, Feb 07: 10, Jul 07: 1, Aug 11: 3, May 14: 4, Jul 14: 3

Pub 100-04, 12, 30.6.12

⊙+93563 Injection procedure during cardiac catheterization including imaging supervision, interpretation, and report; for selective coronary angiography during congenital heart catheterization (List separately in addition to code for primary procedure) Ⓝ

RVU Mod	Non-Fac Total	Fac Total	Global Days	51	50	62	80	MUE
	1.69	1.69	ZZZ	0	0	0	0	1

AMA: Dec 11: 11, Aug 11: 3, Jan 13: 6, Dec 14: 6

⊙+93564 Injection procedure during cardiac catheterization including imaging supervision, interpretation, and report; for selective opacification of aortocoronary venous or arterial bypass graft(s) (eg, aortocoronary saphenous vein, free radial artery, or free mammary artery graft) to one or more coronary arteries and in situ arterial conduits (eg, internal mammary), whether native or used for bypass to one or more coronary arteries during congenital heart catheterization, when performed (List separately in addition to code for primary procedure) Ⓝ

RVU Mod	Non-Fac Total	Fac Total	Global Days	51	50	62	80	MUE
	1.78	1.78	ZZZ	0	0	0	0	1

AMA: Dec 11: 11, Aug 11: 3, Jan 13: 6, Dec 14: 6

⊙+93565 Injection procedure during cardiac catheterization including imaging supervision, interpretation, and report; for selective left ventricular or left atrial angiography (List separately in addition to code for primary procedure) Ⓝ

RVU Mod	Non-Fac Total	Fac Total	Global Days	51	50	62	80	MUE
	1.33	1.33	ZZZ	0	0	0	0	1

AMA: Aug 11: 3, Dec 11: 9, Jan 13: 6

● New ▲ Revised ✖ Deleted ⊙ Moderate Sedation ✚ Add-on Codes ⊘ High Risk Denial Ⓐ Age Edit ♀ Female ♂ Male **AMA** *CPT® Assistant* ***MUE*** Medically Unlikely Edit
⊘ Modifier 51 Exempt ⊖ Modifier 63 Exempt ☒ Unlisted **Modifiers:** *See Inside Back Cover* Ⓜ Maternity Ⓐ2–Ⓩ3 ASC Payment Indicators Ⓐ–Ⓨ OPPS Status Indicators

816   CPT © 2015 American Medical Association. All Rights Reserved.   © 2016 DecisionHealth

⊙+93566 Injection procedure during cardiac catheterization including imaging supervision, interpretation, and report; for selective right ventricular or right atrial angiography (List separately in addition to code for primary procedure) N

RVU			Global Days	Modifiers				
Mod	Non-Fac Total	Fac Total			51	50	62	80	MUE
	4.84	1.34	ZZZ	0	0	0	0	1

AMA: Aug 11: 3, Dec 11: 9, Jan 13: 6, May 15: 3

⊙+93567 Injection procedure during cardiac catheterization including imaging supervision, interpretation, and report; for supravalvular aortography (List separately in addition to code for primary procedure) N

RVU			Global Days	Modifiers				
Mod	Non-Fac Total	Fac Total			51	50	62	80	MUE
	4.00	1.52	ZZZ	0	0	0	0	1

AMA: Aug 11: 3, Dec 11: 9, Jan 13: 6

⊙+93568 Injection procedure during cardiac catheterization including imaging supervision, interpretation, and report; for pulmonary angiography (List separately in addition to code for primary procedure) N

RVU			Global Days	Modifiers				
Mod	Non-Fac Total	Fac Total			51	50	62	80	MUE
	4.35	1.37	ZZZ	0	0	0	0	1

AMA: Aug 11: 3, Dec 11: 9, Jan 13: 6

⊙+93571 Intravascular Doppler velocity and/or pressure derived coronary flow reserve measurement (coronary vessel or graft) during coronary angiography including pharmacologically induced stress; initial vessel (List separately in addition to code for primary procedure) N

RVU			Global Days	Modifiers				
Mod	Non-Fac Total	Fac Total			51	50	62	80	MUE
	0.00	0.00	ZZZ	0	0	0	0	1
26	2.77	2.77	ZZZ	0	0	0	0	1
TC	0.00	0.00	ZZZ	0	0	0	0	1

AMA: Nov 98: 33, Apr 00: 2, Mar 08: 4, Aug 11: 3, Dec 14: 6, May 15: 10

⊙+93572 Intravascular Doppler velocity and/or pressure derived coronary flow reserve measurement (coronary vessel or graft) during coronary angiography including pharmacologically induced stress; each additional vessel (List separately in addition to code for primary procedure) N

RVU			Global Days	Modifiers				
Mod	Non-Fac Total	Fac Total			51	50	62	80	MUE
	0.00	0.00	ZZZ	0	0	0	0	2
26	2.22	2.22	ZZZ	0	0	0	0	2
TC	0.00	0.00	ZZZ	0	0	0	0	2

AMA: Nov 98: 34, Apr 00: 2, Aug 11: 5, Dec 14: 6, May 15: 10

Septal Defect Repair

93580 Percutaneous transcatheter closure of congenital interatrial communication (ie, Fontan fenestration, atrial septal defect) with implant J1

Coding tip: Add intracardiac echocardiography - 93662

RVU			Global Days	Modifiers				
Mod	Non-Fac Total	Fac Total			51	50	62	80	MUE
	28.41	28.41	000	2	0	0	0	1

AMA: Mar 03: 23

Percutaneous transcatheter closure of congenital interatrial communication

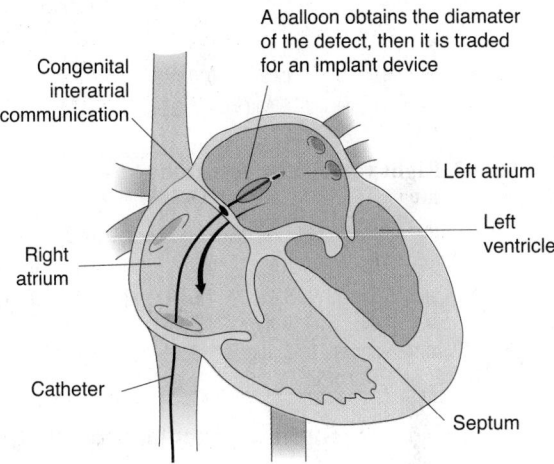

A hole between the atria is closed using a specialized catheter

93581 Percutaneous transcatheter closure of a congenital ventricular septal defect with implant J1

RVU			Global Days	Modifiers				
Mod	Non-Fac Total	Fac Total			51	50	62	80	MUE
	38.75	38.75	000	2	0	0	0	1

AMA: Mar 03: 23, Mar 08: 4

⊙ 93582 Percutaneous transcatheter closure of patent ductus arteriosus J1

RVU			Global Days	Modifiers				
Mod	Non-Fac Total	Fac Total			51	50	62	80	MUE
	19.41	19.41	000	2	0	0	0	1

AMA: Jul 14: 3

⊙ 93583 Percutaneous transcatheter septal reduction therapy (eg, alcohol septal ablation) including temporary pacemaker insertion when performed C

RVU			Global Days	Modifiers				
Mod	Non-Fac Total	Fac Total			51	50	62	80	MUE
	21.94	21.94	000	2	0	0	0	1

Intracardiac Electrophysiological Procedures

Coding Guidance

Placing catheters intravascularly into coronary vessels or chambers of the heart is often necessary for intravascular electrophysiological procedures. Cardiac or selective catheterization codes should not be reported with these procedures. A separately reported cardiac catheterization code may be used when it is medically needed and performed as a distinct service on the same

● New ▲ Revised Deleted ⊙ Moderate Sedation ✛ Add-on Codes ⊘ High Risk Denial Ⓐ Age Edit ♀ Female ♂ Male **AMA** *CPT® Assistant* **MUE** Medically Unlikely Edit
⊘ Modifier 51 Exempt ⊖ Modifier 63 Exempt ✗ Unlisted **Modifiers:** *See Inside Back Cover* Ⓜ Maternity A2-Z3 ASC Payment Indicators A-Y OPPS Status Indicators

© 2016 DecisionHealth CPT © 2015 American Medical Association. All Rights Reserved.

Medicine Procedures

93600 – 93615

day or different patient encounter. Fluoroscopy and ultrasound are not reportable with the procedures described in 93600-93662.

⊘ 93600 Bundle of His recording   J1

Mod	Non-Fac Total	Fac Total	Global Days	51	50	62	80	MUE
	0.00	0.00	000	0	0	0	0	1
26	3.42	3.42	000	0	0	0	0	1
TC	0.00	0.00	000	0	0	0	0	1

AMA: Summer 94: 12, Aug 97: 9, Apr 04: 9, Jul 04: 13, Aug 05: 13, Dec 07: 16, Mar 08: 4, Jul 13: 7, Jun 13: 6, Apr 14: 3

⊘ 93602 Intra-atrial recording   J1

Mod	Non-Fac Total	Fac Total	Global Days	51	50	62	80	MUE
	0.00	0.00	000	0	0	0	0	1
26	3.35	3.35	000	0	0	0	0	1
TC	0.00	0.00	000	0	0	0	0	1

AMA: Summer 94: 12, Aug 97: 9, Apr 04: 9, Jul 04: 13, Aug 05: 13, Jul 13: 7, Jun 13: 6, Apr 14: 3

⊘ 93603 Right ventricular recording   J1

Mod	Non-Fac Total	Fac Total	Global Days	51	50	62	80	MUE
	0.00	0.00	000	0	0	0	0	1
26	3.35	3.35	000	0	0	0	0	1
TC	0.00	0.00	000	0	0	0	0	1

AMA: Summer 94: 12, Aug 97: 9, Apr 04: 9, Jul 04: 13, Aug 05: 13, Jul 13: 7, Jun 13: 6, Apr 14: 3

Right ventricular recording

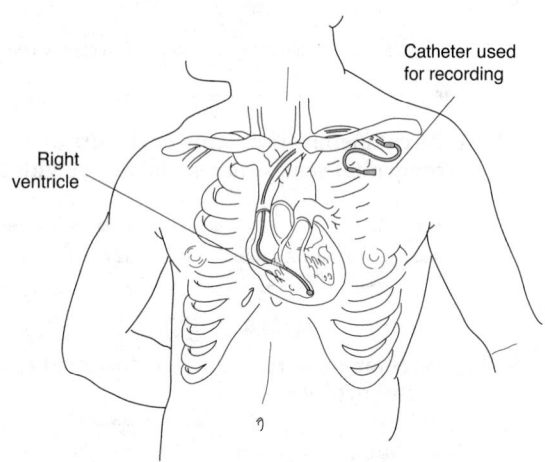

Right ventricle

Catheter used for recording

Recording of the right ventricle, obtained by an electrode-mounted catheter that is fed to the right ventricle with fluoroscopic guidance, and then attached at the other end to an electronic recording device.

⊙+93609 Intraventricular and/or intra-atrial mapping of tachycardia site(s) with catheter manipulation to record from multiple sites to identify origin of tachycardia (List separately in addition to code for primary procedure)   N

Mod	Non-Fac Total	Fac Total	Global Days	51	50	62	80	MUE
	0.00	0.00	ZZZ	0	0	0	0	1
26	8.02	8.02	ZZZ	0	0	0	0	1
TC	0.00	0.00	ZZZ	0	0	0	0	1

AMA: Summer 94: 12, Aug 97: 9, Apr 04: 9, Aug 05: 13, Jul 13: 7, Jun 13: 6, Apr 14: 3

⊘ 93610 Intra-atrial pacing   J1

Mod	Non-Fac Total	Fac Total	Global Days	51	50	62	80	MUE
	0.00	0.00	000	0	0	0	0	1
26	4.75	4.75	000	0	0	0	0	1
TC	0.00	0.00	000	0	0	0	0	1

AMA: Summer 94: 12, Aug 97: 9, Apr 04: 9, Jul 04: 13, Jul 13: 7, Jun 13: 6, Apr 14: 3

⊘ 93612 Intraventricular pacing   J1

Mod	Non-Fac Total	Fac Total	Global Days	51	50	62	80	MUE
	0.00	0.00	000	0	0	0	0	1
26	4.72	4.72	000	0	0	0	0	1
TC	0.00	0.00	000	0	0	0	0	1

AMA: Summer 94: 12, Aug 97: 9, Apr 04: 9, Jul 04: 13, Jul 13: 7, Jun 13: 6, Apr 14: 3

⊙+93613 Intracardiac electrophysiologic 3-dimensional mapping (List separately in addition to code for primary procedure)   N

Mod	Non-Fac Total	Fac Total	Global Days	51	50	62	80	MUE
	11.55	11.55	ZZZ	0	0	0	0	1

AMA: Apr 04: 8, Aug 05: 13, Jul 13: 7, Jun 13: 6, Apr 14: 3

⊙⊘ 93615 Esophageal recording of atrial electrogram with or without ventricular electrogram(s)   J1

Mod	Non-Fac Total	Fac Total	Global Days	51	50	62	80	MUE
	0.00	0.00	000	0	0	0	0	1
26	1.49	1.49	000	0	0	0	0	1
TC	0.00	0.00	000	0	0	0	0	1

AMA: Summer 94: 12, Aug 97: 9, Apr 04: 9, Aug 05: 13, Apr 14: 3

Esophageal recording of atrial electrogram with or without ventricular electrogram

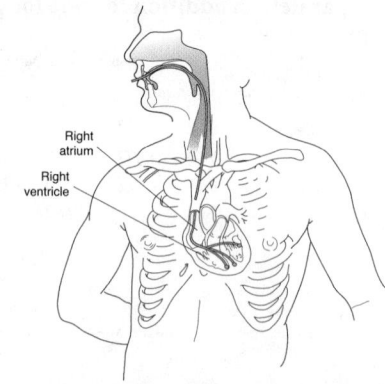

Right atrium

Right ventricle

The physician inserts electrodes into the esophagus via either the mouth or nose, and lowers them until the ideal position is reached to obtain readings from the heart.

● New   ▲ Revised   ✖ Deleted   ⊙ Moderate Sedation   ✚ Add-on Codes   ⊘ High Risk Denial   ⊛ Age Edit   ♀ Female   ♂ Male   **AMA** *CPT® Assistant*   **MUE** Medically Unlikely Edit

⊘ Modifier 51 Exempt   ⊖ Modifier 63 Exempt   ☒ Unlisted   **Modifiers:** *See Inside Back Cover*   Ⓜ Maternity   A2–Z3 ASC Payment Indicators   A–Y OPPS Status Indicators

818   CPT © 2015 American Medical Association. All Rights Reserved.   © 2016 DecisionHealth

⊙⊘**93616** Esophageal recording of atrial electrogram with or without ventricular electrogram(s); with pacing

Mod	RVU Non-Fac Total	Fac Total	Global Days	Modifiers 51	50	62	80	MUE
	0.00	0.00	000	0	0	0	0	1
26	1.86	1.86	000	0	0	0	0	1
TC	0.00	0.00	000	0	0	0	0	1

AMA: Summer 94: 12, Aug 97: 9, Apr 04: 9, Aug 05: 13, Apr 14: 3

⊙⊘**93618** Induction of arrhythmia by electrical pacing

Mod	RVU Non-Fac Total	Fac Total	Global Days	Modifiers 51	50	62	80	MUE
	0.00	0.00	000	0	0	0	0	1
26	6.84	6.84	000	0	0	0	0	1
TC	0.00	0.00	000	0	0	0	0	1

AMA: Summer 94: 12, Aug 97: 9, Oct 97: 10, Apr 99: 10, Jun 00: 5, Nov 00: 9, Apr 04: 9, Jul 04: 13, Aug 05: 13, Dec 07: 16, Jul 13: 7, Jun 13: 6, Apr 14: 3

⊙ **93619** Comprehensive electrophysiologic evaluation with right atrial pacing and recording, right ventricular pacing and recording, His bundle recording, including insertion and repositioning of multiple electrode catheters, without induction or attempted induction of arrhythmia

Mod	RVU Non-Fac Total	Fac Total	Global Days	Modifiers 51	50	62	80	MUE
	0.00	0.00	000	2	0	0	0	1
26	11.68	11.68	000	2	0	0	0	1
TC	0.00	0.00	000	0	0	0	0	1

AMA: Aug 97: 9, Oct 97: 10, Nov 00: 9, Apr 04: 9, Jul 04: 13, Aug 05: 13, Dec 07: 16, Jul 13: 7, Nov 12: 6, Jun 13: 6, Apr 14: 3

⊙ **93620** Comprehensive electrophysiologic evaluation including insertion and repositioning of multiple electrode catheters with induction or attempted induction of arrhythmia; with right atrial pacing and recording, right ventricular pacing and recording, His bundle recording

Mod	RVU Non-Fac Total	Fac Total	Global Days	Modifiers 51	50	62	80	MUE
	0.00	0.00	000	2	0	0	0	1
26	18.54	18.54	000	2	0	0	0	1
TC	0.00	0.00	000	0	0	0	0	1

AMA: Summer 94: 12, Aug 97: 9, Oct 97: 10, Jul 98: 10, Aug 98: 7, Nov 00: 9, Apr 04: 9, Jul 04: 13, Aug 05: 13, Dec 07: 16, Oct 08: 10, Jul 13: 7, Nov 12: 6, Jun 13: 6, Apr 14: 3

⊙+**93621** Comprehensive electrophysiologic evaluation including insertion and repositioning of multiple electrode catheters with induction or attempted induction of arrhythmia; with left atrial pacing and recording from coronary sinus or left atrium (List separately in addition to code for primary procedure)

Mod	RVU Non-Fac Total	Fac Total	Global Days	Modifiers 51	50	62	80	MUE
	0.00	0.00	ZZZ	0	0	0	0	1
26	3.38	3.38	ZZZ	0	0	0	0	1
TC	0.00	0.00	ZZZ	0	0	0	0	1

AMA: Summer 94: 12, Aug 97: 9, Oct 97: 10, Jul 98: 10, Aug 98: 7, Nov 98: 34, Nov 00: 9, Apr 04: 9, Jul 04: 13, Aug 05: 13, Dec 07: 16, Oct 08: 10, Jul 13: 7, Nov 12: 6, Jun 13: 6, Apr 14: 3

⊙+**93622** Comprehensive electrophysiologic evaluation including insertion and repositioning of multiple electrode catheters with induction or attempted induction of arrhythmia; with left ventricular pacing and recording (List separately in addition to code for primary procedure)

Mod	RVU Non-Fac Total	Fac Total	Global Days	Modifiers 51	50	62	80	MUE
	0.00	0.00	ZZZ	0	0	0	0	1
26	4.94	4.94	ZZZ	0	0	0	0	1
TC	0.00	0.00	ZZZ	0	0	0	0	1

AMA: Summer 94: 14, Aug 97: 9, Oct 97: 10, Jul 98: 10, Aug 98: 7, Nov 98: 34, Nov 00: 9, Apr 04: 9, Jul 04: 13, Aug 05: 13, Dec 07: 16, Mar 08: 4, Jul 13: 7, Nov 12: 6, Jun 13: 6, Apr 14: 3

+ **93623** Programmed stimulation and pacing after intravenous drug infusion (List separately in addition to code for primary procedure)

Mod	RVU Non-Fac Total	Fac Total	Global Days	Modifiers 51	50	62	80	MUE
	0.00	0.00	ZZZ	0	0	0	0	1
26	4.59	4.59	ZZZ	0	0	0	0	1
TC	0.00	0.00	ZZZ	0	0	0	0	1

AMA: Summer 94: 14, Aug 97: 9, Nov 00: 9, Aug 05: 13, Dec 07: 16, Oct 08: 10, Apr 14: 3

⊙ **93624** Electrophysiologic follow-up study with pacing and recording to test effectiveness of therapy, including induction or attempted induction of arrhythmia

Mod	RVU Non-Fac Total	Fac Total	Global Days	Modifiers 51	50	62	80	MUE
	0.00	0.00	000	2	0	0	0	1
26	7.60	7.60	000	2	0	0	0	1
TC	0.00	0.00	000	0	0	0	0	1

AMA: Summer 94: 14, Aug 97: 9, Nov 00: 9, Aug 05: 13, Dec 07: 16

⊘ **93631** Intra-operative epicardial and endocardial pacing and mapping to localize the site of tachycardia or zone of slow conduction for surgical correction

Mod	RVU Non-Fac Total	Fac Total	Global Days	Modifiers 51	50	62	80	MUE
	0.00	0.00	000	0	0	0	0	1
26	11.57	11.57	000	0	0	0	0	1
TC	0.00	0.00	000	0	0	0	0	1

AMA: Summer 94: 14, Aug 97: 9, Nov 00: 9, Aug 05: 13, Dec 07: 16

Intra-operative epicardial and endocardial pacing and mapping

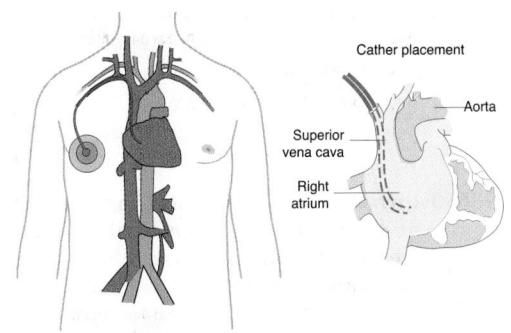

Pacing and mapping is done on the surface and within the heart to localize the site of tachycardia in order to allow correction.

● New ▲ Revised Deleted ⊙ Moderate Sedation + Add-on Codes ⊘ High Risk Denial Ⓐ Age Edit ♀ Female ♂ Male **AMA** *CPT® Assistant* **MUE** Medically Unlikely Edit ⊘ Modifier 51 Exempt ⊖ Modifier 63 Exempt ✕ Unlisted **Modifiers:** *See Inside Back Cover* Ⓜ Maternity A2–Z3 ASC Payment Indicators A–Y OPPS Status Indicators

⊙ **93640** Electrophysiologic evaluation of single or dual chamber pacing cardioverter-defibrillator leads including defibrillation threshold evaluation (induction of arrhythmia, evaluation of sensing and pacing for arrhythmia termination) at time of initial implantation or replacement   **N**

Mod	RVU Non-Fac Total	Fac Total	Global Days	Modifiers 51	50	62	80	MUE
	0.00	0.00	000	2	0	0	0	1
26	5.56	5.56	000	2	0	0	0	1
TC	0.00	0.00	000	0	0	0	0	1

AMA: Summer 94: 14, Aug 97: 9, Apr 99: 10, Nov 99: 50, Nov 00: 9, Aug 05: 13, Jun 12: 3

⊙ **93641** Electrophysiologic evaluation of single or dual chamber pacing cardioverter-defibrillator leads including defibrillation threshold evaluation (induction of arrhythmia, evaluation of sensing and pacing for arrhythmia termination) at time of initial implantation or replacement; with testing of single or dual chamber pacing cardioverter-defibrillator pulse generator   **N**

Mod	RVU Non-Fac Total	Fac Total	Global Days	Modifiers 51	50	62	80	MUE
	0.00	0.00	000	2	0	0	0	1
26	9.45	9.45	000	2	0	0	0	1
TC	0.00	0.00	000	0	0	0	0	1

AMA: Summer 94: 14, Aug 97: 9, Apr 99: 10, Nov 99: 50, Jun 00: 5, Jul 00: 5, Nov 00: 9, Aug 05: 13, Jun 12: 3, Apr 14: 3

⊙ **93642** Electrophysiologic evaluation of single or dual chamber transvenous pacing cardioverter-defibrillator (includes defibrillation threshold evaluation, induction of arrhythmia, evaluation of sensing and pacing for arrhythmia termination, and programming or reprogramming of sensing or therapeutic parameters)   **J1**

Mod	RVU Non-Fac Total	Fac Total	Global Days	Modifiers 51	50	62	80	MUE
	12.14	12.14	000	2	0	0	0	1
26	7.85	7.85	000	2	0	0	0	1
TC	4.29	4.29	000	0	0	0	0	1

AMA: Summer 94: 14, Aug 97: 9, Nov 99: 50, Jun 00: 5, Nov 00: 9, Aug 05: 13, Jul 13: 7, Jun 13: 6, Apr 14: 3

⊙ **93644** Electrophysiologic evaluation of subcutaneous implantable defibrillator (includes defibrillation threshold evaluation, induction of arrhythmia, evaluation of sensing for arrhythmia termination, and programming or reprogramming of sensing or therapeutic parameters)   **N**

Mod	RVU Non-Fac Total	Fac Total	Global Days	Modifiers 51	50	62	80	MUE
	7.88	7.88	000	2	0	0	0	1
26	4.91	4.91	000	2	0	0	0	1
TC	2.97	2.97	000	0	0	0	0	1

⊙ **93650** Intracardiac catheter ablation of atrioventricular node function, atrioventricular conduction for creation of complete heart block, with or without temporary pacemaker placement   **J1**

Mod	RVU Non-Fac Total	Fac Total	Global Days	Modifiers 51	50	62	80	MUE
	17.51	17.51	000	2	0	0	0	1

AMA: Summer 94: 15, Aug 97: 9, Nov 00: 9, Aug 05: 13, Apr 12: 18, May 12: 15

⊙ **93653** Comprehensive electrophysiologic evaluation including insertion and repositioning of multiple electrode catheters with induction or attempted induction of an arrhythmia with right atrial pacing and recording, right ventricular pacing and recording (when necessary), and His bundle recording (when necessary) with intracardiac catheter ablation of arrhythmogenic focus; with treatment of supraventricular tachycardia by ablation of fast or slow atrioventricular pathway, accessory atrioventricular connection, cavo-tricuspid isthmus or other single atrial focus or source of atrial re-entry   **J1**

Mod	RVU Non-Fac Total	Fac Total	Global Days	Modifiers 51	50	62	80	MUE
	24.64	24.64	000	2	0	0	0	1

AMA: Jul 13: 7, Jun 13: 6, Apr 14: 3

⊙ **93654** Comprehensive electrophysiologic evaluation including insertion and repositioning of multiple electrode catheters with induction or attempted induction of an arrhythmia with right atrial pacing and recording, right ventricular pacing and recording (when necessary), and His bundle recording (when necessary) with intracardiac catheter ablation of arrhythmogenic focus; with treatment of ventricular tachycardia or focus of ventricular ectopy including intracardiac electrophysiologic 3D mapping, when performed, and left ventricular pacing and recording, when performed   **J1**

Mod	RVU Non-Fac Total	Fac Total	Global Days	Modifiers 51	50	62	80	MUE
	32.81	32.81	000	2	0	0	0	1

AMA: Jul 13: 7, Jun 13: 6, Apr 14: 3

⊙**+93655** Intracardiac catheter ablation of a discrete mechanism of arrhythmia which is distinct from the primary ablated mechanism, including repeat diagnostic maneuvers, to treat a spontaneous or induced arrhythmia (List separately in addition to code for primary procedure)   **N**

Mod	RVU Non-Fac Total	Fac Total	Global Days	Modifiers 51	50	62	80	MUE
	12.32	12.32	ZZZ	0	0	0	0	2

AMA: Jul 13: 7, Jun 13: 6

⊙ **93656** Comprehensive electrophysiologic evaluation including transseptal catheterizations, insertion and repositioning of multiple electrode catheters with induction or attempted induction of an arrhythmia including left or right atrial pacing/recording when necessary, right ventricular pacing/recording when necessary, and His bundle recording when necessary with intracardiac catheter ablation of atrial fibrillation by pulmonary vein isolation   **J1**

Mod	RVU Non-Fac Total	Fac Total	Global Days	Modifiers 51	50	62	80	MUE
	32.83	32.83	000	2	0	0	0	1

AMA: Jul 13: 7, Jun 13: 6, Apr 14: 3

● New   ▲ Revised   ✖ Deleted   ⊙ Moderate Sedation   ✚ Add-on Codes   ⊘ High Risk Denial   Ⓐ Age Edit   ♀ Female   ♂ Male   **AMA** CPT® Assistant   **MUE** Medically Unlikely Edit
⊘ Modifier 51 Exempt   ⊖ Modifier 63 Exempt   ✗ Unlisted   **Modifiers:** See Inside Back Cover   Ⓜ Maternity   **A2**–**Z3** ASC Payment Indicators   **A**–**Y** OPPS Status Indicators

⊙+**93657** Additional linear or focal intracardiac catheter ablation of the left or right atrium for treatment of atrial fibrillation remaining after completion of pulmonary vein isolation (List separately in addition to code for primary procedure) **N**

RVU			Global Days	Modifiers				
Mod	Non-Fac Total	Fac Total		51	50	62	80	MUE
	12.31	12.31	ZZZ	0	0	0	0	1

AMA: Jul 13: 7, Jun 13: 6, Apr 14: 3

93660 Evaluation of cardiovascular function with tilt table evaluation, with continuous ECG monitoring and intermittent blood pressure monitoring, with or without pharmacological intervention **S**

RVU			Global Days	Modifiers				
Mod	Non-Fac Total	Fac Total		51	50	62	80	MUE
	4.46	4.46	000	2	0	0	0	1
26	2.67	2.67	000	2	0	0	0	1
TC	1.79	1.79	000	0	0	0	0	1

AMA: Nov 12: 6

+ **93662** Intracardiac echocardiography during therapeutic/diagnostic intervention, including imaging supervision and interpretation (List separately in addition to code for primary procedure) **N**

RVU			Global Days	Modifiers				
Mod	Non-Fac Total	Fac Total		51	50	62	80	MUE
	0.00	0.00	ZZZ	0	0	0	0	1
26	4.05	4.05	ZZZ	0	0	0	0	1
TC	0.00	0.00	ZZZ	0	0	0	0	1

AMA: Mar 03: 23

Peripheral Artery Disease Rehabilitation Services

93668 Peripheral arterial disease (PAD) rehabilitation, per session **E**

RVU			Global Days	Modifiers				
Mod	Non-Fac Total	Fac Total		51	50	62	80	MUE
	0.54	0.54	XXX	9	9	9	9	

Noninvasive Physiological Procedures/Studies

93701 Bioimpedance-derived physiologic cardiovascular analysis **Q1**

RVU			Global Days	Modifiers				
Mod	Non-Fac Total	Fac Total		51	50	62	80	MUE
	0.68	0.68	XXX	6	0	0	0	1

AMA: Mar 02: 3, Mar 08: 4

93702 Bioimpedance spectroscopy (BIS), extracellular fluid analysis for lymphedema assessment(s) **S**

RVU			Global Days	Modifiers				
Mod	Non-Fac Total	Fac Total		51	50	62	80	MUE
	3.05	3.05	XXX	6	0	0	0	1

93724 Electronic analysis of antitachycardia pacemaker system (includes electrocardiographic recording, programming of device, induction and termination of tachycardia via implanted pacemaker, and interpretation of recordings) **S**

RVU			Global Days	Modifiers				
Mod	Non-Fac Total	Fac Total		51	50	62	80	MUE
	7.65	7.65	000	6	0	0	0	1
26	6.86	6.86	000	6	0	0	0	1
TC	0.79	0.79	000	6	0	0	0	1

AMA: Summer 94: 23

93740 Temperature gradient studies **Q1**

RVU			Global Days	Modifiers				
Mod	Non-Fac Total	Fac Total		51	50	62	80	MUE
	0.23	0.23	XXX	9	9	9	9	0

93745 Initial set-up and programming by a physician or other qualified health care professional of wearable cardioverter-defibrillator includes initial programming of system, establishing baseline electronic ECG, transmission of data to data repository, patient instruction in wearing system and patient reporting of problems or events **S**

RVU			Global Days	Modifiers				
Mod	Non-Fac Total	Fac Total		51	50	62	80	MUE
	0.00	0.00	XXX	0	0	0	0	1
26	0.00	0.00	XXX	0	0	0	0	1
TC	0.00	0.00	XXX	0	0	0	0	1

93750 Interrogation of ventricular assist device (VAD), in person, with physician or other qualified health care professional analysis of device parameters (eg, drivelines, alarms, power surges), review of device function (eg, flow and volume status, septum status, recovery), with programming, if performed, and report **S**

RVU			Global Days	Modifiers				
Mod	Non-Fac Total	Fac Total		51	50	62	80	MUE
	1.58	1.32	XXX	0	0	0	0	4

AMA: Apr 10: 6

93770 Determination of venous pressure **N**

RVU			Global Days	Modifiers				
Mod	Non-Fac Total	Fac Total		51	50	62	80	MUE
	0.23	0.23	XXX	9	9	9	9	0

93784 Ambulatory blood pressure monitoring, utilizing a system such as magnetic tape and/or computer disk, for 24 hours or longer; including recording, scanning analysis, interpretation and report **B**

RVU			Global Days	Modifiers				
Mod	Non-Fac Total	Fac Total		51	50	62	80	MUE
	1.52	1.52	XXX	6	0	0	0	1

Pub 100-04, 32, 10.1

93786 Ambulatory blood pressure monitoring, utilizing a system such as magnetic tape and/or computer disk, for 24 hours or longer; recording only **Q1**

RVU			Global Days	Modifiers				
Mod	Non-Fac Total	Fac Total		51	50	62	80	MUE
	0.84	0.84	XXX	6	0	0	0	1

Pub 100-04, 32, 10.1

● New ▲ Revised Deleted ⊙ Moderate Sedation ✚ Add-on Codes ⊘ High Risk Denial Ⓐ Age Edit ♀ Female ♂ Male **AMA** CPT® Assistant **MUE** Medically Unlikely Edit
⊘ Modifier 51 Exempt ⊖ Modifier 63 Exempt ⊠ Unlisted **Modifiers:** See Inside Back Cover Ⓜ Maternity A2–Z3 ASC Payment Indicators A–Y OPPS Status Indicators

Medicine Procedures

93788 – 93895

93788 Ambulatory blood pressure monitoring, utilizing a system such as magnetic tape and/or computer disk, for 24 hours or longer; scanning analysis with report ⊗◨Ⅰ

RVU			Global Days	Modifiers				
Mod	Non-Fac Total	Fac Total		51	50	62	80	MUE
	0.15	0.15	XXX	6	0	0	0	1

Pub 100-04, 32, 10.1

93790 Ambulatory blood pressure monitoring, utilizing a system such as magnetic tape and/or computer disk, for 24 hours or longer; review with interpretation and report Ⅿ

RVU			Global Days	Modifiers				
Mod	Non-Fac Total	Fac Total		51	50	62	80	MUE
	0.53	0.53	XXX	0	0	0	0	1

Pub 100-04, 32, 10.1

Other Cardiovascular Procedures

Coding Guidance
Do not report E&M services with comprehensive cardiac rehabilitation unless a completely unrelated, documented, and separately identifiable service is performed.

93797 Physician or other qualified health care professional services for outpatient cardiac rehabilitation; without continuous ECG monitoring (per session) S

RVU			Global Days	Modifiers				
Mod	Non-Fac Total	Fac Total		51	50	62	80	MUE
	0.46	0.25	000	0	0	0	0	2

Pub 100-04, 32, 140.1.1, 140.2.2.4

93798 Physician or other qualified health care professional services for outpatient cardiac rehabilitation; with continuous ECG monitoring (per session) S

RVU			Global Days	Modifiers				
Mod	Non-Fac Total	Fac Total		51	50	62	80	MUE
	0.71	0.40	000	0	0	0	0	2

Pub 100-04, 32, 140.1.1, 140.2.2.4

93799 Unlisted cardiovascular service or procedure ⊗xS

Coding tip: *Use unlisted code 93799 to report nonsurgical septal reduction therapy, intracardiac phonogram*

RVU			Global Days	Modifiers				
Mod	Non-Fac Total	Fac Total		51	50	62	80	MUE
	0.00	0.00	XXX	0	0	0	0	
26	0.00	0.00	XXX	0	0	0	0	
TC	0.00	0.00	XXX	0	0	0	0	

AMA: Mar 98: 11, Mar 02: 10, Nov 05: 15, Apr 09: 9, Oct 11: 7, Nov 11: 11, Jul 10: 10, Dec 13: 18

Pub 100-04, 13, 120

93880 Duplex scan of extracranial arteries; complete bilateral study S

RVU			Global Days	Modifiers				
Mod	Non-Fac Total	Fac Total		51	50	62	80	MUE
	5.74	5.74	XXX	6	2	0	0	1
26	1.14	1.14	XXX	6	2	0	0	1
TC	4.60	4.60	XXX	6	2	0	0	1

AMA: Jun 96: 9, Dec 05: 3

93882 Duplex scan of extracranial arteries; unilateral or limited study S

RVU			Global Days	Modifiers				
Mod	Non-Fac Total	Fac Total		51	50	62	80	MUE
	3.67	3.67	XXX	6	0	0	0	1
26	0.72	0.72	XXX	6	0	0	0	1
TC	2.95	2.95	XXX	6	0	0	0	1

AMA: Jun 96: 9, Dec 05: 3

93886 Transcranial Doppler study of the intracranial arteries; complete study S

RVU			Global Days	Modifiers				
Mod	Non-Fac Total	Fac Total		51	50	62	80	MUE
	7.98	7.98	XXX	6	0	0	0	1
26	1.35	1.35	XXX	6	0	0	0	1
TC	6.63	6.63	XXX	6	0	0	0	1

AMA: Jun 96: 9, Dec 05: 3

93888 Transcranial Doppler study of the intracranial arteries; limited study S

RVU			Global Days	Modifiers				
Mod	Non-Fac Total	Fac Total		51	50	62	80	MUE
	4.17	4.17	XXX	6	0	0	0	1
26	0.73	0.73	XXX	6	0	0	0	1
TC	3.44	3.44	XXX	6	0	0	0	1

AMA: Jun 96: 9, Dec 05: 3

93890 Transcranial Doppler study of the intracranial arteries; vasoreactivity study ◨Ⅰ

RVU			Global Days	Modifiers				
Mod	Non-Fac Total	Fac Total		51	50	62	80	MUE
	8.18	8.18	XXX	6	0	0	0	1
26	1.47	1.47	XXX	6	0	0	0	1
TC	6.71	6.71	XXX	6	0	0	0	1

AMA: Dec 05: 3

93892 Transcranial Doppler study of the intracranial arteries; emboli detection without intravenous microbubble injection ◨Ⅰ

RVU			Global Days	Modifiers				
Mod	Non-Fac Total	Fac Total		51	50	62	80	MUE
	9.46	9.46	XXX	6	0	0	0	1
26	1.74	1.74	XXX	6	0	0	0	1
TC	7.72	7.72	XXX	6	0	0	0	1

AMA: Dec 05: 3

93893 Transcranial Doppler study of the intracranial arteries; emboli detection with intravenous microbubble injection ◨Ⅰ

RVU			Global Days	Modifiers				
Mod	Non-Fac Total	Fac Total		51	50	62	80	MUE
	9.82	9.82	XXX	6	0	0	0	1
26	1.70	1.70	XXX	6	0	0	0	1
TC	8.12	8.12	XXX	6	0	0	0	1

AMA: Dec 05: 3

93895 Quantitative carotid intima media thickness and carotid atheroma evaluation, bilateral E

RVU			Global Days	Modifiers				
Mod	Non-Fac Total	Fac Total		51	50	62	80	MUE
	0.00	0.00	XXX	6	0	0	0	
26	0.00	0.00	XXX	6	0	0	0	
TC	0.00	0.00	XXX	6	0	0	0	

● New   ▲ Revised   ✖ Deleted   ⊙ Moderate Sedation   ✚ Add-on Codes   ⊘ High Risk Denial   Ⓐ Age Edit   ♀ Female   ♂ Male   **AMA** *CPT® Assistant*   **MUE** Medically Unlikely Edit
⊘ Modifier 51 Exempt   ⊖ Modifier 63 Exempt   ⊠ Unlisted   **Modifiers:** *See Inside Back Cover*   Ⓜ Maternity   Ａ2–Ｚ3 ASC Payment Indicators   Ａ–Ｙ OPPS Status Indicators

822   CPT © 2015 American Medical Association. All Rights Reserved.   © 2016 DecisionHealth

Extremity Artery Studies

93922 Limited bilateral noninvasive physiologic studies of upper or lower extremity arteries, (eg, for lower extremity: ankle/brachial indices at distal posterior tibial and anterior tibial/dorsalis pedis arteries plus bidirectional, Doppler waveform recording and analysis at 1-2 levels, or ankle/brachial indices at distal posterior tibial and anterior tibial/dorsalis pedis arteries plus volume plethysmography at 1-2 levels, or ankle/brachial indices at distal posterior tibial and anterior tibial/dorsalis pedis arteries with, transcutaneous oxygen tension measurement at 1-2 levels) **Q1**

RVU			Global Days	Modifiers				
Mod	Non-Fac Total	Fac Total		51	50	62	80	MUE
	2.52	2.52	XXX	6	2	0	0	1
26	0.36	0.36	XXX	6	2	0	0	1
TC	2.16	2.16	XXX	6	2	0	0	1

AMA: Jun 96: 9, Dec 05: 3, Aug 09: 3, Jun 12: 16, Jun 13: 14, Jan 14: 10

Pub 100-04, 16, 120.2; 100-04, 32, 130.1

93923 Complete bilateral noninvasive physiologic studies of upper or lower extremity arteries, 3 or more levels (eg, for lower extremity: ankle/brachial indices at distal posterior tibial and anterior tibial/dorsalis pedis arteries plus segmental blood pressure measurements with bidirectional Doppler waveform recording and analysis, at 3 or more levels, or ankle/brachial indices at distal posterior tibial and anterior tibial/dorsalis pedis arteries plus segmental volume plethysmography at 3 or more levels, or ankle/brachial indices at distal posterior tibial and anterior tibial/dorsalis pedis arteries plus segmental transcutaneous oxygen tension measurements at 3 or more levels), or single level study with provocative functional maneuvers (eg, measurements with postural provocative tests, or measurements with reactive hyperemia) **S**

RVU			Global Days	Modifiers				
Mod	Non-Fac Total	Fac Total		51	50	62	80	MUE
	3.92	3.92	XXX	6	2	0	0	1
26	0.64	0.64	XXX	6	2	0	0	1
TC	3.28	3.28	XXX	6	2	0	0	1

AMA: Jun 96: 9, Jun 01: 10, Dec 05: 3, Aug 09: 3, Jun 12: 16, Jan 14: 10

Pub 100-04, 16, 120.2; 100-04, 32, 130.1

93924 Noninvasive physiologic studies of lower extremity arteries, at rest and following treadmill stress testing, (ie, bidirectional Doppler waveform or volume plethysmography recording and analysis at rest with ankle/brachial indices immediately after and at timed intervals following performance of a standardized protocol on a motorized treadmill plus recording of time of onset of claudication or other symptoms, maximal walking time, and time to recovery) complete bilateral study **S**

RVU			Global Days	Modifiers				
Mod	Non-Fac Total	Fac Total		51	50	62	80	MUE
	4.92	4.92	XXX	6	2	0	0	1
26	0.71	0.71	XXX	6	2	0	0	1
TC	4.21	4.21	XXX	6	2	0	0	1

AMA: Jun 96: 9, Dec 05: 3, Aug 09: 3, Jun 12: 16, Jan 14: 10

93925 Duplex scan of lower extremity arteries or arterial bypass grafts; complete bilateral study **S**

RVU			Global Days	Modifiers				
Mod	Non-Fac Total	Fac Total		51	50	62	80	MUE
	7.38	7.38	XXX	6	2	0	0	1
26	1.12	1.12	XXX	6	2	0	0	1
TC	6.26	6.26	XXX	6	2	0	0	1

AMA: Jun 96: 9, Dec 05: 3

Pub 100-04, 16, 120.2

93926 Duplex scan of lower extremity arteries or arterial bypass grafts; unilateral or limited study **S**

RVU			Global Days	Modifiers				
Mod	Non-Fac Total	Fac Total		51	50	62	80	MUE
	4.34	4.34	XXX	6	0	0	0	1
26	0.69	0.69	XXX	6	0	0	0	1
TC	3.65	3.65	XXX	6	0	0	0	1

AMA: Jun 96: 9, Oct 01: 2, Dec 05: 3

Pub 100-04, 16, 120.2

93930 Duplex scan of upper extremity arteries or arterial bypass grafts; complete bilateral study **S**

RVU			Global Days	Modifiers				
Mod	Non-Fac Total	Fac Total		51	50	62	80	MUE
	5.94	5.94	XXX	6	2	0	0	1
26	1.14	1.14	XXX	6	2	0	0	1
TC	4.80	4.80	XXX	6	2	0	0	1
	5.94	5.94	XXX	6	2	0	0	1
26	1.14	1.14	XXX	6	2	0	0	1
TC	4.80	4.80	XXX	6	2	0	0	1

AMA: Jun 96: 9, Dec 05: 3

Pub 100-04, 16, 120.2

93931 Duplex scan of upper extremity arteries or arterial bypass grafts; unilateral or limited study **S**

RVU			Global Days	Modifiers				
Mod	Non-Fac Total	Fac Total		51	50	62	80	MUE
	3.64	3.64	XXX	6	0	0	0	1
26	0.70	0.70	XXX	6	0	0	0	1
TC	2.94	2.94	XXX	6	0	0	0	1
	3.64	3.64	XXX	6	0	0	0	1
26	0.70	0.70	XXX	6	0	0	0	1
TC	2.94	2.94	XXX	6	0	0	0	1

AMA: Jun 96: 9, Oct 01: 2, Dec 05: 3

Pub 100-04, 16, 120.2

Extremity Vein Studies

93965 Noninvasive physiologic studies of extremity veins, complete bilateral study (eg, Doppler waveform analysis with responses to compression and other maneuvers, phleborheography, impedance plethysmography) **S**

RVU			Global Days	Modifiers				
Mod	Non-Fac Total	Fac Total		51	50	62	80	MUE
	3.38	3.38	XXX	6	2	0	0	1
26	0.49	0.49	XXX	6	2	0	0	1
TC	2.89	2.89	XXX	6	2	0	0	1

AMA: Jun 96: 9, Dec 05: 3

Pub 100-04, 16, 120.2

● New   ▲ Revised   Deleted   ⊙ Moderate Sedation   ✚ Add-on Codes   ⊗ High Risk Denial   Ⓐ Age Edit   ♀ Female   ♂ Male   **AMA** *CPT® Assistant*   **MUE** Medically Unlikely Edit
⃠ Modifier 51 Exempt   ⊖ Modifier 63 Exempt   ⊠ Unlisted   **Modifiers:** *See Inside Back Cover*   Ⓜ Maternity   A2–Z3 ASC Payment Indicators   A–Y OPPS Status Indicators

© 2016 DecisionHealth   CPT © 2015 American Medical Association. All Rights Reserved.   **823**

Medicine Procedures

93970 – 93998

93970 Duplex scan of extremity veins including responses to compression and other maneuvers; complete bilateral study **S**

RVU			Global Days	Modifiers				
Mod	Non-Fac Total	Fac Total		51	50	62	80	MUE
	5.59	5.59	XXX	6	2	0	0	1
26	0.99	0.99	XXX	6	2	0	0	1
TC	4.60	4.60	XXX	6	2	0	0	1

AMA: Jun 96: 9, Dec 05: 3, Jan 12: 13, Feb 12: 11, Oct 14: 6

Pub 100-04, 16, 120.2

93971 Duplex scan of extremity veins including responses to compression and other maneuvers; unilateral or limited study **S**

RVU			Global Days	Modifiers				
Mod	Non-Fac Total	Fac Total		51	50	62	80	MUE
	3.41	3.41	XXX	6	0	0	0	1
26	0.64	0.64	XXX	6	0	0	0	1
TC	2.77	2.77	XXX	6	0	0	0	1

AMA: Jun 96: 9, Oct 01: 2, Mar 03: 21, Dec 05: 3, Apr 11: 13, Jan 12: 13, Feb 12: 11, Jul 10: 6, Oct 14: 6, Aug 15: 8

Pub 100-04, 16, 120.2

Visceral Organ/Penile Vascular Studies

Coding Guidance

Abdominal ultrasound (76700-76775) and abdominal duplex exams will generally be done for differing clinical scenarios, but some instances occur when both types of services may be necessary at the same time. When both services are necessary, report the ultrasound procedure with the appropriate modifier.

93975 Duplex scan of arterial inflow and venous outflow of abdominal, pelvic, scrotal contents and/or retroperitoneal organs; complete study **S**

RVU			Global Days	Modifiers				
Mod	Non-Fac Total	Fac Total		51	50	62	80	MUE
	8.02	8.02	XXX	6	0	0	0	1
26	1.65	1.65	XXX	6	0	0	0	1
TC	6.37	6.37	XXX	6	0	0	0	1

AMA: Apr 96: 11, Jun 96: 9, Dec 05: 3, Mar 15: 10, Jun 14: 15

93976 Duplex scan of arterial inflow and venous outflow of abdominal, pelvic, scrotal contents and/or retroperitoneal organs; limited study **S**

RVU			Global Days	Modifiers				
Mod	Non-Fac Total	Fac Total		51	50	62	80	MUE
	4.62	4.62	XXX	6	0	0	0	1
26	1.13	1.13	XXX	6	0	0	0	1
TC	3.49	3.49	XXX	6	0	0	0	1

AMA: Apr 96: 11, Jun 96: 9, Dec 05: 3, Mar 15: 10

93978 Duplex scan of aorta, inferior vena cava, iliac vasculature, or bypass grafts; complete study **S**

RVU			Global Days	Modifiers				
Mod	Non-Fac Total	Fac Total		51	50	62	80	MUE
	5.43	5.43	XXX	6	0	0	0	1
26	1.13	1.13	XXX	6	0	0	0	1
TC	4.30	4.30	XXX	6	0	0	0	1

AMA: Jun 96: 9, Dec 05: 3

93979 Duplex scan of aorta, inferior vena cava, iliac vasculature, or bypass grafts; unilateral or limited study **Q1**

RVU			Global Days	Modifiers				
Mod	Non-Fac Total	Fac Total		51	50	62	80	MUE
	3.40	3.40	XXX	6	0	0	0	1
26	0.71	0.71	XXX	6	0	0	0	1
TC	2.69	2.69	XXX	6	0	0	0	1

AMA: Jun 96: 9, Dec 05: 3, Jun 14: 15

93980 Duplex scan of arterial inflow and venous outflow of penile vessels; complete study **S**

RVU			Global Days	Modifiers				
Mod	Non-Fac Total	Fac Total		51	50	62	80	MUE
TC	1.68	1.68	XXX	6	0	0	0	1
	3.42	3.42	XXX	6	0	0	0	1
26	1.74	1.74	XXX	6	0	0	0	1

AMA: Jun 96: 9, Dec 05: 3

93981 Duplex scan of arterial inflow and venous outflow of penile vessels; follow-up or limited study **S**

RVU			Global Days	Modifiers				
Mod	Non-Fac Total	Fac Total		51	50	62	80	MUE
	2.08	2.08	XXX	6	0	0	0	1
26	0.63	0.63	XXX	6	0	0	0	1
TC	1.45	1.45	XXX	6	0	0	0	1

AMA: Jun 96: 9, Dec 05: 3

93982 Noninvasive physiologic study of implanted wireless pressure sensor in aneurysmal sac following endovascular repair, complete study including recording, analysis of pressure and waveform tracings, interpretation and report **Q1**

RVU			Global Days	Modifiers				
Mod	Non-Fac Total	Fac Total		51	50	62	80	MUE
	1.22	1.22	XXX	0	0	0	0	1

Extremity Artery-Vein Studies

93990 Duplex scan of hemodialysis access (including arterial inflow, body of access and venous outflow) **Q1**

RVU			Global Days	Modifiers				
Mod	Non-Fac Total	Fac Total		51	50	62	80	MUE
	4.59	4.59	XXX	6	0	0	0	2
26	0.71	0.71	XXX	6	0	0	0	2
TC	3.88	3.88	XXX	6	0	0	0	2

AMA: Jun 96: 9, Dec 05: 3

93998 Unlisted noninvasive vascular diagnostic study **⊗✗Q1**

RVU			Global Days	Modifiers				
Mod	Non-Fac Total	Fac Total		51	50	62	80	MUE
	0.00	0.00	XXX	0	0	1	0	

AMA: Sep 12: 9, Jan 14: 10

● New ▲ Revised ✖ Deleted ⊙ Moderate Sedation ✚ Add-on Codes ⊗ High Risk Denial Ⓐ Age Edit ♀ Female ♂ Male **AMA** *CPT® Assistant* **MUE** Medically Unlikely Edit
⊘ Modifier 51 Exempt ⊖ Modifier 63 Exempt ✗ Unlisted **Modifiers:** *See Inside Back Cover* Ⓜ Maternity A2–Z3 ASC Payment Indicators A–Y OPPS Status Indicators

824 CPT © 2015 American Medical Association. All Rights Reserved. © 2016 DecisionHealth

Pulmonary Services/Procedures

Ventilator Management Services

94002 Ventilation assist and management, initiation of pressure or volume preset ventilators for assisted or controlled breathing; hospital inpatient/observation, initial day   Q3

	RVU		Global Days	Modifiers				
Mod	Non-Fac Total	Fac Total		51	50	62	80	MUE
	2.66	2.66	XXX	0	0	0	0	1

AMA: Feb 07: 10, Mar 07: 10, Apr 07: 3, Jul 07: 1, Nov 08: 5, May 14: 4, Oct 14: 9

Pub 100-04, 12, 30.6.12

94003 Ventilation assist and management, initiation of pressure or volume preset ventilators for assisted or controlled breathing; hospital inpatient/observation, each subsequent day   Q3

	RVU		Global Days	Modifiers				
Mod	Non-Fac Total	Fac Total		51	50	62	80	MUE
	1.90	1.90	XXX	0	0	0	0	1

AMA: Feb 07: 10, Apr 07: 3, Jul 07: 1, Nov 08: 5, May 14: 4

Pub 100-04, 12, 30.6.12

94004 Ventilation assist and management, initiation of pressure or volume preset ventilators for assisted or controlled breathing; nursing facility, per day B

	RVU		Global Days	Modifiers				
Mod	Non-Fac Total	Fac Total		51	50	62	80	MUE
	1.39	1.39	XXX	0	0	0	0	1

AMA: Feb 07: 10, Apr 07: 3, Jul 07: 1, Nov 08: 5

Pub 100-04, 12, 30.6.12

94005 Home ventilator management care plan oversight of a patient (patient not present) in home, domiciliary or rest home (eg, assisted living) requiring review of status, review of laboratories and other studies and revision of orders and respiratory care plan (as appropriate), within a calendar month, 30 minutes or more   M

	RVU		Global Days	Modifiers				
Mod	Non-Fac Total	Fac Total		51	50	62	80	MUE
	2.63	2.63	XXX	9	9	9	9	

AMA: Mar 07: 11, Apr 07: 3, Nov 08: 5, Oct 14: 9

Other Pulmonary Procedures

94010 Spirometry, including graphic record, total and timed vital capacity, expiratory flow rate measurement(s), with or without maximal voluntary ventilation   Q1

	RVU		Global Days	Modifiers				
Mod	Non-Fac Total	Fac Total		51	50	62	80	MUE
	1.01	1.01	XXX	0	0	0	0	1
26	0.24	0.24	XXX	0	0	0	0	1
TC	0.77	0.77	XXX	0	0	0	0	1

AMA: Summer 91: 16, Summer 95: 4, Feb 96: 9, Nov 97: 45, Nov 98: 35, Feb 99: 9, Aug 03: 15, Jul 05: 11, Nov 08: 5, Mar 96: 10, Jan 99: 8, Oct 10: 15, Dec 10: 15, Aug 12: 6, 7, Nov 12: 14, Dec 13: 12, Mar 14: 11

94011 Measurement of spirometric forced expiratory flows in an infant or child through 2 years of age   A Q1

	RVU		Global Days	Modifiers				
Mod	Non-Fac Total	Fac Total		51	50	62	80	MUE
	2.91	2.91	XXX	0	0	0	0	1

AMA: May 10: 7, Aug 12: 6, Dec 13: 12

94012 Measurement of spirometric forced expiratory flows, before and after bronchodilator, in an infant or child through 2 years of age   A Q1

	RVU		Global Days	Modifiers				
Mod	Non-Fac Total	Fac Total		51	50	62	80	MUE
	4.45	4.45	XXX	0	0	0	0	1

AMA: May 10: 7, Aug 12: 6

94013 Measurement of lung volumes (ie, functional residual capacity [FRC], forced vital capacity [FVC], and expiratory reserve volume [ERV]) in an infant or child through 2 years of age   A S

	RVU		Global Days	Modifiers				
Mod	Non-Fac Total	Fac Total		51	50	62	80	MUE
	0.98	0.98	XXX	0	0	0	0	1

AMA: May 10: 7, Aug 12: 6, Dec 13: 12

94014 Patient-initiated spirometric recording per 30-day period of time; includes reinforced education, transmission of spirometric tracing, data capture, analysis of transmitted data, periodic recalibration and review and interpretation by a physician or other qualified health care professional   Q1

	RVU		Global Days	Modifiers				
Mod	Non-Fac Total	Fac Total		51	50	62	80	MUE
	1.59	1.59	XXX	0	0	0	0	1

AMA: Summer 95: 4, Nov 98: 34, Jan 99: 8, Jul 05: 11, Nov 08: 5

94015 Patient-initiated spirometric recording per 30-day period of time; recording (includes hook-up, reinforced education, data transmission, data capture, trend analysis, and periodic recalibration)   Q1

	RVU		Global Days	Modifiers				
Mod	Non-Fac Total	Fac Total		51	50	62	80	MUE
	0.87	0.87	XXX	0	0	0	0	1

AMA: Summer 95: 4, Nov 98: 34, Jan 99: 8, Jul 05: 11, Nov 08: 5

94016 Patient-initiated spirometric recording per 30-day period of time; review and interpretation only by a physician or other qualified health care professional   A

	RVU		Global Days	Modifiers				
Mod	Non-Fac Total	Fac Total		51	50	62	80	MUE
	0.72	0.72	XXX	0	0	0	0	1

AMA: Summer 95: 4, Nov 98: 34, Jan 99: 8, Jul 05: 11, Nov 08: 5

94060 Bronchodilation responsiveness, spirometry as in 94010, pre- and post-bronchodilator administration   S

	RVU		Global Days	Modifiers				
Mod	Non-Fac Total	Fac Total		51	50	62	80	MUE
	1.72	1.72	XXX	0	0	0	0	1
26	0.37	0.37	XXX	0	0	0	0	1
TC	1.35	1.35	XXX	0	0	0	0	1

AMA: Summer 95: 4, Feb 96: 9, Feb 97: 10, Nov 98: 34, Jan 99: 8, Feb 99: 9, Jul 05: 11, Nov 08: 5, Dec 10: 15, Aug 12: 6, 7, Mar 14: 11

● New   ▲ Revised   Deleted   ⊙ Moderate Sedation   ✚ Add-on Codes   ⊘ High Risk Denial   Ⓐ Age Edit   ♀ Female   ♂ Male   **AMA** *CPT® Assistant*   **MUE** Medically Unlikely Edit
⊘ Modifier 51 Exempt   ⊖ Modifier 63 Exempt   ✗ Unlisted   **Modifiers:** *See Inside Back Cover*   Ⓜ Maternity   A2–Z3 ASC Payment Indicators   A–Y OPPS Status Indicators

© 2016 DecisionHealth   CPT © 2015 American Medical Association. All Rights Reserved.

Coding Guidance

Only one unit of service is reportable, regardless of the number of spirometric determinations needed. Report the administration of the agent(s) used with 99070 or the corresponding HCPCS Level II supply code.

94070 Bronchospasm provocation evaluation, multiple spirometric determinations as in 94010, with administered agents (eg, antigen[s], cold air, methacholine) S

RVU			Global Days	Modifiers				
Mod	Non-Fac Total	Fac Total		51	50	62	80	MUE
	1.69	1.69	XXX	0	0	0	0	1
26	0.82	0.82	XXX	0	0	0	0	1
TC	0.87	0.87	XXX	0	0	0	0	1

AMA: Summer 91: 16, Summer 95: 4, Feb 96: 9, Nov 97: 45, Jan 99: 8, Jul 05: 11, Nov 08: 5, Aug 12: 6, Nov 12: 11

94150 Vital capacity, total (separate procedure) ⊘Q1

RVU			Global Days	Modifiers				
Mod	Non-Fac Total	Fac Total		51	50	62	80	MUE
	0.72	0.72	XXX	9	9	9	9	0
26	0.11	0.11	XXX	9	9	9	9	0
TC	0.61	0.61	XXX	9	9	9	9	0

AMA: Summer 95: 4, Feb 96: 9, Jul 05: 11, Nov 08: 5, Dec 10: 15, Aug 12: 6, Mar 14: 11

94200 Maximum breathing capacity, maximal voluntary ventilation Q1

RVU			Global Days	Modifiers				
Mod	Non-Fac Total	Fac Total		51	50	62	80	MUE
	0.71	0.71	XXX	0	0	0	0	1
26	0.16	0.16	XXX	0	0	0	0	1
TC	0.55	0.55	XXX	0	0	0	0	1

AMA: Summer 95: 4, Feb 96: 9, Aug 03: 15, Jul 05: 11, Nov 08: 5, Dec 10: 15, Aug 12: 6, 7, Mar 14: 11

94250 Expired gas collection, quantitative, single procedure (separate procedure) Q1

RVU			Global Days	Modifiers				
Mod	Non-Fac Total	Fac Total		51	50	62	80	MUE
	0.74	0.74	XXX	0	0	0	0	1
26	0.15	0.15	XXX	0	0	0	0	1
TC	0.59	0.59	XXX	0	0	0	0	1

AMA: Summer 95: 4, Feb 96: 9, Jul 05: 11, Nov 08: 5

Coding Guidance

Flow volume loop is included in standard spirometry studies as it is another method for calculating a standard spirometric parameter.

94375 Respiratory flow volume loop Q1

RVU			Global Days	Modifiers				
Mod	Non-Fac Total	Fac Total		51	50	62	80	MUE
	1.11	1.11	XXX	0	0	0	0	1
26	0.42	0.42	XXX	0	0	0	0	1
TC	0.69	0.69	XXX	0	0	0	0	1

AMA: Summer 95: 4, Feb 96: 9, Oct 03: 2, Jul 05: 11, Jul 06: 4, Jul 07: 1, Nov 08: 5, Aug 12: 6, 7, Mar 14: 11

94400 Breathing response to CO2 (CO2 response curve) Q1

RVU			Global Days	Modifiers				
Mod	Non-Fac Total	Fac Total		51	50	62	80	MUE
	1.58	1.58	XXX	0	0	0	0	1
26	0.56	0.56	XXX	0	0	0	0	1
TC	1.02	1.02	XXX	0	0	0	0	1

AMA: Summer 95: 4, Feb 96: 9, Jul 05: 11, Nov 08: 5, Dec 10: 15, Mar 14: 11

94450 Breathing response to hypoxia (hypoxia response curve) Q1

RVU			Global Days	Modifiers				
Mod	Non-Fac Total	Fac Total		51	50	62	80	MUE
	1.93	1.93	XXX	0	0	0	0	1
26	0.57	0.57	XXX	0	0	0	0	1
TC	1.36	1.36	XXX	0	0	0	0	1

AMA: Summer 95: 4, Feb 96: 9, Jul 05: 11, Nov 08: 5

94452 High altitude simulation test (HAST), with interpretation and report by a physician or other qualified health care professional Q1

RVU			Global Days	Modifiers				
Mod	Non-Fac Total	Fac Total		51	50	62	80	MUE
	1.63	1.63	XXX	0	0	0	0	1
26	0.41	0.41	XXX	0	0	0	0	1
TC	1.22	1.22	XXX	0	0	0	0	1

AMA: Jul 05: 11, Nov 08: 5

94453 High altitude simulation test (HAST), with interpretation and report by a physician or other qualified health care professional; with supplemental oxygen titration Q1

RVU			Global Days	Modifiers				
Mod	Non-Fac Total	Fac Total		51	50	62	80	MUE
	2.26	2.26	XXX	0	0	0	0	1
26	0.54	0.54	XXX	0	0	0	0	1
TC	1.72	1.72	XXX	0	0	0	0	1

AMA: Jul 05: 11, Nov 08: 5

⊘ 94610 Intrapulmonary surfactant administration by a physician or other qualified health care professional through endotracheal tube ⒶQ1

RVU			Global Days	Modifiers				
Mod	Non-Fac Total	Fac Total		51	50	62	80	MUE
	1.69	1.69	XXX	0	0	0	0	2

AMA: Apr 07: 3, Jul 08: 7, Nov 08: 5, Dec 10: 15

Coding Guidance

Complex pulmonary stress testing includes several component tests that should not be billed separately: venous access, ECG monitoring, spirometric parameters before, during, and after exercise, oximetry, CO2 production measurements, oxygen consumption, cardiac stress test, and any other component of a simple pulmonary stress test.

94620 Pulmonary stress testing; simple (eg, 6-minute walk test, prolonged exercise test for bronchospasm with pre- and post-spirometry and oximetry) Q1

RVU			Global Days	Modifiers				
Mod	Non-Fac Total	Fac Total		51	50	62	80	MUE
	1.58	1.58	XXX	0	0	0	0	1
26	0.87	0.87	XXX	0	0	0	0	1
TC	0.71	0.71	XXX	0	0	0	0	1

AMA: Summer 95: 4, Feb 96: 9, Nov 98: 35, Jan 99: 8, Mar 04: 10, Jul 05: 11, 13, Apr 07: 3, Jun 07: 11, Nov 08: 5, Nov 12: 14

94621 Pulmonary stress testing; complex (including measurements of CO2 production, O2 uptake, and electrocardiographic recordings) S

RVU			Global Days	Modifiers				
Mod	Non-Fac Total	Fac Total		51	50	62	80	MUE
	4.60	4.60	XXX	0	0	0	0	1
26	1.95	1.95	XXX	0	0	0	0	1
TC	2.65	2.65	XXX	0	0	0	0	1

● New ▲ Revised ✖ Deleted ⊙ Moderate Sedation ➕ Add-on Codes ⊘ High Risk Denial Ⓐ Age Edit ♀ Female ♂ Male **AMA** *CPT® Assistant* **MUE** Medically Unlikely Edit
⊘ Modifier 51 Exempt ⊖ Modifier 63 Exempt ✗ Unlisted **Modifiers:** *See Inside Back Cover* Ⓜ Maternity Ⓐ2–Ⓩ3 ASC Payment Indicators Ⓐ–Ⓨ OPPS Status Indicators

CPT © 2015 American Medical Association. All Rights Reserved. © 2016 DecisionHealth

Medicine Procedures

AMA: Summer 95: 4, Nov 98: 35, Jan 99: 8, Aug 02: 10, Jul 05: 11, Nov 08: 5, Nov 12: 14

▲ **94640 Pressurized or nonpressurized inhalation treatment for acute airway obstruction for therapeutic purposes and/or for diagnostic purposes such as sputum induction with an aerosol generator, nebulizer, metered dose inhaler or intermittent positive pressure breathing (IPPB) device** Q1

RVU			Global Days	Modifiers				
Mod	Non-Fac Total	Fac Total		51	50	62	80	MUE
	0.52	0.52	XXX	0	0	0	0	4

AMA: Summer 95: 4, Feb 96: 9, May 98: 10, Apr 00: 11, Jul 05: 11, Apr 07: 3, Nov 08: 5, Sep 10: 3, Dec 13: 12, Mar 14: 11

94642 Aerosol inhalation of pentamidine for pneumocystis carinii pneumonia treatment or prophylaxis Q1

RVU			Global Days	Modifiers				
Mod	Non-Fac Total	Fac Total		51	50	62	80	MUE
	0.00	0.00	XXX	0	0	0	0	1

AMA: Summer 95: 4, Feb 96: 9, Jul 05: 11, Nov 08: 5

94644 Continuous inhalation treatment with aerosol medication for acute airway obstruction; first hour Q1

RVU			Global Days	Modifiers				
Mod	Non-Fac Total	Fac Total		51	50	62	80	MUE
	1.24	1.24	XXX	0	0	0	0	1

AMA: Apr 07: 3, Nov 08: 5, Mar 14: 11

✚ **94645 Continuous inhalation treatment with aerosol medication for acute airway obstruction; each additional hour (List separately in addition to code for primary procedure)** N

RVU			Global Days	Modifiers				
Mod	Non-Fac Total	Fac Total		51	50	62	80	MUE
	0.40	0.40	XXX	0	0	0	0	2

AMA: Apr 07: 3, Nov 08: 5, Mar 14: 11

94660 Continuous positive airway pressure ventilation (CPAP), initiation and management Q1

RVU			Global Days	Modifiers				
Mod	Non-Fac Total	Fac Total		51	50	62	80	MUE
	1.79	1.08	XXX	0	0	0	0	1

AMA: Fall 92: 30, Spring 95: 4, Summer 95: 4, Feb 96: 9, Jan 99: 10, Aug 00: 2, Oct 03: 2, Jul 05: 11, Jul 06: 4, Feb 07: 10, Jul 07: 1, Nov 08: 5, May 14: 4, Oct 14: 9

Pub 100-04, 12, 30.6.12

94662 Continuous negative pressure ventilation (CNP), initiation and management Q3

RVU			Global Days	Modifiers				
Mod	Non-Fac Total	Fac Total		51	50	62	80	MUE
	1.06	1.06	XXX	0	0	0	0	1

AMA: Fall 92: 30, Spring 94: 4, Summer 95: 4, Feb 96: 9, Aug 00: 2, Jul 05: 11, Feb 07: 10, Jul 07: 1, Nov 08: 5, May 14: 4

Pub 100-04, 12, 30.6.12

94664 Demonstration and/or evaluation of patient utilization of an aerosol generator, nebulizer, metered dose inhaler or IPPB device Q1

RVU			Global Days	Modifiers				
Mod	Non-Fac Total	Fac Total		51	50	62	80	MUE
	0.49	0.49	XXX	0	0	0	0	1

AMA: Summer 95: 4, Feb 96: 9, May 98: 10, Apr 00: 11, Jul 05: 11, Nov 08: 5, Sep 10: 3, Dec 13: 12

94667 Manipulation chest wall, such as cupping, percussing, and vibration to facilitate lung function; initial demonstration and/or evaluation Q1

RVU			Global Days	Modifiers				
Mod	Non-Fac Total	Fac Total		51	50	62	80	MUE
	0.73	0.73	XXX	0	0	0	0	1

AMA: Summer 95: 4, Feb 96: 9, Jul 05: 11, Nov 08: 5, Sep 10: 3, Dec 13: 12, Mar 14: 11

94668 Manipulation chest wall, such as cupping, percussing, and vibration to facilitate lung function; subsequent Q1

RVU			Global Days	Modifiers				
Mod	Non-Fac Total	Fac Total		51	50	62	80	MUE
	0.81	0.81	XXX	0	0	0	

AMA: Summer 95: 4, Feb 96: 9, Jul 05: 11, Sep 10: 3, Dec 13: 12, Mar 14: 11

94669 Mechanical chest wall oscillation to facilitate lung function, per session Q1

RVU			Global Days	Modifiers				
Mod	Non-Fac Total	Fac Total		51	50	62	80	MUE
	0.93	0.93	XXX	0	0	0	0	4

94680 Oxygen uptake, expired gas analysis; rest and exercise, direct, simple Q1

RVU			Global Days	Modifiers				
Mod	Non-Fac Total	Fac Total		51	50	62	80	MUE
	1.62	1.62	XXX	0	0	0	0	1
26	0.36	0.36	XXX	0	0	0	0	1
TC	1.26	1.26	XXX	0	0	0	0	1

AMA: Summer 95: 4, Feb 96: 9, Jul 05: 11

94681 Oxygen uptake, expired gas analysis; including CO2 output, percentage oxygen extracted Q1

RVU			Global Days	Modifiers				
Mod	Non-Fac Total	Fac Total		51	50	62	80	MUE
26	0.28	0.28	XXX	0	0	0	0	1
TC	1.21	1.21	XXX	0	0	0	0	1
	1.49	1.49	XXX	0	0	0	0	1

AMA: Summer 95: 4, Feb 96: 9, Jul 05: 11

94690 Oxygen uptake, expired gas analysis; rest, indirect (separate procedure) Q1

RVU			Global Days	Modifiers				
Mod	Non-Fac Total	Fac Total		51	50	62	80	MUE
	1.41	1.41	XXX	0	0	0	0	1
26	0.11	0.11	XXX	0	0	0	0	1
TC	1.30	1.30	XXX	0	0	0	0	1

AMA: Summer 95: 4, Feb 96: 9, Jul 05: 11

● New ▲ Revised Deleted ⊙ Moderate Sedation ✚ Add-on Codes ⊘ High Risk Denial Ⓐ Age Edit ♀ Female ♂ Male AMA CPT® Assistant MUE Medically Unlikely Edit
⊘ Modifier 51 Exempt ⊖ Modifier 63 Exempt ✖ Unlisted Modifiers: See Inside Back Cover Ⓜ Maternity A2–Z3 ASC Payment Indicators A–Y OPPS Status Indicators
© 2016 DecisionHealth — CPT © 2015 American Medical Association. All Rights Reserved.

Medicine Procedures

94726 – 94775

94726 Plethysmography for determination of lung volumes and, when performed, airway resistance Q1

Mod	RVU Non-Fac Total	Fac Total	Global Days	Modifiers 51	50	62	80	MUE
	1.49	1.49	XXX	0	0	0	0	1
26	0.35	0.35	XXX	0	0	0	0	1
TC	1.14	1.14	XXX	0	0	0	0	1

AMA: Jan 12: 3, Aug 12: 6, May 13: 11

94727 Gas dilution or washout for determination of lung volumes and, when performed, distribution of ventilation and closing volumes Q1

Mod	RVU Non-Fac Total	Fac Total	Global Days	Modifiers 51	50	62	80	MUE
	1.19	1.19	XXX	0	0	0	0	1
26	0.35	0.35	XXX	0	0	0	0	1
TC	0.84	0.84	XXX	0	0	0	0	1

AMA: Jan 12: 3, Aug 12: 6, May 13: 11

94728 Airway resistance by impulse oscillometry ⊝Q1

Documentation Finder: The documentation should show that they are using "sound waves" to assess the patient's airway resistance. The record should show that the patient is breathing normally during testing. You may see the abbreviation IOS to indicate that type of testing.

Mod	RVU Non-Fac Total	Fac Total	Global Days	Modifiers 51	50	62	80	MUE
	1.14	1.14	XXX	0	0	0	0	1
26	0.36	0.36	XXX	0	0	0	0	1
TC	0.78	0.78	XXX	0	0	0	0	1

AMA: Jan 12: 3, Aug 12: 6, May 13: 11, Mar 14: 11

+ 94729 Diffusing capacity (eg, carbon monoxide, membrane) (List separately in addition to code for primary procedure) N

Mod	RVU Non-Fac Total	Fac Total	Global Days	Modifiers 51	50	62	80	MUE
26	0.26	0.26	ZZZ	0	0	0	0	1
TC	1.28	1.28	ZZZ	0	0	0	0	1
	1.54	1.54	ZZZ	0	0	0	0	1

AMA: Jan 12: 3, Aug 12: 6, Dec 13: 12

94750 Pulmonary compliance study (eg, plethysmography, volume and pressure measurements) Q1

Mod	RVU Non-Fac Total	Fac Total	Global Days	Modifiers 51	50	62	80	MUE
	2.27	2.27	XXX	0	0	0	0	1
26	0.32	0.32	XXX	0	0	0	0	1
TC	1.95	1.95	XXX	0	0	0	0	1

AMA: Summer 95: 4, Feb 96: 9, Jul 05: 11

94760 Noninvasive ear or pulse oximetry for oxygen saturation; single determination ⊝N

Documentation Finder: The documentation should show that just one determination was performed to obtain the actual rating – for example, after having the patient on a treadmill for many minutes, the provider tested the patient's oxygen saturation.

Mod	RVU Non-Fac Total	Fac Total	Global Days	Modifiers 51	50	62	80	MUE
	0.09	0.09	XXX	0	0	0	0	1

AMA: Summer 95: 4, Feb 96: 9, Feb 97: 10, Jul 98: 2, Oct 03: 2, Jul 05: 11, Feb 06: 9, Jul 06: 4, Feb 07: 10, Apr 07: 1, Jul 07: 1, Dec 10: 15, May 14: 4

Pub 100-04, 12, 30.6.12; 100-04, 32, 130.1

94761 Noninvasive ear or pulse oximetry for oxygen saturation; multiple determinations (eg, during exercise) ⊝N

Documentation Finder: Your documentation needs to show that multiple determinations were taken such as after exercise or treadmill and then also at rest. Documentation should reflect more than one determination. This code would not be used when also using the critical care codes 99291/99292.

Mod	RVU Non-Fac Total	Fac Total	Global Days	Modifiers 51	50	62	80	MUE
	0.14	0.14	XXX	0	0	0	0	1

AMA: Summer 95: 4, Feb 96: 9, Jul 98: 2, Jun 99: 10, Jul 05: 11, Feb 06: 9, Jul 06: 4, Feb 07: 10, Apr 07: 1, Jun 07: 11, Jul 07: 1, Dec 08: 5, May 14: 4

Pub 100-04, 12, 30.6.12; 100-04, 32, 130.1

94762 Noninvasive ear or pulse oximetry for oxygen saturation; by continuous overnight monitoring (separate procedure) Q3

Mod	RVU Non-Fac Total	Fac Total	Global Days	Modifiers 51	50	62	80	MUE
	0.69	0.69	XXX	0	0	0	0	1

AMA: Summer 95: 4, Feb 96: 9, Jul 98: 2, Oct 03: 2, Jul 05: 11, Feb 06: 9, Jul 06: 4, Feb 07: 10, Apr 07: 1, Jul 07: 1, Dec 08: 5, May 14: 4

Pub 100-04, 12, 30.6.12

94770 Carbon dioxide, expired gas determination by infrared analyzer S

Mod	RVU Non-Fac Total	Fac Total	Global Days	Modifiers 51	50	62	80	MUE
	0.21	0.21	XXX	0	0	0	0	1

AMA: Summer 95: 4, Feb 96: 9, Jul 05: 11, Mar 14: 11

94772 Circadian respiratory pattern recording (pediatric pneumogram), 12-24 hour continuous recording, infant ⊝ⒶS

Mod	RVU Non-Fac Total	Fac Total	Global Days	Modifiers 51	50	62	80	MUE
	0.00	0.00	XXX	0	0	0	0	1
26	0.00	0.00	XXX	0	0	0	0	1
TC	0.00	0.00	XXX	0	0	0	0	1

AMA: Summer 95: 4, Feb 96: 9, Jul 05: 11

94774 Pediatric home apnea monitoring event recording including respiratory rate, pattern and heart rate per 30-day period of time; includes monitor attachment, download of data, review, interpretation, and preparation of a report by a physician or other qualified health care professional B

Mod	RVU Non-Fac Total	Fac Total	Global Days	Modifiers 51	50	62	80	MUE
	0.00	0.00	YYY	0	0	0	0	1

AMA: Apr 07: 3, Mar 08: 4

94775 Pediatric home apnea monitoring event recording including respiratory rate, pattern and heart rate per 30-day period of time; monitor attachment only (includes hook-up, initiation of recording and disconnection) ⊝S

Mod	RVU Non-Fac Total	Fac Total	Global Days	Modifiers 51	50	62	80	MUE
	0.00	0.00	YYY	0	0	0	0	1

AMA: Apr 07: 3, Mar 08: 4

● New   ▲ Revised   ✖ Deleted   ⊙ Moderate Sedation   ✚ Add-on Codes   ⊝ High Risk Denial   Ⓐ Age Edit   ♀ Female   ♂ Male   **AMA** *CPT® Assistant*   **MUE** Medically Unlikely Edit   ⊘ Modifier 51 Exempt   ⊖ Modifier 63 Exempt   ✗ Unlisted   **Modifiers:** *See Inside Back Cover*   Ⓜ Maternity   A2–Z3 ASC Payment Indicators   A–Y OPPS Status Indicators

CPT © 2015 American Medical Association. All Rights Reserved.   © 2016 DecisionHealth

94776 Pediatric home apnea monitoring event recording including respiratory rate, pattern and heart rate per 30-day period of time; monitoring, download of information, receipt of transmission(s) and analyses by computer only   S

RVU			Global Days	Modifiers				
Mod	Non-Fac Total	Fac Total		51	50	62	80	MUE
	0.00	0.00	YYY	0	0	0	0	1

AMA: Apr 07: 3, Mar 08: 4

94777 Pediatric home apnea monitoring event recording including respiratory rate, pattern and heart rate per 30-day period of time; review, interpretation and preparation of report only by a physician or other qualified health care professional   CB

RVU			Global Days	Modifiers				
Mod	Non-Fac Total	Fac Total		51	50	62	80	MUE
	0.00	0.00	YYY	0	0	0	0	1

AMA: Apr 07: 3, Mar 08: 4

94780 Car seat/bed testing for airway integrity, neonate, with continual nursing observation and continuous recording of pulse oximetry, heart rate and respiratory rate, with interpretation and report; 60 minutes   ⊘Ⓐ Q I

RVU			Global Days	Modifiers				
Mod	Non-Fac Total	Fac Total		51	50	62	80	MUE
	1.59	0.65	XXX	0	0	0	1	1

AMA: Aug 12: 6, May 15: 11

+ 94781 Car seat/bed testing for airway integrity, neonate, with continual nursing observation and continuous recording of pulse oximetry, heart rate and respiratory rate, with interpretation and report; each additional full 30 minutes (List separately in addition to code for primary procedure)   ⊘Ⓐ N

RVU			Global Days	Modifiers				
Mod	Non-Fac Total	Fac Total		51	50	62	80	MUE
	0.65	0.25	ZZZ	0	0	0	1	1

AMA: Aug 12: 6, May 15: 11

94799 Unlisted pulmonary service or procedure   ⊗✗Q I

RVU			Global Days	Modifiers				
Mod	Non-Fac Total	Fac Total		51	50	62	80	MUE
	0.00	0.00	XXX	0	0	0	0	
26	0.00	0.00	XXX	0	0	0	0	
TC	0.00	0.00	XXX	0	0	0	0	

AMA: Summer 95: 4, Feb 96: 9, Mar 96: 10, Jul 05: 11, Dec 10: 15, Nov 12: 14, Dec 13: 12, May 15: 11

Pub 100-04, 13, 120

Allergy/Immunology Services/Procedures

Allergy Testing Procedures

Coding Guidance

If both a single percutaneous and/or intracutaneous test (95004, 95027) and sequential and incremental percutaneous and/or intracutaneous tests (95017, 95018, 95027) are performed on the same date, the codes may be reported together if they were for different allergens or different dilutions of the same allergen. The number of separate tests is the number of units of service to be reported. If the provider uses three different solutions in sequential and incremental testing of the same antigen proven positive in a single test, then one unit of service may be reported for the single test, and three units of service for the sequential and incremental test code.

95004 Percutaneous tests (scratch, puncture, prick) with allergenic extracts, immediate type reaction, including test interpretation and report, specify number of tests   Q I

RVU			Global Days	Modifiers				
Mod	Non-Fac Total	Fac Total		51	50	62	80	MUE
	0.19	0.19	XXX	0	0	0	0	

AMA: May 10: 3, Summer 91: 15, Jan 13: 9

Pub 100-04, 12, 200

95012 Nitric oxide expired gas determination   Q I

RVU			Global Days	Modifiers				
Mod	Non-Fac Total	Fac Total		51	50	62	80	MUE
	0.54	0.54	XXX	0	0	0	0	2

AMA: Mar 07: 11, Apr 07: 6, Jan 13: 9, Mar 14: 11

Pub 100-04, 12, 200

95017 Allergy testing, any combination of percutaneous (scratch, puncture, prick) and intracutaneous (intradermal), sequential and incremental, with venoms, immediate type reaction, including test interpretation and report, specify number of tests   Q I

RVU			Global Days	Modifiers				
Mod	Non-Fac Total	Fac Total		51	50	62	80	MUE
	0.22	0.10	XXX	0	0	0	0	

AMA: Jan 13: 9, Jul 15: 9

Pub 100-04, 12, 200

95018 Allergy testing, any combination of percutaneous (scratch, puncture, prick) and intracutaneous (intradermal), sequential and incremental, with drugs or biologicals, immediate type reaction, including test interpretation and report, specify number of tests   Q I

RVU			Global Days	Modifiers				
Mod	Non-Fac Total	Fac Total		51	50	62	80	MUE
	0.58	0.20	XXX	0	0	0	0	19

AMA: Jan 13: 9, Jul 15: 9

Pub 100-04, 12, 200

95024 Intracutaneous (intradermal) tests with allergenic extracts, immediate type reaction, including test interpretation and report, specify number of tests   Q I

RVU			Global Days	Modifiers				
Mod	Non-Fac Total	Fac Total		51	50	62	80	MUE
	0.22	0.03	XXX	0	0	0	0	

AMA: Summer 91: 15, May 10: 3, Jan 13: 9

Pub 100-04, 12, 200

95027 Intracutaneous (intradermal) tests, sequential and incremental, with allergenic extracts for airborne allergens, immediate type reaction, including test interpretation and report, specify number of tests   Q I

RVU			Global Days	Modifiers				
Mod	Non-Fac Total	Fac Total		51	50	62	80	MUE
	0.13	0.13	XXX	0	0	0	0	

AMA: Summer 91: 15, Jun 97: 10, Dec 07: 9, May 10: 3, Jan 13: 9

Pub 100-04, 12, 200

94776 – 95027

● New   ▲ Revised   Deleted   ⊙ Moderate Sedation   ✚ Add-on Codes   ⊘ High Risk Denial   Ⓐ Age Edit   ♀ Female   ♂ Male   **AMA** *CPT® Assistant*   **MUE** Medically Unlikely Edit

⊘ Modifier 51 Exempt   ⊖ Modifier 63 Exempt   ✗ Unlisted   **Modifiers:** *See Inside Back Cover*   Ⓜ Maternity   A2–Z3 ASC Payment Indicators   A–Y OPPS Status Indicators

© 2016 DecisionHealth   CPT © 2015 American Medical Association. All Rights Reserved.   **829**

95028 Intracutaneous (intradermal) tests with allergenic extracts, delayed type reaction, including reading, specify number of tests ⊙Ⅱ

RVU			Global Days	Modifiers				
Mod	Non-Fac Total	Fac Total		51	50	62	80	MUE
	0.38	0.38	XXX	0	0	0	0	

AMA: Summer 91: 14, May 10: 3, Jan 13: 9

Pub 100-04, 12, 200

95044 Patch or application test(s) (specify number of tests) ⊙Ⅱ

Documentation Finder: *The documentation needs to support the actual number of skin patches for the components being tested. Each skin patch typically represents one unit of service. This is usually done for contact allergic dermatitis. Usually you will see 20 to 30 antigens being used in the usual routine screening panel of patch tests. The patches are removed after 48 hours and an initial reading is taken one hour later. The final reading is taken 48 hours later.*

RVU			Global Days	Modifiers				
Mod	Non-Fac Total	Fac Total		51	50	62	80	MUE
	0.16	0.16	XXX	0	0	0	0	

AMA: Summer 91: 15, Spring 94: 31, Jan 13: 9

Pub 100-04, 12, 200

95052 Photo patch test(s) (specify number of tests) ⊙Ⅱ

RVU			Global Days	Modifiers				
Mod	Non-Fac Total	Fac Total		51	50	62	80	MUE
	0.19	0.19	XXX	0	0	0	0	

AMA: Spring 94: 31, Jan 13: 9

Pub 100-04, 12, 200

95056 Photo tests ⊙Ⅱ

RVU			Global Days	Modifiers				
Mod	Non-Fac Total	Fac Total		51	50	62	80	MUE
	1.26	1.26	XXX	0	0	0	0	1

AMA: Summer 91: 16, Jan 13: 9

Pub 100-04, 12, 200

95060 Ophthalmic mucous membrane tests ⊙Ⅱ

RVU			Global Days	Modifiers				
Mod	Non-Fac Total	Fac Total		51	50	62	80	MUE
	0.99	0.99	XXX	0	0	0	0	1

AMA: Summer 91: 16, Jan 13: 9

Pub 100-04, 12, 200

95065 Direct nasal mucous membrane test ⊙Ⅱ

RVU			Global Days	Modifiers				
Mod	Non-Fac Total	Fac Total		51	50	62	80	MUE
	0.72	0.72	XXX	0	0	0	0	1

AMA: Summer 91: 15, Jan 13: 9

Pub 100-04, 12, 200

95070 Inhalation bronchial challenge testing (not including necessary pulmonary function tests); with histamine, methacholine, or similar compounds S

RVU			Global Days	Modifiers				
Mod	Non-Fac Total	Fac Total		51	50	62	80	MUE
	0.86	0.86	XXX	0	0	0	0	1

AMA: Summer 91: 16, Nov 12: 11, Jan 13: 9

Pub 100-04, 12, 200

95071 Inhalation bronchial challenge testing (not including necessary pulmonary function tests); with antigens or gases, specify ⊙Ⅱ

RVU			Global Days	Modifiers				
Mod	Non-Fac Total	Fac Total		51	50	62	80	MUE
	0.99	0.99	XXX	0	0	0	0	1

AMA: Summer 91: 16, Jan 13: 9, Nov 12: 11

Pub 100-04, 12, 200

Ingestion Challenge Test

95076 Ingestion challenge test (sequential and incremental ingestion of test items, eg, food, drug or other substance); initial 120 minutes of testing S

RVU			Global Days	Modifiers				
Mod	Non-Fac Total	Fac Total		51	50	62	80	MUE
	3.29	2.07	XXX	0	0	0	0	1

AMA: Jan 13: 9

Pub 100-04, 12, 200

✛ **95079** Ingestion challenge test (sequential and incremental ingestion of test items, eg, food, drug or other substance); each additional 60 minutes of testing (List separately in addition to code for primary procedure) N

RVU			Global Days	Modifiers				
Mod	Non-Fac Total	Fac Total		51	50	62	80	MUE
	2.34	1.90	ZZZ	0	0	0	0	2

AMA: Jan 13: 9

Allergen Immunotherapy Services

Coding Guidance

Clinical allergen immunotherapy is divided into administration of allergenic extracts only (95115-95117), antigen preparation/provision and administration at the same session (95120-95134), and preparation of antigens for delivery to a different physician for immunotherapy administration (95144-95170). In standard medical practice, performing allergy testing (95004-95079) and immunotherapy (95115-95180) is not done on the same day. Codes from these two ranges should not be reported together.

95115 Professional services for allergen immunotherapy not including provision of allergenic extracts; single injection S

Documentation Finder: *In the documentation, the provider should reference an injection performed during this encounter as this code is for the professional service of administering the allergenic extract.*

RVU			Global Days	Modifiers				
Mod	Non-Fac Total	Fac Total		51	50	62	80	MUE
	0.25	0.25	XXX	0	0	0	0	1

AMA: Fall 91: 19, Spring 94: 30, Summer 95: 4, May 96: 1, Nov 98: 35, Apr 00: 4, Feb 05: 10, 12, Nov 05: 1, Nov 06: 23, Dec 07: 9, Jan 13: 9

Pub 100-04, 12, 200

95117 Professional services for allergen immunotherapy not including provision of allergenic extracts; 2 or more injections S

RVU			Global Days	Modifiers				
Mod	Non-Fac Total	Fac Total		51	50	62	80	MUE
	0.29	0.29	XXX	0	0	0	0	1

AMA: Fall 91: 19, Spring 94: 30, Summer 95: 4, May 96: 1, Aug 96: 10, Nov 98: 35, Apr 00: 4, Feb 05: 10, 12, Nov 05: 1, Nov 06: 23, Dec 07: 9, Jan 13: 9

Pub 100-04, 12, 200

● New   ▲ Revised   ✖ Deleted   ⊙ Moderate Sedation   ✛ Add-on Codes   ⊘ High Risk Denial   Ⓐ Age Edit   ♀ Female   ♂ Male   **AMA** *CPT® Assistant*   *MUE* Medically Unlikely Edit

⊘ Modifier 51 Exempt   ⊖ Modifier 63 Exempt   Ⅺ Unlisted   **Modifiers:** *See Inside Back Cover*   Ⓜ Maternity   Ⓐ2–Ⓩ3 ASC Payment Indicators   Ⓐ–Ⓨ OPPS Status Indicators

CPT © 2015 American Medical Association. All Rights Reserved.   © 2016 DecisionHealth

Medicine Procedures

95120 Professional services for allergen immunotherapy in the office or institution of the prescribing physician or other qualified health care professional, including provision of allergenic extract; single injection   CE

RVU			Global Days	Modifiers				
Mod	Non-Fac Total	Fac Total		51	50	62	80	MUE
	0.00	0.00	XXX	9	9	9	9	

AMA: Fall 91: 19, Spring 94: 30, Summer 95: 4, May 96: 2, Nov 98: 35, Feb 05: 10, 12, Jan 13: 9

Pub 100-04, 12, 200

95125 Professional services for allergen immunotherapy in the office or institution of the prescribing physician or other qualified health care professional, including provision of allergenic extract; 2 or more injections   CE

RVU			Global Days	Modifiers				
Mod	Non-Fac Total	Fac Total		51	50	62	80	MUE
	0.00	0.00	XXX	9	9	9	9	

AMA: Fall 91: 19, Spring 94: 30, Summer 95: 4, May 96: 2, Aug 96: 10, Nov 98: 35, Feb 05: 10, 12, Jan 13: 9

Pub 100-04, 12, 200

95130 Professional services for allergen immunotherapy in the office or institution of the prescribing physician or other qualified health care professional, including provision of allergenic extract; single stinging insect venom   CE

RVU			Global Days	Modifiers				
Mod	Non-Fac Total	Fac Total		51	50	62	80	MUE
	0.00	0.00	XXX	9	9	9	9	

AMA: Fall 91: 19, Summer 95: 4, May 96: 2, Jun 96: 10, Nov 98: 35, Sep 99: 10, Feb 05: 10, 12, Jan 13: 9

Pub 100-04, 12, 200

95131 Professional services for allergen immunotherapy in the office or institution of the prescribing physician or other qualified health care professional, including provision of allergenic extract; 2 stinging insect venoms   CE

RVU			Global Days	Modifiers				
Mod	Non-Fac Total	Fac Total		51	50	62	80	MUE
	0.00	0.00	XXX	9	9	9	9	

AMA: Summer 95: 4, May 96: 2, Jun 96: 10, Nov 98: 35, Sep 99: 10, Feb 05: 10, 12, Jan 13: 9, Fall 91: 19

Pub 100-04, 12, 200

95132 Professional services for allergen immunotherapy in the office or institution of the prescribing physician or other qualified health care professional, including provision of allergenic extract; 3 stinging insect venoms   CE

RVU			Global Days	Modifiers				
Mod	Non-Fac Total	Fac Total		51	50	62	80	MUE
	0.00	0.00	XXX	9	9	9	9	

AMA: Fall 91: 19, Summer 95: 4, May 96: 2, Nov 98: 35, Sep 99: 11, Feb 05: 10, 12, Jan 13: 9

Pub 100-04, 12, 200

95133 Professional services for allergen immunotherapy in the office or institution of the prescribing physician or other qualified health care professional, including provision of allergenic extract; 4 stinging insect venoms   CE

RVU			Global Days	Modifiers				
Mod	Non-Fac Total	Fac Total		51	50	62	80	MUE
	0.00	0.00	XXX	9	9	9	9	

AMA: Fall 91: 19, Summer 95: 4, May 96: 2, Nov 98: 35, Sep 99: 11, Feb 05: 10, 12, Jan 13: 9

Pub 100-04, 12, 200

95134 Professional services for allergen immunotherapy in the office or institution of the prescribing physician or other qualified health care professional, including provision of allergenic extract; 5 stinging insect venoms   CE

RVU			Global Days	Modifiers				
Mod	Non-Fac Total	Fac Total		51	50	62	80	MUE
	0.00	0.00	XXX	9	9	9	9	

AMA: Fall 91: 19, Summer 95: 4, May 96: 2, Nov 98: 35, Sep 99: 11, Feb 05: 10, 12, Jan 13: 9

Pub 100-04, 12, 200

95144 Professional services for the supervision of preparation and provision of antigens for allergen immunotherapy, single dose vial(s) (specify number of vials)   S

RVU			Global Days	Modifiers				
Mod	Non-Fac Total	Fac Total		51	50	62	80	MUE
	0.35	0.09	XXX	0	0	0	0	

AMA: Fall 91: 19, Spring 94: 30, Summer 95: 4, May 96: 11, Nov 98: 35, Feb 05: 10, 11, Jan 13: 9

Pub 100-04, 12, 200

95145 Professional services for the supervision of preparation and provision of antigens for allergen immunotherapy (specify number of doses); single stinging insect venom   S

RVU			Global Days	Modifiers				
Mod	Non-Fac Total	Fac Total		51	50	62	80	MUE
	0.61	0.09	XXX	0	0	0	0	

AMA: Fall 91: 19, Summer 95: 4, May 96: 11, Nov 98: 35, Feb 05: 10, 12, Jan 13: 9

Pub 100-04, 12, 200

95146 Professional services for the supervision of preparation and provision of antigens for allergen immunotherapy (specify number of doses); 2 single stinging insect venoms   S

RVU			Global Days	Modifiers				
Mod	Non-Fac Total	Fac Total		51	50	62	80	MUE
	1.10	0.09	XXX	0	0	0	0	

AMA: Fall 91: 19, Summer 95: 4, May 96: 11, Nov 98: 35, Feb 05: 10, 12, Jan 13: 9

Pub 100-04, 12, 200

● New   ▲ Revised   Deleted   ⊙ Moderate Sedation   ✚ Add-on Codes   ⊘ High Risk Denial   Ⓐ Age Edit   ♀ Female   ♂ Male   **AMA** *CPT® Assistant*   **MUE** Medically Unlikely Edit
⊘ Modifier 51 Exempt   ⊖ Modifier 63 Exempt   ✖ Unlisted   **Modifiers:** *See Inside Back Cover*   Ⓜ Maternity   A2–Z3 ASC Payment Indicators   A–Y OPPS Status Indicators

© 2016 DecisionHealth   CPT © 2015 American Medical Association. All Rights Reserved.   **831**

95147 **Professional services for the supervision of preparation and provision of antigens for allergen immunotherapy (specify number of doses); 3 single stinging insect venoms** S

RVU			Global Days	Modifiers				
Mod	Non-Fac Total	Fac Total		51	50	62	80	MUE
	0.99	0.09	XXX	0	0	0	0	

AMA: May 96: 11, Nov 98: 35, Feb 05: 10, 12, Jan 13: 9, Fall 91: 19, Summer 95: 4

Pub 100-04, 12, 200

95148 **Professional services for the supervision of preparation and provision of antigens for allergen immunotherapy (specify number of doses); 4 single stinging insect venoms** S

RVU			Global Days	Modifiers				
Mod	Non-Fac Total	Fac Total		51	50	62	80	MUE
	1.47	0.09	XXX	0	0	0	0	

AMA: Fall 91: 19, Summer 95: 4, May 96: 11, Nov 98: 35, Feb 05: 10, 12, Jan 13: 9

Pub 100-04, 12, 200

95149 **Professional services for the supervision of preparation and provision of antigens for allergen immunotherapy (specify number of doses); 5 single stinging insect venoms** S

RVU			Global Days	Modifiers				
Mod	Non-Fac Total	Fac Total		51	50	62	80	MUE
	1.98	0.09	XXX	0	0	0	0	

AMA: Fall 91: 19, Summer 95: 4, May 96: 11, Nov 98: 35, Feb 05: 10, 12, Jan 13: 9

Pub 100-04, 12, 200

95165 **Professional services for the supervision of preparation and provision of antigens for allergen immunotherapy; single or multiple antigens (specify number of doses)** S

RVU			Global Days	Modifiers				
Mod	Non-Fac Total	Fac Total		51	50	62	80	MUE
	0.36	0.09	XXX	0	0	0	0	

AMA: Fall 91: 19, Spring 94: 30, Summer 95: 4, May 96: 11, Nov 98: 35, Apr 00: 4, Apr 01: 11, Feb 05: 10, 12, Jun 05: 9, Jan 13: 9

Pub 100-04, 12, 200

95170 **Professional services for the supervision of preparation and provision of antigens for allergen immunotherapy; whole body extract of biting insect or other arthropod (specify number of doses)** S

RVU			Global Days	Modifiers				
Mod	Non-Fac Total	Fac Total		51	50	62	80	MUE
	0.27	0.09	XXX	0	0	0	0	

AMA: Fall 91: 19, Spring 94: 30, Summer 95: 4, May 96: 12, Apr 01: 11, Feb 05: 10, 12, Jun 05: 9, Jan 13: 9

Pub 100-04, 12, 200

95180 **Rapid desensitization procedure, each hour (eg, insulin, penicillin, equine serum)** Q1

RVU			Global Days	Modifiers				
Mod	Non-Fac Total	Fac Total		51	50	62	80	MUE
	3.78	2.87	XXX	0	0	0	0	

AMA: Summer 95: 4, Jan 13: 9

Pub 100-04, 12, 200

95199 **Unlisted allergy/clinical immunologic service or procedure** ⊘✗Q1

Coding tip: *Before assigning unlisted code 95199 for allergy tests, verify that there are no other code(s) listed for the specific tests()/technique(s)*

RVU			Global Days	Modifiers				
Mod	Non-Fac Total	Fac Total		51	50	62	80	MUE
	0.00	0.00	XXX	0	0	0	0	

AMA: Summer 95: 4, Nov 98: 35, Jan 13: 9

Pub 100-04, 12, 200

Endocrinology Services

95250 **Ambulatory continuous glucose monitoring of interstitial tissue fluid via a subcutaneous sensor for a minimum of 72 hours; sensor placement, hook-up, calibration of monitor, patient training, removal of sensor, and printout of recording** V

RVU			Global Days	Modifiers				
Mod	Non-Fac Total	Fac Total		51	50	62	80	MUE
	4.45	4.45	XXX	0	0	0	0	1

95251 **Ambulatory continuous glucose monitoring of interstitial tissue fluid via a subcutaneous sensor for a minimum of 72 hours; interpretation and report** B

RVU			Global Days	Modifiers				
Mod	Non-Fac Total	Fac Total		51	50	62	80	MUE
	1.23	1.23	XXX	0	0	0	0	1

95782 **Polysomnography; younger than 6 years, sleep staging with 4 or more additional parameters of sleep, attended by a technologist** S

Coding tip: *Code 95782 is listed out of numerical order in CPT. Related polysomnography procedures for a patient age 6 years or older - 95808-95811*

RVU			Global Days	Modifiers				
Mod	Non-Fac Total	Fac Total		51	50	62	80	MUE
	28.98	28.98	XXX	0	0	0	0	1
26	3.59	3.59	XXX	0	0	0	0	1
TC	25.39	25.39	XXX	0	0	0	0	1

AMA: Feb 13: 14

95783 **Polysomnography; younger than 6 years, sleep staging with 4 or more additional parameters of sleep, with initiation of continuous positive airway pressure therapy or bi-level ventilation, attended by a technologist** ⊘S

Coding tip: *Code 95783 is listed out of numerical order in CPT. Related polysomnography procedures for a patient age 6 years or older - 95808-95811*

RVU			Global Days	Modifiers				
Mod	Non-Fac Total	Fac Total		51	50	62	80	MUE
	30.46	30.46	XXX	0	0	0	0	1
26	3.98	3.98	XXX	0	0	0	0	1
TC	26.48	26.48	XXX	0	0	0	0	1

AMA: Feb 13: 14, Oct 14: 9

● New   ▲ Revised   ✖ Deleted   ⊙ Moderate Sedation   ✚ Add-on Codes   ⊘ High Risk Denial   Ⓐ Age Edit   ♀ Female   ♂ Male   **AMA** CPT® Assistant   **MUE** Medically Unlikely Edit

⊘ Modifier 51 Exempt   ⊖ Modifier 63 Exempt   ✗ Unlisted   **Modifiers:** *See Inside Back Cover*   Ⓜ Maternity   A 2 – Z 3 ASC Payment Indicators   A –Y OPPS Status Indicators

832

CPT © 2015 American Medical Association. All Rights Reserved.   © 2016 DecisionHealth

Neurological/Neurovascular Services/Procedures

Sleep Studies

95800 Sleep study, unattended, simultaneous recording; heart rate, oxygen saturation, respiratory analysis (eg, by airflow or peripheral arterial tone), and sleep time   S

Coding tip: Code 95800 is listed out of numerical order in CPT. Related unattended sleep study procedures - 95801, 95806

RVU			Global Days	Modifiers				
Mod	Non-Fac Total	Fac Total		51	50	62	80	MUE
	5.02	5.02	XXX	0	0	0	0	1
26	1.47	1.47	XXX	0	0	0	0	1
TC	3.55	3.55	XXX	0	0	0	0	1

AMA: Nov 11: 3, Jan 11: 6, Feb 13: 14

95801 Sleep study, unattended, simultaneous recording; minimum of heart rate, oxygen saturation, and respiratory analysis (eg, by airflow or peripheral arterial tone)   Q1

Coding tip: Code 95801 is listed out of numerical order in CPT. Related unattended sleep study procedures - 95800, 95806

RVU			Global Days	Modifiers				
Mod	Non-Fac Total	Fac Total		51	50	62	80	MUE
TC	1.16	1.16	XXX	0	0	0	0	1
	2.56	2.56	XXX	0	0	0	0	1
26	1.40	1.40	XXX	0	0	0	0	1

AMA: Nov 11: 3, Jan 11: 7, Feb 13: 14

95803 Actigraphy testing, recording, analysis, interpretation, and report (minimum of 72 hours to 14 consecutive days of recording)   Q1

RVU			Global Days	Modifiers				
Mod	Non-Fac Total	Fac Total		51	50	62	80	MUE
	3.99	3.99	XXX	0	0	0	0	1
26	1.24	1.24	XXX	0	0	0	0	1
TC	2.75	2.75	XXX	0	0	0	0	1

AMA: Nov 11: 3

95805 Multiple sleep latency or maintenance of wakefulness testing, recording, analysis and interpretation of physiological measurements of sleep during multiple trials to assess sleepiness   S

RVU			Global Days	Modifiers				
Mod	Non-Fac Total	Fac Total		51	50	62	80	MUE
	12.06	12.06	XXX	0	0	0	0	1
26	1.68	1.68	XXX	0	0	0	0	1
TC	10.38	10.38	XXX	0	0	0	0	1

AMA: Nov 97: 45, 46, Nov 98: 35, Dec 01: 3, Sep 02: 2, 3, Mar 08: 4, Nov 11: 3

Pub 100-02, 15, 70

95806 Sleep study, unattended, simultaneous recording of, heart rate, oxygen saturation, respiratory airflow, and respiratory effort (eg, thoracoabdominal movement)   S

RVU			Global Days	Modifiers				
Mod	Non-Fac Total	Fac Total		51	50	62	80	MUE
	4.75	4.75	XXX	0	0	0	0	1
26	1.73	1.73	XXX	0	0	0	0	1
TC	3.02	3.02	XXX	0	0	0	0	1

AMA: Nov 97: 45, 46, Aug 98: 10, Nov 98: 35, Nov 11: 3, Jan 11: 7, Jul 13: 11, Feb 13: 14

95807 Sleep study, simultaneous recording of ventilation, respiratory effort, ECG or heart rate, and oxygen saturation, attended by a technologist   S

RVU			Global Days	Modifiers				
Mod	Non-Fac Total	Fac Total		51	50	62	80	MUE
	13.51	13.51	XXX	0	0	0	0	1
26	1.77	1.77	XXX	0	0	0	0	1
TC	11.74	11.74	XXX	0	0	0	0	1

AMA: Nov 97: 46, Nov 98: 35, Mar 08: 4, Nov 11: 3, Feb 13: 14

Pub 100-02, 15, 70

Coding Guidance

Polysomnography differs from sleep studies in that it requires sleep staging, which includes both qualitative and quantitative assessments of sleep by standard scoring methods. Polysomnography and sleep study codes are not to be reported together. Polysomnography requires several electroencephalographic (EEG) electrodes, both centrally placed and elsewhere. EEGs for sleep staging are different from diagnostic or continuous monitoring EEG services. EEG testing is not reported with polysomnography, unless a significant, separately identified service is documented.

95808 Polysomnography; any age, sleep staging with 1-3 additional parameters of sleep, attended by a technologist   S

RVU			Global Days	Modifiers				
Mod	Non-Fac Total	Fac Total		51	50	62	80	MUE
	17.79	17.79	XXX	0	0	0	0	1
26	2.49	2.49	XXX	0	0	0	0	1
TC	15.30	15.30	XXX	0	0	0	0	1

AMA: Sep 96: 11, Nov 97: 46, Feb 98: 6, Nov 98: 35, Sep 02: 2, 3, Mar 08: 4, Nov 11: 3, Feb 13: 14

95810 Polysomnography; age 6 years or older, sleep staging with 4 or more additional parameters of sleep, attended by a technologist   S

RVU			Global Days	Modifiers				
Mod	Non-Fac Total	Fac Total		51	50	62	80	MUE
	17.60	17.60	XXX	0	0	0	0	1
26	3.46	3.46	XXX	0	0	0	0	1
TC	14.14	14.14	XXX	0	0	0	0	1

AMA: Feb 98: 6, Nov 98: 35, Sep 02: 2, 3, Nov 11: 3, Feb 13: 14

Pub 100-02, 15, 70

95811 Polysomnography; age 6 years or older, sleep staging with 4 or more additional parameters of sleep, with initiation of continuous positive airway pressure therapy or bilevel ventilation, attended by a technologist   S

RVU			Global Days	Modifiers				
Mod	Non-Fac Total	Fac Total		51	50	62	80	MUE
	18.49	18.49	XXX	0	0	0	0	1
26	3.60	3.60	XXX	0	0	0	0	1
TC	14.89	14.89	XXX	0	0	0	0	1

AMA: Nov 97: 46, Feb 98: 6, Nov 98: 35, Sep 02: 2, 3, Mar 08: 4, Nov 11: 3, Feb 13: 14, Oct 14: 9

Electroencephalogram (EEG)

Coding Guidance

Polysomnography requires several electroencephalographic (EEG) electrodes, both centrally placed and elsewhere. EEGs for sleep staging are different from diagnostic or continuous monitoring EEG services. EEG testing is not reported with polysomnography, unless a significant, separately identified service is documented.

● New   ▲ Revised   Deleted   ⊙ Moderate Sedation   ✚ Add-on Codes   ⊗ High Risk Denial   Ⓐ Age Edit   ♀ Female   ♂ Male   **AMA** *CPT® Assistant*   **MUE** Medically Unlikely Edit
⊘ Modifier 51 Exempt   ⊖ Modifier 63 Exempt   ✗ Unlisted   **Modifiers:** *See Inside Back Cover*   Ⓜ Maternity   A2–Z3 ASC Payment Indicators   A–Y OPPS Status Indicators

95812 Electroencephalogram (EEG) extended monitoring; 41-60 minutes ⓢ

Mod	RVU Non-Fac Total	Fac Total	Global Days	Modifiers 51	50	62	80	MUE
	9.85	9.85	XXX	0	0	0	0	1
26	1.64	1.64	XXX	0	0	0	0	1
TC	8.21	8.21	XXX	0	0	0	0	1

AMA: Winter 94: 18, Nov 98: 35, May 11: 3, 10

95813 Electroencephalogram (EEG) extended monitoring; greater than 1 hour ⓢ

Mod	RVU Non-Fac Total	Fac Total	Global Days	Modifiers 51	50	62	80	MUE
	11.90	11.90	XXX	0	0	0	0	1
26	2.61	2.61	XXX	0	0	0	0	1
TC	9.29	9.29	XXX	0	0	0	0	1

AMA: Winter 94: 18, Nov 98: 35, May 11: 3, 10

Coding Guidance

When a spinal or intracranial procedure uses intraoperative neurophysiological testing, the physician who performs the main surgical service should not report 90000 codes, such as 95822 for intraoperative neurophysiological testing, as they are included in the global package.

95816 Electroencephalogram (EEG); including recording awake and drowsy ⓢ

Mod	RVU Non-Fac Total	Fac Total	Global Days	Modifiers 51	50	62	80	MUE
	10.20	10.20	XXX	0	0	0	0	1
26	1.64	1.64	XXX	0	0	0	0	1
TC	8.56	8.56	XXX	0	0	0	0	1

AMA: Sep 96: 11, Nov 98: 35, Nov 99: 51, Jul 00: 1, May 11: 3

95819 Electroencephalogram (EEG); including recording awake and asleep ⓢ

Mod	RVU Non-Fac Total	Fac Total	Global Days	Modifiers 51	50	62	80	MUE
	11.67	11.67	XXX	0	0	0	0	1
26	1.64	1.64	XXX	0	0	0	0	1
TC	10.03	10.03	XXX	0	0	0	0	1

AMA: Nov 98: 35, Nov 99: 51, Jul 00: 1, May 11: 3

95822 Electroencephalogram (EEG); recording in coma or sleep only ⓢ

Mod	RVU Non-Fac Total	Fac Total	Global Days	Modifiers 51	50	62	80	MUE
	10.51	10.51	XXX	0	0	0	0	1
26	1.64	1.64	XXX	0	0	0	0	1
TC	8.87	8.87	XXX	0	0	0	0	1

AMA: May 13: 8, Nov 98: 35, May 11: 3, Dec 14: 19
Pub 100-02, 15, 70

95824 Electroencephalogram (EEG); cerebral death evaluation only ⓢ

Mod	RVU Non-Fac Total	Fac Total	Global Days	Modifiers 51	50	62	80	MUE
	0.00	0.00	XXX	0	0	0	0	1
26	1.12	1.12	XXX	0	0	0	0	1
TC	0.00	0.00	XXX	0	0	0	0	1

AMA: Nov 98: 35

95827 Electroencephalogram (EEG); all night recording ⓢ

Mod	RVU Non-Fac Total	Fac Total	Global Days	Modifiers 51	50	62	80	MUE
	19.65	19.65	XXX	0	0	0	0	1
26	1.62	1.62	XXX	0	0	0	0	1
TC	18.03	18.03	XXX	0	0	0	0	1

AMA: Nov 98: 35

95829 Electrocorticogram at surgery (separate procedure) Ⓝ

Mod	RVU Non-Fac Total	Fac Total	Global Days	Modifiers 51	50	62	80	MUE
	53.09	53.09	XXX	0	0	0	0	1
26	9.57	9.57	XXX	0	0	0	0	1
TC	43.52	43.52	XXX	0	0	0	0	1

AMA: Nov 98: 35

95830 Insertion by physician or other qualified health care professional of sphenoidal electrodes for electroencephalographic (EEG) recording Ⓑ

Mod	RVU Non-Fac Total	Fac Total	Global Days	Modifiers 51	50	62	80	MUE
	6.93	2.62	XXX	0	0	0	0	1

Muscle/Range of Motion Tests

95831 Muscle testing, manual (separate procedure) with report; extremity (excluding hand) or trunk Ⓐ

Mod	RVU Non-Fac Total	Fac Total	Global Days	Modifiers 51	50	62	80	MUE
	0.86	0.43	XXX	0	0	0	0	5

AMA: Nov 99: 51, Dec 99: 10, Mar 00: 11, Jul 00: 2, Nov 01: 5, Apr 03: 28, Dec 03: 7, Feb 04: 5, May 08: 9, Aug 13: 7

95832 Muscle testing, manual (separate procedure) with report; hand, with or without comparison with normal side Ⓐ

Mod	RVU Non-Fac Total	Fac Total	Global Days	Modifiers 51	50	62	80	MUE
	0.84	0.45	XXX	0	0	0	0	1

AMA: Nov 99: 51, Dec 99: 10, Mar 00: 11, Jul 00: 2, Nov 01: 5, Apr 03: 28, Dec 03: 7, Feb 04: 5, May 08: 9, Aug 13: 7

95833 Muscle testing, manual (separate procedure) with report; total evaluation of body, excluding hands ⊙Ⓐ

Mod	RVU Non-Fac Total	Fac Total	Global Days	Modifiers 51	50	62	80	MUE
	1.05	0.61	XXX	0	0	0	0	

AMA: Nov 99: 51, Dec 99: 10, Jul 00: 2, Nov 01: 5, Jul 02: 2, Apr 03: 28, Dec 03: 7, Feb 04: 5, May 08: 9, Sep 12: 16, Aug 13: 7

● New   ▲ Revised   ✖ Deleted   ⊙ Moderate Sedation   ✚ Add-on Codes   ⊗ High Risk Denial   Ⓐ Age Edit   ♀ Female   ♂ Male   **AMA** *CPT® Assistant*   **MUE** Medically Unlikely Edit
⊘ Modifier 51 Exempt   ⊖ Modifier 63 Exempt   ✗ Unlisted   **Modifiers:** *See Inside Back Cover*   Ⓜ Maternity   Ⓐ2–Ⓩ3 ASC Payment Indicators   Ⓐ–Ⓨ OPPS Status Indicators

834   CPT © 2015 American Medical Association. All Rights Reserved.   © 2016 DecisionHealth

95834 Muscle testing, manual (separate procedure) with report; total evaluation of body, including hands 🔵A

Documentation Finder: Documentation needs to show that manual testing was performed to assess the maximum force a muscle is capable of exerting. This testing is usually performed on muscles that have been impaired. CPT has specified a grading system for this section of codes that should be in the documentation, such as "contractions felt in the muscle" or "antigravity position" where pressure can be placed on the given muscle to see how it holds up to that resistance. Because this is a "separate procedure" designated code, the provider should not be doing any additional work on that same area that would support a given CPT code.

RVU			Global Days	Modifiers				
Mod	Non-Fac Total	Fac Total		51	50	62	80	MUE
	1.44	0.89	XXX	0	0	0	0	

AMA: Nov 99: 51, Dec 99: 10, Jul 00: 2, Nov 01: 5, Apr 03: 28, Dec 03: 7, Feb 04: 5, May 08: 9, Aug 13: 7

Coding Guidance

Do not report codes from the range 95851-95937 when nerve testing, such as electromyography (EMG) or nerve conduction velocity studies, are done to assess paralysis levels during mechanical ventilation or anesthesia.

95851 Range of motion measurements and report (separate procedure); each extremity (excluding hand) or each trunk section (spine) 🔵A

Documentation Finder: In the documentation, you should see reference to degrees that a given joint or section of the spine can be moved. Such examples could state, "right shoulder ROM was 75 degrees." This code would not be reported when performing an E/M service and in the examination, it states "limited ROM." This code is for a specific testing and not part of an examination as it related to an office vist. This is not a timed code. Since this is a "separate procedure" designated code, the provider should not be doing any additional work on that same area that would support a given CPT code.

RVU			Global Days	Modifiers				
Mod	Non-Fac Total	Fac Total		51	50	62	80	MUE
	0.52	0.22	XXX	0	0	0	0	3

AMA: Sep 99: 10, Nov 01: 5, Apr 03: 28, Dec 03: 7, Feb 04: 5, Dec 07: 16, May 08: 9, Aug 13: 7

95852 Range of motion measurements and report (separate procedure); hand, with or without comparison with normal side 🔵A

RVU			Global Days	Modifiers				
Mod	Non-Fac Total	Fac Total		51	50	62	80	MUE
	0.46	0.17	XXX	0	0	0	0	1

AMA: Nov 01: 5, Apr 03: 28, Dec 03: 7, May 08: 9, Aug 13: 7

95857 Cholinesterase inhibitor challenge test for myasthenia gravis 🅂

RVU			Global Days	Modifiers				
Mod	Non-Fac Total	Fac Total		51	50	62	80	MUE
	1.53	0.84	XXX	0	0	0	0	1

AMA: Feb 11: 3

Needle Electromyography

Coding Guidance

When a spinal or intracranial procedure uses intraoperative neurophysiological testing, the physician who performs the main surgical service should not report 90000 codes, such as 95860 or 95861 for intraoperative neurophysiological testing, as they are included in the global package. Biofeedback sessions involve electromyography (EMG) techniques for recording muscle activity. Do not report CPT codes 95860-95872 with biofeedback services that are dependent on EMG during the session. Needle EMG procedures performed with nerve conduction studies are reported with codes 95885-95886. Nerve conduction studies performed without needle EMG on same date of service are reported with codes 95905-95913.

95860 Needle electromyography; 1 extremity with or without related paraspinal areas ⬛Q1

RVU			Global Days	Modifiers				
Mod	Non-Fac Total	Fac Total		51	50	62	80	MUE
	3.45	3.45	XXX	0	0	0	0	1
26	1.47	1.47	XXX	0	0	0	0	1
TC	1.98	1.98	XXX	0	0	0	0	1

AMA: May 13: 8, Nov 97: 46, Jul 00: 2, Apr 02: 2, May 03: 20, Jun 03: 3, Feb 04: 4, Jul 04: 6, Oct 04: 15, Jun 06: 8, Sep 06: 5, Aug 08: 12, Jan 09: 8, Feb 12: 8, Oct 10: 15, Dec 10: 15, Mar 13: 3, Mar 15: 6

95861 Needle electromyography; 2 extremities with or without related paraspinal areas ⬛Q1

RVU			Global Days	Modifiers				
Mod	Non-Fac Total	Fac Total		51	50	62	80	MUE
	4.84	4.84	XXX	0	0	0	0	1
26	2.36	2.36	XXX	0	0	0	0	1
TC	2.48	2.48	XXX	0	0	0	0	1

AMA: May 13: 8, Feb 04: 4, Jul 04: 6, Oct 04: 15, Jun 05: 9, Jun 06: 8, Sep 06: 5, Aug 08: 12, Jan 09: 8, Feb 12: 8, Oct 10: 15, Dec 10: 15, Mar 13: 3, Nov 97: 46, Jul 00: 2, Apr 02: 2, May 03: 20, Jun 03: 3

95863 Needle electromyography; 3 extremities with or without related paraspinal areas 🅂

RVU			Global Days	Modifiers				
Mod	Non-Fac Total	Fac Total		51	50	62	80	MUE
	6.01	6.01	XXX	0	0	0	0	1
26	2.84	2.84	XXX	0	0	0	0	1
TC	3.17	3.17	XXX	0	0	0	0	1

AMA: May 13: 8, Nov 97: 46, Jul 00: 2, Apr 02: 2, May 03: 20, Jun 03: 3, Feb 04: 4, Jul 04: 6, Oct 04: 15, Jun 06: 8, Sep 06: 5, Feb 12: 8, Oct 10: 15, Dec 10: 15, Mar 13: 3

95864 Needle electromyography; 4 extremities with or without related paraspinal areas 🅂

RVU			Global Days	Modifiers				
Mod	Non-Fac Total	Fac Total		51	50	62	80	MUE
	6.78	6.78	XXX	0	0	0	0	1
26	3.07	3.07	XXX	0	0	0	0	1
TC	3.71	3.71	XXX	0	0	0	0	1

AMA: May 13: 8, Nov 97: 46, Jul 00: 2, Jan 02: 11, Apr 02: 2, May 03: 20, Jun 03: 3, Feb 04: 4, Jul 04: 6, Oct 04: 15, Jun 06: 8, Sep 06: 5, Aug 08: 12, Jan 09: 8, Feb 12: 8, Oct 10: 15, Dec 10: 15, Mar 13: 3

95865 Needle electromyography; larynx ⬛Q1

RVU			Global Days	Modifiers				
Mod	Non-Fac Total	Fac Total		51	50	62	80	MUE
	4.08	4.08	XXX	0	2	0	0	1
26	2.41	2.41	XXX	0	2	0	0	1
TC	1.67	1.67	XXX	0	2	0	0	1

AMA: May 13: 8, Sep 06: 5, Dec 07: 16, Jan 09: 8, Jan 14: 6

95866 Needle electromyography; hemidiaphragm 🔵Q1

RVU			Global Days	Modifiers				
Mod	Non-Fac Total	Fac Total		51	50	62	80	MUE
	3.77	3.77	XXX	0	3	0	0	1
26	1.91	1.91	XXX	0	3	0	0	1
TC	1.86	1.86	XXX	0	3	0	0	1

AMA: May 13: 8

Coding Guidance

When a spinal or intracranial procedure uses intraoperative neurophysiological testing, the physician who performs the main surgical service should not

● New   ▲ Revised   Deleted   ⊙ Moderate Sedation   ✚ Add-on Codes   ⊘ High Risk Denial   Ⓐ Age Edit   ♀ Female   ♂ Male   **AMA** *CPT® Assistant*   **MUE** Medically Unlikely Edit

⊘ Modifier 51 Exempt   ⊖ Modifier 63 Exempt   ✘ Unlisted   **Modifiers:** *See Inside Back Cover*   Ⓜ Maternity   A2-Z3 ASC Payment Indicators   A-Y OPPS Status Indicators

© 2016 DecisionHealth   CPT © 2015 American Medical Association. All Rights Reserved.   **835**

report 90000 codes, such as 95867, 95868, or 95870 for intraoperative neurophysiological testing, as they are included in the global package.

95867   Needle electromyography; cranial nerve supplied muscle(s), unilateral   ⊙S

Documentation Finder: Any of the muscles in the neck area or head area should be referenced in the documentation. Some of those muscles might be trapezius muscle, spinal accessory muscles, etc., but they must be placing the probes into those areas on one side (unilateral).

Mod	RVU Non-Fac Total	Fac Total	Global Days	51	50	62	80	MUE
	2.67	2.67	XXX	0	0	0	0	1
26	1.19	1.19	XXX	0	0	0	0	1
TC	1.48	1.48	XXX	0	0	0	0	1

AMA: Apr 02: 2, May 03: 20, Jun 03: 3, Jun 06: 8, Sep 06: 5, Dec 07: 16, Aug 08: 12, Jan 09: 8, May 13: 8, Feb 12: 8, Mar 13: 3

95868   Needle electromyography; cranial nerve supplied muscles, bilateral   S

Documentation Finder: Any of the muscles in the neck area or head area should be referenced in the documentation. Some of those muscles might be trapezius muscle, spinal accessory muscles, etc., but they must be placing the probes on both sides (bilateral).

Mod	RVU Non-Fac Total	Fac Total	Global Days	51	50	62	80	MUE
TC	1.95	1.95	XXX	0	2	0	0	1
	3.75	3.75	XXX	0	2	0	0	1
26	1.80	1.80	XXX	0	2	0	0	1

AMA: Apr 02: 2, May 03: 20, Jun 03: 3, Jun 06: 8, Sep 06: 5, Dec 07: 16, Jan 09: 8, May 13: 8, Feb 12: 8, Mar 13: 3

95869   Needle electromyography; thoracic paraspinal muscles (excluding T1 or T12)   Q1

Mod	RVU Non-Fac Total	Fac Total	Global Days	51	50	62	80	MUE
	2.63	2.63	XXX	0	0	0	0	1
26	0.57	0.57	XXX	0	0	0	0	1
TC	2.06	2.06	XXX	0	0	0	0	1

AMA: Nov 97: 46, Apr 02: 2, May 03: 20, Jun 03: 3, Feb 04: 4, Jun 06: 8, Sep 06: 5, Jan 09: 8, May 13: 8, Feb 12: 8, May 10: 9, Mar 13: 3

95870   Needle electromyography; limited study of muscles in 1 extremity or non-limb (axial) muscles (unilateral or bilateral), other than thoracic paraspinal, cranial nerve supplied muscles, or sphincters   Q1

Mod	RVU Non-Fac Total	Fac Total	Global Days	51	50	62	80	MUE
	2.62	2.62	XXX	0	0	0	0	
26	0.56	0.56	XXX	0	0	0	0	
TC	2.06	2.06	XXX	0	0	0	0	

AMA: Nov 97: 46, Nov 99: 51, Jul 00: 2, Apr 02: 2, May 03: 20, Jun 03: 3, Feb 04: 4, Jul 04: 6, Jun 05: 9, Jun 06: 8, Sep 06: 5, Jan 09: 8, May 13: 8, Feb 12: 8, Mar 13: 3

95872   Needle electromyography using single fiber electrode, with quantitative measurement of jitter, blocking and/or fiber density, any/all sites of each muscle studied   S

Mod	RVU Non-Fac Total	Fac Total	Global Days	51	50	62	80	MUE
	5.55	5.55	XXX	0	0	0	0	
26	4.37	4.37	XXX	0	0	0	0	
TC	1.18	1.18	XXX	0	0	0	0	

AMA: Apr 02: 2, May 03: 20, Jun 03: 3, Sep 06: 5, Jan 09: 8

Chemodenervation Guidance/Ischemic Muscle Testing

✚ 95873   Electrical stimulation for guidance in conjunction with chemodenervation (List separately in addition to code for primary procedure)   N

Mod	RVU Non-Fac Total	Fac Total	Global Days	51	50	62	80	MUE
	2.08	2.08	ZZZ	0	0	0	0	1
26	0.57	0.57	ZZZ	0	0	0	0	1
TC	1.51	1.51	ZZZ	0	0	0	0	1

AMA: Apr 13: 5, Jan 14: 6

Coding Guidance

Muscle chemodenervation will occasionally require needle electromyography (EMG) guidance. When this is reasonable and necessary, code 95874 may be reported in conjunction with codes 64612-64615.

✚ 95874   Needle electromyography for guidance in conjunction with chemodenervation (List separately in addition to code for primary procedure)   N

Mod	RVU Non-Fac Total	Fac Total	Global Days	51	50	62	80	MUE
	2.06	2.06	ZZZ	0	0	0	0	1
26	0.57	0.57	ZZZ	0	0	0	0	1
TC	1.49	1.49	ZZZ	0	0	0	0	1

AMA: Apr 13: 5, Jan 14: 6, Oct 14: 15

95875   Ischemic limb exercise test with serial specimen(s) acquisition for muscle(s) metabolite(s)   S

Mod	RVU Non-Fac Total	Fac Total	Global Days	51	50	62	80	MUE
	3.53	3.53	XXX	0	0	0	0	2
26	1.68	1.68	XXX	0	0	0	0	2
TC	1.85	1.85	XXX	0	0	0	0	2

AMA: Jun 03: 3

✚ 95885   Needle electromyography, each extremity, with related paraspinal areas, when performed, done with nerve conduction, amplitude and latency/velocity study; limited (List separately in addition to code for primary procedure)   N

Coding tip: Code 95885 is listed out of numerical order in CPT. Additional needle electromyography (EMG) services - 95860-95872 and 95886-95887

Mod	RVU Non-Fac Total	Fac Total	Global Days	51	50	62	80	MUE
	1.65	1.65	ZZZ	0	3	0	0	4
26	0.54	0.54	ZZZ	0	3	0	0	4
TC	1.11	1.11	ZZZ	0	3	0	0	4

AMA: May 13: 8, Feb 12: 8, Mar 13: 3, Sep 13: 18, Mar 15: 6

● New   ▲ Revised   ✖ Deleted   ⊙ Moderate Sedation   ✚ Add-on Codes   ⊘ High Risk Denial   Ⓐ Age Edit   ♀ Female   ♂ Male   **AMA** CPT® Assistant   **MUE** Medically Unlikely Edit
⊘ Modifier 51 Exempt   ⊖ Modifier 63 Exempt   ✗ Unlisted   **Modifiers:** See Inside Back Cover   Ⓜ Maternity   A2-Z3 ASC Payment Indicators   A-Y OPPS Status Indicators

+ 95886 Needle electromyography, each extremity, with related paraspinal areas, when performed, done with nerve conduction, amplitude and latency/velocity study; complete, five or more muscles studied, innervated by three or more nerves or four or more spinal levels (List separately in addition to code for primary procedure) **N**

Coding tip: Code 95886 is listed out of numerical order in CPT. Additional needle electromyography (EMG) services - 95860-95872 , 95885 and 95887

Mod	RVU Non-Fac Total	Fac Total	Global Days	Modifiers 51	50	62	80	MUE
TC	1.26	1.26	ZZZ	0	3	0	0	4
	2.57	2.57	ZZZ	0	3	0	0	4
26	1.31	1.31	ZZZ	0	3	0	0	4

AMA: May 13: 8, Feb 12: 8, Mar 13: 3, Sep 13: 18, Mar 15: 6

+ 95887 Needle electromyography, non-extremity (cranial nerve supplied or axial) muscle(s) done with nerve conduction, amplitude and latency/velocity study (List separately in addition to code for primary procedure) **N**

Coding tip: Code 95887 is listed out of numerical order in CPT. Additional needle electromyography (EMG) services - 95860-95872 and 95885-95886

Mod	RVU Non-Fac Total	Fac Total	Global Days	Modifiers 51	50	62	80	MUE
	2.29	2.29	ZZZ	0	3	0	0	1
26	1.08	1.08	ZZZ	0	3	0	0	1
TC	1.21	1.21	ZZZ	0	3	0	0	1

AMA: Feb 12: 8, Jul 12: 12, Mar 13: 3, Jan 14: 8, Mar 15: 6

⊘ 95905 Motor and/or sensory nerve conduction, using preconfigured electrode array(s), amplitude and latency/velocity study, each limb, includes F-wave study when performed, with interpretation and report **Q1**

Mod	RVU Non-Fac Total	Fac Total	Global Days	Modifiers 51	50	62	80	MUE
	1.99	1.99	XXX	0	0	0	0	2
26	0.08	0.08	XXX	0	0	0	0	2
TC	1.91	1.91	XXX	0	0	0	0	2

AMA: Mar 13: 3

95907 Nerve conduction studies; 1-2 studies **S**

Mod	RVU Non-Fac Total	Fac Total	Global Days	Modifiers 51	50	62	80	MUE
	2.70	2.70	XXX	0	0	0	0	1
26	1.52	1.52	XXX	0	0	0	0	1
TC	1.18	1.18	XXX	0	0	0	0	1

AMA: May 13: 8, Sep 13: 18, Mar 13: 3

95908 Nerve conduction studies; 3-4 studies **S**

Mod	RVU Non-Fac Total	Fac Total	Global Days	Modifiers 51	50	62	80	MUE
	3.34	3.34	XXX	0	0	0	0	1
26	1.89	1.89	XXX	0	0	0	0	1
TC	1.45	1.45	XXX	0	0	0	0	1

AMA: May 13: 8, Mar 13: 3, Sep 13: 18, Mar 15: 6

95909 Nerve conduction studies; 5-6 studies **S**

Mod	RVU Non-Fac Total	Fac Total	Global Days	Modifiers 51	50	62	80	MUE
	4.08	4.08	XXX	0	0	0	0	1
26	2.28	2.28	XXX	0	0	0	0	1
TC	1.80	1.80	XXX	0	0	0	0	1

AMA: May 13: 8, Mar 13: 3, Sep 13: 18

95910 Nerve conduction studies; 7-8 studies **S**

Mod	RVU Non-Fac Total	Fac Total	Global Days	Modifiers 51	50	62	80	MUE
TC	2.37	2.37	XXX	0	0	0	0	1
	5.42	5.42	XXX	0	0	0	0	1
26	3.05	3.05	XXX	0	0	0	0	1

AMA: May 13: 8, Mar 13: 3, Sep 13: 18

95911 Nerve conduction studies; 9-10 studies **S**

Mod	RVU Non-Fac Total	Fac Total	Global Days	Modifiers 51	50	62	80	MUE
	6.55	6.55	XXX	0	0	0	0	1
26	3.81	3.81	XXX	0	0	0	0	1
TC	2.74	2.74	XXX	0	0	0	0	1

AMA: May 13: 8, Mar 13: 3, Sep 13: 18

95912 Nerve conduction studies; 11-12 studies **S**

Mod	RVU Non-Fac Total	Fac Total	Global Days	Modifiers 51	50	62	80	MUE
	7.34	7.34	XXX	0	0	0	0	1
26	4.52	4.52	XXX	0	0	0	0	1
TC	2.82	2.82	XXX	0	0	0	0	1

AMA: May 13: 8, Mar 13: 3, Sep 13: 18

95913 Nerve conduction studies; 13 or more studies **S**

Mod	RVU Non-Fac Total	Fac Total	Global Days	Modifiers 51	50	62	80	MUE
	8.39	8.39	XXX	0	0	0	0	1
26	5.35	5.35	XXX	0	0	0	0	1
TC	3.04	3.04	XXX	0	0	0	0	1

AMA: May 13: 8, Mar 13: 3, Sep 13: 18

Autonomic Nervous System Function Testing

Coding Guidance

Autonomic function testing of both parasympathetic function and sympathetic function performed simultaneously and independently is reported with code 95943.

95921 Testing of autonomic nervous system function; cardiovagal innervation (parasympathetic function), including 2 or more of the following: heart rate response to deep breathing with recorded R-R interval, Valsalva ratio, and 30:15 ratio **S**

Mod	RVU Non-Fac Total	Fac Total	Global Days	Modifiers 51	50	62	80	MUE
	2.43	2.43	XXX	0	0	0	0	1
26	1.29	1.29	XXX	0	0	0	0	1
TC	1.14	1.14	XXX	0	0	0	0	1

AMA: Nov 98: 35, 36, Apr 02: 2, Oct 03: 11, Feb 06: 15, Nov 12: 6

● New   ▲ Revised   Deleted   ⊙ Moderate Sedation   ✚ Add-on Codes   ⊘ High Risk Denial   Ⓐ Age Edit   ♀ Female   ♂ Male   **AMA** *CPT® Assistant*   **MUE** Medically Unlikely Edit
⊘ Modifier 51 Exempt   ⊖ Modifier 63 Exempt   ☒ Unlisted   **Modifiers:** *See Inside Back Cover*   Ⓜ Maternity   A2–Z3 ASC Payment Indicators   A–Y OPPS Status Indicators

© 2016 DecisionHealth   CPT © 2015 American Medical Association. All Rights Reserved.   **837**

Medicine Procedures

95922 – 95933

95922 Testing of autonomic nervous system function; vasomotor adrenergic innervation (sympathetic adrenergic function), including beat-to-beat blood pressure and R-R interval changes during Valsalva maneuver and at least 5 minutes of passive tilt ⊙Q1

RVU			Global Days	Modifiers				
Mod	Non-Fac Total	Fac Total		51	50	62	80	MUE
	2.85	2.85	XXX	0	0	0	0	1
26	1.38	1.38	XXX	0	0	0	0	1
TC	1.47	1.47	XXX	0	0	0	0	1

AMA: Nov 98: 35, 36, Apr 02: 2, Jun 03: 11, Feb 06: 15, Nov 06: 23, Dec 08: 4, Nov 12: 6

95923 Testing of autonomic nervous system function; sudomotor, including 1 or more of the following: quantitative sudomotor axon reflex test (QSART), silastic sweat imprint, thermoregulatory sweat test, and changes in sympathetic skin potential ⊙Q1

RVU			Global Days	Modifiers				
Mod	Non-Fac Total	Fac Total		51	50	62	80	MUE
	4.63	4.63	XXX	0	0	0	0	1
26	1.32	1.32	XXX	0	0	0	0	1
TC	3.31	3.31	XXX	0	0	0	0	1

AMA: Nov 98: 35, 36, Apr 02: 2, Feb 06: 15, Nov 12: 6

95924 Testing of autonomic nervous system function; combined parasympathetic and sympathetic adrenergic function testing with at least 5 minutes of passive tilt ⑤

RVU			Global Days	Modifiers				
Mod	Non-Fac Total	Fac Total		51	50	62	80	MUE
	4.21	4.21	XXX	0	0	0	0	1
26	2.54	2.54	XXX	0	0	0	0	1
TC	1.67	1.67	XXX	0	0	0	0	1

AMA: Nov 12: 6

Evoked Potential/Reflex Testing

Coding Guidance

When a spinal or intracranial procedure uses intraoperative neurophysiological testing, the physician who performs the main surgical service should not report 90000 codes, such as 95925-95937 for intraoperative neurophysiological testing, as they are included in the global package.

95925 Short-latency somatosensory evoked potential study, stimulation of any/all peripheral nerves or skin sites, recording from the central nervous system; in upper limbs ⑤

Coding tip: *Short-latency somatosensory evoked potential study upper and lower limbs - 95938*

RVU			Global Days	Modifiers				
Mod	Non-Fac Total	Fac Total		51	50	62	80	MUE
	4.39	4.39	XXX	0	2	0	0	1
26	0.80	0.80	XXX	0	2	0	0	1
TC	3.59	3.59	XXX	0	2	0	0	1

AMA: Nov 98: 35, 36, Apr 02: 2, May 13: 8, Apr 12: 17

95926 Short-latency somatosensory evoked potential study, stimulation of any/all peripheral nerves or skin sites, recording from the central nervous system; in lower limbs ⑤

Coding tip: *Short-latency somatosensory evoked potential study upper and lower limbs - 95938*

RVU			Global Days	Modifiers				
Mod	Non-Fac Total	Fac Total		51	50	62	80	MUE
	3.88	3.88	XXX	0	2	0	0	1
26	0.78	0.78	XXX	0	2	0	0	1
TC	3.10	3.10	XXX	0	2	0	0	1

AMA: May 01: 11, Apr 02: 2, May 13: 8, Apr 12: 17

95927 Short-latency somatosensory evoked potential study, stimulation of any/all peripheral nerves or skin sites, recording from the central nervous system; in the trunk or head ⑤

RVU			Global Days	Modifiers				
Mod	Non-Fac Total	Fac Total		51	50	62	80	MUE
	4.01	4.01	XXX	0	0	0	0	1
26	0.78	0.78	XXX	0	0	0	0	1
TC	3.23	3.23	XXX	0	0	0	0	1

AMA: Apr 02: 2, May 13: 8

95928 Central motor evoked potential study (transcranial motor stimulation); upper limbs ⑤

Coding tip: *Central motor evoked potential study upper and lower limbs - 95939*

RVU			Global Days	Modifiers				
Mod	Non-Fac Total	Fac Total		51	50	62	80	MUE
	6.35	6.35	XXX	0	2	0	0	1
26	2.28	2.28	XXX	0	2	0	0	1
TC	4.07	4.07	XXX	0	2	0	0	1

AMA: May 13: 8

95929 Central motor evoked potential study (transcranial motor stimulation); lower limbs ⑤

Coding tip: *Central motor evoked potential study upper and lower limbs - 95939*

RVU			Global Days	Modifiers				
Mod	Non-Fac Total	Fac Total		51	50	62	80	MUE
	6.39	6.39	XXX	0	2	0	0	1
26	2.29	2.29	XXX	0	2	0	0	1
TC	4.10	4.10	XXX	0	2	0	0	1

AMA: May 13: 8

95930 Visual evoked potential (VEP) testing central nervous system, checkerboard or flash ⑤

RVU			Global Days	Modifiers				
Mod	Non-Fac Total	Fac Total		51	50	62	80	MUE
	3.61	3.61	XXX	0	2	0	0	1
26	0.52	0.52	XXX	0	2	0	0	1
TC	3.09	3.09	XXX	0	2	0	0	1

AMA: May 13: 8, Aug 14: 8

95933 Orbicularis oculi (blink) reflex, by electrodiagnostic testing ⊙Q1

RVU			Global Days	Modifiers				
Mod	Non-Fac Total	Fac Total		51	50	62	80	MUE
	2.12	2.12	XXX	0	0	0	0	1
26	0.89	0.89	XXX	0	0	0	0	1
TC	1.23	1.23	XXX	0	0	0	0	1

AMA: Nov 98: 35, 36, May 13: 8

● New   ▲ Revised   ✖ Deleted   ⊙ Moderate Sedation   ✚ Add-on Codes   ⊗ High Risk Denial   Ⓐ Age Edit   ♀ Female   ♂ Male   **AMA** *CPT® Assistant*   **MUE** Medically Unlikely Edit
⊘ Modifier 51 Exempt   ⊖ Modifier 63 Exempt   ⊠ Unlisted   **Modifiers:** *See Inside Back Cover*   Ⓜ Maternity   Ａ2–Ｚ3 ASC Payment Indicators   Ａ–Ｙ OPPS Status Indicators

838   CPT © 2015 American Medical Association. All Rights Reserved.   © 2016 DecisionHealth

95937   Neuromuscular junction testing (repetitive stimulation, paired stimuli), each nerve, any 1 method   ⓢ

Mod	RVU Non-Fac Total	Fac Total	Global Days	Modifiers 51	50	62	80	MUE
	2.30	2.30	XXX	0	0	0	0	
26	0.98	0.98	XXX	0	0	0	0	
TC	1.32	1.32	XXX	0	0	0	0	

AMA: Nov 98: 35, 36, Apr 02: 2, Jun 06: 8, May 13: 8, Mar 13: 3

95938   Short-latency somatosensory evoked potential study, stimulation of any/all peripheral nerves or skin sites, recording from the central nervous system; in upper and lower limbs   ⓢ

Coding tip: Code 95938 is listed out of numerical order in CPT. Additional short latency somatosensory evoked potential studies - upper limbs only - 95925; lower limbs only - 95926

Mod	RVU Non-Fac Total	Fac Total	Global Days	Modifiers 51	50	62	80	MUE
	9.63	9.63	XXX	0	2	0	0	1
26	1.31	1.31	XXX	0	2	0	0	1
TC	8.32	8.32	XXX	0	2	0	0	1

AMA: Apr 12: 17, 18, May 13: 8, Feb 13: 17

95939   Central motor evoked potential study (transcranial motor stimulation); in upper and lower limbs   ⓢ

Coding tip: Code 95939 is listed out of numerical order in CPT. Additional central motor evoked potential studies - upper limbs only - 95928; lower limbs only - 95929

Mod	RVU Non-Fac Total	Fac Total	Global Days	Modifiers 51	50	62	80	MUE
TC	10.72	10.72	XXX	0	2	0	0	1
	14.12	14.12	XXX	0	2	0	0	1
26	3.40	3.40	XXX	0	2	0	0	1

AMA: Apr 12: 17, 18, May 13: 8

Intraoperative Neurophysiological Testing

Coding Guidance

Codes for continuous intraoperative neurophysiology monitoring in the operating room ,95940 and 95941, are listed out of numerical order in CPT. In CPT, these codes follow nerve conduction studies (codes 95905-95913). Even though some spinal and intracranial procedures use intraoperative neurophysiological testing, CPT codes 95940 and 95941 should not be reported by the same physician who performed the operative procedure or anesthesia, as these services are included in the global package. When a different physician performs the testing, however, it is reportable by the second physician. The physician who performs the main spinal or intracranial surgical service should not report other 90000 codes for the intraoperative neurophysiological testing, either, as they are also included.

➕ 95940   Continuous intraoperative neurophysiology monitoring in the operating room, one on one monitoring requiring personal attendance, each 15 minutes (List separately in addition to code for primary procedure)   Ⓝ Ⓝ

Mod	RVU Non-Fac Total	Fac Total	Global Days	Modifiers 51	50	62	80	MUE
	0.93	0.93	XXX	0	0	0	0	

AMA: Apr 14: 5, 11, May 13: 8, 9, 10

Intraoperative Neurophysiological Testing

➕ 95941   Continuous intraoperative neurophysiology monitoring, from outside the operating room (remote or nearby) or for monitoring of more than one case while in the operating room, per hour (List separately in addition to code for primary procedure)   Ⓒ Ⓝ Ⓘ Ⓝ

Mod	RVU Non-Fac Total	Fac Total	Global Days	Modifiers 51	50	62	80	MUE
	0.00	0.00	XXX	9	9	9	9	

AMA: May 13: 8, Apr 14: 5, 11, Feb 13: 16, Dec 14: 19

95943   Simultaneous, independent, quantitative measures of both parasympathetic function and sympathetic function, based on time-frequency analysis of heart rate variability concurrent with time-frequency analysis of continuous respiratory activity, with mean heart rate and blood pressure measures, during rest, paced (deep) breathing, Valsalva maneuvers, and head-up postural change   ⓢ

Coding tip: Code 95943 is listed out of numerical order in CPT. Additional autonomic function tests - 95921-95924

Mod	RVU Non-Fac Total	Fac Total	Global Days	Modifiers 51	50	62	80	MUE
TC	0.00	0.00	XXX	0	0	0	0	1
	0.00	0.00	XXX	0	0	0	0	1
26	0.00	0.00	XXX	0	0	0	0	1

AMA: Nov 12: 6

Special Electroencephalographic Testing

95950   Monitoring for identification and lateralization of cerebral seizure focus, electroencephalographic (eg, 8 channel EEG) recording and interpretation, each 24 hours   ⓢ

Mod	RVU Non-Fac Total	Fac Total	Global Days	Modifiers 51	50	62	80	MUE
	9.32	9.32	XXX	0	0	0	0	1
26	2.27	2.27	XXX	0	0	0	0	1
TC	7.05	7.05	XXX	0	0	0	0	1

AMA: Nov 98: 35, Feb 11: 3

95951   Monitoring for localization of cerebral seizure focus by cable or radio, 16 or more channel telemetry, combined electroencephalographic (EEG) and video recording and interpretation (eg, for presurgical localization), each 24 hours   ⓢ

Mod	RVU Non-Fac Total	Fac Total	Global Days	Modifiers 51	50	62	80	MUE
	0.00	0.00	XXX	0	0	0	0	1
26	9.08	9.08	XXX	0	0	0	0	1
TC	0.00	0.00	XXX	0	0	0	0	1

AMA: Nov 98: 35, Mar 03: 21, Dec 04: 18, Dec 09: 3, Nov 10: 6, Feb 11: 3, Aug 13: 14, Dec 14: 17

● New   ▲ Revised   Deleted   ⊙ Moderate Sedation   ➕ Add-on Codes   ⊘ High Risk Denial   Ⓐ Age Edit   ♀ Female   ♂ Male   **AMA** *CPT® Assistant*   **MUE** Medically Unlikely Edit
⊘ Modifier 51 Exempt   ⊖ Modifier 63 Exempt   ☒ Unlisted   **Modifiers:** *See Inside Back Cover*   Ⓜ Maternity   Ⓐ2–Ⓩ3 ASC Payment Indicators   Ⓐ–Ⓨ OPPS Status Indicators

© 2016 DecisionHealth   CPT © 2015 American Medical Association. All Rights Reserved.   **839**

95953 Monitoring for localization of cerebral seizure focus by computerized portable 16 or more channel EEG, electroencephalographic (EEG) recording and interpretation, each 24 hours, unattended   S

Mod	RVU Non-Fac Total	Fac Total	Global Days	Modifiers 51	50	62	80	MUE
	11.89	11.89	XXX	0	0	0	0	1
26	4.66	4.66	XXX	0	0	0	0	1
TC	7.23	7.23	XXX	0	0	0	0	1

AMA: Nov 98: 35, Dec 09: 3, Feb 11: 3, Dec 14: 17

95954 Pharmacological or physical activation requiring physician or other qualified health care professional attendance during EEG recording of activation phase (eg, thiopental activation test)   S

Mod	RVU Non-Fac Total	Fac Total	Global Days	Modifiers 51	50	62	80	MUE
	12.83	12.83	XXX	0	0	0	0	1
26	3.56	3.56	XXX	0	0	0	0	1
TC	9.27	9.27	XXX	0	0	0	0	1

AMA: Winter 94: 18, Nov 98: 35

95955 Electroencephalogram (EEG) during nonintracranial surgery (eg, carotid surgery)   N

Mod	RVU Non-Fac Total	Fac Total	Global Days	Modifiers 51	50	62	80	MUE
	6.09	6.09	XXX	0	0	0	0	1
26	1.54	1.54	XXX	0	0	0	0	1
TC	4.55	4.55	XXX	0	0	0	0	1

AMA: Nov 98: 35, Dec 14: 19

95956 Monitoring for localization of cerebral seizure focus by cable or radio, 16 or more channel telemetry, electroencephalographic (EEG) recording and interpretation, each 24 hours, attended by a technologist or nurse   S

Mod	RVU Non-Fac Total	Fac Total	Global Days	Modifiers 51	50	62	80	MUE
	46.24	46.24	XXX	0	0	0	0	1
26	5.44	5.44	XXX	0	0	0	0	1
TC	40.80	40.80	XXX	0	0	0	0	1

AMA: Nov 98: 35, Dec 09: 3, Feb 11: 3

95957 Digital analysis of electroencephalogram (EEG) (eg, for epileptic spike analysis)   N

Mod	RVU Non-Fac Total	Fac Total	Global Days	Modifiers 51	50	62	80	MUE
	8.88	8.88	XXX	0	0	0	0	1
26	2.99	2.99	XXX	0	0	0	0	1
TC	5.89	5.89	XXX	0	0	0	0	1

AMA: Winter 94: 18, Nov 98: 35, Nov 10: 6

95958 Wada activation test for hemispheric function, including electroencephalographic (EEG) monitoring   S

Mod	RVU Non-Fac Total	Fac Total	Global Days	Modifiers 51	50	62	80	MUE
	16.15	16.15	XXX	0	0	0	0	1
26	6.43	6.43	XXX	0	0	0	0	1
TC	9.72	9.72	XXX	0	0	0	0	1

AMA: Nov 98: 35

95961 Functional cortical and subcortical mapping by stimulation and/or recording of electrodes on brain surface, or of depth electrodes, to provoke seizures or identify vital brain structures; initial hour of attendance by a physician or other qualified health care professional   S

Mod	RVU Non-Fac Total	Fac Total	Global Days	Modifiers 51	50	62	80	MUE
	8.32	8.32	XXX	0	0	0	0	1
26	4.62	4.62	XXX	0	0	0	0	1
TC	3.70	3.70	XXX	0	0	0	0	1

AMA: Winter 94: 18, Nov 98: 35, Nov 99: 52, 53, Apr 10: 10, Feb 11: 3, Aug 10: 13

Pub 100-04, 32, 50.4.3

+ **95962** Functional cortical and subcortical mapping by stimulation and/or recording of electrodes on brain surface, or of depth electrodes, to provoke seizures or identify vital brain structures; each additional hour of attendance by a physician or other qualified health care professional (List separately in addition to code for primary procedure)   N

Mod	RVU Non-Fac Total	Fac Total	Global Days	Modifiers 51	50	62	80	MUE
	7.40	7.40	ZZZ	0	0	0	0	
26	4.93	4.93	ZZZ	0	0	0	0	
TC	2.47	2.47	ZZZ	0	0	0	0	

AMA: Winter 94: 18, Nov 98: 35, Nov 99: 52, 53, Apr 10: 10, Feb 11: 3, Aug 10: 13

Pub 100-04, 32, 50.4.3

95965 Magnetoencephalography (MEG), recording and analysis; for spontaneous brain magnetic activity (eg, epileptic cerebral cortex localization)   S

Mod	RVU Non-Fac Total	Fac Total	Global Days	Modifiers 51	50	62	80	MUE
	0.00	0.00	XXX	0	0	0	0	1
26	11.93	11.93	XXX	0	0	0	0	1
TC	0.00	0.00	XXX	0	0	0	0	1

95966 Magnetoencephalography (MEG), recording and analysis; for evoked magnetic fields, single modality (eg, sensory, motor, language, or visual cortex localization)   S

Mod	RVU Non-Fac Total	Fac Total	Global Days	Modifiers 51	50	62	80	MUE
	0.00	0.00	XXX	0	0	0	0	1
26	6.05	6.05	XXX	0	0	0	0	1
TC	0.00	0.00	XXX	0	0	0	0	1

+ **95967** Magnetoencephalography (MEG), recording and analysis; for evoked magnetic fields, each additional modality (eg, sensory, motor, language, or visual cortex localization) (List separately in addition to code for primary procedure)   N

Mod	RVU Non-Fac Total	Fac Total	Global Days	Modifiers 51	50	62	80	MUE
	0.00	0.00	ZZZ	0	0	0	0	3
26	5.27	5.27	ZZZ	0	0	0	0	3
TC	0.00	0.00	ZZZ	0	0	0	0	3

● New   ▲ Revised   ✖ Deleted   ⊙ Moderate Sedation   ✚ Add-on Codes   ⊘ High Risk Denial   Ⓐ Age Edit   ♀ Female   ♂ Male   **AMA** CPT® Assistant   **MUE** Medically Unlikely Edit

⊖ Modifier 51 Exempt   ⊖ Modifier 63 Exempt   ✖ Unlisted   **Modifiers:** See Inside Back Cover   Ⓜ Maternity   A2–Z3 ASC Payment Indicators   A–Y OPPS Status Indicators

CPT © 2015 American Medical Association. All Rights Reserved.   © 2016 DecisionHealth

Neurostimulator Analysis/Programming

95970 Electronic analysis of implanted neurostimulator pulse generator system (eg, rate, pulse amplitude, pulse duration, configuration of wave form, battery status, electrode selectability, output modulation, cycling, impedance and patient compliance measurements); simple or complex brain, spinal cord, or peripheral (ie, cranial nerve, peripheral nerve, sacral nerve, neuromuscular) neurostimulator pulse generator/transmitter, without reprogramming   Q1

RVU			Global Days	Modifiers				
Mod	Non-Fac Total	Fac Total		51	50	62	80	MUE
	1.93	0.69	XXX	0	0	0	0	1

AMA: Nov 98: 36, 37, Sep 99: 1, Nov 99: 53, 54, Aug 05: 7, Sep 05: 10, Oct 12: 15

Pub 100-04, 32, 50.4.3

95971 Electronic analysis of implanted neurostimulator pulse generator system (eg, rate, pulse amplitude, pulse duration, configuration of wave form, battery status, electrode selectability, output modulation, cycling, impedance and patient compliance measurements); simple spinal cord, or peripheral (ie, peripheral nerve, sacral nerve, neuromuscular) neurostimulator pulse generator/transmitter, with intraoperative or subsequent programming   S

RVU			Global Days	Modifiers				
Mod	Non-Fac Total	Fac Total		51	50	62	80	MUE
	1.42	1.16	XXX	0	0	0	0	1

AMA: Nov 98: 36, 37, Sep 99: 1, Nov 99: 53, 54, Aug 05: 7, Apr 11: 11, Oct 10: 14, Dec 10: 14, Oct 12: 15

Pub 100-04, 32, 50.4.3

▲ 95972 Electronic analysis of implanted neurostimulator pulse generator system (eg, rate, pulse amplitude, pulse duration, configuration of wave form, battery status, electrode selectability, output modulation, cycling, impedance and patient compliance measurements); complex spinal cord, or peripheral (ie, peripheral nerve, sacral nerve, neuromuscular) (except cranial nerve) neurostimulator pulse generator/transmitter, with intraoperative or subsequent programming   S

RVU			Global Days	Modifiers				
Mod	Non-Fac Total	Fac Total		51	50	62	80	MUE
	1.66	1.19	XXX	0	0	0	0	1

AMA: Nov 98: 36, 37, Sep 99: 1, Nov 99: 53, 54, Aug 05: 7, Apr 11: 10, Oct 12: 15, Aug 14: 5

Pub 100-04, 32, 50.4.3

✖ 95973 Electronic analysis of implanted neurostimulator pulse generator system (eg, rate, pulse amplitude, pulse duration, configuration of wave form, battery status, electrode selectability, output modulation, cycling, impedance and patient compliance measurements); complex spinal cord, or peripheral (ie, peripheral nerve, sacral nerve, neuromuscular) (except cranial nerve) neurostimulator pulse generator/transmitter, with intraoperative or subsequent programming, each additional 30 minutes after first hour (List separately in addition to code for primary procedure)

95974 Electronic analysis of implanted neurostimulator pulse generator system (eg, rate, pulse amplitude, pulse duration, configuration of wave form, battery status, electrode selectability, output modulation, cycling, impedance and patient compliance measurements); complex cranial nerve neurostimulator pulse generator/ transmitter, with intraoperative or subsequent programming, with or without nerve interface testing, first hour   S

RVU			Global Days	Modifiers				
Mod	Non-Fac Total	Fac Total		51	50	62	80	MUE
	5.87	4.66	XXX	0	0	0	0	1

AMA: Nov 98: 36, 37, Sep 99: 1, Nov 99: 53, 54, Sep 05: 10, Apr 11: 11, Aug 14: 5

+ 95975 Electronic analysis of implanted neurostimulator pulse generator system (eg, rate, pulse amplitude, pulse duration, configuration of wave form, battery status, electrode selectability, output modulation, cycling, impedance and patient compliance measurements); complex cranial nerve neurostimulator pulse generator/ transmitter, with intraoperative or subsequent programming, each additional 30 minutes after first hour (List separately in addition to code for primary procedure)   N

RVU			Global Days	Modifiers				
Mod	Non-Fac Total	Fac Total		51	50	62	80	MUE
	3.16	2.64	ZZZ	0	0	0	0	2

AMA: Nov 98: 36, 37, Sep 99: 1, Nov 99: 53, 54, Sep 05: 10, Apr 11: 11

95978 Electronic analysis of implanted neurostimulator pulse generator system (eg, rate, pulse amplitude and duration, battery status, electrode selectability and polarity, impedance and patient compliance measurements), complex deep brain neurostimulator pulse generator/transmitter, with initial or subsequent programming; first hour   S

RVU			Global Days	Modifiers				
Mod	Non-Fac Total	Fac Total		51	50	62	80	MUE
	7.05	5.48	XXX	0	0	0	0	1

AMA: Aug 05: 7, Aug 14: 5

● New   ▲ Revised   Deleted   ⊙ Moderate Sedation   ✚ Add-on Codes   ⊘ High Risk Denial   Ⓐ Age Edit   ♀ Female   ♂ Male   **AMA** *CPT® Assistant*   **MUE** Medically Unlikely Edit

⊘ Modifier 51 Exempt   ⊖ Modifier 63 Exempt   ✖ Unlisted   **Modifiers:** *See Inside Back Cover*   Ⓜ Maternity   A2–Z3 ASC Payment Indicators   A–Y OPPS Status Indicators

© 2016 DecisionHealth   CPT © 2015 American Medical Association. All Rights Reserved.   **841**

Medicine Procedures

95979 – 96003

+ **95979** Electronic analysis of implanted neurostimulator pulse generator system (eg, rate, pulse amplitude and duration, battery status, electrode selectability and polarity, impedance and patient compliance measurements), complex deep brain neurostimulator pulse generator/transmitter, with initial or subsequent programming; each additional 30 minutes after first hour (List separately in addition to code for primary procedure)   **N**

RVU			Global Days	Modifiers				
Mod	Non-Fac Total	Fac Total		51	50	62	80	MUE
	3.06	2.55	ZZZ	0	0	0	0	

AMA: Aug 05: 7

95980 Electronic analysis of implanted neurostimulator pulse generator system (eg, rate, pulse amplitude and duration, configuration of wave form, battery status, electrode selectability, output modulation, cycling, impedance and patient measurements) gastric neurostimulator pulse generator/transmitter; intraoperative, with programming   **N**

RVU			Global Days	Modifiers				
Mod	Non-Fac Total	Fac Total		51	50	62	80	MUE
	1.32	1.32	XXX	0	0	0	0	1

AMA: Jan 08: 8, Nov 10: 8

95981 Electronic analysis of implanted neurostimulator pulse generator system (eg, rate, pulse amplitude and duration, configuration of wave form, battery status, electrode selectability, output modulation, cycling, impedance and patient measurements) gastric neurostimulator pulse generator/transmitter; subsequent, without reprogramming   **Q1**

RVU			Global Days	Modifiers				
Mod	Non-Fac Total	Fac Total		51	50	62	80	MUE
	0.90	0.51	XXX	0	0	0	0	1

AMA: Jan 08: 8

95982 Electronic analysis of implanted neurostimulator pulse generator system (eg, rate, pulse amplitude and duration, configuration of wave form, battery status, electrode selectability, output modulation, cycling, impedance and patient measurements) gastric neurostimulator pulse generator/transmitter; subsequent, with reprogramming   **Q1**

RVU			Global Days	Modifiers				
Mod	Non-Fac Total	Fac Total		51	50	62	80	MUE
	1.49	1.04	XXX	0	0	0	0	1

AMA: Jan 08: 8

Other Neurological/Neuromuscular Services/Procedures

95990 Refilling and maintenance of implantable pump or reservoir for drug delivery, spinal (intrathecal, epidural) or brain (intraventricular), includes electronic analysis of pump, when performed   **S**

RVU			Global Days	Modifiers				
Mod	Non-Fac Total	Fac Total		51	50	62	80	MUE
	2.60	2.60	XXX	0	0	0	0	2

AMA: Nov 02: 4, Nov 05: 1, Jul 06: 1, Jul 12: 6, Aug 12: 10, 11, 12, 15

95991 Refilling and maintenance of implantable pump or reservoir for drug delivery, spinal (intrathecal, epidural) or brain (intraventricular), includes electronic analysis of pump, when performed; requiring skill of a physician or other qualified health care professional   **S**

RVU			Global Days	Modifiers				
Mod	Non-Fac Total	Fac Total		51	50	62	80	MUE
	3.46	1.14	XXX	0	0	0	0	2

AMA: Nov 05: 1, Jul 06: 1, Jul 12: 6, Aug 12: 10, 11, 12, 15

⊘ **95992** Canalith repositioning procedure(s) (eg, Epley maneuver, Semont maneuver), per day   **A**

RVU			Global Days	Modifiers				
Mod	Non-Fac Total	Fac Total		51	50	62	80	MUE
	1.22	1.06	XXX	0	0	0	0	1

95999 Unlisted neurological or neuromuscular diagnostic procedure   **⊘x Q1**

RVU			Global Days	Modifiers				
Mod	Non-Fac Total	Fac Total		51	50	62	80	MUE
	0.00	0.00	XXX	0	0	0	0	

AMA: Feb 99: 11, Jan 02: 11, Mar 07: 4, Apr 07: 7, Dec 08: 10, Aug 15: 8

Pub 100-04, 13, 120

Motion Analysis Testing

96000 Comprehensive computer-based motion analysis by video-taping and 3D kinematics   **S**

RVU			Global Days	Modifiers				
Mod	Non-Fac Total	Fac Total		51	50	62	80	MUE
	2.70	2.70	XXX	0	2	0	0	1

AMA: Aug 02: 5, Jun 03: 2

96001 Comprehensive computer-based motion analysis by video-taping and 3D kinematics; with dynamic plantar pressure measurements during walking   **⊘S**

RVU			Global Days	Modifiers				
Mod	Non-Fac Total	Fac Total		51	50	62	80	MUE
	3.04	3.04	XXX	0	2	0	0	1

AMA: Aug 02: 5, Jun 03: 2

96002 Dynamic surface electromyography, during walking or other functional activities, 1-12 muscles   **⊘S**

RVU			Global Days	Modifiers				
Mod	Non-Fac Total	Fac Total		51	50	62	80	MUE
	0.61	0.61	XXX	0	2	0	0	1

AMA: Aug 02: 5, Jun 03: 3, Aug 15: 8

96003 Dynamic fine wire electromyography, during walking or other functional activities, 1 muscle   **⊘Q1**

RVU			Global Days	Modifiers				
Mod	Non-Fac Total	Fac Total		51	50	62	80	MUE
	0.51	0.51	XXX	0	2	0	0	1

AMA: Aug 02: 5, Jun 03: 3

● New   ▲ Revised   ✖ Deleted   ⊙ Moderate Sedation   + Add-on Codes   ⊘ High Risk Denial   ⊛ Age Edit   ♀ Female   ♂ Male   **AMA** *CPT® Assistant*   **MUE** Medically Unlikely Edit
⊘ Modifier 51 Exempt   ⊖ Modifier 63 Exempt   **X** Unlisted   **Modifiers:** *See Inside Back Cover*   **M** Maternity   **A2–Z3** ASC Payment Indicators   **A–Y** OPPS Status Indicators

CPT © 2015 American Medical Association. All Rights Reserved.   © 2016 DecisionHealth

96004 Review and interpretation by physician or other qualified health care professional of comprehensive computer-based motion analysis, dynamic plantar pressure measurements, dynamic surface electromyography during walking or other functional activities, and dynamic fine wire electromyography, with written report **B**

RVU			Global Days	Modifiers				
Mod	Non-Fac Total	Fac Total		51	50	62	80	MUE
	3.32	3.32	XXX	0	2	0	0	1

AMA: Aug 02: 5, Jun 03: 3, Aug 15: 8

Functional Brain Mapping Testing

96020 Neurofunctional testing selection and administration during noninvasive imaging functional brain mapping, with test administered entirely by a physician or other qualified health care professional (ie, psychologist), with review of test results and report **N**

RVU			Global Days	Modifiers				
Mod	Non-Fac Total	Fac Total		51	50	62	80	MUE
	0.00	0.00	XXX	0	0	0	0	1
26	4.64	4.64	XXX	0	0	0	0	1
TC	0.00	0.00	XXX	0	0	0	0	1

AMA: Feb 07: 6

Medical Genetics/Genetic Counseling

96040 Medical genetics and genetic counseling services, each 30 minutes face-to-face with patient/family **⊕B**

RVU			Global Days	Modifiers				
Mod	Non-Fac Total	Fac Total		51	50	62	80	MUE
	1.33	1.33	XXX	9	9	9	9	

AMA: Aug 07: 9

Central Nervous System Cognitive Assessment/Testing

Coding Guidance
Codes 96101-96103 are for psychological testing by different performance and interpretation methods. Only when the different techniques are utilized for different tests can two or more codes from this range be reported on the same date of service.

96101 Psychological testing (includes psychodiagnostic assessment of emotionality, intellectual abilities, personality and psychopathology, eg, MMPI, Rorschach, WAIS), per hour of the psychologist's or physician's time, both face-to-face time administering tests to the patient and time interpreting these test results and preparing the report **Q3**

RVU			Global Days	Modifiers				
Mod	Non-Fac Total	Fac Total		51	50	62	80	MUE
	2.25	2.23	XXX	0	0	0	0	

AMA: Oct 11: 4, Sep 10: 9, Jun 14: 3
Pub 100-02, 15, 80.2; 100-04, 12, 210.1

96102 Psychological testing (includes psychodiagnostic assessment of emotionality, intellectual abilities, personality and psychopathology, eg, MMPI and WAIS), with qualified health care professional interpretation and report, administered by technician, per hour of technician time, face-to-face **Q3**

RVU			Global Days	Modifiers				
Mod	Non-Fac Total	Fac Total		51	50	62	80	MUE
	1.79	0.66	XXX	0	0	0	0	

Pub 100-02, 15, 80.2; 100-04, 12, 210.1

96103 Psychological testing (includes psychodiagnostic assessment of emotionality, intellectual abilities, personality and psychopathology, eg, MMPI), administered by a computer, with qualified health care professional interpretation and report **Q1**

RVU			Global Days	Modifiers				
Mod	Non-Fac Total	Fac Total		51	50	62	80	MUE
	0.79	0.76	XXX	0	0	0	0	1

AMA: Oct 11: 10
Pub 100-02, 15, 80.2; 100-04, 12, 210.1

96105 Assessment of aphasia (includes assessment of expressive and receptive speech and language function, language comprehension, speech production ability, reading, spelling, writing, eg, by Boston Diagnostic Aphasia Examination) with interpretation and report, per hour **A**

RVU			Global Days	Modifiers				
Mod	Non-Fac Total	Fac Total		51	50	62	80	MUE
	3.03	3.03	XXX	0	0	0	0	3

AMA: Jul 96: 8, May 05: 1, Nov 09: 10
Pub 100-02, 15, 80.2

96110 Developmental screening (eg, developmental milestone survey, speech and language delay screen), with scoring and documentation, per standardized instrument **⊕E**

RVU			Global Days	Modifiers				
Mod	Non-Fac Total	Fac Total		51	50	62	80	MUE
	0.25	0.25	XXX	9	9	9	9	

AMA: Jul 96: 9, May 05: 1, Nov 09: 10, Aug 15: 5, Jun 14: 3
Pub 100-02, 15, 80.2; 100-04, 12, 210.1

96111 Developmental testing, (includes assessment of motor, language, social, adaptive, and/or cognitive functioning by standardized developmental instruments) with interpretation and report **Q3**

RVU			Global Days	Modifiers				
Mod	Non-Fac Total	Fac Total		51	50	62	80	MUE
	3.65	3.47	XXX	0	0	0	0	

AMA: Jul 96: 9, May 05: 1, Nov 09: 10
Pub 100-02, 15, 80.2; 100-04, 12, 210.1

● New ▲ Revised Deleted ⊙ Moderate Sedation ✚ Add-on Codes ⊘ High Risk Denial ⓐ Age Edit ♀ Female ♂ Male **AMA** *CPT® Assistant* **MUE** Medically Unlikely Edit
⦸ Modifier 51 Exempt ⊖ Modifier 63 Exempt ✗ Unlisted **Modifiers:** *See Inside Back Cover* Ⓜ Maternity **A2–Z3** ASC Payment Indicators **A–Y** OPPS Status Indicators

© 2016 DecisionHealth | CPT © 2015 American Medical Association. All Rights Reserved. | **843**

Medicine Procedures

96116 Neurobehavioral status exam (clinical assessment of thinking, reasoning and judgment, eg, acquired knowledge, attention, language, memory, planning and problem solving, and visual spatial abilities), per hour of the psychologist's or physician's time, both face-to-face time with the patient and time interpreting test results and preparing the report   **Q3**

RVU			Global Days	Modifiers				
Mod	Non-Fac Total	Fac Total		51	50	62	80	MUE
	2.62	2.46	XXX	0	0	0	0	

AMA: Oct 11: 4, Jun 14: 3

Pub 100-02, 15, 80.2; 100-04, 12, 190.3, 210.1

Coding Guidance

Codes 96118-96120 are for neuropsychological testing by different performance and interpretation methods. Only when the different techniques are utilized for different tests can two or more codes from this range be reported on the same date of service.

96118 Neuropsychological testing (eg, Halstead-Reitan Neuropsychological Battery, Wechsler Memory Scales and Wisconsin Card Sorting Test), per hour of the psychologist's or physician's time, both face-to-face time administering tests to the patient and time interpreting these test results and preparing the report   **Q3**

RVU			Global Days	Modifiers				
Mod	Non-Fac Total	Fac Total		51	50	62	80	MUE
	2.76	2.22	XXX	0	0	0	0	

AMA: Oct 11: 4, Sep 10: 9, Jun 14: 3

Pub 100-02, 15, 80.2; 100-04, 12, 210.1

96119 Neuropsychological testing (eg, Halstead-Reitan Neuropsychological Battery, Wechsler Memory Scales and Wisconsin Card Sorting Test), with qualified health care professional interpretation and report, administered by technician, per hour of technician time, face-to-face   **Q3**

RVU			Global Days	Modifiers				
Mod	Non-Fac Total	Fac Total		51	50	62	80	MUE
	2.26	0.67	XXX	0	0	0	0	

Pub 100-02, 15, 80.2

96120 Neuropsychological testing (eg, Wisconsin Card Sorting Test), administered by a computer, with qualified health care professional interpretation and report   **Q3**

RVU			Global Days	Modifiers				
Mod	Non-Fac Total	Fac Total		51	50	62	80	MUE
	1.36	0.74	XXX	0	0	0	0	1

Pub 100-02, 15, 80.2

96125 Standardized cognitive performance testing (eg, Ross Information Processing Assessment) per hour of a qualified health care professional's time, both face-to-face time administering tests to the patient and time interpreting these test results and preparing the report   **A**

RVU			Global Days	Modifiers				
Mod	Non-Fac Total	Fac Total		51	50	62	80	MUE
	3.31	3.31	XXX	5	0	0	0	2

AMA: Oct 11: 4

96127 Brief emotional/behavioral assessment (eg, depression inventory, attention-deficit/hyperactivity disorder [ADHD] scale), with scoring and documentation, per standardized instrument   **Q1**

RVU			Global Days	Modifiers				
Mod	Non-Fac Total	Fac Total		51	50	62	80	MUE
	0.15	0.15	XXX	0	0	0	0	2

AMA: Aug 15: 5

Health and Behavior Assessment/Intervention Services

96150 Health and behavior assessment (eg, health-focused clinical interview, behavioral observations, psychophysiological monitoring, health-oriented questionnaires), each 15 minutes face-to-face with the patient; initial assessment   **Q3**

RVU			Global Days	Modifiers				
Mod	Non-Fac Total	Fac Total		51	50	62	80	MUE
	0.61	0.60	XXX	0	0	0	0	

AMA: Mar 02: 4, Feb 04: 11, Mar 04: 10, May 05: 1, Jun 05: 10, Aug 09: 9, May 13: 12, Sep 14: 15, Jun 14: 3

Pub 100-04, 12, 190.3

96151 Health and behavior assessment (eg, health-focused clinical interview, behavioral observations, psychophysiological monitoring, health-oriented questionnaires), each 15 minutes face-to-face with the patient; re-assessment   **Q3**

RVU			Global Days	Modifiers				
Mod	Non-Fac Total	Fac Total		51	50	62	80	MUE
	0.58	0.57	XXX	0	0	0	0	

AMA: Mar 02: 4, Feb 04: 11, Mar 04: 10, May 05: 1, Jun 05: 10, Aug 09: 9, May 13: 12, Sep 14: 15, Jun 14: 3

Pub 100-04, 12, 190.3

96152 Health and behavior intervention, each 15 minutes, face-to-face; individual   **Q3**

RVU			Global Days	Modifiers				
Mod	Non-Fac Total	Fac Total		51	50	62	80	MUE
	0.56	0.55	XXX	0	0	0	0	

AMA: Mar 02: 4, Feb 04: 11, Mar 04: 10, May 05: 1, Jun 05: 10, Aug 09: 9, May 13: 12, Jun 14: 3, Sep 14: 15

Pub 100-04, 12, 190.3

96153 Health and behavior intervention, each 15 minutes, face-to-face; group (2 or more patients)   **Q3**

RVU			Global Days	Modifiers				
Mod	Non-Fac Total	Fac Total		51	50	62	80	MUE
	0.13	0.13	XXX	0	0	0	0	

AMA: Mar 02: 4, Feb 04: 11, Mar 04: 10, May 05: 1, Jun 05: 10, Aug 09: 9, May 13: 12, Jun 14: 3, Sep 14: 15

Pub 100-04, 12, 190.3

96154 Health and behavior intervention, each 15 minutes, face-to-face; family (with the patient present)   **Q3**

RVU			Global Days	Modifiers				
Mod	Non-Fac Total	Fac Total		51	50	62	80	MUE
	0.55	0.54	XXX	0	0	0	0	

AMA: Mar 02: 4, Feb 04: 11, Mar 04: 10, May 05: 1, Jun 05: 10, Aug 09: 9, May 13: 12, Jun 14: 3, Sep 14: 15

Pub 100-04, 12, 190.3

● New   ▲ Revised   ✖ Deleted   ⊙ Moderate Sedation   ✚ Add-on Codes   ⊘ High Risk Denial   Ⓐ Age Edit   ♀ Female   ♂ Male   **AMA** CPT® Assistant   **MUE** Medically Unlikely Edit
⊘ Modifier 51 Exempt   ⊖ Modifier 63 Exempt   ✗ Unlisted   **Modifiers:** See Inside Back Cover   Ⓜ Maternity   A2-Z3 ASC Payment Indicators   A-Y OPPS Status Indicators

844   CPT © 2015 American Medical Association. All Rights Reserved.   © 2016 DecisionHealth

96155 Health and behavior intervention, each 15 minutes, face-to-face; family (without the patient present)   Ⓔ

RVU			Global Days	Modifiers				
Mod	Non-Fac Total	Fac Total		51	50	62	80	MUE
	0.64	0.64	XXX	9	9	9	9	

AMA: Mar 02: 4, 12, Feb 04: 11, Mar 04: 10, May 05: 1, Jun 05: 10, Aug 09: 9, May 13: 12, Jun 14: 3, Sep 14: 15

Injection/Infusion Services

Hydration

96360 Intravenous infusion, hydration; initial, 31 minutes to 1 hour   Ⓢ

RVU			Global Days	Modifiers				
Mod	Non-Fac Total	Fac Total		51	50	62	80	MUE
	1.61	1.61	XXX	0	0	0	0	1

AMA: May 11: 7, Oct 11: 3, Dec 11: 3, May 10: 8, Oct 13: 3, May 14: 11

✚ 96361 Intravenous infusion, hydration; each additional hour (List separately in addition to code for primary procedure)   Ⓢ

RVU			Global Days	Modifiers				
Mod	Non-Fac Total	Fac Total		51	50	62	80	MUE
	0.43	0.43	ZZZ	0	0	0	0	

AMA: Oct 11: 3, Dec 11: 3, May 10: 8, May 11: 7, Oct 13: 3, May 14: 11

Diagnostic/Therapeutic/Prophylactic Injections and Infusions

96365 Intravenous infusion, for therapy, prophylaxis, or diagnosis (specify substance or drug); initial, up to 1 hour   Ⓢ

RVU			Global Days	Modifiers				
Mod	Non-Fac Total	Fac Total		51	50	62	80	MUE
	1.95	1.95	XXX	0	0	0	0	1

AMA: May 11: 7, Oct 11: 4, Dec 11: 3, May 10: 8

✚ 96366 Intravenous infusion, for therapy, prophylaxis, or diagnosis (specify substance or drug); each additional hour (List separately in addition to code for primary procedure)   Ⓢ

RVU			Global Days	Modifiers				
Mod	Non-Fac Total	Fac Total		51	50	62	80	MUE
	0.53	0.53	ZZZ	0	0	0	0	

AMA: May 11: 7, Dec 11: 3

✚ 96367 Intravenous infusion, for therapy, prophylaxis, or diagnosis (specify substance or drug); additional sequential infusion of a new drug/substance, up to 1 hour (List separately in addition to code for primary procedure)   Ⓢ

RVU			Global Days	Modifiers				
Mod	Non-Fac Total	Fac Total		51	50	62	80	MUE
	0.86	0.86	ZZZ	0	0	0	0	

AMA: May 11: 7, Dec 11: 3

✚ 96368 Intravenous infusion, for therapy, prophylaxis, or diagnosis (specify substance or drug); concurrent infusion (List separately in addition to code for primary procedure)   Ⓝ

RVU			Global Days	Modifiers				
Mod	Non-Fac Total	Fac Total		51	50	62	80	MUE
	0.58	0.58	ZZZ	0	0	0	0	1

AMA: May 11: 7, Dec 11: 3, May 10: 8

96369 Subcutaneous infusion for therapy or prophylaxis (specify substance or drug); initial, up to 1 hour, including pump set-up and establishment of subcutaneous infusion site(s)   Ⓢ

RVU			Global Days	Modifiers				
Mod	Non-Fac Total	Fac Total		51	50	62	80	MUE
	5.41	5.41	XXX	0	0	0	0	1

AMA: May 11: 7

✚ 96370 Subcutaneous infusion for therapy or prophylaxis (specify substance or drug); each additional hour (List separately in addition to code for primary procedure)   Ⓢ

RVU			Global Days	Modifiers				
Mod	Non-Fac Total	Fac Total		51	50	62	80	MUE
	0.42	0.42	ZZZ	0	0	0	0	3

AMA: May 11: 7

✚ 96371 Subcutaneous infusion for therapy or prophylaxis (specify substance or drug); additional pump set-up with establishment of new subcutaneous infusion site(s) (List separately in addition to code for primary procedure)   ⒸⓃ

RVU			Global Days	Modifiers				
Mod	Non-Fac Total	Fac Total		51	50	62	80	MUE
	2.04	2.04	ZZZ	0	0	0	0	1

AMA: May 11: 7

96372 Therapeutic, prophylactic, or diagnostic injection (specify substance or drug); subcutaneous or intramuscular   Ⓢ

Coding tip: *Use 96372 for hormonal therapy injections without antineoplastic agents*

Documentation Finder: *Make sure the documentation shows that the provider is injecting into a muscle, usually biceps or buttock muscles, or that the note references subcutaneous. This code is most used when the medication being injected is for a systemic reason.*

RVU			Global Days	Modifiers				
Mod	Non-Fac Total	Fac Total		51	50	62	80	MUE
	0.71	0.71	XXX	0	0	0	0	

AMA: May 11: 7, May 10: 9, Jan 13: 9, Jan 14: 10

96373 Therapeutic, prophylactic, or diagnostic injection (specify substance or drug); intra-arterial   Ⓢ

RVU			Global Days	Modifiers				
Mod	Non-Fac Total	Fac Total		51	50	62	80	MUE
	0.54	0.54	XXX	0	0	0	0	2

AMA: May 11: 7

96374 Therapeutic, prophylactic, or diagnostic injection (specify substance or drug); intravenous push, single or initial substance/drug   Ⓢ

RVU			Global Days	Modifiers				
Mod	Non-Fac Total	Fac Total		51	50	62	80	MUE
	1.60	1.60	XXX	0	0	0	0	1

AMA: May 11: 7, Oct 11: 3, Dec 11: 4, May 10: 8, Feb 13: 3, Jun 13: 9

● New   ▲ Revised   Deleted   ⊙ Moderate Sedation   ✚ Add-on Codes   ⊘ High Risk Denial   Ⓐ Age Edit   ♀ Female   ♂ Male   **AMA** *CPT® Assistant*   **MUE** Medically Unlikely Edit
⊘ Modifier 51 Exempt   ⊖ Modifier 63 Exempt   ✗ Unlisted   **Modifiers:** *See Inside Back Cover*   Ⓜ Maternity   A2–Z3 ASC Payment Indicators   A–Y OPPS Status Indicators

© 2016 DecisionHealth   CPT © 2015 American Medical Association. All Rights Reserved.

+ 96375 Therapeutic, prophylactic, or diagnostic injection (specify substance or drug); each additional sequential intravenous push of a new substance/drug (List separately in addition to code for primary procedure)   S

Mod	RVU Non-Fac Total	Fac Total	Global Days	Modifiers 51	50	62	80	MUE
	0.63	0.63	ZZZ	0	0	0	0	

AMA: May 11: 7, May 10: 8, Feb 13: 3

+ 96376 Therapeutic, prophylactic, or diagnostic injection (specify substance or drug); each additional sequential intravenous push of the same substance/drug provided in a facility (List separately in addition to code for primary procedure)   ⓒN

Mod	RVU Non-Fac Total	Fac Total	Global Days	Modifiers 51	50	62	80	MUE
	0.00	0.00	ZZZ	9	9	9	9	0

AMA: May 11: 7, Dec 11: 3, May 10: 6, Nov 14: 15

96379 Unlisted therapeutic, prophylactic, or diagnostic intravenous or intra-arterial injection or infusion   ⓒⓍS

Mod	RVU Non-Fac Total	Fac Total	Global Days	Modifiers 51	50	62	80	MUE
	0.00	0.00	XXX	0	0	0	0	

AMA: May 11: 7, Dec 11: 19

Chemotherapy Administration Services

Injection/Intravenous Infusion Chemotherapy Administration

Coding Guidance

Codes 96401-96425 include both the work and practice expenses of code 99211, which may not be reported in addition to chemotherapy administration. Other E&M codes may be reported with modifier 25, if the physician provides a distinctly identifiable, separate E&M service.

96401 Chemotherapy administration, subcutaneous or intramuscular; non-hormonal anti-neoplastic   S

Mod	RVU Non-Fac Total	Fac Total	Global Days	Modifiers 51	50	62	80	MUE
	2.10	2.10	XXX	0	0	0	0	

AMA: Nov 05: 1, Jan 06: 47, Jan 07: 30, May 07: 3, Jun 07: 4, Feb 09: 17, Aug 11: 9, Dec 11: 3

96402 Chemotherapy administration, subcutaneous or intramuscular; hormonal anti-neoplastic   S

Mod	RVU Non-Fac Total	Fac Total	Global Days	Modifiers 51	50	62	80	MUE
	0.91	0.91	XXX	0	0	0	0	2

AMA: Nov 05: 1, Jan 07: 30, May 07: 3, Feb 09: 17, Dec 11: 3

Coding Guidance

Nonspecific lesion injection codes should not be used to report the administration of local anesthesia for another definitive procedure. Codes 96405 and 96406 are not reported together, unless separate groups of lesions are injected with different agents, in which case, a modifier should be attached.

96405 Chemotherapy administration; intralesional, up to and including 7 lesions   S

Mod	RVU Non-Fac Total	Fac Total	Global Days	Modifiers 51	50	62	80	MUE
	2.32	0.86	000	2	0	0	1	1

AMA: Sep 96: 5, Aug 97: 19, Feb 01: 10, Jul 01: 2, Nov 05: 1, Jan 07: 30, May 07: 3, Feb 09: 17

96406 Chemotherapy administration; intralesional, more than 7 lesions   S

Mod	RVU Non-Fac Total	Fac Total	Global Days	Modifiers 51	50	62	80	MUE
	3.29	1.32	000	2	0	0	1	1

AMA: Sep 96: 5, Aug 97: 19, Feb 01: 10, Jul 01: 2, Nov 05: 1, Jan 07: 30, May 07: 3, Feb 09: 17

96409 Chemotherapy administration; intravenous, push technique, single or initial substance/drug   S

Mod	RVU Non-Fac Total	Fac Total	Global Days	Modifiers 51	50	62	80	MUE
	3.11	3.11	XXX	0	0	0	0	1

AMA: Nov 05: 1, Jan 07: 30, May 07: 3, Feb 09: 17, Dec 11: 3, May 10: 8, May 11: 17

+ 96411 Chemotherapy administration; intravenous, push technique, each additional substance/drug (List separately in addition to code for primary procedure)   S

Mod	RVU Non-Fac Total	Fac Total	Global Days	Modifiers 51	50	62	80	MUE
	1.75	1.75	ZZZ	0	0	0	0	

AMA: Nov 05: 1, Jan 07: 30, May 07: 3, Feb 09: 17, Dec 11: 3

96413 Chemotherapy administration, intravenous infusion technique; up to 1 hour, single or initial substance/drug   S

Mod	RVU Non-Fac Total	Fac Total	Global Days	Modifiers 51	50	62	80	MUE
	3.80	3.80	XXX	0	0	0	0	1

AMA: Nov 05: 1, Jan 07: 30, May 07: 3, Sep 07: 3, Dec 07: 15, Feb 09: 17, Dec 11: 4, May 10: 8, May 11: 7

+ 96415 Chemotherapy administration, intravenous infusion technique; each additional hour (List separately in addition to code for primary procedure)   S

Mod	RVU Non-Fac Total	Fac Total	Global Days	Modifiers 51	50	62	80	MUE
	0.80	0.80	ZZZ	0	0	0	0	

AMA: Nov 05: 1, Jan 07: 30, May 07: 3, Sep 07: 3, Dec 07: 15, Feb 09: 17, Dec 11: 3

96416 Chemotherapy administration, intravenous infusion technique; initiation of prolonged chemotherapy infusion (more than 8 hours), requiring use of a portable or implantable pump   S

Mod	RVU Non-Fac Total	Fac Total	Global Days	Modifiers 51	50	62	80	MUE
	3.95	3.95	XXX	0	0	0	0	1

AMA: Nov 05: 1, Jan 07: 30, May 07: 3, Sep 07: 3, Dec 07: 15, Feb 09: 17, Dec 11: 3

● New   ▲ Revised   ✖ Deleted   ⊙ Moderate Sedation   ✚ Add-on Codes   ⊘ High Risk Denial   ⓐ Age Edit   ♀ Female   ♂ Male   **AMA** CPT® Assistant   **MUE** Medically Unlikely Edit
⊘ Modifier 51 Exempt   ⊖ Modifier 63 Exempt   Ⓧ Unlisted   **Modifiers:** See Inside Back Cover   Ⓜ Maternity   A2–Z3 ASC Payment Indicators   A–Y OPPS Status Indicators

846   CPT © 2015 American Medical Association. All Rights Reserved.   © 2016 DecisionHealth

+ 96417 Chemotherapy administration, intravenous infusion technique; each additional sequential infusion (different substance/drug), up to 1 hour (List separately in addition to code for primary procedure) ⓢ

RVU		Global Days	Modifiers				
Mod	Non-Fac Total	Fac Total		51	50	62	80	MUE
	1.76	1.76	ZZZ	0	0	0	0	

AMA: Nov 05: 1, Jan 07: 30, May 07: 3, Jun 07: 4, Feb 09: 17, Aug 11: 9, Dec 11: 3

Intra-Arterial Chemotherapy Administration

96420 Chemotherapy administration, intra-arterial; push technique ⊘ⓢ

RVU		Global Days	Modifiers				
Mod	Non-Fac Total	Fac Total		51	50	62	80	MUE
	2.91	2.91	XXX	0	0	0	0	2

AMA: Aug 97: 19, Nov 98: 37, Nov 99: 54, Feb 01: 10, Jul 01: 2, Nov 05: 1, Jan 07: 30, May 07: 3, Jun 07: 4, Feb 09: 17, Aug 11: 9, Dec 11: 3, Nov 13: 6

96422 Chemotherapy administration, intra-arterial; infusion technique, up to 1 hour ⓢ

RVU		Global Days	Modifiers				
Mod	Non-Fac Total	Fac Total		51	50	62	80	MUE
	4.77	4.77	XXX	0	0	0	0	2

AMA: Dec 96: 10, Aug 97: 19, Nov 98: 37, Feb 01: 10, Jul 01: 2, Nov 05: 1, Jan 07: 30, May 07: 3, Dec 07: 15, Feb 09: 17, Dec 11: 3, Aug 11: 9

+ 96423 Chemotherapy administration, intra-arterial; infusion technique, each additional hour (List separately in addition to code for primary procedure) ⊘ⓢ

RVU		Global Days	Modifiers				
Mod	Non-Fac Total	Fac Total		51	50	62	80	MUE
	2.21	2.21	ZZZ	0	0	0	0	

AMA: Dec 96: 10, Nov 98: 37, Feb 01: 10, Jul 01: 2, Nov 05: 1, Jan 07: 30, May 07: 3, Dec 07: 15, Feb 09: 17, Dec 11: 3

96425 Chemotherapy administration, intra-arterial; infusion technique, initiation of prolonged infusion (more than 8 hours), requiring the use of a portable or implantable pump ⓢ

RVU		Global Days	Modifiers				
Mod	Non-Fac Total	Fac Total		51	50	62	80	MUE
	5.10	5.10	XXX	0	0	0	0	1

AMA: Nov 99: 54, Feb 01: 10, Jul 01: 2, Nov 05: 1, Jan 07: 30, May 07: 3, Jun 07: 4, Feb 09: 17, Aug 11: 9, Dec 11: 3

Other Chemotherapy Administration

96440 Chemotherapy administration into pleural cavity, requiring and including thoracentesis ⓢ

RVU		Global Days	Modifiers				
Mod	Non-Fac Total	Fac Total		51	50	62	80	MUE
	24.08	4.03	000	0	0	0	0	1

AMA: Feb 01: 10, Jul 01: 2, Nov 05: 1, Jan 07: 30, May 07: 3, Jun 07: 4, Feb 09: 17

96446 Chemotherapy administration into the peritoneal cavity via indwelling port or catheter ⓢ

RVU		Global Days	Modifiers				
Mod	Non-Fac Total	Fac Total		51	50	62	80	MUE
	5.66	0.82	XXX	0	0	0	0	1

AMA: Oct 10: 16, Dec 10: 16

96450 Chemotherapy administration, into CNS (eg, intrathecal), requiring and including spinal puncture ⓢ

RVU		Global Days	Modifiers				
Mod	Non-Fac Total	Fac Total		51	50	62	80	MUE
	5.13	2.30	000	0	0	0	0	1

AMA: Feb 01: 10, Jul 01: 2, Nov 05: 1, Jan 07: 30, May 07: 3, Feb 09: 17

96521 Refilling and maintenance of portable pump ⓢ

RVU		Global Days	Modifiers				
Mod	Non-Fac Total	Fac Total		51	50	62	80	MUE
	3.87	3.87	XXX	0	0	0	0	2

AMA: Nov 05: 1, Jan 07: 30, May 07: 3, Feb 09: 17, Dec 11: 3

96522 Refilling and maintenance of implantable pump or reservoir for drug delivery, systemic (eg, intravenous, intra-arterial) ⓢ

RVU		Global Days	Modifiers				
Mod	Non-Fac Total	Fac Total		51	50	62	80	MUE
	3.18	3.18	XXX	0	0	0	0	1

AMA: Jul 06: 1, Jan 07: 30, May 07: 3, Feb 09: 17, Dec 11: 3

Coding Guidance

Flushing or irrigating an implanted vascular access port or device before infusing a chemotherapeutic/nonchemotherapeutic substance is included in the drug administration code. Do not report 96523 in addition.

96523 Irrigation of implanted venous access device for drug delivery systems ◎Ⓘ

RVU		Global Days	Modifiers				
Mod	Non-Fac Total	Fac Total		51	50	62	80	MUE
	0.70	0.70	XXX	0	0	0	0	1

AMA: Jan 07: 30, May 07: 3, Feb 09: 17, Jul 11: 16, Dec 11: 3

Pub 100-04, 12, 30.5

96542 Chemotherapy injection, subarachnoid or intraventricular via subcutaneous reservoir, single or multiple agents ⓢ

RVU		Global Days	Modifiers				
Mod	Non-Fac Total	Fac Total		51	50	62	80	MUE
	3.40	1.20	XXX	0	0	0	0	1

AMA: Aug 97: 19, Jul 01: 2, Nov 05: 1, Jan 07: 30, May 07: 3, Feb 09: 17

96549 Unlisted chemotherapy procedure ⊘xⓢ

RVU		Global Days	Modifiers				
Mod	Non-Fac Total	Fac Total		51	50	62	80	MUE
	0.00	0.00	XXX	0	0	0	0	

AMA: Aug 97: 19, Jul 01: 2, Nov 05: 1, Jan 07: 30, May 07: 3, Jun 07: 4, Oct 10: 16, Dec 10: 16

Photodynamic Therapy Procedures

96567 Photodynamic therapy by external application of light to destroy premalignant and/or malignant lesions of the skin and adjacent mucosa (eg, lip) by activation of photosensitive drug(s), each phototherapy exposure session ◎Ⓘ

RVU		Global Days	Modifiers				
Mod	Non-Fac Total	Fac Total		51	50	62	80	MUE
	3.82	3.82	XXX	0	0	0	0	1

AMA: Aug 03: 15, Aug 09: 7, Mar 10: 10

● New   ▲ Revised   Deleted   ⊙ Moderate Sedation   ✚ Add-on Codes   ⊘ High Risk Denial   Ⓐ Age Edit   ♀ Female   ♂ Male   **AMA** *CPT® Assistant*   ***MUE*** Medically Unlikely Edit
⊘ Modifier 51 Exempt   ⊖ Modifier 63 Exempt   ✗ Unlisted   **Modifiers:** *See Inside Back Cover*   Ⓜ Maternity   A2–Z3 ASC Payment Indicators   A–Y OPPS Status Indicators

© 2016 DecisionHealth   CPT © 2015 American Medical Association. All Rights Reserved.   **847**

+ 96570 Photodynamic therapy by endoscopic application of light to ablate abnormal tissue via activation of photosensitive drug(s); first 30 minutes (List separately in addition to code for endoscopy or bronchoscopy procedures of lung and gastrointestinal tract) **N**

RVU			Global Days	Modifiers				
Mod	Non-Fac Total	Fac Total		51	50	62	80	MUE
	1.65	1.65	ZZZ	0	0	0	1	1

AMA: Nov 99: 54, Sep 00: 5, Oct 11: 11, Apr 13: 8

+ 96571 Photodynamic therapy by endoscopic application of light to ablate abnormal tissue via activation of photosensitive drug(s); each additional 15 minutes (List separately in addition to code for endoscopy or bronchoscopy procedures of lung and gastrointestinal tract) **N**

RVU			Global Days	Modifiers				
Mod	Non-Fac Total	Fac Total		51	50	62	80	MUE
	0.77	0.77	ZZZ	0	0	0	1	3

AMA: Nov 99: 54, Sep 00: 5, Oct 11: 11, Apr 13: 8

Dermatological Procedures

96900 Actinotherapy (ultraviolet light) **Q1**

RVU			Global Days	Modifiers				
Mod	Non-Fac Total	Fac Total		51	50	62	80	MUE
	0.58	0.58	XXX	0	0	0	0	1

AMA: Jul 12: 9

96902 Microscopic examination of hairs plucked or clipped by the examiner (excluding hair collected by the patient) to determine telogen and anagen counts, or structural hair shaft abnormality **N**

RVU			Global Days	Modifiers				
Mod	Non-Fac Total	Fac Total		51	50	62	80	MUE
	0.61	0.59	XXX	9	9	9	9	0

AMA: Nov 97: 46, 47

96904 Whole body integumentary photography, for monitoring of high risk patients with dysplastic nevus syndrome or a history of dysplastic nevi, or patients with a personal or familial history of melanoma **N**

RVU			Global Days	Modifiers				
Mod	Non-Fac Total	Fac Total		51	50	62	80	MUE
	1.78	1.78	XXX	0	0	0	0	1

96910 Photochemotherapy; tar and ultraviolet B (Goeckerman treatment) or petrolatum and ultraviolet B **Q1**

RVU			Global Days	Modifiers				
Mod	Non-Fac Total	Fac Total		51	50	62	80	MUE
	2.02	2.02	XXX	0	0	0	0	1

AMA: Jul 12: 9

96912 Photochemotherapy; psoralens and ultraviolet A (PUVA) **Q1**

RVU			Global Days	Modifiers				
Mod	Non-Fac Total	Fac Total		51	50	62	80	MUE
	2.58	2.58	XXX	0	0	0	0	1

AMA: Jul 12: 9

96913 Photochemotherapy (Goeckerman and/or PUVA) for severe photoresponsive dermatoses requiring at least 4-8 hours of care under direct supervision of the physician (includes application of medication and dressings) **T**

RVU			Global Days	Modifiers				
Mod	Non-Fac Total	Fac Total		51	50	62	80	MUE
	3.70	3.70	XXX	0	0	0	0	1

96920 Laser treatment for inflammatory skin disease (psoriasis); total area less than 250 sq cm **Q1**

RVU			Global Days	Modifiers				
Mod	Non-Fac Total	Fac Total		51	50	62	80	MUE
	4.39	1.91	000	2	0	0	1	1

AMA: Jul 12: 9, Oct 10: 9, May 13: 12

96921 Laser treatment for inflammatory skin disease (psoriasis); 250 sq cm to 500 sq cm **Q1**

RVU			Global Days	Modifiers				
Mod	Non-Fac Total	Fac Total		51	50	62	80	MUE
	4.84	2.15	000	2	0	0	1	1

AMA: Jul 12: 9, Oct 10: 9, May 13: 12

96922 Laser treatment for inflammatory skin disease (psoriasis); over 500 sq cm **Q1**

RVU			Global Days	Modifiers				
Mod	Non-Fac Total	Fac Total		51	50	62	80	MUE
	6.71	3.48	000	2	0	0	1	1

AMA: Oct 10: 9, Jul 12: 9, May 13: 12

● 96931 Reflectance confocal microscopy (RCM) for cellular and sub-cellular imaging of skin; image acquisition and interpretation and report, first lesion **M**

RVU			Global Days	Modifiers				
Mod	Non-Fac Total	Fac Total		51	50	62	80	MUE
	0.00	0.00	YYY	0	0	0	0	1

● 96932 Reflectance confocal microscopy (RCM) for cellular and sub-cellular imaging of skin; image acquisition only, first lesion **Q1**

RVU			Global Days	Modifiers				
Mod	Non-Fac Total	Fac Total		51	50	62	80	MUE
	0.00	0.00	YYY	0	0	0	0	1

● 96933 Reflectance confocal microscopy (RCM) for cellular and sub-cellular imaging of skin; interpretation and report only, first lesion **B**

RVU			Global Days	Modifiers				
Mod	Non-Fac Total	Fac Total		51	50	62	80	MUE
	0.00	0.00	YYY	0	0	0	0	1

+● 96934 Reflectance confocal microscopy (RCM) for cellular and sub-cellular imaging of skin; image acquisition and interpretation and report, each additional lesion (List separately in addition to code for primary procedure) **N**

RVU			Global Days	Modifiers				
Mod	Non-Fac Total	Fac Total		51	50	62	80	MUE
	0.00	0.00	YYY	0	0	0	0	

● New   ▲ Revised   ✖ Deleted   ⊙ Moderate Sedation   ✚ Add-on Codes   ⊘ High Risk Denial   Ⓐ Age Edit   ♀ Female   ♂ Male   **AMA** *CPT® Assistant*   *MUE* Medically Unlikely Edit
⊘ Modifier 51 Exempt   ⊖ Modifier 63 Exempt   ⊠ Unlisted   **Modifiers:** *See Inside Back Cover*   Ⓜ Maternity   A2–Z3 ASC Payment Indicators   A–Y OPPS Status Indicators

+● 96935 Reflectance confocal microscopy (RCM) for cellular and sub-cellular imaging of skin; image acquisition only, each additional lesion (List separately in addition to code for primary procedure)   N

RVU		Global Days	Modifiers				
Mod	Non-Fac Total	Fac Total		51	50	62	80	MUE
	0.00	0.00	YYY	0	0	0	0

+● 96936 Reflectance confocal microscopy (RCM) for cellular and sub-cellular imaging of skin; interpretation and report only, each additional lesion (List separately in addition to code for primary procedure)   N

RVU		Global Days	Modifiers				
Mod	Non-Fac Total	Fac Total		51	50	62	80	MUE
	0.00	0.00	YYY	0	0	0	0

96999 Unlisted special dermatological service or procedure   ⊘x Q 1

RVU		Global Days	Modifiers				
Mod	Non-Fac Total	Fac Total		51	50	62	80	MUE
	0.00	0.00	XXX	0	0	0	0

AMA: Jul 12: 9, May 13: 12

Physical Medicine/Rehabilitation Therapy Services

Coding Guidance
Physical medicine and rehabilitation therapy codes cannot be reported together for the same 15 minute time period and they are excluded from the use of modifier 51. When two procedures are performed in different timed intervals, modifier 59 may be used to report both services, even if they were sequential.

Coding Guidance
Re-evaluation codes 97002, 97004, 97006 are not reported routinely during a planned course of therapy. If there is a change in patient status and re-evaluation is needed, report with modifier 59.

97001 Physical therapy evaluation   A

RVU		Global Days	Modifiers				
Mod	Non-Fac Total	Fac Total		51	50	62	80	MUE
	2.11	2.11	XXX	5	0	0	0

AMA: Nov 97: 47, Feb 00: 11, Sep 01: 10, Oct 02: 11, Dec 03: 4, Feb 04: 5, Apr 05: 13, Aug 06: 11, May 08: 9, Jun 15: 11
Pub 100-02, 15, 80.3

97002 Physical therapy re-evaluation   A

RVU		Global Days	Modifiers				
Mod	Non-Fac Total	Fac Total		51	50	62	80	MUE
	1.18	1.18	XXX	5	0	0	0

AMA: Nov 97: 47, Feb 00: 11, Sep 01: 10, Oct 02: 11, Dec 03: 4, Feb 04: 5, May 08: 9
Pub 100-02, 15, 80.3

97003 Occupational therapy evaluation   A

RVU		Global Days	Modifiers				
Mod	Non-Fac Total	Fac Total		51	50	62	80	MUE
	2.39	2.39	XXX	5	0	0	0

AMA: Nov 97: 47, Oct 02: 11, Feb 04: 5, Aug 06: 11, May 08: 9, Jun 14: 3
Pub 100-02, 15, 80.3

97004 Occupational therapy re-evaluation   A

RVU		Global Days	Modifiers				
Mod	Non-Fac Total	Fac Total		51	50	62	80	MUE
	1.48	1.48	XXX	5	0	0	0

AMA: Nov 97: 47, Oct 02: 11, Feb 04: 5, May 08: 9, Jun 14: 3
Pub 100-02, 15, 80.3

97005 Athletic training evaluation   ⊘E

RVU		Global Days	Modifiers				
Mod	Non-Fac Total	Fac Total		51	50	62	80	MUE
	0.00	0.00	XXX	9	9	9	9

AMA: Jun 02: 9, Feb 04: 5

97006 Athletic training re-evaluation   ⊘E

RVU		Global Days	Modifiers				
Mod	Non-Fac Total	Fac Total		51	50	62	80	MUE
	0.00	0.00	XXX	9	9	9	9

AMA: Jun 02: 9, Feb 04: 5

Supervised Modalities

Coding Guidance
Supervised modality codes 97010-97028 may be reported for the same 15 minute time period as other therapy services.

97010 Application of a modality to 1 or more areas; hot or cold packs   ⊘A

RVU		Global Days	Modifiers				
Mod	Non-Fac Total	Fac Total		51	50	62	80	MUE
	0.17	0.17	XXX	9	9	9	9	0

AMA: Summer 95: 5, Apr 96: 11, Nov 97: 47, Dec 98: 1, Nov 01: 5, Aug 02: 11, Aug 06: 11, Nov 09: 10, Jun 10: 8, Aug 10: 13, Nov 10: 8

97012 Application of a modality to 1 or more areas; traction, mechanical   ⊘A

Documentation Finder: Make sure the documentation references mechanical traction being applied or performed on one or more areas. This does not require the therapist to spend one-on-one time with the patient, nor does time need to be documented. Some key words in the documentation would be degree of traction being applied, angles of the pulling or autotraction and mechanical, computerized or motorized device. Vertebral axial depression (VAD) also would be a term in the documentation to support this code.

RVU		Global Days	Modifiers				
Mod	Non-Fac Total	Fac Total		51	50	62	80	MUE
	0.45	0.45	XXX	5	0	0	0	1

AMA: Summer 95: 5, Apr 96: 11, Nov 97: 47, Dec 98: 1, May 99: 11, Nov 01: 5, Aug 02: 11, Dec 03: 4, Oct 04: 9, Jun 10: 8, Aug 10: 13, Nov 10: 8

97014 Application of a modality to 1 or more areas; electrical stimulation (unattended)   ⊘E

Coding tip: Code 97014 is not appropriate for reporting electrical stimulation to aid in bone healing; use bone stimulation codes 20974-20975.

RVU		Global Days	Modifiers				
Mod	Non-Fac Total	Fac Total		51	50	62	80	MUE
	0.45	0.45	XXX	9	9	9	9	0

AMA: Summer 95: 5, Apr 96: 11, Nov 97: 47, May 98: 10, Nov 01: 5, Jan 02: 11, Apr 02: 18, Aug 02: 11, Dec 03: 4, Nov 09: 10, Aug 11: 6, Jun 10: 8, Aug 10: 13, Nov 10: 8

97016 Application of a modality to 1 or more areas; vasopneumatic devices   A

RVU		Global Days	Modifiers				
Mod	Non-Fac Total	Fac Total		51	50	62	80	MUE
	0.54	0.54	XXX	5	0	0	0	1

AMA: Summer 95: 6, Apr 96: 11, Dec 98: 1, Nov 01: 5, Aug 02: 11, May 05: 14, Jun 10: 8, Aug 10: 13, Nov 10: 8

Medicine Procedures

97018 – 97110

97018 Application of a modality to 1 or more areas; paraffin bath A

RVU			Global Days	Modifiers				
Mod	Non-Fac Total	Fac Total		51	50	62	80	MUE
	0.31	0.31	XXX	5	0	0	0	1

AMA: Summer 95: 6, Apr 96: 11, Dec 98: 1, Nov 01: 5, Aug 02: 11, Nov 09: 10, Jun 10: 8, Aug 10: 13, Nov 10: 8

97022 Application of a modality to 1 or more areas; whirlpool A

RVU			Global Days	Modifiers				
Mod	Non-Fac Total	Fac Total		51	50	62	80	MUE
	0.66	0.66	XXX	5	0	0	0	1

AMA: Summer 95: 6, Apr 96: 11, May 98: 10, Dec 98: 1, Nov 01: 5, Aug 02: 11, Nov 09: 10, Jun 10: 8, Aug 10: 13, Nov 10: 8

97024 Application of a modality to 1 or more areas; diathermy (eg, microwave) A

Documentation Finder: Make sure the documentation has reference to creating heat in the soft tissues by the passage of high frequency electrical currents. This does not require the therapist to spend one-on-one time with the patient, nor does time need to be documented.

RVU			Global Days	Modifiers				
Mod	Non-Fac Total	Fac Total		51	50	62	80	MUE
	0.18	0.18	XXX	5	0	0	0	1

AMA: Summer 95: 6, Apr 96: 11, Dec 98: 1, Nov 01: 5, Aug 02: 11, Nov 09: 10, Jun 10: 8, Aug 10: 13, Nov 10: 8

97026 Application of a modality to 1 or more areas; infrared A

Documentation Finder: Make sure the documentation has reference to using light and heat to rinse the tissue temperature 5 degrees to 10 degrees centigrade in the area of application. This does not require the therapist to spend one-on-one time with the patient, nor does time need to be documented.

RVU			Global Days	Modifiers				
Mod	Non-Fac Total	Fac Total		51	50	62	80	MUE
	0.17	0.17	XXX	5	0	0	0	1

AMA: Summer 95: 6, Apr 96: 11, Dec 98: 1, Nov 01: 5, Aug 02: 11, Nov 09: 10, Feb 10: 12, Jun 10: 8, Aug 10: 13, Nov 10: 8

97028 Application of a modality to 1 or more areas; ultraviolet A

RVU			Global Days	Modifiers				
Mod	Non-Fac Total	Fac Total		51	50	62	80	MUE
	0.21	0.21	XXX	5	0	0	0	1

AMA: Summer 95: 6, Apr 96: 11, Dec 98: 1, Nov 01: 5, Aug 02: 11, Nov 09: 10, Jun 10: 8, Aug 10: 13, Nov 10: 8

Constant Attendance Modalities

97032 Application of a modality to 1 or more areas; electrical stimulation (manual), each 15 minutes A

Coding tip: Code 97032 is not appropriate for reporting electrical stimulation to aid in bone healing; use bone stimulation codes 20974-20975.

RVU			Global Days	Modifiers				
Mod	Non-Fac Total	Fac Total		51	50	62	80	MUE
	0.54	0.54	XXX	5	0	0	0	

AMA: Summer 95: 6, Dec 98: 1, Nov 01: 5, Apr 02: 18, Jul 04: 14, Nov 09: 10, Jun 10: 8, Aug 10: 13, Nov 10: 8

97033 Application of a modality to 1 or more areas; iontophoresis, each 15 minutes A

RVU			Global Days	Modifiers				
Mod	Non-Fac Total	Fac Total		51	50	62	80	MUE
	0.74	0.74	XXX	5	0	0	0	

AMA: Summer 95: 7, Dec 98: 1, Nov 01: 5, Nov 09: 10, Jun 10: 8, Aug 10: 13, Nov 10: 8

97034 Application of a modality to 1 or more areas; contrast baths, each 15 minutes A

RVU			Global Days	Modifiers				
Mod	Non-Fac Total	Fac Total		51	50	62	80	MUE
	0.51	0.51	XXX	5	0	0	0	

AMA: Summer 95: 7, Dec 98: 1, Nov 01: 5, Jun 10: 8, Aug 10: 13, Nov 10: 8

97035 Application of a modality to 1 or more areas; ultrasound, each 15 minutes A

RVU			Global Days	Modifiers				
Mod	Non-Fac Total	Fac Total		51	50	62	80	MUE
	0.35	0.35	XXX	5	0	0	0	

AMA: Summer 95: 7, Sep 96: 10, Dec 98: 1, Nov 01: 5, Nov 09: 10, Jun 10: 8, Aug 10: 13, Nov 10: 8

97036 Application of a modality to 1 or more areas; Hubbard tank, each 15 minutes A

RVU			Global Days	Modifiers				
Mod	Non-Fac Total	Fac Total		51	50	62	80	MUE
	0.93	0.93	XXX	5	0	0	0	

AMA: Summer 95: 7, Dec 98: 1, Nov 01: 5, Nov 09: 10, Jun 10: 8, Aug 10: 13, Nov 10: 8

97039 Unlisted modality (specify type and time if constant attendance) A

RVU			Global Days	Modifiers				
Mod	Non-Fac Total	Fac Total		51	50	62	80	MUE
	0.00	0.00	XXX	0	0	0	0	

AMA: Summer 95: 7, May 98: 10, Dec 98: 1, Jan 00: 10, Nov 01: 5, May 05: 14, Nov 09: 10, Feb 10: 12, Jun 10: 8, Aug 10: 13, Nov 10: 8

Therapeutic Physical Medicine Procedures

97110 Therapeutic procedure, 1 or more areas, each 15 minutes; therapeutic exercises to develop strength and endurance, range of motion and flexibility A

Documentation Finder: Make sure the documentation supports the therapist is working one-on-one with the patient and reflects the total time spent providing exercise to develop strength and endurance. Some of the parameters you may see in the documentation could be work done on a treadmill, using a gymnastic ball, stabilizing exercises, etc. You will see words such as strengthening, endurance, range of motion, etc.

RVU			Global Days	Modifiers				
Mod	Non-Fac Total	Fac Total		51	50	62	80	MUE
	0.91	0.91	XXX	5	0	0	0	

AMA: Summer 95: 7, Feb 97: 10, Nov 98: 37, Dec 99: 11, Mar 05: 11, Apr 05: 14, Aug 05: 11, Dec 05: 8, Mar 06: 15, Aug 06: 11, May 08: 13, Dec 09: 15, May 10: 9, Mar 12: 9, Mar 14: 15, Aug 14: 6

Pub 100-02, 15, 80.3

● New   ▲ Revised   ✖ Deleted   ⊙ Moderate Sedation   ✚ Add-on Codes   ⊘ High Risk Denial   Ⓐ Age Edit   ♀ Female   ♂ Male   **AMA** CPT® Assistant   **MUE** Medically Unlikely Edit
⊘ Modifier 51 Exempt   ⊖ Modifier 63 Exempt   ✗ Unlisted   **Modifiers:** See Inside Back Cover   Ⓜ Maternity   A 2 – Z 3 ASC Payment Indicators   A – Y OPPS Status Indicators

850   CPT © 2015 American Medical Association. All Rights Reserved.   © 2016 DecisionHealth

97112 **Therapeutic procedure, 1 or more areas, each 15 minutes; neuromuscular reeducation of movement, balance, coordination, kinesthetic sense, posture, and/or proprioception for sitting and/or standing activities** Ⓐ

Documentation Finder: Make sure the documentation supports the therapist is working one-on-one with the patient and reflects the total time spent providing neuromuscular re-education with this patient. Some examples that could be found in the documentation could include proprioceptive neuromuscular facilitation (PNF), Feldenkreis, Bobath, BAPS boards and desensitization techniques. Taping also could fall under this CPT code if the taping is being applied to facilitate movement by providing support and the tape is applied specifically to enable less painful use of the shoulder and greater function (i.e., restricting in some movement, facilitating others).

RVU			Global Days	Modifiers				
Mod	Non-Fac Total	Fac Total		51	50	62	80	MUE
	0.95	0.95	XXX	5	0	0	0	

AMA: Summer 95: 7, Feb 97: 10, Apr 05: 14, Aug 05: 11, Mar 06: 15, Aug 06: 11, May 08: 13, Oct 09: 10, May 10: 9, Mar 12: 9, Mar 14: 15

Pub 100-02, 15, 80.3

97113 **Therapeutic procedure, 1 or more areas, each 15 minutes; aquatic therapy with therapeutic exercises** Ⓐ

Documentation Finder: Make sure the documentation supports the therapist is working one-on-one with the patient and reflects the total time spent providing water exercises. Any type of exercise performed in a water environment can support reporting this code. But reference to whirlpool or Hubbard tank work would not support this code.

RVU			Global Days	Modifiers				
Mod	Non-Fac Total	Fac Total		51	50	62	80	MUE
	1.21	1.21	XXX	5	0	0	0	

AMA: Summer 95: 7, Feb 97: 10, Apr 05: 14, Mar 06: 15, Aug 06: 11, Oct 09: 10, May 10: 9, Mar 14: 15

97116 **Therapeutic procedure, 1 or more areas, each 15 minutes; gait training (includes stair climbing)** Ⓐ

Documentation Finder: Make sure the documentation supports the therapist is working one-on-one with the patient and reflects the total time spent providing gait training. Gait training can be described as stair climbing, postural stance, style of walking, etc.

RVU			Global Days	Modifiers				
Mod	Non-Fac Total	Fac Total		51	50	62	80	MUE
	0.80	0.80	XXX	5	0	0	0	

AMA: Summer 95: 8, Sep 96: 7, Feb 97: 10, Jun 03: 3, Apr 05: 14, Mar 06: 15, Aug 06: 11, Oct 09: 10, May 10: 9, Mar 14: 15

Pub 100-02, 15, 80.3

97124 **Therapeutic procedure, 1 or more areas, each 15 minutes; massage, including effleurage, petrissage and/or tapotement (stroking, compression, percussion)** Ⓢ Ⓐ

Documentation Finder: The documentation needs to support that the therapist is working one-on-one with the patient and reflect the total time spent providing therapeutic massage. You should not see any reference to mechanical massage; this is hands on therapy work. Besides the word "massage," you may also see compression, stroking, percussion.

RVU			Global Days	Modifiers				
Mod	Non-Fac Total	Fac Total		51	50	62	80	MUE
	0.74	0.74	XXX	5	0	0	0	

AMA: Summer 95: 8, May 96: 10, Feb 97: 10, Dec 99: 7, Apr 05: 14, May 05: 14, Mar 06: 15, Aug 06: 11, Oct 09: 10, May 10: 9, Mar 14: 15

97139 **Unlisted therapeutic procedure (specify)** ⓈⓧⒶ

RVU			Global Days	Modifiers				
Mod	Non-Fac Total	Fac Total		51	50	62	80	MUE
	0.00	0.00	XXX	0	0	0	0	

AMA: Summer 95: 8, Feb 97: 10, Apr 05: 14, Aug 06: 11, Mar 14: 15

97140 **Manual therapy techniques (eg, mobilization/ manipulation, manual lymphatic drainage, manual traction), 1 or more regions, each 15 minutes** Ⓐ

Documentation Finder: Make sure the documentation supports that the therapist is working one-on-one with the patient and is hands-on. In the documentation, you should find what areas the therapist is applying manual manipulation. Some of those words could be myofascial release, manual traction, passive stretching. Some of the regions documented could be shoulder, lower cervical, upper thoracic area, etc.

RVU			Global Days	Modifiers				
Mod	Non-Fac Total	Fac Total		51	50	62	80	MUE
	0.84	0.84	XXX	5	0	0	0	

AMA: Nov 98: 37, Feb 99: 10, Mar 99: 1, Jul 99: 11, Aug 01: 10, Dec 03: 5, Oct 09: 10, May 09: 9, Mar 14: 15, Mar 15: 10

Coding Guidance

Speech language pathologists do not perform services reported with 97110-97112, 97150, or 97530-97532, which are generally done by physical or occupational therapists.

97150 **Therapeutic procedure(s), group (2 or more individuals)** Ⓐ

Documentation Finder: Make sure the documentation references that therapy procedures are being performed in a group. The patients don't have to be doing all the same modality, but the therapist has to be working with a group. You would report just this code, not the actual therapy modality the patient is working on in the group setting.

RVU			Global Days	Modifiers				
Mod	Non-Fac Total	Fac Total		51	50	62	80	MUE
	0.49	0.49	XXX	5	0	0	0	1

AMA: Summer 95: 8, Dec 96: 10, Feb 97: 10, Oct 99: 10, Nov 99: 54, 55, Dec 99: 11, Apr 05: 14, Aug 06: 11, Mar 14: 15

Pub 100-02, 15, 230

97530 **Therapeutic activities, direct (one-on-one) patient contact (use of dynamic activities to improve functional performance), each 15 minutes** Ⓐ

RVU			Global Days	Modifiers				
Mod	Non-Fac Total	Fac Total		51	50	62	80	MUE
	0.98	0.98	XXX	5	0	0	0	

AMA: Summer 95: 9, Dec 01: 6, Apr 03: 26, Jul 03: 15, Aug 05: 11, May 08: 13, Mar 14: 15

97532 **Development of cognitive skills to improve attention, memory, problem solving (includes compensatory training), direct (one-on-one) patient contact, each 15 minutes** Ⓐ

RVU			Global Days	Modifiers				
Mod	Non-Fac Total	Fac Total		51	50	62	80	MUE
	0.75	0.75	XXX	0	0	0	0	

AMA: Dec 01: 1, Mar 14: 15

● New   ▲ Revised   Deleted   ⊙ Moderate Sedation   ✚ Add-on Codes   ⊘ High Risk Denial   Ⓐ Age Edit   ♀ Female   ♂ Male   **AMA** *CPT® Assistant*   *MUE* Medically Unlikely Edit

⊘ Modifier 51 Exempt   ⊖ Modifier 63 Exempt   ⓧ Unlisted   **Modifiers:** *See Inside Back Cover*   Ⓜ Maternity   Ⓐ2–Ⓩ3 ASC Payment Indicators   Ⓐ–Ⓨ OPPS Status Indicators

© 2016 DecisionHealth   CPT © 2015 American Medical Association. All Rights Reserved.   **851**

97533 Sensory integrative techniques to enhance sensory processing and promote adaptive responses to environmental demands, direct (one-on-one) patient contact, each 15 minutes 🅰

RVU			Global Days	Modifiers				
Mod	Non-Fac Total	Fac Total		51	50	62	80	MUE
	0.82	0.82	XXX	5	0	0	0	

AMA: Dec 01: 1, Mar 14: 15

97535 Self-care/home management training (eg, activities of daily living (ADL) and compensatory training, meal preparation, safety procedures, and instructions in use of assistive technology devices/adaptive equipment) direct one-on-one contact, each 15 minutes 🅰

RVU			Global Days	Modifiers				
Mod	Non-Fac Total	Fac Total		51	50	62	80	MUE
	0.99	0.99	XXX	5	0	0	0	

AMA: Sep 96: 7, Apr 00: 11, Dec 03: 6, Mar 14: 15, Mar 15: 10, Jun 15: 11

97537 Community/work reintegration training (eg, shopping, transportation, money management, avocational activities and/or work environment/ modification analysis, work task analysis, use of assistive technology device/adaptive equipment), direct one-on-one contact, each 15 minutes 🅰

RVU			Global Days	Modifiers				
Mod	Non-Fac Total	Fac Total		51	50	62	80	MUE
	0.85	0.85	XXX	5	0	0	0	

AMA: Sep 96: 7, Dec 03: 6, Mar 14: 15

97542 Wheelchair management (eg, assessment, fitting, training), each 15 minutes 🅰

Coding tip: Use code 97542 for all wheelchair management services

RVU			Global Days	Modifiers				
Mod	Non-Fac Total	Fac Total		51	50	62	80	MUE
	0.87	0.87	XXX	5	0	0	0	

AMA: Sep 96: 8, Mar 14: 15, Jun 15: 11

97545 Work hardening/conditioning; initial 2 hours ⊘🅰

RVU			Global Days	Modifiers				
Mod	Non-Fac Total	Fac Total		51	50	62	80	MUE
	0.00	0.00	XXX	0	0	0	0	1

AMA: Apr 03: 26, Jul 03: 15, May 08: 13, Mar 14: 15

+ 97546 Work hardening/conditioning; each additional hour (List separately in addition to code for primary procedure) ⊘🅰

RVU			Global Days	Modifiers				
Mod	Non-Fac Total	Fac Total		51	50	62	80	MUE
	0.00	0.00	ZZZ	0	0	0	0	2

AMA: Mar 14: 15

Active Wound Care

97597 Debridement (eg, high pressure waterjet with/ without suction, sharp selective debridement with scissors, scalpel and forceps), open wound, (eg, fibrin, devitalized epidermis and/or dermis, exudate, debris, biofilm), including topical application(s), wound assessment, use of a whirlpool, when performed and instruction(s) for ongoing care, per session, total wound(s) surface area; first 20 sq cm or less 🆃

Documentation Finder: *Make sure the documentation supports that they are removing skin and not going deeper into the subcutaneous tissues. The types of tools (i.e., scissors, scalpel) used for the selective debridement also should be noted in the documentation. Documenting the total surface area of the wound being debrided should be documented in square centimeters or in a format where the total square centimeters can be obtained.*

RVU			Global Days	Modifiers				
Mod	Non-Fac Total	Fac Total		51	50	62	80	MUE
	2.12	0.66	000	0	0	0	0	1

AMA: Jun 05: 1, 10, Nov 09: 10, May 11: 3, Sep 11: 11, Jan 12: 8, Jun 10: 8, Mar 12: 11, Nov 10: 9, Oct 12: 3, Jun 14: 11

+ 97598 Debridement (eg, high pressure waterjet with/ without suction, sharp selective debridement with scissors, scalpel and forceps), open wound, (eg, fibrin, devitalized epidermis and/or dermis, exudate, debris, biofilm), including topical application(s), wound assessment, use of a whirlpool, when performed and instruction(s) for ongoing care, per session, total wound(s) surface area; each additional 20 sq cm, or part thereof (List separately in addition to code for primary procedure) 🅽

RVU			Global Days	Modifiers				
Mod	Non-Fac Total	Fac Total		51	50	62	80	MUE
	0.69	0.31	ZZZ	0	0	0	0	

AMA: Jun 05: 1, 10, May 11: 3, Sep 11: 11, Jan 12: 8, Mar 12: 11, Jun 14: 11

97602 Removal of devitalized tissue from wound(s), non-selective debridement, without anesthesia (eg, wet-to-moist dressings, enzymatic, abrasion), including topical application(s), wound assessment, and instruction(s) for ongoing care, per session ⊘🅾🅸

RVU			Global Days	Modifiers				
Mod	Non-Fac Total	Fac Total		51	50	62	80	MUE
	0.00	0.00	XXX	9	9	9	9	0

AMA: May 02: 5, Jun 05: 1, 10, Sep 08: 11, May 11: 4, Aug 11: 7, Jan 12: 9, Mar 12: 11, Dec 12: 15, Jun 14: 11

97605 Negative pressure wound therapy (eg, vacuum assisted drainage collection), utilizing durable medical equipment (DME), including topical application(s), wound assessment, and instruction(s) for ongoing care, per session; total wound(s) surface area less than or equal to 50 square centimeters 🅾🅸

Documentation Finder: *Provider must document both total wound area treated and the type of NPWT device used for appropriate code selection.*

RVU			Global Days	Modifiers				
Mod	Non-Fac Total	Fac Total		51	50	62	80	MUE
	1.16	0.71	XXX	0	0	0	0	1

AMA: Apr 05: 13, Jun 05: 1, 10, May 11: 4, Nov 14: 8

● New   ▲ Revised   ✖ Deleted   ⊙ Moderate Sedation   ✚ Add-on Codes   ⊘ High Risk Denial   ⊛ Age Edit   ♀ Female   ♂ Male   **AMA** *CPT® Assistant*   **MUE** Medically Unlikely Edit
⊘ Modifier 51 Exempt   ⊖ Modifier 63 Exempt   ⊠ Unlisted   **Modifiers:** *See Inside Back Cover*   Ⓜ Maternity   🄰2–🅉3 ASC Payment Indicators   🄰–🅈 OPPS Status Indicators

97606 Negative pressure wound therapy (eg, vacuum assisted drainage collection), utilizing durable medical equipment (DME), including topical application(s), wound assessment, and instruction(s) for ongoing care, per session; total wound(s) surface area greater than 50 square centimeters ▣❶

Documentation Finder: Provider must document both total wound area treated and the type of NPWT device used for appropriate code selection.

RVU			Global Days	Modifiers				
Mod	Non-Fac Total	Fac Total		51	50	62	80	MUE
	1.37	0.77	XXX	0	0	0	0	1

AMA: Apr 05: 13, Jun 05: 1, 10, May 11: 4, Nov 14: 8

97607 Negative pressure wound therapy, (eg, vacuum assisted drainage collection), utilizing disposable, non-durable medical equipment including provision of exudate management collection system, topical application(s), wound assessment, and instructions for ongoing care, per session; total wound(s) surface area less than or equal to 50 square centimeters 🇹

Documentation Finder: Provider must document both total wound area treated and the type of NPWT device used for appropriate code selection.

RVU			Global Days	Modifiers				
Mod	Non-Fac Total	Fac Total		51	50	62	80	MUE
	0.00	0.00	XXX	0	0	0	0	1

AMA: Nov 14: 8

97608 Negative pressure wound therapy, (eg, vacuum assisted drainage collection), utilizing disposable, non-durable medical equipment including provision of exudate management collection system, topical application(s), wound assessment, and instructions for ongoing care, per session; total wound(s) surface area greater than 50 square centimeters 🇹

Documentation Finder: Provider must document both total wound area treated and the type of NPWT device used for appropriate code selection.

RVU			Global Days	Modifiers				
Mod	Non-Fac Total	Fac Total		51	50	62	80	MUE
	0.00	0.00	XXX	0	0	0	0	1

AMA: Nov 14: 8

97610 Low frequency, non-contact, non-thermal ultrasound, including topical application(s), when performed, wound assessment, and instruction(s) for ongoing care, per day ⊘▣❶

RVU			Global Days	Modifiers				
Mod	Non-Fac Total	Fac Total		51	50	62	80	MUE
	3.35	0.45	XXX	0	0	0	0	1

AMA: Jun 14: 11

Physical Medicine Tests/Measurement

97750 Physical performance test or measurement (eg, musculoskeletal, functional capacity), with written report, each 15 minutes ▣

RVU			Global Days	Modifiers				
Mod	Non-Fac Total	Fac Total		51	50	62	80	MUE
	0.93	0.93	XXX	5	0	0	0	

AMA: Summer 95: 5, Feb 97: 10, Aug 98: 11, Mar 00: 11, Nov 01: 5, May 02: 18, Apr 03: 28, Dec 03: 7, Feb 04: 5, Feb 07: 12, May 08: 9, Aug 13: 7

Pub 100-02, 15, 80.3

Coding Guidance
Assistive technology assessment is used with severely impaired patients, such as those with the use of only one limb.

97755 Assistive technology assessment (eg, to restore, augment or compensate for existing function, optimize functional tasks and/or maximize environmental accessibility), direct one-on-one contact, with written report, each 15 minutes ▣

RVU			Global Days	Modifiers				
Mod	Non-Fac Total	Fac Total		51	50	62	80	MUE
	1.01	1.01	XXX	5	0	0	0	

Pub 100-02, 15, 220

Orthotic/Prosthetic Management

97760 Orthotic(s) management and training (including assessment and fitting when not otherwise reported), upper extremity(s), lower extremity(s) and/or trunk, each 15 minutes ▣

RVU			Global Days	Modifiers				
Mod	Non-Fac Total	Fac Total		51	50	62	80	MUE
	1.07	1.07	XXX	5	0	0	0	

AMA: Dec 05: 8, 11, Feb 07: 8

97761 Prosthetic training, upper and/or lower extremity(s), each 15 minutes ▣

RVU			Global Days	Modifiers				
Mod	Non-Fac Total	Fac Total		51	50	62	80	MUE
	0.93	0.93	XXX	5	0	0	0	

AMA: Dec 05: 8, 11, Feb 07: 8

97762 Checkout for orthotic/prosthetic use, established patient, each 15 minutes ▣

RVU			Global Days	Modifiers				
Mod	Non-Fac Total	Fac Total		51	50	62	80	MUE
	1.34	1.34	XXX	5	0	0	0	

AMA: Dec 05: 8, 11, Feb 07: 8

Other Physical Medicine Procedures

97799 Unlisted physical medicine/rehabilitation service or procedure ⊘▣

RVU			Global Days	Modifiers				
Mod	Non-Fac Total	Fac Total		51	50	62	80	MUE
	0.00	0.00	XXX	0	0	0	0	

AMA: Summer 95: 5, Oct 99: 10

Medical Nutrition Therapy Services

97802 Medical nutrition therapy; initial assessment and intervention, individual, face-to-face with the patient, each 15 minutes ▣

RVU			Global Days	Modifiers				
Mod	Non-Fac Total	Fac Total		51	50	62	80	MUE
	0.98	0.92	XXX	0	0	0	0	

AMA: Apr 03: 10, Nov 03: 1, Feb 09: 13

Pub 100-04, 12, 190.3; 100-04, 18, 1.2

Medicine Procedures

97803 – 98940

97803 Medical nutrition therapy; re-assessment and intervention, individual, face-to-face with the patient, each 15 minutes Ⓐ

RVU		Global Days	Modifiers				
Mod	Non-Fac Total	Fac Total		51	50	62	80	MUE
	0.85	0.78	XXX	0	0	0	0	

AMA: Apr 03: 10, Nov 03: 1, Feb 09: 13

Pub 100-04, 12, 190.3; 100-04, 18, 1.2

97804 Medical nutrition therapy; group (2 or more individual(s)), each 30 minutes ⒸⒶ

Documentation Finder: Documentation must show that this is not being performed by the physician/non-physician practitioner (NPP) but is performed by a registered dietitian and other licensed nutrition qualified professionals. Documentation must show the number of minutes as well as the size of the group. Detailed information must be supplied as to what nutritional information was discussed during this group session.

RVU		Global Days	Modifiers				
Mod	Non-Fac Total	Fac Total		51	50	62	80	MUE
	0.44	0.43	XXX	0	0	0	0	

AMA: Apr 03: 10, Nov 03: 1, Feb 09: 13

Pub 100-04, 12, 190.3; 100-04, 18, 1.2

Acupuncture Procedures

97810 Acupuncture, 1 or more needles; without electrical stimulation, initial 15 minutes of personal one-on-one contact with the patient ⒸⒺ

RVU		Global Days	Modifiers				
Mod	Non-Fac Total	Fac Total		51	50	62	80	MUE
	1.03	0.87	XXX	9	9	9	9	

AMA: Jan 05: 16, 17, Jun 05: 5, Jun 06: 20, Aug 06: 4

+ 97811 Acupuncture, 1 or more needles; without electrical stimulation, each additional 15 minutes of personal one-on-one contact with the patient, with re-insertion of needle(s) (List separately in addition to code for primary procedure) ⒸⒺ

RVU		Global Days	Modifiers				
Mod	Non-Fac Total	Fac Total		51	50	62	80	MUE
	0.77	0.72	ZZZ	9	9	9	9	

AMA: Jan 05: 16, Jun 05: 5, Aug 06: 4

97813 Acupuncture, 1 or more needles; with electrical stimulation, initial 15 minutes of personal one-on-one contact with the patient ⒸⒺ

RVU		Global Days	Modifiers				
Mod	Non-Fac Total	Fac Total		51	50	62	80	MUE
	1.10	0.94	XXX	9	9	9	9	

AMA: Jan 05: 16, 18, Jun 05: 5, Jun 06: 20, Aug 06: 4

+ 97814 Acupuncture, 1 or more needles; with electrical stimulation, each additional 15 minutes of personal one-on-one contact with the patient, with re-insertion of needle(s) (List separately in addition to code for primary procedure) ⒸⒺ

RVU		Global Days	Modifiers				
Mod	Non-Fac Total	Fac Total		51	50	62	80	MUE
	0.87	0.79	ZZZ	9	9	9	9	

AMA: Jan 05: 16, Jun 05: 5, Aug 06: 4

Osteopathic Manipulation

Coding Guidance

Per Medicare anesthesia rules, a provider of osteopathic manipulative treatment (OMT) cannot report nerve blocks or epidural injections separately when given for anesthesia or postoperative pain for OMT.

98925 Osteopathic manipulative treatment (OMT); 1-2 body regions involved ⓆⅠ

RVU		Global Days	Modifiers				
Mod	Non-Fac Total	Fac Total		51	50	62	80	MUE
	0.89	0.67	000	0	0	0	0	1

AMA: May 96: 10, Jan 97: 8, 10, Jul 98: 10, Aug 00: 11, Dec 00: 15, Oct 09: 10

98926 Osteopathic manipulative treatment (OMT); 3-4 body regions involved ⓆⅠ

RVU		Global Days	Modifiers				
Mod	Non-Fac Total	Fac Total		51	50	62	80	MUE
	1.29	1.02	000	0	0	0	0	1

AMA: May 96: 10, Jan 97: 8, Aug 00: 11, Dec 00: 15, Oct 09: 10

98927 Osteopathic manipulative treatment (OMT); 5-6 body regions involved ⓆⅠ

RVU		Global Days	Modifiers				
Mod	Non-Fac Total	Fac Total		51	50	62	80	MUE
	1.67	1.34	000	0	0	0	0	1

AMA: May 96: 10, Jan 97: 8, Aug 00: 11, Dec 00: 15, Oct 09: 10

98928 Osteopathic manipulative treatment (OMT); 7-8 body regions involved ⓆⅠ

RVU		Global Days	Modifiers				
Mod	Non-Fac Total	Fac Total		51	50	62	80	MUE
	2.05	1.69	000	0	0	0	0	1

AMA: May 96: 10, Jan 97: 8, Aug 00: 11, Dec 00: 15, Oct 09: 10, Mar 12: 14, May 12: 14

98929 Osteopathic manipulative treatment (OMT); 9-10 body regions involved ⓆⅠ

RVU		Global Days	Modifiers				
Mod	Non-Fac Total	Fac Total		51	50	62	80	MUE
	2.45	2.03	000	0	0	0	0	1

AMA: May 96: 10, Jan 97: 8, 10, Aug 00: 11, Oct 09: 10

Chiropractic Manipulation

Coding Guidance

Medicare will cover chiropractic manipulative treatment (CMT) for five spinal regions. When services covered by codes 97112, 97124, and 97140 are performed in the same spinal region undergoing CMT, they cannot be separately reported. The provider may report these physical medicine codes in a different region other than where the CMT is performed.

98940 Chiropractic manipulative treatment (CMT); spinal, 1-2 regions ⓆⅠ

RVU		Global Days	Modifiers				
Mod	Non-Fac Total	Fac Total		51	50	62	80	MUE
	0.80	0.64	000	0	0	0	0	1

AMA: Jan 97: 7, 11, Feb 99: 10, Dec 00: 15, Mar 06: 15, Dec 07: 16, 17, Oct 09: 10, May 10: 9, Dec 13: 15

● New   ▲ Revised   ✖ Deleted   ⊙ Moderate Sedation   ✚ Add-on Codes   ⊘ High Risk Denial   Ⓐ Age Edit   ♀ Female   ♂ Male   **AMA** *CPT® Assistant*   *MUE* Medically Unlikely Edit
⊘ Modifier 51 Exempt   ⊖ Modifier 63 Exempt   ⊠ Unlisted   **Modifiers:** *See Inside Back Cover*   Ⓜ Maternity   Ⓐ②–Ⓩ③ ASC Payment Indicators   Ⓐ–Ⓨ OPPS Status Indicators

CPT © 2015 American Medical Association. All Rights Reserved.   © 2016 DecisionHealth

98941 Chiropractic manipulative treatment (CMT); spinal, 3-4 regions   ▢Ⅰ

Documentation Finder: Make sure that you see reference to hands-on manipulation. Be aware of what the spinal regions represent and that the documentation supports three to four regions being treated. CMT procedures are performed on five spinal regions:

1. Cervical region (including atlanto-occipital joint, C1 through C7);

2. Thoracic region (including costovertebral and costotransverse joints, T1 through T12);

3. Lumbar region (L1 through L5);

4. Sacral region (including the sacrococcygeal junction); and

5. Pelvic (including sacro-iliac joint, and other pelvic articulations). If C1 and C2, T4 and T5 and L3 and L4 lumbar vertebrae are being manipulated, this code would be used only once as three separate regions were manipulated. You do not report this code per level.

	RVU		Global Days	Modifiers				
Mod	Non-Fac Total	Fac Total		51	50	62	80	MUE
	1.15	0.97	000	0	0	0	0	1

AMA: Jan 97: 7, 11, Mar 97: 10, Feb 99: 10, Dec 00: 15, Mar 06: 15, Dec 07: 16, 17, Oct 09: 10, May 10: 9

98942 Chiropractic manipulative treatment (CMT); spinal, 5 regions   ▢Ⅰ

	RVU		Global Days	Modifiers				
Mod	Non-Fac Total	Fac Total		51	50	62	80	MUE
	1.49	1.32	000	0	0	0	0	1

AMA: Jan 97: 7, 11, Feb 99: 10, Dec 00: 15, Mar 06: 15, Dec 07: 16, 17, Oct 09: 10, May 10: 9

98943 Chiropractic manipulative treatment (CMT); extraspinal, 1 or more regions   ⒸE

	RVU		Global Days	Modifiers				
Mod	Non-Fac Total	Fac Total		51	50	62	80	MUE
	0.77	0.67	XXX	9	9	9	9	

AMA: Jan 97: 7, 11, Mar 97: 10, Feb 99: 10, Dec 00: 15, Mar 06: 15, Dec 07: 16, 17, Oct 09: 10, May 10: 9, Dec 13: 15

Patient Self-Management Education and Training

98960 Education and training for patient self-management by a qualified, nonphysician health care professional using a standardized curriculum, face-to-face with the patient (could include caregiver/family) each 30 minutes; individual patient   ⒸE

	RVU		Global Days	Modifiers				
Mod	Non-Fac Total	Fac Total		51	50	62	80	MUE
	0.79	0.79	XXX	9	9	9	9	

AMA: Apr 13: 3, Nov 13: 3, Oct 14: 3

98961 Education and training for patient self-management by a qualified, nonphysician health care professional using a standardized curriculum, face-to-face with the patient (could include caregiver/family) each 30 minutes; 2-4 patients   ⒸE

	RVU		Global Days	Modifiers				
Mod	Non-Fac Total	Fac Total		51	50	62	80	MUE
	0.38	0.38	XXX	9	9	9	9	

AMA: Aug 07: 9, Aug 08: 3, Feb 09: 13, Apr 13: 3

98962 Education and training for patient self-management by a qualified, nonphysician health care professional using a standardized curriculum, face-to-face with the patient (could include caregiver/family) each 30 minutes; 5-8 patients   ⒸE

	RVU		Global Days	Modifiers				
Mod	Non-Fac Total	Fac Total		51	50	62	80	MUE
	0.28	0.28	XXX	9	9	9	9	

AMA: Aug 07: 9, Aug 08: 3, Feb 09: 13, Apr 13: 3, Nov 13: 3, Oct 14: 3

Non-Face to Face Nonphysician Practitioner Services

Telephone Patient Contact

98966 Telephone assessment and management service provided by a qualified nonphysician health care professional to an established patient, parent, or guardian not originating from a related assessment and management service provided within the previous 7 days nor leading to an assessment and management service or procedure within the next 24 hours or soonest available appointment; 5-10 minutes of medical discussion   ⒸE

	RVU		Global Days	Modifiers				
Mod	Non-Fac Total	Fac Total		51	50	62	80	MUE
	0.39	0.36	XXX	9	9	9	9	

AMA: Apr 13: 3, Oct 13: 11, Nov 13: 3, Oct 14: 3

98967 Telephone assessment and management service provided by a qualified nonphysician health care professional to an established patient, parent, or guardian not originating from a related assessment and management service provided within the previous 7 days nor leading to an assessment and management service or procedure within the next 24 hours or soonest available appointment; 11-20 minutes of medical discussion   ⒸE

	RVU		Global Days	Modifiers				
Mod	Non-Fac Total	Fac Total		51	50	62	80	MUE
	0.76	0.72	XXX	9	9	9	9	

AMA: Apr 13: 3, Oct 13: 11

98968 Telephone assessment and management service provided by a qualified nonphysician health care professional to an established patient, parent, or guardian not originating from a related assessment and management service provided within the previous 7 days nor leading to an assessment and management service or procedure within the next 24 hours or soonest available appointment; 21-30 minutes of medical discussion   ⒸE

	RVU		Global Days	Modifiers				
Mod	Non-Fac Total	Fac Total		51	50	62	80	MUE
	1.12	1.08	XXX	9	9	9	9	

AMA: Apr 13: 3, Oct 13: 11, Nov 13: 3, Oct 14: 3

● New   ▲ Revised   Deleted   ⊙ Moderate Sedation   ✚ Add-on Codes   ⊘ High Risk Denial   Ⓐ Age Edit   ♀ Female   ♂ Male   **AMA** *CPT® Assistant*   *MUE* Medically Unlikely Edit
   ⊘ Modifier 51 Exempt   ⊖ Modifier 63 Exempt   ✗ Unlisted   **Modifiers:** *See Inside Back Cover*   Ⓜ Maternity   A2-Z3 ASC Payment Indicators   A-Y OPPS Status Indicators

© 2016 DecisionHealth   CPT © 2015 American Medical Association. All Rights Reserved.   **855**

Medicine Procedures

98969 – 99060

On-line Assessment/Management

98969 Online assessment and management service provided by a qualified nonphysician health care professional to an established patient or guardian, not originating from a related assessment and management service provided within the previous 7 days, using the Internet or similar electronic communications network ⊖E

RVU			Global Days	Modifiers				
Mod	Non-Fac Total	Fac Total		51	50	62	80	MUE
	0.00	0.00	XXX	9	9	9	9	

AMA: Apr 13: 3, Oct 13: 11, Nov 13: 3, Oct 14: 3

Special Services/Procedures/Reports

Miscellaneous Services/Procedures

99000 Handling and/or conveyance of specimen for transfer from the office to a laboratory ⊖E

RVU			Global Days	Modifiers				
Mod	Non-Fac Total	Fac Total		51	50	62	80	MUE
	0.00	0.00	XXX	9	9	9	9	

AMA: Winter 94: 26, Feb 99: 10, Oct 99: 11, May 02: 19, Aug 06: 6, Sep 06: 15, Jan 07: 30

99001 Handling and/or conveyance of specimen for transfer from the patient in other than an office to a laboratory (distance may be indicated) ⊖E

RVU			Global Days	Modifiers				
Mod	Non-Fac Total	Fac Total		51	50	62	80	MUE
	0.00	0.00	XXX	9	9	9	9	

AMA: Winter 94: 26, May 02: 19, Aug 06: 6, Sep 06: 15, Jan 07: 30

99002 Handling, conveyance, and/or any other service in connection with the implementation of an order involving devices (eg, designing, fitting, packaging, handling, delivery or mailing) when devices such as orthotics, protectives, prosthetics are fabricated by an outside laboratory or shop but which items have been designed, and are to be fitted and adjusted by the attending physician or other qualified health care professional ⊖B

RVU			Global Days	Modifiers				
Mod	Non-Fac Total	Fac Total		51	50	62	80	MUE
	0.00	0.00	XXX	9	9	9	9	0

AMA: Winter 94: 26, May 02: 19, Aug 06: 6, Sep 06: 15, Jan 07: 30

99024 Postoperative follow-up visit, normally included in the surgical package, to indicate that an evaluation and management service was performed during a postoperative period for a reason(s) related to the original procedure ⊖B

RVU			Global Days	Modifiers				
Mod	Non-Fac Total	Fac Total		51	50	62	80	MUE
	0.00	0.00	XXX	9	9	9	9	0

AMA: Winter 94: 26, Sep 97: 10, Aug 98: 5, May 02: 19, Nov 03: 13, Aug 06: 6, Sep 06: 15, Jan 07: 30, Mar 15: 3

99026 Hospital mandated on call service; in-hospital, each hour ⊖E

RVU			Global Days	Modifiers				
Mod	Non-Fac Total	Fac Total		51	50	62	80	MUE
	0.00	0.00	XXX	9	9	9	9	

AMA: Jun 03: 10, Aug 06: 6, Sep 06: 15, Jan 07: 30

99027 Hospital mandated on call service; out-of-hospital, each hour ⊖E

RVU			Global Days	Modifiers				
Mod	Non-Fac Total	Fac Total		51	50	62	80	MUE
	0.00	0.00	XXX	9	9	9	9	

AMA: Jun 03: 10, Aug 06: 6, Sep 06: 15, Jan 07: 30

99050 Services provided in the office at times other than regularly scheduled office hours, or days when the office is normally closed (eg, holidays, Saturday or Sunday), in addition to basic service ⊖B

RVU			Global Days	Modifiers				
Mod	Non-Fac Total	Fac Total		51	50	62	80	MUE
	0.00	0.00	XXX	9	9	9	9	9

AMA: Winter 94: 27, May 02: 19, Jun 03: 10, May 06: 18, Aug 06: 6, Sep 06: 15, Jan 07: 30, Aug 10: 9

Pub 100-04, 13, 70.2

99051 Service(s) provided in the office during regularly scheduled evening, weekend, or holiday office hours, in addition to basic service ⊖B

RVU			Global Days	Modifiers				
Mod	Non-Fac Total	Fac Total		51	50	62	80	MUE
	0.00	0.00	XXX	9	9	9	9	0

AMA: May 06: 18, Aug 06: 6, Sep 06: 15, Jan 07: 30, Aug 10: 9

99053 Service(s) provided between 10:00 PM and 8:00 AM at 24-hour facility, in addition to basic service ⊖B

RVU			Global Days	Modifiers				
Mod	Non-Fac Total	Fac Total		51	50	62	80	MUE
	0.00	0.00	XXX	9	9	9	9	0

AMA: May 06: 18, Aug 06: 6, Sep 06: 15, Jan 07: 30

99056 Service(s) typically provided in the office, provided out of the office at request of patient, in addition to basic service ⊖B

RVU			Global Days	Modifiers				
Mod	Non-Fac Total	Fac Total		51	50	62	80	MUE
	0.00	0.00	XXX	9	9	9	9	0

AMA: Winter 94: 27, May 02: 19, May 06: 18, Aug 06: 6, Sep 06: 15, Jan 07: 30

99058 Service(s) provided on an emergency basis in the office, which disrupts other scheduled office services, in addition to basic service ⊖B

RVU			Global Days	Modifiers				
Mod	Non-Fac Total	Fac Total		51	50	62	80	MUE
	0.00	0.00	XXX	9	9	9	9	0

AMA: Winter 94: 27, May 02: 19, May 06: 18, Aug 06: 6, Sep 06: 15, Jan 07: 30, Aug 10: 9

Pub 100-04, 13, 70.2

99060 Service(s) provided on an emergency basis, out of the office, which disrupts other scheduled office services, in addition to basic service ⊖B

RVU			Global Days	Modifiers				
Mod	Non-Fac Total	Fac Total		51	50	62	80	MUE
	0.00	0.00	XXX	9	9	9	9	0

AMA: May 06: 18, Aug 06: 6, Sep 06: 15, Jan 07: 30

● New   ▲ Revised   ✖ Deleted   ⊙ Moderate Sedation   ✚ Add-on Codes   ⊘ High Risk Denial   Ⓐ Age Edit   ♀ Female   ♂ Male   **AMA** *CPT® Assistant*   *MUE* Medically Unlikely Edit
⊘ Modifier 51 Exempt   ⊖ Modifier 63 Exempt   ✗ Unlisted   **Modifiers:** *See Inside Back Cover*   Ⓜ Maternity   A2–Z3 ASC Payment Indicators   A–Y OPPS Status Indicators

856   CPT © 2015 American Medical Association. All Rights Reserved.   © 2016 DecisionHealth

99070 Supplies and materials (except spectacles), provided by the physician or other qualified health care professional over and above those usually included with the office visit or other services rendered (list drugs, trays, supplies, or materials provided) ⊛B

RVU		Global Days	Modifiers				
Mod	Non-Fac Total	Fac Total		51	50	62	80	MUE
	0.00	0.00	XXX	9	9	9	9	0

AMA: Mar 13: 6, Winter 94: 28, May 98: 10, Jun 99: 10, Jun 00: 11, Jul 01: 2, May 02: 19, Aug 02: 11, Jun 05: 1, Jul 06: 1, Aug 06: 6, Sep 06: 15, Jan 07: 30, 31, Feb 07: 8, Sep 08: 11, May 09: 8, Sep 09: 5, May 10: 10, Jun 10: 8, Sep 10: 11, Apr 12: 10, Nov 12: 11, Dec 13: 12, Mar 14: 11

99071 Educational supplies, such as books, tapes, and pamphlets, for the patient's education at cost to physician or other qualified health care professional ⊛B

RVU		Global Days	Modifiers				
Mod	Non-Fac Total	Fac Total		51	50	62	80	MUE
	0.00	0.00	XXX	9	9	9	9	0

AMA: Winter 94: 28, May 02: 19, Aug 06: 6, Sep 06: 15, Jan 07: 30, Apr 13: 3, Nov 13: 3, Oct 14: 3

Pub 100-04, 13, 70.2

99075 Medical testimony ⊛E

RVU		Global Days	Modifiers				
Mod	Non-Fac Total	Fac Total		51	50	62	80	MUE
	0.00	0.00	XXX	9	9	9	9	

AMA: Winter 94: 28, May 02: 19, Aug 06: 6, Sep 06: 15, Jan 07: 30

99078 Physician or other qualified health care professional qualified by education, training, licensure/regulation (when applicable) educational services rendered to patients in a group setting (eg, prenatal, obesity, or diabetic instructions) ⊛N

RVU		Global Days	Modifiers				
Mod	Non-Fac Total	Fac Total		51	50	62	80	MUE
	0.00	0.00	XXX	9	9	9	9	0

AMA: Winter 94: 28, Jan 98: 12, May 02: 19, Aug 06: 6, Sep 06: 15, Jan 07: 30, Aug 07: 9, Apr 13: 3, Nov 13: 3, Oct 14: 3

99080 Special reports such as insurance forms, more than the information conveyed in the usual medical communications or standard reporting form ⊛B

RVU		Global Days	Modifiers				
Mod	Non-Fac Total	Fac Total		51	50	62	80	MUE
	0.00	0.00	XXX	9	9	9	9	0

AMA: Winter 94: 28, May 02: 19, Aug 06: 6, Sep 06: 15, Jan 07: 30, Apr 13: 3, Nov 13: 3, Oct 14: 3

99082 Unusual travel (eg, transportation and escort of patient) ⊛B

RVU		Global Days	Modifiers				
Mod	Non-Fac Total	Fac Total		51	50	62	80	MUE
	0.00	0.00	XXX	0	0	0	0	1

AMA: May 02: 19, Jan 03: 24, Nov 03: 14, Aug 06: 6, Sep 06: 15, Jan 07: 30

Pub 100-04, 12, 80.3

99090 Analysis of clinical data stored in computers (eg, ECGs, blood pressures, hematologic data) ⊛B

RVU		Global Days	Modifiers				
Mod	Non-Fac Total	Fac Total		51	50	62	80	MUE
	0.00	0.00	XXX	9	9	9	9	0

AMA: Winter 94: 28, May 02: 19, Jun 03: 10, Aug 06: 6, Sep 06: 15, Jan 07: 30, Feb 07: 10, Jul 07: 1, Apr 09: 7, Apr 13: 3, Nov 13: 3, May 14: 4, Oct 14: 3

Pub 100-04, 12, 30.6.12; 100-04, 13, 70.2

99091 Collection and interpretation of physiologic data (eg, ECG, blood pressure, glucose monitoring) digitally stored and/or transmitted by the patient and/or caregiver to the physician or other qualified health care professional, qualified by education, training, licensure/regulation (when applicable) requiring a minimum of 30 minutes of time ⊛N

RVU		Global Days	Modifiers				
Mod	Non-Fac Total	Fac Total		51	50	62	80	MUE
	1.59	1.59	XXX	9	9	9	9	0

AMA: May 02: 19, Jun 03: 10, Aug 06: 6, Sep 06: 15, Jan 07: 30, Apr 09: 7, Dec 09: 6, Apr 13: 3, Nov 13: 3, Oct 14: 3

Anesthesia Qualifying Circumstances

✚ **99100** Anesthesia for patient of extreme age, younger than 1 year and older than 70 (List separately in addition to code for primary anesthesia procedure) ⊛B

RVU		Global Days	Modifiers				
Mod	Non-Fac Total	Fac Total		51	50	62	80	MUE
	0.00	0.00	ZZZ	9	9	9	9	

AMA: Apr 08: 3

✚ **99116** Anesthesia complicated by utilization of total body hypothermia (List separately in addition to code for primary anesthesia procedure) ⊛B

RVU		Global Days	Modifiers				
Mod	Non-Fac Total	Fac Total		51	50	62	80	MUE
	0.00	0.00	ZZZ	9	9	9	9	0

AMA: Apr 08: 3

✚ **99135** Anesthesia complicated by utilization of controlled hypotension (List separately in addition to code for primary anesthesia procedure) ⊛B

RVU		Global Days	Modifiers				
Mod	Non-Fac Total	Fac Total		51	50	62	80	MUE
	0.00	0.00	ZZZ	9	9	9	9	0

AMA: Apr 08: 3

✚ **99140** Anesthesia complicated by emergency conditions (specify) (List separately in addition to code for primary anesthesia procedure) ⊛B

RVU		Global Days	Modifiers				
Mod	Non-Fac Total	Fac Total		51	50	62	80	MUE
	0.00	0.00	ZZZ	9	9	9	9	0

AMA: Mar 01: 10, Apr 08: 3

● New   ▲ Revised   Deleted   ⊙ Moderate Sedation   ✚ Add-on Codes   ⊘ High Risk Denial   Ⓐ Age Edit   ♀ Female   ♂ Male   **AMA** *CPT® Assistant*   **MUE** Medically Unlikely Edit
⊘ Modifier 51 Exempt   ⊖ Modifier 63 Exempt   ⊠ Unlisted   **Modifiers:** *See Inside Back Cover*   Ⓜ Maternity   A2–Z3 ASC Payment Indicators   A–Y OPPS Status Indicators

© 2016 DecisionHealth   CPT © 2015 American Medical Association. All Rights Reserved.   **857**

Conscious Sedation

Coding Guidance

Separate payment may be allowed for moderate conscious sedation provided by the same physician when the medical or surgical procedure performed is not included in Appendix G. No other anesthesia services (e.g. local infiltration, regional blocks, mild or deep sedation, other monitored anesthesia) provided by the same physician performing the medical or surgical procedure are allowed as separately reportable.

⊘ **99143** Moderate sedation services (other than those services described by codes 00100-01999) provided by the same physician or other qualified health care professional performing the diagnostic or therapeutic service that the sedation supports, requiring the presence of an independent trained observer to assist in the monitoring of the patient's level of consciousness and physiological status; younger than 5 years of age, first 30 minutes intra-service time ⊘Ⓐ🅽

RVU		Global Days	Modifiers				
Mod	Non-Fac Total Fac Total		51	50	62	80	MUE
	0.00　　0.00	XXX	0	0	0	0	2

AMA: Feb 06: 9, May 06: 19, 20, Feb 08: 5, Nov 09: 11, Dec 09: 10, Oct 11: 4, Nov 12: 3, Feb 13: 3, May 13: 12, Aug 14: 5
Pub 100-04, 12, 50

⊘ **99144** Moderate sedation services (other than those services described by codes 00100-01999) provided by the same physician or other qualified health care professional performing the diagnostic or therapeutic service that the sedation supports, requiring the presence of an independent trained observer to assist in the monitoring of the patient's level of consciousness and physiological status; age 5 years or older, first 30 minutes intra-service time 🅽

RVU		Global Days	Modifiers				
Mod	Non-Fac Total Fac Total		51	50	62	80	MUE
	0.00　　0.00	XXX	0	0	0	0	2

AMA: Feb 06: 9, May 06: 19, 20, Feb 08: 5, Nov 09: 11, Dec 09: 10, Jul 11: 17, Oct 11: 4, Jul 12: 13, Nov 12: 3, Feb 13: 3, May 13: 12, Aug 14: 5
Pub 100-04, 12, 50

✚ **99145** Moderate sedation services (other than those services described by codes 00100-01999) provided by the same physician or other qualified health care professional performing the diagnostic or therapeutic service that the sedation supports, requiring the presence of an independent trained observer to assist in the monitoring of the patient's level of consciousness and physiological status; each additional 15 minutes intra-service time (List separately in addition to code for primary service) 🅽

RVU		Global Days	Modifiers				
Mod	Non-Fac Total Fac Total		51	50	62	80	MUE
	0.00　　0.00	ZZZ	0	0	0	0	

AMA: Feb 06: 9, May 06: 19, 20, Feb 08: 5, Nov 09: 11, Dec 09: 10, Jul 11: 17, Oct 11: 4, Nov 12: 3, Feb 13: 3, May 13: 12, Aug 14: 5
Pub 100-04, 12, 50

99148 Moderate sedation services (other than those services described by codes 00100-01999), provided by a physician or other qualified health care professional other than the health care professional performing the diagnostic or therapeutic service that the sedation supports; younger than 5 years of age, first 30 minutes intra-service time ⊘Ⓐ🅽

RVU		Global Days	Modifiers				
Mod	Non-Fac Total Fac Total		51	50	62	80	MUE
	0.00　　0.00	XXX	0	0	0	0	2

AMA: Feb 06: 9, May 06: 19, 20, Nov 09: 11, Dec 09: 10, Oct 11: 4, Feb 13: 3, May 13: 12, Aug 14: 5
Pub 100-04, 12, 50

99149 Moderate sedation services (other than those services described by codes 00100-01999), provided by a physician or other qualified health care professional other than the health care professional performing the diagnostic or therapeutic service that the sedation supports; age 5 years or older, first 30 minutes intra-service time 🅽

RVU		Global Days	Modifiers				
Mod	Non-Fac Total Fac Total		51	50	62	80	MUE
	0.00　　0.00	XXX	0	0	0	0	2

AMA: Feb 06: 9, May 06: 19, 20, Nov 09: 11, Dec 09: 10, Oct 11: 4, Feb 13: 3, May 13: 12, Aug 14: 5
Pub 100-04, 12, 50

✚ **99150** Moderate sedation services (other than those services described by codes 00100-01999), provided by a physician or other qualified health care professional other than the health care professional performing the diagnostic or therapeutic service that the sedation supports; each additional 15 minutes intra-service time (List separately in addition to code for primary service) 🅽

RVU		Global Days	Modifiers				
Mod	Non-Fac Total Fac Total		51	50	62	80	MUE
	0.00　　0.00	ZZZ	0	0	0	0	

AMA: Feb 06: 9, May 06: 19, 20, Nov 09: 11, Dec 09: 10, Oct 11: 4, Feb 13: 3, May 13: 12, Aug 14: 5
Pub 100-04, 12, 50

Other Medicine Services/Procedures

99170 Anogenital examination, magnified, in childhood for suspected trauma, including image recording when performed ⊘Ⓐ🆃

RVU		Global Days	Modifiers				
Mod	Non-Fac Total Fac Total		51	50	62	80	MUE
	4.90　　2.53	000	2	0	0	1	1

AMA: Nov 99: 55, Apr 06: 1, Sep 14: 7

● New　▲ Revised　✖ Deleted　⊙ Moderate Sedation　✚ Add-on Codes　⊘ High Risk Denial　Ⓐ Age Edit　♀ Female　♂ Male　**AMA** *CPT® Assistant*　**MUE** Medically Unlikely Edit
⊘ Modifier 51 Exempt　⊖ Modifier 63 Exempt　✗ Unlisted　**Modifiers:** *See Inside Back Cover*　🅼 Maternity　🄰2–🅉3 ASC Payment Indicators　🄰–🆈 OPPS Status Indicators

CPT © 2015 American Medical Association. All Rights Reserved.　　　© 2016 DecisionHealth

99172 Visual function screening, automated or semi-automated bilateral quantitative determination of visual acuity, ocular alignment, color vision by pseudoisochromatic plates, and field of vision (may include all or some screening of the determination[s] for contrast sensitivity, vision under glare) ⊖E

RVU		Global Days	Modifiers				
Mod	Non-Fac Total	Fac Total		51	50	62	80	MUE
	0.00	0.00	XXX	9	9	9	9	

AMA: Feb 01: 7, Mar 05: 1, 3

99173 Screening test of visual acuity, quantitative, bilateral ⊖E

RVU		Global Days	Modifiers				
Mod	Non-Fac Total	Fac Total		51	50	62	80	MUE
	0.09	0.09	XXX	9	9	9	9	

AMA: Nov 99: 55, May 02: 2, Mar 05: 1, 3

▲ **99174** Instrument-based ocular screening (eg, photoscreening, automated-refraction), bilateral; with remote analysis and report ⊖E

RVU		Global Days	Modifiers				
Mod	Non-Fac Total	Fac Total		51	50	62	80	MUE
	0.00	0.00	XXX	9	9	9	9	

AMA: Mar 13: 6

Coding Guidance
The observation time devoted exclusively to monitoring the response to the emetic cannot be included in another timed service code.

99175 Ipecac or similar administration for individual emesis and continued observation until stomach adequately emptied of poison ⊖N

RVU		Global Days	Modifiers				
Mod	Non-Fac Total	Fac Total		51	50	62	80	MUE
	0.48	0.48	XXX	0	0	0	0	1

● **99177** Instrument-based ocular screening (eg, photoscreening, automated-refraction), bilateral; with on-site analysis E

RVU		Global Days	Modifiers				
Mod	Non-Fac Total	Fac Total		51	50	62	80	MUE
	0.00	0.00	XXX	9	9	9	9	1

99183 Physician or other qualified health care professional attendance and supervision of hyperbaric oxygen therapy, per session B

RVU		Global Days	Modifiers				
Mod	Non-Fac Total	Fac Total		51	50	62	80	MUE
	3.13	3.13	XXX	0	0	0	0	1

AMA: Jan 03: 23

Pub 100-04, 32, 30.1

99184 Initiation of selective head or total body hypothermia in the critically ill neonate, includes appropriate patient selection by review of clinical, imaging and laboratory data, confirmation of esophageal temperature probe location, evaluation of amplitude EEG, supervision of controlled hypothermia, and assessment of patient tolerance of cooling C

RVU		Global Days	Modifiers				
Mod	Non-Fac Total	Fac Total		51	50	62	80	MUE
	6.49	6.49	XXX	0	0	0	0	1

99188 Application of topical fluoride varnish by a physician or other qualified health care professional E

RVU		Global Days	Modifiers				
Mod	Non-Fac Total	Fac Total		51	50	62	80	MUE
	0.00	0.00	XXX	0	0	0	0	

99190 Assembly and operation of pump with oxygenator or heat exchanger (with or without ECG and/or pressure monitoring); each hour ⊖C

RVU		Global Days	Modifiers				
Mod	Non-Fac Total	Fac Total		51	50	62	80	MUE
	0.00	0.00	XXX	9	9	9	9	

99191 Assembly and operation of pump with oxygenator or heat exchanger (with or without ECG and/or pressure monitoring); 45 minutes ⊖C

RVU		Global Days	Modifiers				
Mod	Non-Fac Total	Fac Total		51	50	62	80	MUE
	0.00	0.00	XXX	9	9	9	9	1

99192 Assembly and operation of pump with oxygenator or heat exchanger (with or without ECG and/or pressure monitoring); 30 minutes ⊖C

RVU		Global Days	Modifiers				
Mod	Non-Fac Total	Fac Total		51	50	62	80	MUE
	0.00	0.00	XXX	9	9	9	9	1

Coding Guidance
Transfusion service codes, plasmapheresis, or transfusion exchange codes should not be reported with therapeutic phlebotomy.

99195 Phlebotomy, therapeutic (separate procedure) ⊙1

RVU		Global Days	Modifiers				
Mod	Non-Fac Total	Fac Total		51	50	62	80	MUE
	2.81	2.81	XXX	0	0	0	0	2

AMA: Apr 96: 3, Jun 96: 10

99199 Unlisted special service, procedure or report ⊘xB

RVU		Global Days	Modifiers				
Mod	Non-Fac Total	Fac Total		51	50	62	80	MUE
	0.00	0.00	XXX	0	0	0	0	

AMA: Nov 99: 55, Jun 12: 16, Sep 12: 9

Pub 100-04, 18, 150.1, 150.2

Home Health Services/Procedures

99500 Home visit for prenatal monitoring and assessment to include fetal heart rate, non-stress test, uterine monitoring, and gestational diabetes monitoring ⊖♀E

RVU		Global Days	Modifiers				
Mod	Non-Fac Total	Fac Total		51	50	62	80	MUE
	0.00	0.00	XXX	9	9	9	9	

AMA: Oct 03: 7, Jan 07: 30

99501 Home visit for postnatal assessment and follow-up care ⊖♀E

RVU		Global Days	Modifiers				
Mod	Non-Fac Total	Fac Total		51	50	62	80	MUE
	0.00	0.00	XXX	9	9	9	9	

AMA: Oct 03: 7, Jan 07: 30

● New   ▲ Revised   Deleted   ⊙ Moderate Sedation   ✚ Add-on Codes   ⊘ High Risk Denial   Ⓐ Age Edit   ♀ Female   ♂ Male   **AMA** CPT® Assistant   **MUE** Medically Unlikely Edit

⊘ Modifier 51 Exempt   ⊖ Modifier 63 Exempt   ✗ Unlisted   **Modifiers:** See Inside Back Cover   Ⓜ Maternity   A2–Z3 ASC Payment Indicators   A–Y OPPS Status Indicators

99502 Home visit for newborn care and assessment ⊗Ⓐ🄴

RVU			Global Days	Modifiers				
Mod	Non-Fac Total	Fac Total		51	50	62	80	MUE
	0.00	0.00	XXX	9	9	9	9	

AMA: Oct 03: 7, Jan 07: 30

99503 Home visit for respiratory therapy care (eg, bronchodilator, oxygen therapy, respiratory assessment, apnea evaluation) 🄴

RVU			Global Days	Modifiers				
Mod	Non-Fac Total	Fac Total		51	50	62	80	MUE
	0.00	0.00	XXX	9	9	9	9	

AMA: Oct 03: 7, Jan 07: 30

99504 Home visit for mechanical ventilation care 🄴

RVU			Global Days	Modifiers				
Mod	Non-Fac Total	Fac Total		51	50	62	80	MUE
	0.00	0.00	XXX	9	9	9	9	

AMA: Oct 03: 7, Jan 07: 30

99505 Home visit for stoma care and maintenance including colostomy and cystostomy 🄴

RVU			Global Days	Modifiers				
Mod	Non-Fac Total	Fac Total		51	50	62	80	MUE
	0.00	0.00	XXX	9	9	9	9	

AMA: Oct 03: 7, Jan 07: 30

99506 Home visit for intramuscular injections 🄴

RVU			Global Days	Modifiers				
Mod	Non-Fac Total	Fac Total		51	50	62	80	MUE
	0.00	0.00	XXX	9	9	9	9	

AMA: Oct 03: 7, Jan 07: 30

99507 Home visit for care and maintenance of catheter(s) (eg, urinary, drainage, and enteral) 🄴

RVU			Global Days	Modifiers				
Mod	Non-Fac Total	Fac Total		51	50	62	80	MUE
	0.00	0.00	XXX	9	9	9	9	

AMA: Oct 03: 7, Jan 07: 30

99509 Home visit for assistance with activities of daily living and personal care 🄴

RVU			Global Days	Modifiers				
Mod	Non-Fac Total	Fac Total		51	50	62	80	MUE
	0.00	0.00	XXX	9	9	9	9	

AMA: Oct 03: 7, Jan 07: 30

99510 Home visit for individual, family, or marriage counseling 🄴

RVU			Global Days	Modifiers				
Mod	Non-Fac Total	Fac Total		51	50	62	80	MUE
	0.00	0.00	XXX	9	9	9	9	

AMA: Oct 03: 7, Jan 07: 30

99511 Home visit for fecal impaction management and enema administration 🄴

RVU			Global Days	Modifiers				
Mod	Non-Fac Total	Fac Total		51	50	62	80	MUE
	0.00	0.00	XXX	9	9	9	9	

AMA: Oct 03: 7, Jan 07: 30

99512 Home visit for hemodialysis 🄴

RVU			Global Days	Modifiers				
Mod	Non-Fac Total	Fac Total		51	50	62	80	MUE
	0.00	0.00	XXX	9	9	9	9	

AMA: Oct 03: 7, Jan 07: 30

99600 Unlisted home visit service or procedure ⊗x🄴

RVU			Global Days	Modifiers				
Mod	Non-Fac Total	Fac Total		51	50	62	80	MUE
	0.00	0.00	XXX	9	9	9	9	

AMA: Oct 03: 7, Jan 07: 30

Home Infusion Services/Procedures

99601 Home infusion/specialty drug administration, per visit (up to 2 hours) 🄴

RVU			Global Days	Modifiers				
Mod	Non-Fac Total	Fac Total		51	50	62	80	MUE
	0.00	0.00	XXX	9	9	9	9	

AMA: Nov 05: 1

+ 99602 Home infusion/specialty drug administration, per visit (up to 2 hours); each additional hour (List separately in addition to code for primary procedure) 🄴

RVU			Global Days	Modifiers				
Mod	Non-Fac Total	Fac Total		51	50	62	80	MUE
	0.00	0.00	XXX	9	9	9	9	

AMA: Nov 05: 1

Medication Therapy Management

99605 Medication therapy management service(s) provided by a pharmacist, individual, face-to-face with patient, with assessment and intervention if provided; initial 15 minutes, new patient 🄴

RVU			Global Days	Modifiers				
Mod	Non-Fac Total	Fac Total		51	50	62	80	MUE
	0.00	0.00	XXX	9	9	9	9	0

AMA: Apr 13: 3, Nov 13: 3, Oct 14: 3

99606 Medication therapy management service(s) provided by a pharmacist, individual, face-to-face with patient, with assessment and intervention if provided; initial 15 minutes, established patient 🄴

RVU			Global Days	Modifiers				
Mod	Non-Fac Total	Fac Total		51	50	62	80	MUE
	0.00	0.00	XXX	9	9	9	9	0

AMA: Apr 13: 3

+ 99607 Medication therapy management service(s) provided by a pharmacist, individual, face-to-face with patient, with assessment and intervention if provided; each additional 15 minutes (List separately in addition to code for primary service) 🄴

RVU			Global Days	Modifiers				
Mod	Non-Fac Total	Fac Total		51	50	62	80	MUE
	0.00	0.00	XXX	9	9	9	9	0

AMA: Apr 13: 3, Nov 13: 3, Oct 14: 3

● New   ▲ Revised   ✖ Deleted   ⊙ Moderate Sedation   ✚ Add-on Codes   ⊗ High Risk Denial   Ⓐ Age Edit   ♀ Female   ♂ Male   **AMA** *CPT® Assistant*   **MUE** Medically Unlikely Edit
⊘ Modifier 51 Exempt   ⊖ Modifier 63 Exempt   x̶ Unlisted   **Modifiers:** *See Inside Back Cover*   Ⓜ Maternity   A2–Z3 ASC Payment Indicators   A–Y OPPS Status Indicators

860   CPT © 2015 American Medical Association. All Rights Reserved.   © 2016 DecisionHealth

Category II Codes

Category II Procedures

This section of the Procedural Coding Expert is used to report performance measurements with alpha-numeric, five-digit codes, with the last character being the letter F. They are supplemental codes that may, in the future, require less medical record chart abstraction and review. These codes are currently for data collection purposes.

Category II codes are currently used to capture additional information about the encounter, but are not mandatory for reimbursement purposes. However, CMS has developed a voluntary reporting program that provides an incentive payment for successful reporting of selected quality measures using Category II CPT codes and/or HCPCS Level II G-codes in combination with certain Category I procedure codes and ICD-9-CM diagnosis codes as described in the quality measure. This voluntary reporting program is called the Physician Quality Reporting System (previously called the Physician Quality Reporting Initiative

(PQRI)). For more information on the Physician Quality Reporting System, see the CMS website. Category II codes do not have a payment indicator (RVU) associated with them.

The listing of performance measurements are broken down into the following sections:

- Composite measures
- Patient management
- Patient history
- Physical examination
- Diagnostic/screening processes of results
- Therapeutic, preventive, or other interventions
- Follow-up or other outcomes
- Patient safety
- Structural measures

Modifiers

The Category II code modifiers identify circumstances when a service in a measurement was contemplated, but due to specific issues (as described in the modifiers and the expanded descriptions) the services were not provided. These modifiers should only be reported with Category II CPT codes, not with Category I (CPT) or Category III (new technology) codes.

1P **Performance Measure Exclusion Modifier due to Medical Reasons**
Reasons include:
Not indicated (absence of organ/limb, already received/performed, other)
Contraindicated (patient allergic history, potential adverse drug interaction, other)
Other medical reasons

2P **Performance Measure Exclusion Modifier due to Patient Reasons**
Reasons include:
Patient declined
Economic, social, or religious reasons
Other patient reasons

3P **Performance Measure Exclusion Modifier due to System Reasons**
Reasons include:
Resources to perform the services not available
Insurance coverage/payer-related limitations
Other reasons attributable to health care delivery systems

8P **Performance measure reporting modifier – action not performed, reason not otherwise specified.**

Composite/Combined Codes

0001F **Heart failure assessed (includes assessment of all the following components) (CAD):**

Blood pressure measured (2000F)

Level of activity assessed (1003F)

Clinical symptoms of volume overload (excess) assessed (1004F)

Weight, recorded (2001F)

Clinical signs of volume overload (excess) assessed (2002F)

RVU			Global Days	Modifiers				
Mod	Non-Fac Total	Fac Total		51	50	62	80	MUE
	0.00	0.00	XXX	9	9	9	9	

AMA: Oct 05: 1

0005F **Osteoarthritis assessed (OA)**

Includes assessment of all the following components:

Osteoarthritis symptoms and functional status assessed (1006F)

Use of anti-inflammatory or over-the-counter (OTC) analgesic medications assessed (1007F)

Initial examination of the involved joint(s) (includes visual inspection, palpation, range of motion) (2004F)

RVU			Global Days	Modifiers				
Mod	Non-Fac Total	Fac Total		51	50	62	80	MUE
	0.00	0.00	XXX	9	9	9	9	

AMA: Oct 05: 1, 6

0012F **Community-acquired bacterial pneumonia assessment (includes all of the following components) (CAP):**

Co-morbid conditions assessed (1026F)

Vital signs recorded (2010F)

Mental status assessed (2014F)

Hydration status assessed (2018F)

RVU			Global Days	Modifiers				
Mod	Non-Fac Total	Fac Total		51	50	62	80	MUE
	0.00	0.00	XXX	9	9	9	9	

0014F **Comprehensive preoperative assessment performed for cataract surgery with intraocular lens (IOL) placement (includes assessment of all of the following components) (EC):**

Dilated fundus evaluation performed within 12 months prior to cataract surgery (2020F)

Pre-surgical (cataract) axial length, corneal power measurement and method of intraocular lens power calculation documented (must be performed within 12 months prior to surgery) (3073F)

Preoperative assessment of functional or medical indication(s) for surgery prior to the cataract surgery with intraocular lens placement (must be performed within 12 months prior to cataract surgery) (3325F)

RVU			Global Days	Modifiers				
Mod	Non-Fac Total	Fac Total		51	50	62	80	MUE
	0.00	0.00	XXX	9	9	9	9	

0015F **Melanoma follow up completed (includes assessment of all of the following components) (ML):**

History obtained regarding new or changing moles (1050F)

● New ▲ Revised Deleted ⊙ Moderate Sedation ✚ Add-on Codes ⊘ High Risk Denial Ⓐ Age Edit ♀ Female ♂ Male **AMA** CPT® Assistant **MUE** Medically Unlikely Edit
⊘ Modifier 51 Exempt ⊖ Modifier 63 Exempt ⊠ Unlisted **Modifiers:** *See Inside Back Cover* Ⓜ Maternity Ⓐ2-Ⓩ3 ASC Payment Indicators Ⓐ-Ⓨ OPPS Status Indicators

© 2016 DecisionHealth | CPT © 2015 American Medical Association. All Rights Reserved. | **861**

Category II Procedures

0500F – 0525F

Complete physical skin exam performed (2029F)

Patient counseled to perform a monthly self skin examination (5005F)   Ⓔ

Mod	Non-Fac Total	Fac Total	Global Days	51	50	62	80	MUE
	0.00	0.00	XXX	9	9	9	9	

Patient Management Codes

0500F Initial prenatal care visit (report at first prenatal encounter with health care professional providing obstetrical care. Report also date of visit and, in a separate field, the date of the last menstrual period [LMP]) (Prenatal)   ♀Ⓔ

Mod	Non-Fac Total	Fac Total	Global Days	51	50	62	80	MUE
	0.00	0.00	XXX	9	9	9	9	

AMA: Oct 05: 1, 6, Aug 07: 1

0501F Prenatal flow sheet documented in medical record by first prenatal visit (documentation includes at minimum blood pressure, weight, urine protein, uterine size, fetal heart tones, and estimated date of delivery). Report also: date of visit and, in a separate field, the date of the last menstrual period [LMP] (Note: If reporting 0501F Prenatal flow sheet, it is not necessary to report 0500F Initial prenatal care visit) (Prenatal)   ♀Ⓔ

Mod	Non-Fac Total	Fac Total	Global Days	51	50	62	80	MUE
	0.00	0.00	XXX	9	9	9	9	

AMA: Oct 05: 6

0502F Subsequent prenatal care visit (Prenatal) [Excludes: patients who are seen for a condition unrelated to pregnancy or prenatal care (eg, an upper respiratory infection; patients seen for consultation only, not for continuing care)]   ♀Ⓔ

Mod	Non-Fac Total	Fac Total	Global Days	51	50	62	80	MUE
	0.00	0.00	XXX	9	9	9	9	

AMA: Oct 05: 6

0503F Postpartum care visit (Prenatal)   ♀Ⓔ

Mod	Non-Fac Total	Fac Total	Global Days	51	50	62	80	MUE
	0.00	0.00	XXX	9	9	9	9	

AMA: Oct 05: 6

0505F Hemodialysis plan of care documented (ESRD, P-ESRD)   Ⓔ

Mod	Non-Fac Total	Fac Total	Global Days	51	50	62	80	MUE
	0.00	0.00	XXX	9	9	9	9	

0507F Peritoneal dialysis plan of care documented (ESRD)   Ⓔ

Mod	Non-Fac Total	Fac Total	Global Days	51	50	62	80	MUE
	0.00	0.00	XXX	9	9	9	9	

0509F Urinary incontinence plan of care documented (GER)   Ⓜ

Mod	Non-Fac Total	Fac Total	Global Days	51	50	62	80	MUE
	0.00	0.00	XXX	9	9	9	9	

0513F Elevated blood pressure plan of care documented (CKD)   Ⓜ

Mod	Non-Fac Total	Fac Total	Global Days	51	50	62	80	MUE
	0.00	0.00	XXX	9	9	9	9	

0514F Plan of care for elevated hemoglobin level documented for patient receiving Erythropoiesis-Stimulating Agent therapy (ESA) (CKD)   Ⓔ

Mod	Non-Fac Total	Fac Total	Global Days	51	50	62	80	MUE
	0.00	0.00	XXX	9	9	9	9	

0516F Anemia plan of care documented (ESRD)   Ⓔ

Mod	Non-Fac Total	Fac Total	Global Days	51	50	62	80	MUE
	0.00	0.00	XXX	9	9	9	9	

0517F Glaucoma plan of care documented (EC)   Ⓜ

Mod	Non-Fac Total	Fac Total	Global Days	51	50	62	80	MUE
	0.00	0.00	XXX	9	9	9	9	

0518F Falls plan of care documented (GER)   Ⓜ

Mod	Non-Fac Total	Fac Total	Global Days	51	50	62	80	MUE
	0.00	0.00	XXX	9	9	9	9	

0519F Planned chemotherapy regimen, including at a minimum: drug(s) prescribed, dose, and duration, documented prior to initiation of a new treatment regimen (ONC)   Ⓔ

Mod	Non-Fac Total	Fac Total	Global Days	51	50	62	80	MUE
	0.00	0.00	XXX	9	9	9	9	

0520F Radiation dose limits to normal tissues established prior to the initiation of a course of 3D conformal radiation for a minimum of 2 tissue/organ (ONC)   Ⓜ

Mod	Non-Fac Total	Fac Total	Global Days	51	50	62	80	MUE
	0.00	0.00	XXX	9	9	9	9	

0521F Plan of care to address pain documented (COA) (ONC)   Ⓜ

Mod	Non-Fac Total	Fac Total	Global Days	51	50	62	80	MUE
	0.00	0.00	XXX	9	9	9	9	

0525F Initial visit for episode (BkP)   Ⓔ

Mod	Non-Fac Total	Fac Total	Global Days	51	50	62	80	MUE
	0.00	0.00	XXX	9	9	9	9	

● New ▲ Revised ✖ Deleted ⊙ Moderate Sedation ➕ Add-on Codes ⊘ High Risk Denial Ⓐ Age Edit ♀ Female ♂ Male **AMA** *CPT® Assistant* **MUE** Medically Unlikely Edit ⊘ Modifier 51 Exempt ⊖ Modifier 63 Exempt ⓧ Unlisted **Modifiers:** *See Inside Back Cover* Ⓜ Maternity A2-Z3 ASC Payment Indicators A-Y OPPS Status Indicators

862   CPT © 2015 American Medical Association. All Rights Reserved.   © 2016 DecisionHealth

0526F Subsequent visit for episode (BkP) ⓒⓂ

RVU			Global Days	Modifiers				
Mod	Non-Fac Total	Fac Total		51	50	62	80	MUE
	0.00	0.00	XXX	9	9	9	9	

0528F Recommended follow-up interval for repeat colonoscopy of at least 10 years documented in colonoscopy report (End/Polyp) ⓒⓂ

RVU			Global Days	Modifiers				
Mod	Non-Fac Total	Fac Total		51	50	62	80	MUE
	0.00	0.00	XXX	9	9	9	9	

0529F Interval of 3 or more years since patient's last colonoscopy, documented (End/Polyp) ⓒⓂ

RVU			Global Days	Modifiers				
Mod	Non-Fac Total	Fac Total		51	50	62	80	MUE
	0.00	0.00	XXX	9	9	9	9	

0535F Dyspnea management plan of care, documented (Pall Cr) ⓒⒺ

RVU			Global Days	Modifiers				
Mod	Non-Fac Total	Fac Total		51	50	62	80	MUE
	0.00	0.00	XXX	9	9	9	9	

0540F Glucorticoid Management Plan Documented (RA) ⓒⓂ

RVU			Global Days	Modifiers				
Mod	Non-Fac Total	Fac Total		51	50	62	80	MUE
	0.00	0.00	XXX	9	9	9	9	

0545F Plan for follow-up care for major depressive disorder, documented (MDD ADOL) ⓒⒺ

RVU			Global Days	Modifiers				
Mod	Non-Fac Total	Fac Total		51	50	62	80	MUE
	0.00	0.00	XXX	9	9	9	9	

0550F Cytopathology report on routine nongynecologic specimen finalized within two working days of accession date (PATH) ⓒⒺ

RVU			Global Days	Modifiers				
Mod	Non-Fac Total	Fac Total		51	50	62	80	MUE
	0.00	0.00	XXX	9	9	9	9	

0551F Cytopathology report on nongynecologic specimen with documentation that the specimen was non-routine (PATH) ⓒⒺ

RVU			Global Days	Modifiers				
Mod	Non-Fac Total	Fac Total		51	50	62	80	MUE
	0.00	0.00	XXX	9	9	9	9	

0555F Symptom management plan of care documented (HF) ⓒⒺ

RVU			Global Days	Modifiers				
Mod	Non-Fac Total	Fac Total		51	50	62	80	MUE
	0.00	0.00	XXX	9	9	9	9	

0556F Plan of care to achieve lipid control documented (CAD) ⓒⒺ

RVU			Global Days	Modifiers				
Mod	Non-Fac Total	Fac Total		51	50	62	80	MUE
	0.00	0.00	XXX	9	9	9	9	

0557F Plan of care to manage anginal symptoms documented (CAD) ⓒⓂ

RVU			Global Days	Modifiers				
Mod	Non-Fac Total	Fac Total		51	50	62	80	MUE
	0.00	0.00	XXX	9	9	9	9	

0575F HIV RNA control plan of care, documented (HIV) ⓒⒺ

RVU			Global Days	Modifiers				
Mod	Non-Fac Total	Fac Total		51	50	62	80	MUE
	0.00	0.00	XXX	9	9	9	9	

0580F Multidisciplinary care plan developed or updated (ALS) ⓒⒺ

RVU			Global Days	Modifiers				
Mod	Non-Fac Total	Fac Total		51	50	62	80	MUE
	0.00	0.00	XXX	9	9	9	9	

0581F Patient transferred directly from anesthetizing location to critical care unit (Peri2) ⓒⓂ

RVU			Global Days	Modifiers				
Mod	Non-Fac Total	Fac Total		51	50	62	80	MUE
	0.00	0.00	XXX	9	9	9	9	

0582F Patient not transferred directly from anesthetizing location to critical care unit (Peri2) ⓒⒺ

RVU			Global Days	Modifiers				
Mod	Non-Fac Total	Fac Total		51	50	62	80	MUE
	0.00	0.00	XXX	9	9	9	9	

0583F Transfer of care checklist used (Peri2) ⓒⓂ

RVU			Global Days	Modifiers				
Mod	Non-Fac Total	Fac Total		51	50	62	80	MUE
	0.00	0.00	XXX	9	9	9	9	

0584F Transfer of care checklist not used (Peri2) Ⓔ

RVU			Global Days	Modifiers				
Mod	Non-Fac Total	Fac Total		51	50	62	80	MUE
	0.00	0.00	XXX	9	9	9	9	

Patient History Codes

1000F Tobacco use assessed (CAD, CAP, COPD, PV) (DM) ⓒⒺ

RVU			Global Days	Modifiers				
Mod	Non-Fac Total	Fac Total		51	50	62	80	MUE
	0.00	0.00	XXX	9	9	9	9	

AMA: Oct 05: 1, 6

1002F Anginal symptoms and level of activity assessed (NMA-No Measure Associated) ⓒⒺ

RVU			Global Days	Modifiers				
Mod	Non-Fac Total	Fac Total		51	50	62	80	MUE
	0.00	0.00	XXX	9	9	9	9	

AMA: Oct 05: 6

1003F Level of activity assessed (NMA-No Measure Associated) ⓒⒺ

RVU			Global Days	Modifiers				
Mod	Non-Fac Total	Fac Total		51	50	62	80	MUE
	0.00	0.00	XXX	9	9	9	9	

AMA: Oct 05: 6

● New ▲ Revised Deleted ⊙ Moderate Sedation ✚ Add-on Codes ⊘ High Risk Denial Ⓐ Age Edit ♀ Female ♂ Male **AMA** *CPT® Assistant* **MUE** Medically Unlikely Edit
⊗ Modifier 51 Exempt ⊖ Modifier 63 Exempt Ⓧ Unlisted **Modifiers:** *See Inside Back Cover* Ⓜ Maternity Ⓐ2–Ⓩ3 ASC Payment Indicators Ⓐ–Ⓨ OPPS Status Indicators

© 2016 DecisionHealth   CPT © 2015 American Medical Association. All Rights Reserved.   **863**

Category II Procedures

1004F – 1034F

1004F Clinical symptoms of volume overload (excess) assessed (NMA-No Measure Associated) ⊘E

Mod	Non-Fac Total	Fac Total	Global Days	51	50	62	80	MUE
	0.00	0.00	XXX	9	9	9	9	

AMA: Oct 05: 6

1005F Asthma symptoms evaluated (includes documentation of numeric frequency of symptoms or patient completion of an asthma assessment tool/survey/questionnaire) (NMA-No Measure Associated) ⊘E

Mod	Non-Fac Total	Fac Total	Global Days	51	50	62	80	MUE
	0.00	0.00	XXX	9	9	9	9	

AMA: Oct 05: 6

1006F Osteoarthritis symptoms and functional status assessed (may include the use of a standardized scale or the completion of an assessment questionnaire, such as the SF-36, AAOS Hip & Knee Questionnaire) (OA) [Instructions: Report when osteoarthritis is addressed during the patient encounter] ⊘M

Mod	Non-Fac Total	Fac Total	Global Days	51	50	62	80	MUE
	0.00	0.00	XXX	9	9	9	9	

AMA: Oct 05: 6

1007F Use of anti-inflammatory or analgesic over-the-counter (OTC) medications for symptom relief assessed (OA) ⊘E

Mod	Non-Fac Total	Fac Total	Global Days	51	50	62	80	MUE
	0.00	0.00	XXX	9	9	9	9	

AMA: Oct 05: 6

1008F Gastrointestinal and renal risk factors assessed for patients on prescribed or OTC non-steroidal anti-inflammatory drug (NSAID) (OA) ⊘E

Mod	Non-Fac Total	Fac Total	Global Days	51	50	62	80	MUE
	0.00	0.00	XXX	9	9	9	9	

AMA: Oct 05: 6

1010F Severity of angina assessed by level of activity (CAD) ⊘M

Mod	Non-Fac Total	Fac Total	Global Days	51	50	62	80	MUE
	0.00	0.00	XXX	9	9	9	9	

1011F Angina present (CAD) ⊘M

Mod	Non-Fac Total	Fac Total	Global Days	51	50	62	80	MUE
	0.00	0.00	XXX	9	9	9	9	

1012F Angina absent (CAD) ⊘M

Mod	Non-Fac Total	Fac Total	Global Days	51	50	62	80	MUE
	0.00	0.00	XXX	9	9	9	9	

1015F Chronic obstructive pulmonary disease (COPD) symptoms assessed (Includes assessment of at least 1 of the following: dyspnea, cough/sputum, wheezing), or respiratory symptom assessment tool completed (COPD) ⊘E

Mod	Non-Fac Total	Fac Total	Global Days	51	50	62	80	MUE
	0.00	0.00	XXX	9	9	9	9	

1018F Dyspnea assessed, not present (COPD) ⊘E

Mod	Non-Fac Total	Fac Total	Global Days	51	50	62	80	MUE
	0.00	0.00	XXX	9	9	9	9	

1019F Dyspnea assessed, present (COPD) ⊘E

Mod	Non-Fac Total	Fac Total	Global Days	51	50	62	80	MUE
	0.00	0.00	XXX	9	9	9	9	

1022F Pneumococcus immunization status assessed (CAP, COPD) ⊘E

Mod	Non-Fac Total	Fac Total	Global Days	51	50	62	80	MUE
	0.00	0.00	XXX	9	9	9	9	

1026F Co-morbid conditions assessed (eg, includes assessment for presence or absence of: malignancy, liver disease, congestive heart failure, cerebrovascular disease, renal disease, chronic obstructive pulmonary disease, asthma, diabetes, other co-morbid conditions) (CAP) ⊘E

Mod	Non-Fac Total	Fac Total	Global Days	51	50	62	80	MUE
	0.00	0.00	XXX	9	9	9	9	

1030F Influenza immunization status assessed (CAP) ⊘E

Mod	Non-Fac Total	Fac Total	Global Days	51	50	62	80	MUE
	0.00	0.00	XXX	9	9	9	9	

1031F Smoking status and exposure to second hand smoke in the home assessed (Asthma) ⊘E

Mod	Non-Fac Total	Fac Total	Global Days	51	50	62	80	MUE
	0.00	0.00	XXX	9	9	9	9	

1032F Current tobacco smoker or currently exposed to secondhand smoke (Asthma) ⊘E

Mod	Non-Fac Total	Fac Total	Global Days	51	50	62	80	MUE
	0.00	0.00	XXX	9	9	9	9	

1033F Current tobacco non-smoker and not currently exposed to secondhand smoke (Asthma) ⊘E

Mod	Non-Fac Total	Fac Total	Global Days	51	50	62	80	MUE
	0.00	0.00	XXX	9	9	9	9	

1034F Current tobacco smoker (CAD, CAP, COPD, PV) (DM) ⊘E

Mod	Non-Fac Total	Fac Total	Global Days	51	50	62	80	MUE
	0.00	0.00	XXX	9	9	9	9	

● New   ▲ Revised   ✖ Deleted   ⊙ Moderate Sedation   ✚ Add-on Codes   ⊘ High Risk Denial   Ⓐ Age Edit   ♀ Female   ♂ Male   **AMA** CPT® Assistant   **MUE** Medically Unlikely Edit
⊘ Modifier 51 Exempt   ⊖ Modifier 63 Exempt   Ⓧ Unlisted   **Modifiers:** See Inside Back Cover   Ⓜ Maternity   A2–Z3 ASC Payment Indicators   A–Y OPPS Status Indicators

864   CPT © 2015 American Medical Association. All Rights Reserved.   © 2016 DecisionHealth

1035F Current smokeless tobacco user (eg, chew, snuff) (PV) CⒺ

RVU			Global Days	Modifiers				
Mod	Non-Fac Total	Fac Total		51	50	62	80	MUE
	0.00	0.00	XXX	9	9	9	9	

1036F Current tobacco non-user (CAD, CAP, COPD, PV) (DM) (IBD) CⓂ

RVU			Global Days	Modifiers				
Mod	Non-Fac Total	Fac Total		51	50	62	80	MUE
	0.00	0.00	XXX	9	9	9	9	

1038F Persistent asthma (mild, moderate or severe) (Asthma) CⓂ

RVU			Global Days	Modifiers				
Mod	Non-Fac Total	Fac Total		51	50	62	80	MUE
	0.00	0.00	XXX	9	9	9	9	

AMA: Jul 10: 3

1039F Intermittent asthma (Asthma) CⓂ

RVU			Global Days	Modifiers				
Mod	Non-Fac Total	Fac Total		51	50	62	80	MUE
	0.00	0.00	XXX	9	9	9	9	

AMA: Jul 10: 3

1040F DSM-5 criteria for major depressive disorder documented at the initial evaluation (MDD, MDD ADOL) CⒺ

RVU			Global Days	Modifiers				
Mod	Non-Fac Total	Fac Total		51	50	62	80	MUE
	0.00	0.00	XXX	9	9	9	9	

1050F History obtained regarding new or changing moles (ML) CⒺ

RVU			Global Days	Modifiers				
Mod	Non-Fac Total	Fac Total		51	50	62	80	MUE
	0.00	0.00	XXX	9	9	9	9	

1052F Type, anatomic location, and activity all assessed (IBD) CⒺ

RVU			Global Days	Modifiers				
Mod	Non-Fac Total	Fac Total		51	50	62	80	MUE
	0.00	0.00	XXX	9	9	9	9	

1055F Visual functional status assessed (EC) CⒺ

RVU			Global Days	Modifiers				
Mod	Non-Fac Total	Fac Total		51	50	62	80	MUE
	0.00	0.00	XXX	9	9	9	9	

1060F Documentation of permanent or persistent or paroxysmal atrial fibrillation (STR) CⒺ

RVU			Global Days	Modifiers				
Mod	Non-Fac Total	Fac Total		51	50	62	80	MUE
	0.00	0.00	XXX	9	9	9	9	

1061F Documentation of absence of permanent and persistent and paroxysmal atrial fibrillation (STR) CⒺ

RVU			Global Days	Modifiers				
Mod	Non-Fac Total	Fac Total		51	50	62	80	MUE
	0.00	0.00	XXX	9	9	9	9	

1065F Ischemic stroke symptom onset of less than 3 hours prior to arrival (STR) CⒺ

RVU			Global Days	Modifiers				
Mod	Non-Fac Total	Fac Total		51	50	62	80	MUE
	0.00	0.00	XXX	9	9	9	9	

1066F Ischemic stroke symptom onset greater than or equal to 3 hours prior to arrival (STR) CⒺ

RVU			Global Days	Modifiers				
Mod	Non-Fac Total	Fac Total		51	50	62	80	MUE
	0.00	0.00	XXX	9	9	9	9	

1070F Alarm symptoms (involuntary weight loss, dysphagia, or gastrointestinal bleeding) assessed; none present (GERD) CⒺ

RVU			Global Days	Modifiers				
Mod	Non-Fac Total	Fac Total		51	50	62	80	MUE
	0.00	0.00	XXX	9	9	9	9	

1071F Alarm symptoms (involuntary weight loss, dysphagia, or gastrointestinal bleeding) assessed; 1 or more present (GERD) CⒺ

RVU			Global Days	Modifiers				
Mod	Non-Fac Total	Fac Total		51	50	62	80	MUE
	0.00	0.00	XXX	9	9	9	9	

1090F Presence or absence of urinary incontinence assessed (GER) CⓂ

RVU			Global Days	Modifiers				
Mod	Non-Fac Total	Fac Total		51	50	62	80	MUE
	0.00	0.00	XXX	9	9	9	9	

1091F Urinary incontinence characterized (eg, frequency, volume, timing, type of symptoms, how bothersome) (GER) CⒺ

RVU			Global Days	Modifiers				
Mod	Non-Fac Total	Fac Total		51	50	62	80	MUE
	0.00	0.00	XXX	9	9	9	9	

1100F Patient screened for future fall risk; documentation of 2 or more falls in the past year or any fall with injury in the past year (GER) ⊘ⒶⓂ

RVU			Global Days	Modifiers				
Mod	Non-Fac Total	Fac Total		51	50	62	80	MUE
	0.00	0.00	XXX	9	9	9	9	

1101F Patient screened for future fall risk; documentation of no falls in the past year or only 1 fall without injury in the past year (GER) ⊘ⒶⓂ

RVU			Global Days	Modifiers				
Mod	Non-Fac Total	Fac Total		51	50	62	80	MUE
	0.00	0.00	XXX	9	9	9	9	

1110F Patient discharged from an inpatient facility (eg, hospital, skilled nursing facility, or rehabilitation facility) within the last 60 days (GER) CⒺ

RVU			Global Days	Modifiers				
Mod	Non-Fac Total	Fac Total		51	50	62	80	MUE
	0.00	0.00	XXX	9	9	9	9	

● New ▲ Revised Deleted ⊙ Moderate Sedation ✚ Add-on Codes ⊘ High Risk Denial Ⓐ Age Edit ♀ Female ♂ Male **AMA** *CPT® Assistant* **MUE** Medically Unlikely Edit
⊘ Modifier 51 Exempt ⊖ Modifier 63 Exempt 🅧 Unlisted **Modifiers:** *See Inside Back Cover* Ⓜ Maternity A 2 – Z 3 ASC Payment Indicators A – Y OPPS Status Indicators

© 2016 DecisionHealth | CPT © 2015 American Medical Association. All Rights Reserved. | **865**

1111F Discharge medications reconciled with the current medication list in outpatient medical record (COA) (GER) Ⓜ

RVU		Global Days	Modifiers				
Mod	Non-Fac Total	Fac Total		51	50	62	80	MUE
	0.00	0.00	XXX	9	9	9	9

1116F Auricular or periauricular pain assessed (AOE) Ⓔ

RVU		Global Days	Modifiers				
Mod	Non-Fac Total	Fac Total		51	50	62	80	MUE
	0.00	0.00	XXX	9	9	9	9

1118F GERD symptoms assessed after 12 months of therapy (GERD) Ⓔ

RVU		Global Days	Modifiers				
Mod	Non-Fac Total	Fac Total		51	50	62	80	MUE
	0.00	0.00	XXX	9	9	9	9

1119F Initial evaluation for condition (HEP C)(EPI, DSP) Ⓔ

RVU		Global Days	Modifiers				
Mod	Non-Fac Total	Fac Total		51	50	62	80	MUE
	0.00	0.00	XXX	9	9	9	9

1121F Subsequent evaluation for condition (HEP C) (EPI) Ⓔ

RVU		Global Days	Modifiers				
Mod	Non-Fac Total	Fac Total		51	50	62	80	MUE
	0.00	0.00	XXX	9	9	9	9

1123F Advance Care Planning discussed and documented advance care plan or surrogate decision maker documented in the medical record (DEM) (GER, Pall Cr) Ⓜ

RVU		Global Days	Modifiers				
Mod	Non-Fac Total	Fac Total		51	50	62	80	MUE
	0.00	0.00	XXX	9	9	9	9

1124F Advance Care Planning discussed and documented in the medical record, patient did not wish or was not able to name a surrogate decision maker or provide an advance care plan (DEM) (GER, Pall Cr) Ⓜ

RVU		Global Days	Modifiers				
Mod	Non-Fac Total	Fac Total		51	50	62	80	MUE
	0.00	0.00	XXX	9	9	9	9

1125F Pain severity quantified; pain present (COA) (ONC) Ⓜ

RVU		Global Days	Modifiers				
Mod	Non-Fac Total	Fac Total		51	50	62	80	MUE
	0.00	0.00	XXX	9	9	9	9

1126F Pain severity quantified; no pain present (COA) (ONC) Ⓜ

RVU		Global Days	Modifiers				
Mod	Non-Fac Total	Fac Total		51	50	62	80	MUE
	0.00	0.00	XXX	9	9	9	9

1127F New episode for condition (NMA-No Measure Associated) Ⓔ

RVU		Global Days	Modifiers				
Mod	Non-Fac Total	Fac Total		51	50	62	80	MUE
	0.00	0.00	XXX	9	9	9	9

1128F Subsequent episode for condition (NMA-No Measure Associated) Ⓔ

RVU		Global Days	Modifiers				
Mod	Non-Fac Total	Fac Total		51	50	62	80	MUE
	0.00	0.00	XXX	9	9	9	9

1130F Back pain and function assessed, including all of the following: Pain assessment and functional status and patient history, including notation of presence or absence of "red flags" (warning signs) and assessment of prior treatment and response, and employment status (BkP) Ⓔ

RVU		Global Days	Modifiers				
Mod	Non-Fac Total	Fac Total		51	50	62	80	MUE
	0.00	0.00	XXX	9	9	9	9

1134F Episode of back pain lasting 6 weeks or less (BkP) Ⓔ

RVU		Global Days	Modifiers				
Mod	Non-Fac Total	Fac Total		51	50	62	80	MUE
	0.00	0.00	XXX	9	9	9	9

1135F Episode of back pain lasting longer than 6 weeks (BkP) Ⓔ

RVU		Global Days	Modifiers				
Mod	Non-Fac Total	Fac Total		51	50	62	80	MUE
	0.00	0.00	XXX	9	9	9	9

1136F Episode of back pain lasting 12 weeks or less (BkP) Ⓔ

RVU		Global Days	Modifiers				
Mod	Non-Fac Total	Fac Total		51	50	62	80	MUE
	0.00	0.00	XXX	9	9	9	9

1137F Episode of back pain lasting longer than 12 weeks (BkP) Ⓔ

RVU		Global Days	Modifiers				
Mod	Non-Fac Total	Fac Total		51	50	62	80	MUE
	0.00	0.00	XXX	9	9	9	9

1150F Documentation that a patient has a substantial risk of death within 1 year (Pall Cr) Ⓔ

RVU		Global Days	Modifiers				
Mod	Non-Fac Total	Fac Total		51	50	62	80	MUE
	0.00	0.00	XXX	9	9	9	9

1151F Documentation that a patient does not have a substantial risk of death within one year (Pall Cr) Ⓔ

RVU		Global Days	Modifiers				
Mod	Non-Fac Total	Fac Total		51	50	62	80	MUE
	0.00	0.00	XXX	9	9	9	9

1152F Documentation of advanced disease diagnosis, goals of care prioritize comfort (Pall Cr) Ⓔ

RVU		Global Days	Modifiers				
Mod	Non-Fac Total	Fac Total		51	50	62	80	MUE
	0.00	0.00	XXX	9	9	9	9

● New   ▲ Revised   ✖ Deleted   ⊙ Moderate Sedation   ✚ Add-on Codes   ⊘ High Risk Denial   Ⓐ Age Edit   ♀ Female   ♂ Male   **AMA** *CPT® Assistant*   **MUE** Medically Unlikely Edit
⊘ Modifier 51 Exempt   ⊖ Modifier 63 Exempt   ✗ Unlisted   **Modifiers:** *See Inside Back Cover*   Ⓜ Maternity   A2–Z3 ASC Payment Indicators   A–Y OPPS Status Indicators

CPT © 2015 American Medical Association. All Rights Reserved.
© 2016 DecisionHealth

1153F Documentation of advanced disease diagnosis, goals of care do not prioritize comfort (Pall Cr) ⊘E

RVU			Global Days	Modifiers				
Mod	Non-Fac Total	Fac Total		51	50	62	80	MUE
	0.00	0.00	XXX	9	9	9	9	

1157F Advance care plan or similar legal document present in the medical record (COA) ⊘E

RVU			Global Days	Modifiers				
Mod	Non-Fac Total	Fac Total		51	50	62	80	MUE
	0.00	0.00	XXX	9	9	9	9	

1158F Advance care planning discussion documented in the medical record (COA) ⊘M

RVU			Global Days	Modifiers				
Mod	Non-Fac Total	Fac Total		51	50	62	80	MUE
	0.00	0.00	XXX	9	9	9	9	

1159F Medication list documented in medical record (COA) ⊘E

RVU			Global Days	Modifiers				
Mod	Non-Fac Total	Fac Total		51	50	62	80	MUE
	0.00	0.00	XXX	9	9	9	9	

1160F Review of all medications by a prescribing practitioner or clinical pharmacist (such as, prescriptions, OTCs, herbal therapies and supplements) documented in the medical record (COA) ⊘E

RVU			Global Days	Modifiers				
Mod	Non-Fac Total	Fac Total		51	50	62	80	MUE
	0.00	0.00	XXX	9	9	9	9	

1170F Functional status assessed (COA) (RA) ⊘M

RVU			Global Days	Modifiers				
Mod	Non-Fac Total	Fac Total		51	50	62	80	MUE
	0.00	0.00	XXX	9	9	9	9	

1175F Functional status for dementia assessed and results reviewed (DEM) ⊘M

RVU			Global Days	Modifiers				
Mod	Non-Fac Total	Fac Total		51	50	62	80	MUE
	0.00	0.00	XXX	9	9	9	9	

1180F All specified thromboembolic risk factors assessed (AFIB) ⊘E

RVU			Global Days	Modifiers				
Mod	Non-Fac Total	Fac Total		51	50	62	80	MUE
	0.00	0.00	XXX	9	9	9	9	

1181F Neuropsychiatric symptoms assessed and results reviewed (DEM) ⊘M

RVU			Global Days	Modifiers				
Mod	Non-Fac Total	Fac Total		51	50	62	80	MUE
	0.00	0.00	XXX	9	9	9	9	

1182F Neuropsychiatric symptoms, one or more present (DEM) ⊘E

RVU			Global Days	Modifiers				
Mod	Non-Fac Total	Fac Total		51	50	62	80	MUE
	0.00	0.00	XXX	9	9	9	9	

1183F Neuropsychiatric symptoms, absent (DEM) E

RVU			Global Days	Modifiers				
Mod	Non-Fac Total	Fac Total		51	50	62	80	MUE
	0.00	0.00	XXX	9	9	9	9	

1200F Seizure type(s) and current seizure frequency(ies) documented (EPI) ⊘E

RVU			Global Days	Modifiers				
Mod	Non-Fac Total	Fac Total		51	50	62	80	MUE
	0.00	0.00	XXX	9	9	9	9	

1205F Etiology of epilepsy or epilepsy syndrome(s) reviewed and documented (EPI) ⊘E

RVU			Global Days	Modifiers				
Mod	Non-Fac Total	Fac Total		51	50	62	80	MUE
	0.00	0.00	XXX	9	9	9	9	

1220F Patient screened for depression (SUD) ⊘E

RVU			Global Days	Modifiers				
Mod	Non-Fac Total	Fac Total		51	50	62	80	MUE
	0.00	0.00	XXX	9	9	9	9	

1400F Parkinson's disease diagnosis reviewed (Prkns) ⊘M

RVU			Global Days	Modifiers				
Mod	Non-Fac Total	Fac Total		51	50	62	80	MUE
	0.00	0.00	XXX	9	9	9	9	

1450F Symptoms improved or remained consistent with treatment goals since last assessment (HF) E

RVU			Global Days	Modifiers				
Mod	Non-Fac Total	Fac Total		51	50	62	80	MUE
	0.00	0.00	XXX	9	9	9	9	

1451F Symptoms demonstrated clinically important deterioration since last assessment (HF) E

RVU			Global Days	Modifiers				
Mod	Non-Fac Total	Fac Total		51	50	62	80	MUE
	0.00	0.00	XXX	9	9	9	9	

1460F Qualifying cardiac event/diagnosis in previous 12 months (CAD) ⊘M

RVU			Global Days	Modifiers				
Mod	Non-Fac Total	Fac Total		51	50	62	80	MUE
	0.00	0.00	XXX	9	9	9	9	

1461F No qualifying cardiac event/diagnosis in previous 12 months (CAD) ⊘M

RVU			Global Days	Modifiers				
Mod	Non-Fac Total	Fac Total		51	50	62	80	MUE
	0.00	0.00	XXX	9	9	9	9	

1490F Dementia severity classified, mild (DEM) ⊘M

RVU			Global Days	Modifiers				
Mod	Non-Fac Total	Fac Total		51	50	62	80	MUE
	0.00	0.00	XXX	9	9	9	9	

1491F Dementia severity classified, moderate (DEM) ⊘M

RVU			Global Days	Modifiers				
Mod	Non-Fac Total	Fac Total		51	50	62	80	MUE
	0.00	0.00	XXX	9	9	9	9	

● New   ▲ Revised   Deleted   ⊙ Moderate Sedation   ✚ Add-on Codes   ⊗ High Risk Denial   Ⓐ Age Edit   ♀ Female   ♂ Male   **AMA** *CPT® Assistant*   **MUE** Medically Unlikely Edit
⊘ Modifier 51 Exempt   ⊖ Modifier 63 Exempt   ✗ Unlisted   **Modifiers:** *See Inside Back Cover*   Ⓜ Maternity   A2–Z3 ASC Payment Indicators   A–Y OPPS Status Indicators

© 2016 DecisionHealth   CPT © 2015 American Medical Association. All Rights Reserved.

1493F Dementia severity classified, severe (DEM) Ⓜ

Mod	RVU Non-Fac Total	Fac Total	Global Days	Modifiers 51	50	62	80	MUE
	0.00	0.00	XXX	9	9	9	9	

1494F Cognition assessed and reviewed (DEM) Ⓜ

Mod	RVU Non-Fac Total	Fac Total	Global Days	Modifiers 51	50	62	80	MUE
	0.00	0.00	XXX	9	9	9	9	

1500F Symptoms and signs of distal symmetric polyneuropathy reviewed and documented (DSP) Ⓔ

Mod	RVU Non-Fac Total	Fac Total	Global Days	Modifiers 51	50	62	80	MUE
	0.00	0.00	XXX	9	9	9	9	

1501F Not initial evaluation for condition (DSP) Ⓔ

Mod	RVU Non-Fac Total	Fac Total	Global Days	Modifiers 51	50	62	80	MUE
	0.00	0.00	XXX	9	9	9	9	

1502F Patient queried about pain and pain interference with function using a valid and reliable instrument (DSP) Ⓔ

Mod	RVU Non-Fac Total	Fac Total	Global Days	Modifiers 51	50	62	80	MUE
	0.00	0.00	XXX	9	9	9	9	

1503F Patient queried about symptoms of respiratory insufficiency (ALS) Ⓔ

Mod	RVU Non-Fac Total	Fac Total	Global Days	Modifiers 51	50	62	80	MUE
	0.00	0.00	XXX	9	9	9	9	

1504F Patient has respiratory insufficiency (ALS) Ⓔ

Mod	RVU Non-Fac Total	Fac Total	Global Days	Modifiers 51	50	62	80	MUE
	0.00	0.00	XXX	9	9	9	9	

1505F Patient does not have respiratory insufficiency (ALS) Ⓔ

Mod	RVU Non-Fac Total	Fac Total	Global Days	Modifiers 51	50	62	80	MUE
	0.00	0.00	XXX	9	9	9	9	

Physical Examination Codes

2000F Blood pressure measured (CKD)(DM) Ⓜ

Mod	RVU Non-Fac Total	Fac Total	Global Days	Modifiers 51	50	62	80	MUE
	0.00	0.00	XXX	9	9	9	9	

AMA: Oct 05: 1, 6, Aug 07: 1

2001F Weight recorded (PAG) Ⓔ

Mod	RVU Non-Fac Total	Fac Total	Global Days	Modifiers 51	50	62	80	MUE
	0.00	0.00	XXX	9	9	9	9	

AMA: Oct 05: 6

2002F Clinical signs of volume overload (excess) assessed (NMA-No Measure Associated) Ⓔ

Mod	RVU Non-Fac Total	Fac Total	Global Days	Modifiers 51	50	62	80	MUE
	0.00	0.00	XXX	9	9	9	9	

AMA: Oct 05: 6

2004F Initial examination of the involved joint(s) (includes visual inspection, palpation, range of motion) (OA) [Instructions: Report only for initial osteoarthritis visit or for visits for new joint involvement] Ⓔ

Mod	RVU Non-Fac Total	Fac Total	Global Days	Modifiers 51	50	62	80	MUE
	0.00	0.00	XXX	9	9	9	9	

AMA: Oct 05: 6

2010F Vital signs (temperature, pulse, respiratory rate, and blood pressure) documented and reviewed (CAP) (EM) Ⓔ

Mod	RVU Non-Fac Total	Fac Total	Global Days	Modifiers 51	50	62	80	MUE
	0.00	0.00	XXX	9	9	9	9	

2014F Mental status assessed (CAP) (EM) Ⓔ

Mod	RVU Non-Fac Total	Fac Total	Global Days	Modifiers 51	50	62	80	MUE
	0.00	0.00	XXX	9	9	9	9	

2015F Asthma impairment assessed (Asthma) Ⓔ

Mod	RVU Non-Fac Total	Fac Total	Global Days	Modifiers 51	50	62	80	MUE
	0.00	0.00	XXX	9	9	9	9	

2016F Asthma risk assessed (Asthma) Ⓔ

Mod	RVU Non-Fac Total	Fac Total	Global Days	Modifiers 51	50	62	80	MUE
	0.00	0.00	XXX	9	9	9	9	

2018F Hydration status assessed (normal/mildly dehydrated/severely dehydrated) (CAP) Ⓔ

Mod	RVU Non-Fac Total	Fac Total	Global Days	Modifiers 51	50	62	80	MUE
	0.00	0.00	XXX	9	9	9	9	

2019F Dilated macular exam performed, including documentation of the presence or absence of macular thickening or hemorrhage and the level of macular degeneration severity (EC) Ⓜ

Mod	RVU Non-Fac Total	Fac Total	Global Days	Modifiers 51	50	62	80	MUE
	0.00	0.00	XXX	9	9	9	9	

2020F Dilated fundus evaluation performed within 12 months prior to cataract surgery (EC) Ⓔ

Mod	RVU Non-Fac Total	Fac Total	Global Days	Modifiers 51	50	62	80	MUE
	0.00	0.00	XXX	9	9	9	9	

2021F Dilated macular or fundus exam performed, including documentation of the presence or absence of macular edema and level of severity of retinopathy (EC) Ⓔ

Mod	RVU Non-Fac Total	Fac Total	Global Days	Modifiers 51	50	62	80	MUE
	0.00	0.00	XXX	9	9	9	9	

● New   ▲ Revised   ✖ Deleted   ⊙ Moderate Sedation   ➕ Add-on Codes   ⊘ High Risk Denial   Ⓐ Age Edit   ♀ Female   ♂ Male   **AMA** *CPT® Assistant*   **MUE** Medically Unlikely Edit
⊘ Modifier 51 Exempt   ⊖ Modifier 63 Exempt   ✖ Unlisted   **Modifiers:** *See Inside Back Cover*   Ⓜ Maternity   A2–Z3 ASC Payment Indicators   A–Y OPPS Status Indicators

CPT © 2015 American Medical Association. All Rights Reserved.   © 2016 DecisionHealth

2022F Dilated retinal eye exam with interpretation by an ophthalmologist or optometrist documented and reviewed (DM) ⊛M

RVU			Global Days	Modifiers				
Mod	Non-Fac Total	Fac Total		51	50	62	80	MUE
	0.00	0.00	XXX	9	9	9	9	

2024F 7 standard field stereoscopic photos with interpretation by an ophthalmologist or optometrist documented and reviewed (DM) ⊛M

RVU			Global Days	Modifiers				
Mod	Non-Fac Total	Fac Total		51	50	62	80	MUE
	0.00	0.00	XXX	9	9	9	9	

2026F Eye imaging validated to match diagnosis from 7 standard field stereoscopic photos results documented and reviewed (DM) ⊛M

RVU			Global Days	Modifiers				
Mod	Non-Fac Total	Fac Total		51	50	62	80	MUE
	0.00	0.00	XXX	9	9	9	9	

2027F Optic nerve head evaluation performed (EC) ⊛M

RVU			Global Days	Modifiers				
Mod	Non-Fac Total	Fac Total		51	50	62	80	MUE
	0.00	0.00	XXX	9	9	9	9	

2028F Foot examination performed (includes examination through visual inspection, sensory exam with monofilament, and pulse exam - report when any of the 3 components are completed) (DM) ⊛E

RVU			Global Days	Modifiers				
Mod	Non-Fac Total	Fac Total		51	50	62	80	MUE
	0.00	0.00	XXX	9	9	9	9	

2029F Complete physical skin exam performed (ML) ⊛E

RVU			Global Days	Modifiers				
Mod	Non-Fac Total	Fac Total		51	50	62	80	MUE
	0.00	0.00	XXX	9	9	9	9	

2030F Hydration status documented, normally hydrated (PAG) ⊛E

RVU			Global Days	Modifiers				
Mod	Non-Fac Total	Fac Total		51	50	62	80	MUE
	0.00	0.00	XXX	9	9	9	9	

2031F Hydration status documented, dehydrated (PAG) ⊛E

RVU			Global Days	Modifiers				
Mod	Non-Fac Total	Fac Total		51	50	62	80	MUE
	0.00	0.00	XXX	9	9	9	9	

2035F Tympanic membrane mobility assessed with pneumatic otoscopy or tympanometry (OME) ⊛E

RVU			Global Days	Modifiers				
Mod	Non-Fac Total	Fac Total		51	50	62	80	MUE
	0.00	0.00	XXX	9	9	9	9	

2040F Physical examination on the date of the initial visit for low back pain performed, in accordance with specifications (BkP) ⊛E

RVU			Global Days	Modifiers				
Mod	Non-Fac Total	Fac Total		51	50	62	80	MUE
	0.00	0.00	XXX	9	9	9	9	

2044F Documentation of mental health assessment prior to intervention (back surgery or epidural steroid injection) or for back pain episode lasting longer than 6 weeks (BkP) ⊛E

RVU			Global Days	Modifiers				
Mod	Non-Fac Total	Fac Total		51	50	62	80	MUE
	0.00	0.00	XXX	9	9	9	9	

2050F Wound characteristics including size and nature of wound base tissue and amount of drainage prior to debridement documented (CWC) ⊛E

RVU			Global Days	Modifiers				
Mod	Non-Fac Total	Fac Total		51	50	62	80	MUE
	0.00	0.00	XXX	9	9	9	9	

2060F Patient interviewed directly on or before date of diagnosis of major depressive disorder (MDD ADOL) ⊛E

RVU			Global Days	Modifiers				
Mod	Non-Fac Total	Fac Total		51	50	62	80	MUE
	0.00	0.00	XXX	9	9	9	9	

Diagnostic/Screening Processes/Result Codes

3006F Chest X-ray results documented and reviewed (CAP) ⊛E

RVU			Global Days	Modifiers				
Mod	Non-Fac Total	Fac Total		51	50	62	80	MUE
	0.00	0.00	XXX	9	9	9	9	

AMA: Aug 07: 1

3008F Body Mass Index (BMI), documented (PV) ⊛E

RVU			Global Days	Modifiers				
Mod	Non-Fac Total	Fac Total		51	50	62	80	MUE
	0.00	0.00	XXX	9	9	9	9	

3011F Lipid panel results documented and reviewed (must include total cholesterol, HDL-C, triglycerides and calculated LDL-C) (CAD) ⊛E

RVU			Global Days	Modifiers				
Mod	Non-Fac Total	Fac Total		51	50	62	80	MUE
	0.00	0.00	XXX	9	9	9	9	

3014F Screening mammography results documented and reviewed (PV) ⊛M

RVU			Global Days	Modifiers				
Mod	Non-Fac Total	Fac Total		51	50	62	80	MUE
	0.00	0.00	XXX	9	9	9	9	

3015F Cervical cancer screening results documented and reviewed (PV) ♀⊛E

RVU			Global Days	Modifiers				
Mod	Non-Fac Total	Fac Total		51	50	62	80	MUE
	0.00	0.00	XXX	9	9	9	9	

3016F Patient screened for unhealthy alcohol use using a systematic screening method (PV) (DSP) ⊛E

RVU			Global Days	Modifiers				
Mod	Non-Fac Total	Fac Total		51	50	62	80	MUE
	0.00	0.00	XXX	9	9	9	9	

● New   ▲ Revised   Deleted   ⊙ Moderate Sedation   ✚ Add-on Codes   ⊘ High Risk Denial   Ⓐ Age Edit   ♀ Female   ♂ Male   **AMA** *CPT® Assistant*   **MUE** Medically Unlikely Edit
⊘ Modifier 51 Exempt   ⊖ Modifier 63 Exempt   ✗ Unlisted   **Modifiers:** *See Inside Back Cover*   M Maternity   A2–Z3 ASC Payment Indicators   A–Y OPPS Status Indicators

Category II Procedures

3017F – 3046F

3017F Colorectal cancer screening results documented and reviewed (PV) Ⓜ

RVU			Global Days	Modifiers				
Mod	Non-Fac Total	Fac Total		51	50	62	80	MUE
	0.00	0.00	XXX	9	9	9	9	

3018F Pre-procedure risk assessment and depth of insertion and quality of the bowel prep and complete description of polyp(s) found, including location of each polyp, size, number and gross morphology and recommendations for follow-up in final colonoscopy report documented (End/Polyp) Ⓔ

RVU			Global Days	Modifiers				
Mod	Non-Fac Total	Fac Total		51	50	62	80	MUE
	0.00	0.00	XXX	9	9	9	9	

3019F Left ventricular ejection fraction (LVEF) assessment planned post discharge (HF) Ⓔ

RVU			Global Days	Modifiers				
Mod	Non-Fac Total	Fac Total		51	50	62	80	MUE
	0.00	0.00	XXX	9	9	9	9	

3020F Left ventricular function (LVF) assessment (eg, echocardiography, nuclear test, or ventriculography) documented in the medical record (Includes quantitative or qualitative assessment results) (NMA-No Measure Associated) Ⓔ

RVU			Global Days	Modifiers				
Mod	Non-Fac Total	Fac Total		51	50	62	80	MUE
	0.00	0.00	XXX	9	9	9	9	

3021F Left ventricular ejection fraction (LVEF) less than 40% or documentation of moderately or severely depressed left ventricular systolic function (CAD, HF) Ⓜ

RVU			Global Days	Modifiers				
Mod	Non-Fac Total	Fac Total		51	50	62	80	MUE
	0.00	0.00	XXX	9	9	9	9	

3022F Left ventricular ejection fraction (LVEF) greater than or equal to 40% or documentation as normal or mildly depressed left ventricular systolic function (CAD, HF) Ⓜ

RVU			Global Days	Modifiers				
Mod	Non-Fac Total	Fac Total		51	50	62	80	MUE
	0.00	0.00	XXX	9	9	9	9	

3023F Spirometry results documented and reviewed (COPD) Ⓜ

RVU			Global Days	Modifiers				
Mod	Non-Fac Total	Fac Total		51	50	62	80	MUE
	0.00	0.00	XXX	9	9	9	9	

3025F Spirometry test results demonstrate FEV1/FVC less than 70% with COPD symptoms (eg, dyspnea, cough/sputum, wheezing) (CAP, COPD) Ⓔ

RVU			Global Days	Modifiers				
Mod	Non-Fac Total	Fac Total		51	50	62	80	MUE
	0.00	0.00	XXX	9	9	9	9	

3027F Spirometry test results demonstrate FEV1/FVC greater than or equal to 70% or patient does not have COPD symptoms (COPD) Ⓔ

RVU			Global Days	Modifiers				
Mod	Non-Fac Total	Fac Total		51	50	62	80	MUE
	0.00	0.00	XXX	9	9	9	9	

3028F Oxygen saturation results documented and reviewed (includes assessment through pulse oximetry or arterial blood gas measurement) (CAP, COPD) (EM) Ⓔ

RVU			Global Days	Modifiers				
Mod	Non-Fac Total	Fac Total		51	50	62	80	MUE
	0.00	0.00	XXX	9	9	9	9	

3035F Oxygen saturation less than or equal to 88% or a PaO2 less than or equal to 55 mm Hg (COPD) Ⓔ

RVU			Global Days	Modifiers				
Mod	Non-Fac Total	Fac Total		51	50	62	80	MUE
	0.00	0.00	XXX	9	9	9	9	

3037F Oxygen saturation greater than 88% or PaO2 greater than 55 mm Hg (COPD) Ⓔ

RVU			Global Days	Modifiers				
Mod	Non-Fac Total	Fac Total		51	50	62	80	MUE
	0.00	0.00	XXX	9	9	9	9	

3038F Pulmonary function test performed within 12 months prior to surgery (Lung/Esop Cx) Ⓔ

RVU			Global Days	Modifiers				
Mod	Non-Fac Total	Fac Total		51	50	62	80	MUE
	0.00	0.00	XXX	9	9	9	9	

3040F Functional expiratory volume (FEV1) less than 40% of predicted value (COPD) Ⓔ

RVU			Global Days	Modifiers				
Mod	Non-Fac Total	Fac Total		51	50	62	80	MUE
	0.00	0.00	XXX	9	9	9	9	

3042F Functional expiratory volume (FEV1) greater than or equal to 40% of predicted value (COPD) Ⓔ

RVU			Global Days	Modifiers				
Mod	Non-Fac Total	Fac Total		51	50	62	80	MUE
	0.00	0.00	XXX	9	9	9	9	

3044F Most recent hemoglobin A1c (HbA1c) level less than 7.0% (DM) Ⓜ

RVU			Global Days	Modifiers				
Mod	Non-Fac Total	Fac Total		51	50	62	80	MUE
	0.00	0.00	XXX	9	9	9	9	

3045F Most recent hemoglobin A1c (HbA1c) level 7.0-9.0% (DM) Ⓜ

RVU			Global Days	Modifiers				
Mod	Non-Fac Total	Fac Total		51	50	62	80	MUE
	0.00	0.00	XXX	9	9	9	9	

3046F Most recent hemoglobin A1c level greater than 9.0% (DM) Ⓜ

RVU			Global Days	Modifiers				
Mod	Non-Fac Total	Fac Total		51	50	62	80	MUE
	0.00	0.00	XXX	9	9	9	9	

● New ▲ Revised ✖ Deleted ⊙ Moderate Sedation ✚ Add-on Codes ⊘ High Risk Denial Ⓐ Age Edit ♀ Female ♂ Male **AMA** *CPT® Assistant* **MUE** Medically Unlikely Edit
⊘ Modifier 51 Exempt ⊖ Modifier 63 Exempt ✗ Unlisted **Modifiers:** *See Inside Back Cover* Ⓜ Maternity A2–Z3 ASC Payment Indicators A–Y OPPS Status Indicators

CPT © 2015 American Medical Association. All Rights Reserved.   © 2016 DecisionHealth

3048F Most recent LDL-C less than 100 mg/dL (CAD) (DM) ○E

RVU		Global Days	Modifiers				
Mod	Non-Fac Total	Fac Total		51	50	62	80	MUE
	0.00	0.00	XXX	9	9	9	9

3049F Most recent LDL-C 100-129 mg/dL (CAD) (DM) ○E

RVU		Global Days	Modifiers				
Mod	Non-Fac Total	Fac Total		51	50	62	80	MUE
	0.00	0.00	XXX	9	9	9	9

3050F Most recent LDL-C greater than or equal to 130 mg/dL (CAD) (DM) ○E

RVU		Global Days	Modifiers				
Mod	Non-Fac Total	Fac Total		51	50	62	80	MUE
	0.00	0.00	XXX	9	9	9	9

3055F Left ventricular ejection fraction (LVEF) less than or equal to 35% (HF) ○E

RVU		Global Days	Modifiers				
Mod	Non-Fac Total	Fac Total		51	50	62	80	MUE
	0.00	0.00	XXX	9	9	9	9

3056F Left ventricular ejection fraction (LVEF) greater than 35% or no LVEF result available (HF) ○E

RVU		Global Days	Modifiers				
Mod	Non-Fac Total	Fac Total		51	50	62	80	MUE
	0.00	0.00	XXX	9	9	9	9

3060F Positive microalbuminuria test result documented and reviewed (DM) ○M

RVU		Global Days	Modifiers				
Mod	Non-Fac Total	Fac Total		51	50	62	80	MUE
	0.00	0.00	XXX	9	9	9	9

3061F Negative microalbuminuria test result documented and reviewed (DM) ○M

RVU		Global Days	Modifiers				
Mod	Non-Fac Total	Fac Total		51	50	62	80	MUE
	0.00	0.00	XXX	9	9	9	9

3062F Positive macroalbuminuria test result documented and reviewed (DM) ○M

RVU		Global Days	Modifiers				
Mod	Non-Fac Total	Fac Total		51	50	62	80	MUE
	0.00	0.00	XXX	9	9	9	9

3066F Documentation of treatment for nephropathy (eg, patient receiving dialysis, patient being treated for ESRD, CRF, ARF, or renal insufficiency, any visit to a nephrologist) (DM) ○M

RVU		Global Days	Modifiers				
Mod	Non-Fac Total	Fac Total		51	50	62	80	MUE
	0.00	0.00	XXX	9	9	9	9

3072F Low risk for retinopathy (no evidence of retinopathy in the prior year) (DM) ○M

RVU		Global Days	Modifiers				
Mod	Non-Fac Total	Fac Total		51	50	62	80	MUE
	0.00	0.00	XXX	9	9	9	9

3073F Pre-surgical (cataract) axial length, corneal power measurement and method of intraocular lens power calculation documented within 12 months prior to surgery (EC) ○E

RVU		Global Days	Modifiers				
Mod	Non-Fac Total	Fac Total		51	50	62	80	MUE
	0.00	0.00	XXX	9	9	9	9

3074F Most recent systolic blood pressure less than 130 mm Hg (DM), (HTN, CKD, CAD) ○E

RVU		Global Days	Modifiers				
Mod	Non-Fac Total	Fac Total		51	50	62	80	MUE
	0.00	0.00	XXX	9	9	9	9

3075F Most recent systolic blood pressure 130 - 139 mm Hg (DM),(HTN, CKD, CAD) ○E

RVU		Global Days	Modifiers				
Mod	Non-Fac Total	Fac Total		51	50	62	80	MUE
	0.00	0.00	XXX	9	9	9	9

3077F Most recent systolic blood pressure greater than or equal to 140 mm Hg (HTN, CKD, CAD) (DM) ○E

RVU		Global Days	Modifiers				
Mod	Non-Fac Total	Fac Total		51	50	62	80	MUE
	0.00	0.00	XXX	9	9	9	9

3078F Most recent diastolic blood pressure less than 80 mm Hg (HTN, CKD, CAD) (DM) ○E

RVU		Global Days	Modifiers				
Mod	Non-Fac Total	Fac Total		51	50	62	80	MUE
	0.00	0.00	XXX	9	9	9	9

3079F Most recent diastolic blood pressure 80-89 mm Hg (HTN, CKD, CAD) (DM) ○E

RVU		Global Days	Modifiers				
Mod	Non-Fac Total	Fac Total		51	50	62	80	MUE
	0.00	0.00	XXX	9	9	9	9

3080F Most recent diastolic blood pressure greater than or equal to 90 mm Hg (HTN, CKD, CAD) (DM) ○E

RVU		Global Days	Modifiers				
Mod	Non-Fac Total	Fac Total		51	50	62	80	MUE
	0.00	0.00	XXX	9	9	9	9

3082F Kt/V less than 1.2 (Clearance of urea [Kt]/volume [V]) (ESRD, P-ESRD) ○E

RVU		Global Days	Modifiers				
Mod	Non-Fac Total	Fac Total		51	50	62	80	MUE
	0.00	0.00	XXX	9	9	9	9

3083F Kt/V equal to or greater than 1.2 and less than 1.7 (Clearance of urea [Kt]/volume [V]) (ESRD, P-ESRD) ○E

RVU		Global Days	Modifiers				
Mod	Non-Fac Total	Fac Total		51	50	62	80	MUE
	0.00	0.00	XXX	9	9	9	9

3084F Kt/V greater than or equal to 1.7 (Clearance of urea [Kt]/volume [V]) (ESRD, P-ESRD) ○E

RVU		Global Days	Modifiers				
Mod	Non-Fac Total	Fac Total		51	50	62	80	MUE
	0.00	0.00	XXX	9	9	9	9

● New   ▲ Revised   Deleted   ⊙ Moderate Sedation   ✚ Add-on Codes   ⊘ High Risk Denial   Ⓐ Age Edit   ♀ Female   ♂ Male   **AMA** CPT® Assistant   **MUE** Medically Unlikely Edit

⊘ Modifier 51 Exempt   ⊖ Modifier 63 Exempt   ☒ Unlisted   **Modifiers:** See Inside Back Cover   Ⓜ Maternity   A2–Z3 ASC Payment Indicators   A–Y OPPS Status Indicators

© 2016 DecisionHealth   CPT © 2015 American Medical Association. All Rights Reserved.

3085F Suicide risk assessed (MDD, MDD ADOL) ⊙Ⓔ

RVU			Global Days	Modifiers				
Mod	Non-Fac Total	Fac Total		51	50	62	80	MUE
	0.00	0.00	XXX	9	9	9	9	

3088F Major depressive disorder, mild (MDD) ⊙Ⓔ

RVU			Global Days	Modifiers				
Mod	Non-Fac Total	Fac Total		51	50	62	80	MUE
	0.00	0.00	XXX	9	9	9	9	

3089F Major depressive disorder, moderate (MDD) ⊙Ⓔ

RVU			Global Days	Modifiers				
Mod	Non-Fac Total	Fac Total		51	50	62	80	MUE
	0.00	0.00	XXX	9	9	9	9	

3090F Major depressive disorder, severe without psychotic features (MDD) ⊙Ⓔ

RVU			Global Days	Modifiers				
Mod	Non-Fac Total	Fac Total		51	50	62	80	MUE
	0.00	0.00	XXX	9	9	9	9	

3091F Major depressive disorder, severe with psychotic features (MDD) Ⓔ

RVU			Global Days	Modifiers				
Mod	Non-Fac Total	Fac Total		51	50	62	80	MUE
	0.00	0.00	XXX	9	9	9	9	

3092F Major depressive disorder, in remission (MDD) ⊙Ⓔ

RVU			Global Days	Modifiers				
Mod	Non-Fac Total	Fac Total		51	50	62	80	MUE
	0.00	0.00	XXX	9	9	9	9	

3093F Documentation of new diagnosis of initial or recurrent episode of major depressive disorder (MDD) ⊙Ⓔ

RVU			Global Days	Modifiers				
Mod	Non-Fac Total	Fac Total		51	50	62	80	MUE
	0.00	0.00	XXX	9	9	9	9	

3095F Central dual-energy X-ray absorptiometry (DXA) results documented (OP)(IBD) ⊙Ⓜ

RVU			Global Days	Modifiers				
Mod	Non-Fac Total	Fac Total		51	50	62	80	MUE
	0.00	0.00	XXX	9	9	9	9	

3096F Central dual-energy X-ray absorptiometry (DXA) ordered (OP)(IBD) ⊙Ⓔ

RVU			Global Days	Modifiers				
Mod	Non-Fac Total	Fac Total		51	50	62	80	MUE
	0.00	0.00	XXX	9	9	9	9	

3100F Carotid imaging study report (includes direct or indirect reference to measurements of distal internal carotid diameter as the denominator for stenosis measurement) (STR, RAD) ⊙Ⓜ

RVU			Global Days	Modifiers				
Mod	Non-Fac Total	Fac Total		51	50	62	80	MUE
	0.00	0.00	XXX	9	9	9	9	

3110F Documentation in final CT or MRI report of presence or absence of hemorrhage and mass lesion and acute infarction (STR) ⊙Ⓔ

RVU			Global Days	Modifiers				
Mod	Non-Fac Total	Fac Total		51	50	62	80	MUE
	0.00	0.00	XXX	9	9	9	9	

3111F CT or MRI of the brain performed in the hospital within 24 hours of arrival or performed in an outpatient imaging center, to confirm initial diagnosis of stroke, TIA or intracranial hemorrhage (STR) ⊙Ⓔ

RVU			Global Days	Modifiers				
Mod	Non-Fac Total	Fac Total		51	50	62	80	MUE
	0.00	0.00	XXX	9	9	9	9	

3112F CT or MRI of the brain performed greater than 24 hours after arrival to the hospital or performed in an outpatient imaging center for purpose other than confirmation of initial diagnosis of stroke, TIA, or intracranial hemorrhage (STR) ⊙Ⓔ

RVU			Global Days	Modifiers				
Mod	Non-Fac Total	Fac Total		51	50	62	80	MUE
	0.00	0.00	XXX	9	9	9	9	

3115F Quantitative results of an evaluation of current level of activity and clinical symptoms (HF) Ⓔ

RVU			Global Days	Modifiers				
Mod	Non-Fac Total	Fac Total		51	50	62	80	MUE
	0.00	0.00	XXX	9	9	9	9	

3117F Heart failure disease specific structured assessment tool completed (HF) ⊙Ⓔ

RVU			Global Days	Modifiers				
Mod	Non-Fac Total	Fac Total		51	50	62	80	MUE
	0.00	0.00	XXX	9	9	9	9	

3118F New York Heart Association (NYHA) Class documented (HF) Ⓔ

RVU			Global Days	Modifiers				
Mod	Non-Fac Total	Fac Total		51	50	62	80	MUE
	0.00	0.00	XXX	9	9	9	9	

3119F No evaluation of level of activity or clinical symptoms (HF) ⊙Ⓔ

RVU			Global Days	Modifiers				
Mod	Non-Fac Total	Fac Total		51	50	62	80	MUE
	0.00	0.00	XXX	9	9	9	9	

3120F 12-Lead ECG Performed (EM) ⊙Ⓜ

RVU			Global Days	Modifiers				
Mod	Non-Fac Total	Fac Total		51	50	62	80	MUE
	0.00	0.00	XXX	9	9	9	9	

3126f Esophageal biopsy report with a statement about dysplasia (present, absent, or indefinite, and if present, contains appropriate grading) (PATH) Ⓜ

RVU			Global Days	Modifiers				
Mod	Non-Fac Total	Fac Total		51	50	62	80	MUE
	0.00	0.00	XXX	9	9	9	9	

● New   ▲ Revised   ✖ Deleted   ⊙ Moderate Sedation   ✚ Add-on Codes   ⊘ High Risk Denial   Ⓐ Age Edit   ♀ Female   ♂ Male   **AMA** *CPT® Assistant*   **MUE** Medically Unlikely Edit
⊘ Modifier 51 Exempt   ⊖ Modifier 63 Exempt   ⊠ Unlisted   **Modifiers:** *See Inside Back Cover*   Ⓜ Maternity   A2–Z3 ASC Payment Indicators   A–Y OPPS Status Indicators

872   CPT © 2015 American Medical Association. All Rights Reserved.   © 2016 DecisionHealth

3130F Upper gastrointestinal endoscopy performed (GERD) ⊕E

Mod	Non-Fac Total	Fac Total	Global Days	51	50	62	80	MUE
	0.00	0.00	XXX	9	9	9	9	

3132F Documentation of referral for upper gastrointestinal endoscopy (GERD) ⊕E

Mod	Non-Fac Total	Fac Total	Global Days	51	50	62	80	MUE
	0.00	0.00	XXX	9	9	9	9	

3140F Upper gastrointestinal endoscopy report indicates suspicion of Barrett's esophagus (GERD) ⊕E

Mod	Non-Fac Total	Fac Total	Global Days	51	50	62	80	MUE
	0.00	0.00	XXX	9	9	9	9	

3141F Upper gastrointestinal endoscopy report indicates no suspicion of Barrett's esophagus (GERD) ⊕E

Mod	Non-Fac Total	Fac Total	Global Days	51	50	62	80	MUE
	0.00	0.00	XXX	9	9	9	9	

3142F Barium swallow test ordered (GERD) ⊕E

Mod	Non-Fac Total	Fac Total	Global Days	51	50	62	80	MUE
	0.00	0.00	XXX	9	9	9	9	

3150F Forceps esophageal biopsy performed (GERD) ⊕E

Mod	Non-Fac Total	Fac Total	Global Days	51	50	62	80	MUE
	0.00	0.00	XXX	9	9	9	9	

3155F Cytogenetic testing performed on bone marrow at time of diagnosis or prior to initiating treatment (HEM) ⊕M

Mod	Non-Fac Total	Fac Total	Global Days	51	50	62	80	MUE
	0.00	0.00	XXX	9	9	9	9	

3160F Documentation of iron stores prior to initiating erythropoietin therapy (HEM) ⊕M

Mod	Non-Fac Total	Fac Total	Global Days	51	50	62	80	MUE
	0.00	0.00	XXX	9	9	9	9	

3170F Flow cytometry studies performed at time of diagnosis or prior to initiating treatment (HEM) ⊕M

Mod	Non-Fac Total	Fac Total	Global Days	51	50	62	80	MUE
	0.00	0.00	XXX	9	9	9	9	

3200F Barium swallow test not ordered (GERD) ⊕E

Mod	Non-Fac Total	Fac Total	Global Days	51	50	62	80	MUE
	0.00	0.00	XXX	9	9	9	9	

3210F Group A Strep Test Performed (PHAR) ⊕M

Mod	Non-Fac Total	Fac Total	Global Days	51	50	62	80	MUE
	0.00	0.00	XXX	9	9	9	9	

3215F Patient has documented immunity to Hepatitis A (HEP-C) ⊕M

Mod	Non-Fac Total	Fac Total	Global Days	51	50	62	80	MUE
	0.00	0.00	XXX	9	9	9	9	

3216F Patient has documented immunity to Hepatitis B (HEP-C)(IBD) ⊕E

Mod	Non-Fac Total	Fac Total	Global Days	51	50	62	80	MUE
	0.00	0.00	XXX	9	9	9	9	

3218F RNA testing for Hepatitis C documented as performed within 6 months prior to initiation of antiviral treatment for Hepatitis C (HEP-C) ⊕E

Mod	Non-Fac Total	Fac Total	Global Days	51	50	62	80	MUE
	0.00	0.00	XXX	9	9	9	9	

3220F Hepatitis C quantitative RNA testing documented as performed at 12 weeks from initiation of antiviral treatment (HEP-C) ⊕E

Mod	Non-Fac Total	Fac Total	Global Days	51	50	62	80	MUE
	0.00	0.00	XXX	9	9	9	9	

3230F Documentation that hearing test was performed within 6 months prior to tympanostomy tube insertion (OME) E

Mod	Non-Fac Total	Fac Total	Global Days	51	50	62	80	MUE
	0.00	0.00	XXX	9	9	9	9	

3250F Specimen site other than anatomic location of primary tumor (PATH) ⊕M

Mod	Non-Fac Total	Fac Total	Global Days	51	50	62	80	MUE
	0.00	0.00	XXX	9	9	9	9	

3260F pT category (primary tumor), pN category (regional lymph nodes), and histologic grade documented in pathology report (PATH) ⊕M

Mod	Non-Fac Total	Fac Total	Global Days	51	50	62	80	MUE
	0.00	0.00	XXX	9	9	9	9	

3265F Ribonucleic acid (RNA) testing for Hepatitis C viremia ordered or results documented (HEP C) ⊕E

Mod	Non-Fac Total	Fac Total	Global Days	51	50	62	80	MUE
	0.00	0.00	XXX	9	9	9	9	

3266F Hepatitis C genotype testing documented as performed prior to initiation of antiviral treatment for Hepatitis C (HEP C) ⊕E

Mod	Non-Fac Total	Fac Total	Global Days	51	50	62	80	MUE
	0.00	0.00	XXX	9	9	9	9	

● New   ▲ Revised   Deleted   ⊙ Moderate Sedation   ✚ Add-on Codes   ⊘ High Risk Denial   Ⓐ Age Edit   ♀ Female   ♂ Male   **AMA** *CPT® Assistant*   **MUE** Medically Unlikely Edit
⊘ Modifier 51 Exempt   ⊖ Modifier 63 Exempt   ✗ Unlisted   **Modifiers:** *See Inside Back Cover*   Ⓜ Maternity   A2–Z3 ASC Payment Indicators   A–Y OPPS Status Indicators

© 2016 DecisionHealth   CPT © 2015 American Medical Association. All Rights Reserved.

Category II Procedures

3267F – 3294F

3267F Pathology report includes pT category, pN category, Gleason score, and statement about margin status (PATH) ⓈM

Mod	RVU Non-Fac Total	Fac Total	Global Days	Modifiers 51	50	62	80	MUE
	0.00	0.00	XXX	9	9	9	9	

3268F Prostate-specific antigen (PSA), and primary tumor (T) stage, and Gleason score documented prior to initiation of treatment (PRCA) ⓈE

Mod	RVU Non-Fac Total	Fac Total	Global Days	Modifiers 51	50	62	80	MUE
	0.00	0.00	XXX	9	9	9	9	

3269F Bone scan performed prior to initiation of treatment or at any time since diagnosis of prostate cancer (PRCA) ⓈM

Mod	RVU Non-Fac Total	Fac Total	Global Days	Modifiers 51	50	62	80	MUE
	0.00	0.00	XXX	9	9	9	9	

3270F Bone scan not performed prior to initiation of treatment nor at any time since diagnosis of prostate cancer (PRCA) ⓈM

Mod	RVU Non-Fac Total	Fac Total	Global Days	Modifiers 51	50	62	80	MUE
	0.00	0.00	XXX	9	9	9	9	

3271F Low risk of recurrence, prostate cancer (PRCA) ⓈM

Mod	RVU Non-Fac Total	Fac Total	Global Days	Modifiers 51	50	62	80	MUE
	0.00	0.00	XXX	9	9	9	9	

3272F Intermediate risk of recurrence, prostate cancer (PRCA) ⓈE

Mod	RVU Non-Fac Total	Fac Total	Global Days	Modifiers 51	50	62	80	MUE
	0.00	0.00	XXX	9	9	9	9	

3273F High risk of recurrence, prostate cancer (PRCA) ⓈE

Mod	RVU Non-Fac Total	Fac Total	Global Days	Modifiers 51	50	62	80	MUE
	0.00	0.00	XXX	9	9	9	9	

3274F Prostate cancer risk of recurrence not determined or neither low, intermediate nor high (PRCA) ⓈE

Mod	RVU Non-Fac Total	Fac Total	Global Days	Modifiers 51	50	62	80	MUE
	0.00	0.00	XXX	9	9	9	9	

3278F Serum levels of calcium, phosphorus, intact Parathyroid Hormone (PTH) and lipid profile ordered (CKD) ⓈE

Mod	RVU Non-Fac Total	Fac Total	Global Days	Modifiers 51	50	62	80	MUE
	0.00	0.00	XXX	9	9	9	9	

3279F Hemoglobin level greater than or equal to 13 g/dL (CKD, ESRD) ⓈE

Mod	RVU Non-Fac Total	Fac Total	Global Days	Modifiers 51	50	62	80	MUE
	0.00	0.00	XXX	9	9	9	9	

3280F Hemoglobin level 11 g/dL to 12.9 g/dL (CKD, ESRD) ⓈE

Mod	RVU Non-Fac Total	Fac Total	Global Days	Modifiers 51	50	62	80	MUE
	0.00	0.00	XXX	9	9	9	9	

3281F Hemoglobin level less than 11 g/dL (CKD, ESRD) ⓈE

Mod	RVU Non-Fac Total	Fac Total	Global Days	Modifiers 51	50	62	80	MUE
	0.00	0.00	XXX	9	9	9	9	

3284F Intraocular pressure (IOP) reduced by a value of greater than or equal to 15% from the pre-intervention level (EC) ⓈM

Mod	RVU Non-Fac Total	Fac Total	Global Days	Modifiers 51	50	62	80	MUE
	0.00	0.00	XXX	9	9	9	9	

3285F Intraocular pressure (IOP) reduced by a value less than 15% from the pre-intervention level (EC) ⓈM

Mod	RVU Non-Fac Total	Fac Total	Global Days	Modifiers 51	50	62	80	MUE
	0.00	0.00	XXX	9	9	9	9	

3288F Falls risk assessment documented (GER) ⓈM

Mod	RVU Non-Fac Total	Fac Total	Global Days	Modifiers 51	50	62	80	MUE
	0.00	0.00	XXX	9	9	9	9	

3290F Patient is D (Rh) negative and unsensitized (Pre-Cr) E

Mod	RVU Non-Fac Total	Fac Total	Global Days	Modifiers 51	50	62	80	MUE
	0.00	0.00	XXX	9	9	9	9	

3291F Patient is D (Rh) positive or sensitized (Pre-Cr) E

Mod	RVU Non-Fac Total	Fac Total	Global Days	Modifiers 51	50	62	80	MUE
	0.00	0.00	XXX	9	9	9	9	

3292F HIV testing ordered or documented and reviewed during the first or second prenatal visit (Pre-Cr) ⓈE

Mod	RVU Non-Fac Total	Fac Total	Global Days	Modifiers 51	50	62	80	MUE
	0.00	0.00	XXX	9	9	9	9	

3293F ABO and Rh blood typing documented as performed (Pre-Cr) E

Mod	RVU Non-Fac Total	Fac Total	Global Days	Modifiers 51	50	62	80	MUE
	0.00	0.00	XXX	9	9	9	9	

3294F Group B Streptococcus (GBS) screening documented as performed during week 35-37 gestation (Pre-Cr) ⓈE

Mod	RVU Non-Fac Total	Fac Total	Global Days	Modifiers 51	50	62	80	MUE
	0.00	0.00	XXX	9	9	9	9	

● New   ▲ Revised   ✖ Deleted   ⊙ Moderate Sedation   ✚ Add-on Codes   ⊖ High Risk Denial   Ⓐ Age Edit   ♀ Female   ♂ Male   **AMA** CPT® Assistant   **MUE** Medically Unlikely Edit
⊘ Modifier 51 Exempt   ⊖ Modifier 63 Exempt   Ⓧ Unlisted   **Modifiers:** See Inside Back Cover   Ⓜ Maternity   A2–Z3 ASC Payment Indicators   A–Y OPPS Status Indicators

CPT © 2015 American Medical Association. All Rights Reserved.   © 2016 DecisionHealth

3300F American Joint Committee on Cancer (AJCC) stage documented and reviewed (ONC) ⊛M

Mod	Non-Fac Total	Fac Total	Global Days	51	50	62	80	MUE
	0.00	0.00	XXX	9	9	9	9	

3301F Cancer stage documented in medical record as metastatic and reviewed (ONC) ⊛M

Mod	Non-Fac Total	Fac Total	Global Days	51	50	62	80	MUE
	0.00	0.00	XXX	9	9	9	9	

3315F Estrogen receptor (ER) or progesterone receptor (PR) positive breast cancer (ONC) ⊛M

Mod	Non-Fac Total	Fac Total	Global Days	51	50	62	80	MUE
	0.00	0.00	XXX	9	9	9	9	

3316F Estrogen receptor (ER) and progesterone receptor (PR) negative breast cancer (ONC) ⊛M

Mod	Non-Fac Total	Fac Total	Global Days	51	50	62	80	MUE
	0.00	0.00	XXX	9	9	9	9	

3317F Pathology report confirming malignancy documented in the medical record and reviewed prior to the initiation of chemotherapy (ONC) ⊛E

Mod	Non-Fac Total	Fac Total	Global Days	51	50	62	80	MUE
	0.00	0.00	XXX	9	9	9	9	

3318F Pathology report confirming malignancy documented in the medical record and reviewed prior to the initiation of radiation therapy (ONC) E

Mod	Non-Fac Total	Fac Total	Global Days	51	50	62	80	MUE
	0.00	0.00	XXX	9	9	9	9	

3319F 1 of the following diagnostic imaging studies ordered: chest x-ray, CT, Ultrasound, MRI, PET, or nuclear medicine scans (ML) ⊛M

Mod	Non-Fac Total	Fac Total	Global Days	51	50	62	80	MUE
	0.00	0.00	XXX	9	9	9	9	

3320F None of the following diagnostic imaging studies ordered: chest X-ray, CT, Ultrasound, MRI, PET, or nuclear medicine scans (ML) ⊛M

Mod	Non-Fac Total	Fac Total	Global Days	51	50	62	80	MUE
	0.00	0.00	XXX	9	9	9	9	

3321F AJCC Cancer Stage 0 or IA Melanoma, documented (ML) ⊛M

Mod	Non-Fac Total	Fac Total	Global Days	51	50	62	80	MUE
	0.00	0.00	XXX	9	9	9	9	

3322F Melanoma greater than AJCC Stage 0 or IA (ML) ⊛M

Mod	Non-Fac Total	Fac Total	Global Days	51	50	62	80	MUE
	0.00	0.00	XXX	9	9	9	9	

3323F Clinical tumor, node and metastases (TNM) staging documented and reviewed prior to surgery (Lung/Esop Cx) ⊛E

Mod	Non-Fac Total	Fac Total	Global Days	51	50	62	80	MUE
	0.00	0.00	XXX	9	9	9	9	

3324F MRI or CT scan ordered, reviewed or requested (EPI) ⊛E

Mod	Non-Fac Total	Fac Total	Global Days	51	50	62	80	MUE
	0.00	0.00	XXX	9	9	9	9	

3325F Preoperative assessment of functional or medical indication(s) for surgery prior to the cataract surgery with intraocular lens placement (must be performed within 12 months prior to cataract surgery) (EC) ⊛E

Mod	Non-Fac Total	Fac Total	Global Days	51	50	62	80	MUE
	0.00	0.00	XXX	9	9	9	9	

3328F Performance status documented and reviewed within 2 weeks prior to surgery (Lung/Esop Cx) ⊛E

Mod	Non-Fac Total	Fac Total	Global Days	51	50	62	80	MUE
	0.00	0.00	XXX	9	9	9	9	

3330F Imaging study ordered (BkP) ⊛E

Mod	Non-Fac Total	Fac Total	Global Days	51	50	62	80	MUE
	0.00	0.00	XXX	9	9	9	9	

3331F Imaging study not ordered (BkP) ⊛E

Mod	Non-Fac Total	Fac Total	Global Days	51	50	62	80	MUE
	0.00	0.00	XXX	9	9	9	9	

3340F Mammogram assessment category of "incomplete: need additional imaging evaluation" documented (RAD) ⊛M

Mod	Non-Fac Total	Fac Total	Global Days	51	50	62	80	MUE
	0.00	0.00	XXX	9	9	9	9	

3341F Mammogram assessment category of "negative," documented (RAD) ⊛M

Mod	Non-Fac Total	Fac Total	Global Days	51	50	62	80	MUE
	0.00	0.00	XXX	9	9	9	9	

3342F Mammogram assessment category of "benign," documented (RAD) ⊛M

Mod	Non-Fac Total	Fac Total	Global Days	51	50	62	80	MUE
	0.00	0.00	XXX	9	9	9	9	

3343F Mammogram assessment category of "probably benign," documented (RAD) ⊛M

Mod	Non-Fac Total	Fac Total	Global Days	51	50	62	80	MUE
	0.00	0.00	XXX	9	9	9	9	

● New ▲ Revised Deleted ⊙ Moderate Sedation ✛ Add-on Codes ⊘ High Risk Denial Ⓐ Age Edit ♀ Female ♂ Male AMA CPT® Assistant MUE Medically Unlikely Edit
⊗ Modifier 51 Exempt ⊖ Modifier 63 Exempt ⊠ Unlisted Modifiers: See Inside Back Cover Ⓜ Maternity A2–Z3 ASC Payment Indicators A–Y OPPS Status Indicators

3344F Mammogram assessment category of "suspicious," documented (RAD) Ⓜ

Mod	Non-Fac Total	Fac Total	Global Days	51	50	62	80	MUE
	0.00	0.00	XXX	9	9	9	9	

3345F Mammogram assessment category of "highly suggestive of malignancy," documented (RAD) Ⓜ

Mod	Non-Fac Total	Fac Total	Global Days	51	50	62	80	MUE
	0.00	0.00	XXX	9	9	9	9	

3350F Mammogram assessment category of "known biopsy proven malignancy," documented (RAD) Ⓜ

Mod	Non-Fac Total	Fac Total	Global Days	51	50	62	80	MUE
	0.00	0.00	XXX	9	9	9	9	

3351F Negative screen for depressive symptoms as categorized by using a standardized depression screening/assessment tool (MDD) Ⓔ

Mod	Non-Fac Total	Fac Total	Global Days	51	50	62	80	MUE
	0.00	0.00	XXX	9	9	9	9	

3352F No significant depressive symptoms as categorized by using a standardized depression assessment tool (MDD) Ⓔ

Mod	Non-Fac Total	Fac Total	Global Days	51	50	62	80	MUE
	0.00	0.00	XXX	9	9	9	9	

3353F Mild to moderate depressive symptoms as categorized by using a standardized depression screening/assessment tool (MDD) Ⓔ

Mod	Non-Fac Total	Fac Total	Global Days	51	50	62	80	MUE
	0.00	0.00	XXX	9	9	9	9	

3354F Clinically significant depressive symptoms as categorized by using a standardized depression screening/assessment tool (MDD) Ⓔ

Mod	Non-Fac Total	Fac Total	Global Days	51	50	62	80	MUE
	0.00	0.00	XXX	9	9	9	9	

3370F AJCC Breast Cancer Stage 0 documented (ONC) Ⓜ

Mod	Non-Fac Total	Fac Total	Global Days	51	50	62	80	MUE
	0.00	0.00	XXX	9	9	9	9	

3372F AJCC Breast Cancer Stage I: T1mic, T1a or T1b (tumor size < 1 cm) documented (ONC) Ⓜ

Mod	Non-Fac Total	Fac Total	Global Days	51	50	62	80	MUE
	0.00	0.00	XXX	9	9	9	9	

3374F AJCC Breast Cancer Stage I: T1c (tumor size > 1 cm to 2 cm) documented (ONC) Ⓜ

Mod	Non-Fac Total	Fac Total	Global Days	51	50	62	80	MUE
	0.00	0.00	XXX	9	9	9	9	

3376F AJCC Breast Cancer Stage II documented (ONC) Ⓜ

Mod	Non-Fac Total	Fac Total	Global Days	51	50	62	80	MUE
	0.00	0.00	XXX	9	9	9	9	

3378F AJCC Breast Cancer Stage III documented (ONC) Ⓜ

Mod	Non-Fac Total	Fac Total	Global Days	51	50	62	80	MUE
	0.00	0.00	XXX	9	9	9	9	

3380F AJCC Breast Cancer Stage IV documented (ONC) Ⓜ

Mod	Non-Fac Total	Fac Total	Global Days	51	50	62	80	MUE
	0.00	0.00	XXX	9	9	9	9	

3382F AJCC colon cancer, Stage 0 documented (ONC) Ⓜ

Mod	Non-Fac Total	Fac Total	Global Days	51	50	62	80	MUE
	0.00	0.00	XXX	9	9	9	9	

3384F AJCC colon cancer, Stage I documented (ONC) Ⓜ

Mod	Non-Fac Total	Fac Total	Global Days	51	50	62	80	MUE
	0.00	0.00	XXX	9	9	9	9	

3386F AJCC colon cancer, Stage II documented (ONC) Ⓜ

Mod	Non-Fac Total	Fac Total	Global Days	51	50	62	80	MUE
	0.00	0.00	XXX	9	9	9	9	

3388F AJCC colon cancer, Stage III documented (ONC) Ⓜ

Mod	Non-Fac Total	Fac Total	Global Days	51	50	62	80	MUE
	0.00	0.00	XXX	9	9	9	9	

3390F AJCC colon cancer, Stage IV documented (ONC) Ⓜ

Mod	Non-Fac Total	Fac Total	Global Days	51	50	62	80	MUE
	0.00	0.00	XXX	9	9	9	9	

3394F Quantitative HER2 immunohistochemistry (IHC) evaluation of breast cancer consistent with the scoring system defined in the ASCO/CAP guidelines (PATH) Ⓜ

Mod	Non-Fac Total	Fac Total	Global Days	51	50	62	80	MUE
	0.00	0.00	XXX	9	9	9	9	

3395F Quantitative non-HER2 immunohistochemistry (IHC) evaluation of breast cancer (eg, testing for estrogen or progesterone receptors [ER/PR]) performed (PATH) Ⓜ

Mod	Non-Fac Total	Fac Total	Global Days	51	50	62	80	MUE
	0.00	0.00	XXX	9	9	9	9	

● New   ▲ Revised   ✖ Deleted   ⊙ Moderate Sedation   ✚ Add-on Codes   ⊘ High Risk Denial   Ⓐ Age Edit   ♀ Female   ♂ Male   **AMA** *CPT® Assistant*   **MUE** Medically Unlikely Edit

⊘ Modifier 51 Exempt   ⊖ Modifier 63 Exempt   ✗ Unlisted   **Modifiers:** *See Inside Back Cover*   Ⓜ Maternity   A2–Z3 ASC Payment Indicators   A–Y OPPS Status Indicators

876   CPT © 2015 American Medical Association. All Rights Reserved.   © 2016 DecisionHealth

3450F Dyspnea screened, no dyspnea or mild dyspnea (Pall Cr) ⓒⒺ

RVU			Global Days	Modifiers				
Mod	Non-Fac Total	Fac Total		51	50	62	80	MUE
	0.00	0.00	XXX	9	9	9	9	

3451F Dyspnea screened, moderate or severe dyspnea (Pall Cr) ⓒⒺ

RVU			Global Days	Modifiers				
Mod	Non-Fac Total	Fac Total		51	50	62	80	MUE
	0.00	0.00	XXX	9	9	9	9	

3452F Dyspnea not screened (Pall Cr) ⓒⒺ

RVU			Global Days	Modifiers				
Mod	Non-Fac Total	Fac Total		51	50	62	80	MUE
	0.00	0.00	XXX	9	9	9	9	

3455F TB screening performed and results interpreted within six months prior to initiation of first-time biologic disease modifying anti-rheumatic drug therapy for RA (RA) ⓒⓂ

RVU			Global Days	Modifiers				
Mod	Non-Fac Total	Fac Total		51	50	62	80	MUE
	0.00	0.00	XXX	9	9	9	9	

3470F Rheumatoid arthritis (RA) disease activity, low (RA) ⓒⓂ

RVU			Global Days	Modifiers				
Mod	Non-Fac Total	Fac Total		51	50	62	80	MUE
	0.00	0.00	XXX	9	9	9	9	

3471F Rheumatoid arthritis (RA) disease activity, moderate (RA) ⓒⓂ

RVU			Global Days	Modifiers				
Mod	Non-Fac Total	Fac Total		51	50	62	80	MUE
	0.00	0.00	XXX	9	9	9	9	

3472F Rheumatoid arthritis (RA) disease activity, high (RA) ⓒⓂ

RVU			Global Days	Modifiers				
Mod	Non-Fac Total	Fac Total		51	50	62	80	MUE
	0.00	0.00	XXX	9	9	9	9	

3475F Disease prognosis for rheumatoid arthritis assessed, poor prognosis documented (RA) ⓒⓂ

RVU			Global Days	Modifiers				
Mod	Non-Fac Total	Fac Total		51	50	62	80	MUE
	0.00	0.00	XXX	9	9	9	9	

3476F Disease prognosis for rheumatoid arthritis assessed, good prognosis documented (RA) ⓒⓂ

RVU			Global Days	Modifiers				
Mod	Non-Fac Total	Fac Total		51	50	62	80	MUE
	0.00	0.00	XXX	9	9	9	9	

3490F History of AIDS-defining condition (HIV) ⓒⒺ

RVU			Global Days	Modifiers				
Mod	Non-Fac Total	Fac Total		51	50	62	80	MUE
	0.00	0.00	XXX	9	9	9	9	

3491F HIV indeterminate (infants of undetermined HIV status born of HIV-infected mothers) (HIV) ⒶⒺ

RVU			Global Days	Modifiers				
Mod	Non-Fac Total	Fac Total		51	50	62	80	MUE
	0.00	0.00	XXX	9	9	9	9	

3492F History of nadir CD4+ cell count <350 cells/mm3 (HIV) ⓒⒺ

RVU			Global Days	Modifiers				
Mod	Non-Fac Total	Fac Total		51	50	62	80	MUE
	0.00	0.00	XXX	9	9	9	9	

3493F No history of nadir CD4+ cell count <350 cells/mm3 and no history of AIDS-defining condition (HIV) ⓒⒺ

RVU			Global Days	Modifiers				
Mod	Non-Fac Total	Fac Total		51	50	62	80	MUE
	0.00	0.00	XXX	9	9	9	9	

3494F CD4+ cell count <200 cells/mm3 (HIV) ⓒⓂ

RVU			Global Days	Modifiers				
Mod	Non-Fac Total	Fac Total		51	50	62	80	MUE
	0.00	0.00	XXX	9	9	9	9	

3495F CD4+ cell count 200 - 499 cells/mm3 (HIV) ⓒⓂ

RVU			Global Days	Modifiers				
Mod	Non-Fac Total	Fac Total		51	50	62	80	MUE
	0.00	0.00	XXX	9	9	9	9	

3496F CD4+ cell count >500 cells/mm3 (HIV) ⓒⓂ

RVU			Global Days	Modifiers				
Mod	Non-Fac Total	Fac Total		51	50	62	80	MUE
	0.00	0.00	XXX	9	9	9	9	

3497F CD4+ cell percentage <15% (HIV) ⓒⒺ

RVU			Global Days	Modifiers				
Mod	Non-Fac Total	Fac Total		51	50	62	80	MUE
	0.00	0.00	XXX	9	9	9	9	

3498F CD4+ cell percentage >15% (HIV) Ⓔ

RVU			Global Days	Modifiers				
Mod	Non-Fac Total	Fac Total		51	50	62	80	MUE
	0.00	0.00	XXX	9	9	9	9	

3500F CD4+ cell count or CD4+ cell percentage documented as performed (HIV) ⓒⒺ

RVU			Global Days	Modifiers				
Mod	Non-Fac Total	Fac Total		51	50	62	80	MUE
	0.00	0.00	XXX	9	9	9	9	

3502F HIV RNA viral load below limits of quantification (HIV) ⓒⒺ

RVU			Global Days	Modifiers				
Mod	Non-Fac Total	Fac Total		51	50	62	80	MUE
	0.00	0.00	XXX	9	9	9	9	

3503F HIV RNA viral load not below limits of quantification (HIV) ⓒⒺ

RVU			Global Days	Modifiers				
Mod	Non-Fac Total	Fac Total		51	50	62	80	MUE
	0.00	0.00	XXX	9	9	9	9	

● New   ▲ Revised   Deleted   ⊙ Moderate Sedation   ✚ Add-on Codes   ⊘ High Risk Denial   Ⓐ Age Edit   ♀ Female   ♂ Male   **AMA** CPT® Assistant   **MUE** Medically Unlikely Edit
⊘ Modifier 51 Exempt   ⊖ Modifier 63 Exempt   ✗ Unlisted   **Modifiers:** See Inside Back Cover   Ⓜ Maternity   Ⓐ2–Ⓩ3 ASC Payment Indicators   Ⓐ–Ⓨ OPPS Status Indicators

3510F Documentation that tuberculosis (TB) screening test performed and results interpreted (HIV) (IBD) ⓜ

RVU			Global Days	Modifiers				
Mod	Non-Fac Total	Fac Total		51	50	62	80	MUE
	0.00	0.00	XXX	9	9	9	9	

3511F Chlamydia and gonorrhea screenings documented as performed (HIV) ⓒⒺ

RVU			Global Days	Modifiers				
Mod	Non-Fac Total	Fac Total		51	50	62	80	MUE
	0.00	0.00	XXX	9	9	9	9	

3512F Syphilis screening documented as performed (HIV) ⓒⒺ

RVU			Global Days	Modifiers				
Mod	Non-Fac Total	Fac Total		51	50	62	80	MUE
	0.00	0.00	XXX	9	9	9	9	

3513F Hepatitis B screening documented as performed (HIV) ⓒⒺ

RVU			Global Days	Modifiers				
Mod	Non-Fac Total	Fac Total		51	50	62	80	MUE
	0.00	0.00	XXX	9	9	9	9	

3514F Hepatitis C screening documented as performed (HIV) ⓒⒺ

RVU			Global Days	Modifiers				
Mod	Non-Fac Total	Fac Total		51	50	62	80	MUE
	0.00	0.00	XXX	9	9	9	9	

3515F Patient has documented immunity to Hepatitis C (HIV) Ⓔ

RVU			Global Days	Modifiers				
Mod	Non-Fac Total	Fac Total		51	50	62	80	MUE
	0.00	0.00	XXX	9	9	9	9	

3517F Hepatitis B Virus (HBV) status assessed and results interpreted within one year prior to receiving a first course of anti-TNF (tumor necrosis factor) therapy (IBD) ⓜ

RVU			Global Days	Modifiers				
Mod	Non-Fac Total	Fac Total		51	50	62	80	MUE
	0.00	0.00	XXX	9	9	9	9	

3520F Clostridium difficile testing performed (IBD) ⓒⒺ

RVU			Global Days	Modifiers				
Mod	Non-Fac Total	Fac Total		51	50	62	80	MUE
	0.00	0.00	XXX	9	9	9	9	

3550F Low risk for thromboembolism (AFIB) Ⓔ

RVU			Global Days	Modifiers				
Mod	Non-Fac Total	Fac Total		51	50	62	80	MUE
	0.00	0.00	XXX	9	9	9	9	

3551F Intermediate risk for thromboembolism (AFIB) ⓒⒺ

RVU			Global Days	Modifiers				
Mod	Non-Fac Total	Fac Total		51	50	62	80	MUE
	0.00	0.00	XXX	9	9	9	9	

3552F High risk for thromboembolism (AFIB) Ⓔ

RVU			Global Days	Modifiers				
Mod	Non-Fac Total	Fac Total		51	50	62	80	MUE
	0.00	0.00	XXX	9	9	9	9	

3555F Patient had International Normalized Ratio (INR) measurement performed (AFIB) ⓒⒺ

RVU			Global Days	Modifiers				
Mod	Non-Fac Total	Fac Total		51	50	62	80	MUE
	0.00	0.00	XXX	9	9	9	9	

3570F Final report for bone scintigraphy study includes correlation with existing relevant imaging studies (eg, x-ray, MRI, CT) corresponding to the same anatomical region in question (NUC_MED) ⓜ

RVU			Global Days	Modifiers				
Mod	Non-Fac Total	Fac Total		51	50	62	80	MUE
	0.00	0.00	XXX	9	9	9	9	

3572F Patient considered to be potentially at risk for fracture in a weight-bearing site (NUC_MED) ⓒⒺ

RVU			Global Days	Modifiers				
Mod	Non-Fac Total	Fac Total		51	50	62	80	MUE
	0.00	0.00	XXX	9	9	9	9	

3573F Patient not considered to be potentially at risk for fracture in a weight-bearing site (NUC_MED) Ⓔ

RVU			Global Days	Modifiers				
Mod	Non-Fac Total	Fac Total		51	50	62	80	MUE
	0.00	0.00	XXX	9	9	9	9	

3650F Electroencephalogram (EEG) ordered, reviewed or requested (EPI) ⓒⒺ

RVU			Global Days	Modifiers				
Mod	Non-Fac Total	Fac Total		51	50	62	80	MUE
	0.00	0.00	XXX	9	9	9	9	

3700F Psychiatric disorders or disturbances assessed (Prkns) ⓜ

RVU			Global Days	Modifiers				
Mod	Non-Fac Total	Fac Total		51	50	62	80	MUE
	0.00	0.00	XXX	9	9	9	9	

3720F Cognitive impairment or dysfunction assessed (Prkns) ⓜ

RVU			Global Days	Modifiers				
Mod	Non-Fac Total	Fac Total		51	50	62	80	MUE
	0.00	0.00	XXX	9	9	9	9	

3725F Screening for depression performed (DEM) ⓜ

RVU			Global Days	Modifiers				
Mod	Non-Fac Total	Fac Total		51	50	62	80	MUE
	0.00	0.00	XXX	9	9	9	9	

3750F Patient not receiving dose of corticosteroids greater than or equal to 10mg/day for 60 or greater consecutive days (IBD) ⓒⒺ

RVU			Global Days	Modifiers				
Mod	Non-Fac Total	Fac Total		51	50	62	80	MUE
	0.00	0.00	XXX	9	9	9	9	

● New   ▲ Revised   ✖ Deleted   ⊙ Moderate Sedation   ✚ Add-on Codes   ⊘ High Risk Denial   Ⓐ Age Edit   ♀ Female   ♂ Male   **AMA** *CPT® Assistant*   **MUE** Medically Unlikely Edit
⊘ Modifier 51 Exempt   ⊖ Modifier 63 Exempt   ✖ Unlisted   **Modifiers:** *See Inside Back Cover*   Ⓜ Maternity   Ⓐ-2–Ⓩ-3 ASC Payment Indicators   Ⓐ–Ⓨ OPPS Status Indicators

CPT © 2015 American Medical Association. All Rights Reserved.   © 2016 DecisionHealth

3751F Electrodiagnostic studies for distal symmetric polyneuropathy conducted (or requested), documented, and reviewed within 6 months of initial evaluation for condition (DSP) **E**

RVU Mod	Non-Fac Total	Fac Total	Global Days	Modifiers 51	50	62	80	MUE
	0.00	0.00	XXX	9	9	9	9	

3752F Electrodiagnostic studies for distal symmetric polyneuropathy not conducted (or requested), documented, or reviewed within 6 months of initial evaluation for condition (DSP) **E**

RVU Mod	Non-Fac Total	Fac Total	Global Days	Modifiers 51	50	62	80	MUE
	0.00	0.00	XXX	9	9	9	9	

3753F Patient has clear clinical symptoms and signs that are highly suggestive of neuropathy AND cannot be attributed to another condition, AND has an obvious cause for the neuropathy (DSP) **E**

RVU Mod	Non-Fac Total	Fac Total	Global Days	Modifiers 51	50	62	80	MUE
	0.00	0.00	XXX	9	9	9	9	

3754F Screening tests for diabetes mellitus reviewed, requested, or ordered (DSP) **⊖E**

RVU Mod	Non-Fac Total	Fac Total	Global Days	Modifiers 51	50	62	80	MUE
	0.00	0.00	XXX	9	9	9	9	

3755F Cognitive and behavioral impairment screening performed (ALS) **E**

RVU Mod	Non-Fac Total	Fac Total	Global Days	Modifiers 51	50	62	80	MUE
	0.00	0.00	XXX	9	9	9	9	

3756F Patient has pseudobulbar affect, sialorrhea, or ALS-related symptoms (ALS) **E**

RVU Mod	Non-Fac Total	Fac Total	Global Days	Modifiers 51	50	62	80	MUE
	0.00	0.00	XXX	9	9	9	9	

3757F Patient does not have pseudobulbar affect, sialorrhea, or ALS-related symptoms (ALS) **E**

RVU Mod	Non-Fac Total	Fac Total	Global Days	Modifiers 51	50	62	80	MUE
	0.00	0.00	XXX	9	9	9	9	

3758F Patient referred for pulmonary function testing or peak cough expiratory flow (ALS) **⊖E**

RVU Mod	Non-Fac Total	Fac Total	Global Days	Modifiers 51	50	62	80	MUE
	0.00	0.00	XXX	9	9	9	9	

3759F Patient screened for dysphagia, weight loss, and impaired nutrition, and results documented (ALS) **⊖E**

RVU Mod	Non-Fac Total	Fac Total	Global Days	Modifiers 51	50	62	80	MUE
	0.00	0.00	XXX	9	9	9	9	

3760F Patient exhibits dysphagia, weight loss, or impaired nutrition (ALS) **⊖E**

RVU Mod	Non-Fac Total	Fac Total	Global Days	Modifiers 51	50	62	80	MUE
	0.00	0.00	XXX	9	9	9	9	

3761F Patient does not exhibit dysphagia, weight loss, or impaired nutrition (ALS) **⊖E**

RVU Mod	Non-Fac Total	Fac Total	Global Days	Modifiers 51	50	62	80	MUE
	0.00	0.00	XXX	9	9	9	9	

3762F Patient is dysarthric (ALS) **E**

RVU Mod	Non-Fac Total	Fac Total	Global Days	Modifiers 51	50	62	80	MUE
	0.00	0.00	XXX	9	9	9	9	

3763F Patient is not dysarthric (ALS) **E**

RVU Mod	Non-Fac Total	Fac Total	Global Days	Modifiers 51	50	62	80	MUE
	0.00	0.00	XXX	9	9	9	9	

3775F Adenoma(s) or other neoplasm detected during screening colonoscopy (SCADR) **M**

RVU Mod	Non-Fac Total	Fac Total	Global Days	Modifiers 51	50	62	80	MUE
	0.00	0.00	XXX	9	9	9	9	

3776F Adenoma(s) or other neoplasm not detected during screening colonoscopy (SCADR) **M**

RVU Mod	Non-Fac Total	Fac Total	Global Days	Modifiers 51	50	62	80	MUE
	0.00	0.00	XXX	9	9	9	9	

Therapeutic/Preventative/Other Interventional Codes

4000F Tobacco use cessation intervention, counseling (COPD, CAP, CAD, Asthma) (DM) (PV) **⊖E**

RVU Mod	Non-Fac Total	Fac Total	Global Days	Modifiers 51	50	62	80	MUE
	0.00	0.00	XXX	9	9	9	9	

AMA: Oct 05: 1

4001F Tobacco use cessation intervention, pharmacologic therapy (COPD, CAD, CAP, PV, Asthma) (DM) (PV) **⊖E**

RVU Mod	Non-Fac Total	Fac Total	Global Days	Modifiers 51	50	62	80	MUE
	0.00	0.00	XXX	9	9	9	9	

AMA: Oct 05: 6

4003F Patient education, written/oral, appropriate for patients with heart failure, performed (NMA-No Measure Associated) **⊖E**

RVU Mod	Non-Fac Total	Fac Total	Global Days	Modifiers 51	50	62	80	MUE
	0.00	0.00	XXX	9	9	9	9	

AMA: Oct 05: 6

● New   ▲ Revised   Deleted   ⊙ Moderate Sedation   ✚ Add-on Codes   ⊘ High Risk Denial   Ⓐ Age Edit   ♀ Female   ♂ Male   **AMA** *CPT® Assistant*   **MUE** Medically Unlikely Edit
⊘ Modifier 51 Exempt   ⊖ Modifier 63 Exempt   ✗ Unlisted   **Modifiers:** *See Inside Back Cover*   Ⓜ Maternity   A2-Z3 ASC Payment Indicators   A-Y OPPS Status Indicators

© 2016 DecisionHealth   CPT © 2015 American Medical Association. All Rights Reserved.   **879**

4004F Patient screened for tobacco use and received tobacco cessation intervention (counseling, pharmacotherapy, or both), if identified as a tobacco user (PV, CAD) Ⓜ

RVU				Global Days	Modifiers				
Mod	Non-Fac Total	Fac Total			51	50	62	80	MUE
	0.00	0.00	XXX		9	9	9		9

4005F Pharmacologic therapy (other than minerals/vitamins) for osteoporosis prescribed (OP) (IBD) Ⓜ

RVU				Global Days	Modifiers				
Mod	Non-Fac Total	Fac Total			51	50	62	80	MUE
	0.00	0.00	XXX		9	9	9		9

4008F Beta-blocker therapy prescribed or currently being taken (CAD,HF) Ⓜ

RVU				Global Days	Modifiers				
Mod	Non-Fac Total	Fac Total			51	50	62	80	MUE
	0.00	0.00	XXX		9	9	9		9

4010F Angiotensin Converting Enzyme (ACE) Inhibitor or Angiotensin Receptor Blocker (ARB) therapy prescribed or currently being taken (CAD, CKD, HF) (DM) Ⓜ

RVU				Global Days	Modifiers				
Mod	Non-Fac Total	Fac Total			51	50	62	80	MUE
	0.00	0.00	XXX		9	9	9		9

4011F Oral antiplatelet therapy prescribed (CAD) Ⓔ

RVU				Global Days	Modifiers				
Mod	Non-Fac Total	Fac Total			51	50	62	80	MUE
	0.00	0.00	XXX		9	9	9		9

AMA: Oct 05: 6

4012F Warfarin therapy prescribed (NMA-No Measure Associated) Ⓔ

RVU				Global Days	Modifiers				
Mod	Non-Fac Total	Fac Total			51	50	62	80	MUE
	0.00	0.00	XXX		9	9	9		9

AMA: Oct 05: 6

4013F Statin therapy prescribed or currently being taken (CAD) Ⓔ

RVU				Global Days	Modifiers				
Mod	Non-Fac Total	Fac Total			51	50	62	80	MUE
	0.00	0.00	XXX		9	9	9		9

4014F Written discharge instructions provided to heart failure patients discharged home (Instructions include all of the following components: activity level, diet, discharge medications, follow-up appointment, weight monitoring, what to do if symptoms worsen) (NMA-No Measure Associated) ⓈⒶⒺ

RVU				Global Days	Modifiers				
Mod	Non-Fac Total	Fac Total			51	50	62	80	MUE
	0.00	0.00	XXX		9	9	9		9

4015F Persistent asthma, preferred long term control medication or an acceptable alternative treatment, prescribed (NMA-No Measure Associated) Ⓔ

RVU				Global Days	Modifiers				
Mod	Non-Fac Total	Fac Total			51	50	62	80	MUE
	0.00	0.00	XXX		9	9	9		9

4016F Anti-inflammatory/analgesic agent prescribed (OA) (Use for prescribed or continued medication[s], including over-the-counter medication[s]) Ⓔ

RVU				Global Days	Modifiers				
Mod	Non-Fac Total	Fac Total			51	50	62	80	MUE
	0.00	0.00	XXX		9	9	9		9

AMA: Oct 05: 6

4017F Gastrointestinal prophylaxis for NSAID use prescribed (OA) Ⓔ

RVU				Global Days	Modifiers				
Mod	Non-Fac Total	Fac Total			51	50	62	80	MUE
	0.00	0.00	XXX		9	9	9		9

AMA: Oct 05: 6

4018F Therapeutic exercise for the involved joint(s) instructed or physical or occupational therapy prescribed (OA) Ⓔ

RVU				Global Days	Modifiers				
Mod	Non-Fac Total	Fac Total			51	50	62	80	MUE
	0.00	0.00	XXX		9	9	9		9

AMA: Oct 05: 6

4019F Documentation of receipt of counseling on exercise and either both calcium and vitamin D use or counseling regarding both calcium and vitamin D use (OP) Ⓔ

RVU				Global Days	Modifiers				
Mod	Non-Fac Total	Fac Total			51	50	62	80	MUE
	0.00	0.00	XXX		9	9	9		9

4025F Inhaled bronchodilator prescribed (COPD) Ⓜ

RVU				Global Days	Modifiers				
Mod	Non-Fac Total	Fac Total			51	50	62	80	MUE
	0.00	0.00	XXX		9	9	9		9

4030F Long-term oxygen therapy prescribed (more than 15 hours per day) (COPD) Ⓔ

RVU				Global Days	Modifiers				
Mod	Non-Fac Total	Fac Total			51	50	62	80	MUE
	0.00	0.00	XXX		9	9	9		9

4033F Pulmonary rehabilitation exercise training recommended (COPD) Ⓔ

RVU				Global Days	Modifiers				
Mod	Non-Fac Total	Fac Total			51	50	62	80	MUE
	0.00	0.00	XXX		9	9	9		9

4035F Influenza immunization recommended (COPD) (IBD) Ⓔ

RVU				Global Days	Modifiers				
Mod	Non-Fac Total	Fac Total			51	50	62	80	MUE
	0.00	0.00	XXX		9	9	9		9

● New   ▲ Revised   ✖ Deleted   ⊙ Moderate Sedation   ✚ Add-on Codes   ⊘ High Risk Denial   Ⓐ Age Edit   ♀ Female   ♂ Male   **AMA** *CPT® Assistant*   **MUE** Medically Unlikely Edit   ⊘ Modifier 51 Exempt   ⊖ Modifier 63 Exempt   ⌶ Unlisted   **Modifiers:** *See Inside Back Cover*   Ⓜ Maternity   A2–Z3 ASC Payment Indicators   A–Y OPPS Status Indicators

CPT © 2015 American Medical Association. All Rights Reserved.   © 2016 DecisionHealth

4037F Influenza immunization ordered or administered (COPD, PV, CKD, ESRD)(IBD) Ⓔ

RVU			Global Days	Modifiers				
Mod	Non-Fac Total	Fac Total		51	50	62	80	MUE
	0.00	0.00	XXX	9	9	9	9	

4040F Pneumococcal vaccine administered or previously received (COPD) (PV), (IBD) Ⓜ

RVU			Global Days	Modifiers				
Mod	Non-Fac Total	Fac Total		51	50	62	80	MUE
	0.00	0.00	XXX	9	9	9	9	

4041F Documentation of order for cefazolin OR cefuroxime for antimicrobial prophylaxis (PERI 2) Ⓔ

RVU			Global Days	Modifiers				
Mod	Non-Fac Total	Fac Total		51	50	62	80	MUE
	0.00	0.00	XXX	9	9	9	9	

4042F Documentation that prophylactic antibiotics were neither given within 4 hours prior to surgical incision nor given intraoperatively (PERI 2) Ⓜ

RVU			Global Days	Modifiers				
Mod	Non-Fac Total	Fac Total		51	50	62	80	MUE
	0.00	0.00	XXX	9	9	9	9	

4043F Documentation that an order was given to discontinue prophylactic antibiotics within 48 hours of surgical end time, cardiac procedures (PERI 2) Ⓔ

RVU			Global Days	Modifiers				
Mod	Non-Fac Total	Fac Total		51	50	62	80	MUE
	0.00	0.00	XXX	9	9	9	9	

4044F Documentation that an order was given for venous thromboembolism (VTE) prophylaxis to be given within 24 hours prior to incision time or 24 hours after surgery end time (PERI 2) Ⓜ

RVU			Global Days	Modifiers				
Mod	Non-Fac Total	Fac Total		51	50	62	80	MUE
	0.00	0.00	XXX	9	9	9	9	

4045F Appropriate empiric antibiotic prescribed (CAP), (EM) Ⓔ

RVU			Global Days	Modifiers				
Mod	Non-Fac Total	Fac Total		51	50	62	80	MUE
	0.00	0.00	XXX	9	9	9	9	

4046F Documentation that prophylactic antibiotics were given within 4 hours prior to surgical incision or given intraoperatively (PERI 2) Ⓜ

RVU			Global Days	Modifiers				
Mod	Non-Fac Total	Fac Total		51	50	62	80	MUE
	0.00	0.00	XXX	9	9	9	9	

4047F Documentation of order for prophylactic parenteral antibiotics to be given within 1 hour (if fluoroquinolone or vancomycin, 2 hours) prior to surgical incision (or start of procedure when no incision is required) (PERI 2) Ⓔ

RVU			Global Days	Modifiers				
Mod	Non-Fac Total	Fac Total		51	50	62	80	MUE
	0.00	0.00	XXX	9	9	9	9	

4048F Documentation that administration of prophylactic parenteral antibiotic was initiated within 1 hour (if fluoroquinolone or vancomycin, 2 hours) prior to surgical incision (or start of procedure when no incision is required) as ordered (PERI 2) Ⓔ

RVU			Global Days	Modifiers				
Mod	Non-Fac Total	Fac Total		51	50	62	80	MUE
	0.00	0.00	XXX	9	9	9	9	

4049F Documentation that order was given to discontinue prophylactic antibiotics within 24 hours of surgical end time, non-cardiac procedure (PERI 2) Ⓜ

RVU			Global Days	Modifiers				
Mod	Non-Fac Total	Fac Total		51	50	62	80	MUE
	0.00	0.00	XXX	9	9	9	9	

4050F Hypertension plan of care documented as appropriate (NMA-No Measure Associated) Ⓔ

RVU			Global Days	Modifiers				
Mod	Non-Fac Total	Fac Total		51	50	62	80	MUE
	0.00	0.00	XXX	9	9	9	9	

4051F Referred for an arteriovenous (AV) fistula (ESRD, CKD) Ⓔ

RVU			Global Days	Modifiers				
Mod	Non-Fac Total	Fac Total		51	50	62	80	MUE
	0.00	0.00	XXX	9	9	9	9	

4052F Hemodialysis via functioning arteriovenous (AV) fistula (ESRD) Ⓔ

RVU			Global Days	Modifiers				
Mod	Non-Fac Total	Fac Total		51	50	62	80	MUE
	0.00	0.00	XXX	9	9	9	9	

4053F Hemodialysis via functioning arteriovenous (AV) graft (ESRD) Ⓔ

RVU			Global Days	Modifiers				
Mod	Non-Fac Total	Fac Total		51	50	62	80	MUE
	0.00	0.00	XXX	9	9	9	9	

4054F Hemodialysis via catheter (ESRD) Ⓔ

RVU			Global Days	Modifiers				
Mod	Non-Fac Total	Fac Total		51	50	62	80	MUE
	0.00	0.00	XXX	9	9	9	9	

4055F Patient receiving peritoneal dialysis (ESRD) Ⓔ

RVU			Global Days	Modifiers				
Mod	Non-Fac Total	Fac Total		51	50	62	80	MUE
	0.00	0.00	XXX	9	9	9	9	

4056F Appropriate oral rehydration solution recommended (PAG) Ⓔ

RVU			Global Days	Modifiers				
Mod	Non-Fac Total	Fac Total		51	50	62	80	MUE
	0.00	0.00	XXX	9	9	9	9	

4058F Pediatric gastroenteritis education provided to caregiver (PAG) Ⓔ

RVU			Global Days	Modifiers				
Mod	Non-Fac Total	Fac Total		51	50	62	80	MUE
	0.00	0.00	XXX	9	9	9	9	

● New ▲ Revised Deleted ⊙ Moderate Sedation ✚ Add-on Codes ⊘ High Risk Denial Ⓐ Age Edit ♀ Female ♂ Male AMA CPT® Assistant MUE Medically Unlikely Edit
⊘ Modifier 51 Exempt ⊖ Modifier 63 Exempt ⚟ Unlisted Modifiers: See Inside Back Cover Ⓜ Maternity A2-Z3 ASC Payment Indicators A-Y OPPS Status Indicators

© 2016 DecisionHealth CPT © 2015 American Medical Association. All Rights Reserved. 881

4060F Psychotherapy services provided (MDD, MDD ADOL) Ⓔ

Mod	Non-Fac Total	Fac Total	Global Days	51	50	62	80	MUE
	0.00	0.00	XXX	9	9	9	9	

4062F Patient referral for psychotherapy documented (MDD, MDD ADOL) Ⓔ

Mod	Non-Fac Total	Fac Total	Global Days	51	50	62	80	MUE
	0.00	0.00	XXX	9	9	9	9	

4063F Antidepressant pharmacotherapy considered and not prescribed (MDD ADOL) Ⓔ

Mod	Non-Fac Total	Fac Total	Global Days	51	50	62	80	MUE
	0.00	0.00	XXX	9	9	9	9	

4064F Antidepressant pharmacotherapy prescribed (MDD, MDD ADOL) Ⓔ

Mod	Non-Fac Total	Fac Total	Global Days	51	50	62	80	MUE
	0.00	0.00	XXX	9	9	9	9	

4065F Antipsychotic pharmacotherapy prescribed (MDD) Ⓔ

Mod	Non-Fac Total	Fac Total	Global Days	51	50	62	80	MUE
	0.00	0.00	XXX	9	9	9	9	

4066F Electroconvulsive therapy (ECT) provided (MDD) Ⓔ

Mod	Non-Fac Total	Fac Total	Global Days	51	50	62	80	MUE
	0.00	0.00	XXX	9	9	9	9	

4067F Patient referral for electroconvulsive therapy (ECT) documented (MDD) Ⓔ

Mod	Non-Fac Total	Fac Total	Global Days	51	50	62	80	MUE
	0.00	0.00	XXX	9	9	9	9	

4069F Venous thromboembolism (VTE) prophylaxis received (IBD) Ⓔ

Mod	Non-Fac Total	Fac Total	Global Days	51	50	62	80	MUE
	0.00	0.00	XXX	9	9	9	9	

4070F Deep vein thrombosis (DVT) prophylaxis received by end of hospital day 2 (STR) Ⓔ

Mod	Non-Fac Total	Fac Total	Global Days	51	50	62	80	MUE
	0.00	0.00	XXX	9	9	9	9	

4073F Oral antiplatelet therapy prescribed at discharge (STR) Ⓔ

Mod	Non-Fac Total	Fac Total	Global Days	51	50	62	80	MUE
	0.00	0.00	XXX	9	9	9	9	

4075F Anticoagulant therapy prescribed at discharge (STR) Ⓔ

Mod	Non-Fac Total	Fac Total	Global Days	51	50	62	80	MUE
	0.00	0.00	XXX	9	9	9	9	

4077F Documentation that tissue plasminogen activator (t-PA) administration was considered (STR) Ⓔ

Mod	Non-Fac Total	Fac Total	Global Days	51	50	62	80	MUE
	0.00	0.00	XXX	9	9	9	9	

4079F Documentation that rehabilitation services were considered (STR) Ⓔ

Mod	Non-Fac Total	Fac Total	Global Days	51	50	62	80	MUE
	0.00	0.00	XXX	9	9	9	9	

4084F Aspirin received within 24 hours before emergency department arrival or during emergency department stay (EM) Ⓔ

Mod	Non-Fac Total	Fac Total	Global Days	51	50	62	80	MUE
	0.00	0.00	XXX	9	9	9	9	

4086F Aspirin or clopidogrel prescribed or currently being taken (CAD) Ⓜ

Mod	Non-Fac Total	Fac Total	Global Days	51	50	62	80	MUE
	0.00	0.00	XXX	9	9	9	9	

4090F Patient receiving erythropoietin therapy (HEM) Ⓜ

Mod	Non-Fac Total	Fac Total	Global Days	51	50	62	80	MUE
	0.00	0.00	XXX	9	9	9	9	

4095F Patient not receiving erythropoietin therapy (HEM) Ⓔ

Mod	Non-Fac Total	Fac Total	Global Days	51	50	62	80	MUE
	0.00	0.00	XXX	9	9	9	9	

4100F Bisphosphonate therapy, intravenous, ordered or received (HEM) Ⓜ

Mod	Non-Fac Total	Fac Total	Global Days	51	50	62	80	MUE
	0.00	0.00	XXX	9	9	9	9	

4110F Internal mammary artery graft performed for primary, isolated coronary artery bypass graft procedure (CABG) Ⓜ

Mod	Non-Fac Total	Fac Total	Global Days	51	50	62	80	MUE
	0.00	0.00	XXX	9	9	9	9	

4115F Beta blocker administered within 24 hours prior to surgical incision (CABG) Ⓜ

Mod	Non-Fac Total	Fac Total	Global Days	51	50	62	80	MUE
	0.00	0.00	XXX	9	9	9	9	

● New   ▲ Revised   ✖ Deleted   ⊙ Moderate Sedation   ✚ Add-on Codes   ⊘ High Risk Denial   Ⓐ Age Edit   ♀ Female   ♂ Male   **AMA** *CPT® Assistant*   **MUE** Medically Unlikely Edit
⊘ Modifier 51 Exempt   ⊖ Modifier 63 Exempt   🅧 Unlisted   **Modifiers:** *See Inside Back Cover*   Ⓜ Maternity   A2–Z3 ASC Payment Indicators   A–Y OPPS Status Indicators

882   CPT © 2015 American Medical Association. All Rights Reserved.   © 2016 DecisionHealth

4120F Antibiotic prescribed or dispensed (URI, PHAR), (A-BRONCH)   ⓒⓂ

Mod	Non-Fac Total	Fac Total	Global Days	51	50	62	80	MUE
	0.00	0.00	XXX	9	9	9	9	

4124F Antibiotic neither prescribed nor dispensed (URI, PHAR), (A-BRONCH)   ⓒⓂ

Mod	Non-Fac Total	Fac Total	Global Days	51	50	62	80	MUE
	0.00	0.00	XXX	9	9	9	9	

4130F Topical preparations (including OTC) prescribed for acute otitis externa (AOE)   ⓒⓂ

Mod	Non-Fac Total	Fac Total	Global Days	51	50	62	80	MUE
	0.00	0.00	XXX	9	9	9	9	

4131F Systemic antimicrobial therapy prescribed (AOE)   ⓒⓂ

Mod	Non-Fac Total	Fac Total	Global Days	51	50	62	80	MUE
	0.00	0.00	XXX	9	9	9	9	

4132F Systemic antimicrobial therapy not prescribed (AOE)   ⓒⓂ

Mod	Non-Fac Total	Fac Total	Global Days	51	50	62	80	MUE
	0.00	0.00	XXX	9	9	9	9	

4133F Antihistamines or decongestants prescribed or recommended (OME)   ⓒⒺ

Mod	Non-Fac Total	Fac Total	Global Days	51	50	62	80	MUE
	0.00	0.00	XXX	9	9	9	9	

4134F Antihistamines or decongestants neither prescribed nor recommended (OME)   ⓒⒺ

Mod	Non-Fac Total	Fac Total	Global Days	51	50	62	80	MUE
	0.00	0.00	XXX	9	9	9	9	

4135F Systemic corticosteroids prescribed (OME)   Ⓔ

Mod	Non-Fac Total	Fac Total	Global Days	51	50	62	80	MUE
	0.00	0.00	XXX	9	9	9	9	

4136F Systemic corticosteroids not prescribed (OME)   ⓒⒺ

Mod	Non-Fac Total	Fac Total	Global Days	51	50	62	80	MUE
	0.00	0.00	XXX	9	9	9	9	

4140F Inhaled corticosteroids prescribed (Asthma)   ⓒⓂ

Mod	Non-Fac Total	Fac Total	Global Days	51	50	62	80	MUE
	0.00	0.00	XXX	9	9	9	9	

4142F Corticosteroid sparing therapy prescribed (IBD)   ⓒⓂ

Mod	Non-Fac Total	Fac Total	Global Days	51	50	62	80	MUE
	0.00	0.00	XXX	9	9	9	9	

4144F Alternative long-term control medication prescribed (Asthma)   ⓒⓂ

Mod	Non-Fac Total	Fac Total	Global Days	51	50	62	80	MUE
	0.00	0.00	XXX	9	9	9	9	

4145F Two or more anti-hypertensive agents prescribed or currently being taken (CAD, HTN)   ⓒⒺ

Mod	Non-Fac Total	Fac Total	Global Days	51	50	62	80	MUE
	0.00	0.00	XXX	9	9	9	9	

4148F Hepatitis A vaccine injection administered or previously received (HEP-C)   ⓒⓂ

Mod	Non-Fac Total	Fac Total	Global Days	51	50	62	80	MUE
	0.00	0.00	XXX	9	9	9	9	

4149F Hepatitis B vaccine injection administered or previously received (HEP-C, HIV) (IBD)   ⓒⒺ

Mod	Non-Fac Total	Fac Total	Global Days	51	50	62	80	MUE
	0.00	0.00	XXX	9	9	9	9	

4150F Patient receiving antiviral treatment for Hepatitis C (HEP-C)   ⓒⒺ

Mod	Non-Fac Total	Fac Total	Global Days	51	50	62	80	MUE
	0.00	0.00	XXX	9	9	9	9	

4151F Patient not receiving antiviral treatment for Hepatitis C (HEP-C)   ⓒⓂ

Mod	Non-Fac Total	Fac Total	Global Days	51	50	62	80	MUE
	0.00	0.00	XXX	9	9	9	9	

4153F Combination peginterferon and ribavirin therapy prescribed (HEP-C)   ⓒⒺ

Mod	Non-Fac Total	Fac Total	Global Days	51	50	62	80	MUE
	0.00	0.00	XXX	9	9	9	9	

4155F Hepatitis A vaccine series previously received (HEP-C)   ⓒⒺ

Mod	Non-Fac Total	Fac Total	Global Days	51	50	62	80	MUE
	0.00	0.00	XXX	9	9	9	9	

4157F Hepatitis B vaccine series previously received (HEP-C)   ⓒⒺ

Mod	Non-Fac Total	Fac Total	Global Days	51	50	62	80	MUE
	0.00	0.00	XXX	9	9	9	9	

4158F Patient counseled about risks of alcohol use (HEP-C)   ⓒⒺ

Mod	Non-Fac Total	Fac Total	Global Days	51	50	62	80	MUE
	0.00	0.00	XXX	9	9	9	9	

● New   ▲ Revised   Deleted   ⊙ Moderate Sedation   ✚ Add-on Codes   ⊘ High Risk Denial   Ⓐ Age Edit   ♀ Female   ♂ Male   **AMA** *CPT® Assistant*   **MUE** Medically Unlikely Edit

⊘ Modifier 51 Exempt   ⊖ Modifier 63 Exempt   ✗ Unlisted   **Modifiers:** *See Inside Back Cover*   Ⓜ Maternity   Ⓐ2–Ⓩ3 ASC Payment Indicators   Ⓐ–Ⓨ OPPS Status Indicators

4159F Counseling regarding contraception received prior to initiation of antiviral treatment (HEP-C) ⊘E

Mod	Non-Fac Total	Fac Total	Global Days	51	50	62	80	MUE
	0.00	0.00	XXX	9	9	9	9	

4163F Patient counseling at a minimum on all of the following treatment options for clinically localized prostate cancer: active surveillance, and interstitial prostate brachytherapy, and external beam radiotherapy, and radical prostatectomy, provided prior to initiation of treatment (PRCA) ⊘E

Mod	Non-Fac Total	Fac Total	Global Days	51	50	62	80	MUE
	0.00	0.00	XXX	9	9	9	9	

4164F Adjuvant (ie, in combination with external beam radiotherapy to the prostate for prostate cancer) hormonal therapy (gonadotropin-releasing hormone [GnRH] agonist or antagonist) prescribed/administered (PRCA) ⊘M

Mod	Non-Fac Total	Fac Total	Global Days	51	50	62	80	MUE
	0.00	0.00	XXX	9	9	9	9	

4165F 3-dimensional conformal radiotherapy (3D-CRT) or intensity modulated radiation therapy (IMRT) received (PRCA) ⊘E

Mod	Non-Fac Total	Fac Total	Global Days	51	50	62	80	MUE
	0.00	0.00	XXX	9	9	9	9	

4167F Head of bed elevation (30-45 degrees) on first ventilator day ordered (CRIT) ⊘E

Mod	Non-Fac Total	Fac Total	Global Days	51	50	62	80	MUE
	0.00	0.00	XXX	9	9	9	9	

4168F Patient receiving care in the intensive care unit (ICU) and receiving mechanical ventilation, 24 hours or less (CRIT) E

Mod	Non-Fac Total	Fac Total	Global Days	51	50	62	80	MUE
	0.00	0.00	XXX	9	9	9	9	

4169F Patient either not receiving care in the intensive care unit (ICU) OR not receiving mechanical ventilation OR receiving mechanical ventilation greater than 24 hours (CRIT) E

Mod	Non-Fac Total	Fac Total	Global Days	51	50	62	80	MUE
	0.00	0.00	XXX	9	9	9	9	

4171F Patient receiving erythropoiesis-stimulating agents (ESA) therapy (CKD) ⊘E

Mod	Non-Fac Total	Fac Total	Global Days	51	50	62	80	MUE
	0.00	0.00	XXX	9	9	9	9	

4172F Patient not receiving erythropoiesis-stimulating agents (ESA) therapy (CKD) ⊘E

Mod	Non-Fac Total	Fac Total	Global Days	51	50	62	80	MUE
	0.00	0.00	XXX	9	9	9	9	

4174F Counseling about the potential impact of glaucoma on visual functioning and quality of life, and importance of treatment adherence provided to patient and/or caregiver(s) (EC) ⊘E

Mod	Non-Fac Total	Fac Total	Global Days	51	50	62	80	MUE
	0.00	0.00	XXX	9	9	9	9	

4175F Best-corrected visual acuity of 20/40 or better (distance or near) achieved within the 90 days following cataract surgery (EC) ⊘M

Mod	Non-Fac Total	Fac Total	Global Days	51	50	62	80	MUE
	0.00	0.00	XXX	9	9	9	9	

4176F Counseling about value of protection from UV light and lack of proven efficacy of nutritional supplements in prevention or progression of cataract development provided to patient and/or caregiver(s) (NMA-No Measure Associated) ⊘E

Mod	Non-Fac Total	Fac Total	Global Days	51	50	62	80	MUE
	0.00	0.00	XXX	9	9	9	9	

4177F Counseling about the benefits and/or risks of the Age-Related Eye Disease Study (AREDS) formulation for preventing progression of age-related macular degeneration (AMD) provided to patient and/or caregiver(s) (EC) ⊘AM

Mod	Non-Fac Total	Fac Total	Global Days	51	50	62	80	MUE
	0.00	0.00	XXX	9	9	9	9	

4178F Anti-D immune globulin received between 26 and 30 weeks gestation (Pre-Cr) ⊘E

Mod	Non-Fac Total	Fac Total	Global Days	51	50	62	80	MUE
	0.00	0.00	XXX	9	9	9	9	

4179F Tamoxifen or aromatase inhibitor (AI) prescribed (ONC) ⊘M

Mod	Non-Fac Total	Fac Total	Global Days	51	50	62	80	MUE
	0.00	0.00	XXX	9	9	9	9	

4180F Adjuvant chemotherapy referred, prescribed, or previously received for Stage III colon cancer (ONC) ⊘E

Mod	Non-Fac Total	Fac Total	Global Days	51	50	62	80	MUE
	0.00	0.00	XXX	9	9	9	9	

4181F Conformal radiation therapy received (NMA-No Measure Associated) E

Mod	Non-Fac Total	Fac Total	Global Days	51	50	62	80	MUE
	0.00	0.00	XXX	9	9	9	9	

● New   ▲ Revised   ✖ Deleted   ⊙ Moderate Sedation   ✚ Add-on Codes   ⊘ High Risk Denial   Ⓐ Age Edit   ♀ Female   ♂ Male   **AMA** *CPT® Assistant*   **MUE** Medically Unlikely Edit
⊘ Modifier 51 Exempt   ⊖ Modifier 63 Exempt   ⊠ Unlisted   **Modifiers:** *See Inside Back Cover*   M Maternity   A2–Z3 ASC Payment Indicators   A–Y OPPS Status Indicators

4182F Conformal radiation therapy not received (NMA-No Measure Associated) **E**

RVU			Global Days	Modifiers				
Mod	Non-Fac Total	Fac Total		51	50	62	80	MUE
	0.00	0.00	XXX	9	9	9	9	

4185F Continuous (12-months) therapy with proton pump inhibitor (PPI) or histamine H2 receptor antagonist (H2RA) received (GERD) **E**

RVU			Global Days	Modifiers				
Mod	Non-Fac Total	Fac Total		51	50	62	80	MUE
	0.00	0.00	XXX	9	9	9	9	

4186F No continuous (12-months) therapy with either proton pump inhibitor (PPI) or histamine H2 receptor antagonist (H2RA) received (GERD) **E**

RVU			Global Days	Modifiers				
Mod	Non-Fac Total	Fac Total		51	50	62	80	MUE
	0.00	0.00	XXX	9	9	9	9	

4187F Disease modifying anti-rheumatic drug therapy prescribed or dispensed (RA) **M**

RVU			Global Days	Modifiers				
Mod	Non-Fac Total	Fac Total		51	50	62	80	MUE
	0.00	0.00	XXX	9	9	9	9	

4188F Appropriate angiotensin converting enzyme (ACE)/angiotensin receptor blockers (ARB) therapeutic monitoring test ordered or performed (AM) **E**

RVU			Global Days	Modifiers				
Mod	Non-Fac Total	Fac Total		51	50	62	80	MUE
	0.00	0.00	XXX	9	9	9	9	

4189F Appropriate digoxin therapeutic monitoring test ordered or performed (AM) **E**

RVU			Global Days	Modifiers				
Mod	Non-Fac Total	Fac Total		51	50	62	80	MUE
	0.00	0.00	XXX	9	9	9	9	

4190F Appropriate diuretic therapeutic monitoring test ordered or performed (AM) **E**

RVU			Global Days	Modifiers				
Mod	Non-Fac Total	Fac Total		51	50	62	80	MUE
	0.00	0.00	XXX	9	9	9	9	

4191F Appropriate anticonvulsant therapeutic monitoring test ordered or performed (AM) **E**

RVU			Global Days	Modifiers				
Mod	Non-Fac Total	Fac Total		51	50	62	80	MUE
	0.00	0.00	XXX	9	9	9	9	

4192F Patient not receiving glucocorticoid therapy (RA) **M**

RVU			Global Days	Modifiers				
Mod	Non-Fac Total	Fac Total		51	50	62	80	MUE
	0.00	0.00	XXX	9	9	9	9	

4193F Patient receiving <10 mg daily prednisone (or equivalent), or RA activity is worsening, or glucocorticoid use is for less than 6 months (RA) **M**

RVU			Global Days	Modifiers				
Mod	Non-Fac Total	Fac Total		51	50	62	80	MUE
	0.00	0.00	XXX	9	9	9	9	

4194F Patient receiving >/= 10 mg daily prednisone (or equivalent) for longer than 6 months, and improvement or no change in disease activity (RA) **M**

RVU			Global Days	Modifiers				
Mod	Non-Fac Total	Fac Total		51	50	62	80	MUE
	0.00	0.00	XXX	9	9	9	9	

4195F Patient receiving first-time biologic disease modifying anti-rheumatic drug therapy for rheumatoid arthritis (RA) **M**

RVU			Global Days	Modifiers				
Mod	Non-Fac Total	Fac Total		51	50	62	80	MUE
	0.00	0.00	XXX	9	9	9	9	

4196F Patient not receiving first-time biologic disease modifying anti-rheumatic drug therapy for rheumatoid arthritis (RA) **M**

RVU			Global Days	Modifiers				
Mod	Non-Fac Total	Fac Total		51	50	62	80	MUE
	0.00	0.00	XXX	9	9	9	9	

4200F External beam radiotherapy as primary therapy to prostate with or without nodal irradiation (PRCA) **E**

RVU			Global Days	Modifiers				
Mod	Non-Fac Total	Fac Total		51	50	62	80	MUE
	0.00	0.00	XXX	9	9	9	9	

4201F External beam radiotherapy with or without nodal irradiation as adjuvant or salvage therapy for prostate cancer patient (PRCA) **E**

RVU			Global Days	Modifiers				
Mod	Non-Fac Total	Fac Total		51	50	62	80	MUE
	0.00	0.00	XXX	9	9	9	9	

4210F Angiotensin converting enzyme (ACE) or angiotensin receptor blockers (ARB) medication therapy for 6 months or more (MM) **E**

RVU			Global Days	Modifiers				
Mod	Non-Fac Total	Fac Total		51	50	62	80	MUE
	0.00	0.00	XXX	9	9	9	9	

4220F Digoxin medication therapy for 6 months or more (MM) **E**

RVU			Global Days	Modifiers				
Mod	Non-Fac Total	Fac Total		51	50	62	80	MUE
	0.00	0.00	XXX	9	9	9	9	

4221F Diuretic medication therapy for 6 months or more (MM) **E**

RVU			Global Days	Modifiers				
Mod	Non-Fac Total	Fac Total		51	50	62	80	MUE
	0.00	0.00	XXX	9	9	9	9	

● New   ▲ Revised   Deleted   ⊙ Moderate Sedation   ✚ Add-on Codes   ⊘ High Risk Denial   Ⓐ Age Edit   ♀ Female   ♂ Male   **AMA** CPT® Assistant   **MUE** Medically Unlikely Edit
⊘ Modifier 51 Exempt   ⊖ Modifier 63 Exempt   ⊠ Unlisted   **Modifiers:** See Inside Back Cover   Ⓜ Maternity   A2–Z3 ASC Payment Indicators   A–Y OPPS Status Indicators

4230F Anticonvulsant medication therapy for 6 months or more (MM) ⃝E

RVU			Global Days	Modifiers				
Mod	Non-Fac Total	Fac Total		51	50	62	80	MUE
	0.00	0.00	XXX	9	9	9	9	

4240F Instruction in therapeutic exercise with follow-up provided to patients during episode of back pain lasting longer than 12 weeks (BkP) E

RVU			Global Days	Modifiers				
Mod	Non-Fac Total	Fac Total		51	50	62	80	MUE
	0.00	0.00	XXX	9	9	9	9	

4242F Counseling for supervised exercise program provided to patients during episode of back pain lasting longer than 12 weeks (BkP) ⃝E

RVU			Global Days	Modifiers				
Mod	Non-Fac Total	Fac Total		51	50	62	80	MUE
	0.00	0.00	XXX	9	9	9	9	

4245F Patient counseled during the initial visit to maintain or resume normal activities (BkP) ⃝E

RVU			Global Days	Modifiers				
Mod	Non-Fac Total	Fac Total		51	50	62	80	MUE
	0.00	0.00	XXX	9	9	9	9	

4248F Patient counseled during the initial visit for an episode of back pain against bed rest lasting 4 days or longer (BkP) ⃝E

RVU			Global Days	Modifiers				
Mod	Non-Fac Total	Fac Total		51	50	62	80	MUE
	0.00	0.00	XXX	9	9	9	9	

4250F Active warming used intraoperatively for the purpose of maintaining normothermia, or at least 1 body temperature equal to or greater than 36 degrees Centigrade (or 96.8 degrees Fahrenheit) recorded within the 30 minutes immediately before or the 15 minutes immediately after anesthesia end time (CRIT) ⃝E

RVU			Global Days	Modifiers				
Mod	Non-Fac Total	Fac Total		51	50	62	80	MUE
	0.00	0.00	XXX	9	9	9	9	

4255F Duration of general or neuraxial anesthesia 60 minutes or longer, as documented in the anesthesia record (CRIT) (Peri2) ⃝M

RVU			Global Days	Modifiers				
Mod	Non-Fac Total	Fac Total		51	50	62	80	MUE
	0.00	0.00	XXX	9	9	9	9	

4256F Duration of general or neuraxial anesthesia less than 60 minutes, as documented in the anesthesia record (CRIT) (Peri2) ⃝E

RVU			Global Days	Modifiers				
Mod	Non-Fac Total	Fac Total		51	50	62	80	MUE
	0.00	0.00	XXX	9	9	9	9	

4260F Wound surface culture technique used (CWC) ⃝E

RVU			Global Days	Modifiers				
Mod	Non-Fac Total	Fac Total		51	50	62	80	MUE
	0.00	0.00	XXX	9	9	9	9	

4261F Technique other than surface culture of the wound exudate used (eg, Levine/deep swab technique, semi-quantitative or quantitative swab technique) or wound surface culture technique not used (CWC) ⃝E

RVU			Global Days	Modifiers				
Mod	Non-Fac Total	Fac Total		51	50	62	80	MUE
	0.00	0.00	XXX	9	9	9	9	

4265F Use of wet to dry dressings prescribed or recommended (CWC) ⃝E

RVU			Global Days	Modifiers				
Mod	Non-Fac Total	Fac Total		51	50	62	80	MUE
	0.00	0.00	XXX	9	9	9	9	

4266F Use of wet to dry dressings neither prescribed nor recommended (CWC) ⃝E

RVU			Global Days	Modifiers				
Mod	Non-Fac Total	Fac Total		51	50	62	80	MUE
	0.00	0.00	XXX	9	9	9	9	

4267F Compression therapy prescribed (CWC) ⃝E

RVU			Global Days	Modifiers				
Mod	Non-Fac Total	Fac Total		51	50	62	80	MUE
	0.00	0.00	XXX	9	9	9	9	

4268F Patient education regarding the need for long term compression therapy including interval replacement of compression stockings received (CWC) ⃝E

RVU			Global Days	Modifiers				
Mod	Non-Fac Total	Fac Total		51	50	62	80	MUE
	0.00	0.00	XXX	9	9	9	9	

4269F Appropriate method of offloading (pressure relief) prescribed (CWC) ⃝E

RVU			Global Days	Modifiers				
Mod	Non-Fac Total	Fac Total		51	50	62	80	MUE
	0.00	0.00	XXX	9	9	9	9	

4270F Patient receiving potent antiretroviral therapy for 6 months or longer (HIV) ⃝E

RVU			Global Days	Modifiers				
Mod	Non-Fac Total	Fac Total		51	50	62	80	MUE
	0.00	0.00	XXX	9	9	9	9	

4271F Patient receiving potent antiretroviral therapy for less than 6 months or not receiving potent antiretroviral therapy (HIV) ⃝E

RVU			Global Days	Modifiers				
Mod	Non-Fac Total	Fac Total		51	50	62	80	MUE
	0.00	0.00	XXX	9	9	9	9	

4274F Influenza immunization administered or previously received (HIV) (P-ESRD) ⃝E

RVU			Global Days	Modifiers				
Mod	Non-Fac Total	Fac Total		51	50	62	80	MUE
	0.00	0.00	XXX	9	9	9	9	

4276F Potent antiretroviral therapy prescribed (HIV) ⃝E

RVU			Global Days	Modifiers				
Mod	Non-Fac Total	Fac Total		51	50	62	80	MUE
	0.00	0.00	XXX	9	9	9	9	

● New   ▲ Revised   ✖ Deleted   ⊙ Moderate Sedation   ✚ Add-on Codes   ⊘ High Risk Denial   Ⓐ Age Edit   ♀ Female   ♂ Male   **AMA** *CPT® Assistant*   **MUE** Medically Unlikely Edit
⊘ Modifier 51 Exempt   ⊖ Modifier 63 Exempt   ✗ Unlisted   **Modifiers:** *See Inside Back Cover*   Ⓜ Maternity   A2–Z3 ASC Payment Indicators   A–Y OPPS Status Indicators

CPT © 2015 American Medical Association. All Rights Reserved.   © 2016 DecisionHealth

4279F Pneumocystis jiroveci pneumonia prophylaxis prescribed (HIV) E

RVU		Global Days	Modifiers				
Mod	Non-Fac Total	Fac Total		51	50	62	80	MUE
	0.00	0.00	XXX	9	9	9	9	

4280F Pneumocystis jiroveci pneumonia prophylaxis prescribed within 3 months of low CD4+ cell count or percentage (HIV) ⊙E

RVU		Global Days	Modifiers				
Mod	Non-Fac Total	Fac Total		51	50	62	80	MUE
	0.00	0.00	XXX	9	9	9	9	

4290F Patient screened for injection drug use (HIV) ⊙E

RVU		Global Days	Modifiers				
Mod	Non-Fac Total	Fac Total		51	50	62	80	MUE
	0.00	0.00	XXX	9	9	9	9	

4293F Patient screened for high-risk sexual behavior (HIV) ⊙E

RVU		Global Days	Modifiers				
Mod	Non-Fac Total	Fac Total		51	50	62	80	MUE
	0.00	0.00	XXX	9	9	9	9	

4300F Patient receiving warfarin therapy for nonvalvular atrial fibrillation or atrial flutter (AFIB) ⊙E

RVU		Global Days	Modifiers				
Mod	Non-Fac Total	Fac Total		51	50	62	80	MUE
	0.00	0.00	XXX	9	9	9	9	

4301F Patient not receiving warfarin therapy for nonvalvular atrial fibrillation or atrial flutter (AFIB) ⊙E

RVU		Global Days	Modifiers				
Mod	Non-Fac Total	Fac Total		51	50	62	80	MUE
	0.00	0.00	XXX	9	9	9	9	

4305F Patient education regarding appropriate foot care and daily inspection of the feet received (CWC) ⊙E

RVU		Global Days	Modifiers				
Mod	Non-Fac Total	Fac Total		51	50	62	80	MUE
	0.00	0.00	XXX	9	9	9	9	

4306F Patient counseled regarding psychosocial and pharmacologic treatment options for opioid addiction (SUD) E

RVU		Global Days	Modifiers				
Mod	Non-Fac Total	Fac Total		51	50	62	80	MUE
	0.00	0.00	XXX	9	9	9	9	

4320F Patient counseled regarding psychosocial and pharmacologic treatment options for alcohol dependence (SUD) ⊙E

RVU		Global Days	Modifiers				
Mod	Non-Fac Total	Fac Total		51	50	62	80	MUE
	0.00	0.00	XXX	9	9	9	9	

4322F Caregiver provided with education and referred to additional resources for support (DEM) ⊙M

RVU		Global Days	Modifiers				
Mod	Non-Fac Total	Fac Total		51	50	62	80	MUE
	0.00	0.00	XXX	9	9	9	9	

4324F Patient (or caregiver) queried about Parkinson's disease medication related motor complications (Prkns) E

RVU		Global Days	Modifiers				
Mod	Non-Fac Total	Fac Total		51	50	62	80	MUE
	0.00	0.00	XXX	9	9	9	9	

4325F Medical and surgical treatment options reviewed with patient (or caregiver) (Prkns) ⊙M

RVU		Global Days	Modifiers				
Mod	Non-Fac Total	Fac Total		51	50	62	80	MUE
	0.00	0.00	XXX	9	9	9	9	

4326F Patient (or caregiver) queried about symptoms of autonomic dysfunction (Prkns) E

RVU		Global Days	Modifiers				
Mod	Non-Fac Total	Fac Total		51	50	62	80	MUE
	0.00	0.00	XXX	9	9	9	9	

4328F Patient (or caregiver) queried about sleep disturbances (Prkns) ⊙M

RVU		Global Days	Modifiers				
Mod	Non-Fac Total	Fac Total		51	50	62	80	MUE
	0.00	0.00	XXX	9	9	9	9	

4330F Counseling about epilepsy specific safety issues provided to patient (or caregiver(s)) (EPI) ⊙E

RVU		Global Days	Modifiers				
Mod	Non-Fac Total	Fac Total		51	50	62	80	MUE
	0.00	0.00	XXX	9	9	9	9	

4340F Counseling for women of childbearing potential with epilepsy (EPI) ⊙M

RVU		Global Days	Modifiers				
Mod	Non-Fac Total	Fac Total		51	50	62	80	MUE
	0.00	0.00	XXX	9	9	9	9	

4350F Counseling provided on symptom management, end of life decisions, and palliation (DEM) ⊙E

RVU		Global Days	Modifiers				
Mod	Non-Fac Total	Fac Total		51	50	62	80	MUE
	0.00	0.00	XXX	9	9	9	9	

4400F Rehabilitative therapy options discussed with patient (or caregiver) (Prkns) ⊙M

RVU		Global Days	Modifiers				
Mod	Non-Fac Total	Fac Total		51	50	62	80	MUE
	0.00	0.00	XXX	9	9	9	9	

4450F Self-care education provided to patient (HF) ⊙E

RVU		Global Days	Modifiers				
Mod	Non-Fac Total	Fac Total		51	50	62	80	MUE
	0.00	0.00	XXX	9	9	9	9	

4470F Implantable cardioverter-defibrillator (ICD) counseling provided (HF) E

RVU		Global Days	Modifiers				
Mod	Non-Fac Total	Fac Total		51	50	62	80	MUE
	0.00	0.00	XXX	9	9	9	9	

4480F Patient receiving ACE inhibitor/ARB therapy and beta-blocker therapy for 3 months or longer (HF) ⊙E

RVU		Global Days	Modifiers				
Mod	Non-Fac Total	Fac Total		51	50	62	80	MUE
	0.00	0.00	XXX	9	9	9	9	

● New   ▲ Revised   Deleted   ⊙ Moderate Sedation   ✚ Add-on Codes   ⊘ High Risk Denial   Ⓐ Age Edit   ♀ Female   ♂ Male   **AMA** CPT® Assistant   **MUE** Medically Unlikely Edit
⊘ Modifier 51 Exempt   ⊖ Modifier 63 Exempt   ✗ Unlisted   **Modifiers:** See Inside Back Cover   Ⓜ Maternity   A2–Z3 ASC Payment Indicators   A–Y OPPS Status Indicators

Category II Procedures

4481F – 4563F

4481F Patient receiving ACE inhibitor/ARB therapy and beta-blocker therapy for less than 3 months or patient not receiving ACE inhibitor/ARB therapy and beta-blocker therapy (HF)   Ⓒ E

Mod	RVU Non-Fac Total	Fac Total	Global Days	51	50	62	80	MUE
	0.00	0.00	XXX	9	9	9	9	

4500F Referred to an outpatient cardiac rehabilitation program (CAD)   Ⓒ M

Mod	RVU Non-Fac Total	Fac Total	Global Days	51	50	62	80	MUE
	0.00	0.00	XXX	9	9	9	9	

4510F Previous cardiac rehabilitation for qualifying cardiac event completed (CAD)   M

Mod	RVU Non-Fac Total	Fac Total	Global Days	51	50	62	80	MUE
	0.00	0.00	XXX	9	9	9	9	

4525F Neuropsychiatric intervention ordered (DEM)   Ⓒ M

Mod	RVU Non-Fac Total	Fac Total	Global Days	51	50	62	80	MUE
	0.00	0.00	XXX	9	9	9	9	

4526F Neuropsychiatric intervention received (DEM)   Ⓒ M

Mod	RVU Non-Fac Total	Fac Total	Global Days	51	50	62	80	MUE
	0.00	0.00	XXX	9	9	9	9	

4540F Disease modifying pharmacotherapy discussed (ALS)   E

Mod	RVU Non-Fac Total	Fac Total	Global Days	51	50	62	80	MUE
	0.00	0.00	XXX	9	9	9	9	

4541F Patient offered treatment for pseudobulbar affect, sialorrhea, or ALS-related symptoms (ALS)   Ⓒ E

Mod	RVU Non-Fac Total	Fac Total	Global Days	51	50	62	80	MUE
	0.00	0.00	XXX	9	9	9	9	

4550F Options for noninvasive respiratory support discussed with patient (ALS)   Ⓒ E

Mod	RVU Non-Fac Total	Fac Total	Global Days	51	50	62	80	MUE
	0.00	0.00	XXX	9	9	9	9	

4551F Nutritional support offered (ALS)   Ⓒ E

Mod	RVU Non-Fac Total	Fac Total	Global Days	51	50	62	80	MUE
	0.00	0.00	XXX	9	9	9	9	

4552F Patient offered referral to a speech language pathologist (ALS)   Ⓒ E

Mod	RVU Non-Fac Total	Fac Total	Global Days	51	50	62	80	MUE
	0.00	0.00	XXX	9	9	9	9	

4553F Patient offered assistance in planning for end of life issues (ALS)   Ⓒ E

Mod	RVU Non-Fac Total	Fac Total	Global Days	51	50	62	80	MUE
	0.00	0.00	XXX	9	9	9	9	

4554F Patient received inhalational anesthetic agent (Peri2)   Ⓒ M

Mod	RVU Non-Fac Total	Fac Total	Global Days	51	50	62	80	MUE
	0.00	0.00	XXX	9	9	9	9	

4555F Patient did not receive inhalational anesthetic agent (Peri2)   Ⓒ E

Mod	RVU Non-Fac Total	Fac Total	Global Days	51	50	62	80	MUE
	0.00	0.00	XXX	9	9	9	9	

4556F Patient exhibits 3 or more risk factors for post-operative nausea and vomiting (Peri2)   Ⓒ M

Mod	RVU Non-Fac Total	Fac Total	Global Days	51	50	62	80	MUE
	0.00	0.00	XXX	9	9	9	9	

4557F Patient does not exhibit 3 or more risk factors for post-operative nausea and vomiting (Peri2)   Ⓒ E

Mod	RVU Non-Fac Total	Fac Total	Global Days	51	50	62	80	MUE
	0.00	0.00	XXX	9	9	9	9	

4558F Patient received at least 2 prophylactic pharmacologic anti-emetic agents of different classes preoperatively and intraoperatively (Peri2)   Ⓒ M

Mod	RVU Non-Fac Total	Fac Total	Global Days	51	50	62	80	MUE
	0.00	0.00	XXX	9	9	9	9	

4559F At least 1 body temperature measurement equal to or greater than 35.5 degrees Celsius (or 95.9 degrees Fahrenheit) recorded within the 30 minutes immediately before or the 15 minutes immediately after anesthesia end time (Peri2)   Ⓒ M

Mod	RVU Non-Fac Total	Fac Total	Global Days	51	50	62	80	MUE
	0.00	0.00	XXX	9	9	9	9	

4560F Anesthesia technique did not involve general or neuraxial anesthesia (Peri2)   Ⓒ E

Mod	RVU Non-Fac Total	Fac Total	Global Days	51	50	62	80	MUE
	0.00	0.00	XXX	9	9	9	9	

4561F Patient has a coronary artery stent (Peri2)   E

Mod	RVU Non-Fac Total	Fac Total	Global Days	51	50	62	80	MUE
	0.00	0.00	XXX	9	9	9	9	

4562F Patient does not have a coronary artery stent (Peri2)   E

Mod	RVU Non-Fac Total	Fac Total	Global Days	51	50	62	80	MUE
	0.00	0.00	XXX	9	9	9	9	

4563F Patient received aspirin within 24 hours prior to anesthesia start time (Peri2)   E

Mod	RVU Non-Fac Total	Fac Total	Global Days	51	50	62	80	MUE
	0.00	0.00	XXX	9	9	9	9	

● New   ▲ Revised   ✖ Deleted   ⊙ Moderate Sedation   ✚ Add-on Codes   ⊘ High Risk Denial   Ⓐ Age Edit   ♀ Female   ♂ Male   **AMA** *CPT® Assistant*   **MUE** Medically Unlikely Edit
⊘ Modifier 51 Exempt   ⊖ Modifier 63 Exempt   ⊠ Unlisted   **Modifiers:** *See Inside Back Cover*   M Maternity   A2–Z3 ASC Payment Indicators   A–Y OPPS Status Indicators

CPT © 2015 American Medical Association. All Rights Reserved.   © 2016 DecisionHealth

Follow-up/Other Outcome Codes

5005F Patient counseled on self-examination for new or changing moles (ML) ⊚Ⓔ

RVU		Global Days	Modifiers				
Mod	Non-Fac Total	Fac Total		51	50	62	80	MUE
	0.00	0.00	XXX	9	9	9	9

5010F Findings of dilated macular or fundus exam communicated to the physician or other qualified health care professional managing the diabetes care (EC) ⊚Ⓜ

RVU		Global Days	Modifiers				
Mod	Non-Fac Total	Fac Total		51	50	62	80	MUE
	0.00	0.00	XXX	9	9	9	9

5015F Documentation of communication that a fracture occurred and that the patient was or should be tested or treated for osteoporosis (OP) ⊚Ⓜ

RVU		Global Days	Modifiers				
Mod	Non-Fac Total	Fac Total		51	50	62	80	MUE
	0.00	0.00	XXX	9	9	9	9

5020F Treatment summary report communicated to physician(s) or other qualified health care professional(s) managing continuing care and to the patient within 1 month of completing treatment (ONC) ⊚Ⓔ

RVU		Global Days	Modifiers				
Mod	Non-Fac Total	Fac Total		51	50	62	80	MUE
	0.00	0.00	XXX	9	9	9	9

5050F Treatment plan communicated to provider(s) managing continuing care within 1 month of diagnosis (ML) ⊚Ⓜ

RVU		Global Days	Modifiers				
Mod	Non-Fac Total	Fac Total		51	50	62	80	MUE
	0.00	0.00	XXX	9	9	9	9

5060F Findings from diagnostic mammogram communicated to practice managing patient's on-going care within 3 business days of exam interpretation (RAD) ⊚Ⓝ Ⓘ Ⓔ

RVU		Global Days	Modifiers				
Mod	Non-Fac Total	Fac Total		51	50	62	80	MUE
	0.00	0.00	XXX	9	9	9	9

5062F Findings from diagnostic mammogram communicated to the patient within 5 days of exam interpretation (RAD) Ⓔ

RVU		Global Days	Modifiers				
Mod	Non-Fac Total	Fac Total		51	50	62	80	MUE
	0.00	0.00	XXX	9	9	9	9

5100F Potential risk for fracture communicated to the referring physician or other qualified health care professional within 24 hours of completion of the imaging study (NUC_MED) ⊚Ⓔ

RVU		Global Days	Modifiers				
Mod	Non-Fac Total	Fac Total		51	50	62	80	MUE
	0.00	0.00	XXX	9	9	9	9

5200F Consideration of referral for a neurological evaluation of appropriateness for surgical therapy for intractable epilepsy within the past 3 years (EPI) ⊚Ⓔ

RVU		Global Days	Modifiers				
Mod	Non-Fac Total	Fac Total		51	50	62	80	MUE
	0.00	0.00	XXX	9	9	9	9

5250F Asthma discharge plan provided to patient (Asthma) ⊚Ⓔ

RVU		Global Days	Modifiers				
Mod	Non-Fac Total	Fac Total		51	50	62	80	MUE
	0.00	0.00	XXX	9	9	9	9

Patient Safety Codes

6005F Rationale (eg, severity of illness and safety) for level of care (eg, home, hospital) documented (CAP) Ⓔ

RVU		Global Days	Modifiers				
Mod	Non-Fac Total	Fac Total		51	50	62	80	MUE
	0.00	0.00	XXX	9	9	9	9

AMA: Aug 07: 1

6010F Dysphagia screening conducted prior to order for or receipt of any foods, fluids, or medication by mouth (STR) ⊚Ⓔ

RVU		Global Days	Modifiers				
Mod	Non-Fac Total	Fac Total		51	50	62	80	MUE
	0.00	0.00	XXX	9	9	9	9

6015F Patient receiving or eligible to receive foods, fluids, or medication by mouth (STR) ⊚Ⓔ

RVU		Global Days	Modifiers				
Mod	Non-Fac Total	Fac Total		51	50	62	80	MUE
	0.00	0.00	XXX	9	9	9	9

6020F NPO (nothing by mouth) ordered (STR) ⊚Ⓔ

RVU		Global Days	Modifiers				
Mod	Non-Fac Total	Fac Total		51	50	62	80	MUE
	0.00	0.00	XXX	9	9	9	9

▲ **6030F All elements of maximal sterile barrier technique, hand hygiene, skin preparation and, if ultrasound is used, sterile ultrasound techniques followed (CRIT)** ⊚Ⓜ

RVU		Global Days	Modifiers				
Mod	Non-Fac Total	Fac Total		51	50	62	80	MUE
	0.00	0.00	XXX	9	9	9	9

6040F Use of appropriate radiation dose reduction devices OR manual techniques for appropriate moderation of exposure, documented (RAD) ⊚Ⓔ

RVU		Global Days	Modifiers				
Mod	Non-Fac Total	Fac Total		51	50	62	80	MUE
	0.00	0.00	XXX	9	9	9	9

6045F Radiation exposure or exposure time in final report for procedure using fluoroscopy, documented (RAD) ⊚Ⓔ

RVU		Global Days	Modifiers				
Mod	Non-Fac Total	Fac Total		51	50	62	80	MUE
	0.00	0.00	XXX	9	9	9	9

● New ▲ Revised   Deleted ⊙ Moderate Sedation ✚ Add-on Codes ⊘ High Risk Denial ⒶAge Edit ♀ Female ♂ Male **AMA** *CPT® Assistant* **MUE** Medically Unlikely Edit
⊘ Modifier 51 Exempt ⊖ Modifier 63 Exempt ☒ Unlisted **Modifiers:** *See Inside Back Cover* Ⓜ Maternity Ⓐ2–Ⓩ3 ASC Payment Indicators Ⓐ–Ⓨ OPPS Status Indicators

© 2016 DecisionHealth   CPT © 2015 American Medical Association. All Rights Reserved.   **889**

6070F Patient queried and counseled about anti-epileptic drug (AED) side effects (EPI) ⓒⒺ

RVU			Global Days	Modifiers				
Mod	Non-Fac Total	Fac Total		51	50	62	80	MUE
	0.00	0.00	XXX	9	9	9	9	

6080F Patient (or caregiver) queried about falls (Prkns, DSP) ⓒⒺ

RVU			Global Days	Modifiers				
Mod	Non-Fac Total	Fac Total		51	50	62	80	MUE
	0.00	0.00	XXX	9	9	9	9	

6090F Patient (or caregiver) counseled about safety issues appropriate to patient's stage of disease (Prkns) Ⓔ

RVU			Global Days	Modifiers				
Mod	Non-Fac Total	Fac Total		51	50	62	80	MUE
	0.00	0.00	XXX	9	9	9	9	

6100F Timeout to verify correct patient, correct site, and correct procedure, documented (PATH) ⓒⒺ

RVU			Global Days	Modifiers				
Mod	Non-Fac Total	Fac Total		51	50	62	80	MUE
	0.00	0.00	XXX	9	9	9	9	

6101F Safety counseling for dementia provided (DEM) ⓒⓂ

RVU			Global Days	Modifiers				
Mod	Non-Fac Total	Fac Total		51	50	62	80	MUE
	0.00	0.00	XXX	9	9	9	9	

6102F Safety counseling for dementia ordered (DEM) ⓒⓂ

RVU			Global Days	Modifiers				
Mod	Non-Fac Total	Fac Total		51	50	62	80	MUE
	0.00	0.00	XXX	9	9	9	9	

6110F Counseling provided regarding risks of driving and the alternatives to driving (DEM) ⓒⓂ

RVU			Global Days	Modifiers				
Mod	Non-Fac Total	Fac Total		51	50	62	80	MUE
	0.00	0.00	XXX	9	9	9	9	

6150F Patient not receiving a first course of anti-TNF (tumor necrosis factor) therapy (IBD) ⓒⒺ

RVU			Global Days	Modifiers				
Mod	Non-Fac Total	Fac Total		51	50	62	80	MUE
	0.00	0.00	XXX	9	9	9	9	

7010F Patient information entered into a recall system that includes: target date for the next exam specified and a process to follow up with patients regarding missed or unscheduled appointments (ML) ⓒⓂ

RVU			Global Days	Modifiers				
Mod	Non-Fac Total	Fac Total		51	50	62	80	MUE
	0.00	0.00	XXX	9	9	9	9	

7020F Mammogram assessment category (eg, Mammography Quality Standards Act [MQSA], Breast Imaging Reporting and Data System [BI-RADS], or FDA approved equivalent categories) entered into an internal database to allow for analysis of abnormal interpretation (recall) rate (RAD) ⓒⒺ

RVU			Global Days	Modifiers				
Mod	Non-Fac Total	Fac Total		51	50	62	80	MUE
	0.00	0.00	XXX	9	9	9	9	

7025F Patient information entered into a reminder system with a target due date for the next mammogram (RAD) ⓒⓂ

RVU			Global Days	Modifiers				
Mod	Non-Fac Total	Fac Total		51	50	62	80	MUE
	0.00	0.00	XXX	9	9	9	9	

9001F Aortic aneurysm less than 5.0 cm maximum diameter on centerline formatted CT or minor diameter on axial formatted CT (NMA-No Measure Associated) ⓒⒺ

RVU			Global Days	Modifiers				
Mod	Non-Fac Total	Fac Total		51	50	62	80	MUE
	0.00	0.00	XXX	9	9	9	9	

9002F Aortic aneurysm 5.0 - 5.4 cm maximum diameter on centerline formatted CT or minor diameter on axial formatted CT (NMA-No Measure Associated) ⓒⒺ

RVU			Global Days	Modifiers				
Mod	Non-Fac Total	Fac Total		51	50	62	80	MUE
	0.00	0.00	XXX	9	9	9	9	

9003F Aortic aneurysm 5.5 - 5.9 cm maximum diameter on centerline formatted CT or minor diameter on axial formatted CT (NMA-No Measure Associated) ⓒⓂ

RVU			Global Days	Modifiers				
Mod	Non-Fac Total	Fac Total		51	50	62	80	MUE
	0.00	0.00	XXX	9	9	9	9	

9004F Aortic aneurysm 6.0 cm or greater maximum diameter on centerline formatted CT or minor diameter on axial formatted CT (NMA-No Measure Associated) ⓒⓂ

RVU			Global Days	Modifiers				
Mod	Non-Fac Total	Fac Total		51	50	62	80	MUE
	0.00	0.00	XXX	9	9	9	9	

9005F Asymptomatic carotid stenosis: No history of any transient ischemic attack or stroke in any carotid or vertebrobasilar territory (NMA-No Measure Associated) ⓒⒺ

RVU			Global Days	Modifiers				
Mod	Non-Fac Total	Fac Total		51	50	62	80	MUE
	0.00	0.00	XXX	9	9	9	9	

9006F Symptomatic carotid stenosis: Ipsilateral carotid territory TIA or stroke less than 120 days prior to procedure (NMA-No Measure Associated) ⓒⓂ

RVU			Global Days	Modifiers				
Mod	Non-Fac Total	Fac Total		51	50	62	80	MUE
	0.00	0.00	XXX	9	9	9	9	

9007F Other carotid stenosis: Ipsilateral TIA or stroke 120 days or greater prior to procedure or any prior contralateral carotid territory or vertebrobasilar TIA or stroke (NMA-No Measure Associated) ⓒⓂ

RVU			Global Days	Modifiers				
Mod	Non-Fac Total	Fac Total		51	50	62	80	MUE
	0.00	0.00	XXX	9	9	9	9	

● New　　▲ Revised　　✖ Deleted　　⊙ Moderate Sedation　　✚ Add-on Codes　　⊘ High Risk Denial　　Ⓐ Age Edit　　♀ Female　　♂ Male　　**AMA** *CPT® Assistant*　　**MUE** Medically Unlikely Edit
⊘ Modifier 51 Exempt　　⊖ Modifier 63 Exempt　　☒ Unlisted　　**Modifiers:** *See Inside Back Cover*　　Ⓜ Maternity　　A 2–Z 3 ASC Payment Indicators　　A –Y OPPS Status Indicators

CPT © 2015 American Medical Association. All Rights Reserved.　　　　© 2016 DecisionHealth

Category III Procedures

Category III procedures identify new technologies that do not yet have a CPT Level I code. Where a Category III code is available, it must be reported instead of an "unlisted" CPT code. These temporary new technology codes describe emerging technology services and procedures that allow for data collection to determine if a CPT Level I code should be created. If, in five years, the procedure described by the Category III code has not shown efficacy or is not performed with sufficient frequency, the Category III code is deleted without moving the procedure to the Category I section or assigning a Category I code.

Category III codes consist of five digits, and are alphanumeric, with the last character being a "T". This section is not broken down into anatomical sites as with Category I codes. Instead, codes are placed in numerical order as they are developed and introduced into the healthcare market.

0019T Extracorporeal shock wave involving musculoskeletal system, not otherwise specified, low energy A

Mod	Non-Fac Total	Fac Total	Global Days	51	50	62	80	MUE
	0.00	0.00	XXX	0	0	0	0	1

AMA: Jun 05: 6, Mar 06: 1

0042T Cerebral perfusion analysis using computed tomography with contrast administration, including post-processing of parametric maps with determination of cerebral blood flow, cerebral blood volume, and mean transit time N

Mod	Non-Fac Total	Fac Total	Global Days	51	50	62	80	MUE
	0.00	0.00	XXX	0	0	0	0	1

0051T Implantation of a total replacement heart system (artificial heart) with recipient cardiectomy C

Mod	Non-Fac Total	Fac Total	Global Days	51	50	62	80	MUE
	0.00	0.00	XXX	0	0	0	0	1

AMA: Jun 04: 7

0052T Replacement or repair of thoracic unit of a total replacement heart system (artificial heart) C

Mod	Non-Fac Total	Fac Total	Global Days	51	50	62	80	MUE
	0.00	0.00	XXX	0	0	0	0	1

AMA: Jun 04: 7

0053T Replacement or repair of implantable component or components of total replacement heart system (artificial heart), excluding thoracic unit C

Mod	Non-Fac Total	Fac Total	Global Days	51	50	62	80	MUE
	0.00	0.00	XXX	0	0	0	0	1

AMA: Jun 04: 7

+ 0054T Computer-assisted musculoskeletal surgical navigational orthopedic procedure, with image-guidance based on fluoroscopic images (List separately in addition to code for primary procedure) N

Mod	Non-Fac Total	Fac Total	Global Days	51	50	62	80	MUE
	0.00	0.00	XXX	0	0	0	0	2

AMA: May 04: 14, Jun 04: 8

+ 0055T Computer-assisted musculoskeletal surgical navigational orthopedic procedure, with image-guidance based on CT/MRI images (List separately in addition to code for primary procedure) N

Mod	Non-Fac Total	Fac Total	Global Days	51	50	62	80	MUE
	0.00	0.00	XXX	0	0	0	0	2

AMA: May 04: 14, Jun 04: 8

0058T Cryopreservation; reproductive tissue, ovarian 1

Mod	Non-Fac Total	Fac Total	Global Days	51	50	62	80	MUE
	0.00	0.00	XXX	0	0	0	0	1

0071T Focused ultrasound ablation of uterine leiomyomata, including MR guidance; total leiomyomata volume less than 200 cc of tissue ♀ T

Mod	Non-Fac Total	Fac Total	Global Days	51	50	62	80	MUE
	0.00	0.00	XXX	0	0	0	0	1

AMA: Mar 05: 1, 5, Dec 05: 3

0072T Focused ultrasound ablation of uterine leiomyomata, including MR guidance; total leiomyomata volume greater or equal to 200 cc of tissue ♀ T

Mod	Non-Fac Total	Fac Total	Global Days	51	50	62	80	MUE
	0.00	0.00	XXX	0	0	0	0	1

AMA: Mar 05: 1, 5, Dec 05: 3

0075T Transcatheter placement of extracranial vertebral artery stent(s), including radiologic supervision and interpretation, open or percutaneous; initial vessel C

Mod	Non-Fac Total	Fac Total	Global Days	51	50	62	80	MUE
	0.00	0.00	XXX	0	0	0	0	1
26	0.00	0.00	XXX	0	0	0	0	1
TC	0.00	0.00	XXX	0	0	0	0	1

AMA: May 05: 7, Mar 14: 8

+ 0076T Transcatheter placement of extracranial vertebral artery stent(s), including radiologic supervision and interpretation, open or percutaneous; each additional vessel (List separately in addition to code for primary procedure) C

Mod	Non-Fac Total	Fac Total	Global Days	51	50	62	80	MUE
	0.00	0.00	XXX	0	0	0	0	2
26	0.00	0.00	XXX	0	0	0	0	2
TC	0.00	0.00	XXX	0	0	0	0	2

AMA: May 05: 7, Mar 14: 8

0085T Breath test for heart transplant rejection E

Mod	Non-Fac Total	Fac Total	Global Days	51	50	62	80	MUE
	0.00	0.00	XXX	9	9	9	9	

AMA: May 05: 7

● New ▲ Revised Deleted ⊙ Moderate Sedation ✚ Add-on Codes ⊘ High Risk Denial Ⓐ Age Edit ♀ Female ♂ Male **AMA** *CPT® Assistant* **MUE** Medically Unlikely Edit ⦸ Modifier 51 Exempt ⊖ Modifier 63 Exempt ✗ Unlisted **Modifiers:** *See Inside Back Cover* Ⓜ Maternity A2–Z3 ASC Payment Indicators A–Y OPPS Status Indicators

© 2016 DecisionHealth   CPT © 2015 American Medical Association. All Rights Reserved.

+ 0095T Removal of total disc arthroplasty (artificial disc), anterior approach, each additional interspace, cervical (List separately in addition to code for primary procedure) Ⓒ

RVU			Global Days	Modifiers				
Mod	Non-Fac Total	Fac Total		51	50	62	80	MUE
	0.00	0.00	XXX	0	0	0	0	1

AMA: Jun 05: 6, Feb 06: 1

+ 0098T Revision including replacement of total disc arthroplasty (artificial disc), anterior approach, each additional interspace, cervical (List separately in addition to code for primary procedure) Ⓒ

RVU			Global Days	Modifiers				
Mod	Non-Fac Total	Fac Total		51	50	62	80	MUE
	0.00	0.00	XXX	0	0	0	0	1

AMA: Jun 05: 6, Feb 06: 1

✖ 0099T Implantation of intrastromal corneal ring segments

0100T Placement of a subconjunctival retinal prosthesis receiver and pulse generator, and implantation of intra-ocular retinal electrode array, with vitrectomy Ⓙ8Ⓣ

RVU			Global Days	Modifiers				
Mod	Non-Fac Total	Fac Total		51	50	62	80	MUE
	0.00	0.00	XXX	0	0	0	0	2

AMA: Jun 05: 6, Feb 06: 1, Jun 11: 13

0101T Extracorporeal shock wave involving musculoskeletal system, not otherwise specified, high energy ⒼG2Ⓣ

RVU			Global Days	Modifiers				
Mod	Non-Fac Total	Fac Total		51	50	62	80	MUE
	0.00	0.00	XXX	0	0	0	0	1

AMA: Jun 05: 6, Mar 06: 1, Jun 11: 13

0102T Extracorporeal shock wave, high energy, performed by a physician, requiring anesthesia other than local, involving lateral humeral epicondyle ⒼG2Ⓣ

RVU			Global Days	Modifiers				
Mod	Non-Fac Total	Fac Total		51	50	62	80	MUE
	0.00	0.00	XXX	0	0	0	0	2

AMA: Jun 05: 6, Mar 06: 1, Jun 11: 13

✖ 0103T Holotranscobalamin, quantitative

0106T Quantitative sensory testing (QST), testing and interpretation per extremity; using touch pressure stimuli to assess large diameter sensation ⓈⓆⒾ

RVU			Global Days	Modifiers				
Mod	Non-Fac Total	Fac Total		51	50	62	80	MUE
	0.00	0.00	XXX	0	0	0	0	4

AMA: Jun 05: 6, Mar 06: 1, May 11: 10, Jun 11: 13

0107T Quantitative sensory testing (QST), testing and interpretation per extremity; using vibration stimuli to assess large diameter fiber sensation ⓈⓆⒾ

RVU			Global Days	Modifiers				
Mod	Non-Fac Total	Fac Total		51	50	62	80	MUE
	0.00	0.00	XXX	0	0	0	0	4

AMA: Jun 05: 6, Mar 06: 1, May 11: 10, Jun 11: 13

0108T Quantitative sensory testing (QST), testing and interpretation per extremity; using cooling stimuli to assess small nerve fiber sensation and hyperalgesia ⓈⓆⒾ

RVU			Global Days	Modifiers				
Mod	Non-Fac Total	Fac Total		51	50	62	80	MUE
	0.00	0.00	XXX	0	0	0	0	4

AMA: Jun 05: 6, Mar 06: 1, May 11: 10, Jun 11: 13

0109T Quantitative sensory testing (QST), testing and interpretation per extremity; using heat-pain stimuli to assess small nerve fiber sensation and hyperalgesia ⓈⓆⒾ

RVU			Global Days	Modifiers				
Mod	Non-Fac Total	Fac Total		51	50	62	80	MUE
	0.00	0.00	XXX	0	0	0	0	4

AMA: Jun 05: 6, Mar 06: 1, May 11: 10, Jun 11: 13

0110T Quantitative sensory testing (QST), testing and interpretation per extremity; using other stimuli to assess sensation ⓈⓆⒾ

RVU			Global Days	Modifiers				
Mod	Non-Fac Total	Fac Total		51	50	62	80	MUE
	0.00	0.00	XXX	0	0	0	0	4

AMA: Jun 05: 6, Mar 06: 1, May 11: 10, Jun 11: 13

0111T Long-chain (C20-22) omega-3 fatty acids in red blood cell (RBC) membranes ⓈⒶ

RVU			Global Days	Modifiers				
Mod	Non-Fac Total	Fac Total		51	50	62	80	MUE
	0.00	0.00	XXX	9	9	9	9	1

AMA: Jun 05: 6, Mar 06: 1, Jun 11: 13

✖ 0123T Fistulization of sclera for glaucoma, through ciliary body

0126T Common carotid intima-media thickness (IMT) study for evaluation of atherosclerotic burden or coronary heart disease risk factor assessment ⓈⓆⒾ

RVU			Global Days	Modifiers				
Mod	Non-Fac Total	Fac Total		51	50	62	80	MUE
	0.00	0.00	XXX	0	0	0	0	1

AMA: Jun 11: 13

+ 0159T Computer-aided detection, including computer algorithm analysis of MRI image data for lesion detection/characterization, pharmacokinetic analysis, with further physician review for interpretation, breast MRI (List separately in addition to code for primary procedure) ⒼN

RVU			Global Days	Modifiers				
Mod	Non-Fac Total	Fac Total		51	50	62	80	MUE
	0.00	0.00	ZZZ	0	0	0	0	2
26	0.00	0.00	ZZZ	0	0	0	0	2
TC	0.00	0.00	ZZZ	0	0	0	0	2

AMA: Mar 07: 7, Jul 07: 6

● New ▲ Revised ✖ Deleted ⊙ Moderate Sedation ✚ Add-on Codes ⊗ High Risk Denial Ⓐ Age Edit ♀ Female ♂ Male **AMA** *CPT® Assistant* **MUE** Medically Unlikely Edit
Ⓢ Modifier 51 Exempt ⊖ Modifier 63 Exempt Ⓧ Unlisted **Modifiers:** *See Inside Back Cover* Ⓜ Maternity Ⓐ2–Ⓩ3 ASC Payment Indicators Ⓐ–Ⓨ OPPS Status Indicators

CPT © 2015 American Medical Association. All Rights Reserved.

© 2016 DecisionHealth

+ 0163T Total disc arthroplasty (artificial disc), anterior approach, including discectomy to prepare interspace (other than for decompression), each additional interspace, lumbar (List separately in addition to code for primary procedure) ⊘C

RVU			Global Days	Modifiers				
Mod	Non-Fac Total	Fac Total		51	50	62	80	MUE
	0.00	0.00	YYY	0	0	0	0	2

AMA: Jun 07: 1

Pub 100-04, 32, 170.2

+ 0164T Removal of total disc arthroplasty, (artificial disc), anterior approach, each additional interspace, lumbar (List separately in addition to code for primary procedure) C

RVU			Global Days	Modifiers				
Mod	Non-Fac Total	Fac Total		51	50	62	80	MUE
	0.00	0.00	YYY	0	0	0	0	4

AMA: Jun 07: 1

+ 0165T Revision including replacement of total disc arthroplasty (artificial disc), anterior approach, each additional interspace, lumbar (List separately in addition to code for primary procedure) C

RVU			Global Days	Modifiers				
Mod	Non-Fac Total	Fac Total		51	50	62	80	MUE
	0.00	0.00	YYY	0	0	0	0	4

AMA: Jun 07: 1

0169T Stereotactic placement of infusion catheter(s) in the brain for delivery of therapeutic agent(s), including computerized stereotactic planning and burr hole(s) ⊘C

RVU			Global Days	Modifiers				
Mod	Non-Fac Total	Fac Total		51	50	62	80	MUE
	0.00	0.00	XXX	0	0	0	0	1

AMA: Jul 07: 6, May 08: 15, Jul 08: 4

0171T Insertion of posterior spinous process distraction device (including necessary removal of bone or ligament for insertion and imaging guidance), lumbar; single level J 8 J I

RVU			Global Days	Modifiers				
Mod	Non-Fac Total	Fac Total		51	50	62	80	MUE
	0.00	0.00	XXX	0	0	0	0	1

AMA: Dec 13: 17, Oct 14: 15

+ 0172T Insertion of posterior spinous process distraction device (including necessary removal of bone or ligament for insertion and imaging guidance), lumbar; each additional level (List separately in addition to code for primary procedure) N

RVU			Global Days	Modifiers				
Mod	Non-Fac Total	Fac Total		51	50	62	80	MUE
	0.00	0.00	XXX	0	0	0	0	3

+ 0174T Computer-aided detection (CAD) (computer algorithm analysis of digital image data for lesion detection) with further physician review for interpretation and report, with or without digitization of film radiographic images, chest radiograph(s), performed concurrent with primary interpretation (List separately in addition to code for primary procedure) ⊘N

RVU			Global Days	Modifiers				
Mod	Non-Fac Total	Fac Total		51	50	62	80	MUE
	0.00	0.00	XXX	0	0	0	0	1

0175T Computer-aided detection (CAD) (computer algorithm analysis of digital image data for lesion detection) with further physician review for interpretation and report, with or without digitization of film radiographic images, chest radiograph(s), performed remote from primary interpretation N

RVU			Global Days	Modifiers				
Mod	Non-Fac Total	Fac Total		51	50	62	80	MUE
	0.00	0.00	XXX	0	0	0	0	1

0178T Electrocardiogram, 64 leads or greater, with graphic presentation and analysis; with interpretation and report B

RVU			Global Days	Modifiers				
Mod	Non-Fac Total	Fac Total		51	50	62	80	MUE
	0.00	0.00	XXX	0	0	0	0	1

0179T Electrocardiogram, 64 leads or greater, with graphic presentation and analysis; tracing and graphics only, without interpretation and report ⊘Q I

RVU			Global Days	Modifiers				
Mod	Non-Fac Total	Fac Total		51	50	62	80	MUE
	0.00	0.00	XXX	0	0	0	0	1

0180T Electrocardiogram, 64 leads or greater, with graphic presentation and analysis; interpretation and report only B

RVU			Global Days	Modifiers				
Mod	Non-Fac Total	Fac Total		51	50	62	80	MUE
	0.00	0.00	XXX	0	0	0	0	1

✕ 0182T ~~High dose rate electronic brachytherapy, per fraction~~

0184T Excision of rectal tumor, transanal endoscopic microsurgical approach (ie, TEMS), including muscularis propria (ie, full thickness) J I

RVU			Global Days	Modifiers				
Mod	Non-Fac Total	Fac Total		51	50	62	80	MUE
	0.00	0.00	XXX	0	0	0	0	1

AMA: Jun 10: 3

0188T Remote real-time interactive video-conferenced critical care, evaluation and management of the critically ill or critically injured patient; first 30-74 minutes ⊘M

RVU			Global Days	Modifiers				
Mod	Non-Fac Total	Fac Total		51	50	62	80	MUE
	0.00	0.00	XXX	9	9	9	9	

AMA: Aug 11: 10

● New   ▲ Revised   Deleted   ⊙ Moderate Sedation   ✛ Add-on Codes   ⊘ High Risk Denial   Ⓐ Age Edit   ♀ Female   ♂ Male   **AMA** *CPT® Assistant*   **MUE** Medically Unlikely Edit
⊘ Modifier 51 Exempt   ⊖ Modifier 63 Exempt   ✗ Unlisted   **Modifiers:** *See Inside Back Cover*   Ⓜ Maternity   A2–Z3 ASC Payment Indicators   A–Y OPPS Status Indicators

© 2016 DecisionHealth   CPT © 2015 American Medical Association. All Rights Reserved.   **893**

Category III Procedures

0189T – 0207T

✚ **0189T Remote real-time interactive video-conferenced critical care, evaluation and management of the critically ill or critically injured patient; each additional 30 minutes (List separately in addition to code for primary service)** ⓂM

RVU			Global Days	Modifiers				
Mod	Non-Fac Total	Fac Total		51	50	62	80	MUE
	0.00	0.00	XXX	9	9	9	9	

AMA: Aug 11: 10

✚ **0190T Placement of intraocular radiation source applicator (List separately in addition to primary procedure)** ⓒN

RVU			Global Days	Modifiers				
Mod	Non-Fac Total	Fac Total		51	50	62	80	MUE
	0.00	0.00	XXX	0	0	0	0	2

0191T Insertion of anterior segment aqueous drainage device, without extraocular reservoir, internal approach, into the trabecular meshwork; initial insertion G2 J I

Coding tip: Insertion of anterior segment aqueous drainage device without extraocular reservoir; internal approach into the suprachoroidal space - 0253T

RVU			Global Days	Modifiers				
Mod	Non-Fac Total	Fac Total		51	50	62	80	MUE
	0.00	0.00	XXX	0	0	0	0	2

AMA: Dec 12: 14

0195T Arthrodesis, pre-sacral interbody technique, disc space preparation, discectomy, without instrumentation, with image guidance, includes bone graft when performed; L5-S1 interspace ⓒC

RVU			Global Days	Modifiers				
Mod	Non-Fac Total	Fac Total		51	50	62	80	MUE
	0.00	0.00	XXX	0	0	0	0	1

AMA: Jul 13: 3

✚ **0196T Arthrodesis, pre-sacral interbody technique, disc space preparation, discectomy, without instrumentation, with image guidance, includes bone graft when performed; L4-L5 interspace (List separately in addition to code for primary procedure)** ⓒC

RVU			Global Days	Modifiers				
Mod	Non-Fac Total	Fac Total		51	50	62	80	MUE
	0.00	0.00	XXX	0	0	0	0	1

AMA: Jul 13: 3

0198T Measurement of ocular blood flow by repetitive intraocular pressure sampling, with interpretation and report ⓒ O I

RVU			Global Days	Modifiers				
Mod	Non-Fac Total	Fac Total		51	50	62	80	MUE
	0.00	0.00	XXX	0	0	0	0	2

AMA: Mar 11: 10, Aug 12: 9

⊙ **0200T Percutaneous sacral augmentation (sacroplasty), unilateral injection(s), including the use of a balloon or mechanical device, when used, 1 or more needles, includes imaging guidance and bone biopsy, when performed** ⓒG2 T

RVU			Global Days	Modifiers				
Mod	Non-Fac Total	Fac Total		51	50	62	80	MUE
	0.00	0.00	XXX	0	1	0	0	1

AMA: Apr 15: 8

⊙ **0201T Percutaneous sacral augmentation (sacroplasty), bilateral injections, including the use of a balloon or mechanical device, when used, 2 or more needles, includes imaging guidance and bone biopsy, when performed** ⓒG2 T

RVU			Global Days	Modifiers				
Mod	Non-Fac Total	Fac Total		51	50	62	80	MUE
	0.00	0.00	XXX	0	2	0	0	1

AMA: Apr 15: 8

0202T Posterior vertebral joint(s) arthroplasty (eg, facet joint[s] replacement), including facetectomy, laminectomy, foraminotomy, and vertebral column fixation, injection of bone cement, when performed, including fluoroscopy, single level, lumbar spine ⓒC

RVU			Global Days	Modifiers				
Mod	Non-Fac Total	Fac Total		51	50	62	80	MUE
	0.00	0.00	XXX	0	0	0	0	1

✚ **0205T Intravascular catheter-based coronary vessel or graft spectroscopy (eg, infrared) during diagnostic evaluation and/or therapeutic intervention including imaging supervision, interpretation, and report, each vessel (List separately in addition to code for primary procedure)** ⓒN

RVU			Global Days	Modifiers				
Mod	Non-Fac Total	Fac Total		51	50	62	80	MUE
	0.00	0.00	ZZZ	0	0	0	0	

0206T Computerized database analysis of multiple cycles of digitized cardiac electrical data from two or more ECG leads, including transmission to a remote center, application of multiple nonlinear mathematical transformations, with coronary artery obstruction severity assessment ⓒ O I

RVU			Global Days	Modifiers				
Mod	Non-Fac Total	Fac Total		51	50	62	80	MUE
	0.00	0.00	XXX	0	0	0	0	1

0207T Evacuation of meibomian glands, automated, using heat and intermittent pressure, unilateral ⓒ O I

RVU			Global Days	Modifiers				
Mod	Non-Fac Total	Fac Total		51	50	62	80	MUE
	0.00	0.00	XXX	0	0	0	0	2

AMA: May 14: 5

● New   ▲ Revised   ✖ Deleted   ⊙ Moderate Sedation   ✚ Add-on Codes   ⊘ High Risk Denial   Ⓐ Age Edit   ♀ Female   ♂ Male   **AMA** *CPT® Assistant*   **MUE** Medically Unlikely Edit
⊘ Modifier 51 Exempt   ⊖ Modifier 63 Exempt   ✖ Unlisted   **Modifiers:** *See Inside Back Cover*   Ⓜ Maternity   A2-Z3 ASC Payment Indicators   A-Y OPPS Status Indicators

894   CPT © 2015 American Medical Association. All Rights Reserved.   © 2016 DecisionHealth

0208T Pure tone audiometry (threshold), automated; air only

RVU			Global Days	Modifiers				
Mod	Non-Fac Total	Fac Total		51	50	62	80	MUE
	0.00	0.00	XXX	0	0	0	0	1

AMA: Aug 14: 3

0209T Pure tone audiometry (threshold), automated; air and bone

RVU			Global Days	Modifiers				
Mod	Non-Fac Total	Fac Total		51	50	62	80	MUE
	0.00	0.00	XXX	0	0	0	0	1

AMA: Mar 11: 8, Aug 14: 3

0210T Speech audiometry threshold, automated

RVU			Global Days	Modifiers				
Mod	Non-Fac Total	Fac Total		51	50	62	80	MUE
	0.00	0.00	XXX	0	0	0	0	1

AMA: Mar 11: 8

0211T Speech audiometry threshold, automated; with speech recognition

RVU			Global Days	Modifiers				
Mod	Non-Fac Total	Fac Total		51	50	62	80	MUE
	0.00	0.00	XXX	0	0	0	0	1

AMA: Mar 11: 8

0212T Comprehensive audiometry threshold evaluation and speech recognition (0209T, 0211T combined), automated

RVU			Global Days	Modifiers				
Mod	Non-Fac Total	Fac Total		51	50	62	80	MUE
	0.00	0.00	XXX	0	0	0	0	1

AMA: Mar 11: 8, Aug 14: 3

0213T Injection(s), diagnostic or therapeutic agent, paravertebral facet (zygapophyseal) joint (or nerves innervating that joint) with ultrasound guidance, cervical or thoracic; single level

RVU			Global Days	Modifiers				
Mod	Non-Fac Total	Fac Total		51	50	62	80	MUE
	0.00	0.00	XXX	0	1	0	0	1

AMA: Feb 11: 5, Jul 11: 14

+ **0214T** Injection(s), diagnostic or therapeutic agent, paravertebral facet (zygapophyseal) joint (or nerves innervating that joint) with ultrasound guidance, cervical or thoracic; second level (List separately in addition to code for primary procedure)

RVU			Global Days	Modifiers				
Mod	Non-Fac Total	Fac Total		51	50	62	80	MUE
	0.00	0.00	ZZZ	0	1	0	0	1

AMA: Jul 11: 14

+ **0215T** Injection(s), diagnostic or therapeutic agent, paravertebral facet (zygapophyseal) joint (or nerves innervating that joint) with ultrasound guidance, cervical or thoracic; third and any additional level(s) (List separately in addition to code for primary procedure)

RVU			Global Days	Modifiers				
Mod	Non-Fac Total	Fac Total		51	50	62	80	MUE
	0.00	0.00	ZZZ	0	1	0	0	1

AMA: Jul 11: 14

0216T Injection(s), diagnostic or therapeutic agent, paravertebral facet (zygapophyseal) joint (or nerves innervating that joint) with ultrasound guidance, lumbar or sacral; single level

RVU			Global Days	Modifiers				
Mod	Non-Fac Total	Fac Total		51	50	62	80	MUE
	0.00	0.00	XXX	0	1	0	0	1

AMA: Jul 11: 14

+ **0217T** Injection(s), diagnostic or therapeutic agent, paravertebral facet (zygapophyseal) joint (or nerves innervating that joint) with ultrasound guidance, lumbar or sacral; second level (List separately in addition to code for primary procedure)

RVU			Global Days	Modifiers				
Mod	Non-Fac Total	Fac Total		51	50	62	80	MUE
	0.00	0.00	ZZZ	0	1	0	0	1

AMA: Jul 11: 14

+ **0218T** Injection(s), diagnostic or therapeutic agent, paravertebral facet (zygapophyseal) joint (or nerves innervating that joint) with ultrasound guidance, lumbar or sacral; third and any additional level(s) (List separately in addition to code for primary procedure)

RVU			Global Days	Modifiers				
Mod	Non-Fac Total	Fac Total		51	50	62	80	MUE
	0.00	0.00	ZZZ	0	1	0	0	1

AMA: Feb 11: 5, Jul 11: 14

0219T Placement of a posterior intrafacet implant(s), unilateral or bilateral, including imaging and placement of bone graft(s) or synthetic device(s), single level; cervical

RVU			Global Days	Modifiers				
Mod	Non-Fac Total	Fac Total		51	50	62	80	MUE
	0.00	0.00	XXX	0	0	0	0	1

AMA: Jul 11: 18, Nov 10: 8

0220T Placement of a posterior intrafacet implant(s), unilateral or bilateral, including imaging and placement of bone graft(s) or synthetic device(s), single level; thoracic

RVU			Global Days	Modifiers				
Mod	Non-Fac Total	Fac Total		51	50	62	80	MUE
	0.00	0.00	XXX	0	0	0	0	1

AMA: Jul 11: 18, Nov 10: 8

0221T Placement of a posterior intrafacet implant(s), unilateral or bilateral, including imaging and placement of bone graft(s) or synthetic device(s), single level; lumbar

RVU			Global Days	Modifiers				
Mod	Non-Fac Total	Fac Total		51	50	62	80	MUE
	0.00	0.00	XXX	0	0	0	0	1

AMA: Jul 11: 18, Nov 10: 8

● New ▲ Revised Deleted ⊙ Moderate Sedation ✚ Add-on Codes ⊗ High Risk Denial Ⓐ Age Edit ♀ Female ♂ Male **AMA** *CPT® Assistant* **MUE** Medically Unlikely Edit
⊘ Modifier 51 Exempt ⊖ Modifier 63 Exempt ⊠ Unlisted **Modifiers:** *See Inside Back Cover* Ⓜ Maternity A 2–Z 3 ASC Payment Indicators A–Y OPPS Status Indicators

© 2016 DecisionHealth | CPT © 2015 American Medical Association. All Rights Reserved.

Category III Procedures

0222T – 0238T

✚ **0222T** Placement of a posterior intrafacet implant(s), unilateral or bilateral, including imaging and placement of bone graft(s) or synthetic device(s), single level; each additional vertebral segment (List separately in addition to code for primary procedure) ⒸN

RVU			Global Days	Modifiers				
Mod	Non-Fac Total	Fac Total		51	50	62	80	MUE
	0.00	0.00	ZZZ	0	0	0	0	1

AMA: Jul 11: 18, Nov 10: 6

✖ 0223T Acoustic cardiography, including automated analysis of combined acoustic and electrical intervals; single, with interpretation and report

✖ 0224T Acoustic cardiography, including automated analysis of combined acoustic and electrical intervals; multiple, including serial trended analysis and limited reprogramming of device parameter, AV or VV delays only, with interpretation and report

✖ 0225T Acoustic cardiography, including automated analysis of combined acoustic and electrical intervals; multiple, including serial trended analysis and limited reprogramming of device parameter, AV and VV delays, with interpretation and report

0228T Injection(s), anesthetic agent and/or steroid, transforaminal epidural, with ultrasound guidance, cervical or thoracic; single level ⒸG2T

RVU			Global Days	Modifiers				
Mod	Non-Fac Total	Fac Total		51	50	62	80	MUE
	0.00	0.00	XXX	0	1	0	1	1

AMA: Jul 11: 16, Feb 11: 4

✚ **0229T** Injection(s), anesthetic agent and/or steroid, transforaminal epidural, with ultrasound guidance, cervical or thoracic; each additional level (List separately in addition to code for primary procedure) ⒸN

RVU			Global Days	Modifiers				
Mod	Non-Fac Total	Fac Total		51	50	62	80	MUE
	0.00	0.00	XXX	0	1	0	1	

AMA: Jul 11: 16, Feb 11: 4

0230T Injection(s), anesthetic agent and/or steroid, transforaminal epidural, with ultrasound guidance, lumbar or sacral; single level ⒸG2T

RVU			Global Days	Modifiers				
Mod	Non-Fac Total	Fac Total		51	50	62	80	MUE
	0.00	0.00	XXX	0	1	0	1	1

AMA: Jul 11: 16, Nov 11: 11, Feb 11: 4

✚ **0231T** Injection(s), anesthetic agent and/or steroid, transforaminal epidural, with ultrasound guidance, lumbar or sacral; each additional level (List separately in addition to code for primary procedure) ⒸN

RVU			Global Days	Modifiers				
Mod	Non-Fac Total	Fac Total		51	50	62	80	MUE
	0.00	0.00	XXX	0	1	0	1	

AMA: Jul 11: 16, Feb 11: 4

0232T Injection(s), platelet rich plasma, any site, including image guidance, harvesting and preparation when performed ⒸQ1

RVU			Global Days	Modifiers				
Mod	Non-Fac Total	Fac Total		51	50	62	80	MUE
	0.00	0.00	XXX	0	0	0	1	1

AMA: Oct 10: 8, Dec 10: 8, May 12: 11, Oct 12: 14

✖ 0233T Skin advanced glycation endproducts (AGE) measurement by multi-wavelength fluorescent spectroscopy

0234T Transluminal peripheral atherectomy, open or percutaneous, including radiological supervision and interpretation; renal artery ⒸJ1

RVU			Global Days	Modifiers				
Mod	Non-Fac Total	Fac Total		51	50	62	80	MUE
	0.00	0.00	YYY	0	0	0	0	2

AMA: Jul 11: 3

0235T Transluminal peripheral atherectomy, open or percutaneous, including radiological supervision and interpretation; visceral artery (except renal), each vessel ⒸC

RVU			Global Days	Modifiers				
Mod	Non-Fac Total	Fac Total		51	50	62	80	MUE
	0.00	0.00	YYY	0	0	0	0	2

AMA: Jul 11: 3

0236T Transluminal peripheral atherectomy, open or percutaneous, including radiological supervision and interpretation; abdominal aorta ⒸJ1

RVU			Global Days	Modifiers				
Mod	Non-Fac Total	Fac Total		51	50	62	80	MUE
	0.00	0.00	YYY	0	0	0	0	1

AMA: Jul 11: 3

0237T Transluminal peripheral atherectomy, open or percutaneous, including radiological supervision and interpretation; brachiocephalic trunk and branches, each vessel ⒸJ1

RVU			Global Days	Modifiers				
Mod	Non-Fac Total	Fac Total		51	50	62	80	MUE
	0.00	0.00	YYY	0	0	0	0	2

AMA: Jul 11: 3

0238T Transluminal peripheral atherectomy, open or percutaneous, including radiological supervision and interpretation; iliac artery, each vessel ⒸJ8 J1

RVU			Global Days	Modifiers				
Mod	Non-Fac Total	Fac Total		51	50	62	80	MUE
	0.00	0.00	YYY	0	0	0	0	

AMA: Jul 11: 3

✖ 0240T Esophageal motility (manometric study of the esophagus and/or gastroesophageal junction) study with interpretation and report; with high resolution esophageal pressure topography

● New   ▲ Revised   ✖ Deleted   ⊙ Moderate Sedation   ✚ Add-on Codes   ⊗ High Risk Denial   Ⓐ Age Edit   ♀ Female   ♂ Male   **AMA** CPT® Assistant   **MUE** Medically Unlikely Edit
⊘ Modifier 51 Exempt   ⊖ Modifier 63 Exempt   🅇 Unlisted   **Modifiers:** See Inside Back Cover   Ⓜ Maternity   A2–Z3 ASC Payment Indicators   A–Y OPPS Status Indicators

896

CPT © 2015 American Medical Association. All Rights Reserved.   © 2016 DecisionHealth

✗ ~~0241T Esophageal motility (manometric study of the esophagus and/or gastroesophageal junction) study with interpretation and report; with stimulation or perfusion during high resolution esophageal pressure topography study (eg, stimulant, acid or alkali perfusion) (List separately in addition to code for primary procedure)~~

✗ ~~0243T Intermittent measurement of wheeze rate for bronchodilator or bronchial-challenge diagnostic evaluation(s), with interpretation and report~~

✗ ~~0244T Continuous measurement of wheeze rate during treatment assessment or during sleep for documentation of nocturnal wheeze and cough for diagnostic evaluation 3 to 24 hours, with interpretation and report~~

0249T Ligation, hemorrhoidal vascular bundle(s), including ultrasound guidance   G2 T

RVU			Global Days	Modifiers				
Mod	Non-Fac Total	Fac Total		51	50	62	80	MUE
	0.00	0.00	YYY	0	0	0	0	1

0253T Insertion of anterior segment aqueous drainage device, without extraocular reservoir, internal approach, into the suprachoroidal space   G2 J 1

Coding tip: Code 0253T is listed out of numerical order in CPT. Insertion of anterior segment aqueous drainage device without extraocular reservoir: internal approach into the trabecular meshwork - 0191T; external approach - 0192T

RVU			Global Days	Modifiers				
Mod	Non-Fac Total	Fac Total		51	50	62	80	MUE
	0.00	0.00	YYY	0	0	0	0	1

0254T Endovascular repair of iliac artery bifurcation (eg, aneurysm, pseudoaneurysm, arteriovenous malformation, trauma) using bifurcated endoprosthesis from the common iliac artery into both the external and internal iliac artery, unilateral   C

RVU			Global Days	Modifiers				
Mod	Non-Fac Total	Fac Total		51	50	62	80	MUE
	0.00	0.00	YYY	0	0	0	0	2

AMA: Dec 13: 8

0255T Endovascular repair of iliac artery bifurcation (eg, aneurysm, pseudoaneurysm, arteriovenous malformation, trauma) using bifurcated endoprosthesis from the common iliac artery into both the external and internal iliac artery, unilateral; radiological supervision and interpretation   C

RVU			Global Days	Modifiers				
Mod	Non-Fac Total	Fac Total		51	50	62	80	MUE
	0.00	0.00	YYY	0	0	0	0	2
26	0.00	0.00	YYY	0	0	0	0	2
TC	0.00	0.00	YYY	0	0	0	0	2

AMA: Dec 13: 8

✗ ~~0262T Implantation of catheter-delivered prosthetic pulmonary valve, endovascular approach~~

0263T Intramuscular autologous bone marrow cell therapy, with preparation of harvested cells, multiple injections, one leg, including ultrasound guidance, if performed; complete procedure including unilateral or bilateral bone marrow harvest   G2 S

RVU			Global Days	Modifiers				
Mod	Non-Fac Total	Fac Total		51	50	62	80	MUE
	0.00	0.00	XXX	0	0	0	0	1

0264T Intramuscular autologous bone marrow cell therapy, with preparation of harvested cells, multiple injections, one leg, including ultrasound guidance, if performed; complete procedure excluding bone marrow harvest   G2 S

RVU			Global Days	Modifiers				
Mod	Non-Fac Total	Fac Total		51	50	62	80	MUE
	0.00	0.00	XXX	0	0	0	0	1

0265T Intramuscular autologous bone marrow cell therapy, with preparation of harvested cells, multiple injections, one leg, including ultrasound guidance, if performed; unilateral or bilateral bone marrow harvest only for intramuscular autologous bone marrow cell therapy   G2 S

RVU			Global Days	Modifiers				
Mod	Non-Fac Total	Fac Total		51	50	62	80	MUE
	0.00	0.00	XXX	0	0	0	0	1

0266T Implantation or replacement of carotid sinus baroreflex activation device; total system (includes generator placement, unilateral or bilateral lead placement, intra-operative interrogation, programming, and repositioning, when performed)   C

RVU			Global Days	Modifiers				
Mod	Non-Fac Total	Fac Total		51	50	62	80	MUE
	0.00	0.00	YYY	0	0	0	0	1

0267T Implantation or replacement of carotid sinus baroreflex activation device; lead only, unilateral (includes intra-operative interrogation, programming, and repositioning, when performed)   T

RVU			Global Days	Modifiers				
Mod	Non-Fac Total	Fac Total		51	50	62	80	MUE
	0.00	0.00	YYY	0	0	0	0	1

0268T Implantation or replacement of carotid sinus baroreflex activation device; pulse generator only (includes intra-operative interrogation, programming, and repositioning, when performed)   J 1

RVU			Global Days	Modifiers				
Mod	Non-Fac Total	Fac Total		51	50	62	80	MUE
	0.00	0.00	YYY	0	0	0	0	1

● New   ▲ Revised   Deleted   ⊙ Moderate Sedation   ✚ Add-on Codes   ⊘ High Risk Denial   Ⓐ Age Edit   ♀ Female   ♂ Male   **AMA** *CPT® Assistant*   **MUE** Medically Unlikely Edit
⊘ Modifier 51 Exempt   ⊖ Modifier 63 Exempt   ☒ Unlisted   **Modifiers:** *See Inside Back Cover*   Ⓜ Maternity   A2 – Z3 ASC Payment Indicators   A – Y OPPS Status Indicators

© 2016 DecisionHealth   CPT © 2015 American Medical Association. All Rights Reserved.

Category III Procedures

0269T – 0284T

0269T Revision or removal of carotid sinus baroreflex activation device; total system (includes generator placement, unilateral or bilateral lead placement, intra-operative interrogation, programming, and repositioning, when performed)   G2 Q2

RVU			Global Days	Modifiers				
Mod	Non-Fac Total	Fac Total		51	50	62	80	MUE
	0.00	0.00	XXX	0	0	0	0	1

0270T Revision or removal of carotid sinus baroreflex activation device; lead only, unilateral (includes intra-operative interrogation, programming, and repositioning, when performed)   G2 Q2

RVU			Global Days	Modifiers				
Mod	Non-Fac Total	Fac Total		51	50	62	80	MUE
	0.00	0.00	XXX	0	0	0	0	1

0271T Revision or removal of carotid sinus baroreflex activation device; pulse generator only (includes intra-operative interrogation, programming, and repositioning, when performed)   G2 Q2

RVU			Global Days	Modifiers				
Mod	Non-Fac Total	Fac Total		51	50	62	80	MUE
	0.00	0.00	XXX	0	0	0	0	1

0272T Interrogation device evaluation (in person), carotid sinus baroreflex activation system, including telemetric iterative communication with the implantable device to monitor device diagnostics and programmed therapy values, with interpretation and report (eg, battery status, lead impedance, pulse amplitude, pulse width, therapy frequency, pathway mode, burst mode, therapy start/stop times each day)   S

RVU			Global Days	Modifiers				
Mod	Non-Fac Total	Fac Total		51	50	62	80	MUE
	0.00	0.00	XXX	0	0	0	0	1

0273T Interrogation device evaluation (in person), carotid sinus baroreflex activation system, including telemetric iterative communication with the implantable device to monitor device diagnostics and programmed therapy values, with interpretation and report (eg, battery status, lead impedance, pulse amplitude, pulse width, therapy frequency, pathway mode, burst mode, therapy start/stop times each day); with programming   S

RVU			Global Days	Modifiers				
Mod	Non-Fac Total	Fac Total		51	50	62	80	MUE
	0.00	0.00	XXX	0	0	0	0	1

0274T Percutaneous laminotomy/laminectomy (interlaminar approach) for decompression of neural elements, (with or without ligamentous resection, discectomy, facetectomy and/or foraminotomy), any method, under indirect image guidance (eg, fluoroscopic, CT), with or without the use of an endoscope, single or multiple levels, unilateral or bilateral; cervical or thoracic   G2 J1

RVU			Global Days	Modifiers				
Mod	Non-Fac Total	Fac Total		51	50	62	80	MUE
	0.00	0.00	YYY	0	0	0	0	1

AMA: Jan 12: 14, Jul 12: 3, 4

0275T Percutaneous laminotomy/laminectomy (interlaminar approach) for decompression of neural elements, (with or without ligamentous resection, discectomy, facetectomy and/or foraminotomy), any method, under indirect image guidance (eg, fluoroscopic, CT), with or without the use of an endoscope, single or multiple levels, unilateral or bilateral; lumbar   G2 J1

RVU			Global Days	Modifiers				
Mod	Non-Fac Total	Fac Total		51	50	62	80	MUE
	0.00	0.00	XXX	9	9	9	9	1

AMA: Jan 12: 14, Jul 12: 3, 4

Pub 100-04, 32, 330.1, 330.2

0278T Transcutaneous electrical modulation pain reprocessing (eg, scrambler therapy), each treatment session (includes placement of electrodes)   Q1

RVU			Global Days	Modifiers				
Mod	Non-Fac Total	Fac Total		51	50	62	80	MUE
	0.00	0.00	XXX	0	0	0	0	1

0281T Percutaneous transcatheter closure of the left atrial appendage with implant, including fluoroscopy, transseptal puncture, catheter placement(s), left atrial angiography, left atrial appendage angiography, radiological supervision and interpretation   C

RVU			Global Days	Modifiers				
Mod	Non-Fac Total	Fac Total		51	50	62	80	MUE
	0.00	0.00	XXX	0	0	0	0	1

⊙ **0282T** Percutaneous or open implantation of neurostimulator electrode array(s), subcutaneous (peripheral subcutaneous field stimulation), including imaging guidance, when performed, cervical, thoracic or lumbar; for trial, including removal at the conclusion of trial period   J8 J1

RVU			Global Days	Modifiers				
Mod	Non-Fac Total	Fac Total		51	50	62	80	MUE
	0.00	0.00	XXX	0	1	0	0	1

⊙ **0283T** Percutaneous or open implantation of neurostimulator electrode array(s), subcutaneous (peripheral subcutaneous field stimulation), including imaging guidance, when performed, cervical, thoracic or lumbar; permanent, with implantation of a pulse generator   J8 J1

RVU			Global Days	Modifiers				
Mod	Non-Fac Total	Fac Total		51	50	62	80	MUE
	0.00	0.00	XXX	0	1	0	0	1

⊙ **0284T** Revision or removal of pulse generator or electrodes, including imaging guidance, when performed, including addition of new electrodes, when performed   G2 Q2

RVU			Global Days	Modifiers				
Mod	Non-Fac Total	Fac Total		51	50	62	80	MUE
	0.00	0.00	XXX	0	0	0	0	1

● New   ▲ Revised   ✖ Deleted   ⊙ Moderate Sedation   ✚ Add-on Codes   ⊘ High Risk Denial   Ⓐ Age Edit   ♀ Female   ♂ Male   **AMA** *CPT® Assistant*   **MUE** Medically Unlikely Edit
⊘ Modifier 51 Exempt   ⊖ Modifier 63 Exempt   ✗ Unlisted   **Modifiers:** *See Inside Back Cover*   Ⓜ Maternity   A2–Z3 ASC Payment Indicators   A–Y OPPS Status Indicators

898   CPT © 2015 American Medical Association. All Rights Reserved.   © 2016 DecisionHealth

0285T Electronic analysis of implanted peripheral subcutaneous field stimulation pulse generator, with reprogramming when performed   ⊂S

RVU		Global Days	Modifiers				
Mod	Non-Fac Total	Fac Total		51	50	62	80	MUE
	0.00	0.00	XXX	0	0	0	0	1

0286T Near-infrared spectroscopy studies of lower extremity wounds (eg, for oxyhemoglobin measurement)   ⊂N

RVU		Global Days	Modifiers				
Mod	Non-Fac Total	Fac Total		51	50	62	80	MUE
	0.00	0.00	XXX	0	0	0	0	1

AMA: Jun 12: 16

0287T Near-infrared guidance for vascular access requiring real-time digital visualization of subcutaneous vasculature for evaluation of potential access sites and vessel patency   N

RVU		Global Days	Modifiers				
Mod	Non-Fac Total	Fac Total		51	50	62	80	MUE
	0.00	0.00	XXX	0	0	0	0	2

0288T Anoscopy, with delivery of thermal energy to the muscle of the anal canal (eg, for fecal incontinence)   ⊂G2T

RVU		Global Days	Modifiers				
Mod	Non-Fac Total	Fac Total		51	50	62	80	MUE
	0.00	0.00	XXX	0	0	0	0	1

+ 0289T Corneal incisions in the donor cornea created using a laser, in preparation for penetrating or lamellar keratoplasty (List separately in addition to code for primary procedure)   ⊂N

RVU		Global Days	Modifiers				
Mod	Non-Fac Total	Fac Total		51	50	62	80	MUE
	0.00	0.00	ZZZ	0	0	0	0	2

AMA: Aug 12: 15

+ 0290T Corneal incisions in the recipient cornea created using a laser, in preparation for penetrating or lamellar keratoplasty (List separately in addition to code for primary procedure)   ⊂N

RVU		Global Days	Modifiers				
Mod	Non-Fac Total	Fac Total		51	50	62	80	MUE
	0.00	0.00	ZZZ	0	0	0	0	1

AMA: Aug 12: 15

⊙+0291T Intravascular optical coherence tomography (coronary native vessel or graft) during diagnostic evaluation and/or therapeutic intervention, including imaging supervision, interpretation, and report; initial vessel (List separately in addition to primary procedure)   ⊂N

RVU		Global Days	Modifiers				
Mod	Non-Fac Total	Fac Total		51	50	62	80	MUE
	0.00	0.00	ZZZ	0	0	0	0	1

⊙+0292T Intravascular optical coherence tomography (coronary native vessel or graft) during diagnostic evaluation and/or therapeutic intervention, including imaging supervision, interpretation, and report; each additional vessel (List separately in addition to primary procedure)   ⊂N

RVU		Global Days	Modifiers				
Mod	Non-Fac Total	Fac Total		51	50	62	80	MUE
	0.00	0.00	ZZZ	0	0	0	0	1

⊙ 0293T Insertion of left atrial hemodynamic monitor; complete system, includes implanted communication module and pressure sensor lead in left atrium including transseptal access, radiological supervision and interpretation, and associated injection procedures, when performed   ⊂C

RVU		Global Days	Modifiers				
Mod	Non-Fac Total	Fac Total		51	50	62	80	MUE
	0.00	0.00	XXX	0	0	0	0	1

⊙+0294T Insertion of left atrial hemodynamic monitor; pressure sensor lead at time of insertion of pacing cardioverter-defibrillator pulse generator including radiological supervision and interpretation and associated injection procedures, when performed (List separately in addition to code for primary procedure)   ⊂C

RVU		Global Days	Modifiers				
Mod	Non-Fac Total	Fac Total		51	50	62	80	MUE
	0.00	0.00	ZZZ	0	0	0	0	1

0295T External electrocardiographic recording for more than 48 hours up to 21 days by continuous rhythm recording and storage; includes recording, scanning analysis with report, review and interpretation   M

RVU		Global Days	Modifiers				
Mod	Non-Fac Total	Fac Total		51	50	62	80	MUE
	0.00	0.00	XXX	0	0	0	0	1

AMA: Feb 13: 17

0296T External electrocardiographic recording for more than 48 hours up to 21 days by continuous rhythm recording and storage; recording (includes connection and initial recording)   Q1

RVU		Global Days	Modifiers				
Mod	Non-Fac Total	Fac Total		51	50	62	80	MUE
	0.00	0.00	XXX	0	0	0	0	1

AMA: Feb 13: 17

0297T External electrocardiographic recording for more than 48 hours up to 21 days by continuous rhythm recording and storage; scanning analysis with report   Q1

RVU		Global Days	Modifiers				
Mod	Non-Fac Total	Fac Total		51	50	62	80	MUE
	0.00	0.00	XXX	0	0	0	0	1

AMA: Feb 13: 17

● New   ▲ Revised   Deleted   ⊙ Moderate Sedation   ✚ Add-on Codes   ⊘ High Risk Denial   Ⓐ Age Edit   ♀ Female   ♂ Male   **AMA** CPT® Assistant   **MUE** Medically Unlikely Edit
⊘ Modifier 51 Exempt   ⊖ Modifier 63 Exempt   ✗ Unlisted   **Modifiers:** See Inside Back Cover   M Maternity   A2–Z3 ASC Payment Indicators   A–Y OPPS Status Indicators

© 2016 DecisionHealth   CPT © 2015 American Medical Association. All Rights Reserved.

Category III Procedures

0298T – 0310T

0298T External electrocardiographic recording for more than 48 hours up to 21 days by continuous rhythm recording and storage; review and interpretation ▣M

RVU		Global Days	Modifiers				
Mod	Non-Fac Total	Fac Total		51	50	62	80	MUE
	0.00	0.00	XXX	0	0	0	0	1

AMA: Feb 13: 17

0299T Extracorporeal shock wave for integumentary wound healing, high energy, including topical application and dressing care; initial wound ▣R2T

RVU		Global Days	Modifiers				
Mod	Non-Fac Total	Fac Total		51	50	62	80	MUE
	0.00	0.00	XXX	0	0	0	0	1

+ 0300T Extracorporeal shock wave for integumentary wound healing, high energy, including topical application and dressing care; each additional wound (List separately in addition to code for primary procedure) ▣N

RVU		Global Days	Modifiers				
Mod	Non-Fac Total	Fac Total		51	50	62	80	MUE
	0.00	0.00	ZZZ	0	0	0	0	1

⊙ 0301T Destruction/reduction of malignant breast tumor with externally applied focused microwave, including interstitial placement of disposable catheter with combined temperature monitoring probe and microwave focusing sensocatheter under ultrasound thermotherapy guidance ▣G2T

RVU		Global Days	Modifiers				
Mod	Non-Fac Total	Fac Total		51	50	62	80	MUE
	0.00	0.00	XXX	0	0	0	0	1

⊙ 0302T Insertion or removal and replacement of intracardiac ischemia monitoring system including imaging supervision and interpretation when performed and intra-operative interrogation and programming when performed; complete system (includes device and electrode) ▣J8JI

RVU		Global Days	Modifiers				
Mod	Non-Fac Total	Fac Total		51	50	62	80	MUE
	0.00	0.00	YYY	2	0	2	1	1

⊙ 0303T Insertion or removal and replacement of intracardiac ischemia monitoring system including imaging supervision and interpretation when performed and intra-operative interrogation and programming when performed; electrode only ▣J8JI

RVU		Global Days	Modifiers				
Mod	Non-Fac Total	Fac Total		51	50	62	80	MUE
	0.00	0.00	YYY	2	0	0	1	1

⊙ 0304T Insertion or removal and replacement of intracardiac ischemia monitoring system including imaging supervision and interpretation when performed and intra-operative interrogation and programming when performed; device only ▣J8JI

RVU		Global Days	Modifiers				
Mod	Non-Fac Total	Fac Total		51	50	62	80	MUE
	0.00	0.00	YYY	2	0	0	1	1

0305T Programming device evaluation (in person) of intracardiac ischemia monitoring system with iterative adjustment of programmed values, with analysis, review, and report ▣QI

RVU		Global Days	Modifiers				
Mod	Non-Fac Total	Fac Total		51	50	62	80	MUE
	0.00	0.00	XXX	0	0	0	0	1

0306T Interrogation device evaluation (in person) of intracardiac ischemia monitoring system with analysis, review, and report ▣QI

RVU		Global Days	Modifiers				
Mod	Non-Fac Total	Fac Total		51	50	62	80	MUE
	0.00	0.00	XXX	0	0	0	0	1

⊙ 0307T Removal of intracardiac ischemia monitoring device ▣G2Q2

RVU		Global Days	Modifiers				
Mod	Non-Fac Total	Fac Total		51	50	62	80	MUE
	0.00	0.00	YYY	2	0	0	1	1

⊙▲0308T Insertion of ocular telescope prosthesis including removal of crystalline lens or intraocular lens prosthesis ▣J8JI

RVU		Global Days	Modifiers				
Mod	Non-Fac Total	Fac Total		51	50	62	80	MUE
	0.00	0.00	YYY	2	1	0	1	1

AMA: Mar 13: 6

+ 0309T Arthrodesis, pre-sacral interbody technique, including disc space preparation, discectomy, with posterior instrumentation, with image guidance, includes bone graft, when performed, lumbar, L4-L5 interspace (List separately in addition to code for primary procedure) ▣C

RVU		Global Days	Modifiers				
Mod	Non-Fac Total	Fac Total		51	50	62	80	MUE
	0.00	0.00	ZZZ	0	0	0	0	1

0310T Motor function mapping using non-invasive navigated transcranial magnetic stimulation (nTMS) for therapeutic treatment planning, upper and lower extremity ▣S

RVU		Global Days	Modifiers				
Mod	Non-Fac Total	Fac Total		51	50	62	80	MUE
	0.00	0.00	XXX	0	0	0	0	1

✖ 0311T ~~Non-invasive calculation and analysis of central arterial pressure waveforms with interpretation and report~~

● New ▲ Revised ✖ Deleted ⊙ Moderate Sedation ✚ Add-on Codes ⊘ High Risk Denial ⒶAge Edit ♀ Female ♂ Male **AMA** CPT® Assistant **MUE** Medically Unlikely Edit ◎ Modifier 51 Exempt ⊖ Modifier 63 Exempt ✗ Unlisted **Modifiers:** See Inside Back Cover ▣ Maternity A2–Z3 ASC Payment Indicators A–Y OPPS Status Indicators

900 CPT © 2015 American Medical Association. All Rights Reserved. © 2016 DecisionHealth

0312T Vagus nerve blocking therapy (morbid obesity); laparoscopic implantation of neurostimulator electrode array, anterior and posterior vagal trunks adjacent to esophagogastric junction (EGJ), with implantation of pulse generator, includes programming **J1**

RVU		Global Days	Modifiers				
Mod	Non-Fac Total	Fac Total		51	50	62	80	MUE
	0.00	0.00	XXX	0	0	0	0	1

AMA: Jan 13: 11

0313T Vagus nerve blocking therapy (morbid obesity); laparoscopic revision or replacement of vagal trunk neurostimulator electrode array, including connection to existing pulse generator **G2 T**

RVU		Global Days	Modifiers				
Mod	Non-Fac Total	Fac Total		51	50	62	80	MUE
	0.00	0.00	XXX	0	0	0	0	1

AMA: Jan 13: 11

0314T Vagus nerve blocking therapy (morbid obesity); laparoscopic removal of vagal trunk neurostimulator electrode array and pulse generator **G2 Q2**

RVU		Global Days	Modifiers				
Mod	Non-Fac Total	Fac Total		51	50	62	80	MUE
	0.00	0.00	XXX	0	0	0	0	1

AMA: Jan 13: 11

0315T Vagus nerve blocking therapy (morbid obesity); removal of pulse generator **G2 Q2**

RVU		Global Days	Modifiers				
Mod	Non-Fac Total	Fac Total		51	50	62	80	MUE
	0.00	0.00	XXX	0	0	0	0	1

AMA: Jan 13: 11

0316T Vagus nerve blocking therapy (morbid obesity); replacement of pulse generator **J8 J1**

RVU		Global Days	Modifiers				
Mod	Non-Fac Total	Fac Total		51	50	62	80	MUE
	0.00	0.00	XXX	0	0	0	0	1

AMA: Jan 13: 11

0317T Vagus nerve blocking therapy (morbid obesity); neurostimulator pulse generator electronic analysis, includes reprogramming when performed **Q1**

RVU		Global Days	Modifiers				
Mod	Non-Fac Total	Fac Total		51	50	62	80	MUE
	0.00	0.00	XXX	0	0	0	0	1

AMA: Jan 13: 11

0329T Monitoring of intraocular pressure for 24 hours or longer, unilateral or bilateral, with interpretation and report **E**

RVU		Global Days	Modifiers				
Mod	Non-Fac Total	Fac Total		51	50	62	80	MUE
	0.00	0.00	YYY	9	9	9	9	1

AMA: May 14: 5

0330T Tear film imaging, unilateral or bilateral, with interpretation and report **Q1**

RVU		Global Days	Modifiers				
Mod	Non-Fac Total	Fac Total		51	50	62	80	MUE
	0.00	0.00	YYY	9	9	9	9	1

AMA: May 14: 5

0331T Myocardial sympathetic innervation imaging, planar qualitative and quantitative assessment **Z2 S**

RVU		Global Days	Modifiers				
Mod	Non-Fac Total	Fac Total		51	50	62	80	MUE
	0.00	0.00	YYY	9	9	9	9	1

AMA: Jun 14: 15

0332T Myocardial sympathetic innervation imaging, planar qualitative and quantitative assessment; with tomographic SPECT **Z2 S**

RVU		Global Days	Modifiers				
Mod	Non-Fac Total	Fac Total		51	50	62	80	MUE
	0.00	0.00	YYY	9	9	9	9	1

AMA: Jun 14: 15

0333T Visual evoked potential, screening of visual acuity, automated **E**

RVU		Global Days	Modifiers				
Mod	Non-Fac Total	Fac Total		51	50	62	80	MUE
	0.00	0.00	YYY	9	9	9	9	1

AMA: Aug 14: 8

⊙ **0335T** Extra-osseous subtalar joint implant for talotarsal stabilization **G2 T**

RVU		Global Days	Modifiers				
Mod	Non-Fac Total	Fac Total		51	50	62	80	MUE
	0.00	0.00	YYY	9	9	9	9	2

0336T Laparoscopy, surgical, ablation of uterine fibroid(s), including intraoperative ultrasound guidance and monitoring, radiofrequency **G2 J1**

RVU		Global Days	Modifiers				
Mod	Non-Fac Total	Fac Total		51	50	62	80	MUE
	0.00	0.00	YYY	9	9	9	9	1

0337T Endothelial function assessment, using peripheral vascular response to reactive hyperemia, non-invasive (eg, brachial artery ultrasound, peripheral artery tonometry), unilateral or bilateral **Q1**

RVU		Global Days	Modifiers				
Mod	Non-Fac Total	Fac Total		51	50	62	80	MUE
	0.00	0.00	YYY	9	9	9	9	1

● New ▲ Revised Deleted ⊙ Moderate Sedation ✚ Add-on Codes ⊗ High Risk Denial Ⓐ Age Edit ♀ Female ♂ Male **AMA** *CPT® Assistant* **MUE** Medically Unlikely Edit
⊘ Modifier 51 Exempt ⊖ Modifier 63 Exempt ✗ Unlisted **Modifiers:** *See Inside Back Cover* Ⓜ Maternity **A2–Z3** ASC Payment Indicators **A–Y** OPPS Status Indicators

0338T Transcatheter renal sympathetic denervation, percutaneous approach including arterial puncture, selective catheter placement(s) renal artery(ies), fluoroscopy, contrast injection(s), intraprocedural roadmapping and radiological supervision and interpretation, including pressure gradient measurements, flush aortogram and diagnostic renal angiography when performed; unilateral   G2 J1

RVU		Global Days	Modifiers				
Mod	Non-Fac Total	Fac Total		51	50	62	80	MUE
	0.00	0.00	YYY	9	9	9	9	1

0339T Transcatheter renal sympathetic denervation, percutaneous approach including arterial puncture, selective catheter placement(s) renal artery(ies), fluoroscopy, contrast injection(s), intraprocedural roadmapping and radiological supervision and interpretation, including pressure gradient measurements, flush aortogram and diagnostic renal angiography when performed; bilateral   G2 J1

RVU		Global Days	Modifiers				
Mod	Non-Fac Total	Fac Total		51	50	62	80	MUE
	0.00	0.00	YYY	9	9	9	9	1

⊙ **0340T** Ablation, pulmonary tumor(s), including pleura or chest wall when involved by tumor extension, percutaneous, cryoablation, unilateral, includes imaging guidance   G2 T

RVU		Global Days	Modifiers				
Mod	Non-Fac Total	Fac Total		51	50	62	80	MUE
	0.00	0.00	YYY	9	9	9	9	

0341T Quantitative pupillometry with interpretation and report, unilateral or bilateral   N

RVU		Global Days	Modifiers				
Mod	Non-Fac Total	Fac Total		51	50	62	80	MUE
	0.00	0.00	YYY	9	9	9	9	

0342T Therapeutic apheresis with selective HDL delipidation and plasma reinfusion   G2 S

RVU		Global Days	Modifiers				
Mod	Non-Fac Total	Fac Total		51	50	62	80	MUE
	0.00	0.00	YYY	9	9	9	9	

0345T Transcatheter mitral valve repair percutaneous approach via the coronary sinus   C

RVU		Global Days	Modifiers				
Mod	Non-Fac Total	Fac Total		51	50	62	80	MUE
	0.00	0.00	YYY	9	9	9	9	

Pub 100-04, 32, 340, 340.2

+ **0346T** Ultrasound, elastography (List separately in addition to code for primary procedure)   N

RVU		Global Days	Modifiers				
Mod	Non-Fac Total	Fac Total		51	50	62	80	MUE
	0.00	0.00	YYY	9	9	9	9	

0347T Placement of interstitial device(s) in bone for radiostereometric analysis (RSA)   Q1

RVU		Global Days	Modifiers				
Mod	Non-Fac Total	Fac Total		51	50	62	80	MUE
	0.00	0.00	YYY	9	9	9	9	1

AMA: Jun 15: 8

0348T Radiologic examination, radiostereometric analysis (RSA); spine, (includes cervical, thoracic and lumbosacral, when performed)   Q1

RVU		Global Days	Modifiers				
Mod	Non-Fac Total	Fac Total		51	50	62	80	MUE
	0.00	0.00	YYY	9	9	9	9	1

AMA: Jun 15: 8

0349T Radiologic examination, radiostereometric analysis (RSA); upper extremity(ies), (includes shoulder, elbow, and wrist, when performed)   Q1

RVU		Global Days	Modifiers				
Mod	Non-Fac Total	Fac Total		51	50	62	80	MUE
	0.00	0.00	YYY	9	9	9	9	1

AMA: Jun 15: 8

0350T Radiologic examination, radiostereometric analysis (RSA); lower extremity(ies), (includes hip, proximal femur, knee, and ankle, when performed)   Q1

RVU		Global Days	Modifiers				
Mod	Non-Fac Total	Fac Total		51	50	62	80	MUE
	0.00	0.00	YYY	9	9	9	9	1

AMA: Jun 15: 8

0351T Optical coherence tomography of breast or axillary lymph node, excised tissue, each specimen; real-time intraoperative   N

RVU		Global Days	Modifiers				
Mod	Non-Fac Total	Fac Total		51	50	62	80	MUE
	0.00	0.00	YYY	9	9	9	9	5

AMA: Apr 15: 6

0352T Optical coherence tomography of breast or axillary lymph node, excised tissue, each specimen; interpretation and report, real-time or referred   B

RVU		Global Days	Modifiers				
Mod	Non-Fac Total	Fac Total		51	50	62	80	MUE
	0.00	0.00	YYY	9	9	9	9	5

AMA: Apr 15: 6

0353T Optical coherence tomography of breast, surgical cavity; real-time intraoperative   N

RVU		Global Days	Modifiers				
Mod	Non-Fac Total	Fac Total		51	50	62	80	MUE
	0.00	0.00	YYY	9	9	9	9	2

AMA: Apr 15: 6

0354T Optical coherence tomography of breast, surgical cavity; interpretation and report, real-time or referred   B

RVU		Global Days	Modifiers				
Mod	Non-Fac Total	Fac Total		51	50	62	80	MUE
	0.00	0.00	YYY	9	9	9	9	2

AMA: Apr 15: 6

● New   ▲ Revised   ✖ Deleted   ⊙ Moderate Sedation   ✚ Add-on Codes   ⊘ High Risk Denial   Ⓐ Age Edit   ♀ Female   ♂ Male   **AMA** *CPT® Assistant*   ***MUE*** Medically Unlikely Edit
⊘ Modifier 51 Exempt   ⊖ Modifier 63 Exempt   ✗ Unlisted   **Modifiers:** *See Inside Back Cover*   Ⓜ Maternity   A2–Z3 ASC Payment Indicators   A–Y OPPS Status Indicators

CPT © 2015 American Medical Association. All Rights Reserved.   © 2016 DecisionHealth

0355T Gastrointestinal tract imaging, intraluminal (eg, capsule endoscopy), colon, with interpretation and report   **T**

RVU			Global Days	Modifiers				
Mod	Non-Fac Total	Fac Total		51	50	62	80	MUE
	0.00	0.00	YYY	9	9	9	9	1

0356T Insertion of drug-eluting implant (including punctal dilation and implant removal when performed) into lacrimal canaliculus, each   **Q1**

RVU			Global Days	Modifiers				
Mod	Non-Fac Total	Fac Total		51	50	62	80	MUE
	0.00	0.00	YYY	9	9	9	9	4

0357T Cryopreservation; immature oocyte(s)   **Q1**

RVU			Global Days	Modifiers				
Mod	Non-Fac Total	Fac Total		51	50	62	80	MUE
	0.00	0.00	XXX	0	0	0	0	1

▲ **0358T** Bioelectrical impedance analysis whole body composition assessment, with interpretation and report   **Q1**

RVU			Global Days	Modifiers				
Mod	Non-Fac Total	Fac Total		51	50	62	80	MUE
	0.00	0.00	YYY	9	9	9	9	1

0359T Behavior identification assessment, by the physician or other qualified health care professional, face-to-face with patient and caregiver(s), includes administration of standardized and non-standardized tests, detailed behavioral history, patient observation and caregiver interview, interpretation of test results, discussion of findings and recommendations with the primary guardian(s)/caregiver(s), and preparation of report   **V**

RVU			Global Days	Modifiers				
Mod	Non-Fac Total	Fac Total		51	50	62	80	MUE
	0.00	0.00	YYY	9	9	9	9	1

AMA: Jun 14: 4

0360T Observational behavioral follow-up assessment, includes physician or other qualified health care professional direction with interpretation and report, administered by one technician; first 30 minutes of technician time, face-to-face with the patient   **V**

RVU			Global Days	Modifiers				
Mod	Non-Fac Total	Fac Total		51	50	62	80	MUE
	0.00	0.00	YYY	9	9	9	9	1

AMA: Jun 14: 4

+ **0361T** Observational behavioral follow-up assessment, includes physician or other qualified health care professional direction with interpretation and report, administered by one technician; each additional 30 minutes of technician time, face-to-face with the patient (List separately in addition to code for primary service)   **N**

RVU			Global Days	Modifiers				
Mod	Non-Fac Total	Fac Total		51	50	62	80	MUE
	0.00	0.00	ZZZ	9	9	9	9	3

AMA: Jun 14: 4

0362T Exposure behavioral follow-up assessment, includes physician or other qualified health care professional direction with interpretation and report, administered by physician or other qualified health care professional with the assistance of one or more technicians; first 30 minutes of technician(s) time, face-to-face with the patient   **V**

RVU			Global Days	Modifiers				
Mod	Non-Fac Total	Fac Total		51	50	62	80	MUE
	0.00	0.00	YYY	9	9	9	9	1

AMA: Jun 14: 4

+ **0363T** Exposure behavioral follow-up assessment, includes physician or other qualified health care professional direction with interpretation and report, administered by physician or other qualified health care professional with the assistance of one or more technicians; each additional 30 minutes of technician(s) time, face-to-face with the patient (List separately in addition to code for primary procedure)   **N**

RVU			Global Days	Modifiers				
Mod	Non-Fac Total	Fac Total		51	50	62	80	MUE
	0.00	0.00	ZZZ	9	9	9	9	3

AMA: Jun 14: 4

0364T Adaptive behavior treatment by protocol, administered by technician, face-to-face with one patient; first 30 minutes of technician time   **S**

RVU			Global Days	Modifiers				
Mod	Non-Fac Total	Fac Total		51	50	62	80	MUE
	0.00	0.00	YYY	9	9	9	9	1

AMA: Jun 14: 6

+ **0365T** Adaptive behavior treatment by protocol, administered by technician, face-to-face with one patient; each additional 30 minutes of technician time (List separately in addition to code for primary procedure)   **N**

RVU			Global Days	Modifiers				
Mod	Non-Fac Total	Fac Total		51	50	62	80	MUE
	0.00	0.00	ZZZ	9	9	9	

AMA: Jun 14: 6

0366T Group adaptive behavior treatment by protocol, administered by technician, face-to-face with two or more patients; first 30 minutes of technician time   **S**

RVU			Global Days	Modifiers				
Mod	Non-Fac Total	Fac Total		51	50	62	80	MUE
	0.00	0.00	YYY	9	9	9	9	1

AMA: Jun 14: 6

+ **0367T** Group adaptive behavior treatment by protocol, administered by technician, face-to-face with two or more patients; each additional 30 minutes of technician time (List separately in addition to code for primary procedure)   **N**

RVU			Global Days	Modifiers				
Mod	Non-Fac Total	Fac Total		51	50	62	80	MUE
	0.00	0.00	ZZZ	9	9	9	

AMA: Jun 14: 6

● New   ▲ Revised   Deleted   ⊙ Moderate Sedation   + Add-on Codes   ⊘ High Risk Denial   Ⓐ Age Edit   ♀ Female   ♂ Male   **AMA** *CPT® Assistant*   **MUE** Medically Unlikely Edit
⊘ Modifier 51 Exempt   ⊖ Modifier 63 Exempt   ✗ Unlisted   **Modifiers:** *See Inside Back Cover*   Ⓜ Maternity   **A2–Z3** ASC Payment Indicators   **A–Y** OPPS Status Indicators

0368T Adaptive behavior treatment with protocol modification administered by physician or other qualified health care professional with one patient; first 30 minutes of patient face-to-face time **S**

RVU		Global Days	Modifiers				
Mod	Non-Fac Total	Fac Total		51	50	62	80	MUE
	0.00	0.00	YYY	9	9	9	9	1

AMA: Jun 14: 4

+ 0369T Adaptive behavior treatment with protocol modification administered by physician or other qualified health care professional with one patient; each additional 30 minutes of patient face-to-face time (List separately in addition to code for primary procedure) **N**

RVU		Global Days	Modifiers				
Mod	Non-Fac Total	Fac Total		51	50	62	80	MUE
	0.00	0.00	ZZZ	9	9	9	9	

AMA: Jun 14: 4

0370T Family adaptive behavior treatment guidance, administered by physician or other qualified health care professional (without the patient present) **S**

RVU		Global Days	Modifiers				
Mod	Non-Fac Total	Fac Total		51	50	62	80	MUE
	0.00	0.00	YYY	9	9	9	9	1

AMA: Jun 14: 3, 8

0371T Multiple-family group adaptive behavior treatment guidance, administered by physician or other qualified health care professional (without the patient present) **S**

RVU		Global Days	Modifiers				
Mod	Non-Fac Total	Fac Total		51	50	62	80	MUE
	0.00	0.00	YYY	9	9	9	9	1

AMA: Jun 14: 3, 8

0372T Adaptive behavior treatment social skills group, administered by physician or other qualified health care professional face-to-face with multiple patients **S**

RVU		Global Days	Modifiers				
Mod	Non-Fac Total	Fac Total		51	50	62	80	MUE
	0.00	0.00	YYY	9	9	9	9	1

AMA: Jun 14: 8

0373T Exposure adaptive behavior treatment with protocol modification requiring two or more technicians for severe maladaptive behavior(s); first 60 minutes of technicians' time, face-to-face with patient **S**

RVU		Global Days	Modifiers				
Mod	Non-Fac Total	Fac Total		51	50	62	80	MUE
	0.00	0.00	YYY	9	9	9	9	1

AMA: Jun 14: 4, 6, 9

+ 0374T Exposure adaptive behavior treatment with protocol modification requiring two or more technicians for severe maladaptive behavior(s); each additional 30 minutes of technicians' time face-to-face with patient (List separately in addition to code for primary procedure) **N**

RVU		Global Days	Modifiers				
Mod	Non-Fac Total	Fac Total		51	50	62	80	MUE
	0.00	0.00	ZZZ	9	9	9	9	

AMA: Jun 14: 4, 6, 9

0375T Total disc arthroplasty (artificial disc), anterior approach, including discectomy with end plate preparation (includes osteophytectomy for nerve root or spinal cord decompression and microdissection), cervical, three or more levels **C**

RVU		Global Days	Modifiers				
Mod	Non-Fac Total	Fac Total		51	50	62	80	MUE
	0.00	0.00	XXX	0	0	0	0	1

AMA: Apr 15: 7

+ 0376T Insertion of anterior segment aqueous drainage device, without extraocular reservoir, internal approach, into the trabecular meshwork; each additional device insertion (List separately in addition to code for primary procedure) **N**

RVU		Global Days	Modifiers				
Mod	Non-Fac Total	Fac Total		51	50	62	80	MUE
	0.00	0.00	XXX	0	0	0	0	2

0377T Anoscopy with directed submucosal injection of bulking agent for fecal incontinence **G2T**

RVU		Global Days	Modifiers				
Mod	Non-Fac Total	Fac Total		51	50	62	80	MUE
	0.00	0.00	XXX	0	0	0	0	1

0378T Visual field assessment, with concurrent real time data analysis and accessible data storage with patient initiated data transmitted to a remote surveillance center for up to 30 days; review and interpretation with report by a physician or other qualified health care professional **B**

RVU		Global Days	Modifiers				
Mod	Non-Fac Total	Fac Total		51	50	62	80	MUE
	0.00	0.00	XXX	0	0	0	0	1

0379T Visual field assessment, with concurrent real time data analysis and accessible data storage with patient initiated data transmitted to a remote surveillance center for up to 30 days; technical support and patient instructions, surveillance, analysis, and transmission of daily and emergent data reports as prescribed by a physician or other qualified health care professional **Q1**

RVU		Global Days	Modifiers				
Mod	Non-Fac Total	Fac Total		51	50	62	80	MUE
	0.00	0.00	XXX	0	0	0	0	1

● New ▲ Revised ✖ Deleted ⊙ Moderate Sedation ✚ Add-on Codes ⊘ High Risk Denial Ⓐ Age Edit ♀ Female ♂ Male **AMA** CPT® Assistant **MUE** Medically Unlikely Edit
⊘ Modifier 51 Exempt ⊖ Modifier 63 Exempt ✗ Unlisted **Modifiers:** See Inside Back Cover Ⓜ Maternity A2–Z3 ASC Payment Indicators A–Y OPPS Status Indicators

CPT © 2015 American Medical Association. All Rights Reserved.
© 2016 DecisionHealth

0380T Computer-aided animation and analysis of time series retinal images for the monitoring of disease progression, unilateral or bilateral, with interpretation and report Q1

RVU			Global Days	Modifiers				
Mod	Non-Fac Total	Fac Total		51	50	62	80	MUE
	0.00	0.00	XXX	0	0	0	0	1

● **0381T** External heart rate and 3-axis accelerometer data recording up to 14 days to assess changes in heart rate and to monitor motion analysis for the purposes of diagnosing nocturnal epilepsy seizure events; includes report, scanning analysis with report, review and interpretation by a physician or other qualified health care professional M

RVU			Global Days	Modifiers				
Mod	Non-Fac Total	Fac Total		51	50	62	80	MUE
	0.00	0.00	XXX	0	0	0	0	1

Pub 100-04, 32, 290.1.1

● **0382T** External heart rate and 3-axis accelerometer data recording up to 14 days to assess changes in heart rate and to monitor motion analysis for the purposes of diagnosing nocturnal epilepsy seizure events; review and interpretation only M

RVU			Global Days	Modifiers				
Mod	Non-Fac Total	Fac Total		51	50	62	80	MUE
	0.00	0.00	XXX	0	0	0	0	1

● **0383T** External heart rate and 3-axis accelerometer data recording from 15 to 30 days to assess changes in heart rate and to monitor motion analysis for the purposes of diagnosing nocturnal epilepsy seizure events; includes report, scanning analysis with report, review and interpretation by a physician or other qualified health care professional M

RVU			Global Days	Modifiers				
Mod	Non-Fac Total	Fac Total		51	50	62	80	MUE
	0.00	0.00	XXX	0	0	0	0	1

● **0384T** External heart rate and 3-axis accelerometer data recording from 15 to 30 days to assess changes in heart rate and to monitor motion analysis for the purposes of diagnosing nocturnal epilepsy seizure events; review and interpretation only M

RVU			Global Days	Modifiers				
Mod	Non-Fac Total	Fac Total		51	50	62	80	MUE
	0.00	0.00	XXX	0	0	0	0	1

● **0385T** External heart rate and 3-axis accelerometer data recording more than 30 days to assess changes in heart rate and to monitor motion analysis for the purposes of diagnosing nocturnal epilepsy seizure events; includes report, scanning analysis with report, review and interpretation by a physician or other qualified health care professional M

RVU			Global Days	Modifiers				
Mod	Non-Fac Total	Fac Total		51	50	62	80	MUE
	0.00	0.00	XXX	0	0	0	0	1

● **0386T** External heart rate and 3-axis accelerometer data recording more than 30 days to assess changes in heart rate and to monitor motion analysis for the purposes of diagnosing nocturnal epilepsy seizure events; review and interpretation only M

RVU			Global Days	Modifiers				
Mod	Non-Fac Total	Fac Total		51	50	62	80	MUE
	0.00	0.00	XXX	0	0	0	0	1

● **0387T** Transcatheter insertion or replacement of permanent leadless pacemaker, ventricular J8 J1

RVU			Global Days	Modifiers				
Mod	Non-Fac Total	Fac Total		51	50	62	80	MUE
	0.00	0.00	XXX	0	0	0	0	1

AMA: May 15: 3

● **0388T** Transcatheter removal of permanent leadless pacemaker, ventricular G2 T

RVU			Global Days	Modifiers				
Mod	Non-Fac Total	Fac Total		51	50	62	80	MUE
	0.00	0.00	XXX	0	0	0	0	1

AMA: May 15: 3

● **0389T** Programming device evaluation (in person) with iterative adjustment of the implantable device to test the function of the device and select optimal permanent programmed values with analysis, review and report, leadless pacemaker system Q1

RVU			Global Days	Modifiers				
Mod	Non-Fac Total	Fac Total		51	50	62	80	MUE
	0.00	0.00	XXX	0	0	0	0	1

AMA: May 15: 3

● **0390T** Peri-procedural device evaluation (in person) and programming of device system parameters before or after a surgery, procedure or test with analysis, review and report, leadless pacemaker system N N

RVU			Global Days	Modifiers				
Mod	Non-Fac Total	Fac Total		51	50	62	80	MUE
	0.00	0.00	XXX	0	0	0	0	1

AMA: May 15: 3

● **0391T** Interrogation device evaluation (in person) with analysis, review and report, includes connection, recording and disconnection per patient encounter, leadless pacemaker system Q1

RVU			Global Days	Modifiers				
Mod	Non-Fac Total	Fac Total		51	50	62	80	MUE
	0.00	0.00	XXX	0	0	0	0	1

AMA: May 15: 3

● **0392T** Laparoscopy, surgical, esophageal sphincter augmentation procedure, placement of sphincter augmentation device (ie, magnetic band) G2 J1

RVU			Global Days	Modifiers				
Mod	Non-Fac Total	Fac Total		51	50	62	80	MUE
	0.00	0.00	YYY	0	0	0	0	1

● **0393T** Removal of esophageal sphincter augmentation device G2 Q2

RVU			Global Days	Modifiers				
Mod	Non-Fac Total	Fac Total		51	50	62	80	MUE
	0.00	0.00	YYY	0	0	0	0	1

● New ▲ Revised Deleted ⊙ Moderate Sedation ✚ Add-on Codes ⊘ High Risk Denial Ⓐ Age Edit ♀ Female ♂ Male **AMA** *CPT® Assistant* **MUE** Medically Unlikely Edit
⊗ Modifier 51 Exempt ⊖ Modifier 63 Exempt ✗ Unlisted **Modifiers:** *See Inside Back Cover* Ⓜ Maternity A2–Z3 ASC Payment Indicators A–Y OPPS Status Indicators

© 2016 DecisionHealth CPT © 2015 American Medical Association. All Rights Reserved.

● **0394T** High dose rate electronic brachytherapy, skin surface application, per fraction, includes basic dosimetry, when performed   **Z2 S**

RVU		Global Days	Modifiers				
Mod	Non-Fac Total	Fac Total		51	50	62	80	MUE
	0.00	0.00	XXX	0	0	0	0	2

● **0395T** High dose rate electronic brachytherapy, interstitial or intracavitary treatment, per fraction, includes basic dosimetry, when performed   **Z2 S**

RVU		Global Days	Modifiers				
Mod	Non-Fac Total	Fac Total		51	50	62	80	MUE
	0.00	0.00	XXX	0	0	0	0	2

✚● **0396T** Intra-operative use of kinetic balance sensor for implant stability during knee replacement arthroplasty (List separately in addition to code for primary procedure)   **N**

RVU		Global Days	Modifiers				
Mod	Non-Fac Total	Fac Total		51	50	62	80	MUE
	0.00	0.00	XXX	0	0	0	0	2

⊙✚● **0397T** Endoscopic retrograde cholangiopancreatography (ERCP), with optical endomicroscopy (List separately in addition to code for primary procedure)   **N**

RVU		Global Days	Modifiers				
Mod	Non-Fac Total	Fac Total		51	50	62	80	MUE
	0.00	0.00	XXX	0	0	0	0	1

● **0398T** Magnetic resonance image guided high intensity focused ultrasound (MRgFUS), stereotactic ablation lesion, intracranial for movement disorder including stereotactic navigation and frame placement when performed   **E**

RVU		Global Days	Modifiers				
Mod	Non-Fac Total	Fac Total		51	50	62	80	MUE
	0.00	0.00	XXX	0	0	0	0	1

✚● **0399T** Myocardial strain imaging (quantitative assessment of myocardial mechanics using image-based analysis of local myocardial dynamics) (List separately in addition to code for primary procedure)   **N**

RVU		Global Days	Modifiers				
Mod	Non-Fac Total	Fac Total		51	50	62	80	MUE
	0.00	0.00	XXX	0	0	0	0	1

● **0400T** Multi-spectral digital skin lesion analysis of clinically atypical cutaneous pigmented lesions for detection of melanomas and high risk melanocytic atypia; one to five lesions   **N**

RVU		Global Days	Modifiers				
Mod	Non-Fac Total	Fac Total		51	50	62	80	MUE
	0.00	0.00	XXX	0	0	0	0	1

● **0401T** Multi-spectral digital skin lesion analysis of clinically atypical cutaneous pigmented lesions for detection of melanomas and high risk melanocytic atypia; six or more lesions   **N**

RVU		Global Days	Modifiers				
Mod	Non-Fac Total	Fac Total		51	50	62	80	MUE
	0.00	0.00	XXX	0	0	0	0	1

● **0402T** Collagen cross-linking of cornea (including removal of the corneal epithelium and intraoperative pachymetry when performed)   **R2 T**

RVU		Global Days	Modifiers				
Mod	Non-Fac Total	Fac Total		51	50	62	80	MUE
	0.00	0.00	XXX	0	0	0	0	2

● **0403T** Preventive behavior change, intensive program of prevention of diabetes using a standardized diabetes prevention program curriculum, provided to individuals in a group setting, minimum 60 minutes, per day   **E**

RVU		Global Days	Modifiers				
Mod	Non-Fac Total	Fac Total		51	50	62	80	MUE
	0.00	0.00	XXX	0	0	0	0	1

● **0404T** Transcervical uterine fibroid(s) ablation with ultrasound guidance, radiofrequency   **J1**

RVU		Global Days	Modifiers				
Mod	Non-Fac Total	Fac Total		51	50	62	80	MUE
	0.00	0.00	XXX	0	0	0	0	1

● **0405T** Oversight of the care of an extracorporeal liver assist system patient requiring review of status, review of laboratories and other studies, and revision of orders and liver assist care plan (as appropriate), within a calendar month, 30 minutes or more of non-face-to-face time   ♀**B**

RVU		Global Days	Modifiers				
Mod	Non-Fac Total	Fac Total		51	50	62	80	MUE
	0.00	0.00	XXX	0	0	0	0	1

● **0406T** Nasal endoscopy, surgical, ethmoid sinus, placement of drug eluting implant   **N**

RVU		Global Days	Modifiers				
Mod	Non-Fac Total	Fac Total		51	50	62	80	MUE
	0.00	0.00	XXX	0	0	0	0	2

● **0407T** Nasal endoscopy, surgical, ethmoid sinus, placement of drug eluting implant; with biopsy, polypectomy or debridement   **N**

RVU		Global Days	Modifiers				
Mod	Non-Fac Total	Fac Total		51	50	62	80	MUE
	0.00	0.00	XXX	0	0	0	0	2

● New   ▲ Revised   ✖ Deleted   ⊙ Moderate Sedation   ✚ Add-on Codes   ⊗ High Risk Denial   Ⓐ Age Edit   ♀ Female   ♂ Male   **AMA** CPT® Assistant   **MUE** Medically Unlikely Edit
⊘ Modifier 51 Exempt   ⊖ Modifier 63 Exempt   ✗ Unlisted   **Modifiers:** See Inside Back Cover   Ⓜ Maternity   **A2–Z3** ASC Payment Indicators   **A–Y** OPPS Status Indicators

906   CPT © 2015 American Medical Association. All Rights Reserved.   © 2016 DecisionHealth

Anatomical Illustrations

Introduction

Without a strong background in or reference materials regarding human anatomy and physiology, it is more difficult to adequately code medical diagnoses. The following pages can be utilized as a reference for beginning and seasoned coders.

Male Figure
(Anterior View)

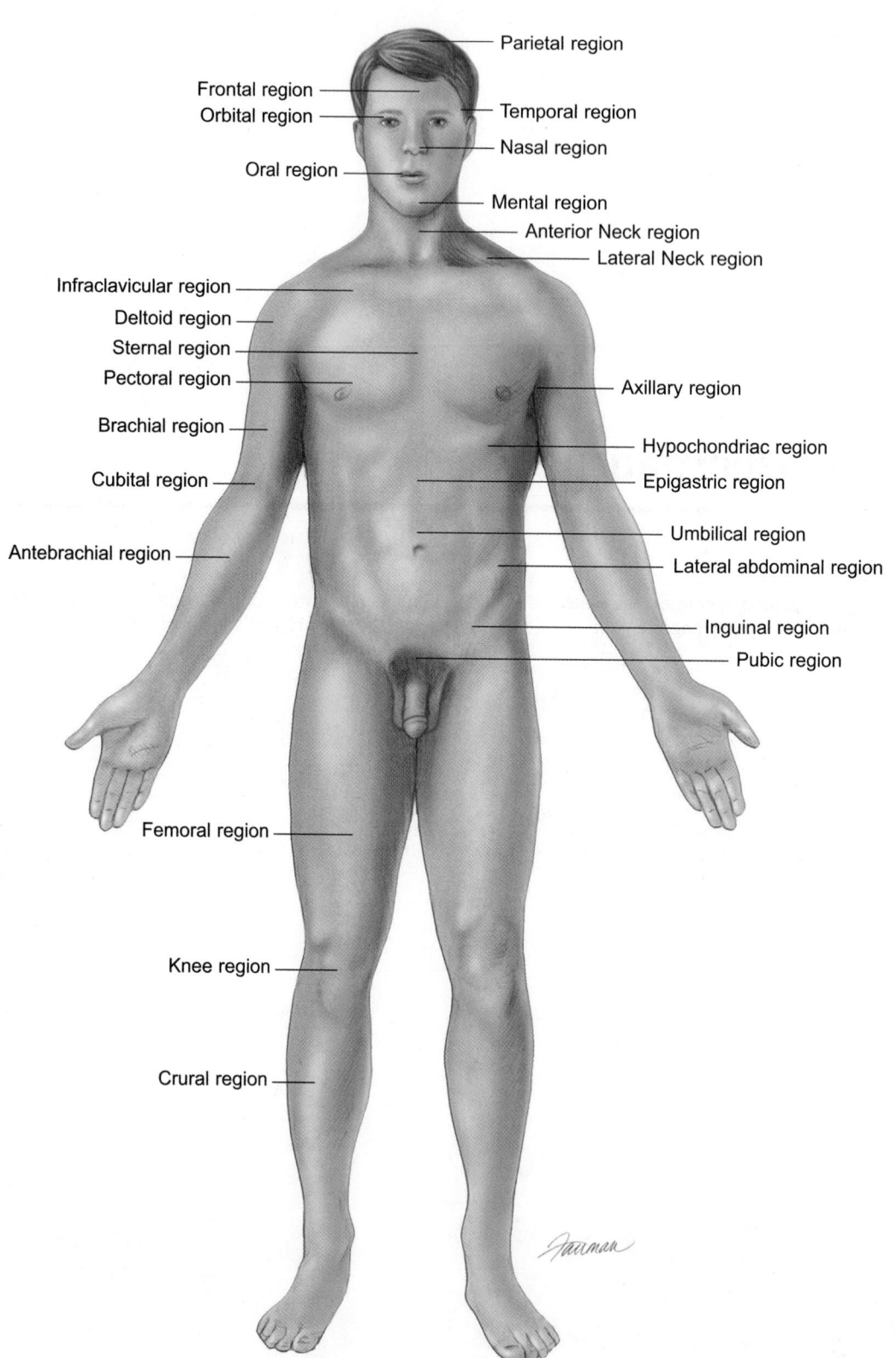

Parietal region

Frontal region

Orbital region

Temporal region

Nasal region

Oral region

Mental region

Anterior Neck region

Lateral Neck region

Infraclavicular region

Deltoid region

Sternal region

Pectoral region

Axillary region

Brachial region

Hypochondriac region

Cubital region

Epigastric region

Umbilical region

Antebrachial region

Lateral abdominal region

Inguinal region

Pubic region

Femoral region

Knee region

Crural region

© Fairman Studios, LLC, 2002. All Rights Reserved.

Female Figure
(Anterior View)

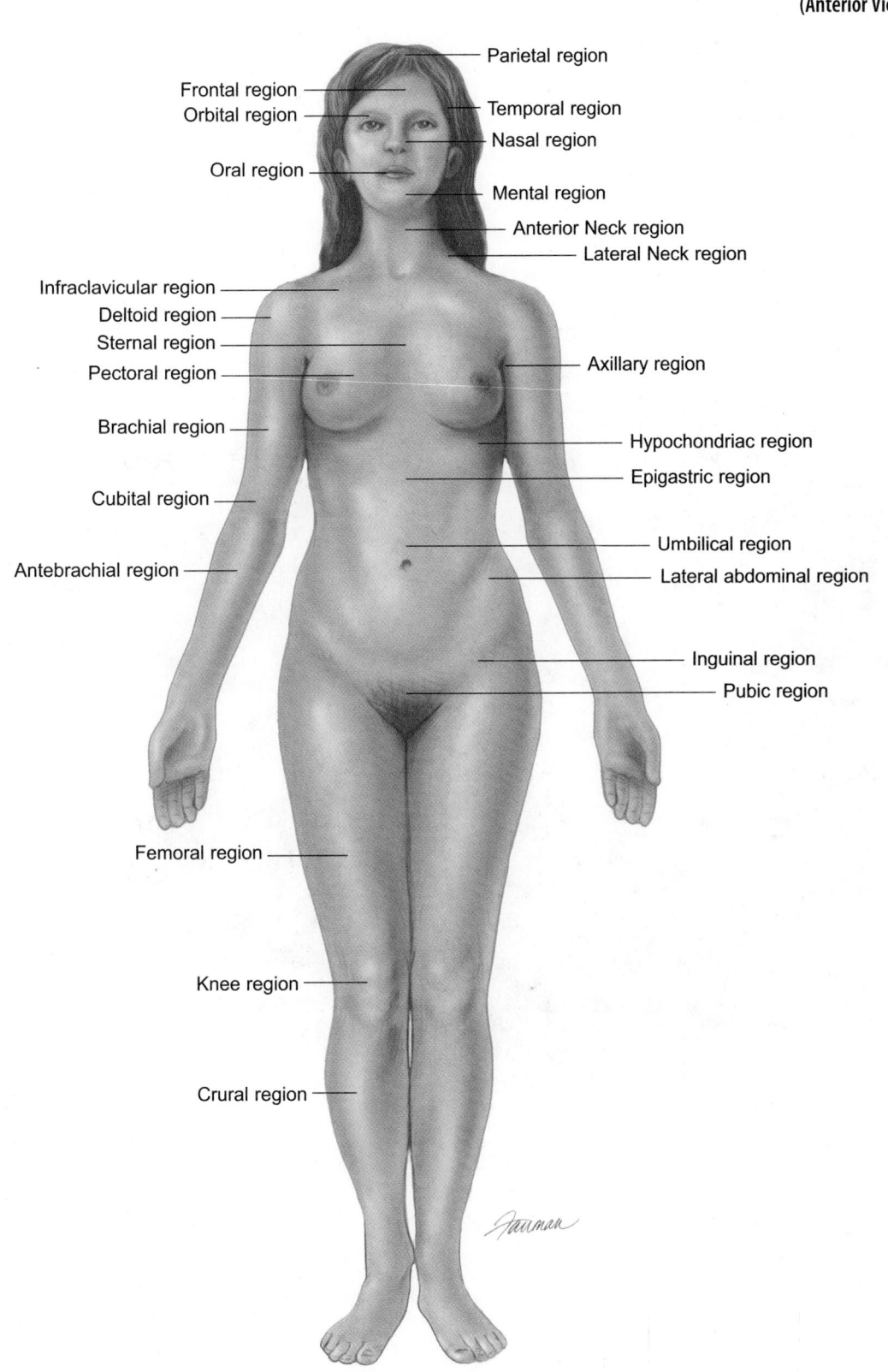

Parietal region

Frontal region

Orbital region

Temporal region

Nasal region

Oral region

Mental region

Anterior Neck region

Lateral Neck region

Infraclavicular region

Deltoid region

Sternal region

Pectoral region

Axillary region

Brachial region

Hypochondriac region

Epigastric region

Cubital region

Umbilical region

Antebrachial region

Lateral abdominal region

Inguinal region

Pubic region

Femoral region

Knee region

Crural region

© Fairman Studios, LLC, 2002. All Rights Reserved.

Anatomical Illustrations

Female Breast

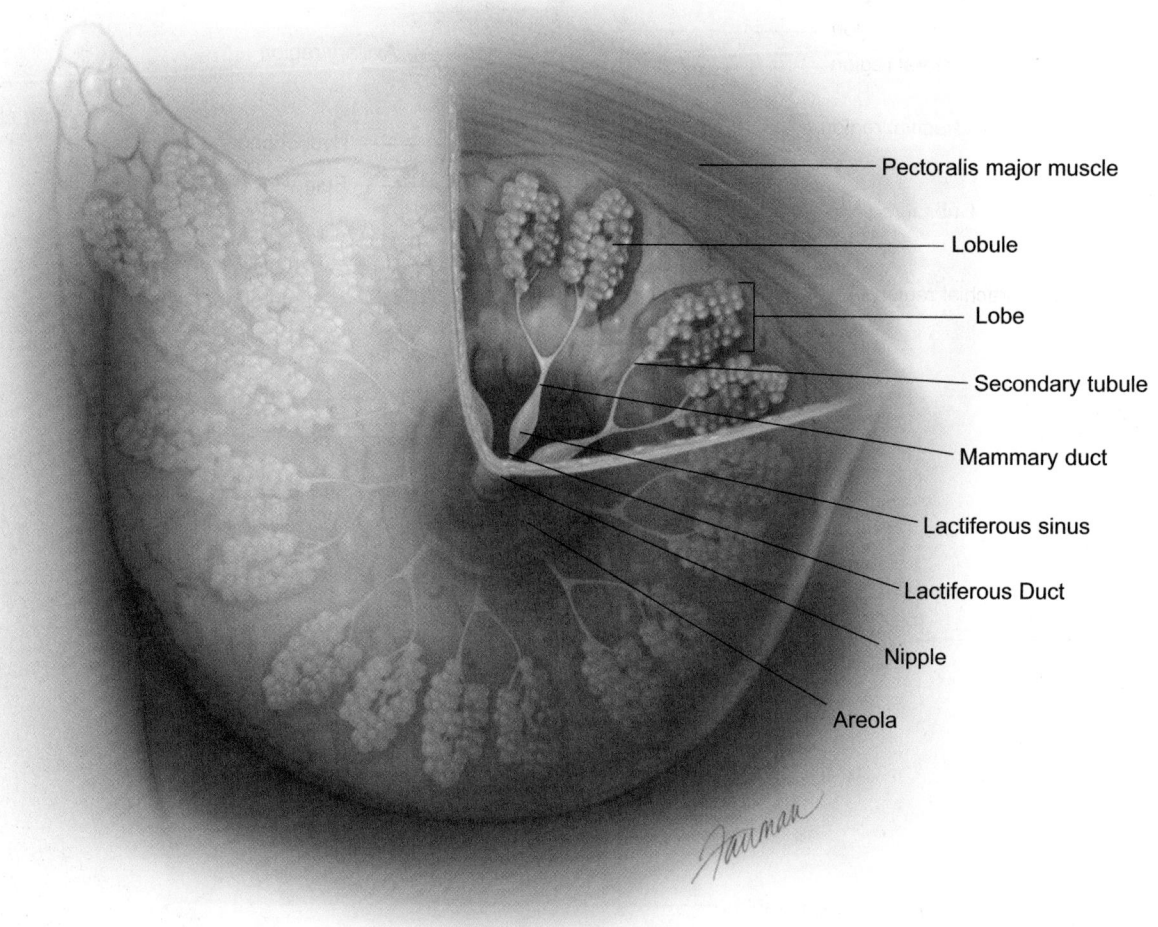

Pectoralis major muscle

Lobule

Lobe

Secondary tubule

Mammary duct

Lactiferous sinus

Lactiferous Duct

Nipple

Areola

© Fairman Studios, LLC, 2002. All Rights Reserved.

Muscular System
(Anterior View)

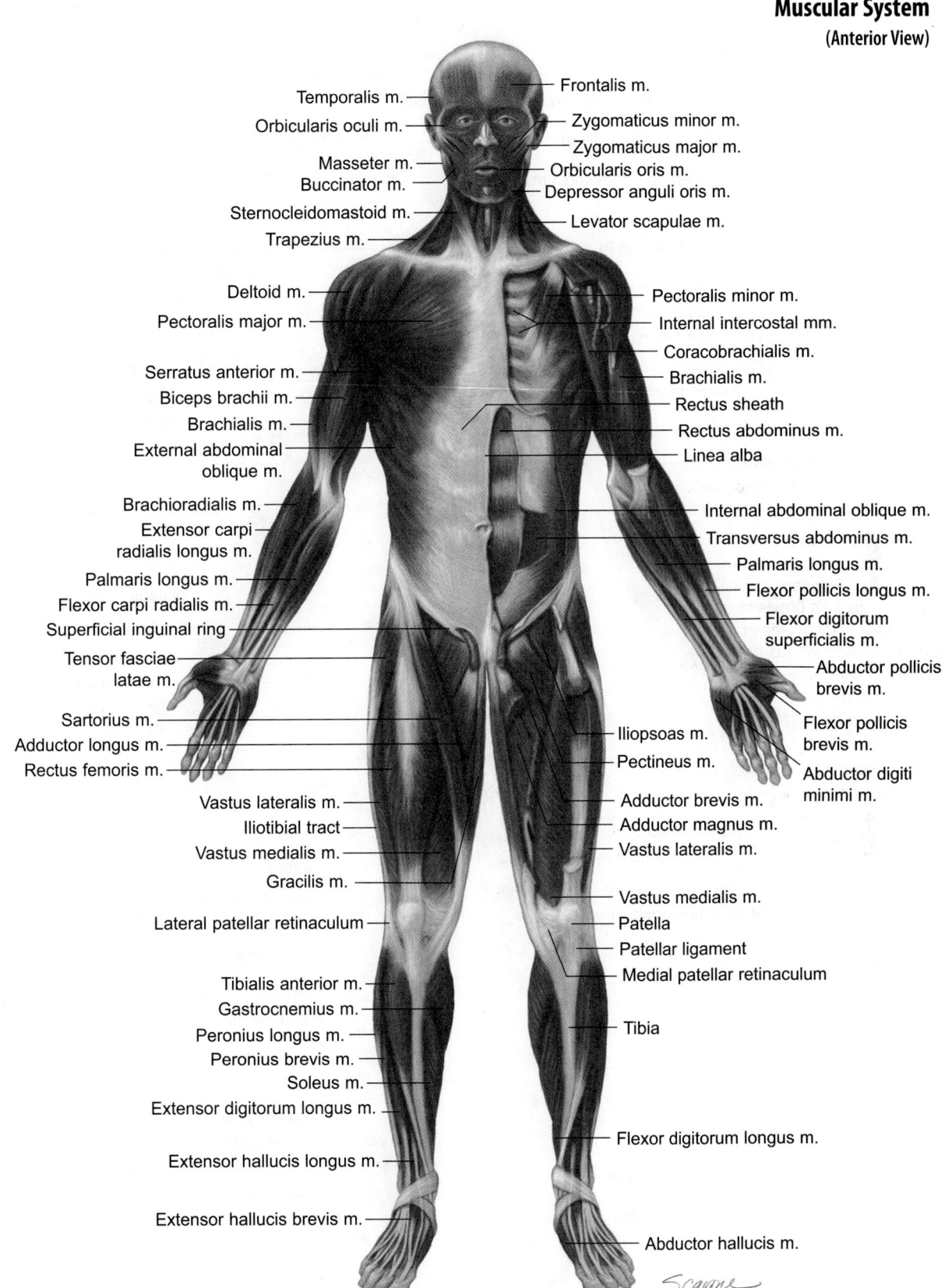

Temporalis m.
Orbicularis oculi m.
Masseter m.
Buccinator m.
Sternocleidomastoid m.
Trapezius m.

Frontalis m.
Zygomaticus minor m.
Zygomaticus major m.
Orbicularis oris m.
Depressor anguli oris m.
Levator scapulae m.

Deltoid m.
Pectoralis major m.

Serratus anterior m.
Biceps brachii m.
Brachialis m.
External abdominal oblique m.

Brachioradialis m.
Extensor carpi radialis longus m.
Palmaris longus m.
Flexor carpi radialis m.
Superficial inguinal ring
Tensor fasciae latae m.

Sartorius m.
Adductor longus m.
Rectus femoris m.

Vastus lateralis m.
Iliotibial tract
Vastus medialis m.
Gracilis m.

Lateral patellar retinaculum

Tibialis anterior m.
Gastrocnemius m.
Peronius longus m.
Peronius brevis m.
Soleus m.
Extensor digitorum longus m.

Extensor hallucis longus m.

Extensor hallucis brevis m.

Pectoralis minor m.
Internal intercostal mm.
Coracobrachialis m.
Brachialis m.
Rectus sheath
Rectus abdominus m.
Linea alba

Internal abdominal oblique m.
Transversus abdominus m.
Palmaris longus m.
Flexor pollicis longus m.
Flexor digitorum superficialis m.
Abductor pollicis brevis m.

Flexor pollicis brevis m.

Iliopsoas m.
Pectineus m.

Abductor digiti minimi m.

Adductor brevis m.
Adductor magnus m.
Vastus lateralis m.

Vastus medialis m.
Patella
Patellar ligament
Medial patellar retinaculum

Tibia

Flexor digitorum longus m.

Abductor hallucis m.

Scavone

© Fairman Studios, LLC, 2002. All Rights Reserved.

Muscular System
(Posterior View)

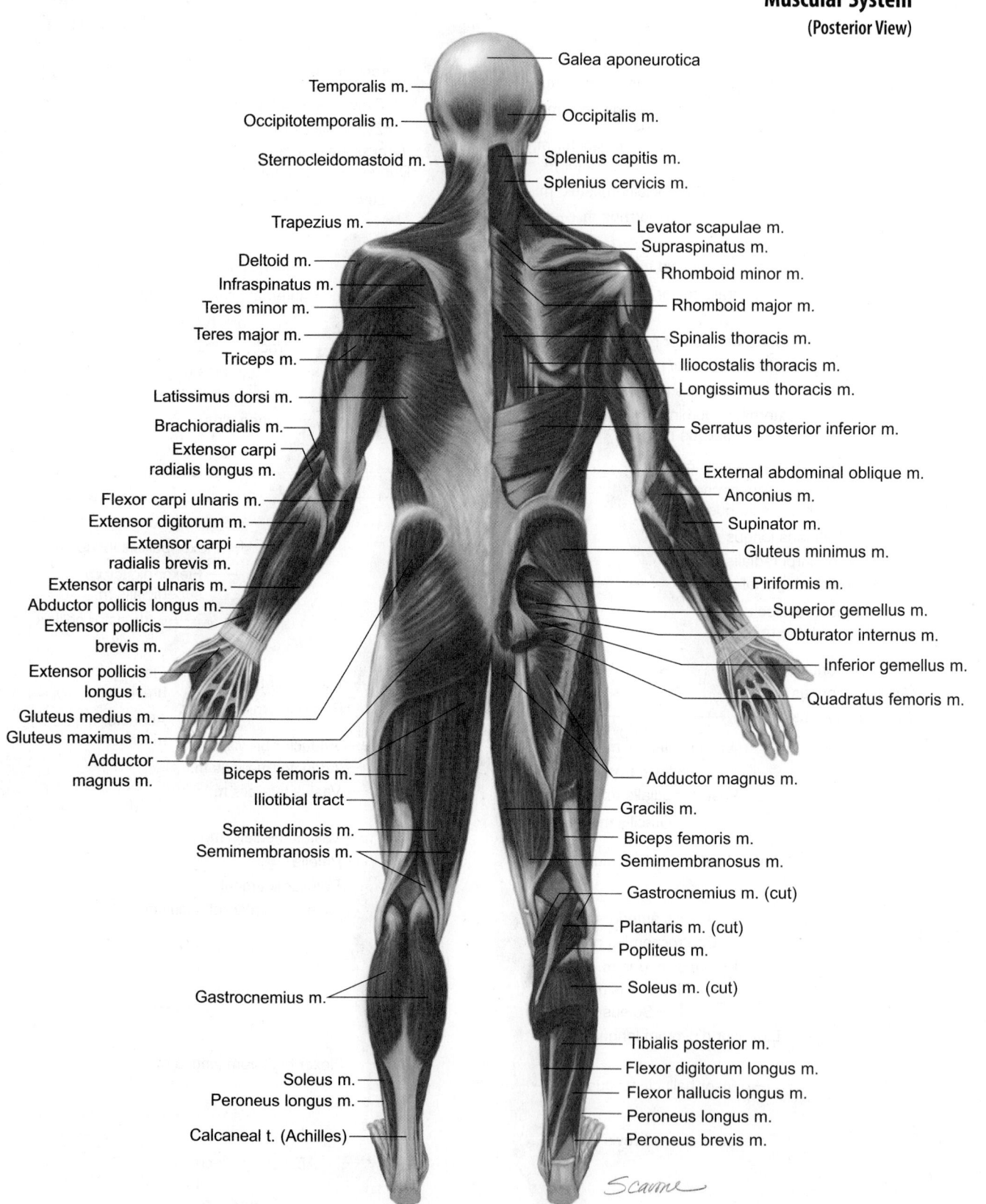

- Galea aponeurotica
- Temporalis m.
- Occipitotemporalis m.
- Occipitalis m.
- Sternocleidomastoid m.
- Splenius capitis m.
- Splenius cervicis m.
- Trapezius m.
- Levator scapulae m.
- Supraspinatus m.
- Deltoid m.
- Rhomboid minor m.
- Infraspinatus m.
- Teres minor m.
- Rhomboid major m.
- Teres major m.
- Spinalis thoracis m.
- Triceps m.
- Iliocostalis thoracis m.
- Longissimus thoracis m.
- Latissimus dorsi m.
- Brachioradialis m.
- Serratus posterior inferior m.
- Extensor carpi radialis longus m.
- External abdominal oblique m.
- Anconius m.
- Flexor carpi ulnaris m.
- Supinator m.
- Extensor digitorum m.
- Extensor carpi radialis brevis m.
- Gluteus minimus m.
- Extensor carpi ulnaris m.
- Piriformis m.
- Abductor pollicis longus m.
- Superior gemellus m.
- Extensor pollicis brevis m.
- Obturator internus m.
- Extensor pollicis longus t.
- Inferior gemellus m.
- Gluteus medius m.
- Quadratus femoris m.
- Gluteus maximus m.
- Adductor magnus m.
- Biceps femoris m.
- Adductor magnus m.
- Iliotibial tract
- Gracilis m.
- Semitendinosis m.
- Biceps femoris m.
- Semimembranosis m.
- Semimembranosus m.
- Gastrocnemius m. (cut)
- Plantaris m. (cut)
- Popliteus m.
- Soleus m. (cut)
- Gastrocnemius m.
- Tibialis posterior m.
- Flexor digitorum longus m.
- Flexor hallucis longus m.
- Soleus m.
- Peroneus longus m.
- Peroneus longus m.
- Peroneus brevis m.
- Calcaneal t. (Achilles)

© Fairman Studios, LLC, 2002. All Rights Reserved.

© 2016 DecisionHealth

Skeletal System
(Anterior View)

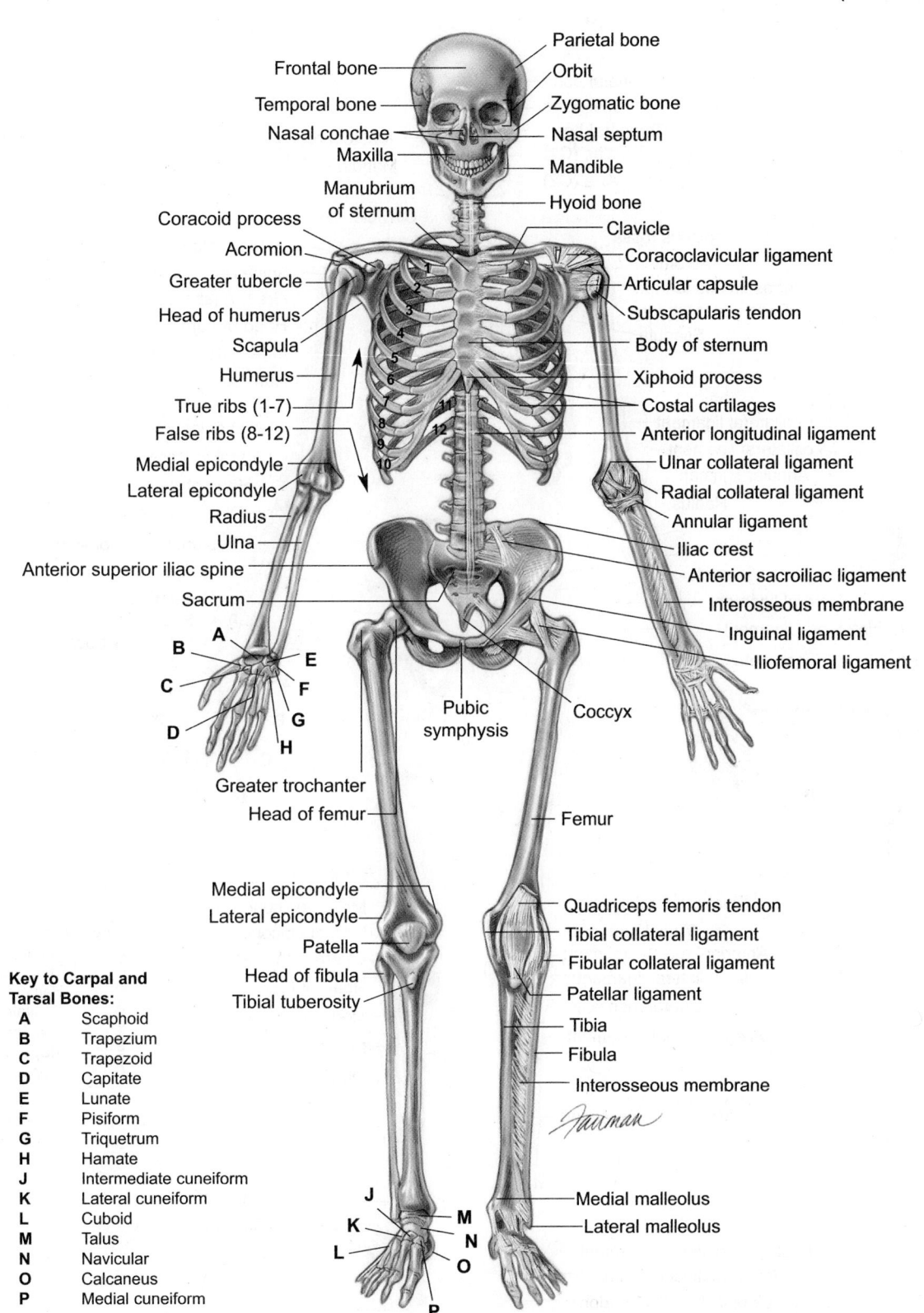

Parietal bone
Frontal bone
Orbit
Temporal bone
Zygomatic bone
Nasal conchae
Nasal septum
Maxilla
Mandible
Manubrium of sternum
Hyoid bone
Coracoid process
Clavicle
Acromion
Coracoclavicular ligament
Greater tubercle
Articular capsule
Head of humerus
Subscapularis tendon
Scapula
Body of sternum
Humerus
Xiphoid process
True ribs (1-7)
Costal cartilages
False ribs (8-12)
Anterior longitudinal ligament
Medial epicondyle
Ulnar collateral ligament
Lateral epicondyle
Radial collateral ligament
Radius
Annular ligament
Ulna
Iliac crest
Anterior superior iliac spine
Anterior sacroiliac ligament
Sacrum
Interosseous membrane
Inguinal ligament
Iliofemoral ligament

A
B
C
E
F
D
G
H

Pubic symphysis
Coccyx

Greater trochanter
Head of femur
Femur

Medial epicondyle
Quadriceps femoris tendon
Lateral epicondyle
Tibial collateral ligament
Patella
Fibular collateral ligament
Head of fibula
Patellar ligament
Tibial tuberosity
Tibia
Fibula
Interosseous membrane

Key to Carpal and Tarsal Bones:

A	Scaphoid
B	Trapezium
C	Trapezoid
D	Capitate
E	Lunate
F	Pisiform
G	Triquetrum
H	Hamate
J	Intermediate cuneiform
K	Lateral cuneiform
L	Cuboid
M	Talus
N	Navicular
O	Calcaneus
P	Medial cuneiform

J
K
L
M
N
O
P

Medial malleolus
Lateral malleolus

© Fairman Studios, LLC, 2002. All Rights Reserved.

Anatomical Illustrations

Skeletal System
(Posterior View)

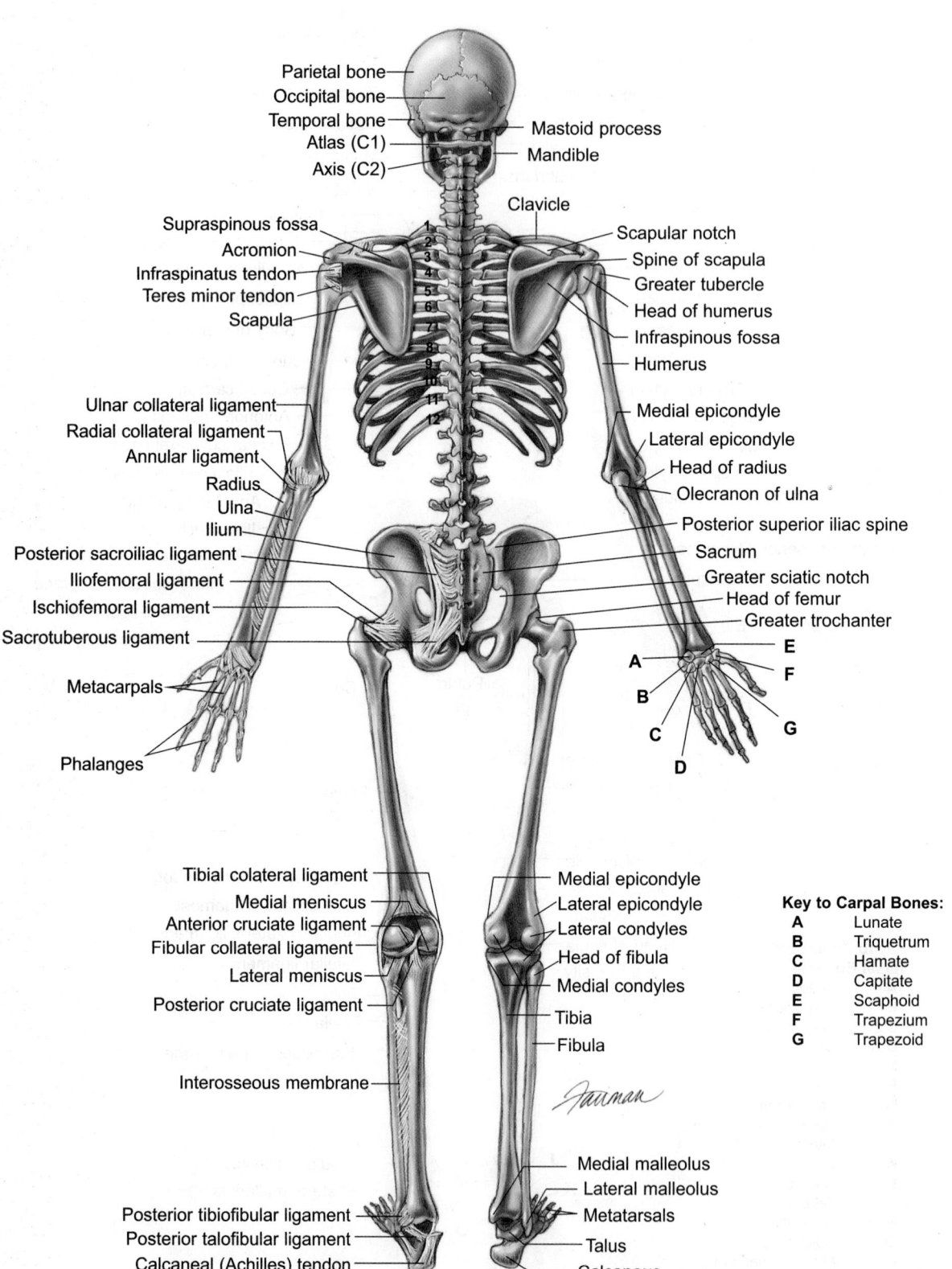

Parietal bone
Occipital bone
Temporal bone
Atlas (C1)
Axis (C2)

Mastoid process
Mandible

Clavicle

Supraspinous fossa
Acromion
Infraspinatus tendon
Teres minor tendon
Scapula

Scapular notch
Spine of scapula
Greater tubercle
Head of humerus
Infraspinous fossa
Humerus

Ulnar collateral ligament
Radial collateral ligament
Annular ligament
Radius
Ulna
Ilium
Posterior sacroiliac ligament
Iliofemoral ligament
Ischiofemoral ligament
Sacrotuberous ligament

Medial epicondyle
Lateral epicondyle
Head of radius
Olecranon of ulna
Posterior superior iliac spine
Sacrum
Greater sciatic notch
Head of femur
Greater trochanter

Metacarpals

Phalanges

A
B
C
D

E
F
G

Tibial colateral ligament
Medial meniscus
Anterior cruciate ligament
Fibular collateral ligament
Lateral meniscus
Posterior cruciate ligament

Medial epicondyle
Lateral epicondyle
Lateral condyles
Head of fibula
Medial condyles
Tibia
Fibula

Interosseous membrane

Key to Carpal Bones:
A   Lunate
B   Triquetrum
C   Hamate
D   Capitate
E   Scaphoid
F   Trapezium
G   Trapezoid

Posterior tibiofibular ligament
Posterior talofibular ligament
Calcaneal (Achilles) tendon

Medial malleolus
Lateral malleolus
Metatarsals
Talus
Calcaneus

© Fairman Studios, LLC, 2002. All Rights Reserved.

Skeletal System
(Vertebral Column – Left Lateral View)

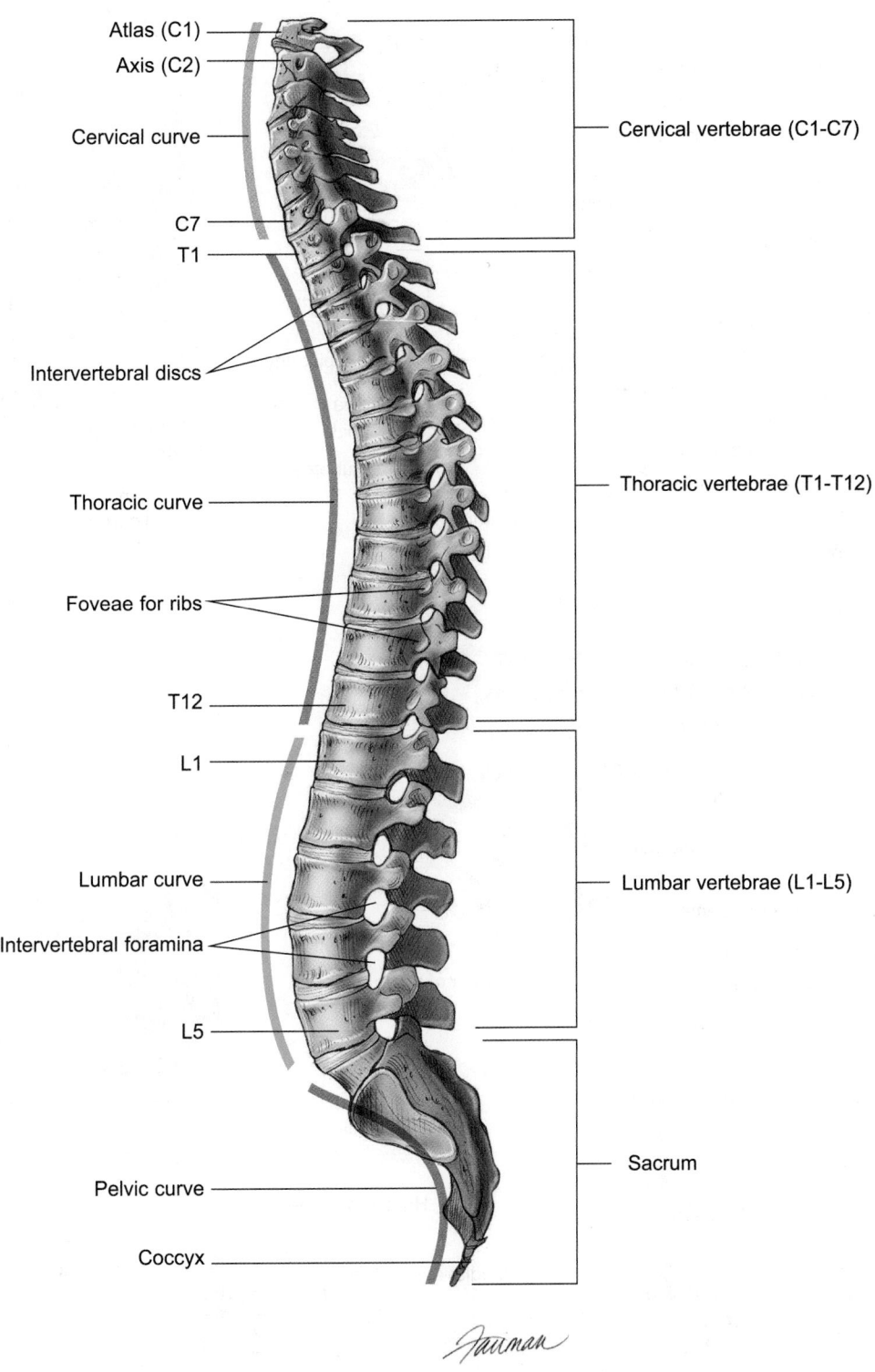

Atlas (C1)

Axis (C2)

Cervical curve

Cervical vertebrae (C1-C7)

C7

T1

Intervertebral discs

Thoracic curve

Thoracic vertebrae (T1-T12)

Foveae for ribs

T12

L1

Lumbar curve

Lumbar vertebrae (L1-L5)

Intervertebral foramina

L5

Sacrum

Pelvic curve

Coccyx

© Fairman Studios, LLC, 2002. All Rights Reserved.

Shoulder and Elbow
(Anterior View)

Scapular notch
Coracoid process
Acromion
Head of humerus
Greater tubercle
Lesser tubercle
Subscapular fossa
Scapula
Humerus
Clavicle

Coracoclavicular ligament
Acromioclavicular ligament
Coracoacromial ligament
Coracohumural ligament
Transverse humeral ligament
Long tendon of biceps
Subscapularis tendon
Articular capsule

Coronoid fossa
Lateral epicondyle
Capitulum
Head of radius
Radial tuberosity
Humerus
Medial epicondyle
Trochlea
Coronoid process
Ulnar tuberosity
Ulna
Radius

Articular capsule
Radial collateral ligament
Annular ligament
Biceps tendon
Ulnar collateral ligament
Anterior ligament
Interosseous membrane
Radius
Ulna

Acromioclavicular ligament
Infraspinatus tendon
Teres minor tendon
Scapula
Humerus
Ulnar collateral ligament
Radial collateral ligament
Annular ligament
Radius
Ulna
Interosseous membrane
Olecranon of ulna

(Posterior View)

Supraspinous fossa
Clavicle
Scapular notch
Acromion
Spine of scapula
Greater tubercle
Head of humerus
Infraspinous fossa

Humerus
Medial epicondyle
Radius
Ulna
Lateral epicondyle
Olecranon fossa
Olecranon process

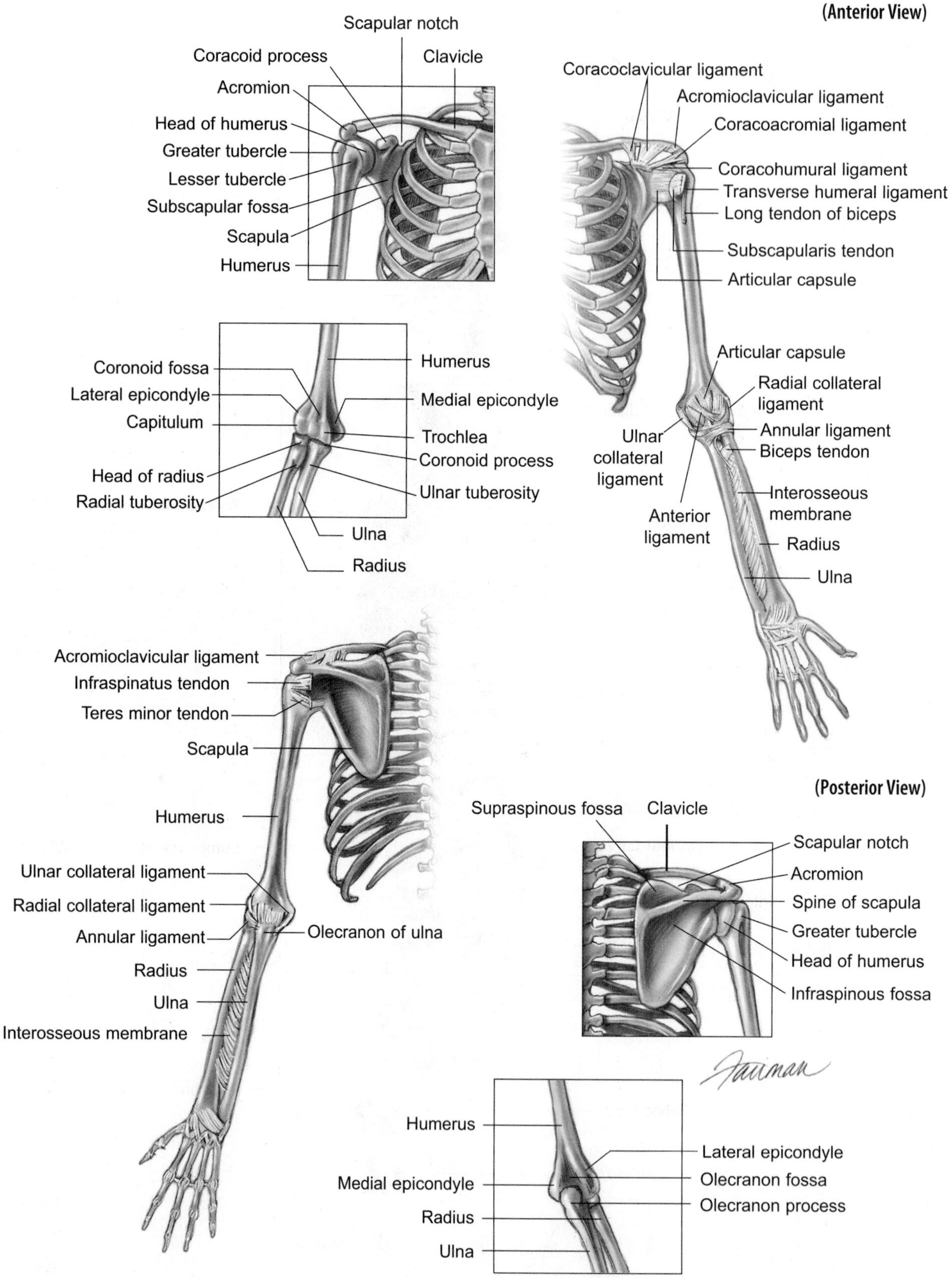

© Fairman Studios, LLC, 2002. All Rights Reserved.

Musculoskeletal System – Hand and Wrist
(Dorsal and Palmar Views)

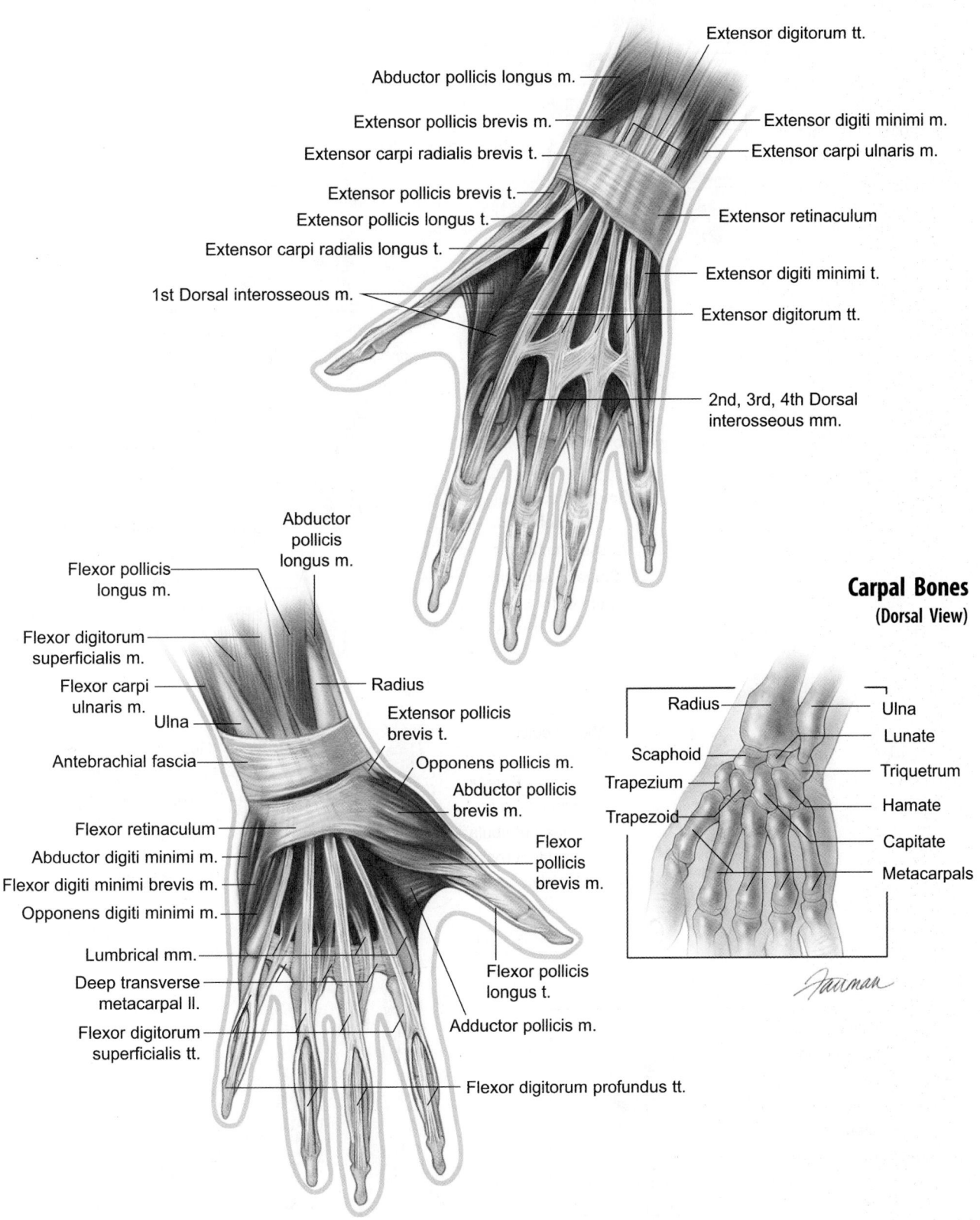

Extensor digitorum tt.

Abductor pollicis longus m.

Extensor pollicis brevis m.

Extensor digiti minimi m.

Extensor carpi radialis brevis t.

Extensor carpi ulnaris m.

Extensor pollicis brevis t.

Extensor pollicis longus t.

Extensor retinaculum

Extensor carpi radialis longus t.

Extensor digiti minimi t.

1st Dorsal interosseous m.

Extensor digitorum tt.

2nd, 3rd, 4th Dorsal interosseous mm.

Abductor pollicis longus m.

Flexor pollicis longus m.

Flexor digitorum superficialis m.

Radius

Flexor carpi ulnaris m.

Extensor pollicis brevis t.

Ulna

Opponens pollicis m.

Antebrachial fascia

Abductor pollicis brevis m.

Flexor retinaculum

Abductor digiti minimi m.

Flexor pollicis brevis m.

Flexor digiti minimi brevis m.

Opponens digiti minimi m.

Lumbrical mm.

Deep transverse metacarpal ll.

Flexor pollicis longus t.

Flexor digitorum superficialis tt.

Adductor pollicis m.

Flexor digitorum profundus tt.

Carpal Bones
(Dorsal View)

Radius

Ulna

Lunate

Scaphoid

Triquetrum

Trapezium

Hamate

Trapezoid

Capitate

Metacarpals

Fairman

© Fairman Studios, LLC, 2002. All Rights Reserved.

Musculoskeletal System – Hip and Knee
(Anterior and Posterior Views)

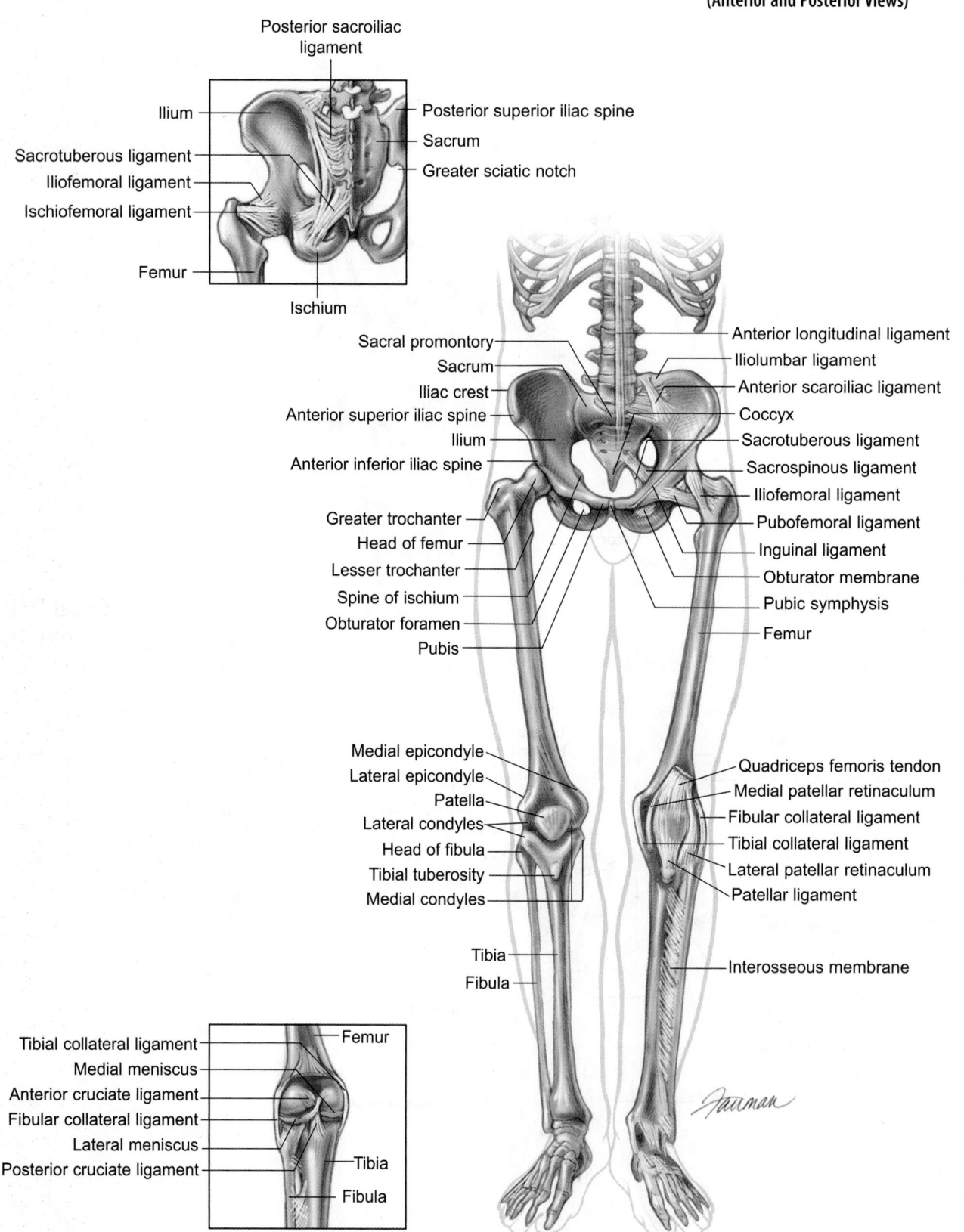

Posterior sacroiliac ligament

Ilium

Sacrotuberous ligament

Iliofemoral ligament

Ischiofemoral ligament

Femur

Ischium

Posterior superior iliac spine

Sacrum

Greater sciatic notch

Sacral promontory

Sacrum

Iliac crest

Anterior superior iliac spine

Ilium

Anterior inferior iliac spine

Greater trochanter

Head of femur

Lesser trochanter

Spine of ischium

Obturator foramen

Pubis

Anterior longitudinal ligament

Iliolumbar ligament

Anterior scaroiliac ligament

Coccyx

Sacrotuberous ligament

Sacrospinous ligament

Iliofemoral ligament

Pubofemoral ligament

Inguinal ligament

Obturator membrane

Pubic symphysis

Femur

Medial epicondyle

Lateral epicondyle

Patella

Lateral condyles

Head of fibula

Tibial tuberosity

Medial condyles

Quadriceps femoris tendon

Medial patellar retinaculum

Fibular collateral ligament

Tibial collateral ligament

Lateral patellar retinaculum

Patellar ligament

Tibia

Fibula

Interosseous membrane

Tibial collateral ligament

Medial meniscus

Anterior cruciate ligament

Fibular collateral ligament

Lateral meniscus

Posterior cruciate ligament

Femur

Tibia

Fibula

© Fairman Studios, LLC, 2002. All Rights Reserved.

Musculoskeletal System – Foot and Ankle

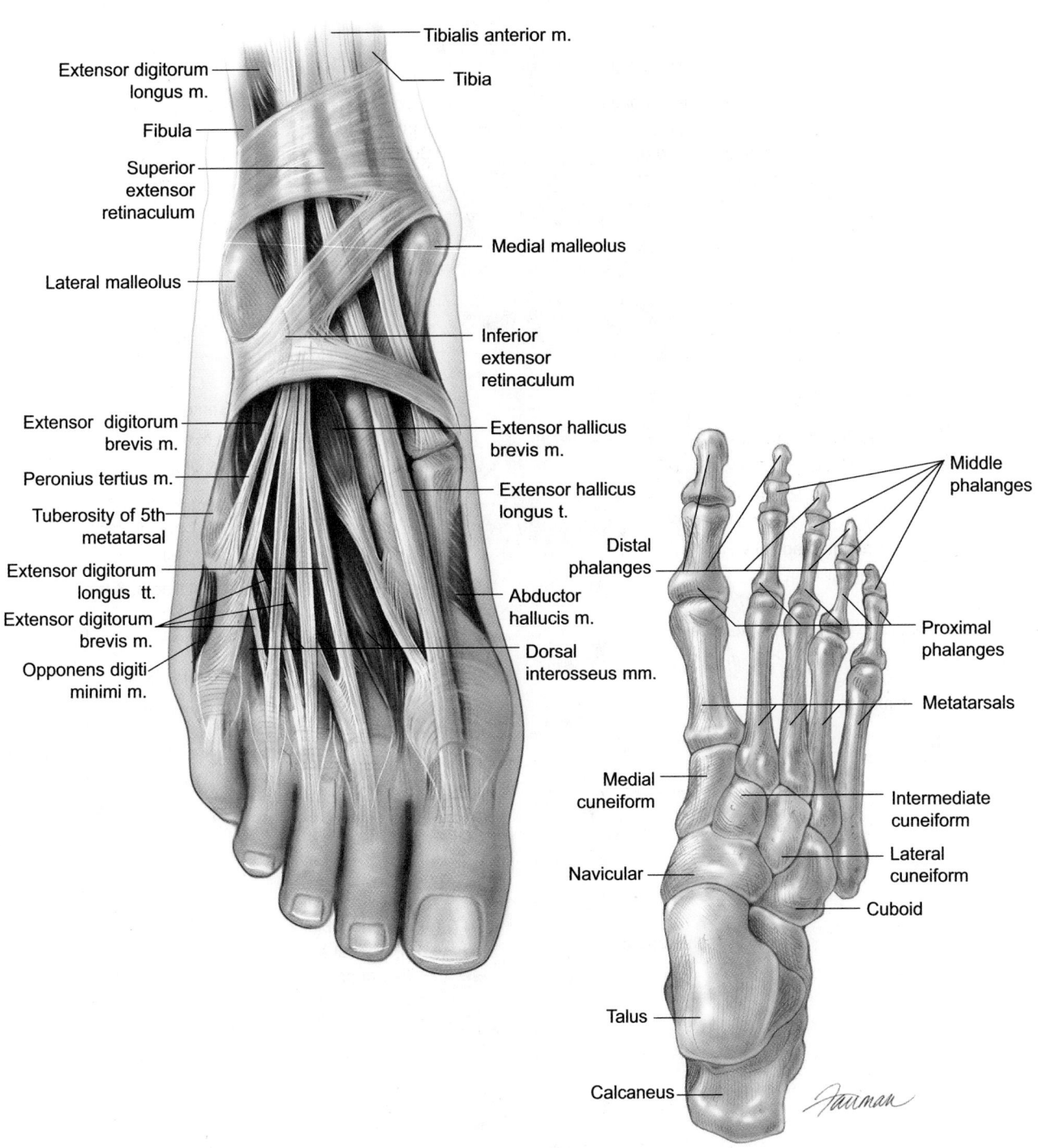

Tibialis anterior m.

Extensor digitorum longus m.

Tibia

Fibula

Superior extensor retinaculum

Medial malleolus

Lateral malleolus

Inferior extensor retinaculum

Extensor digitorum brevis m.

Extensor hallicus brevis m.

Peronius tertius m.

Extensor hallicus longus t.

Tuberosity of 5th metatarsal

Extensor digitorum longus tt.

Abductor hallucis m.

Extensor digitorum brevis m.

Dorsal interosseus mm.

Opponens digiti minimi m.

Middle phalanges

Distal phalanges

Proximal phalanges

Metatarsals

Medial cuneiform

Intermediate cuneiform

Lateral cuneiform

Navicular

Cuboid

Talus

Calcaneus

© Fairman Studios, LLC, 2002. All Rights Reserved.

Vascular System

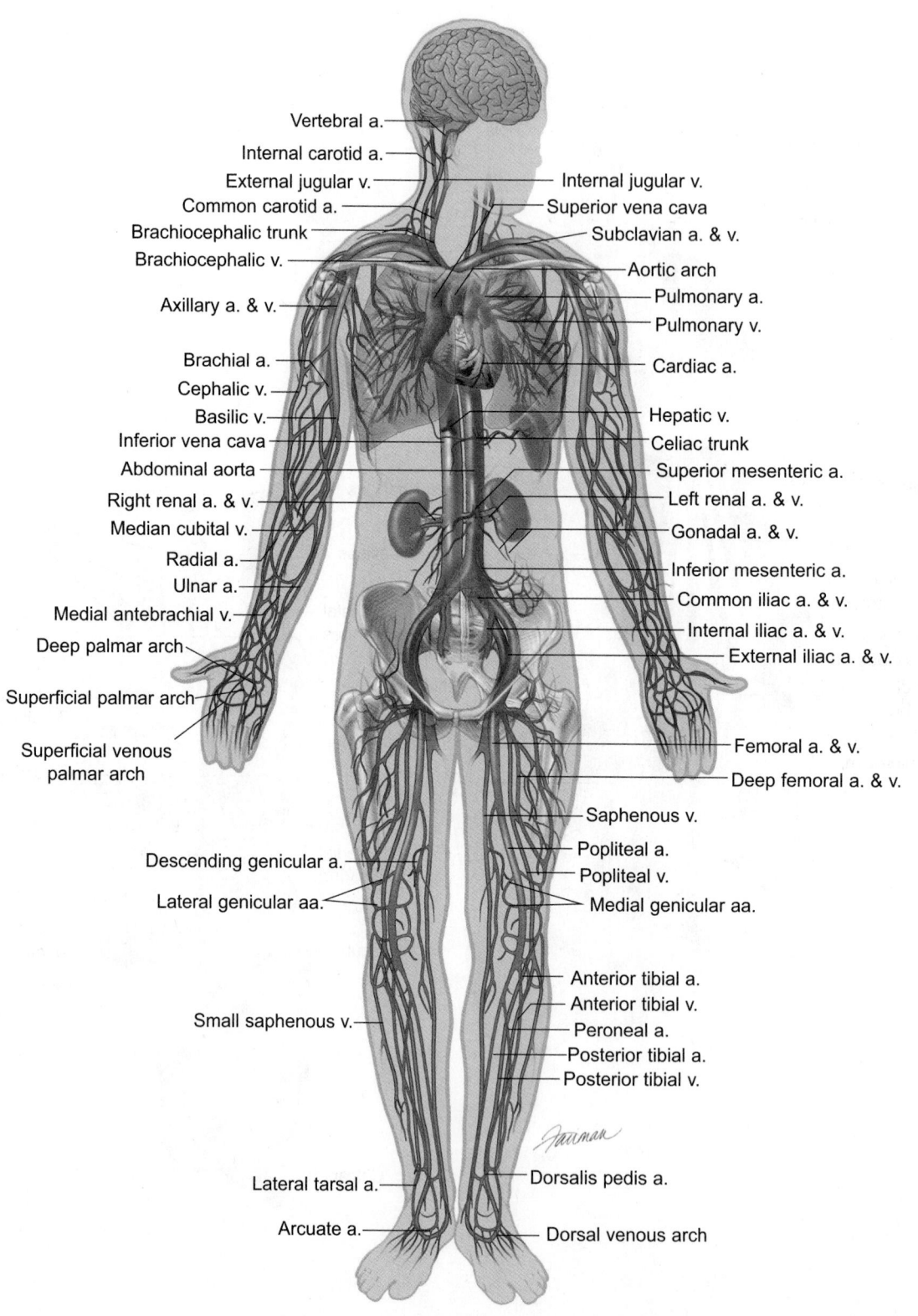

Vertebral a.
Internal carotid a.
External jugular v.
Common carotid a.
Brachiocephalic trunk
Brachiocephalic v.
Axillary a. & v.
Brachial a.
Cephalic v.
Basilic v.
Inferior vena cava
Abdominal aorta
Right renal a. & v.
Median cubital v.
Radial a.
Ulnar a.
Medial antebrachial v.
Deep palmar arch
Superficial palmar arch
Superficial venous palmar arch

Internal jugular v.
Superior vena cava
Subclavian a. & v.
Aortic arch
Pulmonary a.
Pulmonary v.
Cardiac a.
Hepatic v.
Celiac trunk
Superior mesenteric a.
Left renal a. & v.
Gonadal a. & v.
Inferior mesenteric a.
Common iliac a. & v.
Internal iliac a. & v.
External iliac a. & v.
Femoral a. & v.
Deep femoral a. & v.
Saphenous v.
Popliteal a.
Popliteal v.
Medial genicular aa.

Descending genicular a.
Lateral genicular aa.

Small saphenous v.

Anterior tibial a.
Anterior tibial v.
Peroneal a.
Posterior tibial a.
Posterior tibial v.

Lateral tarsal a.
Arcuate a.

Dorsalis pedis a.
Dorsal venous arch

© Fairman Studios, LLC, 2002. All Rights Reserved.

© 2016 DecisionHealth

Heart
(External View)

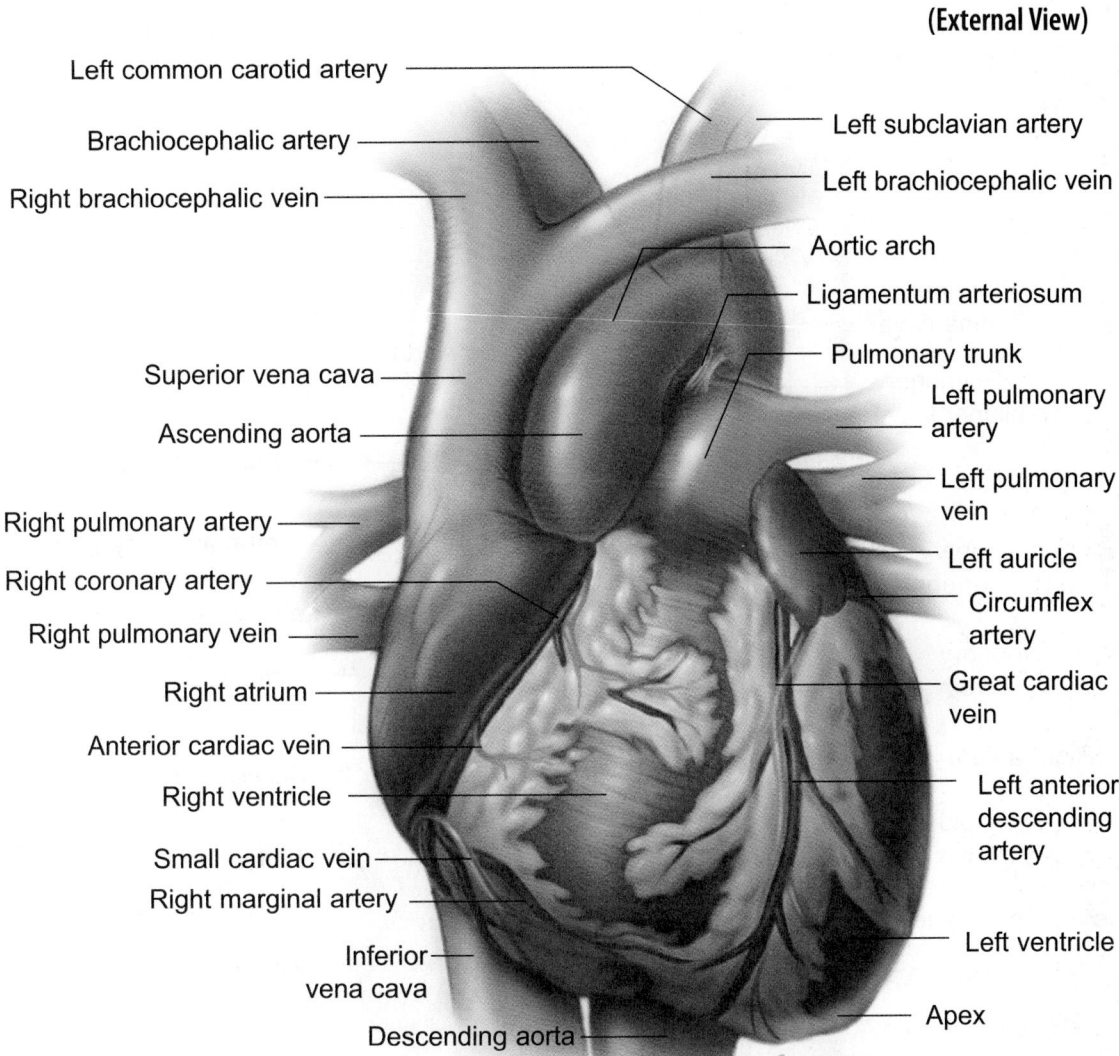

Left common carotid artery

Brachiocephalic artery

Right brachiocephalic vein

Left subclavian artery

Left brachiocephalic vein

Aortic arch

Ligamentum arteriosum

Pulmonary trunk

Superior vena cava

Ascending aorta

Left pulmonary artery

Left pulmonary vein

Right pulmonary artery

Right coronary artery

Right pulmonary vein

Left auricle

Circumflex artery

Great cardiac vein

Right atrium

Anterior cardiac vein

Right ventricle

Left anterior descending artery

Small cardiac vein

Right marginal artery

Inferior vena cava

Left ventricle

Apex

Descending aorta

© Fairman Studios, LLC, 2002. All Rights Reserved.

Heart
(Internal View)

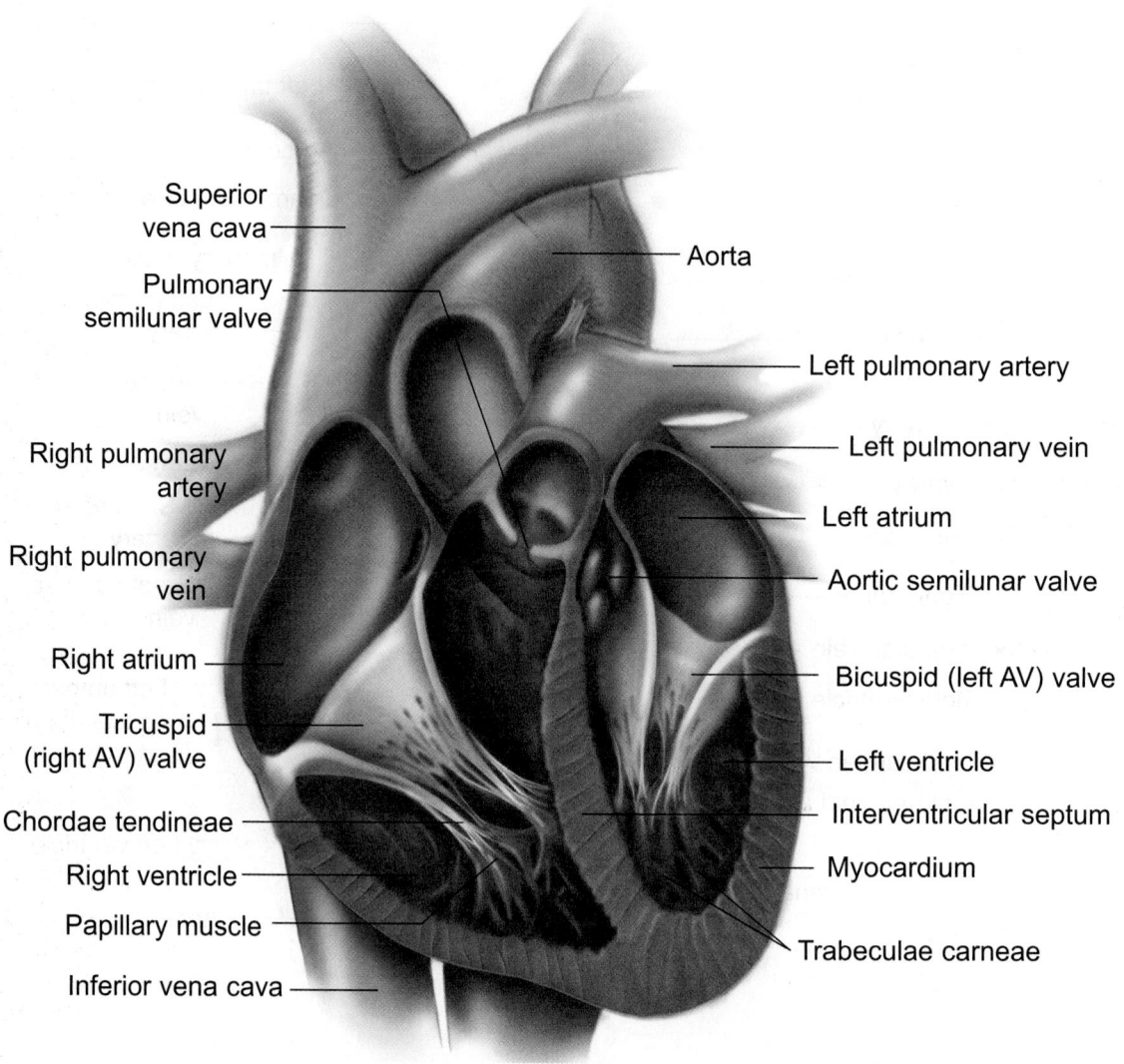

Superior vena cava

Aorta

Pulmonary semilunar valve

Left pulmonary artery

Left pulmonary vein

Right pulmonary artery

Left atrium

Right pulmonary vein

Aortic semilunar valve

Right atrium

Bicuspid (left AV) valve

Tricuspid (right AV) valve

Left ventricle

Chordae tendineae

Interventricular septum

Right ventricle

Myocardium

Papillary muscle

Trabeculae carneae

Inferior vena cava

© Fairman Studios, LLC, 2002. All Rights Reserved.

© 2016 DecisionHealth

Respiratory System

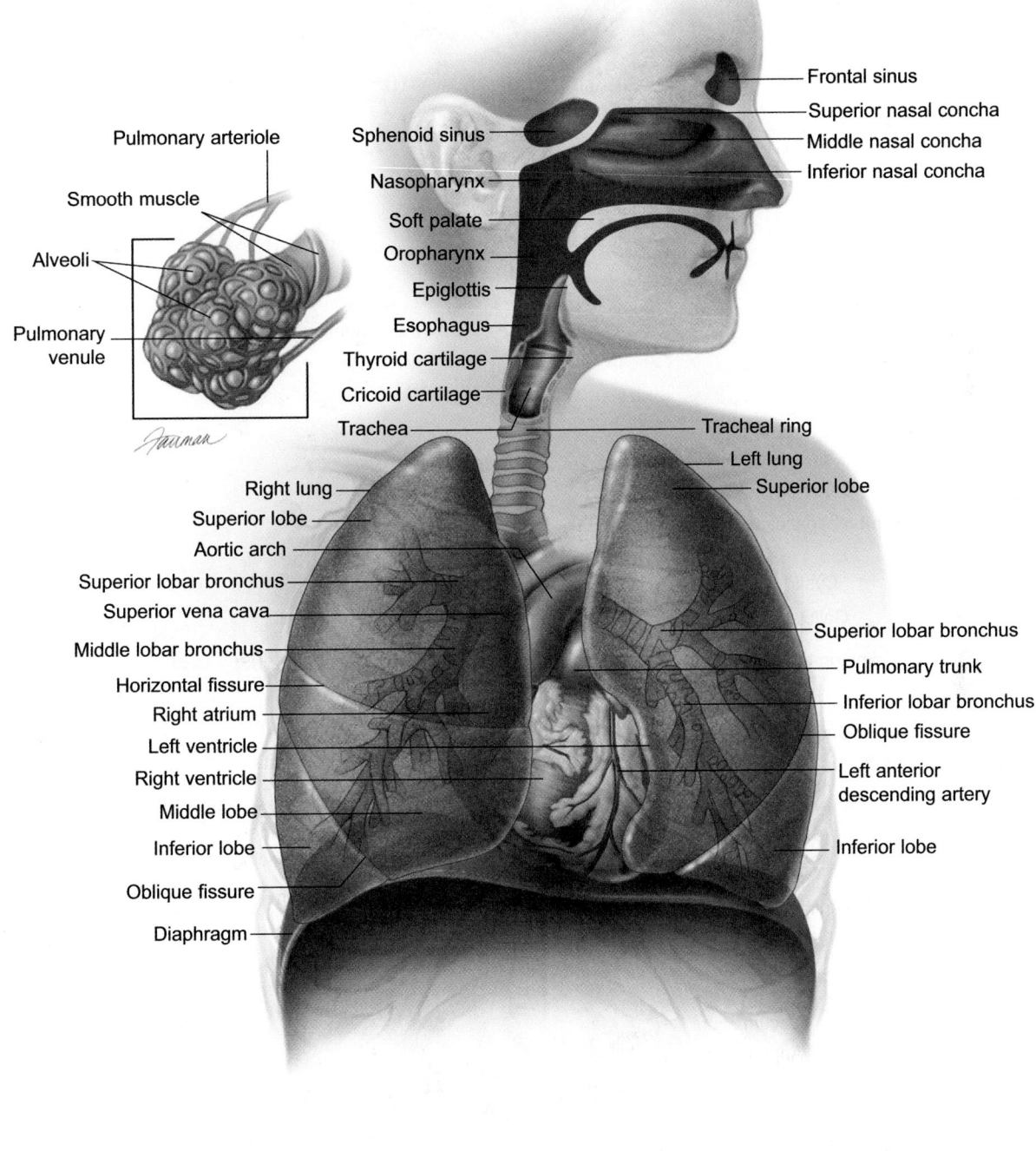

Pulmonary arteriole

Smooth muscle

Alveoli

Pulmonary venule

Frontal sinus
Superior nasal concha
Middle nasal concha
Inferior nasal concha

Sphenoid sinus
Nasopharynx
Soft palate
Oropharynx
Epiglottis
Esophagus
Thyroid cartilage
Cricoid cartilage
Trachea

Tracheal ring
Left lung
Superior lobe

Right lung
Superior lobe
Aortic arch
Superior lobar bronchus
Superior vena cava
Middle lobar bronchus
Horizontal fissure
Right atrium
Left ventricle
Right ventricle
Middle lobe
Inferior lobe
Oblique fissure
Diaphragm

Superior lobar bronchus
Pulmonary trunk
Inferior lobar bronchus
Oblique fissure
Left anterior descending artery
Inferior lobe

© Fairman Studios, LLC, 2002. All Rights Reserved.

Digestive System

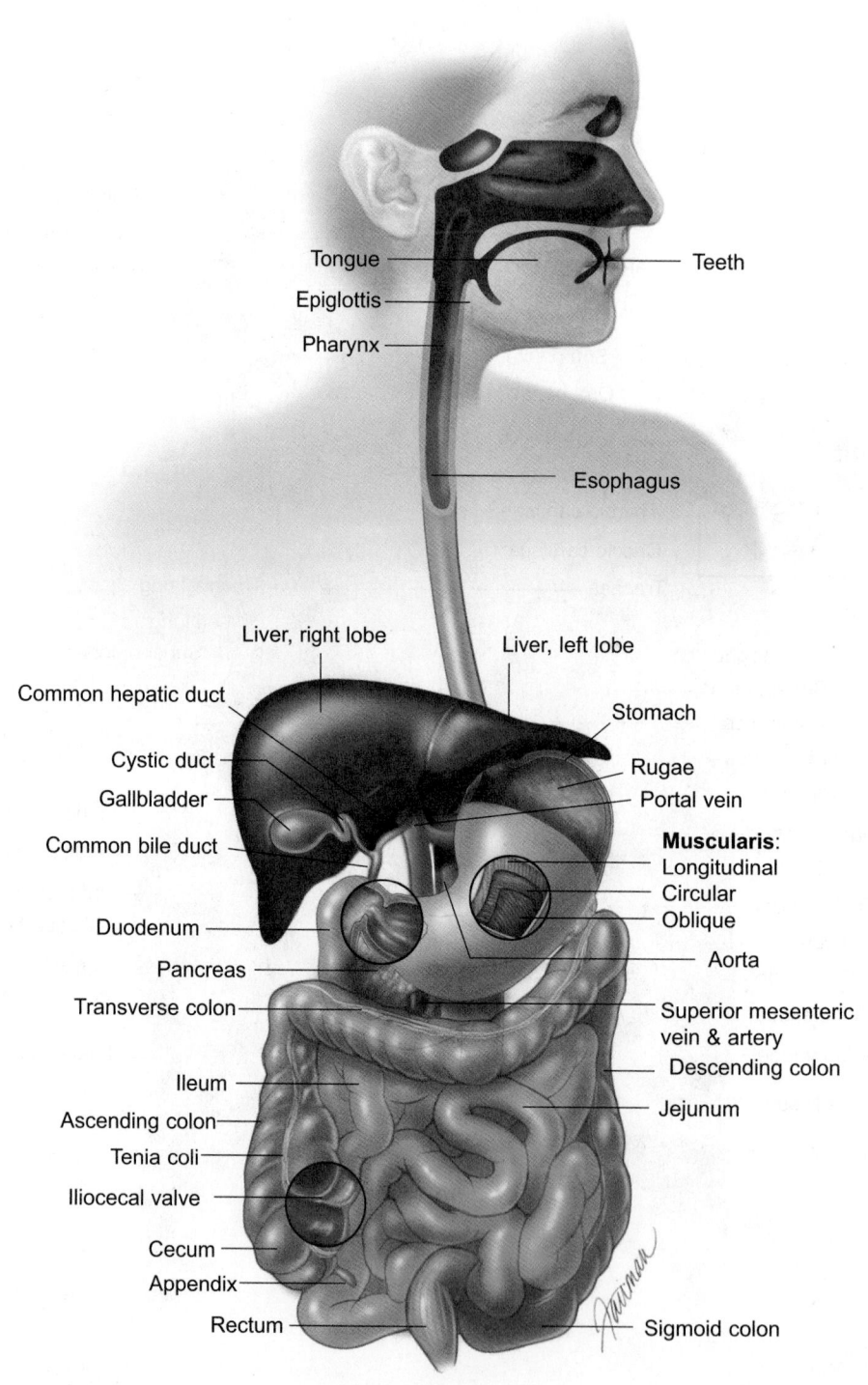

© Fairman Studios, LLC, 2002. All Rights Reserved.

© 2016 DecisionHealth

Nervous System

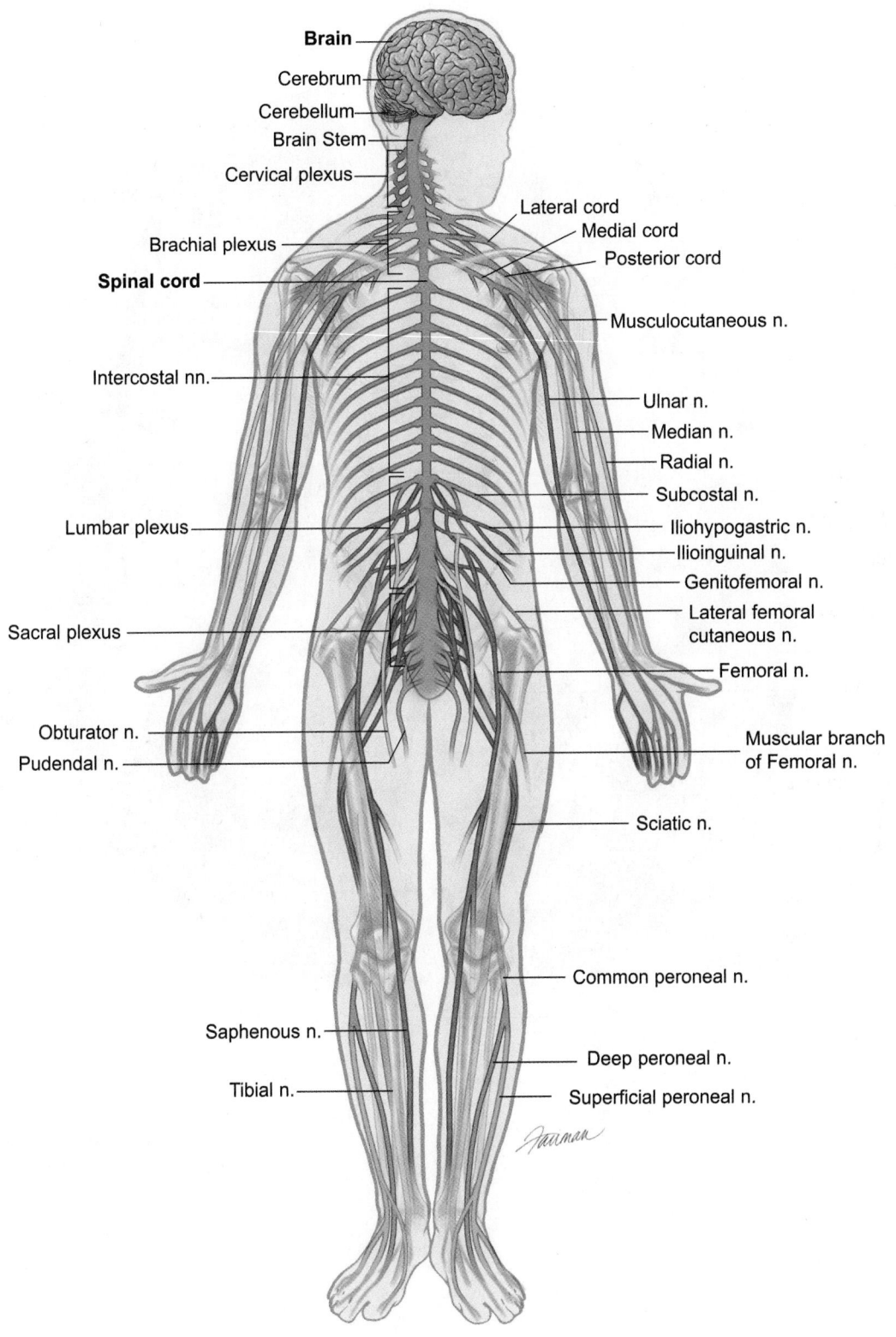

Brain
Cerebrum
Cerebellum
Brain Stem
Cervical plexus
Lateral cord
Medial cord
Brachial plexus
Posterior cord
Spinal cord
Musculocutaneous n.
Intercostal nn.
Ulnar n.
Median n.
Radial n.
Subcostal n.
Lumbar plexus
Iliohypogastric n.
Ilioinguinal n.
Genitofemoral n.
Lateral femoral cutaneous n.
Sacral plexus
Femoral n.
Obturator n.
Pudendal n.
Muscular branch of Femoral n.
Sciatic n.
Common peroneal n.
Saphenous n.
Deep peroneal n.
Tibial n.
Superficial peroneal n.

© Fairman Studios, LLC, 2002. All Rights Reserved.

Brain
(Inferior View)

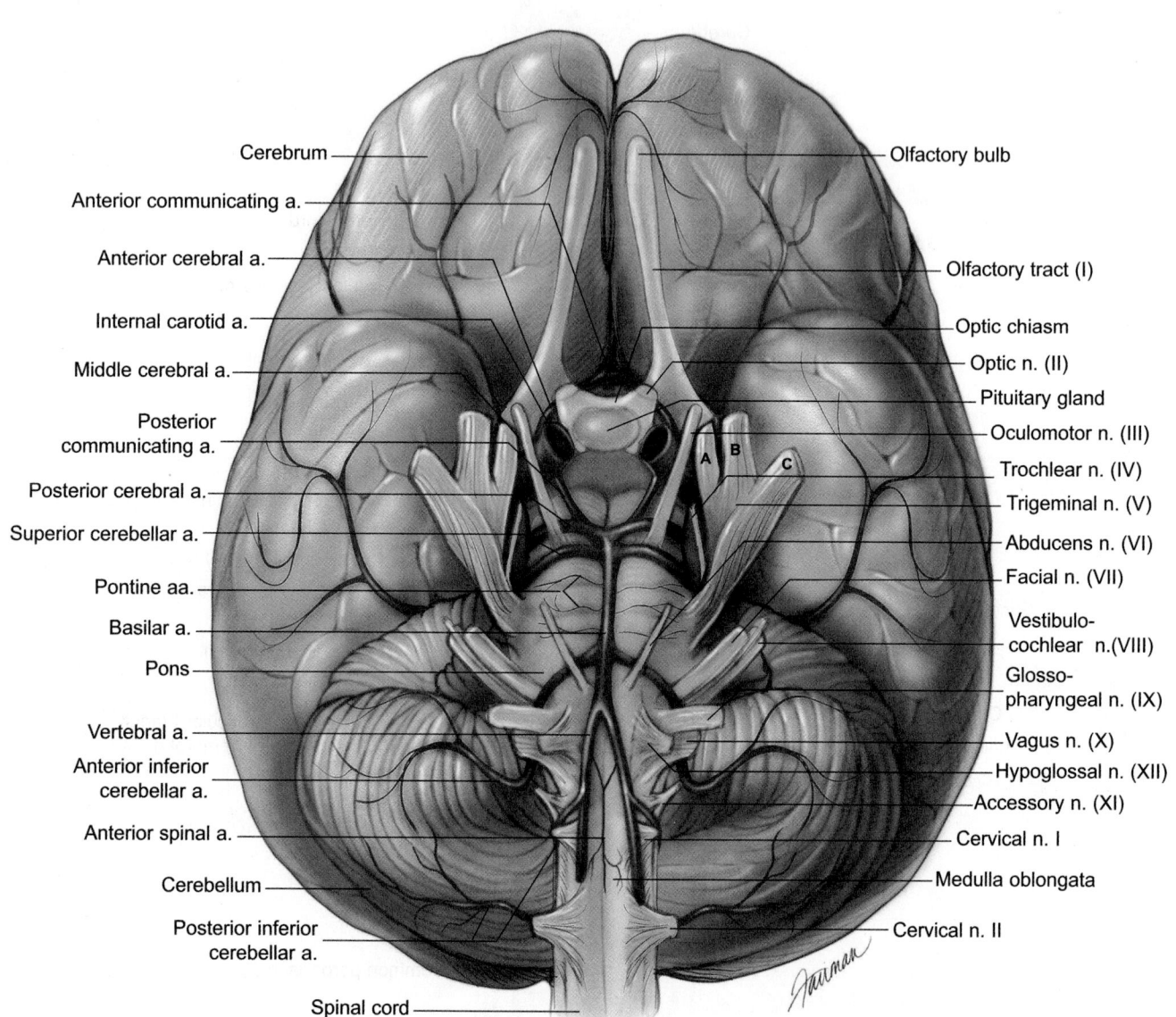

Cerebrum

Anterior communicating a.

Anterior cerebral a.

Internal carotid a.

Middle cerebral a.

Posterior communicating a.

Posterior cerebral a.

Superior cerebellar a.

Pontine aa.

Basilar a.

Pons

Vertebral a.

Anterior inferior cerebellar a.

Anterior spinal a.

Cerebellum

Posterior inferior cerebellar a.

Spinal cord

Olfactory bulb

Olfactory tract (I)

Optic chiasm

Optic n. (II)

Pituitary gland

Oculomotor n. (III)

Trochlear n. (IV)

Trigeminal n. (V)

Abducens n. (VI)

Facial n. (VII)

Vestibulo-cochlear n.(VIII)

Glosso-pharyngeal n. (IX)

Vagus n. (X)

Hypoglossal n. (XII)

Accessory n. (XI)

Cervical n. I

Medulla oblongata

Cervical n. II

Trigeminal Nerve (V) branches:
A Ophthalmic branch
B Maxillary branch
C Mandibular branch

© Fairman Studios, LLC, 2002. All Rights Reserved.

The Right Eye
(Transverse Section)

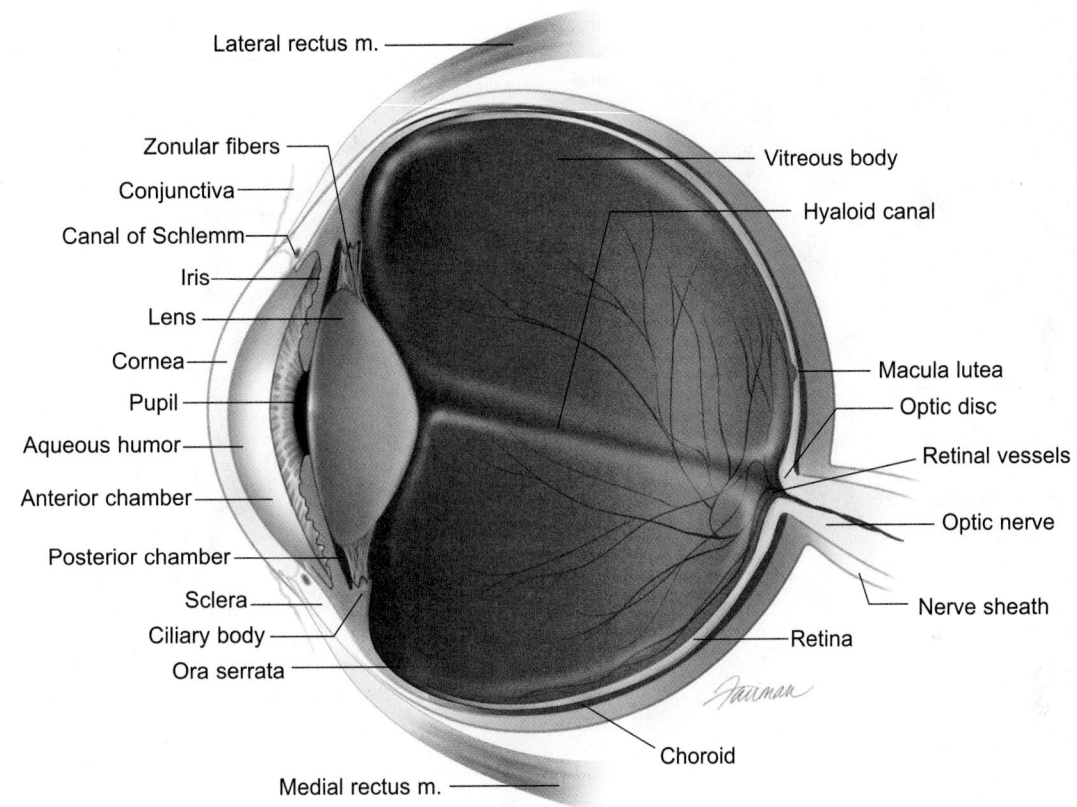

Lateral rectus m.

Zonular fibers

Conjunctiva

Canal of Schlemm

Iris

Lens

Cornea

Pupil

Aqueous humor

Anterior chamber

Posterior chamber

Sclera

Ciliary body

Ora serrata

Medial rectus m.

Vitreous body

Hyaloid canal

Macula lutea

Optic disc

Retinal vessels

Optic nerve

Nerve sheath

Retina

Choroid

© Fairman Studios, LLC, 2002. All Rights Reserved.

The Right Ear

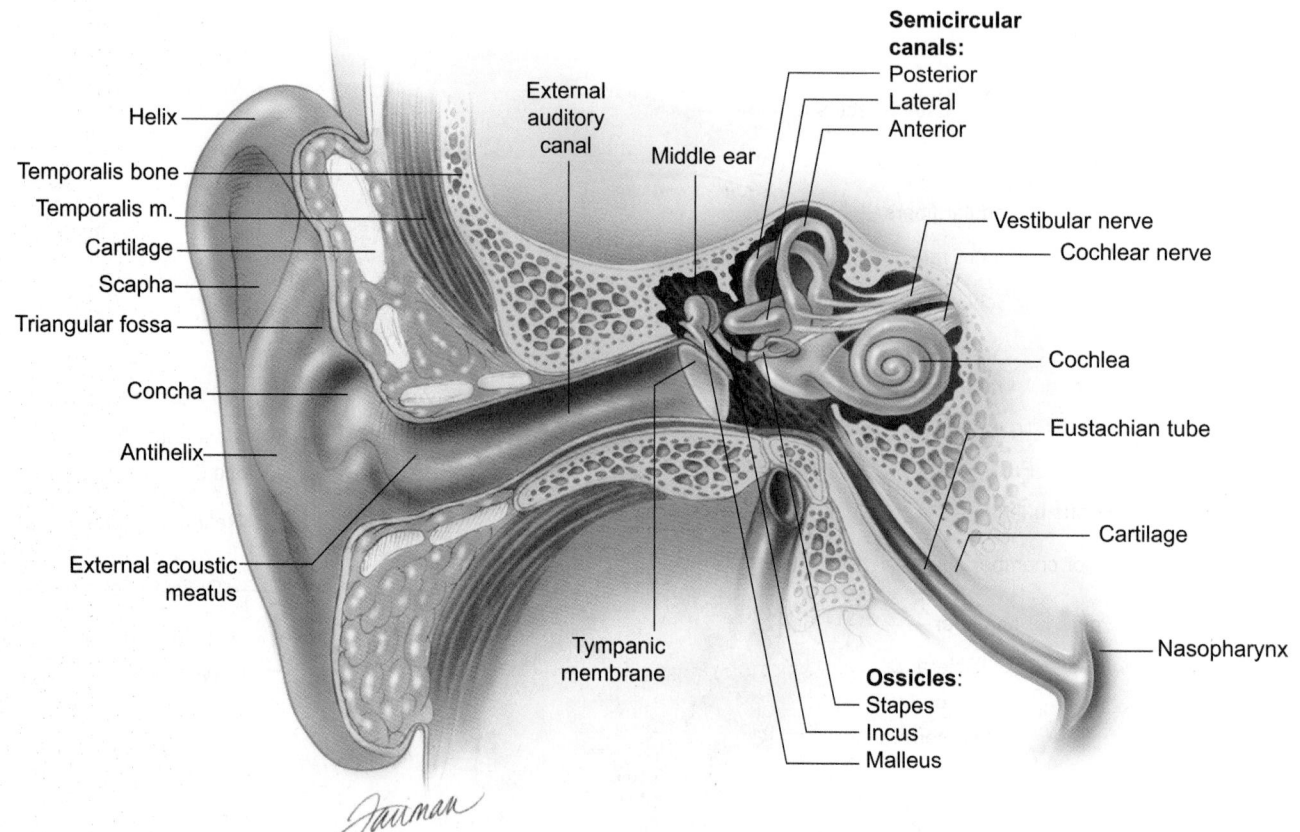

Helix

Temporalis bone

Temporalis m.

Cartilage

Scapha

Triangular fossa

Concha

Antihelix

External acoustic
meatus

External
auditory
canal

Middle ear

Tympanic
membrane

**Semicircular
canals:**
Posterior
Lateral
Anterior

Vestibular nerve

Cochlear nerve

Cochlea

Eustachian tube

Cartilage

Nasopharynx

Ossicles:
Stapes
Incus
Malleus

© Fairman Studios, LLC, 2002. All Rights Reserved.

Urinary System

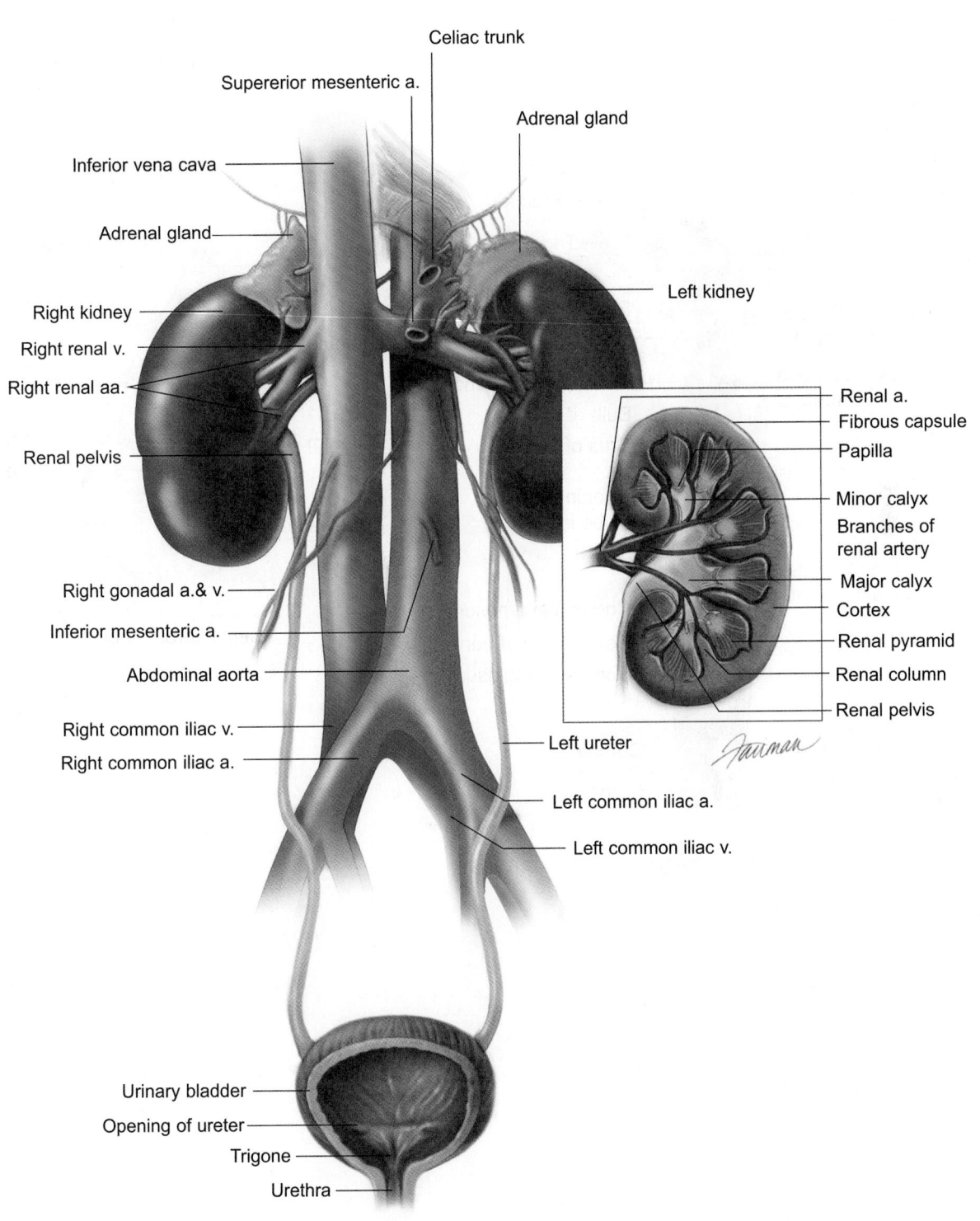

Celiac trunk

Supererior mesenteric a.

Adrenal gland

Inferior vena cava

Adrenal gland

Right kidney

Right renal v.

Right renal aa.

Renal pelvis

Left kidney

Renal a.

Fibrous capsule

Papilla

Minor calyx

Branches of
renal artery

Major calyx

Cortex

Renal pyramid

Renal column

Renal pelvis

Right gonadal a.& v.

Inferior mesenteric a.

Abdominal aorta

Right common iliac v.

Right common iliac a.

Left ureter

Left common iliac a.

Left common iliac v.

Urinary bladder

Opening of ureter

Trigone

Urethra

© Fairman Studios, LLC, 2002. All Rights Reserved.

Male Genital System

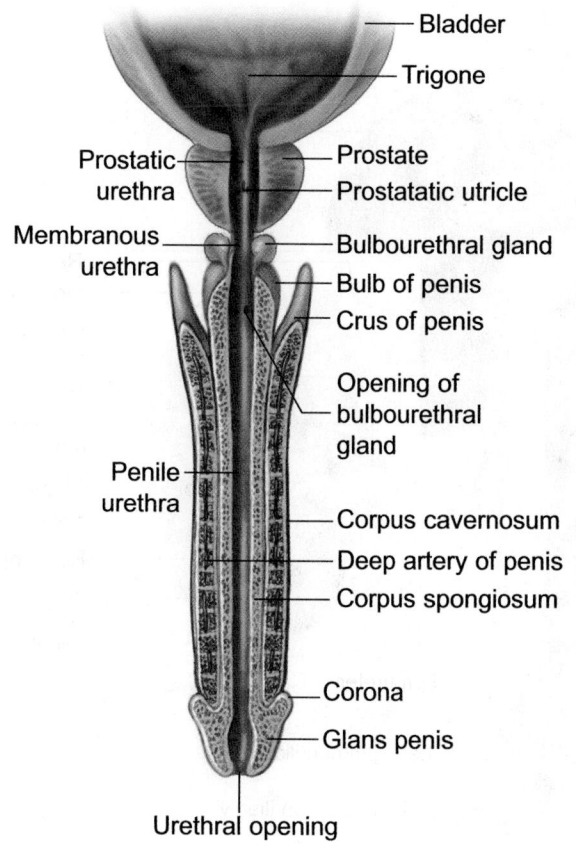

- Bladder
- Trigone
- Prostatic urethra
- Prostate
- Prostatatic utricle
- Membranous urethra
- Bulbourethral gland
- Bulb of penis
- Crus of penis
- Opening of bulbourethral gland
- Penile urethra
- Corpus cavernosum
- Deep artery of penis
- Corpus spongiosum
- Corona
- Glans penis
- Urethral opening

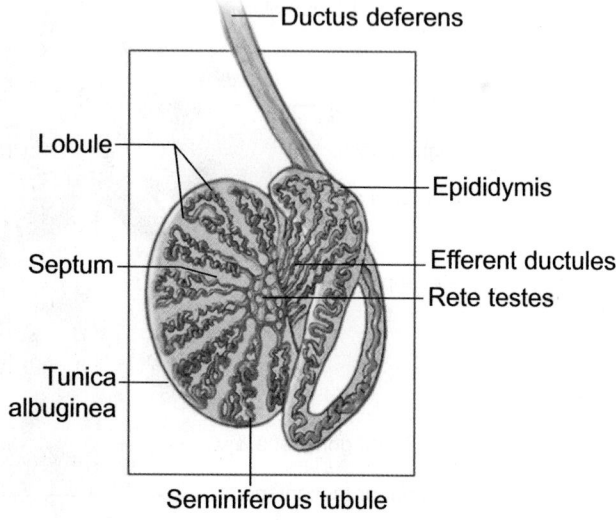

- Ductus deferens
- Lobule
- Epididymis
- Septum
- Efferent ductules
- Rete testes
- Tunica albuginea
- Seminiferous tubule

© Fairman Studios, LLC, 2002. All Rights Reserved.

Male Genital System

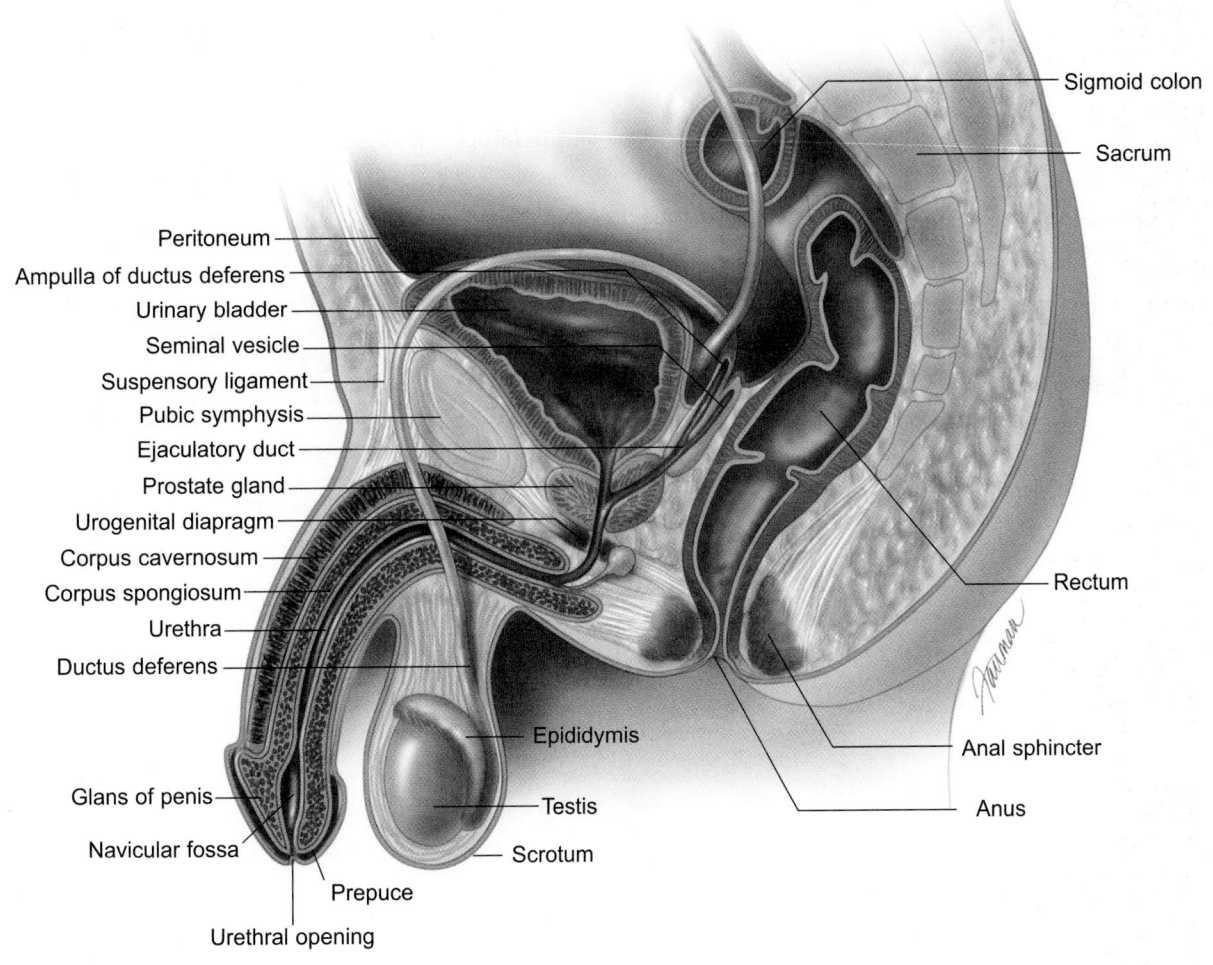

- Sigmoid colon
- Sacrum
- Peritoneum
- Ampulla of ductus deferens
- Urinary bladder
- Seminal vesicle
- Suspensory ligament
- Pubic symphysis
- Ejaculatory duct
- Prostate gland
- Urogenital diapragm
- Corpus cavernosum
- Corpus spongiosum
- Rectum
- Urethra
- Ductus deferens
- Epididymis
- Anal sphincter
- Glans of penis
- Testis
- Anus
- Navicular fossa
- Scrotum
- Prepuce
- Urethral opening

© Fairman Studios, LLC, 2002. All Rights Reserved.

Female Genital System

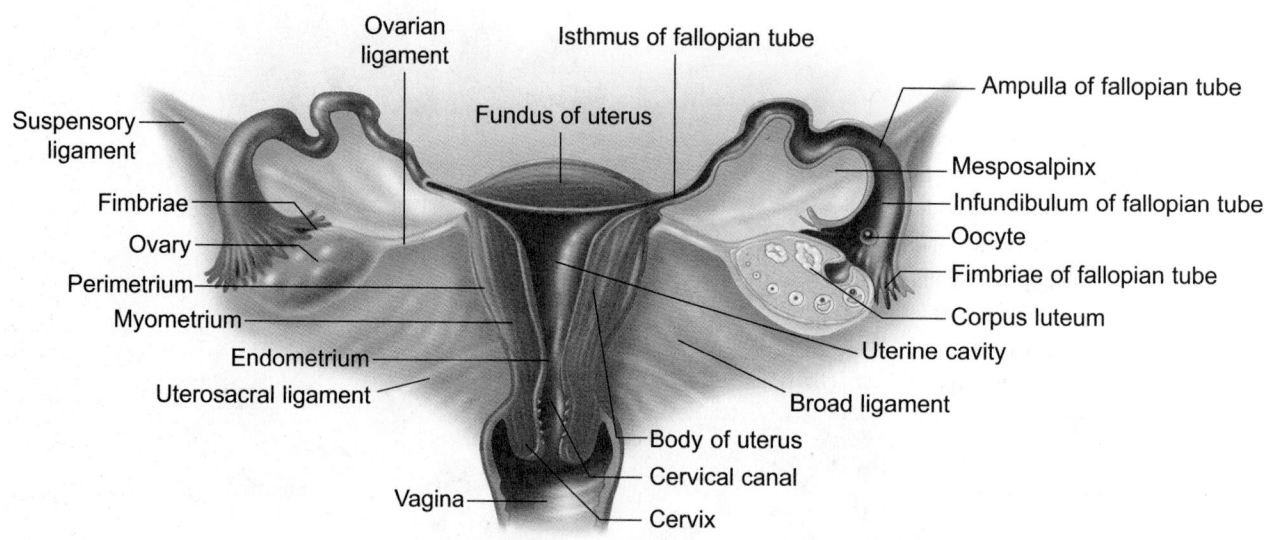

Ovarian ligament

Isthmus of fallopian tube

Ampulla of fallopian tube

Fundus of uterus

Suspensory ligament

Mesposalpinx

Fimbriae

Infundibulum of fallopian tube

Ovary

Oocyte

Perimetrium

Fimbriae of fallopian tube

Myometrium

Corpus luteum

Endometrium

Uterine cavity

Uterosacral ligament

Broad ligament

Body of uterus

Cervical canal

Vagina

Cervix

© Fairman Studios, LLC, 2002. All Rights Reserved.

© 2016 DecisionHealth

Female Genital System

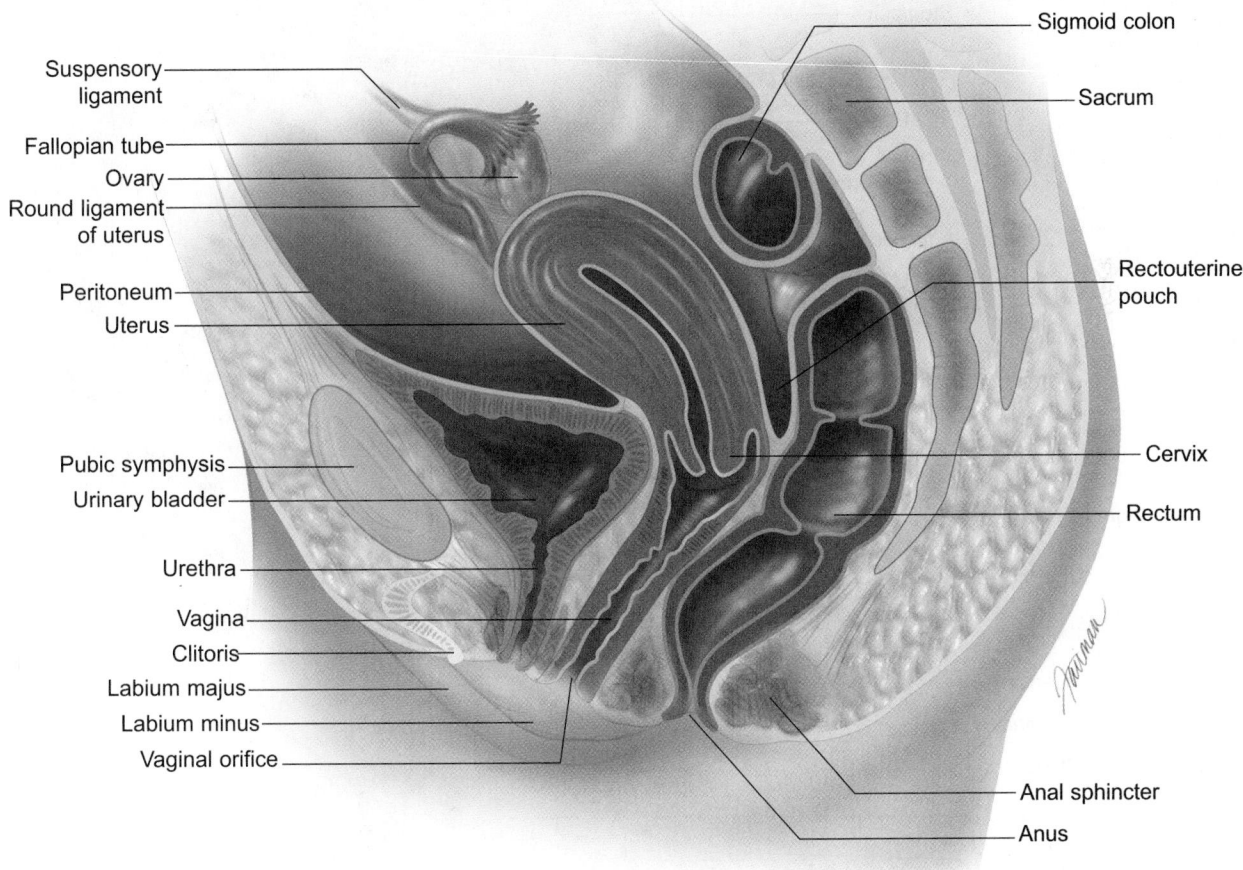

Suspensory ligament

Fallopian tube

Ovary

Round ligament of uterus

Peritoneum

Uterus

Pubic symphysis

Urinary bladder

Urethra

Vagina

Clitoris

Labium majus

Labium minus

Vaginal orifice

Sigmoid colon

Sacrum

Rectouterine pouch

Cervix

Rectum

Anal sphincter

Anus

© Fairman Studios, LLC, 2002. All Rights Reserved.

Female Reproductive System – Pregnancy
(Lateral View)

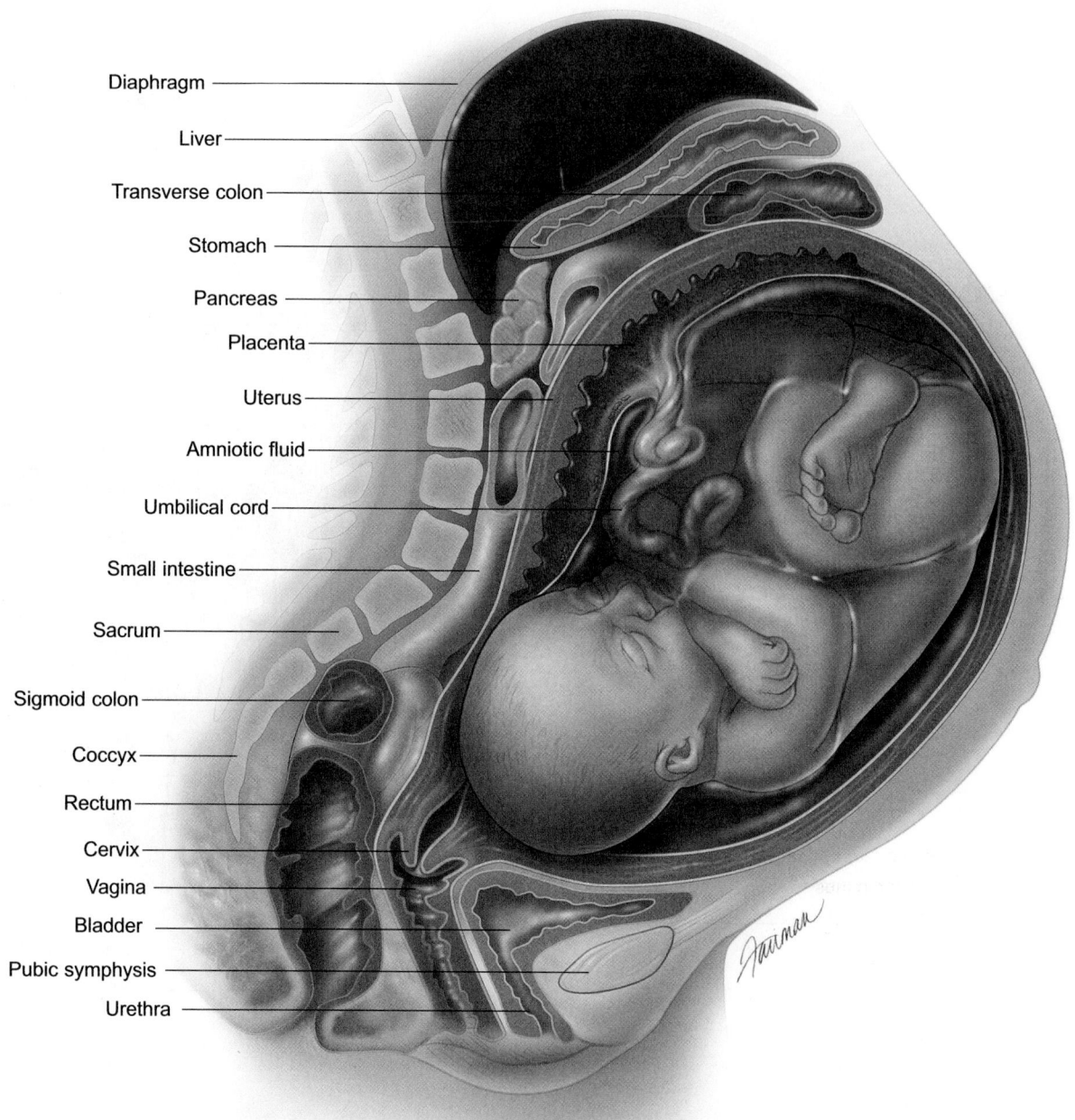

Diaphragm

Liver

Transverse colon

Stomach

Pancreas

Placenta

Uterus

Amniotic fluid

Umbilical cord

Small intestine

Sacrum

Sigmoid colon

Coccyx

Rectum

Cervix

Vagina

Bladder

Pubic symphysis

Urethra

© Fairman Studios, LLC, 2002. All Rights Reserved.

Cerebral Vasculature

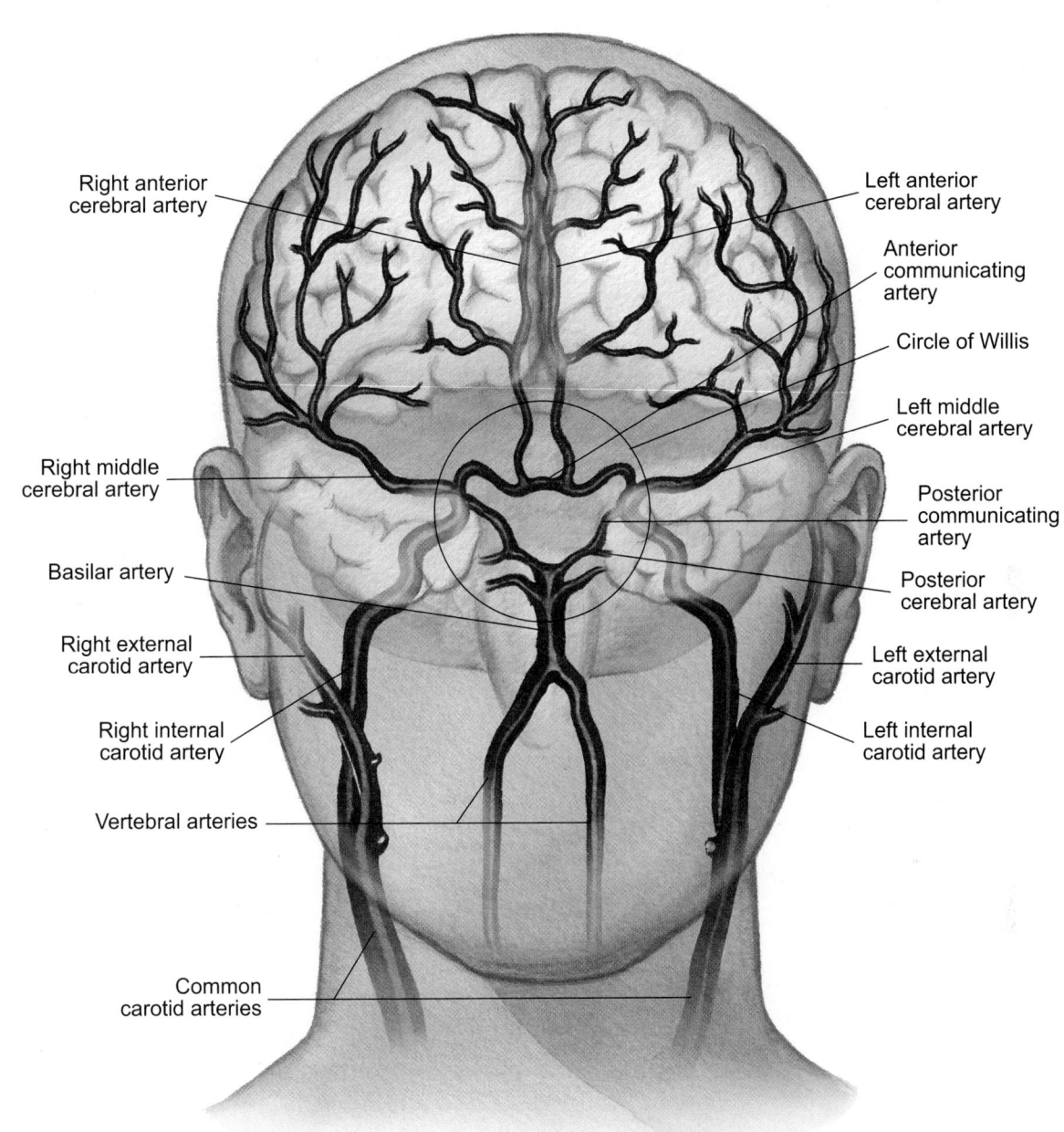

Right anterior cerebral artery

Left anterior cerebral artery

Anterior communicating artery

Circle of Willis

Right middle cerebral artery

Left middle cerebral artery

Posterior communicating artery

Basilar artery

Posterior cerebral artery

Right external carotid artery

Left external carotid artery

Right internal carotid artery

Left internal carotid artery

Vertebral arteries

Common carotid arteries

© BradleyClarkArt.com. All Rights Reserved.

Place of Service (POS) Codes

The following is the current national Place of Service (POS) code set, with facility (F) and non-facility (NF) designations noted for Medicare payment for services on the Physician Fee Schedule. POS codes not applicable for Medicare adjudication are designated N/A.

01 Pharmacy (NF)	A facility or location where drugs and other medically related items and services are sold, dispensed, or otherwise provided directly to patients.	15 Mobile Unit (NF)	A facility/unit that moves from place-to-place equipped to provide preventive, screening, diagnostic, and/or treatment services.
02 Unassigned	N/A	16 Temporary Lodging (NF)	A short-term accommodation such as a hotel, camp ground, hostel, cruise ship or resort where the patient receives care, and which is not identified by any other POS code.
03 School (NF)	A facility whose primary purpose is education.		
04 Homeless Shelter (NF)	A facility or location whose primary purpose is to provide temporary housing to homeless individuals (e.g., emergency shelters, individual or family shelters).	17 Walk-in Retail Health Clinic (N/A)	A walk-in health clinic, other than an office, urgent care facility, pharmacy or independent clinic and not described by any other Place of Service code, that is located within a retail operation and provides, on an ambulatory basis, preventive and primary care services.
05 Indian Health Service Free-standing Facility (N/A)	A facility or location, owned and operated by the Indian Health Service, which provides diagnostic, therapeutic (surgical and nonsurgical), and rehabilitation services to American Indians and Alaska Natives who do not require hospitalization.	18 Place of Employment/ Worksite (N/A)	A location, not described by any other POS code, owned or operated by a public or private entity where the patient is employed, and where a health professional provides on-going or episodic occupational medical, therapeutic or rehabilitative services to the individual.
06 Indian Health Service Provider-based Facility (N/A)	A facility or location, owned and operated by the Indian Health Service, which provides diagnostic, therapeutic (surgical and nonsurgical), and rehabilitation services rendered by, or under the supervision of, physicians to American Indians and Alaska Natives admitted as inpatients or outpatients.	19 Unassigned	N/A
		20 Urgent Care Facility (NF)	Location, distinct from a hospital emergency room, an office, or a clinic, whose purpose is to diagnose and treat illness or injury for unscheduled, ambulatory patients seeking immediate medical attention.
07 Tribal 638 Free-Standing Facility (N/A)	A facility or location owned and operated by a federally recognized American Indian or Alaska Native tribe or tribal organization under a 638 agreement, which provides diagnostic, therapeutic (surgical and nonsurgical), and rehabilitation services to tribal members who do not require hospitalization.	21 Inpatient Hospital (F)	A facility, other than psychiatric, which primarily provides diagnostic, therapeutic (both surgical and nonsurgical), and rehabilitation services by, or under, the supervision of physicians to patients admitted for a variety of medical conditions.
08 Tribal 638 Provider-Based Facility (N/A)	A facility or location owned and operated by a federally recognized American Indian or Alaska Native tribe or tribal organization under a 638 agreement, which provides diagnostic, therapeutic (surgical and nonsurgical), and rehabilitation services to tribal members admitted as inpatients or outpatients.	22 Outpatient Hospital (F)	A portion of a hospital which provides diagnostic, therapeutic (both surgical and nonsurgical), and rehabilitation services to sick or injured persons who do not require hospitalization or institutionalization.
		23 Emergency Room-Hospital (F)	A portion of a hospital where emergency diagnosis and treatment of illness or injury is provided.
09 Prison/ Correctional Facility (NF)	A prison, jail, reformatory, work farm, detention center, or any other similar facility maintained by either Federal, State or local authorities for the purpose of confinement or rehabilitation of adult or juvenile criminal offenders.	24 Ambulatory Surgical Center (F)	A freestanding facility, other than a physician's office, where surgical and diagnostic services are provided on an ambulatory basis.
		25 Birthing Center (NF)	A facility, other than a hospital's maternity facilities or a physician's office, which provides a setting for labor, delivery, and immediate postpartum care as well as immediate care of newborn infants.
10 Unassigned	N/A		
11 Office (NF)	Location, other than a hospital, skilled nursing facility (SNF), military treatment facility, community health center, State or local public health clinic, or intermediate care facility (ICF), where the health professional routinely provides health examinations, diagnosis, and treatment of illness or injury on an ambulatory basis.	26 Military Treatment Facility (F)	A medical facility operated by one or more of the Uniformed Services. Military Treatment Facility (MTF) also refers to certain former U.S. Public Health Service (USPHS) facilities now designated as Uniformed Service Treatment Facilities (USTF).
		27-30 Unassigned	N/A
12 Home (NF)	Location, other than a hospital or other facility, where the patient receives care in a private residence.	31 Skilled Nursing Facility (F)	A facility which primarily provides inpatient skilled nursing care and related services to patients who require medical, nursing, or rehabilitative services but does not provide the level of care or treatment available in a hospital.
13 Assisted Living Facility (NF)	Congregate residential facility with self-contained living units providing assessment of each resident's needs and on-site support 24 hours a day, 7 days a week, with the capacity to deliver or arrange for services including some health care and other services.		
		32 Nursing Facility (NF)	A facility which primarily provides to residents skilled nursing care and related services for the rehabilitation of injured, disabled, or sick persons, or, on a regular basis, health-related care services above the level of custodial care to other than mentally retarded individuals.
14 Group Home (NF)	A residence, with shared living areas, where clients receive supervision and other services such as social and/or behavioral services, custodial service, and minimal services (e.g., medication administration).		

33 Custodial Care Facility (NF)	A facility which provides room, board and other personal assistance services, generally on a longterm basis, and which does not include a medical component.	56 Psychiatric Residential Treatment Center (F)	A facility or distinct part of a facility for psychiatric care which provides a total 24-hour therapeutically planned and professionally staffed group living and learning environment.
34 Hospice (F)	A facility, other than a patient's home, in which palliative and supportive care for terminally ill patients and their families are provided.	57 Non-residential Substance Abuse Treatment Facility (NF)	A location which provides treatment for substance (alcohol and drug) abuse on an ambulatory basis. Services include individual and group therapy and counseling, family counseling, laboratory tests, drugs and supplies, and psychological testing.
35-40 Unassigned	N/A		
41 Ambulance— Land (F)	A land vehicle specifically designed, equipped and staffed for lifesaving and transporting the sick or injured.	58-59 Unassigned	N/A
42 Ambulance— Air or Water (F)	An air or water vehicle specifically designed, equipped and staffed for lifesaving and transporting the sick or injured.	60 Mass Immunization Center (NF)	A location where providers administer pneumococcal pneumonia and influenza virus vaccinations and submit these services as electronic media claims, paper claims, or using the roster billing method. This generally takes place in a mass immunization setting, such as, a public health center, pharmacy, or mall but may include a physician office setting.
43-48 Unassigned	N/A		
49 Independent Clinic (NF)	A location, not part of a hospital and not described by any other Place of Service code, that is organized and operated to provide preventive, diagnostic, therapeutic, rehabilitative, or palliative services to outpatients only.		
		61 Comprehensive Inpatient Rehabilitation Facility (F)	A facility that provides comprehensive rehabilitation services under the supervision of a physician to inpatients with physical disabilities. Services include physical therapy, occupational therapy, speech pathology, social or psychological services, and orthotics and prosthetics services.
50 Federally Qualified Health Center (NF)	A facility located in a medically underserved area that provides Medicare beneficiaries preventive primary medical care under the general direction of a physician.		
51 Inpatient Psychiatric Facility (F)	A facility that provides inpatient psychiatric services for the diagnosis and treatment of mental illness on a 24-hour basis, by or under the supervision of a physician.	62 Comprehensive Outpatient Rehabilitation Facility (NF)	A facility that provides comprehensive rehabilitation services under the supervision of a physician to outpatients with physical disabilities. Services include physical therapy, occupational therapy, and speech pathology services.
52 Psychiatric Facility-Partial Hospitalization (F)	A facility for the diagnosis and treatment of mental illness that provides a planned therapeutic program for patients who do not require full time hospitalization, but who need broader programs than are possible from outpatient visits to a hospital-based or hospital-affiliated facility.	63-64 Unassigned	N/A
		65 End-Stage Renal Disease Treatment Facility (NF)	A facility other than a hospital, which provides dialysis treatment, maintenance, and/or training to patients or caregivers on an ambulatory or home-care basis.
53 Community Mental Health Center (F)	A facility that provides the following services: outpatient services, including specialized outpatient services for children, the elderly, individuals who are chronically ill, and residents of the CMHC's mental health services area who have been discharged from inpatient treatment at a mental health facility; 24 hour a day emergency care services; day treatment, other partial hospitalization services, or psychosocial rehabilitation services; screening for patients being considered for admission to State mental health facilities to determine the appropriateness of such admission; and consultation and education services.	66-70 Unassigned	N/A
		71 State or Local Public Health Clinic (NF)	A facility maintained by either State or local health departments, that provides ambulatory primary medical care under the general direction of a physician.
		72 Rural Health Clinic (NF)	A certified facility which is located in a rural medically underserved area that provides ambulatory primary medical care under the general direction of a physician.
54 Intermediate Care Facility/ Mentally Retarded (NF)	A facility which primarily provides health-related care and services above the level of custodial care to mentally retarded individuals but does not provide the level of care or treatment available in a hospital or SNF.	73-80 Unassigned	N/A
		81 Independent Laboratory (NF)	A laboratory certified to perform diagnostic and/or clinical tests independent of an institution or a physician's office.
55 Residential Substance Abuse Treatment Facility (NF)	A facility which provides treatment for substance (alcohol and drug) abuse to live-in residents who do not require acute medical care. Services include individual and group therapy and counseling, family counseling, laboratory tests, drugs and supplies, psychological testing, and room and board.	82-98 Unassigned	N/A
		99 Other Place of Service (NF)	Other place of service not identified above.

CPT © 2015 American Medical Association. All rights reserved.
© 2016 DecisionHealth

Notes

Notes

Notes

Notes

Notes

Modifiers

A modifier provides the means to report or indicate that a service or procedure that has been performed has been altered by some specific circumstance but not changed in its definition or code. Modifiers also enable health care professionals to effectively respond to payment policy requirements established by other entities.

22	Increased Procedural Services
23	Unusual Anesthesia
24	Unrelated Evaluation and Management Service by the Same Physician or Other Qualified Health Care Professional During a Postoperative Period
25	Significant, Separately Identifiable Evaluation and Management Service by the Same Physician or Other Qualified Health Care Professional on the Same Day of the Procedure or Other Service
26	Professional Component
32	Mandated Services
33	Preventive Services
47	Anesthesia by Surgeon
50	Bilateral Procedure
51	Multiple Procedures
52	Reduced Services
53	Discontinued Procedure
54	Surgical Care Only
55	Postoperative Management Only
56	Preoperative Management Only
57	Decision for Surgery
58	Staged or Related Procedure or Service by the Same Physician or Other Qualified Health Care Professional During the Postoperative Period
59	Distinct Procedural Service
62	Two Surgeons
63	Procedure Performed on Infants less than 4 kg
66	Surgical Team
76	Repeat Procedure or Service by Same Physician or Other Qualified Health Care Professional
77	Repeat Procedure by AnOther Physician or Other Qualified Health Care Professional
78	Unplanned Return to the Operating/Procedure Room by the Same Physician or Other Qualified Health Care Professional Following Initial Procedure for a Related Procedure During the Postoperative Period
79	Unrelated Procedure or Service by the Same Physician or Other Qualified Health Care Professional During the Postoperative Period
80	Assistant Surgeon
81	Minimum Assistant Surgeon
82	Assistant Surgeon (when qualified resident surgeon not available)
90	Reference (Outside) Laboratory
91	Repeat Clinical Diagnostic Laboratory Test
92	Alternative Laboratory Platform Testing
99	Multiple Modifiers

Anesthesia Physical Status Modifiers

P1:	A normal healthy patient
P2:	A patient with mild systemic disease
P3:	A patient with severe systemic disease
P4:	A patient with severe systemic disease that is a constant threat to life
P5:	A moribund patient who is not expected to survive without the operation
P6:	A declared brain-dead patient whose organs are being removed for donor purposes

Modifiers Approved for Ambulatory Surgery Center (ASC) Hospital Outpatient Use

CPT Level I Modifiers

25	Significant, Separately Identifiable Evaluation and Management Service by the Same Physician or Other Qualified Health Care Professional on the Same Day of the Procedure or Other Service
27	Multiple Outpatient Hospital E/M Encounters on the Same Date
50	Bilateral Procedure
52	Reduced Services
58	Staged or Related Procedure or Service by the Same Physician or Other Qualified Health Care Professional During the Postoperative Period
59	Distinct Procedural Service
73	Discontinued Outpatient Hospital/Ambulatory Surgery Center (ASC) Procedure Prior to the Administration of Anesthesia
74	Discontinued Outpatient Hospital/Ambulatory Surgery Center (ASC) Procedure After Administration of Anesthesia
76	Repeat Procedure or Service by Same Physician or Other Qualified Health Care Professional
77	Repeat Procedure by AnOther Physician or Other Qualified Health Care Professional
78	Unplanned Return to the Operating/Procedure Room by the Same Physician or Other Qualified Health Care Professional Following Initial Procedure for a Related Procedure During the Postoperative Period
79	Unrelated Procedure or Service by the Same Physician or Other Qualified Health Care Professional During the Postoperative Period
91	Repeat Clinical Diagnostic Laboratory Test

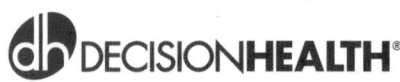

contexo | media

About DecisionHealth

DecisionHealth serves the business and regulatory needs of healthcare practitioners, hospitals, facilities, providers and their administrative staff nationwide. Every year, customers turn to DecisionHealth for solutions to a variety of challenges including medical coding, reimbursement and revenue cycle management, hospital accreditation, payment and billing practices, benchmarks and fee services, compliance and HIPAA privacy laws.

In 2013, DecisionHealth announced the acquisition of Contexo Media, transforming into a one-stop shop for your coding, billing and practice management needs. As an independent entity, unaffiliated with special interest groups and with no conflicting stake in the healthcare industry, DecisionHealth works for you with a single goal in mind: to ensure the financial well-being of healthcare providers.

1-855-CALL-DH1
(1-855-225-5341)

www.codingbooks.com

ISBN-13:978-1-58383-845-7

11495

9 781583 838457

MPB-PCE-16 $114.95 U.S.

Procedural Coding Expert

The *2016 Procedural Coding Expert* empowers accurate, complete professional services coding by putting all valid CPT® codes and descriptions at your fingertips, along with guidance on how the codes will be valued and covered for reimbursement purposes.

This annotated manual has everything you need on a daily basis for proper coding and clean claims. It is ideal for physician practice, hospital, and ambulatory surgery center coders alike.

- Complete list of all valid 2016 CPT® codes with long desciptions and icons
  - New and revised codes have helpful icons
  - Deleted codes are noted with a strikethrough and a valid cross-reference
  - All codes in numeric sequence—unlike most code books, you never find a CPT® code to be out of numeric order in this guide
- Coding Guidance and Coding Tips—simplify code selection with added clarification.
- Documentation Finder—tips highlighting synonyms and/or supporting chart references help align clinical and coding nomenclature to defend medical necessity
- Best-in-class index—code faster with multiple ways to find a procedure, encounter, or test
- More than 650 illustrations—visual insight to interpret clinical notes more effectively
- Also includes:
  - Medicare Pub 100 citations
  - AMA CPT® Assistant citations
  - Facility and Non-Facility Relative Value Units (RVUs)
  - Global Days and MUE Billing Restrictions
  - APC and ASC Payment icons
  - Medicare reimbursement icons
  - Age, Sex, and Maternity icons